Claire B. Wilcox M.D.

Claire B. Wilcox M.D.

SYNOPSIS OF

Diseases of the Chest

SYNOPSIS OF

Diseases of the Chest SECOND EDITION

Richard S. Fraser, MD, CM
Associate Professor of Pathology
McGill University
Royal Victoria Hospital and Montreal Chest Hospital
Montreal, Quebec, Canada

J.A. Peter Paré, MD, CM
Professor Emeritus, Department of Medicine
McGill University
Montreal, Quebec, Canada

Robert G. Fraser, MD
Professor Emeritus, Department of Radiology
University of Alabama
Birmingham, Alabama

P.D. Paré, MD, CM
Professor of Medicine
University of British Columbia and St. Paul's Hospital
Vancouver, British Columbia, Canada

W.B. SAUNDERS COMPANY
A Division of Harcourt Brace & Company
Philadelphia ■ London ■ Toronto ■ Montreal ■ Sydney ■ Tokyo

W.B. SAUNDERS COMPANY
A Division of
Harcourt Brace & Company

The Curtis Center
Independence Square West
Philadelphia, Pennsylvania 19106

Library of Congress Cataloging-in-Publication Data

Synopsis of diseases of the chest/Richard S. Fraser [et al.].
2nd ed.

p. cm.

Rev. ed. of: Synopsis of diseases of the chest/Richard S. Fraser. 1983.

Includes bibliographical references and index.

ISBN 0–7216–3669–1

1. Chest—Diseases.   I. Fraser, Richard S.   II. Paré,
   J. A. Peter. Synopsis of diseases of the chest.
   [DNLM: 1. Thoracic Diseases.   WF 975 S993 1994]

RC941.P28   1994

617.5′4—dc20

DNLM/DLC   93-25873

SYNOPSIS OF DISEASES OF THE CHEST, Second Edition   ISBN 0–7216–3669–1

Printed in the United States of America.

Last digit is the print number: 9   8   7   6   5   4   3   2

This book is dedicated to our wives,
children, grandchildren, and great-grandchild
with apologies for periods of unavailability
over recent years.

Preface

Following the path established by the second edition of *Diagnosis of Diseases of the Chest,* the third edition increased substantially in size, to the extent that it had to be published sequentially in four volumes from 1988 to 1991. This was chiefly the result of new knowledge that had accumulated between the two editions, and was particularly related to a more thorough discussion of the pathogenesis and pathologic characteristics of disease, and the inclusion of a more complete coverage of the CT and MRI characteristics of a variety of conditions. This expansion resulted in almost 3,300 pages and more than 20,000 references, clearly a work that is more likely to be used as a reference than as a text to be studied from cover to cover. While not denying the usefulness of such a reference work, we felt that the information that we had culled from our own experience and from published reports might be beneficial to individuals unwilling to read the entire text. Thus, we decided to create an abbreviated version, or synopsis, of the main work, aimed principally at residents in respiratory medicine or radiology and physicians or surgeons seeking a relatively concise review of the subject.

With minor exceptions, the 21 chapters in this book follow the same order and cover more or less the same material as the major work, features that we hope will make it easy for readers to locate an expanded version of any subject in the four-volume set, if desired. All descriptions of chest disease have been subdivided into etiology and pathogenesis, pathologic characteristics, roentgenographic manifestations, clinical manifestations, and prognosis. Since conventional roentgenography and special-ized imaging techniques play such important roles in the investigation and diagnosis of chest disease, we have retained numerous illustrations, the vast majority of which are derived from the third edition; however, many have been cropped or reduced in size in order to restrict the length of the book to manageable proportions. Although this synopsis is not meant to be a reference text, key references are cited so the interested reader can further pursue a particular subject; as much as possible, we have attempted to update these references to reflect changes since publication of the four-volume set.

As in the previous edition of *Synopsis of Diseases of the Chest,* we invite our readers to inform us of differences of opinion they may have with the contents of this book. It is only through such an interchange of information and opinion that we can hope to establish, on a firm basis, the knowledge necessary for a full understanding of respiratory disease.

RSF
JAPP
RGF
PDP

Acknowledgments

It is not possible to overstate our gratitude to the many individuals who helped produce this book. Donna O'Connor of the Montreal General Hospital, Margaret Stewart of St. Paul's Hospital, Vancouver, and Lynne Hogan of the Hospital of the University of Alabama at Birmingham all had significant input in the typing of manuscript. The photographic work was the accomplishment of the Department of Visual Aids of the Royal Victoria Hospital, Susie Gray and Tony Zagar of the Department of Radiology, University of Alabama, David Mandeville of the University of Saskatchewan Hospital, Stuart Greene of St. Paul's Hospital, and Joseph Donohue and Anthony Graham of Montreal. Special words of thanks are due Joanne Fraser, who graciously performed the tedious task of renumbering and organizing the references for all the chapters, and Ann Paré, who helped collect and sort reference abstracts.

The majority of the radiographic images are of patients of staff members of the Royal Victoria Hospital, the Montreal General Hospital, The Montreal Chest Hospital, the Hospital of the University of Alabama at Birmingham, and the Medical Center of the University of Saskatchewan, Saskatoon. All illustrations of pathology derive from patients in the Montreal General Hospital and the Montreal Chest Hospital. Our indebtedness to our colleagues who were caring for these patients cannot be overemphasized. Special acknowledgment is due Dr. N. Müller, Vancouver, British Columbia, for supplying many of the high-resolution CT images. Throughout our work, we received much support and cooperation from our publisher, particularly from Lisette Bralow, who effectively and sympathetically minimized the obstacles we encountered.

Finally, we would like to acknowledge the patience and understanding displayed by our wives and children throughout our labors. Without their continuous encouragement this book surely would not have been completed, and we acknowledge their many virtues with love.

RSF
JAPP
RGF
PDP

Contents

1

THE NORMAL CHEST

AIRWAYS AND PULMONARY VENTILATION

The lung can be divided into three zones, each with somewhat different but overlapping structural and functional characteristics. The *conductive zone* includes the trachea, bronchi, and membranous (nonalveolated) bronchioles. Since air cannot diffuse through the well-developed walls of these airways, their primary function is to conduct air to the alveolar surface. These structures, along with the pulmonary and bronchial arteries and veins, lymphatic channels, nerves, connective tissues of the peribronchial and perivascular spaces, and the interlobular septa, constitute the nonparenchymatous portion of the lung.

The *transitional zone* consists of the respiratory bronchioles and alveolar ducts, each of which conducts air to the most peripheral alveoli. Unlike the case with airways of the conductive zone, a variable number of alveoli arise from the walls of the airways of the transitional zone, resulting in the additional function of gas exchange.

The *respiratory zone* consists of the alveolar sacs and alveoli themselves, whose primary function is the exchange of gases between air and blood. Together with the structures in the transitional zone, they make up the lung parenchyma.

Anatomy—Conductive Zone

Geometry and Dimensions

In one study of resin casts of human lungs inflated and fixed at a volume of 5 L,[1] investigators measured the length of each branch between two points of bifurcation as well as the diameter at the midpoint of every branch, from an arbitrary diameter of 0.7 mm. One of the interesting findings was a roughly linear relationship between the order number° and the logarithm of the number, diameter, and length of airway branches (Fig. 1–1). Thus, by measuring the slope of the line relating the two, the diameter and length of any order can be predicted by dividing the diam-

eter and length of its parent by 1.4 and 1.49, respectively. Similarly, the number of branches is linearly related to order number, the branching ratio of the entire conductive zone (average number of daughter branches per parent branch) being 2.8.

These "number laws" do not apply precisely at all airway levels; for example, the trachea clearly does not divide 2.8 times, and, in fact, the branching pattern of the proximal conducting system probably is best described as dichotomous, each parent dividing into two branches. However, the branching ratio of 2.8 is precise from orders 6 through 15. Similarly, the diameter law is not applicable throughout the whole airway system; at order 7 (approximately), diminution in airway diameter ceases, and the more distal branches (to order 1) retain the parent's diameter.

Counting distally from the trachea, the number of generations to a 0.7-mm airway ranges from 8 to 25[1]; that is, the route with the shortest path length is reached after 8 divisions, and the one with the longest after 25. It is likely that local spatial constraints are most important in determining these figures. Analysis of the frequency distribution of divisions down to the lobular branches (Fig. 1–2) shows a stepwise increase from division 8 to a peak at 14 and a decrease from 15 to 25.[1] Path lengths proximal to branches 0.7 mm in diameter vary from 7.5 to 21.5 cm, and those distal from 0.2 to 0.9 cm; thus, the overall distance from carina to distal respiratory bronchioles ranges from 7.7 to 22.4 cm. The volume of airways from the carina to 0.7-mm branches has been computed to be about 70 mL[1]; when this is added to the volume of the upper airways from the mouth to the carina (80 mL), the sum is a total volume of conducting airways almost identical to the volume of anatomic dead space as determined by physiologic techniques.

Morphology

The basic morphology of the trachea, bronchi, and membranous bronchioles is the same and consists of a surface epithelium, composed largely of ciliated and secretory cells, and subepithelial tissue containing supportive connective tissue, cells of the inflammatory and immune systems, and glands (Fig. 1–3). The proportion and type of these elements vary considerably with airway order.

Epithelium. The tracheal and proximal bronchial epi-

°In this context, order refers to the level of airway within the conducting system. The terminal bronchiole is considered to be order 1; when two such bronchioles join, they form a single branch of order 2; when two of order 2 join, they form a branch of order 3, and so on.

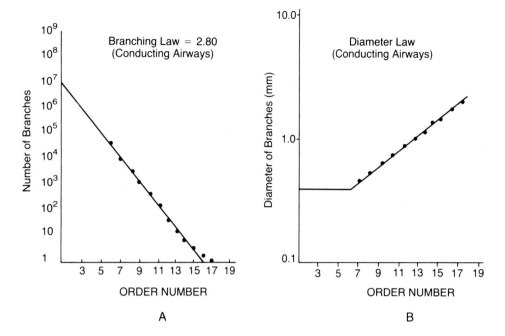

Figure 1–1. Number of Branches *(A)* and Their Diameter *(B)* Plotted Against Their Order Number. *B,* Note that orders 1 through 7 undergo no diameter change—diminution in caliber ceases at order 7, chiefly respiratory bronchioles. (From Cumming G, Horsfield K, Harding LK, et al: Biological branching systems, with special reference to the lung airways. Bull Physiopathol Resp 7: 31, 1971.)

thelium is composed of tall columnar cells and smaller, somewhat triangular basal cells.[2] Since not all cells reach the luminal surface and since their nuclei are situated at varying levels, the epithelium possesses a pseudostratified appearance (Fig. 1–4). This is gradually lost in the distal bronchi and bronchioles as the cells assume a low columnar shape. Ciliated and secretory cells, either goblet or Clara in type, constitute the bulk of the epithelium, with basal, intermediate, lymphoreticular, and neuroendocrine cells interspersed in lesser numbers.

The *ciliated cell* is the most prominent cell type in normal epithelium, being present in numbers three to five times those of goblet cells in the central airways (Fig. 1–5). Columnar in shape, the ciliated cell extends from the luminal surface to the basal lamina, to which it is attached by a thin, tapering base. Cells are also attached firmly to one another at their apical surface by tight junctions, thus forming a barrier physically impermeable to most substances. Emanating from the surface of each cell are approximately 200 to 250 cilia as well as numerous shorter microvilli, which have been hypothesized to function either in the absorption of secretions emanating from more peripheral

airways or in the secretion of a portion of the periciliary mucous layer.[3]

Each cilium is covered by a prolongation of the cell surface membrane and contains a complex structure called

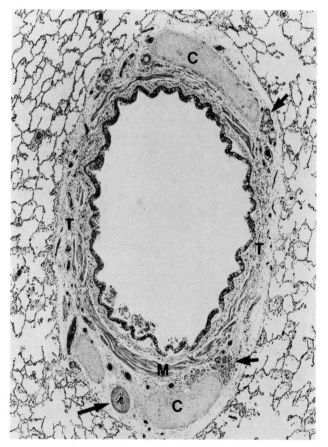

Figure 1–3. Normal Subsegmental Bronchus. C = cartilage plate; T = interstitial connective tissue; M = smooth muscle; short arrows = bronchial glands; long arrow = bronchial artery. (× 30.)

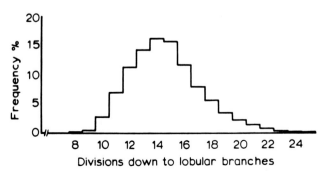

Figure 1–2. Frequency Distribution of the Number of Divisions Down to the Lobular Branches. (From Horsfield K, Cumming G: Morphology of the bronchial tree in man. J Appl Physiol 24: 373, 1968.)

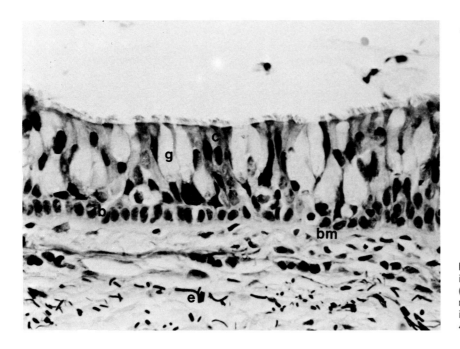

Figure 1–4. Normal Bronchial Epithelium. Ciliated (c), goblet (g), intermediate (i), and basal (b) cells are seen. Note also the thin basement membrane (bm) and scattered elastic fibers (e) in the lamina propria. (Verhoeff-van Gieson; × 425.)

the *axoneme* (Fig. 1–6).[4] This consists of two central microtubules surrounded by nine peripheral doublets, composed, in turn, of two intimately related microtubules termed A and B subfibers. Two small arms, composed of the protein

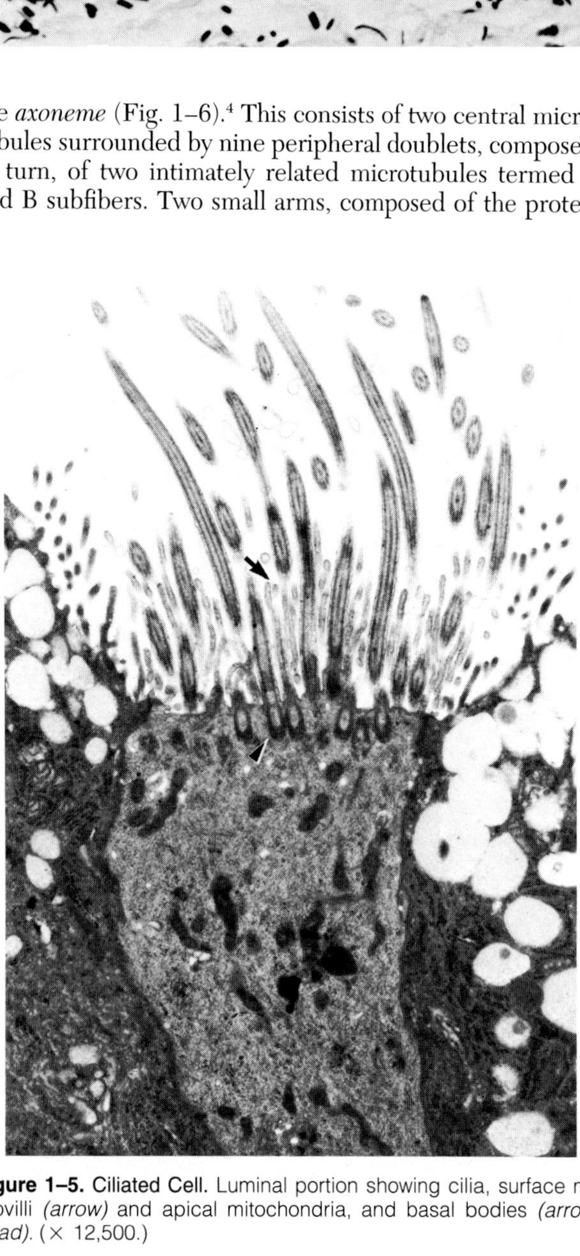

Figure 1–5. Ciliated Cell. Luminal portion showing cilia, surface microvilli *(arrow)* and apical mitochondria, and basal bodies *(arrowhead).* (× 12,500.)

dynein and believed to be the major focus of energy conversion into ciliary movement, project from the A subfiber of one doublet to the B subfiber of the next. Also attached to each A subfiber is a radial spoke that joins it to a central sheath that surrounds the inner microtubules.

Goblet cells (*see* Fig. 1–4) constitute about 20 to 30 per cent of cells in the more proximal airways and decrease in number distally, so that only occasional cells are present in normal bronchioles; in conditions of both acute and chronic airway irritation, however, they may substantially increase in number in the proximal airways and also may appear in bronchioles.[5] The apical portion of the cell is expanded by numerous membrane-bound secretory granules, whereas the basal portion has few organelles and is attenuated as it approaches the basal lamina; this combination results in the typical goblet shape from which the name of the cell is derived.

Basal cells (*see* Fig. 1–4) are relatively small, flattened or triangular cells whose bases are adjacent to the basal lamina; their apices normally do not reach the airway lumen. They are more abundant in the proximal airways, where they form a more or less continuous layer, and gradually diminish in number distally so as to become difficult to identify in bronchioles. Their cytoplasmic contents show little specialization, and there is evidence that the basal cell is a reserve cell from which the epithelium is continuously repopulated.[6] It also has been speculated that these cells function as a scaffold for the attachment of ciliated and goblet cells to the basal lamina.[7]

Intermediate cells (*see* Fig. 1–4) possess somewhat more cytoplasm than do basal cells and show evidence of either ciliogenesis or mucous granule accumulation. They are generally believed to represent a stage of differentiation between the basal cell and either the goblet or the ciliated cell. It also is possible that the secretory form is important in the repair of injured airway epithelium.[8] The response to such injury is rapid; in one study in which the suprabasal epithelium of rat trachea was mechanically damaged, basal cellular mitotic activity reached a peak between 26 and 30

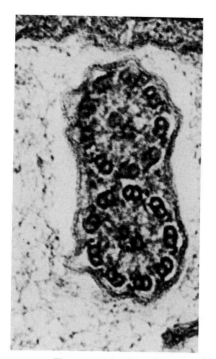

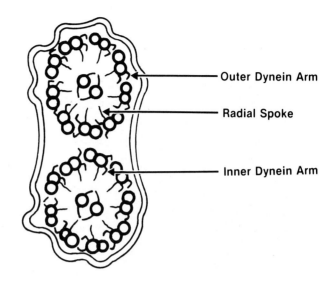

- Outer Dynein Arm
- Radial Spoke
- Inner Dynein Arm

Figure 1–6. Doublet Cilium from Chronic Smoker. Although paired within the same plasma membrane, the individual components of this cilium are normal, showing nine peripheral and two central doublets and the typical arrangement of dynein arms and radial spokes.

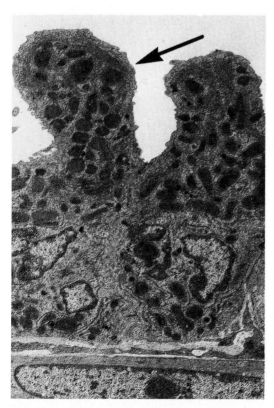

Figure 1–7. Clara Cells. These cells are low columnar in type and possess tongue-shaped cytoplasmic processes *(arrow)* that project into the airway lumen. Nuclei are basal in position, and the apical cytoplasm contains numerous osmiophilic granules. (× 4500.) (From Wang N-S, Huang SN, Sheldon H, et al: Ultrastructural changes of Clara and type II alveolar cells in adrenalin-induced pulmonary edema in mice. Am J Pathol 62: 237, 1971.)

hours postinjury, and the epithelium was virtually reconstituted with ultrastructurally mature cells by 90 hours.[9]

The *Clara cell (nonciliated bronchiolar secretory cell)* is found primarily in bronchioles, in which it makes up the majority of the epithelium along with ciliated cells. It is columnar in shape and bulges into the airway lumen, projecting slightly above the surrounding ciliated cells (Fig. 1–7). In the apical cytoplasm are membrane-bound granules whose contents are believed to form at least part of the surface layer that normally lines the bronchiolar epithelium. Clara cells also function in the regeneration of damaged bronchiolar epithelium[10] and in the secretion of a leukocyte protease inhibitor[11] that may be important in maintaining the integrity of the bronchiolar epithelium.

Neuroendocrine cells (K cells) possess a roughly triangular shape, their bases resting on the basal lamina, and their long, tapering apices pointing toward, but infrequently reaching, the luminal surface. The cytoplasm contains numerous membrane-bound granules with a central, electron-dense core surrounded by a thin, lucent halo (neurosecretory granules) (Fig. 1–8). These are concentrated in the basal portion of the cytoplasm and may contain several biologically active peptides, including calcitonin, gastrin-releasing peptide, and 5-hydroxytryptamine (serotonin).[12] The cells are found more frequently in peripheral airways and in younger individuals, particularly fetuses and neonates, in whom they have been estimated to constitute 1 to 2 per cent of all bronchial epithelial cells.[13]

Several potentially important functions have been hypothesized for pulmonary neuroendocrine cells.[12] Their relative prominence in fetal lungs and their fairly rapid decrease in number after birth have suggested a role in regulation of the fetal or neonatal circulation. In addition,

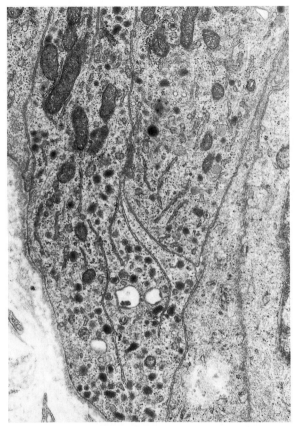

Figure 1–8. Neuroendocrine Cell. Magnified view of base of neuroendocrine cell showing lamina propria and thin basal lamina at bottom left and numerous intracytoplasmic neurosecretory granules. (× 31,000.)

the observation that the cells are the first to differentiate in developing airway epithelium has suggested that they may be important in lung maturation. There is evidence that the cells may increase in number in hypoxic conditions[14]; as a consequence, it also has been speculated that they may be mediators of the pulmonary vascular hypoxic response.

A structure probably related to the solitary neuroendocrine cell and known as the *neuroepithelial body* is found throughout the tracheobronchial and bronchiolar epithelium, especially near branch points. The neuroepithelial body consists of a fairly well-demarcated cluster of 4 to 10 columnar cells, each of which contains neurosecretory granules that have been shown to contain serotonin and other peptides.[15] Although individual cells of the neuroepithelial body resemble solitary neuroendocrine cells, their clustered arrangement and fairly consistent relationship to nerve fibers and possibly capillaries have suggested that the two may have different functions.

Submucosa and Lamina Propria. The subepithelial tissue can be subdivided into a lamina propria, situated between the basal lamina and the muscularis mucosa, and a submucosa, comprising all the remaining airway tissue. The *lamina propria,* more prominent in the trachea and proximal bronchi than in distal airways, consists principally of small blood and lymphatic vessels, a meshwork of fine reticulin fibers continuous with the basal lamina, and elastic tissue. The *submucosa* contains cartilage, muscle, and other supportive connective tissue elements, the major portion of the tracheobronchial glands, lymphatics, bronchial arteries and veins, and various cells related to airway function and defense mechanisms.

Tracheal cartilage is arranged in a series of 16 to 20 horseshoe-shaped rings oriented in a horizontal plane with their open ends directed posteriorly. This U-shaped structure also is present in the main bronchi, but in more distal branches the plates become quite irregular in size and shape. At bronchial division points, they frequently take the shape of a saddle conforming to the branching angle, thus providing extra support at sites of increased turbulence. As the airway proceeds distally, the plates become smaller and less complete until they finally disappear altogether in airways 1 to 2 mm in diameter (bronchioles). With advancing age, the plates often become ossified and may be visible roentgenographically.

The bronchial cartilage plates are tethered together by dense fibroelastic tissue arranged predominantly in a longitudinal direction. At numerous points, particularly in smaller airways, elastic fibers pass obliquely from these longitudinally arranged bundles to intermingle with the elastic tissue of the lamina propria.[16] These obliquely arranged fibers are believed to help transmit to the more rigid and stronger cartilaginous-fibrous tissue the longitudinal tensions that arise in the surface epithelium and the parenchyma as a whole during respiration.

Tracheal muscle is found predominantly in the membranous (posterior) portion, where it is arranged in transverse bundles that are attached to the inner perichondrium. In the intrapulmonary bronchi, there is no such attachment, and the muscle coat lies close to the epithelium adjacent to the lamina propria (Fig. 1–9; *see* also Fig. 1–3, page 3). In the larger airways, the orientation is mainly transverse, as in the trachea, but it soon becomes obliquely oriented and arranged in branching and anastomosing bundles that form irregular spirals down the airway. There is evidence that the relative thickness of the muscle coat expressed as a proportion of airway diameter is greater in peripheral than in proximal airways.[17]

Loose connective tissue containing collagen and reticulin fibers occupies the bulk of the remainder of the submucosa. It is continuous with adjacent periarterial connective tissue, with perivenous connective tissue near the hilum, and, thus by extension, with interlobular and pleural interstitial connective tissue. This interdependence of connective tissue is important in maintaining the overall structure of the lung and in providing a scaffold for the more delicate connective tissue of the parenchyma.

Tracheobronchial glands (*see* Fig. 1–9), specialized extensions of the surface epithelium into the lamina propria and submucosa, are seen exclusively in the trachea and bronchi.[18] The secretory portion of the gland is connected with the airway surface by a collecting duct. Multiple, usually branched, secretory tubules arise from the duct and are lined proximally by plump mucous cells and distally by somewhat flattened serous cells. The precise nature of the secretion of serous cells is not known. However, their electron and light microscopic appearances as well as their content of carbonic anhydrase suggest that their principal secretion is a low-viscosity substance, possibly meant to flush out the secretion of the mucous cells. Serous cells

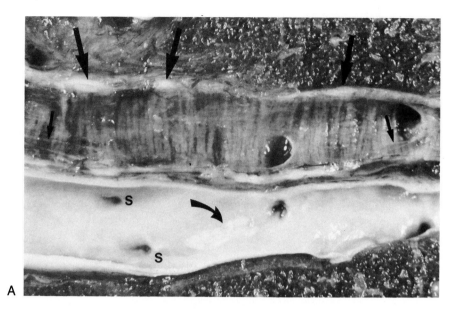

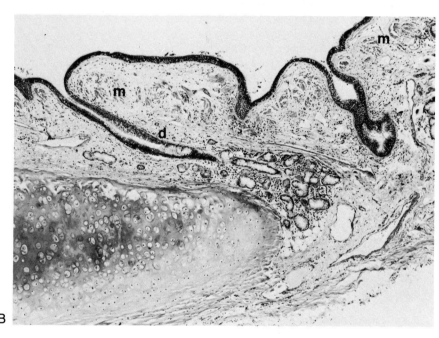

Figure 1–9. Normal Bronchus and Pulmonary Artery. *A,* Longitudinal slice of a small bronchus and adjacent pulmonary artery showing cartilage plates *(long arrows),* more or less circularly oriented smooth muscle bundles, and sparse, relatively thin, longitudinal elastic tissue bundles *(short arrows).* Note the supernumerary artery branches (unassociated with airway branches) (S) and the small focus of mild atherosclerosis *(curved arrow). B,* Histologic section through the bronchial wall showing cartilage plate, muscularis mucosa (m), bronchial gland duct (d), and acini (a). (× 40.)

have also been shown to be a source of lysozyme,[19] lactoferrin,[20] and leukocyte protease inhibitor[11]—substances of importance in local airway defense. There is also evidence that the cells function both in the manufacture of secretory component and in its coupling with and ultimate secretion of dimeric immunoglobulin (IgA).[21]

Many cells concerned with airway defense and other functions are found scattered in the lamina propria and submucosa. Lymphocytes are present both in subepithelial tissue and in the epithelium itself, either singly or in clusters, the latter being variously termed lymphoid nodules, lymphoid aggregates, or *bronchus-associated lymphoid tissue* (BALT).[22] These clusters are not present at birth but appear during the neonatal period and progressively increase in number so as to be found in almost all lungs by the age of 5 years.[23] *Plasma cells,* primarily IgA in type, are commonly found in the tracheobronchial tree, particularly in relation to mucous glands and in the lamina propria close

to the basal lamina.[24] Isolated *macrophages* and *mast cells* are found throughout the lamina propria and submucosa.

Anatomy—Transitional Zone

Geometry and Dimensions

Detailed three-dimensional studies of peripheral pulmonary tissue have shown that the geometry of the airways at this level is much more complex than is usually appreciated by examining two-dimensional histologic sections.[25] Although branching can occur in a more or less symmetric dichotomous fashion, trichotomous and even quadrivial (sometimes asymmetric) divisions of the respiratory bronchioles are frequent. In addition, the number, overall configuration, length, and diameter of airways from terminal bronchiole to alveolar sac are quite variable; for example, the number of generations from the terminal bronchiole to the alveolar sac may be as many as 12 and as few as 2, although 6 to 8 is probably representative of most pathways. This geometric irregularity is probably related, at least in part, to spatial constraints imposed by pleura, interlobular septa, and larger airways and vessels.

The number of alveoli per respiratory bronchiole, alveolar duct, and alveolar sac also exhibits much variation; for example, the mean number of alveoli per alveolar sac has been calculated to range from 3.5 to 29, with most studies documenting about 10.[25] The most realistic estimate of the number of alveoli per alveolar duct is probably 15 to 20.

Morphology

Respiratory bronchioles have a low columnar-to-cuboidal epithelium (composed mostly of ciliated and Clara cells) that gradually decreases in extent as the number of alveoli increases (Fig. 1–10). In the first- and second-order bronchioles, the epithelium is usually complete on one side, overlying a lamina propria and submucosa continuous with that of the terminal bronchiole and containing a prominent pulmonary artery branch. As the number of alveoli increases, the submucosa disappears, but the muscle and elastic tissue continue in fairly prominent bundles in a spi-

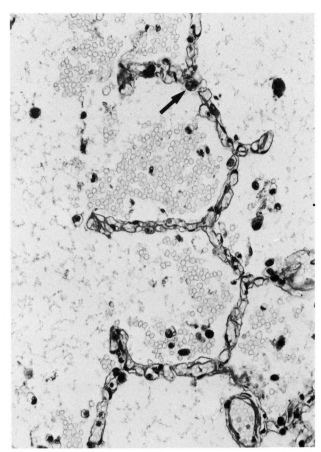

Figure 1–11. Normal Alveoli. Note the minute amount of tissue interposed between airspaces and capillary lumina. The nucleus of a type II cell, or macrophage, is present at the junction of two septa *(arrow)*; type I cells are not clearly evident. (× 350.)

ral fashion surrounding alveolar mouths. In the alveolar duct, bronchiolar epithelium is absent altogether, and only scanty interstitial tissue is present in the adjacent alveolar walls. Alveolar ducts terminate in a series of rounded enclosures called alveolar sacs, from each of which arise multiple alveoli.

Anatomy—Respiratory Zone

Geometry and Dimensions

Alveoli are small, cup-shaped outpouchings of respiratory bronchioles, alveolar ducts, and alveolar sacs that have been likened to the cells of a honeycomb or closely packed bubbles of soap foam (Fig. 1–11). They are demarcated by thin septa (walls) or, at their base in the respiratory bronchioles, by interstitial connective tissue. In general, three septa have a common line of junction at an average angle of 120 degrees, and it is assumed that they are more or less flat if there is no pressure difference between contiguous alveoli. As a result of close packing of several alveoli of adjacent alveolar ducts and sacs, the dome of an alveolus may consist of more than three septa.

The number of alveoli in the human lung is related to body length and varies considerably; in one study of lungs from 32 subjects aged 19 to 85 years, the computed totals ranged from 212×10^6 to 605×10^6 (mean, 375×10^6).[26]

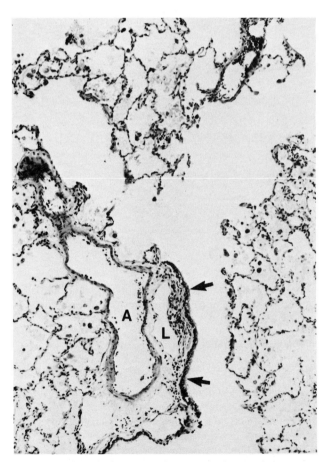

Figure 1–10. Respiratory Bronchioles. One wall of a proximal respiratory bronchiole is completely lined by a low columnar epithelium *(arrows)*. Adjacent to this is a small amount of interstitial tissue, a dilated lymphatic channel (L), and a branch of the pulmonary artery (A). The walls of the distal bronchiolar branches are almost completely alveolated. (× 80.)

In adults, both maximal diameter and depth of the alveolus average 250 to 300 μm.[2] Total alveolar surface area also varies with body size, ranging from 40 to 100 m[2] in one study.[27] In the average adult, it is probably between 70 and 80 m[2].[25]

Morphology

Alveolar septa are composed of a continuous, flattened epithelium covering a thin layer of interstitial tissue. The former consists primarily of two morphologically and functionally distinct cells, termed type I and type II. The interstitium itself contains a variety of cell types as well as a small amount of connective tissue. Although not usually considered a part of the alveolar wall, the alveolar macrophage is, in fact, normally present on the alveolar epithelial surface and may be partly derived from septal interstitial cells; thus, it is convenient to describe its morphology and function here.

Type I Alveolar Epithelial Cell. The type I alveolar cell (membranous pneumocyte) covers approximately 95 per cent of the alveolar surface area and has a total volume twice that of the histologically more obvious type II cell.[28] Its nucleus is small, somewhat flattened, and covered by a thin rim of cytoplasm containing few organelles (Fig. 1–12). The rest of the cytoplasm forms several broad sheets or plates that measure only 0.3 to 0.4 μm in thickness and that extend in all directions for 50 μm or more over the alveolar surface, covering an area measuring approximately 5000 μm[2].[28] The plates are joined firmly to one another and to type II cells by occluding or tight junctions (*see* Fig. 1–12) that are believed to represent a more or less complete barrier to the diffusion of water-soluble substances into the alveolar lumen.[29]

Although at first glance, the morphology of the type I cell suggests a purely passive role in pulmonary function, there is evidence that this might not be the case. The cytoplasm contains fairly numerous pinocytotic vesicles, which have been hypothesized to transport fluid or proteins in either direction across the air-blood barrier and have been thought to be a means of resorbing neonatal or pathologic alveolar fluid.[30] The cells also have been shown to have the ability to ingest intra-alveolar particulate material,[31] although the quantitative significance of this mechanism in relation to total lung particle clearance is probably small in comparison with alveolar macrophages.

Type II Alveolar Epithelial Cell. The type II epithelial cell (granular pneumocyte) is roughly cuboidal in shape and is usually located between type I cells near corners where adjacent alveoli meet. The cytoplasm contains fairly numerous membrane-bound granules filled with electron-dense lamellar material (Fig. 1–13) that is believed to be the source of alveolar surfactant.[32] In tissue fixed by perfusion through the vascular system, surfactant can be seen as a layer of acellular material about 4-nm thick lining the alveolar surface.[33] It consists of two components:[34] (1) a film facing the alveolar airspace, which is composed of densely spaced phospholipids that have a prominent tubular appearance (tubular myelin) (Fig. 1–14); and (2) deep to this film, a layer containing surface-active phospholipids in a different physicochemical configuration and representing the hypophase described by the physiologist. Components of the superficial layer are thought to be recruited from the deeper hypophase during expansion of the lung and may re-enter the hypophase layer at low lung volumes.

In addition to surfactant production, there are several other functions of the type 2 cell. In normal conditions, about 1 per cent are mitotically active and are responsible for renewal of the alveolar surface by differentiation into type I cells.[35] This replicative ability is also important in healing after lung injury, in which the relative cytoplasmic simplicity and large surface area of type I cells makes them particularly susceptible to damage. In such circumstances, type II cells proliferate and temporarily repopulate the alveolar walls, providing epithelial integrity. Providing there is minimal airspace and interstitial damage, the new type 2 cells can then transform into type I cells, completely restoring the normal alveolar surface. There is also evidence that type 2 cells may have a role in local immunoregulation by suppressing lymphocyte proliferation.[36]

Alveolar Septal Interstitium. A more or less continuous basal lamina underlies both type I and type II cells. Over about 50 per cent of its area, it is intimately apposed to the underlying endothelial basal lamina; interstitial connective tissue and endothelial and epithelial cell nuclei are absent from this region of apposition, so that the thickness of the air-blood barrier is determined only by the thin type I cell plate, endothelial cell wall, and fused basement membranes, the whole measuring about 0.5 μm (Fig. 1–15). Elsewhere, endothelial and epithelial basal lamina are separated by an interstitial space of variable width. The alveolar interstitium is, thus, separated into two distinct anatomic compartments, one relatively thin, across which the major portion of gas transfer takes place, and the other thicker.

In addition to the separated basement membranes, the thick portion of the interstitium contains connective tissue and several cell types. The former consists of a proteoglycan matrix in which are embedded elastic and collagen fibers that are intimately intertwined with and provide support for the capillary network. *Elastin* makes up almost 30 per cent of dry lung weight and can stretch to about 140 per cent of its length before breaking[37]; thus, it is of great importance in determining the mechanical properties of the lung. *Collagen*—of which the major types are I and III—is less abundant, constituting only about 15 per cent of dry lung weight[38]; although pulmonary synthesis and degradation have been traditionally believed to occur very slowly, there is evidence that they may be quite rapid. Both the collagen and the elastin of the alveolar septa are continuous with the fibroelastic tissue of the pleura, airways, and interlobular septa, thus forming a complex, three-dimensional connective tissue framework traversing and interconnecting the whole of the lung.

In addition to fibroblasts, the alveolar interstitium contains a variety of other cell types. One, termed the *contractile interstitial cell (myofibroblast)*, shows ultrastructural and immunohistochemical features suggestive of both smooth muscle and fibroblast differentiation.[39] These cells appear to cross the interstitial space and attach to the basement membrane of epithelial and endothelial cells. It has been suggested that their contraction may result in a reduction in capillary blood flow and that this may be the mechanism by which hypoxia causes decreased alveolar perfusion—thus, a possible means for local alveolar $\dot{V}_A/\dot{Q}$

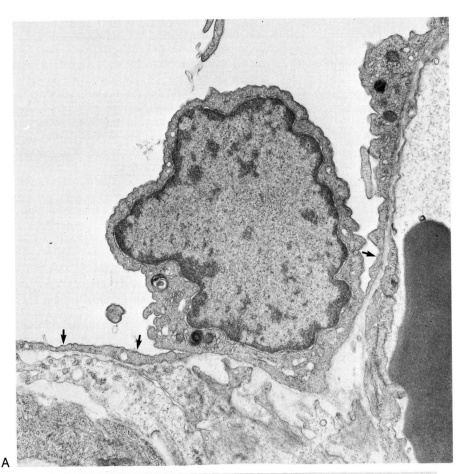

A

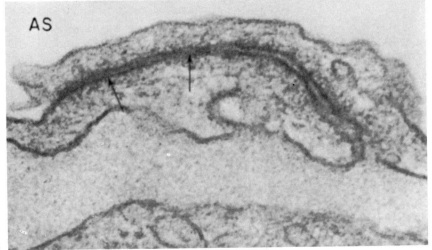

AS

B

Figure 1–12. Type I Alveolar Epithelial Cell. *A,* Low magnification showing the large nucleus and scanty cytoplasm that attenuates on both sides over the alveolar surface *(arrows). B,* High magnification of the junction between two type I cells, showing a cleft extending roughly horizontally inward from the alveolar space (AS). In several areas *(arrows)* the outer leaflets of the plasma membranes appear fused. (*A* courtesy of Dr. Nai-San Wang, McGill University; *B,* from Schneeberger-Kelley EE, Karnovsky MJ: The ultrastructural basis of alveolar-capillary membrane permeability to peroxidase used as tracer. J Cell Biol 37: 781, 1968. Reproduced from the *Journal of Cell Biology,* by copyright permission of the Rockefeller University Press.)

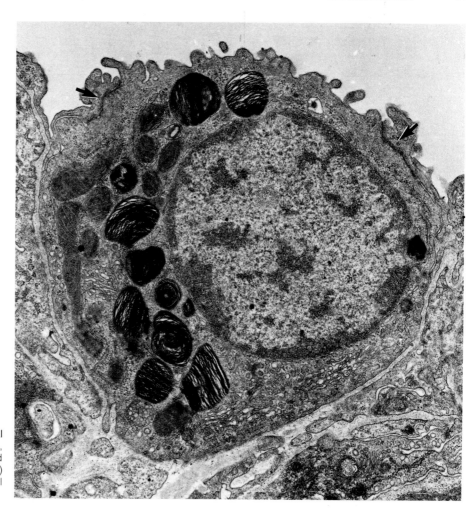

Figure 1–13. Type II Alveolar Epithelial Cell. Note the short surface microvilli, junctions with type I cells *(arrows)*, and lamellated inclusion bodies. (× 20,000.) (Courtesy of Dr. Nai-San Wang, McGill University, Montreal.)

regulation.[39] It also has been proposed that these cells may function as compliance regulators of the interstitial space, increasing resistance to interstitial expansion by edema fluid and thus propelling such fluid from the alveolar interstitium toward peribronchiolar lymphatics, where it may be effectively removed.[40]

Alveolar Macrophage. Pulmonary macrophages may be divided into four groups on the basis of differing anatomic location: (1) the *airway macrophage,* situated within the lumen or beneath the epithelial lining of conducting airways; (2) the *interstitial macrophage,* found either isolated or in relation to lymphoid tissue within interstitial connective tissue throughout the lung; (3) the *intravascular macrophage,* located adjacent to the capillary endothelial cell and possibly functioning as a reticuloendothelial cell similar to that in liver and spleen[41]; and (4) the *alveolar macrophage,* situated on the alveolar surface and within the airspace itself.[42] Although all these cells are morphologically similar, there is evidence that they may represent subpopulations with differing functional capabilities. However, because of its easy accessibility by bronchoalveolar lavage, the alveolar macrophage has been the most extensively studied, and the following discussion deals principally with this cell.

Alveolar macrophages range from 15 to 50 μm in diameter and are situated on the alveolar surface, with a preference for localization at the junctions between adjacent septa. Ultrastructurally, they show prominent surface mi-

crovilli and an abundance of intracytoplasmic, membrane-bound granules of variable appearance, representing primary and secondary lysosomes. Multiple studies have shown that alveolar macrophages are ultimately derived from bone marrow precursors, probably via the peripheral blood monocyte.[42] In addition, there is evidence for a population of alveolar interstitial macrophages that is capable of division and of replenishment or augmentation of the alveolar macrophage population.[43]

The functions of the alveolar macrophage are numerous and complex,[44] and only a brief overview will be given here. They can be considered under three headings: (1) phagocytosis and clearance of unwanted intra-alveolar material, (2) immunologic interactions, and (3) production of inflammatory and other chemical mediators. There is evidence that different subpopulations of macrophages may have different capacities for these functions.[45]

Phagocytosis and Clearance. Alveolar macrophages are motile and, in response to appropriate chemical stimuli, actively accumulate at the site of foreign material. Their surface possesses receptors for the Fc portion of various IgG molecules as well as IgE, IgA, and C3; in association with these and perhaps other opsonins, such as fibronectin, active phagocytosis of foreign material occurs. In addition to inhaled foreign substances, alveolar macrophages ingest and eliminate endogenous pulmonary material, including dead type I and type II cells, alveolar surfactant, and in-

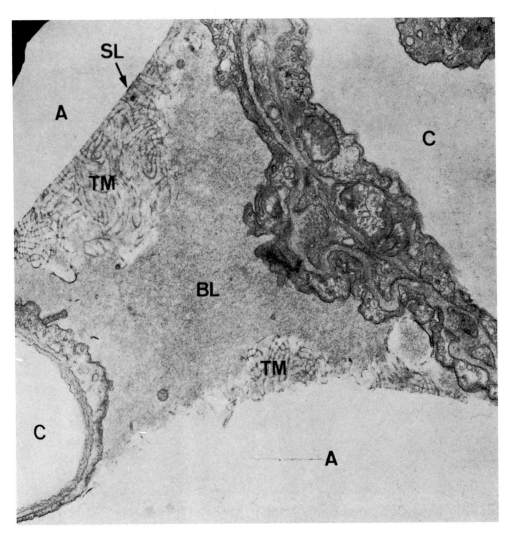

Figure 1–14. A Pore of Kohn. The pore is closed by lining material containing tubular myelin figures (TM) near the air-liquid interface. On the upper side, an osmiophilic outline (SL) is identified. BL = base layer of lining film; A = alveolus; C = capillary. (× 21,060.) (From Gil J, Weibel ER: Improvements in demonstration of lining layer of lung alveoli by electron microscopy. Respir Physiol 8: 13, 1969.)

flammatory exudate that may be produced during pneumonitis.

Although some macrophages containing foreign material enter the alveolar interstitium and either remain there or are transported via lymphatics to regional lymph nodes, there is evidence that few follow this route.[46] Instead, the majority either die within the alveoli or make their way to the terminal bronchioles, where they enter the mucociliary escalator and, along with their ingested material, are carried to the larynx and swallowed or expectorated.

Immunologic Interactions. Alveolar macrophages have important functions in both afferent and efferent immunologic reactions. Inhaled immunogens are phagocytosed and presented to T lymphocytes, which then develop specific immunity. Subsequent antigen presentation, again by macrophages, stimulates the T cells, which in turn leads to both T and B cell and T cell and macrophage interactions. The latter, mediated via lymphokines, results in macrophage activation and is manifested by features such as an increased number of surface receptors, increased amounts of lysosomal enzymes, and increased microbicidal activity. The importance of these interactions is illustrated by the frequency and severity of pulmonary infection in immunocompromised individuals. Macrophage–T lymphocyte interactions may also be important in the pathogenesis of some fibrotic lung diseases.[47]

Production of Mediators. Alveolar macrophages synthesize and probably secrete a variety of substances in both resting and activated conditions.[44] Many of these may have important effects on local pulmonary defense and structural integrity, including *fibronectin*,[48] a variety of proteases and antiproteases (*alpha₁-antitrypsin, alpha₂-macroglobulin, elastases,* and *collagenases*), highly active inflammatory mediators such as *prostaglandins*[49] and *leukotrienes,* and antimicrobial substances such as *lysozyme* and *interferon.*[50]

Various inhaled foreign materials have a deleterious effect on macrophage function. For example, particulates such as silicon dioxide can damage the lysosomal membrane, releasing enzymes into the cytoplasm and resulting in alteration of normal cell function or even cell death. A variety of insoluble compounds, such as nitrogen dioxide and ozone, may penetrate directly to the alveoli, where they damage the macrophage through lipid peroxidation or by chemical combination on the cell membrane of the oxidant gas with susceptible enzymes such as sulfhydryl enzymes.[51] Cigarette smoke also has been found to affect the alveolar macrophage by inhibiting metabolic activity and phagocytosis.[52]

Lung Unit

Of the subdivisions of lung parenchyma that have been proposed as the "fundamental unit" of lung structure, the primary and secondary lobules of Miller and the pulmonary

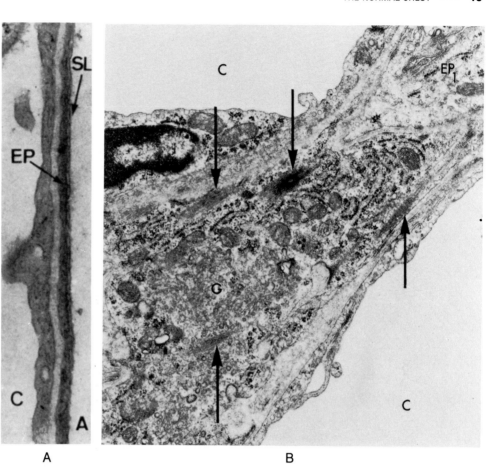

Figure 1–15. The Air-Blood Barrier. *A,* Thin portion. A capillary (C) is present on the left, and the alveolar space (A) on the right. A type I alveolar epithelial cell (EP) is covered by a layer of surfactant (SL). (× 48,420.) (From Gil J, Weibel ER: Respir Physiol 8: 13, 1969.) *B,* Thick portion. Capillaries (C) and epithelial cells (EP) are separated by collagen fibers and a prominent interstitial cell containing a Golgi apparatus (G) and numerous fibrillar bundles *(arrows).* (× 24,000.) (From Kapanci Y, Assimacopoulos A, Irle C, et al: "Contractile interstitial cells" in pulmonary alveolar septa: A possible regulator of ventilation-perfusion ratio? J Cell Biol 60: 375, 1974. Reproduced from the *Journal of Cell Biology,* by copyright permission of the Rockefeller University Press.)

A   B

acinus have gained the widest acceptance. The question of which most accurately represents the anatomic basis of normal and pathologic processes is controversial, since each possesses characteristics that suit one set of circumstances better than another. As we shall attempt to show, however, the one most acceptable for descriptive purposes is the pulmonary acinus.

Primary Pulmonary Lobule

The primary pulmonary lobule consists of all alveolar ducts, alveolar sacs, and alveoli, together with their accompanying blood vessels, nerves, and connective tissues, distal to the last respiratory bronchiole. Since there are approximately 23 million primary lobules in the human lung,[1] it is clear that this unit is too small to be seen roentgenographically when consolidated and, thus, is of no practical roentgenologic significance.

Secondary Pulmonary Lobule

The secondary pulmonary lobule is defined as the smallest discrete portion of the lung that is surrounded by connective tissue septa (Fig. 1–16). It is composed of three to five terminal bronchioles, with their accompanying transitional airways and parenchyma, and has been estimated to contain between 30 and 50 primary lobules. It is irregularly polyhedral in shape and generally ranges from 1 to 2.5 cm in diameter. Although some regard the secondary lobule as the basic unit of lung structure and function and hold that most pulmonary diseases are best considered in terms of this unit's pathology,[53] we take exception to this view for three reasons:

1. The distribution of lobules is not uniform within the lung, being particularly uncommon along the interlobar fissures, the posterior and mediastinal aspects, and the central portion; thus, in disease affecting these regions a lobular distribution is usually impossible to detect.

2. Even when the septa and lobules are visible, their size and extent are not uniform.

3. The secondary lobule seldom is recognizable as a structural unit by standard roentgenography, although it can be identified in both normal and pathologic states by high-resolution computed tomography (HRCT).[54]

Pulmonary Acinus

The acinus can be defined as that portion of the lung distal to a terminal bronchiole, comprising the respiratory bronchioles, alveolar ducts, alveolar sacs, and alveoli.[55] Since it is visible macroscopically, it is reasonable to assume its visibility roentgenologically when completely or partially filled with contrast material or inflammatory exudate. In order to demonstrate this, Gamsu and colleagues progressively opacified segments of normal lungs distal to a wedged catheter with a special tantalum suspension, obtaining sequential roentgenograms on fine-grain film until almost total opacification was achieved.[56] Progressive filling of a single acinus initially produced a rosette appearance and eventually a spherical lesion (Fig. 1–17). Measurements of 25 acini revealed a mean diameter of 7.4 mm (range, 6 to 10 mm) at a volume roughly equivalent to total lung capacity (TLC).

In the light of these observations and of previous discussions of the morphology of the lung parenchyma, we pro-

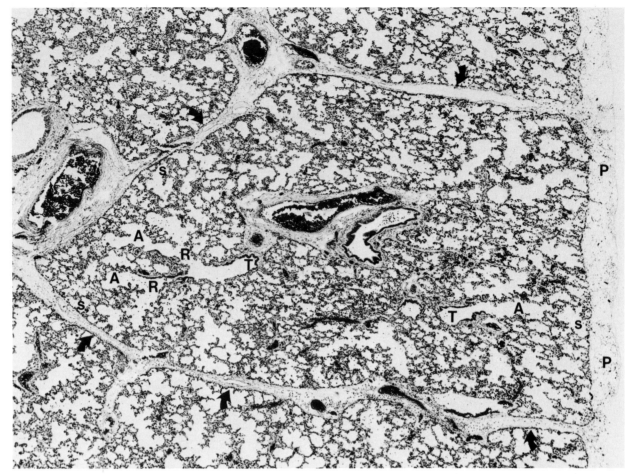

Figure 1–16. Secondary Lobule-Histologic Appearance. A = alveolar duct; *arrows* = interlobular septum; P = pleura; R = respiratory bronchiole; S = alveolar sac; T = terminal bronchiole. (× 6.)

pose three reasons for accepting the acinus as a roentgenologic unit: (1) it is roentgenologically visible; (2) it is recognizable throughout the entire lung; and (3) it provides a useful correlation with function, since it constitutes the gas exchange portion of the lung.

Channels of Peripheral Airway and Acinar Communication

The first and probably the most studied of these structures are small discontinuities in the alveolar septa termed *alveolar pores (pores of Kohn)* (Fig. 1–18). They are round or oval in shape, often situated at the junction of adjacent alveolar septa, and range in diameter from 2 to 10 μm. Because of their rarity in children most authorities believe that they are acquired; it has been suggested that they may result from the desquamation of alveolar epithelial cells, from the action of ventilatory stresses on alveolar walls, or from loss of interstitial connective tissue.[57] By transmission electron microscopy, the pore aperture is usually free of cellular or other material in airway-fixed material; in vascular-perfused tissue, however, it is frequently occluded by a thin film of alveolar surfactant.[58] Since it is probable that vascular-perfused tissue more closely represents the normal state within the alveolar lumen, this observation casts considerable doubt on the significance of the pores in collateral ventilation.

The relationship of *alveolar fenestrae*—discontinuities measuring from 20 to 100 μm in diameter—to alveolar pores is unclear. They are thought by most investigators to represent a pathologic state of the alveolar wall, some believing them to be the earliest stage of pulmonary emphysema. It has also been speculated that alveolar pores may themselves be the precursors of fenestrae.[59] Whatever their relationship, it is possible that these larger discontinuities are of greater significance than alveolar pores in providing a pathway for interacinar communication.

Direct communications between alveoli and respiratory, terminal, and preterminal bronchioles are termed *canals of Lambert* and consist of epithelium-lined tubular structures that, in lungs fixed in deflation, range in diameter from "practically closed" to 30 μm.[60] It is not known whether these "airways" provide solely intra-acinar accessory communications or whether interacinar connections capable of subserving collateral ventilation occur as well.

Roentgenology

Although several systems of bronchial nomenclature have been described, those of Boyden[61] and of Jackson and Huber[62] have been the most widely adopted and remain the generally accepted terminology in North America (Table 1–1). It should be remembered, however, that the pattern of bronchial branching described, although the com-

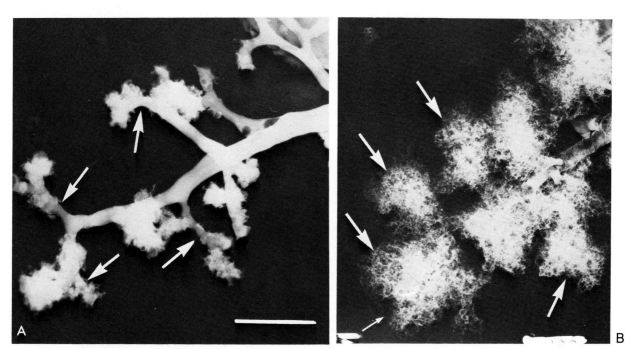

Figure 1–17. Bronchographic Morphology of the Peripheral Airways and Acinus. *A,* Selected area from the periphery of a bronchogram on a normal human lung removed at necropsy and opacified with a tantalum suspension. *Arrows* indicate terminal bronchioles. *B,* Roentgenogram after air-drying of the lung. There has now been further opacification of the intra-acinar airways. *Arrows* indicate partially opacified acini that can be related to the terminal bronchioles in *A.* The bar in *A* represents 5 mm. (From Gamsu G, Thurbeck WM, Macklem PT, et al: Peripheral bronchographic morphology in the normal human lung. Invest Radiol 6: 171, 1971.)

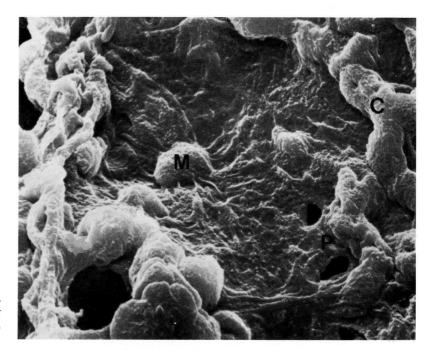

Figure 1–18. Surface of an Alveolus. Note surrounding capillaries (C), a macrophage (M), and alveolar pores (P). (× 3650.) (Courtesy of Dr. Nai-San Wang, McGill University.)

Table 1–1. **NOMENCLATURE OF BRONCHOPULMONARY ANATOMY**

Jackson-Huber	Boyden
Right Upper Lobe	
Apical	B[1]
Anterior	B[2]
Posterior	B[3]
Right Middle Lobe	
Lateral	B[4]
Medial	B[5]
Right Lower Lobe	
Superior	B[6]
Medial basal	B[7]
Anterior basal	B[8]
Lateral basal	B[9]
Posterior basal	B[10]
Left Upper Lobe	
Upper division	
Apical-posterior	B[1&3]
Anterior	B[2]
Lower (lingular) division	
Superior lingular	B[4]
Inferior lingular	B[5]
Left Lower Lobe	
Superior	B[6]
Anteromedial basal	B[7&8]
Lateral basal	B[9]
Posterior basal	B[10]

Modified from Hinshaw HC: Diseases of the Chest. 3rd ed. Philadelphia, WB Saunders, 1969.

monest, is far from standard, there being considerable anatomic variation (*see* page 268). The normal anatomy and common variations of the lower[63] and upper[64] lobe airways have also been described as viewed on thin-section, contiguous CT scans; virtually all segmental bronchi can be identified precisely, thus providing an additional technique whereby bronchial abnormalities may be evaluated. The anatomy of the bronchi in the hila as seen on CT is described farther on (*see* page 38).

Trachea and Main Bronchi

For all intents and purposes, the trachea is a midline structure; a slight deviation to the right after entering the thorax is a normal finding and should not be misinterpreted as evidence of displacement (*see* Fig. 1–19, page 18). The walls of the trachea are parallel except on the left side just above the bifurcation, where the aorta commonly impresses a smooth indentation. The air columns of the trachea, main bronchi, and intermediate bronchus have a smoothly serrated contour, created by the indentations of the cartilage rings in their walls at regular intervals.

In one CT study of 50 subjects without tracheal or mediastinal abnormalities, the length of the intrathoracic trachea ranged from 6 to 9 cm (mean, 7.5 ± 0.8 cm).[64a] The commonest shape was round or oval; a horseshoe shape with a flat posterior tracheal membrane was seen in only 12 subjects, an inverted pear shape in 6, and an almost square configuration in 2. Twenty-two of the 50 subjects had more than one distinct shape at different levels. Assuming a normative range that encompasses three standard deviations from the mean (99.7 per cent of the normal population), in men aged 20 to 79 years the upper limits of normal for coronal and sagittal diameters are 25 mm and 27 mm,

respectively[64b]; in women of the same age, they are 21 mm and 23 mm, respectively. The lower limit of normal for both dimensions is 13 mm in men and 10 mm in women. There are only negligible differences in coronal or sagittal dimensions on roentgenograms exposed at full inspiration and maximal expiration.

The trachea divides into right and left main bronchi at the carina. The angle of bifurcation varies considerably; in one study of 100 normal adult subjects, the range was 35 to 90.5 degrees (mean, 60.8 degrees ± 11.8 degrees).[65] In adults, the course of the right main bronchus distally is more direct than that of the left and is attributable, at least in part, to the pressure on the left wall of the trachea by the aorta. The transverse diameter of the right main bronchus at TLC is greater than that of the left (15.3 mm, compared with 13.0 mm[66]), although its length before the origin of the upper lobe bronchus as measured at necropsy is shorter (average, 2.2 cm, compared with 5 cm on the left[67]).

Lobar Bronchi and Bronchopulmonary Segments

On this and the following pages, the anatomy of the proximal bronchi and bronchopulmonary segments is described and illustrated. Each segmental bronchus is considered separately, preceded by reproductions of a right bronchogram, and corresponding drawings in anteroposterior (AP) (Fig. 1–19) and lateral (Fig. 1–20) projections, and of a left bronchogram similarly depicted (Figs. 1–21 and 1–22).

Right Upper Lobe. The bronchus to the right upper lobe arises from the lateral aspect of the main bronchus approximately 2.5 cm from the carina. It divides at slightly more than 1 cm from its origin, most commonly into three branches designated anterior, posterior, and apical. The branching pattern is particularly variable in relation to the axillary portion of the lobe.

Right Middle Lobe. The intermediate bronchus continues distally for 3 to 4 cm from the takeoff of the right upper lobe bronchus and then bifurcates to become the bronchi to the middle and lower lobes. The middle lobe bronchus arises from the anterolateral wall of the intermediate bronchus, almost opposite the origin of the superior segmental bronchus of the lower lobe; 1 to 2 cm beyond its origin it bifurcates into lateral and medial segments.

Right Lower Lobe. The superior segmental bronchus arises from the posterior aspect of the lower lobe bronchus immediately beyond its origin; thus, it is almost opposite the takeoff of the middle lobe bronchus. The four basal segments of the lower lobe can be readily identified roentgenologically: reference to Figures 1–21 and 1–22 shows that in the frontal projection of a well-filled bronchogram, the order of the basal bronchi from the lateral to the medial aspect of the hemithorax is *anterior-lateral-posterior-medial*. As the patient is rotated into 45-degree oblique and lateral projections, the relationship anterior-lateral-posterior is maintained; hence the mnemonic "ALP."

Left Upper Lobe. About 1 cm beyond its origin from the anterolateral aspect of the main bronchus, the bronchus to the left upper lobe either bifurcates or trifurcates, usually the former. In the bifurcation pattern, the upper division almost immediately divides again into two segmental branches, the apical posterior and anterior. The lower division is the lingular bronchus, which is roughly analogous to the middle lobe bronchus of the right lung. When trifurcation of the left upper lobe bronchus occurs, the apical posterior, anterior, and lingular bronchi originate simultaneously. The lingular bronchus extends anteroinferiorly for 2 to 3 cm before bifurcating into superior and inferior divisions.

Left Lower Lobe. The divisions of the left lower lobe bronchus are similar in name and anatomic distribution to those of the right lower lobe. The one exception lies in the absence of a separate medial basal bronchus, the anterior and medial portions of the lobe being supplied by a single anteromedial bronchus. The mnemonic ALP applies as well to the left lower lobe as to the right for identification of the order of basilar bronchi and their relationship to one another in frontal, oblique, and lateral projections.

Function—Pulmonary Ventilation

The main purpose of breathing is to achieve and maintain alveolar and arterial blood gas homeostasis so that the oxygen demands of the organism are met and the metabolic byproduct, carbon dioxide, is exhaled. This is accomplished by a combination of ventilation (involving movement of gas to and from the alveoli), diffusion (involving movement of oxygen and carbon dioxide across the alveolocapillary membrane), and perfusion (comprising transport of blood within the lung to and from the alveoli). The first of these three processes is discussed in this section; the remaining two are dealt with in the section on the vascular system (*see* page 45).

Composition of Gas in Alveoli

The composition of alveolar gas depends on the amount of oxygen removed and carbon dioxide added by capillary blood and the quantity and composition of the gas that reaches the acinus through the tracheobronchial tree.

Ventilation of the Acinus. Air contains approximately 21 per cent oxygen and 79 per cent nitrogen and, at sea level, has an atmospheric pressure of 760 mm Hg. The partial pressure for O_2 is approximately 160 and for N_2 is 600. As air is inhaled into the tracheobronchial tree, it becomes fully saturated with water vapor at body temperature at a partial pressure of 47 mm Hg, so that the partial pressure of oxygen drops to 150 mm Hg.

The quantity of gas reaching the alveoli (alveolar ventilation [$\dot{V}_A$]) depends on the depth of inspiration (tidal volume [V_T]), the volume of the conducting airways (the anatomic dead space [V_{DS}]), and the number of breaths per minute (f) and can be calculated by the formula:

$$\dot{V}_A \text{ (L/min)} = (V_T - V_{DS}) \times f$$

$\dot{V}_{DS}$ ventilation is not considered alveolar ventilation because at the end of expiration, the dead space is filled with expired air having a composition equivalent to that in the acinus. The V_A portion of each breath (ΔV) is added to the residual alveolar gas (V_O), and rapid diffusive mixing occurs so that gas tensions approach a uniform alveolar concentration. Failure of complete diffusive mixing within the air spaces may occur with acinar enlargement (emphysema) and with a decreased time for mixing.

Alveolar-Capillary Gas Exchange. Blood flow in the pulmonary capillaries affects the composition of alveolar gas by continuous removal of oxygen and addition of carbon dioxide. The ratio of alveolar ventilation to perfusion ($\dot{V}_A/\dot{Q}$) varies within the lung, and the interaction of these two dynamic processes results in fluctuation in alveolar gas tensions not only throughout the respiratory cycle but also from breath to breath, lobe to lobe, and even acinus to acinus.

Mechanics of Acinar Ventilation. The movement of air down the conducting system to the acinus requires force, measured as pressure, to overcome the elastic recoil of the lung parenchyma and chest wall, the frictional resistance to airflow through the tracheobronchial tree, and the inertia of the gas. Since air has very little mass, the inertial component is negligible with normal breathing frequencies; thus, elastic recoil and frictional resistance represent the major portion of the work of breathing.[68]

The force necessary to inflate the lung is provided by contraction of the inspiratory muscles—mainly the diaphragm and, to a lesser extent, the external intercostal muscles. Normally, expiration is a passive phenomenon associated with relaxation of the inspiratory muscles. However, in patients with obstructive airway disease and in normal subjects during periods of increased ventilation, expiratory muscles, especially the abdominals, may be recruited.

Elastic Recoil of Lung Parenchyma and Thoracic Cage. At the end of a quiet breath (functional residual capacity [FRC]), the chest wall recoils outward, exerting a force that is equal and opposite to the force exerted by the lung recoiling inward (Fig. 1–23). These balanced forces result in a negative pleural pressure of approximately 4 to 5 cm H_2O. On inspiration, the respiratory muscles act initially to overcome the elastic recoil of the lungs only. The chest wall actually aids inflation by its outward recoil until a volume of about 70 per cent TLC is reached; at this point, it is inflated beyond its resting position, and the force of muscle contraction is then exerted against the recoil of both lung and chest wall. TLC is reached when the inspiratory force achieved by the muscles is equaled by the combined recoil force of lung and chest wall. It is apparent from Figure 1–23 that as lung volume increases, the elastic recoil of the lung parenchyma increases in a nonlinear fashion.

During deflation of the lung from FRC toward residual volume (RV), the expiratory muscles are aided by the elastic recoil of the lung. As RV is approached, the chest wall becomes more difficult to distort, and it is finally set at the point at which outward recoil of the chest wall equals the force exerted by the expiratory muscles. In older subjects and in patients with obstructive lung disease, this point may not be reached, since the airways may narrow and limit expiration at higher lung volumes.[69]

The relationship between changes in volume and pressure ($\Delta V/\Delta P$) is compliance, which can be calculated for the lung and chest wall either separately or together (respiratory system compliance). The major determinants of the compliance of the lung are the quantity and anatomic arrangement of the collagen and elastic fibers in the parenchyma and airways and the surface tension at the air-fluid interface of the alveolar surface (*see* later). The compliance of the chest wall is determined largely by the rigidity of the rib cage. In normal subjects, the compliance of the respi-

Text continued on page 26

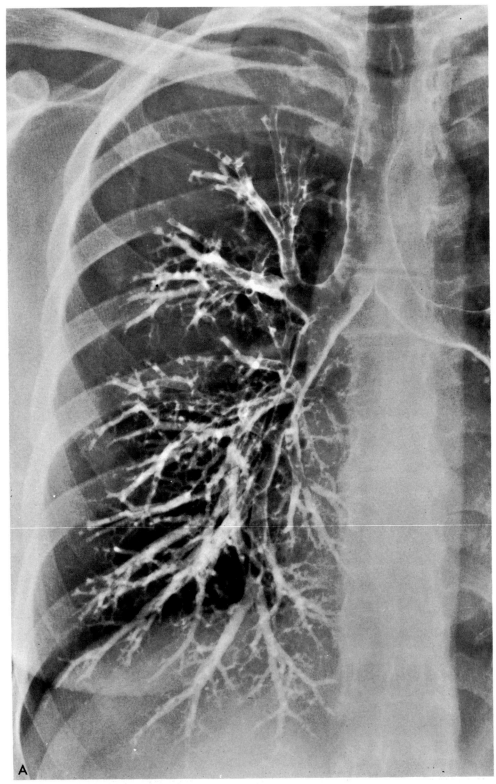

Figure 1–19. Right Bronchial Tree (Frontal Projection). *A,* Normal bronchogram of a 39-year-old woman.

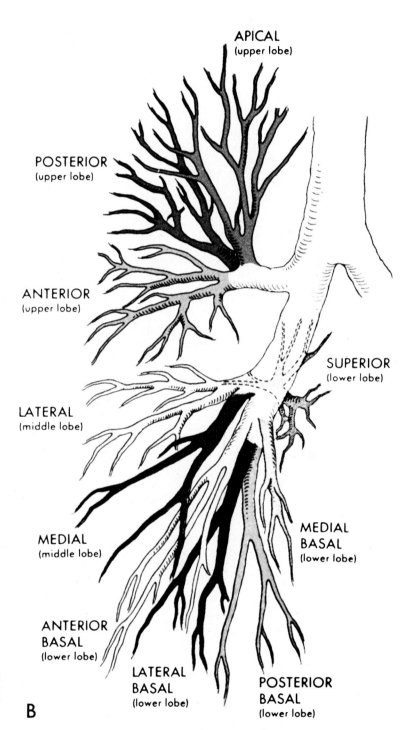

Figure 1–19 *Continued B,* The normal segments of the right bronchial tree in frontal projection. (*B* from Lehman JS, Crellin JA: Med Radiogr Photog 31: 81, 1955. Courtesy of Eastman Kodak Company.)

B

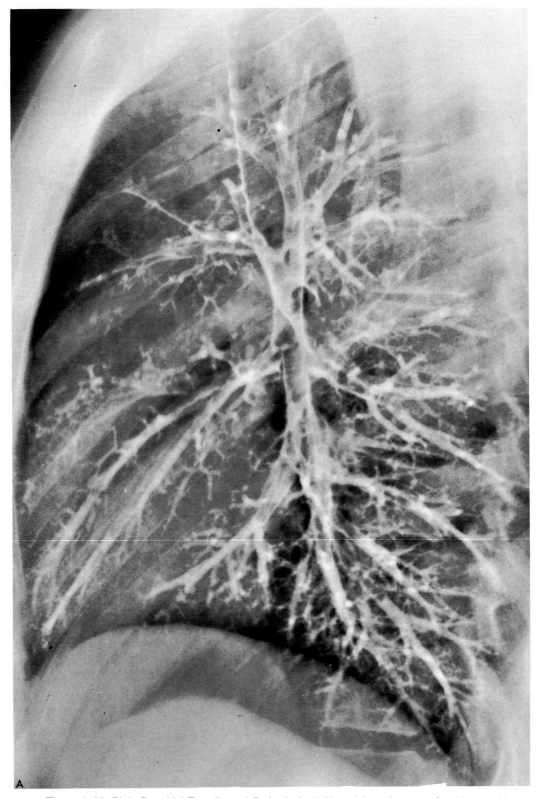

Figure 1–20. Right Bronchial Tree (Lateral Projection). *A,* Normal bronchogram of a 39-year-old woman.

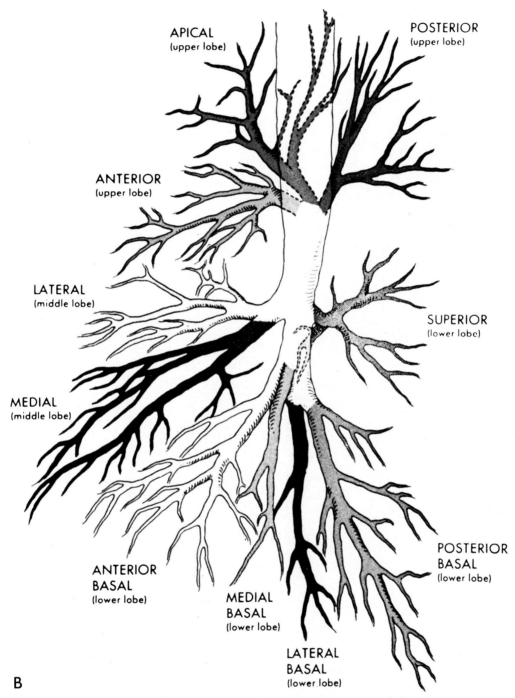

Figure 1–20 *Continued B,* The normal segments of the right bronchial tree in lateral projection. (*B* from Lehman JS, Crellin JA: Med Radiogr Photog 31: 81, 1955. Courtesy of Eastman Kodak Company.)

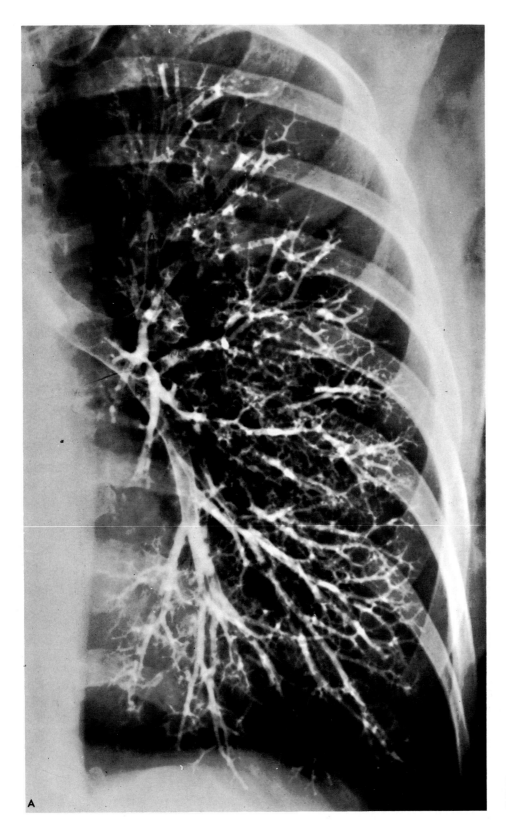

Figure 1–21. Left Bronchial Tree (Frontal Projection). *A,* Normal bronchogram of a 39-year-old woman.

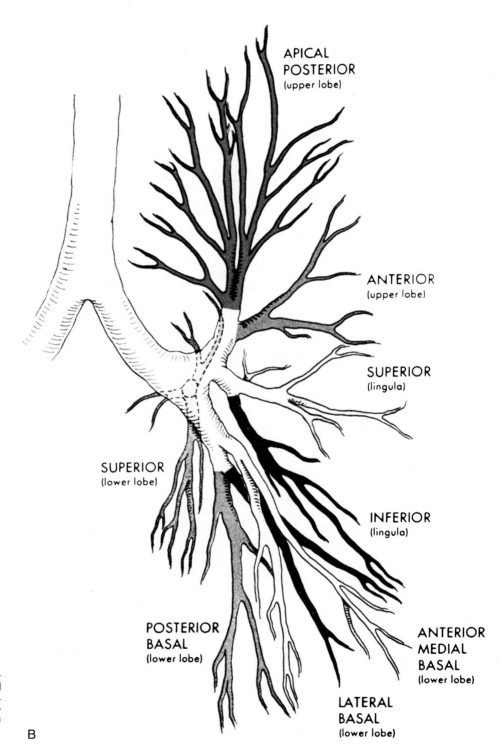

APICAL
POSTERIOR
(upper lobe)

ANTERIOR
(upper lobe)

SUPERIOR
(lingula)

INFERIOR
(lingula)

SUPERIOR
(lower lobe)

POSTERIOR
BASAL
(lower lobe)

LATERAL
BASAL
(lower lobe)

ANTERIOR
MEDIAL
BASAL
(lower lobe)

Figure 1–21 *Continued B,* The normal segments of the left bronchial tree in frontal projection. (*B* from Lehman JS, Crellin JA: Med Radiogr Photog 31: 81, 1955. Courtesy of Eastman Kodak Company.)

B

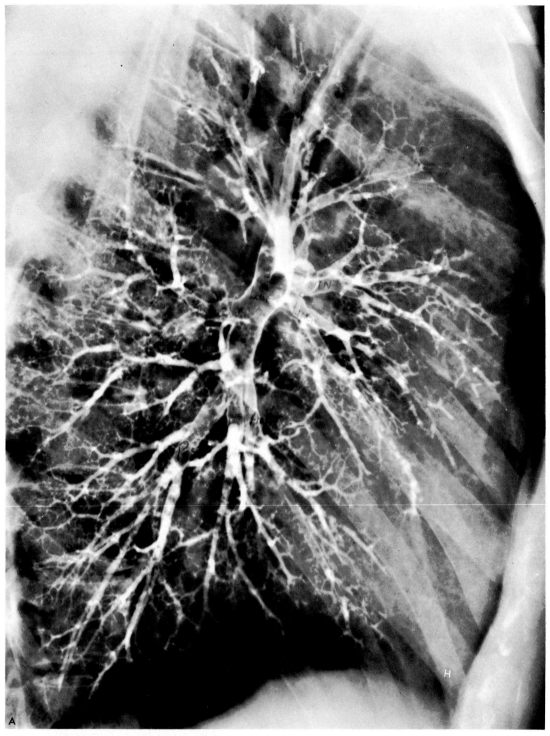

Figure 1–22. Left Bronchial Tree (Lateral Projection). *A,* Normal bronchogram of a 39-year-old woman.

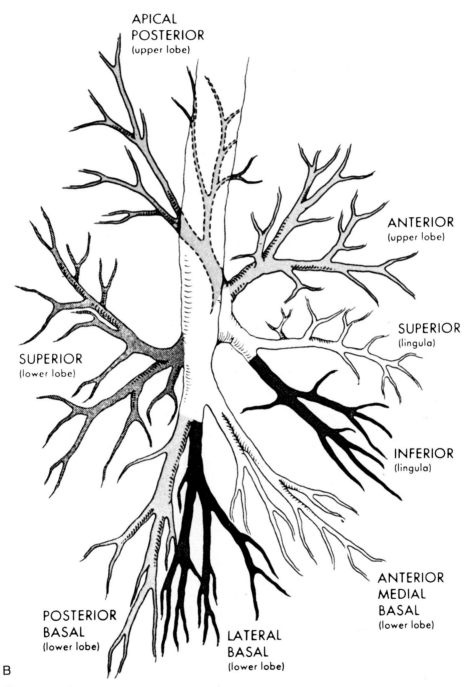

APICAL
POSTERIOR
(upper lobe)

ANTERIOR
(upper lobe)

SUPERIOR
(lingula)

SUPERIOR
(lower lobe)

INFERIOR
(lingula)

ANTERIOR
MEDIAL
BASAL
(lower lobe)

POSTERIOR
BASAL
(lower lobe)

LATERAL
BASAL
(lower lobe)

B

Figure 1–22 *Continued B,* The normal segments of the left bronchial tree in lateral projection. (*B* from Lehman JS, Crellin JA: Med Radiogr Photog 31: 81, 1955. Courtesy of Eastman Kodak Company.)

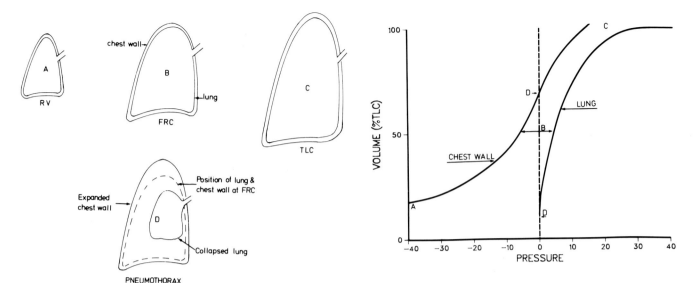

Figure 1–23. The Static Pressure-Volume Relationships of the Lung and Chest Wall. In the right panel, lung and chest wall volumes are plotted against pressure. Transpulmonary pressure (pleural pressure–alveolar pressure) is the appropriate pressure for the lung, whereas transthoracic pressure (pleural pressure–atmospheric pressure) is the appropriate pressure for the chest wall. In the left panel, drawing B shows the relationship of lung and chest wall at FRC; point B below shows that, at FRC, the transpulmonary and transthoracic pressures are equal and opposite in sign. At RV (residual volume) (A in left and right panels), transpulmonary pressure is near zero as the lung deflates toward its resting position, while the transthoracic pressure is very negative because the chest wall becomes stiffer at low lung volumes. At TLC (C in left and right panels), both the lung and the chest wall are expanded beyond their resting position, and both exert recoil favoring deflation. With development of a complete pneumothorax, transpulmonary and transthoracic pressures become zero, and the lung and chest wall assume their unstressed and relaxed positions (D).

ratory system is the major determinant of the work of breathing; in disease states, the work of breathing can be altered by increases or decreases in the compliance of the lung or chest wall. It is apparent from Figure 1–23 that as lung volume increases, the compliance of the lung and chest wall decrease; therefore, hyperinflation increases the work of breathing.

Surface Tension and Surfactant. The surface lining of the lung has unique properties that produce a much lower surface tension than if the alveoli were lined by water or plasma and that cause a reduction in surface tension as the lung is deflated. The substance responsible for these properties is surfactant, 90 per cent of which is composed of phospholipids; the main component of these is dipalmitoyl phosphatidylcholine (DPPC). Surfactant is secreted as a complex of these phospholipids and protein, of which two—apoproteins A and B—have been identified. Although pure phospholipid and the complex of apoprotein and phospholipids have similar capabilities for lowering surface tension, the lipoprotein complex spreads much more readily over the air-liquid interface, and the protein is probably necessary for efficient function.

The functions of surfactant include prevention of alveolar collapse, decrease in the work of breathing, an anti-sticking action that prevents adherence of alveolar walls, and an anti-wetting action that may aid in keeping the alveolar lining layer dry.[70] The forces that tend to decrease alveolar size are surface tension and tissue elasticity. The force generated by tissue elasticity is roughly proportional to lung volume but constitutes only one third of the total lung elastic recoil at TLC; the other two thirds are caused by

surface tension. The pressure due to surface factors can be calculated from the Young-Laplace relationship:

$$P = 2 \gamma/r,$$

where γ is the surface tension of the alveolar air-liquid interface and r is the alveolar radius. Opposed to the lung elastic recoil and surface tension forces that tend to collapse alveoli is the transpulmonary pressure. Mechanical balance is achieved when the transpulmonary pressure equals the pressures generated by elastic recoil and surface tension. With lung deflation, transpulmonary pressure decreases at the same time that alveolar radius is decreasing, a situation that favors alveolar collapse. This is why a substance with the surface tension–lowering ability of surfactant is necessary to achieve alveolar stability.

The reduction in surface tension imparted by surfactant may have an important role in fluid balance in the lung, distinct from its role in the mechanics of breathing. The reduced surface tension counteracts the tendency for fluid to be sucked into alveolar spaces from the capillary lumen.[71] Besides decreasing surface tension as lung volume decreases, surfactant imparts hysteresis to the lung's pressure-volume behavior; thus, at any given lung volume, surface tension and therefore lung elastic recoil are greater during inflation than during deflation. It has been suggested that in addition to alteration in surface forces, lung hysteresis is caused partly by a different sequence of recruitment and derecruitment of alveoli during inflation and deflation.[72]

Surfactant production and secretion are under complex neural, humoral, and chemical control. They are stimulated by an increase in ventilation or in tidal volume[73]; this effect appears to be mediated through the beta-adrenergic system, since this mechanical stimulatory effect can be blocked by propranolol.[74] The ultimate metabolic fate of secreted surfactant is poorly understood. Very little passes directly up the airways; however, some is taken up by alveolar macrophages and transported in them up the mucociliary escalator. In addition, a proportion enters the type I cells (via pinocytotic vesicles) and finds its way back into type II cells, where, presumably, it is reutilized.[70]

Resistance of the Airways. Frictional resistance to air flow through the tracheobronchial tree is the second major factor in the work of breathing and is related to the relationship of pressure to flow (P/V̇). The pressure necessary to produce laminar flow through a tube is described by the formula:

$$\text{Pressure required} \sim \frac{\text{Length} \times \text{Viscosity} \times \text{Flow}}{\text{Radius}^4}$$

It is apparent from this equation that airway radius is the dominant variable in determining resistance; a doubling of airway length would only double the pressure necessary to produce a given flow (i.e., double resistance), whereas a halving of the radius would lead to a 16-fold increase in resistance.

Under conditions of laminar flow, the flow rate is linearly related to pressure; that is, a doubling of pressure is required for a doubling of flow. However, with the development of turbulence and other nonlaminar flow regimes, the relationship becomes nonlinear, and a greater increase in pressure is required to produce a given increment in flow. In addition, with nonlaminar regimes, gas density begins to play a role, resistance decreasing with gases of low density (e.g., a helium and oxygen mixture). In normal individuals during quiet breathing through the mouth, the flow regime is almost totally laminar[75]; however, with breathing through the nose or through narrowed airways and during the increased flow rates of exercise, substantial turbulence may occur, resulting in an increasing proportion of the work of breathing devoted to overcoming resistance.

Total airway resistance represents the sum of the resistances of the various levels of the airway from the larynx and large bronchi down to the respiratory bronchioles. In normal subjects, the major part of total airway resistance is provided by large airways,[76] the relatively small component contributed by the smaller airways being related to their large cross-sectional area. However, in diseases such as asthma and chronic obstructive lung disease, the primary site of increased resistance is the small airways.

Tissue Resistance. Although the major impedance of the lungs and chest wall tissue is elastic, they do provide a small amount of frictional resistance, estimated to be between 5 and 40 per cent of total pulmonary resistance.[77]

Collateral Ventilation

Collateral air flow between lung units can be important in preserving gas exchange capacity and in matching ventilation and perfusion in the presence of airway obstruction.[78] The resistance to airflow through collateral channels (Rcoll) can be measured by wedging a bronchoscope in a peripheral airway and measuring the pressure required to force air through that airway and the collateral channels into the surrounding lung. It varies with several parameters, including inspired gas tension, lung inflation, and anatomic site. Increasing the partial pressure of carbon dioxide (P_{CO_2}) in inspired gas lowers collateral resistance, whereas the response is opposite with a decrease in the partial pressure of inspired oxygen (P_{O_2}). Collateral resistance decreases with lung inflation in a manner similar to the decrease in airway resistance that occurs with lung inflation. In normal lungs, however, collateral flow resistance at FRC is some 50 times greater than resistance to flow through the normal airways.[79]

Function—Respiratory Mucus and Mucus Rheology

The precise definitions of mucus, tracheobronchial secretions, and sputum are sometimes confused. Mucus represents the products derived from secretion of the tracheobronchial glands and epithelial goblet cells, whereas tracheobronchial secretions include the mucus plus other fluid and solutes derived from the alveolar and airway epithelium and the circulation; in normal subjects, the volume of these secretions has been estimated to range from 0.1 to 0.3 mL per kg of body weight, or up to about 10 mL per day.[80] Sputum consists of expectorated or swallowed mucus contaminated by saliva, transudated serum proteins, and inflammatory and desquamated epithelial cells; it is invariably associated with pulmonary disease.

Tracheobronchial secretions have three important roles:[81] (1) clearance of particulate matter deposited within the respiratory tract, (2) protection from microbial infection, and (3) humidification of inspired air and prevention of excessive fluid loss from the airway surface.

Biochemical Characteristics of Tracheobronchial Secretions. The biochemical composition of tracheobronchial secretions can be divided into two portions—a glycoprotein fraction that gives them their characteristic viscoelastic and rheologic properties, and sol-phase proteins that are derived from both local production and transudation from the serum.

The protein and nonmucous glycoprotein content in the sol phase of respiratory secretions has been characterized in sputum from patients and in bronchial lavage fluid from normal subjects.[82] It has been calculated that the quantity of IgG, IgA, transferrin, alpha$_1$-antitrypsin, and ceruloplasmin is greater than expected if transudation alone was the mechanism of their production, suggesting local production and secretion.[83] The excess immunoglobulins are synthesized by plasma cells in the airway submucosa and released into the airway lumen. Other substances that are locally produced include antiproteinases and antimicrobial substances, such as lysozyme and lactoferrin.

Ninety-five to 98 per cent of the weight of normal tracheobronchial secretions is water.[84] The electrolyte composition of the sol phase of airway secretions is similar to that of serum but has important differences; for example, the relative concentration of chloride is significantly higher than in serum, and normal airway secretions appear to be hyperosmolar relative to plasma.

Control of Tracheobronchial Secretions. Since atropine or vagal blockade decreases the basal secretion rate of tracheobronchial secretions to approximately 60 per cent,[85] normal secretion appears to be under a tonic cholinergic stimulation. There also appears to be both beta- and alpha-adrenergic stimulatory influences, and beta-blockade decreases basal secretions as well. Adrenergic stimulation increases secretion from serous cells predominantly, whereas beta-adrenergic stimulation increases chiefly mucous cell secretion; cholinergic stimulation increases secretion from both cell types equally.[86] Hypoxia, stimulation of gastric mechanoreceptors, stimulation of upper airway cough receptors, and a wide variety of irritants, such as ammonia, cigarette smoke, sulfur dioxide, and organic vapors, cause an increase in mucous secretion. Inflammatory mediators such as histamine, the prostaglandins, the leukotrienes, and the neuropeptides substance P and vasoactive intestinal polypeptide are also respiratory mucous secretagogues.

Optimal mucociliary clearance by respiratory tract cilia depends on a proper balance between the volume of the mucous layer and the more fluid and less viscid sol phase through which the rapid recovery stroke of the cilia occurs.[87] Increasing evidence supports the concept that this periciliary sol phase is linked to active ion transport across the epithelium.[88] In the trachea, a sodium-potassium adenosine triphosphatase (ATPase) pump appears to be located on the basal lateral surface of the epithelial cells. It acts by actively excluding sodium and results in chloride's being pumped into the cell and subsequently diffusing, along with water, down its electrochemical gradient across the apical epithelial cell surface into the lumen. This process results in an electrical potential difference across the airway epithelium, the lumen being approximately 30 mV negative relative to the submucosa.

There is evidence that this ion transport mechanism is under neural-humoral control. Pharmacologic alpha-adrenergic stimulation increases both the luminal movement of chloride and water and the submucosal movement of sodium, whereas beta-agonists increase only chloride secretion. Acetylcholine, histamine, prostaglandins, theophylline, and cylic adenosine monophosphate (cAMP) also increase chloride transport.[89] Regional differences in ion and water transport may have relevance in the control of the depth of the sol layer. This is a potentially important effect, since there is a rapid decrease in cross-sectional area of the airways as secretions move proximally (*see later*).

Physical Characteristics of Tracheobronchial Secretions. Few data exist on the controlling mechanisms that affect the viscoelastic properties of mucus. The rate of secretion of mucous glycoprotein and periciliary fluid is presumably important, but changes in the biochemical composition of the secreted mucus and the sol-phase proteins undoubtedly play a role as well. Vagal stimulation and methacholine inhalation tend to increase elasticity and dynamic viscosity at low stimulation frequencies and dose, whereas both viscoelastic characteristics decrease at higher frequencies and concentrations.[81] Beta-adrenergic stimulation imparts a selective stimulation of mucous cells and leads to increased elasticity and dynamic viscosity; by contrast, alpha-adrenergic stimulation selectively stimulates serous cells and results in a more watery mucus.[81] The inhalation of prostaglandin F_2, histamine, or acetylcholine has been shown to produce alterations in the viscoelastic properties of mucus in normal subjects, but these agents also increase the transudation of serum proteins into the bronchial mucus, suggesting altered epithelial fluid permeability.[90] Purulent sputum is more viscous but less elastic than mucoid sputum.[91]

Mucociliary Transport Mechanism. According to the sliding microtubule hypothesis,[92] ciliary movement occurs by means of the coordinated movement of dynein arms of one ciliary doublet along an adjacent doublet, much like going up or down the rungs of a ladder. Since not all doublets move at the same time, this coordinated movement leads to a shortening of some peripheral microtubules relative to those that are either contiguous to or on the opposite side of the cilium. With the internal rigidity that is provided by the radial spokes and the basal anchoring system, the cilium bends in the direction of shortening. The cilia normally lie in a bath of clear serous fluid of low viscosity (sol layer) and propel the mucus (gel layer) that floats on its surface like a raft supported by many hands beneath. During the rapid forward stroke, the cilia probably extend about 1 μm into the mucous layer; during the slower recovery stroke, they bend and move within the relatively less viscous sol layer.

The surface area on which the mucus lies converges about 2000-fold from small airways to the trachea; as a result, some absorption of fluid and acceleration of transport must occur to prevent the plugging of central airways.[87] A combination of an increased number of ciliated cells, an increased length of cilia, and increased ciliary beat frequency also contributes to more efficient clearing of secretions.

The mucociliary clearance rate varies widely in normal subjects and depends on a complex interaction among ciliary beat frequency, the depth of the periciliary sol phase, the quantity and viscoelastic properties of the airway mucus, and the state of hydration. Beta-adrenergic agonists appear to enhance transport rates.[93] High-frequency oscillatory ventilation[94] and dehydration[95] tend to decrease clearance rates, whereas high-frequency chest wall oscillation[96] and rehydration[95] increase them.

Cough. Cough is an important mechanism of respiratory defense and an adjuvant to the clearance of tracheobronchial secretions. It can be initiated voluntarily or involuntarily, the latter by stimulation of irritant receptors in the larynx, trachea, or large bronchi. The procedure begins with an inspiratory maneuver followed by glottic closure. Expiratory muscles then contract to increase pleural, abdominal, and alveolar pressures to a level of 100 mm Hg or more. The glottis is suddenly opened and expiratory flow begins, peaking in 30 to 50 milliseconds with flows at the mouth as high as 12 L per second. Expiratory flow limitation within the thorax occurs as a result of airway collapse and leads to gas velocities that reach three quarters of the speed of sound (1600 to 2400 cm per second). These high velocities produce enormous shear stress on the liquid layer lining the airways and move large amounts of mucus and any incorporated particulate debris proximally. Although cough is most effective in clearing secretions from large airways, calculations suggest that some clearance can occur down to twentieth-generation airways. The greater the depth of the periciliary serous layer and the less viscous it is, the greater is its effectiveness.

PULMONARY VASCULAR SYSTEM

Anatomy

Morphology and Dimensions of the Major Vessels

The conducting and transitional airways are intimately related to the pulmonary vasculature, a branch of the pulmonary artery always accompanying the appropriate bronchial division. In addition to these "conventional" vessels, many accessory ("supernumerary") branches of the pulmonary artery arise at points other than corresponding bronchial divisions and directly penetrate the lung parenchyma. These accessory branches outnumber the conventional ones and originate throughout the length of the arterial tree, most frequently peripherally. Thus, the branching ratio (average number of daughter branches emanating from one parent branch) increases as vessel size decreases; proximally, the ratio is about 3, a value comparable to that of the conducting airways, and distally it rises to about 3.6.[97] The precapillary pulmonary vessels can be conveniently divided into three morphologic types: elastic, muscular, and arteriolar.

Elastic arteries include the main pulmonary artery and its lobar, segmental, and subsegmental branches, extending approximately to the junction of bronchi and bronchioles. Histologically, the large extrapulmonary vessels contain a multilayered latticework of elastic fibers. Within the lung, the number of laminae diminishes so that at a diameter of 500 to 1000 μm, medial elastic tissue is lost altogether, leaving only well-developed internal and external laminae.

Muscular arteries have an external diameter ranging from about 70 to 500 μm and possess a well-developed layer of circularly oriented smooth muscle cells between the elastic laminae. Acinar vessels with recognizable arterial features and most supernumerary arterial branches are of this type. Beyond a diameter of 70 to 80 μm, arteries gradually lose their medial smooth muscle to become arterioles, composed solely of a thin intima and a single elastic lamina that is continuous with the external elastic lamina of arteries. Within the acinus, arterioles continue to divide and accompany their respective branches of the transitional airways as well as giving rise to many accessory branches. These branches as well as those that terminate around the alveolar sacs break up to form the capillary network of the alveoli.

Pericytes are found in alveolar capillaries and arterioles in intimate association with endothelial cells. Their importance and precise function are not clear, but it has been suggested that they may act as either contractile or phagocytic elements.[98] Mast cells also occur in the connective tissue adjacent to pulmonary vessels, where they may function as mediators of hypoxic vasoconstriction.[99]

The pulmonary veins arise from capillaries of the alveolar meshwork and from some of the bronchial capillaries. The larger branches are located within their own interstitial sheath separate from the bronchoarterial bundles. Although their final course is somewhat variable, there are usually two large superior and two large inferior pulmonary veins, the former draining the middle and upper lobes on the right side and the upper lobe on the left, and the latter the lower lobes.

Histologically, pulmonary veins show a variable number of elastic laminae associated with small bundles of smooth muscle cells and collagen. No valves are present; however, regularly spaced annular constrictions, possibly caused by local accumulations of smooth muscle, have been identified in animal veins and have been hypothesized to be capable of influencing blood flow.[100]

Pulmonary Endothelium

Ultrastructurally, endothelial cells are arranged in an interlocking mosaic of platelike processes measuring as little as 0.1 μm in thickness.[101] On the cell surface are numerous small microvilli, which are present at all levels of the vascular system but are most prominent in veins and arteries. These greatly increase the cell surface area and have been shown to react immunochemically with an antibody to angiotensin-converting enzyme,[102] implying a role in metabolic function.

A prominent feature of the capillary endothelial cell is the presence of numerous small pits, or vesicles (*caveolae intracellularis*) (Fig. 1–24).[103] These are located in the thick, non–gas-exchanging part of the cell, either at the luminal or abluminal surface or free in the cytoplasm. Small electron-dense granules, considered to represent enzyme complexes responsible for various metabolic functions, can be seen at the bases of the vesicles. In addition to this role, it is thought that the vesicles function as a transport mechanism for fluid and proteins between blood and interstitial tissue.[104]

Endothelial cells are joined by tight junctions,[101] which appear by transmission electron microscopy as focal areas of fusion of the outer lamellae of adjacent cell membranes. As seen by freeze-fracture techniques, the junctions are less complex than those of the alveolar epithelium; along with evidence provided by autoradiographic tracer studies, this suggests that the main site of solute impermeability in the air-blood barrier is the epithelium. The complexity of the endothelial junctions is variable, being greater in arterioles (which are felt to be relatively impermeable) and less in venules (which are thought to be the major site of vascular fluid leakage).

Geometry and Dimensions of the Alveolar Capillary Network

The pulmonary capillaries form a dense network of interconnecting vessels within the alveolar wall (Fig. 1–25). Their actual arrangement is highly complicated, when one considers the three-dimensional capillary and alveolar geometry under dynamic conditions. In this situation, the shape of the alveolar septa—and the vessels they contain— can be affected by three mechanical factors, each of which can vary in the normal respiratory cycle:[105] (1) tissue force as a result of tension on the interstitial connective tissue transmitted through the connective tissue of the visceral pleura, (2) capillary distending pressure, and (3) alveolar air-fluid surface forces.

The external diameter of capillary segments in fresh lung averages 8.6 μm[106]; allowing 0.3 μm for the average thickness of the capillary endothelial wall, the average internal

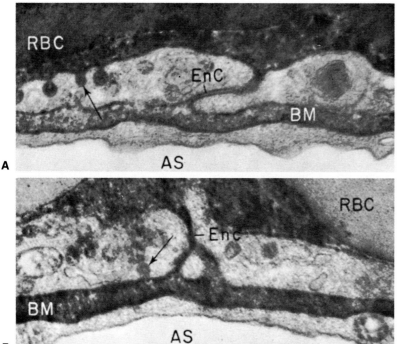

A

B

Figure 1–24. Endothelial Intercellular Cleft. Section of alveolar wall from the lung of a mouse sacrificed 90 seconds after horseradish peroxidase injection. Reaction product in the capillary lumen (indicated by RBC) extends through the endothelial intercellular cleft (EnC) into the adjacent basement membrane (BM). In *A*, the staining of horseradish peroxidase is quite light, whereas in *B* the basement membrane is deeply stained. Reaction product is present in endothelial invaginations (caveolae intracellularae) on both the capillary side *(arrow in A)* and the alveolar side *(arrow in B)* of the cell. (× 46,000.) (From Schneeberger-Kelley EE, Karnovsky MJ: The ultrastructural basis of alveolar-capillary membrane permeability to peroxidase used as tracer. J Cell Biol 37: 781, 1968. Reproduced from the *Journal of Cell Biology,* by copyright permission of the Rockefeller University Press.)

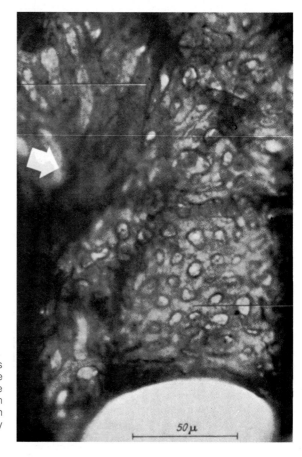

Figure 1–25. Alveolar Capillary Network. The face of an alveolar septum has been stained with periodic acid–Schiff (PAS) to show the complex, sievelike capillary network. A fan-shaped precapillary arteriole *(arrow)* leads into the network. (× 580.) (From Weibel ER, Gomez DM: Architecture of the human lung: Use of quantitative methods establishes fundamental relations between size and number of lung structures. Science 137: 577, 1962. Copyright 1962 by the American Association for the Advancement of Science.)

capillary diameter is thus about 8 μm. (However, these values may vary substantially with both lung volume and capillary pressure.[107]) The axial length of capillary segments ranges from 9 to 13 μm (average, 10.3 μm). Weibel deduced that each alveolus is surrounded by about 1800 to 2000 capillary segments and that the total capillary surface of the lung is about 70 m², only slightly less than that of the alveolar surface.[106]

Intervascular Anastomoses

Because of the lungs' dual blood supply, several combinations of intervascular anastomoses are possible. Those between *bronchial arteries* and *pulmonary veins* are undoubtedly the most frequent and probably represent the normal pathway for the bulk of bronchial venous drainage. *Bronchial artery–pulmonary artery* anastomoses have been shown to occur in the normal lung, but their significance in terms of extent is debated; however, their number and size may increase appreciably in various disease states. Although investigated extensively, the existence of *pulmonary arteriovenous anastomoses* is uncertain; some studies find evidence for their presence, whereas others do not.

Roentgenology—Vasculature

The main pulmonary artery originates in the mediastinum at the pulmonic valve and passes upward, backward, and to the left before bifurcating within the pericardium into the shorter left and longer right pulmonary arteries.

The *right pulmonary artery* courses to the right behind the ascending aorta before dividing behind the superior vena cava and in front of the right main bronchus into ascending (truncus anterior) and descending (interlobar) rami (Fig. 1–26). Although variable, the common pattern is for the ascending artery to subdivide into the segmental branches that supply the right upper lobe, whereas the descending branch ultimately contributes the segmental arteries to the middle and right lower lobes. The first portion of the right interlobar artery is horizontal, interposed between the superior vena cava in front and the intermediate bronchus behind. It then turns sharply downward and backward, assuming a vertical orientation within the major fissure anterolateral to the intermediate and right lower lobe bronchi before giving off the segmental branches— one or two to the middle lobe and usually single branches to each of the five bronchopulmonary segments of the lower lobe.

The *left pulmonary artery,* after passing over the left main bronchus, sometimes gives off a short ascending branch that subsequently divides into segmental branches to the upper lobe; more commonly, however, it continues directly into the vertically oriented left interlobar artery, from which the segmental arteries to the upper and lower lobes arise directly. The left interlobar artery lies posterolateral to the lower lobe bronchus (Fig. 1–27).

Measurement of arterial width can be useful in the diagnosis of diseases affecting the pulmonary vessels,[108] and normal limits have been established. In one study of more than 1000 healthy American adults, the upper limit of the transverse diameter of the right interlobar artery (measured during full inspiration) from its lateral aspect to the air

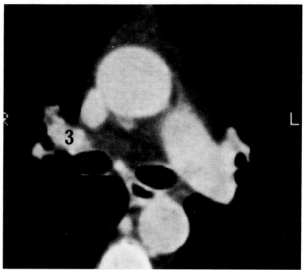

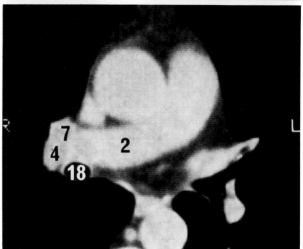

Figure 1–26. Anatomic Features of the Right Pulmonary Artery and Its Major Branches. The right pulmonary artery (2) divides within the pericardium into ascending (3) and descending (4) rami; the latter turns vertically at the hilum, lateral to the intermediate bronchus (18) and posterior to the right superior vein (7). Note that the interlobar artery is thus composed of a short horizontal limb and a longer, obliquely vertical part.

column of the intermediate bronchus was 16 mm in men and 15 mm in women[109]; these figures decreased by 1 to 3 mm in full expiration. In addition to direct measurement, changes in arterial caliber can be estimated by determining the ratio of the transverse diameter of a pulmonary artery to the contiguous bronchus viewed end-on in the perihilar area (the artery-bronchus index). In one study of 1200 tomograms of 250 normal subjects in the supine position,[110] this measurement was independent of age, sex, and body build and provided a more objective assessment of disturbances in pressure and flow in the pulmonary circulation than was possible with direct measurement of the caliber of the artery itself. The mean value of the index was 1.30 immediately distal to the takeoff of the right upper lobe bronchus and 1.40 immediately beyond the origin of the left upper lobe bronchus.

As indicated previously, the course of the *pulmonary veins* is remote from that of the bronchoarterial bundles, so

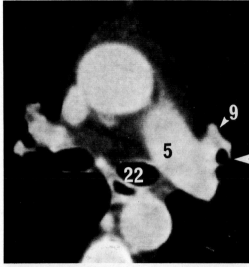

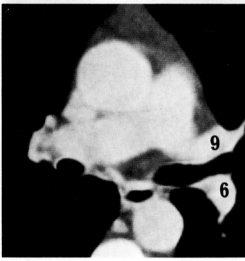

Figure 1–27. Anatomic Features of the Left Pulmonary Artery and Its Major Branches. The left pulmonary artery (5) passes over the left main bronchus (22), forming the interlobar (6) branch. The left superior vein (9) lies medial to the apicoposterior bronchus *(arrowhead)* before it passes into the mediastinum in front of the left upper/main bronchial continuum prior to its entrance into the top of the left atrium.

that in all areas the arteries and their corresponding veins are separated by air-containing lung. Theoretically, this should permit distinction of artery from vein, particularly in the medial third of the lung, where the continuity of the artery with its accompanying bronchus may be more readily distinguished and where the typical course of the larger veins on their way to the mediastinum can be recognized. However, in a pulmonary angiographic study of 50 patients in AP projection, the upper lobe artery and vein were superimposed in 40 to 50 per cent of subjects, the implication being that these vessels could not be distinguished on standard roentgenograms.[111]

Segmental veins from the right upper lobe coalesce to form the *right superior pulmonary vein* (Fig. 1–28), which descends medially into the mediastinum before joining the upper posterior aspect of the left atrium (the superior venous confluence). Along its course caudad, this vessel is intimately associated with the junction of the horizontal and vertical segments of the right interlobar pulmonary artery

and the anteromedial aspect of the middle lobe bronchus. The *middle lobe vein,* after passing under the middle lobe bronchus, usually joins the left atrium at the base of the superior pulmonary venous confluence, although occasionally the three veins on the right (superior, middle, and inferior) remain separate.

On the left, the segmental veins from the upper lobe join to form the *left superior pulmonary vein* (Fig. 1–29), which, after uniting with the lingular vein, courses obliquely downward and medially into the mediastinum. Along its course caudad, this vessel lies medial to the apicoposterior bronchoarterial bundle, anterolateral to the left pulmonary artery, and, finally, anterior to the continuum formed by the left main and upper lobe bronchi. It thus separates these airways from the left atrium before it enters this chamber.

The horizontally oriented lower lobe segmental veins on both sides coalesce medial to the lower lobe bronchi to form the *right* and *left inferior pulmonary veins;* as they attach to the left atrium medially, they form the inferior pulmonary venous confluences (Fig. 1–30). The left inferior pulmonary vein and venous confluence are at the same level as or slightly higher than those on the right and slightly more posterior; this vein may join with the left superior vein to form a common chamber before entering the left atrium. The normal superior and inferior venous confluences are sometimes prominent enough to simulate a mass on a lateral chest roentgenogram, particularly, but not exclusively, on the right.

Roentgenology—Hila

Although the anatomic boundaries defining the hila are somewhat vague,[112] they can be conveniently defined as those areas in the center of the thorax that connect the mediastinum to the lungs. There are three principal roentgenographic techniques for their examination: (1) conventional roentgenograms in posteroanterior (PA) and lateral projections, the method that suffices in the majority of cases; (2) CT; and (3) magnetic resonance imaging (MRI). Each of these techniques possesses distinct advantages and disadvantages; however, since all of them are used to greater or lesser extent in clinical practice, it is necessary to describe the normal features of each.

Conventional Posteroanterior and Lateral Roentgenograms

In PA projection, the *right upper hilar opacity* relates to the ascending pulmonary artery (truncus anterior) and right superior pulmonary vein, including respective branches of each (Fig. 1–31). The end-on opacity and radiolucency, respectively, of the contiguous anterior (occasionally posterior) segmental artery and bronchus can be identified in the majority of normal subjects.[113] A short segment of the upper lobe bronchus, beneath the ascending right pulmonary artery, may sometimes be observed before it trifurcates into the segmental branches serving the upper lobe.

The *lower portion of the right hilum* (see Fig. 1–31) is formed by the vertically oriented interlobar artery, the right superior pulmonary vein superolaterally as it crosses the junction of the horizontal and vertical limbs of the interlo-

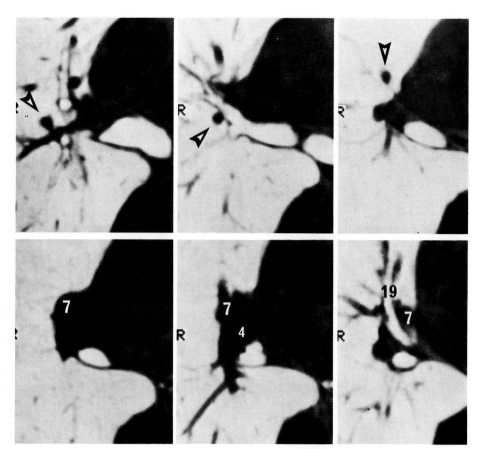

Figure 1–28. Right Superior Pulmonary Vein (RSPV). Sequential CT scans through the right hilum. The RSPV (7) is formed following the union of upper lobe segmental veins *(arrowhead);* so formed, it relates intimately to the horizontal limb of the interlobar artery (4) and the middle lobe bronchus (19) before entering the left atrium. The RSPV and the right interlobar artery form a typical "elephant head-and-trunk" configuration *(middle frame, bottom).*

bar artery, and the respective branches of these vessels. More inferiorly lies the horizontally oriented inferior pulmonary vein. The radiolucent lumen of the intermediate bronchus is invariably identified medial to the interlobar artery. Occasionally, segmental bronchi and arteries in the middle and lower lobes can be seen either in profile or end-on.

The *left superior hilum,* unlike its counterpart on the right, is often partly or completely covered by mediastinal fat and pleura between the aortic arch and the left pulmonary artery, or by a portion of the cardiac silhouette. When it is visible, the upper hilar opacity is formed by the distal left pulmonary artery, the proximal portion of the left interlobar artery, its segmental arterial branches, and the left superior pulmonary vein and its major tributaries (Fig. 1–32). Frequently, the anterior segmental or lingular bronchoarterial bundle can be identified end-on. The proximal left pulmonary artery is almost always higher than the highest point of the right interlobar artery. As suggested by Simon, the reference point for the determination of this relationship is the point at which the right and left superior pulmonary veins cross their respective pulmonary arteries prior to entering the mediastinum.[114]

The *lower portion of the left hilum* is formed by the distal interlobar artery, the lingular artery and vein, and, more caudally, the left inferior pulmonary vein (*see* Fig. 1–32). The air columns of the left upper lobe bronchus, and its superior and inferior (lingular) divisions, and the left lower lobe bronchus may be identified.

The roentgenographic anatomy of the hila in *lateral projection* is complex, since the right and left hilar components

are to a large degree superimposed.[115, 116] The most useful landmarks for the carina are the left pulmonary artery or the proximal third of the intermediate stem line, structures that bear a close approximation to the tracheal bifurcation. The air column of the normally more cephalad right upper lobe bronchus can be identified end-on in 50 per cent of subjects, whereas that of the more caudad left upper lobe bronchus is seen in about 75 per cent (Fig. 1–33).[115] Occasionally (usually in sthenic individuals), the uppermost radiolucency represents the right main bronchus, and the lowermost the left main bronchus.

The orifice of the right upper lobe bronchus is seldom as well circumscribed as that of the left; this is due to the fact that the latter is completely surrounded by vessels (the left pulmonary artery above, the interlobar artery behind, and the mediastinal component of the left superior pulmonary vein in front), whereas the former is devoid of vascular envelopment on its posterior aspect so that aerated upper or lower lobe parenchyma normally abuts its wall. Consequently, clear identification of the right upper lobe bronchial lumen *en face* constitutes highly suggestive evidence that the airway is completely surrounded by soft tissue, most likely enlarged lymph nodes.

The posterior walls of the right main and intermediate bronchi form the anatomic foundation for the *intermediate stem line* (*see* Fig. 1–33), a vertically oriented linear opacity measuring up to 3 mm in width[117] that is visible in 95 per cent of individuals.[115] The posterior walls of these two bronchi are rendered visible by air in their lumina in front and aerated lung parenchyma in the azygoesophageal recess behind. On a well-centered lateral projection, the line tran-

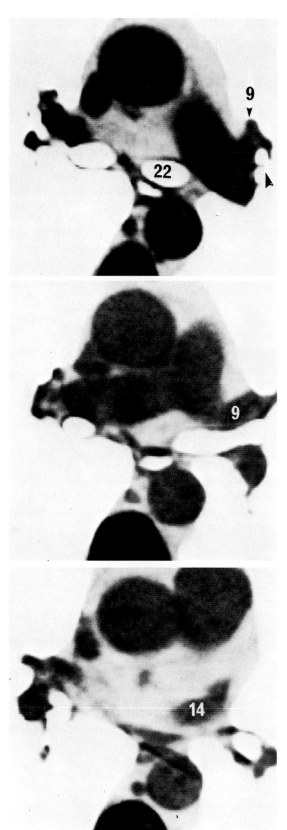

Figure 1–29. Left Superior Pulmonary Vein (LSPV). Sequential CT scans through the left hilum. The LSPV (9) is formed following union of the upper lobe segmental veins; it relates to the apicoposterior bronchus *(arrowhead)* before passing into the mediastinum in front of the left upper/main bronchial continuum (22) prior to its insertion into the superior portion of the left atrium (14).

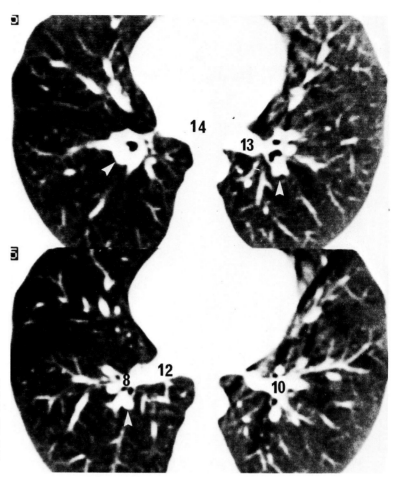

Figure 1–30. Right and Left Inferior Pulmonary Veins and Confluences. In contrast with the vertical orientation of the lower lobe arteries *(arrowheads),* the right (12) and left (13) pulmonary vein confluences, inferior pulmonary veins (8, 10), and their major branches are horizontally oriented in the lower lobes prior to their entry into the left atrium (14). The left inferior pulmonary vein is usually higher and more posterior than the right.

sects the middle or posterior third of the circular, radiolucent left upper lobe bronchus; it terminates caudally at the origin of the superior segmental bronchus of the right lower lobe, slightly proximal to or at the same level as the origin of the middle lobe bronchus anteriorly.

The physical characteristics that render the intermediate stem line visible are also operative to some extent on the left, so that the posterior wall of the left main bronchus and the proximal portion of the left lower lobe bronchus may be profiled as the *left retrobronchial line (see* Fig. 1–33).[118] This short, vertical linear opacity measures 3 mm or less in width and terminates caudally at the origin of the superior segmental bronchus of the left lower lobe. The distinction between the intermediate stem line and the left retrobronchial line is not difficult, bearing in mind that the former is both longer and more anteriorly located than the latter. The anterior and posterior walls of the right lower lobe bronchus can be identified in 8 per cent of individuals, whereas the arcuate configuration of the anterior wall of the left lower lobe bronchus, merging with the orifice of the left upper lobe bronchus, is visible in more than 95 per cent of individuals (Fig. 1–34).[119]

There has been much confusion concerning the nomenclature of the hilar vasculature. One common misrepresentation is to depict the right hilar opacity as the "right pulmonary artery." In reality, the right pulmonary artery is a mediastinal vessel enveloped by other vessels or soft tissue elements, and it is its ascending and descending (interlobar)

branches that compose the true hilar arterial vessels. The right superior pulmonary vein abuts the anterior aspect of the right interlobar artery; consequently, the right hilar complex is composed of the superior vein anteriorly, the ascending and descending arteries posteriorly, and surrounding connective tissue and lymph nodes.

The major portion of the left hilar vasculature is visible behind the intermediate stem line. The top of the left pulmonary artery is seen in 95 per cent of subjects, usually as a sharply marginated opacity above and behind the radiolucency of the left upper lobe bronchus. Immediately posterior to this bronchus is the continuation of the left pulmonary artery, the interlobar artery. The left superior pulmonary vein, like its counterpart on the right, is closely associated with the arterial vasculature of the hilum; however, this vein is not a contour-forming vessel on conventional lateral roentgenograms and thus cannot be identified. Prominence of the left common or superior pulmonary venous confluence can impinge on and displace the left lower lobe bronchus superiorly and posteriorly both in normal subjects and when it becomes dilated as a result of postcapillary pulmonary hypertension.

The right and left inferior pulmonary veins are commonly imaged end-on as a result of their horizontal orientation, creating a nodular opacity below and behind the lower portion of the hila. Fortunately, vessels can usually be identified converging toward the opacity, permitting its distinction from a true parenchymal mass.

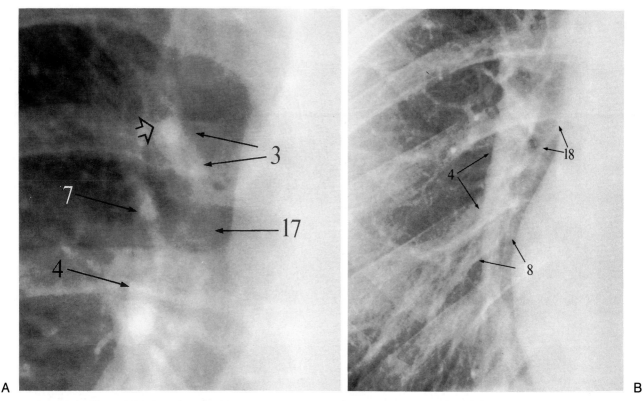

Figure 1–31. Right Hilar Anatomy. A detail view of the right hilum from a conventional PA roentgenogram *(A)* demonstrates the ascending (3) and descending (4) arteries. The right superior pulmonary vein (7) crosses the hilum obliquely to form the typical *V* configuration. The lumen of the right upper lobe bronchus (17) and of the end-on bronchus and the opaque artery *(open arrowhead)* of the anterior segment are shown. Inferiorly *(B)*, the interlobar (4) artery lies lateral to the intermediate bronchus (18). Note that this vessel dominates the roentgenographic anatomy of the lower hilum. The horizontally oriented inferior pulmonary vein (8) lies posteroinferior to the hilum.

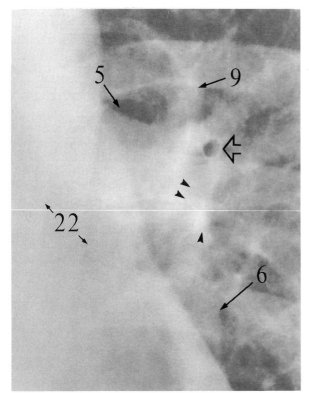

Figure 1–32. Left Hilar Anatomy. A detail view of the left hilum from a PA chest roentgenogram shows the left pulmonary artery (5), the interlobar artery (6), and the left superior pulmonary vein (9). The left main bronchus (22) and its superior *(two arrowheads)* and inferior *(single arrowhead)* divisions are overlapped by the hilar vessels. The end-on bronchus and opaque artery *(single open arrowhead)* of the anterior segment are seen.

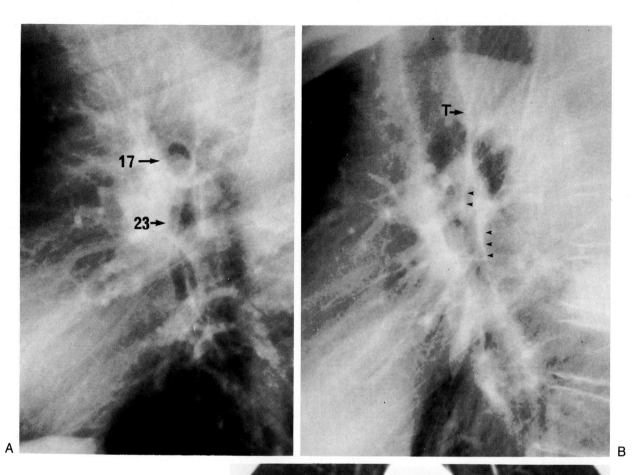

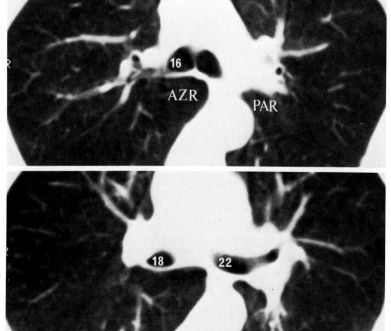

Figure 1–33. Hilar Anatomy Revealed by Conventional Lateral Roentgenograms. *A,* The end-on orifices of the right (17) and left (23) upper lobe bronchi can be easily identified. Although the left hilum is normally located cephalad to the right, the right upper lobe bronchus projects cephalad to its counterpart on the left. *B,* In another subject, a conventional lateral chest roentgenogram demonstrates the posterior tracheal stripe (T), intermediate stem line *(two arrowheads),* and left retrobronchial line *(three arrowheads).* On a true lateral view, the intermediate stem line bisects the orifice of the left upper lobe bronchus. *C,* CT scans through the carina *(top)* and 2 cm caudad *(bottom)* reveal the anatomic prerequisites underlying the features described in *B.* Aerated lung in the azygoesophageal recess (AZR) and the preaortic recess (PAR) abut the posterior wall of the right main (16) and intermediate (18) bronchi and the posterior wall of the left main bronchus (22), respectively.

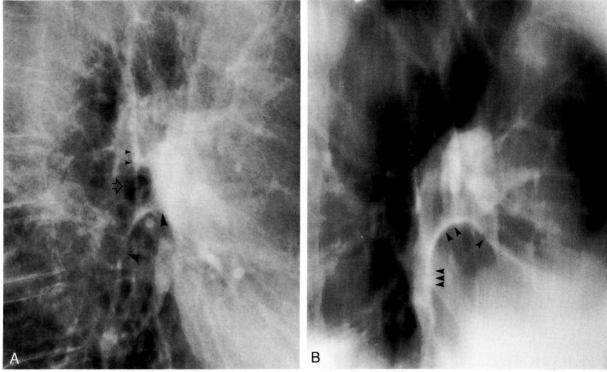

Figure 1–34. Hilar Anatomy in Lateral Projection. *A,* On a detail view from a lateral roentgenogram, there is a curvilinear (reversed comma-shaped) opacity *(large arrowheads)* anteroinferior to the end-on orifice of the distal left main or proximal left upper lobe bronchus *(open arrow);* this opacity represents, in succession, the inferior or anterior wall of the lingular bronchus, the left main bronchus, and the left lower lobe bronchus. The right-sided intermediate stem line *(small arrowheads)* bisects the bronchial lumen. *B,* A conventional lateral linear tomogram through the left hilum reveals the inferior wall of the lingula *(single arrowhead),* anterior wall of the left main bronchus *(two arrowheads),* and anterior wall of the left lower lobe bronchus *(three arrowheads)* as the three components of the line identified in *A.*

Computed Tomography

It is of paramount importance that the radiologist pay meticulous attention to the examination technique when performing CT imaging of the hila. Contrast-enhanced scans are essential in most circumstances, particularly if there is any uncertainty concerning an anatomic feature. The patient should be examined in the supine position during suspended full inspiration. Ten- or five-mm collimated scans with 10-mm spacing are generally adequate, although two or three additional high-resolution scans may be needed to clarify any uncertainty. Anatomic features are best described by a series of horizontal planes or levels through the tracheobronchial tree (Fig. 1–35).[120, 121]

Level I (Supracarinal Trachea). On the right, the circular apical pulmonary artery lies medial to the radiolucent end-on apical bronchus; the apical pulmonary vein is situated lateral to this bronchoarterial bundle. On the left, the apicoposterior bronchus and artery are seen; the apical and anterior veins lie in front and medial to the bronchus and artery.

Level II (Carina/Right Upper Lobe Bronchus). On the right, the upper lobe bronchus divides into the horizontally oriented anterior and posterior segmental bronchi. In front of the main bronchus and upper lobe bronchus is the ascending branch of the right pulmonary artery; its anterior segmental branch parallels the bronchus medially or supe-

riorly. The right superior pulmonary vein is invariably identified immediately lateral to the division of the anterior and posterior segmental bronchi. In some patients, a small vein from the anterior and apical portions of the upper lobe may be seen in front of the ascending artery. On the left, the circular apicoposterior bronchus and artery are situated immediately lateral to the left pulmonary artery. The superior pulmonary vein is located in front of and medial to the bronchus and artery.

Level III (Proximal Intermediate Bronchus/Left Upper Lobe Bronchus). On the right, the intermediate bronchus is covered anteriorly by the horizontal branch of the interlobar artery and laterally by the vertical branch of the same vessel. The superior pulmonary vein abuts the junction between the horizontal and the vertical components of the interlobar artery, creating a typical "elephant head-and-trunk" configuration (*see* Fig 1–28, page 33). On the left, the distal main and upper lobe bronchial continuum is seen. Frequently, the end-on radiolucency of the superior division of the upper lobe bronchus is visible. Medial to the interlobar artery, air in the superior segment of the left lower lobe may abut the posterior wall of the left main bronchus, creating the CT "retrobronchial stripe."[118]

Level IV (Distal Intermediate Bronchus/Lingular Bronchus). On the right, the anatomic features are similar to those of level III. On the left, the proximal portion of the lingular bronchus is separated from the end-on orifice of the lower lobe bronchus by the lingular spur. The superior segmental bronchus to the lower lobe arises posteriorly. The left interlobar artery is situated lateral to the carina or spur separating the lingular bronchus from the lower lobe bronchus. As it enters the mediastinum, the superior pulmonary vein is joined by the lingular vein in front of and medial to the lingular bronchus.

Level V (Middle Lobe Bronchus). On the right the horizontal middle lobe bronchus courses obliquely into the middle lobe, where it divides after a centimeter or so into the medial and lateral segmental bronchi. Behind, divided by a distinct carina or lateral spur, is the orifice of the lower lobe bronchus viewed end-on. The superior segmental bronchus to the lower lobe arises at or slightly superior to this level and passes posterolaterally for a few millimeters before dividing into two subsegmental bronchi. The vertical part of the interlobar artery is situated posterolateral to the middle lobe bronchus and anterolateral to the lower lobe bronchus as it enters lung parenchyma. The middle lobe artery or vein may be identified lateral to the middle lobe bronchus; the termination of the superior pulmonary vein is located anteromedial to this airway (see Fig 1–28, page 33). On the left, the end-on lumen of the lower lobe bronchus is seen medial to the contiguous interlobar artery. Occasionally, a portion of the inferior pulmonary vein may be identified posteromedial to this bronchus.

Level VI (Basilar Lower Lobe Bronchi/Inferior Pulmonary Veins). Segmental bronchi in the lower lobes may be identified in 60 to 90 per cent of cases on the right and 30 to 80 per cent on the left.[122] On the right, the medial segmental bronchus, the first branch to be identified, is characteristically located in front of the horizontal inferior pulmonary vein. The anterior, lateral, and posterior basilar bronchi arise in succession to supply their respective segments. On the left, the anteromedial segmental bronchus is located anterior to the inferior pulmonary vein; the lateral and posterior segmental bronchi may be identified behind this vessel.

Magnetic Resonance Imaging

This technique differs from CT in two important aspects. First, flowing blood within the lumen of vessels provokes little or no signal and hence is perceived as a radiolucency on the MR scan (Fig. 1–36). This "flow-void" phenomenon[123] is particularly advantageous in distinguishing a vessel from a mass that is signal-provoking (e.g., an enlarged lymph node). Such distinction is often difficult or impossible on a non–contrast-enhanced CT study, although the combination of contrast enhancement and dynamic scanning increases the sensitivity and specificity of the CT examination. Second, on both MRI and CT, the lumina of gas-containing bronchi are radiolucent; however, although both procedures are capable of clearly demonstrating the major airways, the superior resolution of CT permits routine demonstration of segmental and subsegmental bronchi, whereas the identification of these smaller airways with MRI is possible in only about 30 per cent of cases.[124]

The frequency with which normal structures of the mediastinum and hila are identified on MRI is as follows: aorta (100 per cent), central pulmonary arteries (100 per cent), arch arteries (100 per cent), mediastinal veins (100 per

Text continued on page 45

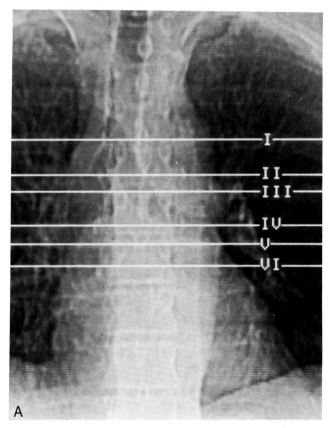

Figure 1–35. Normal CT Hilar Anatomy. *A,* On a scout view of the thorax, the bars indicate the appropriate levels for *B* through *G.*
Illustration continued on following page

A

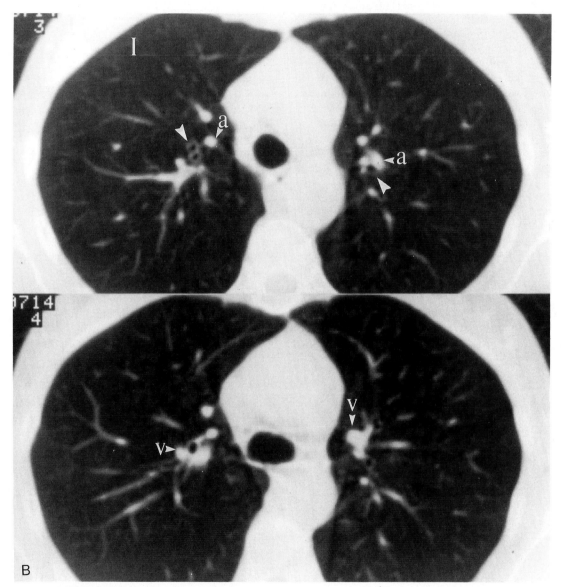

Figure 1–35 *Continued B*, In *level I* (supracarinal trachea), the apical bronchus *(arrowhead)*, artery (a), and vein (v) are depicted on the right and the apicoposterior bronchus *(arrowhead)*, artery (a), and vein (v) on the left.

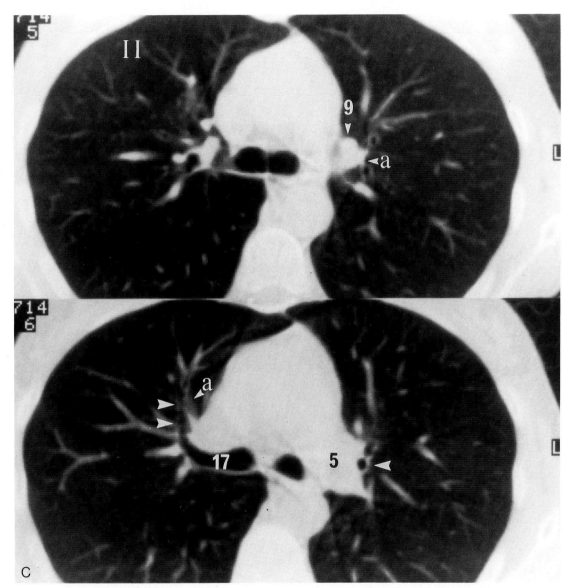

Figure 1–35 *Continued C,* In *level II* (carina/right upper lobe bronchus), the upper lobe bronchus (17), anterior segmental bronchus *(two arrowheads),* and artery (a) are shown on the right; on the left, the apicoposterior bronchus *(arrowhead)* and artery (a) are stationed immediately lateral to the left pulmonary artery (5). The left superior pulmonary vein (9) is located anteromedial to the bronchoarterial bundle.

Illustration continued on following page

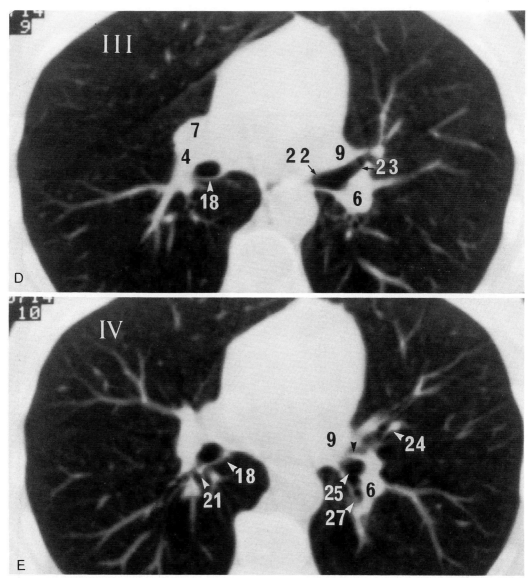

Figure 1–35 *Continued D,* In *level III* (proximal intermediate bronchus/left upper lobe bronchus), on the right, the intermediate bronchus (18) is covered anteriorly and laterally by the interlobar artery (4). The right superior pulmonary vein (7) relates closely to the interlobar artery, creating a typical "elephant head-and-trunk" configuration. On the left, the distal main (22) and upper lobe (23) bronchial continuum is seen. Note the shallow indentation on the anterior and posterior walls of the upper lobe bronchus created by the mediastinal component of the left superior vein (9) and the proximal interlobar artery (6). *E,* In *level IV* (distal intermediate bronchus/lingular bronchus), the intermediate bronchus (18) and the superior segmental bronchus (21) of the lower lobe can be identified on the right, and the lingular bronchus (24) separated by the lingular spur *(arrowhead)* from the end-on orifice of the lower lobe bronchus (25) on the left. The superior segmental bronchus (27) lies posteriorly, the interlobar artery (6) posterolaterally, and the left superior pulmonary vein (9) anteromedially.

Figure 1–35 *Continued F,* In *level V,* the middle lobe bronchus (19) divides into medial (m) and lateral (l) segmental bronchi. The lower lobe bronchus (20) is separated from the middle lobe bronchus by a distinct spur or carina *(arrowheads).* The right superior pulmonary vein (7) lies anteromedial to the middle lobe bronchus and the interlobar artery (4) anterolateral to the lower lobe bronchus. On the left, the interlobar artery (6) lies posterolateral to the lower lobe bronchus (25). *G,* In *level VI* (basilar lower lobe bronchi/inferior pulmonary veins) on the right, the medial (m), anterior (a), lateral (l), and posterior (p) segmental bronchi relate closely to the inferior pulmonary vein (8). On the left, the anteromedial (am), lateral (l) and posterior (p) segmental bronchi relate to the left inferior pulmonary vein (10).

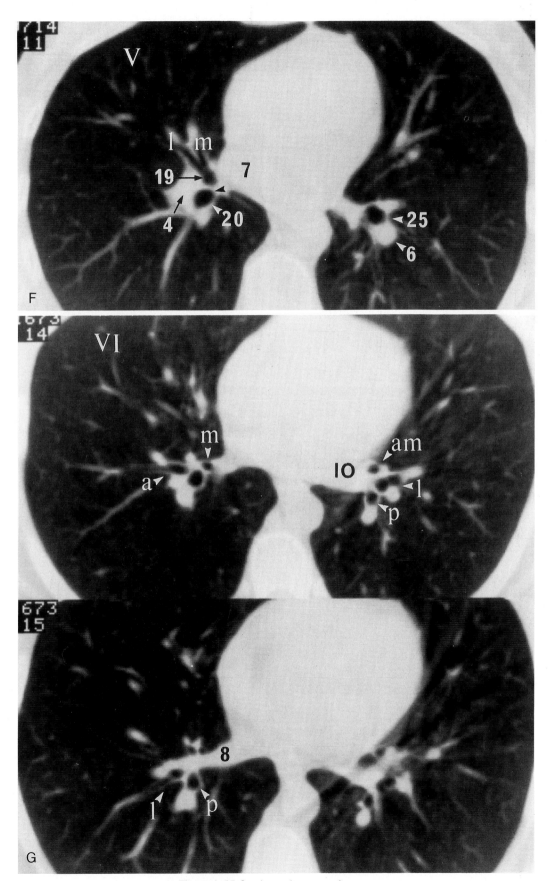

Figure 1–35 *See legend on opposite page*

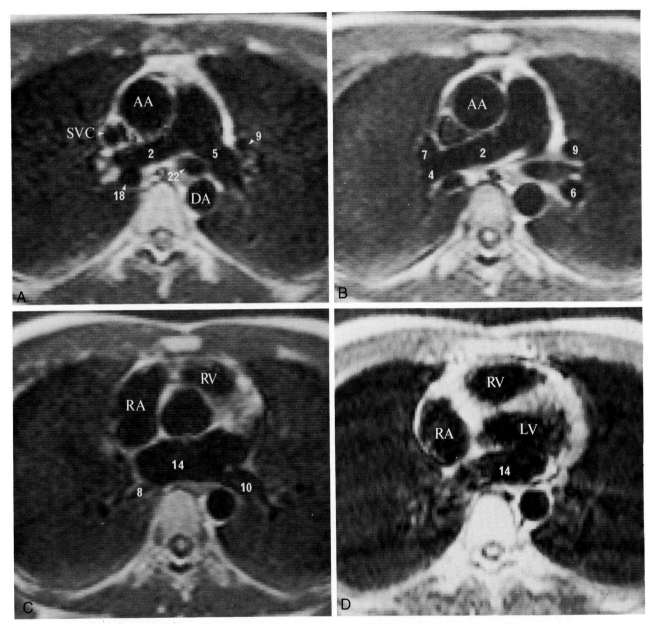

Figure 1–36. Anatomy of the Mediastinum and Hila on Axial Magnetic Resonance Images. Transverse SE 1163/40 scans from cephalad *(A)* to caudad *(D)* from a normal subject. Note that blood within vessels is lucent, since flowing blood provokes little or no signal—the "flow-void" phenomenon. AA, ascending aorta; DA, descending aorta; SVC, superior vena cava; 9, left superior pulmonary vein; 7, right superior pulmonary vein; 2, right pulmonary artery; 5, left pulmonary artery; RB, right main bronchus; 22, left main bronchus; 6, left interlobar artery; 4, right interlobar artery; 18, intermediate bronchus; 14, left atrium; 10, left inferior pulmonary vein; 8, right inferior pulmonary vein; RA, right atrium; RV, right ventricle; LV, left ventricle. (Courtesy of Dr. David Li, University of British Columbia Hospital, Vancouver, B.C.)

cent), lobar bronchi (100 per cent), one to three segmental bronchi (30 per cent), azygos vein or arch (50 per cent), hilar fat (50 per cent), and esophagus (20 per cent). In addition, normal lymph nodes as small as 5 to 10 mm in size can be seen in certain areas of the mediastinum.

Function

Perfusion of the Acinar Unit

Pulmonary blood volume (PBV), the volume of blood within the pulmonary arteries, pulmonary capillaries, and pulmonary veins, is about 500 mL, or 10 per cent of total blood volume in the average normal adult. Capillary blood volume is about 20 to 25 per cent of total PBV and can double during heavy exercise.[125]

Various pressures modify the flow of blood through the capillaries: (1) *mean intravascular pressure*, which is only 14 mm Hg in the main pulmonary artery, despite the fact that it handles the same cardiac output as the systemic circulation; (2) *transmural vascular pressure*, which for extrapulmonary arteries is the intravascular pressure minus intrapleural pressure, for "extra-alveolar" intraparenchymal vessels is intravascular pressure minus interstitial pressure, and for the "alveolar" vessels is intravascular pressure minus alveolar pressure; and (3) *driving pressure*, which in the pulmonary circulation in upright subjects at rest is the difference between arterial and pulmonary venous or left atrial pressures in the lower part of the lung and the difference between arterial and alveolar pressures in the upper part of the lung.

Pulmonary vascular resistance is made up of the arterial, capillary, and venous resistances arranged in series. Although there is some controversy, it is believed that in zone II and III conditions (*see* later) the compliant capillary bed contributes least to total resistance and the arterioles and venules most.[126] The average capillary pressure is probably in the order of 8 to 10 cm H_2O, and since colloidal osmotic pressure is between 25 and 30 mm Hg there is a considerable force keeping fluid within the pulmonary capillaries and maintaining the alveoli dry. Even during maximal exercise when cardiac output increases to 25 to 30 L per minute, the hydrostatic pressure does not increase greatly because of capillary recruitment.

As with the conducting airways, doubling or halving the radius of pulmonary vessels causes a 16-fold change in resistance. When cardiac output increases, vessels widen and closed capillaries open, leading to a fall in resistance. Part of this decrease in resistance with increased flow and driving pressure may be explained by the fact that the pulmonary vascular pressure-flow curve does not have a zero pressure intercept. Put simply, this means that a critical pulmonary artery pressure must be achieved before flow begins.

Factors Influencing Pulmonary Circulation

Gravity. By altering regional vascular transmural pressures and therefore vascular diameters, gravity has a major influence on the distribution of blood flow in the lung.[127] The distribution of flow is governed largely by the relationship among arterial, alveolar, and venous pressures (Fig. 1–37). The lung measures approximately 30 cm from apex to base, and the hilum is positioned at about the midlevel. Since a column of blood 15 cm high is equivalent to a column of mercury 11 mm high, gravity affects the intravascular pressure in the erect subject by decreasing systolic, diastolic, and mean pressures by 11 mm Hg at the apex and by increasing them 11 mm Hg at the base. If pulmonary arterial pressure in the hilar vessels is taken as 20/9 mm Hg, it follows that pressure at the extreme apex will be 9/2, and at the base 31/20. Since the pulmonary veins enter the left atrium at approximately the same level as the pulmonary arteries, there also will be a similar and proportional variation in venous pressure.

These gravity-dependent changes in intravascular pressure result in regional differences in the capillary transmural pressure. Since extraluminal capillary pressure is 0 (atmospheric), apical vessels are virtually closed, at least

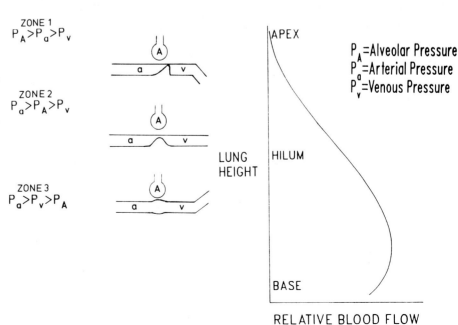

Figure 1–37. Regional Blood Flow in the Lung as Determined by the Relationship Among Alveolar (A), Pulmonary Arterial (a), and Pulmonary Venous (v) Pressures. At the apex, where pulmonary arterial and venous pressures may be subatmospheric, alveolar pressure will compress alveolar microvessels, increase resistance, and decrease flow (zone 1). Lower in the lung, pulmonary arterial pressure exceeds alveolar pressure, but alveolar pressure still exceeds the subatmospheric venous pressure, and vessel caliber and flow depend on the difference between arterial and alveolar pressures (zone 2). Nearer the base of the lung, arterial and venous pressures exceed alveolar pressure, dilating microvessels and further increasing flow (zone 3). At the lung base (zone 4), a region of decreased flow exists that cannot be simply explained by the relationship of Pa, PA, and Pv.

ZONE 1
$P_A > P_a > P_v$

ZONE 2
$P_a > P_A > P_v$

ZONE 3
$P_a > P_v > P_A$

LUNG HEIGHT

APEX

HILUM

BASE

P_A = Alveolar Pressure
P_a = Arterial Pressure
P_v = Venous Pressure

RELATIVE BLOOD FLOW

during diastole; in this region (zone 1), the pulmonary vasculature acts as a Starling resistor in which the pertinent driving pressure is the difference between arterial and alveolar pressures (*see* Fig. 1–37). Farther down the lung, pulmonary artery pressure exceeds alveolar pressure throughout the cardiac cycle, but alveolar pressure still exceeds venous pressure, resulting in a narrowing of capillaries at their downstream venous end (zone 2). Finally, as the lung base is approached, both arterial and venous pressures exceed alveolar pressure, and the vasculature progressively dilates (zone 3). Strangely, at the extreme base of the lung (zone 4), pulmonary vascular resistance increases and blood flow decreases, a phenomenon for which there is no adequate explanation.

Intrapleural Pressure and Lung Volume. The pulmonary vessels may be divided into extra-alveolar and alveolar compartments, based on their response to changes in lung volume.[128] The former comprises the arteries and veins whose extraluminal pressure is equivalent to pleural and/or interstitial pressure; they respond by tending to dilate as lung volume increases. The alveolar compartment includes capillaries, arterioles, and venules; these respond to alveolar pressure as their extraluminal pressure and tend to be compressed as the lung is inflated. Despite this compression, it is possible to perfuse the lung slowly even when alveolar pressure substantially exceeds pulmonary artery pressure. The explanation for this may be related to the presence of vessels situated at alveolar corners, which tend to be stretched and dilated rather than compressed as the lung inflates.[129]

Neurogenic and Chemical Effects. Neurogenic, humoral, blood gas, and blood chemistry changes may result in active vasomotion and modify the pulmonary circulation. This may occur generally throughout the lung or, more importantly, on a regional basis, thus altering blood flow distribution and affecting local ventilation-perfusion relationships.

Hypoxia is one of the most potent stimuli of pulmonary vasoconstriction. This effect is predominantly local, since the vasoconstrictor response is present in denervated lungs and, indeed, in excised perfused lungs.[130] Despite its obvious importance in both the physiologic regulation of blood flow and the pathophysiology of pulmonary hypertensive states, the mechanism of hypoxic vasoconstriction has remained elusive. Most evidence suggests that it is the local alveolar Po_2 that provides the major stimulus, although mixed venous Po_2 may also influence the response.[131] Increased hydrogen ion concentration, whether induced by hypercapnia or metabolic acidosis, also produces pulmonary vasoconstriction by a separate mechanism and interacts with hypoxia in increasing pulmonary arterial pressure.[132]

Although stimulation of sympathetic nerves in animals results in increased pulmonary vascular resistance and decreased compliance of large pulmonary vessels, little is known about the afferent input that could produce such reflex changes.[133] Parenterally administered epinephrine, norepinephrine, serotonin, histamine, and prostaglandin $F_{2\alpha}$ vasoconstrict, whereas beta-agonists and acetylcholine result in vasodilation.[134]

Diffusion of Gas from Acinar Units to Red Blood Cells

Diffusion in the Acinar Unit. There are several factors that affect diffusion of gas in the acinus. As a general rule,

diffusion occurs passively from an area of higher partial pressure to one of lower partial pressure. In addition, in a gaseous medium, a light gas diffuses faster than a heavier one, whereas in a liquid or in tissue the rate of diffusion is dependent largely on the solubility of the particular gas in that medium. Oxygen is slightly lighter than carbon dioxide and, therefore, diffuses more rapidly in acinar gas. In water and tissue, however, carbon dioxide is more soluble than oxygen and diffuses through these media 20 times faster than oxygen. The alveolar ventilation portion of each tidal volume is only about 10 per cent of the gas within the lung at FRC; however, because of the rapid diffusion of oxygen in a gaseous medium, complete mixing of this fresh air with intra-acinar gas is virtually instantaneous in normal lung.

Diffusion Across the Alveolocapillary Membrane. Under resting conditions, oxygen has a driving pressure of approximately 60 mm Hg (Po_2 of alveolar gas minus Po_2 of mixed venous blood [$100 - 40 = 60$ mm Hg]) through the alveolocapillary membrane and almost fully saturates the blood in one third of the time taken by blood to traverse the pulmonary capillaries. However, the amount of *effective* alveolocapillary membrane usually is reduced because of mismatching of capillary circulation with acinar ventilation (*see* later).

The distance for diffusion of gas is increased in pulmonary edema and in the many diseases that thicken the alveolocapillary membrane. Since ventilation-perfusion mismatching is an inevitable accompaniment of such diseases, assessment of the separate contribution of diffusion impairment to arterial hypoxemia may be difficult. In these cases, the arterial oxygen saturation may be normal in patients at rest, despite significant reduction in diffusing capacity; however, exercise elicits hypoxemia because the transit time through capillaries is decreased.

The measurement of the diffusing capacity of oxygen is difficult for a variety of technical reasons; therefore, that for carbon monoxide ($D_{L_{CO}}$) is generally used instead. The three important variables that contribute to the overall diffusing capacity of the lung (D_L) are the alveolocapillary membrane diffusing capacity (Dm), the reaction rate of carbon monoxide with hemoglobin, and the pulmonary capillary blood volume (Vc). Both the Dm and the Vc components of D_L decrease with age, the membrane component first.[135]

Matching Capillary Blood Flow with Ventilation in the Acinus

Ideally, alveolar ventilation and alveolar perfusion should be uniform; that is, each acinus should receive just the right amount of ventilation to oxygenate the hemoglobin completely and remove all the carbon dioxide given off during gas exchange. Despite the fact that this does not occur, even in the normal lung, the concept of an "ideal" ventilation/perfusion ($\dot{V}_A/\dot{Q}$) ratio is useful as a point of reference in judging relationships between ventilation and perfusion within acini and the lung as a whole. When the $\dot{V}_A/\dot{Q}$ ratio is not ideal, it is either because perfusion is reduced relative to ventilation (high $\dot{V}_A/\dot{Q}$) or because ventilation is decreased relative to blood flow (low $\dot{V}_A/\dot{Q}$).

Figure 1–38 shows the theoretic distribution of $\dot{V}_A/\dot{Q}$ ratios in the lung, using a five-compartment model. The central unit (no. 3) corresponds to the "ideal" unit with a

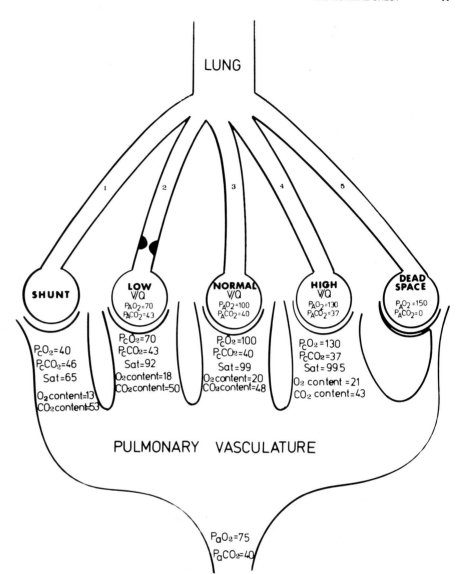

LUNG

| | | | | | | | | | |
|1| |2| |3| |4| |5| |

SHUNT

LOW
V/Q
$P_AO_2=70$
$P_ACO_2=43$

NORMAL
V/Q
$P_AO_2=100$
$P_ACO_2=40$

HIGH
V/Q
$P_AO_2=130$
$P_ACO_2=37$

DEAD SPACE
$P_AO_2=150$
$P_ACO_2=0$

$P_cO_2=40$
$P_cCO_2=46$
Sat=65
O_2content=13
CO_2content=53

$P_cO_2=70$
$P_cCO_2=43$
Sat=92
O_2content=18
CO_2content=50

$P_cO_2=100$
$P_cCO_2=40$
Sat=99
O_2content=20
CO_2content=48

$P_cO_2=130$
$P_cCO_2=37$
Sat=99.5
O_2 content =21
CO_2 content=43

PULMONARY VASCULATURE

$P_aO_2=75$
$P_aCO_2=40$

Figure 1–38. Theoretical Distribution of the $\dot{V}_A/\dot{Q}$ Ratios in the Lung. All possible ventilation-perfusion ratios are depicted here, schematically ranging from unit 1, a shunt with a ventilation-perfusion ratio of 0, to unit 5, pure dead space with a ventilation-perfusion ratio at infinity. Blood coming from unit 1 will have gas tensions identical to that of mixed venous blood, and alveolar gas in unit 5 will have gas tensions that approach that of inspired air. Although the average alveolar P_O_2 in the ventilated and perfused units (2, 3, and 4) is 100 mm Hg, the resultant arterial P_O_2 after blood from all units has mixed is only 75 mm Hg. This $P_{AO_2} - P_{aO_2}$ is caused both by the low oxygen content in the shunted blood and the failure of the overventilated unit 4 to compensate for the underventilated unit 2 with respect to oxygen uptake.

$\dot{V}_A/\dot{Q}$ of 0.9. In this acinus, ventilation is sufficient to achieve an alveolar oxygen tension (P_{AO_2}) of approximately 100 mm Hg. With unimpaired diffusion between alveolar gas and capillary blood, this results in a capillary oxygen tension (P_{cO_2}) of 100 mm Hg in the blood leaving this unit, a level that is sufficient to achieve nearly 100 per cent saturation of the hemoglobin (20 mL O_2 per 100 mL of blood if the hemoglobin concentration is 15 g per dL). The resulting P_{ACO_2} and P_{cCO_2} are each 40 mm Hg, which is sufficient to lower mixed venous carbon dioxide content from 53 to 48 mL per dL.

Unit no. 1 typifies the region with the lowest possible $\dot{V}_A/\dot{Q}$ ratio, with a value of 0, and represents a true intrapulmonary shunt. Capillary blood emerges from such a unit with gas partial pressures and contents identical to those of mixed venous blood (in our example, a P_{cO_2} of 40 mm Hg and a P_{cCO_2} of 46 mm Hg for capillary contents of O_2 = 13 mL per dL and CO_2 = 53 mL per dL). Unit no. 2 has a $\dot{V}_A/\dot{Q}$ ratio somewhere between 0.9 and 0, resulting in alveolar and capillary gas pressures and contents that are less than "ideal" for oxygen and more than "ideal" for carbon dioxide (in our example, a P_{cO_2} of 70 mm Hg and a

P_{cCO_2} of 44 mm Hg). Unit no. 5 typifies true alveolar dead space, representing a region of lung that is ventilated but not perfused ($\dot{V}_A/\dot{Q}$ = infinity); the ventilation to such a unit is completely wasted ventilation, since alveolar gas does not come in contact with capillary blood. Unit no. 4 has a $\dot{V}_A/\dot{Q}$ ratio between 0.9 and infinity, resulting in alveolar and capillary partial pressures that are greater than "ideal" for oxygen and less than "ideal" for carbon dioxide (in our example, a P_{cO_2} of 130 mm Hg and a P_{cCO_2} of 37 mm Hg).

Because of the relationships between the oxygen and carbon dioxide contents of blood and their partial pressures, $\dot{V}_A/\dot{Q}$ mismatch has quite different effects on the efficiency of the lung to take up oxygen and remove carbon dioxide. As shown in Figure 1–39, the O_2 dissociation curve is flat for values of P_O_2 above 70 or 80 mm Hg, so that the overventilated unit (no. 4) cannot make up for the underventilated unit (no. 2) in terms of oxygen uptake. Although the elevated P_O_2 in unit no. 4 results in a slight increase in the amount of dissolved oxygen in the capillary blood, hemoglobin is virtually 100 per cent saturated above a P_O_2 of 100, and since dissolved oxygen can increase only by 0.003

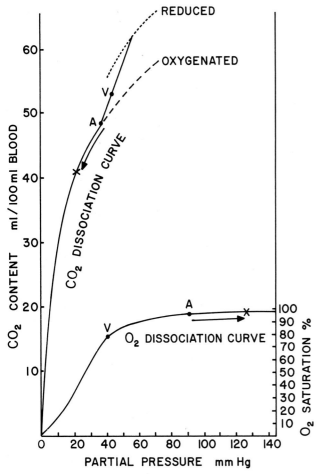

Figure 1–39. The Carbon Dioxide and Oxygen Dissociation Curves of Blood. The arrows (A → X) indicate the effect of doubling the ventilation on both CO_2 content and O_2 content (arterial oxygen saturation). The normal values for both arterial (A) and venous (V) oxygen and carbon dioxide are noted. It can be seen that, at any given PCO_2, reduced blood can carry more carbon dioxide than oxygenated blood. *See* text.

mL per dL of blood per mm Hg rise in PO_2, little gain is achieved by overventilating units. By contrast, overventilated units can compensate for underventilated units in the removal of carbon dioxide. Since the CO_2 dissociation curve is virtually linear over the range of physiologic PCO_2 values, the lowered carbon dioxide content of blood from unit no. 4 can compensate for the greater than "ideal" content in unit no. 2.

When blood from units 1, 2, 3, and 4 mix in the pulmonary veins and left atrium, the resulting PaO_2 will be less than the mean alveolar PO_2 of units 2, 3, and 4, whereas the $PaCO_2$ will be equal to the mean alveolar PCO_2. Put simply, $\dot{V}A/\dot{Q}$ mismatch decreases the efficiency of oxygen and carbon dioxide uptake and removal; in the case of oxygen, this results in a gradient between mean alveolar PO_2 and arterial PO_2 ($PAO_2 - PaO_2$), whereas for carbon dioxide there is none. If a disease process leads to the development of units with low $\dot{V}A/\dot{Q}$ ratios (no. 2) or true shunt (no. 1), arterial hypoxemia and hypercapnia will result. Since both a lowered PO_2 and an increased PCO_2 stimulate increased ventilation, total alveolar ventilation will increase. The alveolar PO_2 in well-ventilated acinar units (no.

4) will rise while the PCO_2 in these units will fall. The excess carbon dioxide retained by blood circulating through the poorly ventilated units (nos. 1 and 2) will be balanced by the supranormal output from the well-ventilated units, thus correcting the hypercapnia. Since increased ventilation cannot completely compensate for the hypoxemia (owing to the oxygen content–partial pressure relationship), PO_2 will remain relatively low.

Figure 1–38 is a simplified model that spans the entire range of possible $\dot{V}A/\dot{Q}$ ratios in five compartments. In fact, a continuous distribution of ratios is likely to exist, and even in the normal lung substantial regional differences in $\dot{V}A/\dot{Q}$ ratios have been demonstrated. This variation is caused largely by gravity.[136] As discussed previously, the effect of gravity is to increase blood flow to the dependent portions of the lung. A gravity-dependent vertical gradient in pleural pressure also results in variation in ventilation and, thus, in regional lung volume; in erect subjects pleural pressure at the lung apex (or anteriorly in the supine position) is more negative than at the base, and the local pleural pressure (Ppl) increases progressively (i.e., becomes less subatmospheric) as the base of the lung is approached. This gradient is approximately 0.25 cm H_2O per cm distance up and down the lung and is similar in different body positions and at different overall lung volumes. Since alveolar pressure is constant up and down the lung, this means that the local transpulmonary pressure also varies in a gravity-dependent fashion. Regional foci of lung parenchyma respond to the local transpulmonary pressure according to their own pressure-volume curves; therefore, at the end of a quiet expiration, acinar units in upper lung regions are more distended and at a higher percentage of their TLC value than are the less well-distended units at the base of the lung.

Despite the gradient in end-expiratory pleural and transpulmonary pressures up and down the lung, the changes in Ppl that occur during tidal breathing are similar at different vertical levels. Thus, because of the general pressure-volume characteristics of the lung (*see* Fig. 1–23, page 26), upper lung units are less well ventilated per unit of lung volume than are acini at the lung base, which are on a steeper portion of their PV curve. Thus, the gravity-dependent pleural pressure gradient results in a regional variation in both lung volume (V_o) and ventilation ($\Delta V/V_o$).

If the increase in $\Delta V/V_o$ from apex to base were directly proportional to the increase in blood flow from apex to base, the $\dot{V}A/\dot{Q}$ ratio would not vary. However, since the effect of gravity on regional perfusion is greater than the effect on regional ventilation, blood flow and ventilation are slightly mismatched even in the normal lung. In the upright posture, the $\dot{V}A/\dot{Q}$ ratio is between 2 and 3 at the lung apex and decreases to between 0.5 and 1 at the base.[137]

Although gravity-dependent variations in pulmonary artery and pleural pressures are the most important factors influencing $\dot{V}A/\dot{Q}$ ratios, other effects may also be involved. For example, at low lung volumes ventilation to the lung bases in the upright position or posterior regions in the supine position may not follow the distribution suggested by regional pleural pressure, since airway closure may occur in these regions.[138] The overall lung volume at which airways in dependent lung regions first close is termed the "closing volume." Since FRC decreases on assuming the supine posture while closing volume does not change, a greater number of dependent airways may close during supine tidal breathing, resulting in a paradoxical decrease in ventilation to dependent lung regions, further $\dot{V}_A/\dot{Q}$ mismatch, and arterial hypoxemia.

Measurement of Ventilation-Perfusion Mismatch

The most commonly used and easily calculated estimate of $\dot{V}_A/\dot{Q}$ mismatch is the alveolar-arterial gradient for oxygen, $P(A\text{-}a)O_2$. Calculation of the $P(A\text{-}a)O_2$ requires knowledge of the mean alveolar PO_2, which can be determined using the simplified alveolar air equation:

$$P_{AO_2} = P_{IO_2} - \frac{P_{aCO_2}}{R} \qquad (1)$$

in which P_{IO_2} is inspired PO_2, R is the ratio of CO_2 production to O_2 consumption (assumed to equal 0.8), and P_{aCO_2} is the arterial PCO_2 (assumed to be equal to P_{ACO_2}).

Once the P_{AO_2} is calculated, the alveolar-arterial gradient for oxygen $P(A\text{-}a)O_2$ can be obtained by comparing P_{AO_2} with measured arterial PO_2:

$$P(A\text{-}a)O_2 = P_{AO_2} - P_{aO_2} \qquad (2)$$

One disadvantage of the $P(A\text{-}a)O_2$ as a measurement of gas exchange is that a given maldistribution of ventilation and perfusion or shunt will result in a different P_aO_2 and calculated $P(A\text{-}a)O_2$ if there is a change in the mixed venous PO_2, the inspired PO_2 or the position of the O_2 dissociation curve.[139] Calculations of venous admixture and shunt provide more accurate estimates of $\dot{V}_A/\dot{Q}$ maldistribution and are less affected by mixed venous and inspired gas tensions; however, they require a sample of mixed venous blood. The same equation is used for calculation of venous admixture and shunt:

$$\frac{\dot{Q}s}{\dot{Q}t} = \frac{C\acute{c}O_2 - CaO_2}{C\acute{c}O_2 - C\bar{v}O_2} \qquad (3)$$

where $\dot{Q}s/\dot{Q}t$ is the venous admixture ratio or shunt if 100 per cent oxygen is breathed, $C\acute{c}O_2$ is the oxygen content of end-capillary blood, CaO_2 is the oxygen content of arterial blood, and $C\bar{v}O_2$ is the oxygen content of mixed venous blood; the equation assumes equilibration between alveolar and capillary PO_2. Ideal capillary PO_2 is calculated using the alveolar air equation (see equation 2). Content is calculated by determining the hemoglobin concentration and assuming that it is identical in venous, arterial, and capillary blood:

$$O_2 \text{ content (mL/100 blood)} =$$
$$(\text{Hgb, g/dL} \times 1.39 \times \% \text{ saturation})$$
$$+ (PO_2 \times 0.003) \qquad (4)$$

where PO_2 is the PO_2 of capillary, arterial, or mixed venous blood; the first term in this equation relates to the oxygen content of hemoglobin, and the second to the quantity of dissolved oxygen. When measurements for this calculation are obtained while the patient is breathing air or a gas mixture containing less than 100 per cent oxygen, the resulting ratio is the venous admixture that is an "as if" shunt, representing the amount of mixed venous blood that would have to be added to capillary blood in order to result in the observed arterial PO_2 and A-a gradient.

Although venous admixture is a more robust estimate of the lung's gas exchange ability, it is also affected by the inspired PO_2 and mixed venous PO_2.[140] Only when pure oxygen is breathed for a time sufficient to wash nitrogen out of the lung completely can a measure be obtained of gas exchange uninfluenced by inspired PO_2 and mixed venous PO_2. The calculation of shunt using equation 3 gives an estimate of only one compartment in the $\dot{V}_A/\dot{Q}$ spectrum. Moreover, the breathing of pure O_2 for a prolonged period can itself increase the intrapulmonary shunt by causing alveolar collapse.

A major advance in the measurement of $\dot{V}_A/\dot{Q}$ mismatch came with the development of a method to measure the "continuous" distribution of $\dot{V}_A/\dot{Q}$ ratios in normal and diseased lungs.[141] The technique involves the intravenous infusion of up to 10 inert gases dissolved in saline; the gases used have a wide range of solubility in blood, and in their passage through the lung enter alveolar gas. The mixed expired and arterial concentration of each gas is measured by gas chromatography when a steady state is achieved; the retention and excretion of each gas can then be calculated and plotted against solubility. From the plot, the distribution of blood flow and ventilation with respect to $\dot{V}_A/\dot{Q}$ ratios can be calculated using a computer. The technique allows measurement of absolute shunt as well as alveolar dead space and also permits calculation of the proportion of perfusion and ventilation to a large number of units of varying $\dot{V}_A/\dot{Q}$ ratio.

Blood Gases and Acid-Base Balance

Blood Gases. The ability of the lung to perform its prime function—the exchange of oxygen and carbon dioxide—is readily determined from analysis of a sample of arterial blood. The oxygen carried in the blood is predominantly attached to hemoglobin and can be calculated using equation 4 above.

In contrast with oxygen, approximately 75 per cent of carbon dioxide is contained in plasma. In the resting subject, while mixed venous blood holds about 15 mL of oxygen per dL of blood at a PO_2 of 40 mm Hg and an oxygen saturation of 75 per cent, its carbon dioxide content is about 52 mL per dL of blood at a PCO_2 of 45 mm Hg. Although the red blood cell carries only 25 per cent of the carbon dioxide, it plays an essential role in the transport of this gas to the lungs; it contains the enzyme carbonic anhydrase, which rapidly hydrates the carbon dioxide passing through the erythrocyte membrane and converts it into carbonic acid, H^+ ions, and bicarbonate ions. The bicarbonate ions (HCO_3^-) quickly permeate the cell membrane and enter the plasma in exchange for chloride ions; in this manner, as bicarbonate, most of the carbon dioxide from the tissues is carried by the blood. Since blood that contains reduced hemoglobin can carry more carbon dioxide than can fully oxygenated blood at the same PCO_2, the circumstances are ideal for the uptake of carbon dioxide in the tissues and for its unloading in the pulmonary capillaries when the hemoglobin has been reoxygenated (see Fig. 1–39).

Arterial hypoxemia may be due to one or more of four mechanisms—diffusion defect, true shunt, ventilation-perfusion inequality, or hypoventilation. A *diffusion defect* results in hypoxemia if there is failure of equilibration of alveolar and capillary P_{O_2} in the brief transit of the red blood cell through the pulmonary capillary bed. It is probable that this mechanism contributes to the hypoxemia seen in emphysema, the increase in hypoxemia that occurs with exercise in patients who have interstitial lung disease, the hypoxemia that develops in some individuals during severe exercise, and the hypoxemia of high altitude. During exercise, the mechanism is probably a decrease in the red blood cell capillary transit time, whereas at high altitudes it is related to a low alveolar P_{O_2}. Since carbon dioxide is about 20 times more soluble than oxygen in water and the tissue membranes, equilibration times are more rapid, and diffusion limitation does not play a role in the genesis of carbon dioxide retention.

A *true shunt* is the primary cause of hypoxemia in cardiogenic and noncardiogenic pulmonary edema and in other conditions characterized by air space consolidation, such as pneumonia. The shunted blood never comes in contact with acinar gas, and for this reason the P_{O_2} of the arterial blood cannot be raised to a normal value (approximately 600 mm Hg) during inhalation of 100 per cent oxygen. In fact, when the shunt handles 10 per cent or more of the cardiac output, the arterial P_{O_2} cannot rise above 400 mm Hg. Other mechanisms that produce hypoxemia can be corrected by the inspiration of 100 per cent oxygen, which replaces nitrogen in even the most poorly ventilated acini.

$\dot{V}A/\dot{Q}$ *inequality* is the commonest cause of hypoxemia that accompanies pulmonary disease. The capillary blood that perfuses underventilated acinar units is not fully saturated and does not release normal amounts of carbon dioxide, since the gradient between the P_{CO_2} of blood and the acinus is reduced. However, because of the differences in the slopes of the dissociation curves, $\dot{V}A/\dot{Q}$ mismatching and shunt tends to affect oxygen transport and arterial P_{O_2} to a greater extent than carbon dioxide transport and P_{CO_2}. Hyperventilation of well-ventilated acini, with consequent reduction in alveolar P_{CO_2}, increases the blood-to-acinus gradient and eliminates more carbon dioxide from these areas. Consequently, in patients with $\dot{V}A/\dot{Q}$ inequality or shunt, P_{CO_2} may be low or normal. However, overventilation of these same units does not make up for the underventilated units in terms of oxygen uptake.

If overall *alveolar ventilation* decreases, carbon dioxide retention occurs as well as alveolar hypoxia and resulting hypoxemia. The hypoxemia associated with hypoventilation does not produce an increased alveolar-arterial gradient for oxygen and thus differs from that caused by diffusion defect, $\dot{V}A/\dot{Q}$ inequality, and shunt. Since hypoventilation often occurs in association with these gas exchange abnormalities, calculation of $P_{AO_2} - P_{aO_2}$ aids in separating the component of hypoxemia related to hypoventilation from that caused by gas exchange problems.

Acid-Base Balance. The hydrogen ion concentration and therefore the pH of the blood is dependent on at least three physicochemical systems:[142] (1) the electrochemical balance of strong ions, electrolytes that are fully dissociated at normal physiologic pH—Na^+, K^+, and Cl^- (since the law of electrical neutrality requires that the electrical charge of all dissolved strong ions equals 0, changes in the concentrations of these ions can influence the degree of dissociation of water and therefore the concentrations of hydrogen and hydroxyl ion in the blood); (2) the buffering capacity of weak electrolytes such as the imidazole group of histidine molecules in tissue proteins, plasma proteins, and hemoglobin (these can accept or donate protons, buffering changes of hydrogen ion concentration in the blood); and (3) most important, the carbon dioxide–bicarbonate system.

The terms alkalemia and acidemia are restricted to situations in which there is a decrease or increase in arterial hydrogen ion concentration above or below the normal range, whereas the terms alkalosis and acidosis are used to describe abnormal processes that would increase or decrease the hydrogen ion concentration of blood if there were no secondary compensatory changes. The interdependence of hydrogen ion concentration, arterial P_{CO_2}, and bicarbonate is illustrated by the Kassirer-Bleich modification of the Henderson-Hasselbalch equation:[143]

$$[H^+] = \frac{24 \times P_{CO_2}}{HCO_3}$$

Examination of this equation shows that the arterial concentration of hydrogen ion is dependent on the *ratio* of arterial P_{CO_2} to arterial bicarbonate: anything that increases the ratio will cause an increase in hydrogen ion concentration (decrease in pH), and anything that decreases the ratio will cause a decrease in hydrogen ion concentration (increase in pH).

Disturbances of acid-base balance can be divided into those that are respiratory in origin and those that are nonrespiratory or metabolic. Respiratory changes in the balance are due to overventilation or underventilation with excess removal or retention of carbon dioxide. Metabolic disturbances are the result of an increase or decrease in noncarbonic acid or a loss or gain of bicarbonate in the extracellular fluid. Acidosis or alkalosis may be "simple"— that is, purely respiratory or metabolic—or mixed, reflecting physiologic disturbances that are both respiratory and metabolic in nature.

Respiratory Acidosis. Respiratory acidosis results from alveolar hypoventilation and may be secondary to (1) decreased central neurogenic drive to breathe; (2) an abnormality of the neural connections between the central nervous system and the respiratory muscles; (3) an abnormality of the respiratory muscles or ribcage; or (4) an abnormality of the airways or lung parenchyma that produces an inordinate increase in the work of breathing.

Respiratory acidosis may be acute or chronic. An acute increase in arterial P_{CO_2} causes a shift of the Henderson equation to the right ($H_2O + CO_2 \rightleftarrows H_2CO_3 \rightleftarrows H^+ + HCO_3^-$), thereby increasing both hydrogen and bicarbonate ion concentrations. The increase in bicarbonate tends to attenuate the increase in hydrogen ion concentration that would have otherwise occurred, limiting the acute change in arterial pH. As a rule of thumb, the increase in bicarbonate associated with acute CO_2 retention is approximately 1 mmol per L for each 10 mm Hg rise in P_{CO_2}. When carbon dioxide retention is prolonged, there is a renal response that consists of the formation and retention of bicarbonate. The process begins immediately, is well developed by 48 hours, and is usually complete within 5 days. During "steady-state" respiratory acidosis there is an approximate 3.5 mmol per L increase in HCO_3^- for each 10 mm Hg increase in P_{CO_2}. This process returns the arterial pH toward normal, but complete compensation does not occur.

Respiratory Alkalosis. Respiratory alkalosis results

from hyperventilation, the commonest cause of which is an anxiety state. Traumatic, infectious, or vascular lesions of the central nervous system, hyperthyroidism, pregnancy, liver failure, and some drugs may produce prolonged respiratory alkalosis. Mild respiratory alkalosis can also be seen in pneumonia, asthma, fibrotic interstitial pulmonary diseases, and the early stages of pulmonary edema. An acute fall in serum bicarbonate occurs with hyperventilation. This change is approximately 2 mmol per L for each 10 mm Hg decrease in PCO_2. With chronic respiratory alkalosis, there is increased renal excretion of bicarbonate, so that pH and hydrogen ion concentration return toward the normal level. As a rule of thumb, there is a 5 mmol per L decrease in bicarbonate for each 10 mm Hg decrease in PCO_2.

Metabolic Acidosis. Metabolic acidosis results from the accumulation of noncarbonic acids in the extracellular fluid or from a loss of bicarbonate ion. It can be further subdivided on the basis of whether or not it results in an elevated anion gap.[144] The latter is the difference in the serum concentrations of sodium and the sum of the chloride and bicarbonate $[Na^+ - (Cl^- + HCO_3^-)]$ and is normally about 12 mmol per L. When there is an accumulation of an anionic acid within the body, the law of electrical neutrality requires that the sum of Cl^- and HCO_3^- plus the added anion equals the concentration of cations. Thus, when there is an accumulation of an unmeasured acid anion, there will be a decrease in Cl^- and HCO_3^- and an increase in the calculated difference between Na^+ and the sum of Cl^- and HCO_3^-.

Compensation for metabolic acidosis occurs by the buffering of the excess of hydrogen ions by hemoglobin, plasma proteins, and phosphate and by a shift of the Henderson equation to the left as bicarbonate combines with the increased hydrogen ion to form carbonic acid (CO_2 + $H_2O \leftarrow H_2O_3 \leftarrow H^+ + HCO_3^-$). The elevated hydrogen ion concentration stimulates the central and peripheral chemoreceptors, augmenting alveolar ventilation and lowering arterial PCO_2. There is a time lag in the respiratory response to metabolic acidosis related to the time required for hydrogen ion and bicarbonate to equilibrate across the blood-brain barrier. In general, maximal respiratory compensation occurs by 12 hours, although the response is insufficient to return the pH to normal. During steady-state metabolic acidosis, the PCO_2 should decrease between 1 and 1.3 mm Hg for every mmol per L decrease in serum bicarbonate concentration.

Metabolic Alkalosis. Metabolic alkalosis results when the hydrogen ion concentration in extracellular fluid is decreased secondary to a loss of acid or an increase in alkali, such as can occur with severe, prolonged vomiting or following prolonged nasogastric suction. Chronic diuretic therapy, excessive exogenous administration of alkali, hyperaldosteronism, Cushing's syndrome, and excessive exogenous steroid administration are additional causes. In pulmonary practice, one of the commonest causes of apparent metabolic alkalosis occurs during treatment of chronic carbon dioxide retention. If artificial ventilation is used to reduce PCO_2 in patients who have chronic CO_2 retention and compensated respiratory acidosis, the patient will be left with an apparent metabolic alkalosis.

The expected respiratory compensation for metabolic alkalosis is a decrease in alveolar ventilation and a rise in alveolar and arterial PCO_2. Although cellular and extracellular buffers make more H^+ available to attenuate the increase in plasma HCO_3^- concentration, it is primarily an increase in PCO_2 that will return the PCO_2-bicarbonate ratio toward normal and stabilize pH. However, the respiratory response to metabolic alkalosis is the least predictable and most variable of the compensatory mechanisms. The arterial PCO_2 often fails to increase or increases much less than would be expected. In some patients, the "failure" to compensate may be related to concomitant respiratory or cardiovascular disorders that independently increase the drive to breathe and counteract the decreased ventilatory drive that is caused by a fall in arterial and cerebrospinal fluid hydrogen ion concentration. As a general rule, one can expect that the arterial PCO_2 will increase by 0.4 to 0.5 mm Hg for each 1 mmol per L increase in serum bicarbonate.

BRONCHIAL CIRCULATION

The bronchial arteries normally arise directly from the aorta or the intercostobronchial trunk and usually number from two to four.[145] The extrapulmonary branches course to the hila, where they form an intercommunicating circular arc around the main bronchi, from which the intrapulmonary arteries radiate. These vessels are situated within the peribronchial connective tissue and extend along the bronchial tree branching with the airways. They have extensive horizontal communications within the peribronchial tissue and also send branches into the bronchial wall to form a similar intercommunicating network in the mucosa. The arteries continue as far as the terminal bronchioles. The bronchial circulation is unique in that it has a dual venous drainage: a portion of the bronchial flow drains in the bronchial veins to the right side of the heart via the azygos and hemiazygos systems, whereas another portion forms extensive anastomoses with the pulmonary circulation at precapillary, capillary, and postcapillary sites and drains into the left atrium via the pulmonary veins.[146]

The bronchial arteries supply the tracheal, bronchial, and bronchiolar walls; the middle third of the esophagus; the visceral pleura over the mediastinal and diaphragmatic surfaces of the lungs (the visceral pleura over the lung convexities being supplied by pulmonary arteries); the outer layers of the aortic arch, pulmonary arteries, and pulmonary veins via the vasa vasorum; the paratracheal, carinal, hilar, and intrapulmonary lymph nodes and lymphoid tissue; the vagus and bronchopulmonary nerves; and, sometimes, the parietal layer of the pericardium and the thymus.[147] In addition to providing blood to all these structures, the bronchial vasculature may have other important functions, including the humidification and warming of inspired air[148] and an emergency backup to maintain nutritive blood flow to the lung when the pulmonary arteries are obstructed.[149]

Because of the relative inaccessibility of the bronchial vessels, very few measurements of flow have been made in humans. Measurements of bronchopulmonary anastomotic flow have been made in patients, the results being highly variable (ranging from 1 per cent to almost 24 per cent of cardiac output); flow is increased in patients who have pulmonary disease.[150]

NONRESPIRATORY FUNCTIONS OF THE LUNG

In addition to respiration, the lungs have several functions that are of considerable importance in the maintenance of well-being. These can be discussed under three headings: metabolism, defense, and certain physical and other related functions.

Physical and Related Functions

The pulmonary capillary network is interposed between the systemic venous and arterial circulations and, in normal circumstances, receives the entire cardiac output. It thus has the capacity to act as a sieve, protecting vital organs on the systemic side of the circulation from various potentially harmful materials. Probably the most important of these are thrombi originating in peripheral veins. Such thrombi are not uncommon, particularly in ill individuals; although most are small and result in no significant pulmonary damage, it is clear that their potential for causing serious harm would be much greater in organs such as the heart or the brain.

Normally occurring tissue elements also can be trapped within the lungs. The commonest of these are megakaryocytes derived from the bone marrow, which are frequently seen in pulmonary capillaries, both in patients with systemic disease and in previously healthy individuals who have died suddenly.[151] The pulmonary capillaries also serve as a storage site for blood leukocytes, resulting in the formation of the so-called "marginated pool," which is two to three times larger than the number of circulating leukocytes.[152] Rather than remaining in the lung, the sequestered cells are delayed in their passage, so that there is a constant turnover of cells within the pool. This sequestration is probably related in part to size. Normal leukocytes are slightly larger than most pulmonary capillaries and so have to be deformed to transit the lung; since leukocytes are 1000 times less deformable than red blood cells, this process is associated with delayed passage through the capillaries.

The lungs also play a role in the excretion of volatile substances other than carbon dioxide, including acetone in diabetes and fasting, methylmercaptan and ammonia in liver cell failure, methanol of unknown source, paraldehyde, and ethanol.

Pulmonary Defense

The entire surface of the conducting airways and lung parenchyma is normally in contact with the external environment. As a result, there is a constant risk of exposure to a variety of potentially harmful substances, including organic and inorganic particles, toxic gases and fumes, and a bewildering array of microorganisms. The defense mechanisms in response to such inhaled or aspirated substances are numerous and complex and, for convenience of discussion, can be divided into those that are specific (related to the immune system) and those that are nonspecific (including particle deposition and clearance, inflammation, and secretion of protective enzymes). The efficiency of many of these defense mechanisms may be impaired by various environmental insults and physiologic conditions, including hypoxia, hyperoxia, acidosis, cigarette smoke, and drugs (particularly corticosteroids and other suppressors of the immune or inflammatory reactions).

Particle Deposition and Clearance. The first line of defense against inhaled or aspirated noxious particles° is clearance; obviously, the faster the lungs can eliminate such substances, the less potential there is for damage. A variety of mechanisms are involved in this process, each of which depends on several factors.

Size and Shape of Inhaled Particles. Four physical processes largely determine particle deposition in the lungs:

1. *Inertial impaction.* This occurs when the momentum of a particle being carried in an air current causes it to impinge on an airway wall when the latter changes direction. This is the principal mechanism by which large particles (from 2 to 100 μm in diameter) are deposited in the respiratory tract,[153] particularly the nose and the nasopharynx. Inertial impaction also occurs within the lungs, especially at the bifurcation of proximal bronchi.

2. *Sedimentation.* Sedimentation is the mechanism by which particles are deposited on airway walls as a result of the influence of gravity; in general, the larger and denser the particle, the more rapid the settling. This is an important mechanism of deposition of particles ranging from 0.5 to 2 μm in diameter and occurs mostly in the bronchi and membranous bronchioles.

3. *Diffusion (Brownian movement).* This causes small particles (mostly less than 0.5 μm in diameter) to move randomly as a result of energy transfer from adjacent gas molecules. Although the vast majority of such particles are exhaled and therefore not retained within the lung, those that do remain are deposited in the alveoli principally by diffusion.

4. *Interception.* The first three mechanisms of deposition relate predominantly to particles that are approximately spherical in shape. When the length-to-diameter ratio of particles increases to 3:1 or greater, they are termed *fibers,* and a fourth mechanism comes into play. Such particulates, especially those with a large cross-sectional diameter such as chrysotile asbestos, are likely to come into contact with and be deposited on the airway wall. By contrast, fibers with a straight configuration and a relatively small diameter tend to travel like a javelin in the center of the airway lumen and can penetrate far into the lung periphery.[154]

The Rate and Pattern of Breathing. Because the majority of large particles are trapped on the nasal mucosa, a greater concentration of such particles tends to reach the lower respiratory tract in individuals engaged in heavy exercise in whom mouth breathing is instituted. However, since the high flow rate that accompanies such exercise enhances inertial impaction, many of these particles are deposited on the proximal airways and do not reach the lung parenchyma itself. Nonetheless, increased ventilation itself results in a greater number of particles reaching the lung in a given period. Since sedimentation is a passive process related to gravity, the rate of settling and deposition

---

°Strictly speaking, the term "particle" refers to a fragment of inanimate organic or inorganic matter; for purposes of this discussion, however, it also includes living organisms (e.g., fungal spores or conidia) and liquid droplets (on which bacteria or viruses may be adherent).

of a particle by this means is dependent on the time the particle resides within the lung. Breathing patterns that are associated with an increase in this time, such as breath holding or quiet breathing, may result in increased deposition by this mechanism.

Distribution of Inhaled Particles. Because ventilation in the erect position is relatively greater in lower than in upper lung regions, it might be predicted that the former would be more susceptible to lung damage from inhaled particles. That this is not always the case, however, is indicated by the predominant involvement of the upper lung zones in patients with silicosis and coal worker's pneumoconiosis. It is unclear to what extent such anatomic predilection for disease is caused by the initial distribution of particles, perhaps influenced by variations in bronchial anatomy[155] or by the phase of the respiratory cycle at which the particles are inhaled. Particle size itself may be important in this respect; in one study, investigators showed that relatively large particles (3.5 μm in diameter) were preferentially deposited in the upper lobes, as compared with particles 1.1 μm in size.[156] As might be expected, intrinsic lung disease such as emphysema also can have an appreciable effect on particle deposition.[157] In addition, particles deposited on both large and small airways can induce bronchospasm, which may influence regional particle distribution.[158]

Concentration of Inhaled Particles. The ability of the lung to cope with potentially harmful particles appears to relate to some extent to the number inhaled. For example, a concentration of fewer than 10 inorganic dust particles of 5 μm or less per mL can be completely eliminated, whereas only about 90 per cent of a concentration of approximately 1000 such particles per mL is removed; the retained 10 per cent can produce a slowly developing pneumoconiosis.

Clearance of Inhaled Particles. Clearance of inhaled or aspirated particles is accomplished by several mechanisms, including transport up the mucociliary escalator (*see* page 28), cough (*see* page 28), phagocytosis by alveolar macrophages (*see* page 11), lymphatic drainage (*see* page 63), and, in the case of some organic particles, destruction within macrophage phagosomes. Regional differences in these mechanisms may explain some of the variation in anatomic localization of disease in different conditions. In addition, differences in the effectiveness of clearance may partly explain differences in susceptibility to certain diseases among individual patients. For example, particles deposited on the airway mucosa are usually transported in tracheobronchial secretions to the pharynx, where they are either expectorated or swallowed; in healthy individuals, the time to clear the airways may be as little as several hours. However, transport is prolonged in some individuals as a result of either inherent individual variation in mucus flow rate,[159] environmental factors such as cigarette smoke,[160] or intrinsic lung disease; such prolongation may predispose to greater particle retention and an increased risk of pulmonary disease.

The majority of particles deposited in the alveoli are probably phagocytosed by alveolar macrophages, which then migrate to the mucociliary escalator, are transported to the pharynx, and are expectorated or swallowed in the same manner as free particles. When the capacity of these macrophages to clear the airspaces in this manner is over-

whelmed by an abundance of particles, disease may ensue. In the case of inorganic particles, there may be penetration directly across the epithelium into the alveolar or peribronchiolar interstitial tissue. Some of these particles are then transported centripetally via peribronchovascular lymphatics to bronchopulmonary and hilar lymph nodes or centrifugally via lymphatics in the interlobular septa to the pleura. Others, however, remain in the interstitial tissue (particularly peribronchiolar), where they may accumulate and eventually cause significant disease.

Inflammation and Secreted Proteins. Polymorphonuclear leukocytes normally are present both in alveolar airspaces and along the conducting airways, albeit in very small numbers. Their role is, presumably, similar to that of the alveolar macrophage, although the substances that they phagocytose and degrade may differ. In addition to these normally occurring cells, an inflammatory reaction is a common result of particle deposition, particularly if clearance mechanisms are inadequate.

Several substances secreted by airway and alveolar epithelial cells or by macrophages, or derived directly from the blood, also have a local nonspecific protective function. These include lysozyme, lactoferrin, interferon, fibronectin, surfactant, and various complement components. In addition, epithelial cells produce substances, such as leukocyte antiprotease, which act to protect the lung from the deleterious side effects of proteolytic enzymes that are probably released normally in small amounts by intrapulmonary inflammatory cells.

The reaction to irritating or noxious gases is somewhat different from that to inhaled particles. The first line of defense is cessation of ventilation; gases that do enter the conducting system are absorbed on the moist surface of the upper airways or are detoxified by dilution.

Pulmonary Immune Mechanisms. Cells of the intrapulmonary immune system are localized at a variety of sites, including lymph nodes and mucosal lymphoid nodules, and as isolated cells in the alveolar and bronchovascular interstitium. Numerous lymph nodes are present in the tissue adjacent to proximal bronchi. They receive lymph with admixed cells and debris from the parenchyma and conducting airways and function both as a repository for foreign particulate material and as a station for antigen processing. The precise function of mucosal lymphoid tissue is unclear; however, it has been suggested that it is a component of a common epithelial mucosal IgA system that includes the gastrointestinal tract and is possibly involved in antigen processing and local IgA production.[161]

All immunoglobulin classes are found in tracheobronchial secretions, although the predominant forms are IgG and IgA.[162] They may be produced and secreted locally (particularly IgA and IgE) or derived from the serum by transudation (IgG). IgA is the most abundant and is present predominantly in dimeric (secretory) form. It is probably produced mostly by B cells in the connective tissue of the lamina propria and tracheobronchial glands. These antibodies have multiple functions, including opsonization and enhanced phagocytosis (particularly IgG), complement activation, toxin neutralization, and microbial agglutination.

Cell-mediated immunity is also undoubtedly important in pulmonary defense, particularly with respect to infection. Bronchoalveolar lavage of normal individuals yields a cellular population composed of about 80 to 85 per cent macrophages and 10 to 15 per cent lymphocytes, of which the great majority are T cells. Most of these appear to be derived from a pool of sensitized lymphocytes in the systemic circulation.[163] Such cells emigrate from pulmonary vessels at the site where an appropriate antigen is deposited and participate either in modulation and enhancement of alveolar macrophage function or in cell-mediated cytotoxicity.

Metabolic Functions

As previously indicated, mast cells are found throughout the lungs in airway, alveolar, and pleural interstitial tissue.[164] They contain several mediators that are stored in granules or are synthesized when the cells are stimulated. Such mediators include

1. vasoactive substances, such as histamine, leukotrienes, platelet activating factor, prostaglandins, and thromboxane A_2 (in general, these agents cause plasma leakage from bronchial and pulmonary vessels and airway smooth muscle contraction);
2. chemotactic factors, such as eosinophil chemotactic factor of anaphylaxis, neutrophil chemotactic factor, leukotriene B, and platelet activating factor (also vasoactive); and
3. a variety of proteoglycans and enzymes, including heparin sulfate, argylsulfatase, tryptase, superoxide dismutase, and chymase.

Mast cells are activated when IgE bound to their surface receptors interacts with specific antigen. The most studied role of the cells in disease has been in allergic bronchoconstriction; however, they probably have a function in many other forms of pulmonary inflammation. They also have been hypothesized to have a role in the regulation of mucous gland secretion, neuropeptide activity, bronchomotor tone, and fibroblast mitogenesis.[164]

The vast endothelial network of the pulmonary capillaries has several metabolic functions. For example, there is evidence that endothelial cells can modulate the coagulability of blood; the lungs contain large amounts of plasmin activator and thrombokinase, the former converting plasminogen to plasmin, and the latter prothrombin to thrombin. The presence of lipoprotein lipases within or on the surface of capillary endothelial cells indicates that the lungs have an enormous capacity for lipolysis. Lipids, especially long-chain fatty acids absorbed by the intestinal tract, enter the bloodstream as chylomicra, which pass up the thoracic duct and through the right side of the heart to the pulmonary vascular bed. The fatty acids released by hydrolysis of lipid ester bonds may be used by tissues, including the lung, both as a substrate for oxidative metabolism and for the formation of complex lipids.

Other biologically active substances, about which even less is known, are stored, transformed, or synthesized in the lungs. Serotonin is metabolized to 5-hydroxyindoleacetic acid and may be taken up by platelets within the lung.[165] The presence in lung tissue of enzymes known to be active in catecholamine synthesis and degradation suggests that the norepinephrine and epinephrine in the walls of bronchi and blood vessels may be produced and rendered inactive at these sites. Both E and F prostaglandins

have been identified in lipid extracts of lung tissue[166]; they appear to act directly on the muscle of bronchi and pulmonary vessels, prostaglandin E causing relaxation and F causing constriction.

Angiotensin-converting enzyme (ACE) is produced largely by pulmonary endothelial cells. It inactivates bradykinin, a powerful hypotensive and edematogenic substance, and simultaneously activates angiotensin II, an equally powerful pressor agent. In animals, ACE activity is inhibited by hypoxia; if this finding can be applied to humans, it may explain the systemic hypertension and pulmonary edema that sometimes occur in lung disease associated with hypoxemia.

DEVELOPMENT AND GROWTH OF THE LUNG

The growth and development of the lung can be divided into intrauterine and postnatal stages. Traditionally, the former itself has been divided into four periods: *embryonic, pseudoglandular, canalicular,* and *terminal sac*[167]; recently, the addition of a fifth, or *alveolar,* phase also has been proposed.[168]

Conducting and Transitional Airways and Alveoli

The *embryonic period* of lung development begins at about 26 days of life with the formation of a ventral diverticulum of the foregut near the junction of the occipital and cervical segments. During the next 2 to 3 days, the diverticulum gives rise to right and left lung buds that progressively elongate and branch, so that by days 32 to 34 the five lobar bronchi have appeared, a point marking the end of the embryonic period.

The *pseudoglandular period* extends from the end of the fifth to the sixteenth week of gestation and is concerned primarily with the development of the bronchial tree. Following the appearance of the five lobar bronchi, branching occurs quickly and more or less dichotomously. Between the tenth and the fourteenth weeks, 65 to 75 per cent of all bronchial branching has occurred, and by the sixteenth week virtually all conducting airways are present. During this period, the airways are blind tubules lined with columnar or cuboidal epithelium—hence the term pseudoglandular (Fig. 1–40).

From the sixteenth to the twenty-fourth or twenty-fifth week of intrauterine life (*canalicular period*), the peripheral portion of the bronchial tree undergoes further development in the form of primitive canaliculi that represent early stages of the acinar airways. At the same time, the mesenchyme adjacent to the canaliculi becomes vascularized through ingrowth of capillaries.

By the twenty-fourth to twenty-fifth week, terminal thin-walled spaces with flattened epithelium, termed saccules, become visible at the ends of the canaliculi. This marks the beginning of the *terminal sac* period, which is traditionally believed to last until birth. (Despite this, alveolar development has been demonstrated as early as 30 weeks of gestation and, in one study, was uniformly present by 36 weeks[168]; it has thus been suggested that the final period of lung development, from 36 weeks to term, be designated the *alveolar phase.*) Acini develop rapidly, so that by the

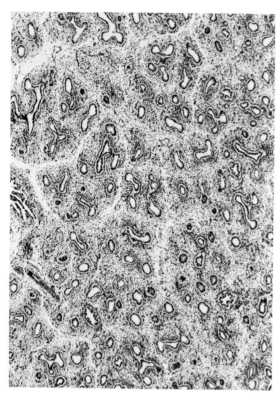

Figure 1–40. Developing Human Lung. Microscopic appearance of lung in the late pseudoglandular period showing branching presumptive airways and relatively abundant mesenchymal tissue. (× 52.)

twenty-eighth week, several generations of respiratory bronchioles open into so-called transitional ducts, with several generations of saccules arising from them. Further intrauterine development consists largely of saccular proliferation and a corresponding decrease in and more organized vascularization of the mesenchyme. At birth, the typical acinus consists of three generations of respiratory bronchioles, one of transitional ducts, and three of saccules.[167]

Throughout the canalicular period, airway epithelium progressively decreases in height so that the entire acinar pathway is eventually lined by a cuboidal or flattened epithelium. At about 28 weeks, differentiation into type I and type II alveolar epithelial cells has begun, and an occasional type II osmiophilic granule can be identified.[169] At this stage, a blood-gas barrier exists that is capable of permitting gas exchange.

During early *postnatal* development, the acinus increases in length, and its components are remodeled, largely as a result of the appearance of alveoli. Thus, terminal bronchioles may be transformed into respiratory bronchioles, and distal respiratory bronchioles into alveolar ducts. The saccules themselves probably develop into both alveolar ducts and alveolar sacs. Although there is little true airway branching after birth, each terminal saccule may generate as many as four additional alveolar sacs,[167] probably by budding. There is general consensus that the majority of alveoli appear during early childhood, probably up to 2 to 4 years of age,[170] and that they enlarge from childhood to adulthood. The age at which alveolar development is completed

is controversial, although it appears most likely that multiplication occurs until at least 8 years of age.[169]

The nature of and factors controlling postpneumonectomy compensatory lung growth are poorly understood. On the basis of animal experiments, it appears that such growth is a result of both cellular and connective tissue proliferation (as opposed to simple hypertrophy or alveolar distention) and that stretch is the initial stimulus.[171]

Vascular System

The pulmonary artery develops from the sixth aortic arch during the early embryonic period. On both sides, the proximal part of the arch develops into the proximal segment of the right and left pulmonary arteries; however, on the right side the distal part loses its connection with the aortic arch, whereas during intrauterine life the distal arch on the left maintains its connection with the aorta as the ductus arteriosus. Branches from both arches grow toward the developing lung buds and become incorporated with them in the future hila.

During the embryonic and pseudoglandular periods, pulmonary arteries develop at approximately the same rate and in the same manner as the airways, so that the majority of preacinar branches are present by the end of the sixteenth week. During the latter part of fetal life, the main feature of arterial development is an increase in vessel diameter and length. In the postnatal stage, there is a small continuing increase in the development of conventional branches until about age 18 months, related to the small increase in acinar airways that occurs during this period.[169] By contrast, a marked increase occurs in the supernumerary branches, corresponding to the prolific alveolar development of early childhood; this continues, although at a decreasing rate, until about 8 years of age.[172]

In the embryonic stage, pulmonary venous blood drains via the splanchnic plexus into the primordia of the systemic venous system. Subsequently, an outpouching of the sinoatrial region of the heart (termed the common pulmonary vein) extends toward and connects with that portion of the splanchnic plexus draining the lungs. Eventually, the common pulmonary vein is incorporated into the left atrial wall and the majority of the splanchnic-pulmonary connections are obliterated, leaving four independent pulmonary veins directly entering the left atrium. As in the arterial system, the postacinar venous pattern is essentially complete halfway through fetal life, and the intra-acinar pattern develops during childhood.[173]

Factors Influencing Development and Growth

Several factors affect lung growth and development, and it is probable that heredity has an important effect on at least some of them.[174] If the lung buds are removed from an animal in an early stage of development and then cultured, the branching process continues, but only if the adjacent mesenchyme is included in the culture medium.[175] The mechanisms responsible for this relationship are unclear; however, it is likely that cell surface interactions are necessary in at least some situations,[176] and it is possible that production of extracellular matrix or locally active chemical mediators are involved.[177]

It is also possible that the nervous system plays an important role in normal lung development. Recent studies have documented pulmonary hypoplasia in animals subjected to intrauterine cervical or phrenic nerve injury[178]; it has been speculated that this effect is mediated by abnormalities of respiratory movement due to denervation.

The role of systemic hormones and locally produced peptides in growth and development, although undoubtedly important, is for the most part poorly understood. Glucocorticoids have a significant effect on the maturation of alveolar type II cells and, thus, on surfactant production. The precise morphologic effects of other hormones, such as thyroxine, insulin, and growth hormone, have not been well demonstrated, although they undoubtedly occur.[179] As mentioned previously, pulmonary neuroendocrine cells have been hypothesized to play a role in airway development, possibly mediated by gastrin releasing peptide.[12]

The effects on lung growth of bronchopulmonary or systemic disease acquired in childhood also are not well understood; however, experimental evidence indicates that a variety of conditions such as viral infection[180] and starvation[181] can have an important influence.

INNERVATION OF THE LUNG

The lung is innervated by fibers that travel in the vagus nerve and in nerves derived from the second to fifth thoracic ganglia of the sympathetic trunk. The vagus contains preganglionic, parasympathetic efferent fibers, nonadrenergic-noncholinergic (NANC) efferent fibers, and afferent fibers from various lung receptors. The sympathetic fibers are largely postganglionic efferent in type.

Small branches of the recurrent laryngeal nerve on the left side and of the vagus itself on the right are distributed directly to the trachea, where they form several plexuses that are most prominent on the posterior wall. After giving off these branches, fibers from the vagus and sympathetic chains enter the hila, join with branches from the cardiac autonomic plexus, and form large posterior and smaller anterior plexuses in the peribronchovascular connective tissue. From these emanate multiple individual peribronchial and perivascular nerve fibers.

Afferent receptors have been divided into three functional groups on the basis of their distribution and physiologic response to various stimuli.

1. *Irritant* or *cough receptors*, located predominantly in central airways, are composed of highly arborized nets with numerous free nerve endings in the airway epithelium.[182] They respond to lung inflation or deflation and to a wide variety of chemical and mechanical stimuli. Their stimulation results in a reflex bronchoconstriction, and their role is probably to inhibit inhalation of toxic material.[183]

2. *Stretch receptors* occur as tendril-like structures closely applied to the surface of individual muscle cells in the airway wall. They are responsible for sending information to the respiratory center regarding lung volume, and their activation contributes to termination of inspiratory neural drive.

3. *Juxtacapillary (J) receptors,* situated in lung parenchyma adjacent to alveolar septa and pulmonary capillaries,[184] are thought to respond to stretching of these structures, such as occurs with lung congestion or interstitial edema.

Stimulation of postganglionic cholinergic efferent fibers increases secretion by the tracheobronchial glands and goblet cells, causes airway smooth muscle contraction and airway narrowing, and results in vascular smooth muscle relaxation and pulmonary vasodilation. All these effects are blocked by atropine. Postganglionic adrenergic fibers innervate pulmonary and bronchial vascular smooth muscle, and stimulation results in constriction. (Although there is no adrenergic innervation of human airway smooth muscle, there are numerous beta$_2$-adrenergic receptors on the muscle[185]; these respond to circulating catecholamines and therapeutically administered beta-agonists by relaxation.)

The third component of the autonomic nervous system, the so-called NANC system, has only recently been demonstrated.[186] Its stimulation causes airway smooth muscle relaxation, and it has been suggested that a defect in the system may be important in the production of nonspecific bronchial hyper-reactivity, a characteristic feature of asthma and other airway diseases.

THE PLEURA

Anatomy

The pleural space is enclosed by the visceral pleura, which covers the lungs, and by the parietal pleura, which lines the chest wall, diaphragm, and mediastinum.[187] The two join at the hila. Although they may come into intimate contact locally, the left and right pleural spaces are normally separate.

The visceral pleura is a thin but strong "membrane" that can be divided histologically into three layers (Fig. 1–41):

1. The *endopleura*, which is composed of a continuous layer of mesothelial cells and a thin underlying network of irregularly arranged collagen and elastic fibers;

2. The *external elastic lamina*, which is primarily responsible for pleural mechanical stability and consists of a thin layer of dense collagen and elastic tissue;

3. The *vascular (interstitial) layer,* which lies beneath the external elastic lamina and consists of loose connective tissue in which lymphatic channels, nerves, and bronchial vessels are situated. It is continuous with the interstitial tissue of the interlobular septa and directly overlays the *internal elastic lamina.* The latter is a thin, elastic-collagen layer that is continuous with the connective tissue of the alveolar septa and surrounds almost the entire lung, effectively connecting the parenchyma to the pleura. The external and internal elastic laminae are only loosely attached and may be readily separated in the connective tissue plane of the vascular layer; in appropriate circumstances, liquid or gas readily accumulates in this region.

The parietal pleura consists of a layer of connective tissue deep to the endothoracic fascia of the chest wall. It is divided into two parts by a fibroelastic band, with the majority of vessels being located in the more external layer.

The blood supply to the parietal pleura is derived from the subclavian, internal mammary, and intercostal arte-

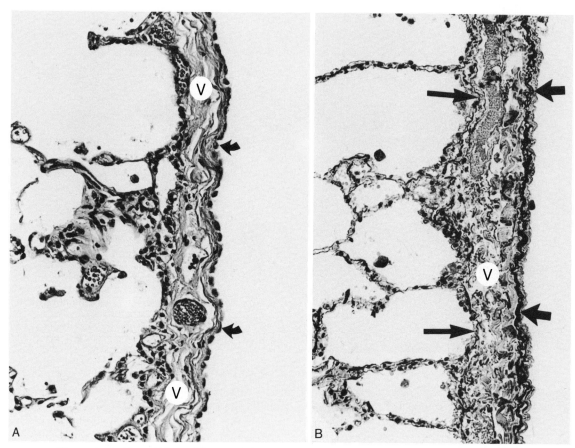

Figure 1–41. Normal Visceral Pleura. *A*, Mesothelial cells *(curved arrows)*. *B*, Vascular layer (V), internal elastic lamina *(long arrows)*, external elastic lamina *(short arrows)*. (*A*, H&E; *B*, Verhoeff–van Gieson; both × 200.)

ries.[188] The origin of the blood supply of the visceral pleura, however, is not as clear. According to some observers, the hilar, apical, mediastinal, and interlobar regions are supplied by the bronchial circulation, the remainder being nourished by the pulmonary arteries; others believe that the blood supply of the costal and diaphragmatic portions is also bronchial in origin.[188] With the exception of the hilar regions (which are drained by bronchial veins), the visceral pleural venous return is via the pulmonary veins.

Mesothelial Cell

Mesothelial cells form a continuous layer over the whole of the visceral and parietal pleural surfaces. Their shape and size are inconstant, the diameter varying directly with transpulmonary pressure (the cells becoming more flattened as the lung expands[187]). When individual cells are stimulated, they enlarge, become cuboidal or columnar in shape, and develop large nuclei with prominent nucleoli; occasionally, these features are sufficient to obscure the distinction between mesothelioma and a reactive process.

Ultrastructurally, mesothelial cells are joined by tight junctions and contain pinocytotic vesicles on both luminal and basal aspects. The cell surface is covered by numerous microvilli (Fig. 1–42) that are typically long and thin, measuring about 0.1 μm in diameter and up to 3 μm in length. Presumably by means of these microvilli and the pinocytotic vesicles, mesothelial cells help regulate the composi-

tion and amount of pleural fluid. It is not certain whether the cells actively synthesize substances found in the fluid or simply transport them from underlying connective tissue cells or blood.[187]

Roentgenology

The combined thickness of the parietal and visceral pleurae over the convexity of the lungs and over the diaphragmatic and mediastinal surfaces normally is insufficient to render them roentgenographically visible, except by HRCT.[189] By contrast, because of the presence of air-containing lung on both sides of the visceral pleura in the interlobar regions, contiguous layers of visceral pleura are visible when the x-ray beam passes tangentially along their surfaces.

Normal Fissures

Fissures form the contact surfaces between pulmonary lobes. Although they may extend to the hilum—resulting in complete lobar separation—commonly they are incomplete. For example, in one study of 100 excised lungs, an incomplete fissure was found between the right lower and upper lobes in 70 per cent of cases, between the right lower and middle lobes in about 45 per cent, between the left lower and upper lobes in about 40 per cent, and between the right upper and middle lobes (minor fissure) in almost

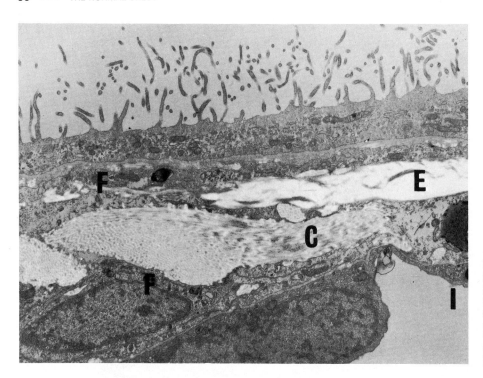

Figure 1–42. Normal Pleura—Ultrastructure. Rabbit visceral pleura, showing fibroblasts (F), elastic (E) and collagen (C) fibers, type I pneumocyte (I), and surface mesothelial cell with numerous elongated microvilli. (× 12,600.) (From Wang N-S: The regional difference of pleural mesothelial cells in rabbits. Am Rev Respir Dis 111: 623, 1974.)

90 per cent.[190] Similar figures have been found in lungs examined by standard or thin-section CT.[191] The incompleteness of interlobar fissures is important, since the parenchymal "bridge" that is established provides a ready pathway for collateral air drift or for the spread of disease to another lobe, creating roentgenographic signs that may give rise to erroneous conclusions.

The *major (oblique) fissures*, which separate the upper (and on the right, the middle lobe) from the lower lobes, begin at or about the level of the fifth thoracic vertebra and extend obliquely downward and forward, roughly paralleling the sixth rib, ending at the diaphragm a few centimeters behind the anterior pleural gutter (Fig. 1–43). Some variation exists in the orientation of the right and left major fissures. In one study of 100 consecutive CT scans of adults, the upper part of each major fissure was oriented with its lateral aspect posterior to its medial aspect (lateral facing).[192] However, in the lower part of the thorax, the lateral aspect of both the right and the left major fissures was normally anterior to the medial aspect (medial facing) (*see* Fig. 1–43); at the level of the carina, the lateral and medial aspects of the fissure were in the coronal plane. Not infrequently, a triangular opacity caused by the presence of adipose tissue is present at the lower end of the major fissures, its base contiguous with the diaphragm and its apex tapering cephalad into the fissure.[193]

The *horizontal (minor) fissure* separates the anterior segment of the right upper lobe from the middle lobe and lies roughly horizontal at about the level of the fourth rib anteriorly. There is considerable variation in its orientation, the anterior aspect generally being lower than the posterior, and the lateral part lower than the medial.[190]

The incidence of completeness of the pleural fissures on conventional roentgenograms is highly variable. This is not difficult to understand considering the underlying anatomic variability, the curved orientation of the fissures, and the

fact that the major fissures are almost always oriented slightly away from the coronal plane. As a result, the major fissures are seldom seen along their entirety on lateral chest roentgenograms. The minor fissure can be identified in about 55[194] to 80[114] per cent of cases by standard roentgenography and in about 80 per cent by thin-section CT.[195] Anatomically, the minor fissure rarely reaches the mediastinum and then only in its anterior portion; despite this, one of the more constant relationships on PA roentgenograms is the fissure's medial termination (or projected termination) at the lateral margin of the interlobar pulmonary artery. A fissure line or interface that projects medial to this point is almost invariably a downward displaced major fissure, providing certain evidence of volume loss in the right lower lobe.

In one investigation of 100 consecutive CT scans of adults,[192] three different manifestations of the right and left major fissures were described: lucent bands, lines, and dense bands (Fig. 1–44). Depending on the level of the scan (upper, middle, or lower thorax), the lucent band form was seen in about 60 to 75 per cent of cases. The linear manifestation was identified at the three levels in 1 to 10 per cent on the right and 1 to 20 per cent on the left. Dense bands were the least common manifestation, being identified in up to 4 per cent on the right and up to 6 per cent on the left. The varying appearance of the major fissures was considered to be related to the plane of the fissure on the cross-sectional image. Thus, a perpendicular fissure (e.g., in the upper thorax) is likely to produce a linear configuration, whereas a more oblique orientation causes a well-defined, dense (ground-glass) band. If the upper part of the major fissure is not quite perpendicular to the cross-sectional image, the smaller vessels at the periphery of the lobes on both sides of the fissure tend to cause the fissure to be displayed as a relatively avascular lucent band.

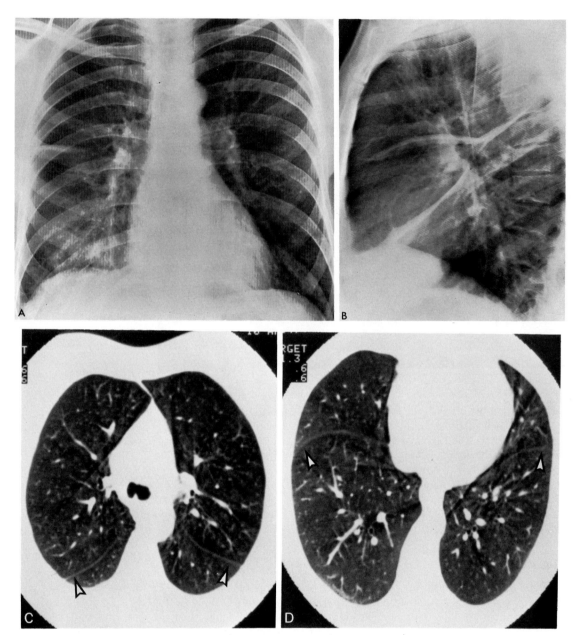

Figure 1–43. Interlobar Fissures, Right Lung. The presence of minimal interlobar effusion renders the fissures clearly visible in PA *(A)* and lateral *(B)* roentgenograms. *C,* A CT scan through the upper thorax reveals the lateral portion of the right and left major fissures *(arrowheads)* to be situated posterior to the anteromedial portion, so-called "lateral facing." *D,* A CT scan through the lower thorax shows that the lateral portion of the major fissures *(arrowheads)* is located anterior to the anteromedial aspect of the major fissures, so-called "medial facing."

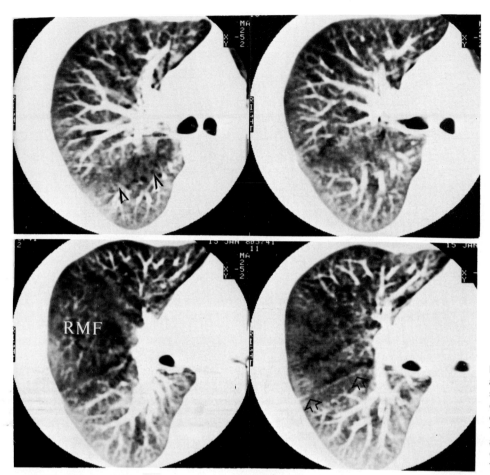

Figure 1–44. CT Appearance of Major and Minor Fissures. Sequential CT scans (10 mm thick; 10-mm spacing) demonstrate the right major fissure as either a lucent band *(arrowheads)* or a thin line *(open arrows)*. The broad, triangular lucency (the right midlung window) identifies the apex of the minor fissure (RMF).

The minor fissure and the plane of the CT scan are more or less tangential to each other, resulting in a lucent area relatively devoid of vessels when compared with the same region in the left lung (the *right midlung window*[196]). It is generally seen on only one or two scans, usually at the level of the intermediate bronchus. In about 45 per cent of cases, it is triangular in shape, its apex at the hilum; in about 10 per cent, it is round or oval (*see* Fig. 1–44), a shape possibly caused by its domelike configuration.

Pulmonary Ligament

The pulmonary ligament consists of a double layer of pleura that drapes caudally from the lung hilum, tethering the medial aspect of the lower lobe to the mediastinum and diaphragm.[197] It is formed by the mediastinal (parietal) pleura as it reflects over the main bronchi and pulmonary arteries and veins onto the surface of the lung as the visceral pleura (Fig. 1–45). The ligament may terminate in a free falciform border anywhere between the inferior pulmonary vein and the superior aspect of the hemidiaphragm (*incomplete form*), or it may extend inferiorly and cover a portion of the medial aspect of the hemidiaphragm (*complete form*). Thus, the pulmonary ligament divides the mediastinal pleural space below the hilum into either complete or incomplete anterior and posterior compartments. The bare area of mediastinum thus created contains a network of connective tissue, small bronchial vessels, lymphatics,

and lymph nodes. The left pulmonary ligament is closely related to the esophagus and is bordered posteriorly by the descending aorta; the shorter, right ligament can be situated anywhere along an arc that extends from the inferior vena cava anteriorly to the azygos vein posteriorly.

Although the pulmonary ligaments are never seen on conventional PA or lateral chest roentgenograms, they are frequently identified on CT.[198] The appearance is variable but usually consists of a small peak or pyramid on the mediastinal surface and a thin linear opacity that extends obliquely posteriorly from the apex of the peak to the lung, marking the intersublobar septum. It is most evident on scans obtained at or just above the level of the hemidiaphragm. Ordinarily, the right ligament is seen at a level slightly higher than the left, and both ligaments can be appreciated on only one or two slices of a series.

Accessory Fissures

Any portion of lung may be partly or completely separated from adjacent portions by an accessory pleural fissure. These fissures, which are present in about 50 per cent of lungs, vary in their degree of development, from superficial slits in the lung surface not more than 1 or 2 cm deep to complete fissures that extend all the way to the hilum. Most are of little more than academic interest roentgenologically. When well developed, however, their recognition is important for three reasons: (1) the lung parenchyma they sub-

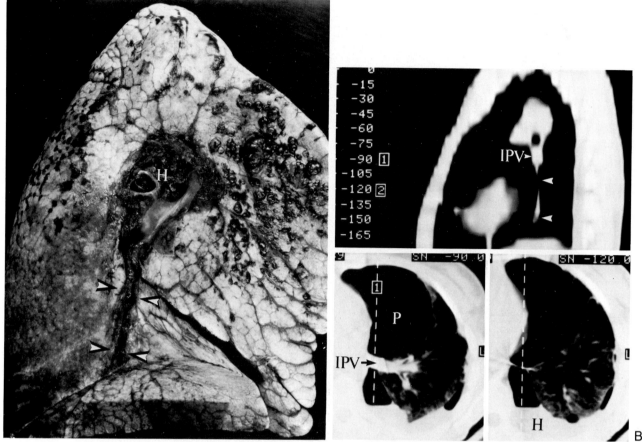

Figure 1–45. The Pulmonary Ligament. *A,* As seen on an inflated postmortem specimen of the left lung viewed from the medial aspect, the mediastinal (parietal) pleura reflects over the hilum superiorly, anteriorly, and posteriorly; caudally these pleural layers are more closely apposed to compose the pulmonary ligament *(arrowheads).* In *B* are a reformatted CT scan *(top)* and representative transverse images *(bottom)* through the plane of the left inferior pulmonary vein (IPV) and 3 cm caudally in a patient with a spontaneous hydropneumothorax (H and P). Note that the vertically oriented septum *(arrowheads)* divides the mediastinal pleural space into anterior and posterior compartments.

tend may be the only site of disease whose spread is prevented by the fissure; (2) a fissure in a specific anatomic location, such as between the superior and the basal segments of the right lower lobe, can be mistaken for the minor fissure between upper and middle lobes and thus create confusion in interpretation; and (3) they are important components of discoid atelectasis *(see* page 229).

Azygos Fissure. This is created by downward invagination of the azygos vein through the apical portion of the right upper lobe (Fig. 1–46).[199] The familiar curvilinear shadow extends obliquely across the upper portion of the right lung and terminates in the "teardrop" shadow caused by the vein itself at a variable distance above the right hilum. Since the azygos vein runs outside the parietal pleura, the fissure is formed by four pleural layers (two parietal and two visceral). Although the bronchial supply of the azygos lobe is variable, either the apical bronchus or its anterior subsegmental branch is always present. The importance of the anomaly roentgenologically lies in the failure of the apical pleural surfaces to separate when pneumothorax is present.

Inferior Accessory Fissure. This fissure is found in 30

to 45 per cent of lungs and separates the medial basal segment from the remainder of the lower lobe; when complete, the isolated lung is termed the inferior accessory or retrocardiac lobe. On the diaphragmatic surface of the lung, the fissure extends laterally from near the pulmonary ligament and then makes a convex arc forward to join the major fissure. On conventional roentgenograms, the fissure line extends superiorly and slightly medially from the inner third of the right or left hemidiaphragm.

Superior Accessory Fissure. This fissure separates the superior segment from the basal segments of the lower lobes, more often on the right (Fig. 1–47). Since it commonly lies horizontally at the same level as the minor fissure, the two may be confused on a frontal roentgenogram, although their separate anatomic positions may be clearly established on lateral or oblique roentgenograms.

Left Minor Fissure. This fissure separates the lingula from the rest of the left upper lobe; in almost all cases, the usual segmental anatomy of the left lung is preserved. One recent study of 2000 consecutive PA and lateral chest roentgenograms identified it in only 32 (1.6 per cent) instances.[200] Its position is usually more cephalad than the

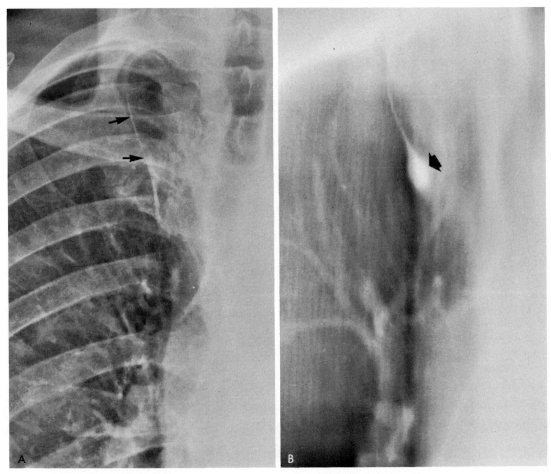

Figure 1–46. Accessory Fissure of the Azygos Vein. *A,* On a standard roentgenogram in PA projection, the fissure can be identified as a curvilinear shadow *(arrows)* extending obliquely across the upper portion of the right lung, its lower end some distance above the right hilum. *B,* A tomographic section with the patient in the supine position permits better perception of the teardrop shadow of the vein *(arrow)* because of distention.

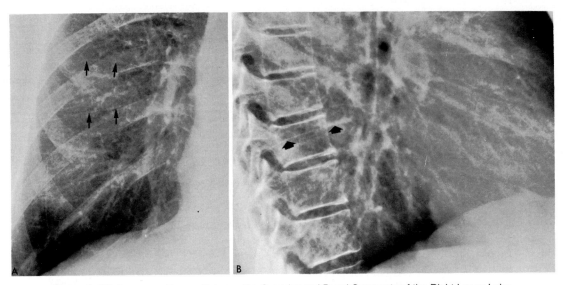

Figure 1–47. Accessory Fissure Between the Superior and Basal Segments of the Right Lower Lobe. *A,* In a PA projection of the lower half of the right lung two horizontal fissures can be identified, the superior *(upper arrows)* representing the normal minor fissure and the inferior *(lower arrows)* representing an accessory fissure between the superior and the basal bronchopulmonary segments of the right lower lobe. *B,* In lateral projection, the accessory fissure is well seen *(arrows).*

right minor fissure, and its lateral end is usually superior to its medial end.

Function

The visceral and parietal pleura form smooth membranes that facilitate the movement of the lungs within the pleural space, chiefly as the result of secretion and absorption of pleural fluid.[201] The amount of fluid in normal humans ranges from less than 1 mL to 20 mL. The dynamics of transudation and absorption of fluid obey the Starling equation and depend on a combination of hydrostatic, colloid osmotic, and tissue pressures. The tissue pressures are not known, but knowledge of the first two suggests that in health, fluid is formed at the parietal pleura and absorbed at the visceral pleura (Fig. 1–48).

The net hydrostatic pressure that forces fluid out of the parietal pleura can be calculated by determining the hydrostatic pressure in systemic capillaries that supply the parietal pleura (30 cm H_2O) and the pleural pressure (−5 cm H_2O at FRC); thus, the net hydrostatic drive is 35 cm H_2O. The osmotic colloid pressure in the systemic capillaries is 34 cm H_2O, and that of the pleura approximately 8 cm H_2O, yielding a net drive of 26 cm colloid osmotic pressure from the pleural space to the capillaries of the parietal pleura. The balance of these forces (35 − 26 cm = 9 cm H_2O) is directed from the parietal pleura to the pleural cavity. The visceral pleura is supplied by pulmonary and bronchial vessels, and the capillary pressure is much lower than systemic capillary pressure (about 11 cm H_2O), so that the net hydrostatic pressure from visceral pleura toward pleural cavity is 16 cm H_2O (11 + 5 cm). The osmotic colloid pressures remain constant, with a pressure of 26 cm H_2O away from the pleural cavity. Thus, the net effect of these forces is a drive of 10 cm H_2O (26 − 16 cm) toward the visceral pleural capillaries. Pleural fluid is also removed by lymphatics that originate in the parietal pleura.

LYMPHATIC SYSTEM

Lymphatics of the Lungs and Pleura

Anatomy

Pleural lymphatics course within the vascular layer, where they form a plexus of channels roughly following the pleural lobular boundaries. Between these channels and joining with them are smaller intercommunicating and blindly ending tributaries that ramify over the pleural surface. The entire network drains into the medial aspect of the lung near the hilum. Although the lymphatic channels are present over the whole of the pleural surface, they are much better developed over the lower than the upper lobes.

Pulmonary lymphatic channels form two major pathways, one in the bronchoarterial and the other in the interlobular septal connective tissue. The bronchoarterial lymphatics originate in the region of the distal respiratory bronchioles (none are present in alveolar interstitial tissue) and run proximally (Fig. 1–49), eventually reaching the bronchial and hilar lymph nodes.[202] The interlobular lymphatics drain partly into the bronchoarterial lymphatics and partly into the pleural system. Numerous funnel-shaped valves direct lymph flow in both pathways. Anastomotic channels connect the interlobular lymphatics with those in the bronchoarterial sheath; they are up to 4 cm long and usually lie approximately midway between the hilum and the periphery of the lung. Distention of these communicating lymphatics and edema in their surrounding connective tissue result in Kerley A lines; similar processes in the interlobular lymphatics and connective tissue result in Kerley B lines.

The lymphatic capillary endothelium rests on a discontinuous basal lamina that is entirely absent for considerable lengths.[202] In some areas, the endothelial cells are joined by intercellular junctions, but in others they are entirely free, leaving significant gaps in vascular integrity. Endothelial cell cytoplasm contains numerous microfilaments, some of which are thought to constitute an actinlike contractile system that possibly regulates the opening or closing of these intercellular gaps. Perilymphatic collagen fibers are in close contact with endothelial cells and basal lamina and have been regarded as a tethering mechanism that keeps the capillaries open. These features—endothelial and basement membrane discontinuities and connective tissue anchoring system—appear to be ideal for the provision of easy and continuous access of interstitial fluid to the capillary lumen.

Function

There is evidence that the flow of lymph through pulmonary lymphatic channels is aided by the "pumping" action of ventilation. For example, in one study of 15 adult

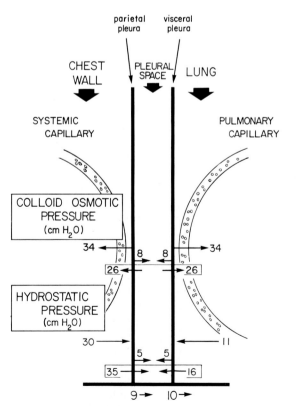

Figure 1–48. Diagrammatic Representation of the Pressures Involved in the Formation and Absorption of Pleural Fluid. *See* text for description.

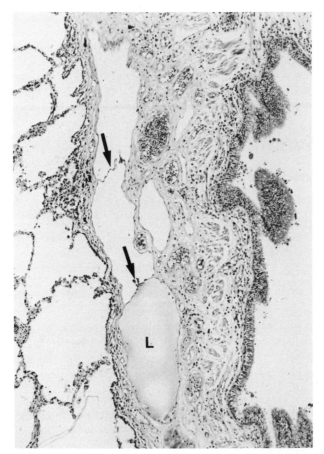

Figure 1–49. Peribronchial Lymphatic Channel. A peribronchiolar lymphatic (L) is distended by fluid (locally lost during tissue processing). Two valves are apparent *(arrows)*. (× 72.)

human lungs removed at necropsy,[203] ethiodized oil injected into pleural lymphatics was shown to fill the deep pulmonary lymphatics; subsequently, when a fixed inflation pressure was maintained, flow did not occur within the lymphatics. Forward flow occurred only during ventilation and appeared to depend on the lung volume at the time the lymphatics were filled. When contrast medium was injected with lung volume maintained at FRC, forward flow occurred within the lymphatics; by contrast, when filling was obtained at a lung volume of 70 per cent TLC, ventilation resulted in no forward movement of contrast medium within lymphatics. The authors suggested that this difference is best explained on the basis of the smaller volume of parenchymal lymphatic segments at high rather than at low lung volumes, reducing the influence of subsequent ventilation.

Thoracic Duct and Right Lymphatic Duct

The thoracic duct, a continuation of the cisterna chyli, enters the thorax through the aortic hiatus of the diaphragm. In the majority of subjects it lies to the right of the aorta and follows its course cephalad; thus, in the lower portion of the thorax it lies roughly in the midline or slightly to one side. At about the level of the carina, it crosses the left main bronchus and runs cephalad in a plane parallel to the left lateral wall of the trachea and slightly posterior to

it. The duct leaves the thorax between the esophagus and the left subclavian artery and runs posterior to the left innominate vein; much of the cephalic one third (the cervical portion) is supraclavicular. It joins the venous system most commonly by emptying into the internal jugular vein and sometimes into the subclavian, innominate, or external jugular veins. The diameter of the normal thoracic duct ranges from 1 to 7 mm[204]; thus, this parameter cannot be used as a single determinant of obstruction. Valves are present in about 85 per cent of cases, primarily in the upper two thirds.

The roentgenologic anatomy of the right lymphatic duct has been poorly documented, since this vessel cannot be suitably opacified and is inconstantly identified. The three trunks—the right jugular, right subclavian, and right mediastinal—often open separately into the jugular, subclavian, and innominate veins, respectively.

Lymph Nodes of the Mediastinum

Intrathoracic lymph nodes may be considered in two categories: (1) a *parietal group*, which resides outside the parietal pleura in extramediastinal tissue and drains the thoracic wall and a variety of extrathoracic structures; and (2) a *visceral group*, which is located within the mediastinum between the pleural membranes and is concerned particularly with the drainage of the intrathoracic tissues. The general organization of mediastinal and hilar lymph nodes has been thoroughly described by several observers.[205, 206]

Parietal Lymph Nodes

The parietal lymph nodes themselves may be divided into three groups.

1. The *anterior parietal* or *internal mammary* nodes are located in the upper thorax behind the anterior intercostal spaces bilaterally, either medial or lateral to the internal mammary vessels (Fig. 1–50). They receive afferent channels from the upper anterior abdominal wall, anterior thoracic wall, anterior portion of the diaphragm, and the medial portion of the breasts. These lymph nodes communicate with the visceral group of the anterior mediastinal nodes and the cervical nodes; their main efferent channel is the right lymphatic duct or thoracic duct.

2. The *posterior parietal* lymph nodes relate to the rib heads in the posterior intercostal spaces (*intercostal nodes*) and to the vertebrae (*juxtavertebral nodes*) (Fig. 1–51). Both groups drain the intercostal spaces, parietal pleura, and vertebral column. They communicate with posterior mediastinal lymph nodes that relate to the descending aorta and the esophagus. Efferent channels drain to the thoracic duct in the upper thorax and to the cisterna chyli in the lower thoracic area.

3. The *diaphragmatic* lymph nodes (Fig. 1–52) are composed of the *anterior (prepericardiac)* group that is located immediately behind the xiphoid and to the right and left of the pericardium anteriorly, the *middle (juxtaphrenic)* group that is located near the phrenic nerves as they meet the diaphragm, and the *posterior (retrocrural)* nodes that reside behind the right and left crura of the diaphragm. The

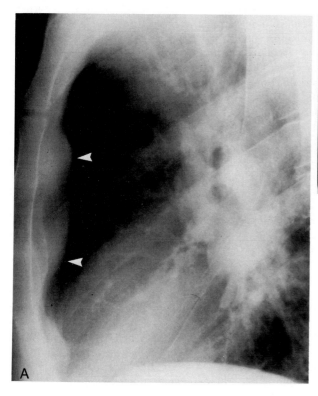

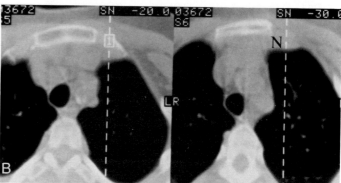

Figure 1–50. Enlargement of Anterior Parietal Lymph Nodes. *A,* A detail view from a conventional lateral chest roentgenogram reveals a smooth, lobulated, homogeneous soft tissue opacity *(arrowheads)* in the retrosternal area caused by enlargement of the anterior parietal (internal mammary) lymph nodes. In *B* are transverse images of a patient with metastatic breast carcinoma. Note the typical semilunar configuration *(arrowheads)* of the enlarged internal mammary nodes (N).

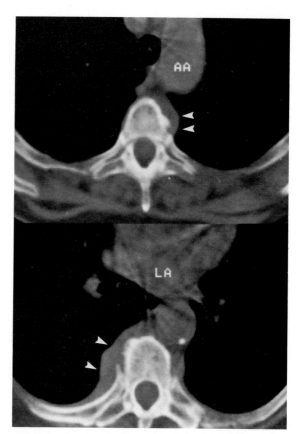

Figure 1–51. Enlargement of Posterior Parietal Lymph Nodes. Transverse CT through the aortic arch (AA) and left atrium (LA) shows lobulated masses related primarily to the costovertebral junctions *(arrowheads).*

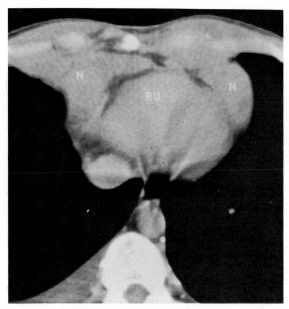

Figure 1–52. Enlargement of Diaphragmatic Lymph Nodes. A CT scan reveals enlarged nodes (N) anterior and lateral to the right ventricle (RV). Note that the enlarged nodes and the heart are iso-dense.

diaphragmatic nodes drain the diaphragm and the antero-superior portion of the liver.

Visceral Lymph Nodes

The visceral lymph nodes also may be divided into three chains.

1. The *anterosuperior mediastinal (prevascular)* nodes are congregated principally along the anterior aspect of the superior vena cava, right and left innominate veins, and ascending aorta (Fig. 1–53). A few nodes also are situated posterior to the sternum in the lower thorax and behind the manubrium anterior to the thymus. These nodes drain most of the structures in the anterior mediastinum, including the pericardium, thymus, diaphragmatic and mediastinal pleura, part of the heart, and the anterior portion of the hila. Efferent channels drain into the right lymphatic or thoracic duct.

2. The *posterior mediastinal* lymph nodes (Fig. 1–54) are located around the esophagus (*periesophageal nodes*) and along the anterior and lateral aspects of the descending aorta (*periaortic nodes*); they are most numerous in the lower portion of the thorax. Their afferent channels arise from the posterior portion of the diaphragm, the pericardium, the esophagus, and directly from the lower lobes of the lungs via the right and left inferior pulmonary ligaments. They communicate with the tracheobronchial nodes, particularly the subcarinal group, and drain chiefly via the thoracic duct.

3. The third and most important member of the visceral nodes is the *tracheobronchial group*. The *paratracheal lymph nodes* (Fig. 1–55) are located in front and to the right and left of the trachea; occasionally, a retrotracheal component is present. The right paratracheal chain is usually the best developed; its lowermost member, the azygos

node, is situated medial to the azygos vein arch in the pretracheal mediastinal fat. These lymph nodes receive afferent channels from the bronchopulmonary and tracheal bifurcation nodes, from the trachea, from the esophagus, and directly from the right and left lungs without diversion through the bronchopulmonary or tracheal bifurcation nodes. Direct communication also exists with the anterior and posterior visceral mediastinal nodes. The efferent channels are the right lymphatic and thoracic ducts.

Lymph nodes situated in the precarinal and subcarinal fat (Fig. 1–56) are commonly referred to as *subcarinal nodes*. On the left, those between the left pulmonary artery and aortic arch are usually designated *aortopulmonary window nodes* (Fig. 1–57); these are arranged in medial, lateral (subpleural), and superior compartments and merge above with the left prevascular chain. Subcarinal lymph nodes receive afferent drainage from the bronchopulmonary nodes, anterior and posterior mediastinal nodes, heart, pericardium, esophagus, and lungs. Efferent drainage is to the paratracheal group, particularly on the right side.

Hilar lymph nodes can be identified on conventional roentgenograms when enlarged (Fig. 1–58); otherwise, they are typically inapparent. According to one CT study, the nodes in the right hilum may be divided into four principal groups—right upper lobe, descending right pulmonary artery, middle lobe, and lower lobe—and in the left hilum into three main groups—left upper lobe, descending pulmonary artery, and lower lobe.[207] Contrast-enhanced CT is indispensable for the precise determination of suspected node enlargement in this area.

The *bronchopulmonary lymph nodes* are numerous but are normally too small to be detected by conventional or CT studies. They are located around the bronchi and vessels, particularly at their points of division. They receive afferent channels from all lobes of the lungs, and their efferent drainage is principally to the hilar nodes.

Imaging Methods in the Evaluation of Mediastinal and Hilar Lymph Nodes

One of the most important advances that CT has made in the investigation of thoracic disease is the ability to image small mediastinal lymph nodes. Although conventional tomography and even standard PA and lateral roentgenography can demonstrate gross lymph node enlargement, both techniques suffer from being unable to distinguish the variable tissue densities within the mediastinum, especially fat and soft tissue. Since adipose tissue is so ubiquitous within the mediastinum and is usually abundant, pathologically enlarged lymph nodes up to 3 cm may be completely enveloped by fat and therefore invisible on conventional studies. Both CT and MRI easily resolve this difficulty.

By CT, a lymph node may be identified as a round or an oval structure of soft tissue density, with or without central or eccentric radiolucent fat, in a location that does not conform to vascular or neural elements. The presence of mediastinal fat greatly facilitates recognition; foci of calcification or lymphangiographic contrast medium serve as more obvious markers.

Genereux and Howie[208] carried out a combined autopsy and CT study that was designed to evaluate the size, num-

Text continued on page 71

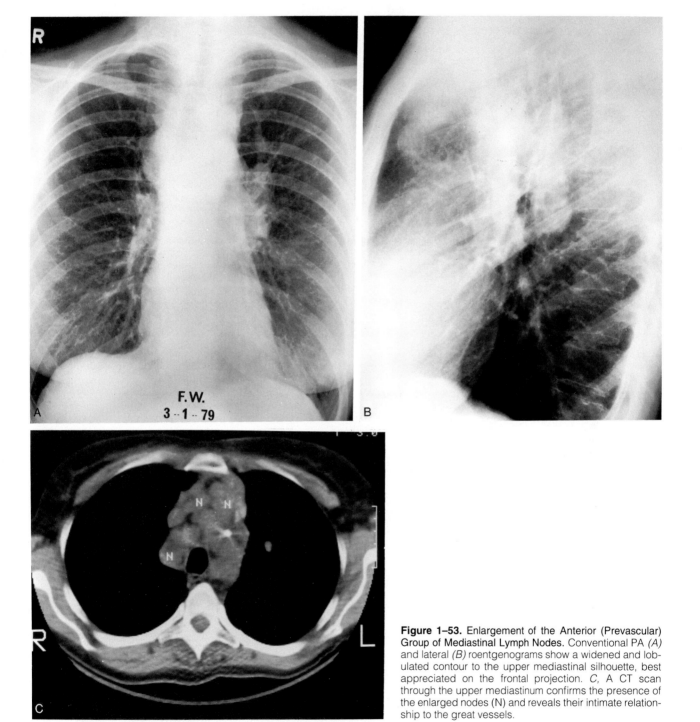

Figure 1–53. Enlargement of the Anterior (Prevascular) Group of Mediastinal Lymph Nodes. Conventional PA *(A)* and lateral *(B)* roentgenograms show a widened and lobulated contour to the upper mediastinal silhouette, best appreciated on the frontal projection. *C,* A CT scan through the upper mediastinum confirms the presence of the enlarged nodes (N) and reveals their intimate relationship to the great vessels.

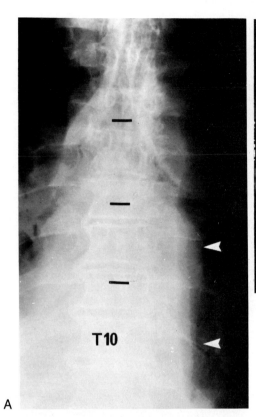

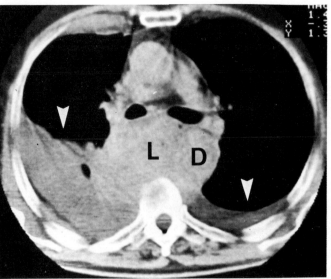

Figure 1–54. Enlargement of Posterior Mediastinal Lymph Nodes. *A*, An AP view of the thoracic spine of a patient with lymphoma reveals slight lobulation of the descending aorta *(arrowheads)*. *B*, An unenhanced CT scan at the level of the middle bar in *A* shows that the descending aorta (D) is isodense with and enveloped by massively enlarged periaortic lymph nodes (L). Bilateral pleural effusions are present *(arrowheads)*. (From Genereux GP: The posterior pleural reflections. AJR 141: 141, 1983. © American Roentgen Ray Society.)

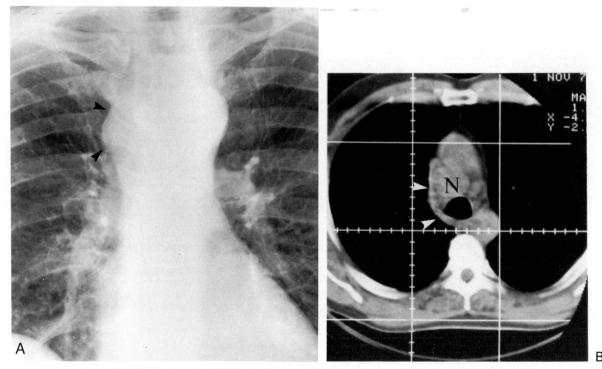

Figure 1–55. Enlargement of the Paratracheal Lymph Nodes. A PA chest roentgenogram *(A)* reveals an abnormal contour of the mediastinum *(arrowheads)* in the right tracheobronchial angle. *B*, A CT scan reveals the mass to be an enlarged azygos lymph node (N) (proved to be caused by metastatic carcinoma from the lung). The azygos vein is displaced *(two arrowheads)* laterally.

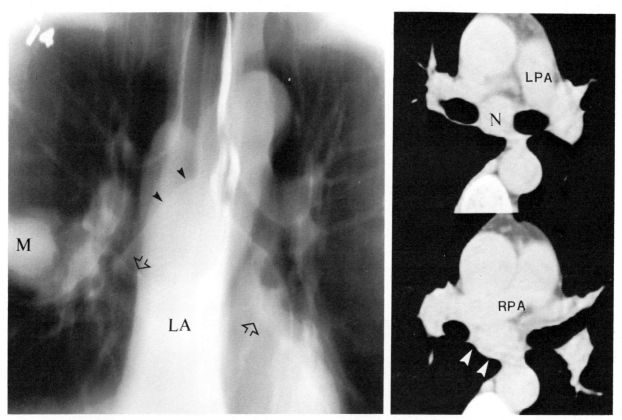

A

B

Figure 1–56. Enlargement of Subcarinal Lymph Nodes. *A,* A conventional AP tomogram in a patient with carcinoma of the middle lobe (M) reveals three important features of subcarinal lymph node enlargement: (1) a soft tissue opacity above the insertion of the inferior pulmonary veins *(open arrows)* into the left atrium (LA); (2) compression and displacement of the barium-filled esophagus to the left; and (3) minimal upward displacement of the right main bronchus *(arrowheads). B,* CT scans through the carina *(top)* and 2 cm caudad *(bottom)* show the abnormal mass to be enlarged lymph nodes (N) in the precarinal-subcarinal compartment. Note that the normal concavity of the azygoesophageal recess interface at this level has been obliterated by the convex nodal mass *(arrowheads).* RPA = right pulmonary artery; LPA = left pulmonary artery. (*A,* From Genereux GP: The posterior pleural reflections. AJR 141: 141, 1983. © American Roentgen Ray Society.)

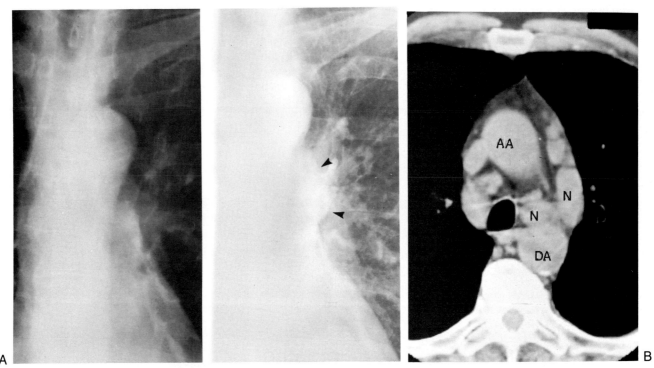

Figure 1–57. Enlargement of Aortopulmonary Lymph Nodes. *A,* Detail views of the left hilar region from PA chest roentgenograms before *(left)* and after *(right)* involvement of the aortopulmonary lymph nodes by Hodgkin's disease in a middle-aged man. Note the typical lobulated contour *(arrowheads)* between the aortic arch and main pulmonary artery. *B,* A CT scan confirms the presence of numerous enlarged nodes (N) in the aortopulmonary window. AA = ascending aorta; DA = descending aorta.

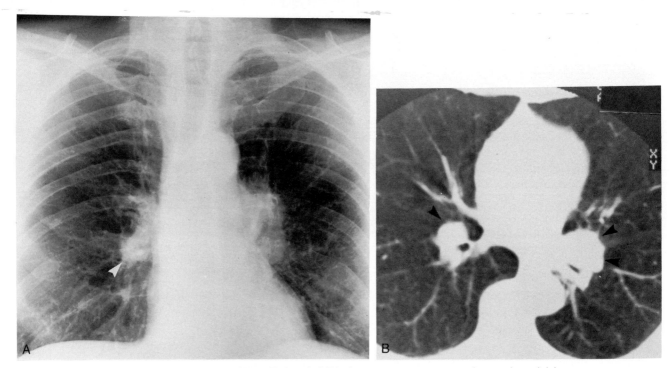

Figure 1–58. Enlargement of Hilar Nodes. *A,* A PA chest roentgenogram reveals an enlarged, lobulated left hilum; the right inferior hilum shows a focal increase in density *(arrowhead)*. These features are consistent with bilateral hilar node enlargement. *B,* A transverse CT scan through the lower hila confirms the presence of bilateral node enlargement *(arrowheads)*. Metastatic small cell carcinoma of the lung.

ber, and location of normal mediastinal lymph nodes. These researchers divided the mediastinum into four zones that related to the left innominate vein, the pretracheal space and right tracheobronchial angle, the precarinal/subcarinal compartment, and the aortopulmonary window. These divisions, designated zones I to IV, were chosen to conform to areas that are most accessible to cervical mediastinoscopy or parasternal mediastinotomy. The number and size of normal mediastinal lymph nodes in each zone as found by these two investigators are shown graphically in Figure 1–59.

In 1985, the American Thoracic Society (ATS) recommended that the terms "mediastinal" and "hilar" be dropped because of a lack of clinical-anatomic specificity and replaced with carefully defined "nodal stations" (Table

1–2 and Fig. 1–60). Using this new ATS scheme, Glazer and associates[209] carried out a CT study of the number and size of normal mediastinal lymph nodes at 11 intrathoracic nodal stations, measuring both the short and the long axis diameters in the transverse plane.

The largest nodes were in the subcarinal and right tracheobronchial regions, where the mean short axis measurement for nodal station 7 was 6.2 mm and for station 10R was 5.9 mm. Upper paratracheal nodes (station 2) were smaller than lower paratracheal (station 4) or tracheobronchial nodes (station 10), a finding that was emphasized in the earlier study by Genereux and Howie. Glazer and colleagues also found that there were more nodes in station 4 than in stations 2 and 10. Finally, these researchers indicated that the threshold size for nodal enlargement de-

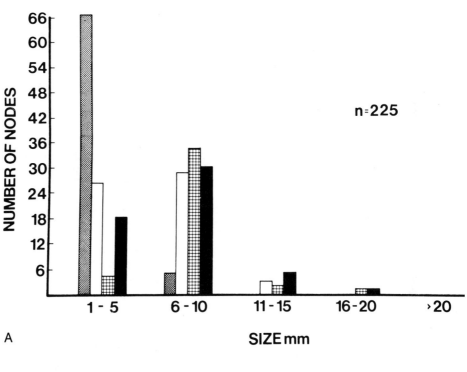

A

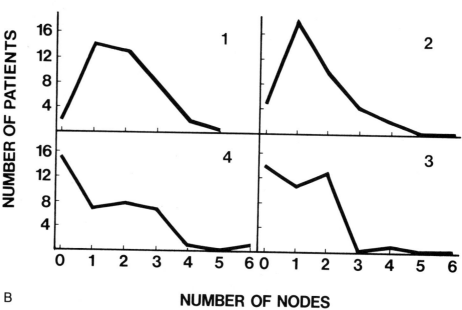

B

Figure 1–59. Size of Normal Mediastinal Lymph Nodes by Zone. *A,* Dotted area represents zone I; solid white, zone II; grid, zone III; and solid black, zone IV. Total number of nodes (n) examined was 225. Note that most of the lymph nodes in zone I are less than 5 mm in diameter, whereas the majority in zones II to IV are in the 6 to 15 mm range. (From Genereux GP, Howie JL: Normal mediastinal lymph node size and number: CT and anatomic study. AJR 142: 1095, 1984. © American Roentgen Ray Society.) *B,* Number of normal mediastinal lymph nodes by zone. Most patients show 1 to 3 nodes per zone. Note that nodes are usually demonstrable in zones 1 and 2, but slightly more than one third of patients show no nodes in zones 3 and 4. (From Genereux GP, Howie JL: Normal mediastinal lymph node size and number: CT and anatomic study. AJR 142: 1095, 1984. © American Roentgen Ray Society.)

Table 1–2. **AMERICAN THORACIC SOCIETY DEFINITIONS OF REGIONAL NODAL STATIONS**

X	**Supraclavicular nodes**
2R	**Right upper paratracheal nodes:** nodes to the right of the midline of the trachea, between the intersection of the caudal margin of the innominate artery with the trachea and the apex of the lung
2L	**Left upper paratracheal nodes:** nodes to the left of the midline of the trachea, between the top of the aortic arch and apex of the lung
4R	**Right lower paratracheal nodes:** nodes to the right of the midline of the trachea, between the cephalic border of the azygos vein and the intersection of the caudal margin of the brachiocephalic artery with the right side of the trachea
4L	**Left lower paratracheal nodes:** nodes to the left of the midline of the trachea, between the top of the aortic arch and the level of the carina, medial to the ligamentum arteriosum
5	**Aortopulmonary nodes:** subaortic and para-aortic nodes, lateral to the ligamentum arteriosum or the aorta or left pulmonary artery, proximal to the first branch of the left pulmonary artery
6	**Anterior mediastinal nodes:** nodes anterior to the ascending aorta or the innominate artery
7	**Subcarinal nodes:** nodes arising caudal to the carina of the trachea but not associated with the lower lobe bronchi or arteries within the lung
8	**Paraesophageal nodes:** nodes dorsal to the posterior wall of the trachea and to the right or left of the midline of the esophagus
9	**Right or left pulmonary ligament nodes:** nodes within the right or left pulmonary ligament
10R	**Right tracheobronchial nodes:** nodes to the right of the midline of the trachea, from the level of the cephalic border of the azygos vein to the origin of the right upper lobe bronchus
10L	**Left peribronchial nodes:** nodes to the left of the midline of the trachea, between the carina and the left upper lobe bronchus, medial to the ligamentum arteriosum
11	**Intrapulmonary nodes:** nodes removed in the right or left lung specimen plus those distal to the mainstem bronchi or secondary carina

Modified from Tisi GM, Friedman PJ, Peters RM, et al: Am Rev Respir Dis 127: 659, 1983.

pended on the particular station under scrutiny; in the upper paratracheal region (station 2), the value of the short axis measurement above which a lymph node was considered enlarged was found to be 7 mm, whereas for nodes residing in the lower paratracheal region (station 4) or around the carina (stations 7 and 10), the figure was 10 to 11 mm. The data comparing the frequency of lymph nodes less than 11 mm in diameter by location in Glazer and associates' study and the Genereux and Howie report are in close agreement (Table 1–3). On the basis of these and other studies, it has been suggested that the optimal size criterion for the diagnosis of malignant mediastinal node enlargement is 10 to 15 mm (short axis measurement).

The recent advent of MRI has raised the possibility that this modality may prove superior to CT in the evaluation of hilar and mediastinal structures. At present, several conclusions can be drawn from studies comparing the techniques:[210, 211] (1) both CT and MRI are capable of defining normal and abnormal lymph nodes, but the superior resolution of CT is better suited for the identification and separation of small (usually normal) lymph nodes; (2) MR images are better for distinguishing mediastinal nodes from vascular structures, even when the CT is contrast-en-

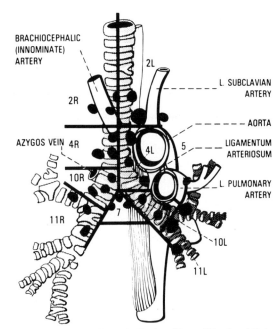

Figure 1–60. American Thoracic Society Map of Regional Pulmonary Nodes. *See* text. (From Tisi GM, Friedman PJ, Peters RM, et al: Am Rev Respir Dis 127: 659, 1983.)

hanced; (3) the sensitivity of CT and that of MRI are comparable in the mediastinum, but the specificity of CT is greater, probably as a result of inferior MRI resolution; and (4) it may be possible in the future to distinguish normal from abnormal lymph nodes on MRI by their T1 characteristics.

Lymphatic Drainage of the Lungs

According to Rouvière, the lungs can be subdivided into three main drainage areas—the superior, middle, and inferior—without correspondence to pulmonary lobes.[212] On the right side, in the superior area, lymph drains directly into the paratracheal and upper bronchopulmonary nodes. The middle zone drains directly into the paratracheal nodes, the subcarinal nodes, and the central group of bronchopulmonary nodes. The inferior zone drains into the inferior bronchopulmonary and bifurcation nodes and the

Table 1–3. **COMPARISON OF FREQUENCY OF LYMPH NODES LESS THAN 11 MM IN DIAMETER BY LOCATION IN TWO STUDIES**

Zone or Station	Genereux & Howie*	Glazer & Associates†
Retroinnominate (I)	72/72 (100%)	
ATS 4R		54/54 (100%)
Pretracheal (II)	55/58 (94.8%)	
ATS 10R		54/55 (98%)
Precarinal/ Subcarinal (III)	38/41 (92.6%)	
ATS 4L, 7, 10L		138/139 (99.2%)
Aortopulmonary (IV)	213/225 (94.6%)	
ATS 5		33/33 (100%)

*Data from Genereux GP, Howie JL: Am J Roentgenol 142: 1095, 1984.
†Data from Glazer GM, Gross BH, Quint LE, et al: Am J Roentgenol 144: 261, 1985.

posterior mediastinal chain. Thus, on the right side, all the lymph drains eventually via the right lymphatic duct.

Rouvière found that, in the left superior area, lymph drains both into the prevascular group of anterior mediastinal nodes and directly into the left paratracheal nodes. The middle zone drains mainly via the bifurcation and central group of bronchopulmonary nodes and partly directly into the left paratracheal group. The inferior zone drains into the bifurcation and inferior bronchopulmonary nodes and into the posterior mediastinal chain. Thus, according to Rouvière, the superior portion and part of the middle zone drain via the left paratracheal nodes into the thoracic duct, and lymph drainage from the remainder of the left lung empties eventually into the right lymphatic duct.

The "crossover" phenomenon was long thought to be of diagnostic and therapeutic importance in diseases originating in the middle or lower portion of the left lung, but more recent investigations have cast some doubt on the validity of the phenomenon in adults. For example, in one study of bilateral prescalene node biopsies in 110 patients with pulmonary carcinoma, the direction of lymphatic spread within the mediastinum was cephalad and usually ipsilateral, irrespective of the location of the primary growth; contralateral spread was uncommon and about equally frequent from either lung.[213] On the strength of these observations, it is reasonable to conclude that prescalene node biopsies should always be performed first on the same side as the pulmonary disease; should this prove negative, contralateral biopsy *occasionally* may be productive.

THE MEDIASTINUM

The mediastinum is an anatomic region bounded by the two lungs on either side, the sternum and vertebral column in front and in back, and the thoracic inlet and diaphragm above and below. For diagnostic and descriptive purposes, it is usually divided into several compartments; the most practical and informative technique for doing this has been the subject of considerable controversy over the years, and several methods have been proposed. The two that we employ in this book and shall describe in some detail are the "traditional" method and the more recent one employed by Heitzman.[112] The former is a reasonable approach, particularly with respect to a consideration of the differential diagnosis of mediastinal masses; in fact, it is this method that we employ in Chapter 19. However, for a thorough understanding of mediastinal *anatomy*, there is little question that the Heitzman method possesses much merit, and we have decided to adopt it for descriptive purposes in this chapter.

Mediastinal Compartments

The Traditional Method

Classic anatomy divides the mediastinum into superior and inferior compartments by an imaginary line extending from the sternal angle to the fourth intervertebral disc; the inferior compartment is further subdivided into prevascular or anterior, cardiovascular or middle, and postvascular or posterior compartments. Since each compartment contains

anatomic structures almost unique to it, many of the afflictions to which the mediastinum is subject tend to occur *predominantly* in one or the other compartment; as a result, this has undoubtedly been the most popular and generally accepted subdivision of the mediastinum over the years.

A modification of the traditional classification is the exclusion of the superior compartment; since it contains structures that are, for the most part, continuous with the compartments below, its separation serves little diagnostic purpose. In this modified classification, the *anterior mediastinal compartment* is bounded anteriorly by the sternum and posteriorly by the pericardium, aorta, and brachiocephalic vessels. It is narrowest anteriorly, where the pleura of the right and left upper lobe converge to form the anterior junction line (*see* later); it broadens posterosuperiorly in an apex-down triangular configuration to form the anterior mediastinal triangle. The anterior mediastinum contains the thymus gland, branches of the internal mammary artery and vein, lymph nodes, the inferior sternopericardial ligament, and variable amounts of fat.

The *middle mediastinal compartment* contains the pericardium and its contents, the ascending and transverse portions of the aorta, the superior and inferior vena cava, the brachiocephalic arteries and veins, the phrenic nerves and upper portion of the vagus nerves, the trachea and main bronchi and their contiguous lymph nodes, and the main pulmonary arteries and veins.

The *posterior mediastinal compartment* is bounded anteriorly by the pericardium and the vertical part of the diaphragm, laterally by the mediastinal pleura, and posteriorly by the bodies of the thoracic vertebrae (although for practical purposes, the paravertebral gutters are included). It contains the descending thoracic aorta, esophagus, thoracic duct, azygos and hemiazygos veins, autonomic nerves, fat, and lymph nodes.

The Heitzman Method

This method differs substantially from the traditional one and includes seven separate anatomic regions:

1. *The thoracic inlet,* a region with a narrow cephalocaudad dimension marking the cervicothoracic junction and lying immediately above and below a transverse plane through the first rib;

2. *The anterior mediastinal compartment,* a region extending from the thoracic inlet to the diaphragm in front of the heart, ascending aorta, and superior vena cava;

3. *The supra-aortic area,* the region behind the anterior mediastinum and above the aortic arch;

4. *The infra-aortic area,* the region behind the anterior mediastinum and below the aortic arch;

5. *The supra-azygos area,* the region behind the anterior mediastinum and above the azygos arch;

6. *The infra-azygos area,* the region behind the anterior mediastinum and below the azygos arch; and

7. *The hila,* the regions containing major bronchi, blood vessels, and lymph nodes in a connective tissue sheath that is continuous with the infra-aortic and infra-azygos areas.

Heitzman justifies the logic of this classification by pointing to the approximately equal sizes of the areas on the right and left sides of the mediastinum separated by a major vascular channel. Further, he states that the aortic and azygos arches actually serve as functional anatomic boundaries in certain disease states, such as in the limitation of the spread of a localized mediastinal abscess. The descriptions that follow of the normal anatomy of the mediastinal compartments have been derived principally from the treatises by Heitzman[112] and by Proto and colleagues.[214, 215]

Thoracic Inlet

The thoracic inlet, or cervicomediastinal continuum, represents the junction between structures at the base of the neck and those of the thorax. It parallels the first rib and thus is higher posteriorly than anteriorly; as a result, an opacity on a PA chest roentgenogram that is effaced on its superior aspect and that projects at or below the level of the clavicles must be situated anteriorly, whereas one that projects above the clavicles is retrotracheal and posteriorly situated.[216]

From front to back (Fig. 1–61), structures occupying the thoracic inlet include the right and left brachiocephalic veins (which join behind the right side of the manubrium to form the superior vena cava), the common carotid arteries (lying immediately anterior to the subclavian arteries and medial to the subclavian veins), the trachea (situated either in the midline or slightly to the right or left immediately behind the great vessels), the esophagus (located behind the trachea and in front of the spine), the recurrent laryngeal nerves on either side of the esophagus, and (sometimes) the upper portion of the thymus.

The spread of disease from the neck into the mediastinum (and *vice versa*) occurs through precise anatomic pathways termed the *cervicothoracic (cervicomediastinal) continuum.*[217] A fascial envelope, the *deep cervical fascia*, surrounds the deep structures of the neck and divides into three layers that define distinct compartments.

1. The posterior layer (*prevertebral fascia*) delineates the prevertebral space and extends from the occipital bone to the thorax, where it becomes continuous with the anterior longitudinal ligament of the spine. Pathologic processes within the prevertebral space of the neck (e.g., an abscess secondary to infectious spondylitis) may extend caudally to the thoracic inlet but usually not below this point because of merging of the prevertebral fascia with the anterior longitudinal ligament.

2. The middle layer (*pretracheal fascia*) lies anterior to the trachea and extends inferiorly from the thyroid gland into the thorax, where it blends with the fascia that surrounds the aorta and pericardium. The pretracheal fascia anteriorly, the prevertebral fascia posteriorly, and the carotid sheaths laterally define the *visceral compartment* of the cervicothoracic continuum; it contains the pharynx, larynx, trachea, and esophagus and is continuous with the mediastinum across the thoracic inlet. Pathologic processes arising in this compartment (e.g., retropharyngeal abscess) can readily spread inferiorly into the mediastinum.

3. At the level of the thyroid gland, the anterior layer of the deep cervical fascia forms the *suprasternal space*, enclosing the submandibular gland, the mastoid process, and the mandible. Infections arising from these structures may enter the suprahyoid space but are generally confined there

by the fascial planes and seldom extend into the mediastinum. However, it is by this route that goiters usually extend from the neck inferiorly to become retrosternal.

Anterior Mediastinal Compartment

The anatomic boundaries and constituents of this compartment were described earlier (*see* page 73). In this section we shall discuss the normal thymus gland and a number of important aspects of roentgenologic anatomy.

The Thymus. The thymus is located in the anterosuperior portion of the mediastinum and extends from a point above the manubrium to the fourth costal cartilage. Posteriorly, it relates to the trachea, left innominate vein, aortic arch and its branches, and the pericardium covering the ascending aorta and main pulmonary artery. On conventional roentgenograms, it is visible only in infants and young children, in whom it fills much of the anterior mediastinal space. Because of this, CT is the commonest technique for imaging the thymus in older individuals. In one extensive CT study of the normal thymus gland of 154 subjects, the following observations were recorded:[218]

1. The gland was recognized in 100 per cent of subjects younger than 30 years of age, in about 75 per cent of subjects between the ages of 30 and 49 years, and in 15 per cent of subjects older than 49 years of age. The maximum thymic size was observed in individuals between 12 and 19 years of age, regression occurring between 20 and 60 years and usually associated with fatty replacement of the parenchyma.

2. About two thirds of normal glands showed an arrowhead configuration, the other third apparently having separate right and left lobes (Fig. 1–62). The shape of the separate lobes was highly variable, being ovoid, elliptic, triangular, or semilunar. The left lobe was almost invariably larger than the right. In about 5 per cent of cases, only a right or left lobe was identified.

3. The CT width (long axis or AP dimension of a lobe) tended to decrease in older patients, although this was not statistically significant. By contrast, the thickness (short axis or transverse dimension of a lobe) displayed a statistically significant decrease between the 6- to 19-year-old and 40- to 49-year-old comparison groups.

4. The CT attenuation values decreased with age: In patients younger than 19 years of age, the gland was isodense, being equal to or higher than the chest wall musculature; in the majority of patients older than 40 years of age, thymic density approached that of fat.

It has been suggested that MRI may permit more accurate assessment of the thymus gland than CT. In one study of the MR characteristics of the normal thymus in 18 patients ranging in age from 5 to 77 years,[219] the thymus was visible in all patients regardless of age and differed from subcutaneous fat in hydrogen density. Although the T_1 relaxation times were much longer than those of fat in patients younger than 30 years of age, this difference decreased with age.

Superior Recesses. As viewed on a PA roentgenogram, the superior recesses are formed by contact of lung with the retromanubrial mediastinum; typically they marginate a V-shaped area, the *anterior mediastinal triangle*, the apex

THE NORMAL CHEST • • • **75**

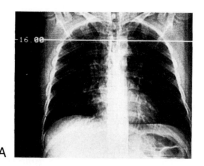

A

List of Anatomic Structures
for Figure 1–61
  1. Manubrium
  2. Left brachiocephalic vein
  3. Right brachiocephalic vein
  4. Calcified lymph node
  5. Innominate artery
  6. Left carotid artery
  7. Trachea
  8. Lymph node
  9. Thoracic duct
  10. Left subclavian artery
  11. Esophagus
  12. Spinal cord

Figure 1–61. Normal Cross-Sectional Anatomy of the Mediastinum at a Level Immediately Cephalad to the Arch of the Aorta. *A,* Scout view indicating level of cut. *B,* CT scan. *C,* Drawing of anatomic structures. Immediately behind the manubrium sterni (1) is the longitudinal shadow of the left brachiocephalic (innominate) vein (2), as it passes from left to right to join the right brachiocephalic vein (3) to form the superior vena cava. Situated in the angle formed by the junction of these two vessels is a tiny, densely calcified lymph node (4). Immediately posterior to and contiguous with the left brachiocephalic vein is the innominate artery to the right (5) and left carotid artery to the left (6). The tracheal air column (7) can be clearly seen immediately posterior to the innominate artery. To the left of the trachea is a collection of mediastinal fat in which are situated a small lymph node (8) and the thoracic duct (9). Also within this fatty tissue posteriorly is the circular image of the left subclavian artery (10). Posterior to the trachea and slightly to the left is the shadow of the esophagus containing a small amount of gas (11). The spinal cord (12) can be readily identified within the spinal canal.

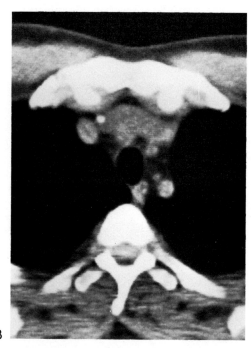

B

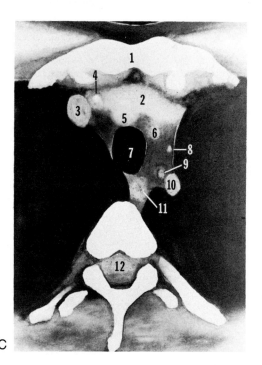

C

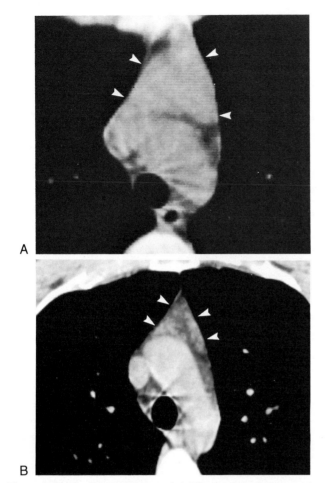

Figure 1–62. The Normal Thymus. *A,* A CT scan through the superior mediastinum of a normal 15-year-old boy reveals a triangular opacity *(arrowheads),* the apex of which points forward while the base abuts the great vessels. CT density is equivalent to that of the chest wall musculature. *B,* A CT scan through the superior mediastinum of an elderly man discloses a thymus *(arrowheads)* composed of isolated nodular opacities and intervening fat (compare the CT density of the gland with the subcutaneous fat).

of which points caudally (Fig. 1–63). Although it has been stated that the right and left boundaries of this triangle are formed by the innominate veins,[112] we tend to agree with Proto and colleagues[214] that each superior recess usually marginates retromanubrial mediastinal fat in front of or contiguous with the innominate veins rather than the veins themselves.

Anterior Junction Line (Anterior Mediastinal Line). As the two lungs approximate anteromedially, they are separated by four layers of pleura and an inconstant quantity of intervening mediastinal adipose tissue, thus forming a septum of variable thickness. As seen on CT, this is a curvilinear opacity that courses vertically from front to back, angling to the right or to the left, and ranging in thickness from 1 mm to more than 3 mm. On a PA chest roentgenogram, the anterior junction line typically is oriented obliquely from upper right to lower left behind the sternum; cephalad, it begins at the apex of the anterior mediastinal triangle and continues caudally for several centimeters before terminating at the apex of the inferior recess. Since the septum dividing the two lungs is variable in

thickness, the resulting opacity may be either a line or a stripe.

Inferior Recess. Inferiorly, the anteromedial portions of the right and left lungs are further separated from each other by the heart and adjacent mediastinal fat; consequently, these lung surfaces in contact with the lower anterior mediastinum form interfaces that marginate an inverted V-shaped area, termed the inferior recess *(see* Fig. 1–63).

Retrosternal Stripe and Cardiac Incisura. On a true lateral roentgenogram of the chest, the relationship between the back of the sternum and the two lungs is normally intimate, creating little or no discernible shadow. However, lung may be excluded from this close contact by mediastinal fat, creating a vertical retrosternal opacity, the *retrosternal stripe* (Fig. 1–64). In one study of 153 normal subjects, its thickness averaged 2.67 mm (±1.38 mm).[220]

On the left side, as the sternum is followed inferiorly, the lung is normally excluded from the anteromedial chest wall by the cardiac apex or the epicardial fat pad or both. This deficiency is termed the *cardiac incisura*; the interface between it and contiguous left lung has a variable appearance, including straight, angular, or rounded *(see* Fig. 1–64). A similar appearance sometimes occurs on the right side as a result of the presence of a fat pad.

Supra-aortic Area

This compartment comprises that portion of the left side of the mediastinum extending from the aortic arch to the thoracic inlet, behind the anterior mediastinum. Structures

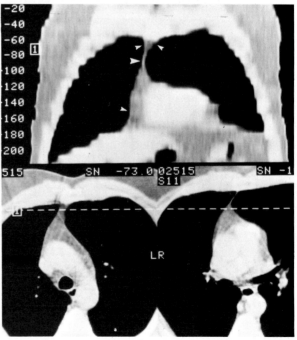

Figure 1–63. Anterior Junction Anatomy. A coronal CT re-formation *(top)* and appropriate transverse images *(bottom)* reveal the superior *(upper arrowheads)* and inferior *(lower arrowhead)* recesses of the anterior junction anatomy. The superior recesses, composed of mediastinal fat, relate closely to the innominate veins. The anterior junction line *(large arrowhead)* separates the superior and inferior recesses.

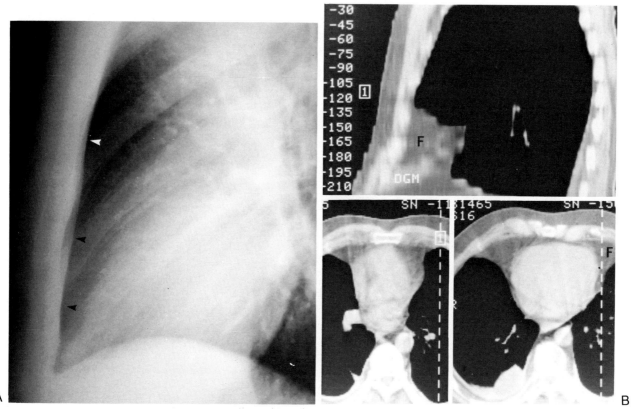

Figure 1–64. Lateral Roentgenographic Anatomy of the Anterior Mediastinum. *A,* A detail view from a lateral chest roentgenogram shows a vertical retrosternal opacity that constitutes the *retrosternal stripe (arrowheads).* This is formed by interposition of fat between the anteromedial portion of the right and left lungs in the anterior mediastinum. *B,* A sagittal CT re-formation slightly to the left of the cardiac apex *(above)* and appropriate transverse images *(below)* show that an opacity frequently identified in the anterior costophrenic sulcus on lateral roentgenograms is formed by paracardiac mediastinal fat (F) contiguous with the cardiac apex. Note that the opacity relates to the epicardial fat pad and not to the cardiac apex. DGM = Diaphragm.

included within it are the left subclavian artery, the left wall of the trachea (visible on PA roentgenograms in about a third of normal subjects[221]), the left superior intercostal vein, and mediastinal fat and lymph nodes. On a lateral roentgenogram of the chest, the area bounded by the posterior wall of the trachea, the top of the aortic arch, and the anterior surface of the thoracic vertebral bodies constitutes the *supra-aortic triangle.*[222]

Left Subclavian Artery. The left subclavian artery arises from the aorta behind the left common carotid artery, passing upward and lateral to the trachea in contact with the left mediastinal pleura. It thus forms an interface with the superomedial left upper lobe that may be identified on a PA roentgenogram as an arcuate opacity (concave laterally) extending from the aortic arch to a point at or just above the medial end of the clavicle *(see* Fig. 1–61). On a lateral chest roentgenogram, the posterior margin of the artery may be identified through the posterior portion of the tracheal air column as a relatively straight opacity coursing obliquely upward toward the neck. The posterior margin of the innominate artery–right subclavian artery complex merges with the posterior wall of the right innominate vein–superior vena cava complex to form a typical sigmoid-shaped interface.

Left Superior Intercostal Vein. Blood from the sec-

ond, third, and fourth intercostal spaces drains into a common vessel, the left superior intercostal vein. In approximately 75 per cent of subjects,[112] this vessel communicates with the accessory hemiazygos vein as it descends along the spine. At T-3 or T-4, the vein arches forward adjacent to the aortic arch to empty into the posterior aspect of the left innominate vein.

In its para-aortic location, the vein can be visualized as the "aortic nipple," a rounded protuberance created by the vein seen end-on as it passes anteriorly adjacent to the aortic knob before entering the left innominate vein. The position of the nipple in relation to the aortic arch may vary from superomedial to inferolateral (Fig. 1–65).[223] The incidence at which it is viewed on PA roentgenograms of erect normal subjects ranges from about 1[224] to 10 per cent.[223]

In normal subjects in the erect position, the vein may attain a diameter of 4.5 mm.[224] As expected, it dilates and becomes more prominent in the supine position and with the Müller maneuver; in fact, it may be seen to best advantage on supine tomography. A variety of disease states that result in increased flow or pressure (or both) within the systemic venous system can cause the vein to dilate, comprising a useful roentgenographic sign analogous to the abnormal distention of the azygos vein in the presence of systemic venous hypertension.

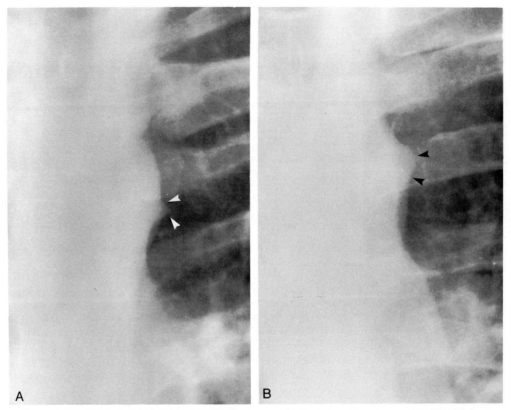

Figure 1–65. The Left Superior Intercostal Vein. *A* and *B*, Detail views from conventional PA chest roentgenograms of two normal adult patients show variations of the "aortic nipple" *(arrowheads)* representing the left superior intercostal vein as it passes anteriorly adjacent to the aortic knob; note that its position may vary from superomedial to inferolateral. In the upright position, the vein appears as a small protuberance along the lateral contour of the aortic arch.

Infra-aortic Area

This compartment of the left side of the mediastinum extends from the aortic arch above to the diaphragm below and from the anterior mediastinal space in front to the paravertebral region behind. The border of the mediastinum cephalad from the diaphragm includes the left ventricle, the left atrial appendage (seldom if ever identifiable as a separate opacity in normal subjects), the left border of the main pulmonary artery, the pleural reflection from the aorta downward onto the main pulmonary artery, and the aortic knob. The general characteristics of the cardiac silhouette are described later. In this section we describe the paraspinal lines and the inferior reflections of pleura off the aortic knob.

Aortopulmonary Window. This consists of the space between the arch of the aorta and the left pulmonary artery; its lateral boundary is the mediastinal pleura and visceral pleura over the left lung, thus creating the aortopulmonary window interface. Within this space are situated fat, the ligament of the ductus arteriosus, the left recurrent laryngeal nerve, and lymph nodes.

Computed tomographic correlation indicates that the interface is formed largely by mediastinal fat residing in front and to the left of the transverse portion of the aortic arch, anterolateral to the left pulmonary artery (Fig. 1–66). Displacement of this interface laterally, particularly as revealed by sequential roentgenograms, should suggest the possibil-

ity of mediastinal pathology, especially lymph node enlargement.

Posterior Pleural Reflections. The right and left paraspinal lines are each about 1 mm wide and appear as linear opacities on an AP thoracic spine film or conventional tomogram.[225] The left line extends from the top or middle of the aortic arch to the level of the ninth to twelfth thoracic vertebrae, depending on the degree of lung inflation (Fig. 1–67). It tends to parallel the lateral margin of the vertebral bodies and may lie anywhere medial to the interface formed by the lung and the descending aorta, although commonly its position is midway between the spine and the aorta. The lateral relationship of the descending aorta to the left paraspinal line exists throughout most of its course, although as the aorta declines toward the midline inferiorly it tends to overlap the paraspinal line. When the aorta elongates as a result of hypertension or atherosclerosis, its left margin is displaced laterally. As a consequence, the left paraspinal line also is displaced to the left, maintaining a relationship roughly halfway between the lateral margin of the aorta and the thoracic spine (Fig. 1–68).

The right paraspinal line is seen less often than the left and usually extends for only two or four vertebral segments at the T-8 to T-12 level before it merges below with the right crus of the diaphragm. Normally, the right line lies within a few millimeters of the vertebrae, reflecting the lesser quantity of paravertebral fat on the right side.

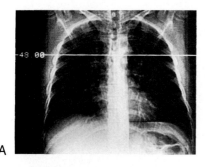

A

List of Anatomic Structures
for Figure 1–66
1. Anterior mediastinal fat
2. Ascending aorta
3. Superior vena cava
4. Trachea
5. Fat in aortopulmonary window
6. Lymph nodes
7. Descending aorta
8. Esophagus
9. Azygos vein

Figure 1–66. Normal Cross-Sectional Anatomy of the Mediastinum at a Level Immediately Caudad to the Arch of the Aorta. *A,* Scout view indicating level of cut. *B,* CT scan. *C,* Drawing of anatomic structures. Immediately posterior to the sternum is a roughly triangular opacity of low attenuation (1) representing an accumulation of fat in the anterior mediastinal septum between the right and left lungs. Posterior to this fatty accumulation is the circular shadow of the ascending aorta (2), to the right of which is the superior vena cava (3). The tracheal air column (4) is readily identified in the midline posterior to the ascending aorta. To the left of the trachea is a rather indistinct zone of relatively low attenuation that represents the upper level of the aortopulmonary window (5); two small lymph nodes (6) can be seen in the lateral portion of the window. The descending aorta (7) relates to the window posteriorly. The shadow of the esophagus (8) is situated directly behind the trachea and close to the right lateral wall of the descending aorta. On the right posterolateral aspect of the trachea is the shadow of the posterior portion of the azygos vein (9) as it begins its horizontal course from the spine toward the superior vena cava.

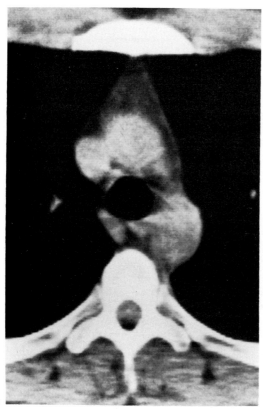

B

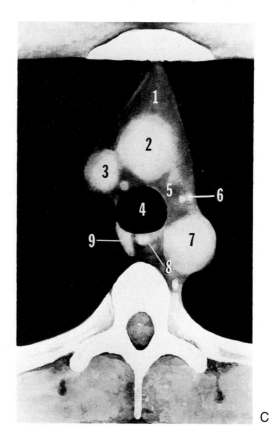

C

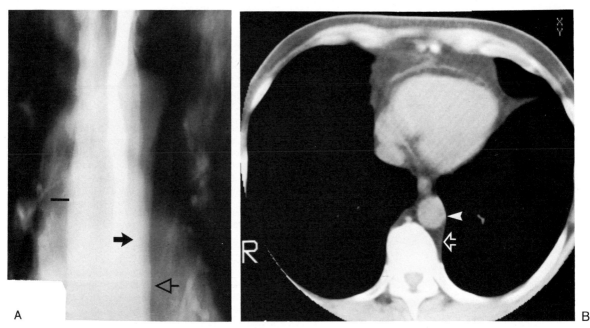

Figure 1–67. The Posterior Pleural Reflections. *A,* On this AP tomogram of the thorax with barium in the esophagus, the left paraspinal line *(black arrow)* and the aortic interface *(open arrow)* are shown; the paraspinal line is depicted as a white line whereas the aortic interface is enhanced by a black line. These lines are Mach bands that are related to the shape of the lung-mediastinal interface rather than to the composition of tissue interposed between the lung and mediastinum. *B,* A transverse CT scan through the posterior mediastinum at the level of the bar depicted in *A* shows that the paraspinal line *(arrow)* relates to the concave interface between the lung and posterior mediastinum behind the aorta; by contrast, the aortic line is caused by the convex shape of the descending aorta *(arrowhead)* as it abuts the lung.

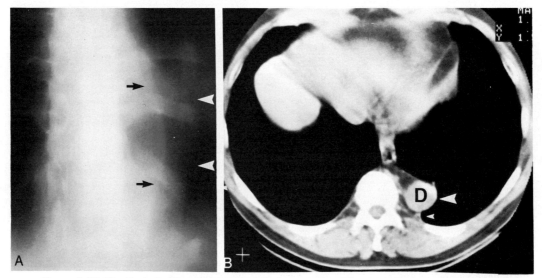

Figure 1–68. The Posterior Pleural Reflections. *A,* A conventional linear tomogram in AP projection through the posterior mediastinum shows the left paraspinal line *(arrows)* to be displaced laterally, closely paralleling the course of the elongated descending aorta *(arrowheads).* *B,* An unenhanced transverse CT scan through the lower thorax reveals posterior and lateral displacement of the descending aorta *(D);* the quantity of fat medial to the aorta is increased. The concave interface between lung and mediastinum behind the aorta *(small arrowhead)* is situated medial to the outer edge of the convex descending aorta *(arrowhead),* creating a concave interface with the lung, thereby accounting for the positive Mach band. (From Genereux GP: The posterior pleural reflections. AJR 141: 141, 1983. © American Roentgen Ray Society.)

A variety of arguments[225] suggest that the paraspinal lines are Mach bands or edge-enhancing phenomena created by the retina in response to strong differences in transmitted illumination.

Supra-azygos Area

The supra-azygos area is that portion of the right side of the mediastinum that extends cephalad from the azygos arch to the thoracic inlet; it is separated from the infra-azygos area by the azygos vein and arch.

The *azygos vein* originates in the upper lumbar region at the level of the renal veins and ascends through the aortic hiatus medial to the right crus of the diaphragm. In the thorax, it pursues a somewhat variable course and may be situated in front, to the right, or, rarely, to the left of the lower eight thoracic vertebrae (Fig. 1–69); it is joined at the T-8 or T-9 level by the hemiazygos vein ascending on the left. At the T-4 or T-5 level, it arches anteriorly and slightly inferiorly and relates intimately to the lateral wall of the esophagus and the right posterior surface of the trachea. It then turns laterally for a short distance before proceeding anteriorly once again, passing over the right main bronchus and truncus anterior and lateral to the right inferior tracheal wall; it finally inserts into the back of the superior vena cava (*see* Fig. 1–69). Along its course, the vein receives tributaries from the fifth to eleventh intercostal veins on the right, the right subcostal vein, the right superior intercostal vein, the right bronchial veins, and the superior and inferior hemiazygos veins.

The *superior hemiazygos vein* begins at the vertebral end of the fourth left intercostal space as the continuation of the fourth posterior intercostal vein; the upper part is often connected to the left superior intercostal vein. It courses downward and forward in relation to T-4 and then descends in close relationship to the left side of the descending aorta as far as the eighth thoracic vertebra. It then bends abruptly to the right and crosses behind the aorta to terminate in the azygos vein.

The *inferior hemiazygos vein* originates from the posterior aspect of the left renal vein or as a continuation of the left subcostal vein or left ascending lumbar vein. It enters the thorax medial to the left crus of the diaphragm and behind the descending aorta and ascends anterolateral to the vertebral column; at the level of T-8 or T-9, it turns abruptly to the right and joins the azygos vein.

Tracheal Interfaces. The trachea normally is bordered on its right lateral aspect and to a variable extent on its anterior and posterior aspects by pleura covering the right upper lobe. This creates a thin stripe of water density, designated the *right tracheal stripe* (Fig. 1–70), that has been identified in two thirds[194] to almost 95 per cent[226] of PA roentgenograms. The thickness of the stripe must be measured above the level of the azygos vein; in one study, the maximum width was 4 mm.[226] An increase in width on serial films is a more important sign of disease than is an enlarged stripe seen on a single examination, since the latter observation may be related simply to an increased amount of paratracheal fat.

A vertically oriented opacity formed by the posterior wall

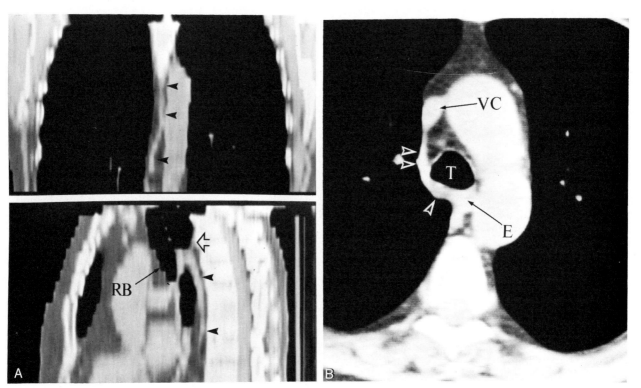

Figure 1–69. The Supra-azygos Area. *A,* Coronal *(top)* and sagittal *(bottom)* CT re-formations demonstrate the course of the azygos vein *(arrowheads).* The azygos arch receives the right superior intercostal vein *(arrow)* and turns forward slightly above the plane of the right upper lobe bronchus (RB). *B,* A CT scan identifies the transverse course of the axygos vein. Note that as it passes forward from its posterior location, it relates, in order, to the esophagus (E), the right posterior tracheal wall (T) *(arrowhead),* and the right upper lobe bronchus *(double arrowheads).* VC = superior vena cava.

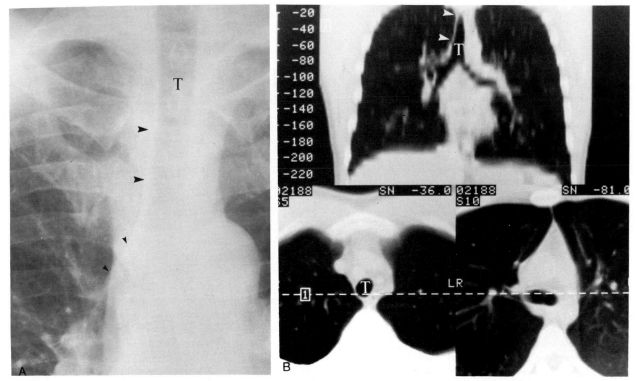

Figure 1–70. The Right Tracheal Stripe. A, A detail view from a PA chest roentgenogram shows a vertically oriented 2-mm linear opacity *(large arrowheads)* that parallels the tracheal air column (T) and is designated the *right tracheal stripe*. The ovoid opacity in the right tracheobronchial angle *(small arrowheads)* represents the third portion of the azygos arch as it passes over the right main and upper lobe bronchi. B, A coronal CT re-formation *(top)* and transverse images *(bottom)* through the middle and lower trachea (T) show minimal areolar tissue between the tracheal wall and the lung *(arrowheads)*; thus, the linear opacity identified in A is caused primarily by the width of the tracheal wall.

of the trachea in contact with right upper lobe parenchyma that inserts into the retrotracheal space may be identified in about 50 per cent of individuals.[227] On well-exposed lateral roentgenograms, it is frequently seen for the entire length of visible trachea and is often continuous inferiorly with the line or stripe formed by the posterior walls of the right main and intermediate bronchi (Fig. 1–71). It has been suggested that this stripe is a manifestation of either the posterior wall of the trachea plus retrotracheal soft tissue or the posterior tracheal wall plus the esophagus[227]; thus, the soft tissue stripe behind the tracheal air column should be considered as either a *posterior tracheal stripe* or a *tracheoesophageal stripe* (Fig. 1–72). The only certain way of distinguishing the two is by CT. However, the tracheoesophageal stripe may be identified as such if a thin vertical radiolucency of fat separates the soft tissue stripe of the trachea from the esophagus, or if the stripe courses through the level of the azygos arch.

As a consequence of the variability in the amount of retrotracheal soft tissue, the position of the esophagus, and the amount of gas within the esophageal lumen, the tracheoesophageal stripe ranges in thickness from 1 to 5.5 mm (mean, 2 mm).[227] The upper limits of normal width for the posterior tracheal stripe are 2 to 3 mm.[228] There is general agreement that a posterior tracheal stripe or tracheoesophageal stripe that measures more than 5 mm in width should be considered abnormal, most commonly as a manifestation of esophageal carcinoma. It is important to remember,

however, that this measurement refers to stripes that can be visualized on plain roentgenograms. In a CT study of 100 normal subjects in which the trachea and its surrounding tissues were studied at the level of the sternal notch and 2 cm caudad, the average thickness of the stripe was found to be 8.4 mm (±3.8 mm), whereas at a CT level 2 cm below the sternal notch the posterolateral tracheal stripe had an average thickness of 6.4 mm (±1.8 mm).[229]

Posterior Junction Anatomy. The apices of the right and left upper lobes contact the mediastinum behind the esophagus anterior to the first and second vertebral bodies. In so doing, they create a V-shaped triangular opacity that constitutes the *posterior mediastinal triangle*; marginating this triangular configuration are the *right* and *left superior recesses* (Fig. 1–73). Caudally, the lungs intrude deeper into a prespinal location posterior to the esophagus and anterior to the third through fifth vertebral bodies, where they form a pleural apposition that, along with any intervening mediastinal tissue, forms the *posterior junction line* (see Fig. 1–73). On a PA roentgenogram, the posterior junction line usually projects through the air column of the trachea; it may be straight or slightly concave to the right. When intervening mediastinal tissue is abundant or a narrowed retroesophageal space precludes lung apposition, the posterior junction line may appear as a distinct stripe.

Below the posterior junction line, the lungs are excluded from the midline by the forward arching of the right and left superior intercostal veins and by the posterior portion

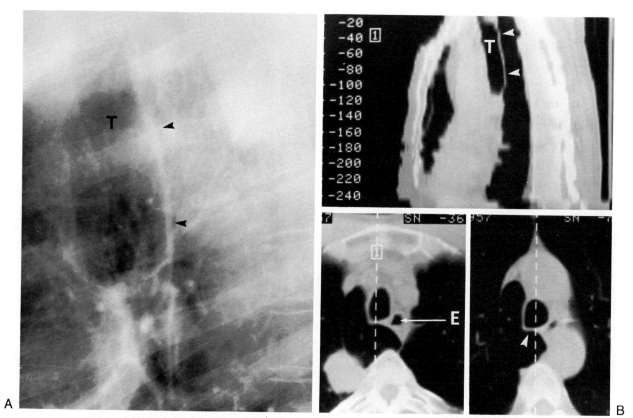

Figure 1–71. The Posterior Tracheal Stripe. *A,* A conventional lateral chest roentgenogram demonstrates a 4-mm wide stripe *(arrowheads)* that parallels the air column of the trachea (T), the *posterior tracheal stripe. B,* A sagittal CT re-formation *(top)* and transverse images *(bottom)* through the trachea (T) at the level of the aortic arch show that the stripe is caused by the posterior wall of the trachea itself *(arrowheads).* Note that in this patient, the esophagus (E) is not contour forming in lateral projection and thus does not contribute to the stripe. Compare with Figure 1–72.

of the azygos arch on the right and the aortic arch on the left. This divergence defines an inverted **V**-shaped opacity that, analogous to the situation superiorly, is marginated by the *right* and *left inferior recesses.* The right inferior recess is usually longer and extends more caudad than the left, reflecting the more caudal location of the azygos arch than the aortic arch.

Right and Left Superior Esophageal Stripes. Air can be identified in the esophagus on the PA roentgenogram of the chest in about one third of normal subjects.[230] When air is present in the upper esophagus, a vertically oriented soft tissue stripe (the *esophageal stripe)* may be identifiable on the right side, left side, or both, provided that the inner and outer margins of both esophageal walls are tangential to the x-ray beam. The commonest site is adjacent to the aortic arch and, in decreasing order of frequency, includes that portion of the esophagus immediately below, above, and medial to the arch (Fig. 1–74).

Azygos Arch. At the level of the aortic arch, the azygos vein is composed of three parts. On AP tomograms, the *posterior* (paraesophageal) *part* is abutted by right upper or lower lobe parenchyma laterally and the esophagus medially. The posterior turn of the azygos vein merges above with that of the right inferior recess and below with the pleura in the cephalad portion of the azygoesophageal recess. The *middle* (retrotracheal) *component* is seen through

the air column of the trachea as an opacity that is angled slightly downward and to the right; it merges laterally with the oval or elliptic shadow of the *anterior component* viewed end-on as it passes forward in the tracheobronchial angle. Depending on the distention of the vessel and the depth of the supra-azygos and infra-azygos recesses, the vein may be identified on a lateral chest roentgenogram or conventional lateral tomogram as a retrotracheal elongated opacity as it passes forward over the right main bronchus (Fig. 1–75). This appearance should not be mistaken for a mass, such as enlarged lymph nodes.

Mensuration of the anterior portion of the azygos vein is important in some diseases, notably portal hypertension, obstruction of the superior vena cava, and systemic venous hypertension. The only point that can be measured accurately on conventional roentgenograms is that in the right tracheobronchial angle as the vein enters the superior vena cava and is viewed roughly tangentially; in this location, it often is visible as a slightly flattened elliptic opacity (Fig. 1–76).

Although there is some dispute, it is reasonable to accept the upper limit of the normal azygos vein diameter in subjects in the erect position as 7 mm or less. A diameter of 7 to 10 mm is seen sometimes in healthy individuals; however, a diameter exceeding 10 mm should be regarded as pathologic, except in pregnant women in whom a maximum

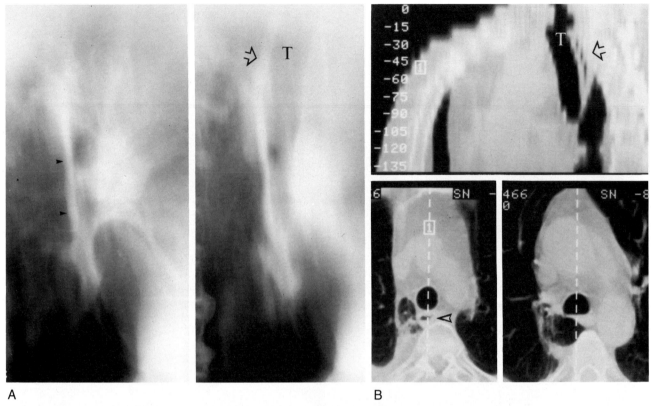

Figure 1–72. The Tracheoesophageal Stripe. *A,* Detail views from conventional linear tomograms in lateral projection disclose a stripe 5 mm in width that extends along the entire length of the tracheal air column (T) *(arrow)* and intermediate stem line *(arrowheads). B,* A sagittal CT re-formation *(top)* and transverse images *(bottom)* show that the linear opacity identified in *A* is caused by a combination of the posterior tracheal wall, mediastinal soft tissue, and gas-containing esophagus *(arrowhead),* thus constituting the *tracheoesophageal stripe (arrow).*

diameter of 15 mm is tolerable (presumably because of hypervolemia).[231] It is important to remember that vascular distention caused by change in body position from erect to recumbent increases the vein's diameter. In one tomographic study of 40 healthy subjects in the supine position, standardization of the maximum diameters to a body weight of 64 kg yielded a mean azygos vein diameter of 14.2 mm; the diameter exceeded 16 mm in only eight subjects.[232] It seems reasonable to employ these figures to indicate normality or otherwise in patients whose roentgenograms must be obtained in a supine position at the bedside.

Vascular Pedicle. A large portion of the mediastinal opacity is caused by the great systemic vessels (*the vascular pedicle*), from which the heart may be considered to "hang."[233] On a frontal chest roentgenogram, the pedicle extends from the thoracic inlet to the top of the heart. On the right, its boundary is formed by the right innominate vein above and the superior vena cava below. The left border of the pedicle is formed by the left subclavian artery above the aortic arch. In essence, the right side of the pedicle is situated anteriorly and is entirely venous, whereas the left side lies more posteriorly and is arterial (Fig. 1–77). The width of the vascular pedicle on PA (or AP) chest roentgenograms (measured from the point at which the superior vena cava crosses the right main bronchus to the point at which the left subclavian artery arises from the aortic arch) is 48 mm (±5 mm).[233]

In two studies investigating the relationship between the

width of the vascular pedicle and total blood volume,[234, 235] vascular pedicle width in patients with dilated neck veins was found to be greater than 62 mm; pedicle width correlated strongly with a change in total blood volume (0.5 cm change in width corresponding to a 1 L change in blood volume). By contrast, the correlation between the azygos vein width and total blood volume was poor, although that between vein width and mean right atrial pressure was stronger.

Infra-azygos Area

Azygoesophageal Recess. As previously described, the azygos vein ascends in the posterior mediastinum in relation to the right side or front of the vertebral column. The esophagus is usually located slightly anterior and to the left of the vein in the prevertebral region, although they are sometimes in contact. Between the esophagus and the azygos vein is a small space into which the right lower lobe parenchyma may intrude to a variable degree. Termed the *azygoesophageal recess,*[236] this space is highly variable in depth, depending largely on the degree of lung inflation and the position of the descending aorta. The recess slopes obliquely from above downward so that the superior component is located posterior to the inferior; consequently, in some subjects the anterior aspect of the azygoesophageal recess may be divided by the right inferior pulmonary vein into well-defined superior and inferior divisions.

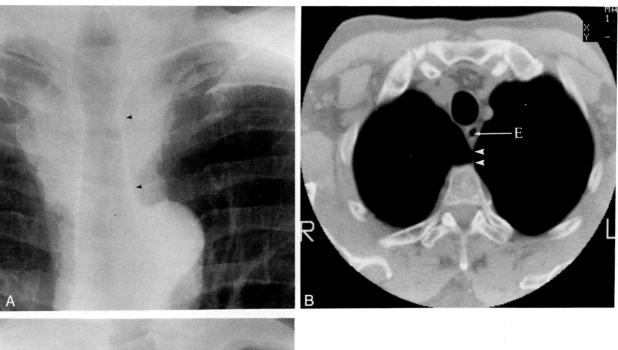

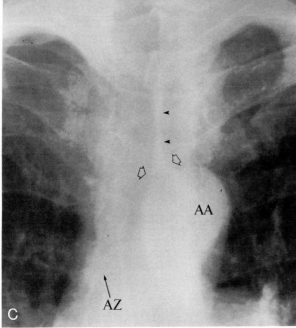

Figure 1–73. Posterior Junction Anatomy. *A,* A detail view of the superior mediastinum from a conventional PA chest roentgenogram demonstrates a thin linear opacity called the *posterior junction line (arrowheads).* It courses obliquely from above downward, slightly to the left of the midline, and relates to thoracic vertebrae 3 to 5. *B,* On a transverse CT scan through the posterior mediastinum above the aortic arch, the right and left upper lobes can be seen to be almost contiguous with each other behind the esophagus (E), separated only by a small amount of mediastinal soft tissue and four layers of pleura *(arrowheads). C,* In a different patient, a detail view from a PA chest roentgenogram demonstrates a somewhat thicker posterior junction line *(arrowheads),* which terminates inferiorly in a triangular opacity whose apex points cephalad and whose base abuts the aortic arch (AA). The right and left interfacers *(arrows)* are designated the *right* and *left inferior recesses.* The right recess extends caudally to cover the azygos arch (AZ), whereas the shorter left recess terminates on the medial aspect of the aortic arch.

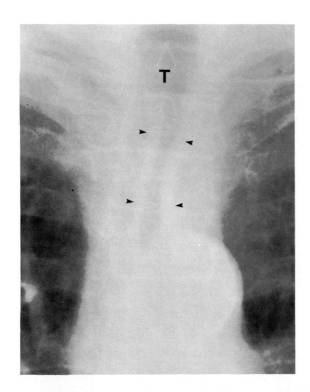

Figure 1–74. The Superior Esophageal Stripes. A detail view from a conventional PA chest roentgenogram shows two vertical stripes *(arrowheads)* projected through the tracheal air column (T). The linear opacities represent the right and left walls of the gas-distended esophagus, designated the *right* and *left superior esophagopleural* or *esophageal stripes.*

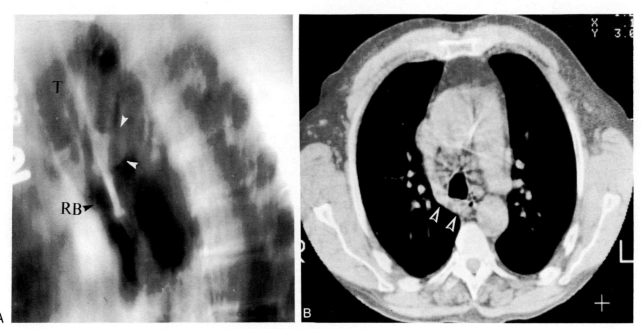

Figure 1–75. The Azygos Vein: Retrotracheal Component. *A,* Conventional lateral tomogram through the trachea (T) reveals a rounded opacity *(arrowheads)* above the right upper lobe bronchus (RB), representing the retrotracheal component of the azygos arch. Its location and shape serve to differentiate it from enlarged lymph nodes. *B,* A CT scan at the level of the azygos arch demonstrates the retrotracheal component *(arrowheads)* abutted by aerated right upper lobe, accounting for the visibility of the vein in this location.

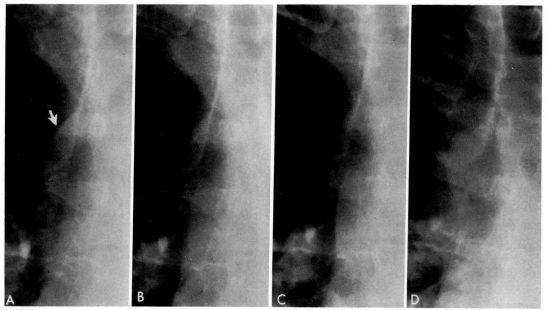

Figure 1–76. Physiologic Variations in Azygos Vein Diameter. Detail views of the region of the right tracheobronchial angle from four PA roentgenograms of a healthy 30-year-old man showing the variations in size of the azygos vein caused by changes in intrathoracic pressure. *A,* At full inspiration with sustained Müller maneuver, vein diameter 13 mm *(arrow); B,* at full inspiration, maintained with glottis open, vein diameter 7 mm; *C,* at full inspiration with sustained Valsalva maneuver, vein diameter 3 mm; *D,* at full expiration with sustained Müller maneuver, vein diameter 17 mm.

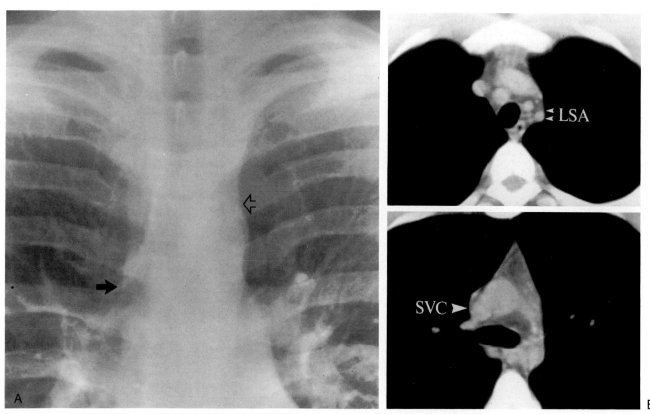

Figure 1–77. The Normal Vascular Pedicle. *A,* A detail view from a conventional PA roentgenogram demonstrates the points for measuring the width of the vascular pedicle (VP). The right (venous) border of the VP is the point at which the superior vena cava crosses the right main bronchus *(closed arrow),* whereas the left border is the point of takeoff of the left subclavian artery from the aorta *(open arrow).* The VP is measured from the superior vena cava to a perpendicular line extended caudally from the left subclavian artery. *B,* A CT scan through the superior mediastinum at the level of the superior vena cava (SVC) *(single arrowhead)* and left subclavian artery (LSA) *(arrowheads)* show that the right border is entirely venous and the left border entirely arterial.

The azygoesophageal recess is frequently identified on well-penetrated PA roentgenograms as an interface that extends from the diaphragm below to the level of the azygos arch above (Fig. 1–78). Its right side is sharply delineated by aerated right lower lobe parenchyma, but its left side is usually of unit density because of contiguity of the azygos vein, esophagus, aorta, and surrounding posterior mediastinal connective tissue. Viewed from above downward on a frontal chest roentgenogram, the configuration of the azygoesophageal recess interface is variable: typically, it presents as a continuous shallow or deep arc concave to the right (Fig. 1–79). Concavity of the superior aspect of the azygoesophageal recess interface is the rule, and any deviation should raise the suspicion of pathology. However, in young adults, a straight or slightly dextroconvex interface may be a normal CT variant.[237]

Esophagopleural Stripe. If gas is present in a distended esophagus, the combined thickness of the right esophageal wall and contiguous pleura may create a vertically oriented linear opacity or stripe known as the *right inferior esophagopleural stripe* (Fig. 1–80). Although there is a potential for the left lung to abut the left wall of the esophagus, it is normally excluded by paraesophageal fat and the descending aorta; when intruding lung does make contact with the gas-distended esophagus, a *left inferior esophagopleural stripe* may be formed.

The Heart

It is beyond the scope of this book to discuss the roentgenology of the heart in detail. However, it is important to recognize that certain deviations in the normal roentgenologic anatomy of the cardiovascular silhouette may give rise to confusion in the interpretation of pulmonary, pleural, or mediastinal disease. In a frontal roentgenogram of the normal chest, the position of the heart in relation to the midline of the thorax depends largely on the patient's build. Assuming roentgenographic exposure with lungs fully inflated, in asthenic patients the heart shadow is almost exactly midline in position, projecting only slightly more to the left; in those of stockier build it lies a little more to the left of midline.

In normal subjects, the transverse diameter of the heart measured on standard roentgenograms is usually in the range of 11.5 to 15.5 cm; it is less than 11.5 cm in approximately 5 per cent and only rarely exceeds 15.5 cm (in very heavy subjects of stocky build, often manual laborers). The custom of trying to assess cardiac size by relating it to the transverse diameter of the chest—i.e., cardiothoracic ratio—is inaccurate. Although 50 per cent is widely accepted as the upper limit of normal for this ratio, in fact it exceeds 50 per cent in at least 10 per cent of normal subjects.[114] Use of this ratio is especially fallacious in patients who have a small heart; in a person with an 8-cm transverse cardiac diameter in a 24-cm thorax, the heart would have to enlarge 4 cm before the cardiothoracic ratio reached the mythic 50 per cent. In our view, it is preferable to evaluate cardiac size subjectively on the basis of experience; alternatively, it is reasonable to assume that a heart whose transverse diameter exceeds 16 cm is enlarged until proved otherwise.

Chiefly as a result of the influence of systole and diastole, both the size and the contour of the heart may vary from one examination to another, even when all examinations are made with an identical degree of lung inflation. In one study of 324 patients for whom PA roentgenograms were obtained in both systole and diastole,[238] the change in transverse cardiac diameter was 0.3 cm or less in 52 per cent, 0.4 to 0.9 cm in 41 per cent, and 1.0 to 1.7 cm in 7 per cent.

Echocardiography has now assumed a major role in the investigation of cardiac abnormalities, and it is likely that MR imaging will play an equally important part in future years (Figs. 1–81 and 1–82).

CONTROL OF BREATHING

The respiratory control system may be divided into four components (Fig. 1–83): (1) afferent inputs to a central respiratory controller; (2) the controller and its central integration; (3) outputs from the respiratory center; and (4) the effectors of the output, the respiratory muscles.

Inputs

There are three major sources of input to the central regulator of respiration: (1) the peripheral and central chemoreceptors, which respond to alterations in arterial Po_2, Pco_2, and hydrogen ion concentration; (2) receptors in the respiratory tract and lungs, which are influenced by lung mechanics; and (3) muscle spindles and tendon organs in the respiratory muscles, which monitor the effectiveness of contraction of the peripheral effector system.

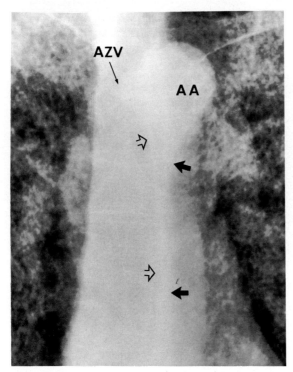

Figure 1–78. The Infra-azygous Area. In a detail view from a conventional PA chest roentgenogram of a middle-aged man with miliary tuberculosis, the concave, deep azygoesophageal recess *(open arrows)* and the straight preaortic recess *(closed arrows)* are shown. The cephalad portion of these two recesses is the azygos arch (AZV) and the aortic arch (AA), respectively.

Text continued on page 94

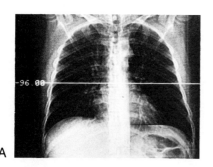

A

List of Anatomic Structures
for Figure 1–79
1. Anterior junction line
2. Right intermediate bronchus
3. Azygos vein
4. Aorta
5. Left upper lobe bronchus
6. Right interlobar artery
7. Left interlobar artery

Figure 1–79. Two Representative CT Scans of the Thorax at Lung Window Settings to Illustrate the Anterior Junction Line, the Azygoesophageal Recess, the Major Hilar Pulmonary Structures, and the Pulmonary Veins. In *A, B,* and *C,* the scan is through the midportion of both hila. Note the slight inclination of the anterior junction line (1) from right to left. The azygoesophageal recess is clearly depicted *(arrows in C),* its anterior boundary being formed by the thin posterior wall of the right intermediate bronchus (2). The small bump on the medial aspect of the azygoesophageal recess represents the azygos vein (3). Seen only in profile is the shadow of the descending thoracic aorta (4). The longitudinal air column in the left hilum is the left upper lobe bronchus (5). The right interlobar artery (6) is directly lateral to the right intermediate bronchus, whereas the left interlobar artery (7) relates to the posterolateral aspect of the left upper lobe bronchus.

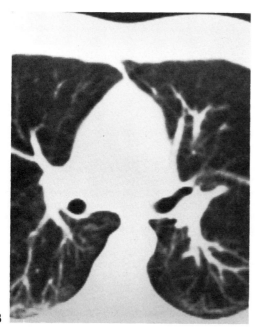

B

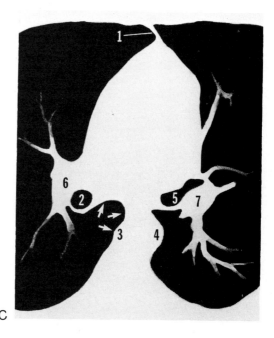

C

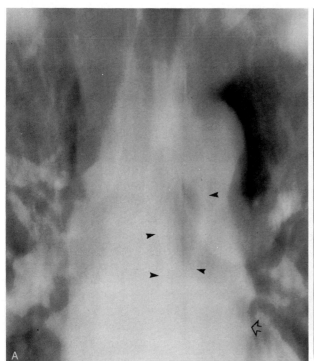

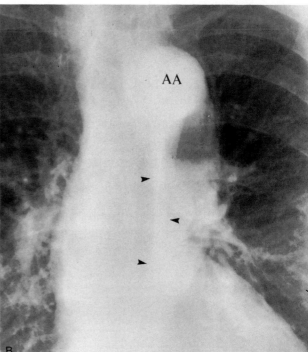

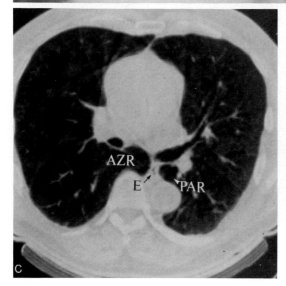

Figure 1–80. The Inferior Esophagopleural Stripes. *A,* An AP linear tomogram through the carina reveals two curvilinear opacities *(arrowheads)* that extend from the infra-aortic region caudally. The opacities converge distally at the level of the left ventricle. Moderate unfolding of the thoracic aorta is present *(arrow)*. The linear opacities represent the right and left wall of the gas-distended esophagus. *B,* A detail view from a PA chest roentgenogram discloses a single thick stripe *(arrowheads)* that extends caudally from the aortic arch (AA). The stripe represents the nondistended esophagus behind the heart, abutted by right and left lower lobe parenchyma in the azygoesophageal and preaortic recesses, respectively. *C,* A transverse CT scan through the carina shows the deep intrusion of the right lower lobe across the midline into the azygoesophageal recess (AZR). On the left, the lower lobe has expanded into the preaortic recess (PAR) behind the left main bronchus and in front of the descending aorta. The two lungs are separated by the septum created by the esophagus (E), mediastinal areolar tissue, and four layers of pleura.

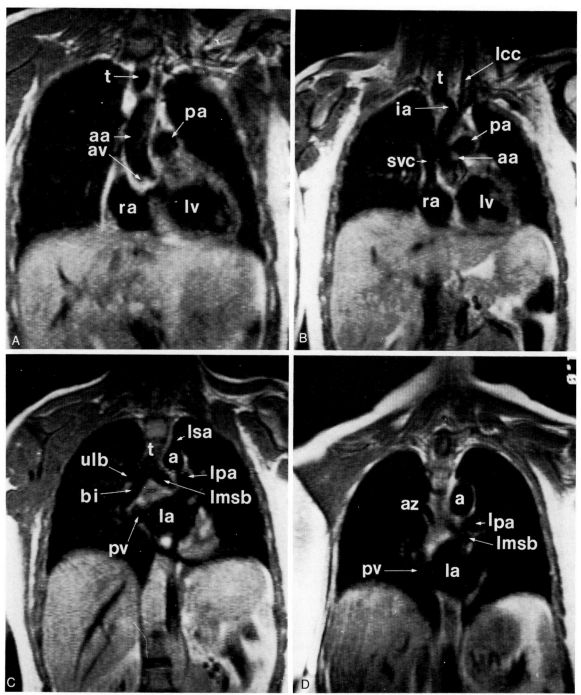

Figure 1–81. Anatomy of the Mediastinum and Hila on Coronal Magnetic Resonance Images. Normal coronal SE 1000/30 scans from anterior *(A)* to posterior *(D)*. *a,* Aorta; *aa,* ascending aorta; *t,* trachea; *av,* aortic valves; *pa,* pulmonary artery; *ra,* right atrium; *lv,* left ventricle; *svc,* superior vena cava; *ta,* truncus anterior; *rpa,* right pulmonary artery; *lpa,* left pulmonary artery; *la,* left atrium; *ivc,* inferior vena cava; *lsa,* left subclavian artery; *ulb,* upper lobe bronchus; *bi,* intermediate bronchi; *lpv,* left pulmonary vein; *lmsb,* left main bronchus; *az,* azygos vein; *ia,* innominate artery; *lcc,* left common carotid artery. (From O'Donovan PB, Ross JS, Sivak SD: Magnetic resonance imaging of the thorax: The advantages of coronal and sagittal planes. AJR 143: 1183, 1984. © American Roentgen Ray Society.)

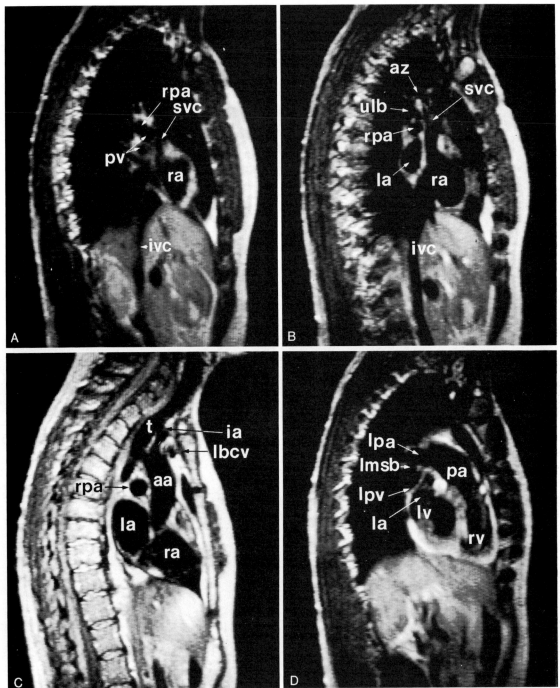

Figure 1–82. Anatomy of the Mediastinum and Hila on Sagittal Magnetic Resonance Images. Normal sagittal SE 1000/30 scans of the hila and mediastinum from right *(A)* to left *(D)*. *aa,* Ascending aorta; *t,* trachea; *pa,* pulmonary artery; *ra,* right atrium; *lv,* left ventricle; *svc,* superior vena cava; *lpa,* left pulmonary artery; *la,* left atrium; *ivc,* inferior vena cava; *ulb,* upper lobe bronchus; *lmsb,* left main bronchus; *az,* azygos vein; *rpa,* right pulmonary artery; *rv,* right ventricle; *lbcv,* left brachiocephalic vein; *lpv,* left pulmonary vein. (See Figure 1–81 for appropriate anatomic designations.) (From O'Donovan PB, Ross JS, Sivak SD, et al: Magnetic resonance imaging of the thorax: The advantages of coronal and sagittal planes. AJR 143: 1183, 1984. © American Roentgen Ray Society.)

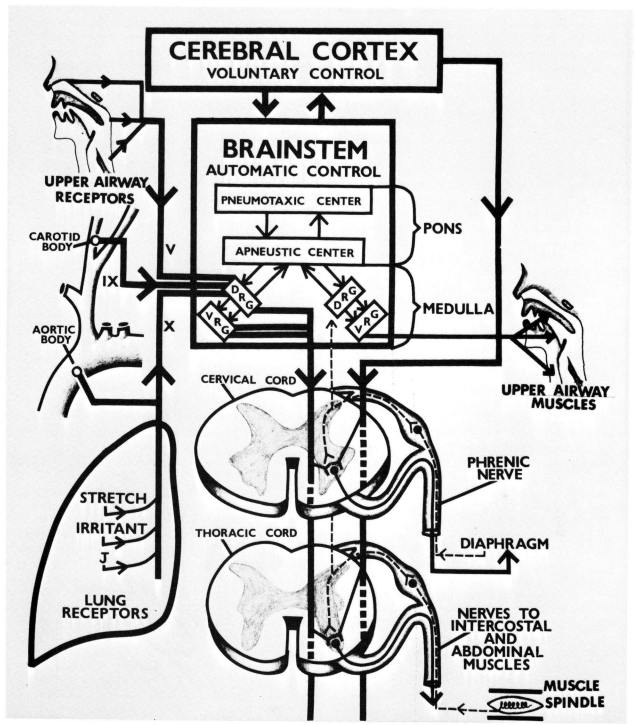

Figure 1–83. The Respiratory Control System. The central respiratory control is shared by voluntary (cerebral) and automatic (brainstem) centers. The efferent fibers for each run in distinct spinal cord pathways, as depicted on the left side of the coronally sectioned spinal cord (*right side* of drawing). A variety of interconnections exist between the cortex and the different components of the brainstem. Afferent fibers ascending the fifth (V), ninth (IX), and tenth (X) cranial nerves from upper airway receptors, peripheral chemoreceptors, and lung receptors connect with the ipsilateral dorsal respiratory group of neurons (DRG). In addition, afferents from Golgi tendon organs in the diaphragm and intercostal muscle spindles travel in the phrenic and intercostal nerves and reach the anterior horn cells as well as ascending to the DRG via the dorsal columns. Respiratory neurons in the DRG are connected with those in the ventral respiratory group (VRG) from which the descending neural output originates. The efferent fibers cross in the brainstem and supply the upper airway muscles via cranial nerves as well as descending in the cord to supply the diaphragm, intercostal, accessory, and expiratory muscles.

Peripheral Chemoreceptors. The carotid body is the major peripheral chemoreceptor.[239] It is composed in part of glomus cells that contain abundant dopamine. Since hypoxia increases dopamine release and synthesis by these cells, it is probable that they act as the chemoreceptive transducers, stimulating postsynaptic afferent nerve endings contained within the carotid body. The organ has an enormous blood supply, receiving as much as 2 L per minute per 100 g of tissue (more than 40 times the flow per gram to the brain); this results in a virtually unchanged PO_2 as the blood passes through the chemoreceptor tissue.

Afferent fibers from the carotid body travel in the glossopharyngeal nerve. Their output is increased not only by hypoxia but also by hypercapnia and changes in pH. The hypoxic and hypercapnic responses are additive, so that both stimuli together result in enhanced response. In addition, enhanced stimulation appears to accompany rapid swings in arterial PO_2 and PCO_2, suggesting that the rate of change of arterial blood gas tension is as important a stimulus as the average level.[240]

In the absence of the peripheral chemoreceptors, hypoxic ventilatory response is abolished, and, in fact, hypoxemia may cause ventilatory depression; however, 85 per cent of the ventilatory response to CO_2 is preserved.

Central Chemoreceptors. The cells that function as central chemoreceptors lie 200 to 500 μm below the surface of the ventrolateral medulla oblongata. Their pertinent stimulus is the hydrogen ion concentration of brain extracellular fluid. Since the blood-brain barrier is freely permeable to carbon dioxide but not to hydrogen or bicarbonate ions, hypercapnic acidosis is a more powerful stimulus to central chemoreceptors than is acute metabolic acidosis. In fact, with the increased circulating hydrogen ion associated with metabolic acidosis, there is stimulation of the peripheral chemoreceptors, resulting in an increase in ventilation and a decrease in PCO_2; thus, there can actually be a paradoxical decrease in cerebrospinal fluid hydrogen ion concentration despite the blood metabolic acidosis.

The higher cerebrospinal fluid pH tends to attenuate the central ventilatory response to metabolic acidosis. Similarly, the acute ventilatory response to hypoxia as a result of stimulation of peripheral chemoreceptors is partly offset by the resulting hypocapnic alkalosis. Changes in cerebrospinal fluid pH occur as hydrogen ion equilibrates across the blood-brain barrier over a period of hours. Thus, if the acidosis is prolonged, there is a progressive fall in cerebrospinal pH to more acid levels, resulting in progressive stimulation of ventilation, so that arterial PCO_2 continues to decrease as metabolic acidosis is sustained.

Receptors in the Respiratory Tract and Lungs. There is afferent input to the respiratory center from receptors at all levels in the respiratory tract, including the nose, the nasopharynx, and the larynx.[241] The tracheobronchial receptors have been the most thoroughly studied and include irritant, stretch, and J receptors. Stimulation of irritant receptors produces rapid shallow breathing and has been implicated in the alterations of breathing pattern seen in patients with airway disease, such as asthma and chronic obstructive pulmonary disease. Pulmonary stretch receptors are responsible for the Hering-Breuer reflex (cessation of respiratory neural drive caused by lung inflation). Stretch receptors respond by increasing their firing frequency with lung inflation or with increases in transpulmonary pressure. Stimulation of "J" receptors causes rapid shallow breathing, laryngeal constriction, hypotension, and bradycardia.

Respiratory Muscle Afferents. The major striated muscle receptors are Golgi tendon organs and muscle spindles. In the diaphragm, the former structure appears to be the more important, muscle spindles being rare. By contrast, muscle spindles predominate in the intercostal muscles, both inspiratory and expiratory, as well as in the accessory muscles of respiration. The precise role of these receptors and their influence on the central respiratory controller is unknown, but a number of studies suggest that they may be important; for example, cutting the dorsal cervical and thoracic roots can lead to temporary respiratory muscle paralysis.[242]

Central Controller

Central control of respiratory rhythm and pattern can originate in the voluntary cortical centers or brainstem automatic centers. Automatic breathing originates in a highly complex accumulation of interconnected nerve cell groups situated in the medulla and the pons. Within the former, the respiratory neurons are grouped in two distinct areas: (1) *the dorsal respiratory group* (DRG), comprising two bilateral aggregates of neurons located near the nucleus of the tractus solitarius and consisting almost exclusively of inspiratory cells; and (2) *the ventral respiratory group* (VRG), which lies close to the nucleus ambiguus and the nucleus retroambigualis and contains both inspiratory and expiratory cells.

It is thought that axons originating in the DRG project to and descend in the contralateral spinal cord and serve as the principal respiratory rhythmic drive to anterior horn cells that innervate the diaphragm and inspiratory intercostals. Axons from the DRG also project to stimulate cells in the VRG, which does not appear to have inherent respiratory rhythmicity or sensory input from peripheral or central chemoreceptors and mechanoreceptors. Axons from the VRG cross and descend in the spinal cord to innervate anterior horn cells in the cervical and thoracic cord; these, in turn, project to the intercostal inspiratory and expiratory muscles as well as to the abdominal and accessory muscles of respiration and the muscles of the upper airway, which are important in maintaining upper airway patency.

Two additional respiratory control centers, the *pneumotaxis center* (PNC) and the *apneustic center* (APC), are located in the pons. Although their activity is not absolutely necessary for the generation of rhythmic respiratory output, they clearly influence and modulate the output of the medullary respiratory center[243]; the rhythm generated from the isolated medulla is slower and of a more gasping nature than that developed when the PNC and the APC are intact.

Inspiration is initiated by a sudden onset of inspiratory motor neuron activity in the DRG followed by a slowly increasing ramp of activity. Inspiratory muscle activation may extend into early expiration to brake expiratory flow. Expiratory neurons are not activated during quiet breathing but may be recruited during increased ventilatory drive.[244]

Although most of our knowledge of central respiratory control involves the automatic brainstem controlling mechanisms, it is clear that the cerebral cortex can influence brainstem mechanisms or bypass them completely to accomplish behavior-related respiratory activity such as speech, cough, and defecation. During voluntary activity, requirements for tone or loudness may override chemical and mechanical inputs; for example, during speech, the response to inhaled carbon dioxide is markedly depressed and the sensation of dyspnea diminished when compared with similar carbon dioxide levels occurring without speech.[245]

Outputs

The basic measurements of outputs used to assess respiratory control are minute ventilation and its components, tidal volume (VT) and respiratory frequency (*f*). Minute ventilation itself can be divided into mean inspiratory flow (VT/Ti) and the ratio of inspiratory time over total respiratory cycle time (Ti/Ttot). It has been proposed that VT/Ti reflects the neural drive while Ti/Ttot is a measure of central timing mechanisms; these measurements have gained wide acceptance in the analysis of respiratory control.[246]

The commonest inputs by which respiratory control is assessed are inhaled carbon dioxide and oxygen, administered in increasing and decreasing concentrations respectively; the responses to added resistive and elastic loads and to exercise also can be measured. In normal subjects, progressive hypercapnia produces a linear increase in ventilation, the slope of the curve varying widely between individuals. With progressive hypoxemia, a parabolic curve of ventilation against PO_2 is generated, with little increase in ventilation until PO_2 falls to between 50 and 60 mm Hg; however, there is also wide variability among individuals in this relationship.

Genetic or acquired alterations in ventilatory response may have profound effects on pulmonary disease. For example, it has been postulated that the genetically determined ventilatory drives to hypoxia and hypercapnia influence the pattern and course of chronic obstructive pulmonary disease; patients with brisk or good responses to carbon dioxide and hypoxia tend to maintain blood gas tensions near normal despite significant airway obstruction (pink puffers), whereas those with depressed ventilatory responses tend to hypoventilate (blue bloaters).[247] Inherited variations in ventilatory drive also may affect the ability of normal subjects to perform various functions; for example, trained endurance athletes have a significantly reduced ventilatory drive to hypoxemia and hypercapnia when compared with normal control subjects, whereas similarly fit, successful high-altitude mountain climbers have significantly increased hypercapnic and hypoxic drive when compared with distance runners.[248]

Control of Ventilation During Exercise

There are four phases in the ventilatory response to exercise. *Phase 1* is an abrupt increase in ventilation that coincides with the start of exercise. This increase occurs prior to any alterations in the gas tensions of mixed venous blood and is termed the "neurogenic component" of the ventilatory response, although the precise neural pathway that mediates the response is unknown. *Phase 2* begins some 10 or 15 seconds following the onset of exercise coincident with alterations in blood gas tensions in mixed

venous blood. The carotid bodies have some role in this phase, since there is a lag in the ventilatory response in patients without carotid bodies. *Phase 3* represents the steady-state response to exercise and is closely linked to carbon dioxide production. Finally, with heavy exercise (*phase 4*) a further increase in ventilation occurs coincident with the metabolic production of lactic acid. This stage in progressive exercise is termed the anaerobic threshold, and at this point ventilation becomes uncoupled from metabolic carbon dioxide production. This final lactic acidosis–induced hyperpnea is mediated by peripheral chemoreceptors.

Compensation for Added Ventilatory Loads

The respiratory muscles act against elastic and resistive loads that may vary greatly under normal physiologic conditions and during disease states. Studies in humans have shown that the decrease in tidal volume that occurs with such added loads is less than would be expected on a purely mechanical basis, indicating that compensatory mechanisms are brought into play to ensure adequate acinar ventilation. The first such mechanism is related to the basic mechanical properties of skeletal muscle. Since the force generated by skeletal muscle is inversely related to its velocity of shortening, an unloaded muscle will shorten rapidly and produce little force; however, with an added load, shortening is slowed and force generation increased, resulting in a tendancy to counteract the expected decrease in tidal volume.

The second mechanism of load compensation involves reflexes initiated by mechanoreceptors in the lung and chest wall, particularly the pulmonary stretch receptors. With an added elastic or resistive load, inspiration is slowed; because pulmonary stretch receptors adapt rapidly with time, their level of activity at any volume during inspiration is decreased; this results in prolonged inspiration, tending to increase tidal volume back toward control levels.[249]

Muscle spindles represent a third mechanism by which load compensation is accomplished. These receptors contain intrafusal fibers that regulate the spindles' stretch and contract in concert with the extrafusal fibers that move the rib cage. This stimulates the gamma afferents, which, through the spinal reflex, enhance motor neuron output to the inspiratory muscles. A final mechanism of load compensation is initiated when central and peripheral chemoreceptors detect changes in the arterial blood gas composition.[249]

Closely related to the topic of load detection and compensation is respiratory sensation and the symptom of dyspnea. Dyspnea (the unpleasant awareness of breathing or respiratory distress) should be distinguished from hyperventilation (defined as a lowered arterial PCO_2) or tachypnea (rapid respiration). The balance of evidence suggests that it occurs when afferent input from respiratory muscles in some way signals an inappropriateness of the central neurogenic drive to breathe and the resulting displacement of the lung and chest wall.[250] It is not caused by alterations in arterial blood gas tensions.

Control of Breathing During Sleep

Sleep has a profound influence on the various aspects of the control of breathing (Table 1–4). Resting ventilation is decreased during slow-wave sleep, with both tidal volume

Table 1–4. EFFECTS OF SLEEP ON BREATHING

	Slow-Wave Sleep	REM Sleep
Alveolar ventilation	Decreased due to ↓ VT and ↓ F	Variable
Arterial PCO₂	↑ 4–6 mm Hg	Variable
Arterial PO₂	↓ 4–8 mm Hg	Variable
Breathing pattern	Stages 1 and 2 periodic Stages 3 and 4 regular	Irregular ↑ F plus ↓ VT
Diaphragmatic contraction	No change	No change
Intercostal contraction	↓	↓ ↓
Upper airway muscle contraction	↓	↓ ↓
Ventilatory response to CO₂	↓	↓ ↓
Ventilatory response to hypoxemia	↓	↓ ↓
Response to lung afferents	↓	↓ ↓
Response to respiratory muscle afferents	↓	↓ ↓

and frequency being less than during wakefulness.[251] During rapid eye movement (REM) sleep, resting ventilation varies as a result of marked irregularity of the breathing pattern, but on the whole hyperventilation rather than hypoventilation is the rule. During stages 1 and 2 of slow-wave sleep, periodic breathing reminiscent of Cheyne-Stokes respiration may occur, changing to a regular pattern during the deeper stages (3 and 4) of slow-wave sleep. The pattern of breathing during REM sleep is characterized as irregular rather than periodic.

The responsiveness of the respiratory control mechanisms to afferent inputs is also profoundly altered during sleep; responsiveness to hypercapnia is decreased during slow-wave sleep and further decreased during REM sleep. The respiratory centers also appear to ignore afferent input from other sources during sleep; pulmonary stretch and irritant receptor discharge, as well as muscle spindle input, are less effective in increasing ventilation and effecting load compensation during sleep.

RESPIRATORY MUSCLES

The respiratory muscles may be divided into four groups with different functions and mechanisms of action—the upper airway muscles,[252] the diaphragm, the intercostal and accessory muscles, and the abdominal muscles.

The diaphragm is the principal muscle of inspiration. It probably acts alone during quiet breathing, with the intercostal and accessory muscles being recruited only when the demand for ventilation increases. However, there is some tonic inspiratory muscle activity in the intercostal muscles in the upright posture, which prevents paradoxical inward movement of the rib cage with diaphragmatic descent. The intercostal muscles include the internal (expiratory) and external (inspiratory) intercostals. The major accessory muscles are the scalenes, the sternomastoids, and the trapezoids. The abdominal muscles include the rectus and transverse abdominis and the external and internal obliques. In healthy individuals, expiration is largely passive, with expiratory muscle activity becoming manifest only

when the minute ventilation exceeds about 50 per cent of the maximal voluntary ventilation.[253]

The Diaphragm

Anatomy

The central portion of the diaphragm (the central tendon) is composed of a broad sheet of decussating muscle fibers, in shape similar to a boomerang, the point of the boomerang being directed toward the sternum and the concavity toward the spine (Fig. 1–84). The costal muscle fibers arise anteriorly from the xiphoid process and around the convexity of the thorax from ribs 7 to 12; posteriorly, the crural fibers arise from the lateral margins of the first, second, and third lumbar vertebrae on the right side, and from the first and second lumbar vertebrae on the left. These fibers converge toward the central tendon and are inserted into it nearly perpendicular to its margin.

Recent evidence suggests that the diaphragm can be considered as two distinct muscles with separate nervous and vascular supplies as well as functions.[254] The costal portion is mechanically in parallel with the intercostal and accessory muscles, and its contraction results in both descent of the diaphragm and elevation of the rib cage; by contrast, the crural portion acts in parallel with the costal diaphragm and in series with the intercostal and accessory muscles, and its contraction results in descent of the diaphragm without elevation of the rib cage (Fig. 1–85).

The diaphragm is composed of three types of muscle fibers: (1) slow-twitch oxidative fatigue-resistant units (type 1); (2) fast-twitch oxidative glycolytic fatigue-resistant units (type 2a); and (3) fast-twitch glycolytic fatiguable units (type 2b). Each type has specific physiologic features and corresponding histochemical profiles[255]; all fibers within individual motor units are of the same type. Normally, type 1 fibers represent approximately 50 per cent of muscle fibers, whereas type 2a represent about 20 per cent, and type 2b about 30 per cent; these percentages could conceivably change with atrophy or training of the respiratory muscles. It is likely that the diaphragm behaves like other skeletal muscles, and that slow-twitch motor units are recruited during low-intensity contractions, such as in sustained quiet breathing, and that fast-twitch units, both fatigue-resistant and fatigue-susceptible, play a greater role with increasing respiratory activity.

The diaphragm receives its blood supply from the phrenic and intercostal arteries and from branches of the internal thoracic (mammary) arteries. The internal mammary and phrenic arteries anastomose to form an arterial circle around the central tendon; this, in turn, gives off branches that form an arcade. A second arterial circle is formed by the intercostals around the insertion of the diaphragm. This diversity of blood supply may be an important factor in the diaphragm's resistance to fatigue.[256] In contrast with limb skeletal muscle, there is no evidence in the diaphragm of blood flow limitation on contractile effort. In fact, the increasing demand for oxygen by the working diaphragm is supplied largely by augmenting the blood flow rather than by increasing the extraction of oxygen from the blood.[257]

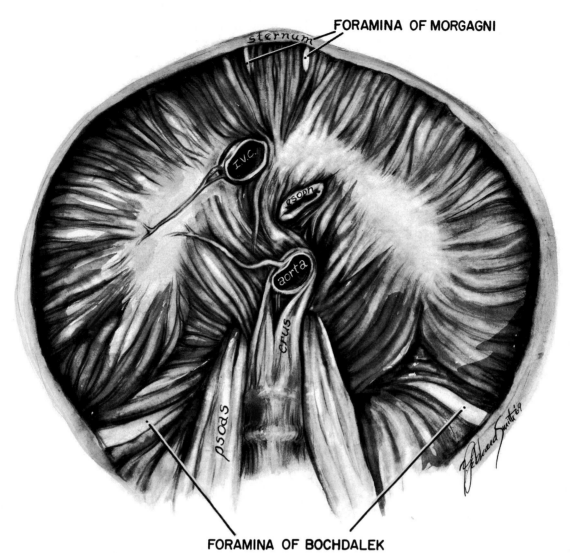

FORAMINA OF MORGAGNI

FORAMINA OF BOCHDALEK

Figure 1–84. Anatomy of the Normal Diaphragm Viewed from Below. *See* text.

Figure 1–85. A Mechanical Model of the Inspiratory Musculature. The bar into which the crural and costal portions of the diaphragm insert represents the central tendon of the diaphragm. The inverted L-shaped structure represents the rib cage. The springs represent the elastic properties of rib cage, lung, and abdomen. The hatched area represents the bony skeleton. The costal and crural portions of the diaphragm are arranged mechanically in parallel. When in parallel, the force applied is the sum of the forces generated by the two muscles, but the displacement (volume change) is equal to the displacement of either muscle. The costal part of the diaphragm is in parallel with the intercostal and accessory muscles, whereas the crural part is in series. When in series, the displacements of the two muscles can be added, while the forces are not summed. The drawing on the right represents more anatomically realistic illustration of the diaphragm, showing separation of costal and crural parts. (From Macklem PT, Macklem DM, De Troyer A: A model of inspiratory muscle mechanics. J Appl Physiol 55: 547, 1983.)

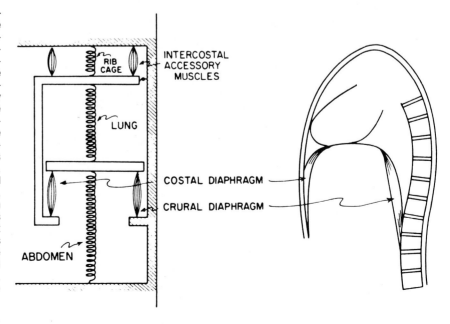

An extensive intradiaphragmatic lymphatic network drains the pleural and peritoneal cavities as well as the diaphragm itself into mediastinal lymph nodes.[258] On the peritoneal surface, small pores 4 to 12 μm in diameter have been demonstrated between the lining mesothelial cells (Fig. 1–86); these appear to provide direct communication between the peritoneal cavity and lymphatic spaces.

The phrenic nerve is the sole motor nerve supply to the diaphragm. It arises chiefly from the fourth cervical nerve but also receives contributions from the third and fifth. At the level of the diaphragm, each phrenic nerve gives off separate branches to the anterior (sternal) region, the anterolateral region, and the crural portion. Hemidiaphragmatic and intercostal muscle innervation has a predominantly contralateral cortical representation. The conduction velocity in the phrenic nerve is high, reaching a maximum of 78 m per second; also, the innervation is dense, each nerve fiber subserving a low number of motor units—an anatomic arrangement that is usually seen in muscles performing precise movements, such as those of the eye. The intercostal motor neurons are located between T-1 and T-12 in the spinal cord and reach the intercostal muscles via the intercostal nerves. Abdominal motor neurons are located between T-11 and L-1.

Roentgenology

Roentgenographic Height of the Normal Diaphragm. In about 95 per cent of normal adults, the level of the cupola of the right hemidiaphragm is projected in a plane ranging from the anterior end of the fifth rib to the sixth anterior interspace; in 40 per cent, it is at the level of the sixth rib anteriorly; in only 5 per cent is it at or below the level of the seventh rib.[259] Generally speaking, the height of the right dome is higher in women, in subjects of heavy build, and in those older than 40 years of age.

Relationship Between the Height of the Right and Left Hemidiaphragms. The tendency for the plane of the right diaphragmatic dome to be about half an interspace higher than the left is well recognized, although in about 10 per cent of normal subjects both are at the same height or the left is higher than the right.[260] The usual lower position of the left hemidiaphragm is caused by the contiguous mass of the heart on this side rather than the presence of the liver under the right hemidiaphragm.[261]

Range of Diaphragmatic Excursion. In a study of inspiratory-expiratory roentgenograms of 350 subjects aged 30 to 80 years without evidence of respiratory disease, we found the mean excursions of the right and left hemidiaphragms to be 3.3 cm and 3.5 cm, respectively (unpublished data), somewhat less than those observed by others; diaphragmatic movement averaged 0.5 cm less in women than in men. Despite the similarity of these mean values, unequal movement of the two hemidiaphragmatic domes in an individual subject is common. For example, in one study of 114 healthy young men, movements were equal in only 10 subjects, being greater on the right in 73 (never by more than 1.9 cm) and greater on the left in 31 (exceeding 1.4 cm in only one case).[260]

It should be emphasized that diaphragmatic excursion of less than 3 cm is not necessarily abnormal. In fact, there is no relationship between diaphragmatic movement and vital capacity; some patients with mean diaphragmatic excursions of less than 3 cm have a vital capacity of more than 5 L.

Physiologic Variations in Diaphragmatic Contour. Scalloping of the diaphragm, in which the normally smooth contour is replaced by smooth, arcuate elevations, occurs in

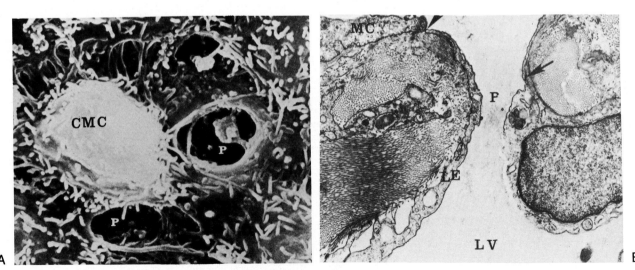

Figure 1–86. Morphologic Characteristics of the Diaphragm. *A,* A scanning electron micrograph shows a surface cuboidal cell (CMC) (possibly a macrophage) and numerous slender mesothelial microvilli. Two intercellular pores (P) are evident. (× 8950.) *B,* A section through a pore (P) viewed by transmission electron microscopy shows processes from two lymphatic endothelial cells (LE) extending onto the peritoneal surface to form intercellular junctions *(arrows)* with the surface mesothelial cells (MC). The close contact between the two cell types provides a direct passageway between the peritoneal cavity and the underlying lymphatic vessels (LV). (× 16,200.) (From Leak LV, Rahil K: Am Rev Respir Dis 119[Suppl]: 8, 1979.)

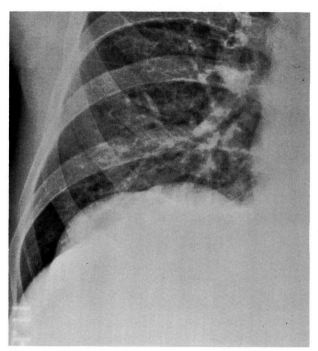

Figure 1–87. Scalloping of the Diaphragm. A roentgenogram of the right hemidiaphragm reveals two smooth arcuate elevations disturbing the normally smooth contour of the dome, a finding of no known significance.

about 5 per cent of individuals (Fig. 1–87). In the majority, it is confined to the right side. The finding is of no clinical significance.

In some subjects, muscle slips originating from the lateral and posterolateral ribs can be identified as short, meniscus-shaped shadows along the lateral half of both hemidiaphragms; these are produced by exceptionally low descent of the diaphragm during inspiration. In the majority of cases, the appearance is caused by severe pulmonary overinflation (Fig. 1–88), as in asthma or emphysema; however, very occasionally it can be seen in healthy young men

and should not be regarded as unequivocal evidence of air trapping in the absence of supportive evidence.

Respiratory Pump

The muscles of ventilation are striated and generally behave in the same fashion as other skeletal muscles. However, they differ in two important respects: (1) they are under voluntary as well as automatic control; and (2) in contrast with the inertial loads facing most other skeletal muscle, they must principally overcome resistive and elastic loads.[253]

The force generated by the contracting diaphragm is a function of the muscle fiber length, the mechanical advantage of the muscle, the loads on the muscle, and the intensity of muscle activation. Like all skeletal muscles, the respiratory muscles have a characteristic length-tension relationship. There is a specific optimal length at which maximal cross-bridging between actin and myosin fibers occurs; at this length, maximal force can be generated with a given stimulation. As the fibers are lengthened or shortened beyond this point, the tension generated by a given stimulus is decreased. Thus, hyperinflation of the lung, as occurs in patients who have obstructive lung disease, decreases the efficiency of the diaphragm by shortening muscle fiber length. The rate of diaphragmatic stimulation is also important in determining its efficiency: diaphragmatic force is maximum in humans when the phrenic nerve is stimulated at a frequency of 100 hertz (Hz); it is reduced to 94 per cent maximum at 50 Hz, 70 per cent maximum at 20 Hz, and 25 per cent maximum at 10 Hz.[262]

When the diaphragm contracts, it not only pushes down on the abdominal viscera and displaces the abdominal wall outward but also lifts and expands the chest cage because of rib articulation and its insertion onto the lower ribs. The mechanical advantage of a dome-shaped muscle such as the diaphragm is related to its radius of curvature; the greater the curvature (the smaller the radius), the more pressure is generated for a given tension (law of Laplace). The abdominal and accessory muscles can act as fixators or positioning

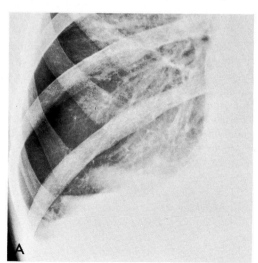
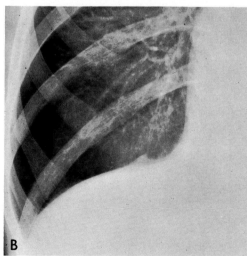

Figure 1–88. Diaphragmatic Muscle Slips. Inspiratory *(A)* and expiratory *(B)* roentgenograms of the lower half of the right hemithorax of a patient with severe emphysema reveal short, meniscus-shaped shadows extending laterally from each hemidiaphragm. These muscle slips are prominent on full inspiration and disappear on expiration.

muscles, which adjust the configuration of the diaphragm, rib cage, and abdomen in such a way as to optimize the curvature and, thus, the efficiency of the diaphragm.[253] This is particularly evident in the upright position, especially during exercise when abdominal muscle contraction during expiration tends to lengthen the diaphragmatic muscle fibers.

Abdominal expiratory muscles can also aid inspiration by decreasing the end-expiratory lung volume below the relaxed volume of the rib cage and abdomen, and then suddenly relaxing at the onset of inspiration; the resulting sudden descent of the diaphragm along its passive length-tension curve represents an energy-independent inspiratory contribution. This strategy is employed by normal subjects in the hyperpnea of carbon dioxide rebreathing and exercise and in patients with bilateral diaphragmatic paralysis.[263] The maneuver is effective in the upright and lateral decubitus positions but ineffective in the supine position, probably accounting for the characteristic increase in dyspnea noted by patients with bilateral diaphragmatic paralysis when they assume the supine posture.[263]

Respiratory Muscle Fatigue

The three major factors that can lead to failure of adequate inspiratory muscle function are decreased neuronal drive, weakness of the respiratory muscle, and fatigue of the muscle. The last two of these are similar, in that the muscles eventually reach a point where the demand placed on them exceeds their capacity to generate force and hence pressure; however, in the case of fatigue, the muscle's capacity can be increased with rest. A failure of central drive with resulting ventilatory respiratory failure occurs in central neurogenic hypoventilation or drug overdosage. Failure related to weakness is seen in neuromuscular disease, such as myasthenia gravis and muscular dystrophy.

Respiratory muscle fatigue is the final common pathway in the majority of patients with respiratory failure related to increased work of breathing; as a result, there has been much interest in its study. The respiratory muscles are the most fatigue-resistant muscles in the body; for example, when intravenous curare is administered in a dose sufficient to completely abolish hand-grip and head-raising, diaphragmatic strength is decreased to only 42 per cent of the control value.[264] In normal humans, respiratory muscle fatigue develops only when the respiratory muscles have to generate more than 40 per cent of their maximal force for prolonged periods.[265]

Recognition of the importance of muscle fatigue in respiratory failure has stimulated an interest in detecting fatiguing muscle before the development of hypercapnia. In the relaxed and supine state, most healthy humans have predominantly abdominal rather than rib cage motion, a finding that is related to breathing with the diaphragm rather than the intercostal muscles.[266] By contrast, normal subjects fatigued from breathing against a high resistance exhibit an interesting sequence of clinical manifestations that correlates with electromyographic evidence of muscle fatigue and the onset of respiratory acidosis. Such individuals are first noted to have very shallow and rapid breathing[267]; this is followed by paradoxical movement of the abdominal wall, the exhausted and flaccid diaphragm being

sucked in by the negative intrapleural pressure created by rib cage expansion. In some patients, alternation between rib cage and abdominal breathing (respiratory alternans) is observed, a presumed homeostatic maneuver that permits resting of one group of muscles while the other works.

CHEST WALL

Soft Tissues

The pectoral muscles form the anterior axillary fold, a structure that normally is visible on PA roentgenograms in both men and women, curving smoothly downward and medially from the axilla to the rib cage. In men, particularly those with heavy muscular development, the inferior border of the pectoralis major may be seen as a downward extension of the anterior axillary fold, passing obliquely across the middle portion of both lungs. In women, this shadow is obscured by the breasts, whose presence and size must be taken into consideration in assessing the density of the lower lung zones.

In many roentgenograms, the shadow of the sternomastoid muscle is visible as a density whose lateral margin parallels the spine in the medial third of the lung apices; it curves downward and laterally to blend with the companion shadow on the superior aspect of each clavicle. The latter shadow, which is 2 to 3 mm thick, parallels the superior aspect of the clavicle; it is formed by the skin and subcutaneous tissue overlaying the clavicles and is rendered visible roentgenologically by the supraclavicular fossae and the tangential direction in which the x-ray beam strikes the clavicles.

Bones

In the absence of pulmonary or pleural disease, deformity of the spine, or congenital anomalies of the ribs themselves, the rib cage should be symmetric. Both the upper and lower borders of the ribs should be sharply defined except in the middle and lower thoracic regions; here, the thin flanges created by the vascular sulci on the inferior aspects of the ribs posteriorly are viewed *en face*, creating a less distinct margin.

Calcification of the rib cartilages is common. It usually begins with the first and is probably never of pathologic significance. The relation between age and costal cartilage calcification differs in men and women: in the former, it is uncommon before the age of 20 years but progressively increases in frequency so that almost 90 per cent of men aged 60 years and over have marginal calcification; by contrast, in women, central calcification is present in 45 per cent of those younger than 20 years of age and in almost 90 per cent older than 60 years.[268]

Thin, smooth shadows of water density that parallel the ribs and measure 1 to 2 mm in diameter project adjacent to the inferior and inferolateral margins of the first and second ribs and to the axillary portions of the lower ribs. These *"companion shadows"* (Fig. 1–89) are caused by visualization in tangential projection of parietal pleura and the soft tissues (principally fat) immediately external to the pleura and should not be interpreted as local pleural thick-

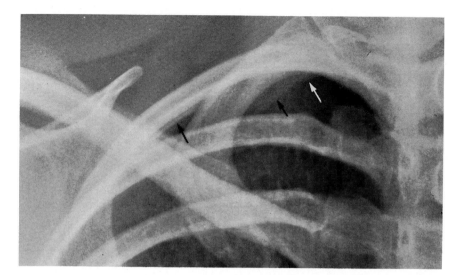

Figure 1–89. Companion Shadows of the Ribs. A magnified view of the apex of the right hemithorax reveals thin, smooth shadows of water density lying roughly parallel to the inferior surfaces of the first and second ribs *(arrows)*. These companion shadows are caused by perception in tangential projection of a combination of parietal and visceral pleura and the soft tissues immediately external to the pleura.

ening. Extrapleural fat is most abundant over the fourth to eighth ribs posterolaterally and relates chiefly to the ribs rather than to the interspaces.[269]

Congenital anomalies of the ribs are relatively uncommon. *Supernumerary ribs* arising from the seventh cervical vertebra have been identified in 1 to 2 per cent of otherwise normal individuals; nearly all are bilateral, although many are asymmetric. Other anomalies, such as hypoplasia of the first rib, bifid or splayed anterior ribs, and, rarely, local fusion of ribs, usually are important only in that they may give rise to an erroneous interpretation of abnormal lung density.

Occasionally, the inferior aspect of the clavicles has an irregular notch or indentation 2 to 3 cm from the sternal articulation; its size and shape vary from a superficial saucer-shaped defect to a deep notch 2 cm wide by 1.0 to 1.5 cm deep. These *rhomboid fossae* (Fig. 1–90) give rise to the costoclavicular, or rhomboid, ligaments that radiate downward to bind the clavicles to the first rib.[270]

The normal *thoracic spine* is straight in frontal projection and gently concave anteriorly in lateral projection. Its roentgenographic density in lateral projection decreases uniformly from above downward, and any deviation from this should arouse suspicion of intrathoracic disease. The lateral and superior borders of the *manubrium* are the only

portions of the sternum visible on frontal projections of the thorax, although the whole of the sternum should be clearly seen tangentially in lateral roentgenograms.

NORMAL CHEST ROENTGENOGRAM

Normal Lung Density

It is readily apparent that the roentgenographic "density" of the lungs is the result of the absorptive powers of each of its component parts—gas, blood, and tissue. Although precise figures for the contributions of blood and tissue vary somewhat, depending on whether results are obtained by anatomic or physiologic methods, data have been compiled that allow a reasonable approximation.

Weibel estimated that the lung parenchyma constitutes 90 per cent of total lung volume.[271] Using a point-counting technique, he also measured the volumetric proportion of the three components of lung parenchyma; air accounted for 92 per cent, and tissue and capillary blood for 8.0 per cent. On the basis of these figures and assuming a total lung volume of 7240 mL, the parenchymal component is approximately 6500 mL (90 per cent of 7240 mL), 500 mL of which consists of tissue and blood (8 per cent of 6500

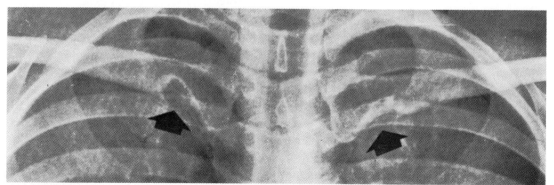

Figure 1–90. Rhomboid Fossae. An irregular notch or indentation is present in the inferior aspect of both clavicles approximately 2 cm from their sternal end *(arrows)*. These fossae give origin to the costoclavicular, or rhomboid, ligaments.

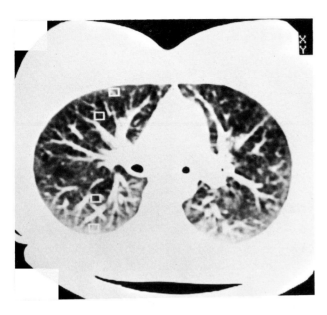

Figure 1–91. Methodology for Attenuation Coefficient Density Evaluation. ROI boxes indicate peripheral and central and anterior and posterior areas in the right lung from which attenuation values are recorded. ROI areas ranged from 0.25 cm² to 0.37 cm² depending on scanner calibration; each contains 35 voxels. Note the remarkable difference in density between anterior and posterior lung regions. (From Genereux GP: Computed tomography and the lung: Review of anatomic and densitometric features with their clinical application. J Can Assoc Radiol 36: 88, June 1985. Reprinted, by permission of the publisher.)

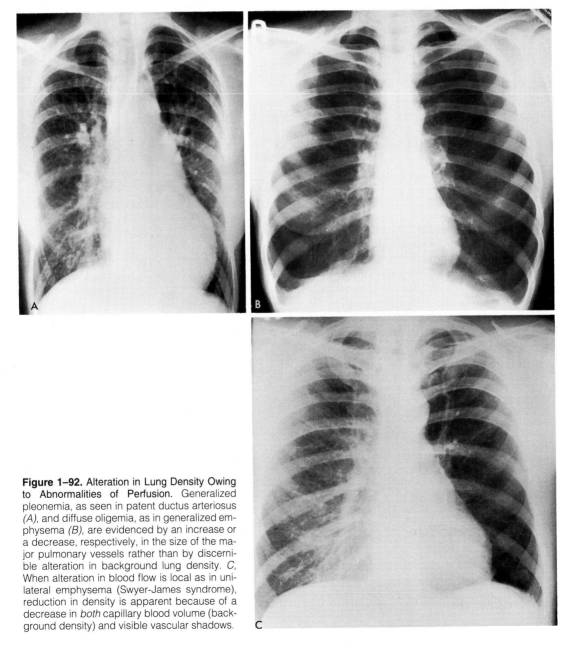

Figure 1–92. Alteration in Lung Density Owing to Abnormalities of Perfusion. Generalized pleonemia, as seen in patent ductus arteriosus *(A)*, and diffuse oligemia, as in generalized emphysema *(B)*, are evidenced by an increase or a decrease, respectively, in the size of the major pulmonary vessels rather than by discernible alteration in background lung density. *C,* When alteration in blood flow is local as in unilateral emphysema (Swyer-James syndrome), reduction in density is apparent because of a decrease in *both* capillary blood volume (background density) and visible vascular shadows.

mL). Thus, *the density of lung parenchyma at TLC is 0.08 (500 g per 6500 mL). It follows that in a chest roentgenogram all the tissue visible in the peripheral 2 cm of the lung or between vascular shadows has a density of 0.08 g per mL.*

The density of lung parenchyma also has been estimated by CT.[272] Such estimation is based on an approximately linear relationship that exists between the attenuation of an x-ray beam of 65 keV (about 120 kVp) and the density of materials of low atomic number (ranging from air to water). Attenuation on a CT scan is commonly expressed in terms of the Hounsfield unit (HU) scale, in which water is 0 HU and air is −1000 HU. With this technique, density has been found to vary between −820 and −840 HU in the majority of subjects (Fig. 1–91).[272]

An attenuation coefficient gradient is normally present between the nondependent and dependent portions of the lung in the supine, prone, and lateral decubitus positions, attributable primarily to the influence of gravity on blood flow. Measurements have shown that the anteroposterior gradient for both lung and blood density is pronounced whereas that for extravascular lung water is small.[273] The average difference between the nondependent and dependent lung parenchyma in subjects studied during quiet respiration is about 110 HU (±45 HU); during inspiratory breath-holding, the average density gradient is about 70 HU (±35 HU).

It is important to appreciate the distinction between pulmonary capillaries and the larger (visible) vessels with respect to their separate contributions to lung density. Although an increase in capillary blood volume is known to occur in conditions such as ventricular septal defect and atrial septal defect, without concomitant alteration in lung volumes, it is doubtful whether the increase in lung density that must result from this increased capillary volume can be appreciated roentgenographically, except by densitometry. Instead, roentgenologic assessment of vascular plethora (pleonemia) in such situations must be based on increases in the size and number of visible pulmonary vessels, both arterial and venous. (These statements apply only to conditions in which perfusion is *uniformly* altered throughout the lungs—for example, in the pleonemia that accompanies intracardiac left-to-right shunt [Fig. 1–92] or in the oligemia of diffuse emphysema.) When reduction in blood flow is *local*, as with lobar emphysema or occasionally with massive pulmonary embolism, alteration in density in the involved area of lung is the result of reduction in *both* capillary blood volume (background density) *and* visible vascular shadows.

Alteration in Lung Density

Alteration in roentgenographic lung density may be due to one of three mechanisms or a combination thereof.

Physiologic Mechanisms. A frequently observed physiologic variation in lung density is the change that may occur from one examination to another in the same subject, depending on depth of inspiration. Such variation is readily explained by comparing the contributions of the three components of the lung to its density. For example, consider a 20-year-old man 170 cm in height, and assume that pulmonary blood volume and tissue volume are reasonably

constant at different degrees of lung inflation. According to the tables of normal values, predicted lung volumes for such a subject are 6.5 L TLC, 3.4 L FRC, and 1.5 L residual volume. Assuming a total maximal tissue volume of 740 mL, average lung density at TLC is 0.10; at FRC, it is almost double (0.18), and at residual volume more than treble (0.33) (Fig. 1–93). Thus, assuming total pulmonary blood volume to be constant at different degrees of lung inflation, it is clear that *lung density is inversely proportional to the amount of contained gas.*

Physical (Technical) Mechanisms. Symmetry of roentgenographic density of the two lungs in a normal subject depends on proper positioning for roentgenography. If the patient is rotated as little as 2 or 3 degrees, the density of the lung closer to the film will be uniformly *greater* than that of the other lung (Fig. 1–94); conversely, the lung that is farthest away from the film will be uniformly blacker, creating a unilateral hyperlucent hemithorax that can sometimes make differential diagnosis difficult. The basis for this effect was demonstrated in a radiographic study of phantoms, in which 80 per cent of the increase in unilateral film blackening resulting from rotation was shown to be caused by asymmetric absorption of the primary x-ray beam, with the remaining 20 per cent being due to scatter radiation.[274] Measurements of chest wall thickness showed that the x-ray beam traversed less tissue on the side of increased film blackening (or conversely more tissue on the side of increased opacity), owing chiefly to the pectoral muscles.

Pathologic Mechanisms. Excluding the contribution to roentgenographic density from the soft tissues of the thoracic wall, and provided physiologic and physical causes are not involved, variation in lung density must be due to an increase or decrease in one or more of the three elements—air, blood, and tissue. In the majority of clinical situations, change in density, whether increased or decreased, local or diffuse, is the result of change in all three. The contribution of each component is discussed in detail in Chapter 4 and in the appropriate sections throughout the text.

Pulmonary Markings

Linear markings are created predominantly by the bronchovascular bundles (Figs. 1–95 and 1–96), structures that fan outward from both hila, tapering gradually as they proceed distally. In the normal state, they are visible up to about 1 to 2 cm from the visceral pleural surface over the convexity of the lung, at which point the lung consists almost entirely of parenchyma and they become invisible.

As indicated in the section dealing with the pulmonary vasculature, the anatomic remoteness of the pulmonary veins from the arteries often renders their distinction possible roentgenographically. In the region of the pulmonary ligaments, especially, these vessels should be readily apparent, since the pulmonary veins in the lower lung zones lie almost horizontally and on a lower plane than the arteries. By contrast, it is probable that in about half of all individuals, superimposition of the upper lobe arteries and veins precludes their distinction on plain roentgenograms in PA projection. When the vessels can be identified separately, the veins that drain the upper lobes always project lateral to their respective arteries—a relationship particularly val-

Text continued on page 110

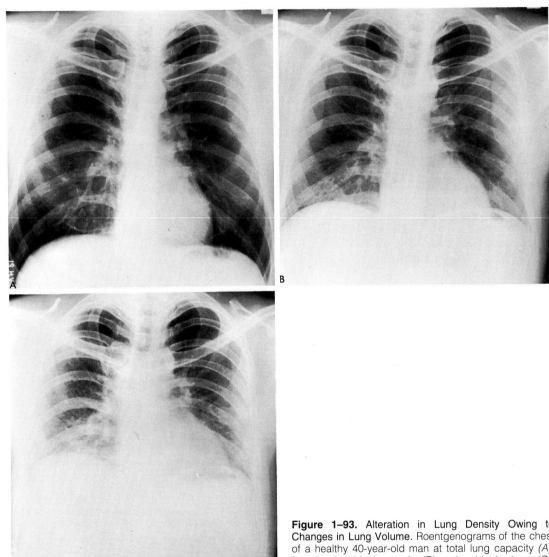

Figure 1–93. Alteration in Lung Density Owing to Changes in Lung Volume. Roentgenograms of the chest of a healthy 40-year-old man at total lung capacity *(A)*, functional residual capacity *(B)*, and residual volume *(C)*.

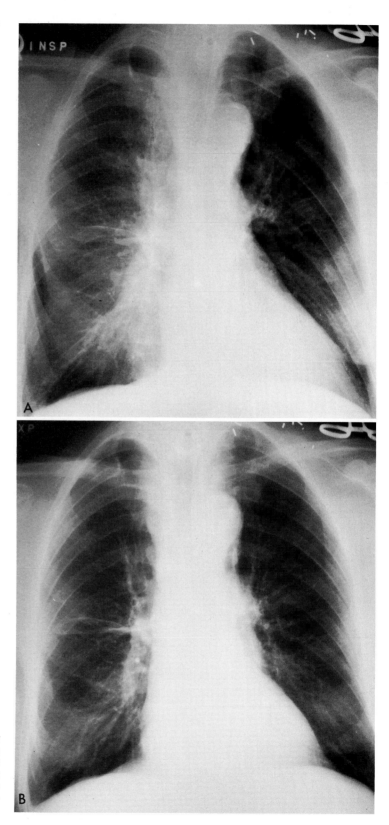

Figure 1–94. Alteration in Lung Density Owing to Improper Positioning. *A,* A roentgenogram of the chest in PA projection was exposed with the patient rotated slightly into the right anterior oblique position, producing an overall increase in density of the right lung compared with the left. In *B,* positioning has been corrected, and the asymmetry has disappeared.

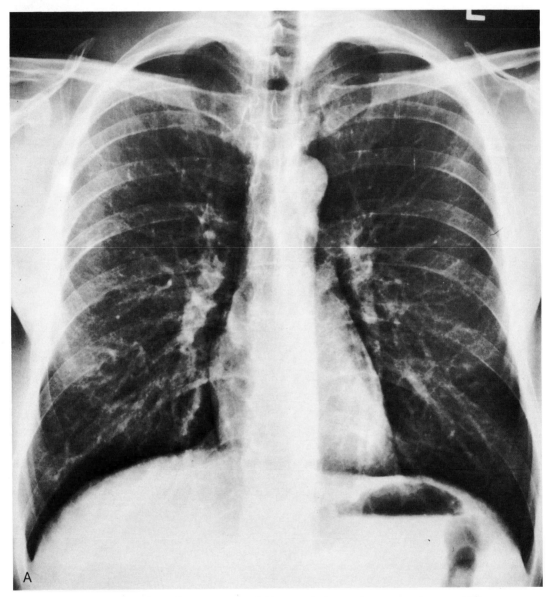

Figure 1–95. Normal Chest Roentgenogram. *A,* Posteroanterior roentgenogram of a normal 28-year-old man.

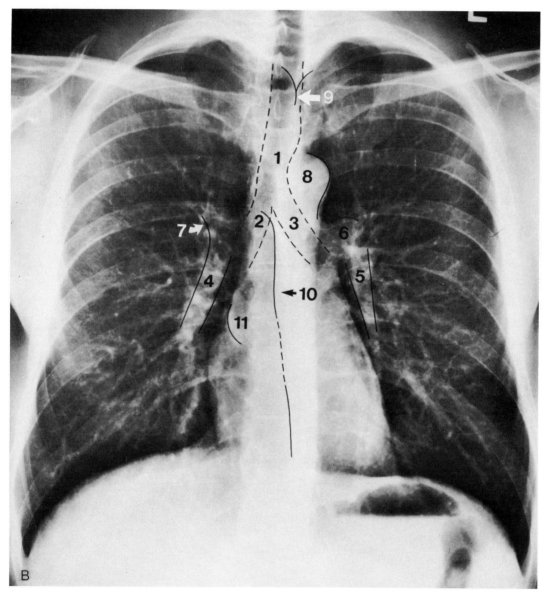

Figure 1–95 *Continued B,* A diagrammatic overlay indicates anatomic structures: 1, trachea; 2, right mainstem bronchus; 3, left mainstem bronchus; 4, right interlobar artery; 5, left interlobar artery; 6, left main pulmonary artery; 7, right superior pulmonary vein; 8, aortic knob; 9, posterior junction line; 10, azygoesophageal recess interface; 11, right pulmonary venous confluence.

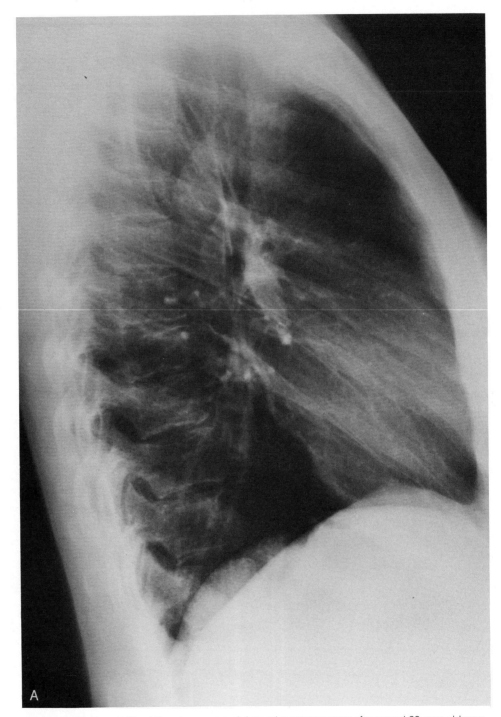

Figure 1–96. Normal Chest Roentgenogram. *A,* Lateral roentgenogram of a normal 28-year-old man.

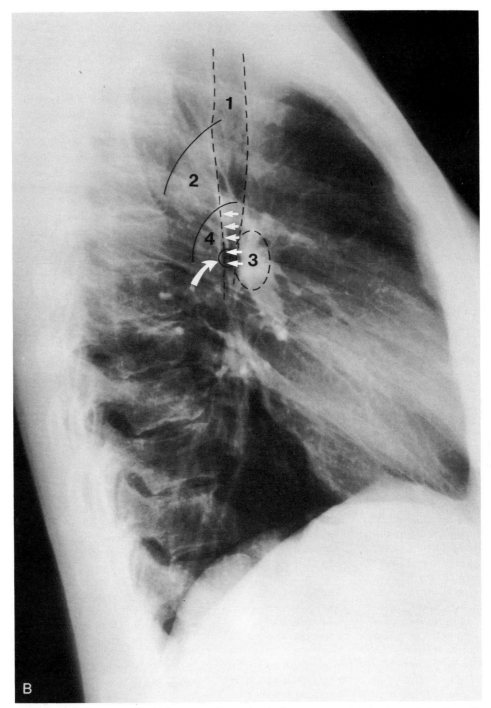

Figure 1–96 *Continued B,* A diagrammatic overlay indicates anatomic structures: 1, trachea; 2, descending arch of the aorta; 3, confluent shadow of the right interlobar artery and right superior pulmonary vein; 4, left interlobar artery. The *curved arrow* points to the circular radiolucency of the left main bronchus, and the *small arrows* to the linear opacity of the posterior wall of the right main and intermediate bronchial continuum.

uable in the right hilar region, in which the superior pulmonary vein forms the lateral aspect of the hilum superiorly and thus produces the upper limb of its concave configuration (*see* Fig. 1–95).

The PA chest roentgenogram of a normal erect subject invariably shows some discrepancy in size of the linear markings in the upper lung zones compared with the lower, owing to less perfusion of the former. In erect subjects, hydrostatic pressure increases pulmonary blood flow progressively from apex to base, a unit volume of lung at the base of the thorax having four to eight times the blood flow of a similar volume at the apex. In recumbent subjects, absence of the influence of gravity renders this discrepancy in vascular size minimal.

Complex interrelationships between transthoracic pressure and pulmonary blood flow occur during inspiration and expiration and during the Valsalva or Müller maneuvers.* During inspiration the blood volume increases in the pulmonary arteries and veins and decreases in the capillaries, changes that can be identified on standard roentgenograms; in one study, the caliber of the right descending pulmonary artery was consistently larger during inspiration than during expiration in normal subjects, the range of difference being 1 to 3 mm.[275]

PERCEPTION IN CHEST ROENTGENOLOGY

Observer Error

The roentgenologic diagnosis of chest disease begins with *identification* of an abnormality on a roentgenogram; that which is not *seen* cannot be appreciated. These statements may appear self-evident, but they express an observation that deserves constant re-emphasis. Many studies of the accuracy of diagnostic procedures have revealed an astonishingly high incidence of both intra- and interobserver error among experienced roentgenologists. For example, in one series the interpreters missed almost one third of roentgenologically positive minifilms and over-read about 1 per cent of negative films.[276] Since these figures are derived from studies by competent, experienced observers, it is clear that no roentgenologist should be lulled into a false sense of security concerning his or her competence to "see" a lesion. This is perhaps particularly important in the area of missed pulmonary cancers.[277]

The reasons for observer error are both subjective and objective and are highly complex; every physician concerned with the interpretation of chest roentgenograms must become familiar with the principles of perception, so that errors are kept to a minimum.[278, 279]

A roentgenogram can be inspected in two ways, each of which may be usefully employed in different situations. Directed search is a method whereby a specific pattern of inspection is carried out, commonly along such lines as thoracic and extrathoracic soft tissues, bony thorax, medias-

tinum, diaphragm, pleura, and, finally, the lungs themselves, the latter usually by individual inspection and comparison of the zones of the two lungs from apex to base. Such a method *must* be employed by roentgenologists-in-training, for it is only through the exercise of this routine during thousands of examinations that the pattern of the normal chest can be recognized. The second method of inspection is free global search, in which the roentgenogram is scanned without a preconceived orderly pattern. This technique is recommended by Tuddenham,[278] who found some objective evidence of its being the method employed by the majority of expert roentgenologists; our experience supports this. However, we consider that discovery of an abnormality during free-search scanning must be followed by an orderly pattern of inspection so that other, less obvious abnormalities are not overlooked.

It is important to view every chest roentgenogram from a distance of at least 6 to 8 ft. The reasons are twofold: (1) the slight nuances of density variation between similar zones of the two lungs can be better appreciated at a distance than from the traditional viewing position; and (2) the visibility of shadows with ill-defined margins is significantly improved by minification. There is also evidence that multiple viewing distances are desirable.[280] An additional means of reducing the frequency of missed lesions is "double viewing"; according to some investigators, dual interpretation by the same observer on two occasions or by two different observers decreases by at least one third the number of positive films missed.[276]

The time during which a roentgenogram is viewed is also important. In one study in which viewing time and the detection of pulmonary lesions were correlated, the following conclusions were reached:[281] (1) a substantial proportion of subtle lung lesions are missed, even with unlimited viewing time; (2) a large proportion of obvious lung cancers are detected with flash viewing; (3) the detectability of lesions decreases considerably as viewing time becomes less than 4 seconds; and (4) differences in detectability are exaggerated by short viewing times.

The enormous increase in the use of roentgenologic services has resulted in a significant increase in the number of examinations each roentgenologist may be required to report. The inevitable result is reader "fatigue" and, consequently, an increased likelihood of error. No experienced roentgenologist denies the diminution in visual and mental acuity that develops during the day when the workload necessitates a heavy reporting schedule. Each individual must set his or her own standards, but two mechanisms may be employed to reduce reader fatigue to a minimum: frequent rest periods away from the viewbox and the establishment of a reasonable maximal number of examinations to be reported each day.

Finally, the atmosphere in which reporting is carried out deserves attention. Quiet surroundings, away from distracting influences, are most desirable for necessary thought and reflection. Viewing facilities should be optimal, the illuminator ideally being regarded as one of the most important pieces of apparatus in any department of roentgenology; despite this, all too often this item is the least expensive in the department, and insufficient attention is paid to such aspects as light intensity and background illumination.

---

*The Valsalva maneuver consists of forced expiration against a closed glottis and the Müller maneuver of inspiration against a closed glottis. For proper hemodynamic effect, pressures of ± 40 to 50 cm H_2O, respectively, should be maintained for 7 to 10 seconds. For roentgenograms to be comparable, both maneuvers should be performed at the same degree of lung inflation, preferably at the end of a quiet inspiration.

Threshold Visibility

In a study in which Lucite discs were employed as test objects,[282] it was found that a structure of unit density must be at least 3 mm in thickness to be roentgenographically visible. By contrast, another investigation found that roentgenologists could locate the shadows of lucite balls regularly if the balls were at least 1 to 2 cm in diameter[283]; balls 0.6 cm in diameter could be located only when projected over intercostal spaces, and those as small as 0.3 cm could be identified only in retrospect. The difference between the figures of the two studies lies in the character of the *border* of the shadow: the 3-mm measurement found in the first investigation applies only to lesions in which borders are sharply defined; lesions with indistinctly defined or beveled margins (e.g., a sphere) must be substantially greater than 3 mm in diameter to be roentgenographically visible.

These limits of visibility apply to individual shadows within the lung rather than to the multiple nodular opacities produced, for example, by miliary tuberculosis. In the latter instance, summation of images becomes important. According to this concept, the wide distribution of a large number of small lesions throughout the lungs allows visibility of individual deposits only when they are *not* summated; when summation does occur, the appreciation of individual deposits is lost through blurring.[284] It should be noted, however, that some investigators believe that objects of subliminal absorption may be brought above threshold by summation of their shadows.[282]

Certain objective reasons for missing lesions during roentgenologic interpretation have been clarified by studies in which postmortem roentgenography of the chest has been correlated with subsequent morphologic study of the lungs. In one such study, the lesions most often missed were small calcified or uncalcified nodules 3 mm or slightly more in diameter in the region of the pleura or subpleural parenchyma.[285] Many nodules of metastatic cancer measuring up to 1 cm in diameter also were not identified. Two areas were identified in which it was difficult to project a lesion so that it was related to air-containing parenchyma without a superimposed confusion of overlaying bones and major blood vessels: over the convexity of the lungs in close proximity to the pleura and rib cage, and in the paramediastinal regions, where the shadows of the aorta, heart, and spine are quite dense. Lesions in close proximity to the diaphragm probably come within the same category. Clearly, it is important to be aware of these relatively "blind" areas in the thorax and to pay particular attention to them in the development of a scanning routine.

Another area of particular importance in the interpretation of chest roentgenograms is the tissue outside the limits of the thorax. The importance to diagnosis of such abnormalities as hepatomegaly or splenomegaly, displacement or alteration in the contour of the gastric air bubble, and calcification within the thoracic soft tissues, liver, or spleen cannot be overstressed. Finally, we have been repeatedly impressed by the information to be gained from thorough inspection of the "corners and borders" of roentgenograms. In most departments, the name and age of the patient is inscribed thereon by photographic imprinting, particulars which should be noted for definite identification; similarly, an appreciation of dextrocardia or transposition of the thoracic and abdominal viscera may depend on the position of the "right" or "left" marker.

References

1. Horsfield K, Cumming G: Morphology of the bronchial tree in man. J Appl Physiol 24: 373, 1968.
2. Gail DB, Lenfant CJM: State of the art: Cells of the lung, biology and clinical implications. Am Rev Respir Dis 127: 366, 1983.
3. Kilburn KH: A hypothesis for pulmonary clearance and its implications. Am Rev Respir Dis 98: 449, 1968.
4. Kuhn C: Ciliated and Clara cells. In Bouhuys A (ed): Lung Cells in Disease. New York, Elsevier North-Holland Biomedical Pr., 1976, p 91.
5. Lumsden AB, McLean A, Lamb D: Goblet and Clara cells of human distal airways: Evidence for smoking-induced changes in their numbers. Thorax 39: 844, 1984.
6. Breuer R, Zajicek G, Christensen TG, et al: Cell kinetics of normal adult hamster bronchial epithelium in the steady state. Am J Respir Cell Mol Biol 2: 51, 1990.
7. Evans MJ, Cox RA, Shami SG, et al: The role of basal cells in attachment of columnar cells to the basal lamina of the trachea. Am J Respir Cell Mol Biol 1: 463, 1989.
8. Inayama Y, Hook GER, Brody AR, et al: The differentiation potential of tracheal basal cells. Lab Invest 58: 706, 1988.
9. Lane BP, Gordon R: Regeneration of rat tracheal epithelium after mechanical injury: I. The relationship between mitotic activity and cellular differentiation. Proc Soc Exp Biol Med 145: 1139, 1974.
10. Evans MJ, Cabral-Anderson LJ, Freeman G: Role of the Clara cell in renewal of the bronchiolar epithelium. Lab Invest 38: 648, 1978.
11. DeWater R, Willems LNA, Van Muijen GNP, et al: Ultrastructural localization of bronchial antileukoprotease in central and peripheral human airways by a gold-labeling technique using monoclonal antibodies. Am Rev Respir Dis 133: 882, 1986.
12. Johnson DE, Georgieff MK: Pulmonary neuroendocrine cells: Their secretory products and their potential roles in health and chronic lung disease in infancy. Am Rev Respir Dis 140: 1807, 1989.
13. Cutz E: Neuroendocrine cells of the lung: An overview of morphologic characteristics and development. Exp Lung Res 3: 185, 1982.
14. Keith IM, Will JA: Hypoxia and the neonatal rabbit lung: Neuroendocrine cell numbers, 5-HT fluorescence intensity, and the relationship to arterial thickness. Thorax 36: 767, 1981.
15. Lauweryns JM, Cokelaere M, Theunynck P: Serotonin producing neuroepithelial bodies in rabbit respiratory mucosa. Science 180: 410, 1973.
16. Krahl VE: Anatomy of the mammalian lung. In Fenn WO, Rahn H (eds): Handbook of Physiology. Section 3, Respiration. Vol 1. Washington, DC, American Physiological Society, 1964, pp 213–284.
17. Ebina M, Yaegashi H, Takahashi T, et al: Distribution of smooth muscles along the bronchial tree: A morphometric study of ordinary autopsy lungs. Am Rev Respir Dis 141: 1322, 1990.
18. Whimster WF, Lord P, Biles B: Tracheobronchial gland profiles in four segmental airways. Am Rev Respir Dis 129: 985, 1984.
19. Mooren HWD, Meyer CJLM, Kramps JA, et al: Ultrastructural localization of the low molecular weight protease inhibitor in human bronchial glands. J Histochem Cytochem 30: 1130, 1982.
20. Wiggins J, Hill SL, Stockley RA: Lung secretion sol-phase proteins: Comparison of sputum with secretions obtained by direct sampling. Thorax 38: 102, 1983.
21. Brandtzaeg P: Mucosal and glandular distribution of immunoglobulin components: Differential localization of free and bound SC in secretory epithelial cells. J Immunol 112: 1553, 1974.
22. Bienenstock J, Clancy RL, Perey DYE: Bronchus-associated lymphoid tissue (BALT): Its relationship to mucosal immunity. In Kirkpatrick CH, Reynolds HY (eds): Immunologic and Infectious Reactions in the Lung. New York, Marcel Dekker, 1976, p 29.
23. Emery JL, Dinsdale F: The postnatal development of lymphoreticular aggregates and lymph nodes in infants' lungs. J Clin Pathol 26: 539, 1973.
24. Soutar CA: Distribution of plasma cells and other cells containing immunoglobulin in the respiratory tract of normal man and class of immunoglobulin contained therein. Thorax 31: 158, 1976.
25. Schreider JP, Raabe OG: Structure of the human respiratory acinus. Am J Anat 162: 221, 1981.

26. Angus GE, Thurlbeck WM: Number of alveoli in the human lung. J Appl Physiol 32: 483, 1972.
27. Thurlbeck WM: The internal surface area of nonemphysematous lungs. Am Rev Respir Dis 95: 765, 1967.
28. Crapo JD, Barry BE, Gehr P, et al: Cell number and cell characteristics of the normal human lung. Am Rev Respir Dis 125: 332, 1982.
29. Bartels H: The air-blood barrier in the human lung: A freeze-fracture study. Cell Tissue Res 198: 269, 1979.
30. Schneeberger EE: The integrity of the air-blood barrier. In Brain JD, Proctor DR, Reid LM (eds): Respiratory Defense Mechanisms. New York, Marcel Dekker, 1977, p 687.
31. Heppleston AG, Young AE: Uptake of inert particulate matter by alveolar cells: An ultrastructural study. J Pathol 111: 159, 1973.
32. Kikkawa Y, Smith F: Biology of disease. Cellular and biochemical aspects of pulmonary surfactant in health and disease. Lab Invest 49: 122, 1983.
33. Kikkawa Y: Morphology of alveolar lining layer. Anat Rec 167: 389, 1970.
34. Gil J, Weibel ER: Improvements in demonstration of lining layer of lung alveoli by electron microscopy. Respir Physiol 8: 13, 1969.
35. Crystal RG: Biochemical processes in the normal lung. In Bouhuys A (ed): Lung Cells in Disease. New York, Elsevier North-Holland Biomedical Pr., 1976, p 17.
36. Paine R III, Mody CH, Chavis A, et al: Alveolar epithelial cells block lymphocyte proliferation in vitro without inhibiting activation. Am J Respir Cell Mol Biol 5: 221, 1991.
37. Starcher BC: Elastin and the lung. Thorax 41: 577, 1986.
38. Laurent GJ: Lung collagen: More than scaffolding. Thorax 41: 418, 1986.
39. Kapanci Y, Assimacopoulos A, Irle C, et al: "Contractile interstitial cells" in pulmonary alveolar septa: A possible regulator of ventilation/perfusion ratio? J Cell Biol 60: 375, 1974.
40. Weibel ER, Bachofen H: Structural design of the alveolar septum and fluid exchange. In Fishman AP, Renkin EM (eds): Pulmonary Edema. Bethesda, MD, American Physiological Society, 1979, p 1.
41. Dehring DJ, Wismar BL: Intravascular macrophages in pulmonary capillaries of humans. Am Rev Respir Dis 139: 1027, 1989.
42. Hocking WG, Golde DW: The pulmonary-alveolar macrophage (first of two parts). N Engl J Med 301: 580, 1979.
43. Adamson IYR, Bowden DH: Role of monocytes and interstitial cells in the generation of alveolar macrophages. II. Kinetic studies after carbon loading. Lab Invest 42: 518, 1980.
44. Sibille Y, Reynolds HY: Macrophages and polymorphonuclear leucocytes in lung defense and injury. Am Rev Respir Dis 141: 471, 1990.
45. Shellito J, Kaltreider HB: Heterogeneity of immunologic function among subfractions of normal rat alveolar macrophages. Am Rev Respir Dis 131: 678, 1985.
46. Lehnert BE, Valdez YE, Stewart CC: Translocation of particles to the tracheobronchial lymph nodes after lung deposition: Kinetics and particle-cell relationships. Exp Lung Res 10: 245, 1986.
47. Kovacs EJ, Delley J: Lymphokine regulation of macrophage-derived growth factor secretion following pulmonary injury. Am J Pathol 121: 261, 1985.
48. Villiger B, Broekelmann T, Kelley D, et al: Bronchoalveolar fibronectin in smokers and nonsmokers. Am Rev Respir Dis 124: 652, 1981.
49. Hsueh W: Prostaglandin biosynthesis in pulmonary macrophages. Am J Pathol 97: 137, 1979.
50. Nugent KM, Glazier J, Monick MM, et al: Stimulated human alveolar macrophages secrete interferon. Am Rev Respir Dis 131: 714, 1985.
51. Green GM: Lung defense mechanisms. Med Clin North Am 57: 547, 1973.
52. Green GM, Carolin D: The depressant effect of cigarette smoke on the in vitro antibacterial activity of alveolar macrophages. N Engl J Med 276: 421, 1967.
53. Heitzman ER, Markarian B, Berger I, et al: The secondary pulmonary lobule: A practical concept for interpretation of chest radiographs. I. Roentgen anatomy of the normal secondary pulmonary lobule. Radiology 93: 507, 1969.
54. Bergin C, Roggli V, Coblentz C, et al: The secondary pulmonary lobule: Normal and abnormal CT appearances. Am J Roentgenol 151: 21, 1988.
55. Hansen JE, Ampaya EP: Human air space shapes, sizes, areas, and volumes. J Appl Physiol 38: 990, 1975.
56. Gamsu G, Thurlbeck WM, Macklem PT, et al: Roentgenographic

57. Takaro T, Gaddy LR, Parra S: Thin alveolar epithelial partitions across connective tissue gaps in the alveolar wall of the human lung: Ultrastructural observations. Am Rev Respir Dis 126: 326, 1982.
58. Takaro T, Price HP, Parra SC: Ultrastructure studies of apertures in the interalveolar septum of the adult human lung. Am Rev Respir Dis 119: 425, 1979.
59. Pump KK: Fenestrae in the alveolar membrane of the human lung. Chest 65: 431, 1974.
60. Lambert MW: Accessory bronchiole-alveolar communications. J Pathol Bacteriol 70: 311, 1955.
61. Boyden EA: Segmental Anatomy of the Lungs. New York, McGraw-Hill, 1955.
62. Jackson CL, Huber JF: Correlated applied anatomy of the bronchial tree and lungs with system of nomenclature. Dis Chest 9: 319, 1943.
63. Naidich DP, Zinn WL, Ettenger NA, et al: Basilar segmental bronchi: Thin-section CT evaluation. Radiology 169: 11, 1988.
64. Lee KS, Bae WK, Lee BH, et al: Bronchovascular anatomy of the upper lobes: Evaluation with thin-section CT. Radiology 181: 765, 1991.
64a. Gamsu G, Webb WR: Computed tomography of the trachea: Normal and abnormal. Am J Roentgenol 139: 321, 1982.
64b. Breatnach E, Abbott GC, Fraser RG: Dimensions of the normal human trachea. Am J Roentgenol 141: 903, 1984.
65. Haskin PH, Goodman LR: Normal tracheal bifurcation angle: A reassessment. Am J Roentgenol 139: 879, 1982.
66. Fraser RG: Measurements of the caliber of human bronchi in three phases of respiration by cinebronchography. J Can Assoc Radiol 12: 102, 1961.
67. Jesseph JE, Merendino KA: The dimensional interrelationships of the major components of the human tracheobronchial tree. Surg Gynecol Obstet 105: 210, 1957.
68. Mead J: Mechanical properties of lungs. Physiol Rev 41: 281, 1961.
69. Islam MS: Mechanisms of controlling residual volume and emptying rate of the lung in young and elderly health subjects. Respiratory 40: 1, 1980.
70. King RJ: Pulmonary surfactant. J Appl Physiol 53: 1, 1982.
71. Albert RK, Lakshminarayan S, Hildebrandt J, et al: Increased surface tension favors pulmonary edema formation in anesthetized dogs' lungs. J Clin Invest 63: 115, 1979.
72. Smaldone GC, Mitzner W, Itoh H: Role of alveolar recruitment in lung inflation: Influence on pressure-volume hysteresis. J Appl Physiol 55: 1321, 1983.
73. Massaro GD, Massaro D: Morphologic evidence that large inflations of the lung stimulate secretion of surfactant. Am Rev Respir Dis 127: 235, 1983.
74. Corbet A, Cregan J, Frink J, et al: Distention-produced phospholipid secretion in postmortem in situ lungs of newborn rabbits: Inhibition by specific beta-adrenergic blockade. Am Rev Respir Dis 128: 695, 1983.
75. Lisboa C, Ross WRD, Jardim J, et al: Pulmonary pressure-flow curves measured by a data-averaging circuit. J Appl Physiol 47: 621, 1979.
76. Macklem PT, Mead J: Resistance of central and peripheral airways measured by a retrograde catheter. J Appl Physiol 22: 395, 1967.
77. Ferris BG, Mead J, Opie LH: Partitioning of respiratory flow resistance in man. J Appl Physiol 19: 653, 1964.
78. Menkes HA, Traystman RJ: Collateral ventilation, lung disease. In Murray J (ed): Lung Disease—State of the Art. New York, American Lung Association, 1978, p 87.
79. Inners CR, Terry PB, Traystman RJ, et al: Effects of lung volume on collateral and airways resistance in man. J Appl Physiol 46: 67, 1979.
80. Keal EE: Physiological and pharmacological control of airway secretion. In Brain JD, Proctor DF, Reid LM (eds): Respiratory Defense Mechanisms—Part I. Lung Biology in Health and Disease. Vol 5. New York, Marcel Dekker, 1977, pp 357–401.
81. King M: Mucus and mucociliary clearance. Basic Resp Dis 11: 1, 1982.
82. Low RB, Davis GS, Giancola MS: Biochemical analyses of bronchoalveolar lavage fluids of healthy human volunteer smokers and non-smokers. Am Rev Respir Dis 118: 863, 1978.
83. Szabo S, Barbu Z, Lakatos L, et al: Local production of proteins in normal human bronchial secretion. Respiration 39: 172, 1980.
84. Lopez-Vidriero MT, Das I, Reid LM: Airway secretion: Source, bio-

chemical and rheological properties. *In* Brain JD, Proctor DF, Reid LM (eds): Respiratory Defense Mechanisms—Part I. Lung Biology in Health and Disease. Vol 5. New York, Marcel Dekker, 1977, p 389.

85. Ueki I, German VF, Nadel JA: Micropipette measurement of airway submucosal gland secretion—autonomic effects. Am Rev Respir Dis 121: 351, 1980.

86. Nadel JA: New approaches to regulation of fluid secretion in airways. Chest 80: 849, 1981.

87. Sleigh MA: The nature and action of respiratory tract cilia. *In* Brain JD, Proctor DF, Reid LM (eds): Respiratory Defense Mechanisms—Part I. Lung Biology in Health and Disease. Vol 5. New York, Marcel Dekker, 1977, pp 247–288.

88. Widdicombe JH, Ueki IF, Bruderman I, et al: The effects of sodium substitution and ouabain on ion transport by dog tracheal epithelium. Am Rev Respir Dis 120: 385, 1979.

89. Widdicombe JH, Welsh MJ: Ion transport by dog tracheal epithelium. Fed Proc 39: 3062, 1980.

90. Lopez-Vidriero MT, Das I, Smith AP, et al: Bronchial secretion from normal human airways after inhalation of prostaglandin F₂, acetylcholine, histamine, and citric acid. Thorax 32: 734, 1977.

91. Adler K, Wooten O, Philippoff W, et al: Physical properties of sputum. III. Rheologic variability and intrinsic relationships. Am Rev Respir Dis 106: 86, 1972.

92. Satir P: How cilia move. Sci Am 231: 45, 1974.

93. Mossberg B, Strandbert K, Camner P: Stimulatory effect of beta-adrenergic drugs on mucociliary transport. Scand J Respir Dis (Suppl) 101: 71, 1977.

94. McEvoy RD, Davies NJ, Hedenstierna G, et al: Lung mucociliary transport during high-frequency ventilation. Am Rev Respir Dis 126: 452, 1982.

95. Chopra SK, Taplin GV, Simmons DH, et al: Effects of hydration and physical therapy on tracheal transport velocity. Am Rev Respir Dis 115: 1009, 1977.

96. King M, Phillips DM, Gross D, et al: Enhanced tracheal mucus clearance with high frequency chest wall compression. Am Rev Respir Dis 128: 511, 1983.

97. Horsfield K: Morphometry of the small pulmonary arteries in man. Circ Res 42: 593, 1978.

98. Weibel ER: On pericytes, particularly their existence on lung capillaries. Microvasc Res 8: 218, 1974.

99. Nadziejko CE, Loud AV, Kikkawa Y: Effect of alveolar hypoxia on pulmonary mast cells in vivo. Am Rev Respir Dis 140: 743, 1989.

100. Schraufnagel DE, Patel KR: Sphincters in pulmonary veins: An anatomic study in rats. Am Rev Respir Dis 141: 721, 1990.

101. Heath D, Smith P: The pulmonary endothelial cell. Thorax 34: 200, 1979.

102. Ryan US, Ryan JW, Whitaker C, et al: Localization of angiotensin-converting enzyme (kininase II). II. Immunocytochemistry and immunofluorescence. Tissue Cell 8: 125, 1976.

103. Smith U, Ryan JW: Substructural features of pulmonary endothelial caveolae. Tissue Cell 4: 49, 1972.

104. Pietra GG, Sampson P, Lanken PN, et al: Transcapillary movement of cationized ferritin in the isolated perfused rat lung. Lab Invest 49: 54, 1983.

105. Assimacopoulos A, Guggenheim R, Kapanci Y: Changes in alveolar capillary configuration at different levels of lung inflation in the rat: An ultrastructural and morphometric study. Lab Invest 34: 10, 1976.

106. Weibel ER: Morphometry of the Human Lung. New York, Academic Press, 1963.

107. Glazier JB, Hughes JMB, Maloney JE, et al: Measurements of capillary dimensions and blood volume in rapidly frozen lungs. J Appl Physiol 26: 65, 1969.

108. Woodring JH: Pulmonary artery–bronchus ratios in patients with normal lungs, pulmonary vascular plethora, and congestive heart failure. Radiology 179: 115, 1991.

109. Chang CH (Joseph): The normal roentgenographic measurement of the right descending pulmonary artery in 1085 cases. Am J Roentgenol 87: 929, 1962.

110. Wójtowicz J: Some tomographic criteria for an evaluation of the pulmonary circulation. Acta Radiol (Diagn) 2: 215, 1964.

111. Burko H, Carwell G, Newman E: Size, location, and gravitational changes of normal upper lobe pulmonary veins. Am J Roentgenol 111: 687, 1971.

112. Heitzman ER: The Mediastinum: Radiologic Correlations with Anatomy and Pathology. St. Louis, CV Mosby, 1977, pp 216–334.

113. Fraser RG, Fraser RS, Renner JW, et al: The roentgenographic diagnosis of chronic bronchitis: A reassessment with emphasis on parahilar bronchi seen end-on. Radiology 120: 1, 1976.

114. Simon G: Principles of Chest X-Ray Diagnosis. 3rd ed. London, Butterworth, 1971.

115. Proto AV, Speckman JM: The left lateral radiograph of the chest. 1. Med Radiogr Photogr 55: 30, 1979.

116. Proto AV, Speckman JM: The left lateral radiograph of the chest. 2. Med Radiogr Photogr 56: 38, 1980.

117. Schnur MJ, Winkler B, Austin JHM: Widening of the posterior wall of the bronchus intermedius: A sign on lateral chest radiographs of congestive heart failure, lymph node enlargement, and neoplastic infiltration. Radiology 139: 551, 1981.

118. Webb WR, Gamsu G: Computed tomography of the left retrobronchial stripe. J Comput Assist Tomogr 7: 65, 1983.

119. Lang EV, Friedman PJ: The anterior wall stripe of the left lower lobe bronchus on the lateral chest radiograph: CT correlative study. Am J Roentgenol 154: 33, 1990.

120. Naidich DP, Khouri NF, Scott WW, et al: Computed tomography of the pulmonary hila: Normal anatomy. J Comput Assist Tomogr 5: 459, 1981.

121. Webb WR, Glazier G, Gamsu G: Computed tomography of the abnormal pulmonary hilum. J Comput Assist Tomogr 5: 485, 1981.

122. Itoh H, Murata K, Todo G, et al: Anatomy of pulmonary lung tissue in the hilum. Jpn J Clin Radiol 29: 1459, 1984.

123. Cohen AM, Creviston S, LiPuma JP, et al: NMR evaluation of hilar and mediastinal lymphadenopathy. Radiology 148: 739, 1983.

124. Gamsu G, Webb WR, Sheldon P, et al: Nuclear magnetic resonance imaging of the thorax. Radiology 147: 473, 1983.

125. Newman F, Smalley BF, Thomson ML: Effect of exercise, body and lung size on CO diffusion in athletes and nonathletes. J Appl Physiol 17: 649, 1962.

126. Hakim TS, Michel RP, Chang HK: Partitioning vascular resistance in dogs by arterial and venous occlusion. J Appl Physiol Respir Environ 52: 710, 1982.

127. West JB: Regional differences in the lung. Chest 74: 426, 1978.

128. Howell JBL, Permutt S, Proctor DF, et al: Effect of inflation of the lung on different parts of the pulmonary vascular bed. J Appl Physiol 16: 71, 1961.

129. Culver BH, Butler J: Mechanical influences on the pulmonary microcirculation. Annu Rev Physiol 42: 187, 1980.

130. Isawa T, Teshima T, Hirano T, et al: Regulation of regional perfusion distribution in the lungs: Effect of regional oxygen concentration. Am Rev Respir Dis 118: 55, 1978.

131. Marshall C, Marshall B: Site and sensitivity for stimulation of hypoxic pulmonary vasoconstriction. J Appl Physiol 55: 711, 1983.

132. Bergofsky EH, Lehr DE, Fishman AP: The effect of changes in hydrogen ion concentration on the pulmonary circulation. J Clin Invest 41: 1492, 1962.

133. Downing SE, Lee JC: Nervous control of the pulmonary circulation. Annu Rev Physiol 42: 199, 1980.

134. Bergofsky EH: Humoral control of the pulmonary circulation. Annu Rev Physiol 42: 221, 1980.

135. Georges R, Sauman G, Loiseau A: The relationship of age to pulmonary membrane conductance and capillary blood volume. Am Rev Respir Dis 117: 1069, 1978.

136. Milic-Emili J: Interregional distribution of inspired gas. Prog Respir Res 16: 33, 1981.

137. West JB, Dollery CT: Distribution of blood flow and ventilation-perfusion ratio in the lung, measured with radioactive CO₂. J Appl Physiol 15: 405, 1960.

138. Engel LA, Grassino A, Anthonisen NR: Demonstration of airway closure in man. J Appl Physiol 38: 1117, 1975.

139. Turek Z, Kreuzer F: Effects of shifts of the O₂ dissociation curve upon alveolar-arterial O₂ gradients in computer models of the lung with ventilation-perfusion mismatching. Respir Physiol 45: 133, 1981.

140. West JB: Ventilation-perfusion inequality and overall gas exchange in computer models of the lung. Respir Physiol 7: 88, 1969.

141. Wagner PD, Saltzman HA, West JB: Measurement of continuous distribution of ventilation-perfusion ratios: Theory. J Appl Physiol 36: 588, 1974.

142. Jones NL: Should we change our approach to acid-base physiology? Ann R Coll Phys Surg Can 23: 235, 1990.

143. Narins RG, Emmett N: Simple and mixed acid-base disorder: A practical approach. Medicine 59: 161, 1980.

144. Emmett M, Nairns RG: Clinical use of the anion gap. Medicine 56: 38, 1977.

145. Cudkowicz L: Bronchial arterial circulation in man: Normal anatomy and responses to disease. *In* Moser KM (ed): Pulmonary Vascular Diseases. New York, Marcel Dekker, 1979, p 111.

146. Murara K, Itoh H, Todo G, et al: Bronchial venous plexus and its communication with pulmonary circulation. Invest Radiol 21: 24, 1986.

147. Botenga ASJ: Selective Bronchial and Intercostal Arteriography. Leiden. HE, Stenfert Kroese, NV, 1970.

148. McFadden ET Jr: Respiratory heat and water exchange: Physiological and clinical implications. J Appl Physiol 54: 331, 1983.

149. Malik AB, Tracy SE: Bronchovascular adjustments after pulmonary embolism. J Appl Physiol 49: 476, 1980.

150. Baile EM, Ling H, Heyworth JR, et al: Bronchopulmonary anastomotic and non-coronary collateral blood flow in humans during cardiopulmonary bypass. Chest 87(6): 749, 1985.

151. Aabo K, Hansen KB: Megakaryocytes in pulmonary blood vessels. I. Incidence at autopsy: Clinicopathological relations especially to disseminated intravascular coagulation. Acta Pathol Microbiol Scand 86: 285, 1978.

152. Hogg JC: Neutrophil kinetics and lung injury. Physiol Rev 67: 1249, 1987.

153. Stuart BO: Deposition of inhaled aerosols. Arch Intern Med 131: 60, 1973.

154. Craighead JE, Mossman BT: The pathogenesis of asbestos-associated diseases. N Engl J Med 306: 1446, 1982.

155. Pinkerton KE, Plopper CG, Mercer RR, et al: Airway branching patterns influence asbestos fiber location and the extent of tissue injury in the pulmonary parenchyma. Lab Invest 55: 688, 1986.

156. Pityn P, Chamberlin MJ, Fraser TM, et al: The topography of particle deposition in the human lung. Respir Physiol 78: 19, 1989.

157. Sweeny TD, Brain JD, Leavitt SA, et al: Emphysema alters the deposition pattern of inhaled particles in hamsters. Am J Pathol 128: 19, 1987.

158. Swartenaren M, Philipson K, Linman L, et al: Regional deposition of particles in human lung after induced bronchoconstriction. Exp Lung Res 10: 223, 1986.

159. Proctor DF, Andersen I, Lundqvist G: Clearance of inhaled particles from the human nose. Arch Intern Med 131: 132, 1973.

160. Bohning DE, Atkins HL, Cohn SH: Long-term particle clearance in man: Normal and impaired. Ann Occup Hyg 26: 259, 1982.

161. Bienenstock J, Befus AD, McDermott M: Mucosal immunity. Monogr Allergy 16: 1, 1980.

162. Burnett D: Immunoglobulins in the lung. Thorax 41: 337, 1986.

163. Kaltreider HB, Byrd PK, Daughety TW, et al: The mechanism of appearance of specific antibody forming cells in lungs of inbred mice after intratracheal immunization with sheep erythrocytes. Am Rev Respir Dis 127: 316, 1983.

164. Caughey GH: The structure and airway biology of mast cell proteases. Am J Respir Cell Mol Biol 4: 387, 1991.

165. Becker KL: The endocrine lung. *In* Becker KL, Gazdar AF (eds): The Endocrine Lung in Health and Disease. Philadelphia, WB Saunders, 1984, p 3.

166. Fanburg BL: Prostaglandins and the lung. Am Rev Respir Dis 108: 482, 1973.

167. Hislop A, Reid L: Development of the acinus in the human lung. Thorax 29: 90, 1974.

168. Langston C, Kida K, Reed M, et al: Human lung growth in late gestation and in the neonate. Am Rev Respir Dis 129: 607, 1984.

169. Thurlbeck WM: Postnatal growth and development of the lung. Am Rev Respir Dis 111: 803, 1975.

170. Thurlbeck WM: Postnatal human lung growth. Thorax 37: 564, 1982.

171. Cagle PT, Thurlbeck WM: Postpneumonectomy compensatory lung growth. Am Rev Respir Dis 138: 1314, 1988.

172. Hislop A, Reid L: Pulmonary arterial development during childhood: Branching pattern and structure. Thorax 28: 129, 1973.

173. Hislop A, Reid L: Fetal and childhood development of the intrapulmonary veins in man: Branching pattern and structure. Thorax 28: 313, 1973.

174. Kida K, Fujino Y, Thurlbeck WM: A comparison of lung structure in male DBA and C57 black mice and their F1 offspring. Am Rev Respir Dis 139: 1238, 1989.

175. Smith BT, Fletcher WA: Pulmonary epithelial-mesenchymal interactions: Beyond organogenesis. Hum Pathol 10: 248, 1979.

176. Adamson IYR, King GM: Sex differences in development of fetal rat lung. II. Quantitative morphology of epithelial-mesenchymal interactions. Lab Invest 50: 461, 1984.

177. Adamson IYR, King GM: L-Azetidine-2-carboxylic acid retards lung growth and surfactant synthesis in fetal rats. Lab Invest 57: 439, 1987.

178. Liggins GC, Vilos GA, Campos GA, et al: The effect of spinal cord transection on lung development in fetal sheep. J Dev Physiol 3: 267, 1981.

179. Pinkerton KE, Kendall JZ, Randall GC, et al: Hypophysectomy and porcine fetal lung development. Am J Respir Cell Mol Biol 1: 319, 1989.

180. Castleman WL: Alterations in pulmonary ultrastructure and morphometric parameters induced by parainfluenza (Sendai) virus in rats during postnatal growth. Am J Pathol 114: 322, 1984.

181. Das RM: The effects of intermittent starvation on lung development in suckling rats. Am J Pathol 117: 326, 1984.

182. Laitinen A: Ultrastructural organization of intraepithelial nerves in the human airway tract. Thorax 40: 488, 1985.

183. Sant'Ambrogio G: Information arising from the tracheobronchial tree of mammals. Physiol Rev 62: 531, 1982.

184. Hung K-S, Hertweck MS, Hardy JD, et al: Electron microscopic observations of nerve endings in the alveolar walls of mouse lungs. Am Rev Respir Dis 108: 328, 1973.

185. Nadel JA, Barnes PJ: Autonomic regulation of the airways. Annu Rev Med 35: 451, 1984.

186. Barnes PJ: The third nervous system in the lung: Physiology and clinical perspective. Thorax 39: 561, 1984.

187. Wang N-S: Anatomy and physiology of the pleural space. Symposium on Pleural Disease. Clin Chest Med 6: 3, 1985.

188. Pistolesi M, Miniati M, Giuntini C: Pleural liquid and solute exchange. Am Rev Respir Dis 140: 825, 1989.

189. Jung-Gi I, Webb WR, Rosen A, et al: Costal pleura: Appearances at high-resolution CT. Radiology 171: 125, 1989.

190. Raasch BN, Carsky EW, Lane EJ, et al: Radiographic anatomy of the interlobar fissures: A study of 100 specimens. Am J Roentgenol 138: 1043, 1982.

191. Glazer HS, Anderson DJ, DiCroce JJ, et al: Anatomy of the major fissure: Evaluation with standard and thin-section CT. Radiology 180: 839, 1991.

192. Proto AV, Ball JB: Computed tomography of the major and minor fissures. Am J Roentgenol 140: 439, 1983.

193. Gale ME, Greif WL: Intrafissural fat: CT correlation with chest radiography. Radiology 160: 333, 1986.

194. Felson B: Chest Roentgenology. Philadelphia, WB Saunders, 1973.

195. Berkmen YM, Auh YH, Davis SD, et al: Anatomy of the minor fissure: Evaluation with thin-section CT. Radiology 170: 647, 1989.

196. Goodman LR, Golkow RS, Steiner RM, et al: The right mid-lung window: A potential source of error in computed tomography of the lung. Radiology 143: 135, 1982.

197. Rabinowitz JG, Cohen BA, Mendleson DS: The pulmonary ligament. Radiol Clin North Am 22: 659, 1984.

198. Rost RC, Proto AV: Inferior pulmonary ligament: Computed tomographic appearance. Radiology 14: 479, 1983.

199. Mata J, Cáceres J, Alegret X, et al: Imaging of the azygos lobe: Normal anatomy and variations. Am J Roentgenol 156: 931, 1991.

200. Austin JHM: The left minor fissure. Radiology 161: 433, 1986.

201. Black LF: The pleural space and pleural fluid. Mayo Clin Proc 47: 493, 1972.

202. Lauweryns JM, Baert JH: Alveolar clearance and the role of the pulmonary lymphatics: State of the art. Am Rev Respir Dis 115: 625, 1977.

203. Hendin AS, Greenspan RH: Ventilatory pumping of human pulmonary lymphatic vessels. Radiology 108: 553, 1973.

204. Rosenberger A, Abrams HL: Radiology of the thoracic duct. Am J Roentgenol 11: 807, 1971.

205. Heitzman ER: Royal College Lecture: Radiologic diagnosis of mediastinal lymph node enlargement. J Can Assoc Radiol 29: 151, 1978.

206. Glazer GM, Gross BH, Quint LE, et al: Normal mediastinal lymph nodes: Number and size according to American Thoracic Society mapping. Am J Roentgenol 144: 261, 1985.

207. Sone S, Higashihara T, Morimoto S, et al: CT anatomy of hilar lymphadenopathy. Am J Roentgenol 140: 887, 1983.

208. Genereux GP, Howie JL: Normal mediastinal lymph node size and number: CT and anatomic study. Am J Roentgenol 142: 1095, 1984.

209. Glazer GM, Orringer MB, Gross BH, et al: The mediastinum in non-small cell lung cancer: CT-surgical correlation. Am J Roentgenol 152: 1101, 1984.
210. Heelan RT, Martini N, Wescott JW, et al: Carcinomatous involvement of the hilum and mediastinum: Computed tomographic and magnetic resonance evaluation. Radiology 156: 111, 1985.
211. Webb WR, Jensen BG, Solitto R, et al: Bronchogenic carcinoma: Staging with MR compared with staging with CT and surgery. Radiology 156: 117, 1985.
212. Rouvière H: Anatomy of the Human Lymphatic System (translated by MJ Tobias). Ann Arbor, MI, Edwards, 1983.
213. Baird JA: The pathways of lymphatic spread of carcinoma of the lung. Br J Surg 52: 868, 1965.
214. Proto AV, Simmons JD, Zylak CJ: The anterior junction anatomy. CRC Crit Rev Diagn Imaging 19: 111, 1983.
215. Proto AV, Simmons JD, Zylak CJ: The posterior junction anatomy. CRC Crit Rev Diagn Imaging 20: 121, 1983.
216. Felson B: The mediastinum. Semin Roentgenol 4: 31, 1969.
217. Oliphant M, Wiot JF, Whalen JP: The cervicothoracic continuum. Radiology 120: 257, 1976.
218. Baron RL, Lee JKT, Sagel SS, et al: Computed tomography of the normal thymus. Radiology 142: 121, 1982.
219. de Geer G, Webb WR, Gamsu G: Normal thymus: Assessment with MR and CT. Radiology 158: 313, 1986.
220. Jemelin C, Candardjis G: Retrosternal soft tissue: Quantitative evaluation and clinical interest. Radiology 109: 7, 1973.
221. Proto AV, Corcoran HL, Ball JB Jr: The left paratracheal reflection. Radiology 171: 625, 1989.
222. Raider L, Landry BA, Brogdon BG: The retrotracheal triangle. Radiographics 10: 1055, 1990.
223. Ball JB Jr, Proto AV: The variable appearance of the left superior intercostal vein. Radiology 144: 445, 1982.
224. Friedman AC, Chambers E, Sprayregen S: The normal and abnormal left superior intercostal vein. Am J Roentgenol 131: 599, 1978.
225. Genereux GP: The posterior pleural reflections. Am J Roentgenol 141: 141, 1983.
226. Savoca CJ, Austin JHM, Goldberg HI: The right paratracheal stripe. Radiology 122: 295, 1977.
227. Proto AV, Speckman JM: The left lateral radiograph of the chest. Med Radiogr Photogr 55(1), 1979.
228. Palayew MJ: The tracheo-esophageal stripe and the posterior tracheal band. Radiology 132: 11, 1979.
229. Kittredge RD: The right posterolateral tracheal band. J Comput Assist Tomogr 3: 348, 1979.
230. Proto AV, Lane EJ: Air in the esophagus: A frequent radiographic finding. Am J Roentgenol 129: 433, 1977.
231. Keats TE, Lipscomb GE, Betts CS III: Mensuration of the arch of the azygos vein and its application to the study of cardiopulmonary disease. Radiology 90: 990, 1968.
232. Doyle FH, Read AE, Evans KT: The mediastinum in portal hypertension. Clin Radiol 12: 114, 1961.
233. Milne ENC, Pistolesi M, Miniati M, et al: The vascular pedicle of the heart and the vena azygos. Part I: The normal subject. Radiology 152: 1, 1984.
234. Pistolesi M, Milne ENC, Miniati M, et al: The vascular pedicle of the heart and the vena azygos. Part II: Acquired heart disease. Radiology 152: 9, 1984.
235. Milne E, Imray TJ, Pistolesi M, et al: The vascular pedicle and the vena azygos. Part III: In trauma—the "vanishing" azygos. Radiology 153: 25, 1984.
236. Heitzman ER, Scrivani JV, Martino J, et al: The azygos vein and its pleural reflections. 1. Normal roentgen anatomy. Radiology 101: 249, 1971.
237. Onitsuka H, Kuhns LR: Dextroconvexity of the mediastinum in the azygoesophageal recess. Radiology 135: 126, 1980.
238. Gammill SL, Krebs C, Meyers P, et al: Cardiac measurements in systole and diastole. Radiology 94: 115, 1970.
239. Lugliani R, Whipp BJ, Seard C, et al: Effect of bilateral carotid body resection on ventilatory control at rest and during exercise in man. N Engl J Med 285: 1105, 1971.
240. Biscoe TJ, Willshaw P: Stimulus-response relationships of the peripheral arterial chemoreceptors. In Hornbein TF, Lenfant C (eds): Regulation of Breathing, Part One. Lung Biology in Health and Disease. New York, Marcel Dekker, 1981.
241. Widdicombe JG: Nervous receptors in the respiratory tract and lungs. In Hornbein TF, Lenfant C (eds): Regulation of Breathing. Part One. Lung Biology in Health and Disease. New York, Marcel Dekker, 1981, p 429.
242. Duron B: Intercostal and diaphragmatic muscle endings and afferents. In Hornbein TF, Lenfant C (eds): Regulation of Breathing, Part One. Lung Biology in Health and Disease. New York, Marcel Dekker, 1981, p 473.
243. Berger AJ, Mitchell RA, Severinghaus JW: Regulation of respiration (second of three parts). N Engl J Med 297: 138, 1977.
244. Martin J, Aubier M, Engel LA: Effects of inspiratory loading on respiratory muscle activity during expiration. Am Rev Respir Dis 125: 352, 1982.
245. Phillipson EA, McClean PA, Sullivan CE, et al: Interaction of metabolic and behavioural respiratory control during hypercapnia and speech. Am Rev Respir Dis 117: 903, 1978.
246. Milic-Emili J: Recent advances in clinical assessment of control of breathing. Lung 160: 1, 1982.
247. Leitch AG: The hypoxic drive to breathing in man. Lancet 1: 428, 1981.
248. Schoene RB: Control of ventilation in climbers to extreme altitude. J Appl Physiol 53: 886, 1982.
249. Cherniak NS, Altose MD: Respiratory responses in ventilatory loading. In Hornbein TF, Lenfant C (eds): Regulation of Breathing, Part Two. Lung Biology in Health and Disease. New York, Marcel Dekker, 1981, p 905.
250. Killian KJ, Campbell EJM: Dyspnea and exercise. Annu Rev Physiol 45: 465, 1983.
251. Douglas NJ, White DP, Pickett CK, et al: Respiration during sleep in normal man. Thorax 37: 840, 1982.
252. Strohl KP: Upper airway muscles of respiration. Am Rev Respir Dis 124: 211, 1981.
253. Sharp JT: Respiratory muscles: A review of old and newer concepts. Lung 157: 185, 1980.
254. De Troyer A, Sampson M, Sigrist S, et al: The diaphragm: Two muscles. Science 213: 237, 1981.
255. Belman MJ, Sieck GS: The ventilatory muscles—fatigue, endurance and training. Chest 82: 761, 1982.
256. Comtois A, Gorczyca W, Grassino A: Microscopic anatomy of the arterial diaphragmatic circulation. Clin Invest Med 7: 81, 1984.
257. Rochester DF, Briscoe AM: Metabolism of the working diaphragm. Am Rev Respir Dis 119: 101, 1979.
258. Leak LV: Gross and ultrastructural morphologic features of the diaphragm. Am Rev Respir Dis 119(Suppl): 3, 1979.
259. Lennon EA, Simon G: The height of the diaphragm in the chest radiograph of normal adults. Br J Radiol 38: 937, 1965.
260. Young DA, Simon G: Certain movements measured on inspiration-expiration chest radiographs correlated with pulmonary function studies. Clin Radiol 23: 37, 1972.
261. Wittenborg MH, Aviad I: Organ influence on the normal posture of the diaphragm: A radiological study of inversions and heterotaxies. Br J Radiol 36: 280, 1963.
262. Moxham J, Morris AJR, Spiro SG, et al: Contractile properties and fatigue of the diaphragm in man. Thorax 36: 164, 1981.
263. Loh L, Goldman M, Newsom-Davis J: The assessment of diaphragm function. Medicine 56: 165, 1977.
264. Gandevia SC, McKenzie DK, Neering IR: Endurance properties of respiratory and limb muscles. Respir Physiol 53: 47, 1983.
265. Derenne J-PH, Macklem PT, Roussos CH: State of the art. The respiratory muscles: Mechanics, control and pathophysiology. Part III. Am Rev Respir Dis 118: 581, 1978.
266. Gilbert R, Auchincloss JH, Peppi D: Relationship of rib cage and abdomen motion to diaphragm function during quiet breathing. Chest 80: 607, 1981.
267. Cohen CA, Zagelbaum G, Gross D, et al: Clinical manifestations of inspiratory muscle fatigue. Am J Med 73: 308, 1982.
268. Navani S, Shah JR, Levy PS: Determination of sex by costal cartilage calcification. Am J Roentgenol 108: 771, 1970.
269. Vix VA: Extrapleural costal fat. Radiology 112: 563, 1974.
270. Shauffer IA, Collins WV: The deep clavicular rhomboid fossa: Clinical significance and incidence in 10,000 routine chest photofluorograms. JAMA 195: 778, 1966.
271. Weibel ER: Morphometrische Analyse von Zahl, Volumen und Oberfläche der Alveolen und Kapillären der menschlichen Lunge. Z Zellforsch Mikrosk Anat 57: 648, 1962.
272. Genereux GP: Computed tomography and the lung: Review of ana-

tomic and densitometric features with their clinical application. Assoc Radiol 36: 88, 1985.

273. Rhodes CG, Wollmer P, Fazio F, et al: Quantitative measurement of regional extravascular lung density using positron emission and transmission tomography. J Comput Assist Tomogr 5: 783, 1981.

274. Joseph AE, de Lacey GJ, Bryant TH, et al: The hypertransradiant hemithorax: The importance of lateral decentering, and the explanation for its appearance due to rotation. Clin Radiol 29: 125, 1978.

275. Chang CH (Joseph): The normal roentgenographic measurement of the right descending pulmonary artery in 1,085 cases. Am J Roentgenol 87: 929, 1962.

276. Garland LH: On the accuracy of diagnostic procedures. Am J Roentgenol 82: 25, 1959.

277. Austin JHM, Romney BM, Goldsmith LS: Missed bronchogenic carcinoma: Radiographic findings in 27 patients with a potentially resectable lesion evident in retrospect. Radiology 182: 115, 1992.

278. Tuddenham WJ: Problems of perception in chest roentgenology: Facts and fallacies. Radiol Clin North Am 1: 277, 1963.

279. Tuddenham WJ: Visual search, image organization, and reader error in roentgen diagnosis: Studies of the psychophysiology of roentgen image perception (Memorial Fund Lecture). Radiology 78: 694, 1962.

280. Shea FJ, Ziskin MC: Visual system transfer function and optimal viewing distance for radiologists. Invest Radiol 7: 147, 1972.

281. Oestmann JW, Greene R, Kushner DC, et al: Lung lesions: Correlation between viewing time and detection. Radiology 166: 451, 1988.

282. Newell RR, Garneau R: The threshold visibility of pulmonary shadows. Radiology 56: 409, 1951.

283. Spratt JS Jr, Ter-Pogossian M, Long RTL: The detection and growth of intrathoracic neoplasms: The lower limits of radiographic distinction of the antemortem size, the duration, and the pattern of growth as determined by direct mensuration of tumor diameters from random thoracic roentgenograms. Arch Surg 86: 283, 1963.

284. Resink JEJ: Is a roentgenogram of fine structures a summation image or a real picture? Acta Radiol 32: 391, 1949.

285. Greening RR, Pendergrass EP: Postmortem roentgenography with particular emphasis upon the lung. Radiology 62: 720, 1954.

2

METHODS OF ROENTGENOLOGIC AND PATHOLOGIC INVESTIGATION

ROENTGENOLOGIC EXAMINATION

The cornerstone of radiologic diagnosis is the plain roentgenogram; all other procedures, including fluoroscopy, conventional and computed tomography (CT), magnetic resonance imaging (MRI), scintigraphy, and special contrast studies, should be regarded as strictly ancillary. Thus, with a few exceptions, to which we refer later on, establishing the *presence* of a disease process by plain roentgenography of the chest should constitute the first step in diagnosis; if this examination does not show clearly the nature and extent of the abnormality, additional studies can be carried out to *complement* the plain roentgenogram.

Conventional Roentgenography

Projections

Roentgenologists vary in their recognition of which projections of the thorax constitute the most satisfactory basic or "routine" views for preliminary evaluation. The great majority, including us, prefer *posteroanterior* and *lateral* projections, views that provide the essential requirement of a three-dimensional inspection of thoracic contents and the chest wall. There are two exceptions to this "routine": (1) bedside roentgenography (in which anything other than a single anteroposterior projection is usually difficult or impossible (*see* later) and (2) roentgenography as a screening procedure, as in mass surveys or as part of the "routine" hospital admission (examinations that are performed on such a colossal scale that it is economically unsound to take more than a single posteroanterior view).

The *lordotic* projection has been advocated for three situations: to improve visibility of the lung apices, superior mediastinum, and thoracic inlet; for locating a lesion by parallax; and for identifying the minor fissure in suspected cases of atelectasis of the right middle lobe.[1, 2] In our opinion, however, much time and money are wasted by performing examinations in this projection when a direct approach such as CT would yield more information.

Oblique studies, with or without prior fluoroscopy, are sometimes useful in locating disease such as pleural plaques; however, in most situations we again prefer to employ more rewarding techniques such as conventional or computed tomography.

Roentgenographic Technique

There are several basic principles of roentgenographic technique.

1. Positioning must be such that the x-ray beam is properly centered, the patient's body is not rotated, and the scapulae are rotated sufficiently anteriorly so as to be projected free of the lungs.

2. Respiration must be fully suspended, preferably at total lung capacity (TLC). In this regard, it is important to note that normal subjects routinely inhale to approximately 95 per cent of TLC without coaxing[3]; thus, such roentgenograms can be of value in estimating lung volume and, by comparison with subsequent roentgenograms, in appreciating increase or decrease in volume as a result of disease.

3. Exposure factors should be such that the resultant roentgenogram permits faint visualization of the thoracic spine and the intervertebral discs, so that lung markings behind the heart are clearly visible; exposure should be the shortest possible that is consistent with the production of adequate contrast.

4. For heavy subjects, appropriate grids must be employed to reduce scatter radiation to a minimum.

Unfortunately, all too frequently technical factors are such that optimal roentgenographic density is achieved over the lungs generally but without adequate penetration of the mediastinum, a result that seriously limits roentgen interpretation. Although the effects of overexposure can be easily overcome by bright illumination,[4] underexposure cannot be compensated for by any viewing technique; because it prevents visualization of vital areas of the thorax, it should not be tolerated in any circumstances. With perseverance, it is always possible to develop roentgenographic techniques that obviate problems of underexposure.

The one that we have employed with consistent success for more than 15 years is based on the output obtainable from a 1000 mA, 3-phase, 12-pulse generator with a maximum rating of 150 kVp. The kVp is fixed at 145, the mA is variable from 400 to 600, and exposure is controlled by phototiming. A time range of 10 to 60 msec establishes the exposure range of 5 to 30 mA for most examinations. A constant focus-film distance of 10 feet is employed, with a fixed 6-inch air gap. This air gap technique interposes a space of 6 inches between the patient and the x-ray film[5]; because the air gap reduces radiation scatter by distance dispersion, no grid is required.

To achieve adequate exposure of the mediastinum while maintaining a proper level of exposure of the lung, we use a tunnel-wedge filter.[6] Wedge filtration has been advocated for equalizing the densities of the thinner apical regions of the chest and the basal regions[7]; in addition to reducing exposure to the apices, it provides increased exposure over the width of the mediastinum. The wedge filter is constructed of layers of 0.003-inch copper foil to a maximum thickness of approximately 0.3 mm; in addition to the advantages just described, it has been shown that a copper filter of 0.32 mm thickness reduces the entrance exposure to the patient by 30 to 40 per cent,[8] a clear advantage in terms of radiation hazard. The filter is mounted over the tube aperture of a rectangular brass cone 61 cm long. This cone, permanently mounted on the x-ray tube, collimates the x-ray beam to a precise 14- by 17-inch area at a distance of 10 feet, precluding excessive field coverage. The film changer system has a multifilm magazine that feeds each film into an evacuated screen-film compression device, thereby producing excellent screen contact during exposure. Completion of the exposure activates photoidentification of the film; this is fed automatically into a 90-second processor, which permits dry film viewing approximately 2 minutes after exposure.

The high-kilovoltage technique[7] has several advantages over that in the standard (60 to 80) kVp range. Because the coefficients of x-ray absorption of bone and soft tissue approximate each other in the higher-kilovoltage ranges, roentgenographic visibility of the bony thorax is reduced with only slight change in the overall visibility of lung structures. Further, the mediastinum is better penetrated, permitting visibility of lung behind the heart and of the many mediastinal lines whose identification is so important to the overall assessment of the chest roentgenogram. This technique can produce images superior in all respects to those obtained with other techniques; in addition to the better penetration of the mediastinum, this method provides a clearer visibility of the pulmonary vasculature and a better appreciation of pulmonary nodules[9] than can be obtained with other techniques. The only possible drawback of the high-kilovoltage technique is the diminished visibility of calcium, resulting from the high coefficient of x-ray absorption; however, in our experience, this has not proved troublesome.

In recent years, a new imaging technique called *scanning equalization radiography* has been developed, in which computer-assisted exposure improves scatter rejection and permits relatively uniform film contrast over all parts of the chest roentgenogram, including the mediastinum and lungs. The pioneering work by Wandtke, Plewes, and colleagues[10–13] has been extended by researchers from the Netherlands, who, in concert with Optical Industries Oldelft, have developed a highly sophisticated multiple-beam scanning equalization system called AMBER (advanced multiple beam equalization radiography).[14–16] The chest roentgenograms made with this unit that we have viewed have shown remarkable clarity and have almost universally shown anatomic structures with greater clarity than conventional roentgenograms.

Inspiratory-Expiratory Roentgenography

Roentgenograms exposed at full inspiration (TLC) and maximal expiration (residual volume) can supply useful information in two specific situations: air trapping and pneumothorax. The former is the main indication. When it is widespread, as in spasmodic asthma or emphysema, diaphragmatic excursion is reduced symmetrically and lung density changes little; in order to demonstrate these features convincingly, however, expiration must be forced, and preferably timed. When air trapping is local, as from bronchial obstruction, the expiratory roentgenogram reveals restricted ipsilateral diaphragmatic elevation, a shift of the mediastinum toward the contralateral hemithorax, and relative absence of density change in involved bronchopulmonary segments (Fig. 2–1).

When pneumothorax is suspected and the visceral-pleural line is not visible on the standard inspiratory roentgenogram or the findings are equivocal, a film taken at full expiration may show the line more clearly. This is because at full expiration (1) the volume of air in the pleural space is relatively greater in relation to the volume of lung, providing better separation of the pleural surfaces, and (2) the relationship of the pleural line to overlying ribs changes.

Roentgenography in the Lateral Decubitus Position

For the lateral decubitus technique, the patient lies on one side and the x-ray beam is oriented horizontally (Fig. 2–2). Because in the majority of instances, the dependent hemithorax is the side being specifically examined, it is desirable to elevate the thorax on a nonabsorbing support such as a foam cushion or mattress. The technique is invaluable for the identification of small pleural effusions: less than 100 mL of fluid may be detected on well-exposed roentgenograms in this position, whereas those taken with the patient erect seldom reveal an effusion of less than 300 mL.[17]

The procedure also is useful in two somewhat less common situations: (1) the presence of a pulmonary cavity, in which it can be used to demonstrate a change in position of an air-fluid level or to ascertain whether a structure that forms part of the cavity represents a freely moving intracavitary loose body such as a fungus ball, and (2) the presence of air trapping, such as that associated with an aspirated foreign body.[18] In this situation, the technique is particularly valuable in infants and young children in whom difficulty in communication may result in poor-quality expiratory roentgenograms. When a child is placed on one side, the dependent hemithorax is splinted, restricting movement of the thoracic cage on that side. As a consequence, in normal children inflation of the dependent lung tends to be less than that of the upper lung; however, when air trapping is present in the dependent lung, the affected lobe or segment tends to remain hyperlucent.

Screening Chest Roentgenography

Though screening chest roentgenography is often performed as part of the "routine" admission work-up in many institutions, its value in this situation is not at all certain. For example, in one study of surgical admissions, investigators carried out clinical screening for factors that would make patients more likely to have abnormal preoperative chest roentgenograms:[19] of the 368 who had no risk factors, only one had an abnormal chest roentgenogram; by contrast, of the 504 patients who had identifiable risk factors, 114 (22 per cent) were found to have serious roentgenographic abnormalities. In another study dealing with a Veterans Administration population known to have a high prev-

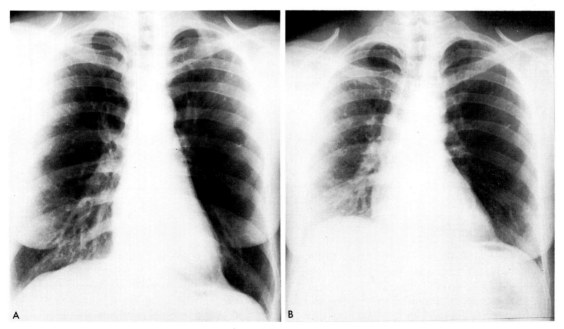

Figure 2–1. Value of Inspiratory-Expiratory Roentgenography in the Assessment of Air Trapping. Posteroanterior roentgenograms in full inspiration *(A)* and expiration *(B)* reveal air trapping in the left lung as evidenced by a shift of the mediastinum to the right, reduction in left hemidiaphragmatic excursion, and a marked discrepancy in overall density of the two lungs. Swyer-James syndrome.

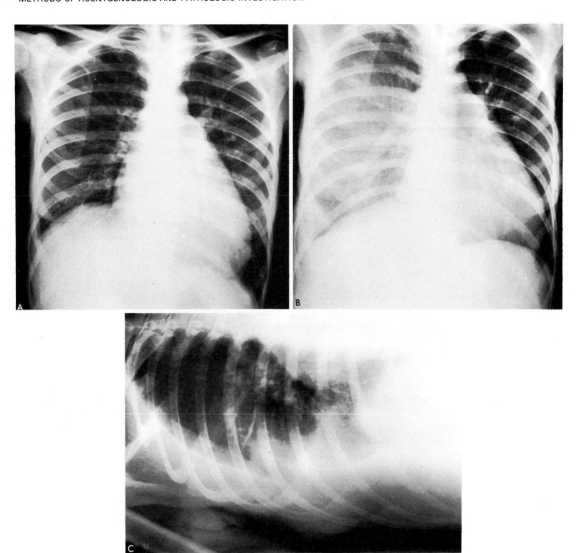

Figure 2–2. Value of Lateral Decubitus Roentgenography in the Assessment of Pleural Effusion. A posteroanterior roentgenogram in the erect position *(A)* reveals what appears to be marked elevation of the right hemidiaphragm. Roentgenography in the supine position *(B)* reveals a marked increase in the density of the right hemithorax, owing to the presence of fluid in the posterior pleural space; the right hemidiaphragm is now viewed in proper perspective, whereas in *A* it was obscured by subpulmonic effusion. A lateral decubitus roentgenogram *(C)* shows the fluid to much better advantage along the costal margin and reveals how much fluid can be accommodated in the subpulmonic space.

alence of cardiopulmonary disease, roentgenographic abnormalities were identified in 106 (36 per cent) of 294 patients[19a]; however, in only 20 of these were the findings new or unexpected, and treatment was changed because of roentgenographic results in only 12 (4 per cent) of the patients.

Reflecting the results of these and other studies, the following recommendations for routine screening chest x-ray examinations were proposed by the American College of Radiology[20] in 1982: (1) All routine prenatal chest x-ray examinations should be discontinued; (2) routine chest roentgenograms should not be required solely because of hospital admission; (3) routine periodic examinations unrelated to job exposure should be discontinued; and (4) mandated chest x-ray examinations as a condition of initial or continuing employment are not justified for tuberculosis detection. Now that the high costs of medical care are

being critically examined, every physician should give careful consideration to these opinions.

Bedside Roentgenography

The number of requests for roentgenographic examination of the chest with mobile apparatus at a patient's bedside has increased enormously in recent years. For example, at the Medical Center, University of Alabama at Birmingham, fully 55 per cent of all roentgenographic examinations of the chest are obtained at the bedside; discussions with colleagues at several other tertiary care institutions suggest that this high figure is not uncommon.

For a variety of reasons, such roentgenograms are almost invariably technically inferior to those obtained in the standard manner in a radiology department. Some of these reasons are uncontrollable, including the patient's supine position, the short focus-film distance, and the limited ability of many bedridden patients to suspend respiration or to achieve full inspiration to TLC. Other factors, however, particularly technical ones employed in the exposure, are subject to control and we and others[21] strongly recommend the use of a high-kilovoltage technique. Currently under investigation and clinical study is the digitization and processing of x-ray exposures on either x-ray film or a specially designed cassette or plate, with the resulting digital image being subject to contrast manipulation on cathode ray tube (CRT) monitors; it is anticipated that this technique will achieve considerable success (*see* later).

In addition to technical reasons, diagnostic error may occur with bedside roentgenograms simply because the patient is in a supine position. Pulmonary blood volume is approximately 30 per cent greater in supine subjects than in erect ones, so pulmonary vascular shadows usually appear larger in the former instance. In the upper lung zones, this dilatation is enhanced by loss of the effects of gravity and consequent increased flow to upper lung zones. This appearance must not be misinterpreted as evidence of pulmonary venous hypertension.

Despite these potential difficulties, it is clear that bedside roentgenography can be of great value in the follow-up of seriously ill persons. For example, in one study of 1132 consecutive bedside roentgenograms obtained on 140 patients admitted to surgical and medical intensive care units, new findings or changes affecting the patient's management were present in 65 per cent of the roentgenograms.[22]

Fluoroscopy

The fluoroscopic screen registers a constant image of the object being examined and thus allows appreciation of the dynamic activity of roentgenographically visible intrathoracic structures. *With few exceptions, the technique should be reserved for this purpose.* Perhaps its major indication is the study of diaphragmatic motion, specifically to establish the presence or absence of paradoxical motion but also to evaluate the presence of expiratory air trapping. Fluoroscopic identification of abnormalities of esophageal position or contour also can be important in roentgenologic diagnosis of pulmonary disease. For example, disturbed esophageal dynamics, as in achalasia or progressive systemic sclerosis, may be the chief indication of the origin of the patchy consolidation seen in aspiration pneumonitis or the diffuse reticular pattern of interstitial fibrosis.

One important exception to the statement regarding dynamic activity concerns the study of the solitary pulmonary nodule (SPN), in which fluoroscopy can be of value in two circumstances: (1) for the precise localization of an SPN for placement of a needle for aspiration biopsy (usually performed with biphase fluoroscopy) and (2) to establish the intrapulmonary location of an SPN when findings from a study of conventional posteroanterior and lateral roentgenograms are inconclusive.

Digital Radiography

Research in the production of digital roentgenographic images of the thorax is progressing along four different lines.[23] The first involves the digitization of the television signal in image-intensified fluorography, a technique that has been employed with limited success in the production of chest images. The approach yields good temporal resolution but degrades the spatial and contrast resolution and provides a limited dynamic range; in addition, it is subject to a variety of distortions and requires a very large intensifying screen sufficient to cover the average chest. This technique is also the basis of digital subtraction angiography (DSA, *see* page 124).

The second method that has achieved some success is digitization and processing of x-ray exposures on a specially designed cassette or plate. This system employs a storage phosphor incorporated into a cassette or high-sensitivity detection plate.[24] During exposure, the receptor stores the x-ray energy and is then scanned by a laser beam, which results in the creation of visible or infrared radiation whose intensity corresponds to the x-ray energy. The resultant luminescence is then converted to digital signals and processed. Subsequently, the digital signals are converted back to analog and reproduced on single-emulsion film by laser camera. The system's image-processing capability provides automated control of image contrast and density and can be extended to effect edge enhancement.[25]

A third method is digital processing of radiographic film, in which a radiograph is digitized using a high-intensity laser scanner; the recorded image data are then subjected to a wide variety of processing options, and images are viewed on a video display terminal.[23] Through the use of a specially designed, energy-selective cassette, this technique also permits dual-energy imaging from two films effectively exposed to different x-ray energy spectra.

The second and third of these techniques provide excellent spatial resolution but suffer from a lack of scatter suppression. Because of the facility for image manipulation and the uncommon necessity for repeat studies, however, they have been shown to be excellent for bedside radiography. In fact, they are now being employed in some centers to provide full departmental digitization.

A fourth approach to digital radiography involves the use of detectors for direct conversion from an analog to a digital electronic signal of x-rays transmitted through a patient. This technique, termed scan projection radiography, is under development by a number of manufacturers who are working in two different but related directions. One employs a pencil beam of x-rays that scans a patient transversely from top to bottom and is capable of producing an image of the chest with an extremely low radiation dose. The second employs a fan beam of x-rays that scans across the patient and is intercepted by a vertical row of scintillation detectors.[26]

Regardless of which of these techniques gains wide clinical application, it is clear that from both technical and economic viewpoints, the time is right for rapid advances to be made in digital chest imaging. In contrast with film, digital methods possess greater sensitivity and latitude, can provide the opportunity for image processing and dual-energy subtraction to enhance diagnostic information,[27–29] and can permit rapid electronic transmission and compact digital storage. In a recently published state of the art paper on digital imaging of the chest[23] in which the experiences of four large teaching centers in the United States were summarized, two major predictions were made: (1) that digital radiography of the chest will completely replace con-

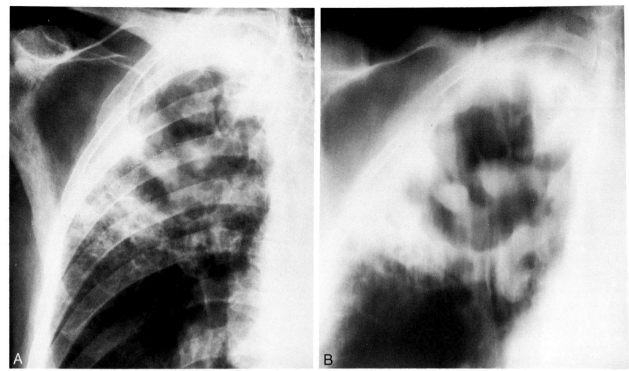

Figure 2–3. Value of Conventional Tomography in the Demonstration of Pulmonary Cavitation. *A*, A detail view from a conventional posteroanterior chest roentgenogram reveals inhomogeneous consolidation in the right upper lobe. *B*, An anteroposterior tomogram through the region of consolidation shows an irregular, thick-walled cavity. *M. tuberculosis* was identified in abundance in the patient's sputum.

ventional film radiography in at least 50 per cent of large teaching hospitals by the turn of the century, a transition that will continue until, by the year 2020, all chest radiography at large medical centers will be digital and (2) that the use of film (hard copy) for imaging of the chest either will disappear completely during the first two decades of the next century or will be reduced to a mere third or less of current film consumption.

Conventional Tomography

Tomography allows selective visibility of a particular layer of tissue to the exclusion of structures lying superficial or deep to it. Regardless of the type of motion employed, the technique involves reciprocal movement of the x-ray tube and film at proportional velocities. The reciprocal motion causes blurring of all structures not continuously in "focus" during excursions of the tube and film, so that the image of only a thin "slice" is recorded in detail on the roentgenogram. The level of tomographic "cut" is controlled by altering the ratio of the tube-object distance to the object-film distance. The thickness of the "cut" is governed by the distance of tube-film travel: the shorter the excursion, the thicker the layer recorded (zonography). Various reciprocal movements of tube and film have been developed, including rectilinear, circular, elliptical, and hypocycloidal.

With the increasing availability and improved technical quality of CT, it is clear that this technique should replace conventional tomography in virtually all situations in which morphologic clarification is required. However, for physi-

cians to whom CT is not available, there are three main indications for standard tomography of the thorax.

The first is the need for precise knowledge of the morphologic characteristics of lesions visible on plain roentgenograms, whose nature is obscured by superimposed images lying superficial and deep to them. Perhaps the best example of this indication is the investigation of pulmonary cavitation (Fig. 2–3), in which tomography can be particularly valuable. For example, in one study of 271 tomograms of 172 patients with pulmonary tuberculosis, tomography revealed cavitation unsuspected on conventional roentgenograms in 10.7 per cent[30]; conversely, in 18.8 per cent, tomography failed to show cavities suspected on plain roentgenograms. Other examples of this indication include identification of calcium in pulmonary nodules and the separation of potentially confusing hilar shadows.

The second use of conventional tomography is to enhance visibility of shadows that on plain roentgenograms are indistinct because of image summation. The principal example of this indication is study of the trachea, proximal bronchi, and pulmonary vasculature; visibility of these structures is very clear by tomography. In addition, posterior oblique tomography at an angle of 55 degrees has been recommended for displaying a clearer outline of the anatomic components of the hila.[31]

The final situation in which conventional tomography might be used is investigation of pulmonary metastases. Although most evidence suggests that the preferred technique in this regard is CT,[32] there is no doubt that full lung tomography also detects metastases not visible on plain roentgenograms in a significant number of cases.[33]

Computed Tomography

The Society for Computed Body Tomography has published a series of indications for body CT[34]; the following, with some modification, represent the recommendations of that organization. They can conveniently be divided into abnormalities affecting the mediastinum, lungs, pleura, and chest wall.

Mediastinum

Evaluation of Abnormalities Identified on Standard Chest Roentgenograms. The differentiation of the cystic or solid nature of mediastinal masses, the localization of such masses relative to other mediastinal structures and to some extent the determination of their composition (e.g., adipose tissue); the assessment of whether mediastinal widening is pathologic or simply an anatomic variation or the result of physiologic fat deposition; the distinction of a solid mass from a vascular anomaly or aneurysm (generally by contrast enhancement); the differentiation of a dilated pulmonary artery from a solid mass in a hilum; the differentiation between lymph node enlargement, vascular abnormality, or anatomic variant in the presence of deformity of the paraspinal line; and finally, determination of the presence and extent of mediastinal tumor in patients with pulmonary carcinoma.

Search for Occult Thymic Lesions. The detection of thymoma or hyperplasia in selected patients with myasthenia gravis when standard chest roentgenograms are negative or suspicious.

Miscellaneous Applications. Assisting in the percutaneous biopsy of mediastinal masses when fluoroscopic guidance is inadequate.

Lungs

Search for Pulmonary Neoplasms. The detection of occult pulmonary metastases when extensive surgery is planned for a known primary neoplasm that has a strong propensity for lung metastases or when a solitary lung metastasis is identified on a chest roentgenogram; the detection of a primary neoplasm in a patient with positive sputum cytology and negative chest roentgenography and fiberoptic bronchoscopy.

Search for Diffuse or Central Calcification. Several investigators have assessed the accuracy of CT in the evaluation of the presence or absence of calcification in solitary pulmonary nodules,[35–39] with variable results; it appears clear, however, that when a special reference phantom is used, the technique can be of great value.

Miscellaneous Applications. Possibly, the early detection of pulmonary emphysema and the determination of its severity.[40]

Pleura

Detection of Pleural Effusion. When its presence may be obscured by a pulmonary opacity and when simpler roentgenographic techniques or ultrasonography fails to clarify the picture.

Determination of the Presence and Extent of

Pleural Neoplasm. In the initial staging of selected patients with pulmonary carcinoma and in the differential diagnosis of postpneumonectomy fibrothorax and recurrent carcinoma.

Miscellaneous Applications. In determining the presence or absence of pleural plaques when conventional roentgenograms are inconclusive.

Chest Wall

Determination of the Extent of Neoplastic Disease. CT can be of value when there is involvement of ribs or thoracic vertebrae; however, in the absence of bone destruction, estimation of chest wall invasion by CT can be notoriously inaccurate (*see* page 477).

In recent years, high-resolution CT has gained considerable fame as a technique capable of demonstrating fine lung structure to better advantage than conventional CT,[41, 42] particularly in persons with chronic diffuse lung disease.[43]

Magnetic Resonance Imaging

When certain atomic nuclei are placed in a magnetic field and stimulated by radio waves of a particular frequency, they re-emit some of the absorbed energy in the form of radio signals. This phenomenon, known as nuclear magnetic resonance, has been increasingly developed for medical purposes in the 1980s and 1990s, and there is no doubt that MRI will have a major impact on the practice of medicine in the future. The physical principles involved in the production of an MR image are highly complex and have been detailed in a number of review articles.[44, 45]

The potential applications of MRI to the diagnosis of disease are numerous.[46] One of the most interesting relates to the concept that MR techniques allow the interpretation of images from a chemical-physiologic, rather than an anatomic point of view. Because chemical and physiologic alterations may precede anatomic changes, MRI becomes an especially attractive diagnostic method. For example, malignant tissue generally has a longer relaxation time than normal tissue (although there is much overlap), suggesting the possibility of earlier and more accurate diagnosis of neoplasms by MRI. The following is a brief summary of the potential applications of MRI for various thoracic diseases.

Hilar Masses and Lymph Nodes. MRI can demonstrate normal and enlarged lymph nodes, in some instances to better advantage than CT. For example, in one retrospective study of 144 patients, MRI and CT gave similar results with abnormal lymph nodes that measured more than 15 mm in diameter, but MRI displayed the nodes better because of its excellent soft tissue contrast resolution.[47] In another investigation of 12 patients with unilateral or bilateral hilar masses, it was possible to differentiate the mass from the hilar vasculature more easily with MRI than with contrast-enhanced CT.[48]

Mediastinal Masses. In one study of 75 patients with mediastinal masses, MRI depicted all masses and demonstrated compromise of vessels and cardiac chambers as a result of the inherent contrast between the masses and cardiovascular structures[49]; in fact, vascular compromise was better assessed with MRI than with CT. It was concluded that, although the anatomic information is comparable to that produced by CT, MRI provides some insight into the composition of the mass. The advantage of coronal and sagittal images of the thorax in the evaluation of mediastinal disease by MRI has been stressed.[50, 51]

Pulmonary Embolism. One experimental study in dogs found that MRI possesses considerable potential for demonstration of relatively small pulmonary emboli.[52]

Pulmonary Edema. In an MRI study of permeability and hydrostatic edema in animals, it was found that the technique can be used to estimate the severity of both types of edema.[53]

Vascular Lesions. Because of the ability of MRI to demonstrate vessels without the use of a contrast agent, it has proved valuable in the diagnosis of vascular lesions involving the mediastinum (e.g., aortic dissection and traumatic aneurysm).[54]

Bronchography

In our view, there is only one indication for bronchography—the investigation of the presence and extent of bronchiectasis—and then only when the clinical state of the patient is such that surgical resection of local disease could be performed with benefit. Whenever such surgery is contemplated, all 19 bronchopulmonary segments must be identified bronchographically, to exclude abnormality in areas in which no changes are apparent on the plain roentgenogram. One cautionary note: Simple dilatation of segmental bronchi without destruction (reversible bronchiectasis) is a frequent concomitant of acute pneumonia and, although temporary, may persist as long as 3 to 4 months. During this period, bronchography may reveal bronchial deformity indistinguishable from irreversible cylindrical bronchiectasis; despite clinical suspicion of chronic disease, therefore, definitive investigation should be postponed for at least 4 months after acute pneumonia.

We emphasize that, in a patient with hemoptysis and a normal chest roentgenogram, bronchography rarely reveals abnormality and seldom is indicated.[55] We believe that the most logical approach to the investigation of these patients should be CT[56]; should this prove unrevealing and if the hemoptysis is potentially life-threatening, one can resort to pulmonary or bronchial arteriography (or both). A similar but more vexing problem develops when sputum cytology findings are repeatedly positive for malignant cells but the plain roentgenographic and bronchoscopic appearances are normal. In such cases, we find bronchography just as unrevealing as in cases of hemoptysis from an unidentified site; as with hemoptysis, we feel that the most logical step in the investigation of these patients is a CT scan. If the scan is normal, watchful waiting is recommended, with plain roentgenograms taken at 3-month intervals or more frequently until either a lesion is demonstrated or the length of the follow-up has reasonably excluded the possibility of neoplasm (false-positive cytologic findings).

The bronchographic techniques most widely used include supraglottic injection, the transglottic catheter method (catheter inserted through the glottis via the nose or mouth), and the percutaneous cricothyroid technique (the medium being administered directly through a needle or by a modified Seldinger technique).

Despite the ease of performing bronchography, it should never be carried out without due consideration for its potential hazards. Apart from the danger of allergic reaction to either the topical anesthesia or the bronchographic medium itself (ranging from bronchospasm through iodism to anaphylaxis and death), bronchography gives rise to a temporary impairment of ventilation and diffusion that should not be disregarded, especially in patients with respiratory insufficiency.[57]

Angiography

Methods for investigating intrathoracic disease that involve intravascular injection of contrast material include pulmonary angiography, aortography, bronchial arteriography, and superior vena cava angiography.

Pulmonary Angiography

The contrast medium can be administered by various routes: (1) by intravenous injection into one arm or both arms simultaneously, through a needle or, preferably, a catheter; (2) via a catheter into the superior vena cava, right atrium, right ventricle, or main pulmonary artery; or (3) by selective injection into the right or left pulmonary artery or one of its branches. Generally speaking, the third technique produces clearer opacification of the pulmonary vascular tree than does venous or intracardiac injection; the superior visibility usually outweighs any disadvantage inherent in the catheterization procedure.

Digital subtraction angiography (DSA) is an imaging modality whose clinical application at the time of writing is somewhat controversial. Although the technique has had considerable success in angiography of the cervical and the abdominal vessels,[58] it has received mixed reviews as a method of examining the pulmonary vasculature. Preliminary studies in both animals[59] and humans[60] have, however, produced promising results, and it is possible that future improvements in equipment design will result in DSA's becoming a safe and reliable technique for the diagnosis of pulmonary embolism.

Undoubtedly, the major use of pulmonary arteriography is in the investigation of thromboembolic disease (Fig. 2–4), in selected cases of which it may be of great diagnostic importance.[61] Other indications include the detection of congenital abnormalities of the pulmonary vascular tree (e.g., agenesis or hypoplasia of a pulmonary artery, arteriovenous malformation, anomalous pulmonary venous drainage, pulmonary venous varix) and occasionally the investigation of pulmonary hemorrhage.[62] When considering the possible use of pulmonary angiography, it must be remembered that the risk of morbidity or mortality is increased in patients with appreciable pulmonary arterial hypertension.

Aortography

The preferred technique is direct percutaneous catheterization of the thoracic aorta[63] with either flooding of the aorta or selective catheterization of a particular vessel. An alternative method is digital subtraction aortography following injection of contrast material into an arm vein or the superior vena cava; this provides satisfactory opacification

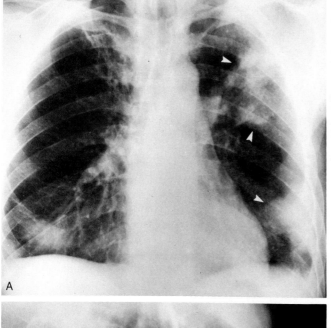

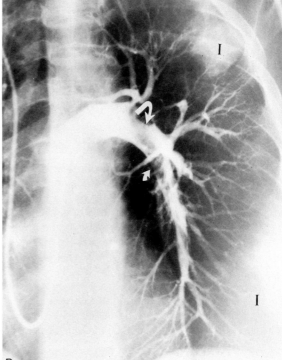

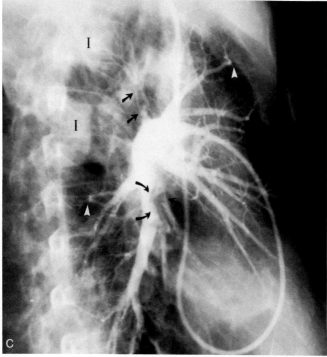

Figure 2–4. Value of Pulmonary Angiography in the Demonstration of Thromboembolism. *A,* A conventional posteroanterior chest roentgenogram discloses multiple areas of consolidation *(arrowheads)* that relate closely to a pleural surface. A selective left pulmonary angiogram in oblique *(B)* and lateral *(C)* projections demonstrates multiple intraluminal filling defects *(arrows)* and amputated peripheral arteries *(arrowheads).*

in selected cases when direct catheterization of the aorta is contraindicated.

When mediastinal widening is observed in a patient who has suffered severe deceleration injuries, it is now generally accepted that CT should be the first investigative procedure performed. If findings are normal, the absence of significant aortic injury can be reasonably assumed. When widening is recognized, emergency aortography is indicated to distinguish purely venous hematoma from major arterial injury and to show the number and sites of arterial lesions. Other indications include the need to precisely identify aortic anomalies, such as patent ductus arteriosus or aortic coarctation, and the need to identify anomalous vessels, such as an artery supplying a sequestered lobe.

Bronchial Arteriography

Most often, optimal opacification of bronchial vessels can be achieved only by selective catheterization, usually via a percutaneous transfemoral approach,[64] the tip of the catheter being wedged into a bronchial artery at the level of the fifth or sixth thoracic vertebra. When the bronchial arteries are markedly hypertrophic and tortuous, in some cases they can be opacified by an aortic flood technique.

The major indication for bronchial arteriography is investigation of severe hemoptysis. In this situation, the technique not only can identify the source of bleeding but also can serve as a means of therapeutic embolization.[65] A number of substances can be employed for occlusion, including

Gianturco coils, Ivalon, Gelfoam, or inflatable balloons (Fig. 2–5). When patients present with cataclysmic hemoptysis, it is important to remember that the nonbronchial systemic vessels also can be the source of bleeding, particularly in patients with chronic infection and pleural fibrosis. In such cases, it may be necessary to perform combined bronchial and subclavian arteriography[66]; selective catheterization of these vessels may demonstrate that either or both supply blood to the lung.

Superior Vena Cava Angiography

This procedure can be carried out by unilateral or simultaneous bilateral arm vein injection or via a catheter inserted into the superior vena cava or one of its large tributary veins. The only indication for its use is the superior vena cava syndrome.

Scintigraphy

Generally speaking, the use of radioactive isotopes in lung studies involves the recording on sensitive devices of the gamma radiation produced by radionuclides injected intravenously into the bloodstream or inhaled into the air spaces.[67] The imaging device that is used most widely is the scintillation, or gamma, camera, which records in a single exposure the flux of gamma radiation from the lungs. A more recent addition to the armamentarium that is said to possess advantages over conventional planar imaging for the diagnosis of pulmonary embolism[68] is the whole-body emission tomographic scanner that images the lungs in a manner analogous to that of the CT scanner.

Quantification of pulmonary scans has received increasing emphasis, particularly for measuring regional pulmonary ventilation and perfusion. A gamma camera-computer system is used; the camera interfaces an analog-to-digital converter, a memory system, and a magnetic tape recorder for data storage, and the data displayed are density changes as a percentage variation from the mean density change[69] or three-dimensional images of pulmonary ventilation and perfusion.[70]

Although the standard scintillation camera is the more popular instrument for quantifying lung function with xenon (^{133}Xe), there is an almost equal trend toward the use of special-purpose multidetector systems. Multiple discrete scintillation detectors cover both front and back of the

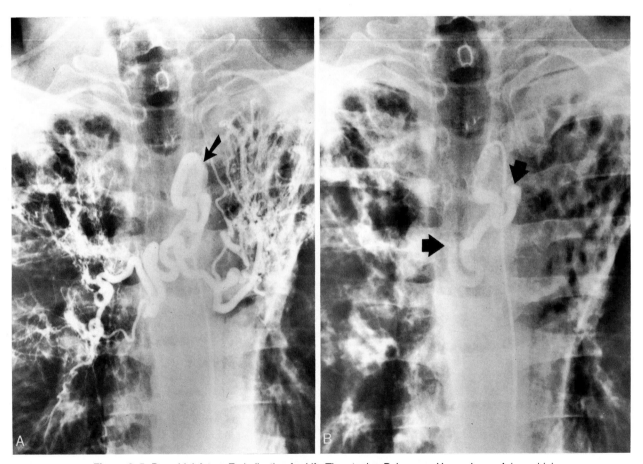

Figure 2–5. Bronchial Artery Embolization for Life-Threatening Pulmonary Hemorrhage. A bronchial artery angiogram *(A)* reveals marked dilatation of the vessel within the mediastinum and a remarkable increase in flow to a partly atelectatic left upper lobe with severe bronchiectasis; note the origin of the bronchial artery from the top of the aortic arch *(arrow)*. This 40-year-old man had cystic fibrosis and presented with hemoptysis amounting to 600 mL during the previous 24 hours. Following the injection of polyvinyl alcohol foam (Ivalon) particles, a repeat injection of contrast medium *(B)* reveals total obstruction of both left and right branches of the bronchial artery *(arrows)* and an absence of flow to the left upper lobe.

chest, resolving each lung into approximately eight regions for assessment of ventilation and perfusion.

The radiopharmaceuticals employed in scintiscanning may be particulate or gaseous, the former having the advantage of allowing more time for scanning. With these substances, an intravenous injection is given of a standard quantity of tagged MAA (macroaggregates of human serum albumin) containing radioactive particles, mostly in the range of 10 to 50 μm in diameter. Being larger than the capillaries, they lodge in the precapillary arterioles. The albumin may be labeled with ^{131}I, ^{99m}Tc, ^{113m}In or radioactive albumin microspheres[71] (the latter are used mainly because of their uniform size).

The gaseous radiopharmaceutical most widely used for studying the pulmonary circulation is ^{133}Xe, which is injected intravenously; while the patient holds his or her breath, a gamma camera picture records perfusion. Since the xenon passes almost instantly into the alveoli, during subsequent respiration the distribution of xenon throughout all areas of ventilated lung, including those poorly perfused, can be recorded. Xenon is cleared from the lungs in 3 to 4 minutes in normally ventilated regions, but clearing is delayed in poorly ventilated regions (i.e., those with air trapping).

Techniques for assessing pulmonary ventilation involve the inhalation of a radioactive gas (e.g., ^{133}Xe or ^{81m}Kr) or a nebulized aerosol of a radioactive material (e.g., albumin labeled with ^{131}I or ^{99m}Tc). For the latter, the particles must be less than 1 μm in diameter to reach the alveoli. A single-breath radioaerosol-inhalation technique has been described that purports to maximize peripheral lung deposition.[72]

The major indication for lung scanning is the investigation of thromboembolic diseases, a condition in which the technique may be diagnostic. This is especially true when the perfusion scan shows one or more defects and the ventilation scan is normal (Fig. 2–6); similarly, a normal lung scan virtually rules out a major pulmonary embolus. It is important to realize, however, that scintigraphic studies are of diagnostic value only when the scan image is compared with the chest roentgenogram; many physiologic and pathologic conditions (e.g., the patient's posture during tracer injection, obesity, cardiomegaly, and cardiac decompensation) alter lung images and must be taken into account for correct interpretation.[73] Since any disease characterized by consolidation or atelectasis or both can diminish pulmonary artery perfusion and since the airless lung can absorb radiation, reduced radioactivity or none on scanning does not necessarily indicate embolism.

In the 1990 Fleischner lecture, Hughes discussed the past, present, and future of radionuclides and the lung,[74] and the interested reader is directed to this excellent review for further information.

Ultrasonography

Ultrasonography has limited applications in the thorax, largely because neither air nor bone transmits sound, instead absorbing or reflecting incoming sonic energy and preventing the collection of information about acoustic interfaces behind ribs or lung tissue. Nevertheless, there are "acoustic windows" in the thorax through which ultrasonography can garner information useful in the investigation of thoracic disease, particularly of the subcostal pleura (via the intercostal spaces), the right hemidiaphragm and contiguous pleura and subphrenic space (via the liver), and mediastinal masses in close proximity to the thoracic cage.

The most important application is assessment of local pleural thickening caused by loculated empyema.[75] Differentiation of liquid from solid pleural collections, which may be exceedingly difficult with standard roentgenographic techniques, often can be achieved easily with ultrasonography (Fig. 2–7), particularly with high-resolution real-time sonographic sector scanning. Furthermore, the technique provides assessment of the amount of fluid loculated in a pleural pocket, indicates the appropriate site for thoracentesis, and simplifies fluid aspiration by permitting insertion of a needle directly through a special transducer. The procedure can be carried out at the patient's bedside with a mobile sonographic apparatus, thus obviating the need for special roentgenographic projections. Pleural fluid in the subpulmonic area of the right hemithorax and collections of fluid in the subphrenic space (subphrenic abscess) can be assessed by ultrasonography. In addition, since the liver is trans-sonic, the right hemidiaphragm is accessible, permitting evaluation of its mobility and determination of fluid collections above and below it.[76]

The acoustic properties of mediastinal masses close to the thoracic cage can be determined, although CT or MRI is undoubtedly the procedure of choice for definitive radiographic diagnosis. Ultrasound studies are limited at present to distinguishing solid masses from cystic ones (e.g., thymoma from pericardial cyst).[77] It must be remembered, however, that some mediastinal neoplasms themselves have a prominent cystic component. Ultrasonography is also useful in localizing pulmonary or mediastinal tumors for percutaneous biopsy.[77a]

PATHOLOGIC EXAMINATION

In many pulmonary diseases, diagnosis is not possible despite the combined use of roentgenographic, clinical, and special laboratory and function studies. In these cases, it is often necessary to obtain cells or tissue for pathologic examination, which in many instances makes a definitive diagnosis possible. The techniques employed to obtain this material, as well as a brief summary of the principles involved in its examination, are discussed in this section.

Cytology

Material for cytologic examination is most often obtained from the lungs by spontaneous or induced expectoration of sputum or by bronchial washing or brushing during endoscopy; it also can be obtained by aspiration of pleural fluid or of tissue within the lung itself. (Pulmonary cells, particularly inflammatory cells, also can be obtained by the technique of bronchoalveolar lavage [see page 149]; however, these are usually analyzed quantitatively and not qualitatively by the cytopathologist.)

Cytology of Tracheobronchial Secretions

Sputum is best collected by having the patient rinse the mouth with water and then expectorate a deep cough specimen into a wide-mouthed collecting jar. The optimal time is considered to be early morning, just after rinsing. Inadequate samples due to insufficient sputum are fairly common[78]; in this situation, it may be helpful to induce deep expectoration by having the patient inhale an aerosolized heated solution of saline, propylene glycol, or sulfur dioxide.[79] It is also important to obtain postbronchoscopic specimens for analysis; the procedure itself leads to repeated deep coughing that may produce diagnostic specimens.

Once collected, sputum is usually processed in one of two ways. In the first, a freshly expectorated sample is brought to the laboratory, where it is smeared evenly over glass slides, immediately fixed, and stained. In the second (Saccomanno's) method,[80] sputum is expectorated into a jar containing 50 per cent ethyl or isopropyl alcohol, which acts as a fixative that permits the collection of specimens over several days. In the laboratory, the sputum-alcohol mixture is blended in a household-type food blender for a short time, which effectively emulsifies the mucus and produces a fluid that can be centrifuged. When the supernatent is discarded, the residual concentrated cellular material is smeared on glass slides and stained. This procedure results in a substantial increase in the number of cells, both benign and malignant, available for examination.[81] Since the number of unsatisfactory and negative specimens decreases as the number of smears increases,[82] at least three slides should be prepared for either technique.

Specimens for cytologic examination are also frequently acquired during bronchoscopy. Those obtained by bronchial brushing are usually smeared directly onto glass slides and rapidly fixed in the endoscopy room. Those derived from bronchial washings can be processed by cytospinning or passed through a membrane filter and, if sufficient in

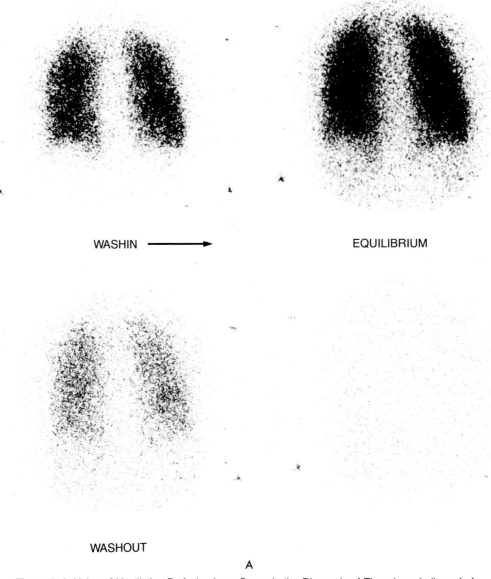

WASHIN ⟶

EQUILIBRIUM

WASHOUT

A

Figure 2–6. Value of Ventilation-Perfusion Lung Scans in the Diagnosis of Thromboembolism. *A,* A xenon-133 posterior inhalation lung scan discloses normal ventilation parameters during the washin, equilibrium, and washout phases.

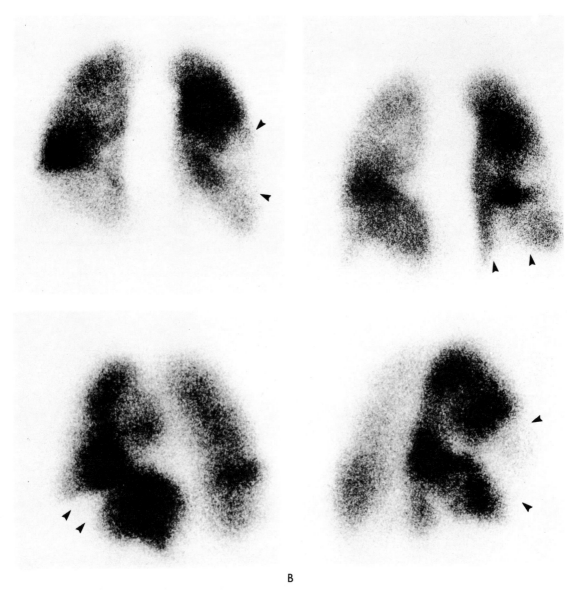

B

Figure 2–6 *Continued B,* Technetium-99m MAA perfusion lung scans in anterior, posterior, and right and left posterior oblique projections identify multiple segmental filling defects throughout both lungs *(arrowheads).* These findings, in concert with the ventilation study, are virtually diagnostic (high probability) of pulmonary thromboembolism.

amount, centrifuged; the cellular residue can then be smeared on a slide or prepared into a cell block for histologic examination.

The principal purpose of cytologic examination of sputum and specimens obtained by bronchial washing and brushing is the detection of malignancy; in large series of patients with confirmed lung cancer, the rate of true-positive findings ranges from 50 to 90 per cent.[83] In many cases, malignant cells derived by one technique will also be identified in specimens from the other two; in a small but important minority, however, the use of the three modes of investigation is complementary.

False-positive results (the reporting of malignant cells in the absence of true neoplasm) are uncommon, being reported in only 1 to 3 per cent of cases in most series. The reasons include evaluation of poorly preserved or inadequately prepared specimens and misinterpretation of reactive epithelial atypia as neoplasia. The latter is most com-

mon in the presence of pneumonia[84] or pulmonary infarction,[85] or in association with cytotoxic drugs.[86]

False-negative results (which have a prevalence of 10 to 50 per cent) are related to inadequate collection and preparation of specimens as well as to sampling problems due to location or size of the tumor. For example, positive cytologic diagnoses are made more often with central than with peripheral neoplasms and with large than with small tumors.[78, 83] Additional samples, particularly of sputum, should always be obtained after a negative result; it has been repeatedly shown that the yield of malignant cells increases with the number of specimens examined. Metastatic neoplasms are less commonly detected than primary lung carcinomas, probably because they involve the pulmonary parenchyma more frequently than the proximal airways; nevertheless, discovery rates of 30 to 50 per cent have been reported.[87]

In benign disease, examination of sputum and bronchial

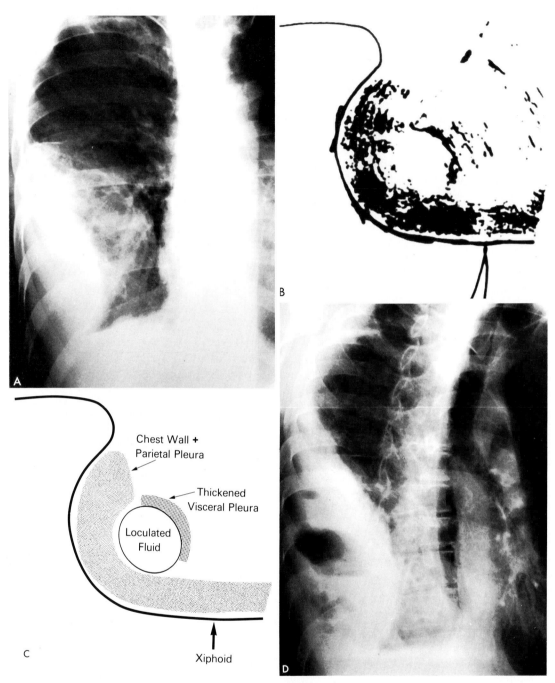

Figure 2–7. Identification of Loculated Empyema by Ultrasonography. An anteroposterior roentgenogram *(A)* reveals a large, homogeneous opacity in the right lower hemithorax whose configuration strongly suggests fluid loculation. An ultrasonic B-scan of the lower chest *(B)* shows a roughly elliptical, sharply demarcated sonolucent space posterolaterally, possessing the typical characteristics of a fluid-filled space. A drawing *(C)* indicates important landmarks. Thoracentesis was carried out, pus withdrawn, and air introduced; an oblique roentgenogram *(D)* reveals the space corresponding to the sonolucent zone in the ultrasound recording. (Courtesy of Dr. Reggie Greene, Massachusetts General Hospital, Boston.)

washings and brushings is usually unrewarding. The most useful application is in the detection of infectious organisms, particularly *Pneumocystis carinii.*

Cytology of Pleural Fluid

If sufficient fluid is available, one portion can be passed through a membrane filter, and another centrifuged to yield a cell-rich residue from which smears or, if possible, a cell block can be made. The latter procedure frequently yields small tissue fragments on which histochemical and immunohistochemical investigations can be performed and may greatly facilitate diagnosis.

The primary objective of diagnostic importance is exclusion or confirmation of malignancy. The prevalence of positive cytologic examination of pleural effusions of malignant origin ranges from 30 to 85 per cent: most series report an accuracy rate of about 50 per cent.[88] As with the cytologic investigation of bronchial secretions, repeated examinations are likely to increase the yield. It should be remembered, however, that when no malignant cells are identified in the effusion of a patient with cancer, it is possible that the effusion is secondary either to pneumonia distal to an obstructing carcinoma or to lymphatic obstruction. A review of the literature in 1981 showed an overall false-positive rate of only 0.4 per cent for several combined series.[89]

In addition to malignant cells, the number and nature of inflammatory and other cells in the effusion may provide valuable clues to the cause. Red blood cell (RBC) counts of more than 10,000 cells per mL are common to all types of effusion and therefore are of no discriminatory value.[88] However, counts exceeding 100,000 cells per mL are often associated with malignant neoplasm, pulmonary infarction, or trauma. A grossly bloody effusion suggests the possibility of a "bloody tap," in which case the RBC count is high only in the first portion of the aspirate.

A large number of neutrophils in pleural fluid usually indicates the presence of bacterial pneumonia, although it can also occur in association with pulmonary infarction, malignant neoplasms, and tuberculosis.[88] An effusion containing 50 per cent lymphocytes or more almost certainly represents either tuberculosis or neoplasm. Most effusions caused by neoplasm contain an admixture of other cell types and thus exhibit a polymorphous cell population. By contrast, the lymphocyte-rich effusion of tuberculosis typically contains a paucity of mesothelial and other mononuclear or polymorphonuclear inflammatory cells.[88] In fact, the cellular uniformity may be so marked as to suggest the possibility of well-differentiated lymphoma.[90]

A pleural effusion that contains a substantial number of eosinophils may or may not be associated with blood eosinophilia and occurs in a variety of conditions. Probably the most common is pleural trauma, such as that encountered in surgery, spontaneous pneumothorax, or transthoracic needle aspiration. The pathogenesis of eosinophilia in these situations may be related to the presence of air in the pleural space. Other conditions occasionally associated with pleural fluid eosinophilia include infections (both fungal and parasitic), immunologic abnormalities such as rheumatoid disease,[91] infarction, and drug hypersensitivity.[92] Tuberculous and neoplastic effusions rarely contain a large number of eosinophils.[91]

Needle Aspiration

In recent years, it has become evident that needle aspiration is a technique with high reliability and minimal discomfort and complications for the patient; it has thus become an important method in the diagnosis of lung cancer. Aspirates can be taken through the chest wall (transthoracic needle aspiration [TTNA]), the bronchial wall (transbronchial needle aspiration), or directly during mediastinoscopy or thoracotomy (intraoperative needle aspiration).

Transthoracic Needle Aspiration. TTNA consists of suction of fluid and cells into a syringe through a narrow-gauge needle inserted percutaneously into lesions in the lung or mediastinum.[93–95] Most clinicians now use needles of 19 to 22 gauge, although some advocate the use of an

ultrathin needle of 24 or 25 gauge, claiming fewer complications and an exceptionally good yield.[96] The prone position is recommended during the procedure, to reduce the possibility of air embolism, and the patient should be instructed to hold his breath during needle insertion. Fluoroscopic television monitoring is usually employed to ensure accurate positioning of the needle within the lesion; CT scanning and ultrasonography have also been used as aids to localization prior to aspiration. When the needle is judged to be inserted properly, it is rotated and withdrawn while vigorous suction is applied. Most investigators stress the importance of making three to six separate aspirations, to optimize the chances of acquiring diagnostic cells.[97]

Aspirated material may be evacuated directly onto glass slides, smeared, and immediately fixed. In addition, the needle can be rinsed with saline and the resulting material either passed through a membrane filter or centrifuged to yield a cell-rich residue that itself can be smeared or fixed and processed into a cell block, a procedure which again substantially increases the chance of finding diagnostic cells.[98] It is desirable to stain smears at the time of the aspiration (in a manner analogous to performing frozen sections on tissue)[99]; this enables rapid assessment of the adequacy of the specimen, so that repeat aspirations may be performed immediately in an attempt to increase the yield.

The two main indications for fine-needle aspiration cytology are diagnosis of pulmonary or mediastinal malignancy and determination of the cause of serious pneumonia; specific guidelines have been proposed by the American Thoracic Society.[100] The procedure should be performed only when noninvasive diagnostic methods have failed, and it is not indicated if there is intention to proceed with resection of a lesion regardless of the results of the test. When cancer is suspected, there are thus three clear indications for TTNA: (1) need to establish a cytologic diagnosis in a patient judged to be unresectable; (2) need to determine cell type in a lesion suspected of representing either a metastasis or a second primary pulmonary carcinoma; and (3) need to establish a diagnosis in a patient who is a poor surgical risk when a positive biopsy finding would permit acceptance of the risk. Contraindications to TTNA include severe pulmonary arterial hypertension, an uncorrectable bleeding disorder (including anticoagulant-induced bleeding diathesis), inability of the patient to tolerate a complicating pneumothorax, and uncontrollable cough.[100]

The procedure itself usually produces little discomfort for the patient. Serious complications are rare and are usually associated with the use of large-bore needles. In a review of the literature to 1982, only 12 deaths were documented; most were caused by hemorrhage.[93] A small pneumothorax is a much more common complication (overall prevalence approximately 30 per cent); however, fewer than a third of these require aspiration of the pleural space. Patients with physiologic or radiologic evidence of obstructive airway disease are at increased risk for this complication.[101] Tumor implantation along the needle track occurs in some cases.[101a]

As with other cytologic techniques, the most important use of TTNA is to establish a diagnosis of malignancy. Recent series indicate that the procedure has an accuracy rate in detecting carcinoma of 85 to 95 per cent[95]; the sensitivity in diagnosing lymphoma is somewhat less.[94] The false-positive rate ranges from 0.5 to 2 per cent,[93] the most common confounding condition being tuberculosis. In addition to simply diagnosing malignancy, TTNA enables differentiation of metastatic from primary lung carcinoma in a substantial number of cases.

Although the principal application of TTNA is in the determination of malignancy and its cell type, a specific diagnosis of a benign condition is also possible, the frequency varying from about 10 to 70 per cent of all benign lesions, depending on the series.[95] Our own experience is consistent with the former figure.[102] The most frequent benign condition identified by TTNA is infection, particularly by *Mycobacterium tuberculosis* or abscess-forming bacteria; in fact, when TTNA is performed because of suspicion of an underlying infection, the yield of a specific diagnosis is as great as 67 per cent.[103] Obviously, culture of aspirated material is the most important aspect of tissue analysis in these cases, and material for this purpose should always be submitted to the microbiology laboratory when there is a suspicion that a lesion might be of infectious origin. Many benign neoplastic and non-neoplastic lesions also can be definitively diagnosed by TTNA,[102] including hamartomas, amyloidosis, thymomas, posterior mediastinal neurogenic tumors, and lipomas.

Transbronchial Needle Aspiration. Although needle aspiration of mediastinal and parahilar lesions may be carried out percutaneously, a transbronchial approach is becoming increasingly popular.[104, 105] Transbronchial needle aspiration may be accomplished through either a rigid or a flexible fiberoptic bronchoscope and has been used both in establishing a primary diagnosis and in the staging of known lung carcinoma.

Biopsy

In some cases of malignancy and in many cases of benign disease, cytologic investigations alone do not provide a definitive diagnosis. In this circumstance, tissue biopsy is usually necessary, and it can be accomplished by a number of techniques, each of which has its own type and rate of complications as well as diagnostic yield. The following discussion outlines the principles involved in deciding which technique is most appropriate for any particular patient and clinical situation. Before discussing specific techniques, however, it is appropriate to emphasize several features common to all.

1. Despite the fact that reported instances of death are rare and that morbidity is seldom serious, every method of obtaining tissue can result in complications; patients at high risk are those with pulmonary hypertension, bleeding diathesis, bullae, or limited respiratory reserve.

2. When considering the merits of a particular technique, it is necessary to take into account the experience of its proponents, who generally obtain results superior to those of less experienced investigators; in fact, the various techniques by a single investigator have been compared infrequently.

3. Although biopsy is usually performed to obtain material for histologic study, in many cases it is essential that some tissue also be processed for bacteriologic and mycologic analysis; this is especially important for specimens obtained by open lung biopsy.

4. It is important to remember that a biopsy samples only a small portion of a particular disease process. Thus, because of possible variations in the distribution and severity of disease, especially when it is diffuse, the findings from one biopsy specimen cannot necessarily be extrapolated to all regions.

5. Finally, it must be stressed that correlation of clinical, roentgenologic, and pathologic findings is likely to provide a far more precise diagnosis than anyone alone is capable of producing, and close cooperation between the respective specialists should be encouraged.

Bronchial Abnormalities, Including Tumors

The principal value of bronchoscopic biopsy is in the diagnosis of malignancy and the establishment of cell type.[106] Overall diagnostic yield from tumors that are bronchoscopically visible is 90 to 95 per cent with the flexible fiberoptic bronchoscope.[107] In addition to malignancy, a diagnosis of sarcoidosis also can often be confirmed by bronchial wall biopsy. The method itself is considered in greater detail on page 149.

Lung

Transbronchial Biopsy. Transbronchial biopsy (TBB) has been proved to be of value in the diagnosis of sarcoidosis, lymphangitic carcinomatosis, and diffuse opportunistic infections caused by organisms such as fungi and *P. carinii;* however, in other forms of noninfectious pneumonitis and fibrosis and in bacterial pneumonia its yield is relatively low.[108, 109] Complications such as pneumothorax (caused in many cases by biopsy of visceral pleura) and minor hemorrhage are not infrequent; however, except in the patient with limited functional reserve or coagulation abnormality (in whom the procedure should be performed with caution, if at all) complications are rarely serious.[109a]

Transthoracic Needle Biopsy. Although microscopic fragments of lung or tumor tissue are sometimes obtained with TTNA (especially with larger-bore needles), a true core of tissue can be procured only with a cutting needle. Three techniques have been used: punch biopsy, trephine drill biopsy, and suction-excision biopsy.[110, 111]

The needle originally designed for punch biopsy, the Vim-Silverman, consists of an inner, split, cutting needle that is driven into the lung, and an outer needle that is inserted over and compresses the cutting blades. Both needles are rotated 180 degrees and then removed, with a thin sliver of tissue trapped between the blades. A number of modifications of the type and gauge of needle employed have been introduced over the years.[112] Although satisfactory lung specimens have been obtained in approximately 80 per cent of cases, a precise tissue diagnosis can be expected in only 65 per cent, and in half this number if the diagnosis of nonspecific pulmonary fibrosis is excluded.[110] The procedure results in pneumothorax in 20 to 25 per cent of patients and in hemoptysis in 10 to 15 per cent[110]; hemorrhage is usually more severe and the mortality rate is undoubtedly higher than in TTNA.

Trephine biopsy employs a high-speed drill with an outside diameter of 2.1 to 3.0 mm; it can be performed more rapidly and is less painful than the conventional form of cutting needle biopsy. Diagnostic biopsies have been reported in 65[110] to 90[113] per cent of cases. Pneumothorax, subcutaneous empyhysema, and hemorrhage (hemoptysis or hemothorax) have been estimated to occur in 15 to 30 per cent of patients.[113]

Although some investigators espouse the virtues of transthoracic needle biopsy,[114] all three procedures are gradually being replaced by TTNA, not only because it is associated with a significantly lower complication rate[110] but also because the diagnostic yield of TTNA is better than[114a] or comparable to[115] that of the cutting techniques. There is some evidence, however, that cutting needle biopsy still may be useful in selected lesions, particularly those that are benign or lymphoproliferative.[116]

Thoracoscopic Biopsy. In addition to the evaluation of pleural disease (*see* later), thoracoscopy also can be used to obtain specimens of lung parenchyma. Since these tend to be larger than those obtained by transbronchial biopsy, the technique has theoretical advantages. In the few reported series of patients with diffuse interstitial disease, the diagnostic yield has ranged from 90 to 100 per cent.[117, 118] Despite these encouraging reports, further experience is required before this procedure can be accepted as an alternative diagnostic approach to open lung biopsy.

Open Lung Biopsy. Open lung biopsy (OLB) is recommended particularly for cases of chronic diffuse lung disease; it is also useful in some cases of acute and, presumably infectious, disease when other, less invasive, procedures have been unproductive. The chest is opened through a standard thoracotomy incision or through a limited incision large enough to allow removal of a fragment of tissue measuring 2 to 3 cm in diameter. When a small incision is used, pulmonary parenchyma is ballooned out by exerting positive pressure on the lung, a clamp is applied, and the tissue is removed; this technique is particularly applicable when the disease is so diffuse that any portion of the lung is likely to reveal it. When disease is more confined, a full thoracotomy incision is recommended, because it enables the surgeon to examine the lung and choose the best region for biopsy.

Selection of the appropriate site for biopsy is clearly of paramount importance. Areas of discrete disease should be removed *en bloc* if small enough to be included in the specimen; if more extensive disease is present, the biopsy should include an area of transition between abnormal and apparently normal lung. Samples from more than one site should be taken if surgically feasible. The tips of the lingula and middle lobe are common sites of chronic vascular changes and fibrosis and should be avoided[119]; similarly, it is unwise to biopsy very abnormal areas, since these often show end-stage disease of unrecognizable origin.[120] In general, the biopsy specimens should be submitted to a pathologist as soon as possible after excision. Portions may then be selected for special examination, and frozen sections can be performed to provide a preliminary diagnosis or to assess adequacy of biopsy material.

In experienced hands the complication rate is low. In one review of 502 patients subjected to OLB for the diagnosis of chronic interstitial lung disease, the mortality rate was 0.3 per cent, and the complication rate 2.5 per cent.[120] However, a review of 2290 cases in the literature showed mortality and complication rates to be 1.8 and 7.0 per cent, respectively,[121] figures that are probably more realistic estimates of the true incidence. As might be expected, patients in respiratory failure at the time of biopsy are at increased risk.[121a]

Pleura

Needle Biopsy. The most common method of obtaining fragments of pleural tissue for histologic examination is transthoracic needle biopsy (TTNB), a procedure that can be performed at the same time as thoracentesis. The two needles most commonly used are the Cope and the Abrams; success with these instruments depends largely on the skill of the operator, judicious selection of patients, and the number of biopsies taken.[122] After local anesthesia, the thoracentesis needle is introduced gradually through the chest wall, and fluid is withdrawn (20 mL is usually sufficient for diagnostic purposes, although more may need to be drained to decompress the pleural space). When the fluid has been removed, the biopsy needle is withdrawn slowly, with some pressure on the needle toward the side containing the biopsy notch. As the parietal pleura slips into the notch, withdrawal of the needle is suddenly interrupted; the cutting cylinder is then rotated, and the needle containing the specimen withdrawn.

The chief value of TTNB of the pleura is in the diagnosis of cancer and tuberculosis.[123] Since granulomatous disease other than tuberculosis seldom involves the pleura, the finding of necrotizing or non-necrotizing granulomas is usually accepted as an indication of tuberculous infection, even when microorganisms are not identified. The diagnostic yield in patients with neoplastic involvement of the pleura ranges from 40 to 75 per cent (average, about 60 per cent).[122] Sensitivity in the diagnosis of tuberculosis is somewhat higher, ranging from 70 to 90 per cent.[122]

Apart from pneumothorax, complications are rare and usually mild; they include hemorrhage into the chest wall and pleural cavity, mediastinal and subcutaneous emphysema, and the development of carcinoma along a needle track.

Thoracoscopic Biospy. Thoracoscopy (pleuroscopy) is a procedure in which the pleura is directly examined visually.[124] After the induction of pneumothorax, an endoscope (preferably a rigid bronchoscope) is inserted through an incision in an intercostal space, and the pleura inspected; biopsy of the parietal pleura or visceral pleura and underlying lung can be performed through the same or a second opening in the thoracic cage. The procedure can be performed with local anesthesia on an outpatient basis. The technique can also be carried out using a video display (videothoracoscopy) and a double-lumen endoscope, through which instruments for limited surgical procedures can be introduced.[124a]

There is good evidence that thoracoscopic biopsy is the diagnostic method of choice in the investigation of patients with persistent pleural effusion in whom a diagnosis has not been established by cytology and needle biospy.[124] It is a less traumatic procedure than open pleural biopsy, and the yield of positive diagnoses is remarkably good. In one series of 102 patients it had a sensitivity of 91 per cent, specificity of 100 per cent, and negative predictive value of 93 per cent for the diagnosis of malignancy[124]; follow-up of patients with adequate visualization of the pleural space and an unequivocally benign biopsy showed that almost all had a clinically benign course. Complications are uncommon.

Open Biopsy. Because of the increased morbidity and added risk of general anesthesia that we consider to be essential for direct pleural biopsy, even with a limited thoracotomy incision, we reserve open pleural biopsy for cases when needle biopsy or thoracoscopic biopsy has not yielded a specific diagnosis in a patient with an effusion.

Mediastinum

The two procedures most often used to obtain tissue from the mediastinum are mediastinoscopy and open biopsy. The main indications for these techniques are the need to stage and (less often) to diagnose pulmonary carcinoma. Primary mediastinal neoplasms also can be diagnosed by these means, as can certain benign conditions, such as sarcoidosis.

Mediastinoscopy. This procedure is carried out through an incision in the suprasternal notch; the soft areolar tissues are dissected along the trachea, and biopsy material is removed under direct vision through an instrument similar to that used for pediatric esophagoscopy. The space explored is the upper half of the mediastinum, including tissues around the intrathoracic portion of the trachea, the tracheal bifurcation, and the proximal part of the major bronchi. Since lymph nodes lower in the mediastinum, particularly those in the subcarinal and aortopulmonary regions, are not as accessible to the mediastinoscope as those in the upper portion, an "extended" mediastinoscopy (performed by carefully dissecting the soft tissues anterior to the aorta) is sometimes employed.

The principal value of mediastinoscopy is that it tells the surgeon whether or not to attempt curative resection of pulmonary carcinoma. If the procedure fails to reveal lymph node metastases, resectability of lung tissue at thoracotomy is almost ensured, being reported in more than 90 per cent of patients.[125] On the other hand, mediastinoscopy is of considerable value in reducing the number of thoracotomies at which disease is found to be unresectable: for example, in one study, unnecessary thoracotomies decreased from 25 to 8 per cent.[126] Complications are uncommon and usually not serious; one review of the literature estimated their prevalence at 3 to 4 per cent.[127] The most important is hemorrhage; a laryngeal nerve, usually the left recurrent, occasionally is injured.

Open Biopsy. This procedure permits direct inspection of mediastinal lymph nodes through the usual thoracotomy incision or limited mediastinotomy.[128] It has the advantage over mediastinoscopy of permitting more extensive exploration of the mediastinum and more accurate assessment of neoplastic extension to the hila. It is particularly advocated for mediastinal exploration in left-sided tumors; because of the barrier produced by the arch of the aorta on the left, standard mediastinoscopy results in a lower positive yield for neoplasms of the left lung than of the right.[129]

Scalene Lymph Nodes

Scalene lymph node biopsy consists of the removal of tissue lying on the scalene group of muscles in the supraclavicular fossa, including the medial fat pad. Its main application is in the determination of spread beyond the thorax in cases of proven or suspected pulmonary carcinoma. Although *in experienced hands* it is a relatively minor procedure, it should not be relegated to inexperienced members of the house staff. Major complications occur in as many as 5 per cent of patients[130] and include local large vessel injury, lymphatic fistulas, Horner's syndrome, and infection extending into the mediastinum.

Scalene lymph nodes that are palpable almost always contain pathologic tissue; in one review of the literature,[131] palpable nodes were involved by neoplasm in 475 (83 per cent) of 576 cases of pulmonary carcinoma. As expected, the positive yield is not nearly as high when scalene nodes are not palpable; in the same review, biopsy of nonpalpable nodes was positive in only 452 (20 per cent) of 2254 patients with pulmonary carcinoma.

Summary and Recommendations

In an attempt to summarize the indications for the use of specific techniques to obtain material for pathologic examination, it must be emphasized that no specific rules apply to every situation. Each patient must be considered individually, and the merits of all the variables must be weighed before making a decision. Despite this, the following general recommendations should apply in all situations.

1. The procedure with the least risk and discomfort to the patient should have the highest priority. Thus, an invasive procedure is not indicated if a diagnosis can be established by simpler, noninvasive techniques, such as sputum culture or cytology.

2. Biopsy usually is not indicated if the possibility of malignancy has been reasonably excluded by certain clinical findings or roentgenographic signs. For example, both calcification within a solitary pulmonary nodule and confirmation of no change in the size of a solitary nodule over time imply a benign process. Special procedures to establish the presence of such calcification should be performed before any invasive procedure is attempted. Similarly, a concerted search for previous roentgenograms should be made.

3. The patient's general condition must be such that it does not by itself contraindicate the procedure. For example, TTNA of a small peripheral nodule for purposes of diagnosis alone might be justified in a patient with severe chronic obstructive pulmonary disease for whom thoracotomy and surgical resection would not be feasible, but the patient should have enough breathing reserve to tolerate a possible complicating pneumothorax.

4. It is important to recognize that the confidence that is placed in any particular technique is proportional to the ability to exclude false results. Apart from inherent deficiencies in the method itself, this ability is determined largely by the expertise of the persons performing the procedure and interpreting the results, and it clearly varies among different institutions and individuals. The value of a particular method should thus be questioned when it is associated with an appreciable number of false-negative or false-positive results.

5. The patient's age and clinical history may be of major importance in deciding whether or not to biopsy. For example, a history of exposure to carcinogens, such as ciga-

rette smoke and radioactive materials, should increase the suspicion of a malignant process.

6. The presence or absence of signs and symptoms of disease elsewhere in the body is an essential factor; for example, entirely different approaches are needed in the investigation of multiple pulmonary nodules in a patient with polyarthritis, in one with a large renal mass, and in one with nasal ulceration and hematuria.

7. Finally, the time course of the disease process is an important consideration. We have seen patients whose roentgenograms revealed a lesion of unknown cause for which biopsy was being considered for definitive diagnosis; however, the lesion had either shrunk or disappeared altogether on roentgenograms obtained a few days later. In many instances, therefore, it is advisable to delay an invasive procedure for at least a week, particularly when a lesion is likely to be infectious.

A discussion of the indications for and techniques of biopsy can be related to six basic roentgenographic patterns of pulmonary disease.

Solitary Pulmonary Nodule (Tumor 3 cm or Less in Diameter)

A lesion of 3 cm or smaller in a patient younger than 30 years of age is almost certainly benign; biopsy is not warranted even if previous roentgenograms are unavailable for comparison or an earlier film did not show a similar opacity. In such cases, however, roentgenograms should be obtained every 3 months for at least a year to confirm the benign nature of the lesion.

In patients older than 30 years of age, particularly those aged 40 to 60 years, a solitary, noncalcified lesion must be regarded as cancer until proved otherwise. If previous roentgenograms are not available for comparison or if such roentgenograms fail to reveal a lesion or show a smaller lesion than is now apparent, the patient should be investigated initially by examination of multiple sputum specimens and by bronchoscopy with washings and brushings (although these are often of little or no value). Skin tests, complement-fixation tests, and a history of possible exposure to known pathogens, such as *Coccidioides immitis*, may be highly significant. If these investigations are negative and if there is no evidence of metastatic disease in the mediastinum or elsewhere, in most cases we recommend proceeding directly to thoracotomy. It should be emphasized that a search for a primary neoplasm elsewhere, on the assumption that a solitary nodule might be metastatic, is almost invariably unrewarding and should not be undertaken unless there is clinical evidence of disease outside the thorax.

If a patient with a solitary pulmonary nodule refuses surgery or has a history of an extrathoracic neoplasm that might reasonably be considered a primary, or if surgery is contraindicated by severe impairment of lung function or evidence of metastatic disease, there is reasonable justification for an invasive procedure such as TTNA. The rationale in each of these circumstances is twofold: to exclude rare benign conditions that can simulate malignancy and to help establish prognosis.

Solitary Pulmonary Mass (Tumor Larger Than 3 cm in Diameter)

Since larger nodules are more likely to be malignant, the age-related conservative approach just described for some patients is not warranted, and management should proceed as described for a nodule in the 40- to 60-year age group. If cavitation is present in a lesion of this size, the cause may be infectious even in the absence of fever, constitutional symptoms, or leukocytosis. Since such lesions are usually caused by anaerobic organisms, a therapeutic trial of penicillin may be indicated if the clinical history is compatible with such a diagnosis.

Segmental Consolidation of Lung Parenchyma, Usually Associated with Loss of Volume

In most cases, segmental consolidation of parenchyma is due to an endobronchial lesion causing atelectasis and obstructive pneumonitis. Bronchoscopy with brushings, washings, and biopsy usually establishes the diagnosis.

Multiple Pulmonary Nodules

In many patients with multiple pulmonary nodules, the diagnosis is apparent without resort to pathologic investigation. The majority of patients have either an established primary neoplasm elsewhere (the pulmonary lesions representing metastases) or an infection, usually tuberculous or fungal. Positive skin reactions to specific antigens or a history of residence or travel in an endemic zone may be helpful in establishing the latter diagnosis. If these investigations are unproductive, we believe that a direct approach by TTNA is the procedure of first choice. In most cases, this yields adequate material for culture or cytologic identification of a specific organism. In patients with an established primary malignancy, pathologic confirmation of the metastatic nature of multiple pulmonary nodules is usually unnecessary. In the occasional case in which such confirmation is considered important, cytologic examination of expectorated sputum is straightforward, and findings are positive in some cases. Failing a definitive answer by this technique, TTNA is again the procedure of choice.

When metastases and infective granulomatous processes have been excluded, the remaining diagnostic possibilities are rather limited and include abnormalities such as Wegener's granulomatosis, rheumatoid nodules, and pyemic abscesses. In many persons with these diseases, careful attention to signs and symptoms of extrathoracic disease and to laboratory findings may enable one to make a confident diagnosis; often, however, open lung biopsy is necessary.

Acute Diffuse Pulmonary Disease

The great majority of patients who exhibit acute diffuse pulmonary disease are immunocompromised hosts. Such patients are likely to be receiving immunosuppressive drugs, corticosteroids, chemotherapeutic agents, and/or antibiotics, and a drastic reduction in dosage or complete withdrawal of medications frequently results in clinical and roentgenologic improvement. An early decision to take this action, before the onset of severe dyspnea and hypoxemia, permits assessment of roentgenologic response before it becomes necessary to subject the patient to an invasive diagnostic procedure. If resolution does occur, it can be assumed either that there has been an improvement in host defenses, with consequent control of infection, or that the disease was the result of a drug reaction. If clearing does not occur, the cause of the diffuse pulmonary disease is probably an opportunistic micro-organism. In most such instances, an immediate invasive procedure is indicated for diagnosis, and we recommend that bronchoscopy with TBB and ancillary procedures such as bronchoalveolar lavage should be performed first; if these prove negative, open lung biopsy can be performed.

Chronic Diffuse Pulmonary Disease

This roentgenographic pattern usually indicates predominant involvement of either the interstitium or the airspaces (more often the former), and onset is usually insidious. Some patients are asymptomatic, in which case it is debatable whether an invasive diagnostic procedure is justified; however, there are many patients whose progressive disease has produced symptoms and whose roentgenographic pattern and clinical picture are inconclusive. In this situation, unless the patient is too old or too ill to warrant the slight risk, biopsy is mandatory to establish the diagnosis of a potentially treatable condition. Open lung biopsy is usually the procedure of choice, although thoracoscopic and transbronchial biopsy are of value in some circumstances (particularly if there is a suspicion of sarcoidosis or lymphangitic spread of carcinoma). Occasionally, patients become so disabled by dyspnea that we hesitate to recommend open biopsy. In such circumstances, we recommend transbronchial biopsy as a first step; should this prove unrewarding, open lung biopsy can then be performed if absolutely necessary.

Examination of Excised Lobes and Whole Lungs

Pulmonary lobes that have been surgically excised or whole lungs that have been removed at surgery or at autopsy can be examined by a variety of techniques. To some extent, the method of examination depends on the suspected nature of the underlying disease; for example, injection of the pulmonary artery with contrast medium might be the procedure of choice in a case of suspected arteriovenous fistula. However, such special techniques are impractical and unnecessary as a routine, and in the great majority of cases the most appropriate method of investigation is inflation and fixation of the lung with liquid formalin, followed by serial slicing.

The easiest and most widely utilized method of fixation is to distend the lung to apparent full inflation with formalin introduced into the bronchi under positive pressure. This is conveniently accomplished by elevating a formalin-filled container above the lung, the most suitable maximal pressure head being about 25 to 30 cm. After inflation, the most proximal airways are clamped, and the lung or lobe is left overnight in a large vat of formalin to be examined the following morning. Following inspection of the pleural surface, the lung is cut with a sharp knife in even sections 1 to

1.5 cm thick. The slices are then laid out on a cutting board for detailed examination.

Several techniques have been advocated to obtain specimens suitable for special investigations such as morphometric analysis and radiologic-pathologic correlation. In one widely used method,[132] a mixture of formalin, polyethylene glycol, and alcohol is insufflated into the bronchi. After fixation (about 48 hours), the lung is dried by blowing air through the bronchus for some time. This produces adequately preserved specimens from which excellent gross and histologic correlation with radiologic patterns can be appreciated (Fig. 2–8).[133]

Special Pathologic Techniques

Examination of the Pulmonary Vasculature and Airways

The most satisfactory substance for pulmonary angiography is the Schlesinger mass,[134] the basic ingredient of which is gelatin that is kept liquid at room temperature by potassium iodide and that solidifies on addition of formalin. Barium sulfate or other radiopaque material can be added to obtain roentgenographic visibility, and dyes can be used to define different components of the vasculature. Bronchography can be performed using either the Schlesinger mass or fine-particle barium, tantalum, or lead insufflated into the bronchial tree.

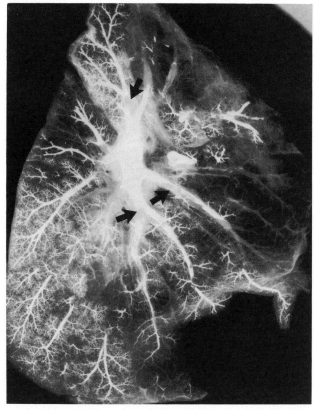

Figure 2–8. Postmortem Pulmonary Angiogram Demonstrating Thromboemboli. Roentgenogram of a 1-cm slice of the left lung shows multiple filling defects in the proximal vessels *(arrows)*; small vessels are normal, although in some there is a lack of contrast material. The specimen was injected via the pulmonary artery with barium gelatin mixture, fixed with an ethylene glycol–alcohol solution, and air-dried.

Electron Microscopy

It is usually unnecessary to examine pulmonary tissue or cells by electron microscopy for diagnostic purposes; nevertheless, in some instances the procedure is helpful—and occasionally indispensable—in establishing a precise diagnosis.

In *transmission electron microscopy* (TEM), an electron beam is focused on an ultrathin section of tissue and an image is produced by collecting the transmitted electrons on a screen or photographic plate. Because of the necessity for a small tissue specimen, one of the major limitations of the technique is related to sampling. Careful handling and fixation of tissue is essential, since autolysis rapidly results in ultrastructural changes that can obscure proper interpretation, especially in diseased lungs.[135] Tissue fragments should be small (1 mm or smaller) to allow for adequate fixative penetration. In addition to tissue specimens, fluid or cells obtained by bronchoalveolar lavage or by aspiration of pleural fluid or pulmonary or mediastinal tumors can also be processed for TEM.

TEM has its greatest use in the diagnosis of pulmonary neoplasms. Occasionally, it is the definitive diagnostic technique in such tumors as carcinoid tumor, small cell carcinoma, and tracheobronchial gland carcinomas,[136] especially when only small amounts of tissue are available from transbronchial biopsy or TTNA. Typing of pulmonary sarcoma is often aided by ultrastructural findings, and most neoplasms with a sarcomatous appearance should be examined in this fashion before a specific diagnosis is applied. TEM is also useful in differentiating mesothelioma from metastatic carcinoma and occasionally can be helpful in distinguishing primary from metastatic lung carcinoma[137] and lymphoma from carcinoma.

The use of TEM in non-neoplastic pulmonary disease is less helpful. Although usually not necessary, it sometimes aids in confirming the diagnosis of viral infection and metabolic abnormalities such as amyloidosis and alveolar proteinosis. Intracytoplasmic "X bodies" are characteristic of the Langerhans' cells of eosinophilic granuloma, and their identification also may help confirm the diagnosis of this disease. The technique is essential for the identification and characterization of the dyskinetic cilia syndrome.

The primary diagnostic use of *scanning electron microscopy* in pulmonary disease is in the study of the pneumoconioses. With this technique, particulate material can be identified, and its composition precisely analyzed. Since the different images derived from the procedure can be correlated, it can provide accurate information about the location of specific particulates within cells or tissues.

Immunochemistry

The development of techniques for the immunochemical demonstration of tissue antigens has been one of the major advances in diagnostic pathology in recent years, and the great variety of applications is only beginning to be appreciated.

Immunofluorescence tests are performed by applying an antibody conjugated with fluorescein dye to a tissue section. After washing, the tissue is examined with a fluorescent microscope, enabling appreciation of the fluorescent antibody-antigen complex. In the lung, the technique has had its widest application in the study of immune-mediated abnormalities, especially Goodpasture's syndrome[138]; when this diagnosis is suspected, tissue should always be taken and examined by immunofluorescence.

Immunoenzymatic techniques involve the conjugation of a diagnostic antibody with an enzyme (most frequently peroxidase), the application of this combination to a tissue section, and the addition of a substrate (e.g., diaminobenzidine in the case of peroxidase) that reacts with the enzyme to produce a visible compound. Although these techniques have been used in the study of immune-mediated lung disease and for the identification of micro-organisms, their major application has been in the diagnosis of pulmonary and mediastinal neoplasms. A variety of antibodies have been developed in attempts to characterize subtypes of pulmonary carcinoma more precisely,[139] to distinguish neoplasms such as mesothelioma from metastatic adenocarcinoma[140] or mediastinal lymphoma from thymoma,[141] and to differentiate reactive from truly neoplastic epithelial cells.[142] Other applications include distinguishing metastatic from primary pulmonary neoplasms, identification of bronchioloalveolar cell carcinoma, and the precise characterization of pulmonary sarcomas.

Molecular Biology

The exciting and rapidly progressing field of molecular biology is certain to contribute in important ways to both the investigation and the diagnosis of pulmonary disease. Although procedures such as the polymerase chain reaction and gene rearrangement techniques are likely to be especially relevant in the diagnosis of infection[143, 144] and neoplasia,[145] their use in other forms of disease is virtually ensured.

References

1. Zinn B, Monroe J: The lordotic position in fluoroscopy and roentgenography of the chest. Am J Roentgenol 75: 682, 1956.
2. Rundle FF, DeLambert RM, Epps RG: Cervicothoracic tumors: A technical aid to their roentgenologic localization. Am J Roentgenol 81: 316, 1959.
3. Crapo RO, Montague T, Armstrong J: Inspiratory lung volume achieved on routine chest films. Invest Radiol 14: 137, 1979.
4. Tuddenham WJ: Problems of perception in chest roentgenography: Facts and fallacies. Radiol Clin North Am 1: 277, 1963.
5. Jackson FI: The air-gap technique, and an improvement by anteroposterior positioning for chest roentgenography. Am J Roentgenol 92: 688, 1964.
6. Wilkinson GA, Fraser RG: Roentgenography of the chest. Appl Radiol 4: 41, 1975.
7. Lynch PA: A different approach to chest roentgenography: Triad technique (high kilovoltage, grid, wedge filter). Am J Roentgenol 93: 965, 1965.
8. Rossi RP, Harnisch G, Hendee WR: Reduction of radiation exposure in radiography of the chest. Radiology 144: 909, 1982.
9. Kelsey CA, Moseley RD, Mettler FA, et al: Comparison of nodule detection with 70-kVp and 120-kVp chest radiographs. Radiology 143: 609, 1982.
10. Wandtke JC, Plewes DP, Vogelstein E: Scanning equalization radiography of the chest: Assessment of image quality. Am J Roentgenol 145: 973, 1985.
11. Plewes DB, Wandtke JC: A scanning equalization system for improved chest radiography. Radiology 142: 765, 1982.
12. Wandtke JC, Plewes DB, McFaul JA: Improved pulmonary nodule

detection with scanning equalization radiography. Radiology 169: 23, 1988.

13. Wandtke JC, Plewes DB: Comparison of scanning equalization and conventional chest radiography. Radiology 172: 641, 1989.
14. Vasbloem H, Kool LJS: AMBER: A scanning multiple-beam equalization system for chest radiography. Radiology 169: 29, 1988.
15. Ravin CE: Advanced multiple-beam equalization radiography (AMBER): Early clinical experience. *In* Peppler WW, Alter A (eds): Proceedings of the Chest Imaging Conference 1987. Madison, WI, Medical Physics Publishing, 1988, p 60.
16. Chotas HG, Van Metter RL, Johnson GA, et al: Small object contrast in AMBER and conventional chest radiography. Radiology 180: 853, 1991.
17. Rigler LG: Roentgen diagnosis of small pleural effusion: A new roentgenographic position. JAMA 96: 104, 1931.
18. Capitanio MA, Kirkpatrick JA: The lateral decubitus film: An aid in determining air-trapping in children. Radiology 103: 460, 1972.
19. Rucker L, Frye EB, Staten MA: Usefulness of screening chest roentgenograms in preoperative patients. JAMA 250: 3209, 1983.
19a. Hubbell FA, Greenfield S, Tyler JL, et al: Special article: The impact of routine admission chest x-ray films on patient care. N Engl J Med 312: 209, 1985.
20. Harris JH: Referral criteria for routine screening chest x-ray examinations. Am Coll Radiol Bull 38: 17, 1982.
21. Tabrisky J, Herman MW, Torrance DJ, et al: Mobile 240 kVp phototimed chest radiography. Am J Roentgenol 135: 395, 1980.
22. Henschke CI, Pasternack GS, Schroeder S, et al: Bedside chest radiography: Diagnostic efficacy. Radiology 149: 23, 1983.
23. Fraser RG, Sanders C, Barnes GT, et al: Digital imaging of the chest. Radiology 171: 297, 1989.
24. Sherrier RH, Chotas HG, Johnson A, et al: Image optimization in a computed-radiography/photostimulable-phosphor system. J Digit Imaging 2: 212, 1989.
25. Schaefer CM, Greene R, Llewellyn HJ, et al: Interstitial lung disease: Impact of postprocessing in digital storage phosphor imaging. Radiology 178: 733, 1991.
26. Fraser RG, Breatnach E, Barnes GT: Digital radiography of the chest: Clinical experience with a prototype unit. Radiology 148: 1, 1983.
27. Oestmann JW, Greene R, Rhea JT, et al: "Single-exposure" dual-energy digital radiography in the detection of pulmonary nodules and calcifications. Invest Radiol 24: 517, 1989.
28. Ergun DL, Mistretta CA, Brown DE, et al: Single-exposure dual-energy computed radiography: Improved detection and processing. Radiology 174: 243, 1990.
29. Fraser RG, Hickey NM, Niklason LT, et al: Calcification in pulmonary nodules: Detection with dual-energy digital radiography. Radiology 160: 595, 1986.
30. Favis EA: Planigraphy (body section radiography) in detecting tuberculous pulmonary cavitation. Dis Chest 27: 668, 1955.
31. Janower ML: Fifty-five degree posterior oblique tomography of the pulmonary hilum. J Can Assoc Radiol 19: 158, 1978.
32. Curtis AM, Ravin CE, Collier PE, et al: Detection of metastatic disease from carcinoma of the breast: Limited value of full-lung tomography. Am J Roentgenol 134: 253, 1980.
33. Sindelar WF, Bagley DH, Felix EL, et al: Lung tomography in cancer patients: Full-lung tomograms in screening for pulmonary metastases. JAMA 240: 2060, 1978.
34. Society for Computed Body Tomography: Special report: New indications for computed body tomography. Am J Roentgenol 133: 115, 1979.
35. Shin MS, Ho H-J: Computed tomographic evaluation of solitary pulmonary nodules in chest roentgenograms. CT 6: 947, 1982.
36. Godwin JD, Speckman JM, Fram EK, et al: Distinguishing benign from malignant pulmonary nodules by computed tomography. Radiology 144: 349, 1982.
37. Levi C, Gray JE, McCullough EC, et al: The unreliability of CT numbers as absolute values. Am J Roentgenol 139: 443, 1982.
38. Cann CE, Gamsu G, Birnberg FA, et al: Quantification of calcium in solitary pulmonary nodules using single- and dual-energy CT. Radiology 145: 493, 1982.
39. Zerhouni EA, Stitik FP, Siegelman SS, et al: CT of the pulmonary nodule: A cooperative study. Radiology 160: 319, 1986.
40. Rosenblum LJ, Mauceri RA, Wellenstein DE, et al: Computed tomography of the lung. Radiology 129: 521, 1978.
41. Bessis L, Callard P, Gotheil C, et al: High-resolution CT of parenchymal lung disease: Precise correlation with histologic findings. Radiographics 12: 45, 1992.
42. Remy-Jardin M, Remy J, Deffontaines C, et al: Assessment of diffuse infiltrative lung disease: Comparison of conventional CT and high resolution CT. Radiology 181: 157, 1991.
43. Müller NL: Clinical value of high-resolution CT in chronic diffuse lung disease. Am J Roentgenol 157: 1163, 1991.
44. Pykett IL, Newhouse JH, Buonanno FS, et al: Nuclear magnetic resonance: Principles of nuclear magnetic resonance imaging. Radiology 143: 157, 1982.
45. Mitchell MR, Partain CL, Price RR, et al: NMR: State of the art in medical imaging: Reflections from National Cancer Institute/Bowman Gray/Vanderbilt International Symposium. Appl Radiol July/Aug: 19, 1982.
46. Webb WR: MRI of the chest. Current applications and possible uses. Appl Radiol Nov/Dec: 69, 1986.
47. Dooms GC, Hricak H, Crooks LE, et al: Magnetic resonance imaging of the lymph nodes: Comparison with CT. Radiology 153: 719, 1984.
48. Webb WR, Gamsu G, Stark DD, et al: Magnetic resonance imaging of the normal and abnormal pulmonary hila. Radiology 152: 89, 1984.
49. von Schulthess GK, McMurdo K, Tscholakoff D, et al: Mediastinal masses: MR imaging. Radiology 158: 289, 1986.
50. Webb WR, Gamsu G, Crooks LE: Multisection sagittal and coronal magnetic resonance imaging of the mediastinum and hila. Radiology 150: 475, 1984.
51. O'Donovan PB, Ross JS, Sivak ED, et al: Magnetic resonance imaging of the thorax: The advantages of coronal and sagittal planes. Am J Roentgenol 143: 1183, 1984.
52. Gamsu G, Hirji M, Moore EH, et al: Experimental pulmonary emboli detected using magnetic resonance. Radiology 153: 467, 1984.
53. Schmidt HC, Tsay DG, Higgins CB: Pulmonary edema: An MR study of permeability and hydrostatic types in animals. Radiology 158: 297, 1986.
54. Amparo EG, Higgins CB, Hoddick W, et al: Magnetic resonance imaging of aortic disease: Preliminary results. Am J Roentgenol 143: 1203, 1984.
55. Forrest JV, Sagel SS, Omell GH: Bronchography in patients with hemoptysis. Am J Roentgenol 126: 597, 1976.
56. Naidich DP, Funt S, Ettenger NA, et al: Hemoptysis: CT-bronchoscopic correlations in 58 cases. Radiology 177: 357, 1990.
57. Suprenant E, Wilson A, Bennett L, et al: Changes in regional pulmonary function following bronchography. Radiology 91: 736, 1968.
58. Meany TF, Weinstein MA, Buonocore E, et al: Digital subtraction angiography of the human cardiovascular system. Am J Roentgenol 135: 1153, 1980.
59. Hirji M, Gamsu G, Webb WR, et al: EKG-gated digital subtraction angiography in the detection of pulmonary emboli. Radiology 152: 19, 1984.
60. Ludwig JW, Verhoeven LAJ, Kersbergen JJ, et al: Digital subtraction and angiography of the pulmonary arteries for the diagnosis of pulmonary embolism. Radiology 147: 639, 1983.
61. Ferris EJ, Stanzler RM, Rourke JA, et al: Pulmonary angiography in pulmonary embolic disease. Am J Roentgenol 100:355, 1967.
62. Wagner RB, Baeza DR, Stewart JE: Active pulmonary hemorrhage localized by selective pulmonary angiography. Chest 67: 121, 1975.
63. Seldinger SI: Catheter replacement of the needle in percutaneous arteriography: A new technique. Acta Radiol 39: 368, 1953.
64. Botenga ASJ: Selective Bronchial and Intercostal Arteriography. Leiden, HE Stenfert Kroese, NV, 1970.
65. Vujic I, Pule R, Hungerford GD, et al: Angiography and therapeutic blockade in the control of hemoptysis: The importance of nonbronchial systemic arteries. Radiology 143: 19, 1982.
66. North LB, Boushy SF, Houk VN: Bronchial and intercostal arteriography in non-neoplastic pulmonary disease. Am J Roentgenol 107: 328, 1969.
67. Mishkin FS, Brashear RE: Use and Interpretation of the Lung Scan. Springfield, IL, Charles C Thomas, 1971.
68. Khan O, Ell PJ, Jarritt PH, et al: Radionuclide section scanning of the lungs in pulmonary embolism. Br J Radiol 54: 586, 1981.
69. Potchen EJ, Evens RG, Hill R, et al: Regional pulmonary function in man: Quantitative transmission radiography as an adjunct to lung scintiscanning. Am J Roentgenol 108: 724, 1970.
70. Goodrich JK, Jones RH, Coulam CM, et al: Xenon-133 measurement of regional ventilation. Radiology 103: 611, 1972.
71. Rhodes BA, Stern HS, Buchanan JA, et al: Lung scanning with ^{99m}Tc microspheres. Radiology 99: 613, 1971.

72. Elam DA, Poe ND: A single-breath radioaerosol-inhalation technique. Radiology 145: 542, 1982.

73. Poe ND, Swanson LA, Taplin GV: Physiological factors affecting lung scan interpretations. Radiology 89: 66, 1967.

74. Hughes JMB: Fleischner lecture: Radionuclides and the lung: Past, present and future. Am J Roentgenol 155: 455, 1990.

75. Doust BD, Baum JK, Maklad NF, et al: Ultrasonic evaluation of pleural opacities. Radiology 114: 135, 1975.

76. Lewandowski BJ, Winsberg F: Sonographic demonstration of the right paramediastinal pleural space. Radiology 145: 127, 1982.

77. Goldberg BB: Mediastinal ultrasonography. J Clin Ultrasound 1: 114, 1973.

77a. Yang PC, Chang DB, Yu CJ, et al: Ultrasound-guided core biopsy of thoracic tumors. Am Rev Respir Dis 146(3): 763, 1992.

78. Ng ABP, Horak GC: Factors significant in the diagnostic accuracy of lung cytology in bronchial washing and sputum samples. II. Sputum samples. Acta Cytol 27: 397, 1983.

79. Fontana RS, Carr DT, Woolner LB, et al: An evaluation of methods of inducing sputum production in patients with suspected cancer of the lung. Mayo Clin Proc 37: 113, 1962.

80. Saccomanno G, Saunders RP, Ellis H, et al: Concentration of carcinoma or atypical cells in sputum. Acta Cytol 7: 305, 1963.

81. Ellis HD, Kernosky JJ: Efficiency of concentrating malignant cells in sputum. Acta Cytol 7: 372, 1963.

82. Russell WO, Neidhardt HW, Mountain CF, et al: Cytodiagnosis of lung cancer: A report of a four-year laboratory, clinical, and statistical study with a review of the literature on lung cancer and pulmonary cytology. Acta Cytol 7: 1, 1963.

83. Ng APB, Horak GC: Factors significant in the diagnostic accuracy of lung cytology in bronchial washing and sputum samples. I. Bronchial washings. Acta Cytol 27: 391, 1983.

84. Johnston WW: Ten years of respiratory cytopathology at Duke University Medical Center. III. The significance of inconclusive cytopathologic diagnoses during the years 1970 to 1974. Acta Cytol 26: 759, 1982.

85. Bewtra C, Dewan N, O'Donahue WJ Jr: Exfoliative sputum cytology in pulmonary embolism. Acta Cytol 27: 489, 1983.

86. Koss LG, Melamed MR, Mayer K: The effect of busulfan on human epithelia. Am J Clin Pathol 44: 385, 1965.

87. Kern WH, Schweizer CW: Sputum cytology of metastatic carcinoma of the lung. Acta Cytol 20: 514, 1976.

88. Light RW, Frozan YS, Ball WC Jr: Cells in pleural fluid: Their value in differential diagnosis. Arch Intern Med 132: 854, 1973.

89. Kutty CPK, Remeniuk E, Varkey B: Malignant-appearing cells in pleural effusion due to pancreatitis: Case report and literature review. Acta Cytol 24: 412, 1980.

90. Spieler P: The cytologic diagnosis of tuberculosis in pleural effusions. Acta Cytol 23: 374, 1979.

91. Campbell GD, Webb WR: Eosinophilic pleural effusion: A review with the presentation of seven new cases. Am Rev Respir Dis 90: 194, 1964.

92. Petusevsky ML, Faling J, Rocklin RE, et al: Pleuropericardial reaction to treatment with dantrolene. JAMA 242: 2772, 1979.

93. Sterrett G, Whitaker K, Glancy J: Fine-needle aspiration of lung, mediastinum and chest wall. A clinicopathologic exercise. Pathol Annu 17(Pt 2): 197, 1982.

94. Westcott JL: Percutaneous transthoracic needle biopsy. Radiology 169: 593, 1988.

95. Perlmutt LM, Johnston WW, Dunnick NR: Percutaneous transthoracic needle aspiration: A review. Am J Roentgenol 152: 451, 1989.

96. Zavala DC, Schoell JE: Ultra-thin needle aspiration of the lung in infectious and malignant disease. Am Rev Respir Dis 123: 125, 1981.

97. Jereb M, Us-Krasovec M: Thin needle biopsy of chest lesions: Time-saving potential. Chest 78: 288, 1980.

98. Smith MJ, Kini SR, Watson E: Fine-needle aspiration and endoscopic brush cytology: Comparison of direct smears and rinsings. Acta Cytol 24: 456, 1980.

99. Pak HY, Yokota S, Teplitz RL, et al: Rapid staining techniques employed in fine-needle aspirations of the lung. Acta Cytol 25: 178, 1981.

100. The American Thoracic Society. Guidelines for percutaneous transthoracic needle biopsy. Am Rev Respir Dis 140: 255, 1989.

101. Fish GD, Stanley JH, Miller KS, et al: Postbiopsy pneumothorax: Estimating the risk by chest radiography and pulmonary function tests. Am J Roentgenol 150: 71, 1988.

101a. Hix WR, Aaron BL: Needle aspiration in lung cancer. Risk of tumor implantation is not negligible. Chest 97: 516, 1990.

102. Fraser RS: Transthoracic needle aspiration—the benign diagnosis. Arch Pathol Lab Med 115: 751, 1991.

103. Conces DJ Jr, Clark SA, Tarver RD, et al: Transthoracic aspiration needle biopsy: Value in the diagnosis of pulmonary infections. Am J Roentgenol 152: 31, 1989.

104. Mehta AC, Kavuru MS, Meeker DP, et al: Transbronchial needle aspiration for histology specimens. Chest 96: 1228, 1989.

105. Wang KP, Terry P, Marsh B: Bronchoscopic needle aspiration biopsy of paratracheal tumors. Am Rev Respir Dis 118: 17, 1978.

106. Zisholtz BM, Eisenberg H: Lung cancer cell type as a determinant of bronchoscopy yield. Chest 84: 428, 1983.

107. Popovich J Jr, Kvale PA, Eichenhorn MS, et al: Diagnostic accuracy of multiple biopsies from flexible fiberoptic bronchoscopy—a comparison of central versus peripheral carcinoma. Am Rev Respir Dis 125: 521, 1982.

108. Haponik EF, Summer WR, Terry PB, et al: Clinical decision making with transbronchial lung biopsies: The value of nonspecific histologic examination. Am Rev Respir Dis 125: 524, 1982.

109. Puksa S, Hutcheon MA, Hyland RH: Usefulness of transbronchial biopsy in immunosuppressed patients with pulmonary infiltrates. Thorax 38: 146, 1983.

109a. Hernández Blasco L, Sanchez Hernández IM, Villena Garrido V, et al: Safety of the transbronchial biopsy in outpatients. Chest 99: 562, 1991.

110. Vitums VC: Percutaneous needle biopsy of the lung with a new disposable needle. Chest 62: 717, 1972.

111. Castillo G, Ahmad M, Vanordstrand HS, et al: Trephine drill biopsy of the lung. Cleveland Clinic experience. JAMA 228: 189, 1974.

112. Kremp RE, Klatte EC, Collins RD: Technical considerations of percutaneous pulmonary biopsy. Radiology 100: 285, 1971.

113. Morgenroth A, Pfeuffer HP, Austgen M, et al: Six years' experience with perthoracic core needle biopsy in pulmonary lesions. Thorax 44: 177, 1989.

114. Strobel SL, Keyhani-Rofagha S, O'Toole RV, et al: Nonaspiration-needle smear preparations of pulmonary lesions: A comparison of cytology and histology. Acta Cytol 29: 1047, 1985.

114a. Yazdi HM, MacDonald LL, Hickey NM: Thoracic fine-needle aspiration biopsy versus fine-needle cutting biopsy: A comparative study of 40 patients. Acta Cytol 32: 635, 1988.

115. Todd TRJ, Weisbrod G, Tao LC, et al: Aspiration needle biopsy of thoracic lesions. Ann Thorac Surg 32: 154, 1981.

116. Goralnik CH, O'Connell DM, El Yousef SJ, et al: CT-guided cutting-needle biopsies of selected chest lesions. Am J Roentgenol 151: 903, 1988.

117. Boutin C, Viallat JR, Cargnino P, et al: Thoracoscopic lung biopsy: Experimental and clinical preliminary study. Chest 82: 44, 1982.

118. Dijkman JH, van der Meer JWM, Bakker W, et al: Transpleural lung biopsy by the thoracoscopic route in patients with diffuse interstitial pulmonary disease. Chest 82: 76, 1982.

119. Newman SL, Michel RP, Wang N-S: Lingular lung biopsy: Is it representative? Am Rev Respir Dis 132: 1084, 1985.

120. Gaensler EA, Carrington CB: Open biopsy for chronic diffuse infiltrative lung disease: Clinical, roentgenographic and physiological correlations in 502 patients. Ann Thorac Surg 30: 411, 1980.

121. Wall CP, Gaensler EA, Carrington CB, et al: Comparison of transbronchial and open biopsies in chronic infiltrative lung diseases. Am Rev Respir Dis 123: 280, 1981.

121a. Wagner JD, Stahler C, Knox S, et al: Clinical utility of open lung biopsy for undiagnosed pulmonary infiltrates. Am J Surg 164(2): 104, 1992.

122. Mungall IPF, Cowen PN, Cooke NT, et al: Multiple pleural biopsy with the Abrams needle. Thorax 35: 600, 1980.

123. The American Thoracic Society: Guidelines for thoracentesis and needle biopsy of the pleura. Am Rev Respir Dis 140: 257, 1989.

124. Menzies R, Charbonneau M: Thoracoscopy for the diagnosis of pleural disease. Ann Intern Med 114: 271, 1991.

124a. Coltharp WH, Arnold JH, Alford WC Jr, et al: Videothoracoscopy: Improved technique and expanded indications. Ann Thorac Surg 53(5): 776, 1992.

125. Mediastinoscopy (Editorial). Lancet 1: 1219, 1972.

126. Marchand P: Mediastinoscopy. S Afr Med J 46: 285, 1972.

127. Hájek M, Homan van der Heide JN: Early detection of mediastinal spread of pulmonary carcinoma by mediastinoscopy. Thorax 25: 720, 1970.

128. Evans DS, Hall JH, Harrison GK: Anterior mediastinotomy. Thorax 28: 444, 1973.

129. Deneffe G, Lacquet LM, Gyselen A: Cervical mediastinoscopy and anterior mediastinotomy in patients with lung cancer and radiologically normal mediastinum. Eur J Respir Dis 64: 613, 1983.

130. Skinner DB: Scalene-lymph-node biopsy: Reappraisal of risks and indications. N Engl J Med 268: 1324, 1963.

131. Brantigan JW, Brantigan CO, Brantigan OC: Biopsy of nonpalpable scalene lymph nodes in carcinoma of the lung. Am Rev Respir Dis 107: 962, 1973.

132. Sutinen S, Pääkkö P, Lahti R: Post-mortem inflation, radiography and fixation of human lungs: A method for radiological and pathological correlations and morphometric studies. Scand J Respir Dis 60: 29, 1979.

133. Pääkkö P, Sutinen S, Lahti R: Pattern recognition in radiography of excised air-inflated human lungs. I. Circulatory disorders in nonemphysematous lungs. Eur J Respir Dis 62: 33, 1981.

134. Schlesinger MJ: New radiopaque mass for vascular injection. Lab Invest 6: 1, 1957.

135. Bachofen M, Weibel ER, Roos B: Postmortem fixation of human lungs for electron microscopy. Am Rev Respir Dis 111: 247, 1975.

136. Heard BE, Dewar A, Firmin RK, et al: One very rare and one new tracheal tumour found by electron microscopy: Glomus tumour and acinic cell tumour resembling carcinoid tumours by light microscopy. Thorax 37: 97, 1982.

137. Posalaky Z, McGinley D, Posalaky IP: Electron microscopic identification of the colorectal origins of tumor cells in pleural fluid. Acta Cytol 25: 45, 1981.

138. Beechler CR, Enquist RW, Hunt KK, et al: Immunofluorescence of transbronchial biopsies in Goodpasture's syndrome. Am Rev Respir Dis 121: 869, 1980.

139. Lehto VP, Stenman S, Miettinen M, et al: Expression of a neural type of intermediate filament as a distinguishing feature between oat cell carcinoma and other lung cancers. Am J Pathol 110: 113, 1983.

140. Corson JM, Pinkus GS: Mesothelioma: Profile of keratin proteins and carcinoembryonic antigen: An immunoperoxidase study of 20 cases and comparison with pulmonary adenocarcinomas. Am J Pathol 108: 80, 1982.

141. Battifora H, Sun T-T, Bahu RM, et al: The use of antikeratin antiserum as a diagnostic tool: Thymoma versus lymphoma. Hum Pathol 11: 635, 1980.

142. Biyoudi-Vouenze R, Tazi A, Hance AJ: Abnormal epithelial cells recovered by bronchoalveolar lavage: Are they malignant? Am Rev Respir Dis 142: 686, 1990.

143. Cagle PT, Buffone G, Holland VA, et al: Semiquantitative measurement of cytomegalovirus DNA in lung and heart-lung transplant patients by in vitro DNA amplification. Chest 101: 93, 1992.

144. de Lassence A, Lecossier D, Pierre C, et al: Detection of mycobacterial DNA in pleural fluid from patients with tuberculous pleurisy by means of the polymerase chain reaction: Comparison of two protocols. Thorax 47: 265, 1992.

145. Kavura MS, Tubbs R, Miller ML, et al: Immunocytochemistry and gene rearrangement in the diagnosis of lymphoma in an idiopathic pleural effusion. Am Rev Respir Dis 145: 209, 1992.

3

METHODS OF CLINICAL, LABORATORY, AND FUNCTIONAL INVESTIGATION

CLINICAL HISTORY

The most important part of any clinical history is the patient's description of the symptoms, which should be listened to with care. When the patient has finished, the physician should ask for any pertinent information about past illnesses and personal habits, where the patient has lived and traveled, and the occupational history. Finally, since lung disease frequently is only one manifestation of a more general process or is secondary to a disease involving other organs, an account of the function of other body systems is essential.

Symptoms of Respiratory Disease

The principal symptoms of respiratory disease are cough (with or without expectoration), shortness of breath, chest pain, and hemoptysis.

Cough and Expectoration

Cough is a defensive mechanism designed to rid the conducting passages of mucus and foreign material. As a symptom of pulmonary disease, therefore, it is often present in patients who aspirate or who have chronic airway irritation from substances such as tobacco smoke. Because it stimulates airway irritant receptors, local bronchial disease such as carcinoma is also commonly manifested in this manner.

It is useful to consider a cough as being dry or productive. The former often develops in the early stages of viral infections of both upper and lower respiratory tracts and may be an early symptom of left-sided heart failure. Although cough also may be a nervous habit (in which case it is usually recognized as such by the patient or the family), it is important to realize that it may be a symptom of asthma, even when it is not associated with wheezing or dyspnea and when routine pulmonary function tests are normal.[1] Asthmatics with this presentation can be identified by the demonstration of bronchial hyperreactivity with inhalational challenge tests or by amelioration of the cough following administration of bronchodilators.[2]

Some coughs, particularly those associated with acute bacterial infection, are productive in the early stage of disease. In addition, most dry coughs eventually become productive if they persist long enough. The character and quantity of expectorated material in these cases may suggest the diagnosis. It usually is clear and mucoid when the stimulus is viral infection or a foreign substance such as smoke. The patient with chronic bronchitis also usually expectorates mucoid material, but with "colds" it may be yellow or green and sometimes slightly blood-streaked. Saccular bronchiectasis gives rise to copious, purulent, and often blood-streaked expectoration every day. The gelatinous, "rusty" expectoration formerly associated with pneumococcal pneumonia has been seen rarely since the advent of antibiotics, and bacterial pneumonia is now more commonly manifested by thick, yellow or greenish sputum. A foul or fetid odor indicates infection from anaerobic organisms, usually associated with abscess formation. Bronchial tree casts, consisting of inspissated mucus, are seen in cases of bronchitis, asthma, or mucoid impaction, the last often in association with allergic aspergillosis.

Knowledge of the time of occurrence of the cough also may be useful in diagnosis. Most people with a chronic cough complain that it is worse when they lie down at night; this is particularly true of those who have bronchiectasis or a postnasal drip from chronic sinusitis. The patient with chronic bronchitis or bronchiectasis characteristically expectorates on arising in the morning. Spasms of coughing caused by asthma or left-sided heart failure frequently occur at night and may waken the patient. A cough during or shortly after eating suggests aspiration into the tracheobronchial tree.

The association of a cough with other symptoms may be highly suggestive of a specific disease process. For example, if it occurs suddenly during an acute febrile episode and is associated with hoarseness, viral laryngotracheobronchitis is very likely the cause. When it is accompanied by stridor, there is likely intrinsic or extrinsic obstruction to the upper respiratory passages, most often caused by carcinoma. A persistent local wheeze during expiration also often indicates an intrinsic bronchial lesion such as carcinoma. A generalized wheeze usually implies acute bronchospasm, although rarely an endotracheal or mediastinal lesion in the region of the carina may be responsible.

It is important to remember that any change in the character of a chronic cough may have significant implications, particularly in the patient with chronic bronchitis caused by cigarette smoking, for whom such an event often indicates the development of malignancy.

Shortness of Breath

The subjective impression of shortness of breath (dyspnea) includes several sensations[3] and occurs in a variety of settings. The anxious patient "unable to take a deep breath," the patient with emphysema having difficulty in tying shoelaces, and the athlete who has just run 100 m in less than 10 seconds are each experiencing different types of breathing difficulty with vastly different implications. Thus, in assessing the significance of dyspnea, the physician must obtain not only a thorough description of the sensation but also an account of the circumstances that tend to precipitate this sensation and its association with other symptoms.[3a]

A detailed description is most useful in differentiating organic causes of shortness of breath from functional (psychoneurotic) dyspnea. The latter, which is related to tension or anxiety, is the commonest cause of shortness of breath; it is said to occur in 10 per cent of patients seen by specialists in internal medicine![4] Usually, it is described as an inability to take a deep breath or "to get air down to the bottom of the lungs." Patients often spontaneously demonstrate by taking a deep breath; if not, it is helpful to ask them to breathe as they do when short of breath. They will respond by taking a deep breath and, as history-taking continues, may unconsciously repeat the sighing respirations from time to time. In dyspnea of organic cause, on the other hand, the sensation is more difficult to describe; patients may say they are "short-winded" or "puff" and on request demonstrate hyperpnea, breathing more deeply and perhaps more rapidly than normal. Patients who are short of breath at rest and not during exercise almost invariably have functional dyspnea; however, it must be remembered that the patient with spasmodic asthma may be able to engage in strenuous exercise without shortness of breath in the intervals between periodic attacks of extreme dyspnea.

Other features also indicate an organic basis for dyspnea. For example, inability to lie flat because of a feeling of suffocation or waking during the night with shortness of breath strongly suggests organic disease, particularly left ventricular failure, but also asthma, bronchitis, or emphysema. Platypnea is dyspnea worsened by assuming an erect position and is associated with postural arterial oxygen desaturation (orthodeoxia); it is usually related to a shunt, either cardiac or pulmonary.[5] Shortness of breath only during exertion also is strong evidence of organic disease. Some patients do not complain of undue dyspnea during exertion but state that it develops afterward, while they are at rest. Often, this indicates some form of left-sided heart failure, but it may be caused by chronic bronchitis or asthma in which bronchospasm or an increase in bronchial secretions is precipitated by exercise.

The relationship of dyspnea to other symptoms also is very important in assessing its significance. In patients with chronic bronchitis or emphysema, dyspnea that develops during exertion often is preceded by a long history of cough and expectoration. By contrast, the person who has been in good health and who develops dyspnea suddenly usually has pneumothorax. Acute dyspnea also may occur with pneumonia or diffuse bronchiolitis, but in these conditions there are usually premonitory symptoms of fever and cough, with or without evidence of infection of the upper respiratory tract. The sudden onset of dyspnea, often with obvious hyperpnea and tachycardia, in an ill or a postoperative patient should raise the possibility of pulmonary embolism.

During pregnancy, dyspnea is physiologic[6] and probably results from a combination of the hyperventilation produced by increased circulating progesterone and an elevated diaphragm. It should cause concern only if it develops abruptly in pre-eclampsia, when it may be caused by pulmonary edema, or during the third trimester, when pulmonary embolism must be ruled out.

Chest Pain

Pain within the thorax can be discussed conveniently according to its three principal sites of origin: pleura, mediastinum, and chest wall.[7]

Pleural Pain. Because both the lung and the visceral pleura lack sensory apparatus to detect it, pulmonary disease may progress to an advanced stage without producing even minor chest pain. The parietal pleura, on the other hand, is richly supplied with sensory nerves, which can be stimulated by inflammation or stretching of the membrane. Pain may vary from lancinating discomfort during slight inspiratory effort to a less severe but still sharp pain that may "catch" the patient at the end of a maximal inspiration. Pleural pain often disappears or is reduced to a dull ache during expiration or breath holding. Pressure over the intercostal muscles in the area of pain may not elicit discomfort; when it does, the pain typically is mild compared with the sensation during breathing. This is in contrast with chest wall pain, which usually is associated with a palpable region of tenderness, often a very small area.

Except when it involves the diaphragm, the diseased area of pleura (which often is secondary to a pulmonary parenchymal lesion) typically underlies the area in which pain is perceived. The central part of the diaphragm is innervated by the phrenic nerve, and the sensory afferent fibers enter the cervical cord mainly in the third and fourth cervical posterior nerve roots; hence, irritation of this portion of the pleura is referred to the neck and the upper part of the shoulder. The outer parts of the diaphragmatic pleura are supplied by lower intercostal nerves, which enter the thoracic cord in the seventh to twelfth dorsal posterior nerve roots; thus, irritation of this portion causes referred pain in the lower thorax.

Mediastinal Pain. The trachea, esophagus, heart, aorta, and many lymph nodes are situated in the mediastinum, and disease involving any of these may cause pain in that region. It also should be borne in mind that inflammation or neoplastic infiltration of the mediastinal soft tissue itself may cause local discomfort. The commonest retrosternal pain is that due to myocardial ischemia; typically, this is described as "squeezing," "pressing," or "choking" and may extend to the neck or down the left arm or both arms. It may be closely simulated in other conditions, including massive pulmonary embolism, pulmonary hypertension, acute pericarditis, and dissecting aneurysm of the aorta. Esophageal disease may give rise to "burning" pain and usually is clearly related to the ingestion of food. Those who have regurgitation of gastric secretions complain that the pain is worse when they recline and may be relieved when they stand. A common retrosternal sensation, which presumably originates in sensory nerve endings of the tracheal mucosa, is the painful rawness under the sternum experienced by patients with infection of the upper respiratory tract and dry, hacking cough.

Chest Wall Pain. Pain originating in the chest wall is common and may be caused by disease in muscles, nerves, or bones. When it appears to originate in intercostal muscle, there may be a history of trauma that produced strain or even tearing; in our experience, such trauma is frequently caused by acute infection of the tracheobronchial tree, accompanied by dry, often paroxysmal, cough. Despite this, there is often no obvious precipitating cause. Pain related to muscle injury may be differentiated from parietal pleural pain by limited exacerbation (if any) during deep inspiration, its association with tenderness to palpation in the painful area, its aggravation by coughing or trunk movement, and its persistence between paroxysms of coughing.

Radicular pain is caused by pressure or inflammation of the posterior nerve root. It follows the specific intercostal nerve distribution and radiates around the chest from behind or, in some cases, is localized to one area. Usually, it is described as dull and aching and is made worse by movement, particularly coughing. It may be caused by a protruding intervertebral disc, rheumatoid spondylitis, malignant disease involving the vertebrae, or inflammatory or malignant disease within the spinal cord. A variety of intercostal nerve root pain whose origin may be difficult to identify in the early stages is that due to herpes zoster; it is usually described as "burning," most often over a wide area unilaterally along the pathway of one or more intercostal nerves.

After muscle, the skeleton is probably the commonest source of chest wall pain. When the pain is confined to vertebral and paravertebral areas, it is usually caused by inflammatory or neoplastic disease of the vertebrae, and percussion over the vertebral spines may elicit local tenderness. Rib fractures are a common cause of chest wall pain; in addition to rib fractures due to accidental trauma are those that result from prolonged episodes of severe coughing. The costochondral junctions of the ribs may be the site of perichondritis, often associated with tenderness and swelling (Tietze's syndrome); usually the pain is persistent and described as "gnawing" or "aching." Rib pain caused by malignancy often is appreciable before a mass develops; at first, it tends to be poorly localized but later becomes a dull, boring ache over the affected area.

A relatively innocuous, transitory pain of undetermined origin has been described by the name "precordial catch." It is a severe, sharp pain that occurs at rest or during mild activity over the left side of the chest, usually at the cardiac apex, and lasts from 30 seconds to 5 minutes.[8] It comes on suddenly during inspiration, and the invariable reaction is a brief suspension of respiration; subsequently, breathing is maintained at a shallow level while the pain disappears gradually. Its onset often is associated with poor posture, improvement in which sometimes relieves the pain. The condition is very common, and its importance lies solely in its differentiation from other chest pain of more serious consequence.

Hemoptysis

Bleeding from the lower respiratory tract most often originates in the bronchial wall. Usually it is from bronchial vessels themselves; occasionally, the source is a major pulmonary artery, in which case hemorrhage is likely to be sudden and massive. It is important to note that in most cases it is not the actual quantity of blood lost that is important prognostically; in fact, "aspiration" of blood into bronchi ipsilateral and contralateral to the site of hemorrhage is much more significant, and most patients who die likely do so by asphyxiation rather than exsanguination. The commonest airway diseases responsible for hemoptysis are bronchitis and carcinoma.[8a]

Bleeding from the lung itself usually is caused by a local process, such as infarction, infection (particularly tuberculosis), and Wegener's granulomatosis. Less often, it is more or less diffuse within the lung parenchyma, in which case it is usually due to an immune disorder (e.g., Goodpasture's syndrome and the leukocytoclastic vasculitis of systemic lupus erythematosus or Wegener's granulomatosis) or an abnormality of coagulation. Although bleeding caused by the last-named condition can occur as an isolated phenomenon, it is important to remember that it also may be the first indication of underlying bronchopulmonary disease (particulary infection) in a patient with a coagulation disorder.

The amount of hemorrhage is of little value in establishing its cause, but its character may suggest the underlying disease process. For example, simple streaking of mucoid material often occurs in bronchitis, although it may denote a more serious condition such as tuberculosis or carcinoma. When the sputum is frankly bloody and does not contain mucoid or purulent material, it is more likely due to pulmonary infarction than to pneumonia, particularly if it persists unchanged for several days. Bloody material mixed with pus should suggest pneumonia or lung abscess in acute illness and bronchiectasis in chronic disease. Finally, when the blood is diluted, giving it a pink and sometimes frothy appearance, pulmonary edema from left heart failure should be suspected.

In assessing the patient with "hemoptysis," it must be remembered that bleeding may originate from the upper respiratory tract or the esophagus. This usually can be distinguished clinically from true hemoptysis; when there is doubt as to the source of bleeding, the patient should be assumed to have lung disease and should be examined accordingly.

Even with minor hemoptysis, a chest roentgenogram and cultures for *Mycobacteria* are indicated. If posteroanterior and lateral views of the thorax are negative, bronchoscopy also should be performed in any patient with a history of smoking; otherwise, it is not mandatory, although even in nonsmokers, some studies indicate that a specific diagnosis may be made.[9, 10] Computed tomography also may provide a diagnosis and should probably be performed if available.[10a] In the majority of patients with hemoptysis who have a normal chest roentgenogram and bronchoscopic examination, the hemoptysis ceases within 6 months with no serious cause detected.[11] In contrast with the rigid bronchoscopy advisable in patients who are actively and copiously bleeding, flexible fiberoptic bronchoscopy is the proper approach to those with mild hemoptysis and those who have stopped bleeding.

"Massive hemoptysis" has been variously defined as 600 mL of blood expectorated in 24 hours[12] or 48 hours,[13] more than 500 mL in a single expectoration, or 1000 mL in smaller increments over a period of several days.[14] It is a controversial problem in management. As a general rule, once the site of bleeding is determined and the appropriate bronchus occluded by a Fogarty catheter, lobar resection is indicated. An alternative method of treatment, which appears to be growing in popularity, is bronchial artery embolization (*see* page 569); however, recurrent bleeding after this procedure is common.[15, 16]

Miscellaneous Symptoms

Sudden onset of *hoarseness* almost always indicates intrinsic laryngeal disease due to viral infection, trauma, allergic edema, or inhalation of noxious fumes.[17] Chronic hoarseness also is most likely to be caused by primary laryngeal disease and should prompt examination of the vocal cords to exclude serious conditions such as carcinoma. The commonest pulmonary cause of persistent hoarseness is unilateral abductor paralysis, usually caused by extension of carcinoma into the aortopulmonary window with involvement of the recurrent laryngeal nerve.

Fever should suggest infectious pneumonia, particularly when the chest roentgenogram reveals an airspace or segmental opacity; if the pneumonia is accompanied by a shaking chill, it is likely pneumococcal in origin. However, it must be remembered that fever may also occur with a variety of other pulmonary diseases, including carcinoma, connective tissue disease, and pulmonary infarction.

Confusion, irrationality, and even *coma* may occur as a result of underlying pulmonary disease, particularly in elderly persons; precipitating diseases include pneumonia, fat embolism or thromboembolism, and carcinoma. In the appropriate clinical settings, it is important to rule out infectious or metastatic lesions of the meninges or cerebrum.

Halitosis is most commonly caused by some disorder of the oral cavity, but it may be a major clue to an anaerobic pulmonary infection.

Past Illnesses and Personal History

Thorough questioning about the patient's medical history and personal habits is an essential part of the initial evaluation of any lung disease. Knowledge derived from such examination may greatly alter the differential diagnosis; for example, respiratory symptoms or an abnormal chest roentgenogram may simply represent previous active lung disease that has left its imprint on the pulmonary parenchyma, or a lung lesion may be a belated metastasis from a primary malignancy elsewhere that was removed many years earlier. In addition to other diseases, patients should be questioned about their therapy; many acute and chronic bacterial and mycotic infections occur in patients receiving long-term antibiotic or corticosteroid therapy; lipid pneumonia may follow use of nose drops or laxatives containing mineral oil, and respiratory failure may be wholly or partly attributable to recent sedation.

The patient's personal habits also may provide important clues to diagnosis. A history of cigarette smoking is clearly important in evaluating suspected cases of pulmonary carcinoma, and knowledge of sexual orientation or illicit drug use may suggest the possibility of an opportunistic infection. A history of contact with other persons who had pulmonary disease may be a useful aid in diagnosis, particularly with respect to infection. Tuberculosis is the most serious disease in this regard, but viral and *Mycoplasma* infections also may be spread through members of a household. The personal history is not complete without inquiry about contact with animals, domestic and wild. This pertains not only to patients with allergies, whose bronchospasm may be due to a household pet, but also, for example, to those with an acute pneumonic lesion who may have contracted ornithosis from a sick pet bird or tularemia from skinning a wild rabbit.

Family History

Some pulmonary diseases have a familial incidence, presumably because they are genetic. They include cystic fibrosis, emphysema due to alpha$_1$-antiprotease deficiency, a hereditary form of fibrosing alveolitis (familial fibrocystic pulmonary dysplasia), and dyskinetic ciliary syndrome. Most of these diseases are uncommon and may be recognized only when a positive family history is elicited.

Occupational and Residential History

Pulmonary disease may result from inhalation of a variety of inorganic and organic dusts and fumes, at work or in the environment. These diseases include the pneumoconioses, chemical-induced bronchitis, bronchiolitis, asthma, and the extrinsic allergic alveolitides. Such conditions are common enough that a thorough occupational history should be a mandatory part of the initial investigation of all lung diseases. Inhaled particulate and chemical material (particularly asbestos) is also important in the pathogenesis of pulmonary and pleural malignancies; knowledge of exposure to these substances is useful not only in diagnosis but also in potential workers' compensation cases.

Questioning about recent travel and country of origin is also necessary, particularly in the assessment of possible pneumonia; diagnosis of many fungal and parasitic diseases is aided by the discovery that a patient has lived or traveled in an endemic area.

Systemic Inquiry

Since pulmonary disease may be only one manifestation of a systemic disease process, inquiry about all body systems is essential. In some instances, the mere fact that certain other organs or tissues are involved may suggest the diagnosis; for instance, the patient with diffuse interstitial lung disease who has Raynaud's phenomenon and difficulty in swallowing almost certainly has progressive systemic sclerosis. On the other hand, pulmonary disease itself may be the cause of systemic symptoms that may be a clue to diagnosis. This is particularly so of neoplasms; for example, paraneoplastic symptoms of cerebral or muscle disease may suggest the presence of a small cell carcinoma. Similarly, a diagnosis of chronic pulmonary insufficiency and respiratory failure may be made after eliciting a history of headache, confusion, tremor, twitching, or somnolence.[18]

PHYSICAL EXAMINATION

Modern roentgenographic imaging techniques and laboratory studies have not replaced the physician's eyes, ears, and hands; rather, they should be regarded as additional, valuable diagnostic methods, complementary to the technique of physical examination and providing information it cannot. This cannot be overemphasized: circumstances will arise in which the physician may have to depend on his or her senses to make decisions concerning therapy that may fundamentally affect the patient's life. These may occur in the home, where roentgenography is unavailable, or even in the hospital, when the patient is too sick to be moved or there is a need for an immediate decision, such as to remove air in the case of tension pneumothorax.

As with symptoms, it must be remembered that the chest roentgenogram may be normal when there is serious and advanced pulmonary disease detectable only by physical examination; conversely, roentgenography may reveal severe disease when physical findings are absent.

Method of Examination and Significant Chest Signs

The front of the thorax is best examined when the patient is supine, and the back when the patient is sitting or standing; patients who are too weak to sit upright unaided should be supported by someone standing at the foot of the bed and holding their hands. It is important to keep in mind that examination of the chest is a comparative exercise:

each region of one side is compared with the corresponding area on the other side; this rule applies equally for inspection, palpation, percussion, and auscultation.

Inspection

The thoracic cage first should be inspected for evidence of deformity, and the skin for color, evidence of collateral venous circulation, and scars. The respiratory rate may be a valuable indicator of early respiratory dysfunction and should be noted.[19]

Movement of the chest wall also should be observed, particularly in an attempt to detect asymmetry between the two sides. A local lag during inspiration may not be obvious during quiet breathing, and for this reason the patient should be asked to take a deep breath as the movements of the chest cage on the two sides are compared. A lag during inspiration or an area of diminished movement seen or felt that involves all or part of a hemithorax may be the only physical sign of disease of the lung or pleura. It indicates loss of elasticity of the underlying tissues or compensatory spasm of intercostal and diaphragmatic musculature in the vicinity, a reflex response reducing pain on movement. This sign is present in acute diseases such as atelectasis, pneumonia, and pleurisy; it also may indicate a chronic or inactive fibrotic process of the lung or pleura, in which case it often is associated with scoliosis of the dorsal spine (with the concavity to the diseased side). When the loss of volume is considerable, whether owing to an acute or chronic process, there may be a shift of the mediastinum; this is detectable as displacement of the apical cardiac impulse and the trachea toward the involved side. With fibrosis, and particularly with atelectasis, the lower intercostal spaces may be abnormally sucked in during inspiration.

Of even greater importance than establishing asynchrony between the two hemithoraces is the assessment of respiratory muscle function. This is best done by observing the relative contribution of diaphragmatic and intercostal muscles in the normal breathing cycle with the patient in the supine position. In this situation, in-drawing of the abdominal wall on inspiration, or cyclic preponderance of abdominal and thoracic movement, suggests paralysis or fatigue of the diaphragm and constitutes a clear indication of the cause of dyspnea or of impending ventilatory failure.

Palpation

A suspected lag detected on inspection of the chest may be confirmed by placing a hand on each hemithorax while the patient breathes deeply. The relative contribution of the respiratory muscles also can be assessed by palpation of the abdominal, intercostal, and accessory muscles during inspiration. The apical cardiac impulse and the trachea should be palpated. A shift from normal position indicates loss of volume or a relative increase in volume of one hemithorax in comparison with the other. The left parasternal region also should be palpated to determine whether a heave is present, denoting right ventricular hypertrophy.

Percussion

The chest wall is then percussed, once again comparing corresponding areas on the two sides. Since the degree of resonance is influenced by the thickness of the chest wall and the volume of lung underlying the percussing finger, "normal" percussion findings differ not only from patient to patient but also from area to area in one patient. It should be stressed that the lung tissue assessed by the percussing finger is only the superficial 5 cm; no matter how much force is used, the central portion of the lung remains silent.

In the presence of pleuropulmonary disease, the percussion note varies from the impaired resonance heard over an area of pneumonia in which there is partial consolidation, to the dullness over a completely consolidated or collapsed segment or lobe, to the extreme dullness or flatness that indicates a large accumulation of pleural fluid. At the other end of the spectrum, the note is hyper-resonant in cases of emphysema and pneumothorax and sometimes is tympanic over a large superficial cavity or pneumothorax. An unusual form, known as skodaic resonance, is heard sometimes over a partly compressed upper lung region when the lower portion is collapsed by pleural effusion; the note has a "boxy" quality, and the mechanism of its production is unknown.

Auscultation

The quality and intensity of the breath sounds, as well as the presence or absence of adventitious noises, are ascertained by listening with the bell or diaphragm held firmly against the chest while the patient breathes quietly and then deeply. The quality and intensity of breath sounds vary from region to region, even in normal subjects, depending on the thickness of the chest wall, the proximity of larger bronchi to the chest wall, and the depth of respiration. In the axillae or at the lung bases, a vesicular sound that has been likened to the rustle of wind in the trees is heard during inspiration and often early in expiration. The sound of air flow has a somewhat different quality over the trachea and upper retrosternal area; the pitch is higher, and expiration is clearly audible and lasts longer than the inspiratory phase. Between the scapulae and anteriorly under the clavicles, particularly on the right side, the breath sounds assume characteristics of both vesicular and bronchial air flow and are described as bronchovesicular.

The mechanism of production of breath sounds is not thoroughly understood. In one study in which the intensity of breath sounds at the mouth was measured while such adventitious sounds as wheezing and stridor were eliminated, the sound of breathing was found to be generated by turbulent flow in the upper respiratory tract[20]; when turbulent flow was reduced by the inspiration of helium, breath sounds were eradicated. The "vesicular breathing" heard at the lung bases is believed to be caused by both a dampening effect of the spongy lung tissue and the entry of air from thousands of narrow terminal bronchioles into acinar units.[21]

Many factors may contribute to reduction or complete abolition of vesicular breathing. In some patients, it simply may be difficult to hear breath sounds because of an excess of subcutaneous fat, the presence of fluid or air in the pleural cavity, or shallow breathing due to weakness or neuromuscular disease. In other cases, there is significant bronchopulmonary disease, such as obstruction of a lobar or segmental bronchus or edema or fibrosis of interstitial tissue, both of which diminish air entry. Complete destruction of acinar units, as in emphysema, may have the same effect.

The quality of breath sounds changes from vesicular to bronchovesicular or bronchial when underlying parenchyma partly or completely loses its air content. This occurs in pneumonia and in nonobstructive atelectasis and is explained by the observation that consolidated or airless lung tissue is an excellent conductor of high-pitched, prolonged expiratory sounds that emanate from adjacent bronchi.

In addition to breath sounds, the voice sounds also may provide clues to pathologic changes. Normally these are soft and barely audible; in the presence of consolidation or nonobstructive atelectasis, however, they become more distinct and are audible over the involved area when the patient whispers *ninety-nine*. In some cases, when large accumulations of fluid compress the lower portion of the lung, the voice sounds have a nasal quality over the upper lung (analogous to skodaic resonance on percussion).

Adventitious sounds are abnormal sounds whose nomenclature is not standard and thus is somewhat confusing. Our approach is descriptive and simple and is similar to that accepted by many physicians. The sounds may be divided into those that have their origin in the airways and those that indicate disease of the pleura and mediastinum.

Rales (crackles)[22] are discontinuous noises that may be fine (usually at the end of inspiration, as air enters the acinar unit), medium (often during both inspiration and expiration, as air flows by an excess of fluid in the smaller bronchi), or coarse (low-pitched, bubbling sounds that result from the accumulation of secretions in larger bronchi and the trachea). They are present more often during inspiration, when air flow is faster. They may be elicited during a rapid, deep breath, or—particularly when they are fine—during a deep breath after maximal expiration ended by a cough (post-tussive rales). Fine rales are sometimes detected at the lung bases at the end of a deep inspiration in normal subjects; however, when they are persistent and occur in "showers," they indicate disease, such as pulmonary edema and pneumonia. In cases of diffuse interstitial disease associated with general loss of lung volume, rales have a high-pitched, superficial quality; they do not disappear on coughing and may represent the passage of air into innumerable atelectatic units, the resulting sound being intensified by adjacent airless pulmonary parenchyma.

Other adventitious sounds that originate in the bronchopulmonary tree are high-pitched (sibilant) and low-pitched (sonorous) continuous noises termed *rhonchi*. (A wheeze is the sound of a rhonchus heard by the physician without the aid of a stethoscope or which the patient himself can detect. The term "wheezing respirations" is used sometimes to denote the persistent inspiratory and expiratory rhonchi, usually of the musical, sibilant variety, heard all over the chest during bronchospasm.) Rhonchi indicate partial obstruction of the bronchial lumen by mucus, edema, spasm, or neoplasm. They are louder during expiration, when the bronchial passages are narrower, but may be heard in both phases. Those not appreciated during quiet breathing may become audible when the rate of air flow is increased during fast, deep breathing or when the bronchi are narrowed during maximal expiration. A particular form of rhonchus or wheeze is known as *stridor*. It is an especially loud

musical sound of constant pitch[23] and is caused by obstruction in the larynx or trachea; it may be heard during inspiration or expiration or throughout the entire respiratory cycle.

Another group of adventitious sounds represents manifestations of pleural disease. A *friction rub* is caused by a fibrinous exudate on adjacent parietal and visceral pleural surfaces. It may be caused by trauma, neoplasm, or inflammation of the pleura itself or by an underlying pulmonary neoplasm, infarct, or pneumonia; characteristically, it disappears when fluid forms and separates the two pleural surfaces. During both inspiration and expiration, and particularly in areas where excursion of the thoracic cage is greatest, a rubbing, rasping, or leathery sound may be heard as the visceral lining moves against the parietal lining. The noise usually is associated with pain. Its disappearance during breath holding, but not during coughing, distinguishes it from rhonchi due to partial bronchial obstruction, which it may closely resemble.

A second pleural sound was originally described by Hamman[24] as a crunching or clicking sound over the lower retrosternal area, synchronous with the heartbeat, which he thought was pathognomonic of air in the mediastinum. In fact, it is now believed to be most commonly associated with a left pneumothorax,[25] although it occasionally indicates roentgenologically undetectable collections of air in the mediastinum.

Clinical examination of the heart is essential in every case of suspected pulmonary disease. Abnormalities affecting either the parenchyma or the pulmonary vasculature may cause pulmonary arterial hypertension; this is evidenced by right ventricular heave, accentuated second pulmonic sound, or pulmonic or tricuspid regurgitant murmurs. In a minority of cases of diffuse pulmonary edema secondary to mitral stenosis or acute left ventricular decompensation, convincing roentgenographic evidence of cardiac enlargement is absent; in such cases, a mitral valve murmur, severe arterial hypertension, or clinical signs of left ventricular strain suggest the cause of the edema. Pulsus paradoxus, an abnormality usually associated with cardiac tamponade, may be observed in patients with obstructive pulmonary disease, particularly severe asthma, and with massive pulmonary embolism. It also may be found when the intrathoracic pressure swing is excessive, as may occur with obstruction of either upper or lower airways or even in some normal young subjects.

Extrathoracic Manifestations of Pulmonary Disease

The diagnosis of pulmonary disease may be aided by the detection on physical examination of extrapulmonary abnormalities. The skin and the endocrine and central nervous systems are most commonly involved. Endocrinopathies and a variety of other paraneoplastic manifestations are particularly frequent in pulmonary carcinoma (see page 474). The sections that follow are concerned with clubbing and cyanosis, one or both of which are associated with many cases of pulmonary or pleural disease.

Clubbing and Hypertrophic Osteoarthropathy

The term "clubbing" refers to a swelling of the soft tissue of the distal portions of the fingers and toes. Hypertrophic osteoarthropathy (HOA) is an osteitis localized principally to the phalanges and distal portions of the arms and legs. Although the two conditions often coexist, clubbing not uncommonly occurs in the absence of osteoarthropathy, and the latter occasionally occurs without clubbing.

There are four generally accepted criteria for clubbing: (1) increased bulk of the distal phalanx; (2) angle between the nail and the proximal skin greater than 180 degrees; (3) sponginess of the nailbed when pressure is applied to the nail; and (4) increased nail curvature. When all these changes are present, or when at least one is severe, clubbing is readily recognizable. Unfortunately, the detection of clubbing at an early stage is highly subjective, its recognition subject to considerable interobserver variation.

The pathogenesis of clubbing is not known. In some patients, blood flow to the digits is increased,[26] probably related to opening of arteriovenous anastamoses (Sucquet-Hoyer canals). It has been suggested that some vasodilator substance that is normally inactivated escapes into the systemic circulation in the presence of pulmonary disease, making this shunting possible.[27] As with HOA, there is evidence that tumor-related growth hormone may be a factor in some cases of pulmonary carcinoma.[27a] Why clubbing is such a prominent feature of some pulmonary diseases (e.g., idiopathic fibrosing alveolitis) and not others is unclear.

The main symptom of HOA is deep-seated, burning pain in the distal parts of the extremities. Edema, warmth, and tenderness of the hands, wrists, feet, and lower legs are usually present; synovial effusions may develop. Roentgenography reveals subperiosteal new bone formation, chiefly of the distal bones of the extremities and some consider this finding essential to diagnosis.[28] Radionuclide bone scanning may show evidence of disease elsewhere, such as in the scapulae and patellae.[29]

HOA is virtually pathognomonic of visceral (although not always pulmonary) disease, the primary organ of involvement having either vagal or glossopharyngeal innervation.[27] Malignant chest neoplasms account for 90 per cent of cases of HOA of pulmonary origin, the majority being primary.[30] Osteoarthropathy is usually detected before or at the time of diagnosis of the underlying disease, but occasionally it may become manifest years later.[31]

As with clubbing, the pathogenesis of HOA is not fully understood. It is generally agreed that the earliest change is a localized overgrowth of vascular connective tissue, followed by subperiosteal new bone formation. Blood flow to the extremities is increased, particularly in the areas of osteoarthropathy. In the great majority of cases, this increase appears to be secondary to a reflex mechanism, the vagus nerve serving as the afferent pathway. The efferent pathway is unknown but is considered to be hormonal rather than neuronal[27]; implicated substances include estrogen[32] and growth hormone.[33] The disorder usually resolves with removal of an associated lung tumor.

In some cases, HOA is not associated with demonstrable disease elsewhere in the body. This unusual condition, known as pachydermoperiostosis, has an autosomal mode of inheritance with marked variability in expressivity, males being more severely affected than females.[34]

Cyanosis

Cyanosis is a blue or bluish-gray discoloration of the skin and mucous membranes caused by excessive blood concentration of reduced hemoglobin. It is most obvious in the nailbeds or buccal mucosa and may be due to inadequate saturation of arterial blood leaving the left side of the heart, excessive slowing of flow in the peripheral capillaries, or both. The estimated volume of reduced hemoglobin that must be present before cyanosis is visible is 5 g per dL; therefore, this sign is never present in patients with severe anemia. Cyanosis may be central (hypoxemic), in which case it is associated with pulmonary or cardiac disease, or peripheral, when the mechanism is related to sluggish blood flow and excessive removal of oxygen by the tissues.

The central variety is commonest in patients with emphysema and indicates that many acinar units have low alveolar ventilation-perfusion ratios; in other words, a large part of underventilated lung is perfused with venous blood. In other lung diseases, such as severe airspace pneumonia with circulatory collapse, both central and peripheral factors undoubtedly play a part; the venous blood in pulmonary capillaries encounters airless acini, and the same blood stagnates in systemic capillaries. Probably both factors also are responsible for the cyanosis so common in patients who have diffuse interstitial pulmonary disease with clubbing; even when they have only mild arterial oxygen unsaturation, the nailbeds are definitely dusky blue. Cardiac conditions associated with right-to-left shunt may engender a central form of cyanosis, but they can be differentiated from pulmonary conditions by the clinical findings and the results of pulmonary function tests.

Peripheral cyanosis is either paroxysmal and precipitated by cold, as in Raynaud's disease, or general and prolonged, in which case it is often associated with systemic hypotension. The latter form is commoner in primary heart disease than lung disease, but may occur in association with cor pulmonale and hypoxemia.

When cyanosis is central in origin the nailbeds usually are deep blue or blue-gray, and the skin is warm, whereas peripheral cyanosis is usually associated with cold, clammy skin and dusky, livid nailbeds. Despite this, it is not possible, on appearance alone, to distinguish with certainty between central and peripheral cyanosis; in questionable cases, the degree of oxygen saturation of arterial blood will give the answer.

When the pathogenesis of cyanosis is obscure, methemoglobinemia or sulfhemoglobinemia should be considered. Rarely, methemoglobinemia is primary and congenital; more commonly, the coffee-colored pigment results from the administration of drugs, including nitrates, chlorates, quinones, aniline dyes, sulfonamide derivatives, acetanilid, and phenacetin. The diagnosis may be confirmed by spectroscopic analysis to identify the absorption bands.

SPECIAL DIAGNOSTIC PROCEDURES

Endoscopic Examination

Laryngoscopy

Laryngoscopy should be performed in any patient who complains of a persistent, dry, hacking or brassy cough, particularly when this is associated with hoarseness. The vocal cords should be well visualized, not only to exclude a local lesion but also to detect paralysis that would account for the hoarseness. In the latter instance, roentgenography may reveal a mediastinal lesion, implying involvment of the recurrent laryngeal nerve.

Bronchoscopy

Bronchoscopy can be performed with either a rigid or a flexible fiberoptic bronchoscope (FFB). The former is preferred by many for investigation of massive hemoptysis and by some for endoscopic examination of children, particularly for the removal of foreign bodies and as a means of inserting the FFB.[35] In most other situations, however, fiberoptic bronchoscopy is the procedure of choice; the great visual range of the flexible scope represents a distinct advantage of this instrument over the rigid instrument, especially in the upper lobes.[36]

There appears to be general agreement that atropine sulfate is indicated prior to bronchoscopy; this drug not only reduces bronchial secretions but also prevents bradycardia and reflex bronchoconstriction produced by stimulation of vagal nerve endings.[37] Some form of sedation is commonly advocated and almost certainly is to be recommended for children; however, it is questionable whether it is needed in adults.[38] Local anesthesia is preferred, certainly in adults,[39] since it allows for cooperation of the patient during the procedure. Since an essential feature of most bronchoscopies is bronchial washing or lavage to obtain secretions from the bronchial tree, it should be borne in mind that some local anesthetics have antibacterial action; for example, tetracaine (Pontocaine) severely inhibits cultural growth of *Mycobacterium tuberculosis*, and lidocaine (Xylocaine) is said to inhibit the growth of fungi and nontuberculous bacteria.[40]

Ideally, fluoroscopic and resuscitative facilities should be available in a special room set aside for endoscopic procedures, but the FFB has a role to play in emergency situations at the bedside, notably in the intensive care unit.[41] Hypoxic patients should be given supplemental oxygen during the procedure; a special adapter is available to prevent air leak for patients who are being artificially ventilated.[42]

A major indication for bronchoscopy is suspected pulmonary carcinoma, in which case it may be used both for diagnosis (when accompanied by biopsy, washings, and brushings) and to help the surgeon determine the extent of disease before possible resection. Other situations in which bronchoscopy is diagnostically useful include hemoptysis, selected cases of interstitial lung disease (especially sarcoidosis and lymphangitic carcinomatosis), infection (particularly tuberculosis and some opportunistic disorders such as *Pneumocystis carinii* pneumonia), and rejection of a lung transplant.[43]

The risk inherent in the bronchoscopic examination itself appears slight; most complications, of which the major ones are hemorrhage and pneumothorax, follow biopsy procedures. The hemodynamic effects are substantial, however, and are probably related largely to a reflex sympathetic discharge caused by mechanical irritation of the larynx and bronchi. In one study of 10 patients, there were mean increases in systemic arterial pressure of 30 per cent, in heart rate of 43 per cent, in cardiac index of 28 per cent, and in pulmonary artery occlusion pressure of 86 per cent[44]; the arterial partial pressure of oxygen (PaO_2) fell an average of 7 mm Hg during bronchial suctioning and in the post-bronchoscopy period. Cardiac arrhythmias are common and correlate with the passage of the bronchoscope through the vocal cords and with the hypoxemia consequent to suctioning.[45] Reported mortality rates are 0.01 per cent[46] to 0.1 per cent.[47]

Esophagoscopy

Pulmonary disease, particularly aspiration pneumonia, may occur in association with esophageal lesions, and diagnosis may be facilitated by direct endoscopic examination of the esophagus. In addition, when the source of expectorated blood is not known, direct viewing of the lower esophagus may be indicated to inspect for bleeding varices.

Bronchoalveolar Lavage

In recent years, the technique of bronchoalveolar lavage (BAL) has been much utilized by pulmonary investigators, particularly in studies of the pathogenesis of disease but also in an attempt to improve diagnosis and to identify predictors of prognosis. The technique we recommend involves injection of 100 to 300 mL of normal saline (in 20-mL aliquots) through a bronchoscope wedged into the lingular or middle lobe bronchus. Fluid is then aspirated back into the scope and sent to the laboratory, where inflammatory and immune mediator cells are identified and counted, and specific proteins analyzed. BAL is also the standard technique for diagnosis of *Pneumocystis carinii* pneumonia.

In healthy nonsmokers, a typical BAL cell population consists of about 90 per cent macrophages, 9 per cent lymphocytes, and fewer than 1 per cent polymorphonuclear leukocytes (although the number of the last-named cells may increase as a result of the BAL itself[47a]). Of the lymphocytes, more than 90 per cent are T cells, of which approximately 50 per cent are helper (CD4) cells and 25 per cent are suppressor (CD8) cells, and fewer than 10 per cent are B cells. Eosinophils are usually sparse; when they constitute more than 5 per cent they are likely to be associated with interstitial lung disease, acquired immunodeficiency sydrome (AIDS), eosinophilic pneumonia, or drug toxicity.[47b]

Pulmonary function tests performed before and after BAL have shown that small-volume lavage (100 to 200 mL) does not significantly reduce function in normal subjects (although it may in patients with pulmonary disease such as sarcoidosis)[47c]; large-volume BAL (approximately 500 mL) may cause decrements in function even in normal subjects. Serious complications are very uncommon[47d]; low-grade fever, pneumonitis, bleeding, and bronchospasm occur in a minority of individuals.

Procedures for Microbiologic Diagnosis

Pleuropulmonary infection is one of the commonest forms of thoracic disease, and appropriate collection and handling of material for culture is thus essential in the diagnostic work-up of many patients. In addition to smears and cultures, the results of serologic and skin tests are often helpful, and sometimes essential, in making a specific diagnosis of an infectious agent.

Collection of Material for Culture

Sputum. All patients who are acutely ill with pneumonia when admitted to the hospital should be encouraged to cough and spit into a sputum container as soon as possible. If they are unable to expectorate because of the severity of their illness, inhalation of an aerosolized solution of propylene glycol, sulfur dioxide, or distilled water may stimulate a cough productive of diagnostic specimens; this method is particularly useful for patients with tuberculosis or AIDS who are incapable of spontaneous expectoration. The fresh sputum should be smeared on a slide, stained with Gram stain (and, if appropriate, acid-fast and silver stains), and inoculated on a culture medium. In cases of suspected nontuberculous bacterial pneumonia, the choice of antibiotic should be made on the basis of the Gram stain, without waiting for culture and sensitivity results. This does not mean that one can diagnose the pathogen of pneumonia by the smear alone; subsequent culture may reveal a pathogen different from that suspected from the preliminary smear. However, since patients with severe acute pneumonia may die before the results of culture are known, this smear represents the most dependable method of making a tentative diagnosis and instituting appropriate therapy.

Because many patients who are admitted to the hospital with pneumonia have been given antibiotics before admission, significant pathogens are often not identified on culture. When a patient fails to respond to antibiotic therapy appropriate for the pathogen that was originally detected, further cultures should be grown, as another pathogenic agent, perhaps one acquired in the hospital, may be responsible.

Swabs of the pharynx or nasopharynx, which frequently are taken from patients suspected of having a viral disease, should be placed immediately in a liquid solution containing salt and either gelatin or bovine albumin, with or without antibiotics.[48] This material should be delivered immediately to the laboratory for inoculation; when preparation must be delayed for a few hours the specimen should be kept at $-40°C$ or, if the delay will be longer, at $-70°C$.

Tracheal Aspiration and Lavage. Since potential pathogens may inhabit the oropharynx and upper respiratory tract without causing disease, it is evident that positive cultures of a pathogenic organism do not necessarily signify that it is the cause of pneumonia. When growth is heavy or pure, it is more likely that the bacterium is responsible; however, even in this situation, definitive diagnosis is not ensured unless the cultured organism is one known not to occur as a commensal in the oropharynx (e.g., *M. tuberculosis*). The combination of sputum washing and quantitative culture appears to be a valid method of increasing diagnostic accuracy, but the time consumed in carrying out these two procedures makes such methods impractical for most laboratories on a routine basis.[49]

Because of these limitations, attention has been directed to bypassing the upper respiratory passages and obtaining material directly from the trachea or more distal airways. One procedure for doing this, transtracheal aspiration,[50] has largely been abandoned, not only because of an unacceptable number of false-positive and false-negative results but, more important, because of the inherent risk of severe complications (e.g., hemorrhage, cardiac arrythmias, and subcutaneous and mediastinal emphysema) and occasional fatalities.[51] In its place, there has been a tendency to turn to transbronchial biopsy, bronchial washings and brushings, transthoracic needle aspiration (TTNA), or open lung biopsy as safer and more productive methods of establishing the cause of obscure pneumonias.

Transbronchial Biopsy. Obtaining specimens for smear and culture through the bronchoscope carries the same risk of contamination by oropharyngeal organisms as does sputum expectoration. In an attempt to obviate this contamination, telescopic or sheathed catheters with a sterile sampling brush have been passed through the fiberoptic bronchoscope, which may have its distal orifice plugged.[52] When the desired site of sampling is reached, the plug is extruded, and the inner catheter and brush advanced 3 to 4 cm before the specimen is collected. Using this technique, some investigators have shown a good yield of presumed pathogens with few false-positive results[53]; however, other workers have not been as successful.[54]

Transthoracic Needle Aspiration and Open Lung Biopsy. Although TTNA plays its greatest role in the diagnosis of nodules or masses, its value in determining the cause of severe airspace pneumonia that has eluded diagnosis by all other means, is also appreciable.[55] Despite this, since the diagnostic yield is greater[56] and complications not more evident following open lung biopsy, the latter procedure is probably preferable in seriously ill patients.

Stool. Microscopic examination of slides of fecal material is indicated in many parasitic diseases of the lungs; viruses also may often be isolated in stool. Centrifugation-filtration methods can be used to concentrate parasites or eggs.[57]

Blood. In every case of fulminating pneumonia a culture should be made at the height of fever, using an aseptic technique. For suspected viral lung disease, blood should be drawn early in the disease; part of the aliquot should be used for culture, and part for identifying antibodies to pathogens (*see* later discussion).

Pleural Effusion. In most cases, the site of removal of pleural fluid is determined by the roentgenographic appearance and by the area of maximum dullness identified on physical examination. If the amount of pleural fluid is small or if the fluid is loculated, ultrasonography is the method of choice to guide thoracentesis.[58] In the majority of cases, initial thoracentesis should be combined with biopsy of the parietal pleura. When the diagnosis has been positively established (e.g., the effusion is considered to be secondary to pneumonia or is grossly a transudate in a patient with cardiac, liver, or renal failure), pleural biopsy is not required.

Complications from thoracentesis are rare; however, when that procedure is done in conjunction with biopsy they are commoner and may be serious (*see* page 133). The amount of fluid withdrawn depends on the circumstances; the chief indications for complete removal are to afford a clearer view of the underlying lung or to relieve dyspnea. It is unwise to remove fluid too rapidly from patients who are in heart failure or who have severe anemia, since acute pulmonary edema is likely to develop; only a limited amount should be removed at any one time, and use of a vacuum bottle is contraindicated.

Serologic and Skin Testing

Blood and skin testing are particularly useful in the diagnosis of pulmonary infections. Since they are based on the presence of immunity to a specific organism, a reaction that typically takes a week or longer to develop, they are most valuable in the convalescent or chronic stage of disease.

Serologic Testing. Serologic testing is most often used to determine the causative pathogen in various bacterial, viral, mycotic, and parasitic diseases. In the great majority of instances, it is dependent on the development in the patient's serum of antibodies that cause agglutination, precipitation, or complement fixation to specific antigens. Although very high titers on one occasion may strongly suggest a specific etiologic agent, rising or falling titers in serial or paired tests performed at some interval constitute much stronger evidence. In addition, in cases of pneumonia in which a bacterium has been cultured in the sputum, the test can be carried out within a few days of onset of the illness; a high titer confirms the causative role of the bacterium.

Serologic tests are valuable in the diagnosis of several fungal infections, particularly coccidioidomycosis and histoplasmosis. The most useful in histoplasmosis is the complement fixation (CF) test, using both histoplasmin and a saline suspension of yeast form as antigens. With these two antigens, positive results are obtained in approximately 95 per cent of culturally proven cases of progressive pulmonary disease and in 55 to 80 per cent of those with disseminated disease[59]; in 85 per cent of active cases of nondisseminated histoplasmosis the titer is higher than 1:16.[60]

In coccidioidomycosis, screening is recommended with agar gel (double diffusion as well as a latex particle agglutination test); positive reactors to either of these should be tested by CF and tubular precipitin. The CF test is used primarily to determine whether the disease is disseminated; a titer above 1:16 suggests this complication. Precipitins may be detected within 1 to 3 weeks after the onset of primary infection; the CF test, however, is not usually positive until 4 to 6 weeks after infection, by which time the precipitin test usually has reverted to negative.

Serologic tests also may assist in the diagnosis of several parasitic diseases; for example, amebiasis may be detected by both gel diffusion precipitin and indirect hemagglutination tests, and a rise in antibody titer is the surest way of establishing the presence of toxoplasmosis. Hydatid disease is almost always associated with the production of antibodies, recognized to best advantage by an indirect hemagglutination test; rupture of a cyst often results in a rise in titer.[61]

In addition to these specific antibodies, nonspecific cold agglutination antibodies and antibodies to *Streptococcus* MG are found in approximately 50 per cent of patients with *Mycoplasma pneumoniae* infection and constitute strong evidence of this disease. However, cold agglutinins sometimes develop in other infectious diseases involving the lungs.

Skin Tests. Skin tests may be divided into those used to detect hypersensitivity to allergens (which typically produce immediate reactions) and those used to diagnose bacterial, fungal, and parasitic diseases (which usually give rise to delayed reactions).

Immediate Reactivity. Scratch or intradermal tests are used to detect atopy, seasonal and perennial rhinitis, and asthma, using common inhalants such as pollens, molds, dusts, and danders; foods and drugs are used when the patient's history indicates specific sensitivity. The tests are particularly useful when they confirm a history indicating specific allergy and form the basis of a desensitization program.

Skin Tests for Bacteria, Fungi, and Parasites. Skin tests of value for diagnosing bacterial infections are those used in suspected mycobacterial disease and tularemia.

The material used for mycobacterial skin testing, known as purified protein derivative (PPD), is obtained from filtrates of heat-killed cultures of bacilli that have grown on a synthetic medium. Different lots and forms of the protein are designated by letters; for example, an international PPD-tuberculin is designated PPD-S. Commonly used PPDs of nontuberculous (atypical) organisms are PPD-Y (*Mycobacterium kansasii*), PPD-G (scotochromogen "Gause"), PPD-B (*Mycobacterium intracellulare*), and PPD-F (*Mycobacterium fortuitum*). Injected material is traditionally measured in tuberculin units (TU), one of which is equivalent to 0.00002 mg of PPD.

Intermediate-strength PPD (5 TU) is usually employed for diagnostic skin testing for tuberculosis. However, if the clinical and roentgenographic findings strongly suggest active disease, only 1 TU should be used initially, since sensitive persons may have severe reactions.[62] If a patient fails to react to intermediate-strength PPD, a second strength (250 TU) can be used, although a positive reaction at this strength is less significant.

The skin test is carried out by injecting the PPD solution intradermally on the volar aspect of the forearm. It should be read on the second or third day after injection, a reaction being indicated by an area of induration, which is measured perpendicularly to the long axis of the forearm and recorded in millimeters. A measurement of 10 mm or larger is considered positive, 5 to 9 mm doubtful, and less than 5 mm negative.[63] A positive reaction is strong evidence that a patient has or has had tuberculosis. False-positive reactions are rare and, in some cases, represent cross-reactions caused by infection from nontuberculous mycobacteria. Several studies indicate that the larger the size of the tuberculin reaction the greater the risk of clinical tuberculosis in the future.[64, 65]

The major drawback of the tuberculin test lies in the considerable incidence of false-negative reactions. These may be caused by (1) faulty technique of administration of PPD; (2) faulty interpretation of the reaction; (3) lack of potency of the injected material; or (4) diminished immune response[66] (which can itself be due to several causes). Patients infected with *M. tuberculosis* typically show negative reactions during the first weeks of infection while cell-mediated hypersensitivity is developing. Various acute exanthemata, particularly measles, transiently depress the tuberculin reaction. In addition, a more permanent diminution or complete loss of delayed skin hypersensitivity may occur in chronic diseases, such as sarcoidosis, lymphoma, leukemia, amyloidosis, hypothyroidism, and carcinoma.[67] Therapy itself may affect the reaction, particularly in early disease[62]; in addition, corticosteroids may render previously positive reactors negative. Finally, it is generally accepted that the reaction to tuberculin may wane with advancing age.

Cross-reactions to mycobacterial PPD occur between antigenically related strains. A patient who reacts to PPD-S, particularly in the doubtful range (5 mm), may have a nontuberculous mycobacterial infection, in which case simultaneous testing with appropriate nontuberculous antigens may be of value.[64] Patients with a larger reaction to PPD-S than to nontuberculous mycobacterial PPD are much more likely to have tuberculosis, especially if induration exceeds 10 mm in diameter. However, the contrary is not true; many patients whose cultures are positive for nontuberculous organisms manifest stronger reactions to PPD-S than to nontuberculous mycobacterial PPD.[68]

Skin tests are of limited value in other bacterial diseases. An exception is *tularemia*, the diagnosis of which can be confirmed by intradermal injection of antigen and subsequent documentation of a reaction within 5 days of the onset of disease; the test is both sensitive and specific for the disease. Skin tests also aid in the diagnosis of many fungal infections, including *histoplasmosis, coccidioidomycosis, paracoccidioidomycosis,* and *sporotrichosis*[59]; however, because of the high incidence of false-positive and false-negative reactions, *North American blastomycosis* cannot be detected by this means.

Skin tests in patients with parasitic infestation produce varied reactions. In *trichinosis,* the injection of an antigen prepared from extracts of ground dry trichinae produces an immediate reaction if administered after the third week of illness. Both immediate and delayed reactions occur when the Casoni test is performed in patients with *hydatid disease.* Skin tests also are of value in diagnosing *filariasis* and *toxoplasmosis,* although positive results may not be obtained in the latter disease until several months after onset.

Biochemical Tests of Pleural Fluid

Identification of a pleural effusion as either a *transudate* or an *exudate* is important in diagnosis and is done most reliably by determining several biochemical parameters. For example, in one study of 150 pleural effusions, Light and associates[69] classified 47 effusions as transudates and 103 as exudates. Biochemically, there were three differentiating characteristics: (1) a fluid-serum protein ratio greater than 0.5; (2) pleural fluid lactic dehydrogenase (LDH) greater than 200 IU; and (3) a fluid-serum LDH ratio greater than 0.6:1. All but one of the clinically diagnosed exudates had at least one of these characteristics, whereas only one transudate had any. These investigators concluded that the simultaneous use of both protein and LDH levels in pleural fluid analysis permits better differentiation of transudates from exudates than does use of just one.

Determination of other substances can also help distinguish between transudates and exudates. For example, in one study of pleural fluid glucose,[70] all but one transudate had levels exceeding 95 mg per dL. In another investigation of 183 studied patients with simultaneous blood and pleural fluid pH determinations,[71] all 36 transudates were found to have a pH above 7.30; 46 of 147 exudates had a pH of less than 7.30 in the presence of a normal blood pH. The measurement of pH also may be helpful in distinguishing tuberculous from malignant effusions. In one study, a pH below 7.30 was highly suggestive of tuberculosis, whereas values greater than 7.40 usually indicated malignancy.[72] When neoplastic effusions had been present for some time, however, pH values tended to fall, presumably as a result of thickening of the pleural membrane that caused an efflux block of H^+.

Pleural fluid does not have the buffering capacity of blood, so small changes in $H+$ concentration are more apparent.[71] Such changes can be caused by several mechanisms. Acid may be produced in the pleura itself or in the pleural membranes by the action of bacteria and leukocytes on glucose (with the production of CO_2 and lactate) and by direct production by tumor cells and red blood cells. Probably a more important contributor to acid-base balance is the state of the serosal membrane, which, when thickened, tends to block the efflux of H^+.

A variety of other substances that may be useful in determining the specific cause of a pleural effusion are discussed in greater detail in Chapter 18.

Hematologic Procedures in Pulmonary Disease

Polycythemia frequently occurs in association with chronic hypoxemia due to pulmonary disease. Although anemia is uncommon, it may develop with chronic infection, widespread malignancy, and some diseases of presumed immune-mediated pathogenesis, such as idiopathic pulmonary hemorrage. In the last condition, it may be noted even before the patient expectorates blood; in this situation, its association with a roentgenogram showing a diffuse acinar pattern constitutes an important diagnostic pointer.

Determination of the total and differential leukocyte count is of obvious importance in the differential diagnosis of lung disease. Leukocytosis in excess of 15,000 white cells per milliliter, with a predominance of polymorphonuclear cells, is strong evidence of bacterial rather than viral pneumonia. It must be remembered, however, that fulminating bacterial pneumonia may be associated with normal or even low white blood cell counts. A precipitous decrease in total leukocyte count in peripheral blood has been found to correlate with the subsequent development of adult respiratory distress syndrome in patients at risk for this disorder. When the differential count shows eosinophilia, the diagnosis is usually asthma, drug reaction, parasite infestation, connective tissue disease, or malignancy.

Electrocardiography

An electrocardiogram is of fundamental importance in differentiating myocardial infarction from acute massive pulmonary embolism. It is also useful in indicating lung disease as a cause of heart failure in patients who might otherwise be considered to be suffering from coronary artery insufficiency or myocardial disease. The electrocardiographic abnormalities of diffuse lung disease[73] must be familiar to physicians who specialize in this field.

PULMONARY FUNCTION TESTS

Pulmonary function tests are an essential part of the investigation of many respiratory diseases. The choice of which ones should be performed in a given setting depends on the purpose of the study, of which there are five principal types: (1) resolving whether symptoms and signs such as dyspnea, cough, and cyanosis are of respiratory origin; (2) managing and following the progression of disease or response to therapy in patients with recognized pulmonary disorders; (3) assessing the risk of developing pulmonary dysfunction and complications as a result of therapeutic interventions such as operative procedures and drugs; (4) quantifying the degree of disability in environmental or occupational lung disease; and (5) carrying out epidemiologic surveys of population groups suspected of having acquired pulmonary disease as a result of exposure to dusts or fumes.

Tests that assess pulmonary function may be conveniently considered in three levels of increasing sophistication (Table 3–1). First is measurement of vital capacity and maximal expiratory flow rates by spirometry and assessment of the gas-exchanging ability of the lungs by measurement of arterial saturation by oximetry. The second level includes measurement of arterial blood gas tensions, assessment of the subdivisions of lung volume using the helium dilution technique, and estimation of the diffusing capacity of the lung. At the third level are more sophisticated tests for assessing lung mechanics, respiratory control, ventilation and perfusion properties of the lung, bronchial reactivity, and exercise performance.

Whatever the level of sophistication, all lung function tests must be interpreted and correlated with clinical and roentgenologic data; without this added information, interpretation of tests is subject to much variability among readers.[74]

Predicted Normal Values of Pulmonary Function

Interpretation of the results of pulmonary function tests is based on the degree of deviation from predicted normal values. These are calculated from regression equations that take into account known attributes that contribute to variations of lung function, including age, sex, height, weight, and race. Genetic and environmental factors that affect lung function are responsible for much of the wide range of values among normal persons.

Ideally, the normal range for a test should encompass 95 per cent of values in a population; in practice, however, a difference of ±20 per cent from the mean predicted value is used for many lung function tests. When interpreting a test as abnormal, it is important to remember that the interindividual variation in lung function can differ greatly

between tests; for example, in a normal population the forced expiratory flow ($FEF_{25\%-75\%}$) and the maximal inspiratory and expiratory pressures (measurement of which is highly effort dependent) can vary as much as 30 to 50 per cent. Tests must also be interpreted with caution for patients at the extremes of age, as for them prediction equations for lung function are often inaccurate.

Although one use of pulmonary function testing is to compare the values obtained from an individual with those of a normal population, following the progress of a patient over time or assessing response to short- or long-term therapy has the advantage of using the patient's own values as a control, thus permitting greater accuracy in detecting changes in lung function. The detection of a significant change, or the lack of change, in any test over time or in response to an intervention is dependent on the intrinsic variability of the test. This variability can be measured as the coefficient of variation of repeated tests, defined as the standard deviation of repeated tests divided by the mean. The coefficient of variation varies widely among lung function tests but, in general, is much narrower than the 95 per cent confidence limits observed in the population (Table 3–2).[75]

Lung Volumes

Lung volumes and capacities may be appreciated by studying the diagram in Figure 3–1. There are four volumes: (1) tidal volume (TV), the amount of gas moved in and out of the lung with each respiratory cycle; (2) residual volume (RV), the amount remaining in the lung after maximal expiration; (3) inspiratory reserve volume (IRV), the additional gas that may be inspired after the end of a quiet inspiration; and (4) expiratory reserve volume (ERV), the additional amount of gas that may be expired from the resting or end-expiratory level. There are also four capacities: (1) total lung capacity (TLC), the gas contained in the lung at the end of maximal inspiration; (2) vital capacity (VC), the amount that can be expired after a maximal inspiration or inspired after a maximal expiration; (3) inspiratory capacity (IC), the amount of gas that can be inspired from the end of a quiet expiration; and (4) functional residual capacity (FRC), the volume of gas remaining in the lung at the end of a quiet expiration.

Vital Capacity

Vital capacity is usually measured as forced vital capacity (FVC), the amount of gas that can be forcefully exhaled after complete inspiration. In patients with obstructive pulmonary disease, the FVC may be less than the inspired vital capacity by as much as 1 L, as a result of dynamic compression of airways, gas trapping on expiration, and failure to detect expired volume at low flow rates.[76] By themselves, the VC and FVC are not very useful measures of pulmonary function, but when combined with measurement of the volume of gas exhaled during the first second of expiration (FEV_1), they yield an invaluable indicator of respiratory disease, the FEV_1/FVC. Calculation of this ratio allows separation of ventilatory abnormalities into "restrictive" or "obstructive" patterns; in patients with obstructive pulmonary disease, the FVC is relatively well maintained in rela-

Table 3–1. TESTS OF LUNG FUNCTION

Level 1
  Spirometry and peak flow (FEV_1, FVC, FEV_1/FVC)
  Bronchodilator response
  Oximetry
Level 2
  Arterial blood gas tensions
  Subdivisions of lung volume
  Lung diffusing capacity
Level 3
  Pulmonary and airway resistance
  Lung pressure-volume curves
  Measures of respiratory muscle strength (PI_{max} and PE_{max})
  Measures of ventilatory response to hypoxia and hypercapnia
  Measures of bronchial responsiveness
  Stage I, II, and III exercise tests

Table 3–2. **INTER- AND INTRAINDIVIDUAL VARIATION IN LUNG FUNCTION IN NORMAL SUBJECTS**

Test	Percentage of Variation Between Individuals	Percentage of Variation Within an Individual
Forced vital capacity (FVC)	± 20–25[75a]	± 6–16[75b, 75c]
Forced expiratory volume in one second (FEV₁)	± 20–22[75a]	± 7–18[75b, 75c]
FEV₁/FVC	± 14[75a]	
Peak expiratory flow rate (PEFR)		± 13–28[75b, 75c]
Forced expiratory flow between 75 and 25%	± 40–60[75a]	
Vital capacity (FEF₂₅₋₇₅)		
Functional residual capacity (FRC):		
By helium dilution	± 20[75d]	
By body plethysmography		± 4[75e]
Density dependence of maximal expiratory flow:		
Δ Vmax 50 breathing 80% He + 20% O₂		± 22[75f]
Volume of isoflow breathing 80% He + 20% O₂		± 100[75g]
Pressure-volume curves:		
PLmax	± 19[75h]	± 11[75i]
PL90%	± 14[75h]	± 9[75i]
Cstat	± 9[75h]	± 15[75i]
logk		± 6[75i]
Diffusing capacity		
DLCOSB	± 21[75j]	± 3–11[75k]
DLCOSB/VA	± 25[75j]	
Closing volume % vital capacity	± 60[75l]	
Closing capacity % TLC	± 23[75l]	

tion to the FEV₁, whereas in restrictive disease the FEV₁ may be nearly normal, and the FVC definitely decreased.

Functional Residual Capacity, Residual Volume, and Total Lung Capacity

Functional residual capacity is determined chiefly by the balance between the outward recoil of the chest wall and the inward recoil of the lung, although both inspiratory muscle activity during expiration and flow limitation during tidal breathing can increase FRC above its static value. Residual volume is determined by the balance between expiratory muscle strength and the stiffness of the chest wall. Total lung capacity is determined by the balance between inspiratory muscle strength and the elastic recoil of the lung and chest wall.

FRC, RV, and TLC can be determined by either inert gas inhalation techniques or body plethysmography. In the closed-circuit inert gas method, the patient breathes from a spirometer of known volume containing helium of known concentration. At the beginning of the study, helium concentration in the lungs is zero; as the patient breathes in and out, the gas mixes between spirometer and lungs until the concentration of helium is the same in both. FRC is calculated by the equation:

$$FRC = \frac{\text{Spirometer volume} \times \text{Initial He concentration}}{\text{Final He concentration}}$$

RV and TLC are calculated by subtracting ERV and adding IC, respectively. The inert gas techniques are subject to error because they do not detect trapped gas, which does not communicate with the tracheobronchial tree; thus, they can seriously underestimate FRC, particularly in patients

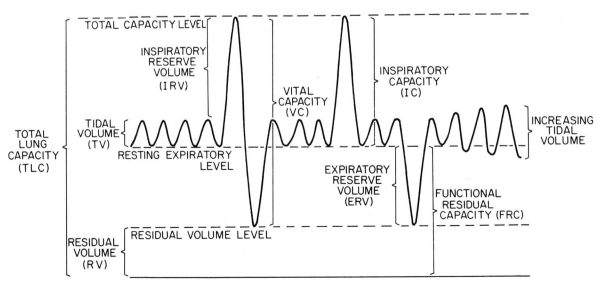

Figure 3–1. Lung Volumes and Capacities.

with severe obstructive lung disease, bullae, or other intra-thoracic noncommunicating accumulations of gas.

The other major method of measuring FRC is based on Boyle's law and employs a body plethysmograph (body box). Boyle's law states that the product of the volume and pressure of gas is constant at constant temperature ($V_1 \times P_1 = V_2 \times P_2$). To measure FRC plethysmographically, the airway is closed at FRC, and the subject pants against the closed airway, thus generating changes in mouth and pleural pressure and small increases and decreases in lung volume due to compression and decompression of thoracic gas. The relationship between changes in thoracic gas volume and mouth pressure ($\Delta V/\Delta P$) can be calibrated so that intrathoracic volume can be derived; in addition, RV and TLC may be obtained by having the subject perform a VC maneuver immediately after measurement of FRC. This method has the advantage that all gas subjected to the swings in intrathoracic pressures is measured, whether or not it communicates with the tracheobronchial tree.

Recent studies have shown that plethysmographic FRC may be overestimated in patients who have airway obstruction, because of a failure of mouth pressure to accurately reflect mean intrathoracic pressure[77]; however, this artifact can be overcome if patients pant at a rate slower than 60 breaths per minute. The determination of TLC based on posteroanterior and lateral chest roentgenograms has been shown to be highly accurate and can be accomplished by experienced workers in less than 5 minutes.[78]

Forced Expiratory Volume and Flow

The forced expiratory maneuver is the most widely used and standardized test of lung function. Three to five measurements are usually obtained, and the test that has the highest sum of FEV_1 and FVC is chosen for analysis.[79, 80] Expired volume is plotted against time (Fig. 3–2) to yield a typical spirogram from which FEV_1, FVC, and $FEF_{25\%-75\%}$ can be derived. Expired volume also can be plotted against the instantaneous expiratory flow rate to yield a flow-volume curve (see Fig. 3–2). Flow at specific percentages of the forced expired vital capacity, such as $\dot{V}max_{50}$ and $\dot{V}max_{25}$, can be determined from the flow-volume curve.

The usefulness of forced expiration as a test of lung function stems largely from the fact that it is relatively effort independent and is highly reproducible. Despite this, submaximal efforts can result in paradoxically high values for FEV_1/FVC and $FEF_{25\%-75\%}$, especially in patients with obstructive pulmonary disease.[81] When measured correctly, the FEV_1 and FVC have an extremely narrow coefficient of variation in normal subjects (± 5 per cent); however, in obstructed patients this increases to approximately 12 per cent when measurements are made on the same day.[75]

Compared with FVC and FEV_1, there is a much higher coefficient of variation for repeated measurements of $FEF_{25\%-75\%}$, $\dot{V}max_{50}$, and $\dot{V}max_{25}$,[82, 83] variability that increases with the degree of pulmonary dysfunction.[84] There is also more variation between individuals for $FEF_{25\%-75\%}$ and $\dot{V}max_{50}$ than for FEV_1 and FVC; the 95 per cent confidence limits for FEV_1 and FVC are generally considered to be 20 per cent, whereas, in order for $FEF_{25\%-75\%}$ and $\dot{V}max_{50}$ to be judged abnormal, values should be more than 40 per cent below predicted.[83]

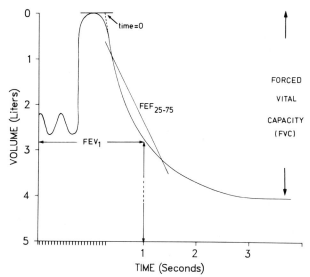

Figure 3–2. Measurement of Ventilatory Volumes. Volume in liters is plotted against time in seconds while the subject forcibly exhales from total lung capacity. The volume versus time slope is back-extrapolated to 0 time, and the expired volume in 1 second (FEV_1) is measured and compared with predicted values as well as to the measured forced vital capacity (FVC). The FEV_1/FVC ratio serves as a volume-independent measure of expiratory airflow obstruction. The average flow over the middle half of the forced expiratory volume ($FEF_{25\%-75\%}$) is obtained as the slope of the volume-time plot between 25 and 75 per cent of the FVC.

Bronchodilator Response

Spirometry is used to assess bronchodilator responsiveness. A 70 per cent increase in peak flow, a 15 per cent increase in FEV_1, a 12 per cent increase in FVC, and/or a 45 per cent increase in $FEF_{25\%-75\%}$ are required to conclude that there is a beneficial effect from a bronchodilator.[85] Since FVC may improve more than FEV_1, the FEV_1/FVC is a poor estimate.[86]

Density Dependence of Maximal Expiratory Flow

Maximal expiratory flow increases after patients are equilibrated with a low-density gas mixture such as 80 per cent helium and 20 per cent oxygen (HeO_2), and measurement of the magnitude of this increase has been advocated as a test of the major site of airflow obstruction.[87] Since the helium-oxygen mixture is less dense than air, there is decreased resistance in central airways, where flow is normally turbulent; by contrast, the gas has no effect on resistance in small airways because of their enormous cross-sectional area and low linear flow velocity. In theory, therefore, patients who have central airflow obstruction will show improvement in maximal flow on HeO_2 and those who have small airway obstruction will show little or no effect. The magnitude of the HeO_2 effect can be calculated as the fractional improvement in $\dot{V}_{max}$ breathing HeO_2.

Despite these theoretical considerations, measurements of density dependence of maximal flow have proved disappointing as a screening test, both because of marked variability and poor reproducibility[88] and because of questions concerning the basic assumptions underlying the test.[89] Along with measurements of inspiratory and expiratory flow-volume curves, however, density dependence of maximal expiratory flow can be useful in the diagnosis of upper airway obstruction,[90] a subject considered in greater detail in Chapter 11.

Maximal Voluntary Ventilation

Maximal voluntary ventilation (MVV) is the ventilation that can be achieved with 15 seconds of maximal effort. Its measurement is influenced by the properties of the lung and airways and correlates with FEV_1, but it is also influenced by inspiratory muscle strength.[91]

Small Airway Tests

Epidemiologic studies have shown that tests of small airway function, such as the single-breath nitrogen washout curve, the density dependence of maximal expiratory flow measured using a helium-oxygen mixture, and measurements of airflow at low lung volumes are abnormal in an appreciable number of asymptomatic smokers.[92] Although controversy still exists regarding the value of such tests in screening for early abnormalities of small airway function,[93] it appears most likely that they do not offer advantages over simple spirometry in detecting the progression of airflow obstruction.[94]

Pressure-Volume Characteristics of the Lung

Lung compliance is the relationship between the volume of air inhaled and the pressure needed to overcome the elastic recoil of the lung. To measure it, a complete pressure-volume curve of the lung is obtained by plotting lung volume against the transpulmonary pressure (PL) over a range of volumes from TLC to FRC or lower. PL is measured by a transducer that compares mouth pressure to esophageal pressure measured with a thin-walled balloon positioned in the midesophagus. Pressure-volume data are collected during quasistatic deflation from TLC or with stepwise interruption of expiratory flow from TLC. Compliance is calculated as the volume change divided by the transpulmonary pressure change over the relatively linear portion of the pressure-volume curve, near FRC.

$$\text{Compliance} = \frac{\Delta \text{ Volume}}{\Delta \text{ Pressure}}$$

Measurement of compliance has the disadvantage of being dependent on lung size, making comparison between individuals difficult. To circumvent this, a number of investigators have suggested fitting the pressure-volume data to an exponential equation[95]:

$$V = A - Be^{-kP}$$

where A is the theoretical maximal lung volume achievable at infinite transpulmonary pressure, B is the difference between A and lung volume at a transpulmonary pressure of zero, P is transpulmonary pressure, and k is the shape constant that reflects the overall compliance of the lung, reagardless of lung size. An increased k value correlates with the severity of emphysema measured morphologically, and a decreased k value has been reported in some cases of interstitial fibrosis.[96]

In addition to compliance, other parameters derived from the pressure-volume curve also reflect the elastic recoil properties of the lung (Fig. 3–3). The maximal elastic recoil pressure that the patient can generate at TLC (PL_{max}) reflects the elastic recoil properties of the lung as well as the inspiratory muscle strength. Elastic recoil pressures at various percentages of TLC (PL_{90}, PL_{80}, PL_{70}, and so on) also can be determined.

Dynamic Compliance

Although the compliance of the lung is normally measured during static maneuvers, dynamic compliance (Cdyn) can be measured during breathing as volume change divided by the changes in transpulmonary pressure at points of zero flow. In normal subjects, Cdyn is very similar to static compliance over the tidal volume range and does not vary with respiratory frequencies up to 100 breaths per minute; however, if there is uneven peripheral airway obstruction, Cdyn decreases as breathing frequency increases, and this test has been advocated as a measure of patchy small airway obstruction.[97] Despite this, it has not gained wide acceptance clinically because it requires expensive equipment, technical expertise, and the placement of an esophageal pressure catheter.[98]

Resistance

Resistance is pressure divided by flow (R = P/V). With respect to the lungs, three forms can be measured:

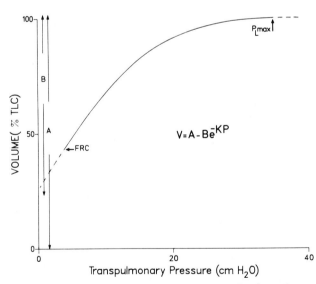

Figure 3–3. Elastic Recoil Properties of the Lung. A schematic pressure volume curve of the lung, in which lung volume as a percentage of TLC (predicted or actual) is plotted against transpulmonary pressure. The pressure volume behavior may be described using various measurements from the P-V curve, including maximal elastic recoil (PLmax), elastic recoil pressure at various percentages of TLC (PL90, PL60, and so on), and compliance—the slope of the $\Delta V/\Delta P$ plot in the relatively linear range near FRC. These all have the disadvantage of describing only a portion of the curve. The whole curve can be fitted to an exponential function,[508] in which V = volume, A = the theoretic maximal lung volume at infinite transpulmonary pressure, B = the volume difference between A and the 0 transpulmonary pressure intercept, P = transpulmonary pressure, and k = the exponent that describes the shape of the P-V curve.

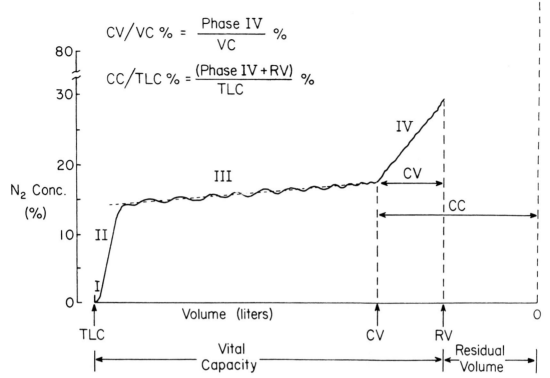

Figure 3–4. The Single Breath Nitrogen Washout. In this test, expired nitrogen concentration (vertical axis) is plotted against expired volume starting at total lung capacity (TLC) and ending at residual volume (RV). Phase I represents dead space gas with 0 nitrogen; phase III represents alveolar nitrogen concentration; the slope of phase III is increased with unevenness of distribution of ventilation. Phase IV begins at closing volume (CV) and represents the increasing contribution of gas from nitrogen-rich nondependent lung regions after basilar regions have closed.

1. Airway resistance (Raw) is the difference between mouth and alveolar pressure divided by flow and is measured in a constant volume body plethysmograph. It also can be expressed as its reciprocal, conductance (Gaw); since both measurements vary with lung volume, they can be expressed as specific resistance (SRaw = Raw × Volume) and specific conductance (SGaw = Gaw/Volume).

2. Pulmonary resistance (RL) is obtained by dividing the difference between mouth and esophageal pressure by flow. Since the pressure difference between the mouth and the pleural space during breathing reflects both the resistive and the elastic properties of the lung, the portion of the transpulmonary pressure swing due to elastic recoil must be subtracted in order to measure the true pressure-flow relationship.[99]

3. Respiratory system resistance (Rrs) is measured by forced oscillation during tidal breathing. Small pulses of flow are generated at the mouth by a loudspeaker, and the relationship between the output of the loudspeaker and the resultant flow can be analyzed to give values for total respiratory system resistance.[98]

Distribution of Inspired Gas and Closing Volume

Single-breath nitrogen washout is a measure of the distribution of inspired gas. The test is carried out by having the patient inhale a VC breath of pure oxygen, beginning the inhalation from residual volume and maintaining the inspiratory flow rate at less than 0.5 L per second. During the subsequent slow exhalation (flow 0.5 L per second) from TLC back to RV, the expired nitrogen concentration measured at the mouth is plotted against the expired volume on an XY recorder or oscilloscope. There are four phases to the changes in volume and nitrogen concentration during progressive exhalation (Fig. 3–4): phase 1 represents the emptying of dead space, which contains pure oxygen and no nitrogen; phase 2 represents the rapid increase in nitrogen, which occurs with the arrival of alveolar gas at the mouth; phase 3, called the alveolar plateau, is the slow, slight rise of nitrogen concentration that occurs as the alveolar gas is exhaled; and phase 4 is the abrupt increase in nitrogen concentration that occurs as residual volume is approached and which represents the onset of dependent airway closure.

Closing volume is the volume above RV at which phase 4 begins, and closing capacity is closing volume plus residual volume. The slope of the alveolar plateau reflects the uniformity of alveolar ventilation and is calculated for the linear portion of the alveolar plateau, expressed as percentage change per liter. The upward-sloping plateau normally found is related to the asynchronous emptying of lung units with different starting nitrogen concentrations. In disease, premature airway closure produces an elevated closing volume and closing capacity; the upward slope of phase 3 is exaggerated owing to regional differences in the distribution of the inhaled oxygen and asynchronous emptying of lung units. Measurement of closing volume and the slope of phase 3 have been proposed as sensitive screening tests of early airway dysfunction[100] but have not gained wide application.

Diffusing Capacity

The diffusing capacity for carbon monoxide (DLCO) is computed as follows:

$$\text{DLCO} = \frac{\text{mL of CO taken up by capillary blood/min}}{\text{Mean alveolar PCO} - \text{Mean capillary PCO}}$$

The amount of CO taken up by capillary blood is calculated by subtracting the product of the expired volume and the CO concentration of expired gas from the product of inspired volume and the CO concentration of inspired gas. The mean alveolar PCO is estimated by obtaining a sample of expired gas after the dead space has been cleared and mean capillary PCO is assumed to be zero.

Several techniques for measuring diffusing capacity with carbon monoxide have been devised,[101–103] the main differences among them being the length of time that the gas is kept in the lungs and the method of determining the mean alveolar PCO. The single-breath method is most widely used. The test is done by having the subject exhale to RV and then take a greater than 90 per cent vital capacity breath of a gas containing 0.3 per cent carbon monoxide, 10 per cent helium, 21 per cent oxygen, and the balance nitrogen. After rapid inspiration of the gas, the breath is held for about 10 seconds near TLC, the first liter of expired gas is discarded, and the next liter (representative of alveolar gas) is collected and analyzed for helium and carbon monoxide. The helium dilution is used to calculate the alveolar volume (VA) as well as the initial concentration of carbon monoxide in the alveolar space. The test can be repeated at brief intervals; two results that agree within 5 per cent are required.[104]

The DLCO is dependent on lung volume. For example, following pneumonectomy or with the chest wall restriction that occurs in conditions such as kyphoscoliosis, a patient may have a reduced DLCO without intrinsic gas exchange abnormality in the remaining or restricted lung.[105] This has led to the suggestion that specific diffusing capacity (the diffusing capacity divided by the alveolar volume at which it is measured [DL/VA]) is a more accurate measurement; this is abbreviated KCO in the United Kingdom.[106]

The diffusing capacity is influenced by factors that alter the alveolar capillary membrane and the pulmonary capillary blood volume (Table 3–3). Since the transfer of carbon monoxide is diffusion- (and not perfusion-) limited, the pulmonary capillary blood volume (VC) rather than pulmonary blood flow is important. In order to calculate the blood volume component of diffusing capacity, VC is multiplied by the kinetic constant θ, which is the rate of combination of carbon monoxide and red blood cells. The membrane and VC × θ contributions to diffusing capacity can be calculated separately by measuring the diffusing capacity with different inspired partial pressures of oxygen. In normal subjects, the two components contribute approximately equally to the measured DLCO.

A variety of factors influence VC and θ and thus, indirectly, DLCO. The θ value is directly affected by the oxygen saturation of hemoglobin and the presence of carboxyhemoglobin associated with smoking or industrial exposure.

Table 3–3. FACTORS AFFECTING DIFFUSING CAPACITY

Alveolar Capillary Membrane
 Lung volume
 Surface area
 "Thickness"
Pulmonary Capillary Blood Volume
  (Blood volume × Hgb concentration)
 Position: increased DLCO standing → sitting → lying
 Müller or Valsalva maneuvers during breath hold
 Hemoglobin concentration
 Hemoglobin affinity for oxygen
Distribution of Ventilation Relative to Perfusion
 Affects steady-state method especially
 Affects FCO least
Back Pressure of Carbon Monoxide
 Cigarette smoking

Smokers can have a level of carboxyhemoglobin as high as 10 per cent, so this must be considered when interpreting test results. Factors that increase or decrease hemoglobin concentration also affect the DLCO, and a number of correction factors for anemia and polycythemia have been suggested. One commonly employed adjustment is to increase or decrease the predicted DLCO by 1.4 per cent for each per cent change in hematocrit above or below 44 per cent.[107]

Acute changes in pulmonary capillary blood volume also can alter measured DLCO; for example, the recruitment of pulmonary vascular bed during exercise results in a substantial increase in DLCO within seconds.[108] DLCO also increases when one breathes through an inspiratory resistance, presumably as a result of increased capillary blood volume caused by negative intrathoracic pressure. It is important to recognize that an increased DLCO is not caused solely by increased *capillary* blood; it also may be markedly increased in patients with intra-alveolar hemorrhage, and the measurement of DLCO has been recommended for the diagnosis of this condition.[109]

Ventilation-Perfusion Ratios

Methods for the assessment of disturbances of ventilation-perfusion ratios are described in Chapter 1 (*see* page 49). The most commonly employed technique involves calculation of the alveolar-arterial gradient for oxygen using the simplified alveolar air equation. An increase in "physiologic" dead space can be measured with the Bohr equation, and venous admixture or true intrapulmonary shunt can be calculated. Radionuclides are commonly used in the study of regional ventilation-perfusion inequality; the multiple inert gas technique provides the most accurate description of the distribution of ventilation-perfusion ratios in the lung, although it does not provide regional information.

Respiratory Control

Alveolar hypoventilation accompanied by an elevated arterial PCO_2 and the resultant fall in arterial PO_2 is the final common pathway of many pulmonary disorders. The clinical challenge is to determine why hypoventilation has occurred: is the patient hypoventilating because he or she *will not* breathe sufficiently or *cannot* breathe sufficiently?[110]

The first step in the investigation of "can't versus won't" is measurement of lung volumes and flow rates, as hypoventilation due to increased work of breathing does not occur unless there is a reduction to less than 25 per cent of the predicted value. If hypoventilation is present with adequate ventilatory reserve, more detailed investigation of respiratory control is warranted.

It is difficult to quantify respiratory center output. The measurement that most accurately reflects central neural drive is an electrical neurogram of the phrenic nerve, but this is a difficult and invasive test and is rarely used. As a result, several other techniques have been proposed.

Ventilatory Response Curves

The ventilatory response to carbon dioxide can be measured with a steady state or rebreathing technique.[111] The most widely used method involves rebreathing of carbon dioxide.[112] The subject breathes from a bag containing CO_2 at approximately the level of mixed venous P_{CO_2} (7 per cent). The mixed venous, arterial, and alveolar P_{CO_2} concentrations come into equilibrium within 30 to 60 seconds, and thereafter a linear increase in CO_2 concentration of 3 to 6 mm Hg per minute occurs, owing to endogenous production of carbon dioxide. The results are expressed as the slope of the ventilatory response, $\Delta V/\Delta P_{CO_2}$, and the relationship is linear with an intercept on the CO_2 axis, which reflects the starting arterial P_{CO_2} (Fig. 3–5). The range of ventilatory response to CO_2 is remarkably wide among normal subjects; there is an approximate 16-fold

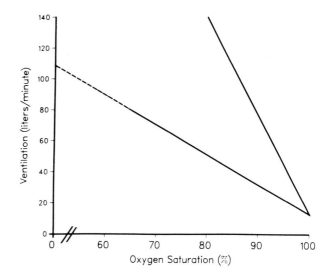

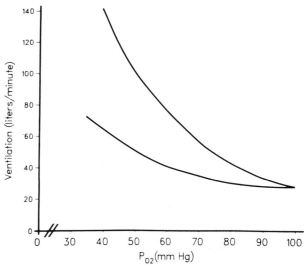

Figure 3–6. The Ventilatory Response to Hypoxemia. The ventilatory response to hypoxemia is tested by plotting ventilation versus changes in oxygen saturation *(upper panel)* or P_{O_2} *(lower panel)*. A wide range of normal responses is shown by these two representative curves, which are at the upper and lower limits of normal responses. The advantage of using O_2 saturation as the independent variable is that linear relationships are produced that allow easier comparison within or between subjects.

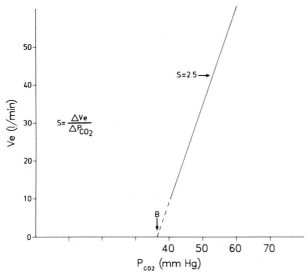

Figure 3–5. The CO_2 Ventilatory Response Curve. The ventilatory response curve to increasing levels of CO_2 serves as a measure of respiratory chemosensitivity. A linear relationship between ventilation and end-tidal CO_2 is observed with the rebreathing method, and chemosensitivity is quantified as the slope of the curve

$$\frac{\Delta \dot{V}e}{\Delta P_{CO_2}}$$

A normal curve in which the $\Delta \dot{V}e/\Delta P_{CO_2}$ is 2.5 L per minute per mm Hg is depicted. There is a wide range of normal for this slope, and the relationship can be changed by alterations in central drive, neuromuscular function, or respiratory system impedance.

variation (between 0.57 and 8.17 L per minute per mm Hg rise in CO_2[113]).

The ventilatory response to hypoxia can be assessed by plotting changes in ventilation as a function of decreasing arterial or end-tidal P_{O_2} or as a function of arterial oxygen saturation measured using an oximeter.[113] The relationship of ventilation with P_{O_2} results in a curvilinear plot (Fig. 3–6); ventilation changes little until P_{O_2} values of approximately 50 or 60 mm Hg, then increases steeply. The relationship of ventilation and saturation is linear, allowing easier quantitation.

The range of normal ventilatory response to hypoxemia is also extremely wide, with a mean value of 1.47 L per minute per cent fall in arterial saturation; 80 per cent of normal subjects have a slope between 0.6 and 2.75.[113]

Mouth Occlusion Pressures

The ventilatory response to CO_2 and O_2 depends heavily on the impedance of the respiratory system. Thus, a patient might have a normal neural output from a normally functioning respiratory center, but the translation of that neural output to ventilation might be impaired purely for mechanical reasons. Measuring the pressure at the mouth 100 msec after an occluded breath represents an attempt to overcome this problem.[114] The technique is performed while the patient is breathing tidally at rest or during various stages of measuring a ventilatory response curve to hypoxia or hypercapnia. Periodically, and unknown to the subject, the mouthpiece is temporarily occluded for at least 100 msec at the onset of inspiration.[114] Although a patient who has a stiff lung or narrowed airways may develop a high occlusion pressure, that pressure would produce only a small change in volume; by contrast, in a normal subject only a small change in pressure is required to produce a volume change equivalent to tidal volume. Thus, pressure is a more direct indicator of the drive to breathe than is ventilation. Using this technique, studies have shown that patients with ventilatory impairment may have normal or even supranormal drive, the decreased ventilation being attributable solely to the increased impedance of the respiratory system.[115]

Breathing Pattern Analysis

Ventilation at rest or during stimulated breathing can be divided into a flow component and a timing component:

$$V_E = V_T/T_i \times T_i/T_{tot}$$

where V_T/T_i is the mean inspiratory flow (tidal volume divided by inspiratory time), and T_i/T_{tot} is the duty cycle (ratio of inspiratory time to total respiratory cycle time). Increase in ventilation can be achieved by increasing the inspiratory flow rate V_T/T_i and keeping T_i/T_{tot} constant, or by increasing T_i/T_{tot} and keeping V_T/T_i constant. The V_T/T_i component is thought to reflect neural output from the respiratory center, whereas the T_i/T_{tot} relationship reflects the timing element.[116]

Electromyography

Respiratory center output can be measured by electromyography of the diaphragm or other respiratory muscles. Recordings are made with surface electrodes placed on the fifth, sixth, and seventh intercostal spaces, close to the costochondral junctions, or with an esophageal electrode.[117] The technique has several disadvantages, particularly that it is invasive and is one step removed from the electrical output of the respiratory center.

Respiratory Muscle Performance

The final step in the assessment of respiratory control involves measurement of neurologic output as reflected in respiratory muscle performance. The simplest means of testing inspiratory and expiratory muscle strength is to measure maximal inspiratory and expiratory pressures (P_{Imax} and P_{Emax}) at the mouth. The technique involves having a subject make maximal inspiratory and maximal expiratory efforts against a closed mouthpiece in which a small leak has been constructed to avoid glottic closure and generation of pressure with the buccal and oropharyngeal muscles. The pressures generated depend on the lung volume at which the test is performed, since this influences the length-tension relationship of various respiratory muscles. Thus, maximal inspiratory pressure is generated near RV and maximal expiratory pressures near TLC when expiratory muscles are lengthened.[118]

Measurement of P_{Imax} and P_{Emax} gives an overall estimate of respiratory muscle performance, but measurement of maximal transdiaphragmatic pressure (P_{dimax}) gives a specific estimate of diaphragm strength. This measurement is obtained by comparing pleural to gastric pressure during maximal inspiratory effort against a closed mouthpiece and has proved useful in the detection of bilateral or unilateral diaphragmatic paralysis.[119]

Inhalation Challenge Tests

Inhalation challenge tests can be broadly categorized into nonspecific and specific types. Nonspecific tests include those involving aerosol challenge with nebulized agonists, such as methacholine and histamine, and those designed to produce cooling and drying of the airway mucosa by exercise and isocapnic hyperventilation. Specific challenge tests involve inhalation of allergens to which the subject is known or suspected to be sensitive or exposure to dust or environmental agents that provoke idiosyncratic lung responses in some individuals.

Nonspecific Inhalation Challenge

All the techniques employed to measure nonspecific bronchial reactivity (NSBR) pharmacologically involve the inhalation of an aerosol containing a known bronchoconstrictive agent. Inhalation is begun with a weak concentration or dose of agonist, and the dose is progressively increased; an index of airway narrowing is measured at each step, so that a dose-response relationship can be constructed. A variety of techniques for delivering agonists and measuring the response and expressing the results have been developed (Table 3–4). The most widely used and carefully standardized one employs nebulized histamine or methacholine (probably the agent of choice) delivered with a face mask during tidal breathing; 2-minute inhalations of increasing concentrations of histamine or methacholine are followed by measurements of FEV_1. Doubling concentrations of agonist are administered, and the test is stopped either when there is at least a 20 per cent fall in FEV_1 or when the highest concentration of agonist is reached. The level of nonspecific reactivity is calculated as the concentration of inhaled agonist that results in a 20 per cent fall in FEV_1 (PC_{20}).[120]

In stable patients, measurements of PC_{20} show remarkable reproducibility over time. They are universally lower than 8 mg per mL in asthmatic patients, whereas in subjects with normal pulmonary function and negative history they are invariably greater than 16 mg per mL. This allows clear separation of patients with reactive airway disease from normal subjects, although patients with chronic bron-

Table 3–4. **TESTS OF NONSPECIFIC BRONCHIAL REACTIVITY**

	Agonist	Method of Administration	Measured Variable	Expression of Results
Cockcroft et al[°°]	Histamine or methacholine	Face mask with nose clip, 2-min inhalations, tidal breathing, Wright nebulizer	FEV_1 before and after each concentration until FEV_1 has decreased 20% or greater	Provocative concentration producing a 20% fall in FEV_1 (PC_{20})
Chai et al[°]	Histamine or methacholine	Devilbiss 646 nebulizer and Rosenthal French dosimeter	FEV_1 after each dose until decreased 20% or greater	Provocative dose producing a 20% fall in FEV_1 (Pd_{20})
Yan et al[†]	Histamine	Handheld Devilbiss No. 40 glass nebulizer, bulb squeezed by technician	FEV_1 60 sec after each dose until 20% fall in FEV_1 recorded	Pd_{20} (cumulative dose calculation)
Orehek et al[‡]	Carbachol	Different concentration of carbachol solution nebulized into spirometer. Varying breath number	Specific airway resistance and specific airway conductance after each dose	Sensitivity = D25 dose causing a 25% rise (cumulative) Reactivity—arithmetic relationship of dose vs. specific airway conductance (%)

°Chai et al. J Allergy Clin Immunol 56:323, 1975.
†Yan et al. Thorax 38:760, 1983.
‡Orehek et al. Am Rev Respir Dis 115:937, 1977.
°°Cockcroft et al. Clin Allergy 7:235, 1977.

chitis, cystic fibrosis, or other chronic airway diseases may have intermediate values. Thus, in doubtful cases, the test can substantiate a diagnosis of asthma and is particularly helpful when baseline spirometry is normal and in patients whose primary complaint is cough. In patients with asthma, measurements of bronchial reactivity correlate well with the severity of symptoms and the need for medication.[120]

Bronchial reactivity can change over time; for example, intensive therapy can result in a decrease in NSBR, whereas exposure to allergens or occupational sensitizers can increase it. Serial measurements of PC_{20} can be obtained to assess the efficacy of treatment or the detrimental effect of exposure.

Specific Inhalation Challenge

Specific inhalation challenge tests are performed on individuals who have, or are suspected of having, allergy or sensitivity to specific allergens or chemicals. They are less well standardized than nonspecific challenge tests; in addition, they are time-consuming and can induce severe and prolonged responses that can be hazardous. For these reasons, these tests are rarely indicated in clinical practice and should be reserved for special cases being investigated in larger centers where there are experts in the methods. Inhalation challenge testing with agents suspected of causing allergic alveolitis or occupational asthma, however, may be important in establishing proof of specific sensitivity to these agents and may be required for compensation purposes.

Exercise-Induced Bronchoconstriction and Isocapnic Hyperventilation

With the demonstration that the bronchoconstriction associated with exercise is caused by breathing cool, dry air, techniques to measure the bronchial responsiveness to such air during isocapnic hyperventilation have been developed.[121] Patients are asked to hyperventilate from a source

of dry air, either cold or at room temperature, and isocapnia is maintained by adding carbon dioxide to the inspired gas to maintain a constant end-tidal carbon dioxide content. Expiratory flow is measured with progressively increasing levels of hyperventilation, and the level of ventilation or the calculated respiratory heat loss that produces a given drop in FEV_1 can be calculated in a fashion similar to the way PC_{20} is calculated. More recently, it has been demonstrated that patients with reactive airway disease show bronchoconstriction on inhalation of ultrasonically nebulized hyper- or hypotonic water mist; this has been suggested as an additional nonspecific bronchial irritant for quantification of bronchial reactivity.[122]

References

1. Corrao WM, Braman SS, Irwin RS: Chronic cough as the sole presenting manifestion of bronchial asthma. N Engl J Med 300: 633, 1979.
2. Irwin RS, Curley FJ, French CL: Chronic cough. The spectrum and frequency of causes, key components of the diagnostic evaluation, and outcome of specific therapy. Am Rev Respir Dis 141: 640, 1990.
3. Simon PM, Schwartzstein RM, Weiss JW, et al: Distinguishable types of dyspnea in patients with shortness of breath. Am Rev Respir Dis 142: 1009, 1990.
3a. Becklake MR: Organic or functional impairment: Overall perspective. Am Rev Respir Dis 129: 896, 1984.
4. Rice RL: Symptom patterns of the hyperventilation syndrome. Am J Med 8: 691, 1950.
5. Harrow AS, Levin DC: Platypnea and orthodeoxia: Surgically corrected dyspnea with recurrence. J Okla State Med Assoc 82: 563, 1989.
6. Weinberger SE, Weiss ST, Cohen WR, et al: Pregnancy and the lung. Am Rev Respir Dis 121: 559, 1980.
7. Schneider RR, Seckler SG: Evaluation of acute chest pain. Med Clin North Am 65: 53, 1981.
8. Lichstein E, Seckler SG: Evaluation of acute chest pain. Med Clin North Am 57:1481, 1973.
8a. Santiago S, Tobias J, Williams AJ: A reappraisal of the causes of hemoptysis. Arch Intern Med 151: 2449, 1991.
9. Heaton RW: Should patients with haemoptysis and a normal chest x-ray be bronchoscoped? Postgrad Med J 63: 947, 1987.
10. Poe RH, Israel RH, Marin MG, et al: Utility of fiberoptic bronchos-

copy in patients with hemoptysis and a nonlocalizing chest roentgenogram. Chest 93: 70, 1988.

10a. Millar AB, Boothroyd AE, Edwards D, Hetzel MR: The role of computed tomography (CT) in the investigation of unexplained haemoptysis. Respir Med 86(1): 39, 1992.

11. Adelman M, Haponik EF, Bleeker ER, et al: Cryptogenic hemoptysis: Clinical features, bronchoscopic findings, and natural history in 67 patients. Ann Intern Med 102: 829, 1985.

12. Conlan AA, Hurwitz SS, Krige L, et al: Massive hemoptysis. Review of 123 cases. J Thorac Cardiovasc Surg 85: 120, 1983.

13. Crocco JA, Rooney JJ, Fankushen DS, et al: Massive hemoptysis. Arch Intern Med 121: 495, 1968.

14. Bredin CP, Richardson PR, King TKC, et al: Treatment of massive hemoptysis by combined occlusion of pulmonary and bronchial arteries. Rev Respir Dis 117: 969, 1978.

15. Katoh O, Kishikawa T, Yamada H, et al: Recurrent bleeding after arterial embolization in patients with hemoptysis. Chest 97: 541, 1990.

16. Sweezey NB, Fellows KE: Bronchial artery embolization for severe hemoptysis in cystic fibrosis. Chest 97: 1322, 1990.

17. Ludman H: ABC of ENT: Hoarseness and stridor. Br Med J 282: 715, 1981.

18. Austen FK, Carmichael MW, Adams RD: Neurologic manifestations of chronic pulmonary insufficiency. N Engl J Med 257: 579, 1957.

19. Gravelyn TR, Weg JG: Respiratory rate as an indicator of acute respiratory dysfunction. JAMA 244: 1123, 1980.

20. Forgacs P, Nathoo AR, Richardson HD: Breath sounds. Thorax 26: 288, 1971.

21. LeBlanc P, Macklem PT, Ross WR: Breath sounds and distribution of pulmonary ventilation. Am Rev Respir Dis 102: 10, 1970.

22. Forgacs P: Crackles and wheezes. Lancet 2: 203, 1967.

23. Forgacs P: The functional basis of pulmonary sounds. Chest 73: 399, 1978.

24. Hamman L: Spontaneous mediastinal emphysema. Bull Johns Hopkins Hosp 64: 1, 1939.

25. Scadding JG, Wood P: Systolic clicks due to left-sided pneumothorax. Lancet 2: 1208, 1939.

26. Racoceanu SN, Mendlowitz M, Suck AF, et al: Digital capillary blood flow in clubbing. ^{85}Kr studies in hereditary and acquired cases. Ann Intern Med 75: 933, 1971.

27. Schneerson JM: Digital clubbing and hypertrophic osteoarthropathy: The underlying mechanisms. Br J Dis Chest 75: 113, 1981.

27a. Gosney MA, Gosney JR, Lye M: Plasma growth hormone and digital clubbing in carcinoma of the bronchus. Thorax 45: 545, 1990.

28. Thiede WH, Banaszak EF: Selective bronchial catheterization. N Engl J Med 286: 526, 1972.

29. Ali A, Tetalman MR, Fordham EW, et al: Distribution of hypertrophic pulmonary osteoarthropathy. Am J Roentgenol 134: 771, 1980.

30. Coury C: Hippocratic fingers and hypertrophic osteoarthropathy: A study of 350 cases. Br J Dis Chest 54: 202, 1960.

31. Perkins PJ: Delayed onset of secondary hypertrophic osteoarthropathy. Am J Roentgenol 130: 561, 1978.

32. Ginsberg J, Brown JB: Increased oestrogen excretion in hypertrophic pulmonary osteoarthropathy. Lancet 2: 1274, 1961.

33. Greenberg PB, Beck C, Martin TJ, et al: Synthesis and release of human growth hormone from lung carcinoma in cell culture. Lancet 1: 350, 1972.

34. Rimoin DL: Pachydermoperiostosis (idiopathic clubbing and periostosis): Genetic and physiologic considerations. N Engl J Med 272: 923, 1965.

35. Oho K, Kato H, Ogawa I, et al: Present status of bronchoscopy in Japan. Br J Dis Chest 75: 409, 1981.

36. Rodenstein D, Stanescu D, Francis C: Demonstration of failure of body plethysmography in airway obstruction. J Appl Physiol 52: 949, 1982.

37. Belen J, Neuhaus A, Markowitz D, et al: Modification of the effect of fiberoptic bronchoscopy on pulmonary mechanics. Chest 79: 516, 1981.

38. Pearce SJ: Fiberoptic bronchoscopy: Is sedation necessary? Br Med J 281: 779, 1980.

39. Mitchell DM, Emerson CJ, Collyer J, et al: Fiberoptic bronchoscopy: Ten years on. Br Med J 281: 360, 1980.

40. Conte BA, LaForet EG: The role of the topical anesthetic agent in modifying bacteriologic data obtained by bronchoscopy. N Engl J Med 267: 957, 1962.

41. Barrett CR Jr: Flexible fiberoptic bronchoscopy in the critically ill patient. Methodology and indications. Chest 73(Suppl): 746, 1978.

42. Barrett CR Jr, Vecchione JJ, Bell ALL Jr: Flexible fiberoptic bronchoscopy for airway management during acute respiratory failure. Am Rev Respir Dis 109: 429, 1974.

43. Higenbottam T, Stewart S, Penketh A, et al: Transbronchial lung biopsy for the diagnosis of rejection in heart-lung transplant patients. Transplantation 46: 532, 1988.

44. Lundgren R, Haggmark S, Reiz S: Hemodynamic effects of flexible fiberoptic bronchoscopy performed under topical anesthesia. Chest 82: 295, 1982.

45. Katz AS, Michelson EL, Stawicki J, et al: Cardiac arrhythmias: Frequency during fiberoptic bronchoscopy and correlation with hypoxemia. Arch Intern Med 141: 603, 1981.

46. Credle WF Jr, Smiddy JF, Elliott RC: Complications of fiberoptic bronchoscopy. Am Rev Respir Dis 109: 67, 1974.

47. Lukomsky GI, Ovchinnikov AA, Bilal A: Complications of bronchoscopy: Comparison of rigid bronchoscopy under general anesthesia and flexible bronchoscopy under topical anesthesia. Chest 79: 316, 1981.

47a. Von Essen SG, Robbins RA, Spurzem JR, et al: Bronchoscopy with bronchoalveolar lavage causes neutrophil recruitment to the lower respiratory tract. Am Rev Respir Dis 144: 848, 1991.

47b. Allen JN, Davis WB, Pacht ER: Diagnostic significance of increased bronchoalveolar lavage fluid eosinophils. Am Rev Respir Dis 142: 642, 1990.

47c. Tilles DS, Goldenheim PD, Ginns LC, et al: Pulmonary function in normal subjects and patients with sarcoidosis after bronchoalveolar lavage. Chest 89: 244, 1986.

47d. Strumpf IJ, Feld MK, Cornelius MJ, et al: Safety of fibreoptic bronchoalveolar lavage in evaluation of interstitial lung disease. Chest 80: 268, 1981.

48. Horstmann DM, Hsiung GD: Principles of diagnostic virology. In Horsfall FL, Tamm I (eds): Viral and Rickettsial Infections of Man. 4th ed. Philadelphia, JB Lippincott, 1965, p 405.

49. Bartlett JG, Finegold SM: Bacteriology of expectorated sputum with quantitative culture and wash technique compared to transtracheal aspirates. Am Rev Respir Dis 117: 1019, 1978.

50. Bartlett JG, Rosenblatt JE, Finegold SM: Percutaneous transtracheal aspiration in the diagnosis of anaerobic pulmonary infection. Ann Intern Med 79: 535, 1973.

51. Spencer DC, Beaty HN: Complications of transtracheal aspiration. N Engl J Med 286: 304, 1972.

52. Joshi JH, Wang K-P, DeJongh CA, et al: A comparative evaluation of 2 fiberoptic bronchoscopy catheters: The plugged telescoping catheter versus the single sheathed nonplugged catheter. Am Rev Respir Dis 126: 860, 1982.

53. Villers D, Derriennic M, Raffi F, et al: Reliability of the bronchoscopic protected catheter brush in intubated and ventilated patients. Chest 88: 527, 1985.

54. Bordelon JY Jr, Legrand P, Gewin WC, et al: The telescoping plugged catheter in suspected anaerobic infections: A controlled series. Am Rev Respir Dis 128: 465, 1983.

55. Castellino RA, Blank N: Etiologic diagnosis of focal pulmonary infection in immunocompromised patients by fluoroscopically guided percutaneous needle aspiration. Radiology 132: 563, 1979.

56. Haverkos HW, Dowling JN, Pasculle AW, et al: Diagnosis of pneumonitis in immunocompromised patients by open lung biopsy. Cancer 52: 1093, 1983.

57. Manson-Bahr PH: Manson's Tropical Diseases. A Manual of the Diseases of Warm Climates. 16th ed. London, Baillière, Tindall, and Cassell, 1966.

58. Janik JS, Nagaraj HS, Groff DB: Thoracoscopic evaluations of intrathoracic lesions in children. J Thorac Cardiovasc Surg 83: 408, 1982.

59. Buechner HA, Seabury JH, Campbell CC, et al: The current status of serologic, immunologic and skin tests in the diagnosis of pulmonary mycoses. Report of the committee on fungus diseases and subcommittee on criteria for clinical diagnosis—American College of Chest Physicians. Chest 63: 259, 1973.

60. Buechner HA: Clinical aspects of fungus diseases of the lungs including laboratory diagnosis and treatment. In Banyai AL, Gordon BL (eds): Advances in Cardiopulmonary Diseases. Vol 3. Chicago, Year Book, 1966, p 123.

61. Hydatid disease. Br Med J 4: 448, 1970.

62. Egsmose T: The effect of an exorbitant intracutaneous dose of 200 micrograms PPD tuberculin compared with 0.02 micrograms PPD tuberculin. Am Rev Respir Dis 102: 35, 1970.

63. National Tuberculosis Association: Diagnostic Standards and Classification of Tuberculosis. New York, National Tuberculosis Association, 1969, pp 61–63.

64. Comstock GW, Furcolow ML, Greenberg RL, et al: The tuberculin skin test: A statement by the Committee on Diagnostic Skin Testing, American Thoracic Society. Am Rev Respir Dis 104: 769, 1971.

65. Edwards LB, Acquaviva FA, Livesay VT: Identification of tuberculous infected. Dual tests and density of reaction. Am Rev Respir Dis 108: 1334, 1973.

66. Schachter EN: Tuberculin negative tuberculosis. Am Rev Respir Dis 106: 587, 1972.

67. Tuberculin anergy. Br Med J 4: 573, 1970.

68. Hsu KH: Diagnostic skin test for mycobacterial infections in man. Chest 64: 1, 1973.

69. Light RW, MacGregor MI, Luchsinger PC, et al: Pleural effusions: The diagnostic separation of transudates and exudates. Ann Intern Med 77: 507, 1972.

70. Light RW, Ball WC Jr: Glucose and amylase in pleural effusions. JAMA 225: 257, 1973.

71. Good JT Jr, Taryle DA, Maulitz RM, et al: The diagnostic value of pleural fluid pH. Chest 78: 55, 1980.

72. Light RW, MacGregor MI, Ball WC Jr, et al: Diagnostic significance of pleural fluid pH and Pco_2. Chest 64: 591, 1973.

73. Spodick DH: Electrocardiographic studies in pulmonary disease. I. Electrocardiographic abnormalities in diffuse lung disease. II. Establishment of criteria for the electrocardiographic inference of diffuse lung disease. Circulation 20: 1067, 1959.

74. Carey J, Huseby J, Culver B, et al: Variability in interpretation of pulmonary function tests. Chest 76: 389, 1979.

75. Pennock B, Rogers R, McCaffree DR: Changes in measured spirometric indices—what is significant? Chest 80: 97, 1981.

75a. Knudson R, Lebowitz M, Holberg C, et al: Changes in the normal maximal expiratory flow volume curve with growth and aging. Am Rev Respir Dis 127: 725, 1983.

75b. Pennock B, Rogers R, McCaffree DR: Changes in measured spirometric indices—what is significant? Chest 80: 97, 1981.

75c. Lam S, Abboud R, Chan-Yeung M: Use of maximal expiratory flow-volume curve with air and helium-oxygen in the detection of ventilatory abnormalities in population surveys. Am Rev Respir Dis 123: 234, 1981.

75d. Goldman HI, Becklake MR: Respiratory function tests: Normal values at median altitudes and the prediction of normal results. Am Rev Tuberc 79: 457, 1959.

75e. Garcia J, Hunninghake G, Nugent K: Thoracic gas volume measurement: Increased variability in patients with obstructive ventilatory defects. Chest 85: 272, 1984.

75f. Loveland M, Corbin R, Ducic S, et al: Evaluation of the analysis and variability of the helium response. Bull Eur Physiopathol Respir 14: 551, 1978.

75g. Zeck R, Solliday N, Celic L, et al: Variability of the volume of isoflow. Chest 79: 269, 1981.

75h. Colebatch H, Greaves I, Ng C: Exponential analysis of elastic recoil and aging in healthy males and females. J Appl Physiol 47: 683, 1979.

75i. McCuaig C, Vessal S, Coppin C, et al: Variability in measurements of pressure volume curves in normal subjects. Am Rev Respir Dis 131: 656, 1985.

75j. Crapo R, Morris A: Standardized single-breath normal values for carbon monoxide diffusing capacity. Am Rev Respir Dis 123: 185, 1981.

75k. Hathaway EH, Tashkin DP, Simmons MS: Intraindividual variability in serial measurements of DLCO and alveolar volume over one year in eight healthy subjects using three independent measuring systems. Am Rev Respir Dis 140: 1818, 1989.

75l. Buist A, Ross B: Predicted values for closing volumes using a modified single-breath nitrogen test. Am Rev Respir Dis 107: 744, 1973.

76. Hughes J, Hutchinson D: Errors in the estimation of vital capacity from expiratory flow-volume curves in pulmonary emphysema. Br J Dis Chest 76: 279, 1982.

77. Begin P, Peslin R: Plethysmographic measurements of thoracic gas volume. Back to assumptions. Bull Eur Physiopathol Resp 19: 247, 1983.

78. O'Brien R, Drizd T: Roentgenographic determination of total lung capacity: Normal values from a national population survey. Am Rev Respir Dis 128: 949, 1983.

79. Peslin R, Bohadana A, Hannhart B, et al: Comparison of various methods for reading maximal expiratory flow-volume curves. Am Rev Respir Dis 119: 271, 1979.

80. Medical Section, American Thoracic Society of the American Lung Association: ATS statement, Snowbird workshop on standardization of spirometry. Am Rev Respir Dis 119: 831, 1979.

81. Suratt P, Hooe D, Owens D, et al: Effect of maximal versus submaximal expiratory effort on spirometric values. Respiration 42: 233, 1981.

82. Whitaker C, Chinn D, Lee W: Statistical reliability of indices derived from the closing volume and flow volume traces. Bull Eur Physiopathol Respir 14: 237, 1978.

83. Lam S, Abboud R, Chan-Yeung M: Use of maximal expiratory flow-volume curve with air and helium-oxygen in the detection of ventilatory abnormalities in population surveys. Am Rev Respir Dis 123: 234, 1981.

84. Rossoff L, Csima A, Zamel N: Reproducibility of maximum expiratory flow in severe chronic obstructive pulmonary disease. Bull Eur Physiopathol Respir 15: 1129, 1979.

85. Sourk R, Nugent K: Bronchodilator testing—confidence intervals derived from placebo inhalations. Am Rev Respir Dis 128: 153, 1983.

86. Girard M, Light W: Should the FVC be considered in evaluating response to bronchodilator? Chest 84: 87, 1983.

87. Hutcheon M, Griffin P, Levison H, et al: Volume of isoflow. A new test in detection of mild abnormalities of lung mechanics. Am Rev Respir Dis 110: 458, 1974.

88. Li K, Tan L, Chong P, et al: Between-technician variation in the measurement of spirometry with air and helium. Am Rev Respir Dis 124: 196, 1981.

89. Mink S, Wood L: How does HeO_2 increase maximum expiratory flow in human lungs? J Clin Invest 66: 720, 1980.

90. Lavelle T Jr, Rotman H, Weg J: Isoflow-volume curves in the diagnosis of upper airway obstruction. Am Rev Respir Dis 117: 845, 1978.

91. Aldrich T, Arora N, Rocheseter D: The influence of airway obstruction and respiratory muscle strength on maximal voluntary ventilation in lung disease. Am Rev Respir Dis 126: 195, 1982.

92. Buist AS, Ghezzo NR, Anthonisen RM, et al: Relationship between the single-breath N_2 test and age, sex and smoking habit in three North American cities. Am Rev Respir Dis 120: 305, 1979.

93. Macklem PT, Becklake M: Is screening for chronic limitation of airflow desirable? Chest 74: 607, 1978.

94. Van de Woestijne KP: Are the small airways really quiet? Eur J Respir Dis 63: 19, 1982.

95. Knudson R, Kaltenborn W: Evaluation of lung elastic recoil by exponential curve analysis. Respir Physiol 46: 29, 1981.

96. Paré PD, Brooks LA, Bates J, et al: Exponential analysis of the lung pressure volume curve as a predictor of pulmonary emphysema. Am Rev Resp Dis 126: 54, 1982.

97. Woolcock AJ, Vincent NJ, Macklem PT: Frequency dependence of compliance as a test for obstruction in the small airways. J Clin Invest 48: 1097, 1969.

98. Cutillo A, Renzetti A Jr: Mechanical behaviour of the respiratory system as a function of frequency in health and disease. Bull Eur Physiopathol Respir 19: 293, 1983.

99. Mead J, Whittenberger JL: Physical properties of human lungs measured during spontaneous respiration. J Appl Physiol 5: 779, 1953.

100. McCarthy DS, Spencer R, Greene R, et al: Measurement of "closing volume" as a simple and sensitive test for early detection of small airway disease. Am J Med 52: 747, 1972.

101. Russell N, Bagg L, Dobrzynski J: Clinical assessment of a rebreathing method for measuring pulmonary gas transfer. Thorax 38: 212, 1983.

102. Graham B, Mink J, Cotton D: Improved accuracy and precision of single-breath CO diffusing capacity measurements. J Appl Physiol 55: 1306, 1981.

103. Cotton D, Newth C, Portner P, et al: Measurement of single-breath CO diffusing capacity by continuous rapid CO analysis in man. J Appl Physiol 46: 1149, 1979.

104. Make B, Miller A, Epler G, et al: Single breath diffusing capacity in the industrial setting. Chest 82: 351, 1982.

105. Siegler D, Zorab P: The influence of lung volume on gas transfer in scoliosis. Br J Dis Chest 76: 44, 1982.

106. Ayers L, Ginsberg M, Fein J, et al: Diffusing capacity, specific diffusing capacity and interpretation of diffusion defects. West J Med 123: 255, 1975.

107. Mohsenifar Z, Brown H, Schnitzer B, et al: The effect of abnormal levels of hematocrit on the single breath diffusing capacity. Lung 160: 325, 1982.

108. Fisher J, Cerny F: Characteristics of adjustment of lung diffusing capacity to work. J Appl Physiol 52: 1124, 1982.

109. Hallenberg C, Holden W, Menzel T, et al: The clinical usefulness of a screening test to detect static pulmonary blood using a multiple breath analysis of diffusing capacity. Am Rev Respir Dis 119: 349, 1979.

110. Lopata M, Lourenco R: Evaluation of respiratory control. Clin Chest Med 1: 33, 1980.

111. Cherniack N, Dempsey J, Fencl V, et al: Workshop on assessment of respiratory control in humans. 1. Methods of measurement of ventilatory responses to hypoxia and hypercapnia. Am Rev Respir Dis 115: 177, 1977.

112. Read D: A clinical method for assessing the ventilatory response to carbon dioxide. Aust Ann Med 16: 20, 1967.

113. Rebuck A, Slutsky A: Measurement of ventilatory responses to hypercapnia and hypoxia. *In* Hornbein TF, Lenfant C (eds): Regulation of Breathing. Part II. Lung Biology in Health and Disease. New York, Marcel Dekker, 1981, p 745.

114. Whitelaw W, Derenne JP, Milic-Emili J: Occlusion pressure as a measure of respiratory centre output in conscious man. Respir Physiol 23: 181, 1975.

115. Zackon H, Despas P, Anthonisen N: Occlusion pressure responses in asthma and chronic obstructive pulmonary disease. Am Rev Respir Dis 114: 917, 1976.

116. Milic-Emili J: Recent advances in clinical assessment of control of breathing. Lung 160: 1, 1982.

117. Milic-Emili J, Whitelaw W, Grassino A: Measurement and testing of respiratory drive. *In* Hornbein TF, Lenfant C (eds): Regulation of Breathing, Part II. Lung Biology in Health and Disease. New York, Marcel Dekker, 1981, p 675.

118. Ringqvist T: The ventilatory capacity in healthy subjects: An analysis of causal factors with special reference to the respiratory forces. Scand J Clin Lab Invest 18(Suppl 88): 5, 1966.

119. Lisboa C, Contreras G, Pertuze J, et al: Inspiratory muscle function in diaphragmatic hemiparalysis. Am Rev Respir Dis 131: A327, 1985.

120. Cockcroft D, Killian D, Mellon J, et al: Bronchial reactivity to inhaled histamine. A method and clinical survey. Clin Allergy 7: 235, 1977.

121. O'Byrne P, Ryan G, Morris M, et al: Asthma induced by cold air and its relation to non-specific bronchial responsiveness to methacholine. Am Rev Respir Dis 125: 281, 1982.

122. Anderson S, Schoeffel R, Finney M: Evaluation of ultrasonically nebulized solutions for provocation testing in patients with asthma. Thorax 38: 284, 1983.

4

ROENTGENOLOGIC SIGNS IN THE DIAGNOSIS OF CHEST DISEASE

The integration of information obtained from systematic interpretation of the chest roentgenogram and careful analysis of the clinical status of the patient yields a high degree of diagnostic accuracy in most chest diseases. Although the final assessment must take into account the patient's history, physical examination, laboratory tests, and pulmonary function studies, the roentgenologist should glean as much information as possible from an objective assessment of the roentgenogram *before* attempting clinical correlation. A systematic approach to roentgenologic interpretation is of cardinal importance. Appreciation of signs such as the size,

number, and density of pulmonary lesions, their homogeneity, sharpness of definition, and anatomic location and distribution, as well as the presence or absence of cavitation or calcification, is needed for an understanding of the pathogenesis of the disease and leads to a reasonable differential diagnosis.

The roentgenographic characteristics of specific disease entities are given in the relevant chapters. This chapter describes *basic roentgen signs* as they indicate the *fundamental nature* of disease. It is subdivided into three major sections: disease associated with increased roentgeno-

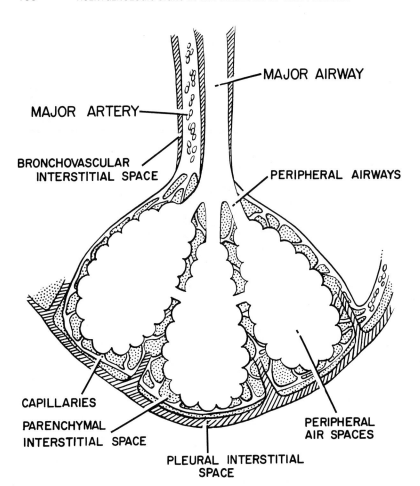

MAJOR AIRWAY

MAJOR ARTERY

BRONCHOVASCULAR
INTERSTITIAL SPACE

PERIPHERAL AIRWAYS

CAPILLARIES

PARENCHYMAL
INTERSTITIAL SPACE

PLEURAL INTERSTITIAL
SPACE

PERIPHERAL
AIR SPACES

Figure 4–1. Diagrammatic Representation of the Lung. This diagram depicts the components of the lung that are involved in the majority of pulmonary diseases—the large and small airways, the peripheral airspaces (including communicating channels), the arteries, veins, and capillaries, and the bronchovascular, pleural, and parenchymal interstitial space. Throughout the chapter this diagram of the normal lung is reproduced alongside diagrams depicting disturbances in morphology.

graphic density, disease associated with decreased roentgenographic density, and diseases of the pleura. Since a knowledge of the pathogenesis and pathology of a disease process is necessary to an understanding of the roentgenographic images it creates, wherever possible we relate the signs to their gross and microscopic morphologic characteristics and to the mechanisms of these changes (Fig. 4–1).

LUNG DISEASES THAT INCREASE ROENTGENOGRAPHIC DENSITY

The various anatomic structures of the lung can be considered to comprise two functional units: that concerned with conduction (airways, blood vessels, and lymphatics) and that concerned with gas exchange (the lung parenchyma, made up of peripheral airspaces, accompanying vessels, and extravascular interstitial tissue). Excluding the vascular system, it is obvious that any pulmonary disease that increases density in the lung periphery involves change in one or both of two components, the airspaces and extravascular interstitial tissue. Although most conditions that produce an increase in roentgenographic density involve both components, it is helpful to divide diseases into three general groups, depending on which is *predominantly* affected: (1) *airspaces,* the "air" being replaced by liquid, cells, or a combination of the two (consolidation) or absorbed and not replaced (atelectasis); (2) *interstitial tissues*; and (3) *combined airspaces and interstitial tissues.*

Predominantly Airspace Disease
Parenchymal Consolidation

In this situation, the air within the acinus is replaced, usually by a substance of unit density consisting of liquid, cells, or a combination of the two (Fig. 4–2). Typically, many contiguous acini are involved, producing an opacity of homogeneous density varying in size from a few centimeters to a whole lobe. Sometimes, however, individual shadows that measure approximately 7 mm in diameter can be identified, coinciding roughly with the size and configuration of single acini.

Roentgenologic Criteria of Airspace Disease

These criteria are closely related and depend on displacement of air from the acinus by either *intrinsic* or *extrinsic* means. Accumulation of edema fluid, blood, or tissue elements within the acinar airspaces exemplifies the intrinsic mechanism, whereas massive encroachment on the distal airspaces by certain expanding interstitial disorders explains the extrinsic pathogenesis. Both of these mechanisms can appear in an almost pure form, exemplified respectively by idiopathic pulmonary hemorrhage and lymphoma. On the other hand, there are conditions such as desquamative interstitial pneumonia, in which both the interstitium and airspaces are involved simultaneously; in such cases, either an airspace or an interstitial pattern can predominate.

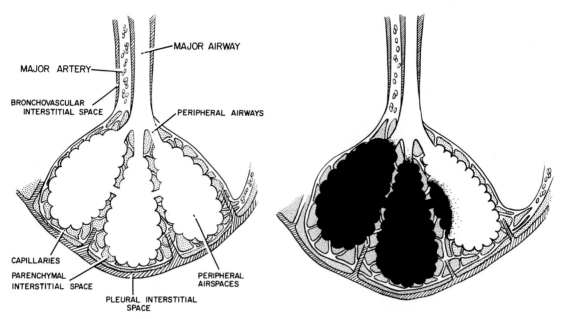

Figure 4–2. The Lung Diagram: Peripheral Airspace Consolidation. Exudate has filled two of the airspaces and is flowing into the third via communicating channels. Volume is unaffected, and the airways are patent. The parenchymal interstitial tissue is increased in amount around the consolidated airspaces.

The Acinar Shadow. On conventional roentgenograms, the classic acinar shadow has two features: a nodular shape 4 to 10 mm in diameter and poor margination (Fig. 4–3) (although the lesion remains discrete enough to permit individual identification). Although computed tomographic (CT) scans are capable of defining the characteristic signs of an airspace-filling process, they cannot reliably reveal individual acinar shadows, a deficiency related to the decreased spatial resolution of CT relative to conventional roentgenography.[1]

A second relatively discrete opacity, termed the *subacinar shadow* (*see* Fig. 4–3), possesses the same general characteristics as the acinar opacity except that multiple small radiolucencies caused by air within bronchioles can be identified within its confines. Invariably, the subacinar shadow is identified on a background of minute (smaller than 1 mm) opacities, descriptively termed "stippling," "granularity," or "ground-glass."

Although we feel that the acinus should be accepted as the basic unit of lung structure for roentgenologic description, this does not imply that *individual* acinar shadows must be identified roentgenographically for a pulmonary shadow to qualify as an airspace-filling disease; in fact, this is the exception rather than the rule. In an experimental study in which silicone rubber compound was injected into peripheral air spaces by micropuncture, Raskin and Herman[2] showed rapid dissemination of the medium throughout the secondary lobule via collateral channels, with little respect for acinar boundaries; although a few individual acini could be identified, the only border limiting dissemination of the injected material was the connective tissue of the interlobular septum. As discussed previously, however, such limitation of dispersion would apply predominantly in the lung periphery (where interlobular septa are relatively frequent) and not in central lung areas (where they are rare).

It is not entirely clear why some disease processes (e.g., endobronchial spread of tuberculosis) and not others (undoubtedly the majority) appear to respect acinar boundaries, although viscosity of the filling medium must play some role. In addition, there are two mechanisms by which, theoretically, liquid might remain localized to an acinus for some time without passing into surrounding parenchyma.[3] First, in normal lungs, resistance to flow is considerably greater in collateral channels than in peripheral airways,[4] a difference that would tend to account for retention of fluid in peripheral airways within the acinus. Second, the terminal bronchiole, being situated at the outlet of the acinus, is the narrowest portion of the entire bronchial tree and, as such, would tend to resist passage of fluid.

The causes of diffuse airspace disease include (1) alveolar edema, either cardiogenic or permeability in type; (2) the inflammatory exudate associated with an acute infection; (3) bleeding into the acini from any cause; (4) aspiration of blood or lipid; (5) neoplastic infiltration, most often by bronchioloalveolar cell carcinoma or lymphoma; and (6) idiopathic conditions such as alveolar proteinosis.

Coalescence of Acinar Shadows. Although important to identify, typical acinar and subacinar nodules are uncommonly visualized. This is because the two most frequent conditions in which they occur—pulmonary edema and infectious pneumonia—both tend to spread through bronchioles and collateral pathways into adjacent airspaces, resulting in coalescence as they proceed. Since all areas of the lung are seldom affected simultaneously and to the same degree, the result is an irregular zone of consolidation with ill-defined borders. Similar disease in nearby or remote acini can result in homogeneous nonsegmental consolidation of major areas of parenchyma.

Distribution Characteristics. A characteristic feature of diseases associated with airspace consolidation is failure to respect segmental boundaries. In widely disseminated

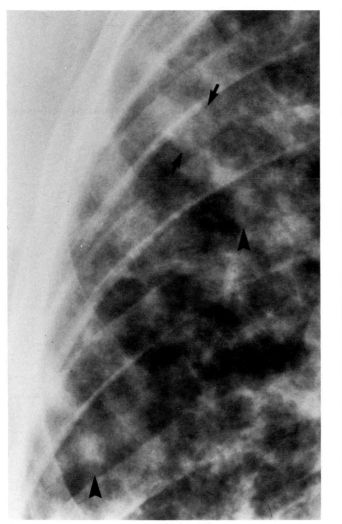

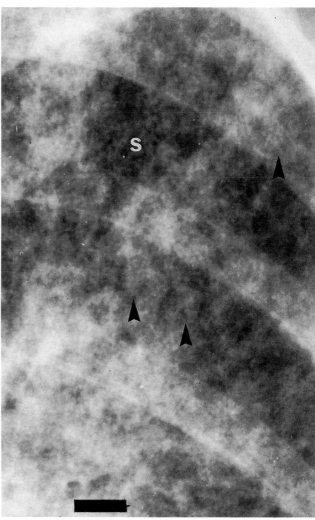

A   B

Figure 4–3. Varieties of Airspace Opacities. *A,* A detail view of the right lung from a posteroanterior chest roentgenogram of a patient with bronchioloalveolar carcinoma. The acinar opacity *(arrowheads)* is characterized by poor margination, nodular shape, and size of 4 to 8 mm. Confluence of several acinar nodules creates a larger airspace opacity *(between arrows).* (Arrowhead length = .6 cm.) *B,* A detail view of the left lung from a posteroanterior chest roentgenogram of a patient with acute airspace edema. The subacinar opacities *(arrowheads)* differ from the acinar shadows depicted in *A* by the presence within them of more radiolucencies. Concomitant background stippling (S) is a prominent feature. (Bar represents 1 cm.) (From Genereux GP: Pattern recognition in diffuse lung disease: A review of theory and practice. Med Radiogr Photogr 61:2, 1985.)

disease, such as pulmonary edema, lack of segmental distribution is not unexpected. Even in localized disease, however, intersegmental spread occurs; for example, in acute pneumococcal pneumonia, infection is propagated throughout the lung periphery via channels of collateral ventilation. Consequently, such diseases are *nonsegmental* in distribution, an observation of importance in establishing the pathogenesis of the disease process and, thereby, in suggesting an etiologic diagnosis (Fig. 4–4). By contrast, processes that are propagated via the vascular or tracheobronchial tree without such spread usually display a striking *segmental* distribution (Fig. 4–5).

Margination. The edge of an airspace-filling process is often characterized by poor margination (*see* Fig. 4–4). This feature is a consequence of the spreading and coalescing wave of consolidation that partly fills acinar components in an irregular fashion so that the x-ray beam fails to detect

a sharp border between involved and uninvolved parenchyma. The clearest example of this phenomenon is the "butterfly" or "bat's wing" appearance of acute airspace edema (Fig. 4–6).

The Air Bronchogram. Consolidation of lung parenchyma, with little or no involvement of conducting airways, creates an important roentgenographic abnormality, aptly named the *air bronchogram* sign (*see* Fig. 4–4).[5] Two situations must exist for this to be identified: the airways must contain air (the bronchus cannot be completely occluded at its origin) and the air content of surrounding lung parenchyma must be markedly reduced or nil.

The commonest process underlying the formation of an air bronchogram is parenchymal consolidation. In acute airspace pneumonia, for example, consolidation usually begins in subpleural parenchyma, the exudate rapidly spreading centrifugally to surround airways as it advances toward

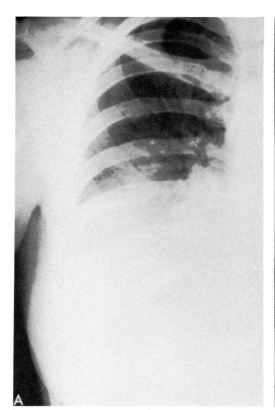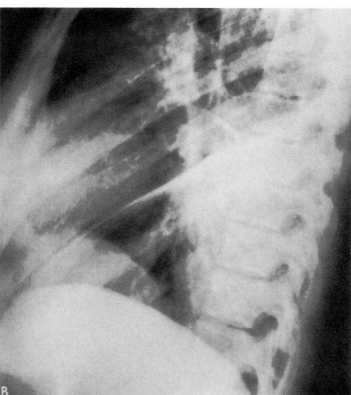

Figure 4–4. Acute Airspace Pneumonia—*Streptococcus pneumoniae.* Views of the right lung from posteroanterior *(A)* and lateral *(B)* roentgenograms reveal extensive consolidation of the lower lobe, a portion of the anterior segment being the only region of lung unaffected. An air bronchogram is visible in the lateral projection. There is little loss of volume.

the hilum. Since the consolidation is entirely parenchymal, air in the bronchi is not displaced. This produces contrast between the air within the bronchial tree and the surrounding airless parenchyma, so that normally invisible airways become roentgenographically visible. This can be identified especially well on CT (Fig. 4–7).

It is important to recognize that although an air bronchogram is an almost invariable finding in airspace consolidation from whatever cause, it can also be seen in other states, particularly atelectasis. As discussed farther on, four mechanisms can result in atelectasis, the commonest being bronchial obstruction; in such circumstances, an air bronchogram cannot exist, since the distal parenchyma no longer communicates with the mouth. However, in the other three types of atelectasis—relaxation, cicatrization, and adhesive—bronchi are not obstructed, and since the parenchyma surrounding air-containing bronchi contains little or no air, an air bronchogram is anticipated. For example, the collapsed lung behind a large pneumothorax invariably shows an air bronchogram, as does the adhesive atelectasis that occurs in acute radiation pneumonitis and hyaline membrane disease.

The Air Bronchiologram. The identification of minute radiolucencies within a focus of airspace consolidation, best exemplified by the subacinar nodule, is an important sign and relates histopathologically to incompletely filled bronchioles. Although these microscopic structures normally are not identifiable on conventional roentgenograms, when the acinus becomes partly consolidated some are rendered visible. The demonstration of such radiolucencies is analogous

to an air bronchogram and carries the same pathogenic implications.

Time Factor. The rapidity with which consolidation resolves can be of great importance in determining the etiology of airspace disease. For example, an airspace pattern that clears over a period of hours or several days is certain evidence of pulmonary edema or hemorrhage. By contrast, airspace disease that persists over time, sometimes for weeks or months, is usually caused by conditions such as bronchioloalveolar carcinoma, lymphoma, or alveolar proteinosis.

Absence of Atelectasis. In airspace consolidation, maintenance of lung volume is understandable when one considers its pathogenesis. In the first place, air in the acini is replaced by an equal or almost equal quantity of liquid or tissue. Second, since the process is predominantly parenchymal, airways leading to affected portions of lung remain patent; thus, there is no reason for collapse to occur before exudate fills the air spaces. Again, there are occasional exceptions to this rule; for example, in pulmonary infarction, volume is often diminished by causes other than airway obstruction, such as surfactant deficit.

Parenchymal Atelectasis

In its pure form, atelectasis may be regarded conceptually as the antithesis of consolidation: in the former, air is absorbed and not replaced, and in the latter, air is replaced by liquid or cells of approximately equal volume. Thus, from a roentgenologic point of view, the major difference

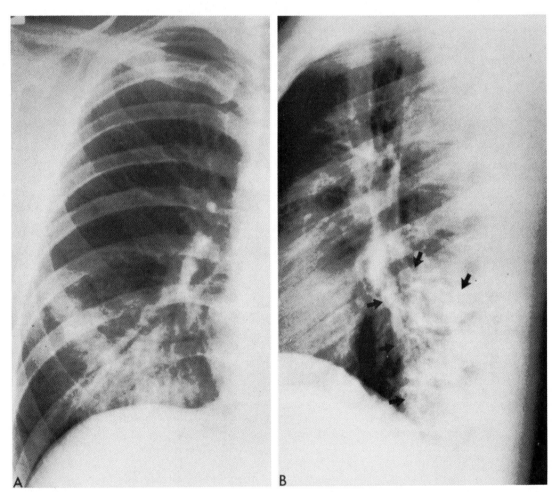

Figure 4–5. Acute Bronchopneumonia—*Streptococcus pyogenes.* Views of the right lung from posteroanterior *(A)* and lateral *(B)* roentgenograms show patchy consolidation of the posterior basal segment of the right lower lobe. The consolidation is inhomogeneous and possesses a roughly triangular configuration in lateral projection *(arrows in B)*, indicating a true segmental distribution.

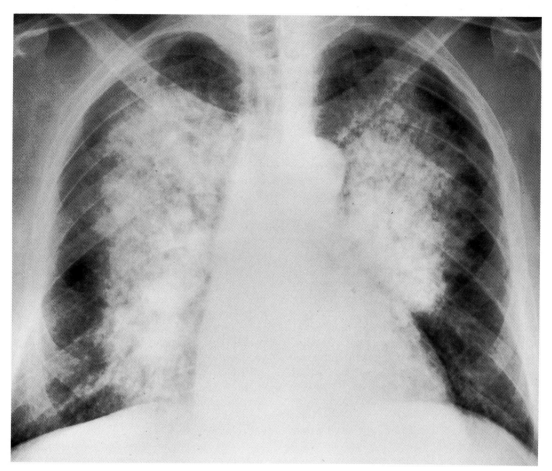

Figure 4–6. The "Bat's Wing" Pattern of Pulmonary Edema. A posteroanterior roentgenogram demonstrates consolidation of the parahilar and "medullary" portions of both lungs, creating a bat's wing or "butterfly" appearance; the "cortex" of both lungs is relatively unaffected. The margins of the edematous lung are rather sharply defined. The consolidation is fairly homogeneous and is associated with a well-defined air bronchogram on both sides. This 59-year-old man had suffered a massive myocardial infarct 48 hours previously.

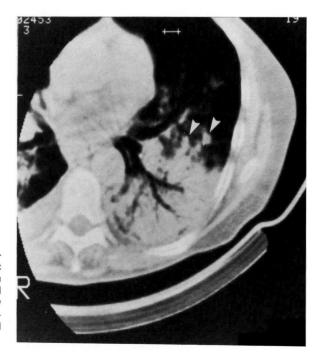

Figure 4–7. An Air Bronchogram Associated with Parenchymal Consolidation. A CT scan through the left lower zone from a woman with idiopathic pulmonary hemorrhage reveals confluent, poorly defined consolidation in the lower lobe and lingula. A prominent air bronchogram is present. Several opacities *(arrowheads)* conform in size to acinar opacities but do not show the typical intra-acinar features of air-containing bronchioles. (From Genereux GP: Pattern recognition in diffuse lung disease: A review of theory and practice. Med Radiogr Photogr *61:* 2, 1985.)

is one of volume: in consolidation, volume is normal; in atelectasis, it is reduced.

The terminology of pulmonary atelectasis is controversial. Etymologically, the word is derived from the Greek words *ateles* (incomplete) and *ektasis* (stretching). The interpretation placed on this by the semantic purist is that "incomplete stretching" is necessarily a neonatal phenomenon and cannot be applied to a state that develops after full inflation has occurred. We prefer to use the word in its broad sense, to denote *diminished air within the lung associated with reduced lung volume*. It is important to note that this definition simply implies loss of volume, not increase in roentgenographic density. Since this concept considers atelectasis essentially in terms of lung volume, it is necessary for an understanding of the pathogenesis of atelectasis and of its classification to consider the mechanisms that keep the lung expanded.

As described in Chapter 1, the lungs have a natural tendency to collapse and do so when removed from the chest. While the lungs are in the thoracic cavity, however, this tendency is opposed by the chest wall; at functional residual capacity (FRC), the tendency for the lung to collapse and for the chest wall to expand are equal and opposite. In the presence of pneumothorax or pleural effusion, the outward retraction force of the chest wall is removed, the lung retracts, and its volume decreases; this is *passive or relaxation atelectasis*. A similar mechanism occurs at the edge of a local space-occupying lesion within the lung: because of its inherent elastic recoil properties, the parenchyma for some distance contiguous with a mass or cyst is reduced in volume. Although this mechanism of volume loss has been termed "compression atelectasis," from a conceptual point of view we consider it preferable to regard it as a variant of passive atelectasis.

In a static system, the volume attained by the lung depends upon the balance between an applied force and the opposing elastic forces. It follows that when the lung is stiffer than normal, that is, when compliance is decreased, lung volume is decreased. This classically occurs with pulmonary fibrosis and is called *cicatrization atelectasis*.

The pressure-volume behavior of the lung also depends upon the forces acting at the air-tissue interface of the alveolar wall; as alveoli diminish in volume, the surface tension of the interface is diminished by surfactant. When the action of surfactant is deficient or absent, as occurs in hyaline membrane disease of the newborn, there is widespread collapse of alveoli. This type of atelectasis has been referred to as microatelectasis or nonobstructive atelectasis, but we shall refer to it as *adhesive atelectasis*.

The commonest form of atelectasis, and the most complex, is caused by the resorption of gas from the alveoli, as occurs in acute bronchial obstruction; this type of atelectasis is best termed *resorption atelectasis*.

Resorption Atelectasis. This form of atelectasis occurs when communication between alveoli and trachea is obstructed (Fig. 4–8). The mechanism of resorption is fairly straightforward. Since the partial pressure of gases is lower in mixed venous blood than in alveolar air, the partial pressures of alveolar gases equilibrate with alveolar pressure as blood passes through the capillaries. The alveoli diminish in volume according to the quantity of oxygen absorbed, their pressure remaining atmospheric; consequently, the partial pressures of carbon dioxide and nitrogen in the alveoli rise relative to those of capillary blood, and both gases diffuse into blood to maintain equilibrium. Thus, alveolar volume is further reduced, with a consequent rise in the alveolar-capillary blood Po_2 gradient; oxygen diffuses into capillary blood, and this cycle is repeated until all alveolar gas is absorbed.

In a previously healthy lobe whose bronchus is acutely obstructed, all air disappears within 18 to 24 hours.[6] Since oxygen is absorbed selectively much more rapidly than nitrogen, when a lobe is filled with oxygen at the moment of occlusion (a situation that might obtain during anesthesia), collapse occurs much more rapidly and should be roentgenographically apparent within an hour. In fact, it has been shown that the rate at which a lung collapses after an airway is blocked is 60 times faster when oxygen rather than air is breathed.[7]

It is important to realize that resorption atelectasis is not

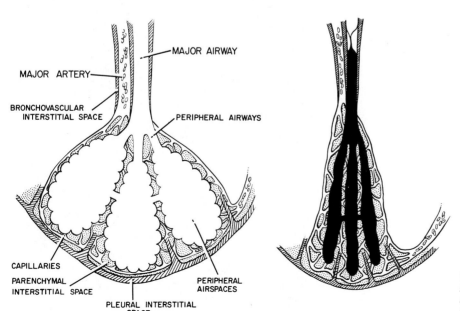

Figure 4–8. The Lung Diagram: Resorption Atelectasis. The major airway is obstructed, and the peripheral airways and airspaces are airless and collapsed.

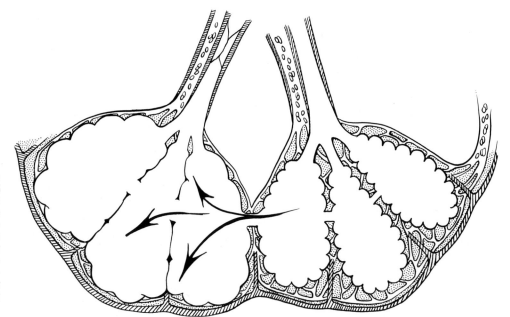

Figure 4–9. The Lung Diagram: Collateral Ventilation Associated with Air Trapping. The airway on the left is obstructed, that on the right patent; the parenchyma distal to the obstructed airway is being ventilated by collateral air drift. The diagram depicts a situation in which air enters the obstructed segment more easily than it leaves, thus resulting in air trapping.

the inevitable or only accompaniment of bronchial obstruction, nor is obstruction of a major bronchus the only cause of resorption atelectasis. The effect of obstruction of the airways depends on the site and extent of bronchial or bronchiolar obstruction, the rapidity of the obstructing process, the pre-existing condition of the lung tissue, and the extent of collateral ventilation. The last-named is particularly important in influencing the development and ultimate degree of atelectasis. There is both anatomic and physiologic evidence to support the presence of collateral ventilation between acini, lobar segments, and (because of the frequency of incomplete fissures) even entire lobes (see pages 14 and 27). Such ventilation is often sufficient to prevent or limit the degree of atelectasis. If collateral ventilation is such a potent force in preventing parenchymal collapse, however, one might ask, under what circum-

stances does collapse occur? This depends chiefly on the site of airway obstruction. If it is in a lobar bronchus, the development of atelectasis is readily explained by the absence of a parenchymal bridge from the involved lobe to a contiguous lobe; if the obstruction is in a segmental or subsegmental bronchus, collapse must be caused by something that *prevents* collateral ventilation, such as inflammatory exudate (Fig. 4–9).[8]

Even excluding the effect of collateral ventilation, the end result of chronic bronchial obstruction (e.g., that associated with carcinoma) is not necessarily a collapsed lobe; in fact, most often it leads to consolidation (obstructive pneumonitis) severe enough to limit loss of volume (Figs. 4–10 and 4–11). It should be emphasized that the pathologic features of obstructive pneumonitis consist of a combination of bronchiectasis with mucous plugging and par-

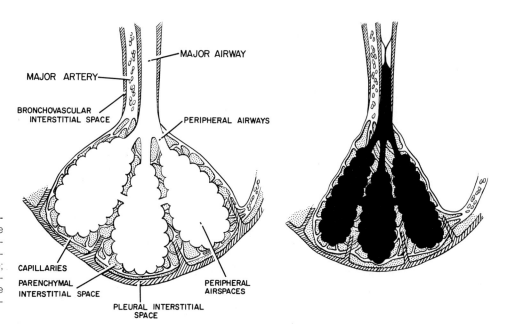

Figure 4–10. The Lung Diagram: Obstructive Pneumonitis. Although the major airway is completely obstructed, loss of volume of the peripheral airspaces is only moderate; accumulated fluid and alveolar macrophages within the airspace have prevented the complete collapse depicted in Figure 4–8.

MAJOR AIRWAY

MAJOR ARTERY

BRONCHOVASCULAR INTERSTITIAL SPACE

PERIPHERAL AIRWAYS

CAPILLARIES

PARENCHYMAL INTERSTITIAL SPACE

PERIPHERAL AIRSPACES

PLEURAL INTERSTITIAL SPACE

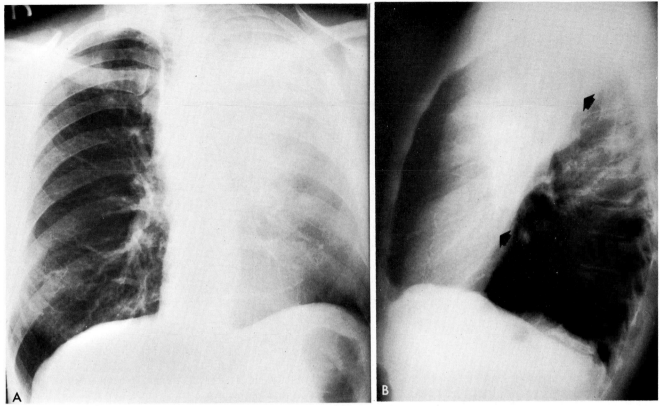

Figure 4–11. **Obstructive Pneumonitis.** Posteroanterior *(A)* and lateral *(B)* roentgenograms reveal homogeneous opacification of the left upper lobe; there is no air bronchogram. The chief fissure *(arrows)* is not displaced forward, and the only signs indicating loss of volume are slight mediastinal shift and hemidiaphragmatic elevation. Collapse was prevented by the accumulation of fluid and alveolar macrophages within distal airspaces and chronic inflammatory cells and fibrous tissue within the interstitium—obstructive pneumonitis. Squamous cell carcinoma.

enchymal inflammation and fibrosis; in the majority of cases, the inflammation is caused not by bacterial infection but by retention of normal epithelial secretions distal to the point of obstruction.[9] When infection does occur, it is almost always superimposed on underlying noninfectious parenchymal changes, and usually it is not possible to determine whether or not infection is present from the roentgenologic findings alone.

Although assessment of volumetric reduction necessarily is rough, it might reasonably be stated that 24 to 48 hours after complete bronchial occlusion in a patient breathing room air, the volume of a pulmonary lobe seldom is reduced more than 50 per cent. Since a completely collapsed lung (as in total pneumothorax) occupies a space no larger than a man's fist, obviously a large amount of fluid must be exuded into the substance of a lobe for its volume to be reduced by only 50 per cent. If obstruction persists and the obstructed lobe remains sterile, volumetric readjustment occurs within the hemithorax; excess edema fluid and blood within the affected lobe gradually are reabsorbed and fibrous tissue increases in amount. The collapsed lobe eventually comes to occupy the smallest possible volume; in fact, it may be so small that it is almost invisible roentgenographically, and then the diagnostician must rely heavily on evidence provided by compensatory phenomena *(see* later).

Passive Atelectasis. This term denotes pulmonary collapse in the presence of a space-occupying intrathoracic

process such as pneumothorax or hydrothorax (Fig. 4–12). Provided the pleural space is without adhesions, collapse of any portion of lung is proportional to the amount of air or fluid in the adjacent pleural space. In upright human beings, the tendency for air to pass to the upper portion of the pleural space results in a relatively greater degree of collapse of upper lobe tissue than of lower. This fact can be employed to advantage in the identification of a small pneumothorax, which is more easily demonstrated with the patient in the lateral decubitus position, using a horizontal roentgen beam.

It might be thought logical that shrinkage of a lung to half its normal projected area would double its roentgenologic density. That this is not so is illustrated by the difficulty commonly experienced in identifying the lung edge in any case of spontaneous pneumothorax, even of moderate degree *(see* Fig. 4–12). In fact, as a lung shrinks in a pneumothorax, its density does not increase notably until its projected area is reduced to about one tenth its normal area at total lung capacity.[10] The probable explanation for this anomalous situation is twofold: first, the reduction in lung volume is approximately balanced by reduction in blood content, net roentgenographic density being altered only slightly; and second, air in the pleural space both anteriorly and posteriorly serves as a nonabsorbing medium, contributing to the overall radiolucency of the roentgenographic image.

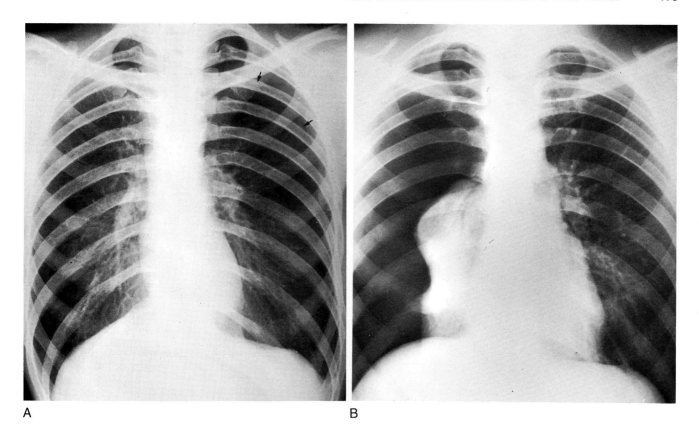

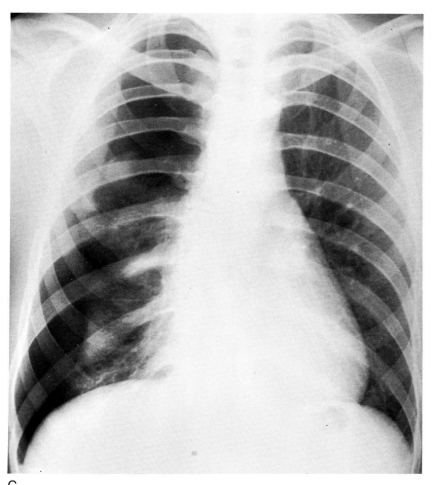

Figure 4–12. Three Cases of Spontaneous Pneumothorax Revealing Different Manifestations. *A,* A posteroanterior roentgenogram reveals a small left pneumothorax (*arrows* point to the visceral pleural line). Note increased size of left hemithorax as a result of the removal of the influence of the lung's elastic recoil on the chest wall. In *B,* note the small volume occupied by a whole lung when totally collapsed. The well-defined air bronchogram indicates airway patency. *C* reveals a moderate right pneumothorax; despite the fact that the right lung has been reduced in volume by approximately 50 per cent, its density differs little from that of the left lung. *See* text.

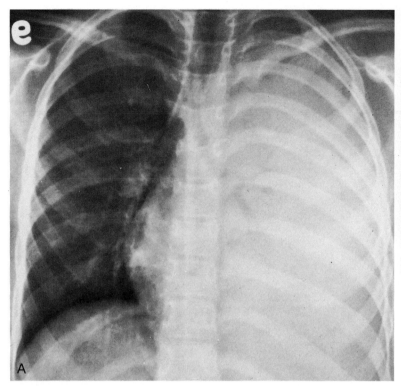

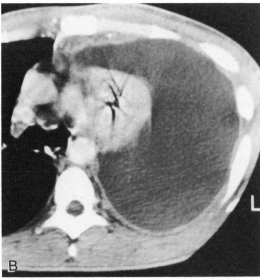

Figure 4–13. Relaxation Atelectasis in the Presence of a Massive Pleural Effusion. *A,* An air bronchogram is clearly visible within the opacity caused by a massive left pleural effusion, analogous to the atelectasis that accompanies a large pneumothorax. *B,* A CT scan reveals the small size of the collapsed lung; note the air bronchogram.

Even when pneumothorax-induced collapse is total, the lung mass is not completely airless: the lobar and larger segmental bronchi are sufficiently stable structurally to resist collapse. Therefore, they remain air-filled and, although reduced in caliber, should be apparent as an air bronchogram. For obvious reasons, it is essential that this sign be sought carefully in any case of total or almost total pneumothorax; absence of an air bronchogram should immediately arouse suspicion of endobronchial obstruction. The response of the lung to a massive pleural effusion is similar to that of a pneumothorax of the same volume: the lung

undergoes passive atelectasis, which, if complete, should be associated with an identifiable air bronchogram (Fig. 4–13).

A thin zone of passive atelectasis is also common adjacent to a pulmonary mass; in most cases, however, the airless lung is contiguous with tissue of identical density, and roentgenographic differentiation of the basic lesion from adjacent collapsed tissue is impossible. Only when the loss of volume is contiguous with a zone of relative radiolucency, such as a bulla, is the atelectatic lung recognizable as a distinct shadow of increased density (Fig. 4–14). Even then, the wall of a bulla may be no more than a hairline

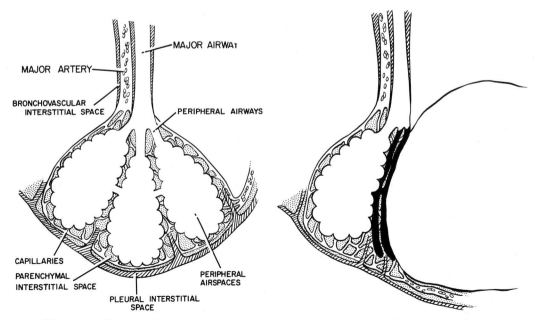

Figure 4–14. The Lung Diagram: Compression Atelectasis. A large "bulla" situated on the right has permitted relaxation of contiguous parenchyma, resulting in focal atelectasis.

shadow, indicating the extremely small volume of completely collapsed lung parenchyma. Generally speaking, therefore, atelectasis of this type is seldom of roentgenologic significance as a cause of increased density.

An unusual form of passive atelectasis has been described under the name *round or helical atelectasis*.[11, 12] On conventional roentgenograms, the lesion presents as a fairly homogeneous, ill-defined, pleural-based opacity that measures up to 7 cm in diameter, most commonly situated in the posterior portion of a lower lobe (Fig. 4–15). The bronchovascular bundles in the vicinity of the opacity are gathered together and appear curvilinear as they pass toward it (the comet tail sign). Lung parenchyma below or lateral to the opacity may be strikingly oligemic. The typical CT appearance consists of a rounded subpleural opacity that is densest at its periphery, the more central (hilar) aspect showing an air bronchogram.[13] Contiguous pleural thickening due to fibrosis is invariably present. As in standard roentgenograms, vessels and bronchi curve into the lesion, resulting in a blurred central margin. Although the lesion has been considered to be caused by folding of the lung secondary to pleural effusion,[12] we consider it likely that the majority of cases are caused by pleural fibrosis, which contracts as it develops, resulting in compression of contiguous lung parenchyma (Fig. 4–16).[14]

Adhesive Atelectasis. Adhesive atelectasis is a controversial and poorly understood process in which there is alveolar collapse in the presence of patent airways ("nonobstructive" atelectasis). The best examples are the respiratory distress syndrome of the newborn, acute radiation pneumonitis, and viral pneumonia (Fig. 4–17). In each of these conditions, atelectasis may be a prominent feature and may be related, at least in part, to inactivation or absence of surfactant.[15] It is likely that adhesive atelectasis also plays a part in loss of volume postoperatively and accounts for the marked venoarterial shunting that may occur even when the chest roentgenogram is relatively normal.

The frequency with which patients who have undergone cardiac bypass surgery develop a left lower lobe opacity in the postoperative period is truly astounding, and, to the best of our knowledge, it has never been adequately explained. The opacity is characteristically homogeneous except for the air bronchogram that is almost always observed. Although signs of atelectasis are seldom convincing, partly as a result of the technical quality of the examination (anteroposterior [AP] projection, supine position at the patient's bedside), we have assumed that the combination of airlessness of the lower lobe and an air bronchogram indicates that the probable mechanism is adhesive atelectasis due to surfactant deficit. Characteristically, patients do not manifest signs or symptoms of acute pneumonia, so that diagnosis is more or less excluded.

Cicatrization Atelectasis. As the term implies, the pathologic process in cicatrization atelectasis is fibrosis. The increase in collagen leads to a decrease in air per unit lung volume (and a corresponding increase in roentgenographic density) as a result of both decreased lung compliance and increased tissue. The roentgenologic signs depend upon whether the process is local or general.

Localized disease is best exemplified by chronic infection, often granulomatous in nature, and epitomized by long-standing fibrocaseous tuberculosis. In this condition, parenchymal fibrosis results not only in atelectasis but also, by traction on airway walls, in bronchiectasis (Figs. 4–18 and 4–19). The roentgenologic signs are as might be expected (Fig. 4–20): a segment or lobe occupying a volume smaller than normal, with a density rendered inhomogeneous by dilated, air-containing bronchi and irregular strands of fibrous tissue extending from the collapsed lung to the hilum. The compensatory signs of chronic loss of volume are usually evident: local mediastinal shift (frequently manifested by a sharp deviation of the trachea when segments of the upper lobe are involved), displacement of the hilum (which may be severe in upper lobe disease), and compensatory overinflation of the remainder of the affected lung.

Generalized fibrotic disease of the lungs also may be associated with loss of volume (Fig. 4–21). In chronic interstitial pulmonary fibrosis, for example, involvement of the interstitial space results in widespread reduction in the volume of air-containing parenchyma; this may be evidenced roentgenologically by elevation of the diaphragm and overall reduction in lung size. In our experience, this gradual reduction in thoracic volume in cases of diffuse interstitial disease is a useful indicator of the fibrotic nature of the pathologic process (Fig. 4–22).

Roentgenologic Signs of Atelectasis

The roentgenologic signs of atelectasis may be both *direct* and *indirect,* the latter consisting chiefly of compensatory phenomena.

Direct Signs. Since we define atelectasis simply as loss of lung volume, the only direct sign is *displacement of interlobar fissures.* Such displacement is one of the most dependable and easily recognized signs of atelectasis (*see* Figs. 4–17 and 4–19); for each lobe, the position and configuration of the displaced fissures are predictable for a given loss of volume. These features are considered further in relation to patterns of lobar and segmental collapse.

Indirect Signs. Although local increase in density is a common manifestation of pulmonary atelectasis, it is not essential to the definition and therefore cannot be construed as a direct sign; nevertheless, it is undoubtedly the most important indirect sign of atelectasis. Other indirect signs are caused primarily by processes that compensate for the reduction in intrapleural pressure—diaphragmatic elevation, mediastinal shift, approximation of ribs, and overinflation of the remainder of the lung (Fig. 4–23). The part played by each compensatory mechanism in any given situation is somewhat unpredictable; all four may operate fairly equally, or one or two may predominate to the exclusion of others. Which mechanism predominates is dictated largely by the anatomic position of the collapsed lobe; however, one general rule deserves emphasis: the more acute the atelectasis, the greater the predominance of diaphragmatic and mediastinal displacement (*see* Fig. 4–23); the more chronic the collapse, the more compensatory overinflation predominates (*see* Fig. 4–19).

Elevation of the Hemidiaphragm. Hemidiaphragmatic elevation is always a more prominent feature of lower than of upper lobe collapse (compare Figs. 4–23A and B). Elevation tends to occur in the area contiguous with the lobe involved—posterior elevation in lower lobe collapse and anterior elevation in middle lobe or lingular collapse (al-

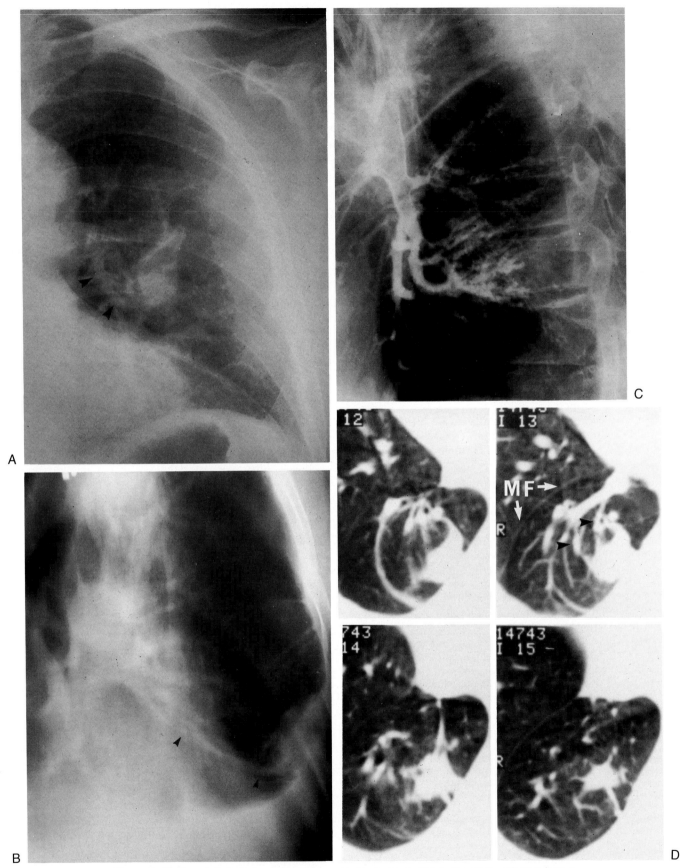

Figure 4–15. Round Atelectasis—Roentgenographic Features. *A,* Detail view of the left lung from a conventional posteroanterior roentgenogram reveals a triangular opacity in the left upper lobe. Note the curvilinear course of pulmonary vessels *(arrowheads)* as they relate to the inferior aspect of the lesion. A conventional oblique tomogram *(B)* and bronchogram *(C)* again show typical curvilinear displacement of the bronchovascular bundles *(arrowheads)* as they converge on the inferior margin of the subpleural mass ("comet-tail" sign). CT scans with lung window technique *(D)* through the mass demonstrate once more displacement of the nearby bronchovascular bundles *(arrowheads)*. The major fissure (MF) is displaced posteromedially, indicating loss of volume of the right lower lobe.

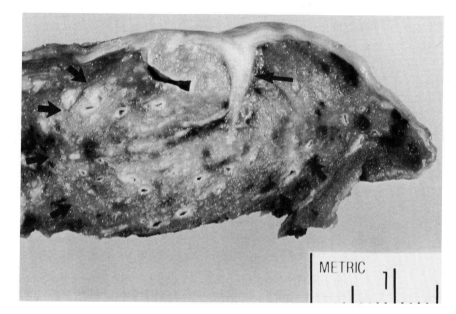

Figure 4–16. Round Atelectasis: Gross Appearance. A slice of an uninflated lower lobe from a patient with roentgenographic evidence of typical round atelectasis shows a poorly defined, vaguely elliptical focus of atelectasis *(short arrows)* that blends imperceptibly with normal lung. The overlying visceral pleura is fibrotic and focally invaginates into the underlying parenchyma *(long arrow).* (From Menzies R, Fraser R: Round atelectasis: Pathologic and pathogenetic features. Am J Surg Pathol *11*: 674, 1987.)

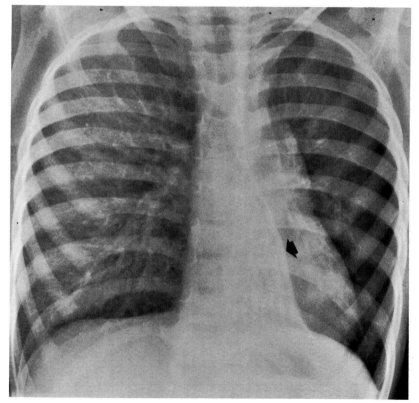

Figure 4–17. Adhesive Atelectasis. The left lower lobe is completely collapsed (*arrow* points to the interface between the displaced major fissure and the overinflated upper lobe). Despite the severe atelectasis, a well-defined air bronchogram can be clearly identified out to the periphery. Bronchoscopy showed no evidence of bronchial obstruction. Patient is a 3½-year-old girl approximately 2 years following acute adenoviral pneumonia of the left lung; the lobe eventually re-expanded spontaneously. (Courtesy of the Winnipeg Children's Hospital.)

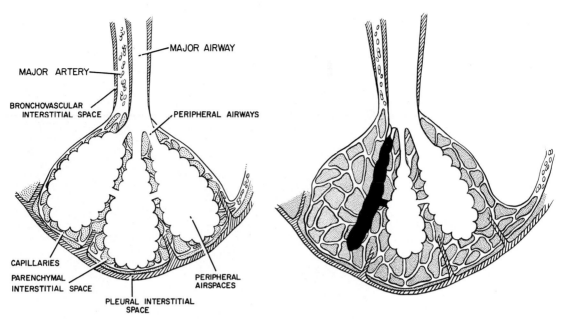

Figure 4–18. The Lung Diagram: Local Cicatrization Atelectasis. The interstitial space is increased in amount and density (fibrosis). The left airspace is totally obliterated, whereas those to the right show different degrees of loss of volume. The major airway is dilated (bronchiectasis), as is the peripheral airway on the right (bronchiolectasis).

though, in the latter two situations, diaphragmatic displacement is seldom severe).

Mediastinal Displacement. The normal mediastinum is a surprisingly mobile structure and reacts promptly to a difference in pressure between the two halves of the thorax (see Fig. 4–23). The anterior and middle mediastinal compartments are less stable than the posterior one and, therefore, shift to a greater extent. The degree of shift is usually greatest in the region of major pulmonary collapse; thus tracheal and upper mediastinal displacement is a feature of upper lobe atelectasis and may be negligible when the lower lobes are involved; in the latter instance, the inferior mediastinum exhibits the greatest displacement.

Local displacement occurs in the three weakest areas of the mediastinum, where the two lungs are separated only by loose connective tissue: (1) *the anterior mediastinal compartment,* at the level of the first three or four costal cartilages, limited anteriorly by the sternum and posteriorly by the great vessels; (2) *the posterosuperior mediastinum,* at the level of the third to fifth thoracic vertebrae, limited anteriorly by the esophagus and trachea and posteriorly by the vertebral column (the supra-aortic triangle); and (3) *the posteroinferior mediastinum,* limited anteriorly by the heart and posteriorly by the vertebral column and aorta (the retrocardiac space). Roentgenologic appreciation of anterior mediastinal displacement is usually easy, through identification of the displaced anterior junction line. The curvilinear opacity of the apposed pleural surfaces is usually visible on a posteroanterior roentgenogram, protruding into the involved hemithorax. In lateral projection, the anterior mediastinum appears exceptionally radiolucent and increased in depth. Appreciation of displacement of the posterior mediastinal weak areas may be more difficult; these portions of the mediastinal septum normally form the posterior junction line and azygoesophageal recess interface, respectively.

Compensatory Overinflation. Overinflation of the remainder of the ipsilateral lung is one of the most important and reliable indirect signs of atelectasis (see Fig. 4–19). It seldom occurs rapidly and, in the early stages of lobar collapse, usually is diagnostically less helpful than the other compensatory phenomena, such as diaphragmatic elevation and mediastinal displacement. As the period of collapse lengthens, however, overinflation becomes more prominent and the diaphragmatic and mediastinal changes regress.

Roentgenologic evidence of compensatory overinflation may be extremely subtle. Although it is often possible to appreciate the increase in lung translucency resulting from the greater air-blood ratio, this may be difficult; recognition may be enhanced by viewing the roentgenogram from a distance of several feet or through minification lenses. Clearly, more reliable evidence of overinflation is supplied by the *alteration in vascular markings* resultant upon the increased lung volume (see Fig. 4–19); the vessels are more widely spaced and sparser than in the normal contralateral lung.

When only a relatively small volume of one lung is collapsed, compensatory overinflation is usually restricted to the remainder of that lung, at least insofar as it is apparent roentgenographically. When larger amounts of one lung become atelectatic, the tendency is greater for the contralateral lung to overinflate; this may progress so far that the opposite lung displaces the mediastinum, either generally or locally.

When an entire lung becomes atelectatic consequent upon obstruction of a main bronchus, the resultant loss of volume of the hemithorax must be compensated for largely by overinflation of the contralateral lung (similar to the situation after pneumonectomy; Fig. 4–24). The resulting mediastinal shift may be large; since the mediastinum is less stable anteriorly than elsewhere, the anterior septum is rotated laterally and posteriorly and the normal lung over-

Text continued on page 187

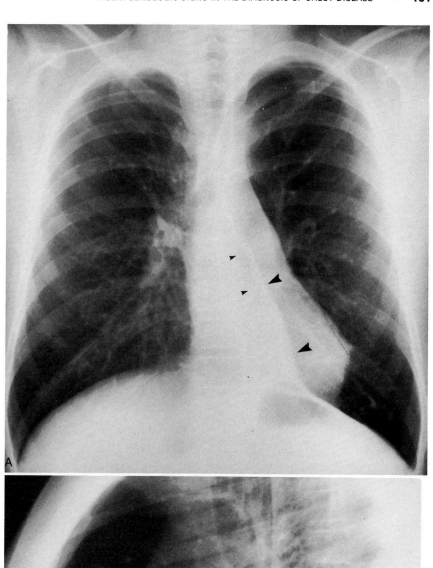

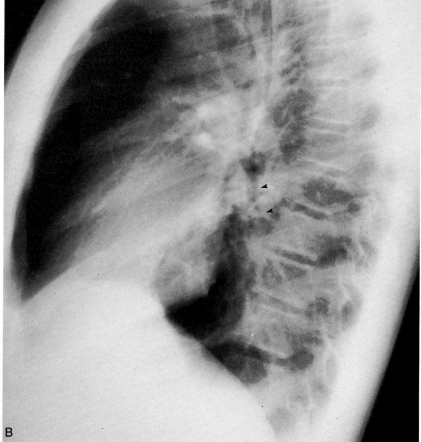

Figure 4–19. Cicatrization Atelectasis Associated with Bronchiectasis. Conventional posteroanterior *(A)* and lateral *(B)* chest roentgenograms disclose total atelectasis of the left lower lobe *(large arrowheads* point to the interface between the collapsed lobe and the overinflated upper lobe). A faint air bronchogram is present *(small arrowheads)*. Note absence of visibility of the left interlobar artery.

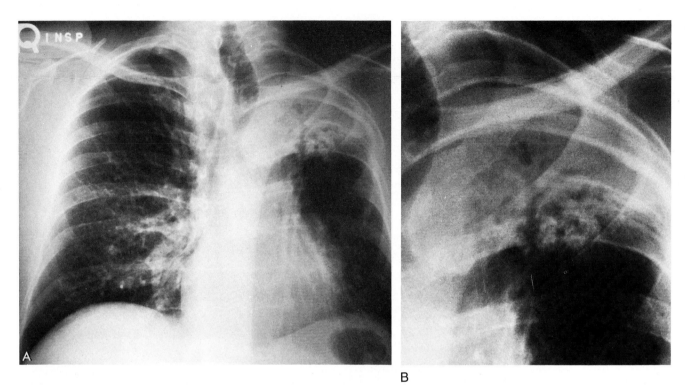

Figure 4–20. Local Cicatrization Atelectasis: Postirradiation Fibrosis. *A,* A posteroanterior roentgenogram reveals considerable loss of volume on the left upper lung, with displacement of the trachea to the left, approximation of the left upper ribs, and elevation of the left hilum. *B,* A magnified view shows a prominent air bronchogram in an otherwise homogeneous opacity.

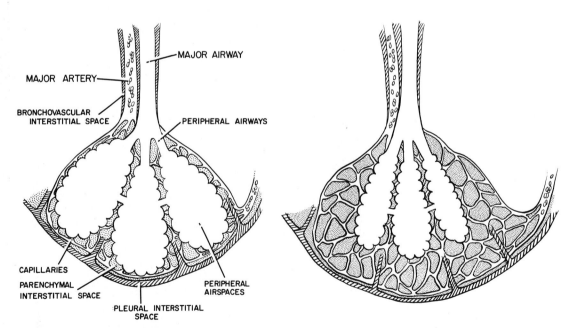

Figure 4–21. The Lung Diagram: General Cicatrization Atelectasis. There is a marked increase in interstitial tissue with uniform reduction in the volume of all airspaces as a result of cicatrization. The dilatation of the major airway seen in local cicatrization atelectasis is not a prominent part of the picture, although peripheral airway dilatation may occur.

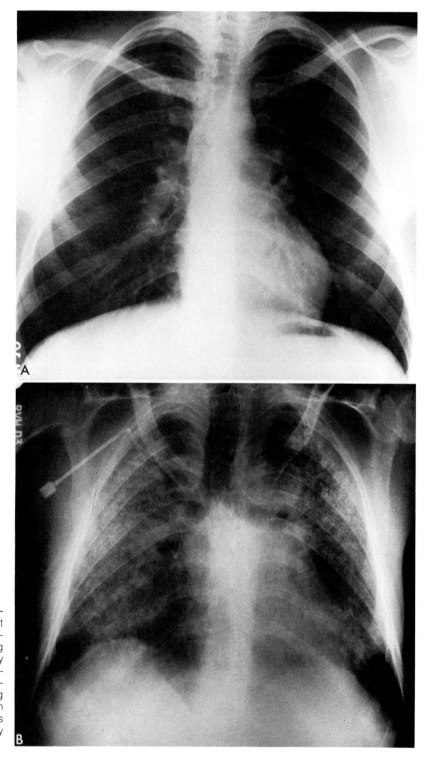

Figure 4–22. General Cicatrization Atelectasis Secondary to Intravenous Talcosis of Drug Abuse. At the time of the normal chest roentgenogram illustrated in *A,* this 19-year-old man had been taking large doses of dissolved methadone intravenously for more than 2 years. Six years later, a roentgenogram *(B)* reveals diffuse interstitial disease throughout both lungs associated with severe loss of lung volume as evidenced by elevation of the diaphragm and smallness of the thoracic cage. This represents diffuse interstitial fibrosis caused by intravenously injected talc.

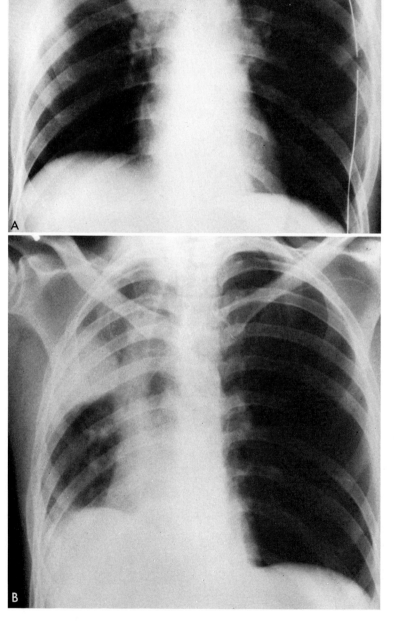

Figure 4–23. Roentgenologic Signs of Atelectasis. *A,* A roentgenogram of the chest in anteroposterior projection, supine position, reveals partial atelectasis of the right upper lobe; the concave lower margin is formed by the upward displaced horizontal fissure; the right hemidiaphragm is slightly elevated. *B,* Twenty-four hours later, the right upper lobe collapse is clearing, but the diaphragmatic elevation has increased, and the mediastinum has shifted markedly to the right; note the approximation of ribs. These signs indicate acute obstruction of the right intermediate bronchus with progressing collapse of the middle and lower lobes. Twenty-four hours later, posteroanterior *(C)* and lateral *(D)* views reveal the right middle and lower lobes to be virtually airless; the right upper lobe has completely re-expanded. The roughly horizontal interface in *C* is the major fissure, not the minor, as might intuitively be thought: in the lateral projection, note that the upper portion of the major fissure has swung downward to a roughly horizontal position *(arrows),* thus making it tangential to the x-ray beam and creating the sharp interface in posteroanterior projection. Following this examination, a mucous plug was removed from the intermediate bronchus bronchoscopically.

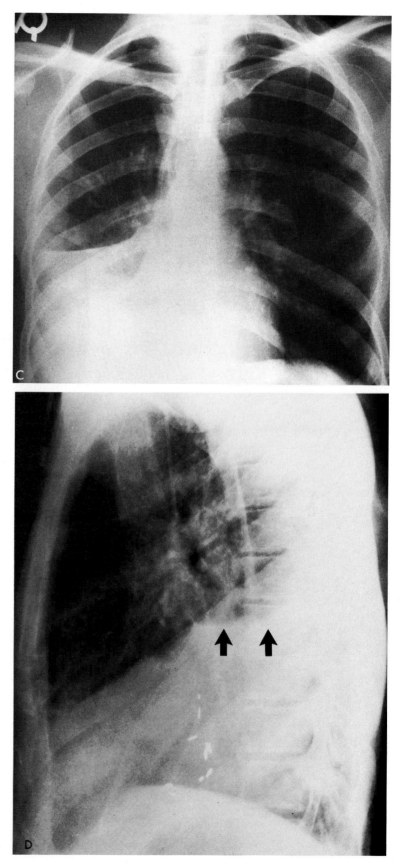

Figure 4–23 *Continued*

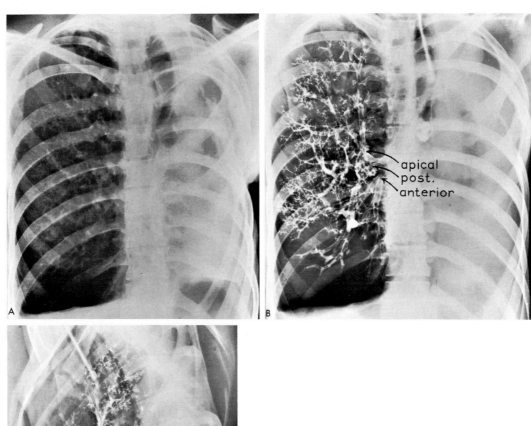

Figure 4–24. Compensatory Overinflation: The One-Lobe Thorax. Over a span of several years, thoracotomy was performed on this 28-year-old woman on three different occasions for advanced incapacitating bronchiectasis: on the first, the left lower lobe and lingula were removed; on the second, the left upper lobe; and on the third, the right middle and lower lobes. At the time of each thoracotomy, the bronchial tree was found to be normal bronchographically in those areas subsequently affected. A right bronchogram (B and C) reveals only three segmental bronchi of the right upper lobe, at least one of which shows moderately advanced bronchiectasis.

inflates to such an extent that it occupies the whole anterior portion of the thorax. Thus, the heart and the collapsed lung are displaced into the posterior portion of the ipsilateral hemithorax. In such circumstances the roentgenologic appearance in lateral projection is distinctive (*see* Fig. 4–24).[16] The margin of the collapsed lung may be sharply delineated where it comes in contact with the opposite overinflated lung; such an appearance makes it easier to distinguish massive collapse from massive unilateral pneumonic consolidation or pleural effusion (Fig. 4–25).

Displacement of the Hila. The hila are often displaced in the presence of atelectasis, more predictably in collapse of the upper than of the lower lobes and usually more markedly the more chronic the atelectasis (*see* Fig. 4–20). It is important to assess the position of the air columns of the trachea and major bronchi in lateral projection as an indication of collapse[17]; on a well-aligned lateral roentgenogram of the chest, the trachea, both main bronchi, and both upper lobe bronchi are in vertical alignment, and any alteration in this relationship should be considered abnor-

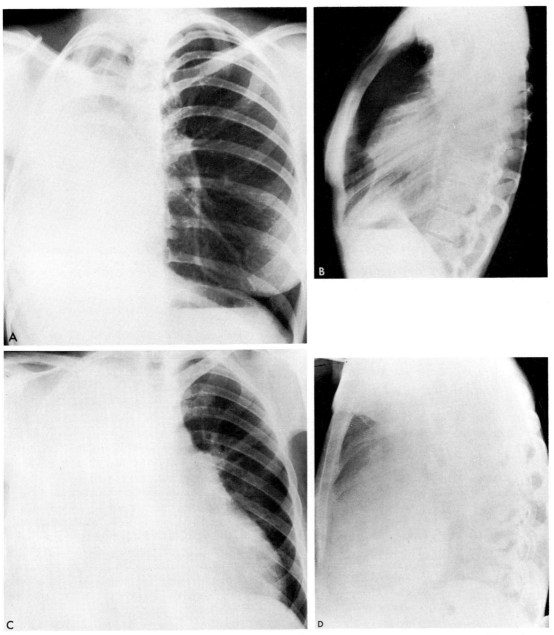

Figure 4–25. Comparison of Massive Collapse and Massive Pleural Effusion. Roentgenograms of the chest in posteroanterior and lateral projections (*A* and *B*) of a patient whose right lung has been removed (analogous to total right pulmonary collapse) reveals marked shift of the mediastinum into the posterior portion of the right hemithorax, with herniation of the overinflated left lung across the midline into the anterior right chest (note the clear retrosternal space). In *C* and *D* (roentgenograms of another patient), a massive right pleural effusion has resulted in a shift of the mediastinum to the left; in lateral projection the opacity is more or less homogeneous (the uniform filter effect). Compare the appearance of the retrosternal space in the two patients.

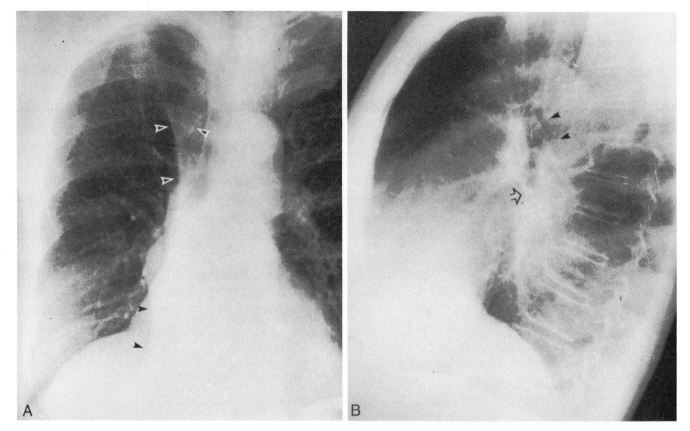

Figure 4–26. Posterior Displacement of the Intermediate Bronchus Associated with Atelectasis of the Right Lower Lobe. *A*, In posteroanterior projection, the right lower lobe is collapsed and airless *(small arrowheads* point to the interface between the downward-displaced major fissure and the overinflated right upper and middle lobes). The anterior junction line and mediastinal triangle *(arrowheads)* are displaced to the right. Note that the right interlobar artery is no longer visible because of silhouetting by the airless lower lobe. *B*, In lateral projection, collapse of the lower lobe is manifested by a vague triangular opacity overlying the lower thoracic vertebrae, and by posterior displacement of the air column of the intermediate bronchus *(arrowheads)*. Normally, this bronchus is aligned with the tracheal air column, slightly in front of the anterior wall of the left lower lobe bronchus *(open arrow)*.

mal. Since the upper lobes are situated mainly anteriorly, atelectasis of these lobes displaces their respective main bronchi forward; similarly, with atelectatic lower lobes, the posterior position of these lobes displaces their major bronchi backward (Fig. 4–26). We have seen this sign repeatedly in cases of lower lobe collapse but seldom very clearly when the upper lobes are affected. Posterior displacement of the left main bronchus can also result from dilatation of the left atrium in cases of pulmonary venous hypertension.[18]

Absence of Visibility of an Interlobar Artery. A cardinal sign of lower lobe collapse is loss of visibility of the interlobar artery; since the lung parenchyma adjacent to the artery is airless, the air-tissue interface is lost and the vessel becomes invisible *(see* Fig. 4–19). This sign is particularly valuable on the left side, where pleural effusion sometimes creates a triangular shadow in the posterior paravertebral zone that simulates total left lower lobe atelectasis. Preservation of the shadow of the interlobar artery establishes the pleural origin of the opacity, whereas its obliteration indicates lobar collapse.

Changes in the Chest Wall. Although approximation of ribs as a sign of smallness of a hemithorax may be of some value in cases of chronic loss of volume, in our experience

it is the least dependable of all compensatory signs. Even a slight degree of rotation of the patient at the time of roentgenography may produce an asymmetry of the two sides of the rib cage that renders assessment of abnormal approximation difficult or even hazardous. The difficulty may be compounded further by alterations in rib angulation, produced by even minor degrees of scoliosis.

Absence of an Air Bronchogram. As a general rule, *resorption atelectasis* cannot be present if air is visible in the bronchial tree, at least on conventional roentgenograms; if bronchial obstruction is severe enough to cause absorption of air from the parenchyma of the affected lobe, it also causes absorption of gas from the airways. Particularly when pneumonitis behind the obstruction is so severe that consolidation exceeds atelectasis, absence of an air bronchogram is a roentgenologic sign of vital importance. Indeed, it may be the only aid in distinguishing an obstructing carcinoma from a consolidative process such as acute airspace pneumonia. An exception to this general rule is confluent bronchopneumonia, (e.g., as from *Staphylococcus aureus*), in which a lobe or segment becomes homogeneously opaque and the bronchi are filled with inflammatory exudate; obviously, an air bronchogram would not be anticipated. One further caveat: the rule regarding absence of an air bronchogram in cases of resorption atelectasis or pneumonitis applies to conventional posteroanterior (PA) and lateral roentgenograms only. It is remarkable in such cases how often CT scans through affected lung parenchyma reveal air within obstructed airways that is not visible on conventional roentgenograms (Fig. 4–27).

The preceding statements apply only to atelectasis produced by resorption and not by the other three mechanisms (passive, adhesive, and cicatrization). In the first two particularly, an air bronchogram is virtually always present.

Patterns of Lobar and Segmental Atelectasis

Before describing the specific features of atelectasis, it is important to emphasize that, regardless of the severity of collapse, the visceral pleural surface usually attempts to maintain contact with the parietal pleura over either the convex or mediastinal surface of the hemithorax, provided the pleural space is intact (i.e., no pneumothorax or hydrothorax; Fig. 4–28A). There are several noteworthy exceptions to this rule. Occasionally in lower lobe atelectasis (see Fig. 4–28B) and frequently in middle lobe atelectasis (see Fig. 4–28C), the convex pleural contact may be lost as the lobe retracts toward the hilum. The resultant shape is partly affected by the semirigid components of the lung (bronchi, arteries, and veins), which can be crowded together in very close apposition in one plane but have a limited capacity to foreshorten. Thus, any pulmonary lobe in its fully inflated state may be likened to a pyramid with its apex at the hilum and its base contiguous with the parietal pleura[19]; as the lobe loses volume, two surfaces of the pyramid approximate, the end result of total atelectasis being a flattened triangle, or triangular "pancake," whose apex and base tend to maintain contiguity with the hilum and parietal pleura, respectively.

In most cases, the degree of collapse of a lobe is governed largely by the amount of fluid and cells it contains, the resultant roentgenographic image varying from a consolidated lobe in which there is only minimal loss of volume to a state of total lobar collapse. Therefore, the anatomicospatial relationships in each lobe are described from a state of normal volume through all stages to total atelectasis. In the descriptions that follow, we have borrowed freely from the publications of several workers, our findings having been fundamentally similar to their observations.[19–21]

Total Pulmonary Atelectasis. When an entire lung collapses because of obstruction of a main bronchus, the compensatory phenomena are identical in character to those that develop with less severe pulmonary collapse but greater in degree and, in some respects, less readily apparent (Fig. 4–29). Elevation of the ipsilateral hemidiaphragm is recognizable only on the left side, the stomach bubble indicating its position. The hemithorax usually exhibits retraction. It is on the mediastinum, however, that the most important effect is exerted. As the normal contralateral lung overinflates, the whole mediastinum moves to the affected side, the greatest shift occurring anteriorly, where the mediastinum is most mobile. As the overinflated lung moves across the midline, it displaces the heart, aorta, and collapsed lung posteriorly. Depth and radiolucency of the retrosternal airspace are increased and the posterior portion of the thorax shows a general increase in roentgenographic

density (see Fig. 4–29). If the overinflated normal lung has rotated sufficiently so as to come in contact with the collapsed lung, the interface between the two may become evident. In posteroanterior projection, the uniform opacity caused by the superimposed cardiovascular structures and collapsed lung is interrupted by the radiolucency of overinflated contralateral lung that has passed across the midline of the thorax. The margin of the overinflated lung is usually visible extending into the involved hemithorax.

It is important to assess the retrosternal space in lateral projection to differentiate complete pulmonary collapse from massive pulmonary consolidation or massive pleural effusion (see Fig. 4–25).[16] In the latter conditions, the anterior mediastinum is little altered in appearance, although its density may be increased; in total unilateral collapse, however, the anterior mediastinum is increased not only in depth but also in radiolucency. Lubert and Krause[16] refer to the "uniform-filter effect" observed in total pulmonary consolidation and massive pleural effusion, in which x-rays passing through the thorax in lateral projection are absorbed uniformly, preventing identification of a specific roentgenographic shadow.

Lobar Atelectasis. The patterns created by atelectasis of the right and left upper lobes differ and therefore are described separately; the lower lobes have almost identical patterns and are considered together.

Right Upper Lobe. The minor fissure and the upper half of the major fissure approximate by shifting upward and forward, respectively (Fig. 4–30). Both fissures become gently curved as seen on lateral projection; the minor fissure assumes a concave configuration inferiorly, whereas the major fissure may be convex, concave, or flat.[21] The minor fissure shows roughly the same curvature in PA projection. As volume diminishes further, the visceral pleural surface sweeps upward over the apex of the hemithorax, so that the lobe comes to assume a flattened shape contiguous with the superior mediastinum. When completely collapsed, its volume is so small that in PA projection its shadow creates no more than a slight widening of the superior mediastinum (see Fig. 4–30). In lateral projection, the collapsed lobe may appear as an indistinctly defined triangular shadow with its apex at the hilum and its base contiguous with the parietal pleura just posterior to the extreme apex of the hemithorax (the mediastinal "wedge"). The collapsed lobe is usually contiguous with the mediastinum so that no air shadow separates them; occasionally, however, an overinflated lower lobe is interposed between the mediastinum and the medial edge of the atelectatic upper lobe, a feature seen much more often with left upper lobe atelectasis (see later).[21]

The *juxtaphrenic peak* sign consists of a small, sharply defined triangular opacity that projects upward from the medial half of the hemidiaphragm at or near the highest point of the dome (see Fig. 4–30). Although it is sometimes associated with upper lobe atelectasis,[22] we have seen classic peaks in patients *without* appreciable collapse and regard it as a sign of questionable value.

Left Upper Lobe. The principal difference between collapse of the left and right upper lobes is the usual absence of a minor fissure on the left, on which side all lung tissue anterior to the major fissure is involved (see Fig. 4–11). This fissure, which is slightly more vertical than the major

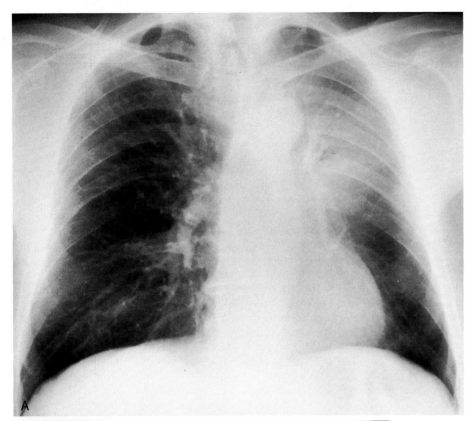

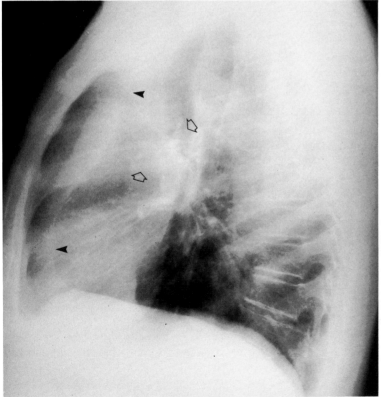

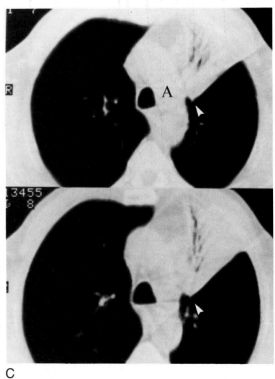

Figure 4–27. Severe Left Upper Lobe Atelectasis. Posteroanterior *(A)* and lateral *(B)* chest roentgenograms reveal the medial-to-lateral decrease in roentgenographic density characteristic of severe left upper lobe atelectasis. On the lateral projection, the serpentine interface between the collapsed upper lobe and overinflated lower lobe *(arrowheads)* relates closely to the anterior chest margin; a vague mediastinal wedge is seen extending upward and forward from the hilum *(arrows)*. Note the clarity with which the posterior portion of the aortic arch can be seen. C, Transverse CT scans at the level of the aortic arch *(A)* disclose a triangular or peaked appearance to the posteromedial fissural surface *(arrowheads)* between the atelectatic upper lobe and the overinflated lower lobe (the Luftsichel). Note the presence of an air bronchogram despite its absence on the conventional roentgenograms.

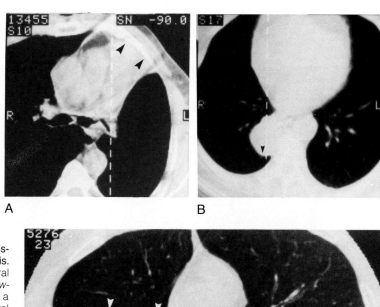

Figure 4–28. Variation in the Relationship Between the Visceral and the Parietal Pleura in the Presence of Atelectasis. *A,* A sagittal CT image in left upper lobe atelectasis: visceral and parietal pleural contiguity is maintained anteriorly *(arrowheads). B,* In contrast with this case, a sagittal CT image in a patient with right lower lobe atelectasis reveals the visceral pleura *(arrowhead)* to have lost all contact with the parietal pleura of the posterior chest wall but not the mediastinum. Similarly, a transverse CT scan *(C)* of a patient with middle lobe atelectasis *(arrowheads)* shows the visceral pleura over the convex (anterior) surface of the lobe to have lost contact with the parietal pleura; however, a thin linear opacity was visible between the lateral point of the collapsed lobe and the chest wall, conceivably caused by contact between the upper and the lower lobes.

fissure on the right, is displaced forward in a plane roughly parallel to the anterior chest wall, a relationship depicted particularly well on lateral roentgenograms (*see* Fig. 4–27). As volume loss increases, the fissure moves farther anteriorly and medially, until on lateral projection the shadow of the lobe is no more than a broad linear opacity contiguous with and parallel to the anterior chest wall (Fig. 4–31). The contiguity of the collapsed lobe with the anterior mediastinum obliterates the left cardiac border in frontal projection (the silhouette sign). The apical segment tends to move downward and forward, the space it vacates being occupied by the overinflated superior segment of the lower lobe; the apex of the hemithorax thus contains aerated lung (Fig. 4–32).

Sometimes the overinflated superior segment inserts itself medially between the apex of the atelectatic upper lobe and the mediastinum, creating a sharp interface with the medial edge of the collapsed lobe. This feature, the *Luftsichel* in the German literature,[23] is more often seen on the left than on the right.[21] CT assessment of the atelectatic lobe in such circumstance almost invariably shows a triangular or peaked appearance to the posteromedial fissural surface between the atelectatic upper lobe and the hyperexpanded lower lobe (*see* Fig. 4–32B).

Middle Lobe. The diagnosis of atelectasis of the middle lobe is one of the easiest to make on a lateral roentgenogram and one of the most difficult on PA projection (Fig. 4–33). With progressive loss of volume, the minor fissure and the lower half of the major fissure approximate, and they are almost in contact when collapse is complete. The resultant triangular pancake of tissue has its apex at the

hilum and its base apparently contiguous with the parietal pleura over the anterolateral convexity of the thorax. CT may demonstrate that this is largely spurious, since the visceral pleura can be retracted completely from the anterior chest wall (*see* Fig. 4–33). In lateral projection, middle lobe atelectasis appears as a broad linear opacity, at times no more than 2 or 3 mm wide; sometimes it is almost horizontal in orientation, whereas on other occasions it may run obliquely, at times paralleling the plane of the major fissure.[24] As Heitzman has emphasized in personal communication, should the thinnest portion of the collapsed lobe be situated some distance from the hilum, thus creating an hourglass configuration, a central mass should be sought as the cause of the atelectasis. In posteroanterior projection there may be no discernible increase in density, the only evidence of disease being obliteration of part of the right cardiac border (the silhouette sign) owing to contiguity of the right atrium with the medial segment of the collapsed lobe.

The CT depiction of right middle lobe atelectasis is characteristic and consists of a broad triangular or trapezoidal opacity with the apex directed toward the hilum (*see* Fig. 4–33). The anterior margin of the collapsed lobe tends to retract towards the hilum while the overinflated right upper lobe parenchyma intrudes anteromedially.

Lower Lobes. The configuration adopted by the lower lobes in the presence of atelectasis is modified by the fulcrumlike effect exerted by the hilum and pulmonary ligament,[25] the fissures approximating in such a manner that the upper half of the major fissure swings downward and the lower half backward (Fig. 4–34). This displacement is

Text continued on page 198

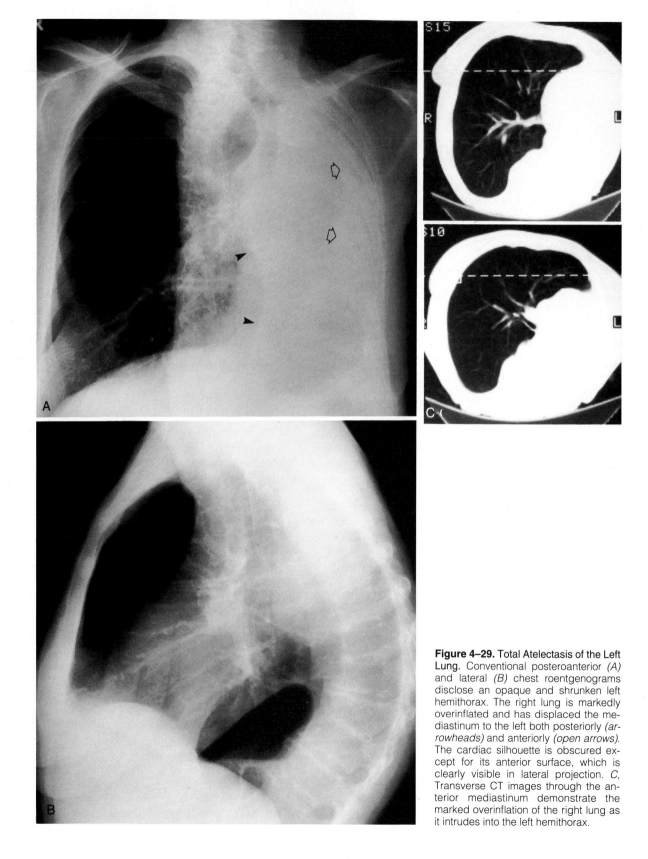

Figure 4–29. Total Atelectasis of the Left Lung. Conventional posteroanterior *(A)* and lateral *(B)* chest roentgenograms disclose an opaque and shrunken left hemithorax. The right lung is markedly overinflated and has displaced the mediastinum to the left both posteriorly *(arrowheads)* and anteriorly *(open arrows)*. The cardiac silhouette is obscured except for its anterior surface, which is clearly visible in lateral projection. *C,* Transverse CT images through the anterior mediastinum demonstrate the marked overinflation of the right lung as it intrudes into the left hemithorax.

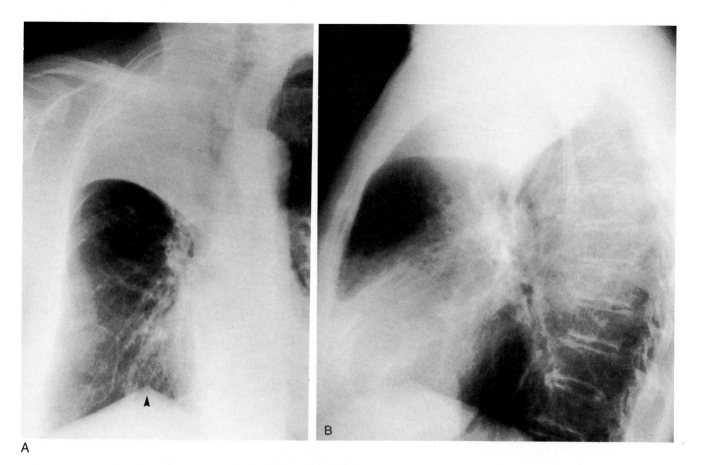

A

B

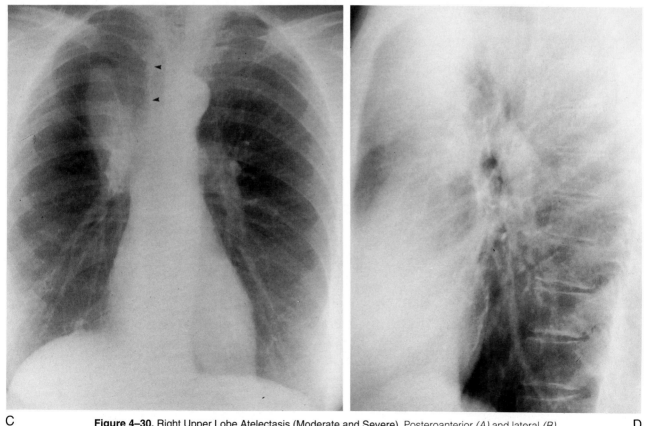

C

D

Figure 4–30. Right Upper Lobe Atelectasis (Moderate and Severe). Posteroanterior *(A)* and lateral *(B)* chest roentgenograms reveal moderate loss of volume of the right upper lobe evidenced by elevation of the minor fissure and anterior displacement of the upper half of the major fissure. A small "juxta-phrenic peak" is present *(arrowhead)*. Similar views in another patient *(C* and *D)* show a homogene-ous opacity extending superiorly from an elevated right hilum. The trachea is displaced minimally to the right, but the tracheal stripe is maintained *(arrowheads)*. Note the slight lucency immediately lateral to the trachea. This appearance is analogous to the "luftsichel" characteristic of left upper lobe atelectasis *(see* Fig. 4–32) and is a manifestation of severe atelectasis of the right upper lobe.

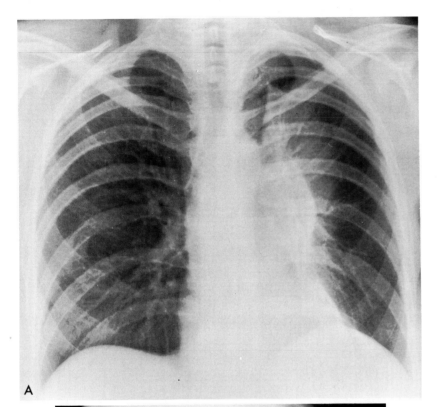

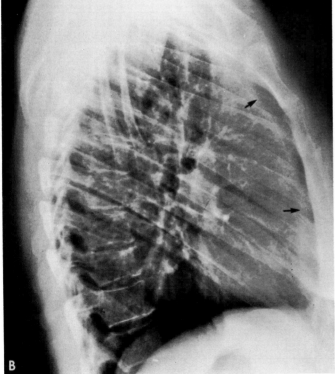

Figure 4–31. Atelectasis of the Left Upper Lobe (Severe). The homogeneous shadow created by the almost complete collapse of the left upper lobe occupies the anteromedial portion of the left hemithorax contiguous to the mediastinum. *A,* In posteroanterior projection, the apex of the hemithorax is occupied by the overinflated lower lobe. *B,* In lateral projection, the chief fissure has swept far anteriorly and can be identified as a rather indistinctly defined interface paralleling the anterior chest wall *(arrows).*

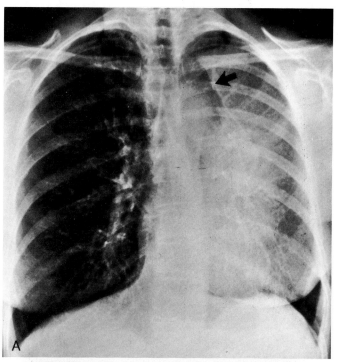

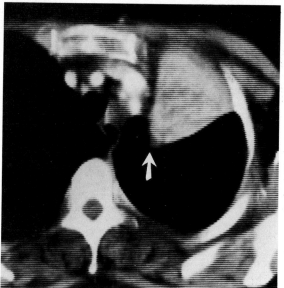

Figure 4–32. Left Upper Lobe Atelectasis with Luftsichel. A postero-anterior *(A)* roentgenogram reveals a common configuration of left upper lobe atelectasis; note the sharp air-tissue interface *(arrow)* representing the tongue of overinflated lower lobe inserted between the mediastinum and the airless upper lobe. *B,* A CT scan shows a V-shaped posterior extremity of the collapsed lobe, an *arrow* pointing along the interface that creates Luftsichel.

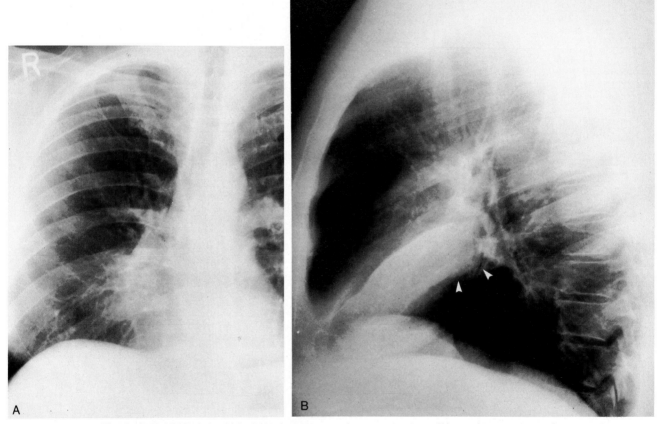

Figure 4–33. Middle Lobe Atelectasis. A posteroanterior roentgenogram *(A)* reveals a vague opacity in the right lower hemithorax obliterating the right cardiac border; a lateral projection of the same patient *(B)* shows the characteristic triangular opacity of middle lobe atelectasis. Note the convex inferior configuration of the major fissure at the hilum *(arrowheads)* indicative of an underlying mass. A CT scan of this patient is illustrated in Figure 4–28C, page 191.

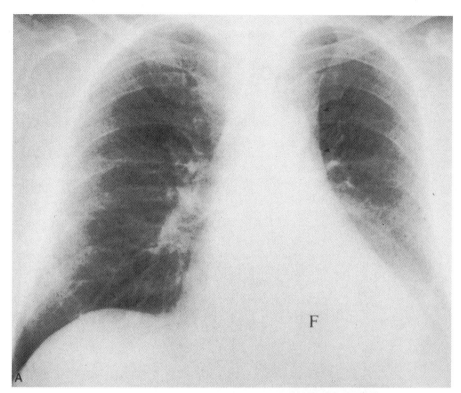

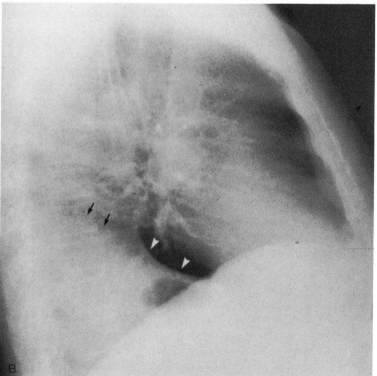

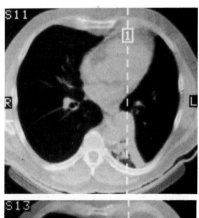

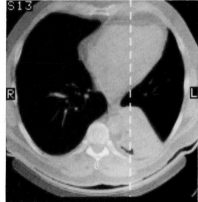

Figure 4–34. Left Lower Lobe Atelectasis. Conventional posteroanterior *(A)* and lateral *(B)* roentgenograms disclose an opacity behind the heart on the left. The left hemidiaphragm is elevated as indicated by the position of the gas-filled gastric fundus (F). In lateral projection, the lower half of the major fissure can be seen to be displaced posteriorly *(arrowheads)*, and the upper half inferiorly *(arrows). C,* Transverse CT images reveal a sharp demarcation between the atelectatic lower lobe and the hyperexpanded upper lobe. Note that the lobe has relocated posteromedially following rotation in a clockwise fashion around the hilum and pulmonary ligament.

best appreciated in lateral projection when the lobe is only partly atelectatic and the major fissure is tangential to the x-ray beam and thus visible as a well-defined interface. During its downward displacement, the upper half of the fissure usually becomes clearly evident in posteroanterior projection as a well-defined interface extending obliquely downward and laterally from the region of the hilum (Fig. 4–35).[26] As collapse progresses, the lobe moves posteromedially to occupy a position in the posterior costophrenic gutter and medial costovertebral angle. Because the flat surface of the triangular pancake lies against the mediastinum, the thickness of tissue traversed by the roentgen beam in lateral projection may be insufficient to cast a shadow (see Fig. 4–19); in fact, when atelectasis is severe the only abnormal feature may be a subtle increase in the radiographic density of the lower thoracic vertebrae (normally, the vertebrae become progressively more radiolucent from above downward).

The *mediastinal wedge*, consisting of the major bronchi and vessels, may be apparent as a narrow triangular band of increased density extending downward and posteriorly from the hilum. Provided that exposure factors ensure adequate penetration of the heart, the collapsed lobe should be plainly visible in frontal projection as a diminutive triangular or rounded opacity in the costovertebral angle (see Fig. 4–35).[25] As noted previously, the interlobar artery is not identifiable because of obscuration by contiguous airless lung.

Combined Lobar Atelectasis. Since involvement of the two lobes of the left lung results in total pulmonary collapse, atelectasis of two lobes simultaneously produces a distinctive roentgenographic pattern only in the right lung.

Combined Right Middle and Lower Lobe Atelectasis. The major and minor fissures are displaced downward and backward so that the resultant opacity occupies the posteroinferior portion of the hemithorax; this appearance is virtually indistinguishable from that of atelectasis of the lower lobe alone. On a PA roentgenogram the density created by the collapsed lobes may completely obliterate the shadow of the right dome of the diaphragm and can possess an upper surface that is concave or convex upward[20]; in the former situation, the appearance can be confused with pleural effusion unless absence of the shadow of the interlobar artery is recognized.

Combined Right Upper and Middle Lobe Atelectasis. Because of the independent and relatively remote origin of the lobar bronchi of the right upper and middle lobes, such an occurrence is rare. Although it has been seen in association with primary and metastatic neoplasms and inflammatory disease, it is likely that mucous plugs are a contributing factor in most cases. As the situation is analogous to atelectasis of the left upper lobe, the roentgenographic appearance is similar, particularly in lateral projection (Fig. 4–36).

Segmental Atelectasis. Segmental atelectasis is invariably caused by airway obstruction, the resulting roentgenographic appearance thus being a combination of both loss of volume and obstructive pneumonitis (Fig. 4–37). Although this statement also probably applies to many cases of subsegmental atelectasis, it is conceivable that the linear opacities commonly observed in the lung bases (discoid atelectasis) are caused at least partly by surfactant deficit.

Predominantly Interstitial Disease

This heading covers the multitude of pulmonary diseases characterized by predominant involvement of the interstitial tissues of the lung. Conceptually, these diseases are the antithesis of the alveolar consolidative processes, in that alveolar airspaces are largely preserved and it is the tissues surrounding them that are increased in volume. Although this concept is useful in diagnosis, it is important to realize that any interstitial process may also affect the adjacent airspaces. For example, in the desquamative phase of fibrosing alveolitis, the morphologic picture is not one of simple thickening of alveolar walls but also of an abundance of macrophages within the alveoli; thus, the disease affects both interstitium and airspaces. Those who question the logic of dividing diffuse lung disease into interstitial and airspace patterns[27] assert that, because the majority of diseases affect both anatomic compartments to some degree, the distinction is arbitrary. We submit that the division is nevertheless valid if one accepts the concept of *predominant* involvement: an acinar pattern indicates *predominant* involvement of the parenchymal airspaces, and a nodular or reticular pattern indicates *predominant* involvement of the interstitium. If this is borne in mind, pattern recognition becomes a logical and useful technique in roentgenologic interpretation.

Concepts of Roentgenologic Anatomy

The interstitial space of the lungs and pleura can conveniently be divided into two anatomically continuous but conceptually distinct components: (1) the *axial interstitial space*, consisting of the connective tissue around the airways, pulmonary arteries and veins, and within the pleura and interlobular septa, and (2) the *parenchymal interstitial space*, which lies between the alveolar and capillary basement membranes.

The distinction between these two compartments is of some value, because their individual involvement usually produces recognizable roentgenographic patterns and has different diagnostic implications. For example, studies of rapidly frozen dog lungs in which pulmonary venous pressures have been raised by graded levels have shown a definite sequence of fluid accumulation in various compartments of the lung (Fig. 4–38).[28] Fluid appears first in the interstitial connective tissue compartment around the large blood vessels and airways; thickening of the alveolar wall follows, but it is not until the axial interstitial compartment is well-filled that alveolar edema appears. It is this anatomic localization in the perivascular and interlobular septal interstitium that produces the typical roentgenographic pattern of loss of the normal sharp definition of the pulmonary vascular markings and thickening of the interlobular septa (B lines of Kerley; Fig. 4–39). Fluid that accumulates in the *parenchymal* interstitial tissues in these circumstances produces little or no discernible roentgenographic change because of its minimal amount. Thus, the pattern of roentgenologic abnormality in the early phase of pulmonary edema shows predominantly axial interstitial tissue involvement; only when alveolar filling by fluid occurs is there roentgenographic evidence of parenchymal abnormality. A similar distribution of disease occurs with lymphangitic

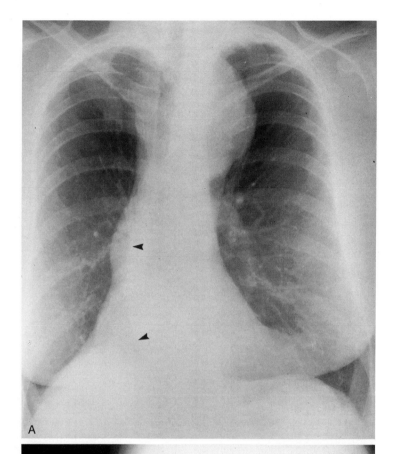

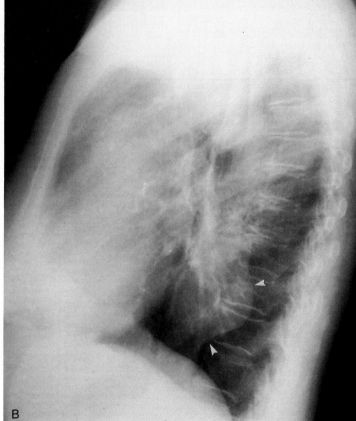

Figure 4–35. Right Lower Lobe Atelectasis. Posteroanterior *(A)* and lateral *(B)* chest roentgenograms of a 65-year-old woman reveal an aortic arch aneurysm that was confirmed by angiography. The right hemithorax is somewhat smaller than the left, and the mediastinum is displaced slightly to the right. An opacity is visible *(arrowheads)* behind the heart extending from approximately the level of the hilum to a point slightly above the right hemidiaphragm. The right hilum is diminished in size, and the right interlobar artery cannot be identified because of incorporation into the opacity of the collapsed lobe. In lateral projection, a sharply defined opacity *(arrowheads)* extends from the inferior aspect of the hilum to a point a few centimeters above the right hemidiaphragm. A CT scan on this patient is illustrated in Figure 4–28B *(see* page 191).

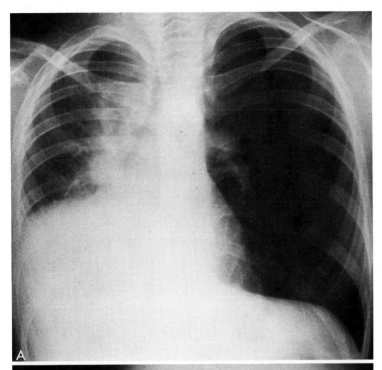

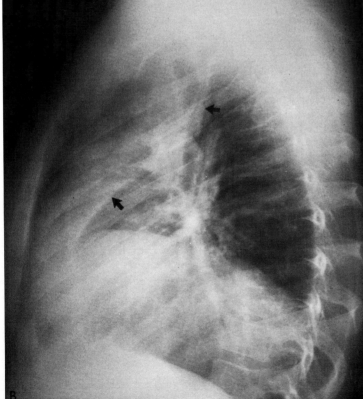

Figure 4–36. Atelectasis of the Right Upper and Middle Lobes Combined. Posteroanterior *(A) and lateral (B)* roentgenograms reveal a pattern of collapse that is virtually identical to the one seen in the left upper lobe. The collapsed lobes relate to the anteromedial aspect of the hemithorax; thus, in lateral projection *(B)*, the major fissure is seen to be displaced forward *(arrows)*. The apex of the right hemithorax is occupied by the overdistended lower lobe. Compensatory signs of diaphragmatic elevation and mediastinal shift are readily apparent. The patient is a 12-year-old boy with spasmodic asthma; a mucous plug impacted in the right upper lobe bronchus was coughed up spontaneously; the right middle lobe collapse was chronic and irreversible (chronic "right middle lobe syndrome").

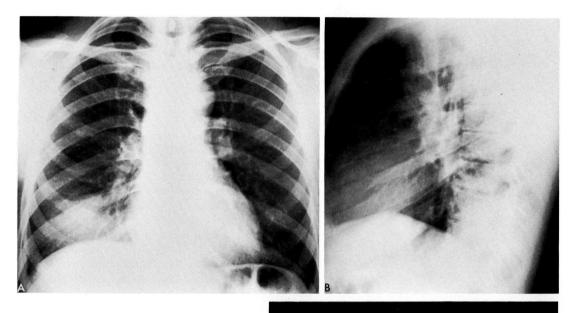

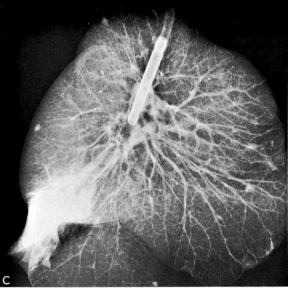

Figure 4–37. Segmental Atelectasis and Consolidation, Posterior Basal Segment, Right Lower Lobe. Posteroanterior (A) and lateral (B) roentgenograms reveal a homogeneous opacity localized to the posterior bronchopulmonary segment of the right lower lobe; no air bronchogram is present. The process is both consolidative and atelectatic, the latter evidenced by posterior displacement of the major fissure. A lateral roentgenogram of the resected lung (C) shows the precise segmental nature of the disease. Squamous cell carcinoma of the posterior basal bronchus.

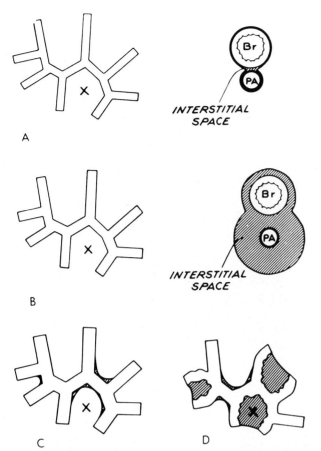

Figure 4–38. Schematic Representation of the Sequence of Fluid Accumulation in Acute Pulmonary Edema. *A,* Normal lung (alveolar wall and alveoli on the left, bronchovascular bundle on the right); *B,* interstitial edema in which fluid accumulated preferentially in the loose interstitial space around the conducting blood vessels and airways without affecting the alveolar walls; *C,* early alveolar edema showing loose interstitial spaces filled and fluid overflowing into alveoli, preferentially at the corners at which the curvature is greatest; *D,* alveolar flooding in which individual alveoli have reached a critical configuration at which existing inflation pressure can no longer maintain stability and the alveolar gas volume rapidly passes to a new configuration with much reduced curvature. (Slightly modified from Staub NE, Nagano H, Pearce ML: Pulmonary edema in dogs, especially the sequence of fluid accumulation in lungs. J Appl Physiol 22: 227, 1967, with permission.)

spread of carcinoma, some pneumoconioses, sarcoidosis, and some forms of lymphoma.

It is probable that the same situation occurs in other types of interstitial disease in which the alveolar wall is widened without much associated distortion of lung architecture; because of their minute size, it is most unlikely that an increase in alveolar wall thickness can produce individually identifiable roentgenographic opacities. As with interstitial pulmonary edema that widens the alveolar wall, however, it is possible that such an abnormality could result in a ground-glass opacity over the lungs, although it is more likely that minor involvement, even if diffuse, is associated with a normal chest roentgenogram.

A number of studies have shown that CT can be useful in the assessment of patients with interstitial lung disease.[29, 30] By eliminating superimposition of structures, it allows a better assessment of the type, distribution, and severity of parenchymal abnormalities; in fact, a characteristic appearance may be seen on CT even in patients whose chest roentgenogram is normal or shows only nonspecific findings. For example, in one study comparing the accuracy of chest roentgenography and CT in the prediction of specific diagnoses in patients with chronic diffuse lung disease, three observers made a confident diagnosis in 23 per cent of roentgenograms and 49 per cent of CT scans; the diagnosis was correct in 77 and 93 per cent of readings, respectively.[31] Despite this apparent benefit, the basic concepts for the interpretation of the CT image and for the assessment of patterns of disease are similar to those of the roentgenogram, so they are considered together.

Roentgenographic Patterns of Diffuse Interstitial Disease

There are four basic roentgenographic patterns of interstitial disease: reticular, nodular, reticulonodular, and linear. Although reticular and nodular patterns exist in pure forms, it is probable that most interstitial diseases show mixed reticulonodular architecture. It is logical that in a reticular network, particularly if it is coarse, many linear densities are seen *en face* and thus appear as a reticular pattern roentgenographically; however, many also must be seen on end, in which case they simulate nodules. Because of this obvious visual effect, it might appear reasonable to designate all these diseases reticulonodular; however, as we discuss later on, the distinction between reticular and nodular diseases not only has certain morphologic significance but also may be important in relation to the effects each may exert on pulmonary function.

Before discussing specific roentgenographic manifestations of diffuse interstitial lung disease, it is desirable to specify the roentgenologic changes common to all, without which the purely interstitial site of involvement should be doubted. Since the disease is anatomically interstitial, the acini contain some air, although their volume may be reduced by effects such as fibrosis. Therefore, *diffuse interstitial disease must produce inhomogeneous roentgenographic density*; in most cases this feature alone distinguishes interstitial disease from airspace disease. Second, and for the same reason, the airways seldom are involved significantly, so that, by and large, there is nothing to prevent air from reaching the lung parenchyma. Thus, *volume reduction due to airway obstruction is not a prominent feature of interstitial disease*.

Reticular Pattern. A reticular pattern is an array of curvilinear opacities that can be likened to a net of variable mesh size. The precise pattern of reticulation depends upon several variables, the two most important being the degree of thickening of the interstitial space and the effect that the interstitial involvement exerts on parenchymal airspaces (Fig. 4–40). It is useful to describe a reticular pattern according to the size of the net meshwork; accordingly, the terms fine, medium, and coarse, although arbitrary, are in wide use and appear to be generally acceptable. *Fine* reticulation simulates a very fine mesh and might be likened to that seen in a nylon stocking. At the opposite end of the spectrum, *coarse* reticulation is characterized by cystic spaces, 5 to 10 mm in diameter ringed by soft tissue. Between these two extremes lies *medium* reticulation (Fig.

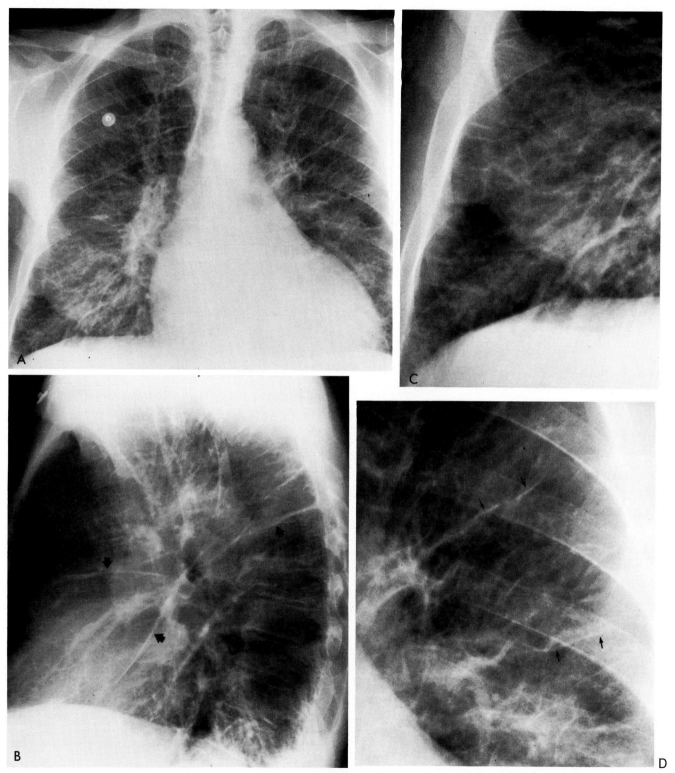

Figure 4–39. Interstitial Pulmonary Edema. Posteroanterior *(A)* and lateral *(B)* roentgenograms reveal multiple linear opacities throughout both lungs, seen to better advantage in magnified views of the right lower *(C)* and left upper *(D)* lungs. These lines consist of a combination of long septal lines (Kerley A), predominantly in the midlung zones *(arrows in D)*, and shorter peripheral septal lines (Kerley B). In lateral projection *(B)*, the interlobar fissures are very prominent *(arrows)*, representing pleural edema.

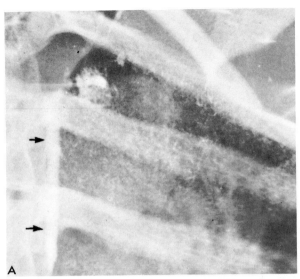 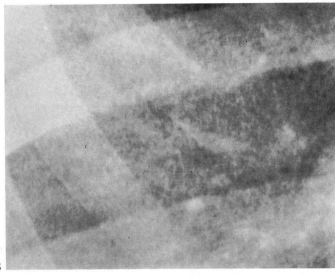

Figure 4–40. The Reticulonodular Pattern. *A,* A magnified view of the apex of the left upper lobe approximately 1½ hours following the injection of 7 mL of Lipiodol into the lymphatics of each leg reveals a fine network of shadows of high density. This network is caused by the presence of contrast medium in the microvascular circulation of the lung. The thoracic duct can be identified on the left *(arrows).* Twenty-four hours later a fine stippled pattern is present, distributed diffusely and evenly *(B).*

4–41), characterized by 3- to 5-mm cystic spaces. The designation "honeycomb" pattern should be reserved for cystic spaces in the medium and coarse categories.

On CT, fine reticulation (Fig. 4–42) is manifested by an amorphous ground-glass opacity or a fine granular pattern. The latter is uncommon and is invariably seen on a background of ground-glass opacity. Medium and coarse reticulation correlate closely with conventional roentgenograms (*see* Fig. 4–42); indeed, CT may demonstrate these gross changes more clearly.[32]

Nodular Pattern. A nodular pattern is produced when discrete, more or less spherical lesions accumulate within the interstitium. The interstitial nodule differs fundamentally from its airspace counterpart in that it is homogeneous, well-defined, and of variable size. The last-named feature permits further subdivision: micronodular (smaller than 1 mm), small (1 to 3 mm), medium (3 to 5 mm), and large (larger than 5 mm).

Nodular interstitial disease of the lungs is perhaps best epitomized by hematogenous dissemination of an infection

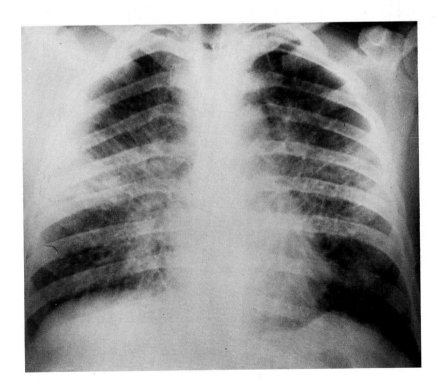

Figure 4–41. Interstitial Non-Hodgkin's Lymphoma. A posteroanterior roentgenogram reveals extensive involvement of both lungs by lymphoma manifested by a rather coarse reticular pattern. The severity of interstitial abnormality is reflected in a loss of definition of vascular markings throughout both lungs, reminiscent of severe interstitial edema.

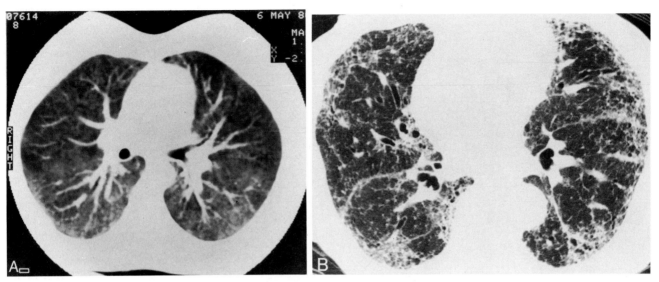

Figure 4–42. CT of a Reticular Interstitial Pattern. *A,* An unenhanced CT scan through the upper and lower lobes of a patient with fibrosing alveolitis demonstrates an amorphous increase in density (ground-glass pattern) and micronodularity. *B,* A high-resolution CT scan (1.5 mm collimation) through the lower lung zones of another patient with the same disease reveals a reticular pattern located predominantly in subpleural lung regions. *(A from Genereux GP: Pattern recognition in diffuse lung disease: A review of theory and practice. Med Radiogr Photogr 61: 2, 1985.)*

such as tuberculosis (Fig. 4–43). Since the infecting organisms reach the lung via the circulation and are trapped in the capillaries, they must be purely interstitial in location (at least in early disease). The tubercles grow in a roughly spherical fashion, creating a micronodular or small nodular pattern. Other diseases that involve the lungs by hematog-

enous dissemination, such as metastatic carcinoma and intravenous talcosis of drug abuse, can have an identical appearance. In addition, certain inhalation diseases such as silicosis and idiopathic conditions such as sarcoidosis are characterized by the formation of discrete nodular lesions within the interstitial space. The pathogenesis of nodule

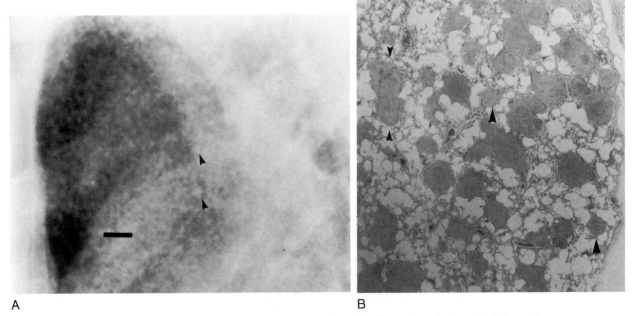

A

B

Figure 4–43. Nodular Interstitial Pattern. *A,* In a patient with miliary tuberculosis, a detail view of the retrosternal lung from a lateral chest roentgenogram shows isolated and confluent small nodular opacities; some of the nodules are denser *(arrowheads)* than others, presumably as a result of summation. (Bar denotes 1 cm.) *B,* A histologic section of the biopsy specimen from this patient discloses isolated *(large arrowheads)* and confluent *(between small arrowheads)* granulomas. (From Genereux GP: Pattern recognition in diffuse lung disease: A review of theory and practice. Med Radiogr Photogr 61: 2, 1985. © Eastman Kodak Company.)

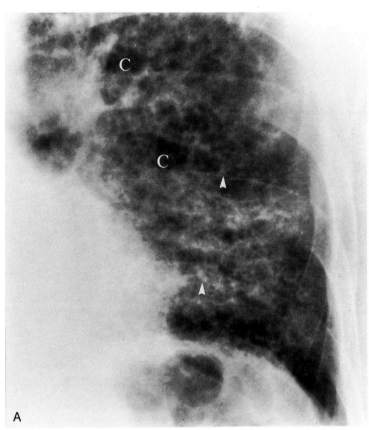
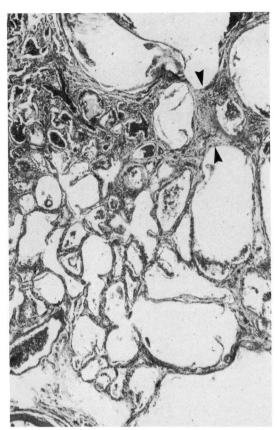

Figure 4–44. Reticulonodular Interstitial Pattern. *A,* A detail view of the left lower lung zone from a posteroanterior chest roentgenogram of a young man with end-stage fibrosing alveolitis shows apparent nodulation *(arrowheads)* and cystic spaces (C). *B,* A representative histologic section of lung from this patient at autopsy discloses typical features of "end-stage" lung; no true nodules are seen. The pseudonodulation seen on the roentgenogram apparently results from tangential projection of the x-ray beam along the path of the curvilinear opacities *(between arrowheads).* (From Genereux GP: Pattern recognition in diffuse lung disease: A review of theory and practice. Med Radiogr Photogr 61: 1, 1985. © Eastman Kodak Company.)

formation in these conditions is not as obvious as in those associated with hematogenous dissemination. The mechanism presumably involves a relatively greater accumulation of the agent in one site than another; the factors involved in this process are unclear.

On CT, small, medium, and large nodules can be readily identified (*see* Fig. 4–43), whereas micronodularity creates an amorphous opacity or fine granularity indistinguishable from the CT pattern of fine reticulation.

Reticulonodular Pattern. Although more or less diffuse thickening of the axial interstitial tissues usually presents roentgenographically as a reticular pattern, orientation of some linear opacities parallel to the x-ray beam sometimes suggests a nodular component in addition to the reticular one (Fig. 4–44). Although in any given situation a reticulonodular pattern can be produced by this mechanism, it can also result from an admixture of nodular deposits and diffuse thickening throughout the interstitium as, for example, in sarcoidosis or lymphangitic spread of carcinoma. The CT depiction of reticulonodularity reflects the pattern seen on conventional roentgenograms.

Linear Pattern. A linear pattern results from thickening of tissues in the bronchoarterial bundles. Undoubtedly, the commonest cause of this is chronic airway disease such as bronchiectasis or severe chronic bronchitis; occasionally,

asthma is responsible. A similar pattern can be caused by lymphangitic spread of carcinoma. On CT, the bronchoarterial bundles in the upper (and to a lesser degree the lower) lobes tend to be oriented perpendicular to the transverse plane of the scan; as a consequence, thickening of these structures is exquisitely demonstrable. However, the tomographic nature of the study, coupled with the plane of the scan, means that the thickening is portrayed as either well-defined, nodular opacities or tubular branching opacities. In cases of obstructive airway disease, emphysematous spaces of varying size should be obvious in addition to the basic pattern.

The "Honeycomb" Pattern. Pathologically, the term "honeycomb pattern" refers to an advanced stage of pulmonary interstitial fibrosis in which normal lung parenchyma is replaced by cystic spaces separated by a variable amount of fibrous tissue (Fig. 4–45). In order to have some diagnostic value, we feel that the roentgenographic correlate of this pattern should be restricted to those cases in which the cystic spaces range in diameter from 5 to 10 mm. Although others have recommended that the term be employed to describe multiple focal lucencies of *any* size,[33] such use leads to its application to a great variety of roentgenographic patterns—too many in our estimation—and seems to sink us into a semantic morass of little utility.

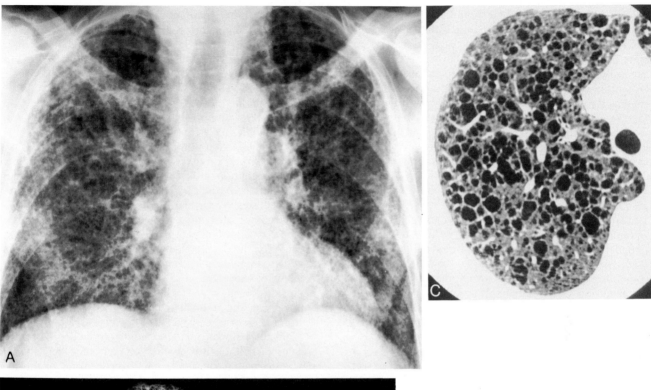

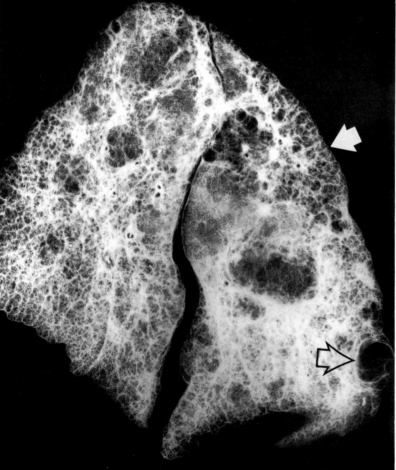

Figure 4–45. Advanced Fibrosing Alveolitis with Honeycombing. A posteroanterior roentgenogram *(A)* reveals a coarse reticular pattern without anatomic predominance. Honeycomb changes are present in several areas. A roentgenogram of a 1-cm-thick slice of left lung removed at autopsy *(B)* shows the honeycombing well *(solid arrows)* and also reveals a large subpleural bulla in the lower lobe *(open arrow)*. A high-resolution CT scan from another patient *(C)* shows similar extensive honeycomb change.

The roentgenographic pattern of honeycombing, as defined above, may be produced by a limited number of diseases, including eosinophilic granuloma, fibrosing alveolitis, rheumatoid disease, lymphangioleiomyomatosis, progressive systemic sclerosis, asbestosis, and sarcoidosis. Anatomic predominance of the pattern aids in the differential diagnosis; for example, eosinophilic granuloma and sarcoidosis often show a predilection for the upper lung zones, whereas the remainder of the diseases tend to have lower zone predominance. It is clear from this short list that restriction of the term "honeycomb lung" to the pattern described here reduces the diagnostic possibilities to relatively few, especially if one takes into account anatomic bias. We submit that this is the only way to bring some order to the confusion that surrounds diffuse interstitial lung disease.

In addition to cystic spaces, the conventional chest roentgenogram reveals decreased, normal, or increased lung volume, depending on the degree of fibrosis and the presence or absence of concomitant airway disease. For example, when fibrosis is dominant and severe, the lungs are typically shrunken and poorly inflated; by contrast, when there is obstructive bronchiolar disease, as in some cases of eosinophilic granuloma, sarcoidosis, and pulmonary lymphangioleiomyomatosis, lung volume tends to be increased.

Modifying Influences. Certain secondary effects sometimes produced by diffuse interstitial disease may considerably modify the basic roentgenographic pattern. For example, emphysema, either secondary to bronchiolar obstruction or compensatory to pulmonary fibrosis, may distort the pulmonary architecture and render the original disease pattern unrecognizable; the combination of conglomerate shadows and emphysema in advanced silicosis exemplifies this situation. Similarly, cicatrization associated with diffuse interstitial fibrosis can reduce lung volume severely. Such modifying influences usually occur in relation to fairly definite etiologic and pathogenic circumstances and, therefore, may help one differentiate the many diseases in which the interstitium is diffusely affected.

Combined Airspace and Interstitial Disease

In many pulmonary diseases, the roentgenologic and pathologic changes include a composite of the three basic abnormalities: consolidation, atelectasis, and interstitial thickening. The commonest combinations are (1) interstitial disease and airspace consolidation and (2) all three abnormalities together.

The pattern of combined airspace consolidation and interstitial disease is best exemplified by pulmonary edema secondary to pulmonary venous hypertension. The roentgenographic manifestations of interstitial involvement are largely those of a change in the axial interstitium (fluid within the bronchovascular sheath increasing the size and reducing the definition of lung markings) and within the interlobular septa (causing Kerley B lines). The roentgenographic manifestations of parenchymal consolidation consist of discrete and confluent "acinar" opacities characteristic of airspace-filling processes. Another example of combined involvement of this type is acute pneumonitis of *Mycoplasma* or viral etiology. This infection tends to be local rather than general in distribution and characteristically causes acute

interstitial inflammation, creating early in its course a pattern of fine to medium reticulation in segmental distribution. This "pure" interstitial involvement is often short lived, the inflammatory reaction soon extending into parenchymal airspaces and resulting in consolidation. Since involvement of the conducting airways is relatively insignificant, loss of volume is negligible in the acute stage of the disease.

The combination of airspace consolidation, atelectasis, and interstitial disease is best exemplified by acute bronchopneumonia, for example, of staphylococcal origin (Fig. 4–46). The infection primarily involves bronchial and bronchiolar walls and produces acute bronchitis and bronchiolitis with distention of the bronchovascular interstitial sheath by an inflammatory exudate. Intraluminal mucopurulent material leads to irregular airway obstruction, resulting in focal areas of atelectasis. Adjacent areas of lung parenchyma may show no abnormality or may overinflate to compensate for the focal atelectasis. Extension of the infection into the parenchyma leads to patchy airspace consolidation; because of this mechanism of spread, the involvement is necessarily segmental. The resultant roentgenographic pattern depicts the interstitial involvement, patchy zones of peripheral airspace consolidation, atelectasis, and normal or overinflated parenchyma. Depending on the degree of consolidation, volume loss in the segment may be slight or moderate; overall density is uneven as a result of the foci of normal or overinflated parenchyma.

General Signs in Diseases That Increase Roentgenographic Density

In addition to the basic signs already described, several others may aid in assessing a pathologic process in the lungs. The signs are described in general terms only, the intention being to indicate the mechanisms by which they are produced and the significance of each in roentgenologic interpretation.

Characteristics of the Border of a Pulmonary Lesion

The *sharpness of definition* of a consolidative process within the lung gives some indication of the nature of its marginal tissues and of its etiology. Acute airspace pneumonia (e.g., that caused by *Streptococcus pneumoniae*) that has extended to an interlobar pleural surface has a sharply defined contour along that border; where it does not abut against a fissure its margin is less distinct, since it is formed by a spreading zone of consolidation. Regardless of the etiology and extent of acinar consolidation, however, the margin between consolidated lung and contiguous air-containing parenchyma has the same definitive character whether the lesion is a small focus of exudative tuberculosis or a massive area of consolidation produced by *Klebsiella pneumoniae*.

Sharpness or definition also can be a clue in the distinction between neoplasia and a non-neoplastic consolidative process. For example, the margin of a fibrotic granulomatous lesion generally is sharply defined, whereas the margin of an infiltrative cancer tends to be indistinct and fuzzy. Conclusions based on this feature must be made with caution, however. In one study of 155 solitary lung lesions, 58

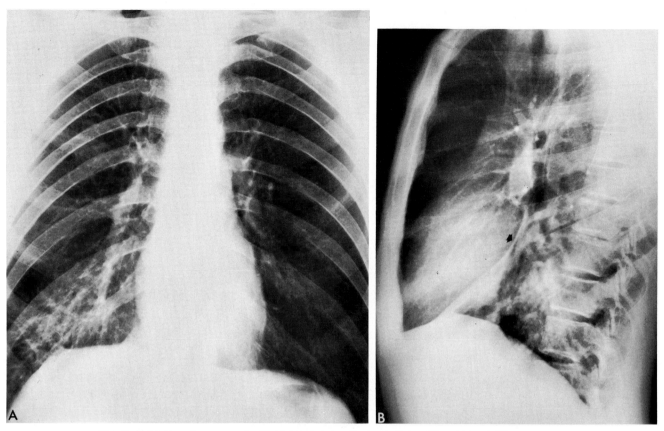

Figure 4–46. Bronchopneumonia, Right Lower Lobe. Posteroanterior *(A)* and lateral *(B)* roentgeno-grams reveal patchy consolidation of the anterior and lateral basal segments of the right lower lobe. Posterior bowing of the chief fissure *(arrow)* indicates some loss of volume. The inhomogeneous nature of the disease suggests combined airspace consolidation, focal atelectasis, and focal compensatory overinflation.

of 80 primary carcinomas (73.5 per cent) had indistinctly defined margins and the remaining 22 were well defined.[34] Of 20 lesions of infectious etiology, 15 had ill-defined margins and 5 were well defined. Only the 40 benign lesions had sharply defined margins in all cases.[34] It may be concluded, therefore, that although the sharpness of definition of a pulmonary opacity gives *some* indication of its nature, it cannot be a sign of *absolute* value in distinguishing benign from malignant lesions (Fig. 4–47).

The *smoothness of contour* (as distinct from nodularity or lobulation) has a significance that is in many respects similar to that of sharpness of definition. In general, it suggests a benign lesion, whereas nodularity or lobulation indicates malignancy (*see* Fig. 4–47). It is likely that "umbilication" or notching of the border of a solitary pulmonary nodule, which has been described as a sign of malignancy, is merely a manifestation of lobulation. As with sharpness of definition, umbilication is not an infallible sign of malignancy; for example, in one study it was identified in 16 of 22 cases of tuberculoma.[35]

"Satellite lesions" are small, punctate opacities close to a larger lesion, usually a solitary peripheral nodule. They are thought to suggest an infectious cause, particularly tuberculosis, having been found in almost 10 per cent of patients with this disease. Although their presence is very suggestive of a benign process, again it is not absolutely reliable; in

one study of 280 cases of pulmonary carcinoma, they were identified in three instances.[36]

The contour of an opacity that relates to the pleura, either over the convexity of the thorax or contiguous with the mediastinum or diaphragm, can provide a useful clue as to whether the process is intra- or extrapulmonary in origin. A mass that originates within the pleural space or extrapleurally displaces the pleura and underlying lung inward so that the angle formed by the margins of the mass and the chest wall is obtuse (Fig. 4–48); by contrast, an intrapulmonary mass tends to relate to contiguous pleura with an acute angle. It should be obvious that these general rules apply when such lesions are viewed tangentially; when viewed *en face,* an extrapleural mass is indistinctly defined because of the obtuse angle of its margins, whereas an intrapulmonary mass tends to be more sharply defined.

Change in Position of Interlobar Fissures

Displacement of a fissure toward a zone of increased density constitutes the only direct sign of atelectasis. An equally valuable but less frequent sign is displacement of an interlobar fissure in the opposite direction from the involved lobe—in other words, bulging of the fissure. Clearly, this is evidence of expansion of the involved lobe; since diseases of increased density capable of increasing the

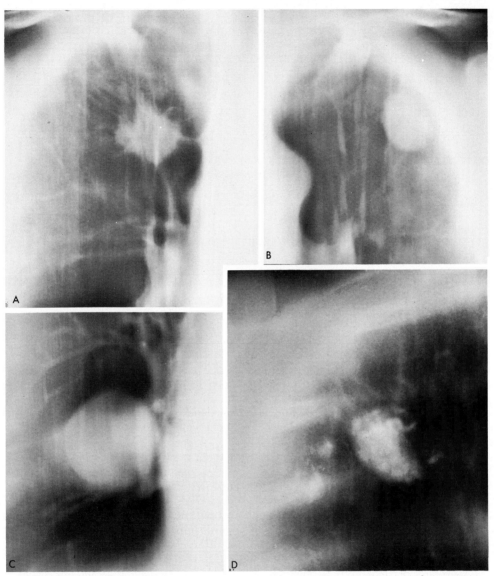

Figure 4–47. Characteristics of the Border of Four Different Pulmonary Nodules Observed Tomographically. *A,* Shaggy, lobulated border of a primary adenocarcinoma; *B,* a smooth, nonlobulated contour of a primary adenocarcinoma; *C,* a smooth, nonlobulated border of a solitary metastasis from embryonal carcinoma of the testis; *D,* a sharply defined, somewhat lobulated contour of a histoplasmoma, with several satellite lesions situated laterally; both the larger nodule and the satellite lesions are calcified.

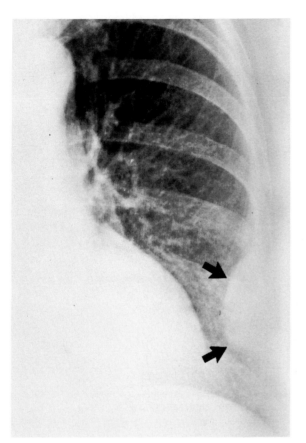

Figure 4–48. Localized Fibrous Tumor. A view of the left lung from a posteroanterior roentgenogram reveals a sharply defined opacity in the axillary region inferiorly *(arrows)*. The mass is homogeneous and possesses a broad pleural base. Note the obtuse angle the mass makes with the pleural surface, indicating its extrapulmonary location.

volume of a lobe are relatively few, recognition of such displacement frequently permits a specific etiologic diagnosis.

Bulging of fissures occurs most often in acute pulmonary infections in which there is an abundant exudate, the commonest of which are caused by *K. pneumoniae, S. pneumoniae, Mycobacterium tuberculosis,* and *Yersinia pestis.* An acute lung abscess also often expands a lobe, particularly when air trapping by a check-valve mechanism in a communicating airway distends the abscess cavity (Fig. 4–49). In addition to these infectious causes, any space-occupying mass within a lobe may displace a fissure if it occupies significant volume or if it is contiguous with the fissure; pulmonary carcinoma is undoubtedly the commonest of these masses.

Fissures are ordinarily an efficient barrier to interlobar spread of parenchymal disease. A few diseases, however, have a propensity for crossing pleural boundaries, thus creating a sign invaluable for differential diagnosis. Undoubtedly the commonest cause of pleural transgression is mycotic or actinomycotic infection, particularly the latter. This process can occur not only across interlobar fissures but also across the visceral and parietal pleural layers over the convexity of the lung, resulting in abscesses and osteomyelitis in the chest wall. Pulmonary tuberculosis also may transgress pleural boundaries, particularly in children; pulmonary carcinoma does so relatively uncommonly. One ca-

veat to the unwary: these statements apply to *complete* interlobar fissures; when fissures are incomplete, disease can extend directly from one lobe to a contiguous lobe via communicating channels, and the differential diagnosis contains more possibilities.

Cavitation

A cavity can be defined as a gas-containing space within the lung surrounded by a wall greater than 1 mm thick (a gas-containing space possessing a wall 1 mm or thinner is a bulla). The presence of a fluid level is not necessary to the definition, nor is size of the cavity relevant. The terms "cavity" and "abscess" are not synonymous. An intrapulmonary abscess without communication with the bronchial tree is roentgenographically opaque; only when the abscess communicates with the bronchial tree, allowing air to replace necrotic material, should the term "cavity" be applied.

The great majority of pulmonary cavities are caused by tissue necrosis followed by expulsion of necrotic material into the bronchial tree. Exceptions are uncommon but include ruptured bronchial or echinococcal cysts (whose contents were originally mucus or fluid rather than necrotic tissue) and an infected cystic space such as a bulla.

The roentgenographic demonstration of pulmonary cavitation is often simple; for example, if the cavity contains fluid, as is frequently the case, the identification of a fluid level is clearly pathognomonic. In some cases, however, confident identification is not easy. The greatest diagnostic difficulty occurs when cavities are small or are situated either among an inhomogeneous group of opacities or in anatomic regions that are ordinarily difficult to see, such as the paramediastinal zones. In these latter circumstances, conventional tomography or CT may be essential to confirm the diagnosis or, perhaps more commonly, to identify cavitary disease that was not even remotely suspected on conventional roentgenograms.

Occasionally, lesions interpreted as cavities on premortem roentgenograms are found at necropsy to contain no air and to have no communication with the bronchial tree. Such pseudocavities are uncommon, but it is important to be aware of them. Histologically, the center of these lesions is composed of necrotic tissue; it is assumed that some chemical change occurs within it, rendering its lipid content sufficiently high to cause a relatively radiolucent shadow roentgenographically that simulates cavitation. Although this phenomenon is generally regarded as a feature of granulomas,[37] it should *not* be regarded as an unequivocal sign of a benign process.

Although the nature of cavity formation within specific disease groups varies considerably, in most cases the general patterns give some indication of the underlying etiology (Fig. 4–50). The roentgenographic features that should be noted in any case of cavitary lung disease include the thickness of the cavity wall, the smoothness or irregularity of its inner lining, the presence and character of its contents, and whether lesions are solitary or multiple. The following examples indicate prevailing patterns; in each category there are occasional exceptions to the general rule.

Cavity Wall. The wall of the cavity usually is thick in acute lung abscess (*see* Fig. 4–49), primary (Fig. 4–51) and metastatic carcinoma, and Wegener's granulomatosis, and

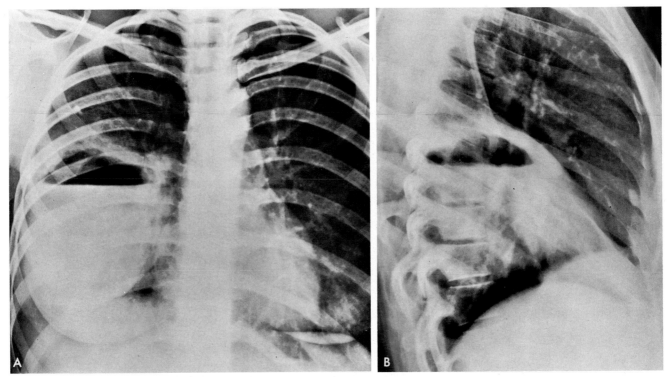

Figure 4–49. Bulging of Interlobar Fissures: Acute Staphylococcal Lung Abscess. Roentgenograms in posteroanterior *(A)* and lateral *(B)* projections reveal a large abscess in the right lower lobe producing upward bulging of the major fissure.

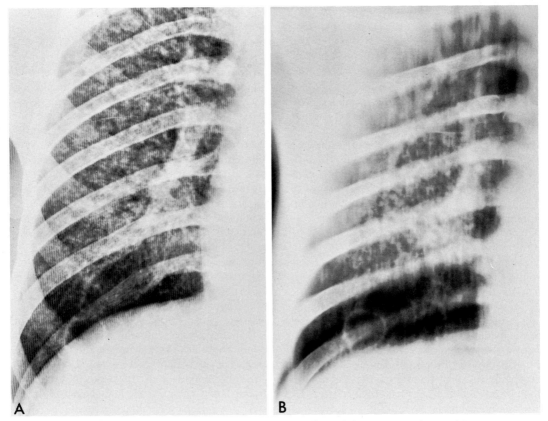

Figure 4–50. Tuberculous Lung Cavity with Bronchogenic Spread. A posteroanterior roentgenogram *(A)* and anteroposterior tomogram *(B)* of the right lung reveal a well-defined, thin-walled cavity in the base of the right lower lobe. Multiple poorly defined shadows possessing the typical characteristics of acinar lesions can be identified throughout much of the right lung, representing bronchogenic spread from the tuberculous cavity. This combination of changes constitutes almost certain evidence of a tuberculous etiology. (Courtesy of the Montreal Chest Hospital Center.)

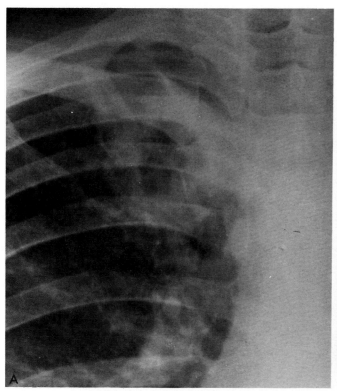
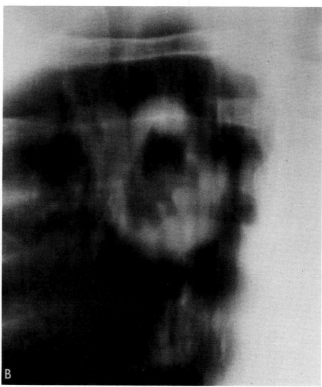

Figure 4–51. Cavitated Pulmonary Carcinoma. Views of the upper half of the right lung from a posteroanterior roentgenogram (A) and an anteroposterior tomogram *(B)* reveal a rather poorly defined cavitated mass. The thickness of the wall and irregular nodular character of the inner lining are highly suggestive of carcinoma. Squamous cell cancer.

almost invariably is thin in infected bullae and post-traumatic cysts. Assessment of wall thickness is especially helpful in distinguishing benign from malignant lesions. For example, in one study of 65 solitary pulmonary cavities, all those in which the thickest part of the cavity wall was 1 mm were benign; of the lesions whose thickest measurement was 4 mm or less, 92 per cent were benign; among cavities that were 5 to 15 mm in their thickest part, benign and malignant lesions were equally represented; finally, when the cavity wall was thicker than 15 mm, 92 per cent of lesions were malignant.[38] According to this study, and in our own experience, measurement of the thickest part of a cavity wall provides a more reliable indication of the benign or malignant character of a lesion than does measurement of the thinnest part.

Character of Inner Lining. The inner lining is usually irregular and nodular in carcinoma (*see* Fig. 4–51), shaggy in acute lung abscess, and smooth in most other lesions.

Nature of Contents. In the majority of cases the contents are liquid, resulting in a flat, smooth fluid level with no distinctive characteristics. In certain diseases, however, the appearance of the contents may be so typical as to be highly suggestive of a specific diagnosis. For example, either an intracavitary fungus ball (Fig. 4–52) or blood clot may form a freely mobile, spherical or lobulated intracavitary mass. Even more characteristic is the appearance sometimes seen in a ruptured echinococcus cyst, in which the membranes float on top of the fluid within the cyst and create the characteristic *water lily* sign, or the *sign of the camalote* (a water plant found in South American rivers; Fig. 4–53).[39]

Multiplicity of Lesions. Some cavitary lesions, such as primary pulmonary carcinoma and acute lung abscess, are characteristically solitary; others are usually multiple, for example, metastatic neoplasm, Wegener's granulomatosis, and acute pyemic abscesses.

Calcification

Intrathoracic calcification is an important diagnostic feature of pulmonary disease. In the majority of cases it is dystrophic (calcium deposition in damaged or dead tissue); less commonly, it is metastatic (calcification of vital tissues). Although the latter is frequent in cases of severe hypercalcemia, it is seldom roentgenographically visible. In addition to the simple tissue deposition of calcium, lamellar bone also can be identified roentgenographically or pathologically in some cases, and then the term "ossification" should be employed.

It is convenient to consider intrathoracic calcification or ossification under five headings, depending on its anatomic location and distribution: local parenchymal, widespread parenchymal, lymph node, pleural, and other.

Local Parenchymal Calcification. The commonest form of pulmonary calcification is a healed primary granulomatous lesion (Ghon focus), consisting of a single, often densely calcified focus, 5 to 20 mm in diameter situated anywhere in the lungs (Fig. 4–54). (Strictly speaking, the term "Ghon focus" refers to the primary parenchymal lesion of tuberculosis; however, since it is often impossible to be certain of the cause of these calcified foci, the term is widely used to refer to all such lesions.) The Ghon focus is

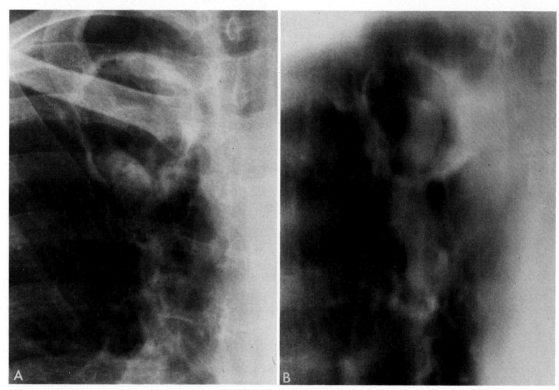

Figure 4–52. Intracavitary Fungus Ball. Views of the upper half of the right lung from a posteroanterior roentgenogram *(A)* and an anteroposterior tomogram *(B)* reveal a rather thin-walled but irregular cavity in the paramediastinal zone. Situated within it is a smooth oblong shadow of homogenous density whose relationships to the wall of the cavity change from the erect *(A)* to the supine *(B)* positions. The cavity was of tuberculous etiology, and the loose body was an aspergilloma.

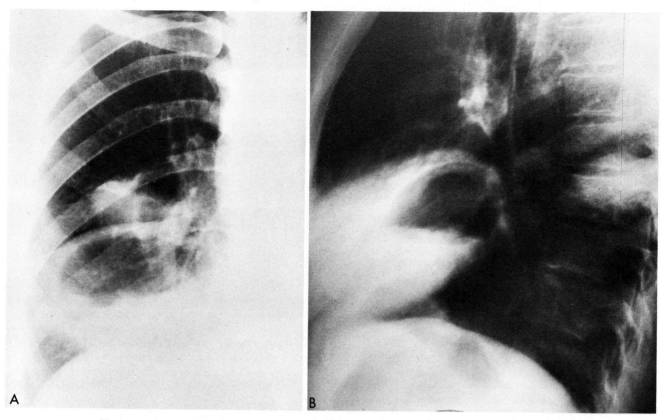

Figure 4–53. Hydatid Cyst with Bronchial Communication. Views of the right lung from posteroanterior *(A)* and lateral *(B)* roentgenograms reveal a large mass in the right middle lobe and a smaller mass in the superior segment of the right lower lobe; the middle lobe mass contains a large central cavity with a prominent air-fluid level, the latter possessing an irregular, lumpy configuration caused by floating membranes from a collapsed echinococcal cyst (the water lily sign, or sign of the camalote). (Courtesy of the Jean Talon Hospital, Montreal.)

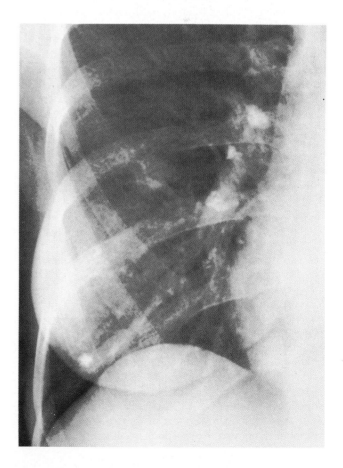

Figure 4–54. The Ranke Complex. A view of the lower half of the right lung from a posteroanterior roentgenogram reveals a solitary, densely calcified nodule just above the right costophrenic sulcus (the Ghon focus); the calcification is homogeneous although irregular. Situated in the right hilum are three or four lymph nodes containing scattered punctate calcium deposits.

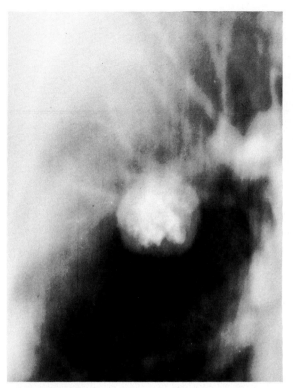

Figure 4–55. Calcification in Pulmonary Hamartoma. A conventional linear tomogram in anteroposterior projection shows a 3-cm, well-defined nodule in the anterior segment of the right upper lobe. The lesion contains a large central area of so-called "popcorn-ball" calcification characteristic of hamartoma.

usually part of a duo (the Ranke complex), the other component being calcified hilar- or mediastinal-drainage lymph nodes. Identification of the Ranke complex fairly conclusively establishes previous infection, most frequently caused by histoplasmosis (at least in areas where it is endemic), less often tuberculosis, occasionally coccidioidomycosis, and rarely other fungal infections. Deciding on the correct cause may be aided by the roentgenographic demonstration of multiple punctate calcifications in the spleen, which are almost always due to histoplasmosis.

The character of the calcification within a solitary pulmonary nodule also may be an important indicator of its etiology. For example, a small *central nidus* is the sign of a granulomatous lesion in most cases (although it also occurs in some hamartomas); *lamination* is almost pathognomonic of a granuloma, usually histoplasmoma, and is the most reliable sign of a benign lesion; *popcorn-ball* calcification is characteristic of hamartoma (Fig. 4–55); and *multiple punctate foci* throughout a lesion may be seen in either granulomas or hamartomas.[40]

Identification of calcification within a solitary pulmonary nodule is important, since it is the most reliable single piece of evidence that a lesion is benign.[40] This is probably related to duration of the lesion rather than to an intrinsic difference in tissue composition; although calcium is deposited in necrotic tissue of both granulomatous and neoplastic lesions, in most cases carcinoma becomes manifest clinically or roentgenographically before sufficient calcium accumulates to be visible. Although calcification is indicative of a benign process in the vast majority of cases, there are a number of noteworthy exceptions, including (1) a periph-

eral primary carcinoma engulfing an existing calcified granuloma, in which case the calcification is usually eccentric; (2) a solitary metastasis, most often from osteogenic sarcoma or chondrosarcoma, in which calcification (or, more often, ossification) occurs as a natural component of the neoplasm; and (3) the occasional instance of a primary pulmonary carcinoma (usually a peripheral adencarcinoma) that, because of the presence of psammoma bodies or dystrophic calcification, presents with diffuse punctate deposits of calcium.[41]

In the investigation of solitary pulmonary nodules, both conventional tomography and CT can sometimes permit identification of calcification not seen or only suggested on plain roentgenograms. In addition, dual-energy digital radiography has been shown to be a highly reliable quantitative technique in the assessment of the calcium content of pulmonary nodules (Fig. 4–56).[42] Preliminary investigations indicate that, in distinguishing benign from malignant lesions on the basis of calcium content, the accuracy of dual-energy is in all instances comparable, and in some instances superior, to that of conventional radiography, conventional tomography, and CT.

Diffuse Parenchymal Calcification. Diffuse parenchymal calcification may be caused by several conditions, but the pattern in each is usually distinctive. For example, the tiny punctate *calcispherytes* of alveolar microlithiasis present a unique, virtually unmistakable roentgenographic image. Multiple nodular foci of calcification or ossification occur in various conditions, including silicosis, mitral stenosis (Fig. 4–57),[43] and certain healed disseminated infectious diseases such as histoplasmosis and varicella pneumonitis.[44] The multiple foci of ossification seen in mitral stenosis usually can be differentiated from the calcification of healed infectious disease by their size (the former measure up to 8 mm in diameter, whereas the latter seldom exceed 2 to 3 mm) and occasionally by the presence of bony trabeculae. Scattered foci of calcification or ossification, sometimes possessing a reticular pattern, can also be idiopathic.[45]

Extensive metastatic pulmonary calcification may occur in cases of longstanding hypercalcemia associated with chronic renal disease and secondary hyperparathyroidism, and in other diseases, such as diffuse myelomatosis, in which the serum calcium level is chronically elevated. It shows remarkable predilection for apical and subapical lung zones, a feature attributed to the high $\dot{V}/\dot{Q}$ ratio that exists in the upper lung zones as compared with the lower ones.[46] The calcific nature of the pulmonary opacities can be readily confirmed by CT or dual-energy radiography or by scanning with bone imaging agents such as technetium 99m (^{99m}Tc) diphosphonate[47]; diffuse uptake of gallium 67 also has been observed.[48]

Lymph Node Calcification. Foci of calcification in lymph nodes are usually amorphous and irregularly distributed throughout the node (*see* Fig. 4–54). Most often, calcification results from healed granulomatous infection, usually tuberculosis or histoplasmosis, and constitutes part of the Ranke complex. Although calcified hilar or mediastinal lymph nodes are usually an incidental finding of little or no clinical significance, they may erode a contiguous airway, causing broncholithiasis with resultant hemoptysis and chronic cough (Fig. 4–58).

"Eggshell" calcification is an uncommon but distinctive

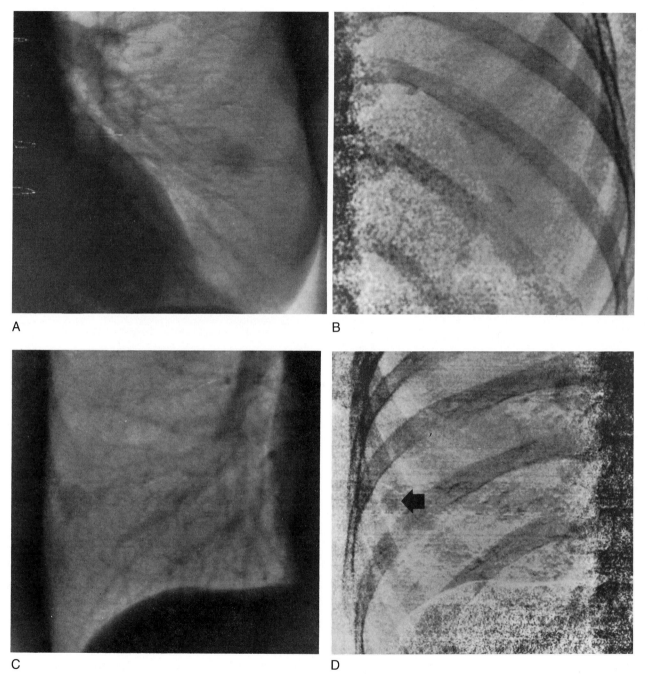

Figure 4–56. Evaluation of the Calcium Content of Solitary Pulmonary Nodules by Dual-Energy Digital Radiography. A digital image of the left lower lobe with bones subtracted *(A)* reveals a solitary pulmonary nodule of soft tissue density. On a bone image (soft tissues subtracted) *(B)*, the lesion is no longer visible and thus is not calcified. Proved adenocarcinoma. Compare these appearances with images of the right lower lobe of a different patient who had had a right mastectomy several years previously: the nodule on the soft tissue image *(C)* looks much the same as the nodule in *A;* however, on the bone image *(D)*, a focus of calcification is visible *(arrow)* that measures about 6 mm less than the nodule in *C*. Presumed histoplasmoma (being followed).

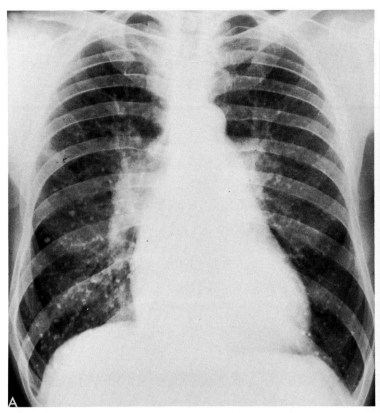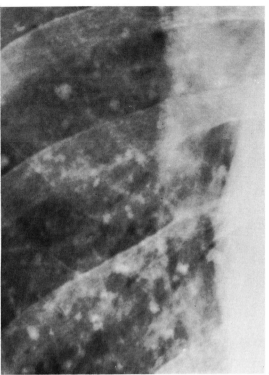

Figure 4–57. Pulmonary Ossification in Mitral Stenosis. A posteroanterior roentgenogram *(A)* of a 46-year-old man with long-standing mitral stenosis and severe pulmonary arterial hypertension reveals multiple, densely calcified nodular shadows ranging in diameter from 1 to 5 mm, situated predominantly in the lower half of the right lung *(B)*. Lesions of this type and localization are highly suggestive (if not diagnostic) of long-standing mitral stenosis.

variety of nodal calcification that appears as a dense ring around the periphery of a lymph node. The bronchopulmonary and hilar nodes are affected most frequently, but involvement of mediastinal and even retroperitoneal nodes can occur. Eggshell calcification is very suggestive of either silicosis or coal workers' pneumoconiosis, although it has been described also in sarcoidosis, Hodgkin's disease (following irradiation), infections such as blastomycosis and histoplasmosis, progressive systemic sclerosis, and amyloidosis.[49]

Pleural Calcification. Pleural calcification is most often the result of a remote hemothorax, pyothorax, or tuberculous effusion, in which case it commonly is associated with thickening of the pleura over the entire lung surface (Fig. 4–59). The calcification usually takes the form of a broad continuous sheet or of multiple discrete plaques. It usually extends from about the level of the midthorax posteriorly, around the lateral lung margin in a generally inferior direction, roughly paralleling the chief fissure. Characteristically, the calcium is deposited on the inner surface of the thickened pleura; as a result, a thick tissue layer of unit density exists between the calcium and the thoracic wall.

Pleural calcification also is a common manifestation of asbestos exposure (Fig. 4–60). The roentgenologic characteristics are sufficiently different from those of calcification secondary to empyema or hemothorax that there should be no difficulty distinguishing the two. The calcification usually occurs in fibrous plaques, commonly along the diaphragm

bilaterally; it almost always occurs in the parietal pleura, whereas when secondary to pyothorax or hemothorax it is usually confined to the visceral pleura. The mediastinal pleura may be involved, but calcification of the interlobar pleura is very uncommon.

Calcification in Other Sites. Calcification or ossification of the cartilage plates of the trachea and major bronchi appears to be a physiologic concomitant of aging; curiously, it is far more common in elderly women than in men.[50] It also may appear in younger patients with hypercalcemia and hyperphosphatemia. In contrast to this innocuous calcification of degenerative or metastatic origin is the rare condition known as tracheobronchopathia osteochondroplastica, in which nodules or spicules of cartilage and bone develop in the submucosa of the trachea and bronchi and may occasion symptoms of chronic obstructive pulmonary disease.

Calcification of the walls of the central pulmonary arteries occurs in a large percentage of patients with severe long-standing pulmonary arterial hypertension, particularly those with a left-to-right shunt.

Distribution of Disease Within the Lungs (Anatomic Bias)

For several reasons, some known and others obscure, many lung diseases tend to develop only or predominantly

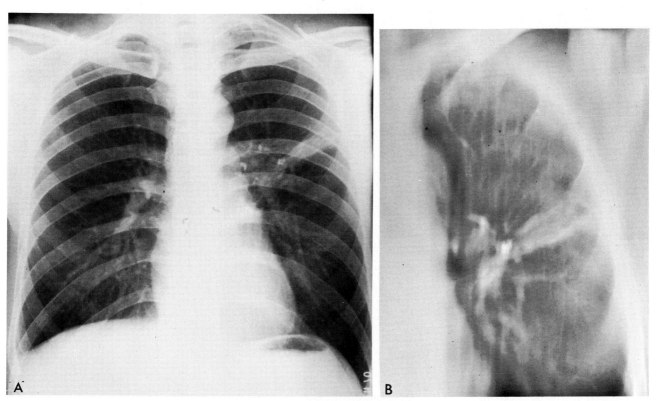

Figure 4–58. Broncholith Associated with Focal Atelectasis and Pneumonitis, Left Upper Lobe. A broad band shadow can be seen in both the posteroanterior roentgenogram (A) and the anteroposterior tomogram (B), extending in a roughly horizontal plane from the lateral aspect of the left hilum to the axillary visceral pleura. The shadow is of variegated density, suggesting the presence of air within dilated airways. The calcific density at the medial aspect of the shadow is a broncholith that is partially obstructing the affected bronchus. Presumed histoplasmosis.

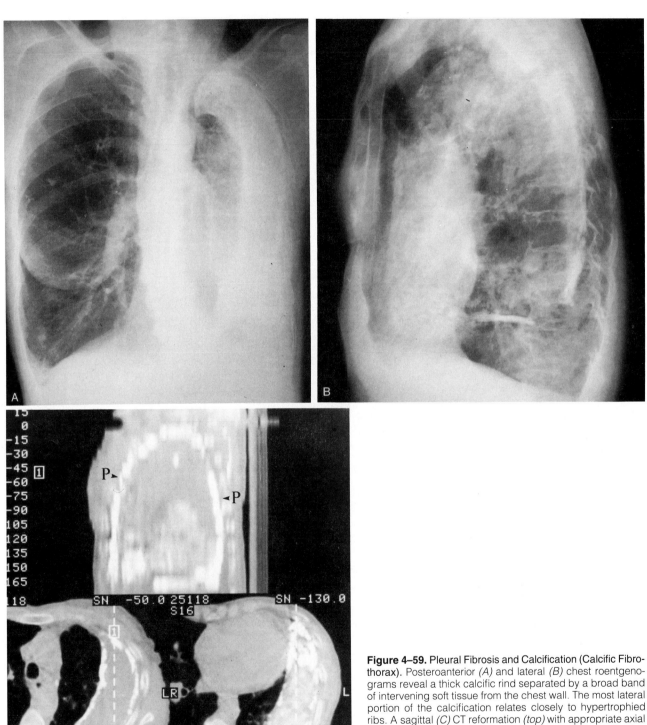

Figure 4–59. Pleural Fibrosis and Calcification (Calcific Fibro-thorax). Posteroanterior *(A)* and lateral *(B)* chest roentgeno-grams reveal a thick calcific rind separated by a broad band of intervening soft tissue from the chest wall. The most lateral portion of the calcification relates closely to hypertrophied ribs. A sagittal *(C)* CT reformation *(top)* with appropriate axial CT scans *(bottom)* illustrate a thick mantle of calcification delineating the visceral and parietal (P) pleura; the tissue between the pleural layers is both fibrous and calcific in nature. The patient is a middle-aged woman with a history of previous tuberculous empyema.

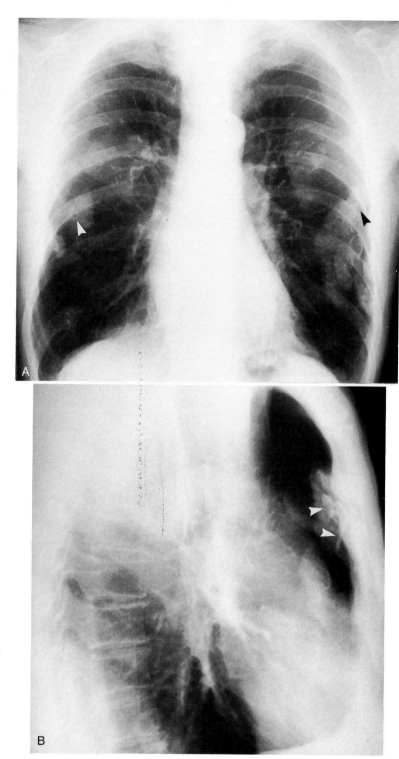

Figure 4–60. Pleural Calcification. Posteroanterior *(A)* and lateral *(B)* chest roentgenograms reveal numerous peripheral masses or plaques bilaterally with roentgenographic characteristics of pleural or extrapleural lesions. The plaques are congregated along the midaxillary and anterior portions of the thorax; many contain linear or mottled calcifications *(arrowheads)*. This appearance is virtually diagnostic of asbestos-related pleural disease.

in certain anatomic locations. Knowledge of such anatomic bias is of obvious diagnostic importance.

Aspiration pneumonia is a typical example in which the influence of gravity largely establishes the anatomic distribution of disease. If aspiration occurs when the patient is supine (during the postoperative period, for instance), the upper lobes are involved more often than the lower ones, and their posterior portions more frequently than the anterior ones; conversely, if aspiration occurs when the patient is erect, involvement of the lower lobes predominates. Whether the patient is recumbent or erect, aspiration occurs more readily into the right lung than the left, because of the more direct origin of the right main bronchus from the trachea.

It is possible that gravity also plays a significant role in the pathogenesis of pneumococcal pneumonia. In an ingenious series of experiments on dogs, the anatomic site in which pneumonia developed could be controlled by altering the position of a dog's thorax so that bacteria-laden exudate flowed into specific segments under the influence of gravity.[51] That this effect is operative in humans is supported by the tendency of acute airspace pneumonia to occur predominantly in the posterior portions of lobes.

Pulmonary infarction occurs much more frequently in lower than in upper lobes, an anatomic bias that undoubtedly reflects the disparity in blood flow to the base and apex of the lung in erect humans. For the same reason, metastatic carcinoma occurs more frequently in lower lobes. By contrast, primary pulmonary carcinoma has an unexplained predilection for upper lung zones; for example, in one study of 250 cases,[52] the ratio of upper to lower lobe origin was approximately 2.5:1. Cavitation of pulmonary carcinoma also is much more likely to occur in the upper than the lower lobes; it has been postulated that this tendency may be due to the normal stresses in the lung apex, which are three to four times greater than in the base.[53]

Pulmonary tuberculosis provides a singular opportunity to employ anatomic bias in differential diagnosis. In postprimary tuberculosis in adults, susceptibility of the apical and posterior bronchopulmonary segments of the upper lobes and the superior segment of the lower lobes is well recognized; for example, these three segments were involved in *all* 100 cases in one series.[54] The reason for this remarkable localization is unclear; however, these segments of lung are characterized by a high $\dot{V}/\dot{Q}$ ratio and relatively high P_{O_2} levels, possibly favoring growth of mycobacteria. The rarity with which the anterior bronchopulmonary segment of an upper lobe is affected *to the exclusion of other segments* is sufficient to make the diagnosis of postprimary tuberculosis in this area extremely unlikely (only one case was reported in the series cited above). For reasons that are unclear, primary tuberculosis shows an anatomic bias opposite that of the postprimary form.

Diffuse lung disease frequently shows an anatomic bias, a factor that may be important to differential diagnosis. For example, reticulation of asbestosis, fibrosing alveolitis, and connective tissue diseases such as progressive systemic sclerosis and rheumatoid disease typically show a predominant basal distribution. Conversely, upper lobe predilection is shown by silicosis, sarcoidosis, eosinophilic granuloma, and the progressive massive fibrosis of complicated silicosis and coal workers' pneumoconiosis.

Roentgenologic Localization of Pulmonary Disease (the Silhouette Sign)

The anatomic location of the great majority of pulmonary diseases that increase local density can be established pre-

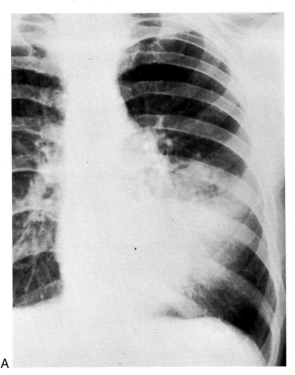
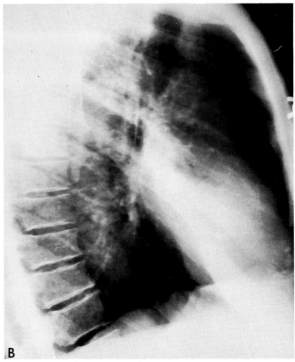

Figure 4–61. The Silhouette Sign. Posteroanterior *(A)* and lateral *(B)* roentgenograms reveal obliteration of the left heart border by a shadow of homogeneous density situated within the lingula; such obliteration inevitably indicates lingular disease (provided there is adequate roentgenographic exposure). Squamous cell carcinoma of the lingular bronchus with distal obstructive pneumonitis.

cisely from posteroanterior and lateral roentgenograms. In two situations, however, this may be difficult: (1) when one or more segments of both lungs are involved, with resultant confusion of superimposed shadows in lateral projection, and (2) when only an anteroposterior projection of the chest is available for evaluation (for example, in the immediate postoperative period or when a patient is too ill for standard roentgenography). In these circumstances, the silhouette sign is particularly useful.[19, 20]

This sign has its basis in the fact that the mediastinal and diaphragmatic contours normally are rendered roentgenographically visible by their contrast with contiguous air-containing lung. Thus, when air is replaced by an opacity situated in any portion of lung adjacent to a mediastinal or diaphragmatic border, that border can no longer be seen roentgenographically (Fig. 4–61). The corollary is that an opacity within the lungs that does *not* obliterate the mediastinal or diaphragmatic contour cannot be situated within lung contiguous to these structures. Clearly, this sign is apparent only when structures have been adequately penetrated; for example, in an underpenetrated roentgenogram, massive consolidation of the right lower lobe prevents identification of the right border of the heart, merely because the flux of roentgen rays is of insufficient penetration to reproduce the heart shadow through the lower lobe opacity, despite the presence of air-containing lung contiguous with the heart.

The silhouette sign is perhaps of most use in distinguishing middle lobe and lingular disease from lower lobe disease; however, in many other sites it may indicate the precise anatomic location, for example, obliteration of the aortic knuckle on the left side by airlessness of the apical posterior segment of the left upper lobe, obliteration of the ascending arch of the aorta and of the superior vena cava by consolidation of the anterior bronchopulmonary segment of the right upper lobe, or obliteration of the left paraspinal line by contiguous airless lung in the posterior gutter.

Although this sign is used chiefly to localize pulmonary disease, we have found it almost as useful for identifying disease processes. For example, on a posteroanterior roentgenogram the increased density produced by total collapse of the right middle lobe may be impossible to appreciate subjectively; however, the silhouette sign almost invariably accompanies such collapse (apparent as loss of sharp definition of the right heart border) and should strongly suggest that there is disease in the right middle lobe (a lateral projection is confirmatory). (An uncommon exception to this "rule" is severe pectus excavatum, which occasionally is associated with loss of definition of the right heart border.) Similarly, it may be very difficult to identify minor consolidation or atelectasis in a posterior basal segment of a lower lobe; however, invisibility of the posterior portion of the hemidiaphragm in lateral projection often permits identification of disease in this segment.

The Time Factor in Roentgenologic Diagnosis

In both acute and chronic lung diseases, roentgenographic signs may overlap or be so nonspecific that only differential diagnostic possibilities can be suggested at the first examination; if the diagnosis cannot be established by

integrating the clinical evidence and results of laboratory and pulmonary function tests, serial films showing changes over the subsequent days, weeks, or months often provide valuable clues.

Such changes are particularly useful in acute lung disease. For example, in thromboembolic disease, consolidation that clears within 4 to 7 days indicates pulmonary hemorrhage without necrosis; by contrast, persistence of the opacity with progressive retraction and loss of volume supports the presence of tissue death. The rapidity with which diffuse interstitial pulmonary edema may appear and disappear (often within hours) allows immediate differentiation from irreversible interstitial disease, which it may otherwise closely mimic. Similarly, it is surprising how frequently a small area of parenchymal consolidation in an upper lobe, roentgenographically typical of exudative tuberculosis, disappears in a few days, indicating a less significant etiology.

The relationship between roentgenograms taken at different times is also important in more chronic disease. This is perhaps best exemplified by the concept of doubling time of pulmonary nodules (Fig. 4–62). Since some benign lesions such as hamartoma and histoplasmoma may grow slowly, increase in size *per se* cannot be the sole consideration in deciding a nodule's benign or malignant nature. Of much greater value is an estimate of the *rate* of growth, as determined by measuring the doubling time.° For example, in one study of 218 pulmonary nodules of which 177 were malignant and 41 benign, virtually all nodules with a doubling time of 7 days or less were benign[55]; if metastatic choriocarcinoma, testicular neoplasms, and osteogenic sarcoma were eliminated, the doubling time for benign lesions increased to 11 days. At the other end of the scale, almost all nodules whose volume doubled in 465 days or more were benign.

Linear Opacities

A linear opacity (line shadow, linear shadow, band shadow) can be defined as "a shadow resembling a line; hence, any elongated opacity of approximately uniform width." The term embraces the normal vascular markings and interlobar fissures as well as many opacities of various causes seen from time to time in roentgenograms of the chest. Such opacities can be considered in six categories: (1) septal lines, (2) tubular shadows (bronchial wall shadows), (3) linear opacities extending from parenchymal lesions to the hila or visceral pleura, (4) parenchymal scarring, (5) line shadows of pleural origin, and (6) long horizontal or obliquely oriented linear opacities occurring at or near the lung bases.

Septal Lines. Septal lines (commonly referred to as *Kerley A, B, and C lines*) are caused by thickening of the interstitial tissue in the interlobular septa and around deep parenchymal veins and anastomotic lymphatic channels. Although this thickening may be due to lymphatic distention alone, most often it is caused predominantly by accumula-

---

°Doubling in this context refers to volume, not diameter. Assuming a nodule to be spherical, multiply its diameter by 1.25 to obtain the diameter of a sphere whose volume is double (e.g., the volume of a nodule 2 cm in diameter is doubled when its diameter reaches 2.5 cm).

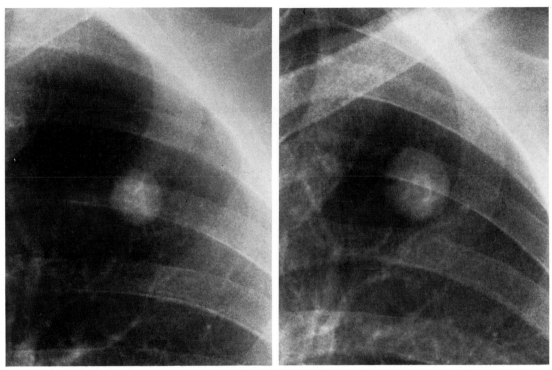

A   B

Figure 4–62. Solitary Nodule: Enlarging Histoplasmoma. In 1969 *(A),* a solitary nodule in the left upper lobe of this 61-year-old asymptomatic man measured 17 mm in diameter; it was sharply defined and showed no convincing evidence of calcification. Two years later *(B),* the diameter of the lesion had reached 21 mm, representing almost a doubling of volume. A central nidus of calcification could now be clearly identified. Proved histoplasmoma.

tion of fluid or tissue in the interstitial space itself.[56] Depending on the disease process that causes them, the lines may be reversible (as in pulmonary edema) or irreversible (as in pneumoconiosis or lymphangitic carcinoma).

Kerley A lines are straight or almost straight linear opacities, seldom more than 1 mm thick and 2 to 6 cm long. Their course bears no definite relationship to the anatomic distribution of bronchoarterial bundles (Fig. 4–63). Unlike Kerley B lines, they never extend to the visceral pleura, although medial extension is usually to a hilum. Although it was originally thought these lines were produced by anastomotic lymphatic channels crossing from perivenous to peribronchial sites, more recent investigations suggest that they represent bands of connective tissue deep in the lung in which run both veins and anastomotic lymphatics.[56]

Kerley B lines are located in the periphery of the lung, where they lie roughly perpendicular to the pleural surface *(see* Fig. 4–39). They are short and straight, seldom being more than 1 mm thick and 2 cm long. Their outer ends invariably abut the visceral pleura, although this relationship may not be apparent on posteroanterior roentgenograms. Care is needed to avoid mistaking small vascular shadows in the lung periphery for Kerley B lines; the former branch, the latter never do.

B lines are caused by increased fluid or tissue in the interlobular septa; because of this location, they are sometimes referred to as septal lines. One of the commonest causes is interstitial pulmonary edema secondary to pulmonary venous hypertension. In such circumstances, the influ-

ence of gravity on pulmonary hemodynamics gives rise to interlobular septal edema predominantly in the lower portions of the lungs; thus, B lines are seen to best advantage just above the costophrenic angles on posteroanterior roentgenograms. When the edema is transient, septal lines appear and disappear sporadically with each episode of decompensation; with repeated insults of this character, or in the presence of chronic and severe pulmonary venous hypertension, fibrosis within the interlobular septa gives rise to permanent B lines.

In other diseases, the anatomic distribution of B lines may be entirely different. For example, in pneumoconiosis, sarcoidosis, lymphangitic carcinomatosis, and lymphoma *(see* Fig. 4–41) in which gravity is not an influence, septal lines may be visible anywhere in the lung periphery where septa normally occur—along most of the axillary portion of the lung up to the apex and in the retrosternal space.

Kerley C Lines consist of pyramidal linear opacities projected on the anterior portion of both lungs, their size and configuration corresponding to secondary lobules. Although they are reputed to be caused by engorgement of pleural lymphatics, it is difficult to believe that a single layer of lymphatics projected *en face* could conceivably cast a roentgenographic shadow. Rather, it is likely they are caused by the superimposition of many Kerley B lines in the anterior and posterior portions of the lungs.[57]

Tubular Shadows (Bronchial Wall Shadows). The air column of the trachea, main bronchi, right intermediate bronchus, and left lower lobe bronchus normally is visible

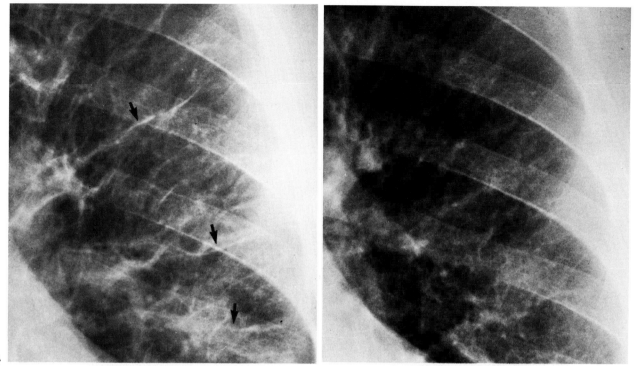

Figure 4–63. Line Shadows: Kerley A Lines. A view of the left lung from a posteroanterior roentgeno-gram *(A)* reveals a coarse network of linear strands widely distributed throughout the lung. Several long line shadows measuring up to 4 cm in length can be identified in the central zone *(arrows)*, extending medially to the hilum but not laterally to the pleura. The orientation of these lines does not conform to the distribution of bronchovascular bundles. These are Kerley A lines and represent edema of central pulmonary septa. A roentgenogram made several days later *(B)* shows complete clearing of the pulmonary edema.

on well-exposed roentgenograms. Where these structures are in contact with air-containing parenchyma their walls also are visible, their thickness being sufficient to cast a roentgenographic shadow that typically is tubular. Beyond the immediate confines of the hila, however, airway walls are so thin that neither they nor the bronchial air columns should be visible normally (except when viewed end-on [*see later*]); thus, when tubular shadows are identified outside the hilar limits, they usually constitute a sign of disease. Such tubular shadows are double-line shadows that may be parallel or slightly tapered as they proceed distally. They always follow the bronchovascular distribution and may branch in a manner characteristic of the bronchial tree. Morphologically, they are caused predominantly by thick-ened bronchial walls due to fibrosis and an inflammatory infiltrate.

The most common cause of tubular shadows is bron-chiectasis (Fig. 4–64), in which the line shadows are usually multiple and measure 1 mm or slightly more in width. The width of the air column separating them depends on the severity of the bronchial dilatation. Because chronic bron-chiectasis is often associated with atelectasis, multiple tubular shadows may be crowded together with little air-containing parenchyma separating them. This typical ap-pearance can be altered in two situations, each of which has the same significance as the more classic appearance: (1) when one of the paired lines is contiguous with a vessel, in which case it casts no roentgenographic shadow; and (2) when the airway becomes filled with retained mucus or

pus, the tubular appearance thus being transformed into a homogeneous, bandlike, often branching, opacity, which has been termed the "gloved finger" shadow (Fig. 4–65).[58]

Tubular shadows can occasionally be identified as an iso-lated abnormality, usually in the right lower lobe, in persons without bronchiectasis (Fig. 4–66). As in the latter disease, their walls may be parallel; not infrequently, however, they taper in much the same fashion as a normal bronchus. Colloquially referred to by the British as "tram lines," in our experience they occur most often in cases of chronic bronchitis; one study[59] documented them in 45 per cent of 185 patients with this disease.

Bronchial walls also can be identified in the parahilar zones of a large percentage of healthy individuals when they are viewed end-on (Fig. 4–67).[60] The resulting shad-ows range in diameter from 3 to 7 mm and represent segmental or subsegmental bronchi in the anterior bron-chopulmonary segment of an upper lobe or the superior bronchopulmonary segment of a lower lobe. The reason for the visibility of a bronchial wall when *en face* as opposed to end-on is related to the different absorptive power of its tissue "in tangent." Since the image of the tangential wall thickness fades off at the margins, loss of definition pre-cludes accurate appreciation of total wall thickness; in con-trast, when the same tube is viewed end-on, a substantially greater amount of tissue is traversed by the x-ray beam, particularly at its periphery, thus reducing the effect of subliminal absorption.

Linear Opacities Extending from Parenchymal Le-

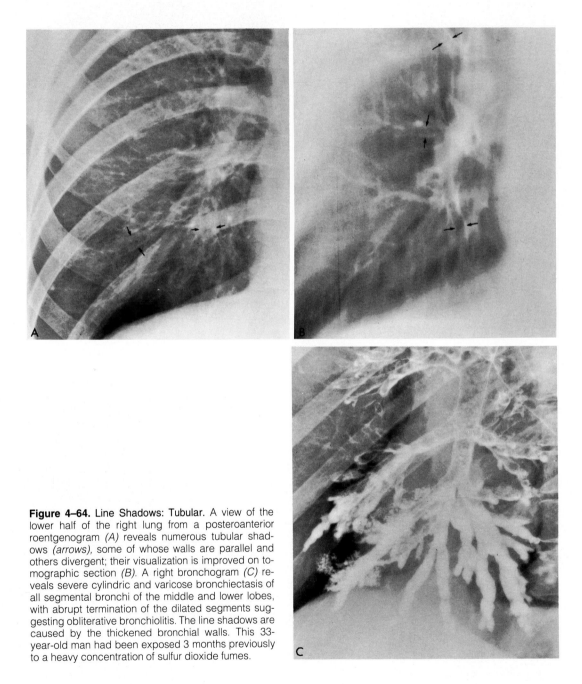

Figure 4–64. Line Shadows: Tubular. A view of the lower half of the right lung from a posteroanterior roentgenogram *(A)* reveals numerous tubular shadows *(arrows)*, some of whose walls are parallel and others divergent; their visualization is improved on tomographic section *(B)*. A right bronchogram *(C)* reveals severe cylindric and varicose bronchiectasis of all segmental bronchi of the middle and lower lobes, with abrupt termination of the dilated segments suggesting obliterative bronchiolitis. The line shadows are caused by the thickened bronchial walls. This 33-year-old man had been exposed 3 months previously to a heavy concentration of sulfur dioxide fumes.

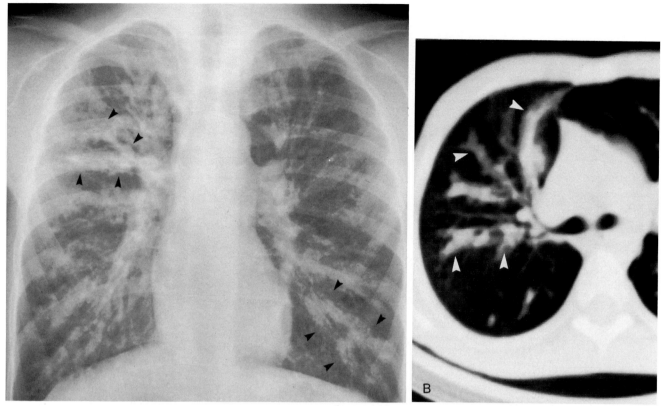

Figure 4–65. Cystic Fibrosis with Bronchiectasis and Mucoid Impaction. *A,* A posteroanterior chest roentgenogram reveals tubular, branching opacities *(arrowheads),* most numerous in the right upper and left lower lobes. *B,* A transverse CT scan through the carina reveals similar branching opacities *(arrowheads)* in the anterior and posterior segments of the right upper lobe. The opacities are caused by mucous plugs in ectatic bronchi and are characteristic of cystic fibrosis.

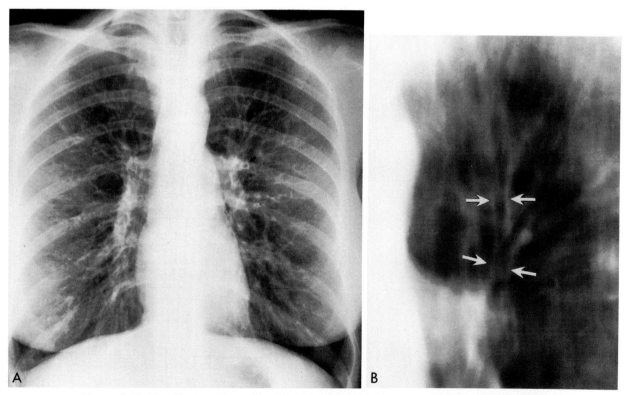

Figure 4–66. Line Shadows Caused by Thickened Bronchial Walls: Tram Lines. A posteroanterior roentgenogram *(A)* reveals prominent markings throughout both lungs. In the left upper zone, parallel or slightly tapering line shadows can be identified in the bronchial distribution of the left upper lobe, seen to better advantage on the anteroposterior tomogram in *B (arrows).* These "tram lines" represent thickened bronchial walls.

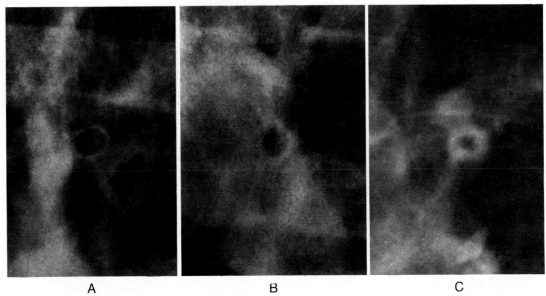

A   B   C

Figure 4–67. Bronchial Wall Thickening as Assessed from Parahilar Bronchi Viewed End-On. Views of the left parahilar zone from posteroanterior roentgenograms of three different patients, showing a normal bronchus (A), a bronchus with moderate wall thickening (B), and a bronchus with marked wall thickening (C). (From Fraser RG, Fraser RS, Renner JW, et al: The roentgenologic diagnosis of chronic bronchitis: a reassessment with emphasis on parahilar bronchi seen end-on. Radiology 120: 1, 1976.)

sions to the Hila or Visceral Pleura. Line shadows of varying width are often visible extending from a parenchymal opacity to the hilum. Although their course may be interrupted, it usually conforms to the pattern of vascular distribution, establishing the anatomic location of the opacities within bronchovascular bundles. Since these shadows may be present in both infectious and neoplastic lesions, they are of no value in differential diagnosis.

When a parenchymal mass is situated near the periphery of the lung, a line shadow also is sometimes visible extending from the mass to the visceral pleura, commonly caused by local in-drawing of the pleura itself (Fig. 4–68). Al-

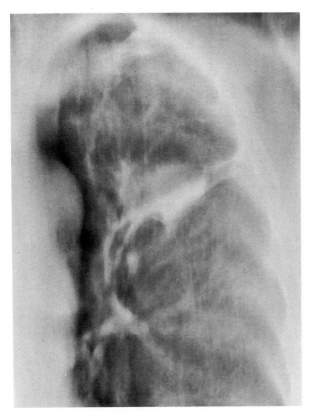

Figure 4–68. Line Shadows: Communication Between a Peripheral Mass and the Visceral Pleura. A view of the upper half of the left lung from an anteroposterior tomogram reveals a rather indistinctly defined homogeneous mass lying in the midlung zone. A prominent line shadow extends from the lateral margin of the mass to the pleura, resulting in a V-shaped deformity of the pleura caused by indrawing. Note also the prominent linear opacity extending medially to the hilum, presumably representing fibrosis and inflammation in the region of lymphatic drainage. Proved histoplasmosis.

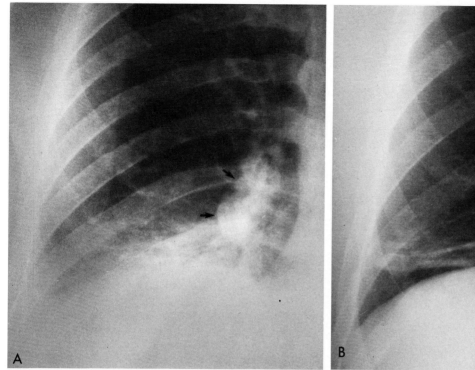
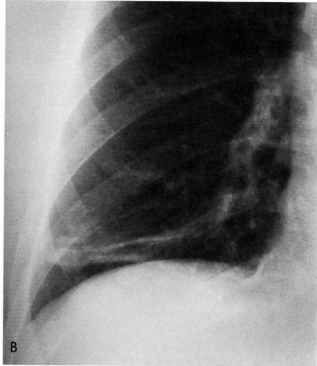

Figure 4–69. Linear Scarring Secondary to Pulmonary Embolism. A view of the right lung in antero-posterior projection *(A)* reveals bulging and "knuckling" of the right interlobar artery *(arrows)*. A homogeneous opacity is situated in distal lung parenchyma, obscuring the right hemidiaphragm. This combination of changes is highly suggestive of pulmonary embolism and infarction. Ten days later, a detail view of the right lower zone *(B)* demonstrated a horizontally oriented linear opacity at the right base that subsequently underwent little change in appearance over the next several months.

though this so-called *tail sign* has been regarded as an indicator of malignancy, particularly adenocarcinoma,[61] there is now convincing evidence that it represents an entirely nonspecific feature of peripherally located pulmonary lesions and cannot be used to differentiate a benign from a malignant process.[62]

Parenchymal Scarring. A segment of lung that was the site of infectious disease and has undergone healing through fibrosis may present as a linear shadow. Several opacities may be fairly closely grouped, commonly extending from the hilum to the visceral pleural surface and diverging slightly toward the periphery. In many cases, there is compensatory overinflation of adjacent lung parenchyma. Healed upper lobe postprimary tuberculosis is a common example of this type of shadow.

The line shadow created by healed pulmonary infarction represents fibrous scarring secondary to lung necrosis (Fig. 4–69). It always extends to a pleural surface, a relationship that has been suggested to be caused, at least in part, by indrawing of the pleura by the scar.[63] The same mechanism could be invoked to explain the linear opacities characterized as discoid atelectasis (*see* later).

Line Shadows of Pleural Origin. Roentgenographic visibility of fissures not normally seen in a particular projection may be important evidence of otherwise invisible disease. For example, when a lower lobe loses volume, the upper portion of the major fissure sweeps downward and medially and at a certain stage becomes visible on postero-anterior roentgenograms as an obliquely oriented shadow extending inferiorly and laterally from the lateral aspect of

the mediastinum above the hilum, across the shadow of the hilum, to end near the lateral costophrenic sulcus. This evidence of atelectasis may be present even when the density in the lower lobe is not increased.

Thickening of an interlobar fissure, especially if more or less uniform, is caused more often by pleural edema than by pleural effusion. Because the pleural connective tissue layer is continuous with the interlobular septa, when edema fluid accumulates in the latter sites (Kerley B lines) it also collects in the pleural interstitial space. In such circumstances, it not only thickens the interlobar fissures but also widens the pleural layer along the lung's convex surface.

Fibrous pleural thickening over the anterior or posterior lung surfaces occasionally gives rise to rather broad linear opacities usually situated near the lung bases (Fig. 4–70). These line shadows tend to appear rather "stringy" and commonly are oriented in a horizontal or oblique plane. Their true nature is usually apparent from their association with other signs of pleural fibrosis (such as obliteration of the costophrenic angle).

Another important indicator of disease is the "double" pleural line seen along either side of the mediastinum in cases of pneumomediastinum; the line shadow is created by the combined thicknesses of parietal and visceral pleura dislocated laterally by mediastinal gas.

Discoid Atelectasis. Few would dispute that, of all pathologic linear opacities observed on chest roentgenograms, the most common are those that tend to occur in the lung bases and that for many years have been called discoid atelectasis (platelike atelectasis, Fleischner's lines,

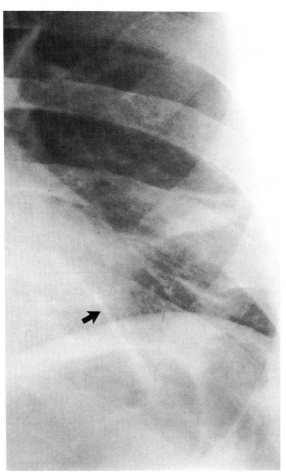

Figure 4–70. Line Shadows: Pleural Thickening. Several irregular line shadows of varying thickness and length are present over the lower portion of the left lung. Most of these are caused by irregular thickening of the pleura over the posterior portion of the left lower lobe (one line shadow indicated by an *arrow* follows the bronchovascular distrubtion and is caused by parenchymal scarring).

lated to several mechanisms. The opacities are almost invariably associated with conditions that diminish diaphragmatic excursion, such as intra-abdominal inflammatory disease. Such conditions may promote atelectasis by several means: (1) restriction of diaphragmatic excursion leading to decreased ventilation of the lungs, especially in the bases; (2) inhibition of coughing by the pain and discomfort it engenders, resulting in accumulation of bronchial secretions in the dependent portions of the lungs and obstruction of small airways; (3) stagnation of secretions and the development of pneumonia, leading to obstruction of channels of collateral ventilation by inflammatory exudate; and (4) reduction in surfactant production resulting from diminished perfusion secondary to decreased ventilation. Of considerable interest in the study cited above[64] was the observation that in 9 of the 10 patients, prominent interlobular septa were observed, either within or bordering the zone of atelectasis, suggesting that the absence of collateral ventilation due to intrinsic anatomic features also may be important.

Although many line shadows termed discoid atelectasis probably represent true atelectasis as described above, it is possible that some of them have another anatomic basis. In the late 1960s, Simon[65, 66] attributed horizontally or obliquely oriented opacities in the middle and lower lung zones to thrombosed arteries or veins, more commonly the latter. In recent years, we have observed many cases in which line shadows have an anatomic distribution similar to that reported by Simon; the major clues to their nature are their anatomic position (which shows little or no relation-

platter atelectasis). These linear opacities of unit density range from 1 to 3 mm in thickness and from 4 to 10 cm in length and are situated in the middle and lower lung zones, most commonly the latter (Fig. 4–71). Although usually oriented in a roughly horizontal plane, they may be obliquely oriented, depending on the zone of lung affected; in midlung zones particularly, they may be angled more than 45 degrees to the horizontal. They may be single or multiple, unilateral or bilateral.

The anatomic basis of discoid atelectasis was elucidated in a correlative roentgenologic-pathologic study of 10 patients whose last antemortem roentgenogram exhibited a linear opacity characteristic of the abnormality and who subsequently were examined at autopsy.[64] All 10 cases revealed subpleural parenchymal collapse combined with invagination of overlying pleura. The atelectasis was either deep to incomplete fissures or extended to pre-existing pleural clefts, but in either case the surface of the lung appeared folded in at the site of linear atelectasis. This frequent association with congenital pleural clefts, indentations, scars, and incomplete fissures suggested that discoid atelectasis may develop preferentially at sites of pre-existing pleural invagination.

The pathogenesis of discoid atelectasis is probably re-

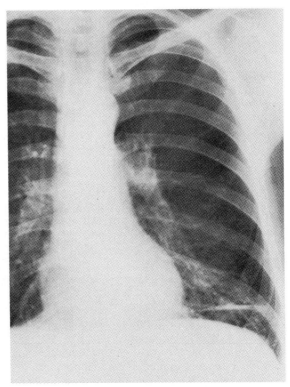

Figure 4–71. Line Shadows: Discoid Atelectasis. A view of the left lung from a posteroanterior roentgenogram reveals a line shadow measuring 3 mm in width and 9 cm in length situated in a plane just above the left hemidiaphragm and roughly horizontal in position. Two days postoperative laparotomy; the line had disappeared 4 days later.

ship to bronchovascular distribution) and the position of their medial extremity (which coincides with the left atrium). They range in thickness from 2 to 10 mm, and, in our experience, just as frequently follow the distribution of a major upper lobe vein as of veins draining the middle or lower zones. Although there is as yet incomplete pathologic correlation, we suspect that at least some of these shadows are the result of pulmonary venous thrombosis.

LUNG DISEASES THAT DECREASE ROENTGENOGRAPHIC DENSITY

Pulmonary diseases that cause a decrease in roentgenographic density (increase in translucency) can be considered in the same manner as those that increase density; just as density may be increased by a change in the relative amounts of air, blood, and interstitial tissue, so may decreased density result from alteration of these three elements. It is emphasized that here we are dealing with the diseases of the *lung* that cause reduced roentgenographic density and not of the thorax as a whole. Any assessment of chest roentgenograms must take into consideration the contribution that abnormalities of *extrapulmonary tissue* might make to reduced density. Thus, certain pleural diseases (e.g., pneumothorax) and some congenital and acquired abnormalities of the chest wall (e.g., congenital absence of the pectoral muscles, mastectomy, neuromuscular disorders that affect one side of the thorax) produce unilateral radiolucency that easily might be mistaken for pulmonary disease unless this possibility is continuously borne in mind.

The reduction of normal lung density in diseases that increase translucency may be very slight, and as a consequence the roentgenologist is faced with the apparent paradox of trying to classify a group of diseases on the basis of a sign that, at best, is extremely subtle. The reasons by which this approach may be justified are two.

1. In *generalized* diseases of the lung characterized by diffuse pulmonary overinflation (for example, emphysema), general reduction in density or increased "translucency" traditionally is cited as a reliable roentgenologic sign. In fact, the validity of this sign is questionable. For many reasons, the most cogent of which is the wide variation in exposure factors that characterizes much chest roentgenography, the impression of increased translucency is not only unreliable as a sign of overinflation but also may be false, particularly in healthy young men with a large total lung capacity. In such situations, reliance must be placed on the *secondary signs* (e.g., low, flat diaphragm) that are an integral part of these diseases; then, recognition of the overall pattern of roentgenographic change permits the *inference* that lung density must be reduced, allowing inclusion in this broad category of disease.

2. In *localized* diseases that reduce roentgenographic density (e.g., lobar emphysema or a large bulla), the story is entirely different. These conditions produce a region of lung in which the density change can be compared with the density in the remainder of the same lung or in the opposite lung, thereby supplying the dependable criterion of contrast. Thus, this group of local diseases can be classified according to absolute change in density, an advantage lacking in generalized disease.

Accepting that diseases that reduce density are characterized by an altered ratio of the three components of air, blood, and interstitial tissue, four combinations of changes can reduce lung density. On the basis of this classification and using the roentgenologic signs to be described, one can fairly confidently diagnose most cases of pulmonary disease that result in decreased density.

Increased Air but Unchanged Blood and Tissue (Fig. 4–72). This group of diseases is exemplified by obstructive overinflation without lung destruction. It may be *local* (e.g., compensatory overinflation secondary to pulmonary resection or atelectasis) or *general* (e.g., spasmodic asthma).

Increased Air with Decreased Blood and Tissue (see Fig. 4–72). This group is epitomized by diffuse emphysema. Not only are the lungs overinflated but also the capillary bed is reduced owing to destruction of alveolar walls. Bullae and thin-walled cysts are examples of local diseases this category.

Normal Amount of Air but Decreased Blood and Tissue (see Fig. 4–72). *Local* diseases in this group include lobar or unilateral emphysema and pulmonary embolism without infarction. (In both conditions, however, the volume of air also may be reduced: in the former because of incomplete maturation of lung parenchyma and in the latter because of surfactant deficit.) *Generalized* abnormalities include diseases characterized by diminished pulmonary artery flow (e.g., tetralogy of Fallot) and those that affect the peripheral vascular system (e.g., primary pulmonary hypertension and multiple peripheral pulmonary thromboemboli).

Reduction in All Three Components (see Fig. 4–72). This condition is rare and probably relates to only one abnormality or variants thereof—unilateral pulmonary artery agenesis. Usually, the lung is reduced in volume and derives its vascular supply solely from the systemic circulation; the resultant density is usually, but not always reduced.

Roentgenologic Signs

Alteration in Lung Volume

With the exception of the reduction in lung volume that occurs in unilateral pulmonary artery agenesis, unilateral or lobar emphysema (Swyer-James syndrome), partly obstructing endobronchial lesions, and pulmonary embolism without infarction, all lung diseases in which there is decreased density and alteration in lung volume are characterized by overinflation. Before considering the roentgenologic signs of overinflation, therefore, it is well to review briefly the mechanisms that keep the lung expanded and the alterations in these mechanisms that increase lung volume.

As discussed previously, the lung has a natural tendency to collapse and does so when removed from the chest. This tendency stems from its inherent elastic recoil properties, which are partly related to connective tissue fibers and partly to alveolar surface tension. When the lung's elastic properties are deranged, as in emphysema, the organ inflates beyond its normal maximal volume; this constitutes *overinflation*. Similarly, the lung's compliance—the change in volume per unit change in pressure—is increased; in other words, a given pressure will produce a greater volume

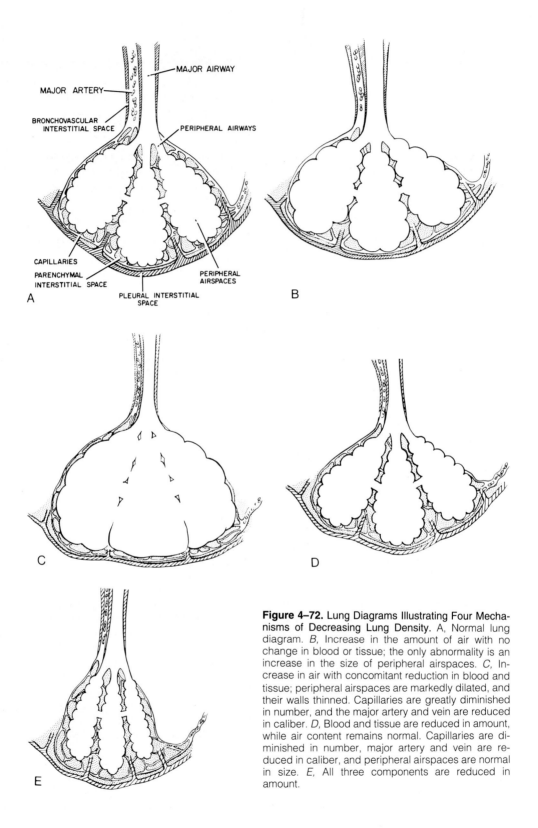

Figure 4–72. Lung Diagrams Illustrating Four Mechanisms of Decreasing Lung Density. A, Normal lung diagram. B, Increase in the amount of air with no change in blood or tissue; the only abnormality is an increase in the size of peripheral airspaces. C, Increase in air with concomitant reduction in blood and tissue; peripheral airspaces are markedly dilated, and their walls thinned. Capillaries are greatly diminished in number, and the major artery and vein are reduced in caliber. D, Blood and tissue are reduced in amount, while air content remains normal. Capillaries are diminished in number, major artery and vein are reduced in caliber, and peripheral airspaces are normal in size. E, All three components are reduced in amount.

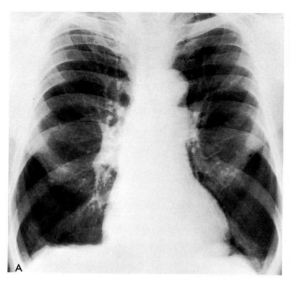
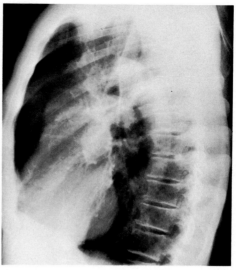

Figure 4–73. Diffuse Emphysema. A posteroanterior roentgenogram of the chest in inspiration *(A)* reveals a low position and somewhat flattened contour of both hemidiaphragms. In lateral projection *(B)*, the superior aspect of the diaphragm is concave rather than convex, and the retrosternal air-spaces somewhat deepened. The lungs are generally oligemic.

change than in normal lung. It is important to recognize that this loss of elastic recoil is the major, if not the only, factor that permits the lung to overinflate. The loss of recoil may be irreversible, as in emphysema, or temporary and reversible, as in asthma; in any event, *unequivocal roentgenographic evidence of pulmonary overinflation implies loss of elastic recoil.* The roentgenologic signs of overinflation depend on whether the process is general or local.

General Excess of Air. Signs to be observed include changes in the diaphragm, the retrosternal space, and the cardiovascular silhouette (Fig. 4–73); by far the most important of these are related to the diaphragm. In the severe overinflation of diffuse emphysema, the diaphragm is characteristically depressed at total lung capacity, often to the level of the seventh rib anteriorly and the eleventh interspace or twelfth rib posteriorly. In addition, the normal "dome" configuration is flattened, particularly as viewed in lateral projection. The severity of flattening may be of value in differential diagnosis, being invariably most marked in emphysema; in fact, overinflation in this condition may render the diaphragmatic contour actually concave rather than convex upward (*see* Fig. 4–73), a sign we have seen only occasionally in other diseases. (In adult patients with asthma, the upper surface is nearly always convex; however, in infants and children it may be associated with remarkable depression of diaphragmatic domes.) The low position of the diaphragm in severe overinflation increases the angle of the costophrenic sinuses, sometimes to almost 90 degrees.

Diseases that show evidence of overinflation at TLC also invariably result in overinflation at smaller lung volumes, a process related at least in part to air trapping. Limited diaphragmatic excursion during respiration is a reliable sign of such air trapping, particularly but not exclusively in emphysema; whereas the average range of diaphragmatic excursion in normal subjects is 3 to 4 cm, the range in emphysema may be no more than 1 to 2 cm (*see* Fig. 4–73).

Other roentgenographic features are not nearly as useful in detecting overinflation as are those related to the diaphragm. Identification in lateral projection of separation of

the cardiovascular structures from the sternum indicates increase in the depth of the retrosternal air space and is a sign that has been employed by some[67] to indicate overinflation; however, we have found it a poor discriminant of normal and overinflated lungs.[68]

Alteration in the size and contour of the thoracic cage is a variable and usually undependable sign of excess air in the lungs. Although the barrel-shaped chest is commonly regarded as indicative of emphysema, often its roentgenologic expression as an increase in the anteroposterior diameter of the chest is inconspicuous. Both anterior bowing of the sternum and increased thoracic kyphosis are unreliable roentgenologic signs in assessment of excess air in the lungs.[69]

When the diaphragm is depressed, the cardiac silhouette tends to be elongated, narrow, and positioned centrally. This configuration also is of little value as a roentgenologic sign; however, it may create difficulty in the assessment of right ventricular enlargement.

Local Excess of Air. Overinflation of a segment or of one or more lobes, the remainder of the lungs being normal, can occur with or without air trapping. In our experience, the former phenomenon has few causes, for example, lobar hyperinflation in infants (*see* Fig. 5–10; page 269)[70] and congenital atresia of the apicoposterior segmental bronchus of the left upper lobe (Fig. 4–74). Although overinflation of lung distal to an endobronchial lesion as a result of check-valve obstruction is frequently cited as an important sign in the early diagnosis of bronchogenic carcinoma, in our experience, and in others', it is a rare manifestation.[71] In fact, the volume of lung behind a partly obstructing endobronchial lesion is almost invariably *reduced* at TLC (*see* page 459).

Overinflation *without air trapping* is a compensatory process, in which parts of the lung fill a larger volume than normal in response to loss of volume elsewhere in the thorax. This may occur after surgical removal of lung tissue or as a result of atelectasis or parenchymal scarring in another portion of lung; in any event, the remaining lung

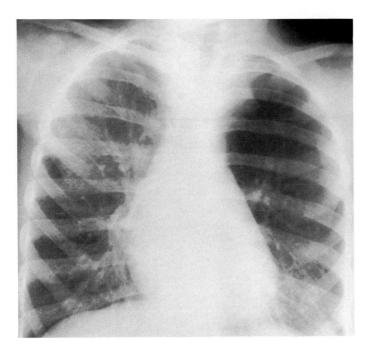

Figure 4–74. Congenital Bronchial Atresia of the Left Upper Lobe. A conventional posteroanterior chest roentgenogram demonstrates striking overinflation and oligemia of the upper two thirds of the left lung; the mediastinum is displaced slightly to the right. The resected left upper lobe showed severe emphysema of the anterior and apical segments, accompanied by mucoid impaction distal to a totally atretic bronchus. The posterior segment was supplied by a single patent bronchus. (Reprinted from, by permission of the publisher, Genereux GP: Bronchial atresia: A rare cause of unilateral lung hypertranslucency. J Can Assoc Radiol 22:71, 1971.)

contains more than its normal complement of air. Since there is no airway obstruction, the roentgenologic signs are different from those of conditions in which air trapping plays a significant role. Thus, it is important to consider the roentgenologic signs of local excess of air under two headings, static and dynamic, according to the presence or absence of airway obstruction.

Static Signs. By static is implied the changes apparent on standard roentgenograms exposed at total lung capacity. There are three signs in this situation.

ALTERATION IN LUNG DENSITY. The fact that the excess of air is local permits comparison with normal density in the remainder of the lung or in the contralateral lung; thus, in contrast to those diseases with generalized excess of air, altered density is a significant and reliable sign. The increased translucency is caused chiefly by a relative increase in air as compared to blood; blood flow to the affected lung may be normal or reduced, the only difference being that, in the latter circumstance, translucency is even more pronounced.

In the case of a partly obstructing endobronchial lesion, the situation is somewhat different. As indicated above, our experience dictates that the volume of lung behind a partly obstructing endobronchial lesion is almost invariably reduced at TLC (Fig. 4–75); despite this smaller volume, however, the density of affected parenchyma typically is *less* than that of the opposite lung, rather than greater as might be anticipated. This is because a reduction in perfusion results from hypoxic vasoconstriction in response to alveolar hypoventilation. The overall effect is an increase in translucency, despite the reduction in volume.

ALTERATION IN VOLUME. The volume of the affected lung depends entirely on whether the excess of air is compensatory or is caused by airway obstruction. Since compensatory overinflation is the expansion of lung tissue beyond its normal volume to fill a limited space, the volume that the expanded lung tissue occupies cannot exceed the volume for which it compensates.

The main sign of increased volume is displacement of structures contiguous with the overinflated lung, the degree varying with the amount and location of affected parenchyma. If in a lower lobe, the hemidiaphragm may be depressed and the mediastinum shifted to the contralateral side; if in an upper lobe, the mediastinum may be displaced and the thoracic cage expanded; if a whole lung is involved, the hemithorax in general is enlarged, the diaphragm is depressed, the mediastinum shifted, and the thoracic cage enlarged. One of the more reliable signs of *lobar* overinflation is outward bulging of the interlobar fissure.

ALTERATION IN VASCULAR PATTERN. The linear markings throughout the affected lung are splayed out in a distribution consistent with the extent of overinflation, and their angles of bifurcation are increased. Provided blood flow is maintained at normal or almost normal levels, vessel caliber is little altered.

Dynamic Signs. The term "dynamic" implies changes that occur during respiration; these are most readily apparent on fluoroscopy, although many can be seen equally clearly on roentgenograms exposed during full inspiration and maximal expiration.

When local increase in translucency is caused by compensatory overinflation, the volume of the overinflated lobe decreases during expiration proportionately with the normal lung tissue; airway obstruction being absent, the affected lung parenchyma deflates normally. Since the overinflated lung tissue contains more air than normal at total lung capacity, it still contains a greater than normal complement of air at residual volume and, therefore, is still relatively more translucent.

In the presence of partial airway obstruction, roentgenologic signs are vastly different from those seen in compensatory overinflation. During expiration, air is trapped within the affected lung parenchyma and volume changes little, whereas the remainder of the lung deflates normally. The roentgenologic signs depend on both the volume and the anatomic location of affected lung. Because there is negli-

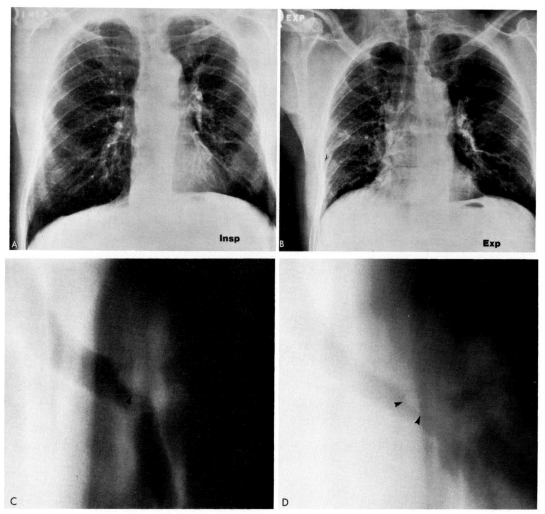

Figure 4–75. Small Cell Carcinoma, Left Main Bronchus, with Expiratory Air Trapping. *A,* A postero-anterior roentgenogram exposed at full inspiration reveals decreased size of the left lung compared with the right. Despite this loss of volume, no opacities can be identified in the left lung to suggest collapse or airlessness. Left lower lobe vessels are obviously smaller than corresponding vessels on the right, indicating reduced perfusion. *B,* A roentgenogram exposed at maximal expiration reveals little change in the volume of the left lung from inspiration, indicating air trapping; by contrast, the right hemidiaphragm has elevated considerably and the mediastinum has swung to the right, indicating good air flow from the right lung. Tomograms of the left main bronchus in inspiration *(C)* and expiration *(D)* reveal a smooth, well-defined soft tissue mass protruding into the air column of the bronchus near its bifurcation *(arrowheads):* the caliber of the bronchial air column is markedly reduced on expiration.

gible change in the amount of air within the obstructed lung parenchyma during expiration, density is little altered and the contrast between affected areas and normally deflated lung is maximally accentuated at residual volume. Since the overinflated parenchyma occupies space within the hemithorax, contiguous structures are displaced away from the affected lobe during expiration; the mediastinum shifts toward the contralateral side and elevation of the hemidiaphragm is restricted. Distribution of the vessels within the overinflated lobe changes little. These dynamic changes are particularly impressive fluoroscopically: when the patient breathes deeply and rapidly, the mediastinum swings like a pendulum, away from the lesion during expiration and back to the midline during inspiration. The extent of diaphragmatic excursion and of reduction in size of the thoracic cage are diminished on the ipsilateral side.

It cannot be overemphasized that evidence of local excess of air may be extremely subtle on roentgenograms exposed at full inspiration (*see* Fig. 4–75); when such changes are even remotely suspected, the dynamics should be studied.

Alteration in Vasculature

Like overinflation, alteration in lung vasculature may be either general or local. As the roentgenologic signs of the two types differ somewhat, it is again desirable to describe them separately.

General Reduction in Vasculature. Diffuse pulmonary oligemia is characterized by a reduction in caliber of the arterial tree throughout the lungs. As pointed out in Chapter 1, appreciation of such vascular change is a subjective process based on a thorough familiarity with the normal. Although such an assessment admittedly is subject to observer error, to our knowledge it has not been replaced by any method that provides an accurate, objective evaluation, with the possible exceptions of roentgen densitometry and CT.

Since reduction in the size of peripheral vessels constitutes the main criterion of diagnosis of all diseases in this category, resort to secondary signs is necessary to distinguish one from another. There are two ancillary signs of major importance: the size and configuration of the central hilar vessels and the presence or absence of general pulmonary overinflation. The following examples serve to indicate how these signs may be useful in differential diagnosis. Three combinations of changes are possible.

Small Peripheral Vessels, No Overinflation, and Normal or Small Hila. This combination indicates reduced pulmonary blood flow from central causes and is virtually pathognomonic of cardiac disease, usually congenital anomalies such as tetralogy of Fallot, Ebstein's anomaly, and, occasionally, isolated pulmonic stenosis (Fig. 4–76). The same combination is seen occasionally in certain acquired conditions, such as pericardial tamponade and inferior vena caval obstruction.

Small Peripheral Vessels, No Overinflation, and Enlarged Hilar Pulmonary Arteries. This combination may result from peripheral or central causes. The *peripheral* conditions include primary pulmonary hypertension, multiple peripheral emboli, and pulmonary hypertension secondary to chronic schistosomiasis. In each of these, the major

changes apparent roentgenographically are the consequence of pulmonary arterial hypertension—enlargement of the hilar pulmonary arteries and diminution of the peripheral vessels. The commonest cause of *central* origin is massive pulmonary artery embolism without infarction. In this situation, the reduction in peripheral pulmonary artery flow results from mechanical obstruction in the large hilar vessels, the latter being ballooned out by thrombus within; severe cardiac enlargement caused by acute cor pulmonale is usually present (Fig. 4–77).

Small Peripheral Vessels, General Pulmonary Overinflation, and Normal or Enlarged Hilar Pulmonary Arteries. This combination is virtually pathognomonic of diffuse emphysema (Fig. 4–78). Enlargement of the hilar pulmonary arteries may be present but is not essential to the diagnosis. It indicates pulmonary arterial hypertension resulting from chronically increased vascular resistance and usually is seen only in the late stages of the disease. In such circumstances, the rapid tapering of pulmonary vessels distally is accentuated by the hilar enlargement.

Local Reduction in Vasculature. The same three combinations of changes apply as in general reduction in vasculature, the major difference being their effects on pulmonary hemodynamics. The affected portion of lung may be segmental, lobar, or multilobar.

Small Peripheral Vessels, Normal or Subnormal Inflation, and Normal or Small Hilum. This combination is epitomized by lobar or unilateral hyperlucent lung (Swyer-James or Macleod's syndrome) (Fig. 4–79), an abnormality characterized by normal or slightly reduced lung volume at total lung capacity, severe airway obstruction during expiration, greatly reduced circulation (oligemia), and a diminutive hilum. The increased vascular resistance in affected areas results in redistribution of blood flow to the contralateral lung or unaffected lobes.

Roentgenographic changes identical to those of Swyer-James syndrome may result from a clinically more important situation. Consider an endobronchial lesion that is incompletely obstructing the lumen of a main bronchus. The reduced ventilation of distal parenchyma results in local hypoxia, which leads to reflex vasoconstriction and consequent reduced perfusion of affected bronchopulmonary segments. The volume of affected lung generally is reduced rather than increased. Since the endobronchial lesion invariably causes expiratory air trapping, it may be extremely difficult roentgenologically to differentiate it from the less significant Swyer-James syndrome. Therefore, whenever this combination of changes is present, it is imperative to exclude an endobronchial lesion (preferably by bronchoscopy).

A picture somewhat similar to that produced by Swyer-James syndrome may be seen in patients with unilateral pulmonary artery agenesis, in which the pulmonary artery is interrupted in the region of the hilum so that the lung is devoid of pulmonary artery perfusion.[72] On plain roentgenograms, the two may be distinguished by the virtual absence of a hilar shadow in pulmonary artery agenesis and a diminutive hilar shadow in Swyer-James syndrome; in addition, in the former there is no expiratory airway obstruction.

Small Peripheral Vessels, Normal or Subnormal Lung Volume, and Enlarged Hilar Pulmonary Arteries (or an Enlarged Hilum). This combination is nearly al-

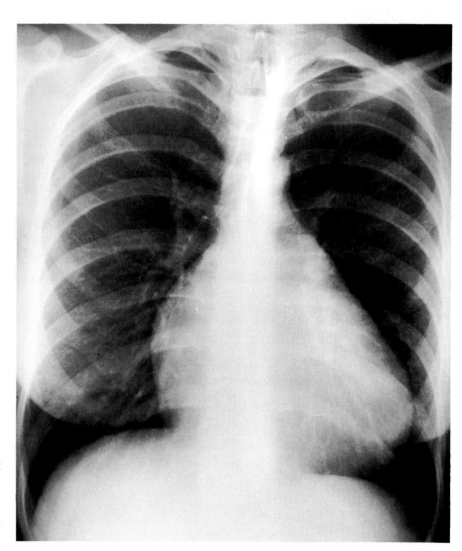

Figure 4–76. Diffuse Oligemia Without Overinflation: Ebstein's Anomaly. The peripheral pulmonary markings are diminished in caliber, and the hila are diminutive; the lungs are not overinflated. The contour of the markedly enlarged heart is consistent with Ebstein's anomaly.

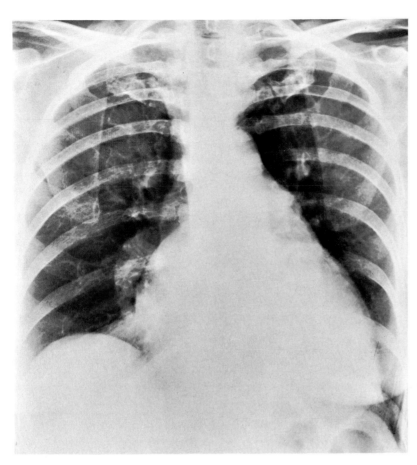

Figure 4–77. Diffuse Oligemia Without Overinflation: Massive Pulmonary Artery Thromboembolism Without Infarction. Marked oligemia of both lungs is associated with moderate enlargement of both hila and rapid tapering of the pulmonary arteries as they proceed distally. The cardiac contour is typical of cor pulmonale. There is no overinflation.

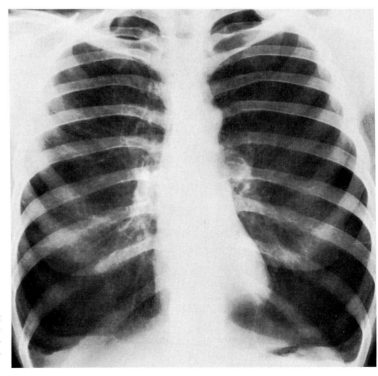

Figure 4–78. Diffuse Oligemia with Generalized Overinflation: Emphysema. The peripheral vasculature of the lungs is markedly diminished. Despite the severe oligemia, the hilar pulmonary arteries are not dilated. The lungs are severely overinflated.

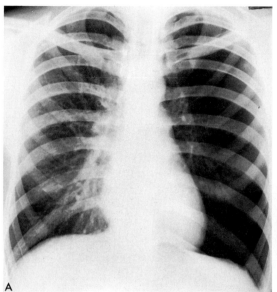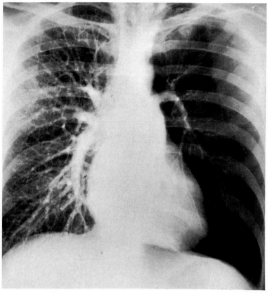

A

B

Figure 4–79. Unilateral Hyperlucent Lung: Swyer-James or Macleod's Syndrome. A posteroanterior roentgenogram exposed at TLC *(A)* reveals a marked discrepancy in the radiolucency of the two lungs, the left showing severe oligemia. The left hilar shadow is diminutive. The left lung appears to be of approximately normal volume compared with the right. A roentgenogram in full expiration *(not illustrated)* revealed severe air trapping in the left lung. In a pulmonary angiogram *(B),* the discrepancy of blood flow to the two lungs is readily apparent; note that the left pulmonary artery is present although diminutive (differentiating the condition from congenital absence of the left pulmonary artery).

ways caused by pulmonary artery embolism without infarction (Fig. 4–80). Since bronchial obstruction is not a feature, there is no overinflation; on the contrary, lung volume is often reduced owing to surfactant loss and reflex bronchoconstriction. A similar roentgenographic picture may be produced by neoplastic obstruction of a pulmonary artery; the hilar enlargement is caused by the original lesion rather than by a distended vessel, although the overall roentgenographic appearance may be the same.

Small Peripheral Vessels, Overinflation, and Normal Hilar Pulmonary Arteries. The roentgenographic appearance of the vascular deficiency of emphysema is often local rather than general, one or a combination of individual lobes being predominantly affected. The involved portions of lung show a combination of overinflation and severe oligemia; less involved areas tend to be pleonemic as a result of redistribution of blood to them caused by the increased resistance to pulmonary blood flow in emphysematous areas. Since the absence of increased vascular resistance in uninvolved lung prevents the development of pulmonary artery hypertension, the hilar pulmonary arteries do not enlarge.

Bullae

A bulla is an air-containing space that ranges in size from 1 cm in diameter to the volume of a whole hemithorax and that possesses a smooth, typically avascular wall no thicker than 1 mm. The space may be unilocular or separated into several compartments by thin septa (Fig. 4–81). Bullae can arise in three circumstances: (1) *de novo,* typically in asso-

ciation with surrounding normal lung tissue; (2) as part of diffuse emphysema, in which case they are characteristically very thin walled, small, and scattered wide throughout the subpleural zone; and (3) secondary to other disease, usually infectious and commonly associated with much parenchymal scarring (Fig. 4–82). In the third circumstance, the bulla is associated with a variable amount of disease in adjacent parenchyma. In addition to a localized area of hyperlucency caused by the absence of lung parenchyma, secondary signs may be present, depending on the size of the bulla; for example, when a huge bulla occupies most of the volume of one hemithorax (Fig. 4–83), signs of air trapping are apparent at small lung volumes.

A large air-containing space of an entirely different nature is the pneumatocele (Fig. 4–84). This is a complication of acute pneumonia, usually caused by *S. aureus* in infants and children; it often develops rapidly and almost invariably resolves completely. Its pathogenesis is believed to relate either to check-valve obstruction of a small bronchus or bronchiole, with distention of the lung distal to the obstruction, or to local necrosis of a bronchial wall with dissection of air into the bronchovascular interstitial space.[73]

ROENTGENOLOGIC SIGNS OF PLEURAL DISEASE

Involvement of the pleura is a common feature of many intrathoracic diseases; roentgenographic manifestations consist predominantly of effusion, fibrosis, neoplastic infiltration, and pneumothorax.

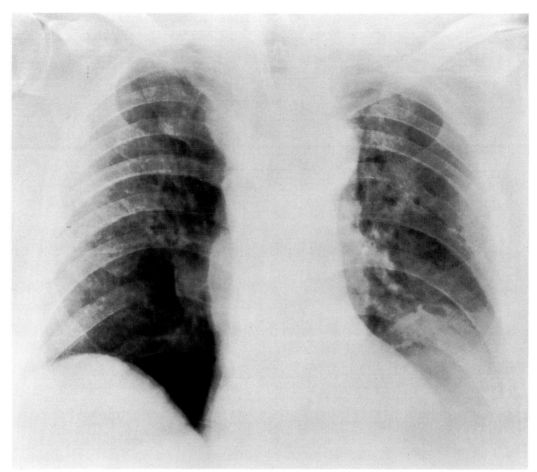

Figure 4–80. Lobar Oligemia Without Overinflation: Thromboembolism without Infarction. An antero-posterior roentgenogram exposed in the supine position demonstrates marked increase in the radio-lucency of the lower half of the right lung. The vascular markings are diminshed in caliber, and the descending branch of the right pulmonary artery is dilated and sharply defined; this vessel tapers rapidly as it proceeds distally. Lobar oligemia as a result of thromboembolism without infarction constitutes Westermark's sign.

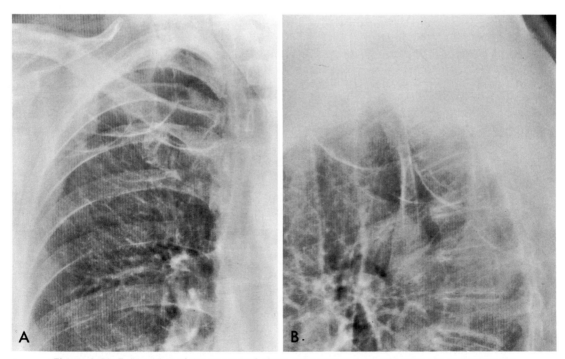

Figure 4–81. Bullae. View of the upper half of the right lung in posteroanterior *(A)* and lateral *(B)* projections reveal several cystic spaces in the lung apex sharply separated from contiguous lung by curvilinear, hairline shadows.

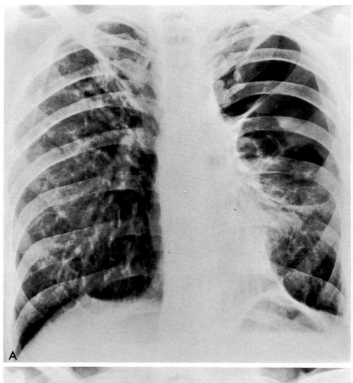

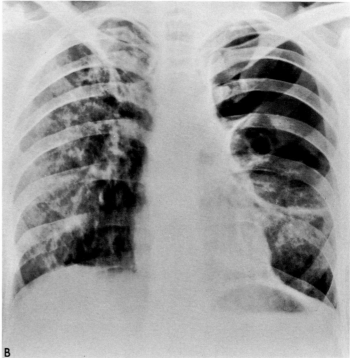

Figure 4–82. Bulla Associated with Pulmonary Scarring. A posteroanterior roentgenogram exposed at TLC *(A)* demonstrates a large, well-defined cystic space occupying the upper half of the left hemithorax, sharply demarcated from contiguous lung. There is extensive bilateral parenchymal disease due to chronic fibroproductive tuberculosis. A roentgenogram exposed at RV *(B)* reveals marked air trapping within the bulla; in fact, by actual measurement, the space is larger at RV than at TLC. *See* text. (Courtesy of the Montreal Chest Hospital Center.)

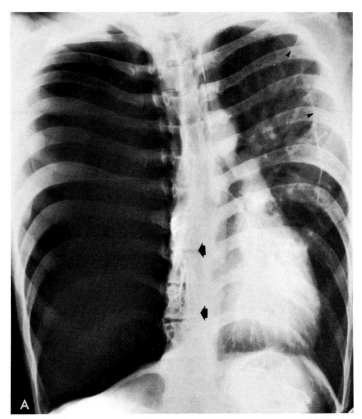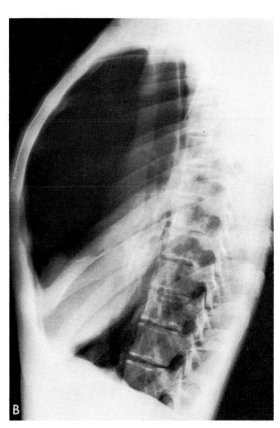

Figure 4–83. Huge Bulla. *A,* An anteroposterior roentgenogram of the chest following bronchography reveals a huge air sac completely filling and overdistending the right hemithorax and extending across the anterior mediastinal septum almost as far as the left axillary pleura (the line shadow indicated by *arrowheads* is formed by four layers of pleura). The right lung is compressed into a small nubbin of tissue situated in the midline; note the markedly crowded right bronchial tree *(thick arrows).* In lateral projection *(B),* extension of the bulla across the midline has resulted in marked increase in depth of the retrosternal airspace and posterior displacement of the heart and major vessels.

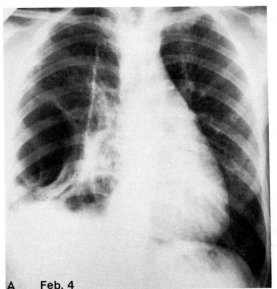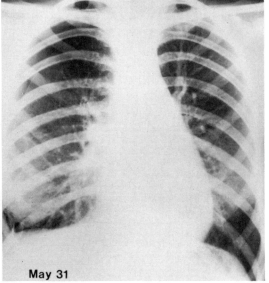

Figure 4–84. Pneumatocele Formation in Acute Staphylococcal Pneumonia. This 16-year-old girl was admitted to the hospital with an acute respiratory illness. Her original roentgenogram *(A)* reveals an inhomogeneous opacity in the lower portion of the right lung associated with a large cystic space (pneumatocele) laterally and several smaller air-containing spaces inferiorly. The mediastinum is shifted to the left. Several weeks later *(B),* much of the parenchymal reaction in the right lung had resolved, and the large pneumatocele originally identified had almost completely disappeared.

Roentgenologic Signs of Pleural Effusion

Although reported figures for the amount of pleural fluid required for roentgenographic demonstration in the erect subject range from 250 to 600 mL, it is important to realize that a substantially smaller amount may be identifiable in the lateral decubitus position in a small but significant percentage of normal individuals. For example, in one study utilizing a modification of the lateral decubitus projection with a horizontal x-ray beam, pleural fluid was identified in 15 of 120 healthy adults (12.5 per cent).[74] Thoracentesis performed on some of these subjects showed that the smallest amount of fluid identifiable by this technique was 3 to 5 mL; the largest amount was 15 mL. In another investigation using cadavers, 5-mL increments of saline or plasma were injected into the pleural space[75]; even 5 mL of fluid was clearly visible on roentgenograms exposed with subjects in the unmodified lateral decubitus position, and increasing amounts caused incremental increases in density. These studies are of obvious practical importance, insofar as they indicate that small amounts of pleural fluid may be demonstrated roentgenographically in the absence of disease.

Typical Distribution of Free Pleural Fluid

It will be recalled from the discussion on the physiology of the pleura that lung tissue has a natural tendency to recoil but is prevented from doing so beyond a certain point by the chest wall's tendency to expand outward with an equal, opposite force. Thus, in the normal state, intimate contact between the visceral and parietal pleural surfaces is maintained. When liquid or gas is introduced into the pleural space, however, the lung can recoil inward toward its fixed mooring at the hilum. The site of retraction depends on the position of the liquid or gas within the pleural space: in the upright subject, the effect of gravity causes gas to rise and liquid to fall in the pleural space, resulting in retraction of the upper portions of the lung in the former instance and of the lower portions in the latter. The different roentgenographic appearances of the two media are due to the fact that one is radiopaque and the other radiolucent; for example, if a roentgenogram was taken of a patient with a pleural effusion of 1 L, in a 90-degree headdown position, the form of the lung would be roughly the same as if 1 L of gas was present and the patient was erect (Fig. 4–85).

These two influences, gravity and elastic recoil, are the major forces that control the location of free fluid in the pleural space.[76] Fluid gravitates first to the base of the hemithorax, where it comes to lie between the inferior surface of the lung and the hemidiaphragm (Fig. 4–86), particularly posteriorly, where the pleural sinus is deepest. With increasing amounts, the fluid spills out into the costophrenic sinuses posteriorly, laterally, and eventually anteriorly; with further accumulation, it spreads upward in mantlelike fashion around the convexity of the lung, tapering gradually as it assumes a higher position in the thorax.

On the basis of this description, it is easy to imagine the typical roentgenographic appearance of pleural effusion. Consider the hypothetical situation of a moderate pleural effusion (1000 mL) (Fig. 4–87): such an amount of fluid completely obscures the hemidiaphragm and the costo-

phrenic sinuses and extends upward around the anterior, lateral, and posterior thoracic wall to about the midportion of the hemithorax. Because the mediastinal surface of the lung possesses relatively less elastic recoil because of its fixation at the hilum and pulmonary ligament, less fluid accumulates along this surface than around the convexity. Thus, in posteroanterior projection, the opacity of the fluid is high laterally and curves gently downward and medially, with a smooth, meniscus-shaped upper border, to terminate along the midcardiac border. In lateral projection, since the fluid has ascended along the anterior and posterior thoracic wall to roughly an equal extent, the upper surface of the fluid opacity will be semicircular, being high anteriorly and posteriorly and curving smoothly downward to its lowest point in the midaxillary line. Comparison of the maximal height of the fluid opacity in the posteroanterior and lateral projections shows that this height is identical posteriorly, laterally, and anteriorly; that is, the top of the fluid accumulation is *horizontal*. The meniscus shape is caused by the fact that the layer of fluid is not deep enough to cast a discernible shadow when viewed *en face*.[76]

Since the distribution of fluid within the pleural space tends to obey the law of gravity, and since the lung tends to maintain its shape as it shrinks, the first place fluid accumulates in the erect patient is between the inferior surface of the lower lobe and the diaphragm. In effect, the lung is "floating" on a layer of fluid (*see* Fig. 4–86). If the amount of fluid is small, it may occupy only this position, without spilling over into the costophrenic sinuses. In such circumstances, the configuration of the hemidiaphragm is maintained and the appearance on posteroanterior and lateral roentgenograms suggests no more than slight elevation of that hemidiaphragm. Bearing in mind the individual variation in the height of the diaphragm in normal subjects, it is readily apparent that small accumulations of fluid in the pleural space can easily be missed roentgenologically.

When the amount of fluid in the infrapulmonary pleural space reaches a certain level, it spills over into the posterior costophrenic sinus and obliterates that sinus as viewed in lateral roentgenographic projection. The normally sharp costophrenic angle is abolished by a shallow, homogeneous shadow whose upper surface is meniscus-shaped. With increasing amounts of fluid, the roentgenologic signs develop in predictable fashion: obliteration of the lateral and eventually anterior costophrenic sulci, and extension of fluid up the chest wall in its typical mantle distribution.

The effects on the thorax as a whole of the accumulation of large amounts of fluid in the pleural space depend largely on the condition of the ipsilateral lung. Even small amounts of fluid produce relaxation atelectasis of contiguous lung, in much the same manner as air does in pneumothorax. When pleural effusion is massive, collapse of the ipsilateral lung may be almost complete. Despite severe atelectasis, however, the overall effect of a massive effusion almost invariably is that of a space-occupying process, with enlargement of the ipsilateral hemithorax, displacement of the mediastinum to the contralateral side, and severe depression and flattening of the ipsilateral hemidiaphragm; in fact, the hemidiaphragm may be depressed so severely as to be concave superiorly (Fig. 4–88).[77]

When one hemithorax is totally opacified, appreciation of the balance of forces between the two sides of the thorax is of obvious importance. If the mediastinum shows no shift

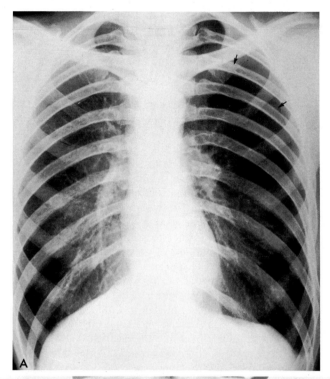

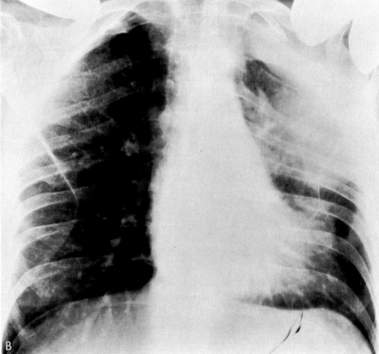

Figure 4–85. Similarity in the Effects on the Lung of Pneumothorax and Hydrothorax. *A,* A posteroanterior roentgenogram of the chest (erect position) reveals a small left pneumothorax (visceral pleural line at *arrows*). *B,* The roentgenogram of another patient with a moderate pleural effusion on whom roentgenography was carried out in a 45-degree Trendelenburg position. The effects on the lung in these two situations are almost identical.

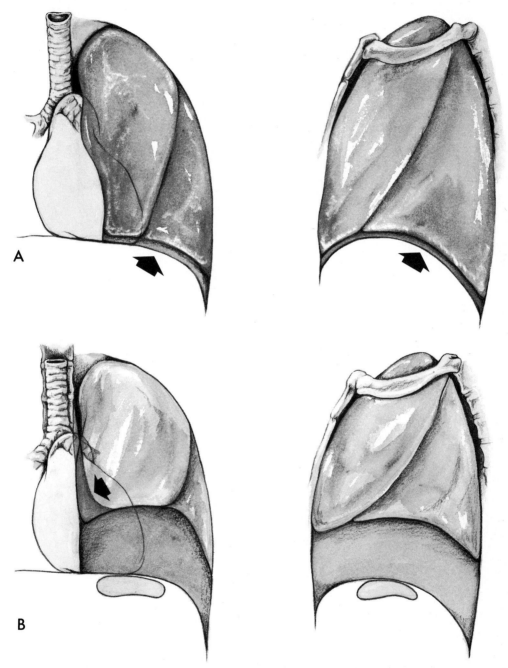

Figure 4–86. Intrapulmonary Accumulation of Pleural Fluid. These drawings depict two degrees of infrapulmonary effusion: in *A*, the situation is "typical" in that it represents the *usual* anatomic location of small amounts of fluid (up to 300 mL); in *B*, the amount of fluid is large (e.g., 1500 mL), and the local infrapulmonary accumulation thus "atypical." *See* text.

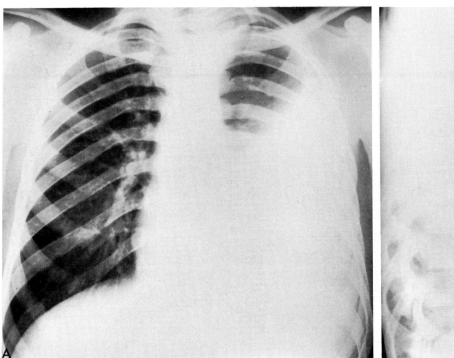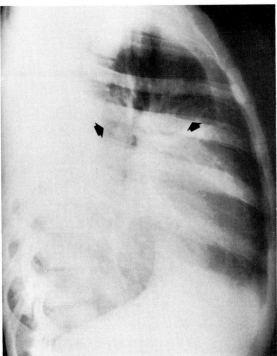

Figure 4–87. Large Pleural Effusion: Typical Appearance. Posteroanterior *(A)* and lateral *(B)* roentgenograms exposed in the erect position demonstrate uniform opacification of the lower two thirds of the left hemithorax. The upper level of the fluid is meniscus-shaped in both projections *(arrows on B)*. Note that only the right hemidiaphragm is visualized in lateral projection, the left being obscured by fluid (the silhouette sign).

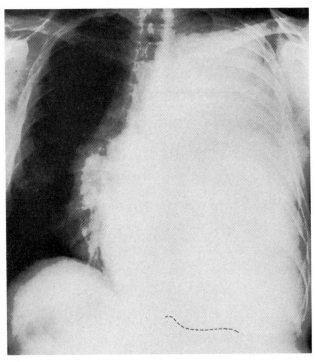

Figure 4–88. Massive Effusion, Underlying Lung Normal. A posteroanterior roentgenogram reveals total opacification of the left hemithorax by a massive pleural effusion. The mediastinum is displaced to the right. The stomach bubble *(dotted line)* is displaced far inferiorly, and its upper surface is concave rather than convex, suggesting that the hemidiaphragm possesses the same contour.

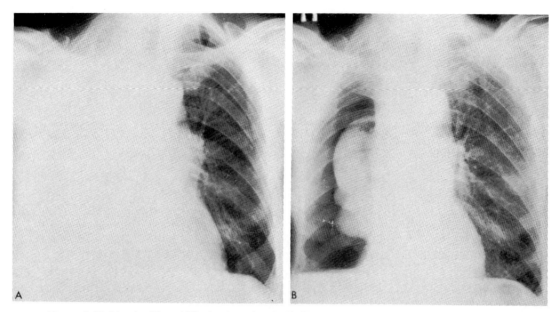

Figure 4–89. Massive Pleural Effusion Associated with Obstructive Atelectasis of the Underlying Lung. A posteroanterior roentgenogram *(A)* shows total opacification of the right hemithorax; in contrast to the situation in Figure 4–88, the mediastinum is central in position. Following removal of almost all the fluid and replacement with an equal quantity of air, the right lung *(B)* can be seen to be totally collapsed and airless. In such a situation, the absence of an air bronchogram constitutes absolute evidence of endobronchial obstruction. At thoracotomy, stenosis of the intermediate stem bronchus was found to be caused by compression by enlarged lymph nodes replaced by adenocarcinoma.

and the hemidiaphragm is only slightly depressed, the presence of antecedent disease within the ipsilateral lung (other than simple relaxation atelectasis) can be stated with absolute certainty (Fig. 4–89). The conclusion *must* be that the balance of forces between effusion (a space-occupying process) and parenchymal disease (which reduces volume) ensures that the volume of the hemithorax is not greater than normal. The possibility of an obstructing endobronchial lesion (e.g., pulmonary carcinoma with pleural metastases) is obvious. In fact, total opacification of one hemithorax without mediastinal or diaphragmatic displacement is highly suggestive of either this diagnosis or malignant mesothelioma (*see* later).

It should be remembered that the descriptions of pleural fluid distribution given above relate to roentgenograms of erect patients. In the supine position, fluid occupies the pleural space from the lung apex to base and appears roentgenographoically as a more or less diffuse haze over the whole hemithorax.

Atypical Distribution of Free Pleural Fluid

It is important to realize that the lung tends to maintain its traditional shape at all stages of collapse, a characteristic termed "form elasticity."[78] In fact, when pneumothorax is present or the thoracic cage is opened (at thoracotomy or necropsy), the shape of the lung in its completely collapsed state is a miniature replica of its shape in the fully distended form (*see* Fig. 4–12, page 175). The effect is the same when pleural effusion or pneumothorax is present, except that the collapse may be local rather than general.

The typical arrangement of fluid in the pleural space requires that the underlying lung be free from disease and thus capable of preserving its shape even while recoiling

from the chest wall; that is, it is able to maintain its form elasticity. An alteration in this uniform recoiling tendency is the influence by which most if not all atypical distribution of pleural fluid can be explained (excluding the restriction of free movement occasioned by pleural adhesions). The precise mechanism by which this occurs is not clear; however, some experimental evidence suggests that parenchymal disease, particularly atelectasis, in any portion of the lung modifies the elastic recoil of that portion locally so that pleural fluid is attracted to it. For example, in one study in which atelectasis was produced in selected lobes of dog lungs, it was shown that when lower lobes were collapsed, fluid injected into the pleural space tended to move to the area of maximal parenchymal distortion, where negative pleural pressure was greatest.[79] In the presence of upper lobe collapse, however, free pleural fluid tended to remain in its "typical" location in an infrapulmonary position. Regardless of the mechanism whereby fluid accumulates in atypical locations within the pleural space, there is little doubt that in the majority of cases it relates to underlying pulmonary disease. Thus, the major roentgenologic significance of atypical pleural effusion is that it *alerts the physician to the presence of both parenchymal and pleural disease.*

The roentgenographic appearance of atypical pleural fluid accumulation in disease affecting individual lobes has been described in detail.[76] One example will illustrate the possible variations. In lower lobe disease, fluid tends to accumulate posteromedially. In posteroanterior projection, the opacity tends to be higher on the mediastinal than on the axillary border, its upper surface curving downward and laterally toward the lateral costophrenic sulcus (simulating the shadow of combined atelectasis and consolidation of the right middle and lower lobes). In lateral projection, the

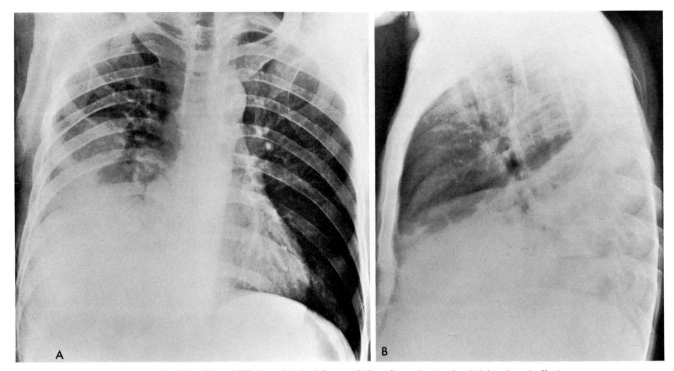

Figure 4–90. Right Pleural Effusion, Atypical Accumulation. A moderate-sized right pleural effusion identified on posteroanterior *(A)* and lateral *(B)* roentgenograms does not possess typical meniscus-shaped upper border in either projection; it is high posteriorly and low anteriorly so as to simulate consolidation of the middle and lower lobes (particularly as visualized in lateral projection). Right lower lobe pneumonia with effusion.

upper border of the density roughly parallels the major fissure, beginning high in the thorax posteriorly and curving downward and anteriorly, toward the anterior costophrenic gutter, which may be clear and sharp (Fig. 4–90).

Since roentgenography of the patient in any position other than the erect detects any change in distribution of *free* pleural fluid, examination in the supine or, preferably, lateral decubitus position will show displacement of the fluid over the posterior or lateral pleural space, respectively. The nature of these unusual opacities can thus be clarified in questionable cases (e.g., an effusion simulating lower lobe consolidation). In addition, these procedures permit clearer identification and more accurate assessment of the underlying parenchymal disease.

There is disagreement whether an *infrapulmonary pleural effusion* (subpulmonic, diaphragmatic effusion) should be considered atypical, since this is the site where effusion first accumulates "normally." Usually, increasing amounts of fluid spill over into the costophrenic sulci and produce the roentgenologic signs described. Occasionally, however, fluid continues to accumulate in an infrapulmonary location without spilling into the costophrenic sulci or extending up the chest wall, producing a roentgenographic configuration in the erect subject that closely simulates diaphragmatic elevation (thus the designation "pseudodiaphragmatic contour") (*see* Fig. 4–86). The fluid accumulation may be unilateral or bilateral; when unilateral, it occurs more commonly on the right.[80]

The pathogenesis of infrapulmonary pleural effusions is not known. They occur in such multifarious conditions (inflammatory, cardiovascular, traumatic, neoplastic, renal) that it is impossible to ascribe a pathogenic role to the underlying cause of the effusion. The biochemical nature and specific gravity of the fluid have no significance, since the effusion may be either an exudate or a transudate. Loculation secondary to fibrous pleural adhesions also is not important, since appropriate positioning of the patient invariably shows the fluid spread over the free pleural space.

Some roentgenologic characteristics are common to most cases of infrapulmonary effusion,[76] and any combination of these warrants confirmatory roentgenographic study in lateral decubitus position to confirm the presence of fluid. All these signs refer to changes observed on posteroanterior and lateral roentgenograms of the erect patient.

1. In posteroanterior projection the peak of the pseudo-diaphragmatic configuration is lateral to that of the normal hemidiaphragm, being situated near the junction of the middle and the lateral thirds rather than near the center (Fig. 4–91); it slopes down sharply toward the lateral costophrenic recess.

2. On the left side, the pseudodiaphragmatic contour is separated farther than normal from the gastric air bubble (*see* Fig. 4–91); the hemidiaphragm and the bubble normally are within 1 cm of each other, although it is important to view the relationship in both posteroanterior and lateral projection.

3. Both the lateral and the posterior costophrenic sulci may be sharp and clear, although in many cases the posterior gutter appears blunted because fluid has spilled over into it.

4. In lateral projection, a characteristic configuration is frequently seen anteriorly, where the convex upper margin

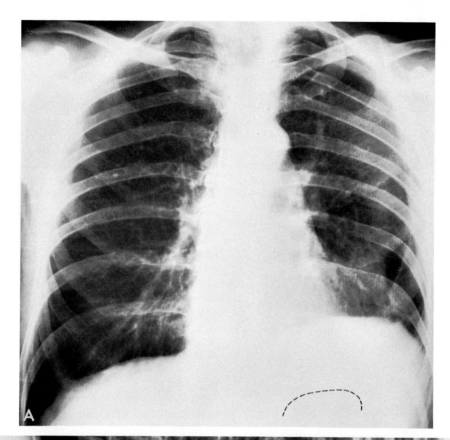

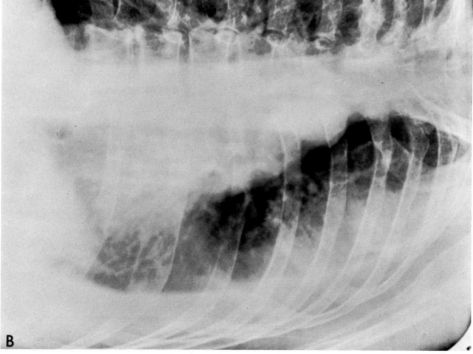

Figure 4–91. Infrapulmonary Pleural Effusion. A posteroanterior roentgenogram exposed in the erect position *(A)* shows a high left pseudodiaphragm whose peak is more laterally situated than that of a normal hemidiaphragm. It is situated several centimeters from the stomach bubble *(dotted line)*. The costophrenic sulcus is sharp. A roentgenogram exposed in the left lateral decubitus position with a horizontal x-ray beam *(B)* shows the fluid to have extended along the axillary lung zone.

of the fluid meets the major fissure. In many cases the contour anterior to the fissure is flattened, this segment descending abruptly to the costophrenic angle. A small amount of fluid is usually apparent in the lower end of the chief fissure where it joins the infrapulmonary collection.

5. In posteroanterior projection, a triangular opacity may be observed in the left paramediastinal zone, its apex approximately halfway up the mediastinum and its base contiguous with the pseudodiaphragmatic contour inferiorly (*see* Fig. 4-86*B*). This shadow, which represents mediastinal extension of the infrapulmonary fluid collection behind the pulmonary ligament, was observed in 8 of 39 patients in one study[80]; since it is situated posteriorly, it obliterates the left paraspinal line. It must not be mistaken for left lower lobe atelectasis, which it closely resembles; identification of the left interlobar artery permits ready distinction.

6. Fluoroscopic examination usually reveals no impairment of diaphragmatic excursion during respiration.

Lateral decubitus roentgenography with a horizontal beam should be performed in all cases, both to confirm the diagnosis and to permit more accurate assessment of the quantity of fluid than is possible with the patient erect. Sonography can also be useful in identifying subpulmonic collections of fluid; the examination should be carried out with the patient erect rather than supine.[81]

Loculation of Pleural Fluid

Loculated effusions may occur anywhere in the pleural space, either between parietal and visceral pleura over the periphery of the lung or between visceral layers in the interlobar fissures. Encapsulation is caused by adhesions between contiguous pleural surfaces and, therefore, tends to occur during or following episodes of pleuritis, often pyothorax or hemothorax. Over the convexity of the thorax, the loculated effusion appears as a smooth, sharply demarcated, homogeneous opacity protruding into the hemithorax and compressing contiguous lung (Fig. 4–92). Ultrasonography or CT helps establish its precise location for subsequent diagnostic or therapeutic thoracentesis; CT is especially advantageous in distinguishing pleural from pulmonary lesions, particularly when complex combined disease is present.[82]

Interlobar loculated effusions are typically elliptical when viewed tangentially, and their extremities blend imperceptibly with the interlobar fissure. In some conditions, particularly cardiac decompensation, the effusion may simulate a mass roentgenographically and be misdiagnosed as a pulmonary neoplasm (Fig. 4–93); however, its distinctive configuration in either posteroanterior or lateral projection should establish the diagnosis. These fluid accumulations tend to absorb spontaneously when heart failure is relieved and, therefore, have acquired the epithet "vanishing tumor" (phantom tumor, pseudotumor). In one series of 41 cases,[83] the effusion was localized to the right horizontal fissure in 78 per cent.

Roentgenologic Signs of Pleural Thickening

After effusion, thickening is the most common roentgenographic manifestation of pleural disease. It is most often caused by fibrosis or neoplasia. Fibrous thickening of the pleural line over the convexity of the thorax and occasionally in the interlobar fissures is fairly common. The thickness of the pleural line may increase to 1 to 10 mm, usually after an episode of pleuritis and almost always as a result of fibrosis of the visceral pleural surface. The major exception is the pleural plaque, an abnormality that occurs almost invariably on the parietal pleura in association with asbestos exposure.

Although sometimes local, pleural fibrosis is more often uniform over the whole lung surface, appearing as a line of unit density separating air-containing lung from contiguous ribs. Calcification may or may not be present. The costophrenic recesses often are partly or completely obliterated, particularly laterally, and roentgenography in the lateral decubitus position may be necessary to differentiate such fibrous thickening from a small pleural effusion. In cases of pleural thickening, however, the blunted costophrenic angle usually is sharply angulated rather than meniscus shaped, and the posterior gutter usually is not obliterated; often the two can be distinguished on this evidence alone.

One rather common form of local pleural fibrosis is a curved shadow of unit density in the apex of one or both lungs, in the concavity formed by the first and second ribs (Fig. 4–94). Called the apical cap, it is caused by a combination of both pleural and subpleural parenchymal fibrosis. Although of no clinical importance, it is sometimes erroneously ascribed to tuberculosis and is discussed further on page 881.

Pleural neoplasms also may be local or diffuse. The former form may arise from either the parietal or visceral pleural surface, over the convexity of the lung or from an interlobar fissure. In the latter situation, it may simulate an intrapulmonary nodule or an encapsulated interlobar effusion; in either case, CT should help establish the true nature of the lesion. When they arise from the convexity of the lung, these solitary tumors may be either sessile or pedunculated, but in either event they almost invariably form an obtuse angle with the chest wall when viewed in profile; this obtuse angle usually distinguishes them from lesions that arise within the lung parenchyma, which tend to form an acute angle with the chest wall.

Roentgenologic Signs of Pneumothorax

The discussion earlier in this section on the influence on underlying lung of fluid within the pleural space applies as well to gas. The only difference is in the manner in which gravity affects the media: in erect patients, air rises to the apex of the hemithorax and causes relaxation atelectasis of the upper portion of the lung whereas fluid falls to the bottom and permits atelectasis of the lower lobe. When pneumothorax is present, the weight of the lung in its gaseous surroundings causes it to drop to its most dependent position, slung by its fixed attachment at the pulmonary ligament. For this reason, a pneumothorax must be large to produce collapse of the whole lung.

The roentgenologic diagnosis of pneumothorax can be made only by identification of the visceral pleural line, a process that can be very difficult on roentgenograms exposed at total lung capacity. As previously discussed (*see* page 174), roentgenographic density of a collapsing lung changes little until volume is much reduced; this renders this sign useless for diagnostic purposes in virtually all cir-

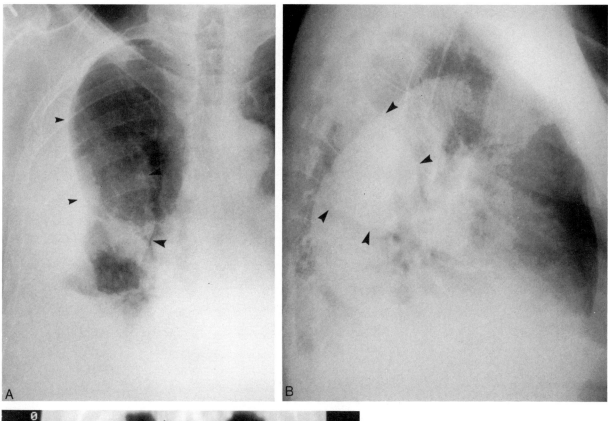

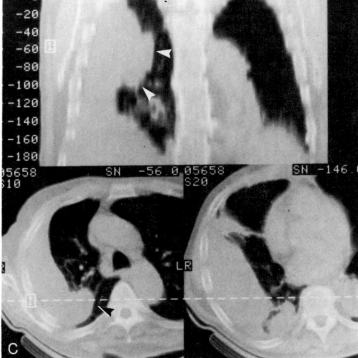

Figure 4–92. Loculated Pleural Effusion. Detail views of the right hemithorax from posteroanterior *(A)* and lateral *(B)* roentgenograms demonstrate a serpentine opacity that relates to the lateral *(small arrowheads)* and posterior interlobar *(large arrowheads)* pleura. Coronal CT reformations *(top)* through the opacity posteriorly *(C)* with appropriate axial CT images *(bottom)* reveal the contributions to the features shown in *A* and *B* by the posterior interlobar *(large arrowheads)* and lateral *(small arrowheads)* components of the encapsulated empyema.

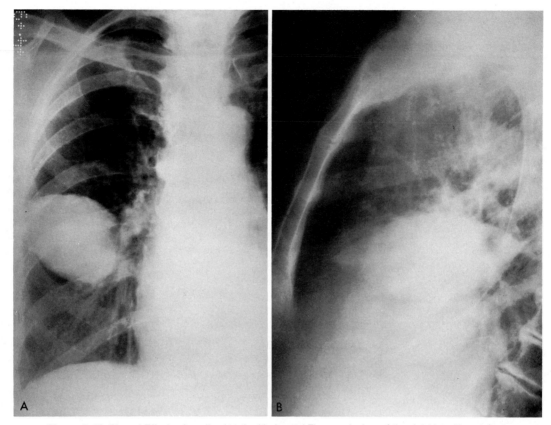

Figure 4–93. Pleural Effusion Localized to the Horizontal Fissure. A view of the right hemithorax from a posteroanterior roentgenogram *(A)* reveals a sharply defined opacity of homogeneous density in the right midlung zone. In lateral projection *(B),* the true nature of the opacity can be appreciated: the mass is elliptical in shape, its pointed extremities being situated anteriorly and posteriorly in keeping with the position of the minor fissure. This unusual collection of pleural fluid developed during a recent episode of cardiac decompensation. With appropriate therapy, it disappeared completely in 3 weeks; thus the designation "vanishing tumor."

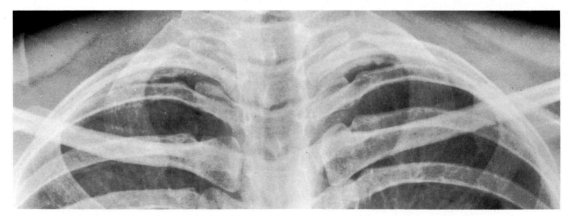

Figure 4–94. Apical Pleural Thickening. A view of the apical zones from a posteroanterior roentgenogram reveals irregular symmetric thickening of the apical pleura. The irregularity serves to differentiate this thickening from companion shadows of the ribs.

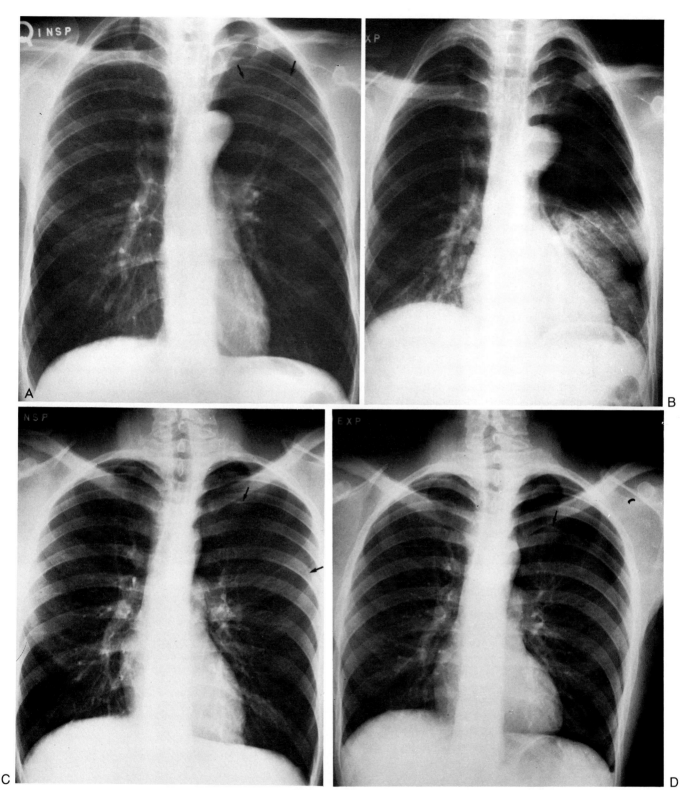

Figure 4–95. Inspiratory-Expiratory Roentgenograms in Spontaneous Pneumothorax Showing Difference in Response to a Closed and an Open Pleural Defect. A posteroanterior roentgenogram exposed at full inspiration *(A)* shows a 10 per cent left pneumothorax (the visceral pleural surface is indicated by *arrows*). On expiration *(B)*, the volume of the left lung has diminished markedly, suggesting that its air has been expelled via the tracheobronchial tree and that the pleural defect therefore must be either closed or exceedingly small. The possibility that air was escaping from the lung *into* the pleural space (thus enlarging the pneumothorax) was excluded by exposing a third film at TLC, which had an appearance identical to that in *A*. A posteroanterior roentgenogram from another patient exposed at full inspiration *(C)* shows a 10 to 15 per cent left pneumothorax (the visceral pleura is indicated by *arrows*). On expiration *(D)*, the volume of the pneumothorax and of the left lung have reduced roughly proportionately, suggesting that equilibrium is present between the two compartments and that the pleural defect thus is open.

cumstances. When pneumothorax is strongly suspected clinically, however, but a pleural line is not identified (possibly obscured by an overlying rib), gas in the pleural space can be detected by either of two procedures. One is roentgenography with the patient erect in full expiration. The rationale is that lung volume is reduced although the volume of gas in the pleural space is constant, thus providing a smaller surface of visceral pleura in contact with air. The other is roentgenography in the lateral decubitus position with a horizontal x-ray beam, the rationale in this situation being that air rises to the highest point in the hemithorax and is more clearly visible over the lateral chest wall than over the apex, where confluence of overlying bony shadows may obscure fine linear shadows.

In the majority of clinical settings, patients with suspected pneumothorax are radiographed in the erect position, in which case the upper portion of the lung is collapsed. When patients must be examined in the supine position, gas in the pleural space rises to the highest point in the hemithorax, which is in the vicinity of the diaphragm.[84] Depending on the size of the pneumothorax, the result can be an exceptionally deep radiolucent costophrenic sulcus,[85] a lucency over the right or left upper quadrant,[86] or a much sharper than normal appearance of the hemidiaphragm, with or without a visible visceral pleural line above the hemidiaphragm.[87]

Inspiration-expiration roentgenography also may be employed in the assessment of the size of the pleural defect in spontaneous pneumothorax. If the defect is closed or very small, the expiratory roentgenogram shows a marked change in volume of the ipsilateral lung because air has been expired via the tracheobronchial tree (Fig. 4–95). If the defect is open, volume change in the ipsilateral lung is minimal, as communication persists between the pleural space and the lung parenchyma. Such information should help referring physicians decide whether insertion of a chest tube is necessary.

Tension Pneumothorax and Hydropneumothorax

On the evidence supplied by roentgenograms of the chest at total lung capacity, detection of increased pressure in a pneumothorax (tension pneumothorax) can be exceedingly difficult, especially if the pneumothorax is complete and collapse of the ipsilateral lung total. Shift of the mediastinum away from the side of a pneumothorax of any size is inevitable, pressure in the contralateral (normal) hemithorax being relatively more negative; such a shift must not be mistaken for evidence of tension pneumothorax. In fact, tension pneumothorax should be regarded as a clinical state characterized by cardiorespiratory embarrassment rather than a radiographic abnormality.

It is important to realize that increased pressure in a pneumothorax develops only occasionally and in a very specific anatomic situation. For the volume of a pneumothorax to increase, air must flow from the lung parenchyma (where pressure is atmospheric) through the pleural defect and into the pleural space. Obviously, such flow cannot occur if pleural pressure is greater than atmospheric, or under tension. Thus, for a pneumothorax to increase in volume, pressure within the pleural space must be relatively negative *during inspiration*: if a check-valve mechanism exists, al-

lowing air to enter the pleural space during inspiration but preventing its egress during expiration, pressure within the pleural space will be positive during the latter phase of respiration. Thus, tension pneumothorax could be qualified appropriately by the term *expiratory*.

The presence of both gas and fluid in the pleural space *(hydropneumothorax)* should be immediately apparent on roentgenograms exposed with the patient in the erect position, by dint of the almost invariable air-fluid level. Loculated forms appear as single or multiple collections, some of which may contain an air-fluid level.

References

1. Genereux GP: CT of acute and chronic distal airspace (alveolar) disease. Semin Roentgenol 19: 211, 1984.
2. Raskin SP, Herman PG: A new experimental model to study flow patterns in the distal airways (abstract). Invest Radiol 8: 263, 1973.
3. Gamsu G, Thurlbeck WM, Macklem PT, et al: Roentgenographic appearance of the human pulmonary acinus. Invest Radiol 6: 171, 1971.
4. Hogg JC, Macklem PT, Thurlbeck WM: The resistance of collateral channels in excised human lungs. J Clin Invest 48: 421, 1969.
5. Felson B: Chest Roentgenology. Philadelphia, WB Saunders, 1973.
6. Coulter WW Jr: Experimental massive pulmonary collapse. Dis Chest 18: 146, 1950.
7. Rahn H: The role of N$_2$ gas in various biological processes, with particular reference to the lung. Harvey Lect 55: 173, 1960.
8. Fleischner FG: Linear shadows in the lung field. In Rabin CB (ed): Roentgenology of the Chest. Springfield, IL, Charles C Thomas, 1958.
9. Burke M, Fraser R: Obstructive pneumonitis: A pathologic and pathogenetic reappraisal. Radiology 166: 699, 1988.
10. Dornhorst AC, Pierce JW: Pulmonary collapse and consolidation: The role of collapse in the production of lung field shadows and the significance of segments in inflammatory lung disease. J Fac Radiol 5: 276, 1954.
11. Schneider HJ, Felson B, Gonzalez LL: Rounded atelectasis. Am J Roentgenol 134: 225, 1980.
12. Hanke R, Kretzschmar R: Round atelectasis. Semin Roentgenol 15: 174, 1980.
13. McHugh K, Blaquiere RM: CT features of rounded atelectasis. Am J Roentgenol 153: 257, 1989.
14. Menzies R, Fraser R: Round atelectasis. Pathologic and pathogenetic features. Am J Surg Pathol 11: 674, 1987.
15. Sutnick AI, Soloff LA: Atelectasis with pneumonia. A pathophysiologic study. Ann Intern Med 60: 39, 1964.
16. Lubert M, Krause GR: Total unilateral pulmonary collapse: A study of the roentgen appearance in the lateral view. Radiology 67: 175, 1956.
17. Whalen JP, Lane EJ Jr: Bronchial rearrangements in pulmonary collapse as seen on the lateral radiograph. Radiology 93: 285, 1969.
18. Lane EJ Jr, Whalen JP: A new sign of left atrial enlargement: Posterior displacement of the left bronchial tree. Radiology 93: 279, 1969.
19. Lubert M, Krause GR: Patterns of lobar collapse as observed radiographically. Radiology 56: 165, 1951.
20. Lubert M, Krause GR: Further observations on lobar collapse. Radiol Clin North Am 1: 331, 1963.
21. Khoury MB, Godwin JD, Halvorsen RA Jr, et al: CT of obstructive lobar collapse. Invest Radiol 20: 708, 1985.
22. Kattan KR, Eyler WR, Felson B: The juxtaphrenic peak in upper lobe collapse. Semin Roentgenol 15: 187, 1980.
23. Webber M, Davies P: The Luftsichel: An old sign in upper lobe collapse. Clin Radiol 32: 271, 1981.
24. Raasch BN, Heitzman ER, Carsky EW, et al: A computed tomographic study of bronchopulmonary collapse. RadioGraphics 4: 195, 1984.
25. Cohen BA, Rabinowitz JG, Mendleson DS: The pulmonary ligament. Radiol Clin North Am 22: 659, 1984.
26. Friedman PJ: Radiology of the superior segment of the lower lobe. A regional perspective, introducing the B6 bronchus sign. Radiology 144: 15, 1982.
27. Felson B: A new look at pattern recognition of diffuse pulmonary disease. Am J Roentgenol 133: 183, 1979.

28. Staub NC, Nagano H, Pearce ML: Pulmonary edema in dogs, especially the sequence of fluid accumulation in lungs. J Appl Physiol 22: 227, 1967.
29. Müller NL, Miller RR: State of the art: Computed tomography of chronic diffuse infiltrative lung disease. Part 1. Am Rev Respir Dis 142: 1206, 1990.
30. Müller NL, Miller RR: State of the art: Computed tomography of chronic diffuse infiltrative lung disease. Part 2. Am Rev Respir Dis 142: 1440, 1990.
31. Mathieson JR, Mayo JR, Staples CA, et al: Chronic diffuse infiltrative lung disease: Comparison of diagnostic accuracy of CT and chest radiography. Radiology 171: 111, 1989.
32. Burgen CJ, Mller NL: CT in the diagnosis of interstitial lung disease. Am J Roentgenol 145: 505, 1985.
33. Friedman PG: The concept of alveolar and interstitial disease. In Potchen EJ (ed): Current Concepts in Radiology. St. Louis, CV Mosby, 1972, pp 64–106.
34. Bateson EM: An analysis of 155 solitary lung lesions illustrating the differential diagnosis of mixed tumours of the lung. Clin Radiol 16: 51, 1965.
35. Drevvatne T, Frimann-Dahl J: Peripheral bronchial carcinomas: A radiological and pathological study. Br J Radiol 34: 180, 1961.
36. Steele JD: The Solitary Pulmonary Nodule. Springfield, IL, Charles C Thomas, 1964.
37. Bancks N, Zornoza J: Pseudocavitary granulomas of the lung. Am J Roentgenol 127: 251, 1976.
38. Woodring JH, Fried M, Chuang VP: Solitary cavities of the lung: Diagnostic implications of cavity wall thickness. Am J Roentgenol 135: 1269, 1980.
39. Bloomfield JA: Protean radiological manifestations of hydatid infestation. Australas Radiol 10: 330, 1966.
40. Good CA: The solitary pulmonary nodule: A problem of management. Radiol Clin North Am 1: 429, 1963.
41. Stewart JG, MacMahon H, Vyborny CJ, et al: Dystrophic calcification in carcinoma of the lung: Demonstration by CT (case report). Am J Roentgenol 148: 29, 1987.
42. Fraser RG, Hickey NM, Nicklason LT, et al: Dual-energy digital radiography in the detection of calcification in pulmonary nodules. Radiology 160: 595, 1986.
43. Galloway RW, Epstein EJ, Coulshed N: Pulmonary ossific nodules in mitral valve disease. Br Heart J 23: 297, 1961.
44. Abrahams EW, Evans C, Knyvett AF, et al: Varicella pneumonia: A possible cause of subsequent pulmonary calcification. Med J Aust 2: 781, 1964.
45. Felson B, Schwarz J, Lukin RR, et al: Idiopathic pulmonary ossification. Radiology 153: 303, 1984.
46. Jost RG, Sagel SS: Metastatic calcification in the lung apex. Am J Roentgenol 133: 1188, 1979.
47. Rosenthal DI, Chandler HL, Azizi F, et al: Uptake of bone imaging agents by diffuse pulmonary metastatic calcification. Am J Roentgenol 129: 871, 1977.
48. Auerbach JM, Ho J: Gallium-67 uptake in the lung associated with metastatic calcification. Am J Roentgenol 136: 605, 1981.
49. Gross BH, Schneider HJ, Proto AV: Eggshell calcification of lymph nodes: An update. Am J Roentgenol 135: 1265, 1980.
50. Salzman E: Lung Calcifications in X-ray Diagnosis. Springfield, IL, Charles C Thomas, 1968.
51. Robertson OH, Hamburger M: Studies on the pathogenesis of experimental pneumococcus pneumonia in dogs. II. Secondary pulmonary lesions. Their production by intratracheal and intrabronchial injection of fluid pneumonic exudate. J Exp Med 72: 275, 1940.
52. Garland LH: Bronchial carcimona. Lobar distribution of lesions in 250 cases. Calif Med 94: 7, 1961.
53. West JB: Regional Differences in the Lung. New York, Academic Press, 1977, pp 313–319.
54. Lentino W, Jacobson HG, Poppel MH: Segmental localization of upper lobe tuberculosis: The rarity of anterior involvement. Am J Roentgenol 77: 1042, 1957.
55. Nathan MH, Collins VP, Adams RA: Differentiation of benign and malignant pulmonary nodules by growth rate. Radiology 79: 221, 1962.
56. Trapnell DH: The differential diagnosis of linear shadows in chest radiographs. Radiol Clin North Am 11: 77, 1973.
57. Heitzman ER, Ziter FM Jr, Makarian B, et al: Kerley's interlobular septal lines: Roentgen pathologic correlation. Am J Roentgenol 100: 578, 1967.
58. Simon G: Principles of Chest X-ray Diagnosis. 3rd ed. London, Butterworth, 1971.
59. Bates DV, Gordon CA, Paul GI, et al: Chronic bronchitis: Report on the third and fourth stages of the co-ordinated study of chronic bronchitis in the Department of Veterans Affairs, Canada. Med Serv J Can 22: 5, 1966.
60. Fraser RG, Fraser RS, Renner JW, et al: The roentgenographic diagnosis of chronic bronchitis: A reassessment with emphasis on parahilar bronchi seen end-on. Radiology 120: 1, 1976.
61. Rigler LG: Personal communication, 1965.
62. Hill CA: "Tail" signs associated with pulmonary lesions: Critical reappraisal. Am J Roentgenol 139: 311, 1982.
63. Reid L: [Quoted by Simon G, as a personal communication.] Br J Radiol 43: 327, 1970.
64. Westcott JL, Cole S: Plate atelectasis. Radiology 155: 1, 1985.
65. Simon G: The cause and significance of some long line shadows in the chest radiograph. Proc R Soc Med 58: 861, 1965.
66. Simon G: Further observations on the long line shadows across a lower zone of lung. Br J Radiol 43: 327, 1970.
67. Sutinen S, Christoforidis AJ, Klugh GA, et al: Roentgenologic criteria for the recognition of nonsymptomatic pulmonary emphysema: Correlation between roentgenologic findings and pulmonary pathology. Am Rev Respir Dis 91: 69, 1965.
68. Thomson KR, Eyssen GE, Fraser RG: Discrimination of normal and overinflated lungs and prediction of total lung capacity based on chest film measurements. Radiology 119: 721, 1976.
69. Christie RV: Emphysema of the lungs. Br Med J 1: 105, 1944.
70. Reid JM, Barclay RS, Stevenson JG, et al: Congenital obstructive lobar emphysema. Dis Chest 49: 359, 1966.
71. Byrd RB, Miller WE, Carr DT, et al: The roentgenographic appearance of squamous cell carcinoma of the bronchus. Mayo Clin Proc 43: 327, 1968.
72. Kieffer SA, Amplatz K, Anderson RC, et al: Proximal interruption of a pulmonary artery: Roentgen features and surgical correction. Am J Roentgenol 95: 592, 1965.
73. Quigley MJ, Fraser RS: Pulmonary pneumatocele: Pathology and pathogenesis. Am J Roentgenol 150: 1275, 1988.
74. Müller R, Löfstedt S: The reaction of the pleura in primary tuberculosis of the lungs. Acta Med Scand 122: 105, 1945.
75. Moskowitz H, Platt RT, Schachar R, et al: Roentgen visualization of minute pleural effusion: An experimental study to determine the minimum amount of pleural fluid visible on a radiograph. Radiology 109: 33, 1973.
76. Fleischner FG: Atypical arrangement of free pleural effusion. Radiol Clin North Am 1: 347, 1963.
77. Mulvey RB: The effect of pleural fluid on the diaphragm. Radiology 84: 1080, 1965,
78. Naidich DP, Zerhouni EA, Siegelman SS: Lobar collapse. In Computed Tomography of the Thorax. New York, Raven Press, 1984, p 111.
79. Peterson JA: Recognition of infrapulmonary pleural effusion. Radiology 74: 34, 1960.
80. Dunbar JS, Favreau M: Infrapulmonary pleural effusion with particular reference to its occurrence in nephrosis. J Can Assoc Radiol 10: 24, 1959.
81. Connell DG, Crothers G, Cooperberg PL: The subpulmonic pleural effusion: Sonographic aspects. J Can Assoc Radiol 33: 101, 1982.
82. Pugatch RK, Faling LJ, Robbins AH, et al: Differentiation of pleural and pulmonary lesions using computed tomography. J Comput Assist Tomog 2: 601, 1978.
83. Higgins JA, Juergens JL, Bruwer AJ, et al: Loculated interlobar pleural effusion due to congestive heart failure. Arch Intern Med 96: 180, 1955.
84. Tocino IM, Miller MH, Fairfax WR: Distribution of pneumothorax in the supine and semirecumbent critically ill adult. Am J Roentgenol 144: 901, 1985.
85. Gordon R: The deep sulcus sign. Radiology 136: 25, 1980.
86. Rhea JT, vanSonnenberg E, McLoud TC: Basilar pneumothorax in the supine adult. Radiology 133: 595, 1979.
87. Ziter FMH, Westcott JL: Supine subpulmonary pneumothorax. Am J Roentgenol 137: 699, 1981.

5

PULMONARY ABNORMALITIES OF DEVELOPMENTAL ORIGIN

For purposes of discussion, developmental anomalies of the trachea, lungs, and major pulmonary vessels can be divided into two groups, depending on the predominant anlage affected: (1) those originating in the primitive foregut or its derivative, the lung bud *(bronchopulmonary or foregut anomalies)*, and (2) those arising from the sixth aortic arch or venous radicles and their derivatives *(pulmo-* *nary vascular anomalies)*. Despite the convenience of this division and the use of specific terms for various anatomic patterns, it should be appreciated that conditions in both groups overlap and, in some instances, it is virtually impossible to categorize an anomaly precisely.[1] In fact, it has been proposed that many of the anomalies represent part of a continuum of maldevelopment rather than distinct entities.[2]

Because of their serious pulmonary or cardiovascular complications and their not infrequent association with other congenital abnormalities, many developmental pulmonary anomalies are discovered in neonates or infants. Some malformations, however, such as intralobar sequestration and bronchial cyst, typically do not occasion signs and symptoms until much later in life. In addition, some abnormalities that normally present in infancy, occasionally are manifested much later.[3] Thus, although most common in infancy and childhood, developmental anomalies should always be considered in the differential diagnosis of adult pulmonary and mediastinal disease, especially in younger individuals.

BRONCHOPULMONARY ANOMALIES

Pulmonary Agenesis, Aplasia, and Hypoplasia

According to Boyden,[4] there are three degrees of arrested pulmonary development: (1) *agenesis*, in which there is complete absence of one or both lungs, with no trace of bronchial or vascular supply or of parenchymal tissue; (2) *aplasia*, in which there is suppression of all but a rudimentary bronchus, which ends in a blind pouch, with no evidence of pulmonary vasculature or parenchyma; and (3) *hypoplasia*, in which the gross morphology of the lung is essentially normal but in which there is a decrease in the number or size of airways, vessels, and alveoli. In practice, an etiologic, pathogenic, or clinical distinction between agenesis and aplasia is seldom apparent, and the two conditions are usually considered together.[5, 6] Hypoplasia, however, is often associated with other congenital anomalies, many of which are thought to be of importance in the pathogenesis of the condition, and it is likely that it represents an abnormality that is qualitatively different from either agenesis or aplasia. Hypoplasia typically involves the whole lung; when it affects only one lobe, it usually is accompanied by anomalies of the ipsilateral pulmonary artery and anomalous pulmonary venous drainage, the three abnormalities constituting the hypogenetic lung syndrome (*see* page 277).

Etiology and Pathogenesis. Unilateral pulmonary agenesis (aplasia) has occasionally been described in twins and in infants with chromosome abnormalities, suggesting a genetic basis for the anomaly.[6] The possibility that twinning itself might be a factor in some cases also has been suggested.[6]

Hypoplasia of the lung can be regarded as *primary* (without obvious associated etiologic factors) or *secondary* (when it occurs with other congenital anomalies that may be implicated in its pathogenesis).[7] Several potential mechanisms underlie these complicating anomalies.

Decreased volume of the ipsilateral hemithorax is the most frequent associated abnormality and can itself have several causes. The most common is a space-occupying mass within the pleural cavity, usually abdominal contents displaced through a congenital diaphragmatic hernia.[8] A variety of musculoskeletal deformities of the thoracic cage[8] and abnormalities of diaphragmatic development[9] also have been associated; although these also may act by reducing the size of the thoracic cavity, it is possible that decreased

intrauterine respiratory movements caused by diminished chest wall compliance or decreased muscle mass[10] may be of greater importance (*see* later).

Another relatively common group of developmental anomalies associated with pulmonary hypoplasia involves the kidney and urinary tract. Of these, Potter's syndrome (renal agenesis, abnormal facies, limb abnormalities, and pulmonary hypoplasia) is the most frequent. It has been suggested that the presence of oligohydramnios in these conditions leads to hypoplasia as a result of thoracic compression by the closely applied uterine wall.[8] Although this may occur to some extent, the occasional cases in which both renal and pulmonary abnormalities are present and amniotic fluid is either normal or excessive in amount[8] suggest that other factors may be more important. One such factor might be decreased *intrapulmonary* fluid; experimental studies in rabbits have suggested that this may occur in lung hypoplasia associated with oligohydramnios.[11] Since such fluid normally exerts positive pressure within the developing lung, its deficiency could result in the loss of an internal template about which the lung can form.

Several investigations have shown appreciable lung hypoplasia in animals subjected to intrauterine cervical cord injury or bilateral phrenic nerve section.[12, 13] Thus, it has been speculated that the central nervous system may have an important role in lung development, possibly by maintaining normal fetal respiratory movements. It is conceivable, therefore, that some neurologic abnormality could result in human pulmonary hypoplasia. It is also possible that a decrease in respiratory movements, at least in part, may be the mechanism by which a thoracic mass or a deformed thoracic cage induces hypoplasia.

Although the mechanisms just described are likely important in the majority of cases of pulmonary hypoplasia, it is clear that others also must exist; several authors have described fairly consistent associations between the anomaly and conditions such as Down's syndrome[14] and rhesus isoimmunization[15] that are not clearly related to the previously discussed pathogenetic mechanisms.

Primary hypoplasia may be more common than is generally recognized.[16] By definition unassociated with other anomalies, it may represent an intrinsic defect in lung development. Conceivably, an unrecognized abnormality in central nervous system (CNS) control of fetal respiratory movements also might be a causative factor.

Pathologic Characteristics. Hypoplastic lungs typically are smaller and weigh less than normal for age. Although there is variation in the severity and type of morphologic abnormality, the most consistent finding is a decrease in the number of airway generations, ranging from about 50 to 75 per cent of normal.[17, 18] In addition, there is frequently a decrease in the number of alveoli, estimated by one group[18] to be about 60 to 70 per cent; this is often associated with a decrease in alveolar size. Some studies have shown normal airway and alveolar maturation for gestational age; in others, the appearance is immature.[19] Abnormalities of the pulmonary arterial system also have been identified.

Roentgenographic Manifestations. The principal roentgenographic finding in cases of agenesis, aplasia, or severe hypoplasia is total or almost total absence of aerated lung in one hemithorax. The markedly reduced volume is indicated by approximation of the ribs, elevation of the ipsilateral hemidiaphragm, and shift of the mediastinum (Fig. 5–1). In most cases, the contralateral lung is greatly overinflated and displaced, along with the anterior mediastinal septum, into the involved hemithorax.[20] Conventional tomography or (preferably) computed tomography (CT)[21] and angiography may be required to establish the degree of underdevelopment[22] or to differentiate agenesis from other conditions that may closely mimic it roentgenographically, such as total atelectasis, severe bronchiectasis with collapse, and advanced fibrothorax.

Clinical Manifestations. Clinical findings in pulmonary hypoplasia depend on the severity of altered growth and the presence of other congenital malformations, particularly of the kidneys, diaphragm, and the thoracic cage itself. Physical examination characteristically reveals asymmetry of the two sides of the thorax, reduction in respiratory movement, and absence of air entry into the affected side. Patients with aplasia manifest similar findings.

Both agenesis and aplasia appear to predispose to respiratory infection,[8, 23] and many patients die before their tenth birthday, particularly in the neonatal period. Despite this, survival into adulthood, sometimes without symptoms, is clearly possible; in a review of the literature published after 1954, 24 of 36 patients with pulmonary agenesis were alive in 1968.[23] The number of individuals who survive with hypoplasia, especially the less severe form, is undoubtedly much greater.

Bronchopulmonary Sequestration

Bronchopulmonary sequestration is a pulmonary malformation in which a portion of lung parenchyma has no communication with the tracheobronchial tree and receives its blood supply via a systemic artery. The anomaly may be *intralobar* or *extralobar*: the first type is contiguous with normal lung parenchyma and within the same visceral pleural envelope; the latter is enclosed within its own pleural membrane, usually close to a normal lung but sometimes within or below the diaphragm. Although it is discussed here as a specific entity, sequestration possesses anatomic features that overlap with those of a variety of other congenital anomalies, and the distinctiveness of the condition has been questioned.[24, 25]

Pathogenesis. The most widely accepted pathogenetic theory considers sequestration to represent a developmental anomaly of tracheobronchial branching with persistence and localized development of a separated branch fragment and retention of its embryonic systemic vascular supply.[26] The location of the sequestration may reflect the time at which the developmental aberration occurs. Fragments of the developing bronchial tree that separate at an early stage from the primitive lung bud or from a separate foregut diverticulum may acquire a separate pleural investment and develop within the mediastinum or outside the thorax, thus forming an extralobar sequestration. By contrast, separated bronchial fragments of the partially developed lung might be expected to continue their development within the lung itself, thus becoming the intralobar form. The relatively frequent communication of extralobar sequestrations with the esophagus[27] supports this hypothesis.

The developmental mechanisms that underlie the abnormal blood supply to the sequestered lung are not clear.

Normally, when the pulmonary artery elaborates from the sixth embryonic arch and invaginates its branches into the primitive pulmonary anlage, the branches of the splanchnic plexus that initially supply the lung bud regress and remain only as the bronchial arteries. According to the standard theory, additional branches persist, resulting in the anomalous systemic arterial supply to the sequestered lung. The reason for this hypothesized persistence may be failure of normal pulmonary vascular ingrowth caused by the abnormal position of the sequestered branch fragment.

Although most investigators believe that bronchopulmonary sequestration represents a developmental anomaly, some have proposed that the intralobar form is in fact an acquired lesion, pathogenetically distinct from the extralobar variety. According to Stocker and Malczak,[28] the initial event in the formation of intralobar sequestration is focal bronchial obstruction, possibly caused by infection or foreign body aspiration. Persistence of the obstruction (or perhaps the effects of an associated infectious pneumonitis) leads to the characteristic cystic and fibrotic changes in lung parenchyma. In addition, these authors propose that the initial inflammatory process interrupts pulmonary artery blood flow to the affected lung segment; hypertrophy of systemic arteries (small branches of which are normally present in the pulmonary ligament of some individuals) then results in the "anomalous" vascular supply.

Intralobar Sequestration

The incidence of intralobar sequestration is low; in one review of the literature to 1975, only 400 cases were identified.[29] In approximately two thirds of cases, the sequestered lung is situated in the paravertebral gutter within the posterior bronchopulmonary segment of the left lower lobe; in most others, it occupies the same anatomic region of the right lower lobe. The abnormality is infrequently associated with other anomalies, the most common being esophageal diverticula, diaphragmatic hernia, and a variety of skeletal and cardiac defects.[29]

Pathologic Characteristics. Grossly, the abnormal tissue is usually well demarcated from surrounding lung parenchyma and consists of one or more cystic spaces with a variable amount of intervening, more solid tissue (Fig. 5–2). The cysts are filled with mucus or, when infection is present, with pus. Microscopically, they resemble dilated bronchi, with respiratory epithelium and occasional mural cartilage plates. The amount of intervening parenchymal tissue varies from scanty to abundant and in uncomplicated cases shows changes of obstructive pneumonitis.

The abnormal tissue invariably derives its arterial supply from the aorta or one of its branches, most commonly the descending thoracic aorta; although usually solitary, multiple tributary vessels can be seen. Typically, the anomalous vessel enters the lung by way of the lower part of the pulmonary ligament and is much larger than would be expected for the volume of tissue supplied. The venous drainage is almost always via the pulmonary venous system, producing a left-to-left shunt.

Roentgenographic Manifestations. The roentgenographic appearance is dependent largely on the volume of lung tissue sequestered and the presence or absence of infection. In instances in which no communication exists

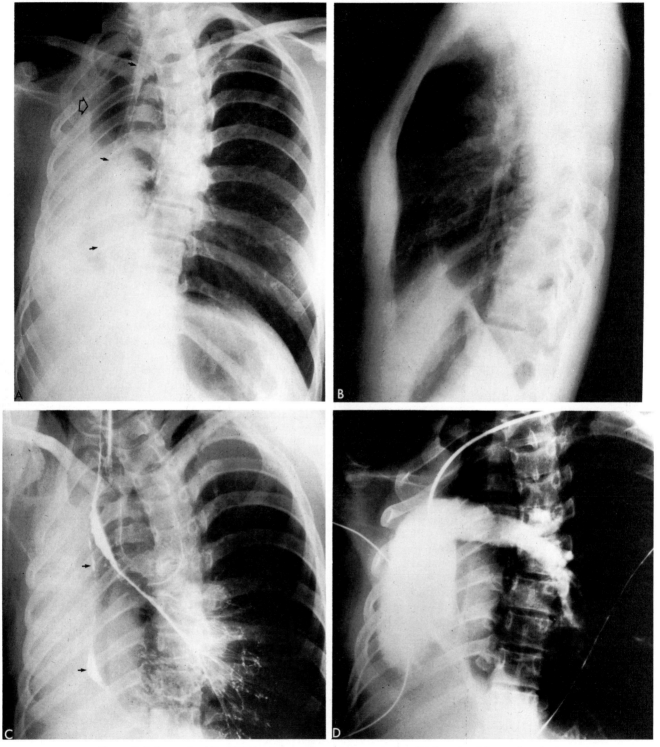

Figure 5–1. Agenesis of the Right Lung. In posteroanterior projection *(A)*, there is evidence of marked displacement of the mediastinum to the right, both the heart and esophagus being entirely within the right hemithorax (the latter indicated by the position of the nasogastric tube—*solid arrows*). The left lung is severely overinflated, as indicated by the displaced anterior mediastinal septum in postero-anterior projection *(open arrow)* and by the large retrosternal airspace in lateral projection *(B)*. A bronchogram *(C)* shows no vestige of a right main bronchus *(arrows* point to contrast medium in the displaced esophagus). A pulmonary angiogram *(D)* reveals total absence of a right pulmonary artery. (Courtesy of Dr. David Stephen, Royal Prince Albert Hospital, Sydney, Australia.)

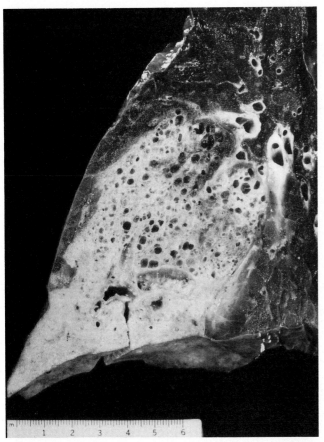

Figure 5–2. Intralobar Bronchopulmonary Sequestration. The posterior basal region of this resected left lower lobe shows a poorly defined area of consolidation containing numerous cystic spaces measuring 1 to 5 mm; its blood supply originated in the abdominal aorta.

between the sequestered lung and normal lung, the anomalous tissue appears as a homogeneous, sharply defined, lobulated mass of unit density in the posterior portion of a lower lobe, almost invariably contiguous with the hemidiaphragm. The cystic nature of the mass can usually be readily demonstrated by either CT[30] or magnetic resonance imaging (MRI).[31] Characteristically, the bronchoarterial and venous bundles of the normal lung are displaced away from or festooned around the periphery of the sequestered lobe (Fig. 5–3), a feature that is revealed particularly well by conventional tomography or CT.[30] Calcification has been reported occasionally.[32, 33]

When infection has resulted in communication with the bronchial tree, the roentgenographic presentation consists of an air-containing cystic mass, with or without fluid levels (Fig. 5–4).[34] The cysts can be single or multiple and vary in size. The pneumonia usually affects the surrounding parenchyma, and the cystic nature of the mass may not be manifested until it resolves. The size of the lesion can vary considerably with time, depending on the amount of gas and fluid within it; in fact, an infected sequestered segment can exhibit a rapidly changing roentgenologic pattern over a very short time.[35] Air trapping within the sequestered segment can occur on expiration, a feature that has recently been shown on dynamic, ultrafast, high-resolution CT scans.[36]

The anomalous systemic vessel feeding the sequestered lung usually is not visible without the aid of aortography, although occasionally it can be seen on CT scans.[30] Imaging methods for the investigation of pulmonary sequestration were recently reviewed.[37, 38]

Clinical Manifestations. Most patients are asymptomatic until an acute respiratory infection develops; in many cases, this does not happen until adulthood.[29] Then, signs and symptoms are those of acute lower lobe pneumonia; the basic defect becomes apparent only through roentgenologic observation of the sequence of changes during resolution of the infection. Infections are usually caused by pyogenic bacteria. Differential diagnosis includes bronchiectasis, lung abscess, and hernia of Bochdalek. Preoperative diagnosis by aortography is important in view of the hazards involved in severing the anomalous systemic vessel during surgical resection.

Extralobar Sequestration

Extralobar pulmonary sequestration is less common than the intralobar variety; in the review of sequestration cited previously, only 123 cases were identified up to 1975.[29]

The abnormality is related to the left hemidiaphragm in 90 per cent of cases; it may be situated between the inferior surface of the lower lobe and the diaphragm, below the diaphragm, within the substance of the diaphragm, or even in the mediastinum. As in intralobar sequestration, the systemic arterial supply is commonly from the aorta, usually the abdominal portion or one of its branches. In contrast to the intralobar variety, however, venous drainage is usually via the systemic venous system—the inferior vena cava, the azygos or hemiazygos veins, or the portal system—creating a left-to-right shunt. Also in contrast to intralobar sequestration, the extralobar anomaly is seen most often in neonates and in many cases is associated with other congenital anomalies, particularly eventration or paralysis of the ipsilateral hemidiaphragm (in approximately 60 per cent of cases[8]) and left diaphragmatic hernia (in approximately 30 per cent[29]).

Morphologically, the sequestered tissue is completely enclosed in a pleural sac. The cut surface reveals spongy, tan-colored tissue with irregularly arranged vessels, often more prominent at one end of the specimen. Airways are usually few in number and parenchymal tissue often appears immature.

Since the sequestered pulmonary tissue is enveloped in its own pleural sac, the chances of its becoming infected are very small, unless there is communication with the gastrointestinal tract.[26] Consequently, the chief mode of presentation in patients without other significant congenital anomalies is as a homogeneous soft tissue mass in an asymptomatic individual. As with intralobar sequestration, the systemic arterial supply to this anomaly should be determined before surgery is undertaken.

Congenital Bronchial Cysts

Like bronchopulmonary sequestration, bronchial (bronchogenic) cysts are believed to represent localized portions of the tracheobronchial tree that become separated from adjacent airways during the branching process. Unlike the latter, however, they do not undergo further development.

Figure 5–3. Intralobar Bronchopulmonary Sequestration. Conventional posteroanterior *(A)* and lateral *(B)* chest roentgenograms demonstrate a well-defined mass of unit density *(arrowheads)* in the posteromedial portion of the right lower lobe. *C,* Following resection of the lower lobe, a catheter was inserted into the aberrant artery *(small arrowheads)* supplying the lower lobe sequestrum and contrast medium injected. The right interlobar artery was also opacified *(large arrowhead)*, revealing the arterial festooning that characterizes this condition.

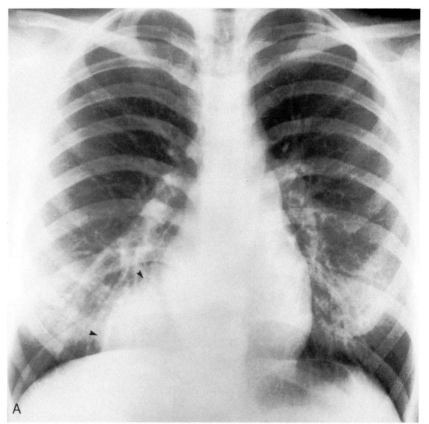

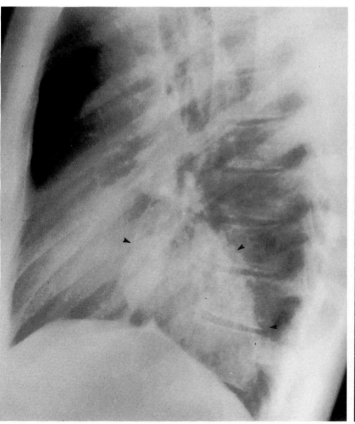

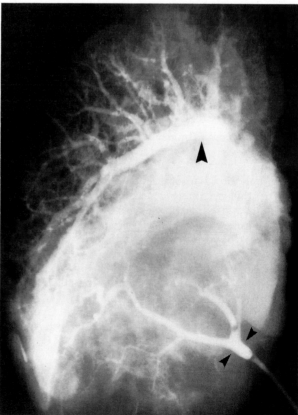

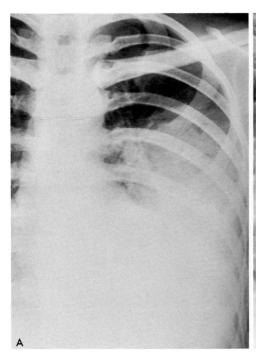
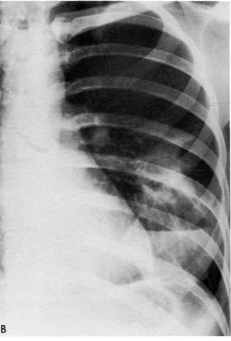

Figure 5–4. Intralobar Pulmonary Sequestration. A view of the left hemithorax from a posteroanterior roentgenogram *(A)* reveals massive airspace consolidation of the lower two thirds of the left lung; note the air bronchogram in the upper portion of the consolidation. Three weeks later *(B)*, there is almost complete resolution of the pneumonia, but there remains a rather well-defined mass lying contiguous to the left hemidiaphragm and possessing a prominent air-fluid level. At thoracotomy, an anomalous systemic vessel was seen to enter the sequestered mass from the diaphragm.

They can thus be considered as representing one end of a spectrum of pathogenetically similar conditions, including extralobar and intralobar sequestration, and, possibly, congenital cystic bronchiectasis. About 75 to 85 per cent of cysts are located in the mediastum and only 15 to 25 per cent in the lung.[39, 40]

The great majority of bronchial cysts probably develop between the twenty-sixth and the fortieth day of intrauterine life, during the most active period of airway development. As in bronchopulmonary sequestration, the timing of the abnormal budding may determine the eventual location of the cyst: if it occurs at an early stage when there is little tissue surrounding the developing airways, the anomalous bud is likely to remain in the mediastinum or hilum; if later, the abnormal branch is more apt to be surrounded by already developed lung and thus to have an intrapulmonary location.

Pathologic Characteristics. Bronchial cysts are usually solitary, thin-walled, unilocular, and roughly spherical. They are filled with either mucoid or serous fluid and do not communicate with the tracheobronchial tree unless they become infected, in which case the cyst fluid may be replaced by pus or by pus and air.

Histologically, the cyst wall typically is lined by respiratory or metaplastic squamous epithelium and contains cartilage, smooth muscle, and sometimes seromucinous bronchial-type glands (Fig. 5–5).[41] The presence of these structures, especially cartilage, is essential to the establishment of the developmental nature of the cyst. Although intrapulmonary cysts that do not contain cartilage and glands in their wall may represent true bronchial cysts, the walls of healed abscess cavities may contain very little fibrous tissue and have the capacity to epithelialize with a ciliated pseudostratified epithelium. On the other hand, the epithelium and portions of the wall of a true congenital cyst may be destroyed if the cyst becomes secondarily infected, so that their absence does not exclude a congenital origin

in the presence of inflammation. In practice, therefore, it may be impossible to differentiate an infected intrapulmonary congenital cyst from an acquired infected bulla or abscess solely on morphologic criteria; in these cases, historical or prior roentgenographic evidence may be necessary for precise classification.

Although the morphologic features of mediastinal bronchial cysts are much less likely to be altered by infection, precise diagnosis also may be difficult. Since esophageal epithelium is ciliated and pseudostratified in early development and since seromucinous glands similar to bronchial glands may exist in the normal esophagus, it is possible that a mediastinal cyst that does not contain cartilage and that is situated posteriorly may be of esophageal derivation.[41] Because of these potential diagnostic difficulties, mediastinal cysts that contain only respiratory-type epithelium without additional structures that indicate bronchial origin are probably best classified imprecisely as simple cysts.

Pulmonary Bronchial Cysts

The typical roentgenographic appearance is a sharply circumscribed, solitary, round or oval shadow of unit density in the medial third of a lower lobe. Serial roentgenography usually shows little change in the size and shape of the mass with time, although slow growth can sometimes be observed over a period of years. Characteristically, the lesions do not communicate with the tracheobronchial tree until they become infected, which occurs eventually in about 75 per cent of cases. When communication is established, the cyst contains air, with or without fluid (Fig. 5–6)[42]; in such cases, the usual sharp definition of the shadow may be obscured by consolidation of surrounding parenchyma, the true nature of the cyst becoming apparent only when the pneumonitis has resolved.

In adults, the majority of uninfected pulmonary bronchial cysts occasion no symptoms and are discovered by

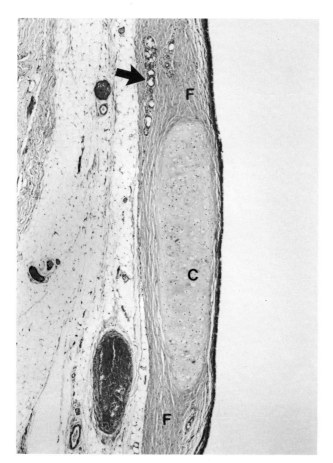

Figure 5–5. Mediastinal Bronchial Cyst. Histologic section of the wall of a mucus-filled mediastinal cyst shows cartilage (C), seromucinous glands (*arrow*), and fibrous tissue (F). At this magnification, the respiratory epithelial lining is evident only as a dark line to the right of the cartilage. (× 40.)

accident on a screening chest roentgenogram. Symptoms, of which hemoptysis is perhaps the most common, almost invariably relate to infection in and around the cyst. Communication between a cyst and the tracheobronchial tree may incorporate a check-valve mechanism that may result in rapid expansion of the cyst.[43]

Mediastinal Bronchial Cysts

Although these cysts may be found anywhere in the mediastinum,[42] the majority are situated in the vicinity of the carina, often attached by a stalk to one of the major airways. They are also relatively common adjacent to the pericardium, usually between the root of the aorta and the superior vena cava; at this site, they may displace the mediastinal vessels and the heart.[44]

The cysts are usually solitary and present roentgenographically as clearly defined masses of homogeneous density just inferior to the carina and often protruding slightly to the right, overlapping the right hilar shadow (Fig. 5–7). The majority are oval or round, although the shape may vary with inspiration and expiration. Calcification of the cyst wall is uncommon.[41] Barium opacification reveals posterior displacement of the esophagus and anterior displacement of the lower trachea, an appearance that may simulate aber-

rant origin of the left pulmonary artery from the right. On CT scanning, the cysts can be confused with solid masses, their content of turbid, mucoid material producing CT numbers of high attenuation.[45]

Mediastinal bronchial cysts may become very large without causing symptoms, although those in the carinal area may cause pressure symptoms even when quite small and roentgenographically invisible.[46] In infants and children particularly, signs and symptoms of upper airway obstruction may simulate asthma, a vascular ring (sling), tracheal or bronchial stenosis, an aspirated foreign body, or bronchiolitis.[47] Symptoms include dyspnea on effort, stridor, and persistent cough.

Transthoracic[48] and transbronchial[49] needle aspiration, with or without cystography, have been advocated as useful diagnostic procedures in some cases.

Congenital Bronchiectasis

Congenital bronchiectasis is much rarer than the acquired disease, and, in fact, its very existence has been questioned.[50] According to Spencer,[51] however, such cases do exist and show tubular dilatation of almost all bronchi in a lobe or lung, extending to a level just beneath the pleural surface. Microscopically, the bronchi end abruptly in a small amount of peripheral parenchymal tissue, which is itself abnormal, containing only scattered alveoli, abnormal bundles of smooth muscle, and small areas of lymphangiectasis. Spencer[51] feels that these changes represent a combination of large airway infection, incomplete bronchial branching, and failure of peripheral lung development.

Williams and colleagues[52] have described a series of patients with bronchiectasis that became manifest in infancy or early childhood. Histologic analysis of some of these cases showed a severe quantitative deficiency of cartilage in segmental and subsegmental airways. Although the authors considered the bronchiectasis to be secondary to a defect in cartilage development, others have questioned this interpretation and feel that the bronchiectasis may, in fact, be acquired.[5]

Congenital Adenomatoid Malformation

Congenital adenomatoid malformation consists of an intralobar mass of disorganized pulmonary tissue that can exist with or without gross cyst formation. When present, the cysts can usually be shown to communicate with normal airways; vascularization is by way of the pulmonary circulation. A 1980 review of 159 cases[53] found that the majority (62 per cent) presented in the first month of life and that 24 per cent became manifest in the first 5 years of life. Occasional cases have been discovered in adults.[54]

The etiology and pathogenesis are unknown. The anomaly is considered by some to represent a hamartoma,[55] whereas others feel that it results from localized arrested development of the fetal bronchial tree.[56]

The lesion has been divided into three morphologic subtypes. *Type I*, or the cystic form, consists of one or more large cystic spaces with a variable number of smaller cysts occupying the intervening parenchyma. This is the commonest type, constituting 29 of 55 cases in two series.[53, 57] *Type II*, or the intermediate form (21 of 55 cases), is com-

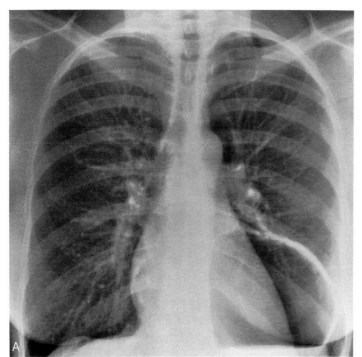

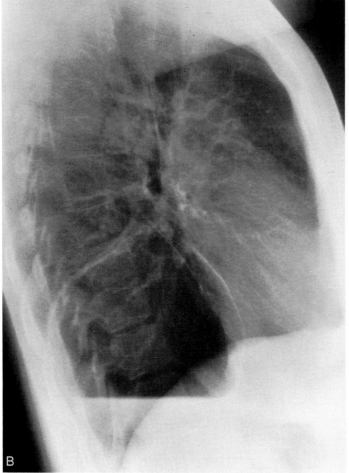

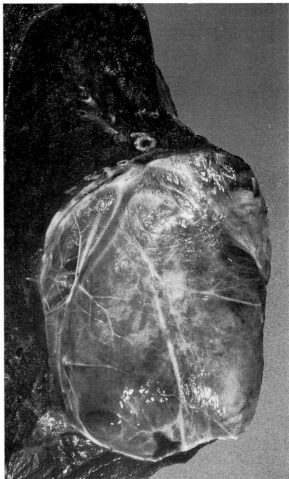

Figure 5–6. Congenital Bronchial Cyst. Posteroanterior *(A)* and lateral *(B)* roentgenograms reveal a large cystic space in the left lower lobe containing a prominent fluid level. The cyst wall measures a maximum of 3 mm in width. The resected specimen *(C)* shows a smooth-surfaced cystic space with vessels coursing over it.

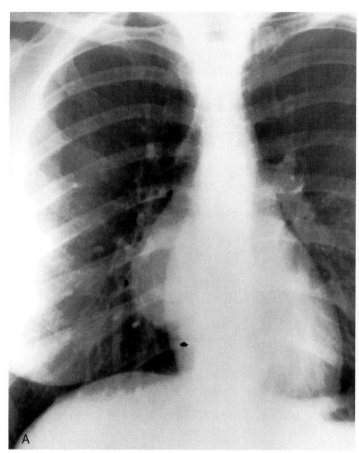
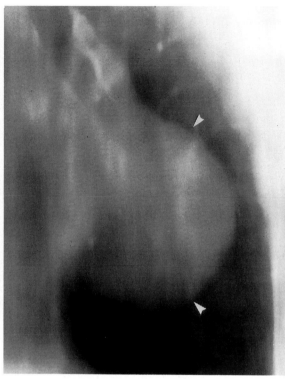

A

B

Figure 5–7. Mediastinal Bronchial Cyst. A conventional posteroanterior chest roentgenogram *(A)* discloses a homogeneous soft tissue mass beneath the carina *(arrowheads)*. A conventional lateral tomogram *(B)* shows the sharp definition of the lesion *(arrowheads)*. The anatomic location, shape, and roentgenographic features are highly suggestive of a mediastinal bronchial cyst.

posed of numerous, evenly spaced cysts, measuring 1 to 10 mm. *Type III*, or the solid form, is least common, accounting for only five of 55 cases, and is manifested by bulky, more-or-less solid masses of tissue without gross cyst formation.

Roentgenologically, the lesion most commonly presents as a mass composed of numerous air-containing cysts scattered irregularly through tissue of unit density (Fig. 5–8). It is space occupying, expanding the ipsilateral hemithorax and shifting the mediastinum to the contralateral side. Occasionally, one cyst may preferentially expand, creating a single lucent area,[57] an appearance that may be confused with that of diaphragmatic hernia and with neonatal lobar hyperinflation.[53] The cysts may contain fluid or air, or both, and fluid levels may be seen; only rarely does fluid completely fill the cysts, resulting in complete roentgenographic opacification. Owing to the absence of cystic spaces in the type III lesion, roentgenograms reveal only a large homogeneous mass.[58]

Clinically, the majority of patients present with increasing respiratory distress in the neonatal period[53]; a minority (most older than 1 month) present with cough and fever, with or without recurrent respiratory infections. In one series, a large proportion of patients with type II lesions had coexistent congenital anomalies that often masked pulmonary symptoms.[57]

Congenital Tracheobronchial Stenosis

Several intrinsic anomalies of the tracheobronchial tree can result in airway narrowing. Abnormalities of the cartilaginous skeleton can occur either alone or in association with a variety of systemic osteocartilaginous defects.[5] *Localized absence of tracheal cartilage* usually results in tracheomalacia, with resultant expiratory airway obstruction and repeated bouts of bronchopneumonia. *Incomplete segmentation of the tracheal cartilage rings* results in defective formation of the posterior membranous sheath and transformation of the trachea into a cartilaginous tube; when tapered caudally, this forms the so-called funnel or carrot-shaped trachea. Similar cartilaginous abnormalities occasionally occur within lobar or segmental bronchi and result in localized airway narrowing.[59] Other causes of bronchial stenosis include atresia (*see* later), hypoplasia,[60] and occlusive fibrous webs.[61] All these anomalies usually manifest themselves early in the neonatal period by respiratory distress, stridor, or recurrent pneumonia; often they are associated with other visceral anomalies.

Congenital Bronchial Atresia

This anomaly consists of atresia or stenosis of a lobar, segmental, or subsegmental bronchus at or near its origin;

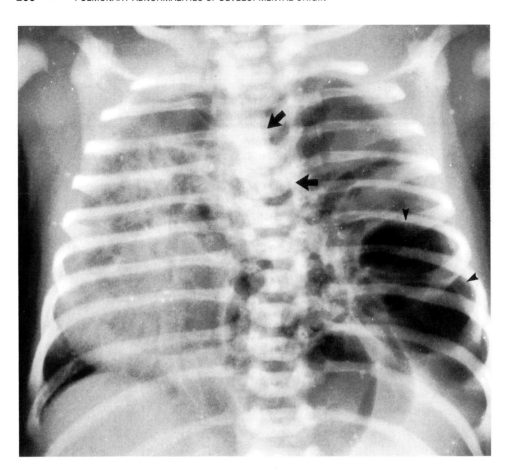

Figure 5–8. Congenital Adenomatoid Malformation of the Lung and Diaphragmatic Hernia. An anteroposterior chest roentgenogram of a male infant reveals a gas-filled lucency in the left lower hemithorax caused by the gastric fundus *(arrowheads)* protruding through a congenital diaphragmatic hernia. Projected superiorly and medially is a vaguely defined cystic and solid lesion *(arrows)* overlying the thoracic spine that was shown at surgery to represent an adenomatoid malformation of the left lung.

the apicoposterior segmental bronchus of the left upper lobe is most commonly affected. The condition is rare: a 1987 review documented only 86 cases.[62] The mean age at the time of diagnosis is 17 years, and approximately two thirds of patients are male.[62]

Two pathogenetic theories have been proposed.[63] In one, an island of multiplying cells at the tip of a bronchial bud loses its connection with the bud itself but continues to branch independently, resulting in a normal distal bronchial branch pattern without a connection between distal and central airways. In the other, a localized intrauterine interruption of the bronchial artery blood supply results in bronchial wall ischemia and secondary luminal obliteration.

Pathologically, the bronchial tree peripheral to the point of obliteration is patent and the complement of airways normal or nearly so. Typically, one or more bronchi are distended with mucus (mucocele). In most cases, dissection fails to find a communication between the proximal and distal airways; occasionally, a septum or fibrous cord separates the two.[62]

Static posteroanterior and lateral roentgenograms typically reveal an area of hyperlucency involving a portion of lung, usually less than the total volume of the affected lung. The hyperlucency results from a combination of oligemia and an increase in the volume of air within the affected parenchyma due to collateral ventilation (Fig. 5–9). Adjacent normal lung parenchyma and mediastinum may be compressed and displaced. The mucocele can be linear, ovoid, or branched or can appear as a cyst. It is characteristically situated close to the hilum, where it forms the apex

of a roughly triangular zone of oligemia and overinflation. Dynamic inspiratory and expiratory films reveal air trapping that is indistinguishable from that caused by a partly obstructing endobronchial lesion; however, endobronchial lesions are rarely, if ever, associated with overinflation of affected bronchopulmonary segments at total lung capacity, an almost invariable finding in bronchial atresia. The oligemia, overinflation, and mucocele can all be exquisitely demonstrated by CT.[21]

Congenital bronchial atresia is usually asymptomatic, the anomaly being discovered on a screening chest roentgenogram; about 20 per cent of patients present with a history of recurrent pneumonia.[62]

Neonatal Lobar Hyperinflation (Congenital Lobar Emphysema)

Neonatal lobar hyperinflation is characterized by severe overinflation of a pulmonary lobe, which invariably presents in infancy and causes marked respiratory distress. The terminology of the condition is somewhat confusing. Although many cases undoubtedly are associated with developmental anomalies, and therefore should be regarded as truly congenital, others are related to acquired bronchial obstruction.[64, 65] Nevertheless, the two possess identical roentgenologic and clinical features. For these reasons, it is probably preferable to employ the designation "neonatal" or "infantile," rather than congenital. In addition, although the use of the term "emphysema" is well established in the literature, the relative importance of this condition versus simple

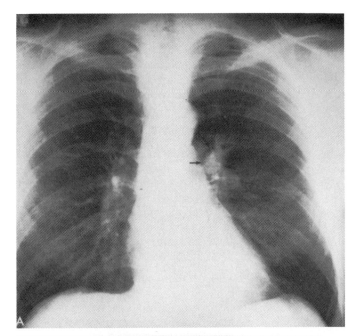

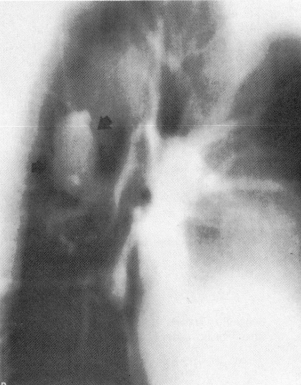

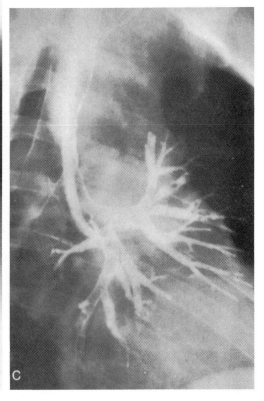

Figure 5–9. Congenital Atresia of the Apicoposterior Segmental Bronchus of the Left Upper Lobe. A posteroanterior roentgenogram *(A)* reveals increased radiolucency, overinflation, and sparse vascularity (oligemia) of the upper half of the left lung. An oval mass of homogeneous density is present just above and behind the left hilum, seen to better advantage on a lateral tomogram *(B)* (*arrows* in both *A* and *B*). A left bronchogram *(C)* shows only the lingular and anterior segmental bronchi arising from the left upper lobe bronchus, there being no evidence of an apicoposterior bronchus. The elliptic mass relates to the expected position of origin of the apicoposterior bronchus and represents inspissated mucus within the lumen of the affected bronchus distal to atresia. The affected bronchopulmonary segment is air-containing as a result of collateral air drift from contiguous, normally ventilated segments. Oligemia is the result of hypoxic vasoconstriction secondary to diminished ventilation.

hyperinflation is not well established, and the word "emphysema" should be used with this understanding; in fact, we prefer that it be replaced with the more nonspecific descriptor "hyperinflation."

Etiology, Pathogenesis, and Pathologic Characteristics. The cause and pathogenesis of the overinflation are varied, and the abnormality should probably be regarded as a clinicopathologic syndrome rather than a specific disease entity. The primary defect can be situated either in the lobar airways, in which case it produces partial obstruction and secondary overinflation, or in the pulmonary parenchyma. The former situation has been documented in about 50 per cent of cases[65] and can be considered in three pathogenetic groups.

1. *Extrinsic airway compression,* estimated to account for about 7 per cent of all cases,[66] can result from a variety of abnormalities. Probably the most common is an anomalous vessel, such as a large ductus arteriosus, an anomalous pulmonary vein, or a left pulmonary artery that arises on the right.

2. *Intramural abnormalities* have been documented in

about two thirds of cases with a presumed obstructive pathogenesis[65] and are invariably characterized by a deficiency of the cartilaginous skeleton with resultant airway collapse and secondary parenchymal overinflation.

3. *Intraluminal obstruction* may be either developmental or acquired, the former consisting of mucosal folds or localized bronchostenosis,[65] and the latter of mucus plugs[65] or granulation tissue.[64]

Although theoretically an intrinsic abnormality of the pulmonary parenchyma is a possible cause of neonatal lobar hyperinflation, it has rarely been documented.[67] In one morphometric study of single lobes resected from three infants, the number of alveoli was found to be increased in each case. In one, they were increased fivefold but of normal size; the number and structure of the airways and vessels were normal for the infant's age, suggesting that the condition represented gigantism of the pulmonary acinus. In the other two patients, the alveoli were increased not only in number but also in size and it was hypothesized that the large airspaces may have been caused by an abnormality in alveolar multiplication after birth.

Approximately 50 per cent of reported cases of neonatal lobar hyperinflation have not been associated with any of the above-mentioned morphologic findings. It is possible that this deficiency is simply a technical matter, since careful morphometric studies are necessary to show alveolar size differences and since airway microdissection techniques and special stains are usually necessary to identify intramural cartilaginous abnormalities; in many case reports, none of these procedures was carried out.

Roentgenographic Manifestations. The roentgenographic manifestations are distinctive, and usually there is little difficulty in diagnosis. There is a distinct predilection for the upper lobes (particularly the left)[68, 69]; the lower lobes are rarely affected. The cardinal features are overinflation and air trapping, the former manifested by markedly increased volume of the affected lobe, even at total lung capacity, depression of the ipsilateral hemidiaphragm, and displacement of the mediastinum into the contralateral hemithorax (Fig. 5–10). The distended lobe may lead to compression atelectasis of the lung's other lobes.[70] Vascular markings in the affected lobe tend to be widely separated and attenuated, the lobe appearing more radiolucent than other lung tissue. Identification of vascular markings is important, permitting differentiation from a large bulla.

Infrequently, the overinflated lobe shows uniformly increased density rather than translucency, an appearance postulated to be caused by impairment of fluid drainage secondary to bronchial obstruction.[71] The roentgenographic manifestations resemble those of the usual form of lobar hyperinflation, except that the affected lobe is opaque rather than radiolucent. The fluid may be cleared within 24 hours or clearing may take as long as 2 weeks; the appearance of the thorax then is typical of the usual form of lobar hyperinflation.

Clinical Manifestations. Respiratory distress develops in at least half the patients during the first month of life, and in only 5 per cent does it develop after 6 months of age[5]; a small percentage of patients are asymptomatic. Physical examination may reveal thoracic asymmetry caused by unilateral overinflation; in addition, the percussion note is increased, breath sounds are much reduced, rales and a local wheeze may be audible, and the respiratory rate is increased.

In some cases the course is rapidly progressive and ends in death unless the lobe is resected; in many, however, the clinical and roentgenographic manifestations resolve spontaneously without the need for thoracotomy.[72]

Anomalies of Tracheobronchial Branching

Many variations in tracheobronchial branching have been described.[5, 6] Some represent an isolated alteration of normal bronchial development, whereas others are associated with anomalies in other organs or tissues and are discovered early in neonatal life or after stillbirth or abortion as part of a spectrum of abnormalities. In addition to numerous minor segmental and subsegmental branching variations,[4, 73] there are four anomalies of the major bronchi:

1. More than one (or occasionally no) lobar or segmental bronchi.[73]
2. Abnormal origin of lobar bronchi, the commonest being tracheal origin of the right upper lobe bronchus, creating the so-called *tracheal or pre-eparterial bronchus.*[4]
3. *Bronchial isomerism,* in which the pattern of bronchial branching as well as pulmonary lobation is identical in the two lungs. This may be an isolated finding but is frequently associated with a variety of cardiac, splenic, and other anomalies.[74]
4. The so-called *pig bronchus,* consisting of a supernumerary airway that usually arises from the inferior wall of the right main or intermediate bronchus.

Although most of these anomalies are of little or no functional or clinical significance, occasional examples are associated with secondary pathologic effects. For example, in one study of 1500 bronchograms, seven cases were identified in which the left apicoposterior bronchus had its origin from the left main bronchus[75]; four of the seven patients showed roentgenographic evidence of airway obstruction isolated to the bronchopulmonary territory of this bronchus. Similar effects may be produced by an ectopic right bronchus originating from the trachea or right main bronchus.[76]

Congenital Tracheoesophageal and Bronchoesophageal Fistulae

Extralaryngeal communication of the normal (nonsequestered) tracheobronchial tree is most often seen as a tracheoesophageal fistula. Two clinicopathologic subtypes—with and without esophageal atresia—have been described. The former, in which the esophagus ends blindly in a dilated pouch, is by far the more common.[77] The blind (proximal) esophageal ending causes regurgitation and aspiration of oropharyngeal secretions and milk, resulting in cough and pneumonia. The condition is thus invariably detected in the neonatal period.

Congenital tracheal and bronchial communication also can occur with an otherwise normal esophagus, the incidence being about 3 per cent of all tracheoesophageal and bronchoesophageal fistulae.[78] In these cases, survival to adult life without detection of the abnormality is not uncommon because of the lack of early signs and symptoms

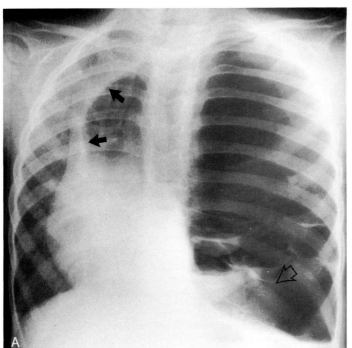
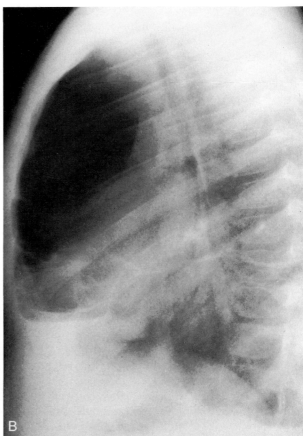

Figure 5–10. Neonatal Lobar Hyperinflation. Anteroposterior *(A)* and lateral *(B)* chest roentgenograms disclose a markedly overinflated and hyperlucent left upper lobe displacing the mediastinum into the right hemithorax, particularly anteriorly *(arrows)*. The left lower lobe *(open arrow)* is severely compressed and displaced posteromedially.

due to aspiration.[77] In addition to the absence of a blind pouch, certain anatomic features of the fistula are probably important in explaining the frequent mildness of respiratory symptoms. Typically, the fistulae are obliquely oriented, the esophageal end being distal to the upper airway communication; more importantly, occlusive membranes and mucosal folds at the esophageal origin of the fistulae may act as check-valves,[79] possibly aided by contraction of mural smooth muscle during swallowing.[80]

Chest roentgenograms of neonates with tracheoesophageal fistula and esophageal atresia frequently show acute airspace pneumonia consistent with aspiration. In older patients without esophageal atresia, evidence of repeated pulmonary insults, such as bronchiectasis, may be present. The diagnosis of fistula is best confirmed by identification of ingested contrast medium within the tracheobronchial tree.

In neonates, symptoms of tracheoesophageal fistula are usually prominent: excessive "salivation" (representing drooling of normal oropharyngeal secretions) and choking upon feeding. When a fistula is not associated with esophageal atresia, careful questioning often reveals a history of symptoms or of recurrent pneumonia for many years.[80] Younger adults may be suspected of having cystic fibrosis or asthma and older patients of having chronic obstructive pulmonary disease. Neither bronchography nor esophagoscopy is of much value in diagnosis in adult patients, al-

though bronchoscopy may reveal the orifice of the communication.

In adults, the prognosis is good following reparative surgery. Similarly, in otherwise healthy term babies who have a blind proximal esophageal pouch, the survival rate after surgery is over 90 per cent. Some infants who have undergone successful surgery are still prone to acute and chronic respiratory complications, presumably as a result of gastroesophageal reflux secondary to an incompetent lower esophageal sphincter,[81] which in turn may be related to a congenital defect of the intrinsic nerve complex of the trachea and esophagus.[82]

Miscellaneous Bronchopulmonary Anomalies

Accessory pulmonary tissue may be defined as the presence of lung parenchyma over and above the normal complement of left and right lungs, supplied by branches of the pulmonary arterial and venous systems and connected by an airway to some portion of the tracheobronchial tree. Individual lobes, and occasionally whole lungs, can be completely enclosed in their own pleural cavity.[83] The nature of the anomaly is best demonstrated by angiography.

Horseshoe lung is a rare congenital malformation in which an isthmus of pulmonary parenchyma extends from the right lung base across the midline behind the pericardium and fuses with the base of the left lung.[84] The majority of cases are associated with the hypogenetic lung (scimitar) syndrome (*see* page 277). The diagnosis can be made by pulmonary angiography, which reveals a branch of the right pulmonary artery originating from its proximal but inferior aspect and coursing into the left hemithorax.

Communication between the biliary tree and the carina or mainstem bronchi (*bronchobiliary fistula*) usually results in neonatal pneumonia and the production of greenish, bile-containing sputum[85]; occasionally, it is detected in adults.[3]

ANOMALIES OF THE PULMONARY ARTERIES

Absence of the Main Pulmonary Artery

Absence of the main pulmonary artery can be manifested by a variety of anatomic patterns.[86] In some cases, the artery is atretic, either in its proximal portion or over its entire length, a residual fibrous cord marking its usual position. In such cases, the right and left main pulmonary arteries persist in their normal sites and are connected to the aorta by a ductus.

In other cases, all morphologic evidence of a main pulmonary artery is lost, and a single great artery arises from a common semilunar heart valve, invariably in association with a ventricular septal defect (persistent truncus arteriosus). Independent pulmonary arteries thus are absent, and pulmonary blood supply is derived from branches of the single trunk vessel at systemic pressure.[87] Four anatomic subtypes have been defined.[88] In the first three, one or two pulmonary vessels arise from the common trunk in its early portion. Type IV, believed to represent a complete failure of development of the sixth aortic arch, lacks all evidence of pulmonary arterial growth. Pulmonary blood supply is derived solely from bronchial arteries. The prognosis is poor: most patients are stillborn or die in infancy with pulmonary hypertension.

Proximal Interruption (Absence) of the Right or Left Pulmonary Artery

Although rare examples of complete absence of both intra- and extrapulmonary artery branches have been described,[51] this anomaly is better designated proximal *interruption* of the right or left pulmonary artery, since the vessels in the lung are usually intact and patent.[89] When the interruption is on the right, pulmonary blood flow is from markedly hypertrophic bronchial arteries or from an anomalous artery that arises from the ascending aorta, aortic arch, or right innominate or subclavian arteries. When the interruption is on the left, vascular supply to the lung is usually from the descending aorta, left innominate or subclavian arteries, or hypertrophic bronchial arteries.[87]

Careful inspection of right-sided anomalous vessels frequently reveals focal stenotic or atretic segments that are histologically similar to the ductus arteriosus; thus, it has been suggested that vessels arising in this location represent (in part) persistence of the right ductus, the stenosis being a normal attempt at duct closure.[90]

The ipsilateral lung is hypoplastic, and its volume reduced (Fig. 5–11). Despite this, it usually is hyperlucent, a finding that, when taken in conjunction with the diminutive hilar shadow, may lead to the erroneous diagnosis of Swyer-

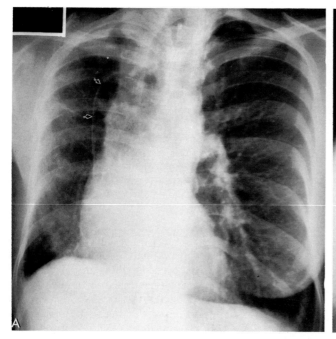
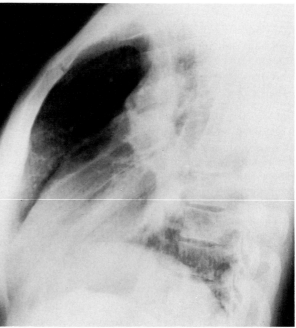

Figure 5–11. Proximal Interruption of the Right Pulmonary Artery. A posteroanterior roentgenogram *(A)* reveals moderate elevation of the right hemidiaphragm and shift of the mediastinum to the right, indicating considerable loss of volume of the right lung. A right hilar shadow cannot be identified and the vascularity of the right lung is markedly reduced in amount and atypical in pattern. The overinflated left lung is displaced into the right hemithorax, as indicated by the anterior junction line *(arrows)*; note the deep retrosternal airspace in lateral projection *(B)*. (Courtesy of Dr. Richard Lesperance, Montreal Chest Hospital Center.)

James syndrome. Differentiation is usually possible by roentgenography in full expiration: patients with Swyer-James syndrome show ipsilateral air trapping owing to bronchiolar obstruction, a sign that is absent in cases of proximal interruption of a pulmonary artery. If further confirmation is required, either V̇/Q̇ scanning or pulmonary arteriography should provide easy differentiation.

Patients have been divided clinically into three groups.[91] The first two usually present in infancy with cardiac decompensation or pulmonary arterial hypertension; many patients die in infancy. The third group has an isolated arterial interruption without pulmonary hypertension; patients may be seen first as adults because of hemoptysis or an abnormal screening chest roentgenogram.[92] The condition must be distinguished from chronic thromboembolism of a main pulmonary artery, which it may closely resemble.[93]

Anomalous Origin of the Left Pulmonary Artery from the Right

In this condition, an aberrant left pulmonary artery passes posteriorly and to the right until it reaches the right side of the distal trachea or right main bronchus; it then turns sharply to the left and passes between the esophagus and trachea in its course to the left hilum (thus the designation "pulmonary sling"). The intimate relationship of this vessel to the right main bronchus and trachea results in their compression and various obstructive effects on the right or both lungs.

The pathogenic mechanism has been hypothesized to be faulty development or reabsorption of the ventral portion of the left sixth aortic arch, leaving the developing left pulmonary plexus to connect with the right sixth aortic arch (subsequently the right pulmonary artery).[94]

Conventional chest roentgenograms may reveal an anterior impression on the distal trachea, and sometimes an extra paratracheal opacity.[95] The demonstration of local posterior displacement of the barium-filled esophagus in the region of the lower trachea makes the diagnosis virtually certain; if necessary, this can be confirmed by pulmonary angiography or CT (Fig. 5–12).

Airway obstruction usually is manifested shortly after birth, as the infant almost invariably exhibits stridor and, often, feeding problems and respiratory tract infections.[96] Occasional patients are asymptomatic, and several cases have been discovered in adults.[95] Associated congenital defects, usually cardiovascular or tracheobronchial ones, are common[95]; of particular interest is tracheal stenosis caused by incomplete septation of the cartilaginous rings ("funnel" trachea). It has been emphasized that bronchoscopy should be performed prior to surgery in any patient with anomalous origin of the left pulmonary artery from the right, to establish whether respiratory difficulty might be caused by such an intrinsic tracheal anomaly rather than by the vascular anomaly per se.[97]

Pulmonary Artery Stenosis or Coarctation

This rare anomaly is characterized by single or multiple coarctations of the pulmonary arteries, commonly with poststenotic dilatation. The stenoses may be short or long, peripheral or central, unilateral or bilateral. Patients have

been separated into two groups on the basis of the location of stenosis[98]: in type 1, the stenosis affects a main branch or proximal branches of the pulmonary artery, whereas in type 2 it involves one or more peripheral branches. Associated cardiovascular anomalies (including infundibular, valvular, or supravalvular pulmonic stenosis and atrial septal defect) are more common with type 1 lesions.

Familial incidence of the anomaly[99] and its association with the Ehlers-Danlos syndrome[100] have been reported. Its occurrence in association with maternal rubella is well documented.[101]

Roentgenographically, the pulmonary vasculature may appear normal, diminished, or increased, depending on the presence and nature of associated malformations (Fig. 5–13). In those instances in which pulmonary artery stenosis is the only anomaly or a major one, roentgenography may reveal poststenotic dilatation of affected pulmonary artery branches, diffuse pulmonary oligemia, and signs of pulmonary arterial hypertension and cor pulmonale. Without selective pulmonary angiography the precise nature of the abnormality may be obscure, so this procedure is essential to diagnosis.

The clinical picture in patients with type 1 anomalies is usually that of the associated cardiovascular abnormalities. With type 2 lesions, the pulmonic second sound is accentuated and a continuous murmur usually is audible bilaterally over the upper part of the chest anteriorly, radiating to the neck and back[98]; however, when stenosis is severe, flow may be so reduced that the lesions are acoustically silent.

Congenital Aneurysms of the Pulmonary Arteries

Aneurysms of the central pulmonary arteries, commonly accompanied by congenital cardiovascular anomalies and present at birth, usually are the result of disturbed hemodynamics created by pulmonary valve stenosis. This type of poststenotic dilatation affects the left pulmonary artery much more commonly than the right; in fact, enlargement of the main pulmonary artery and its left branch in conjunction with a normal right hilum should strongly suggest the diagnosis of pulmonary valve stenosis.

Physical findings include a systolic ejection murmur (attributable to the stenosis of the pulmonary valve orifice in relation to the increased caliber of the main pulmonary artery) and accentuation of the second pulmonic sound (possibly caused by the proximity of the dilated pulmonary artery to the anterior chest wall rather than by pulmonary hypertension). The abnormality is compatible with a normal life span.[102]

Direct Communication of the Right Pulmonary Artery with the Left Atrium

This rare congenital malformation is characterized by direct communication between a branch of the right pulmonary artery and the left atrium without intervening lung parenchyma.[103] The right lung itself can be normal, the anomalous artery appearing as a supernumerary vessel arising from an otherwise unremarkable right pulmonary artery; occasionally, however, there is aplasia or severe hypoplasia of the lower lobe.

The pathogenesis is uncertain. Aplasia of the lower lobe

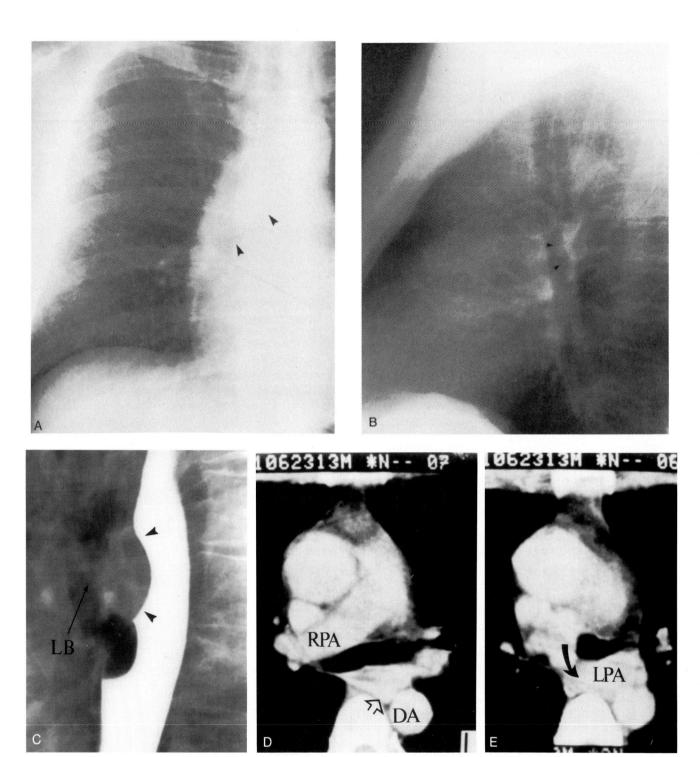

Figure 5–12. Anomalous Origin of the Left Pulmonary Artery from the Right. Conventional posteroanterior *(A)* and lateral *(B)* chest roentgenograms reveal an abnormal mediastinal opacity on the PA view *(small arrowheads)* overlying the right side of the cardiac silhouette. On the lateral projection, the normal right hilar vascular shadow and the intermediate stem line are not seen; note also the impression on the posterior aspect of an airway *(small arrowheads)*. A lateral projection of the chest with barium in the esophagus *(C)* reveals the left pulmonary artery impressing the left main bronchus anteriorly (LB) and the esophagus posteriorly *(arrowheads)*. CT scans through the right pulmonary artery (RPA) *(D)* and at level more cephalad *(E)* reveal the left pulmonary artery (LPA) arising from the right pulmonary artery from which it passes behind the left main bronchus before entering the left hilum. The esophagus *(open arrow)* lies anteromedial to the descending aorta (DA) behind the anomalous pulmonary artery. (*From* Stone DN, Bein ME, and Garris JB: Anomalous left pulmonary artery: Two new adult cases. AJR 135: 1259–1263, 1980, with permission of the authors and editor.)

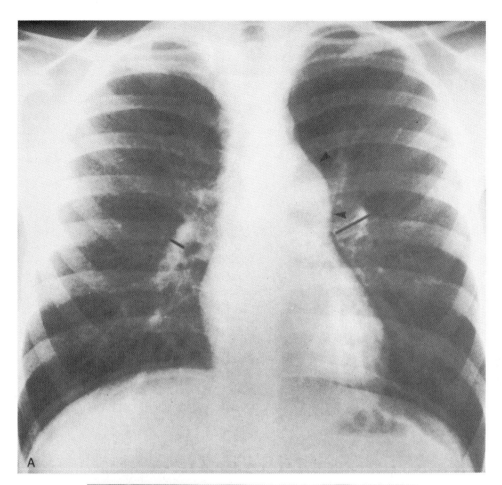

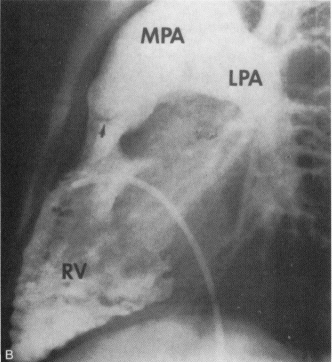

Figure 5–13. Pulmonary Valve Stenosis with Poststenotic Arterial Dilatation. A conventional postero-anterior chest roentgenogram *(A)* demonstrates a prominent main pulmonary artery *(arrowheads)* and a sharp discrepancy between the size of the right and left interlobar arteries at comparable levels *(oblique bars)*. The midlung vasculature is normal on both sides. A right ventricular (RV) angiogram *(B)* in lateral projection reveals dilatation of the right ventricle. The pulmonic valve leaflets *(arrow)* are thickened and domed, indicating stenosis. Note the poststenotic dilatation of the main pulmonary artery (MPA) and the proximal portion of the left interlobar artery (LPA).

in some cases suggests that the malformation represents persistence of the interlobar or lower lobe artery in the absence of peripheral portions of the pulmonary vascular bed. This explanation is clearly inappropriate for cases in which the right lung is normal.

Roentgenography typically reveals a round opacity 2 to 3 cm in diameter in the right hemithorax adjacent to the left atrium[104]—the enlarged abnormal vessel. Angiography is necessary for definitive diagnosis. The diagnosis usually is made in infancy or childhood, but occasional cases have been reported in older individuals.[105] These patients complain of dyspnea and may exhibit cyanosis and clubbing. In most cases, the condition can be corrected relatively easily by ligating or dividing the aberrant vessel.

ANOMALIES OF THE PULMONARY VEINS

Congenital Pulmonary Venous Stenosis or Atresia

Congenital obstruction of one or more pulmonary veins can be caused by compression by an intrathoracic mass or by intrinsic abnormalities of the veins themselves. In addition, some cardiac anomalies such as cor triatriatum can result in venous obstruction that is clinically indistinguishable from the other two forms.

The intrinsic anomaly is characterized by stenosis or atresia of one or more pulmonary veins, typically localized at the venoatrial junction.[106] The stenosis can be caused by a primary abnormality of either the atrium or the veins themselves, the former consisting of endocardial thickening at the mouth of the vein and the latter of medial muscular hypertrophy, intimal fibrosis, or a combination of the two.

In patients without associated cardiovascular anomalies, roentgenographic manifestations consist of signs of pulmonary venous hypertension, with or without arterial hypertension and right ventricular enlargement. In an infant who presents with hemoptysis, the presence of asymmetric vascularity and a unilateral reticular pattern in a normal-sized or small lung should suggest the diagnosis of localized stenosis; confirmation can be obtained by a pulmonary arteriogram that reveals a small ipsilateral pulmonary artery, pruned peripheral branches, stasis of contrast medium, and nonopacification of draining pulmonary veins.[107, 108]

Clinically, the most common symptoms are failure to thrive, fatigue, dyspnea, recurrent respiratory infections, and hemoptysis.[109] In most cases of isolated stenosis, the condition is recognized in the first 3 years of life; occasional individuals have survived to adolescence before the diagnosis is made.[110] As might be expected, common vein atresia is invariably recognized in the neonatal period.

Varicosities of the Pulmonary Veins

This rare abnormality may be either congenital or acquired. It consists of abnormal tortuosity and dilatation of one or more pulmonary veins just before they enter the left atrium.[111] The congenital form is thought to form during the period of transition from splanchnic to pulmonary venous drainage, although the reason for the localized dilatation at that time is not understood.[112] Histologically, the majority of cases in which the vein has been studied have shown normal structure, and an intrinsic defect of the ves-

sel wall does not seem a likely explanation. Acquired varicosities are invariably associated with mitral valve disease and are usually located on the right side, a unilaterality that can be attributed to the anatomy of the mitral valve, whose plane is directed posteriorly, superiorly, and to the right.

In most cases, the lesion is apparent roentgenologically as one or more round or oval homogeneous opacities, somewhat lobulated but well defined, in the medial third of either lung (Fig. 5–14). On the left, the lingular vein usually is involved; on the right, the affected vein is a branch of the inferior pulmonary vein in the region of the medial basal segment of the right lower lobe.[113] The differential diagnosis includes all masses in the lungs. CT can establish the vascular nature of the lesion.[114] In cases of venous varicosity, opacification on angiograms is apparent only in the venous phase, whereas in arteriovenous fistula it occurs in the arterial phase also.[115] The varicosities may opacify more slowly than normal pulmonary veins and, because of sluggish flow, may clear more slowly.[116]

Pulmonary venous varicosities usually are not recognized until the patient reaches adulthood, and they seldom give rise to symptoms. Hemoptysis and some fatalities due to rupture have been reported.[116]

Anomalous Pulmonary Venous Drainage

This abnormality occurs when a portion of the pulmonary venous blood drains directly into the right heart or systemic venous system. It may be partial or total. (The special situation in which a single anomalous vein drains the right lung and is associated with other right-sided anomalies is considered separately as the hypogenetic lung syndrome ([see page 277].) Both forms produce an extracardiac left-to-right shunt; in addition, a total anomalous connection provides a right-to-left shunt through an obligatory septal defect.

Although the anatomy of the anomalous connections is highly variable, drainage may be considered in four groups:[117] (1) *supracardiac*, usually to a persistent left superior vena cava and thence to the left innominate vein (approximately 55 per cent of cases); (2) *cardiac*, in which a direct connection is established with the right atrium or coronary sinus (30 per cent of cases); (3) *infradiaphragmatic*, there being a common vein that extends below the diaphragm to join the portal vein or one of its radicles (15 per cent of cases); and (4) *mixed* (approximately 5 per cent of cases). In most cases, the pathogenesis is probably a failure of connection between the primitive pulmonary splanchnic plexus and the common pulmonary vein derived from the atrium.[117]

The *partial anomaly* incorporates the venous drainage from part or all of one lung via one or more pulmonary veins. Although the anomalous vein may be visible on plain roentgenograms, a more precise characterization of the anomaly can often be achieved by CT.[118, 119] Despite this, pulmonary angiography is usually necessary to confirm the diagnosis and to elucidate the specific anatomic variations (Fig. 5–15).

Since there is usually no significant obstruction to blood flow, pulmonary vascular changes and congestive heart failure develop late in the course of the disease, if at all.[120] When present, symptoms and signs are identical to those of atrial septal defect and include a widely split second

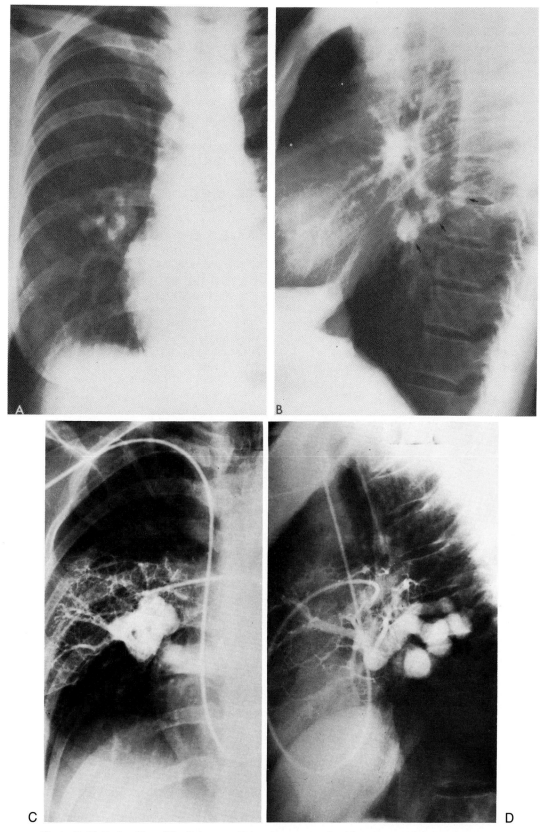

Figure 5–14. Varicosities of the Pulmonary Veins. Posteroanterior *(A)* and lateral *(B)* roentgenograms of this asymptomatic 39-year-old woman reveal a somewhat lobulated opacity projected in the plane of the right hilum and situated slightly posterior to it *(arrows* in *B).* The anterior segmental artery of the right upper lobe was selectively catheterized and contrast medium injected; during the venous phase of the injection *(C* and *D),* dense opacification of several spherical vascular spaces occurred, draining via large dilated veins into the left atrium. (Courtesy of Dr. W. Beamish, University of Alberta Hospital, Edmonton, Alberta.)

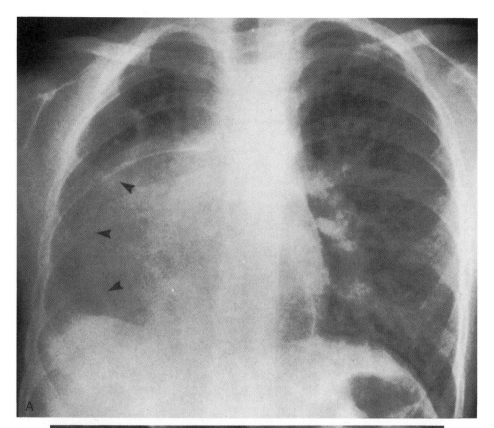

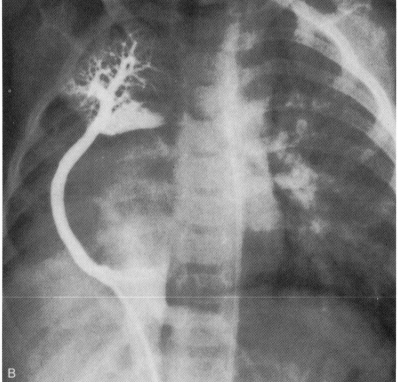

Figure 5–15. Anomalous Pulmonary Venous Return. A posteroanterior chest roentgenogram *(A)* shows a broad curvilinear vessel *(arrowheads)* in the right lung. The heart is displaced to the right, and the right lung is of small volume compared with the left. A pulmonary angiogram revealed a normal complement of pulmonary arteries on both sides. Selective catheterization of the anomalous vessel via the inferior vena cava *(B)* shows an anomalous vein that drains into the hepatic venous system. Although this vein possesses the typical configuration of a scimitar, this patient does not manifest all the anomalies usually associated with the hypogenetic lung (scimitar) syndrome (*see* Fig. 5–16).

heart sound, a systolic ejection murmur, and gallop rhythm. Since pulmonary venous blood mixes with systemic venous blood at or before the right atrium, oxygen saturation tends to be identical in all heart chambers and the two major vessels; in the absence of severe pulmonary hypertension, this may be a clue to the presence of the anomaly. Echocardiography may greatly assist in diagnosis.[121]

Total anomalous pulmonary venous drainage is a relatively uncommon developmental abnormality.[117] In addition to an atrial septal defect or patent ductus arteriosus, at least one of which is necessary for survival, other cardiovascular anomalies are frequently associated,[122] as are syndromes of deranged bronchial anatomy and splenic abnormalities.[123] Pulmonary veins often join directly behind the heart to form a common, somewhat dilated sac before communicating with the systemic venous system.[117] Clinical and pathologic manifestations can result from the large left-to-right shunt (in which case there is frequently pulmonary arterial and right ventricular dilatation) or from obstruction to venous blood flow (the latter caused by drainage of the entire pulmonary blood flow through the hepatic portal circulation, intrinsic stenosis of the abnormal common pulmonary vein, compression of the anomalous common vein between the left main pulmonary artery and the left main bronchus, or a small atrial septal defect).

Roentgenographic features are variable. Cases with communication at the supracardiac or cardiac level usually are characterized by severe pulmonary pleonemia[124]; those with significant pulmonary venous obstruction and hypertension show a characteristic roentgenographic combination of interstitial pulmonary edema and a normal-sized heart.

The majority of patients with total anomalous pulmonary venous drainage die in infancy[125]; even with surgical correction, the mortality rate is about 40 per cent.[126] Patients who survive to adulthood characteristically have a large septal defect and a short anomalous pathway, drainage being directly into the superior vena cava or right atrium.[127]

ANOMALIES OF BOTH ARTERIES AND VEINS

Hypogenetic Lung (Scimitar) Syndrome

The hypogenetic lung syndrome consists of hypoplasia of the right lung and right pulmonary artery, anomalies of the right bronchial tree, and anomalous pulmonary venous drainage from the right lung to the inferior vena cava. Occasionally, there is also extension of a portion of the right lung across the midline into the left hemithorax and cardiac dextroposition. The hypogenetic right lung is supplied partly or completely by systemic arteries, producing a left-to-right shunt. Associated cardiovascular anomalies are frequent, the most common being atrial septal defect (present in 25 per cent of one series[128]).

Although the pathogenesis is unclear, the multiple associated pulmonary anomalies suggest that the condition most likely represents a basic developmental derangement of the entire lung bud early in embryogenesis. In some patients with tetralogy of Fallot,[129] however, and in pigs with experimental unilateral ligation of a pulmonary artery,[130] the number and size of alveoli are decreased. It is possible, therefore, that the abnormal parenchymal development

may be related, at least in part, to hypoplasia of the pulmonary artery. Why the combination of changes is so consistently located on the right side is unknown.

The syndrome shows considerable morphologic variation. Bronchial anomalies are common, particularly isomerism (identical right and left branching patterns).[131] Diverticula are also frequent and may be related to recurrent bronchopulmonary infections in later life.[132] The anomalous systemic artery usually arises from the aorta and runs to the lower lobe. Its vascular distribution does not overlap with the territory of either pulmonary or bronchial arteries; however, its branching pattern is similar to that of the pulmonary arteries, and it is the sole vascular supply for the pulmonary parenchyma.[132] The pattern of venous drainage is also inconstant; most commonly, however, the entire right lung is drained by the anomalous vein.[133]

In most cases, the anomalous vein is visible roentgenologically as a broad, gently curved shadow descending to the diaphragm just to the right of the heart. The shadow is shaped like a scimitar, thus the designation *scimitar syndrome* (Fig. 5–16).[134, 135] Although the diagnosis usually can be made on a conventional posteroanterior roentgenogram, CT can confirm the diagnosis when necessary.[136, 137]

Some patients have cardiorespiratory symptoms, similar in many respects to those of large left-to-right shunts with pulmonary arterial hypertension; others have repeated bronchopulmonary infections or hemoptysis. A systolic murmur of moderate intensity may be heard along the left sternal border, and the electrocardiogram characteristically shows features of right-sided myocardial hypertrophy. Despite these findings, there is evidence that the prognosis is good for most patients, even without surgical correction of the anomalies.[137a]

Congenital Arteriovenous Fistula

Congenital pulmonary arteriovenous fistula (arteriovenous aneurysm, arteriovenous malformation, "angioma," "hemangioma") is considered by most authors to be caused by a defect in the terminal capillary loops that results in dilatation and the formation of thin-walled vascular sacs.[138] Some 40 to 65 per cent of patients have arteriovenous communications elsewhere, including the skin, mucous membranes, and other organs. This condition, known as *hereditary hemorrhagic telangiectasia* or Rendu-Osler-Weber disease,[139] is of simple, dominant transmission and not sex-linked. Although it is assumed that the vascular defects are present at birth, they are seldom manifested clinically until adult life when the vessels have been subjected to pressure over several decades.[140]

Pathologic Characteristics. Grossly, pulmonary arteriovenous fistulae appear as more or less spherical, vascular masses ranging in diameter from 1 mm to several centimeters just beneath the pleura or adjacent to bronchovascular bundles (Fig. 5–17). The few cases examined by corrosion cast technique have shown the fistulae to be supplied and drained by several vessels, the draining veins usually being somewhat larger than the feeding arteries. The intervening vessels may be few and markedly ectatic, resembling a cyst, or numerous and more or less uniform in diameter, resulting in a complex branching mass resembling a Medusa's head. Vascular walls are typically thin, especially in the

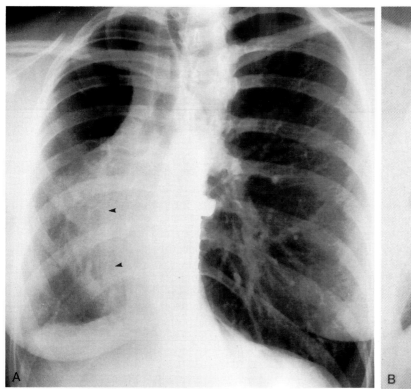
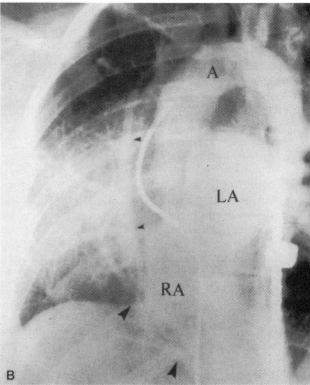

Figure 5–16. The Hypogenetic Lung (Scimitar) Syndrome. A conventional posteroanterior chest roentgenogram *(A)* reveals a small right hemithorax. The pulmonary vasculature of the right lung is diminutive and disorganized while that of the left lung is normal. A large vascular shadow *(small arrowheads)*, coursing caudally from the midlung zone toward the cardiophrenic angle, can be identified through a dextroposed cardiac silhouette. A pulmonary arteriogram performed with the catheter tip in the main pulmonary artery demonstrated an absent right pulmonary artery; the left was normal. During the levo phase of the study *(B)*, venous return from the right lung is entirely through the anomalous veins *(small arrowheads)* to the inferior vena cava and right atrium (RA). Note the small vessels in the cardiophrenic angle *(large arrowheads)* that were subsequently shown by aortography to represent aberrant arterial supply to the right lung from the aorta. (A = aorta; LA = left atrium.)

larger vessels, a characteristic that presumably is the cause of parenchymal hemorrhage.

Roentgenographic Manifestations. Pulmonary arteriovenous fistulae are most common in the lower lobes[141] and are single in about two thirds of cases.[142] The classic appearance is a round or oval homogeneous opacity of unit density, somewhat lobulated in contour but sharply defined, most often in the medial third of the lung, and ranging from smaller than 1 cm to several centimeters in diameter (Fig. 5–18). Calcification, which has been reported in some cases,[140] probably is due to the presence of phleboliths. Approximately a third of patients have multiple lesions in the lungs; some resected specimens contain small fistulae not apparent on plain roentgenograms,[142] a point of obvious importance when resection of a known fistula is contemplated.

Identification of the feeding and draining vessels, which is essential to the diagnosis, is often difficult with plain roentgenograms. On conventional tomography or CT, however, the major artery and vein usually can be distinguished fairly easily, the artery relating to the hilum and the vein deviating from the course of the artery toward the left atrium.[143] Despite this, angiography usually is needed to

confirm the diagnosis and is obviously essential before embolotherapy is attempted.[144, 145] Care must be exercised in obtaining angiographic visualization of all portions of both lungs; it is not enough to perform selective angiography of the lung in question, as lesions may be present in the contralateral lung and may not be visible on plain roentgenograms (Fig. 5–18). In fact, multiple tiny fistulae have been demonstrated in patients with normal plain roentgenograms,[140] notably in asymptomatic siblings of patients with proven fistulae and in patients in whom the diagnosis was suspected clinically because of polycythemia and cyanosis.[146]

Clinical Manifestations. The fistulae occur twice as frequently in women as in men and usually are not recognized until the third or fourth decade of life. Patients may be asymptomatic but often complain of hemoptysis or dyspnea.[141, 147] Signs include cyanosis, finger clubbing, and a continuous murmur or bruit audible over the lesion.

Because of the strong association with hereditary telangiectasia, extrathoracic manifestations of disease also are fairly common. Epistaxis, telangiectasis in the skin or mucous membranes, and upper or lower gastrointestinal tract hemorrhage can be seen. Symptoms referable to the CNS

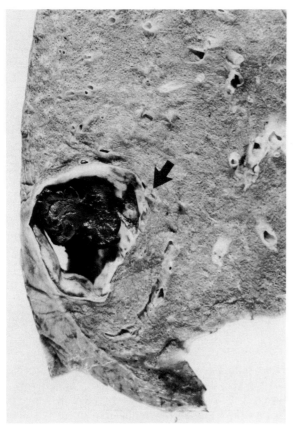

Figure 5–17. Pulmonary Arteriovenous Malformation. A magnified view of a lower lobe shows a well-circumscribed, subpleural cystic space filled with blood clot. A portion of the feeder pulmonary artery is evident at the right *(arrow)*. Histologic sections showed the "cyst" wall to have a variable appearance, focally resembling pulmonary artery and focally pulmonary vein.

are present in many patients. Though they are attributable to intracerebral aneurysms in some cases, in many they are related to complications of the pulmonary aneurysms, such as metastatic abscess, hypoxemia, cerebral embolus, and cerebral thrombosis from secondary polycythemia.[141]

Arterial blood gas analysis and cardiac catheterization may provide useful data in confirming the diagnosis: PO_2 and arterial oxygen saturation are decreased, cardiac output is increased, and pulmonary artery pressure is normal.[141] The electrocardiogram usually is normal, a sign useful in distinguishing it from congenital heart disease. Although the majority of patients have polycythemia,[141] repeated hemorrhage from the nose or lungs may cause anemia.

The prognosis generally is good. Embolotherapy has been found to be a safe and effective treatment[144] and surgical resection also has been employed with some success[148]; measurement of PaO_2 during occlusion of the pulmonary arterial branch may be employed to predict the outcome of resection.[149]

MISCELLANEOUS VASCULAR ANOMALIES

Anomalies of the Heart and Great Vessels Resulting in Increased Pulmonary Blood Flow

These anomalies include atrial and ventricular septal defect, patent ductus arteriosus, and an aorticopulmonary

window. The left-to-right shunt results in some degree of increased pulmonary blood flow, which may be recognizable roentgenologically as increased size and amplitude of pulsation in the central and peripheral pulmonary arteries.

Anomalies of the Heart and Great Vessels Resulting in Decreased Pulmonary Blood Flow

By far the most common cause of general pulmonary oligemia due to diminished flow is a congenital anomaly of the right ventricular outflow tract (isolated pulmonic stenosis, tetralogy of Fallot with pulmonary atresia, type IV persistent truncus arteriosus, or Ebstein's anomaly). The caliber of the pulmonary vessels generally reflects the severity of the flow decrease, the hila usually being diminutive and the peripheral vessels correspondingly small (except with valvular pulmonic stenosis, in which poststenotic dilatation may enlarge the main or left pulmonary artery shadow). The reduction in flow throughout the lungs is more or less uniform, although both physiologic[150] and roentgenologic[151] studies have shown discrepancies of flow through the two upper zones in patients with isolated pulmonary stenosis or tetralogy of Fallot.

Since decreased pulmonary circulation always increases bronchial collateral flow,[152] the pulmonary vascular pattern throughout the lungs may be formed partly or wholly by a greatly hypertrophied bronchial arterial system. This extensive systemic arterial supply is particularly evident in tetralogy of Fallot and in type IV persistent truncus arteriosus. The extent of collateral circulation is best appreciated by selective bronchial arteriography, although the anomalous supply usually is large enough to permit roentgenologic visualization during aortic flooding or even during the levogram phase of angiocardiography. Absence of a pulmonary artery and the presence of atypical vessels arising from the aorta may be detected by tomography in frontal and lateral projections.[153]

Systemic Arterial Supply to the Lung

A portion of lung may be supplied by a systemic artery arising from the aorta or one of its branches. This is most often seen in association with other anomalies, such as bronchopulmonary sequestration, hypogenetic lung syndrome, or proximal interruption of a pulmonary artery. Occasionally, however, it occurs in the absence of these conditions, either in the form of a systemic-pulmonary vascular fistula[154] or as a localized systemic supply of otherwise normal lung.[87, 155] In the latter situation, a large systemic artery supplies a portion of one lung, invariably one or more basal segments of a lower lobe. Additional pulmonary artery supply to the affected segments may or may not be present, but the tracheobronchial tree and the main pulmonary artery and its branches to other lobes are normal. The etiology and pathogenesis are unknown; however, because of the frequent involvement of the basal lung segments, it is possible that abnormal development of one or more of the pulmonary ligament arteries may be implicated.[28]

The chest roentgenogram shows normal or increased vascular markings[156]; ipsilateral rib notching may be present.[157] Because of the high pressure, pulmonary angiography may

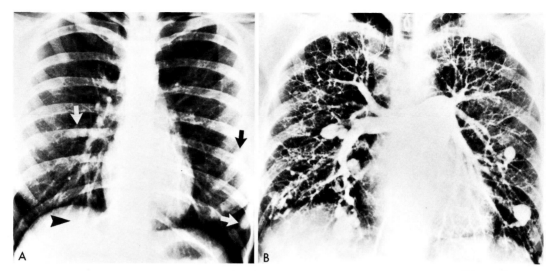

Figure 5–18. Pulmonary Arteriovenous Malformations. A posteroanterior roentgenogram *(A)* reveals several fairly sharply defined nodular opacities in both lungs *(arrows).* Note that the opacity in the right lower lobe *(arrowhead)* appears to possess an intimate relationship to vessels. A pulmonary angiogram during the arterial phase *(B)* reveals many more large arteriovenous communications than are evident on the standard roentgenogram.

reveal no filling or incomplete filling of the segments served by the systemic vessel.[157]

Patients may present in infancy or early childhood with a chest murmur or cardiac decompensation due to a large left-to-left shunt.[158] The anomaly also may cause no symptoms but may become evident on a screening chest roentgenogram or at autopsy.

Systemic-pulmonary vascular fistulae may involve either normal or anomalous systemic arterial branches, and the communication may involve pulmonary veins or arteries, usually in the basal segment of one of the lower lobes.[154] Patients may be asymptomatic, or they may suffer recurrent hemoptysis; a murmur may be audible over the defect. Morphologic and angiographic studies have shown a complex arrangement of intercommunicating vessels.

Similar systemic-pulmonary vascular fistulae may be acquired, usually in association with obliteration of the pleural space by fibrous tissue as a result of infection, trauma, or surgery.[159] In these cases, pleuritis is accompanied by extension of systemic vessels from the chest wall across the pleura into contiguous lung parenchyma; such transgression probably occurs very frequently, especially if the underlying lung has been damaged by infection (e.g., in bronchiectasis) (Fig. 5–19). Occasionally, significant symptoms may derive from the resultant shunt.[160]

Aortography is usually necessary to make a definitive diagnosis of all these conditions. As with bronchopulmonary sequestration, preoperative recognition of the systemic vessel may prevent potentially fatal hemorrhage at thoracotomy.

Congenital Pulmonary Lymphangiectasia

As the name implies, this condition consists of dilatation of the pulmonary lymphatics, which in its severest degree reaches cystic proportions. It can be divided into four groups.[161, 162] In the first, patients have a concomitant cardiac anomaly, which appears to be associated with ob-

structed pulmonary venous return, hemodynamic factors tending to keep the lymphatics dilated.

Group two comprises patients whose lymphangiectasia is not associated with cardiac anomalies. This form is thought to result from abnormal development of the lung between the fourteenth and the twentieth weeks of gestation. During the early part of this phase, the pulmonary lymphatics are large in relation to the remainder of the lung, whereas by the eighteenth to twentieth weeks the lung's connective tissue elements normally diminish and the lymphatics become much narrower. It has been postulated that lymphangiectasia in this group represents a failure of the lymphatics to undergo regression while lung parenchyma continues to grow.[163]

In the third group,[164] the pulmonary abnormality is associated with lymphangiectasia in other viscera, especially the intestine (Noonan's syndrome). Retroperitoneal and mediastinal lymphatics also may be affected, and hemangiomas of bone and other sites may be present.

Finally, three cases have been described[162] that came to medical attention because of an abnormal chest roentgenogram, the changes being limited to one or two lobes and the mediastinum. The late presentation, absence of symptoms, and lobar localization all are features seen infrequently in the other groups and suggest the possibility of a fourth variant.

Morphologic changes are similar in all patients.[165] Grossly, the lungs show numerous small cystic spaces, which can measure up to 5 mm in diameter. Microscopically, the elongated "cysts" are lined by a flattened endothelium and are located within interstitial connective tissue of the bronchovascular bundles or interlobular septa. Adjacent lung parenchyma may show evidence of compression but is otherwise unremarkable.

The roentgenographic changes in all groups are highly variable. Typically, there is marked prominence of interstitial markings in the form of Kerley A and B lines; however, in some patients, the changes consist of no more than

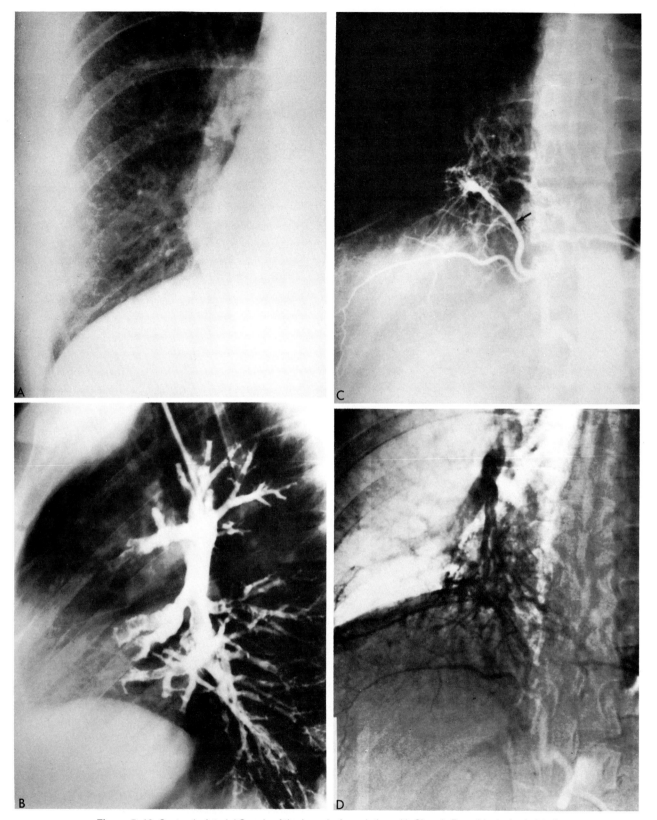

Figure 5–19. Systemic Arterial Supply of the Lung in Association with Chronic Bronchiectasis. A detail view of the lower half of the right lung from a posteroanterior roentgenogram *(A)* reveals loss of visibility of the right heart border caused by airlessness of contiguous middle lobe parenchyma. This 25-year-old woman complained of chronic productive cough, and a bronchogram *(B)* revealed severe bronchiectasis of the right middle lobe, the anterior basal segment of the right lower lobe, and probably of the anterior segment of the right upper lobe. An abdominal aortogram *(C)* reveals opacification of a large branch of the right phrenic artery *(arrow),* which divides into a multitude of smaller radicles that enter the medial portion of the right lung. In a later phase *(D),* segments of the right pulmonary artery have been opacified, indicating systemic to pulmonary artery anastomoses. (Courtesy of Dr. W. Beamish, University Hospital, Edmonton, Alberta.)

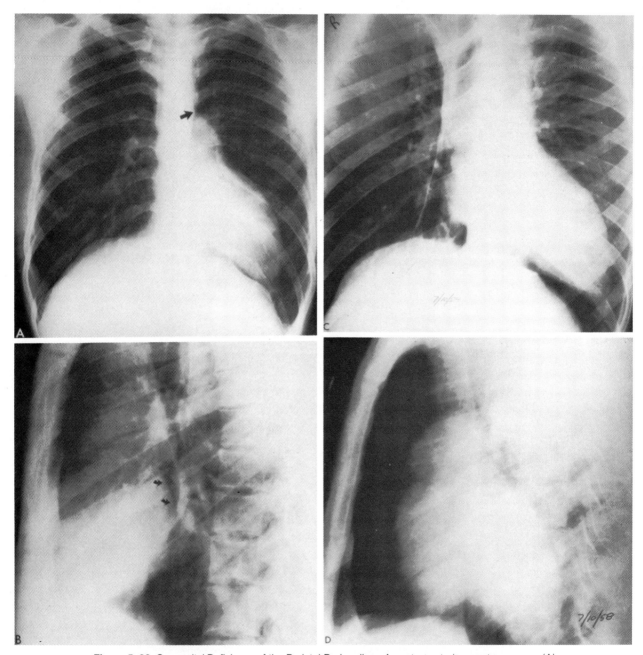

Figure 5–20. Congenital Deficiency of the Parietal Pericardium. A posteroanterior roentgenogram *(A)* shows a shift of the heart to the left and three convexities along the elongated left heart border—the aortic knob, the pulmonary artery segment, and the ventricular segment. The main pulmonary artery is unusually prominent and a radiolucent cleft separates it from the aortic knob *(arrow)*. In lateral projection *(B)*, the anterior surface of the main pulmonary artery is exceptionally well seen, as is the posterior wall of the left atrium *(arrows)*. Following introduction of 500 mL of air into the left pleural space, a lateral decubitus roentgenogram with the left side down *(C)* shows gas separating the heart from the diaphragm. In addition, gas has passed to the right side of the heart, creating a linear opacity which represents the combined thickness of the right side of the pericardium and adjacent mediastinal pleura separating the right pericardial space from the right lung. A lateral roentgenogram of the chest with the patient supine *(D)* shows the heart to have fallen away from the anterior chest wall and diaphragm owing to the lack of support of the left side of the pericardium. (From Ellis K, Leeds NE, Himmelstein A: Am J Roentgenol *82*:125, 1959.)

patchy areas of pneumonia, atelectasis, and focal overinflation.

Congenital lymphangiectasia in the first two groups is almost invariably fatal and usually becomes evident at birth.[161] In Noonan's syndrome, pulmonary involvement may be less severe and associated with a better prognosis.[164]

CONGENITAL DEFICIENCY OF THE PARIETAL PERICARDIUM

Congenital absence of the parietal pericardium may be complete or partial and is usually discovered when a portion of heart herniates through the defect into the left hemithorax. It is readily recognizable on standard chest roentgenograms from the following features (Fig. 5–20):[166] (1) a shift of the heart to the left; (2) an unusual cardiac silhouette, with an elongated left heart border and three convexities: the aortic knob, a long, prominent, sharply demarcated pulmonary artery segment, and a left ventricular segment; (3) a band of radiolucency between the aortic knob and the main pulmonary artery; and (4) a band of radiolucency between the left hemidiaphragm and the base of the heart, caused by interposed air-containing lung (roentgenograms of the patient in the supine position may be necessary to reveal this last sign). Although some investigators have confirmed the diagnosis by demonstrating pneumopericardium after inducing diagnostic pneumothorax, this procedure is not required for diagnosis and may in fact be hazardous.[166] The diagnosis can be established with ease by CT.[167] Echocardiography can be useful in excluding associated cardiovascular anomalies,[168] although it is not diagnostic of the pericardial deficiency itself.

Patients may be asymptomatic or may complain of nonspecific anterior chest pain brought on by exercise or by lying on the left side and of mild shortness of breath on exertion.[166] The apical impulse is in the left axilla, and there is a sustained left ventricular thrust. Electrocardiography characteristically reveals right axis deviation and clockwise rotation of the QRS complex.[166]

Complete absence of the parietal pericardium is a benign condition quite compatible with a normal life span; partial absence, however, may be fatal as a result of herniation of the left ventricle.[166]

References

1. Bailey PV, Tracy T Jr, Connors RH, et al: Congenital bronchopulmonary malformations. Diagnostic and therapeutic considerations. J Thorac Cardiovasc Surg 99: 597, 1990.
2. Panicek DM, Heitzman ER, Randall PA, et al: The continuum of pulmonary developmental anomalies. RadioGraphics 7: 747, 1987.
3. De Carvalho CRR, Barbas CSV, Guarnieri RM, et al: Congenital bronchobiliary fistula: First case in an adult. Thorax 43: 792, 1988.
4. Boyden EA: Developmental anomalies of the lungs. Am J Surg 89: 79, 1955.
5. Landing BH: Congenital malformations and genetic disorders of the respiratory tract (larynx, trachea, bronchi, and lungs). State of the art. Am Rev Respir Dis 120: 151, 1979.
6. Warkany J: The lung. In Warkany M (ed): Congenital Malformations. Chicago, Year Book, 1971, p 604.
7. Swischuk LE, Richardson CJ, Nichols MM, et al: Bilateral pulmonary hypoplasia in the neonate. Am J Roentgenol 133: 1057, 1979.
8. Page DV, Stocker JT: Anomalies associated with pulmonary hypoplasia. Am Rev Respir Dis 125: 216, 1982.
9. Goldstein JD, Reid LM: Pulmonary hypoplasia resulting from phrenic nerve agenesis and diaphragmatic amyoplasia. J Pediatr 97: 282, 1980.
10. Liggins GC, Vilos GA, Campos GA, et al: The effect of bilateral thoracoplasty on lung development in fetal sheep. J Develop Physiol 3: 275, 1981.
11. Adzick NS, Harrison MR, Glick PL, et al: Experimental pulmonary hypoplasia and oligohydramnios: Relative contributions of lung fluid and fetal breathing movements. J Pediatr Surg 19: 658, 1984.
12. Liggins GC, Vilos GA, Campos GA, et al: The effect of spinal cord transection on lung development in fetal sheep. J Develop Physiol 3: 267, 1981.
13. Fewell JE, Lee CC, Kitterman JA: Effects of phrenic nerve section on the respiratory system of fetal lambs. J Appl Physiol 51: 293, 1981.
14. Cooney TP, Thurlbeck WM: Pulmonary hypoplasia in Down's syndrome. N Engl J Med 307: 1170, 1982.
15. Chamberlain D, Hislop A, Hey E, et al: Pulmonary hypoplasia in babies with severe rhesus isoimmunization: A quantitative study. J Pathol 122: 43, 1977.
16. Swischuk LE, Richardson CJ, Nichols MM, et al: Primary pulmonary hypoplasia in the neonate. Pediatrics 95: 573, 1979.
17. Hislop A, Hey E, Reid L: The lungs in congenital bilateral renal agenesis and dysplasia. Arch Dis Child 54: 32, 1979.
18. Kitagawa M, Hislop A, Boyden EA, et al: Lung hypoplasia in congenital diaphragmatic hernia. A quantitative study of airway, artery, and alveolar development. Br J Surg 58: 342, 1971.
19. George DK, Cooney TP, Chiu BK, et al: Hypoplasia and immaturity of the terminal lung unit (acinus) in congenital diaphragmatic hernia. Am Rev Respir Dis 136: 947, 1987.
20. Soulen RL, Cohen RV: Plain film recognition of pulmonary agenesis in the adult. Chest 60: 185, 1971.
21. Mata JM, Cáceres J, Lucaya J, et al: CT of congenital malformations of the lung. RadioGraphics 10: 651, 1990.
22. Steinberg I, Stein HL: Angiocardiography in diagnosis of agenesis of a lung. Am J Roentgenol 96: 991, 1966.
23. Maltz DL, Nadas AS: Agenesis of the lung. Presentation of eight new cases and review of the literature. Pediatrics 42: 175, 1968.
24. Clements BS, Warner JO, Shinebourne EA: Congenital bronchopulmonary vascular malformations: Clinical application of a simple anatomical approach in 25 cases. Thorax 42: 409, 1987.
25. Sade RM, Clouse M, Ellis FH: The spectrum of pulmonary sequestration. Ann Thorac Surg 18: 644, 1974.
26. Gerle RD, Jaretzi A III, Ashley CA, et al: Congenital bronchopulmonary-foregut malformation: Pulmonary sequestration communicating with the gastrointestinal tract. N Engl J Med 278: 1413, 1968.
27. Hruban RH, Shumway SJ, Orel SB, et al: Congenital bronchopulmonary foregut malformations. Intralobar and extralobar pulmonary sequestrations communicating with the foregut. Am J Clin Pathol 91: 403, 1989.
28. Stocker JT, Malczak HT: A study of pulmonary ligament arteries. Relationship to intralobar pulmonary sequestration. Chest 86: 611, 1984.
29. Savic B, Birtel FJ, Tholen W, et al: Lung sequestration: Report of seven cases and review of 540 published cases. Thorax 34: 96, 1979.
30. Ikezoe J, Murayama S, Godwin JD, et al: Bronchopulmonary sequestration: CT assessment. Radiology 176: 375, 1990.
31. Naidich DP, Rumancik WM, Ettenger NA, et al: Congenital anomalies of the lungs in adults: MR diagnosis. Am J Roentgenol 151: 13, 1988.
32. Craig L, Coblentz MD, Chen JT, et al: Calcified intralobar pulmonary sequestration. J Can Assoc Radiol 39: 290, 1988.
33. Samuels T, Morava-Protzner I, Youngson B, et al: Case reports. Calcification in bronchopulmonary sequestration. J Can Assoc Radiol 40: 106, 1989.
34. Sumbas PN, Hatcher CR Jr, Abbott OA, et al: An appraisal of pulmonary sequestration: Special emphasis on unusual manifestations. Am Rev Respir Dis 406: 99, 1969.
35. O'Connell DJ, Kelleher J: Congenital intrathoracic bronchopulmonary foregut malformations in childhood. J Can Assoc Radiol 30: 103, 1979.
36. Stern EJ, Webb WR, Warnock ML, et al: Bronchopulmonary sequestration: Dynamic, ultrafast, high-resolution CT evidence of air trapping. Am J Roentgenol 157: 947, 1991.
37. Felker RE, Tonkin ILD: Imaging of pulmonary sequestration. Am J Roentgenol 154: 241, 1990.
38. Felson B: Pulmonary sequestration revisited. Med Radiogr Photogr 64: 1988.

39. St-Georges R, Deslauriers J, Duranceau A, et al: Clinical spectrum of bronchogenic cysts of the mediastinum and lung in the adult. Ann Thorac Surg 52: 6, 1991.
40. Reed JC, Sobonya RE: Morphologic analysis of foregut cysts in the thorax. Am J Roentgenol 120: 851, 1974.
41. Salyer DC, Salyer WR, Eggleston JC: Benign developmental cysts of the mediastinum. Arch Pathol Lab Med 101: 136, 1977.
42. Rogers LF, Osmer JC: Bronchogenic cyst: A review of 46 cases. Am J Roentgenol 91: 273, 1964.
43. Dahmash NS, Chen JT, Ravin CE, et al: Unusual radiologic manifestations of bronchogenic cyst. South Med J 77: 762, 1984.
44. Steinberg I: Angiocardiography in the differential diagnosis of pericardial and mediastinal tumors. Am J Roentgenol 84: 409, 1960.
45. Mendelson DS, Rose JS, Efremidis SC, et al: Bronchogenic cysts with high CT numbers. Am J Roentgenol 140: 463, 1983.
46. Eraklis AJ, Giscom NT, McGovern JB: Bronchogenic cysts on the mediastinum in infancy. N Engl J Med 281: 1150, 1969.
47. Cohen SR, Geller KA, Birns JW, et al: Foregut cysts in infants and children. Diagnosis and management. Ann Otol Rhinol Laryngol 91: 622, 1982.
48. Zimmer WD, Kamida CB, McGough PF, et al: Mediastinal duplication cyst. Chest 90: 772, 1986.
49. Schwartz AR, Fishman EK, Wang KP: Diagnosis and treatment of a bronchogenic cyst using transbronchial needle aspiration. Thorax 41: 326, 1986.
50. Warkany J: The trachea and bronchi. In Warkany J (ed): Congenital Malformations. Chicago, Year Book, 1971, p 599.
51. Spencer H: Pathology of the Lung (Excluding Pulmonary Tuberculosis). 4th ed. Vol 1. New York, Pergamon, 1985.
52. Williams HE, Landau LI, Phelan PD: Generalized bronchiectasis due to extensive deficiency of bronchial cartilage. Arch Dis Child 47: 423, 1972.
53. Miller RK, Sieber WK, Yunis EJ: Congenital adenomatoid malformation of the lung. A report of 17 cases, and review of the literature. In Sommers SC, Rosen PP (eds): Pathology Annual, Part I. New York, Appleton-Century-Crofts, 1980, p 387.
54. Avitabile AM, Greco MA, Hulnick DH, et al: Congenital cystic adenomatoid malformation of the lung in adults. Am J Surg Pathol 8: 193, 1984.
55. van Dijk C, Wagenvoort CA: The various types of congenital adenomatoid malformation of the lung. J Pathol 110: 131, 1973.
56. Bale PM: Congenital cystic malformation of the lung. A form of congenital bronchiolar ("adenomatoid") malformation. Am J Clin Pathol 71: 411, 1979.
57. Stocker JT, Madewell JE, Drake RM: Congenital cystic adenomatoid malformation of the lung. Classification and morphologic spectrum. Hum Pathol 8: 155, 1977.
58. Fasanelli S, Bellusi A, Patti GL, et al: Congenital cystic adenomatoid malformation. Unusual presentation. Rays (Roma) 5: 43, 1980.
59. Gupta TGCM, Goldberg SJ, Lewis E, et al: Congenital bronchomalacia. Am J Dis Child 115: 88, 1968.
60. Chang N, Hertzler JH, Gregg RH, et al: Congenital stenosis of the right mainstem bronchus. A case report. Pediatrics 41: 739, 1968.
61. Wallace JE: Two cases of congenital web of a bronchus. Arch Pathol 39: 47, 1945.
62. Jederlinic PJ, Sicilian LS, Baigelman W, et al: Congenital bronchial atresia. A report of 4 cases and a review of the literature. Medicine 66: 73, 1987.
63. Reid L: The Pathology of Emphysema. London, Lloyd-Luke, 1967.
64. Miller KE, Edwards DK, Hilton S, et al: Acquired lobar emphysema in premature infants with bronchopulmonary dysplasia: An iatrogenic disease? Radiology 138: 589, 1981.
65. Murray GF: Congenital lobar emphysema. Surg Gynecol Obstet 124: 611, 1967.
66. Kruse RL, Lynn HB: Lobar emphysema in infants. Mayo Clin Proc 44: 525, 1969.
67. Hislop A, Reid L: New pathological findings in emphysema of childhood. I. Polyalveolar lobe with emphysema. Thorax 25: 682, 1970.
68. Staple TW, Hudson HH, Hartman AF Jr, et al: The angiographic findings in four cases of infantile lobar emphysema. Am J Roentgenol 97: 195, 1966.
69. Reid JM, Barclay RS, Stevenson JG, et al: Congenital obstructive lobar emphysema. Dis Chest 49: 359, 1966.
70. Mandelbaum I, Heimburger I, Battersby JS: Congenital lobar obstructive emphysema: Report of eight cases and literature review. Ann Surg 162: 1075, 1965.
71. Fagan CJ, Swischuk LE: The opaque lung in lobar emphysema. Am J Roentgenol 114: 300, 1972.
72. Roghair GD: Nonoperative management of lobar emphysema: Long-term follow-up. Radiology 102: 125, 1972.
73. Atwell SW: Major anomalies of the tracheobronchial tree with a list of the minor anomalies. Dis Chest 52: 611, 1967.
74. Landing BH, Lawrence TYK, Payne VC Jr, et al: Bronchial anatomy in syndromes with abnormal visceral situs, abnormal spleen and congenital heart disease. Am J Cardiol 28: 456, 1971.
75. Rémy J, Smith M, Marache P, et al: La bronche-tracheale-gauche pathogene. (Pathogenetic left tracheal bronchus. A review of the literature in connection with four cases.) J Radiol Electrol 58: 41, 1977.
76. Hosker HSR, Clague HW, Morritt GN: Ectopic right upper lobe bronchus as a cause of breathlessness. Thorax 42: 473, 1987.
77. Black RJ: Congenital tracheo-oesophageal fistula in the adult. Thorax 37: 61, 1982.
78. Salzberg AM: Congenital malformations of the lower respiratory tract. Respiratory disorders in the newborn. In Kendig EL, Chernick V (eds): Disorders of the Respiratory Tract. Philadelphia, WB Saunders, 1983, p 183.
79. Kameya S, Umeda Y, Mizuno K, et al: Congenital esophagobronchial fistula in the adult. Am J Gastroenterol 79: 589, 1984.
80. Osinowo O, Harley HRS, Janigan D: Congenital broncho-oesophageal fistula in the adult. Thorax 38: 138, 1983.
81. Shermeta DW, Whitington PF, Seto DS, et al: Lower esophageal sphincter dysfunction in esophageal atresia: Nocturnal regurgitation and aspiration pneumonia. J Pediatr Surg 12: 871, 1977.
82. Nakazato Y, Wells TR, Landing BH: Abnormal tracheal innervation in patients with esophageal atresia and tracheoesophageal fistula: Study of the intrinsic tracheal nerve plexuses by a microdissection technique. J Pediatr Surg 21: 838, 1986.
83. Brownlee RT, Dafoe CS: Complete reduplication of the right lung. J Thorac Cardiovasc Surg 55: 653, 1968.
84. Freedom RM, Burrows PE, Moes CAF: "Horseshoe" lung: Report of five new cases. Am J Roentgenol 146: 211, 1986.
85. Levasseur P, Navajas M: Congenital tracheobiliary fistula. Ann Thorac Surg 44: 318, 1987.
86. Edwards JE, McGoon DC: Clinicopathologic correlations. Absence of anatomic origin from heart of pulmonary arterial supply. Circulation 47: 393, 1973.
87. Ellis K: Developmental abnormalities in the systemic blood supply to the lungs. Am J Roentgenol 156: 669, 1991.
88. Collett RW, Edwards JE: Persistent truncus arteriosus: A classification according to anatomic types. Surg Clin North Am 29: 1245, 1949.
89. Pool PE, Vogel JHK, Blount SG Jr: Congenital unilateral absence of a pulmonary artery. The importance of flow in pulmonary hypertension. Am J Cardiol 1: 706, 1962.
90. Kauffman SL, Yao AC, Webber CB, et al: Origin of the right pulmonary artery from the aorta. A clinical-pathologic study of two types based on caliber of the pulmonary artery. Am J Cardiol 19: 741, 1967.
91. Bahler RC, Carson P, Traks E, et al: Absent right pulmonary artery. Problems in diagnosis and management. Am J Med 46: 64, 1969.
92. Ko T, Gatz MG, Reisz GR: Congenital unilateral absence of a pulmonary artery: A report of two adult cases. Am Rev Respir Dis 141: 795, 1990.
93. Moser KM, Olson LK, Schlusselberg M, et al: Chronic thromboembolic occlusion in the adult can mimic pulmonary artery agenesis. Chest 95: 503, 1989.
94. Gallo P, Fazzari F, La Magra C, et al: Facio-auriculo-vertebral anomalad and pulmonary artery sling. A hitherto undescribed but probably non-causal association. Pathol Res Pract 173: 172, 1981.
95. Gumbiner CH, Mullins CE, McNamara DG: Pulmonary artery sling. Am J Cardiol 45: 311, 1980.
96. Lincoln JCR, Deverall PB, Stark J, et al: Vascular anomalies compressing the oesophagus and trachea. Thorax 24: 295, 1969.
97. Landing BH: Syndromes of congenital heart disease with tracheobronchial anomalies. Edward BD Neuhauser Lecture, 1974. Am J Roentgenol 123: 679, 1975.
98. Baum D, Khoury GH, Ongley PA, et al: Congenital stenosis of the pulmonary artery branches. Circulation 29: 680, 1964.
99. McDonald AH, Gerlis LM, Somerville J: Familial arteriopathy with associated pulmonary and systemic arterial stenoses. Br Heart J 31: 375, 1969.

100. Lees MH, Menashe VD, Sunderland CO, et al: Ehlers-Danlos syndrome associated with multiple pulmonary artery stenoses and tortuous systemic arteries. J Pediatr 75: 1031, 1969.
101. Esterly JR, Oppenheimer EH: Vascular lesions in infants with congenital rubella. Circulation 36: 544, 1967.
102. Trell E: Pulmonary arterial aneurysm. Thorax 28: 644, 1973.
103. Lekuona I, Cabrera A, Inguanzo R, et al: Direct communication between the right pulmonary artery and the left atrium. Thorax 41: 78, 1986.
104. Krause DW, Kuehn HJ, Sellers RD, et al: Roentgen sign associated with an aberrant vessel connecting right main pulmonary artery to left atrium. Radiology 111: 177, 1974.
105. Ohara H, Ito K, Kohguchi N, et al: Direct communication between the right pulmonary artery and the left hilum: A case report. J Thorac Cardiovasc Surg 77: 742, 1979.
106. Mortensson W, Lundstrm N-R: Congenital obstruction of the pulmonary veins at their atrial junctions. Review of the literature and a case report. Am Heart J 87: 359, 1974.
107. Belcourt CL, Roy DL, Nanton MA, et al: Stenosis of individual pulmonary veins: Radiologic findings. Radiology 161: 109, 1986.
108. Adey CK, Soto B, Shin MS: Congenital pulmonary vein stenosis: A radiographic study. Radiology 161: 113, 1986.
109. Swischuk LE, L'Heureux P: Unilateral pulmonary vein atresia. Am J Roentgenol 135: 667, 1980.
110. Vogel M, Ash J, Rowe R, et al: Congenital unilateral pulmonary vein stenosis complicating transposition of the great arteries. Am J Cardiol 54: 166, 1984.
111. Asayama J, Shiguma R, Katsume H, et al: Pulmonary varix. Angiology 35: 735, 1984.
112. Ben-Menachem Y, Kuroda K, Kyger ER III, et al: The various forms of pulmonary varices. Report of three new cases and review of the literature. Am J Roentgenol 125: 881, 1975.
113. Steinberg I: Pulmonary varices mistaken for pulmonary and hilar disease. Am J Roentgenol 101: 947, 1967.
114. Borkowski GP, O'Donovan PB, Troup BR: Pulmonary varix: CT findings. J Comput Assist Tomogr 5: 827, 1981.
115. Bryk D, Levin EJ: Pulmonary varicosity. Radiology 85: 834, 1965.
116. Steinberg I: Pulmonary varices mistaken for pulmonary and hilar disease. Am J Roentgenol 101: 947, 1967.
117. Darling RC, Rothney WB, Craig JM: Total pulmonary venous drainage into the right side of the heart. Lab Invest 6: 44, 1957.
118. Greene R, Miller SW: Cross-sectional imaging of silent pulmonary venous anomalies. Radiology 159: 279, 1986.
119. Pennes DR, Ellis JH: Anomalous pulmonary venous drainage of the left upper lobe shown by CT scans. Radiology 159: 23, 1986.
120. Kissner DG, Sorkin RP: Anomalous pulmonary venous connection: Medical therapy. Chest 89: 752, 1986.
121. Tajik AJ, Gau GT, Schattenberg TT: Echocardiogram in total anomalous pulmonary venous drainage: Report of case. Mayo Clin Proc 47: 247, 1972.
122. Brody H: Drainage of the pulmonary veins into the right side of the heart. Arch Pathol 33: 221, 1942.
123. Petersen RC, Edwards WD: Pulmonary vascular disease in 57 necropsy cases of total anomalous pulmonary venous connection. Histopathology 7: 487, 1983.
124. Elliott LP, Schiebler GL: A roentgenologic-electrocardiographic approach to cyanotic forms of heart disease. Pediatr Clin North Am 18: 1133, 1971.
125. Gathman GE, Nadas AS: Total anomalous pulmonary venous connection. Clinical and physiologic observations of 75 pediatric patients. Circulation 42: 143, 1970.
126. Bove EL, DeLaval MR, Taylor JFN, et al: Infradiaphragmatic total anomalous pulmonary venous drainage: Surgical treatment and long-term results. Ann Thorac Surg 31: 544, 1981.
127. Singh R, Weisinger B, Carpenter M, et al: Total anomalous pulmonary venous return, surgically corrected in two patients beyond 40 years of age. Chest 60: 38, 1971.
128. Kiely B, Filler J, Stone S, et al: Syndrome of anomalous venous drainage of the right lung to the inferior vena cava. A review of 67 reported cases and three new cases in children. Am J Cardiol 20: 102, 1967.
129. Johnson RJ, Haworth SG: Pulmonary vascular and alveolar development in tetralogy of Fallot: A recommendation for early correction. Thorax 37: 893, 1982.
130. Haworth SG, McKenzie SA, Fitzpatrick ML: Alveolar development after ligation of left pulmonary artery in newborn pig: Clinical relevance to unilateral pulmonary artery. Thorax 36: 938, 1981.
131. Mathey J, Galey JJ, Logeais Y, et al: Anomalous pulmonary venous return into inferior vena cava and associated bronchovascular anomalies (the scimitar syndrome). Thorax 23: 398, 1968.
132. Halasz NA, Halloran KH, Liebow AA: Bronchial and arterial anomalies with drainage of the right lung into the inferior vena cava. Circulation 14: 826, 1956.
133. Bessolo RJ, Maddison FE: Scimitar syndrome: Report of a case with unusual variations. Am J Roentgenol 103: 572, 1968.
134. Roehm JOF Jr, Jue KL, Amplatz K: Radiographic features of the scimitar syndrome. Radiology 86: 856, 1966.
135. Coni NK, Cowan GO, Fessas C: The scimitar syndrome. Br J Radiol 41: 62, 1968.
136. Godwin JD, Tarver RD: Scimitar syndrome: Four new cases examined with CT. Radiology 159: 15, 1986.
137. Olson MA, Becker GJ: The scimitar syndrome: CT findings in partial anomalous pulmonary venous return. Radiology 159: 25, 1986.
137a. Dupuis C, Charaf LA, Brevière GM, et al: The "adult" form of the scimitar syndrome. Am J Cardiol 70(4): 502, 1992.
138. Prager RL, Laws KH, Bender HW Jr: Arteriovenous fistula of the lung. Ann Thorac Surg 36: 231, 1983
139. Revill D, Matts SGF: Pulmonary arteriovenous aneurysm in hereditary telangiectasia. Br J Tuberc 52: 222, 1959.
140. Hodson CH, Burchell HB, Good CA, et al: Hereditary hemorrhagic telangiectasia and pulmonary arteriovenous fistula: Survey of a large family. N Engl J Med 261: 625, 1959.
141. Moyer JH, Glantz G, Brest AN: Pulmonary arteriovenous fistulas. Physiologic and clinical considerations. Am J Med 32: 417, 1962.
142. Abbott OA, Haebich AT, Van Flent WE: Changing patterns relative to the surgical treatment of pulmonary arteriovenous fistulas. Am Surg 25: 674, 1959.
143. Remy J, Remy-Jardin M, Wattinne L, et al: Pulmonary arteriovenous malformations: Evaluation with CT of the chest before and after treatment. Radiology 182: 809, 1992.
144. White RI Jr, Lynch-Nyhan A, Terry P, et al: Pulmonary arteriovenous malformations: Techniques and long-term outcome of embolotherapy. Radiology 169: 663, 1988.
145. White RI Jr: Pulmonary arteriovenous malformations: How do we diagnose them and why is it important to do so? Radiology 182: 633, 1992.
146. MacNee W, Buist TA, Finlayson ND, et al: Multiple microscopic pulmonary arteriovenous connections in the lungs presenting as cyanosis. Thorax 40: 316, 1985.
147. Gomes MMR, Bernatz PE: Arteriovenous fistula: A review and ten-year experience at the Mayo Clinic. Mayo Clin Proc 45: 81, 1970.
148. Brown SE, Wright PW, Renner JW, et al: Staged bilateral thoracotomies for multiple pulmonary arteriovenous malformations complicating hereditary hemorrhagic telangiectasia. J Thorac Cardiovasc Surg 83: 285, 1982.
149. Harrow EM, Beach PM, Wise JR Jr, et al: Pulmonary arteriovenous fistula. Preoperative evaluation with a Swan-Ganz catheter. Chest 73: 92, 1978.
150. Dollery CT, West JB, Wilcken DEL, et al: A comparison of the pulmonary blood flow between left and right lungs in normal subjects and patients with congenital heart disease. Circulation 24: 617, 1961.
151. Wilson WJ, Amplatz K: Unequal vascularity in tetralogy of Fallot. Am J Roentgenol 100: 318, 1967.
152. Turner-Warwick M: Systemic arterial patterns in the lung and clubbing of the fingers. Thorax 18: 238, 1963.
153. Richter K: Anomalous systemic arteries to the lung visualized by tomography. Am J Roentgenol 95: 629, 1965.
154. Brundage BH, Gomez AC, Cheitlin MD, et al: Systemic artery to pulmonary vessel fistulas: Report of two cases and a review of the literature. Chest 62: 19, 1972
155. Flisak ME, Chandrasekar AJ, Marsan RE, et al: Systemic arterialization of lung without sequestration. Am J Roentgenol 138: 751, 1982.
156. Painter RL, Billig DM, Epstein I: Brief recordings: Anomalous systemic arterialization of the lung without sequestration. N Engl J Med 279: 866, 1968.
157. Piessens J, De Geest H, Kesteloot H, et al: Anomalous collateral systemic pulmonary circulation to a normal lung. Chest 59: 222, 1971.
158. Litwin SB, Plauth WH Jr, Nadas AS: Anomalous systemic arterial supply to the lung causing pulmonary artery hypertension. N Engl J Med 283: 1098, 1970.
159. Webb WR, Jacobs RP: Transpleural abdominal systemic artery-pulmonary artery anastomosis in patients with chronic pulmonary infection. Am J Roentgenol 129: 233, 1977.

160. Syme J: Systemic to pulmonary arterial fistula of the chest wall and lung following lobectomy. Australas Radiol 19: 326, 1975.
161. Felman AH, Rhatigan RM, Pierson KK: Pulmonary lymphangiectasia: Observation in 17 patients and proposed classification. Am J Roentgenol 116: 548, 1972.
162. Wagenaar SS, Swierenga J, Wagenvoort CA: Late presentation of primary pulmonary lymphangiectasis. Thorax 33: 791, 1978.
163. Laurence KM: Congenital pulmonary cystic lymphangiectasis. J Pathol Bacteriol 70: 325, 1955.
164. Noonan JA, Walters LR, Reeves JT: Congenital pulmonary lymphangiectasis. Am J Dis Child 120: 314, 1970.
165. Laurence KM: Congenital pulmonary lymphangiectasis. J Clin Pathol 12: 62, 1959.
166. Morgan JR, Rogers AK, Forker AD: Congenital absence of the left pericardium. Clinical findings. Ann Intern Med 74: 370, 1971.
167. Baim RS, MacDonald IL, Wise DJ, et al: Computed tomography of absent left pericardium. Radiology 135: 127, 1980.
168. Nicolosi GL, Borgioni L, Alberti E, et al: M-Mode and two-dimensional echocardiography in congenital absence of the pericardium. Chest 81: 610, 1982.

6

INFECTIOUS DISEASE OF THE LUNGS

GENERAL CONSIDERATIONS

Pneumonia is the most frequent life-threatening infectious disease.[1] In the United States, it is the fifth commonest cause of mortality, accounting for an estimated 55,000 deaths annually,[2] and in autopsy studies it has been identified in as many as 40 per cent of cases.[3] Many of these infections occur in persons with other significant pulmonary or extrathoracic disease; however, previously healthy individuals, particularly children and the aged, are also affected and may have significant morbidity.[4]

Although the most appropriate discussion of pneumonia follows a microbiologic classification, in order to better un-

derstand the roentgenologic and clinical manifestations it is useful to consider the disease in two other ways: that related to the mechanisms and morphologic appearance of infection and that related to the particular clinical or environmental setting in which the pneumonia is contracted.

Mechanisms of Infection

Organisms can enter the lung and cause infection by way of the tracheobronchial tree or pulmonary vasculature, or by direct spread from the mediastinum or across the diaphragm or chest wall. Although there is overlap between these different situations, each possesses certain characteristics sufficiently distinctive to allow pathologic and roentgenographic identification in most cases.

Infection Via the Tracheobronchial Tree

Infection via the tracheobronchial tree—by far the most frequent route—occurs most commonly by aspiration or inhalation of microorganisms.° Occasionally, it develops by direct physical implantation from an infected source, such as a bronchoscope,[5] or by extension of infection into an airway from a focus of parenchymal disease, such as occurs in tuberculosis.

Coughing or sneezing by an individual who is either colonized or infected with a microorganism produces a myriad of water-mucus droplets that are laden with bacteria or virus particles. On exposure to air, the droplets rapidly lose water and become "droplet nuclei." Inhaled nuclei measuring 1 to 2 μm in diameter are likely to be deposited on bronchiolar or alveolar epithelium, where they provide a potential focus for infection. Although such infection occurs most frequently by person-to-person transmission, it should be emphasized that this does not necessarily imply direct contact between infected and healthy individuals; the droplets may remain suspended in air for a considerable period of time, and prolonged exposure to contaminated air may result in infection.[6] In addition to the transmission of organisms via droplet nuclei, the reproductive structures of some microorganisms, such as the conidia of *Histoplasma capsulatum* or *Coccidioides immitis*, themselves may be inhaled as air-borne particles originating in contaminated soil.

"Aspiration" pneumonia occurs most often from contaminated oropharyngeal secretions or gastric contents. The normal adult oropharyngeal flora consists of an astounding variety of microorganisms,[7] most of which are commensals of low virulence that rarely, if ever, lead to pulmonary disease; however, some—such as *Actinomyces israelii* and a variety of anaerobes—can cause significant pulmonary infection. In addition to these relatively innocuous agents, the upper airways of chronically or critically ill hospitalized patients frequently become colonized by virulent organisms, especially gram-negative bacteria. In this circumstance, aspiration of only a small amount of contaminated saliva or nasal secretions may lead to pneumonia. There is evidence that asymptomatic aspiration occurs with ease in many normal people[8]; undoubtedly, it occurs with much greater frequency in individuals who have a decreased level of consciousness or who have neuromuscular or esophageal disease or intubation devices that interfere with normal deglutition.

Colonization of the lower respiratory tract is also an important precursor of pulmonary infection. Almost invariably, this occurs in association with underlying chronic pulmonary disease such as bronchiectasis or a parenchymal cavity. In many of these cases (e.g., an *Aspergillus* fungus ball or airway colonization by a nontuberculous myobacterial species), the implicated organism remains a saprophyte,

°Although the words "aspiration" and "inhalation" are commonly used interchangeably, we prefer to employ the former in relation to solid or liquid material (e.g., foreign bodies, saliva, and gastric contents) and the latter in relation to gaseous material, with or without microscopic particulate matter (e.g., bacteria and dust).

without tissue invasion. However, in other cases (e.g., airway colonization by *Pseudomonas* species in cystic fibrosis), there is frequently chronic active infection with progressive or recurrent episodes of tissue destruction.

Pneumonia acquired via the tracheobronchial tree may be divided into three types: airspace (lobar) pneumonia, bronchopneumonia, and interstitial pneumonia. Although it is not always possible to fit an individual case into one of these three categories using roentgenographic data, a specific pattern may be recognized with sufficient frequency to be of value in suggesting an etiology and in permitting prompt institution of potentially appropriate therapy.

Airspace Pneumonia. Airspace (lobar) pneumonia is characteristic of pneumococcal (*Streptococcus pneumoniae*) infection. The most important pathogenetic feature appears to be the rapid production of abundant edema with relatively minimal cellular reaction. In the early stages, the fluid exudate tends to be localized in the periphery of the lung beneath the visceral pleura. As it increases in amount, it flows directly from alveolus to alveolus and acinus to acinus via communicating channels. Thus, the disease comes to occupy a confluent portion of the lung parenchyma, limited only by pleural boundaries, and, eventually, by the host's cellular inflammatory reaction. Pathologically, this appears as a uniform consolidation that is relatively sharply demarcated from adjacent uninvolved parenchyma (Fig. 6–1). Before the development of effective antibiotic therapy, the pneumonic process frequently progressed to consolidation of an entire lobe or lobes (hence the designation "lobar" pneumonia). With current therapy, however, this outcome is very uncommon, and the term "airspace pneumonia" is more often employed to reflect the less extensive involvement.

The roentgenographic pattern of airspace pneumonia reflects the pathologic features described previously: homogeneous, nonsegmental consolidation of lung parenchyma, almost invariably abutting the visceral pleura, either interlobar or over the convexity (Fig. 6–2). Where the consolidation is not related to the pleura, its margin usually is fairly well defined. Larger bronchi within the area of consolidation usually remain air-containing, thus creating an air bronchogram. The lack of respect for segmental boundaries is of major importance in differentiating acute airspace pneumonia from bronchopneumonia. These typical roentgenographic features may be altered in the presence of underlying disease; for example, the inflammatory exudate may not fill emphysematous spaces, resulting in a sponge-like appearance of the consolidated lung parenchyma (Fig. 6–3).

The clinical diagnosis of acute airspace pneumonia often is suggested by cough, expectoration, chills and fever, and particularly pleural pain. Physical examination of the chest usually reveals only fine rales and decreased breath sounds, indicating the location of the disease. The classic signs of parenchymal consolidation—inspiratory lag, impaired percussion, bronchial breathing, fine rales, and whispering pectoriloquy—are heard much less often than formerly, presumably because the prompt institution of antibiotic therapy prevents the majority of cases from progressing to an advanced stage.

Bronchopneumonia. Bronchopneumonia (lobular pneumonia) is exemplified by infection by *Staphylococcus aureus* and many gram-negative bacteria. It differs from

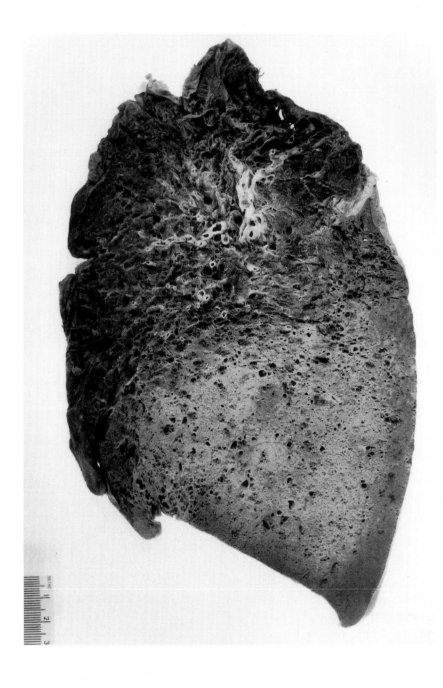

Figure 6–1. Acute Airspace (Lobar) Pneumonia—*Klebsiella pneumoniae.* Slice of left lung showing homogeneous consolidation of almost the entire lower lobe; severe apical emphysema is also present.

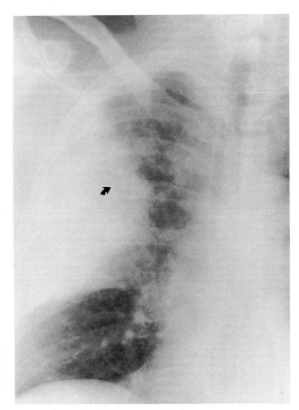

Figure 6–2. Acute Airspace Pneumonia—*S. pneumoniae.* A detail view of the right lung from a posteroanterior chest roentgenogram discloses dense consolidation in the axillary portion of the right upper lobe. The irregular margin of the lesion superomedially and a faint air bronchogram *(curved arrow)* define the more typical signs of an airspace lesion.

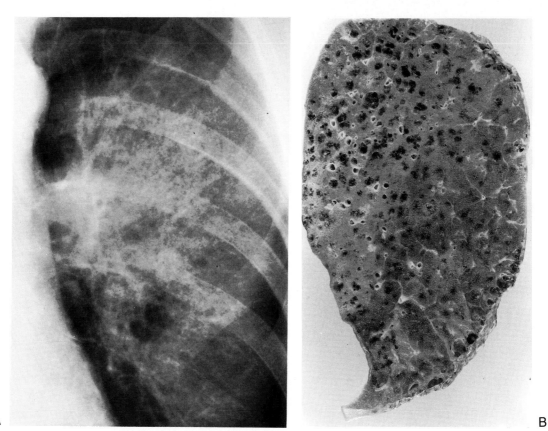

A

B

Figure 6–3. Acute Airspace Pneumonia Superimposed on Emphysema. *A,* A view of the left midlung zone from a posteroanterior roentgenogram reveals a poorly defined opacity in the superior segment of the left lower lobe. Instead of the homogeneous opacity characteristic of acute airspace pneumonia, this consolidation contains a large number of small radiolucencies. *B,* A slice of an upper lobe from another patient shows essentially homogeneous consolidation of the apical and posterior lung parenchyma. Within this region, there are numerous well-defined emphysematous spaces unaffected by the pneumonia. Such incomplete consolidation is responsible for the appearance in *A.*

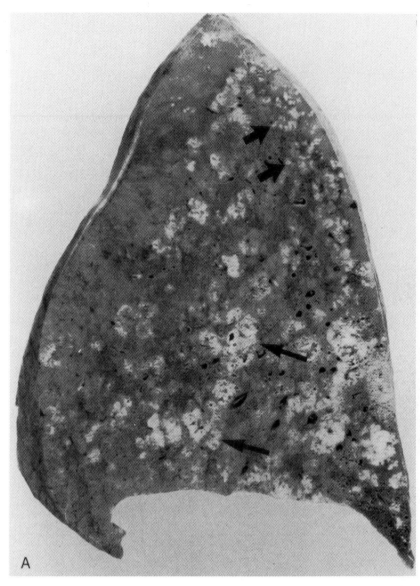

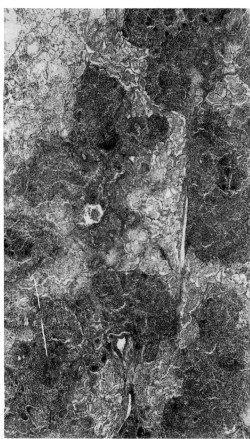

Figure 6–4. Acute Bronchopneumonia—*Pseudomonas aeruginosa. A,* Slice of left lower lobe showing patchy consolidation throughout the lung parenchyma. In some areas *(short arrows),* there is a discrete, finely branching pattern, indicating early infection confined to a bronchiolar location. In other sites *(long arrows),* there is confluent pneumonia; despite the more solid appearance, an underlying nodularity is easily appreciated. *B,* Histologic appearance of the area indicated by long arrows in *A* shows extensive parenchymal consolidation, representing confluence of infection originating about several bronchioles. The patchy nature of the process is still identifiable. (× 12.)

airspace pneumonia by the relatively rapid exudation of numerous polymorphonuclear leukocytes that serve to limit the spread of organisms, at least initially. Since the infection usually occurs at multiple foci at the same time, typically in relation to terminal bronchioles and proximal respiratory bronchioles, this results in a distinctly patchy appearance of the disease (Fig. 6–4). With progression, the inflammatory reaction may spread to involve the lung parenchyma between the distal airways, giving rise to confluent bronchopneumonia.

Roentgenographically, acute bronchopneumonia typically is manifested by parenchymal consolidation that is segmental in distribution (Fig. 6–5). In the early stages, it is patchy in appearance, but with progression to confluence it tends to appear homogeneous. Unlike airspace pneumonia, an exudate commonly fills the larger airways, and some degree of segmental atelectasis may accompany the consolidation. In addition, an air bronchogram is seldom apparent.

Symptoms in acute bronchopneumonia do not differ re-

liably from those of acute airspace infection. In contrast with some cases of airspace pneumonia, however, physical examination usually does not reveal bronchial breathing, whispering pectoriloquy, or abundant rales.

Interstitial Pneumonia. Interstitial pneumonia, caused principally by viruses and *Mycoplasma pneumoniae,* has two morphologic forms, depending to some extent on the chronicity of the process.

1. Relatively long-standing or insidious infection is manifested predominantly by lymphocytic infiltration of airway walls and alveolar septa without significant airspace abnormality (Fig. 6–6*A*).

2. More acute and frequently severe disease is often characterized by a histologic pattern known as diffuse alveolar damage, in which there is alveolar interstitial thickening by edema, capillary congestion, and an inflammatory cellular infiltrate; type II cell hyperplasia; and the development of a proteinaceous exudate within airspaces (*see* Fig.

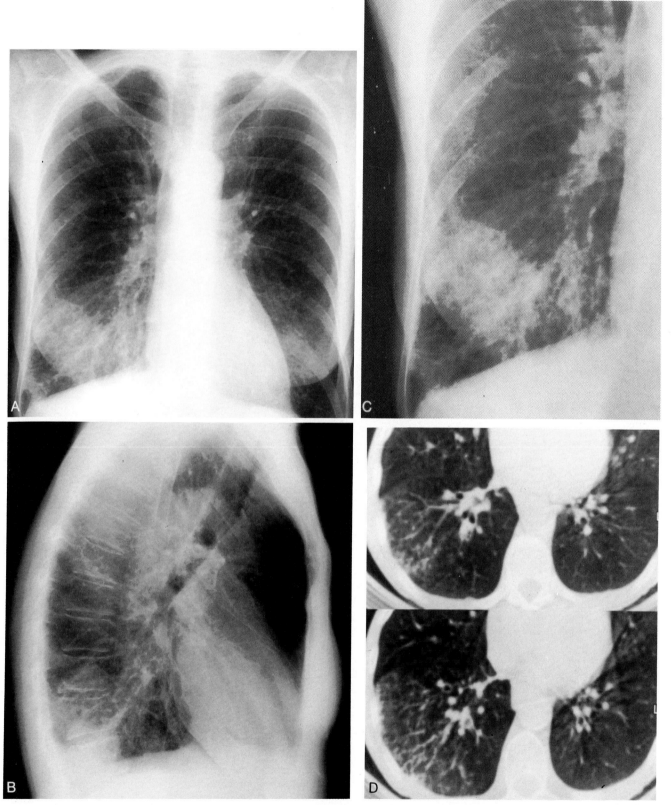

Figure 6–5. Acute Bronchopneumonia—*Staphylococcus aureus.* Posteroanterior *(A)* and lateral *(B)* chest roentgenograms disclose a triangular area of inhomogeneous consolidation in the right lower lobe. A detail view of the right lower zone *(C)* shows thickening and loss of definition of the broncho-vascular bundles, areas of more confluent consolidation, and septal lines in the costophrenic angle. The last feature is seen occasionally in acute bronchopneumonia and is caused by distention of lymphatics and interstitial tissue of interlobular septa by inflammatory edema. Contiguous CT scans through the lower lobes *(D)* reveal a fan-shaped area of increased attenuation and nodulation along the course of the three basal segments.

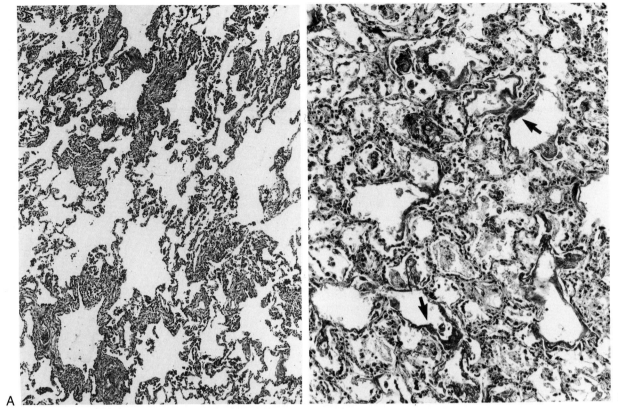

A   B

Figure 6–6. Interstitial Pneumonia: Morphologic Types. *A,* An open lung biopsy from a patient with cytomegalovirus infection shows more or less diffuse interstitial thickening by a lymphocytic infiltrate; the airspaces are unaffected. *B,* A section from another patient with acute herpes zoster pneumonia shows mild interstitial thickening, extensive type II cell hyperplasia, and proteinaceous material within airspaces (diffuse alveolar damage). Well-defined hyaline membranes are present *(arrows).* (*A* × 48; *B* × 100.)

6–6*B*). In alveolar ducts and respiratory bronchioles, this exudate frequently appears as relatively thin layers of densely eosinophilic material (hyaline membranes). Thus, although primarily an interstitial process, disease of this variety typically evolves to affect adjacent airspaces.

As might be expected from this discussion, roentgenographic findings in interstitial pneumonitis vary with the severity of disease. In the early stages, these may be a "ground-glass" or fine reticular pattern; with progression of disease, patchy or, occasionally, diffuse airspace consolidation may be evident (Fig. 6–7).

In patients with interstitial pneumonitis, there is usually a paucity of symptoms and signs. Nonproductive cough and fever may occur, and occasionally pleural pain may be felt. A decrease in the normal intensity of breath sounds may be appreciated, but bronchial breathing is extremely uncommon.

Infection Via the Pulmonary Vasculature

Infection by way of the pulmonary vasculature often occurs in conjunction with extrapulmonary infection; sometimes (particularly in tuberculous or fungal disease), the primary focus of infection is the lung itself. Whatever the source, the pathogenesis of this variety of pneumonia is related to the entry into the blood of relatively large numbers of organisms and their subsequent deposition in the

lung parenchyma. It is probable that most of the organisms exit the circulation from pulmonary arterioles, venules, or capillaries; since these vessels are present more or less uniformly throughout the lung parenchyma, the pattern of involvement tends to be patchy and random in distribution at the acinar level. However, because of preferential gravity-related blood flow to the dependent portions of the lung, infection tends to show considerable basal predominance. A nodular appearance of the individual foci of infection is typical (Fig. 6–8).

Clinically, the presence of fever helps distinguish this pattern of infection from other diseases that present with a nodular pattern on chest roentgenography.

Infection by Direct Spread

Direct spread across the chest wall or diaphragm or from the mediastinum may occur in association with penetrating thoracic wounds or by extension of infection from an extrapulmonary source, such as a subphrenic abscess. In these cases, the pulmonary disease usually is localized to an area contiguous with the extrapulmonary source of infection and often takes the form of an abscess.

Clinical and Environmental Setting of Pneumonia

In addition to the pathologic and roentgenologic patterns just described, it is useful to consider cases of pneumonia

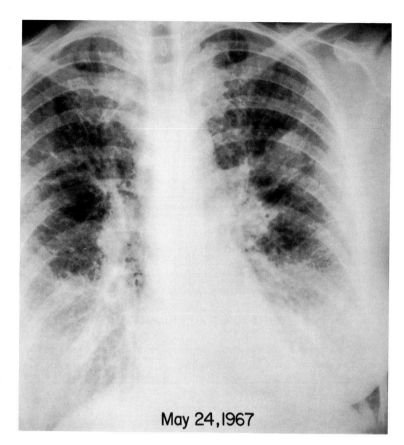

May 24,1967

Figure 6–7. Acute Interstitial and Airspace Pneumonia—*Mycoplasma pneumoniae.* A posteroanterior chest roentgenogram reveals thickening of the bronchovascular bundles and a ground-glass opacity throughout both lungs.

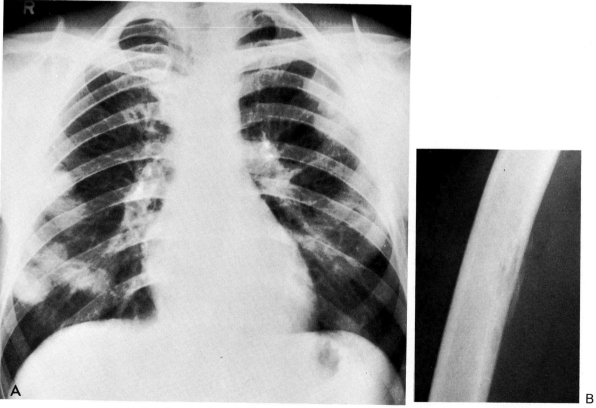

Figure 6–8. Multiple Nodules: Pyemic Abscesses. A posteroanterior roentgenogram *(A)* reveals several sharply defined nodules ranging from 2 to 3 cm in diameter situated predominantly in the right lower lobe and the left upper lobe. The masses are homogeneous in density and show no evidence of cavitation (although cavitation eventually occurred in the majority). A lateral view of the midshaft of the right femur *(B)* shows an irregular area of rarefaction in the cortex, associated with subperiosteal new bone formation along the posterior aspect. *Staphylococcus aureus* was cultured from the sputum and from pus obtained from the thigh at incision and drainage.

in three clinical and environmental groups: (1) those that are acquired in the community by otherwise healthy individuals or by patients with underlying disease that does not profoundly affect pulmonary defense; (2) those that develop in the hospital in the same individuals (nosocomial pneumonias); and (3) those that develop in either location in an individual with deficient defense mechanisms (the compromised host).

Community-Acquired Pneumonia

Community-acquired pneumonia is caused most often by *Mycoplasma pneumoniae*, *Streptococcus pneumoniae*, *Legionella pneumophila*, *Haemophilus influenzae*, *Chlamydia pneumoniae*, anaerobic bacteria, and viruses.[9, 9a] (It is important to remember that this statement refers principally to relatively developed countries, such as those in North America and Europe, since the specific organisms that cause community-acquired pneumonia vary with different areas of the world; for example, in regions where melioidosis is endemic, *Pseudomonas pseudomallei* has been reported to be the commonest organism.[10])

Of the organisms listed previously, *S. pneumoniae* is probably the commonest cause of pneumonia in patients admitted to the hospital; *M. pneumoniae* is generally regarded as the second most frequent.[11] Although *H. influenzae* causes pneumonia primarily in young children, it seems to be increasing in frequency in older children and adults, perhaps because the early administration of antibiotics prevents the development of protective antibodies. *Staphylococcus aureus* more commonly causes pneumonia in hospitalized patients but should be suspected during influenza epidemics, in alcoholics, and in debilitated persons recently discharged from the hospital or in contact with such patients.[12] A considerable number of community-acquired pneumonias in both developed and relatively undeveloped countries also are caused by anaerobic organisms.[13]

Recurrent pneumonia in patients outside the hospital usually denotes some underlying disease[14]; roughly one half of such patients have chronic bronchitis, bronchiectasis, or congestive heart failure, and the other half have extrathoracic illnesses, most commonly alcoholism, diabetes mellitus, chronic sinusitis, or extrapulmonary malignancy. Although most pneumonias in alcoholics are pneumococcal, *Klebsiella* and *H. influenzae* should always be considered seriously in the differential diagnosis.

Hospital-Acquired Pneumonia

Hospital-acquired pneumonias are those that develop in an institutional environment and were neither present nor incubating at the time of admission. They have been estimated to occur in 0.5 to 5.0 per cent of inpatients[15] and are particularly common in mechanically ventilated patients in intensive care units.[16] Causal organisms are typically gram-negative bacteria that have the tendency to colonize the oropharynx and gastrointestinal tract. Such organisms are infrequent commensals in healthy persons, the carrier rate being estimated to range from 2 to 10 per cent. However, in hospitalized patients who are not critically ill, the carrier rate has been found to approximate 30 to 40 per cent, and

in chronically or severely incapacitated in-hospital patients it is as high as 60 to 75 per cent. Colonization is the result largely of contact spread from contaminated hospital personnel or equipment. The persons at greatest risk are the elderly with underlying disease and patients who are malnourished or who have been inappropriately treated with broad-spectrum antibiotics.[17]

Hospital-acquired pneumonia can be difficult to diagnose, since bacterial colonization by no means implies infection and since the symptoms and signs of underlying disease tend to mask the superimposed insult. The infection is also much more serious than that acquired in the community; this is due, in part, to the impaired resistance of acutely or chronically ill patients and, perhaps more important, to the virulence of the causal organisms.

During the past three decades there has been a marked change in the specific organisms responsible for nosocomial pneumonia. Bacteria implicated in the 1950s—*S. pneumoniae*, *H. influenzae*, and β-hemolytic streptococci—became rare in the 1960s, being replaced by penicillinase-producing *S. aureus* and, to a lesser extent, gram-negative organisms. By the mid-1970s, the latter organisms, particularly *P. aeruginosa* and the Enterobacteriaceae, became the predominant offenders, although *S. aureus* remains an important problem.[18] Multiple infecting organisms may be identified in 20 to 40 per cent of cases.[16]

Pneumonia in the Compromised Host

Congenital disorders of immune function, either cell mediated or humoral, are often associated with an increased incidence of pulmonary infection. This may be manifested as bronchiectasis or recurrent pneumonia, or both, depending somewhat on the underlying disease. For example, immunoglobulin deficiency, particularly of some of the subclasses of IgG, is commonly associated with bronchiectasis.[19] (Interestingly, selective IgA deficiency, although frequent, often is not complicated by bronchiectasis.[20]) Bronchiectasis may also develop in acquired disorders of humoral immunity, such as in chronic lymphocytic leukemia associated with hypogammaglobulinemia[21]; however, pneumonia, usually caused by bacteria, is a commoner complication. A well-recognized cause of humoral immunoincompetence is hyposplenism resulting from either splenectomy or infarction, in most cases secondary to sickle cell anemia.[22] The consequent immunoglobulin deficiency causes an impairment of opsonization and, to some extent, a curtailment of splenic phagocytic function, permitting opportunistic infection with a variety of bacteria (particularly *S. pneumoniae*) and protozoa.

Impaired function or deficiency of phagocytic cells of the inflammatory system is also an important predisposing factor to opportunistic pulmonary infection. In many cases, disorders of phagocytic function are secondary to a systemic abnormality such as connective tissue or myeloproliferative disease. In addition, there are several specific disorders of phagocytic function, such as chronic granulomatous disease of childhood, that occur as an isolated process and that may cause significant pulmonary disease. With few exceptions, neutropenia alone does not compromise the host; however, when it is accompanied by a sparsity of mononuclear phagocytes—as in bone marrow failure and in drug-induced "agranulocytosis," in which all phagocytes are depressed—infectious complications may be severe. In addition, its development in cases of agammaglobulinemia or autoimmune disease compounds the susceptibility to infection.

Acquired Immunodeficiency Syndrome (AIDS)

The prevalence of this modern plague has increased exponentially since it was first reported in 1983, so that by May 1993 more than 270,000 cases had been reported in the United States alone.[23] The disease has been described in homosexuals, drug addicts, hemophiliacs who received factor VIII concentrate, residents of Haiti and equatorial Africa, transfusion recipients, female sexual partners of men with AIDS, and infants in high-risk households. In industrialized countries, the majority of cases occur in the first two groups.

Although the precise etiology and pathogenesis of AIDS remain controversial, it is widely believed that the cause is the human immunodeficiency virus (HIV). This virus selectively infects cells that express the CD4 membrane glycoprotein, particularly T lymphocytes, cells of the monocyte-macrophage lineage, and neuronal cells.[24] Such infected cells may be either destroyed or functionally impaired, resulting in a characteristic set of immunologic abnormalities: lymphopenia, a reduction in T-helper cells, a reversal of the T cell helper-to-suppressor ratio, cutaneous anergy, and hypergammaglobulinemia. The characteristic opportunistic infections in patients with AIDS occur in those with CD4 cell counts of 200 to 250 cells per mL or less,[25] particularly in those with a rapidly increasing viral burden.[24] In fact, according to the 1992 classification of the Centers for Disease Control in the United States, a count of fewer than 200 CD4 cells in an HIV-positive individual is diagnostic of AIDS.

HIV has been isolated from a variety of tissues and body secretions, including blood, saliva, and bronchoalveolar lavage (BAL) fluid.[26] At the time of writing, however, diagnosis of HIV infection is based largely on highly sensitive and specific methods of detecting antibody to the virus—enzyme-linked immunosorbent assay (ELISA) and Western blot testing with HIV antigen; the former has been found to have a specificity of 99.8 per cent and a sensitivity of 97 per cent.[27]

Following infection by HIV, patients become asymptomatic and may remain so for variable periods of time. Subsequently, some present with persistent generalized lymphadenopathy (PGL), with or without constitutional symptoms or complicating infections. A minority of patients present with the full-blown clinical picture of AIDS, including opportunistic infections, neoplasms, or both, and are readily identified on that basis alone.

A detailed discussion of the varied pathologic, roentgenographic, and clinical manifestations of AIDS is beyond the scope of this text, and the following discussion concerns only the features related to the lungs. Because the condition is commonly seen by chest physicians and radiologists, consideration is also given to noninfectious complications. A more detailed discussion of specific diseases can be found elsewhere in the appropriate section of the text and in several review articles.[28–31]

Pneumocystis Carinii. Pneumonia caused by this organism is the commonest clinically recognized infection in patients with AIDS,[29] and its presence is considered diagnostic of the syndrome in an individual who is HIV-positive. Although the infection has many features in common with that in individuals without AIDS, there are also important and fairly frequent differences. For example, affected patients with AIDS have substantially more cysts and fewer polymorphonuclear leukocytes in BAL fluid than do patients without AIDS.[32] In addition, unusual pathologic manifestations, such as necrosis, vascular invasion, and the presence of a granulomatous inflammatory reaction, are common.[33]

Atypical roentgenographic manifestations have been found in as many as 10 per cent of cases. For example, in contrast with the commoner diffuse reticular and airspace patterns, predominant upper lobe involvement is sometimes seen, particularly in association with the use of prophylactic aerosol medication.[34] The formation of parenchymal cysts is also an unusual but increasingly recognized complication, particularly on computed tomography (CT). These range from one to several centimeters in diameter and are most commonly multiple, thin-walled, and located in the upper lobes (Fig. 6–9).[35] Pneumothorax is a common complication.[36] Pathologic examination has shown that at least some "cysts" represent areas of necrotizing *Pneumocystis* pneumonia. Hilar and mediastinal lymph node calcification has been described with *P. carinii* infection, presumably also reflecting the presence of necrosis.[37]

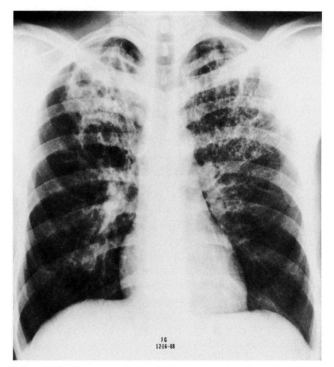

Figure 6–9. *Pneumocystis Carinii* Pneumonia Manifested as Upper Lobe Cavitary Lesions. A posteroanterior roentgenogram reveals a large cavity in the right upper lobe surrounded by a wall of moderate thickness. Smaller cavities with thinner walls are present elsewhere in this lobe and in the left upper lobe. Although a number of patchy opacities are associated with the cavities in both upper lobes, the lower half of each lung shows no evidence of disease. A 23-year-old man with AIDS presenting with fever and a productive cough of several days' duration.

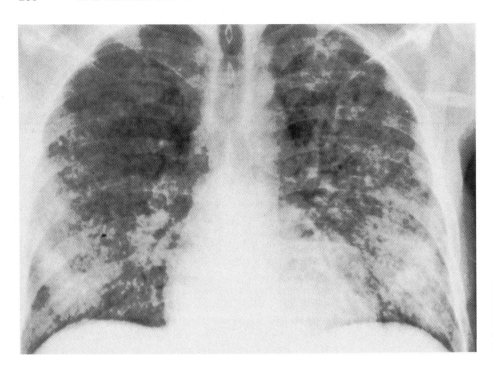

Figure 6–10. Disseminated Histoplasmosis in AIDS. An anteroposterior roentgenogram in the supine position demonstrates widespread, discrete, and confluent nodular opacities ranging in diameter from 2 to 4 mm.

P. carinii pneumonia in patients with AIDS tends to develop insidiously and progress relatively slowly compared with the infection in other compromised hosts[29]; recurrence of disease after therapy is common. The infection should be suspected if the alveolar-to-arterial (A-a) gradient for oxygen shows a considerable increase, even with a normal chest roentgenogram. In patients with signs or symptoms of extrathoracic disease, the possibility of extrapulmonary dissemination should be considered, particularly in those who have received prophylactic therapy; reported sites include lymph nodes (especially mediastinal), bone marrow, liver, spleen, skin (particularly around the head), the upper respiratory tract (e.g., the sinuses), and central nervous system.[29]

Fungi. Cryptococcosis occurs in about 10 per cent of patients[29]; although it most often causes meningoencephalitis, concomitant involvement of the lungs is common.[38] An interstitial pattern is said to be the most frequent roentgenographic manifestation.[29] Rapidly disseminating and often fatal infection with *Histoplasma capsulatum*[39] or *Coccidioides immitis*[40] may occur in patients residing in endemic areas. Roentgenographic manifestations in both conditions usually consist of diffuse reticulonodular or nodular opacities (Fig. 6–10). Infection in these cases may be difficult to recognize pathologically, the reaction consisting only of aggregates of macrophages similar to those seen in *Mycobacterium avium-intracellulare* infection (*see* later). In contrast with many other diseases with compromised pulmonary defense, pulmonary infection by *Aspergillus* species is infrequent in AIDS.[41]

Cytomegalovirus. This is the commonest infectious agent identified in the lungs at autopsy of patients with AIDS and has been detected in BAL fluid in about 20 per cent of patients during life.[42] However, clinically or roentgenographically evident disease is infrequent, and it is likely that many cases in which the organism is identified represent simply a carrier state in which the virus is present but not pathogenic. When disease does occur, pathologic and roentgenographic features are similar to those of cytomegalovirus infection in other situations, except that the number of organisms tends to be much greater.

Mycobacteria. *M. avium-intracellulare* is a common opportunistic organism in patients with AIDS, having been identified in more than 50 per cent of cases at autopsy in some series.[28] Despite this, it is a relatively uncommon cause of disease during life, apparently existing in many individuals more as a saprophyte than as a true pathogen. For reasons that are unclear, the organism is responsible for more than 95 per cent of all nontuberculous mycobacterial infections in AIDS.[28] The presenting features of the disease are usually nonspecific and include chronic diarrhea and malabsorption, wasting, progressive anemia, and obstructive jaundice. Respiratory symptoms and chest radiographic abnormalities are usually absent, even when the organism is cultured from specimens obtained from the lower respiratory tract.

Recently, it has become evident that infection with *M. tuberculosis* also is a relatively frequent complication of HIV infection, particularly in Haitians and Africans,[43] but also in whites.[44] In patients who are HIV-positive without the clinical features of AIDS, the manifestations are similar to those in immunocompetent individuals.[28] However, in patients with AIDS, the disease shows several important differences: it is more likely to be extrapulmonary and to be accompanied by spread to the central nervous system,[45] less likely to be cavitated, and more likely to resemble primary, rather than postprimary, tuberculosis.[46] Of importance from a diagnostic point of view is the observation that the tuberculin skin test reaction is often negative.

Pathologically, a granulomatous inflammatory reaction is frequently absent, particularly with *M. avium-intracellulare* infection of lymph nodes but also with *M. tuberculosis* pulmonary infection. Instead, there is an accumulation of macrophages with abundant, somewhat vacuolated cytoplasm; acid-fast stain demonstrates the macrophages to be stuffed with the organism.

Other Bacteria. In addition to the relatively unusual opportunistic organisms described previously, patients with AIDS appear to be at increased risk for infection from commoner, or garden variety, bacteria, particularly *S. pneumoniae* and *H. influenzae*.[47, 48] As might be expected in any debilitated patient who is dying in the hospital, bacteria such as *Staphylococcus aureus*, *Pseudomonas aeruginosa*, and other gram-negative bacteria are common at autopsy. Infection with organisms of the order Actinomycetales, particularly *Nocardia asteroides*, also occurs with increased frequency and is usually widely disseminated.

Kaposi's Sarcoma. This is a common complication of AIDS and is the presenting manifestation of the disease in as many as one third of patients.[30] It is particularly frequent in homosexual and bisexual men. Lesions occur most often in the skin and oropharyngeal mucosa but can develop anywhere, including the lungs and pleura. In fact, pleuropulmonary involvement has been identified in many patients at autopsy, although clinical and radiographic evidence of disease is not apparent in most. However, in patients with known extrapulmonary Kaposi's sarcoma who present with respiratory symptoms, approximately one third will prove to have pulmonary involvement.[30]

Within the thorax, tumor usually is located in mediastinal, hilar, or bronchopulmonary lymph nodes or in peribronchovascular, septal, or pleural connective tissue. Lymph node involvement may result in compression of airways, leading to partial and, occasionally, complete obstruction. Similar occlusion also may occur by growth of airway mucosal plaques. These are fairly common in both trachea and proximal bronchi and appear endoscopically as bright red or purplish, elevated lesions 0.5 to 2 cm in diameter. Tumor growth also may occur into the lung parenchyma, resulting in nodules or masses that may occasionally occupy an entire lobe. Parenchymal hemorrhage related to the tumor may be severe enough to be fatal. Pleural infiltration is frequent and commonly is associated with effusion, which can be clear or hemorrhagic.[49]

Roentgenographic manifestations consist of bilateral nodules of variable size (reflecting predominant parenchymal involvement) or a coarse reticular or linear pattern (corresponding to interstitial disease). Mediastinal or hilar lymph node enlargement, pleural effusion (usually bilateral), and airspace opacities (representing parenchymal hemorrhage) are seen variably. The commonest pulmonary symptoms are dyspnea and nonproductive cough; hemoptysis and chest pain occur less often.[30] Fever is present in many patients.

Lymphoproliferative Disorders. A parenchymal interstitial infiltrate composed of lymphocytes, plasma cells, and immunoblasts, characteristic of *lymphoid interstitial pneumonia* (LIP), is occasionally seen in patients with AIDS. It has been speculated that it represents a tissue response to Epstein-Barr virus or HIV pulmonary infection[50] or an immune response associated with HLA-DR5.[51] Although predominantly a feature of childhood AIDS—in which group it is diagnostic of the disease in an HIV-positive individual—the complication also has been reported with increas-

ing frequency in adults.[52] In children, LIP appears to overlap with another pathologic condition termed *pulmonary lymphoid hyperplasia*, in which the lymphocyte proliferation occurs as nodules localized to the airway mucosa.[30]

Roentgenographic manifestations of LIP consist of a diffuse reticular or reticulonodular pattern[52]; evidence of mediastinal lymph node enlargement is seen occasionally, usually in patients with pulmonary lymphoid hyperplasia. In contrast with diffuse infectious pulmonary disease in HIV-positive individuals, the reticular or reticulonodular pattern of LIP shows a surprisingly stable appearance over time.[53] The major symptoms are progressive dyspnea and cough; basal rales are common. Systemic lymph node enlargement and hepatosplenomegaly are frequent.

Non-Hodgkin's lymphoma is the second most frequent AIDS-related malignancy; in fact, in an HIV-positive person, it is diagnostic of the disease. Although the tumor most commonly affects the central nervous system, it may also be generalized and occasionally involves the lungs and thoracic lymph nodes.[54] Hilar or mediastinal lymph node enlargement is not a common feature of progressive generalized lymphadenopathy,[55] and its presence should alert the physician to the possibility of Kaposi's sarcoma or lymphoma.

Microbiologic Considerations

In some cases, when a pathogen (or potential pathogen such as an opportunistic organism) is grown on sputum culture, the clinical history is inconsistent with the picture usually attributed to that organism. There are several reasons for such an inconsistency. For example, before admission to the hospital the patient may have received antibiotics without prior bacteriologic study, and such therapy may eliminate the responsible pathogen (in many cases *S. pneumoniae*).[56] Similarly, antibiotic therapy may alter the upper respiratory tract flora and enable resistant organisms to multiply, leading the physician to the erroneous conclusion that the resistant organism is responsible for the disease process. Finally, it should be remembered that even healthy subjects may harbor pathogenic bacteria in their upper respiratory tract; thus, isolation of a specific pathogen does not necessarily indicate the etiology of pulmonary disease, and bacteriologic findings must be interpreted in the light of clinical features and roentgenographic patterns.

The use of multiple or ancillary diagnostic microbiologic procedures can help obviate this uncertainty and can considerably influence the yield of definitive diagnoses. For example, repeated heavy growth of the same organism on culture of purulent expectorated material obviously strengthens the likelihood of that organism's being etiologically responsible for the disease. Quantitative cultures may be useful in recognizing true pathogens; similarly, immunofluorescent determination of antibody-coating of bacteria, although requiring a week or more to develop, can support evidence for pathogenicity and is particularly valuable in patients who have received antibiotics.[57]

Failure to isolate a bacterial pathogen from the sputum of patients with pneumonia usually leads to a diagnosis of viral or mycoplasmal pneumonia. In a small percentage of these cases, the diagnosis is confirmed by subsequent isolation of the organism or by a rise in titer of an antibody to a specific virus during the convalescent period. In addition, a significant number of pneumonias in which aerobic cultures fail to show an accepted pathogen are due to anaerobic infection; this should be suspected when the history suggests the possibility of aspiration of oropharyngeal contents and roentgenography demonstrates cavitation.

When considering the etiology of a pneumonia, it is also important to remember that more than one agent may be responsible. This is particularly relevant in immunocompromised patients, such as those with AIDS. In addition, in many apparently nonimmunocompromised individuals, bacterial pneumonia appears to follow a viral infection. In many of these cases, the viral infection is predominantly limited to the upper respiratory tract[58]; in others, however, it appears that the bacterial infection is a direct complication of pulmonary viral infection. This has been particularly well demonstrated for the development of staphylococcal pneumonia after influenza and for the development of bronchopneumonia from various organisms after measles.[59] The propensity for the development of such superinfection is related to a number of factors, including a deficiency of mucociliary clearance,[60] impairment of alveolar macrophage phagocytosis and bactericidal efficiency,[61] and the enhancement of bacterial adherence to damaged epithelium.[62]

GRAM-POSITIVE AEROBIC BACTERIA

Streptococcus Pneumoniae

Streptococcus pneumoniae is a gram-positive facultative anaerobe that is usually arranged in pairs and is surrounded by a well-developed capsule. It has been estimated to be present as a commensal in approximately 20 per cent of the population.[63] On the basis of chemical differences and polysaccharide composition, about 90 antigenic variants have been identified; the great majority of the pneumonias are caused by types 8, 4, 5, 12, 3, 1, 7, and 9.[64] Specific serotypes are related, to some extent, to both the development and the severity of disease. For example, type 3 appears to show a predilection for the elderly, in whom it is often accompanied by bacteremia and usually by pneumonia with a high mortality rate.[64] By contrast, pneumococcal bacteremia in children seems to carry little risk of death, presumably because the pneumococcal types to which they are susceptible are relatively less virulent.

Pneumococcal pneumonia accounts for as many as 15 to 20 per cent of pneumonias in otherwise healthy adults[65]; in these patients, the disease is generally mild and clinically similar to nonbacterial pneumonias. By contrast, pneumonia is commoner and tends to be severer in indigent persons and in individuals who lack a spleen[66] or who have chronic underlying disease, such as alcoholism, renal failure, lymphoproliferative disorders or leukemia, sickle cell disease,[67] and uncontrolled diabetes mellitus.[68] Infections are commonest during the winter and early spring, and their incidence distinctly increases during influenza epidemics.

Pathogenesis and Pathologic Characteristics

The development of pneumococcal pneumonia is thought to be related, in part, to the presence of the organism's capsule, which is both hydrophilic and acidic; these features render it resistant to phagocytosis and allow it to multiply relatively freely outside cells. Complement also may play a role in its pathogenesis by inducing the early fluid exudate: preparations of pneumococcal cell walls activate the alternative complement pathway,[69] and levels of late complement components are depressed in active pneumococcal disease.[70] Activated complement factors also may act in controlling infection by facilitating opsonization and phagocytosis of organisms by polymorphonuclear leukocytes, although these processes by themselves do not appear to be sufficient. More important in this regard are the development of type-specific antibody production and the presence of macrophages during the stage of resolution.

Whatever the mechanism, the production of abundant, relatively acellular edema fluid during the initial stage of infection is felt to be responsible for the development of the typical solid parenchymal consolidation seen in pneumococcal pneumonia, the disease spreading from alveolus to alveolus and acinus to acinus by flow of fluid through alveolar pores or small airways. Pathologic findings in early disease thus consist of alveolar capillary dilatation and congestion and abundant alveolar edema containing numerous organisms and only occasional leukocytes. Subsequently, alveolar spaces become filled with leukocytes, and extracellular microorganisms become sparse. Histologic evidence of tissue necrosis is usually absent. With time, leukocytes decrease in number and are replaced by macrophages.

In patients who survive the acute infection, complete histologic resolution is the rule, although occasionally the fibrinopurulent exudate organizes rather than resorbs, resulting in fibrosis of affected lung parenchyma. The high incidence of resolution probably is related to several factors, including the lack of toxins produced by the pneumococcus, an increase in serum and lung fluid antiproteases during the infection,[71] and, possibly, the ability of damaged alveolar epithelial cells to regenerate.[72]

Roentgenographic Manifestations

The roentgenographic pattern of acute pneumococcal pneumonia is characteristically one of acute airspace pneumonia, most frequently confined to one lobe and consisting of homogeneous consolidation of lung parenchyma (see Fig. 4–4, page 169). Since the consolidation begins in the peripheral airspaces, it almost invariably abuts a visceral pleural surface, either interlobar or over the convexity. Where it is not related to a visceral pleural surface, its margin usually is fairly well defined. An air bronchogram is very common, and its absence should cast doubt on the diagnosis unless the consolidation is confined to the periphery of the lung where airways are too small to be clearly identifiable.

Since the pathologic process is one of replacement of air by inflammatory exudate, loss of volume is either slight or absent during the acute stage of the disease; during resolution, however, some degree of atelectasis is common and presumably is caused by exudate within airways and resultant obstruction. Cavitation is rare, although massive pulmonary "gangrene" or abscess formation may occur; it is probable that most such cases represent mixed infections, particularly with anaerobic organisms.[73] In contrast with its frequency before the advent of antibiotics, roentgenographically demonstrable pleural effusion is seen less commonly today.

In our experience, resolution can be fairly rapid with appropriate therapy, complete clearing being roentgenologically apparent within 10 to 14 days. However, others have reported disappearance of roentgenographic changes after as long as 8 to 10 weeks, particularly in the elderly and in patients with alcoholism or obstructive lung disease.[74]

Occasionally, the roentgenographic pattern is segmental and inhomogeneous, conforming to the usual pattern of acute bronchopneumonia. In addition, the homogeneity of consolidation may be altered by the presence of a multitude of small air-containing "holes," representing emphysematous spaces that have escaped consolidation (*see* Fig. 6–3, page 291). It is worth remembering, however, that in some instances unusual roentgenographic patterns are attributed in error to pneumococcal infection on the basis of sputum cultures alone, the real etiologic agent being undetected.[63]

Clinical Manifestations

The usual clinical presentation is abrupt, with fever, shaking chills, cough, slight expectoration, and intense pleural pain. On close questioning, many patients admit the presence of an upper respiratory tract infection before the onset of the more dramatic symptoms. Temperature may be as high as 41°C. The cough may be nonproductive at first but soon produces bloody, "rusty," or greenish material. Debilitated and alcoholic patients may be deeply cyanosed, and shock may ensue rapidly. Physical examination may reveal signs of pulmonary consolidation, and in many cases a friction rub is audible over the affected lung.

Complications occur less often now than before the advent of antibiotics; meningitis and empyema are seen in fewer than 10 per cent of cases, and pericarditis, jaundice, and disseminated intravascular coagulation are present only occasionally. Perhaps the commonest complication nowadays is superinfection, usually by gram-negative organisms and typically in patients who have received huge doses of penicillin or a combination of antibiotics.

Laboratory Findings

A pure growth of S. *pneumoniae* on blood culture or the identification of pneumococcal polysaccharide antigen by counterimmunoelectrophoresis or coagulation is diagnostic[75]; however, since the organism is a common commensal in the oropharynx, a positive result of a smear or culture of expectorate cannot be accepted as absolute confirmation of the diagnosis. The reported incidence of negative sputum culture results in patients with pneumococcal pneumonia proved by positive blood cultures is as high as 45 per cent.[76] Some investigators advocate obtaining a brush specimen via a protective catheter[77] or a transthoracic needle aspirate[78] to achieve a higher diagnostic sensitivity and specificity.

The white blood cell count usually is over 20,000 cells per mL, in a range of 10,000 to 40,000. Polymorphonuclear leukocytosis, with many band forms, is common; however, leukopenia develops in many extremely ill patients. Analysis of arterial blood gas may show mild or even severe hypoxemia. In most cases, the partial pressure of carbon dioxide (P_{CO_2}) is reduced, and the minute ventilation indicates hyperventilation with small tidal volume.

Prognosis

The mortality rate in bacteremic pneumococcal pneumonia has been estimated to be 10[79] to 20[79a] per cent; however, the rate for nonhospitalized patients with less severe disease must be considerably less. Older age, underlying lung disease, multilobar involvement, extrapulmonary disease, serotype 3, and the presence of bacteremia individually and in combination worsen the prognosis. Prompt institution of antibiotic therapy also appears to be a key factor in outcome; however, the incidence of resistance to antibiotics such as penicillin[80] appears to be increasing and undoubtedly influences the outcome adversely in individual cases. The prophylactic use of polyvalent pneumococcal polysaccharide vaccine is of some benefit[81]; unfortunately, those in most need of protection—the elderly, the debilitated, and the compromised—are the least likely to produce antibodies.

Streptococcus Pyogenes

Until the advent of antibiotics, *Streptococcus pyogenes* (Lancefield group A β-hemolytic streptococcus) was the commonest cause of bronchopneumonia, particularly after attacks of measles, pertussis, and influenza. Nowadays, pneumonia caused by the organism is seldom seen, although cases are still reported following influenza[82] and as a complication of childhood exanthems.[83] Infection is most frequent during the winter.

In most respects, the roentgenographic characteristics are indistinguishable from those of acute staphylococcal pneumonia; unlike this, however, the tendency to form pneumatoceles or pyopneumothorax is absent. The onset of pneumonia is usually abrupt, with pleural pain, shaking chills, fever, and cough productive of purulent and often blood-tinged material; signs of pleural effusion are usually detectable. Complications include residual pleural thickening and bronchiectasis (especially in children in whom the disease develops in conjunction with an exanthem).

Other Streptococci

In addition to S. *pneumoniae* and S. *pyogenes*, a variety of other streptococci occasionally cause pleuropulmonary disease. Lancefield group B organisms (S. *agalactiae*) in particular can cause serious infection, especially in infants (in whom the birth canal appears to be the chief reservoir of infection[84]) and in adults with diabetes or in patients receiving antibiotic therapy.[85]

Staphylococcus Aureus

Staphylococcus aureus is a gram-positive coccus that characteristically appears on smear in irregular clumps or grapelike clusters. It has replaced *Streptococcus pyogenes* as the commonest cause of bronchopneumonia, frequently complicating viral infection (particularly influenza) or developing in hospitalized patients whose resistance has been lowered by disease or recent surgery. Those receiving antibiotic therapy, particularly with multiple drugs, and those with a prolonged hospital stay are most susceptible. The emergence of this organism as an important and often virulent pathogen is related largely to its ability to develop antibiotic resistance and to the contamination of the hospital environment. *Staphylococcus aureus* is also a relatively frequent cause of tracheitis in children, in whom it appears to occur either as a complication of viral infection or, possibly, as a primary infectious agent.[86]

Pathologic Characteristics

Most cases of pneumonia occur by inhalation or aspiration of organisms into the distal airways. Occasionally, they occur as a result of hematogenous spread from an infected site elsewhere in the body, frequently from pelvic veins or an intravenous catheter.

The pathologic findings in staphylococcal bronchopneumonia depend on the rapidity of the disease process and may be conveniently grouped into three forms: acute hemorrhagic (fulminating), acute purulent, and chronic organizing. The first of these is commonly associated with influenza, although it also may occur sporadically without underlying disease. Microscopically, the parenchyma shows extensive intra-alveolar edema and hemorrhage, with relatively sparse polymorphonuclear leukocytic infiltration and little or no evidence of tissue necrosis. Organisms abound within the edema fluid. It is possible that this appearance is associated with a massive production of bacterial toxins, since similar microscopic changes have been identified in rabbits injected intratracheally with filtrates of bacterial toxin.[87]

The acute purulent variety of pneumonia is the commonest form and appears as a typical bronchopneumonia, frequently associated with abscess formation. As the disease progresses, individual microabscesses enlarge and coalesce, producing one or more macroscopically visible abscesses (Fig. 6–11). Drainage of necrotic material may lead to cavity formation. The chronic organizing form of the disease is characterized by variably severe fibrosis in the lung parenchyma around the abscess cavities.

Staphylococcal tracheitis is manifested by acute inflammation and ulceration of the larynx, trachea, and proximal bronchi. Frequently, there are pseudomembranes or large amounts of thick mucus and inflammatory exudate, which can significantly occlude the airway lumen.

Roentgenographic Manifestations

The typical appearance of staphylococcal bronchopneumonia is parenchymal consolidation, usually segmental in distribution. Depending on the severity of involvement, the process may be patchy or homogeneous; the latter represents confluent bronchopneumonia and, in our experience, is the commoner presentation. Acute inflammatory exudate fills the airways, so that some loss of volume may accompany the consolidation; for the same reason, an air bronchogram is seldom observed, and its presence should cast some doubt on the diagnosis.

The roentgenographic pattern differs somewhat in children and adults. In the former, consolidation tends to develop very rapidly, usually involves a whole lobe, and may be multilobar. An additional distinctive characteristic is the development of pneumatoceles (*see* page 239), which are reported to occur in about 50 per cent of patients.[88] These air-containing spaces are commonly thin-walled and may be enormous—the size of a hemithorax or larger—in which case they may simulate a large pneumothorax. Many contain fluid levels. They usually appear during the first week of the pneumonia and always disappear spontaneously within weeks or months.

In adults, the disease is bilateral in more than 60 per cent of cases.[89] Abscess formation with subsequent communication with the bronchial tree and the appearance of fluid-containing cavities is fairly common. These are usually solitary and characteristically have a very irregular shaggy inner wall (Fig. 6–12). Pneumatocele formation is very uncommon. Pleural effusion or empyema occurs in approximately 50 per cent of patients.

In pneumonia caused by hematogenous spread of organisms from a distant site, the roentgenographic appearance is one of multiple nodular masses throughout the lungs, sometimes with poorly defined borders (*see* Fig. 6–8, page 295). Occasionally, they are confluent and resemble homogeneous consolidation.

Clinical Manifestations

In children and adults who acquire the infection following influenza and in the very occasional case in which the disease develops outside the hospital in an otherwise healthy subject, the onset is abrupt, with pleural pain, cough, and the expectoration of purulent yellow or brown material, sometimes streaked with blood. By contrast, when infection develops in the hospital, the onset often is insidious and is characterized by cough, fever, and the expectoration of purulent, blood-streaked material but rarely by chest pain and chills. Signs of consolidation (bronchial breathing, patchy areas of rales, rhonchi, and decreased breath sounds) may be evident, usually with signs of pleural

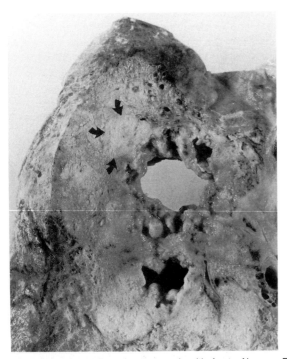

Figure 6–11. Confluent Bronchopneumonia with Acute Abscess Formation—*Staphylococcus aureus.* Magnified view of lower lobe showing extensive consolidation of the superior segment associated with multifocal areas of necrosis *(arrows)*. Drainage of some of the latter via the airways has led to two irregular walled cavities.

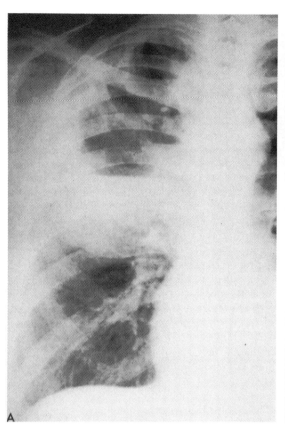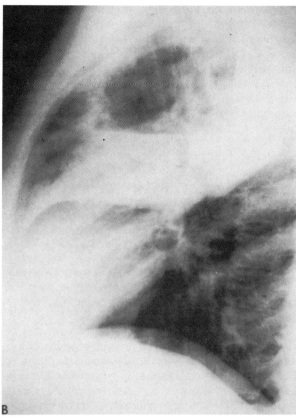

Figure 6–12. Acute Lung Abscess—*Staphylococcus Aureus*. Posteroanterior *(A)* and lateral *(B)* roentgenograms reveal massive consolidation of most of the right upper lobe, a huge ragged cavity being evident in its center. Volume of the lobe has been increased, as indicated by the posterior bulging of the major fissure.

effusion. In children, large pneumatoceles may give rise to a hyper-resonant percussion note.

The clinical features of tracheitis resemble those of croup, with cough, stridor, and difficulty in swallowing.[86] Laryngoscopy or bronchoscopy should be performed, and a patent airway established, since the condition may be rapidly fatal.

The white blood cell count usually is elevated to between 15,000 and 25,000 cells per mL, with polymorphonuclear leukocytosis; however, leukopenia may be present in severely ill patients. Since the organism is a normal inhabitant of the upper respiratory tract in some individuals, demonstration in sputum contaminated by oropharyngeal secretions is not conclusive evidence of infection. Positive results from blood cultures have been obtained in as many as 50 per cent of patients, but septicemia is probably less common than in acute pneumococcal pneumonia.

The complications include meningitis, metastatic abscesses (particularly in the brain and kidneys), and acute endocarditis (which may develop in patients without valvular disease). Pleural effusion may be serous but more commonly is purulent, particularly in infants and children. In fact, in these individuals, empyema, pneumothorax, and pyopneumothorax are so frequent that they should be considered manifestations of the disease rather than complications.

Bacillus Anthracis

Bacillus anthracis, the causative organisms of anthrax, is a large, spore-forming rod that is gram-positive and encapsulated. The spores are found in decaying soil and organic matter, in which they germinate under appropriate conditions and are ingested by herbivorous livestock, such as goats, sheep, and cattle. Humans are infected most commonly by direct contact (resulting in cutaneous disease), less often by ingestion of contaminated meat, and, rarely, by inhalation of spores. Thus, the disease tends to occur in individuals such as farmers, veterinarians, and butchers. In industrialized societies, anthrax is predominantly an occupational disease of persons involved in the handling of contaminated, imported hides in the textile, tannery, and wool industries.

Pathogenesis and Pathologic Characteristics

After inhalation, the spores reach the alveoli, where they are engulfed by macrophages that pass via the lymphatics to hilar lymph nodes. Here, they germinate into the vegetative form of the organism, which is then thought to pass via efferent lymphatic channels into the blood circulation. The pathologic manifestations in the lungs and in other body organs are thus related to septicemia rather than to a direct action of the spore itself. Microscopic findings consist of hemorrhagic edema of hilar and mediastinal lymph nodes and lung parenchyma; typically, bacilli can be easily identified. The pathogenesis of the edema may be related to a toxin complex produced by the organism that has a direct noxious effect on vascular endothelium.[90]

Roentgenographic Manifestations

The characteristic roentgenologic finding is mediastinal widening resulting from lymph node enlargement; this is of particular diagnostic significance if it develops acutely in a patient with a history of occupational or other exposure. Patchy, nonsegmental opacities may develop throughout the lungs; sanguinous pleural effusion is common.

Clinical Manifestations

The commonest clinical manifestation of anthrax is a localized cutaneous papule, vesicle, or ulcer at the site of the initial infection. Adjacent soft tissue hemorrhage and edema may be massive. Gastrointestinal infection is manifested by rapidly developing ascites and watery diarrhea. The initial symptoms following the inhalation of spores are nonspecific, consisting of mild fever, myalgia, nonproductive cough, and frequently a sensation of precordial oppression. The second (septicemic) stage of disease, which begins abruptly within a few days, is characterized by acute dyspnea, cyanosis, tachycardia, fever, and sometimes shock. Diffuse diaphoresis and subcutaneous edema of the chest and neck may develop, and stridor may result from compression of the airways by enlarged lymph nodes. Expectorated material usually is bloody and frothy. Most patients die within 24 hours after onset of the second stage.

The diagnosis cannot await positive culture results and must be made on the basis of a history of acute febrile illness in a person potentially exposed to anthrax spores and showing mediastinal widening roentgenographically.

Listeria Monocytogenes

Listeria monocytogenes is a gram-positive, motile rod that is widely distributed in nature and can be found occasionally in the upper airways, genitalia, and lower gastrointestinal tract of asymptomatic human carriers. Most cases of adult human infection are sporadic and are not associated with an identifiable infectious source; transmission is believed to occur from ingestion of or direct contact with contaminated food or animal products, or from contact with human carriers.

Listeriosis occurs predominantly in neonates, pregnant women, immunocompromised hosts (usually with lymphoreticular malignancy[91]), and older patients with underlying chronic debilitating disease. In adults, infection usually takes the form of meningitis, frequently associated with septicemia, with subsequent pulmonary or pleural involvement in a minority of cases.

Corynebacterium Species

Corynebacteria are gram-positive bacilli or coccobacilli that, when cultured, are usually judged to be commensals or contaminants. The major exception is *C. diphtheriae*, which causes pharyngitis associated with a classic membrane that can extend to the larynx, resulting in upper airway obstruction[92]; the organism has not been reported to cause pneumonia.

GRAM-NEGATIVE AEROBIC BACTERIA

Klebsiella, Enterobacter, and Serratia Species

This section describes three genera—*Klebsiella, Enterobacter,* and *Serratia,* which are sometimes grouped together on the basis of colony morphology and biochemical characteristics. The most important member of the group is *Klebsiella,* an encapsulated, nonmotile organism that is ubiquitous in the environment, particularly in water. Depending on the classification scheme used, three to six species or subspecies can be identified. *Klebsiella pneumoniae* (the commonest and most pathogenic) is introduced into the gastrointestinal tract by ingestion of contaminated water and food; when it develops, pulmonary infection usually follows colonization at this site. Such infection occurs predominantly in men in the sixth decade of life, many of whom are alcoholics.[93] Chronic bronchopulmonary disease and, to a lesser extent, diabetes mellitus also appear to predispose to infection.[94]

The genus *Enterobacter* contains motile species but is otherwise similar to *Klebsiella* and can be grouped with the latter in routine laboratory testing. Pathogenic organisms (most often *E. aerogenes* and sometimes *E. cloacae*) cause a bronchopneumonia that is usually nosocomial.[95]

Serratia marcescens is a common saprophyte of soil, water, and sewage.[96] Most infections are hospital acquired by elderly, debilitated patients, the majority of whom have been receiving antibiotic therapy.

Pathologic Characteristics

Klebsiella pneumoniae infection most commonly involves the posterior portion of an upper lobe or the superior portion of a lower lobe and is usually unilateral. In fulminant cases, disease often takes the form of airspace pneumonia (*see* Fig. 6–1, page 290); in more indolent ones, abscess formation and cavitation are common and may be massive.[97] The pathologic features of *S. marcescens* and *Enterobacter* pneumonia are typically those of necrotizing bronchopneumonia, with microabscess and macroabscess formation.

Roentgenographic Manifestations

As an acute airspace pneumonia, *Klebsiella* pneumonia shows the same general roentgenographic features as acute pneumococcal pneumonia: homogeneous parenchymal consolidation containing an air bronchogram but showing no precise segmental distribution (unless a whole lobe is involved—which occurs in many cases). Three additional features of acute *Klebsiella* pneumonia aid its differentiation from pneumococcal disease: (1) a tendency for the formation of such voluminous inflammatory exudate that the volume of affected lung becomes supranormal, with

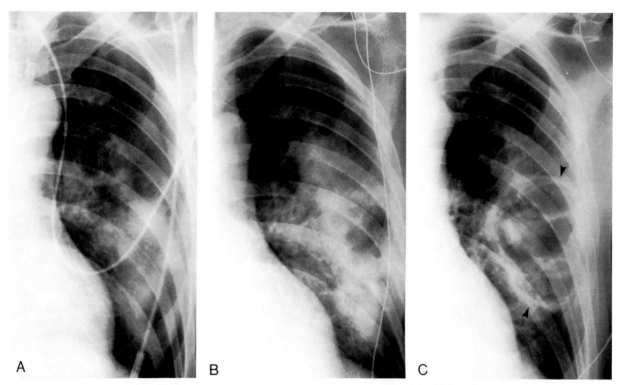

Figure 6–13. Acute Lung Abscess—*Klebsiella Pneumoniae. A,* A view of the left lung from a postero-anterior chest roentgenogram discloses a poorly defined area of airspace consolidation in the lower lobe. *B,* Three days later, the consolidation is more extensive, and several radiolucencies have appeared, indicating necrosis and bronchial communication. *C,* Five days later, the several cavities have coalesced to form a smoothly contoured multiloculated abscess *(arrowheads).*

resultant bulging of interlobar fissures; (2) a tendency to abscess and cavity formation if the patient survives the initial 48 hours (Fig. 6–13); and (3) a greater frequency of pleural effusion and empyema. In some cases the acute disease undergoes only partial resolution and passes into a chronic phase with cavitation and persistent positive cultures for *K. pneumoniae.* In this circumstance, the roentgenographic picture closely simulates that of fibrocaseous tuberculosis.

The roentgenographic features of *Enterobacter* and *S. marcescens* infection are those of bronchopneumonia; in the elderly, particularly, the pneumonia may cavitate.[98]

Clinical Manifestations

The onset of *Klebsiella* pneumonia usually is abrupt, with prostration, pain on breathing, cyanosis, moderate fever, and severe dyspnea; expectoration usually is greenish, purulent, and blood-streaked, and occasionally brick-red and gelatinous.[94] Malaise, chills, and shortness of breath may be present for some time, but on admission to the hospital many patients are in shock. The physical signs usually are those of parenchymal consolidation.

The white blood cell count usually is moderately elevated; when it is normal or reduced, the prognosis is most unfavorable. Bacteremia has been reported to occur in about 25 per cent of cases.[94]

The mortality from *Klebsiella-Enterobacter-Serratia* infection associated with bacteremia is approximately 50 per cent, death usually occurring within 48 hours of the onset of the disease.

Escherichia Coli

Escherichia coli is an uncommon cause of pneumonia that chiefly affects debilitated patients with chronic lung disease or with extrapulmonary diseases, such as diabetes mellitus or renal or cardiovascular failure.[99] Roentgenographically, the usual pattern is one of acute airspace pneumonia; involvement is usually multilobar, with a strong lower lobe anatomic bias. Cavitation is uncommon, but pleural effusion is frequent.

Clinically, pulmonary infection is characterized by the abrupt onset of fever, chills, dyspnea, pleuritic pain, cough, and expectoration of yellow sputum. Gastrointestinal symptoms, including nausea, abdominal pain, dysphagia, diarrhea, and vomiting, may be present. A presumptive diagnosis requires a predominant or pure growth of *E. coli* on sputum culture; occasional colonies are of little significance, particularly in patients receiving antibiotic therapy.

Salmonella Species

Pulmonary infection caused by *Salmonella* species can occur by aspiration of infected gastrointestinal contents or by seeding during bacteremia. Patients who are immunosuppressed[100] or who have disseminated malignancy[101] are predisposed. Pathologic and roentgenographic characteristics depend largely on the mode of infection—aspiration of organisms causing bronchopneumonia and bacteremic seeding resulting in diffuse, often bilateral disease possessing a nodular (sometimes miliary) appearance. Cavitation and pleural effusion (empyema) are common. Clinically, the course of the disease usually is prolonged, with chills, fever, and pleural pain; cough is often nonproductive, but purulent sputum may be expectorated eventually.

Proteus Species

Organisms of the genus *Proteus* are widely distributed in nature and may be isolated from the feces of healthy humans. A variety of strains exist, of which the commonest is *P. mirabilis*. Many affected patients have chronic lung disease, and some have chronic extrathoracic disease such as diabetes mellitus and alcoholism.[102] Both pathologically and roentgenographically, the picture is one of acute airspace pneumonia, often with abscess formation, similar to that of *Klebsiella* pneumonia. Clinically, the onset and course of disease tend to be more insidious than is usual in the other gram-negative pneumonias.

Yersinia Pestis

Yersinia pestis, the agent responsible for plague, is a small, somewhat pleomorphic, nonmotile coccobacillus. Although it is a parasite primarily of wild rodents, of which more than 200 susceptible species have been identified, domestic animals, such as dogs and cats, are also at risk. Transmission of the disease occurs from animal to animal and from animal to human by fleas or ticks, which abandon their host on its death. Disease may also be transmitted by inhalation from individuals with pneumonic plague (*see later*).

In endemic areas—which include southern and East Africa, parts of South America, China and Russia, and the western United States—sporadic disease (sylvatic plague) occurs in individuals such as small animal veterinarians and farmers or trappers who come in contact with rural animals.[103] Occasionally, and far more ominously, the disease spreads to urban rats, from which epidemics of human infection may result. In the United States from 1974 to 1983, an average of 19 cases were reported to the Centers for Disease Control each year, mainly from California and Oregon; most patients were children and adolescents younger than 19 years of age.[104]

Pathogenesis and Pathologic Characteristics

Yersinia bacilli circulating in the blood of infected rodents are ingested by feeding fleas. Bacteria multiply within the flea's midgut, sometimes to such an extent as to block the entire gut; when the flea bites another animal, organisms become mixed with ingested blood and are regurgitated into the wound. In humans, the initial site of infection gives rise within 1 to 5 days to a local skin lesion, usually on the legs, although this is not always appreciated. Regional lymph nodes become enlarged and extremely tender, and the overlying skin becomes firm and purplish, forming the characteristic buboes of *bubonic plague*. The disease may then enter a septicemic phase with involvement of the lungs (*secondary pneumonic plague*), from which air-borne person-to-person transmission of organisms may lead directly to pneumonia (*primary pneumonic plague*).

Morphologically, plague pneumonia is characterized by confluent pneumonia in which there is severe intra-alveolar hemorrhage and edema; in patients who survive long enough, an infiltrate of polymorphonuclear leukocytes and macrophages develops. Alveolar necrosis is prominent, and organisms are abundant.

Roentgenographic Manifestations

The roentgenographic pattern is one of nonsegmental, homogeneous parenchymal consolidation, which may be extensive; cavitation does not occur. In one review, the roentgenographic manifestations in the more severely involved patients simulated those of the adult respiratory distress syndrome.[105] Pleural effusion may be present. Hilar and paratracheal lymph node enlargement is common and, occasionally, may be the sole intrathoracic manifestation.[106]

Clinical Manifestations

Plague pneumonia is typically fulminating, with high fever, dyspnea, cyanosis, and a rapid downhill course. Cough and the expectoration of bloody, frothy material may occur. Pleural pain is common. Terminally, disseminated intravascular coagulation often develops, manifested by cutaneous petechiae and, eventually, by massive ecchymoses (the black death). Most patients have mild to moderate leukocytosis.

The diagnosis should be suspected from the combination of confluent pneumonia, enlarged mediastinal lymph nodes, tender enlarged peripheral lymph nodes, and a history of contact with rats or other rodents. It may be confirmed by culture of sputum, blood, or material aspirated from an enlarged lymph node. However, antibiotic therapy must be initiated on the basis of the appropriate clinical presentation in a patient residing in an endemic area; it is hazardous to await the results of culture.[104] Until the advent of antibiotics, plague pneumonia was invariably fatal within 2 to 4 days; nowadays, appropriate therapy results in complete resolution in the majority of cases.

Pasteurella Multocida

Pasteurella multocida is a gram-negative rod or coccobacillus that principally infects animals. Most patients in whom the organism is isolated give a history of animal contact—infection is especially common in farmers—and have chronic obstructive lung disease or bronchiectasis.[107] Sometimes, such isolation is simply a reflection of colonization of the abnormal lung, but occasional cases have been associated with exacerbation of underlying disease, presumably related to an acute *Pasteurella* bronchitis. The organism may also cause bronchopneumonia, often associated with empyema and sometimes with an abscess.[108]

Haemophilus Influenzae

Haemophilus influenzae is a pleomorphic, nonmotile, coccobacillus that may or may not be encapsulated. Encapsulated strains are divided into six types, a to f, on the basis of antigenic differences in capsular polysaccharide; type b and, less commonly, types e and f are relatively common pathogens in otherwise healthy individuals.[109] Nonencapsulated strains also may cause acute purulent exacerbations in patients with chronic bronchitis[110] and pneumonia in compromised hosts.[111] Children, especially those between the ages of 2 months and 3 years, are particularly prone to infection. In adults, infection occurs most often in patients with underlying bronchopulmonary disease, alcoholism, diabetes mellitus, anatomic or functional asplenia, or an immunoglobulin defect.[112]

Infection may occur in a variety of forms, including epiglottitis, tracheitis, bronchitis, bronchiolitis, and bronchopneumonia. Roentgenographically, the latter usually occurs in the lower lobes and may be bilateral; occasionally there is acute airspace pneumonia simulating that caused by *S. pneumoniae*.[113] Pneumonia is rarely associated with abscess formation but frequently with pleural effusion.

In infants particularly, infection may be very severe, with extreme dyspnea, high fever, and cyanosis resulting from acute bronchiolitis. Pneumonia caused by typable organisms tends to have a fulminant course, the duration of illness at presentation being only 1.5 days, compared with 5 days for patients whose organisms are nontypable.[111]

The mortality rate from bacteremic *H. influenzae* pneumonia has been estimated to be about 25 per cent,[114] a figure probably related to the frequent presence of underlying disease. Another important factor in determining the prognosis is antibiotic resistance, which has increased dramatically over the years and is now seen with penicillin, chloramphenicol, and a variety of other agents.[115]

Pseudomonas Aeruginosa

Pseudomonas aeruginosa is a nonencapsulated rod that has become one of the most dreaded and frequent causes of hospital-acquired pneumonia. The organism shows a great propensity to multiply in liquid media, even in some of the "antiseptic" solutions generally used for "sterilization" of aspiration equipment. Thus, some patients acquire the infection from contamination of saline, soap, creams, jellies, or other substances used in the care of tracheostomy sites or as repositories for suction catheters.[116] Other persons who develop pneumonia have been in contact with a heavily infected source, such as patients with wounds, burns, urinary tract infections and, paticularly, respiratory tract infections. The bacillus also may be cultured from the sputum or throat swabs of healthy individuals or patients without evidence of pulmonary disease, particularly those who have recently received antibiotic therapy.

Most infections develop in persons who have underlying chronic disease, including obstructive lung disease, congestive heart failure, diabetes mellitus, alcoholism, and renal failure.[117] Patients in intensive care units who have recently undergone surgery and are receiving broad-spectrum antibiotics while being ventilated also are particularly prone to colonization and pneumonia.[118] In addition, patients with cystic fibrosis are frequently colonized with the organism,[119] and exacerbations of the disease may be caused by the development of pneumonia. Although the organism is usually aspirated, it can also gain entry into the body directly by way of the bloodstream, usually secondary to contamination at the site of an indwelling catheter.

Pathogenesis

The organism produces a variety of exotoxins and enzymes, including proteases, phospholipase, hemolysin, and exotoxin A.[119a] The last named causes a block of protein synthesis, an action identical to that of diphtheria toxin. Although experimentally the toxin is quite potent in this regard, the mechanism by which it relates to the production of human disease is not well understood. In addition to the production of exotoxins, the organism possesses a cell envelope that contains endotoxin activity similar to that of other gram-negative bacilli.

Some strains of *Pseudomonas* have an extracellular capsulelike "slime" layer as a result of the production of the mucopolysaccharide alginate.[120] Such strains are seen particularly in patients with cystic fibrosis, in whom *in vivo* transformation of "rough" commensals into "smooth" (mucoid) forms is associated with the acquisition of virulence and a relatively poor prognosis. It is not certain whether these effects are a result of the alginate itself—possibly related to decreased effectiveness of macrophage phagocytosis or to an immunologic response[120]—or to other intrinsic changes in the organism.

Pathologic Characteristics

The morphologic appearance of *Pseudomonas* pneumonia acquired via the airways is one of typical bronchopneumonia, often with microabscess formation. By contrast, the lungs of patients that become infected in the course of *P. aeruginosa* bacteremia characteristically show multiple, more or less well-defined nodules scattered throughout the parenchyma.[121] Microscopically, a few of these nodules are abscesses; however, the majority show only coagulative necrosis of lung parenchyma associated with prominent bacterial invasion of the walls of small to medium-sized pulmonary arteries and veins. This histologic appearance suggests that these lesions are caused by diffusion of bacterial toxins into the surrounding lung parenchyma and are analogous to similar nodules of invasive aspergillosis (*see* page 349).

Roentgenographic Manifestations

The roentgenographic manifestations of acute *P. aeruginosa* pneumonia closely resemble those of acute staphylococcal infection.[117] There are two main roentgenographic patterns of parenchymal abnormality; in each, there is a definite lower lobe predilection. Disease is bilateral in the majority of patients.

The first pattern is that of typical bronchopneumonia manifested in the early stages by poorly defined, patchy shadows of homogeneous density that extend rapidly, often despite vigorous antibiotic therapy, and coalesce; ultimately, the major portions of both lungs are massively consolidated (Fig. 6–14). Abscess formation and cavitation are common. The second pattern is that of widespread patchy or nodular shadows diffusely throughout both lungs, reflecting bacteremia. In most series, pleural effusion has not been a prominent feature, although small effusions may be identified in many cases.[122]

In addition to acute pneumonia of other cause, the main conditions to be considered in differential diagnosis include adult respiratory distress syndrome (the majority of these patients are mechanically ventilated), cardiogenic pulmonary edema, and pulmonary embolism and infarction.

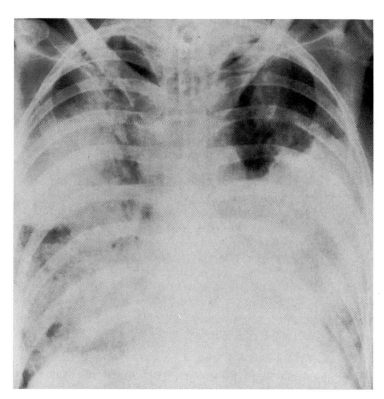

Figure 6–14. Acute Airspace Pneumonia—*Pseudomonas Aeruginosa.* This 38-year-old woman was admitted to the hospital in a deep coma as a result of an overdose of barbiturates; she had been placed on high doses of corticosteroids and antibiotics and required continuous artificial ventilation. Several days after admission, an anteroposterior roentgenogram demonstrated massive airspace consolidation of all lobes of both lungs, the superior portion of the left upper lobe being least involved. An air bronchogram was present in all areas.

Clinical Manifestations

The onset of bronchopneumonia is typically abrupt, with chills, fever, severe dyspnea, and cough productive of copious yellow-green, occasionally blood-streaked, sputum. Pleural pain is infrequent. Bradycardia is the rule. The white blood cell count usually is normal in the early stages but commonly rises to an average of about 20,000 cells per mL. The diagnosis usually is made by repeated culture of a heavy growth of *P. aeruginosa* in the sputum or blood.

In the bacteremic form of the disease, diagnosis may be extremely difficult during the early stages, and only the appearance of circulatory collapse or the typical skin lesions of ecthyma gangrenosum may suggest the etiology. Positive blood culture may antedate by several days discovery of the organism in the sputum. Leukopenia with neutropenia is common.[122]

Pseudomonas Cepacia

Pseudomonas cepacia has become recognized in recent years as an uncommon but important pulmonary pathogen, particularly in patients with cystic fibrosis.[123] Colonization and infection also occur occasionally in patients without cystic fibrosis, invariably in the hospital and often in association with contaminated disinfectant solutions or equipment such as ventilators.[124] Pathologic and roentgenographic features are those of bronchopneumonia, commonly necrotizing and with abscess formation. Patients usually present with high fever and leukocytosis and progress to severe respiratory failure; there is a tendency to develop septicemia and a uniform resistance to antibiotics.

Pseudomonas Pseudomallei

Pseudomonas pseudomallei is a relatively short, nonencapsulated rod that is the causative agent of melioidosis. The disease occurs principally in rodents, cats, and dogs and is endemic throughout southeast Asia[125] and northern Australia.[126] In North America, sporadic cases have been discovered principally in veterans from Vietnam and in refugees from Southeast Asia.

Human infection occurs predominantly in adult men during the wet season, presumably because of contact of damaged skin with infected muddy or stagnant ground water (where the organisms can be found). Underlying disease, particularly diabetes mellitus, increases susceptibility. There have been reports of asymptomatic service personnel returning from Vietnam in whom the infection has recurred months to years later, usually concomitant with other illnesses or surgical procedures.[127]

The disease exists in two clinicopathologic forms: an acute septicemic illness with multiorgan involvement and high mortality, and a chronic illness with a relatively indolent course. Pathologically, the acute variety is characterized by variably sized abscesses that can involve virtually any organ but most frequently the lungs, liver, and spleen[128]; organisms are abundant. The chronic form of disease consists of stellate or serpiginous granulomas similar to those found in lymphogranuloma venereum[128]; organisms typically are difficult to identify.

Roentgenographically, the acute form is characterized by irregular nodular opacities, 1 to 2 cm in diameter, widely disseminated throughout both lungs. These have indistinct borders and tend to enlarge, coalesce, and cavitate as the disease progresses.[129] In advanced disease, chest roentgenograms may reveal local groups of confluent shadows resembling homogeneous consolidation of one or more lobes. The chronic form of the disease simulates tuberculosis and often is associated with cavitation, without hilar lymph node enlargement.[130]

The onset of acute melioidosis is usually abrupt but may be preceded by a brief period of malaise, anorexia, and diarrhea. High fever, chills, cough, expectoration of purulent blood-streaked material, dyspnea, and pleuritic pain may be followed rapidly by evidence of bacteremic dissemination resulting in death within a few days. In chronic cases, patients usually present with fever, productive cough, and weight loss.[131] Pleuritic chest pain and hemoptysis are often present. A history of previous residence in or travel to an endemic area can usually be obtained.

The white blood cell count may be normal or may show moderate leukocytosis with neutrophilia. There is no specific skin test; however, a negative reaction to PPD is important in the differential diagnosis of tuberculosis.

Legionellaceae

This family of weakly staining, gram-negative coccobacilli contains several species that may be distinguished by microbiologic and serologic criteria. The organism that was responsible for the original outbreak of legionnaires' disease and that accounts for the great majority of cases of legionellosis has been designated *Legionella pneumophila* serogroup 1. At least 12 other serogroups exist and may cause disease similar to that seen with serogroup 1.[132] Most patients infected by *L. pneumophila* develop pneumonia that is usually severe and associated with evidence of liver, renal, or central nervous system disturbances. In addition, a grippelike syndrome unaccompanied by lower respiratory tract involvement is sometimes seen, a manifestation commonly referred to as Pontiac fever.

A variety of other species of *Legionella* are also recognized, most of which affect immunocompromised hosts and cause pneumonia that closely resembles that caused by *L. pneumophila*. (Some microbiologists do not consider the species *dumoffii*, *gormanii*, and *micdadei* to be members of the genus *Legionella* and recognize two genera in addition to *Legionella*: Fluoribacter [*F. dumoffii* and *F. gormanii*] and Tatlockia [*T. micdadei*].)

Culture isolation of all these organisms directly from sputum is not feasible because of overgrowth of oropharyngeal commensals on the media.[133] However, they can be isolated from BAL and pleural fluid, blood, and lung tissue.

Epidemiology

Infection by *L. pneumophila* is common; in the United States, the incidence of pneumonia has been estimated to be between 50,000[134] and 250,000 cases[135] per year, and studies of patients hospitalized with pneumonia show an incidence of legionellosis of 10[136] to 25 per cent.[137] In addition, in some areas there is evidence of a fairly high prevalence of prior infection; for example, in an analysis of serum specimens from 4320 healthy residents of New York City, in which *L. pneumophila* serogroup 1 was used as antigen, almost 25 per cent of subjects were found to have a titer of 1:64 or greater.[138]

Legionella organisms possess an affinity for water and have been isolated from various natural and artificial water sources, including hot water storage tanks, showerheads, mixing valves, and taps.[139] In fact, *L. pneumophila* appears to have a particular predisposition to flourish in hot water distribution systems. When disease occurs in outbreaks, bacteria are frequently recovered from air-conditioning cooling towers and evaporative condensers.[140] It is likely that *Legionella* bacilli derived from all these sources reach the lung by inhalation of aerosolized water. To the best of our knowledge, there have been no clinical episodes that suggest person-to-person spread of the disease.

Legionnaires' disease shows a propensity for older men, the male-to-female ratio being 2 or 3 to 1.[141] Many cases occur in patients with pre-existing disease; malignancy (particularly hairy-cell leukemia[142]), renal failure, and transplantation are the commonest conditions associated with nosocomial infection, and chronic lung disease and malignancy are most frequent in patients who become infected in the community.[143]

Pathogenesis and Pathologic Characteristics

Despite the protean clinical manifestations that characterize legionnaires' disease and the occasional positive blood culture result, bacteria usually are confined to the lungs at necropsy. Although this suggests that the impaired function of extrathoracic tissues is caused by a diffusible bacterial product such as endotoxin, one group of investigators who applied accepted methods of assessing endotoxicity found that *Legionella* was only mildly endotoxic.[144] There is experimental evidence that pulmonary damage is caused by a protease secreted by the organism.[145]

Pathologically, the typical appearance is that of a bronchopneumonia which, when seen at autopsy, is usually extensive and confluent. Macroscopic abscess formation has been noted in as many as 25 per cent of cases in some series.[146] Microscopically, alveolar airspaces are more or less uniformly filled with a mixture of polymorphonuclear leukocytes, macrophages, fibrin, and necrotic debris; leukocytoclasis is typically prominent. Organizing pneumonia and interstitial fibrosis may be seen in patients with protracted or clinically resolved infection.

The *Legionella* bacillus is weakly gram negative and is difficult to identify in tissue by this feature alone. It may be seen to better advantage with the Gimenez or Dieterle silver impregnation stains; however, the most reliable methods of identifying the organism are direct immunofluorescence or immunohistochemistry.[147]

Roentgenographic Manifestations

The characteristic roentgenographic pattern is one of airspace consolidation, initially peripheral and sublobar, similar to that seen in acute *S. pneumoniae* pneumonia (Fig. 6–15).[148] Subsequently, the focus of consolidation enlarges to involve an entire lobe or to involve contiguous lobes on the ipsilateral side.[149] Progression of the pneumonia is usually rapid, most of a lobe becoming involved within 3 or 4 days, often despite the institution of appropriate antibiotic therapy. This latter feature is seldom seen in acute airspace pneumonia caused by *S. pneumoniae*.

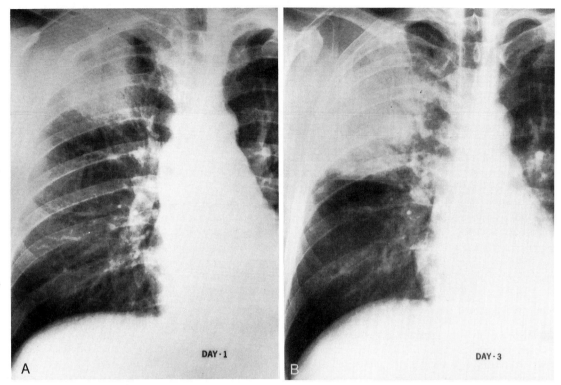

Figure 6–15. Acute Airspace Pneumonia—*Legionella pneumophila.* On the day of admission of this 69-year-old man, a posteroanterior roentgenogram *(A)* revealed homogeneous consolidation of the axillary portion of the right upper lobe; an air bronchogram was clearly apparent. On the assumption that this represented acute *S. pneumoniae* pneumonia, penicillin therapy was instituted, but 2 days later a roentgenogram *(B)* showed marked worsening, a situation that seldom occurs with infection by this organism. *Legionella pneumophila* was recovered from the sputum.

In most cases, the pneumonia is unilateral and unilobar when first seen; however, there is a tendency to bilateral involvement particularly at the peak of the disease. There is a distinct lower lobe predilection.[149] In immunocompetent patients, abscess formation with subsequent cavitation is surprisingly infrequent[150]; however, it is common in immunocompromised patients. Pleural effusion may occur at the peak of the illness. Hilar or mediastinal lymph node enlargement is not a feature.

With appropriate therapy, roentgenographic resolution may be fairly rapid but is often prolonged and tends to lag far behind clinical improvement. For example, in one group of 10 patients, it took up to 8 weeks, with a mean of 5 weeks.[151]

Clinical Manifestations

The usual presenting symptoms are nonproductive cough, a high and unremitting fever, malaise, myalgia, rigors, confusion, headaches, and diarrhea.[149] As the infection progresses, dyspnea and pleural pain may develop. In time, cough may become productive and may be associated with hemoptysis. The combination of acute pleural pain and hemoptysis may suggest a diagnosis of pulmonary embolism.

Symptoms reflecting the involvement of other organs, notably the gastrointestinal, renal, and central nervous systems, are much commoner in legionnaires' disease than in pneumonia caused by other organisms.[152] Patients complain of watery diarrhea and occasionally of abdominal pain. Hematuria and proteinuria may be present; renal failure is usually associated with shock. Bilirubin levels may be elevated. Many patients become confused and even obtunded; in addition to this encephalopathy, other neuromuscular disturbances include myositis, cerebellar dysfunction, neurogenic bladder, and peripheral neuropathy.

The white blood cell count is usually fewer than 15,000 cells per mL with a shift to the left. Lymphopenia is frequent, the count often being 1000 cells per mL or less. Hyponatremia is common, and muscle and liver enzyme levels may be elevated.

Confirmation of the diagnosis requires positive culture, a positive direct or indirect (IFA) immunofluorescent test, a positive hemagglutination test for antibody, or the detection of antigen by ELISA or radiommunoassay. IFA is the technique that has been employed in most cases, demonstration of a fourfold rise in antibody to a titer of at least 1:128 between acute and convalescent phase sera generally being considered necessary for confirmation of infection.[153] A titer of 1:256 on a single specimen has been accepted by some as presumptive evidence of infection in the presence of an appropriate clinical illness, at least in epidemic situations. Seroconversion occurs within 3 weeks of infection in 60 to 90 per cent of culture-proven cases, and the sensitivity of IFA is approximately 90 per cent[153]; however, because of the proven cross-reactivity with other organisms, the specificity is somewhat less.[154] The microagglutination test, which employs heat-killed antigen, is simple, sensitive, and apparently specific.[155] Radioimmunoassay and ELISA methods are used mainly to detect antigen in urine specimens and also appear to be highly specific.[156]

Pneumonia caused by *Legionella* organisms is a serious disease: approximately one third of patients require assisted ventilation, and one fifth die. However, when erythromycin therapy is administered, the case fatality rate is closer to 5 per cent.[153] The pneumonia shows a greater tendency to organize than do other bacterial pneumonias, and patients may be left with some diminution in respiratory reserve and a reduction in diffusing capacity.[157]

Neisseria Meningitidis

Neisseria meningitidis is a gram-negative diplococcus that may be a commoner cause of pneumonia than is generally accepted, both because it is eradicated rapidly by antibiotics and because it is difficult to culture from expectorated material. Most cases of pneumonia occur in adults with evidence of prior adenovirus[158] or influenza virus infection.[159] Young recruits in military service appear to be most susceptible, perhaps because of the greater likelihood of their having close contact with carriers of *N. meningitidis* and of their acquiring viral infections.

Chest roentgenograms show a pattern of acute airspace pneumonia, although disease in some cases has been described as segmental in distribution.[158] Bilateral pulmonary involvement and pleural effusion may occur; cavitation has not been described. In the majority of cases, the pathologic features are those of bronchopneumonia.

The typical history is of gradually increasing fever for 2 to 3 weeks, followed by pleural pain. The infection may be overwhelming, with leukopenia and death within a few days, despite presumably adequate therapy.

Moraxella Catarrhalis

This organism (*Branhamella catarrhalis, Neisseria catarrhalis*) is a gram-negative diplococcus that has only recently been accepted as a pathogen in the upper and lower respiratory tracts. Pulmonary infection usually occurs in patients with underlying disease, especially those with chronic obstructive lung disease who are receiving corticosteroid therapy[160] or who are deficient in immunoglobulins.[161] There is a distinct seasonal incidence in the winter and early spring.[162]

Clinical disease takes the form of an acute tracheobronchitis or bronchopneumonia. In one report, the commonest radiographic pattern was one of interstitial or mixed interstitial and airspace opacities superimposed on pre-exisitng lung disease.[162] In most patients, the infection is mild, complications such as pleural effusion, empyema, and septicemia being uncommon.

Acinetobacter Calcoaceticus

Acinetobacter calcoaceticus is an encapsulated, gram-negative coccobacillus that is ubiquitous in the environment and can be cultured from the skin of approximately 25 per cent of healthy persons. There is a significant association of colonization and infection with endotracheal tubes, tracheostomies, chest tubes, and vascular and urinary catheters, particularly in patients in the intensive care unit who are

receiving antibiotics.[163] The organism can cause an acute bacteremic pneumonia that is often fatal; most affected patients are immunocompromised.[164] The chest roentgenogram may show airspace pneumonia or bronchopneumonia; pleural effusion or empyema is present in about 50 per cent of cases.[164]

Bordetella Pertussis

The genus *Bordetella* is usually held to contain three species—*B. pertussis, B. parapertussis,* and *B. bronchiseptica*—the first two of which cause whooping cough (pertussis) and the last being primarily an animal pathogen. All organisms are very small, gram-negative coccobacilli; only *B. pertussis* is encapsulated.

In nonimmunized populations, pertussis typically occurs in epidemics affecting infants and children younger than 2 years of age. Although it is generally assumed that the disease has been largely eradicated through immunization, it has been suggested that immunity may not be very long lasting and that the disease may be occurring more frequently in adults.[165] It has even been proposed that adults are the major source of infection for children.[166]

The bacilli are noninvasive and are found in airways adherent to cilia. Although a variety of toxins are produced, including lymphocytosis-promoting factor and possibly a neurotoxin, the pathogenesis of the disease is not well understood. Pathologically, there is bronchitis and bronchiolitis associated with a mononuclear inflammatory infiltrate. Intraluminal mucus is characteristically abundant, resulting in partial or complete airway obstruction.

Roentgenographic manifestations in one study of 556 children included various combinations of atelectasis (about 50 per cent of cases), segmental consolidation (usually in the lower lobes or middle lobe, about 25 per cent), and hilar lymph node enlargement (30 per cent).[167] A fairly common but not distinctive feature of the pulmonary disease is its tendency to conglomerate contiguous with the heart, obscuring the cardiac borders.

The clinical picture in children consists of paroxysmal cough ending in a characteristic whoop and vomiting. The diagnosis may be more difficult to make in adults, since they are less likely to have the full-blown "whoop" and may manifest little more than a prolonged or a short-lived paroxysmal cough.[166] When disease develops in vaccinated individuals, the coughing spasms are less severe, and the course less prolonged.[168] Moderate to severe lymphocytosis is often present. Diagnosis depends on positive culture results from nasopharyngeal swabs on Bordet-Gengou medium; fluorescent antibody studies and ELISA[169] may be useful in questionable cases.

Although bronchiectasis was a frequent complication of pertussis in the preantibiotic era, recent follow-up studies have indicated that patients are more subject to respiratory infections than control subjects, without evidence of significant bronchiectasis.[170] Deterioration in lung function has been detected in some studies[170] but not in others.[171]

Francisella Tularensis

Francisella tularensis is a gram-negative, nonmotile bacillus that is responsible for tularemia. The disease is commonest in rodents and small mammals, with insects such as ticks, deer flies, and mosquitoes acting as both reservoirs and vectors. Humans can be infected by direct penetration of the organism into an open sore on the hands, by the bite of insect vectors, by the ingestion of contaminated water or meat, or by the inhalation of culture material in the laboratory. Cases tend to occur in the late winter hunting season (during skinning of infected animals such as rabbits and muskrats) and in middle to late summer (following an insect bite).

Infection is manifested by several clinical forms of disease, including localized skin ulcers, pharyngitis, and conjunctivitis, each of which may be associated with regional lymph node enlargement, as well as the so-called typhoidal form, which is associated with bacteremia and occurs chiefly following the ingestion of contaminated meat. When pulmonary disease occurs, it usually develops as a result of hematogenous dissemination of organisms. It is commonest in association with skin ulcers—in which it develops in about one third of patients—and in the typhoidal form—in which it occurs in about three quarters.

Pathologically, affected lungs are the site of multiple nodules that show coagulative necrosis and are associated with a largely mononuclear inflammatory infiltrate. True granuloma formation has been found occasionally in regional lymph nodes and in the pleura.[172] Typically, organisms are difficult to identify.

Roentgenographically, the typical appearance is one of airspace consolidation, usually patchy and occasionally lobar or segmental.[173] Cavitation appears to be relatively uncommon. Hilar lymph node enlargement, usually ipsilateral, occurs in 25 to 50 per cent of cases; pleural effusion occurs with about the same frequency.

Clinical manifestations include peripheral cutaneous ulcers, enlarged draining lymph nodes, and typhoidlike symptoms. Pulmonary signs and symptoms are nonspecific. An appropriate exposure history may be fairly easy to elicit, as in the case of a butcher or a hunter with a history of recently skinning wild rabbits or muskrats, or a patient who reports being bitten recently by a tick. However, such exposure is not always clear,[173a] and a surprising number of cases have been detected in cities by astute observers who question the possibility of recent animal contact in parks, zoos, and adjacent wooded suburbs.

The white blood cell count usually is normal or low, but mild leukocytosis may occur. Diagnostic cultures can be derived from skin lesions, lymph nodes, or sputum; blood culture is rarely positive. Serial agglutination tests also may yield a positive diagnosis, the antibody titer rising 8 to 10 days after onset of infection. A highly specific tuberculinlike delayed reaction skin test has been reported.[174]

SPIROCHETES

Leptospira Interrogans

Leptospira interrogans is an aerobic, very slender (0.1 μm) spirochete that may be divided antigenetically into about 170 serotypes. For practical purposes, these are usually accumulated into larger serogroups, of which four (*L. icterohaemorrhagiae, L. canicola, L. pomona,* and *L. autumnalis*) are responsible for most cases of human disease. The organism is widely distributed in nature, primarily as a saprophyte or parasite of rodents and domestic animals. In natural hosts, the infection is usually mild and nonfatal, the organisms residing in renal convoluted tubules from which they are constantly shed into the urine. Human infection usually results from contact with contaminated water or damp soil and is most prevalent in the tropics.

In industrialized countries, leptospirosis was formerly seen chiefly in workers in occupations such as sewer work, rice and sugar cane cultivation, farming, and slaughtering. A 1973 report, however, described approximately 60 per cent of cases in children, students, and housewives, and only 16 per cent in patients occupationally exposed.[175] This change may reflect increasingly frequent acquisition of the disease from family pets.

Although pulmonary involvement in leptospirosis usually is overshadowed by the more dramatic symptoms and signs of kidney and liver failure (Weil's disease), roentgenographically evident pulmonary abnormalities have been documented in as many as 25 per cent of patients.[176] The pattern has been described as one of bilateral nodules progressing to confluent consolidation and/or a ground-glass opacity.[177] Pathologic correlation has shown that these abnormalities usually represent hemorrhage and edema, although lung abscess has been reported.

Patients often present with conjunctivitis and muscle tenderness; other manifestations include headaches, chills, nausea and vomiting, pyuria, hematuria, and hepatomegaly. Signs of meningitis, usually aseptic, may be evident, and in severe cases hemorrhage may occur into the gastrointestinal tract or skin. Respiratory involvement is manifested by cough and, occasionally, hemoptysis. The diagnosis may be confirmed by the culture of organisms from blood and urine and by serologic testing.

ANAEROBIC BACTERIA

Although anaerobic pulmonary disease can occur in individuals in excellent health at the time of onset, more often it develops in patients with underlying disease, particularly conditions such as periodontitis and gingivitis, which are associated with proliferation of anaerobic organisms in the oral cavity. For obvious reasons, diseases predisposing to aspiration of oral cavity secretions are also strong risk factors for the development of anaerobic lung infection. Thus, alcoholism has been reported in 40 to 75 per cent of cases, and about 25 per cent of patients give a specific history of compromised consciousness associated with conditions such as general anesthesia, acute cerebrovascular accident, epileptic seizures, and drug ingestion. Dysphagia also is a predisposing factor, commonly in association with multiple sclerosis, vascular or malignant brain disease, or esophageal disease.

Immunosuppressed patients and those with chronic obstructive pulmonary disease are not particularly at risk for inhalational anaerobic infection, provided that there are no additional predisposing factors; however, this is not true for *Bacteroides* bacteremic infection which commonly occurs in patients who are already ill.[178]

The incidence of anaerobic pleuropulmonary infection has undoubtedly decreased in developed countries with improved oral hygiene and the early institution of antibiotic therapy. On the other hand, in developing countries a protracted, relapsing, cavitating infection presumably caused by anaerobic organisms and known as "chronic destructive pneumonia" is being recognized more frequently.[179]

Etiology and Pathogenesis

Virtually all anaerobic infections are endogenous, the major sources being the oropharynx and paranasal sinuses. A few cases are associated with bacteremia, in which circumstances the source of infection is often the gastrointestinal or genitourinary tracts, the latter usually in women. In descending order of frequency, causative organisms include the gram-negative bacilli *Bacteroides* and *Fusobacterium*, gram-negative cocci *Peptococcus* and *Peptostreptococcus*, gram-positive spore-forming rods such as *Clostridium*, and gram-positive non–spore-forming bacilli (*Actinomyces*).[180] Almost all infections are mixed, with, on average, three bacterial species being obtained per case. Isolates are exclusively anaerobic in 30 to 50 per cent of cases, and in the remainder, anaerobic organisms are mixed with facultative and, occasionally, aerobic bacteria.

Two groups of organisms warrant specific comments. Members of the family Bacteroidaceae (*Fusobacterium nucleatum*, *F. necrophorum*, and *Bacteroides* species) can cause pharyngitis and septicemia with subsequent lung abscesses, a syndrome that occurs particularly in young adults (*see* later). *Bacteroides fragilis* bacteremia, however, is usually associated with abdominal surgery or with gynecologic or obstetric conditions; early invasion of regional veins is a hallmark of these infections, with consequent thrombophlebitis and, in many cases, pulmonary emboli.[181] Members of the *Clostridium* genus, usually *C. perfringens*, can cause pleuropulmonary infection either as primary disease or in association with bacteremia following attempted criminal abortion. The former usually occurs in patients with underlying pulmonary or cardiac disease or as a secondary infection in association with pulmonary thromboemboli.[182]

In addition to pulmonary infection, anaerobic bacteria are a common cause of empyema. In one study at three hospitals equipped with anaerobic research laboratories,[183] the organisms were recovered from pleural fluid in 63 (76 per cent) of 83 adult patients who had not received antimicrobial therapy or undergone thoracic surgery. As with lung infection, most empyemas are mixed, the number of species per case in the study previously cited averaging 2.6.

Pathologic Characteristics

The pathologic findings of anaerobic bacterial infection are those of a confluent bronchopneumonia, frequently associated with extensive hemorrhage and abscess formation (Fig. 6–16). Colonies of bacteria and fragments of aspirated foreign material can sometimes be identified in the necrotic foci.

Roentgenographic Manifestations

Roentgenographic manifestations are those of pneumonia or empyema or both; in one review of the presenting findings in 69 patients, disease was found to be confined to the lung parenchyma in 50 per cent, to the pleura in 30 per

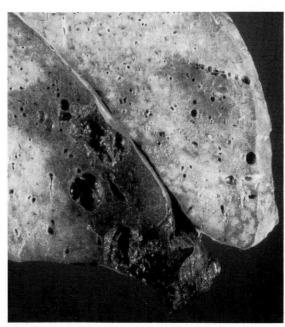

Figure 6–16. Anaerobic Bacterial Pneumonia. A magnified view of anterior basal aspect of the left lower lobe shows extensive hemorrhage associated with multiple shaggy-walled cavities. Although the location is somewhat unusual, the appearance is otherwise typical of anaerobic bacterial lung infection.

cent, and to both the parenchyma and the pleura in the remaining 20 per cent.[184] The anatomic distribution of pneumonia reflects gravitational flow: disease is commonest in the posterior segments of the upper lobes or superior segments of the lower lobes when aspiration occurs in the recumbent position, or the basal segments of the lower lobes when the person is erect; the anterior segments of the upper lobes are involved less often, and the middle lobe and lingula rarely. The right lung is affected approximately twice as often as the left.

The typical roentgenographic pattern is segmental homogeneous consolidation (Fig. 6–17); occasionally, there is a peripheral mass that simulates pulmonary carcinoma. Like others,[185] we have occasionally seen hilar or mediastinal lymph node enlargement associated with an anaerobic abscess; this can be particularly confusing when the abscess is situated distal to a pulmonary carcinoma. In perhaps the majority of instances, extensive necrosis has occurred by the time of the original chest roentgenogram, apparent as single or multiple thick-walled irregular cavities in posterior lung regions. An air-fluid level is common, and there may be consolidation in the surrounding parenchyma. Resolution of the lung abscesses may be very slow, an average closure time of 65 days being noted in one series.[180]

When anaerobic infection is blood-borne, the disease usually is localized to the lower lobes in the form of patchy or confluent nonsegmental, homogeneous consolidation, generally with cavitation.[186]

Empyema tends to progress very rapidly. As indicated previously, many cases occur without recognizable pulmonary disease, and almost all require surgical drainage.[184] Empyema caused by *Bacteroides fragilis* or *Clostridium perfringens* may be associated with gas production and resultant pyopneumothorax.[187]

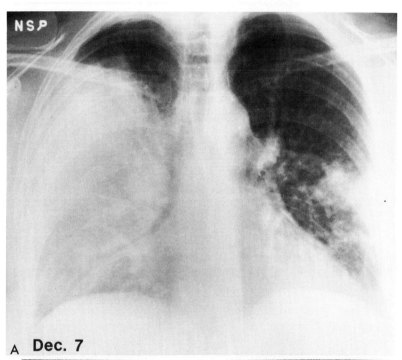

A   **Dec. 7**

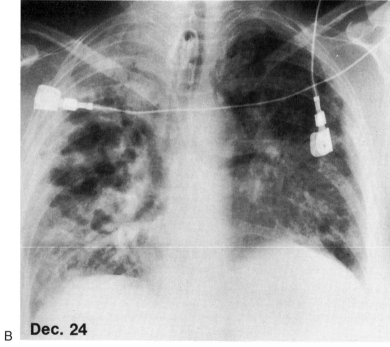

B   **Dec. 24**

Figure 6–17. Massive Airspace Pneumonia with Abscess Formation Caused by Anaerobic Organisms. The first examination *(A)* of this extremely ill, 45-year-old female alcoholic revealed massive, homogeneous consolidation of the right lower lobe and patchy consolidation of the left lung. During the next 2 weeks, a large, ragged, thick-walled cavity had appeared in the right lung *(B);* irregular masses protruded into the cavity.

Clinical Manifestations

In contrast with the acute and often fulminating pneumonias caused by aerobic organisms, anaerobic pulmonary infection tends to have a protracted, insidious course, the mean duration of symptoms being 2 to 3 weeks. In fact, patients may be virtually asymptomatic. Fever is present in 70 to 80 per cent of cases but is usually low grade. Chills are common in *Bacteroides* and *Fusobacterium* bacteremia, in which they are associated with high fever, diaphoresis, and malaise,[181] but are rare in other forms of disease. In the initial stages of infection, cough is frequently nonproductive, and the expectorated material, if any, is seldom putrid. When cavitation occurs, however, expectoration increases and becomes putrid in 40 to 75 per cent of cases. Pleural pain occurs in approximately 50 per cent of patients, and hemoptysis in 25 per cent.[188] Physical findings are nonspecific; clubbing is common in chronic infection.

An unusual type of anaerobic infection known as Lemierre's syndrome was recognized fairly frequently a half century ago and has recently reappeared. The causative agent is a member of either the *Fusobacterium* or the *Bacteroides* genus, and young adults appear to be particularly susceptible. The primary focus occurs in the pharynx, from which septicemic spread occurs, often to bones and joints but also to the lungs and pleura.[189]

Laboratory Findings

In most cases, the leukocyte count is mildly to moderately elevated, although it may be within normal limits. Leukocytosis is particularly common in *Bacteroides* bacteremia.[181] Anemia, commonly accompanied by weight loss, testifies to the frequent chronicity of the infection.[188]

The pleomorphic character of organisms on Gram stain, particularly the presence of both gram-positive and gram-negative bacilli, and a subsequent lack of aerobic growth should alert the physician to the possibility of anaerobic infection. Cultures of expectorated material are of no value in diagnosis, since they are invariably contaminated by mouth flora. To be considered conclusively pathogenic, organisms must be isolated from a closed space such as the pleural cavity, a subcutaneous or intra-abdominal abscess, or the blood. In addition, provided that aseptic precautions are taken, transthoracic needle aspiration (TTNA) should also be accepted as a dependable source of pathogens.

Prognosis

With early diagnosis and the prompt institution of penicillin therapy or, if *Bacteroides* sp. is present, clindamycin, the prognosis of anaerobic pulmonary infections is usually excellent. However, in patients with large cavities, multiple abscesses, or inadequately drained empyema, a prolonged and sometimes lethal course may ensue.[188] With response to therapy, cavity closure occurs steadily but may take many months to complete. Long-term follow-up using bronchography and tomography has shown residual cystic and bronchiectatic abnormalities for as long as 7 years after an otherwise satisfactory response to therapy.[190] These residual abnormalities do not constitute an indication for surgical resection, since reinfection does not occur.

MYCOBACTERIA

Mycobacteria are nonmotile, rod-shaped bacteria that usually cannot be distinguished from one another on the basis of morphology alone. In the majority of species, growth in culture specimens is slow, ranging from 3 to 8 weeks, and is related to an unusually long doubling time. The organisms are strictly aerobic, and a decrease in the ambient oxygen concentration results in a substantial decrease in the growth rate.[191] In comparison with other bacteria, they possess an exceptionally high lipid content, a feature that explains many of their properties, including resistance to drying, alcohol, alkali, some germicides, and acids. The acid-fast quality is especially important in laboratory identification, since mycobacteria that have been stained bright red with carbolfuchsin are able to resist decoloration by strong acid solutions.

The genus contains many species, including saprophytic, parasitic, and pathogenic forms. In humans, by far the commonest and most important pathogens are *M. leprae* (the cause of leprosy) and *M. tuberculosis*, the latter being responsible for 95 to 99 per cent of pulmonary mycobacterial infections. Although disease caused by other mycobacteria is sometimes referred to as tuberculosis, use of this term usually implies infection caused by *M. tuberculosis*.

Mycobacterium bovis, formerly a relatively common cause of disease, particularly in children and often involving the lymph nodes, gastrointestinal tract, and bones, has all but disappeared from North America; however, it is still associated with local outbreaks of disease[192] and has been reported as causing 1 to 3 per cent of mycobacterial disease in humans in the United Kingdom.[193] Pulmonary involvement occurs chiefly by dissemination from extrapulmonary foci. The pathologic and roentgenographic manifestations in the lungs are identical to those of *M. tuberculosis*.

The bacille Calmette-Guérin (BCG) represents an attenuated and relatively avirulent strain of *M. bovis* that has been widely used as a vaccine in the prophylaxis of tuberculosis and, more recently, as an immunostimulant in the treatment of various neoplasms. In both situations, it can cause pathologic or roentgenographic abnormalities, sometimes associated with appreciable clinical manifestations.[194, 195] Several other nontuberculous mycobacteria—so-called atypical, anonymous, or unclassified forms—are also recognized as infrequent causes of pulmonary disease. The pathologic and roentgenographic changes they produce are similar to those of *M. tuberculosis*; however, their epidemiology differs, as they are commonly associated with underlying pulmonary disease or with an immunocompromised state (particularly AIDS).

Mycobacterium Tuberculosis

Tuberculosis is a disease of great social and economic importance. It has been estimated that there are at least 500 million people throughout the world who are infected with tubercle bacilli, of whom 20 million are believed to be sputum-positive, and 600,000 to 3 million to die each year. Between 8 and 10 million new cases of active disease may develop annually.[196]

Although worldwide in distribution, the disease shows significant regional differences in both incidence and prevalence, predominantly as a result of differences in socioeconomic status. At the turn of the century, it was the commonest cause of death in the United States. However, subsequent progress in diagnosis, therapy, and public hygiene greatly reduced both the incidence of infection and the mortality rate, so that in 1979, only 28,000 patients with tuberculosis were reported (12.7 per 100,000 population)[197]; this compares with case rates of 200 to more than 400 per 100,000 in developing countries. In the mid-1980s, however, the incidence rose by 2.6 per cent, related largely to an increase in the number of cases in people with AIDS.[198]

Despite the effective therapeutic and prophylactic use of drugs, tuberculosis in developed countries is still present in socioeconomically disadvantaged areas, where the incidence may approach that of developing nations. This observation is at least partly related to habitation in overcrowded dwellings, which probably accentuates the risk by allowing for increased frequency of contact between infected and noninfected individuals. In North America, for example, the incidence of infection is much higher in the slum areas of large metropolitan centers and in prisons and men's shelters[199] than in the continent as a whole. Infection is also more likely to develop in situations of relative crowding, even in the absence of an effect of poverty; thus, the risk of infection is elevated in schools, children's day care centers, ships, and nursing homes.[200, 201]

Certain groups, especially Inuits, Native Americans, Afro-Americans, and immigrants to North America and Europe,[202] have been noted to have increased infection and disease rates compared with whites. The extent to which these observations are related to inherited factors or are simply a reflection of socioeconomic or other environmental conditions is not certain; however, the dramatic decline in tuberculosis in some of these groups after institution of appropriate prophylactic and therapeutic regimens suggests that socioeconomic factors are prominent.

Development of Infection

The development of infection with *M. tuberculosis* (in contrast with the development of clinically significant disease) occurs most commonly in children and adolescents. In the majority of cases, it is acquired by inhalation of droplet nuclei carrying the organisms; usually this means repeated or constant contact with a person whose sputum is positive for the bacilli. The risk of infection in these cases is related not only to the degree of infectiousness of the source individual but to the defenses of the exposed individual and the frequency of contact between the two.

The degree of source infectiousness itself is associated with several variables, including the extent and nature of the tuberculous disease and the frequency of coughing. The development of pulmonary cavities is the single most important factor in this regard, since their presence results not only in increased oxygen supply to the tubercle bacilli, which can then multiply relatively rapidly, but also in an easy exit route to the outside atmosphere. Appropriate treatment of cavitary tuberculosis is also important, since it quickly renders the sputum noninfectious. After 2 weeks of therapy, the number of bacilli is reduced by 95 per cent and, after 4 weeks, by almost 100 per cent.[203]

The effect of host factors on the acquisition of infection is poorly understood. As indicated previously, infection is commoner in certain racial groups, suggesting that heredity may play an important role; however, it seems likely that socioeconomic factors are more important than genetic ones in determining this effect.

Development of Disease

Clinically evident tuberculosis has been estimated to develop in only 5 to 15 per cent of individuals who are infected with the organism.[204] This may be manifested either by progression of the original focus of infection (*primary* or *progressive primary tuberculosis*) or by the appearance of pulmonary or extrapulmonary disease months or years after the initial infection (*postprimary tuberculosis*). Most active disease in adults represents reactivation of an endogenous focus acquired in childhood; however, in areas in which eradication of infection has been most successful, adults are increasingly being seen with primary tuberculosis.[205] Although the possibility of development of the disease is believed to exist for the lifetime of an infected individual, the risk is greatest during the first 2 years following infection, during which period the incidence has been estimated to be about 4 per cent per year.[206]

The precise mechanisms by which the course of tuberculosis is altered from one of subclinical infection to one of clinically significant disease are not well understood, but a number of risk factors have been identified. As is the case with the development of infection, the most important factors seem to be low socioeconomic status and overcrowded living conditions. In the United States, the patient with active tuberculosis has been characterized as a male at the bottom of the socioeconomic scale, between 35 and 65 years of age, living alone or homeless, and probably an alcoholic or a drug addict.[207] Such individuals often can be found living in skid-row hostels or large city prisons.

Age also is important in determining the likelihood of development of the disease. Case rates among tuberculin reactors tend to be high in the early years of life, then decrease sharply to a low at 10 to 12 years of age, increase again to a peak in late adolescence and early adult life, and then decrease once more to a relatively low level that persists to old age.[197] Since the absolute number of individuals infected increases with age and since older people are less likely to be kept under surveillance, activation in the older age group represents a frequent source of tuberculous infection.[208] In fact, the diagnosis of tuberculosis in these individuals is sometimes made only at autopsy.[209]

Ethnic origin is an additional important predictor of clinically significant tuberculosis; however, as with development of infection, it may be more related to socioeconomic status or environmental factors than to an intrinsic racial predisposition. Whatever the pathogenesis, increasing immigration from developing countries will undoubtedly affect the incidence of tuberculosis in industrialized nations; for example, of the 500,000 refugees who immigrated to the United States from Southeast Asia during the 1970s, 60 per cent had a positive PPD reaction and 1 to 2 per cent had active tuberculosis.[202]

Genetic factors appear to play a major role in susceptibility and resistance to tuberculous infection in some animals,[210] and these factors may also influence the development of active tuberculosis in humans. For example, concordance for tuberculosis has been found to be significantly higher among monozygotic than dizygotic twins,[211] and in one study strong evidence was provided in favor of HLA DR2-associated susceptibility[212]; however, other investigators have found conflicting results.

A number of diseases and surgical procedures are associated with an increased incidence of tuberculosis, including silicosis,[213] diabetes mellitus,[214] chronic renal failure (particularly in patients on dialysis),[215] chronic interstitial lung disease,[216] pulmonary alveolar proteinosis,[217] gastrectomy,[218] jejunoileal bypass performed for the treatment of obesity,[219] and pulmonary carcinoma[220] (although we believe that in most cases coexistence with the latter disease is coincidental). *Mycobacterium tuberculosis* has been isolated from the sputum of more patients thought to have sarcoidosis—particularly blacks[221]—than can be accounted for by chance. Whatever the pathogenetic relationship between these two conditions, if any, it is recommended that patients with persisting pulmonary sarcoidosis should be watched closely for the development of tuberculosis.

Immunocompromised patients also are prone to developing tuberculosis. In fact, the disease develops with sufficient frequency in patients receiving corticosteroid, chlorambucil, and azathioprine therapy to warrant prophylactic use of isoniazid for positive reactors to PPD.[222] The incidence of tuberculosis is greater in patients with AIDS compared with healthy individuals and appears to be increasing (*see* page 298); infection by multiple-drug–resistant organisms is particularly concerning.[222a]

Primary Pulmonary Tuberculosis

Patients who are exposed to the tubercle bacillus for the first time have pathologic, roentgenologic, and clinical features different from those who have reactivation of previous disease; as a consequence, it is logical to consider the disease processes under the separate headings of primary and postprimary tuberculosis. It should be remembered, however, that the pathologic and roentgenologic changes produced by postprimary tuberculosis are conditioned by hypersensitivity and acquired immunity; since these qualities of tissue reaction usually develop 1 to 3 weeks after the onset of the initial infection, patterns of postprimary disease can develop during the primary infection itself.

Primary pulmonary tuberculosis occurs predominantly in children and is particularly prevalent in geographic areas in which control measures are inadequate. However, as indicated earlier, since reduction in the incidence of tuberculosis has resulted in an increased nonsensitized population, the primary form of disease is becoming commoner in adults.[205]

Pathogenesis and Pathologic Characteristics

Mycobacterium tuberculosis produces no known exotoxins or endotoxins and shows no effective resistance to phagocytosis. Virulence has been related to growth in culture in the form of cords of bacilli arranged in parallel, which in turn correlates with the presence of trehalose 6, 6′-dimycolate, commonly known as cord factor. In its puri-

fied form, this substance is associated with a variety of experimental effects, including lethality for mice, chemotaxis and stimulation of macrophages, activation of the alternative complement pathway, and, possibly, the induction of granulomas.[223] Sulfatides—trehalose glycolipids related chemically to cord factor—have been shown to inhibit fusion of lysosomes with phagosomes, and it has been suggested that this may be important in promoting intracellular survival of the organism.[223] Production of catalase also is associated with virulence, as illustrated by the fact that isoniazid-resistant strains that typically lack this enzyme are not pathogenic for guinea pigs[224]; however, the relationship to pathogenesis is not understood.

Whatever the molecular mechanisms, a feature of primary importance in the development of disease is the ability of the organism to survive and multiply within macrophages, and to persist for months or years in unfavorable conditions in an inactive but viable state within tissue. The interplay between survival capacity of the bacillus and the efficiency with which macrophages kill it largely determines the presence and extent of infection. The development of disease, as manifested pathologically by necrosis and, eventually, fibrosis, appears to be determined principally by a hypersensitivity reaction mediated by lymphocytes. Although this reaction is of some benefit to the host in that it localizes and destroys a substantial number of bacteria, it also possesses the major disadvantage of causing tissue destruction.

Persons usually acquire primary pulmonary tuberculosis by inhaling droplet nuclei laden with bacilli that are kept air-borne by air currents normally present in any room. These bacilli are deposited in transitional airways and alveoli, usually in a subpleural location, where they multiply and incite an inflammatory reaction. Although macrophages are able to ingest and, to a limited extent, contain the organisms, in most cases they are unable to kill them. In a short time, however, they undergo morphologic and functional alterations to become more efficient epithelioid cells and begin to aggregate into multiple more or less discrete granulomas (Fig. 6–18).

After 1 to 3 weeks (coinciding with the development of hypersensitivity), granulomas are well formed, and their central portions undergo necrosis. At first, this is patchy; as disease progresses, however, individual necrotic foci tend to enlarge and coalesce, resulting in relatively large areas of necrotic debris completely surrounded by a layer of epithelioid histiocytes and multinucleated giant cells (*see* Fig. 6–18). These, in turn, are surrounded by zones of mononuclear cells—both lymphocytes and blood-derived monocytes—and fibroblasts. This inflammatory reaction serves to localize the tubercle bacilli within a discrete region of the lung parenchyma and, in most cases, to prevent further spread of the disease. At this point, the inflammatory focus is often grossly visible, the central necrotic material being soft, white, and crumbly in texture (similar to ripe goat cheese); this appearance, known as *caseation necrosis*, is characteristic of most forms of tuberculous necrosis.

The initial site of parenchymal infection in primary tuberculosis is termed the *Ghon focus*. As disease progresses, this can either enlarge or undergo healing. In the latter event, which is by far the more frequent, fibroblasts at the periphery of the necrotic foci proliferate and form collagen, resulting in a fibrous capsule that completely surrounds the

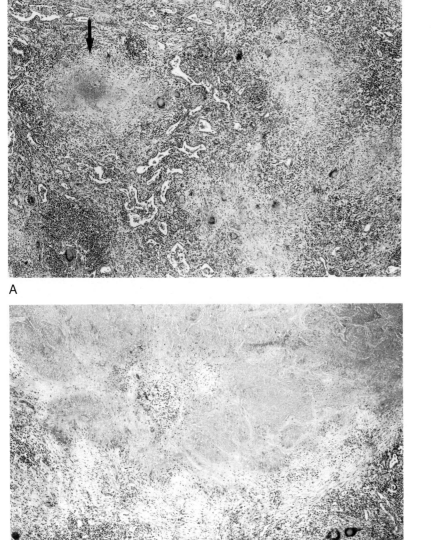

A

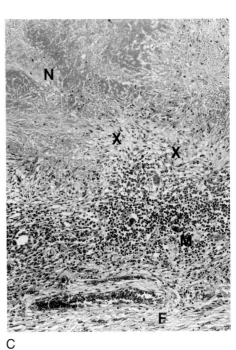

C

B

Figure 6–18. Tuberculosis—Development of Granulomatous Inflammation. *A,* Early stage, showing multiple foci of granulomatous inflammation surrounded by a mononuclear inflammatory infiltrate. Necrosis is apparent in the center of some granulomas *(arrow). B,* More advanced disease, showing confluent necrosis delineated by a zone of granulomatous inflammatory tissue. *C,* Magnified view of the latter region showing zones of necrosis (N), epithelioid histiocytes (X), mononuclear cells (M), and fibrosis (F). (*A* × 40; *B* × 40; *C* × 100.)

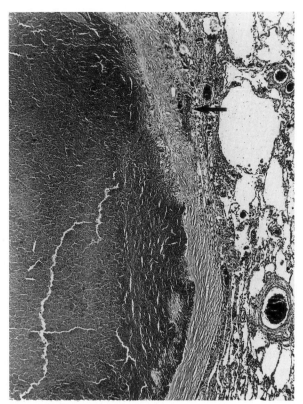

Figure 6–19. Inactive Tuberculous Granuloma. A well-developed fibrous capsule surrounds abundant granular necrotic material. Apart from occasional clusters of lymphocytes *(arrow)*, evidence of inflammation is absent. Although this nodule was caused by *M. tuberculosis,* an identical histologic appearance is seen with *Histoplasma capsulatum* and other fungi. (× 25.)

necrotic material (Fig. 6–19). With time, dystrophic calcification commonly develops and is often of sufficient degree to be visible roentgenographically. Despite the fact that the disease is totally inactive at this stage, viable organisms frequently remain within the encapsulated necrotic tissue and serve as a potential focus for reactivation in later life.

During the early phase of the infection, extension of organisms to regional lymph nodes via lymphatic channels is common, the combination of Ghon focus and affected lymph nodes being known as the *Ranke complex* (Fig. 6–20). The course of the disease in lymph nodes is similar to that of the parenchymal lesion, consisting of granulomatous inflammation and necrosis followed by fibrosis and calcification; however, the degree of inflammatory reaction typically is greater in lymph nodes than in the parenchyma. In fact, node enlargement may be sufficient to compress adjacent airways and result in bronchial occlusion and atelectasis, the latter resolving with the decrease in inflammation that accompanies healing. (Airway compression may also occur with chronic inactive tuberculosis, in which case it is associated with lymph node fibrosis and the development of bronchiectasis.) In addition, fragments of calcified, necrotic material may erode through a bronchial wall and come to lie within the airway lumen, causing broncholithiasis (*see* page 687).

Organisms also gain access to the bloodstream and extrapulmonary tissues via efferent nodal lymphatics or pulmonary vessels in the vicinity of a Ghon focus. Although such

hematogenous dissemination is probably common,[225] clinical manifestations of miliary or extrapulmonary tuberculosis in primary disease are usually absent, presumably as a result of the limited number of disseminated organisms and the adequacy of host defense. Nevertheless, this systemic dispersal of organisms is extremely important, since the minute areas of infection it establishes remain as potential foci of tuberculous reactivation months or years later.

Although healing is the rule in primary tuberculosis, in a small number of patients, local parenchymal disease progresses, either at the Ghon focus or elsewhere in the lung (usually the apical or posterior segments of the upper lobes). This is called *progressive primary tuberculosis* and is similar in both its morphology and its course to postprimary tuberculosis. It develops most commonly in infants younger than 1 year of age and has been estimated to occur in as many as 10 per cent of cases in adolescents and young adults.[226]

Roentgenographic Manifestations

Roentgenographic manifestations of primary tuberculous infection within the thorax can be discussed conveniently

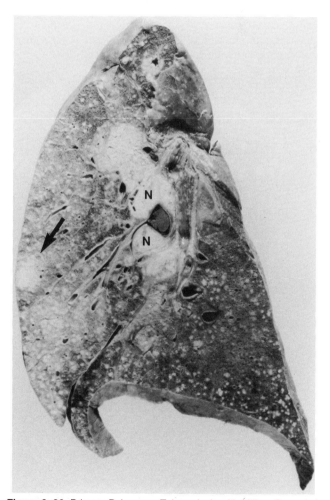

Figure 6–20. Primary Pulmonary Tuberculosis with Miliary Spread. A slice of the right lung shows a 1.5-cm focus of consolidated parenchyma in the subpleural region of the lower portion of the upper lobe (Ghon focus) *(arrow).* Peribronchial lymph nodes (N) are enlarged and show extensive caseous necrosis. The remainder of the lung shows a myriad of round, 1- to 2-mm, white nodules, representing hematogenous dissemination and miliary disease.

under four headings: the pulmonary parenchyma, the mediastinal and hilar lymph nodes, the tracheobronchial tree, and the pleura. Many of the observations to be described were documented in a report by Weber and associates in 1968 based on a study of 83 cases of childhood tuberculosis.[227]

Pulmonary Parenchyma. In Weber and coworkers' study, the upper lobes were affected slightly more often than the lower, but there were no significant differences between left and right lungs or between anterior and posterior segments. In contrast with the distribution in children, primary disease in adults shows a higher incidence of lower lobe involvement.[228] These differences in anatomic distribution of parenchymal disease in reported series probably derive from differences in the character of the parenchymal abnormality; the distribution previously described in children applies to the parenchymal consolidation that occurs in acute pneumonia and not to atelectasis.

The typical roentgenographic appearance is that of airspace consolidation, ranging in diameter from 1 to 7 cm (Fig. 6–21). The consolidation tends to be homogeneous in density and to have ill-defined margins, except where it abuts a fissure. Cavitation is a rare manifestation in infants and children living in communities in which there is a high prevalence of tuberculosis[227]; however, it is relatively frequent in communities in which the disease has been introduced comparatively recently (Fig. 6–22).[229] Evidence of miliary spread is very uncommon.

Complete resolution without residua is roentgenographi-cally apparent in the majority of cases, usually within 6 months to 2 years after institution of therapy; however, 15 of 47 patients (32 per cent) followed long enough by Weber and associates had residual scarring.[227]

Mediastinal and Hilar Lymph Nodes. Hilar or paratracheal lymph node enlargement is common and is the roentgenographic finding that clearly distinguishes primary from postprimary tuberculosis. Of the 83 cases studied by Weber and colleagues, 80 showed roentgenographic evidence of hilar or paratracheal lymph node enlargement, or both; in 13 of the 80 cases, it was bilateral and hilar, and in 33 it was unilateral and both hilar and paratracheal, predominantly on the right side. Although lymph node enlargement as a manifestation of primary tuberculosis is much commoner in children, it may also be the presenting roentgenographic abnormality in adults, occasionally without evidence of pulmonary abnormality.[230]

Decrease in the size of enlarged lymph nodes usually parallels clearing of the active parenchymal infection and is associated with resolution of any atelectasis. However, a considerable number of children who have had atelectasis during the active stage of the disease have residual bronchographic evidence of distortion and dilatation of the bronchial tree in the affected areas.[227]

Although calcification in both the Ghon focus and the draining lymph nodes is an almost invariable pathologic finding in chronic disease, it was surprisingly uncommon in Weber and colleagues' series. Of the 58 patients with adequate follow-up, calcification was identified in the pulmo-

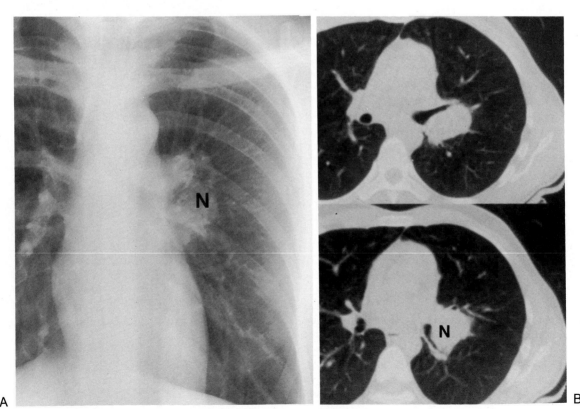

A   B

Figure 6–21. Primary Pulmonary Tuberculosis. A posteroanterior chest roentgenogram *(A)* reveals left hilar lymph node enlargement (N) and a vague opacity in the left apex, probably representing a primary parenchymal focus (Ghon lesion). CT scans through the left upper and lower hilum *(B)* confirm the presence of enlarged lymph nodes (N).

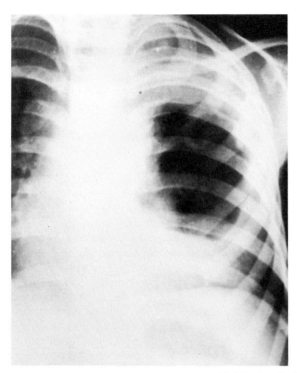

Figure 6–22. Primary Pulmonary Tuberculosis with Massive Cavitation. An anteroposterior roentgenogram of this black South African child reveals massive consolidation of the left upper lobe containing a huge ragged cavity in its center. *Mycobacterium tuberculosis* was recovered from gastric washings. (Courtesy of Baragwanath Hospital and the University of Witwatersrand, Johannesburg, South Africa.)

nary lesion in only 10 (17 per cent) and in the lymph nodes in 21 (36 per cent). If these figures are truly representative, it is apparent how seldom chest roentgenography can detect the primary Ranke complex, indicating previous tuberculous infection (Fig. 6–23).

Tracheobronchial Tree. Atelectasis caused by tuberculous tracheobronchial disease was identified in 25 patients (30 per cent) in Weber and associates' series. The anatomic distribution of collapse showed a two-to-one right-sided predominance. Characteristically, it affects the anterior segment of an upper lobe or the medial segment of the middle lobe, a distribution probably reflecting the anatomic relationships of lymph nodes to the bronchial tree on the right side. Although atelectasis is less common in adults, when it occurs it also tends to involve the anterior segment of the upper lobes and simulates bronchogenic carcinoma.[231]

The Pleura. Pleural effusion has been reported in 10 per cent of children[227] and as many as 40 per cent of adults.[226] In eight of Weber and associates' nine cases it was mild to moderate in degree and was associated with roentgenographic evidence of pulmonary disease. As a manifestation of tuberculosis, pleural effusion is said to be particularly common among adolescents and young adults and usually reflects primary infection.[232]

Clinical Manifestations

Very few patients with primary pulmonary tuberculosis manifest symptoms and signs. When they do occur, symptoms consist of fever, cough, anorexia, weight loss, excessive

perspiration, chest pain, lethargy, and dyspnea.[227] Erythema nodosum is an occasional manifestation, more commonly in Europe than in North America. More severe symptoms may develop as a result of progressive primary pulmonary disease or may be caused by spread of the disease to extrathoracic locations, including the meninges.

The decision to categorize a case of tuberculosis as primary is usually based on recent tuberculin conversion associated with roentgenographic evidence of bronchopulmonary or mediastinal lymph node enlargement or pleural effusion. Since pleural fluid and sputum are usually negative on smear and culture, the diagnosis of tuberculous effusion is best confirmed by histopathology or culture of pleural tissue obtained by needle or thoracoscopic biopsy.

Postprimary Tuberculosis

Pathogenesis and Pathologic Characteristics

Postprimary tuberculosis tends to be localized initially to the apical and posterior segments of the upper lobes. It has been postulated that this is related to the relatively high Po_2 in these zones, as a result of a high ventilation-perfusion ratio,[233] or to impaired lymphatic drainage resulting from decreased pulmonary arterial blood flow.[191] Whatever the mechanism, it is believed that the vast majority of disease that arises in these locations is caused by reactivation

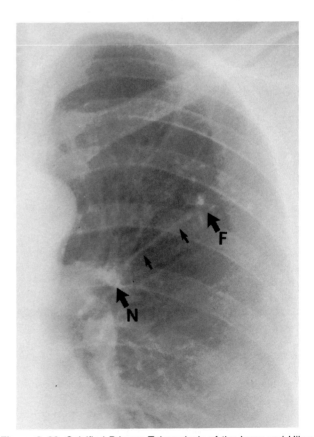

Figure 6–23. Calcified Primary Tuberculosis of the Lung and Hilum (Ranke Complex). A detail view of the left upper lung and hilum reveals multiple small calcific nodules representative of healed Ghon foci *(arrow F)*. Lymph nodes are faintly calcified in the upper hilum *(arrow N)*. The linear opacity that extends from the lung foci to the hilum *(small arrows)* is consistent with a scar.

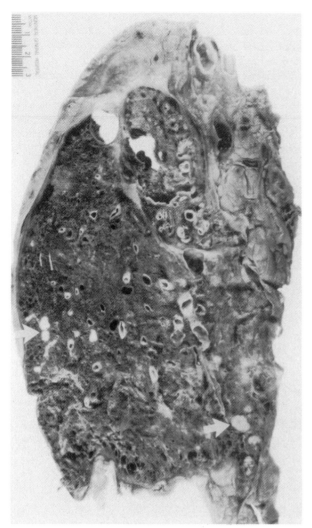

Figure 6–24. Chronic Fibrocaseous Tuberculosis. Gross specimen of the right lung shows severe atelectasis and destruction of the upper lobe associated with a large cavity. Note the well-circumscribed foci of necrotic tissue in the lower and middle lobes *(arrows)*, representing prior endobronchial spread.

of viable but dormant organisms transmitted hematogenously during the primary infection.

Pathologically, the sequence of events is similar to that of the primary infection, except that necrosis probably occurs more rapidly as a result of the presence of hypersensitivity. In addition, in contrast with primary tuberculosis in which fibrosis and healing are the rule, postprimary disease tends to progress, foci of inflammation and necrosis enlarging to occupy ever greater portions of lung parenchyma (Fig. 6–24). During this process, communication with airways is frequent, resulting in drainage of necrotic material and cavity formation.

As in primary tuberculosis, the course of the disease from this point on depends largely on the interplay between host response and the virulence of the organism. When host factors prevail, there is gradual healing with the formation of localized or extensive, often calcified parenchymal scars, frequently accompanied by adjacent emphysema and bronchiectasis. Such changes may occur alone but are seen most often in association with residual, well-demarcated foci of necrotic parenchyma (an appearance known as "chronic

fibrocaseous tuberculosis") (Fig. 6–25). The necrotic foci vary from 1 mm to several centimeters in diameter and either develop and maintain communication with the tracheobronchial tree (thus forming a chronic cavity) or fail to communicate and are filled with caseous material (forming a "tuberculoma"). The development of a fungus ball (usually caused by *Aspergillus* species) within a chronic cavity is a rather frequent complication (*see* page 344).

When the virulence of the organism overpowers host defenses, the disease progresses, either locally—by gradual expansion of the region of necrosis and inflammation—or remotely in other parts of the lung or body—by spread of bacteria via the airways, lymphatics, or bloodstream. Endobronchial spread of liquefied necrotic material from a cavity may result in tuberculous infection in the same lobe or in other lobes of either lung. Such infection occurs initially in the region of the proximal acinar airways and usually causes a typical granulomatous inflammatory reaction, resulting in the appearance of multiple parenchymal nodules ("acinar" or "acinonodose" tuberculosis) (Fig. 6–26). In some individuals, however, the large amounts of tuberculoprotein that suddenly occupy the acini may cause an exudative inflammatory reaction in the absence of a significant granulomatous component; this is associated with widespread parenchymal necrosis and rapid destruction of whole lobules ("tuberculous pneumonia").

Dissemination of organisms by way of the lymphatics or pulmonary vasculature may result in miliary tuberculosis of the lungs, liver, spleen, bone marrow, and many other organs. In the lungs, the appearance is that of a multitude of nodules measuring 1 to 2 mm in diameter and scattered

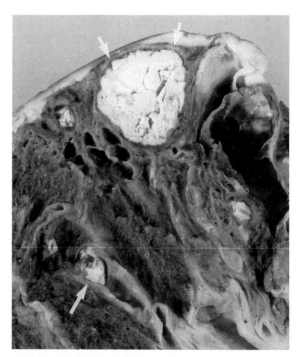

Figure 6–25. Inactive Fibrocaseous Tuberculosis. Apical portion of left upper lobe showing extensive parenchymal fibrosis and bronchiectasis. A 2-cm, well-defined nodule of caseous necrotic material ("tuberculoma") is present in the apex. Its inactive nature is indicated by the well-defined fibrous capsule *(short arrows)* completely surrounding the periphery. Smaller foci of necrosis representing remote granulomatous inflammation are also present, and a 5-mm broncholith is seen in a subsegmental airway *(long arrow)*. (Bar = 0.5 cm.)

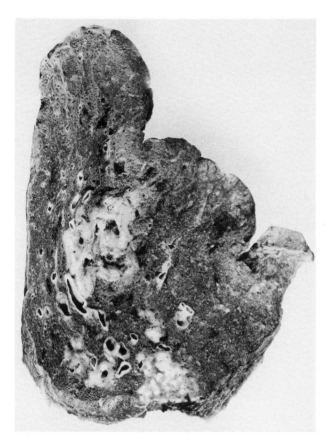

Figure 6–26. Postprimary Tuberculosis with Early Endobronchial Spread. Right upper lobe showing irregular consolidation with small areas of early cavitation. Note the foci of bronchopneumonia confined predominantly to a single lobule in the inferior aspect.

more or less randomly throughout the parenchyma and on the pleura (Fig. 6–27). The nodules tend to be slightly larger in the apices than in the bases and are usually about the same size and of the same histologic age, implying a single episode of dissemination. Sometimes, however, both active and partly or completely healed foci may be observed at the same time, suggesting repeated or protracted episodes of hematogenous spread.[234] It is important to remember that the lungs may be the site of miliary tuberculosis without evidence of a pulmonary source of the infection, dissemination having occurred from an extrapulmonary location; the frequency of such an event has increased since the advent of antituberculous chemotherapy.[234]

Involvement of the tracheobronchial tree is frequent and may be related either to chronic disease (with the development of bronchiectasis) or to acute infection. The latter occurs especially when the disease is rapidly progressive or extensive.[235] In most cases, it develops by spread of organisms within the airway lumen or along peribronchial lymphatic channels from an area of cavitation or localized pneumonia. Although airway involvement is usually associated with obvious parenchymal disease, active bronchial infection occasionally persists as peripheral disease heals, thus providing a potential source of bacteria-laden sputum in the absence of significant roentgenographic abnormality.

Bronchiectasis in postprimary tuberculosis may develop by two mechanisms: (1) most commonly, by destruction and fibrosis of lung parenchyma, resulting in retraction and irreversible bronchial dilatation; and (2) cicatricial bronchostenosis secondary to localized endobronchial infection, as described previously. Since the vast majority of cases of postprimary tuberculosis affect apical and posterior segments of an upper lobe, bronchiectasis is usually found in

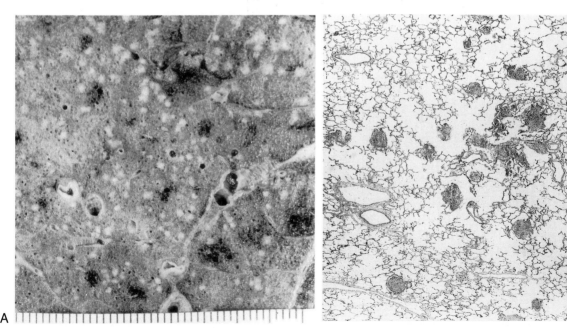

Figure 6–27. Miliary Tuberculosis. *A,* Close-up view of lower lobe showing numerous uniform 0.5- to 1-mm nodules scattered randomly throughout the lung parenchyma. Such a distribution implies hematogenous dissemination. *B,* Histologic appearance showing well-defined foci of granulomatous inflammation within alveolar airspaces. (× 10.)

these sites; because of adequate bronchial drainage, symptoms are usually minimal ("bronchiectasis sicca").

Vascular disease is also common in postprimary tuberculosis. Pulmonary arteries and veins in an area of active tuberculous infection may show vasculitis and thrombosis, and an acid-fast stain should be performed on any necrotizing granulomatous pulmonary vasculitis to exclude a tuberculous etiology. Occasionally, a small to medium-sized artery is contiguous with the fibrous capsule of a cavity wall, usually in a tangential fashion, and undergoes localized dilatation (Rasmussen's aneurysm).[236] Subsequent rupture may result in hemoptysis and, occasionally, death.

Roentgenographic Manifestations

As indicated previously, a characteristic manifestation of postprimary tuberculosis is a tendency for disease to develop in the apical and posterior segments of the upper lobes. Only rarely is disease situated *solely* in the anterior segment,[237] a useful clue in differentiating tuberculosis from other granulomatous diseases, such as histoplasmosis, which often affect the anterior segment. The right lung is involved more often than the left. The lower lobes are affected in 5 to 10 per cent of patients.[238]

Several roentgenographic patterns may be identified, corresponding to the description of pathogenesis given previously. The CT features of these patterns have recently been reviewed.[239]

Local Exudative Tuberculosis. The roentgenographic pattern is one of airspace (acinar) consolidation, patchy or confluent in nature (Fig. 6–28). Individual opacities are indistinctly defined and homogeneous, and there is frequently an accentuation of the bronchovascular markings leading to the ipsilateral hilum.[240] The shadows may disappear rapidly following the institution of chemotherapy, al-

though in some cases the disease worsens roentgenographically following initiation of therapy and then clears.[241] Hilar or mediastinal lymph node enlargement is very uncommon, but its presence should not necessarily exclude the diagnosis.[242]

Cavitation occurs in about 50 per cent of patients.[240] The wall of an untreated cavity may be variably thin or thick, and smooth or internally nodular (Fig. 6–29). A fluid level has been reported in approximately 20 per cent of cases in some series,[240] although our own experience suggests that it is rare. With adequate therapy, the cavity may disappear; sometimes its wall becomes paper thin, and it persists as an air-filled cystic space.

Chronic Fibrocaseous Tuberculosis. In this form, the relatively poor definition of the exudative lesion is replaced by a more sharply defined shadow, usually somewhat irregular and angular in contour. Although the shadow may be homogeneous, its density is no greater than that of the exudative lesion; thus, the terms "soft" and "hard" to describe the shadows of pulmonary tuberculosis are meaningless. Healing occurs by replacement of the tuberculous granulation tissue by fibrous tissue; the resultant cicatrization may result in considerable loss of volume. If the reduction in volume of affected lung is sufficient, compensatory signs become evident in elevation of the ipsilateral hilum, overinflation of the rest of the affected lung, and, in some cases, bulla formation.

Bronchogenic Spread and Tuberculous Bronchopneumonia. As discussed previously, when necrotic material liquefies and communicates with the bronchial tree, disease may disseminate widely to other bronchopulmonary segments and establish new foci of infection (Fig. 6–30).[243] Characteristically, such dissemination leads to the formation of multiple small acinar shadows, an appearance that is highly suggestive of bronchogenic spread. Extension of the disease through surrounding airspaces may result in a pattern of airspace pneumonia indistinguishable from that caused by *Streptococcus pneumoniae*. Clues to tuberculosis as the cause are the finding of a cavity in the ipsilateral or contralateral lung, or of fairly discrete acinar shadows in parts of the lung remote from the massive consolidation; we have rarely seen the latter in acute airspace pneumonia of other cause.

Miliary Tuberculosis. Miliary tuberculosis is manifested by numerous, widely and uniformly distributed, discrete pinpoint opacities (Fig. 6–31). The interval between dissemination and the development of roentgenographically discernible disease is probably 6 weeks or more, during which time the foci are too small to permit identification. When first visible, the opacities measure little more than 1 mm in diameter; in the absence of adequate therapy, they may reach 3 to 5 mm before the patient dies. By this time, they may have become almost confluent, presenting a "snowstorm" appearance. With appropriate treatment, roentgenographic clearing may be extremely rapid, usually faster than in nonhematogenous pulmonary tuberculosis and without residua.[244, 245]

Three additional features are worth noting: (1) few patients die from miliary tuberculosis without demonstrable abnormality on the chest roentgenogram[245]; (2) although the source of dissemination of tubercle bacilli sometimes is apparent clinically or roentgenographically, at least in adults, in many cases the primary focus is not obvious, even

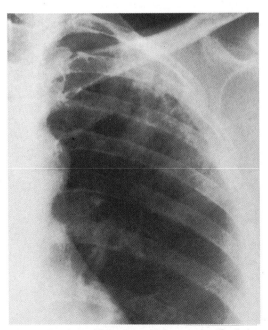

Figure 6–28. Exudative Pulmonary Tuberculosis (Postprimary). A view of the upper half of the left hemithorax from a posteroanterior roentgenogram reveals shadows of inhomogeneous density extending into the axillary portion of the left upper lobe.

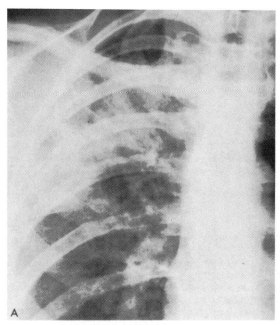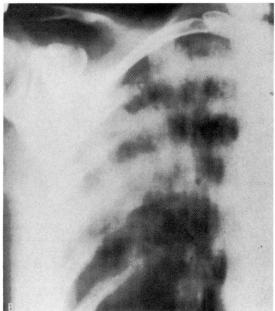

Figure 6–29. Exudative Pulmonary Tuberculosis with Cavitation. Views of the upper half of the right hemithorax from a posteroanterior roentgenogram *(A)* and an anteroposterior tomogram *(B)* show inhomogeneous consolidation of much of the right upper lobe. A fairly large cavity is present, possessing a smooth, although somewhat nodular, inner lining.

at necropsy[245]; and (3) although not widely recognized, the adult respiratory distress syndrome is clearly an occasional complication.[246]

Tuberculous Bronchiectasis and Bronchostenosis. The only distinctive feature of tuberculous bronchiectasis is its tendency to be localized to the apical and posterior segments of an upper lobe. Hemoptysis occurs in some cases, and it has been shown on bronchograms that bronchial dilatation is twice as frequent in patients with this symptom than in patients who do not have hemoptysis.[247]

As indicated earlier, tuberculous bronchitis is common in active disease; occasionally, associated granulation tissue may accumulate in sufficient quantity to cause a polypoid endobronchial mass that can result in atelectasis and obstructive pneumonitis.[248] Fibrosis and bronchostenosis as a result of healing may have the same effect, and both conditions may be misinterpreted as pulmonary carcinoma.[235] CT may be of value in the differential diagnosis.[249]

Tuberculoma. This appears as a round or oval opacity most commonly situated in an upper lobe, the right more often than the left. Most range from 1 to 4 cm in diameter and are smooth and sharply defined; up to 25 per cent are smooth and lobulated.[250] Small, discrete shadows in the immediate vicinity of the main lesion—"satellite" lesions—may be identified in as many as 80 per cent of cases. There may be irregular thickening of the wall of the draining bronchus and, in a small percentage of patients, actual bronchostenosis. The majority of these lesions remain stable for a long time, and many calcify; however, the larger the lesion, the more likely it is to be active (Fig. 6–32).

Pleural Disease. Although pleural effusion is more often thought of as occurring in primary tuberculosis, in one series it was equally common in both primary and postprimary forms.[251] Pleural disease may also take the form of a bronchopleural fistula, either from rupture of a cavity in a patient with active tuberculosis or secondary to empyema.[252]

Clinical Manifestations

Most cases of postprimary tuberculosis come to medical attention following the discovery of disease on a screening chest roentgenogram. On investigation, the great majority prove to be inactive. In fact, many patients do not have a history suggestive of prior active disease, although some will recall a severe bout of "pneumonia" with a rather protracted course and persistent pleuritic pain and fever, usually not documented by chest roentgenography. Most cases of *active tuberculosis* are recognized when patients are referred for roentgenographic examination by their physicians or when routine chest roentgenograms are obtained while the patient is in the hospital.[253]

Clinically apparent disease develops in 2 to 3 per cent of tuberculin-positive persons with normal chest roentgenograms.[254] The yield of active cases of tuberculosis among contacts is almost restricted to those who have been exposed to smear-positive individuals. Annual check-ups of patients considered to have inactive disease reveal reactivation so infrequently that they should be discontinued, the exception being those with other risk factors.[255]

When present, symptoms are usually nonspecific and do not direct the attention of the patient or the physician to the lungs; the commonest are tiredness, weakness, anorexia, and weight loss. A history of contact, usually in the family, is common. Direct questioning may elicit a history of the recent onset of unproductive or mildly productive cough that has persisted since an upper respiratory tract infection and that is occasionally associated with hemoptysis. In some, the initial complaint is pleuritic chest pain, frequently with fever. Hoarseness, usually a manifestation

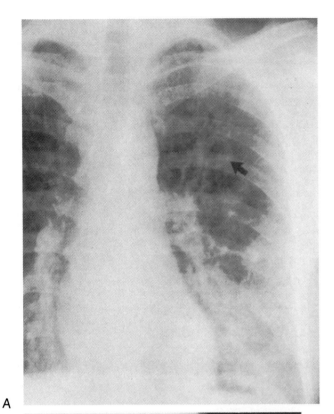

A

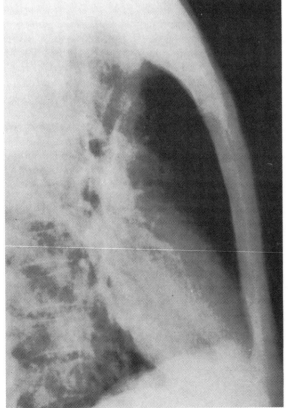

B

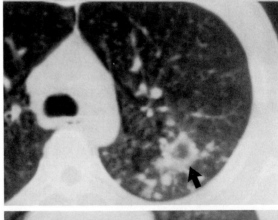

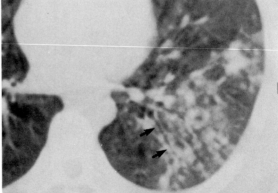

C

Figure 6–30. Tuberculous Cavitation with Bronchogenic Spread. Posteroanterior *(A)* and lateral *(B)* chest roentgenograms reveal a 2.7-cm, thin-walled cavity *(arrow)* in the left upper lobe; small nodular and linear opacities are present cephalad. There is extensive patchy and confluent airspace consolidation in the left lower lobe. The right lung was normal. CT scans through the upper and lower lobes *(C)* show the thin-walled cavity *(arrow)* surrounded by several smaller noncavitated nodules. Discrete and confluent foci of airspace consolidation containing an air bronchogram *(small arrows)* are present throughout much of the lower lobe, representing bronchogenic spread from the upper lobe cavity.

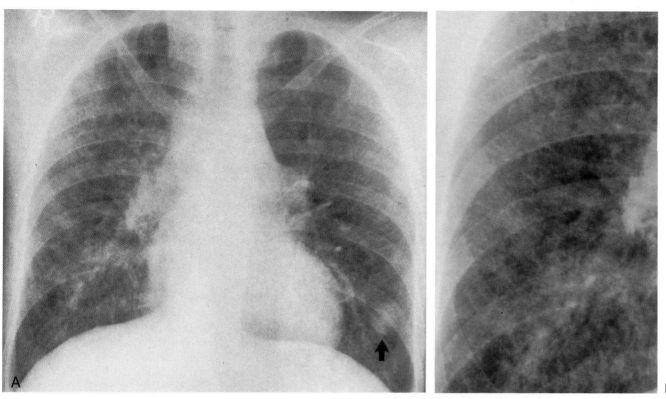

Figure 6–31. Miliary Tuberculosis. A posteroanterior *(A)* chest roentgenogram reveals diffuse, bilateral interstitial lung disease, more marked in the right than in the left lung and in the upper than in the lower lobes. The pattern is micronodular or fine reticulonodular. A 3-cm nodule *(arrow)* is present in the left lower lobe, possibly containing a small cavity. A detail view of the right lung *(B)* shows a multitude of discrete and confluent nodular opacities, ranging in diameter from 1 to 3 mm.

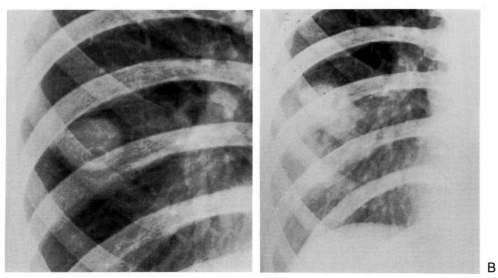

Figure 6–32. Tuberculoma with Reactivation. A view of the right lung from a posteroanterior roentgenogram *(A)* reveals an oval shadow measuring approximately 3 cm in diameter; a small, calcific ring shadow can be identified in the center of the lesion. The surrounding lung parenchyma is normal. Two years later, the patient developed an abrupt onset of an acute respiratory illness; a roentgenogram at that time *(B)* revealed "breakdown" of the tuberculoma with the development of acute airspace disease in the surrounding parenchyma; proven exudative tuberculosis.

of laryngeal involvement, indicates active disease and, in most cases, is associated with a positive sputum culture. Shortness of breath is uncommon and usually indicates long-standing extensive disease.

One third to one half of patients with active tuberculosis are febrile when first seen. The fever is usually low grade and occurs in the afternoon or evening. Its presence correlates with cavitation and far-advanced, smear-positive disease. One third of patients become apyrexic within 2 days of the initiation of therapy, and another one third become apyrexic during the second week; the remaining third, usually those with the more advanced disease, remain febrile beyond the second week of treatment.[256]

With a few exceptions, physical examinations is unrewarding. If an apical lesion is identified on the chest roentgenogram, post-tussive rales on auscultation strongly suggest activity. In patients with recent endobronchial dissemination, rales and rhonchi may be heard extensively over both lungs; diffuse rhonchi may indicate tuberculous bronchitis. When onset of the disease is characterized by pain on respiration, a friction rub or signs of pleural effusion or pneumothorax may be heard. Occasionally, clinical findings suggest lymph node compression or direct infection of mediastinal structures.[257]

Miliary tuberculosis presents a clinical picture different from that of other types of pulmonary involvement. The onset is usually insidious; in one series, the mean duration of symptoms was almost 16 weeks, and more than half the patients had had symptoms for more than 8 weeks.[258] Cough, weight loss, weakness, anorexia, and night sweats are common. Headache and abdominal pain suggest spread to the meninges and peritoneum. Tuberculin testing with 5 TU is negative in at least 25 per cent of patients. Without treatment, the major cause of death is respiratory failure, a complication that may obscure the diagnosis.[259]

As discussed previously, hematogenous dissemination is a frequent complication of primary tuberculosis; although clinical evidence of involvement of other tissues and organs is rare during the initial infection, symptoms and signs may subsequently develop. In at least 75 per cent of cases, the chest roentgenogram shows an abnormality compatible with tuberculosis.[260] In the United States, patients with extrapulmonary tuberculosis are often elderly or black or have AIDS; they commonly present with pyrexia of unknown origin, and many have miliary pulmonary disease.

Perhaps the commonest form of extrapulmonary tuberculosis in adults is genitourinary, and the discovery of pyuria, hematuria, and albuminuria in a patient who has had pulmonary tuberculosis or who shows roentgenographic evidence of a healed pulmonary lesion should suggest tuberculosis as a possible cause. Tuberculosis of the female genital system usually occurs as salpingitis and oophoritis, manifested by pelvic pain and menstrual disturbances. It should be noted, however, that menstrual disorders are frequent in pulmonary tuberculosis without genital involvement, and their presence does not necessarily mean extension of the disease. Although formerly common in children, bone and joint involvement, from hematogenous dissemination or from direct extension via the lymphatic system from the pleura to the thoracic and lumbosacral spine (Pott's disease), is rarely seen today.

Tuberculous meningitis causes headache, somnolence,

irritability, vomiting, and sometimes neck stiffness. Involvement of the upper respiratory and gastrointestinal tracts used to be fairly common in patients with advanced pulmonary disease caused by *M. tuberculosis* or *M. bovis* but has now been largely eradicated by chemotherapy. Nevertheless, tuberculous laryngitis continues to be reported, and is almost invariably associated with far advanced pulmonary tuberculosis.[261] The gastrointestinal tract is usually affected in the ileocecal area or around the rectum, the latter being associated with perianal or ischiorectal abscesses[262]; peritonitis occurs occasionally. Biopsy of the liver reveals granulomas in about 25 per cent of patients with tuberculosis, but this involvement is seldom associated with clinical or biochemical evidence of hepatic dysfunction.[263]

Laboratory Findings

Tuberculin Skin Test. Roentgenographic manifestations of other diseases may closely mimic pulmonary tuberculosis, and skin tests should always be performed in any suspicious case. A negative tuberculin test with 5 TU of stabilized PPD in a person without overwhelming tuberculosis or underlying disease makes the diagnosis unlikely (*see* page 151).

Bacteriologic Investigation. Although definitive diagnosis of pulmonary tuberculosis requires culture of the organism, a smear showing acid-fast bacilli is virtually diagnostic in a patient with clinical and roentgenographic findings suggestive of the disease. (Smear-negative, culture-positive tuberculosis occurs in approximately 25 per cent of all patients and in 5 to 10 per cent of patients with far advanced cavitary disease.[264]) Sputum is the most valuable source of organisms; specimens obtained immediately after bronchoscopy are particularly useful. When a diagnosis of tuberculosis is suspected and sputum is not available, bronchoscopy may be highly productive for both smear and culture diagnosis,[265] usually from brushings or washings but sometimes from biopsy specimens.[266]

Although positive cultures are obtained in about two thirds of patients with miliary tuberculosis, the seriousness of this form of the disease may necessitate that the diagnosis be made by the combination of roentgenographic pattern and pyrexia, with confirmation by transbronchial or even open lung biopsy after initiation of therapy. The detection of tubercle bacilli in suspected cases by bone marrow aspiration or biopsy has been disappointing, ranging from 16 to 33 per cent.[258]

Cytopathologic Examination. Although cytologic examination of sputum or bronchial washings and brushings is occasionally useful because it directs clinical attention to the possibility of tuberculosis, it is seldom rewarding as a primary diagnostic method. Specimens obtained by TTNA are more productive[267]; however, when interpreting the results of TTNA, one must always remember that the most frequent cause of false-positive diagnosis of malignancy in these specimens is tuberculosis.

Hematologic and Biochemical Investigation. The leukocyte count in tuberculosis is usually within normal limits, but may be increased to 10,000 to 15,000 cells per mL. In miliary disease, there is often a shift to the left with a relative polymorphonuclear leukocytosis and lymphocytopenia.[258] Anemia has been reported in 60 per cent of patients,[265] particularly in the presence of chronic pulmonary or miliary disease.

Hypercalcemia may occur but is uncommon[269]; it may be masked by accompanying hypoalbuminemia and may not be recognized until the patient shows improvement while receiving treatment for the tuberculosis itself. Many patients have been receiving supplemental vitamin D. Hyponatremia develops in some cases of pulmonary tuberculosis but is commoner in tuberculous meningitis.[258] It may represent the effect of inappropriate antidiuretic hormone secretion; however, one study of circulating vasopressin suggested that it may be the result of a "down-setting" of osmoregulation.[270]

Increased levels of the acute phase reactants, serum amyloid A protein and C-reactive protein, have been found in pulmonary tuberculosis associated with lung destruction. In susceptible people and in the presence of long-standing disease, amyloidosis may develop.

Serologic and Molecular Biologic Investigation. A variety of antibodies are produced by patients with tuberculosis. These may be detected in cerebrospinal fluid, serum, and BAL fluid by ELISA,[271] a procedure that may prove useful in diagnosing active disease in patients who are smear-negative and in distinguishing sarcoidosis from tuberculosis.[272] The use of the polymerase chain reaction to detect mycobacterial deoxyribonucleic acid (DNA) also may prove to be of great diagnostic benefit, particularly with specimens such as pleural fluid in which the number of infecting organisms may be relatively small.[273]

Pulmonary Function Tests. In the absence of chronic bronchitis and emphysema, patients with pulmonary tuberculosis—even when this is advanced—show little impairment of respiratory function. Since the disease interferes equally with ventilation and perfusion, ventilation-perfusion abnormalities do not develop.[274] Pulmonary function tests are useful in assessing patients before surgery and to determine objectively the degree of disability in patients with diffuse chronic destructive tuberculosis. In miliary tuberculosis, pulmonary function tests show a diffuse restrictive pattern and a reduction in the diffusing capacity. With treatment and restoration of the chest roentgenogram to normal, the diffusing capacity may remain considerably below predicted normal values.[275]

Prognosis

Antibiotic therapy has greatly altered the natural course of pulmonary tuberculosis. Although the incidence of the disease has shown an almost linear decrease in every industrialized country during the last century, the death rate did not alter appreciably until the introduction of chemotherapy.[276] Using rifampicin and isoniazid, the treatment period has been shortened to 9 months or less; bacterial conversion takes place within 2 months in about 80 per cent of patients, treatment failure occurs in fewer than 8 per cent, and relapse occurs in fewer than 2 per cent.[205]

Resistance to drugs used to treat patients with tuberculosis continues to be a major concern in the management of the disease. It is important to differentiate between "true primary resistance"—resistant organisms cultured from patients not previously treated with antibiotics—and an acquired resistance in patients previously treated.[277] Acquired

resistance—a major problem in developing countries because of high rates of default and meager facilities for treatment—ranges from 2 to 7 per cent in the United States, the incidence of rifampicin resistance being similar to that of isoniazid.[278] These figures contrast with the 25 to 50 per cent incidence of resistance estimated from various Asian countries, usually to isoniazid.[277]

Patients who die with active tuberculosis are usually elderly and chronically ill from associated disease, but they are equally likely to succumb from the tuberculosis (often not recognized) as from the underlying illness.[279] Some patients die suddenly of massive pulmonary hemorrhage.

Nontuberculous Mycobacteria

A small but increasing proportion of pleuropulmonary mycobacterial infections are caused by organisms other than *M. tuberculosis* or *M. bovis*; these are referred to variously as "anonymous," "atypical," "chromogenic," or "unclassified" mycobacteria but are perhaps best designated "nontuberculous" (NTM).[280] Features common to these organisms include ready growth of almost all strains on culture at 25 or 37°C and nonpathogenicity for guinea pigs (in contrast with *M. tuberculosis,* which grows only at 37°C and is highly pathogenic for guinea pigs). Based on culture characteristics—morphology, presence or absence of pigment, and rate of growth—they are traditionally classified into four groups (Table 6–1).

Although NTM are most frequently isolated in tropical and subtropical areas, they are of worldwide distribution.[280] Their natural habitat varies somewhat with the species but is often water, soil, or dust; *M. marinum* has been found in fish and fresh and salt water contaminated by fish, and *M. scrofulaceum* has been cultured from milk and other dairy products. The natural habitat of *M. kansasii* is not known, although it has occasionally been isolated from water and animals.

Nontuberculous mycobacterial infection of the lungs is a disease of adults rather than children, the incidence being highest in men older than 50 years of age.[281] Infection may be acquired by inhalation, by ingestion, by direct inoculation following trauma, or through iatrogenic means, such as syringe needles, bronchoscopes, or surgical skin incisions. Animal-to-human or human-to-human transmission has not been convincingly documented, although familial aggregations of group I disease have been reported occasionally, suggesting the possibility of interhuman transmission.[282]

In many cases—particularly those in which the patient is not obviously immunocompromised—underlying chronic lung disease appears to be a predisposing factor. The commonest are chronic bronchitis and emphysema, healed tuberculosis or fungal disease, bronchiectasis, and silicosis. NTM have been shown experimentally to favor a lipid medium for growth,[283] suggesting a rationale for cases of pulmonary infection caused by the *M. fortuitum-chelonei* complex in patients with mineral oil aspiration. Of increasing importance has been the realization that immunodepressed individuals, particularly those with AIDS and hairy-cell leukemia,[284] are prone to NTM infections.

Because of the lack of governmental requirement for case reporting and the difficulty in distinguishing between infection and colonization in some cases, it is difficult to be

Table 6–1. **NONTUBERCULOUS MYCOBACTERIA**

Runyon Group	Organisms	Pulmonary Disease*	Comments	Selected References
I. Photochromogens	*M. kansasii*	Common	Occasionally cervical lymphadenitis	287
	M. simiae	Rare	—	611
	M. marinum	No	Skin disease	
II. Scotochromogens	*M. scrofulaceum*	Rare	Cervical lymphadenitis; sometimes grouped with *M. avium-intracellulare* as the MAIS complex	
	M. szulgai	Uncommon		612
	M. gordonae	Uncommon		613
III. Nonphotochromogens	*M. avium-intracellulare*	Common	Cervical lymphadenitis in children; disseminated or local pulmonary disease in individuals with AIDS; progressive cavitary disease in individuals without AIDS	614, 615
	M. xenopi	Uncommon, but increasing in frequency		616
	M. nonchromogenicum (M. terrae) complex	Uncommon		617
	M. malmoense	Uncommon		618
	M. ulcerans	No		
IV. Rapid Growers	*M. fortuitum*	Rare	Sometimes grouped with *M. chelonei (M. fortuitum-chelonei* complex)	619, 621
	M. chelonei	Rare	Usually skin abscesses	
Unclassified Organisms	*M. asiaticum*	Rare		622
	M. thermoresistible	Rare		623

*Frequency relates to relative incidence of infection in the group of nontuberculous mycobacteria.

precise about the incidence of NTM infection. It has been estimated, however, that in the United States in 1980 there were approximately 700 cases of disease caused by group I organims, 60 by group II, and 2000 by group III.[285] Since the report appeared of *M. avium-intracellulare* infection in persons with AIDS in the 1980s, the incidence of group III infection has undoubtedly increased markedly. Whatever the precise incidence, it appears that both the absolute number of cases and the proportion of mycobacterial disease caused by NTM are steadily increasing.[286] However, there is considerable geographic variation in both the incidence and the particular variety of NTM disease. For example, *M. kansasii* is more prevalent in the midwestern United States than elsewhere, whereas *M. avium-intracellulare* is more commonly identified in the southeastern United States (at least in patients without AIDS). The organisms also have a propensity to colonize patients with cystic fibrosis.[286a]

In contrast with the situation with *M. tuberculosis* whose isolation signifies disease, isolation of NTM from sputum frequently represents only environmental contamination or colonization of the respiratory tract. (An exception may be *M. kansasii*, which usually proves to be pathogenic.[287]) Clinical studies that support the concept of colonization include those that have documented the ability to eradicate the organism with intensive bronchial hygiene[288] and those that show that some patients whose clinical condition remains stable have repeated positive cultures despite treatment.[289] Suggested criteria for diagnosing a culture-positive patient as having true infection include (1) culture of at least two sputum or bronchial lavage specimens yielding the same NTM organism; (2) the appearance of new symptoms or a change in existing symptoms in relation to the first isolation of the organism; (3) an abnormal chest roentgenogram con-

sistent with mycobacterial disease; (4) an absence of other pathogens in the sputum; (5) an absence of other diseases that might account for the patient's illness; and (6) a skin test with an NTM antigen causing induration at least 5 mm larger than the reaction to an equivalent dose of PPD-S.

Pathologic Characteristics

In most cases, gross and histologic characteristics of pulmonary disease caused by NTM are similar to those of *M. tuberculosis*, with granulomatous inflammation and a variable degree of caseation necrosis (Fig. 6–33).[290] A definitive histologic diagnosis of the nontuberculous nature of the disease in these cases is usually difficult if not impossible. The exception lies in cases in which patients are immunocompromised, in which the typical histologic characteristics may be altered. This is particularly noteworthy in some children and in patients with AIDS who are infected with *M. avium-intracellulare*, in whom aggregates of macrophages stuffed with organisms are associated with minimal or absent granulomatous reaction and necrosis.

Occasionally, lung biopsy specimens from patients who apparently are not immunocompromised reveal nonspecific chronic inflammation without a granulomatous component and yet grow NTM on culture.[290] Although the significance of this occurrence is not clear, it is probably best to consider the positive culture a result of colonization or contamination while recognizing the possibility that the histologic reaction itself may be atypical.

Roentgenographic Manifestations

The roentgenographic pattern of pulmonary disease caused by NTM cannot be accurately differentiated from

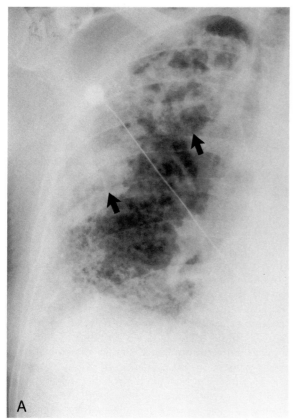

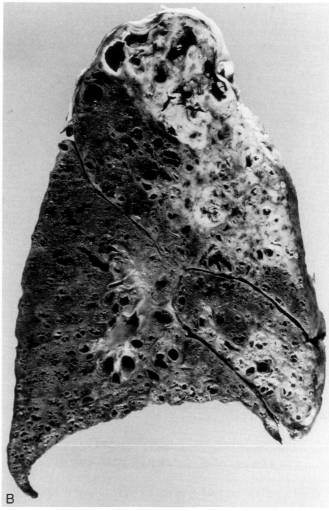

Figure 6–33. *Mycobacterium Xenopi* Pneumonia Superimposed on Idiopathic Fibrosing Alveolitis. *A,* A view of the right lung from an anteroposterior chest roentgenogram discloses inhomogeneous consolidation *(superolateral to arrows)* in the right upper lobe. Elsewhere in both lungs, there is a medium and coarse reticulonodular pattern consistent with diffuse interstitial fibrosis. *B,* Right lung at autopsy showing fibrosing alveolitis with "honeycomb" appearance in the basal aspect of the lower lobe. In addition, the upper and middle lobes show extensive consolidation (white tissue in illustration). Spaces within the consolidated regions represent combined cavitation and cysts related to the underlying interstitial fibrosis.

that produced by *M. tuberculosis,*[291] although the changes usually indicate advanced disease (*see* Fig. 6–33). In studies of 187 cases of pulmonary *M. kansasii* infection[292] and 114 cases of *M. intracellulare* infection (in patients without AIDS),[293] the features that characterized the disease in both groups were as follows:

1. In virtually all patients, the disease was located in the apical or posterior segments of the upper lobes.
2. The disease was bilateral in 66 per cent of patients with *M. intracellulare* infection and in 40 per cent of those with *M. kansasii* disease. In both groups, unilateral disease was twice as common on the right as on the left.
3. Cavitation was seen in 90 to 95 per cent of cases, the cavities usually being multiple and often measuring over 4 cm.
4. Scarring and volume loss occurred in roughly two thirds of both groups.
5. Endobronchial spread was observed in an astounding 80 per cent of the cases of *M. intracellulare* disease and about 65 per cent of those with *M. kansasii* infection.
6. Both pleural effusion and lymph node enlargement were very uncommon in both groups.

Although it is not possible to be definitive about the tuberculous or nontuberculous etiology of any particular case, several findings have been observed more commonly in NTM infection. For example, cavities tend to be thin-walled in NTM disease and are generally smaller than those caused by *M. tuberculosis.*[294] In addition, a single thin-walled cavity or a single circumscribed shadow containing multiple lucencies is more likely to be caused by *M. kansasii* than by *M. tuberculosis.*[295] Other features that seem to be more suggestive of NTM infection include a paucity of so-called exudative lesions, a rarity of hematogenous dissemination, and a strong association with pre-existing pulmonary disease, particularly emphysema and pneumoconiosis.

Clinical Manifestations

The clinical picture of pulmonary disease caused by NTM also is indistinguishable from that of tuberculosis, although middle-aged and elderly persons appear to be more commonly affected. Infection becomes disseminated in a small number of patients, almost all of whom are immunoincompetent as a result of therapy or underlying disease. Such dissemination is almost invariably fatal.[296] Pulmonary involvement is common in this complication, with a miliary roentgenographic pattern in most patients and parenchymal consolidation in about one quarter.

Antigens have been isolated from group I photochromogens (PPD-Y), group II scotochromogens (PPD-G), group III nonphotochromogens (PPD-B), and various strains of rapid growers. Most investigators believe that the high cross-reactivity (low specificity) with PPD-S renders them unreliable as indicators of specific infections.[297] At present it is perhaps wise to assume that a reaction to a nontuberculous mycobacterial antigen represents infection with these mycobacteria only when the induration is 5 mm larger than that from a simultaneous test with other antigens.

Many reports indicate that NTM infection tends to progress if untreated[298] and that the response to chemotherapy is often poor (with the exception of cases caused by *M. kansasii*, which tend to show a good response to even short-course chemotherapy[299]). However, a recent report from a nonreferral community hospital described a response to therapy in 90 per cent of patients treated with intent to cure[300]; it was suggested that the relatively poor therapeutic results of other series may be a reflection of more advanced disease in referral settings.

FUNGI AND ACTINOMYCES

Fungi may cause pulmonary disease by several mechanisms and in a variety of clinical settings. Some organisms (e.g., *Histoplasma capsulatum* and *Coccidioides immitis*) are primary pathogens that most frequently infect healthy individuals. They are found in specific geographic areas and usually cause mild infection evidenced only by the development of positive skin tests. Fulminant primary infection or chronic pulmonary disease, with or without systemic dissemination, are very uncommon but may cause significant morbidity and may occasionally be fatal (particularly in immunocompromied patients). A second group of organisms (e.g., *Aspergillus* and *Candida* species) are opportunistic invaders that chiefly affect immunocompromised hosts or individuals with underlying pulmonary disease; in these situations, they may be present as saprophytes (e.g., a fungus ball) or as invasive organisms that cause tissue destruction. In addition, some fungi (particularly *Aspergillus* species) may cause disease by means of a hypersensitivity reaction without actually invading tissue.

The order Actinomycetales contains a number of genera that show characteristics suggestive of fungi, including the formation of mycelia, extensive branching in a fungal pattern in tissue, and the frequent production of chronic necrotizing and fibrosing disease. For these reasons, these species are often categorized with the true fungi for purposes of discussion, and this custom will be followed here. Despite this, their ultrastructural and biochemical characteristics, as well as their sensitivity to "ordinary" antibiotics and insensitivity to antifungal agents such as amphotericin B, indicate that they are bacteria, not fungi.

Histoplasma Capsulatum (Histoplasmosis)

Histoplasmosis is a disease of varied clinical and roentgenographic manifestations usually caused by the dimorphic fungus *Histoplasma capsulatum*. Its natural habitat is soil that contains a high nitrogen content, usually derived from the guano of birds or bats. Thus, areas such as chicken houses, starling and pigeon roosts, and bat-infested caves or attics commonly are associated with outbreaks of infection.[301] Situations in which clouds of dust are raised, such as bulldozing of roosting sites or cleaning of bat-infested attics, are particularly hazardous. Animal-to-human and person-to-person transmission are not known to occur.

Although the organism is of worldwide distribution, most reports of the disease have come from North America, particularly the Ohio, Mississippi, and St. Lawrence river valleys, which are regarded as endemic areas. The disease is also relatively common in southern Mexico and Central America; however, it is rare in Europe, Australia, and Japan. In endemic areas, a substantial proportion of the population may be shown to be infected: the histoplasmin skin test is positive in as many as 80 per cent of individuals,[302] and postmortem examinations have revealed splenic calcification in 50 per cent of cases,[303] representing remote granulomas derived from hematogenous dissemination during primary infection. Even in endemic areas, however, the infection is unevenly distributed, probably reflecting "point sources" of heavily contaminated soil.[304] Although most commonly an infection of otherwise healthy individuals, it is important to remember that disease occurs with increased frequency and is more virulent in immunocompromised patients, particularly those with AIDS.[39]

Pathogenesis and Pathologic Characteristics

In contrast with tuberculosis, hypersensitivity (and presumably immunity) in histoplasmosis is not permanent, and recurrent infections probably occur in many individuals residing in an endemic area, either unassociated with symptoms or having a clinical picture resembling that of the original episode. Thus, the terms "primary" and "postprimary" as applied to tuberculosis are not suitable to a classification of histoplasmosis.

From clinical and radiographic points of view, histoplasmosis may be conveniently divided into asymptomatic and symptomatic infection, the latter, in turn, being subdivided into several acute syndromes, chronic histoplasmosis, and disseminated disease. It is likely that these varied forms of disease are dependent on a combination of the size of the air-borne inoculum and on the state of the host's immunity. The latter appears to be particularly important. It determines the length of the incubation period, nonimmunized individuals developing symptoms about 2 weeks after exposure, whereas those with immunity become symptomatic in as short a period as 3 days. In addition, there is evidence that the pathogenesis of some second infections (reinfections) and of the chronic form of disease may be related more to the body's immune reaction (i.e., a form of hypersensitivity pneumonitis) than to tissue damage induced directly by the organism.[301, 305]

In appropriate environmental conditions, the mycelia of

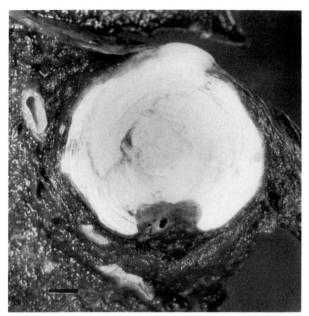

Figure 6–34. Histoplasmoma. Well-circumscribed subpleural nodule showing prominent laminations. (Bar = 5 mm.)

H. capsulatum produce microconidia measuring 2 to 5 μm in diameter that are inhaled and deposited on distal airways. An initial acute inflammatory exudate is followed in 1 or 2 weeks by granulomatous inflammation, necrosis, and the beginning of fibrosis. In most cases, healing is rapid, leaving only small areas of encapsulated, necrotic parenchyma as residua (*see* Fig. 6–19, page 319). Occasionally, individual foci of necrosis coalesce and enlarge, resulting in larger foci of disease (histoplasmomas) (Fig. 6–34). Calcification is frequent.

Regional lymph node involvement is invariable during the initial infection. Complications are similar to those of primary tuberculosis and include atelectasis and obstructive pneumonitis (Fig. 6–35) and bronchiectasis (both caused by airway compression) and broncholithiasis (*see* page 687). Blood-borne dissemination also occurs early in the initial infection, giving rise to small extrapulmonary foci of granulomatous inflammation, particularly in the liver and spleen. Such hematogenous spread seldom results in clinically significant disease; however, foci of necrosis may subsequently undergo calcification, becoming visible roentgenographically as markers of prior disease.

In disseminated histoplasmosis, organisms may be found in many organs but are particularly numerous in the spleen, liver, bone marrow, lymph nodes, gastrointestinal tract, and adrenal glands. The inflammatory reaction is variable, consisting of well-formed granulomas in cases in which there are relatively few organisms and a protracted course, and a virtual absence of response in cases with numerous organisms and a rapid course.[301]

In tissue sections, organisms usually cannot be identifed with hematoxylin and eosin (H&E) stain except when they are within macrophages as part of disseminated disease. When present in necrotic tissue, they are best seen with silver stain.

Asymptomatic Histoplasmosis

Estimates from endemic areas indicate that 95 to 99 per cent of infections are not associated with symptoms, even with retrospective inquiry of recognized histoplasmin converters.[306] Despite this, chest roentgenograms of histoplasmin converters have revealed pulmonary parenchymal opacities, with or without hilar lymph node enlargement, in 10 to 25 per cent of these subclinical episodes.[306] The lack of symptoms probably reflects a low intensity of exposure in a nonimmunized person or a moderate-sized inoculum in one who has immunity.

Symptomatic Histoplasmosis

Acute Histoplasmosis. The abrupt onset of symptoms in a patient with clinical and laboratory evidence of *H. capsulatum* infection is best designated acute histoplasmosis. Under this diagnostic umbrella are several syndromes.

"Flulike" Disease. Symptoms of "flulike" disease consist of fever and headache, usually associated with chills, cough, and retrosternal discomfort, the last-named probably being caused by mediastinal lymph node enlargement.[306] In most cases, physical examination of the chest is normal. Hepatosplenomegaly may develop in children but is rare in adults. Erythema nodosum may be present, usually in young white women, and is sometimes associated

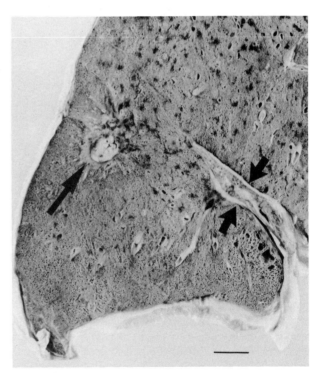

Figure 6–35. Chronic (Inactive) Histoplasmosis with Middle Lobe Collapse. A slice of right lung shows a focus of necrotic tissue surrounded by irregular strands of fibrous tissue in the superior segment of the lower lobe *(long arrow)*. This represents the initial site of infection (analogous to the Ghon focus of tuberculosis). The right middle lobe *(short arrows)* shows marked collapse and fibrosis as a result of spread of infection to peribronchial lymph nodes and obstruction of the middle lobe bronchus. (Bar = 1 cm.)

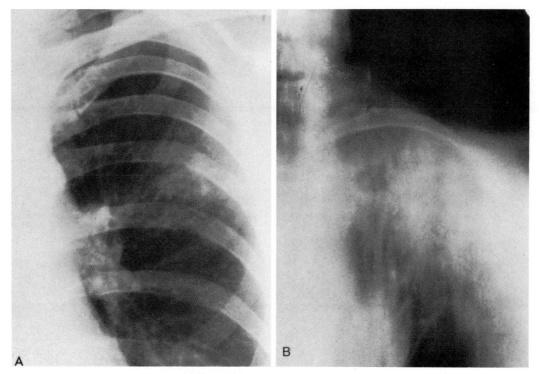

Figure 6–36. Acute Histoplasmosis. Approximately 1 year earlier, this 54-year-old man had had a resection of his left upper lobe for a lesion thqt proved pathologically to be active histoplasmosis. At the time of the roentgenograms illustrated, he returned with symptoms and signs of active pulmonary infection. A posteroanterior roentgenogram *(A)* and an anteroposterior tomogram *(B)* revealed extensive airspace consolidation. Bronchial brushing recovered *Histoplama capsulatum* organisms.

with arthralgia[307]; in such cases, the diagnosis is often evident through awareness of an ongoing miniepidemic. Chest roentgenography may reveal one or more ill-defined nonsegmental opacities, more often in lower than in upper zones, with or without hilar lymph node enlargement.

Acute Pulmonary Histoplasmosis. Acute pulmonary histoplasmosis overlaps with the "flulike" syndrome and may be diagnosed when clinical and roentgenographic findings suggest localization in the lungs. It is characterized roentgenographically by homogeneous parenchymal consolidation of nonsegmental distribution and, thus, may simulate acute bacterial airspace pneumonia (Fig. 6–36). Unlike the latter, however, the disease tends to clear in one area and appear in another. Hilar lymph node enlargement is common.[308] Symptoms include cough with mucopurulent sputum and sometimes hemoptysis, headaches, pleuritic pain, and pain in the limbs and back.

Acute Diffuse Nodular Disease. This is the "epidemic" form of the disease that typically develops in groups of heavily exposed individuals. Following such exposure, the roentgenogram may show no abnormalities for a week or more despite the presence of symptoms; eventually, however, widely disseminated, fairly discrete nodular shadows appear throughout the lungs, individual lesions measuring up to 3 or 4 mm in diameter. Hilar lymph node enlargement is present in the majority of cases.[309] The pulmonary shadows may clear completely in 2 to 8 months or may fibrose and persist. Symptoms may be very mild, and, in fact, exposure may not be recognized until calcified nodules are identified many years later (Fig. 6–37). On the other

hand, overwhelming exposure may result in severe illness and death.[310]

Patients who have been previously infected with *H. capsulatum* and who are heavily re-exposed may have a different reaction from that described above. In these individuals, it has been hypothesized that the incubation period is reduced to 3 to 5 days and the inflammatory reaction is

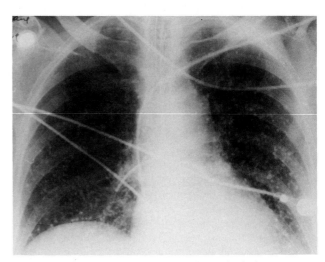

Figure 6–37. Healed Disseminated Histoplasmosis. A chest roentgenogram in anteroposterior projection reveals a multitude of tiny calcific nodules evenly distributed throughout both lungs. Proved at autopsy to be inactive histoplasmosis;. the patient had no respiratory symptoms.

altered because of strong immunity. According to Goodwin and coworkers,[306] such acquired host resistance prevents necrosis and limits the tissue response to minute foci of granulomatous inflammation that are seen on chest roentgenograms as miliary lesions unassociated with hilar node enlargement. These lesions usually clear completely without roentgenographic residua or loss of pulmonary function.

Histoplasmoma. A histoplasmoma is probably the commonest roentgenographic manifestation of pulmonary histoplasmosis.[311] It is usually a solitary, sharply defined, nodular shadow, seldom more than 3 cm in diameter. In most cases the lesion is in a lower lobe, often with satellite lesions nearby; many calcify, producing the "target" lesion that is virtually pathognomonic of the abnormality (Fig. 6–38). Hilar lymph node calcification is common. Serial roentgenograms over months or years may reveal moderate growth, even of calcified nodules, to a point where a metastatic neoplasm may be considered.[312] In this situation, it has been postulated that the original focus of histoplasmosis develops a fibrous capsule that progressively enlarges as a reactive phenomenon,[313] similar to that seen in chronic sclerosing mediastinitis (*see* later).

Lymph Node Involvement. In addition to the common nodal involvement in association with parenchymal disease, histoplasmosis sometimes is manifested by unilateral or bilateral enlargement of hilar, mediastinal, or intrapulmonary lymph nodes in the absence of other roentgenographic abnormalities.[311] This form of disease is particularly common in children.[308] Most patients are asymptomatic during the active phase of the disease; however, with healing and subsequent fibrosis, extrinsic pressure of enlarged nodes on the airways, particularly the middle lobe bronchus, may cause obstruction and resulting distal infection or atelectasis.[308]

Chronic Histoplasmosis. In contrast with acute disease, which typically subsides without treatment in weeks to months, *H. capsulatum* also occasionally causes chronic pulmonary disease, particularly in patients with underlying emphysema, and may lead to a variety of clinical syndromes resulting from granulomatous inflammation and fibrosis within the mediastinum.

Chronic Pulmonary Histoplasmosis. Roentgenographic manifestations of chronic pulmonary histoplasmosis consist of segmental or subsegmental areas of consolidation in the upper lobes that frequently outline centrilobular emphysematous spaces (Fig. 6–39); thick-walled bullae sometimes contain fluid levels. Serial chest roentgenograms tend to show progressive loss of volume associated with increased prominence of linear opacities; infected bullae may disappear completely or may gradually increase in size. The appearance of such chronic cavitary disease simulates postprimary tuberculosis.[314]

Clinically, the disease tends to be associated with cough and expectoration, which in some cases are likely the result of the underlying chronic obstructive pulmonary disease rather than the infection itself. Patients who develop cavitary disease may complain of weight loss, deep-seated chest pain, hemoptysis, and general malaise, or they may remain asymptomatic. The organism may be grown on culture of sputum in only about one in three patients with noncavitary disease; by contrast, about 50 to 70 per cent of patients are culture-positive in the cavitary form. Serologic tests are positive in 75 to 90 per cent of cases.

As indicated previously, it has been suggested that the pathogenesis of some cases of chronic pulmonary histoplasmosis is related to an immunologic reaction.[301] Although many of these cases are undoubtedly accompanied by a deterioration in lung function, there is evidence that this form of disease is not as serious as one might anticipate if it were a true infection, and dissemination is rare. Other cases, however, represent chronic necrotizing infection similar to tuberculosis; although data are sparse, it is likely that the prognosis in patients with this form of disease is worse.

Chronic Mediastinal Histoplasmosis. Histoplasmosis may occur in mediastinal lymph nodes, with subsequent development of a matted mass that may encroach on any mediastinal structure but particularly the esophagus and pericardium. Pericarditis usually occurs in young adults and is often associated with pleural effusion, usually left-sided. It may result in tamponade or calcification of the pericardium, with or without cardiac constriction. Enlarged posterior mediastinal lymph nodes may encroach on the esophagus and displace or partially obstruct it. Healing of the affected lymph nodes may result in periesophageal fibrosis and traction diverticula. Encroachment is more likely to occur in the occasional patient who develops sclerosing mediastinitis (*see* page 897). CT scanning is essential for elucidation of the structural defects occasioned by this fibrous reaction.[315]

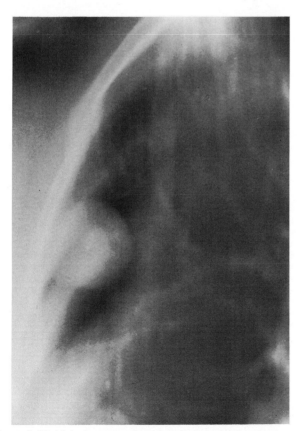

Figure 6–38. Histoplasmoma. An anteroposterior tomogram shows a sharply demarcated, circular shadow measuring 2.8 cm in diameter situated just deep to the visceral pleura. The density is homogeneous except for a central, punctate deposit of calcium (the "target" lesion). (Courtesy of Dr. Max J. Palayew, Jewish General Hospital, Montreal.)

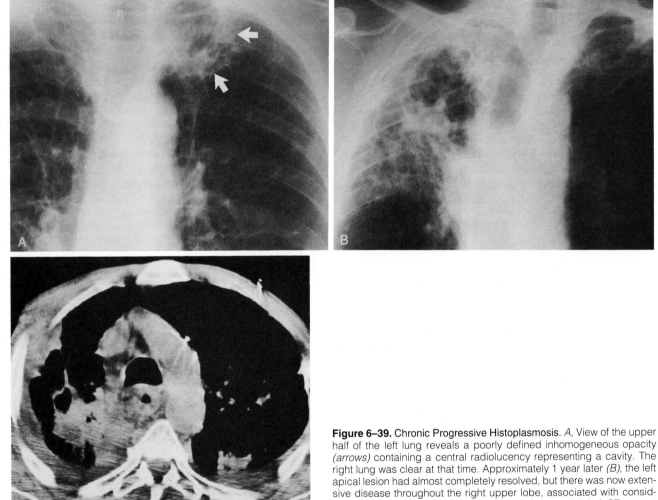

Figure 6–39. Chronic Progressive Histoplasmosis. *A,* View of the upper half of the left lung reveals a poorly defined inhomogeneous opacity *(arrows)* containing a central radiolucency representing a cavity. The right lung was clear at that time. Approximately 1 year later *(B),* the left apical lesion had almost completely resolved, but there was now extensive disease throughout the right upper lobe, associated with considerable loss of volume (note the tracheal shift to the right). A CT scan at the level of the aortic arch *(C)* shows a large homogeneous opacity abutting the posterior mediastinum and containing a well-defined cavity in its anterior portion. *Histoplasma capsulatum* was identified by culture and biopsy.

Disseminated Histoplasmosis. This is a rare variety of histoplasmosis that has been subdivided into three types.[316] In the first (acute) form, lymph nodes, liver, spleen, bone marrow, and adrenal glands are most prominently affected. This is the severest type of infection and occurs most frequently in infants and young children. Its course is measured in weeks. The clinical findings include high persistent fever, prominent hepatosplenomegaly, anemia, leukopenia, and thrombocytopenia; in 25 per cent of patients, there is interstitial pneumonia.

The subacute variety of disease occurs in both children and adults and has a clinical course that runs for months; the symptoms and signs include moderate fever, mild to moderate hepatosplenomegaly, anemia, leukopenia, thrombocytopenia, abdominal pain (caused by gastrointestinal ulceration), and sometimes evidence of Addison's disease, meningitis, focal cerebritis, and endocarditis.

Chronic disseminated histoplasmosis is a relatively mild form of disease that is associated with little or no fever, an absence of hepatosplenomegaly, and no evidence of bone marrow suppression. Patients are almost invariably adult, and the time course is one of months to years. The diagnosis is often made following the discovery of an oropharyngeal ulcer, which is found on examination of the biopsy specimen to be an accumulation of histiocytes containing *H. capsulatum*. Specific organ involvement may result in Addison's disease, meningitis, or endocarditis.

Laboratory Findings

The diagnosis of pulmonary histoplasmosis is seldom made by the identification of the organism in smears of expectorated material or pleural fluid, and in suspected cases these should be cultured; growth usually takes 2 to 4 weeks. Cultures are rarely positive in asymptomatic individuals or in the presence of benign self-limited disease, even in patients who are acutely ill from exposure to a heavy inoculum[301]; during the early pneumonic form of the disease or in the presence of thin-walled cavities, growth is successful in one of three patients or fewer. However, in the presence of thick-walled cavities, culture of sputum is positive in 50 to 70 per cent of cases.[301] Positive results on smear and culture in the presence of symptomatic disseminated histoplasmosis vary with the severity of the disease. In the acute severe form, blood and bone marrow smears, appropriately stained, will usually be diagnostic; the incidence decreases to 50 per cent in subacute and 20 per cent in chronic forms of the disease.

The white blood cell count usually is normal but may increase to 13,000 cells per mL in patients with the acute epidemic form and to 20,000 cells per mL in cases of cavitary disease. Leukopenia, anemia, and thrombocytopenia develop in approximately 50 per cent of patients with symptomatic disseminated disease but rarely in those with other varieties.

As measured by the histoplasmin skin test, cutaneous hypersensitivity develops in almost all patients with asymptomatic or self-limited acute infection, in 75 to 80 per cent of those with chronic pulmonary disease, and in 30 to 50 per cent of patients with symptomatic disseminated disease.[301] It becomes positive 2 to 4 weeks after infection and remains positive for 10 years or more after the initial expo-

sure.[301] Although useful in epidemiologic studies, the test serves little or no purpose in the diagnosis of the disease in the individual patient.

There is some disagreement on the usefulness of the various serologic tests for establishing a diagnosis of *H. capsulatum* infection, at least in areas of high endemicity. It is likely that most authorities would accept a fourfold rise in titer in serial determinations as being significant; however, in contrast with other infectious diseases, this is observed in only a minority of patients believed to have active disease.[317] Many would accept a yeast-phase titer of 1:32 as indicating activity. There are several methods for detecting serum antibodies, and most experts agree that the use of multiple tests, with both mycelial and yeast antigens, increases diagnostic accuracy.[318] Test results become positive about a month after initial infection. A rise in titer is detectable in 95 per cent of mild subclinical or symptomatic cases[301]; 75 per cent of patients with chronic pulmonary histoplasmosis have titers in the suggestive range (<1:32), but in only 25 per cent will the titer be 1:32 or greater. Only 10 per cent of patients with residual solitary nodules have yeast-phase antigen titers of 1:32 or more.[319] Lower titers are found in patients with disseminated disease, titers above 1:8 being present in 60 to 70 per cent.[320]

Coccidioides Immitis (Coccidioidomycosis)

Coccidioidomycosis is a highly infectious disease caused by the dimorphic fungus *Coccidioides immitis*.[321, 322] In its natural habitat (soil), the organism grows as a mycelium of septate hyphae that, when mature, produces numerous 2- to 5-μm arthrospores. These are freed as the mycelium fragments and are quite resistant to drying and highly virulent.

The majority of infections occur in endemic areas by inhalation of arthrospores, so that the risk of acquiring the disease is greatest during dry and windy conditions in which soil is disturbed. Although coccidioidomycosis commonly infects a variety of domestic animals, animal-to-human spread is not believed to occur. Similarly, the disease is probably not transmitted from person to person. The incubation period ranges from 1 to 4 weeks.

The disease is almost exclusively found in the western hemisphere, principally in its endemic areas in the southwestern United States (particularly the San Joaquin Valley), northern Mexico, Venezuela, Paraguay, Argentina, Colombia, Guatemala, and Honduras. The incidence of infection is very high in endemic areas: 25 per cent of newly arrived persons may be expected to have positive skin tests at the end of 1 year, and 50 per cent at the end of 4 years. It has been estimated that in the United States there are as many as 100,000 new cases per year.[321]

Skin reactivity is long-lived but does wane with time, thus permitting exogenous reinfection in endemic areas. However, reactivation of quiescent disease has been documented,[321] and it is generally accepted that some cases of late onset, clinically active dissemination are the result of a loss of immunocompetence in individuals who experienced dissemination during primary infection. The majority of infections that develop outside endemic zones are believed to be related to recent travel within an endemic area, although reactivation of quiescent disease also may occur.

The natural history of coccidioidomycosis is characterized by a variety of pathologic, roentgenographic, and clinical patterns that may be considered under the headings of primary, persistent primary, chronic progressive, and disseminated disease. Of 6000 patients who acquire the infection, approximately 2000 can be expected to be symptomatic; 60 (1 per cent) of these will have illness lasting weeks or months, and in only one patient will the disease become disseminated.

Primary Coccidioidomycosis

Within the lung, inhaled arthrospores develop into spherules that rapidly induce a polymorphonuclear leukocyte reaction in a pattern of typical bronchopneumonia. Although this reaction may persist, with time granulomatous inflammation also ensues. In the majority of cases, the pneumonic focus remains relatively small and undergoes resolution, leaving only small scars as residua. In severer cases, consolidation may be extensive, involving a whole lobe or lung, and is associated with necrosis and cavitation. In these cases, airway involvement in the form of ulcerative bronchitis and bronchiolitis is often prominent, and bronchiectasis may ensue if the patient survives. In tissue sections stained with H&E or silver, spherules measure 20 to 40 μm in diameter, have a thick capsule, and contain characteristic endospores.

Roentgenographically, the parenchymal consolidation develops mainly in the lower lobes and may be homogeneous or mottled, segmental or nonsegmental (Fig. 6–40). Small pleural effusions occur in about 20 per cent of cases, almost invariably in association with parenchymal disease.[323] Hilar lymph node enlargement occurs in about 20 per cent of cases, seldom in the absence of parenchymal involvement.

When present, symptoms consist of fever, cough, chest pain, and sometimes a toxic generalized erythematous rash. On physical examination, rales and rhonchi may be heard, but signs of consolidation are rare. This form of disease almost invariably remains confined to the lungs and clears spontaneously in 2 or 3 weeks. A more specific syndrome occurs in 5 to 20 per cent of patients with symptomatic coccidioidomycosis, sometimes in minor epidemics,[324] and is commonly known as "valley fever." It consists of erythema nodosum or erythema multiforme, arthralgia, and sometimes eosinophilia and influenzalike symptoms. These findings are noted at the onset of skin test reactivity, and in fact these patients are usually very sensitive to coccidioidin. The presence of the syndrome should suggest the diagnosis in endemic areas.

Persistent Primary Coccidioidomycosis

Primary disease that persists longer than 6 weeks is designated persistent primary coccidioidomycosis[322] and may take two roentgenographic forms: (1) one or more nodules

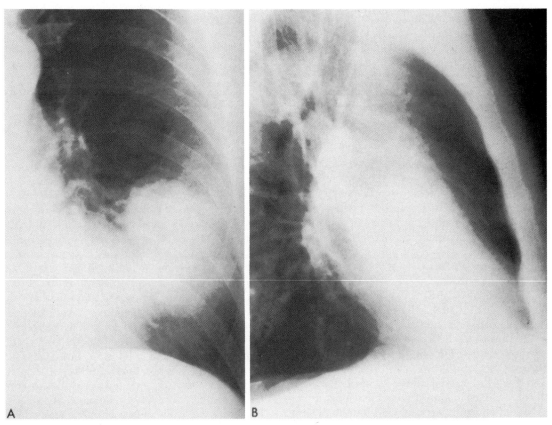

Figure 6–40. Coccidioidomycosis. Views of the left lung from posteroanterior (A) and lateral (B) roentgenograms reveal homogeneous consolidation of much of the lingular segment of the left upper lobe. A faint air bronchogram could be identified on the original roentgenograms but does not reproduce well. The upper border of the consolidation is sharply circumscribed, resembling a mass. (Courtesy of Montreal Chest Hospital Center.)

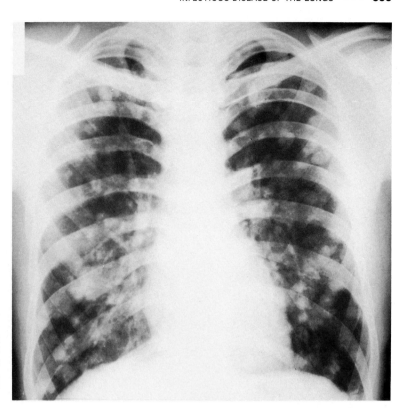

Figure 6–41. Nodular Coccidioidomycosis. A posteroanterior roentgenogram reveals multiple sharply circumscribed nodules distributed randomly throughout both lungs and ranging from 3 to 15 mm in diameter. There is no evidence of calcification or cavitation. The patient is a 25-year-old asymptomatic male, resident of Arizona. (Courtesy of Dr. Paul Capp, University of Arizona Medical Center, Tucson.)

that may persist indefinitely, and (2) progressive pneumonia that may spread to involve large portions of the lungs and may prove fatal.

Nodular lesions (coccidioidomas) represent localized foci of completely or partially resolved pneumonia. Morphologically, they are similar to the residual nodular lesions of tuberculosis and consist of a central zone of necrotic tissue surrounded by a variably well-developed fibrous capsule. Roentgenographically, they range in diameter from 0.5 to 5 cm and are usually single but may be multiple (Fig. 6–41). They tend to occur in the middle and upper lung zones and, in contrast with tuberculosis, may develop in the anterior segment of an upper lobe.[325]

Cavities may develop as a result of necrosis in an area of pneumonia or by excavation of a nodule. Those formed by the latter method have been reported in 10 to 15 per cent of cases[323] and are usually single and located in the upper lobes. They may be thin- or thick-walled; the former have a tendency to change size,[326] possibly reflecting check-valve communication with the bronchial tree.

Almost all patients with coccidioidomas are asymptomatic, even in the presence of cavitation. They are most often found incidentally, sometimes months or years after the patient has left an endemic area, and are investigated to exclude the possibility of malignancy. In contrast, persistent coccidioidal pneumonia is commonly accompanied by hemoptysis, fever, cough, and expectoration, especially when cavitation occurs.

Chronic Progressive Coccidioidomycosis

This form of coccidioidomycosis constitutes fewer than 1 per cent of cases of pulmonary disease and is characterized by an insidious development and a prolonged course of up

to 15 years (average, 5 years).[322] It can occur either in temporal continuity with primary coccidioidomycosis or after a variable time interval during which the infection has apparently been stable and unaccompanied by clinical evidence of activity. Roentgenographic changes resemble those of chronic cavitary tuberculosis. Symptoms include cough, weight loss, fever, hemoptysis, chest pain, and dyspnea. Dark-skinned individuals[327] and patients with insulin-dependent diabetes mellitus[328] appear to be at increased risk for developing this type of infection, but they respond well to treatment; most fatalities occur in patients who are immunocompromised.

Disseminated Coccidioidomycosis

Disseminated coccidioidomycosis may occur as a complication of the primary illness or as a result of reactivation of latent disease in susceptible individuals. The course may be chronic and insidious or rapidly fatal, the latter usually in association with primary disease. Dissemination shows considerable male predominance and a predilection for blacks and Filipinos; pregnant women are also susceptible, especially during the third trimester. Although disease may affect any organ of the body, either alone or in combination, the principal sites of involvement are the skin, bones, joints, kidneys, and meninges.[322] The latter site is affected in as many as 70 per cent of patients and is almost invariably associated with a fatal outcome.

In patients who die of disseminated disease, pulmonary involvement is the rule and is usually extensive. A miliary pattern may occur and represents widespread hematogenous dissemination (Fig. 6–42); it appears most often early in the course of the infection and seldom more than 2 months after onset.[329] Symptoms are often minimal and consist of mild fever, dyspnea, and cachexia.

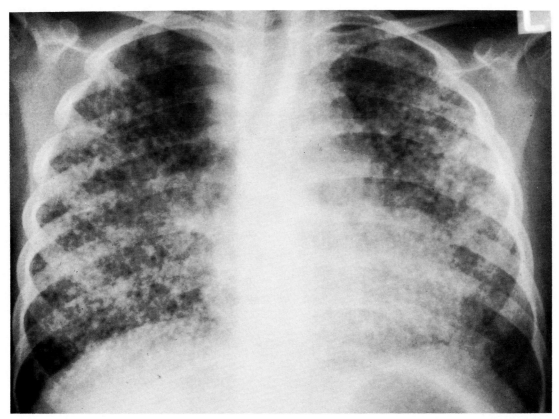

Figure 6–42. Miliary Coccidioidomycosis. Multiple punctate opacities measuring up to 2 mm in diameter are scattered widely throughout both lungs, in some areas being so numerous as to be almost confluent. This child had acute leukemia and was receiving antineoplastic therapy. (Courtesy of Dr. Paul Capp, University of Arizona Medical Center, Tucson.)

Laboratory Findings

Using 10 per cent potassium hydroxide, wet mounts of sputum, pus, gastric washings, or exudates from cutaneous lesions may reveal the large mature spherules that contain endospores. When sputum is unavailable or examination is not diagnostic, flexible fiberoptic bronchoscopy has proved to be a valuable procedure for obtaining material.[330]

The hemoglobin value is decreased in many cases of disseminated disease. The white blood cell count is normal or moderately elevated in most patients, often with a significant degree of eosinophilia, particularly in those with erythema nodosum.

Serologic tests using tube precipitation (TP), latex particle agglutination (LPA), and immunodiffusion (using heated coccidioidin, IDTP) are invaluable for screening, becoming positive 1 to 3 weeks after exposure. The LPA test is more sensitive but less specific than TP; however, neither provides positive results in cerebrospinal fluid of patients with meningitis.[321] A complement fixation reaction becomes positive in the cerebrospinal fluid in most patients who develop meningitis and is diagnostic of dissemination; seropositivity occurs in 50 per cent of patients within 4 weeks and in 90 per cent within 8 weeks.[331] Serum complement fixation titers sustained above 1:16 to 1:32 are unusual in uncomplicated primary coccidioidomycosis and indicate a high risk for progressive primary or disseminated infection.[331]

Skin testing can be done with either spherulin (antigen prepared from the sporangium) or coccidioidin (antigen from mycelial filtrate), the former being the more sensitive.[332] In the benign nondisseminated form of the disease the skin test is positive in virtually all patients within 3 weeks of the onset of infection; it may revert to negative within 2 years but may remain positive for as long as 10 years. Patients with disseminated disease are often anergic, and the reaction may be negative; in fact, a combination of a negative skin test and a complement factor titer greater than 1:16 is practically pathognomonic of disseminated disease.

Blastomyces Dermatitidis (North American Blastomycosis)

North American blastomycosis is caused by the dimorphic fungus *Blastomyces dermatitidis* that occurs as a mycelium in culture and presumably in its natural habitat, and as a yeast at 37°C. In tissue, the yeasts are round or oval in shape, usually measure 8 to 15 μm in diameter, and possess thick walls.

The term "North American blastomycosis" is actually a misnomer, since the disease is considered to be endemic in several regions of Africa.[333] Nevertheless, it occurs most commonly in the Western Hemisphere, mainly the central and southeastern United States, where endemic areas include the Ohio, Mississippi, and Missouri river valleys and the western shore of Lake Michigan.[334]

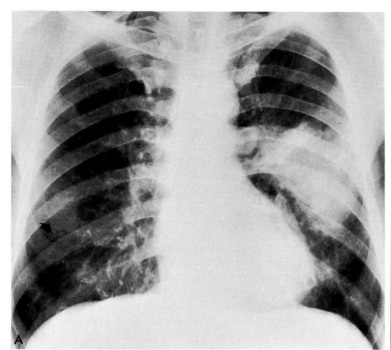
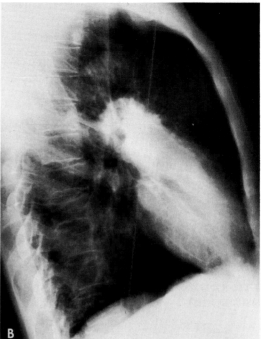

Figure 6–43. North American Blastomycosis. One month prior to admission of this 55-year-old man, a right lower molar tooth had been extracted, followed by the development of swelling below the right eye. Two weeks before admission, he developed a painful swelling of the right side of his chest in the anterior axillary line. On admission, roentgenograms of the chest in posteroanterior (A) and lateral (B) projections demonstrated a large, poorly defined shadow of homogeneous density in the lingula; the consolidation is nonsegmental and shows no evidence of an air bronchogram. In addition, the posteroanterior roentgenogram reveals destruction of the anterior portion of the right fifth rib (arrow). *Blastomyces dermatitidis* was cultured from a 24-hour sputum collection.

The lack of sensitivity and specificity of skin tests and serology in the detection of infection by *B. dermatitidis* and the inability to uncover point sources of outbreaks have prevented an accurate determination of the incidence of the disease; however, clinically evident blastomycosis is uncommon. Middle-aged men are most often affected, the male predominance being 6:1 to 15:1. Although the natural habitat of the organism is not certain, wooded areas appear to be a common site of acquisition of the disease. Infection is believed to occur most often by inhalation of air-borne spores. Occasional cases may represent endogenous reactivation.[335] Most authorities consider *B. dermatitidis* to be a primary pathogen rather than an opportunist; despite this, the disease probably occurs with increased frequency in immunocompromised hosts.[336]

Pathologic Characteristics. The pathologic appearance of acute blastomycosis is usually that of bronchopneumonia. The initial histologic reaction in the lungs is exudative, but this is followed rapidly by mononuclear cell infiltration and, in many instances, by granuloma formation. Progression of disease is manifested by coalescence of separate areas of pneumonia, necrosis, and cavity formation. Airway involvement in the form of ulcerative bronchitis is fairly common.[337] Fibrotic or calcified nodules that represent areas of healed infection are found infrequently at autopsy.

Roentgenographic Manifestations. The commonest pattern is one of acute airspace pneumonia, most often nonsegmental (Fig. 6–43); consolidation is usually homogeneous but may be patchy. The upper lobes are affected more frequently than the lower in a ratio of about 3:2. The next commonest presentation is in the form of a mass, either single or multiple[338]; when solitary, it may mimic primary carcinoma, especially when associated with unilateral lymph node enlargement or bone destruction. The incidence of cavitation ranges from about 15 to 35 per cent.[339] Interstitial disease, hilar and mediastinal lymph node enlargement, and pleural effusion are uncommon; however, pleural thickening without free effusion appears to be a fairly frequent manifestation.[340] Overwhelming infection, usually accompanied by a roentgenographic pattern of miliary dissemination,[341] may be associated with the adult respiratory distress syndrome.[342] CT may be helpful in clarifying the distribution of disease.[342a]

Clinical Manifestations. Experience with miniepidemics indicates that many infected individuals are asymptomatic.[343] Some, however, present with a "flulike" syndrome, usually in the presence of an abnormal chest roentgenogram, or with signs and symptoms of acute pneumonia with pleurisy. As in coccidioidomycosis, erythema nodosum occasionally develops. Rales and rhonchi may be heard in some patients, but signs of parenchymal consolidation are seldom apparent.

Chronic pulmonary disease resembling tuberculosis may follow acute infection or may be the initial form of presentation. The organisms may remain confined to the lungs or may disseminate, most commonly to skin, bone, and the genitourinary tract. In fact, skin lesions are as common as lung lesions and tend to resemble neoplasms.

Laboratory Findings. The leukocyte count is usually normal or only moderately raised but, when disease is extensive, may exceed 30,000 cells per mL. Anemia may develop in cases of chronic disease.

The yeast-phase complement fixation test and serologic and skin tests, using mycelial and yeast antigens, are of no practical value in most cases. Cross-reactions with histoplasmin and coccidioidin are frequent, and a positive blastomycin skin test result should be considered significant only when the reaction is stronger than that to histoplasmin and coccidioidin. Encouraging results have been reported of the use of a double immunodiffusion assay[344] and an enzyme immunoassay[345] for the detection of serum antibody to the A antigen of *B. dermatitidis*.

Organisms may be identified by microscopic examination after 10 per cent potassium hydroxide digestion; perhaps because of the frequency of airway involvement, they are particularly likely to be found in sputum specimens.[346]

Paracoccidioides Brasiliensis (South American Blastomycosis)

South American blastomycosis (paracoccidioidomycosis) is caused by the dimorphic fungus *Paracoccidioides (Blastomyces) brasiliensis*. In tissue, the organism consists predominantly of yeasts that are round to oval in shape and quite variable in diameter, ranging from 2 μm for recently separated buds up to 60 μm for mature mother cells.

The disease is found principally in South and Central America, most commonly in Brazil, Colombia, Venezuela, Peru, Ecuador, and Paraguay. Patients whose disease is recognized in North America or Europe have invariably had prior visits to an endemic area.[347] Clinical disease shows a striking male predominance and is seen most commonly in persons between 25 and 45 years of age.

The natural habitat of the organism is believed to be the soil, and farmers, manual laborers, and other workers engaged in rural occupations are particularly affected. Many cases, however, have been reported in city dwellers and professionals who have not had direct or continued contact with soil.[348] The majority of infections are probably caused by inhalation, resulting in primary pneumonia and secondary systemic dissemination.[349] Animal-to-human and person-to-person transmission have not been documented.

Pathologic Characteristics. Pathologically, pulmonary South American blastomycosis can take a variety of forms, including (1) multiple smooth or lobulated nodules that may become confluent and resemble fibrocaseous tuberculosis, with or without cavitation; (2) solitary paracoccidioidomas; (3) very occasionally, rapidly progressive necrosis and inflammation similar to acute bacterial pneumonia, usually in patients receiving immunosuppressive therapy; and (4) miliary nodules, representing hematogenous spread. Histologic findings consist of a combination of granulomatous and suppurative inflammation.

Roentgenographic Manifestations. The roentgenographic patterns of pulmonary disease are indistinguishable from those of other mycotic infections. In the benign and often asymptomatic form of the primary disease, transient airspace opacities may appear in middle lung zones. Paracoccidioidomas—single or multiple, solid or cavitary—represent a more stable but persistent form of the disease.[350]

Perhaps the most commonly recognized type is one of progressive disease that is often confused with tuberculosis.[351] In this variety, lower lobes are more frequently involved than upper, and cavitation occurs in the minority. Hilar lymph node enlargement may occur in any form of pulmonary parenchymal involvement.

Clinical Manifestations. The results of studies of skin tests clearly indicate that infection is usually asymptomatic.[352] Most clinically documented cases have occurred in patients with dissemination and mucocutaneous manifestations.[353] It should be remembered, however, that in immunosuppressed patients, an acute, progressive, and sometimes fatal pneumonia may develop.

Cryptococcus Neoformans (Cryptococcosis)

In the vast majority of cases, cryptococcosis is caused by *Cryptococcus neoformans*, a unimorphic fungus that exists in yeast form both in its natural habitat and in animals and humans. Although rather pleomorphic, the organisms are usually round to oval in shape and from 5 to 10 μm in diameter in tissue. The majority of strains possess a well-defined capsule that becomes visible as a pericellular halo with India ink preparations and standard tissue mucin stains.

The organism has been found in a variety of natural habitats, of which the most important is dried pigeon excreta. Although it is widely believed that most cases of disease are acquired by inhalation of the organism from these droppings, only occasionally does a history of repeated exposure to pigeons appear to be associated with an increased risk of cryptococcal disease. There is no evidence of transmission from animal to human or person to person. Although cryptococcosis can occur in otherwise normal hosts, it is seen much more frequently in patients with chronic pulmonary disease, those with lymphoproliferative or autoimmune disorders who are receiving chemotherapy or corticosteroid therapy, or those with AIDS.

Pathogenesis and Pathologic Characteristics. Although usually found in tissue as an encapsulated yeast measuring 5 to 10 μm in diameter, there is evidence that many naturally occurring organisms are considerably smaller and lack a capsule.[354] Since the cryptococcal capsule is capable of inhibiting leukocytic phagocytosis to an appreciable extent—in fact, virulence may be correlated with the presence of capsular material[355]—it has been suggested that in the normal host, inhaled capsule-deficient forms are rapidly destroyed by leukocytes. In contrast, in cases in which leukocyte function is impaired, there may be sufficient time for encapsulated forms to be produced locally; since these are resistant to phagocytosis, proliferation and disease may then ensue. Despite these observations, disease is occasionally caused by capsule-deficient forms,[356] and it is likely that other factors such as inoculum size and unidentified virulence factors are also important in the pathogenesis of disease.

Pathologically, pulmonary cryptococcosis may occur in several forms,[357] including (1) relatively well-defined, solitary or multiple nodules that may be solid or cavitated; (2) ill-defined areas of parenchymal consolidation that may involve part or all of the lobe; and (3) widely disseminated parenchymal nodules measuring 1 to 2 mm, representing

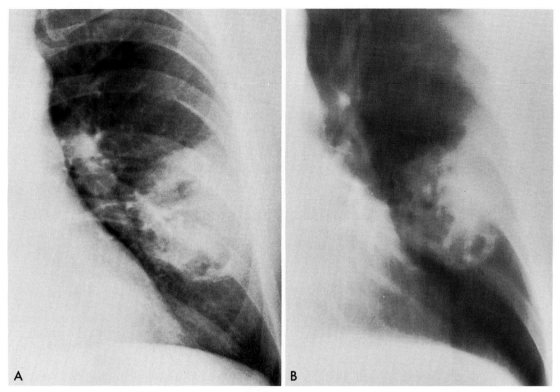

Figure 6–44. Localized Pulmonary Cryptococcosis. Views of the left hemithorax from a posteroanterior roentgenogram *(A)* and an anteroposterior tomogram *(B)* reveal a well-defined mass situated in the axillary portion of the left lower lobe; its lateral aspect abuts the visceral pleura. Several irregular areas of radiolucency are present throughout the mass, representing multiple foci of cavitation. The appearance of the mass is quite characteristic of cryptococcosis, although the cavitation is somewhat unusual. *Cryptococcus neoformans* was cultured from the sputum.

miliary hematogenous spread. As with other fungal infections, the inflammatory reaction is quite variable and may be predominantly granulomatous or suppurative, or a combination of the two. The organisms stain poorly but are recognizable with H&E; they are best identified with silver or mucin stains.

Roentgenographic Manifestations. The commonest roentgenographic manifestation is a fairly well-defined nodule or mass ranging from 2 to 10 cm in diameter (Fig. 6–44).[358] It is usually single and characteristically pleural based. An alternative presentation is a localized area of less well-defined airspace consolidation, usually confined to one lobe[359]; the consolidation may be segmental or nonsegmental in distribution. Cavitation is relatively uncommon compared with other mycoses. Widely disseminated disease may give rise to a miliary pattern or to multiple, diffuse, ill-defined opacities. Hilar and mediastinal lymph node enlargement is unusual. Similarly, pleural effusion is uncommon and usually connotes dissemination of the organism in a patient with underlying disease.[360]

Clinical Manifestations. The initial lung infection often does not occasion symptoms and is probably recognized infrequently. When present, symptoms are usually mild and include cough, scanty mucoid sputum, and, in some cases, chest pain and low-grade fever. Physical examination occasionally reveals rales and rhonchi but seldom signs of consolidation. Dissemination occurs to the central nervous system (commonly causing a low-grade meningitis and sometimes with a normal chest roentgenogram), cutaneous

and mucocutaneous tissues, bones, and, less commonly, the viscera.

In otherwise healthy patients, cryptococcosis is usually confined to the lungs and resolves spontaneously. In immunoincompetent patients, however, dissemination is common and usually occurs weeks to months after the onset of pneumonia; few patients survive without fungicidal therapy.

Laboratory Findings. Although the organism is not a common saprophyte in humans, in perhaps the majority of patients positive culture cannot be definitely considered to indicate disease.[361] A presumptive diagnosis can be made when *C. neoformans* is identified in sputum or bronchial washings in association with roentgenographic evidence of disease. A positive diagnosis is made by appropriate staining or culture of material obtained by transbronchial biopsy, TTNA, or open lung biopsy or by the detection of cryptococcal antigen in the serum; in such circumstances, sputum cultures are usually unrewarding.

Although the various serologic tests used to detect antibody to *C. neoformans* are neither specific nor sensitive, the complement fixation test appears to be more sensitive than either a modified latex fixation or a slide agglutination test.[362] Skin tests are not very helpful because of cross-reactivity with other fungi.[363]

Candidiasis

Candidiasis is caused by fungi of the genus *Candida*, of which *C. albicans* is the most important pathogen. However, in the immunocompromised host, other species are implicated fairly frequently, and the incidence appears to be increasing.[364] In tissue, all species occur as pseudohyphae and yeasts, the latter 2 to 4 μm in diameter.

Candida organisms are common human saprophytes, *C. albicans* being found normally in the gastrointestinal tract and mucocutaneous regions, and a variety of non-*albicans* species being found on the skin. Their numbers are held in check naturally by saprophytic bacteria. Conditions in which the composition of the normal flora is altered—such as antibiotic therapy—are thus likely to lead to overgrowth of *Candida* species and to potential infection. An immunocompromised state is also an important predisposing factor in many infections. In these situations, candidiasis occurs most often in the form of local mucocutaneous infection (oropharynx, vagina, and skin). When clinically significant visceral or disseminated disease develops, it is usually in infants, the elderly, or patients debilitated by chronic disease.

Pulmonary candidiasis can occur as a primary infection acquired by aspiration of organisms from the oral cavity, in which case the pattern is that of a bronchopneumonia associated with a variably intense suppurative response.[365] The infection may remain limited to the lungs or may disseminate. Pulmonary disease also may be part of a systemic hematogenous infection associated with multiorgan involvement and a primary extrapulmonary site (usually the gastrointestinal tract); in these cases, the lungs contain multiple randomly distributed nodules.

The characteristic roentgenographic abnormality is airspace consolidation, sometimes with an interstitial component.[366] Patchy, homogeneous, poorly defined opacities may be bilateral or unilateral. Pleural effusion may develop, but cavitation and hilar or mediastinal lymph node enlargement are uncommon. A diffuse nodular pattern and cavitation in consolidated lung and the formation of an acute "mycetoma"[367] may also occur.

Candidiasis should be suspected in compromised hosts with acute or chronic pulmonary disease showing repeated pure sputum cultures for *Candida* and a positive blood culture, antigenemia, or an increasing titer of anti-*Candida* antibodies.[368] However, since the organism is ordinarily a respiratory tract saprophyte, and transient candidemia can occur without tissue dissemination, conclusive diagnosis requires demonstration of the organism in tissue. Disseminated disease is often a terminal event in debilitated and immunocompromised patients, many of whom are receiving antibiotic, corticosteroid, and/or immunosuppressive therapy.

Aspergillosis

Aspergillosis is a disease of worldwide distribution caused by species of the dimorphic fungus *Aspergillus*. Although approximately 300 species have been described,[369] only a relatively small number have been associated with human disease, the most important being *A. fumigatus*. Other species occasionally pathogenic for humans are *A. niger*, *A. flavus*, and *A. glaucus*.

In the mycelial phase, the organisms occur as septate, rather uniform hyphae, 2 to 4 μm in diameter, with characteristic dichotomous branching at an angle of 45 degrees.

Reproduction occurs by the formation of conidiophores that contain terminal expanded vesicles that produce chains of spores (conidia).

The organisms are extremely hardy and ubiquitous in the environment, having been found in soil, water, and decaying organic material of many types. In most instances, infection is believed to occur by inhalation of air-borne conidia derived from these sites. In addition, the organisms have been isolated in several nosocomial settings, such as ventilation apparatus and opened parenteral medications, in which they have been associated with outbreaks of clinical aspergillosis.[369] There is no evidence of transmission from animal to person or from person to person. Although there is no seasonal predilection for invasive or saprophytic disease, it is generally accepted that episodes of allergic bronchopulmonary aspergillosis are commoner during periods of high atmospheric *Aspergillus* spore counts, which tend to occur during the winter.[370]

Pathogenesis

Aspergillus species produce a variety of toxins, including an endotoxin and several proteases.[369] Although the precise mechanisms by which any of these may be involved in the pathogenesis of disease are not known, the ability of different species and strains to produce them may at least partly explain their variable pathogenicity.[371]

Adequate host defense is clearly important in preventing *Aspergillus* infection. Situations such as a chronic tuberculous cavity, in which clearance of inhaled conidia by the mucociliary escalator is likely to be impaired, are associated with an increased risk of saprophytic disease. Of even greater importance are intact inflammatory and immune systems; for example, granulocytopenia and acute leukemia are strongly associated with the development of invasive aspergillosis. In addition, there is evidence that alveolar macrophages can prevent germination of conidia by phagocytosing and killing them and that defense against invasion is dependent on this mechanism.[372] Of some interest is the observation that intact defense does not appear to be solely determined by the host: there is evidence that spores of *A. fumigatus* produce substances that inhibit both phagocytosis[373] and the production of reactive oxygen intermediates[374] by host phagocytes.

Disease caused by *Aspergillus* organisms may occur by three mechanisms:[374a] (1) saprophytic infestation, usually of preformed parenchymal cavities (aspergilloma); (2) a hypersensitivity reaction, characterized by such entities as allergic bronchopulmonary aspergillosis (ABPA) and extrinsic allergic alveolitis; and (3) invasive, usually necrotizing disease, most often acute and rapidly lethal but sometimes chronic. These three forms of aspergillosis are not mutually exclusive; for example, saprophytic or allergic disease occasionally becomes invasive, and ABPA sometimes is associated with an aspergilloma. Nevertheless, as a rule, each tends to remain true and is associated with significantly different pathologic, radiographic, and clinical features.

Saprophytic Aspergillosis

Saprophytic aspergillosis is characterized by mycelial growth unassociated with invasion of viable tissue. By far the commonest form is the fungus ball or "mycetoma," an abnormality that may be defined as a conglomeration of intertwined fungal hyphae together with fibrin, mucus, and cellular debris within a pulmonary cavity or ectatic bronchus. Many fungal species may cause such a lesion.[375] When a specific organism is identified, however, it is almost always *Aspergillus,* and the term "aspergilloma" is often used to describe these lesions, even in the absence of culture or other proof of etiology.

An aspergilloma most often arises in association with chronic cavitary disease, particularly tuberculosis—of which approximately 25 per cent of patients have a history[375]—and, somewhat less frequently, sarcoidosis[376] and bronchiectasis of unknown cause. Other less common predisposing conditions include chronic fungal cavities, bronchial cysts, chronic bacterial abscesses, and cavitary carcinoma.

Pathologically, an aspergilloma characteristically consists of a round to oval-shaped mass of yellowish or brown granular material (representing fungal hyphae) situated within a cavity surrounded by a fibrous wall of variable thickness (Fig. 6–45). The latter contains chronic inflammatory cells and blood vessels, most of which represent branches of the bronchial arteries and veins and are the source of hemoptysis. An acute inflammatory or granulomatous reaction at the junction of the wall and the mycetoma is seen occasionally, but actual tissue invasion of the organism is not evident.

Roentgenographically, the lesion consists of a solid, rounded mass of unit density within a spherical or ovoid cavity, separated from the wall of the cavity by an airspace of variable size and shape (Fig. 6–46). It occurs much more commonly in upper than in lower lobes, probably because it so frequently occupies a tuberculous cavity. Cavities are usually thin-walled; however, thickening of the walls has been described as an early roentgenographic sign of *Aspergillus* colonization, antedating the formation of a fungus ball.[377] Characteristically, the fungus ball moves when the patient changes position. Calcification of the mycelial mass may be apparent as scattered small nodules, as a fine rim around the periphery of the mass, or as an extensive process involving the greater part of the mycelial ball. The size of the ball may change or may remain constant for many years.

Not all mycetomas possess features that permit easy roentgenographic identification. Some are irregular in shape, conforming to an elongated bronchiectatic cavity; in these cases, change in the position of the patient may not be accompanied by a concomitant movement of the fungus ball. In other cases, the mycelial mass may grow to fill a cavity completely, effectively obliterating the airspace necessary for its recognition roentgenologically. CT can sometimes reveal a spongelike appearance of an otherwise solid mass, even to the point of showing a fairly prominent air-containing space in the center of the mass.[378]

Clinically, cough and expectoration are common, and hemoptysis has been reported in 50 to 95 per cent of cases.[379] The diagnosis is usually readily apparent from the roentgenographic features; if confirmation is necessary, invasive procedures such as surgical excision, TTNA, or bronchial washings of the affected lobe are usually required. The diagnosis also may be suggested by the finding of a positive precipitin test.

The prognosis is good in the majority of patients. Occasionally, hemoptysis necessitates bronchial artery embolization or surgical resection; rarely, it is sufficient to cause death. The lesions undergo spontaneous lysis in 5 to 10 per cent of cases.[380]

Hypersensitivity Aspergillosis

Although hypersensitivity reactions to *Aspergillus* organisms may take the form of extrinsic allergic alveolitis or Löffler's syndrome, by far the commonest manifestation is a somewhat variable clinicopathologic entity known as allergic bronchopulmonary aspergillosis (ABPA). In this condition, the fungus resides in the patient's airways, producing a continual supply of fresh antigen that is responsible for the presence of precipitating antibodies, an immediate and often delayed skin sensitivity, the production of IgE, and both bronchial wall and blood eosinophilia. This combination of findings strongly suggests that the fungus is playing more than a saprophytic role. Most patients with ABPA are atopic; in fact, in some series as many as 25 per cent of asthmatics who manifest immediate skin reactivity to *A. fumigatus* have ABPA.[381] For unknown reasons, patients with cystic fibrosis are also susceptible to ABPA; in fact, ABPA may be an important factor in the rapid clinical deterioration of some patients with this disease.[382]

Pathologically, segmental and proximal subsegmental airways are dilated and filled with thick inspissated mucus, which usually contains numerous eosinophils and fragmented fungal hyphae.[383] The adjacent bronchial walls typically contain lymphocytes, plasma cells, and fairly numerous eosinophils; there is seldom evidence of fungal invasion. In many cases, the histologic pattern of bronchocentric granulomatosis is seen in smaller airways (*see* page 417).

The characteristic roentgenographic pattern of ABPA is homogeneous, fingerlike shadows of unit density in a precise bronchial distribution, usually involving the upper lobes and almost always in the segmental and more central subsegmental bronchi rather than the main, lobar or peripheral bronchi (Fig. 6–47).[384] These bifurcating opacities have been variously described, according to their orientation on the roentgenogram, as having a "gloved-finger," inverted Y or V, or "cluster-of-grapes" appearance. Although the impacted bronchi may relate to atelectatic areas, in our experience this is often notable by its absence, a fact attributable to collateral air drift. The shadows tend to be transient but may persist unchanged for weeks or even months or may enlarge. In the former situation, they tend to recur in the same segmental bronchi, suggesting that bronchial damage predisposes to further episodes.[384] Resolution of the mucoid impaction may reveal cylindrical or saccular bronchiectasis (Fig. 6–48); such dilated bronchi may contain a fluid level[385] or, occasionally, a true aspergilloma.[386] Pleural disease is very uncommon.

Clinically, acute episodes of ABPA are sometimes associated with increased cough, hemoptysis, fever, pleuritic pain, wheezing, and dyspnea.[387] Just as often, however, there is little change in the state of the patient, and the incident is not recognized unless a chest roentgenogram is obtained or serum IgE levels are monitored. With recurrent attacks, almost half the patients expectorate plugs, and

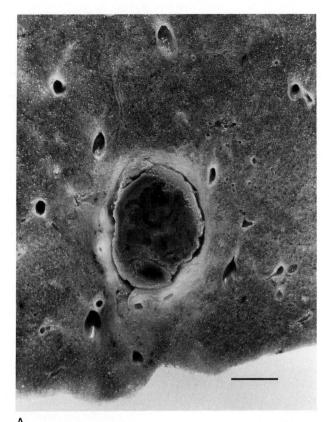

A

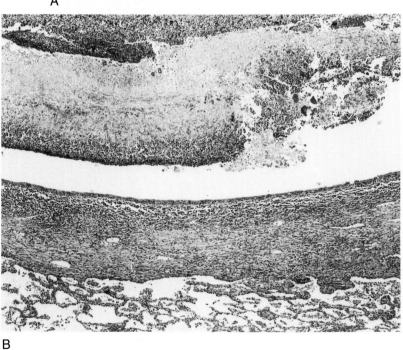

B

Figure 6–45. Aspergilloma. *A,* Magnified view of the basal aspect of a left lower lobe shows a somewhat laminated mass that resembles a thrombus within a thin-walled cavity. *B,* A section through the cavity wall shows fibrosis, chronic inflammation, and an intact epithelial lining. The fungus ball itself consists of scattered polymorphonuclear leukocytes and numerous hyphae (barely visible at this magnification). The patient is a 26-year-old woman with hemoptysis; the etiology of the cavity was not determined. (Bar = 0.5 cm; *B* × 40.)

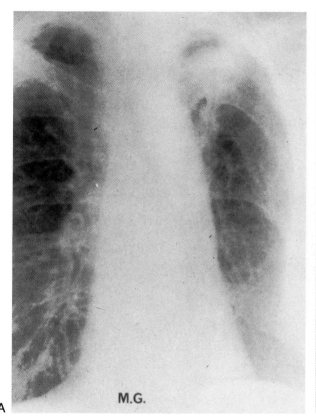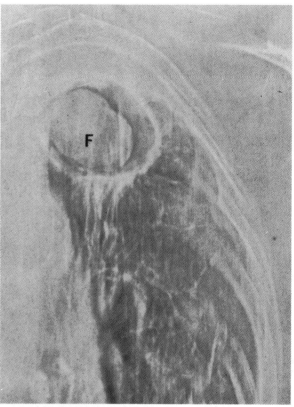

A

B

Figure 6–46. Aspergilloma in a Tuberculous Cavity. *A,* A posteroanterior chest roentgenogram demonstrates a left apical opacity consisting of a well-defined homogeneous mass. An air crescent around the opacity is suggested. The left hilum is elevated as a result of upper lobe fibrosis secondary to long-standing tuberculosis. The sixth and eighth left ribs and part of the lower lobe were surgically excised many years previously for bronchiectasis. An anteroposterior xerotomogram *(B)* demonstrates to excellent advantage a fungus ball (F) within the well-defined, thin-walled cavity. A prominent apical fibrotic cap is also seen.

a slightly lesser number produce sputum suggesting the development of bronchiectasis.[388]

Patterson and colleagues[389] recognize five stages or categories of ABPA that they feel aid in its management:

1. An acute stage characterized by typical roentgenographic manifestations and by laboratory evidence of *Aspergillus* sensitivity.

2. A stage of remission in which corticosteroid therapy results in control of asthma, clearing of the chest roentgenogram, and a decrease in levels of IgE and in eosinophilia.

3. A stage in which exacerbations may occur and may not be symptom-producing, manifested only by a rise in IgE levels and by roentgenographic evidence of mucous plugging.

4. A stage characterized by corticosteroid-dependent asthma. Even with complete control of asthma, however, acute exacerbations of ABPA may occur, and despite the prednisone therapy the majority of patients will show a rise in precipitins, in specific IgE and IgG, and in total IgE.

5. A fibrotic stage, the result of long-standing ABPA and characterized by bronchiectasis and functional obstruction unresponsive to corticosteroids.

A variety of laboratory findings are useful in diagnosis. Eosinophilia of blood (>1000 cells per mL) and sputum is common in adults, although often absent in children.[389]

Levels of total serum IgE are almost always elevated, constituting a reliable screening test for acute attacks.[390] Levels of serum IgE and IgG antibodies to *Aspergillus* are also typically raised. Delayed and immediate skin reactivity may be present to intracutaneous tests with *Aspergillus* antigen, and sputum culture may be positive for *Aspergillus* species.

Most patients with ABPA whose disease remits on steroid therapy will show subsequent exacerbations.[387] Although it has been well established that unrecognized episodes of ABPA can result in irreversible airway obstruction, severe bronchiectasis, pulmonary fibrosis, and even death, some studies have shown little clinical deterioration in the majority of cases. The necessity of monitoring patients with periodic serum sampling for IgE has been emphasized,[391] an increase usually occurring before roentgenographic evidence of mucous plugging. Functional disability has been shown to be related to the chronicity of the disease; in 11 of 17 patients with stage 5 disease (as defined previously) who survived for 5 years, respiratory impairment was mild to moderate in seven and severe in four.[392]

Invasive Aspergillosis

The term "invasive aspergillosis" implies extension of *Aspergillus* organisms into viable tissue, usually associated with necrosis. This form of disease almost always develops

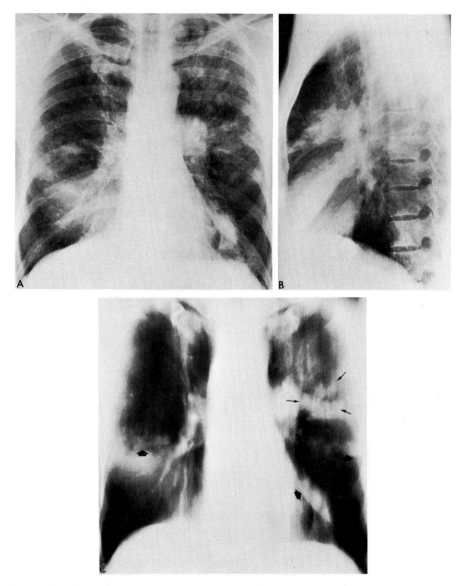

Figure 6–47. Allergic Bronchopulmonary Aspergillosis. Posteroanterior *(A)* and lateral *(B)* roentgeno-grams reveal extensive bilateral pulmonary disease, all lobes of the lung being affected by a process possessing an unusual mixed pattern. In the left upper lobe, the pattern appears to be one of airspace consolidation, confluent shadows of homogeneous density being associated with an air bronchogram; the medial segment of the right middle lobe shows a combination of atelectasis and consolidation; broad areas of consolidation extend into the anterior basal segment of the left lower lobe and the anterior segment of the left upper lobe. A full lung tomogram in anteroposterior projection *(C)* shows numerous broad-band shadows bilaterally, each measuring approximately 1 cm in diameter and extending in a distribution compatible with the bronchovascular bundles *(thick arrows)*; in the mid-portion of the left lung, one possesses a Y configuration *(thin arrows)*. These band shadows are caused by inspissated mucus within markedly dilated bronchi. Note that with the exception of the right middle lobe, all impacted bronchi are unassociated with consolidation or atelectasis of the lung distal to them, presumably as a result of effective collateral air drift.

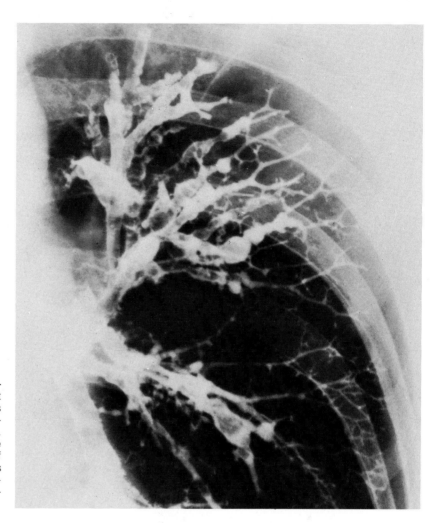

Figure 6–48. Bronchogram in Allergic Bronchopulmonary Aspergillosis. A bronchogram of the left lung in a patient with established ABPA reveals irregular dilatation of the segmental and subsegmental branches of the left upper lobe bronchus. Contrast medium that has passed beyond the bronchiectatic segments has opacified airways of normal appearance. This proximal bronchiectasis is characteristic of mucoid impaction, with or without hypersensitivity bronchopulmonary aspergillosis.

in patients whose host defenses are impaired, most commonly as a result of cancer and its therapy.[393] Patients with acute leukemia who are in relapse and have granulocytopenia are particularly susceptible, accounting for 50 to 70 per cent of cases.[394] Disease often develops when patients are receiving corticosteroid, immunosuppressive, or antineoplastic therapy, or antibiotic therapy directed against a gram-negative organism.

Pulmonary involvement occurs in the vast majority of cases of invasive aspergillosis and may take several forms, including tracheobronchitis, necrotizing bronchopneumonia, and "hemorrhagic infarction." Dissemination outside the thorax occurs in 25 to 50 per cent of patients, chiefly to the gastrointestinal tract, brain, liver, kidneys, and heart.

Bronchitis (and less often tracheitis) is a relatively uncommon manifestation in which infection is limited principally to the larger airways with little, if any, extension of organisms into surrounding pulmonary parenchyma or blood vessels.[395] Pathologically, there is focal or diffuse mucosal ulceration, often associated with pseudomembranes or large intraluminal plugs of mucus and hyphae. Patchy areas of atelectasis related to the mixed mucus-mycelial plugs may be the only roentgenographic abnormality. Clinically, patients manifest dyspnea, wheezing, cough, and hemoptysis.

Aspergillus bronchopneumonia may develop secondary to bronchitis, as described previously, or, more commonly,

in a fashion analogous to bacterial bronchopneumonia. The roentgenographic pattern is one of patchy airspace consolidation without specific features.[393] Clinically, patients characteristically present with unremitting fever that responds poorly or not at all to antibiotic therapy; sometimes there is an initial response and then failure. Dyspnea and tachypnea occur in cases of more extensive disease.

Probably the commonest manifestation of invasive pulmonary aspergillosis is "hemorrhagic infarction." Pathologically, this can possess two patterns:[396] a relatively well-defined nodule with a pale or yellowish center and hemorrhagic rim (Fig. 6–49) or a less well-defined, roughly wedge-shaped, pleural-based hemorrhagic area resembling a typical thromboembolic infarct. Although the latter appearance probably reflects vascular occlusion and true ischemic necrosis, it is unlikely that the former has the same pathogenesis; its characteristic spherical appearance suggests that locally produced toxins diffusing into adjacent lung parenchyma may be of greater importance. Histologically, both patterns show coagulative necrosis and adjacent intra-alveolar hemorrhage. Characteristically, there is extensive vascular permeation and apparent occlusion of small to medium-sized arteries by fungal hyphae; thrombus may or may not be present.

The roentgenographic pattern consists of single or multiple areas of homogeneous consolidation, sometimes in the form of so-called round pneumonia.[397] Cavitation is com-

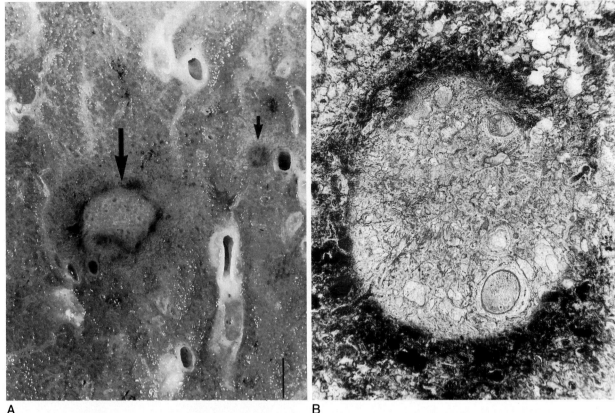

Figure 6–49. Nodular "Infarction" Caused by *Aspergillus*. *A,* Magnified view of lung parenchyma shows a roughly circular focus of necrosis surrounded by a well-defined hemorrhagic rim *(long arrow).* Note that the underlying lung architecture is easily distinguished, implying coagulative necrosis. A smaller focus is present below *(short arrow).* (Bar = 5 mm.) *B,* Corresponding histologic appearance confirming that central pallor corresponds to necrotic lung parenchyma. (*B,* × 16.)

mon (Fig. 6–50) and is sometimes manifested by an unusual and almost distinctive pattern consisting of "air crescents" partly or completely surrounding a central homogeneous mass.[398] This "air crescent sign," which can develop from 1 day to 3 weeks after the appearance of the initial roentgenographic abnormality, results from separation of a fragment of necrotic lung infiltrated by fungus from adjacent viable parenchyma. Occasionally, the characteristically patchy pneumonia extends to involve an entire lobe, roentgenographically simulating acute airspace pneumonia.[399] Both CT[400] and magnetic resonance imaging (MRI)[401] may be of assistance in roentgenographic evaluation.

Clinically, patients with this form of invasive aspergillosis present with fever, dyspnea, and nonproductive cough. Hemoptysis may occur, but it is rarely massive. Pleuritic chest pain is common.[393] Thrombosis of large vessels may suggest a diagnosis of acute thromboembolic disease.

In addition to these acute forms of invasive aspergillosis, there is evidence for a more chronic variety characterized by slowly progressive upper lobe disease that may spread to the contralateral lung and invade the mediastinum, pleural space, or chest wall (chronic necrotizing pulmonary aspergillosis).[402] Most patients are elderly and have a history of previous resectional surgery, radiation therapy, pulmonary infarction, inactive mycobacterial disease, chronic obstructive pulmonary disease, or pneumoconiosis. Cough and expectoration, fever, weight loss, and an increased

white blood cell count may be present. Distant spread is uncommon.

The diagnosis of invasive aspergillosis should be suspected in any patient with an organ transplant, acute leukemia, or other lymphoreticular or hematologic disease associated with granulocytopenia when fever does not respond to broad-spectrum antibiotics. It may be difficult to prove. Sputum is unavailable in many cases, and even when present, its culture is positive in fewer than 10 per cent of patients.[397] To compound matters, positive sputum culture often reflects simple colonization. Nevertheless, in the appropriate clinical setting, repeated positive sputum cultures have been found to be a reliable method of diagnosis.[403] Culture and histochemical staining of cytocentrifuged material obtained by BAL has been reported to have a high diagnostic yield[404]; however, blood cultures are almost never positive. In the final analysis, definitive diagnosis often requires open lung biopsy, a procedure that is not without hazard in these very ill patients with low platelet counts.

Invasive aspergillosis in any form has a poor prognosis, with progression of pulmonary disease and/or dissemination leading to death in many patients. The importance of early diagnosis lies in the well-documented fact that patients treated at this stage are the only ones to survive. For this reason there seems to be general agreement that when the diagnosis is strongly suspected, empiric treatment with one or more fungicides should be initiated promptly.

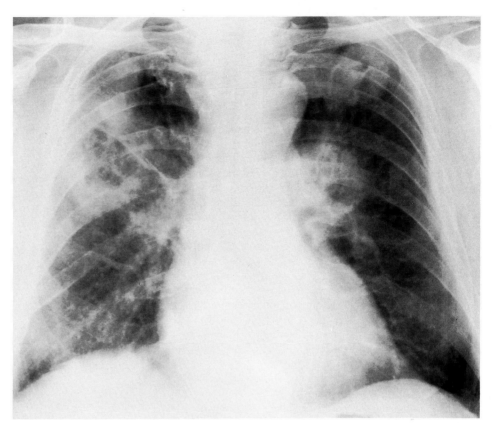

Figure 6–50. Acute Invasive Aspergillosis. This 70-year-old man was admitted to the hospital with the diagnosis of pemphigus vulgaris, which required high doses of corticosteroid therapy for control. He was also diabetic. Within 3 weeks of the beginning of corticosteroid therapy, he developed a cough productive of moderate amounts of mucopurulent sputum that, over a brief period of time, became copious in amount and blood-tinged. This posteroanterior roentgenogram reveals large, thick-walled cavities in both lungs, possessing irregular shaggy inner linings. *Aspergillus fumigatus* was cultured both from the sputum and from creamy pus aspirated directly from one of the cavities.

Mucormycosis

Mucormycosis (phycomycosis, zygomycosis) is caused by fungi of the order Mucorales, which includes a variety of species in the genera *Rhizopus, Rhizomucor, Mucor, Absidia, Saksenaea,* and *Cunninghamella.* The pathologic and roentgenographic features of thoracic disease caused by all species are similar. In tissue the organisms appear as broad (5 to 20 μm), frequently irregular, nonseptate hyphae that branch at varying angles up to 90 degrees. In nature, the hyphae produce large sporangia that liberate sporangiospores into the air, from which it is believed that most human infections are acquired.

The fungi are ubiquitous and worldwide in distribution. They are commonly found in decaying organic material, such as fruit or bread, and are frequent laboratory contaminants. There are no age, sex, or occupational risk factors. Infection occurs almost invariably in patients with underlying disease, particularly during treatment with corticosteroids or antibiotics; the commonest primary diseases are diabetes (especially when associated with ketoacidosis), lymphoma, and leukemia.

Pathologically, pulmonary mucormycosis is similar to the nodular, hemorrhagic form of invasive aspergillosis. Vascular invasion is common and may result in parenchymal hemorrhage or infarction, with or without cavitation. Roentgenographically, lung involvement usually takes the form of segmental and homogeneous opacification (reflecting vascular obstruction) or solitary or multiple nodules.[405] Cavitation is frequent and may be associated with a crescent sign identical to that in invasive aspergillosis.[406]

Patients usually are very ill with fever, chest pain, and bloody sputum. The diagnosis may be difficult to make and may require transbronchial or open lung biopsy. Although the overall prognosis is grave, some success may be achieved with control of diabetes and a reduction or cessation of immunosuppressive therapy.

Geotrichum Candidum (Geotrichosis)

Geotrichosis is caused by *Geotrichum candidum,* a ubiquitous yeastlike fungus that in nature is found in soil, sewage, animal excreta, and a variety of dairy and spoiled food products. In the lungs, the organism is detected most frequently as a saprophyte in the sputum of patients with chronic pulmonary disease. True infection—which is rare and is believed to be derived from endogenous saprophytic organisms—has been divided into two forms. The bronchial type is associated with symptoms of bronchitis or asthma, occasionally with eosinophilia.[407] Bronchoscopy reveals yellow-white plaques, similar to those of oral candidiasis, adherent to the airway mucosa. Invasion of underlying parenchyma does not occur. By contrast, in the bronchopulmonary form of the disease, tissue invasion may be extensive; fever and hemoptysis are present in most cases. In both bronchial and bronchopulmonary disease, purulent expectoration may be copious, and the sputum may be very gelatinous.[408]

The bronchial form of the disease may show no roentgenographic abnormalities or merely an accentuation of basal pulmonary markings.[407] Bronchopulmonary disease usually is manifested by parenchymal consolidation, predominantly in the upper lobes and frequently associated with thin-walled cavities. A skin test and an agglutination test are available and are useful in diagnosis.[407]

Sporothrix Schenckii (Sporotrichosis)

Sporotrichosis is caused by *Sporothrix (Sporotrichum) schenckii*, a dimorphic fungus of worldwide distribution that has been isolated from soil, peat moss, decaying vegetable matter, and a variety of other substances. The disease is usually acquired by direct inoculation into the skin through a scratch from thorns, splinters, grasses, or other contaminated objects. In many cases, such inoculation is related to a specific occupation; for example, in the United States farmers, laborers, florists, and horticulturalists are especially vulnerable. Although most patients are not immunocompromised, particularly when disease is confined to the skin, alcoholics appear to be unusually susceptible.[409]

Sporotrichosis has a variety of clinical forms, including lymphocutaneous (by far the most frequent), mucocutaneous, extracutaneous (usually musculoskeletal), and disseminated. Respiratory disease is usually primary and presumably results from inhalation of spores; occasionally it represents dissemination from cutaneous lesions. The organism also may exist as a simple pulmonary colonist.[410]

The typical histologic pattern consists of necrotic tissue surrounded by a granulomatous inflammatory infiltrate containing numerous giant cells. Organisms may be scanty and difficult to identify with certainty.

Roentgenographically, pulmonary sporotrichosis closely resembles postprimary tuberculosis and, as a result, is probably frequently misdiagnosed. Changes include isolated nodular masses that may cavitate, leaving thin-walled cavities.[409] Hilar lymph node enlargement occurs in many cases and may cause bronchial obstruction[411]; bronchopulmonary and mediastinal lymph node enlargement may be present in the absence of parenchymal disease. A diffuse reticulonodular pattern has also been described.[412]

Clinical manifestations in the cutaneous form of the disease consist of a pustule on the hand or arm accompanied by enlargement of regional lymph nodes. Pulmonary involvement may be associated with severe malaise, cough, and fever. In disseminated disease, the joints may be tender and swollen. Anemia and polymorphonuclear leukocytosis may develop.

Serologic tests are highly specific and should be considered in any case of chronic cavitary disease when acid-fast organisms are not found. Skin test reactions to sporotrichin may be helpful in some cases, although they may be positive in individuals without active disease.[413]

Pseudoallescheriasis

Pseudoallescheriasis (allescheriasis, monosporidiosis, petriellidiosis) is caused by a ubiquitous soil- and sewage-inhabiting fungus that, in its perfect form, is known as *Pseudoallescheria boydii*.[414] A substantial number of cases have been described in farmers and other persons from rural settings. In tissue, the organism appears as septate hyphae similar to *Aspergillus* species, from which it usually cannot be confidently distinguished by morphology alone.

In the lungs, the organism occurs most frequently as a colonizer in association with immunosuppressive or corticosteroid therapy or with chronic fibrotic disease, such as tuberculosis, sarcoidosis, and ankylosing spondylitis.[415] The roentgenographic pattern is one of cavitation, sometimes accompanied by a fungus ball.[416] Clinically, affected patients may be asymptomatic or may suffer repeated hemoptysis; sometimes the only symptoms and signs are those of the underlying disease. The organism must be cultured for certain diagnosis.

Actinomycosis

Actinomycosis is caused by several species of the family Actinomycetaceae, of which the most important is *Actinomyces israelii*. The organisms occur as branching filaments about 0.2 to 0.3 μm in diameter that are pleomorphic in shape. They are anaerobic or microaerophilic and form mycelia that, in tissue, characteristically occur as granules that range in diameter from 40 to 400 μm ("sulfur granules"). Microscopically, these are round to oval, slightly lobulated, basophilic masses, in the center of which organisms can be identified as Gram- and silver-positive filaments. Granules are present in the majority of *Actinomyces* infections, and their presence in the sputum or in exudate from sinus tracts is highly suggestive of the diagnosis.

The organisms are normal inhabitants of the human oropharynx, and in the majority of cases pulmonary infection is believed to be acquired by aspiration of contaminated secretions from this site. Most infections occur in persons who are not immunocompromised.

Pathogenesis and Pathologic Characteristics

The pathogenesis of actinomycosis is not well understood. The organism produces no known toxins, and the presence of granules has not been shown to inhibit phagocytosis or other host defense mechanisms. Differences in the inflammatory reaction to the organisms in experimental animals have suggested that such features as "rough" versus "smooth" growth or specific cell surface structures may be involved in the greater pathogenicity of *A. israelii* compared with other *Actinomyces* species.[418]

Pathologically, chronic pulmonary actinomycosis is characterized by multiple abscesses interconnected by granulating sinus tracts.[419] Pleural fibrosis and adhesions are frequent, and the infection sometimes extends across the pleura into the chest wall or, less commonly, into the mediastinum. Histologically, the abscesses are composed of an outer rim of granulation tissue surrounding masses of polymorphonuclear leukocytes that contain typical actinomycotic granules. The adjacent lung parenchyma shows a variable degree of fibrosis and chronic nonspecific inflammation.

Roentgenographic Manifestations

The typical pattern in acute actinomycosis consists of airspace pneumonia, without recognizable segmental distribution, commonly in the periphery of the lung and with a predilection for the lower lobes (Fig. 6–51). The subsequent course depends largely on whether antibiotic therapy is instituted. With appropriate therapy, most cases resolve without complications. If therapy is not instituted, one or more lung abscesses commonly develop, and the infection may extend into the pleura (with consequent empyema) and thence into the chest wall, with osteomyelitis of the ribs and abscess formation in these areas. Although such extension is characteristic of actinomycosis, it is not unique

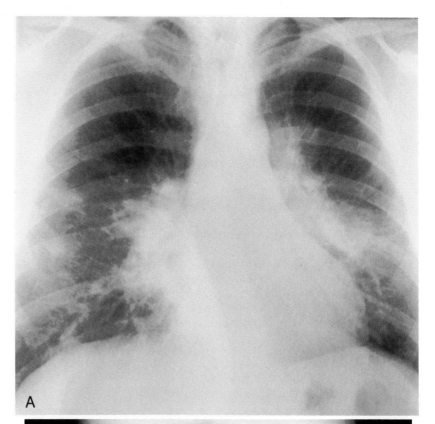

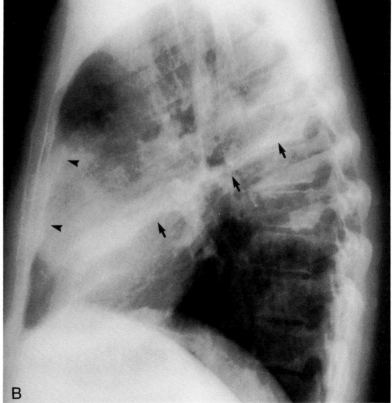

Figure 6–51. Pleuropulmonary Actinomycosis. Posteroanterior *(A)* and lateral *(B)* chest roentgenograms reveal bilateral airspace consolidation involving predominantly the medial segment of the middle lobe and the superior segment of the left lower lobe. The pleura is slightly thickened anteriorly *(arrowheads)*, as is the right major fissure *(arrows)*, representing pleural transgression; the chest wall was not affected.

to this disease—it may also occur in blastomycosis, cryptococcosis, and, of course, tuberculosis. CT can facilitate the diagnosis in questionable cases, particularly in demonstrating cavitation or central areas of low attenuation not apparent on conventional roentgenograms.[420]

Frequently, actinomycosis also presents as a mass that simulates pulmonary carcinoma.[421] Since resolution usually requires prolonged antibiotic therapy, such a lesion may undergo initial remission following institution of therapy, only to exacerbate when therapy has been withdrawn too early. In those patients in whom the pleuropulmonary disease becomes chronic, extensive fibrosis in and about the lung may become a prominent roentgenographic feature,[422] the result being severe distortion of normal anatomic structures.

Clinical Manifestations

Symptoms include cough, initially dry but often becoming productive of purulent, blood-streaked sputum. Pain on breathing may develop as the infection spreads to the pleura and chest wall. Examination of the chest may reveal signs of consolidation and, in some cases, a soft tissue mass. Complicating sinus tracts may result in a bronchocutaneous fistula, mediastinitis, or pericarditis. Dissemination to extrapulmonary sites may occur.[417]

The leukocyte count usually is normal or moderately increased. As the disease progresses, weight loss, anemia, and finger clubbing may occur. The development of pleural effusion almost certainly indicates empyema.[423]

Nocardiosis

Nocardiosis is caused by species of the family Nocardiaceae, of which the most important cause of human pulmonary disease is *Nocardia asteroides*. The organisms are aerobic and non–spore-forming and, in tissue, appear as delicate branching filamentous hyphae. "Sulfur granules" such as those seen in actinomycosis are rarely found and then almost invariably in association with cutaneous and subcutaneous disease.[424]

Nocardia species are common natural inhabitants of soil throughout the world, and most cases of pulmonary disease are believed to be acquired by direct inhalation of organisms from this source. Person-to-person transmission is rare, but there is little doubt that it happens, miniepidemics having occurred in renal transplant units.[425] Instances in which the organism has been identified in the sputum of apparently healthy persons with normal chest roentgenograms[426] and in patients with chronic obstructive pulmonary disease[427] have suggested that in some cases it may be present as a saprophyte.

Nocardiosis may occur as a primary pulmonary disease, in which form it may be commoner than is generally recognized, particularly in some parts of the world.[428] In industrialized countries, however, *N. asteroides* is now more frequently recognized as an opportunistic invader in patients with chronic disease, particularly lymphoma, and, for reasons not well understood, pulmonary alveolar proteinosis[429] and systemic lupus erythematosus in men.[430]

Pathologically, nocardiosis may be manifested by homogeneous consolidation of part or all of a lobe, relatively well-circumscribed nodules or a large multiloculated abscess. Microscopically, the disease is characterized by microabscesses or macroabscesses within which organisms can usually be identified with appropriate stains.

The roentgenologically apparent changes vary but, in most respects, are similar to those of actinomycosis. The most frequent manifestation is airspace pneumonia, usually homogeneous and nonsegmental, but sometimes patchy and inhomogeneous; cavitation is frequent. As with actinomycosis, the infection may extend into the pleural space and cause empyema. Solitary nodules have occasionally been reported.[431]

Cough, purulent sputum (sometimes blood-streaked), pleural pain, and night sweats are the usual symptoms. Examination may reveal rales over the affected area and signs of consolidation or pleural effusion in some cases. The course is usually chronic; however, in patients with lowered resistance, acute, fulminating pneumonia may develop.[431] The infection may spread to other areas of the body, most often the brain or subcutaneous tissue.

The white blood cell count usually is moderately elevated, with neutrophilia; lymphocytosis or leukopenia develops in a few cases. Animal inoculation and serologic tests do not aid diagnosis.

MYCOPLASMA PNEUMONIAE, VIRUSES, CHLAMYDIAE, AND RICKETTSIAE

Many respiratory tract infections caused by these organisms begin in the upper respiratory passages. Some, including certain enteroviruses and the chickenpox and measles viruses, propagate there and disseminate throughout the body, usually without producing lower respiratory tract symptoms. Others typically remain confined to the respiratory mucosa, where they cause a spectrum of disease ranging from mild, virtually asymptomatic rhinitis to acute laryngotracheobronchitis (croup), tracheobronchitis, bronchiolitis, bronchopneumonia, and "primary atypical pneumonia."* Although specific respiratory viruses tend to produce fairly well-defined clinical syndromes, each may cause any form of upper or lower respiratory tract infection, depending on the virulence and dose of the organism and the host's resistance.

The diagnosis of viral pneumonia is often one of exclusion and is based on an absence of sputum production, a failure to culture pathogenic bacteria, a relatively benign clinical presentation, a white blood cell count that is normal or only slightly elevated, a chest roentgenogram that reveals localized interstitial disease, and a lack of response to antibiotic therapy. Radioimmunoassay methods to detect virus antigen may be employed to provide an early presumptive diagnosis.[432] Confirmation requires culture of the organism or a fourfold rise in a specific antibody titer. Use of the

---

*The term "primary atypical pneumonia" was used at one time to describe a form of pneumonia that differed clinically and roentgenographically from bacterial pneumonia. Since the initial descriptions, it has become clear that most cases are caused by *Mycoplasma pneumoniae*, with a lesser number resulting from viruses, Chlamydiae, and Rickettsiae. Although initially the term served some purpose by describing a disorder of unknown etiology, it is logical that with the discovery of its various specific etiologies, it should be discarded as superfluous.

highly specific and sensitive polymerase chain reaction also may prove to be helpful in diagnosing early infection.

Mycoplasma Pneumoniae

The mycoplasmas (pleuropneumonia-like organisms [PPLO]) are the smallest free-living organisms that can be cultured on artificial media. In experimental and human infections they tend to be filamentous or rod-shaped. At one end is a specialized terminal structure that is believed to be necessary for attachment of the organism to epithelial surfaces.[433] Of the nine species that have been recognized, only *M. pneumoniae* has been consistently associated with human respiratory disease; other species cultured from the respiratory tract are usually considered as commensals.[434]

M. pneumoniae is generally accepted as the commonest cause of clinically evident nonbacterial pneumonia, having been estimated to account for 10 to 33 per cent of all pneumonias in civilian populations[435] and for approximately one third of pneumonias in marine recruits.[436] Infections occur throughout the year, with a peak during the autumn and early winter. Disease is commonest in children, adolescents, and young adults.

Infection is believed to be acquired by droplet inhalation. A "carrier state" after recovery from active infection may persist for several months, and spread of infection occurs after prolonged contact in close communities; schoolchildren are probably the major sources of infection. Local outbreaks may occur within a family or other close groups such as military inductees.[436a] More widespread epidemics occur occasionally.[437] The incubation period is 1 to 3 weeks.

Pathogenesis and Pathologic Characteristics

The pathogenesis of *M. pneumoniae* infection is poorly understood and may be related to several mechanisms. The organism is initially localized along the tracheobronchial epithelium, where it is in intimate contact with the surface of ciliated cells.[433] Both scanning and transmission electron microscopic studies of infected tracheal organ cultures[438] have revealed cytopathologic changes, suggesting a direct toxic action by the organism; however, the responsible toxin has not been identified. The possibility that tissue damage is related to the local effects of enzymes and oxygen free radicals released from macrophages has also been proposed.[439]

Immune mechanisms not only play a protective role in *M. pneumoniae* infection but also are implicated in the pathogenesis of disease itself.[438] This concept is supported by the observations that immunodeficient animals and patients appear to be resistant to the development of *Mycoplasma* pneumonia and that protection against infection is afforded by antithymocyte serum and corticosteroid therapy.[440]

Pathologic findings consist principally of a mononuclear inflammatory infiltrate within bronchial and bronchiolar walls; epithelial necrosis may develop, in which case polymorphonuclear leukocytes also may be present. A mononuclear cell infiltrate and type II cell hyperplasia occur to a variable degree in adjacent parenchyma. In severe disease, an airspace exudate may occur.

Roentgenographic Manifestations

The patterns of acute *Mycoplasma* pneumonia are indistinguishable from those of many viral pneumonias and consist of interstitial or airspace opacities or a combination of both. In the early stages, the interstitial inflammation causes a rather fine reticular pattern, followed by signs of airspace consolidation of patchy distribution (Fig. 6–52).[441] With resolution—which usually occurs in 1 to 3 weeks[442]—the process is reversed, the airspace consolidation disappearing first.

In one study of 100 patients, two distinct clinical and roentgenographic presentations were recognized.[443] The largest group (48 patients) presented with symptoms of short duration characteristic of acute pneumonia, including nonpleuritic chest pain, cough, myalgias, and fever. Roentgenologically, there was segmental or lobar consolidation associated with an air bronchogram and sometimes with atelectasis; pleural effusion was evident on erect posteroanterior and lateral roentgenograms of nine patients (19 per cent).

The second group (28 patients) presented with symptoms of malaise, lethargy, and dyspnea ranging in duration from 1 to 4 weeks; in contrast with the first group, most of these patients were afebrile and were free from cough, myalgia, and chest pain. Roentgenologically, they manifested a diffuse, bilateral reticulonodular pattern, sometimes associated with septal (Kerley B) lines; none showed lobar or segmental consolidation. Pleural effusion was observed in only one patient. The remaining 24 patients (group 3) had clinical and roentgenographic manifestations midway between the other two groups and were not easily categorized one way or the other.

Clinical Manifestations

Clinically, pneumonia caused by *M. pneumoniae* is usually more prolonged and more severe than that caused by viruses, lasting 2 to 3 weeks.[444] Rarely—usually in association with underlying disease such as sickle cell anemia[445]—it is fulminant and fatal. Symptoms include cough (usually nonproductive but often associated with mucoid or purulent expectoration when illness is prolonged), headache, malaise, and fever. Upper respiratory tract involvement, characterized by sore throat and nasal symptoms, is present in about 50 per cent of cases. Physical examination of the lungs usually reveals rales and decreased breath sounds at the lung bases, and signs of frank consolidation may occur.

Extrapulmonary manifestations of *M. pneumoniae* infection are perhaps commoner than was once thought and may be increasing in frequency.[446] Many are serious, particularly those that involve the central nervous system, such as meningoencephalitis and transverse myelitis. Perhaps the most frequent complication is Stevens-Johnson syndrome (severe erythema multiforme associated with a systemic reaction, including high fever, stomatitis, and ophthalmia). Other complications include hemagglutination or hemolysis, peripheral venous thrombosis with subsequent pulmonary thromboembolic disease (most often in patients with very high titers of cold agglutinins),[447] arthritis and arthralgia,[448] and pericarditis and myocarditis.[449] These typically become evident 2 to 3 weeks after the initial infection, suggesting an immunologic mechanism in pathogenesis.

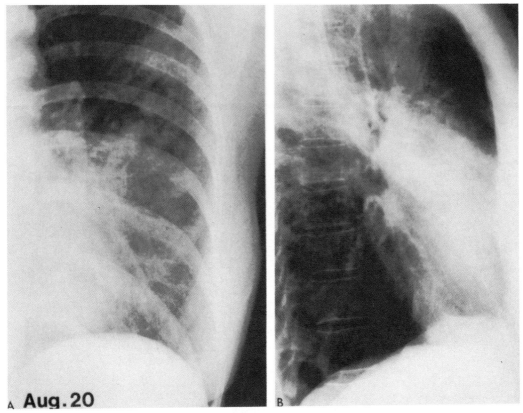

Figure 6–52. Acute Pneumonia Caused by *Mycoplasma Pneumoniae.* Views of the left lung from posteroanterior *(A)* and lateral *(B)* roentgenograms reveal patchy airspace consolidation in the lingular and posterior segments of the left upper lobe. The consolidation is not homogeneous, as would be anticipated in acute bacterial pneumonia due to, for example, *Streptococcus pneumoniae.* Immuno-fluorescence microscopy of sputum revealed *M. pneumoniae* organisms.

Despite this impressive list, *M. pneumoniae* pneumonia is usually a mild disease, with most patients recovering quickly without residual pulmonary abnormality. In a minority, diffuse pulmonary disease results in pulmonary dysfunction, either restrictive[450] or obstructive.[451]

Laboratory Findings

The white blood cell count is usually normal; however, in one quarter to one third of patients levels above 10,000 cells per mL have been recorded.[447] Since the organism takes approximately 1 week and sometimes longer to culture, and since clinical recovery is well under way in most patients by this time, culture commonly is useful only to confirm the diagnosis; when positive specimens are obtained, they are almost invariably from the throat, sputum, or BAL fluid.[452]

M. pneumoniae infection is the commonest respiratory cause of cold agglutinin production, being present in significant titer in about 50 per cent of cases.[444] However, cold agglutinins also develop in viral pneumonia, and, in fact, approximately one quarter of cold agglutinin–positive pneumonias are not caused by *M. pneumoniae.*[436] Of much greater diagnostic value are techniques that show specific antibodies to the organism, including complement fixation, radioimmunoassay, and ELISA.[453] A more rapid and reliable method of early diagnosis may be available with the use of monoclonal antibodies.[454]

Viruses

Influenza Virus

Influenza viruses are divided into three groups—A, B, and C—on the basis of internal membrane and nucleoprotein antigens. Group A, in turn, may be divided into a variety of subtypes related to the presence of two structurally, functionally, and genetically distinct surface glycoproteins, hemagglutinin (H) and neuraminidase (N). The virus may be isolated by culture of sputum in monkey kidney cells or chick embryo, growth occurring in 3 to 21 days; immunofluorescence techniques may be used to identify infected cells before the virus is sufficiently concentrated to give a positive result by complement fixation.

Although the influenza A virus generally has been considered to be an obligate human parasite transmitted from person to person by droplet infection, it is now evident that the virus that caused the Hong Kong epidemic of 1968 can infect a wide range of animals, and it seems likely that transmission of such infection is from human sources. In addition, there is evidence for transmission of disease from animal to human.[455] These findings raise the possibility that animals act as a reservoir for viral influenza and a milieu for genetic recombination, leading to new strains of influenza A virus in humans.

Influenza may occur in pandemics, in epidemics, or sporadically. Almost all severe epidemics and all pandemics are caused by type A viruses. Outbreaks of type B disease also may occur but are less frequent, more localized, and commoner in schoolchildren than in the general population[455a]; sporadic cases of clinical influenza are usually mild and are caused by type C organisms.[456]

Influenza virus predominantly infects persons from 5 years of age to early adulthood. The incubation period is 24 to 48 hours, allowing rapid spread of the disease. It is very contagious, and during epidemics and pandemics a large proportion of the population contracts the infection. Antibody formation to specific strains by either infection or vaccination confers immunity for 1 to 2 years. In addition to strain-specific hemagglutination inhibition antibody, there appears to be a naturally acquired immunity to influenza type A infection, which may last as long as 25 years.[457]

Pneumonia is an uncommon but dreaded complication of influenza infection; although often localized and of only mild to moderate severity, it may be overwhelming and fatal within 24 hours. Although infection with the virus alone may be responsible, in many cases this clinical course is caused by bacteria. In the 1918–1919 influenza pandemic, hemolytic *Streptococcus* was a common cause of such superinfection. In the pandemic of 1957–1958 and the Hong Kong influenza epidemic of 1968, the causative organism was *Staphylococcus aureus*. Infection also predisposes to pneumococcal pneumonia.[458]

Most cases of pneumonia are recognized during epidemics or pandemics; when endemic, they are often misdiagnosed or undiagnosed. At greatest risk are elderly persons in nursing homes,[455a] 25 to 50 per cent of whom will develop influenzal infection when the virus is introduced. Many patients who develop pneumonia are judged to be otherwise healthy[459]; however, about two thirds have a predisposing condition such as mitral stenosis, chronic bronchitis, diabetes, nephrosis, or pregnancy.

Pathologic Characteristics. The lungs of patients who die of influenza pneumonia are bulky, heavy, and dusky red, and the cut surface exudes frothy, blood-tinged fluid. The airway walls are usually markedly congested, and the lumina contain hemorrhagic fluid. Microscopically, the parenchyma shows capillary congestion and a variably severe interstitial mononuclear inflammatory infiltrate. Alveolar airspaces are frequently filled with a combination of red blood cells, edema, and fibrin; type II cell hyperplasia and hyaline membranes may be prominent.[460] Interstitial fibrosis may develop as a residuum.

In a high proportion of cases, the virus may be isolated from postmortem lung parenchyma or airway epithelial specimens; however, it has been shown that it may be detected with a greater degree of accuracy and sensitivity by immunofluoresence than by culture.[461] Inclusions representing viral aggregates cannot be seen with routine light microscopy.

Roentgenographic Manifestations. Involvement may be local or general. The former usually is in the form of segmental consolidation, which may be homogeneous or patchy, most commonly in the lower lobes, and either unilateral or bilateral. Serial chest roentgenograms may show poorly defined patchy areas of consolidation, 1 to 2 cm in diameter, which rapidly become confluent. In one series the disease was unilateral and bilateral in approximately equal incidence, and widely disseminated in roughly a quarter of the latter cases.[462] Roentgenographically there was

diffuse, patchy airspace disease resembling pulmonary edema (Fig. 6–53). Pleural effusion is comparatively rare. Resolution averages about 3 weeks.

Clinical Manifestations. The clinical manifestations depend, to some extent, on the age of the person infected:[463] in young children croup is common, in young adults a systemic influenza syndrome predominates, and in older patients there is a tendency for the development of lower respiratory tract disease. The typical manifestations of the systemic syndrome are a dry cough, pain in the back and leg muscles, chills, headache, conjunctivitis, and a temperature of 38.5°C or more for 3 to 5 days. As in other viral infections involving mucous membranes, the production of purulent expectoration does not necessarily signify a superimposed bacterial infection. Rhinorrhea and pharyngitis are seldom apparent, and gastrointestinal symptoms occur in a minority of patients. Neuromuscular complications include Reye's syndrome, Guillain-Barré syndrome, myositis, and myoglobinuria.

Three forms of respiratory tract disease have been described.[464] The mildest is believed to represent bronchiolitis and produces no roentgenographic abnormality; patients may have hemoptysis and local or diffuse rales, and rhonchi may be audible. The second form is commoner and occurs when bacterial superinfection develops within 2 weeks after the initial viral infection; in this situation, patients expectorate purulent sputum, which may be rusty or bloody, and may complain of pleural pain. The third form is a more fulminating pneumonia, which develops within 12 to 36 hours after the initial symptoms and may be caused by the virus alone or by staphylococcal superinfection. Patients are extremely ill, with dyspnea and cyanosis developing rapidly.

Laboratory Findings. The white blood cell count is usually normal in uncomplicated influenza, but leukopenia develops in some cases and, when severe, indicates a poor prognosis. Overwhelming infection commonly results in a neutrophilia of 20,000 cells per mL or more. The influenza group responsible for infection may be identified by complement-fixation testing, and the subgroup by the demonstration of specific hemagglutination inhibition, neutralization, or antineuraminidase antibodies. One method of rapid diagnosis consists of treating nasal smears directly with fluorescent antibody to influenza viruses prepared in guinea pigs.[465]

The majority of patients with mild, uncomplicated influenza have small airway obstruction, as evidenced by slightly but consistently decreased flow rates at low lung volumes and an increased A-a gradient for oxygen.[466]

Parainfluenza Virus

Parainfluenza virus may be subdivided into four antigenic types. Infections by types 1 and 2 occur predominantly in the winter months and can achieve epidemic proportions.[467] By contrast, parainfluenza virus type 3 causes sporadic infection that does not have a seasonal pattern of incidence. Disease is believed to be transmitted by inhalation of organisms in droplet nuclei.

The organisms cause predominantly mild upper respiratory tract disease and pharyngitis; in adults, they are responsible for a small percentage of cases of coryza and in infants and young children for the majority of cases of

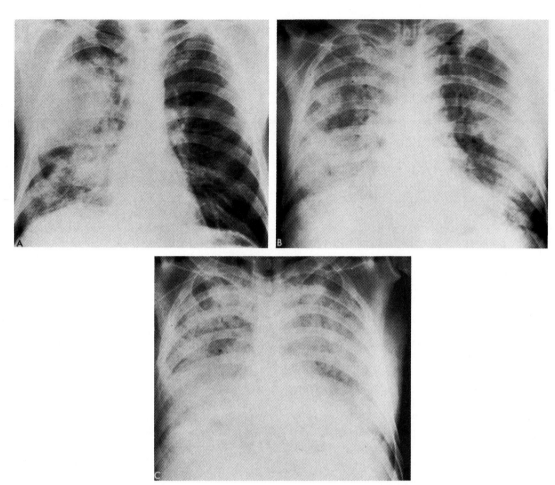

Figure 6–53. Acute Influenza Virus Pneumonia. A posteroanterior roentgenogram on the day of admission of this 32-year-old man *(A)* reveals extensive homogeneous airspace consolidation of the right upper lobe, with patchy shadows of airspace consolidation of the right lower lobe; the left lung is clear. Two days later *(B)*, consolidation of the right lower lobe has become almost uniform, and there has occurred extension of the airspace disease throughout the whole of the left lung; at this time, the roentgenographic appearance would be compatible with diffuse pulmonary edema. Twenty-four hours later *(C)*, both lungs are almost completely consolidated, the only visible air being present within the bronchial tree (a diffuse air bronchogram). Shortly after admission, the patient became comatose and never regained consciousness. A hemagglutination inhibition test was positive to a titer of 1:160 for influenza A_2, Hong Kong variant; respiratory syncytial virus and influenza virus were cultured from the blood, the sputum, and directly from the lung at necropsy. (Courtesy of St. Mary's Hospital, Montreal.)

severe croup. Some cases of lower respiratory tract disease also are caused by the virus, particularly in immunocompromised persons.[468] As with influenza, parainfluenza virus infection predisposes to bacterial superinfection.

Pathologic characteristics of human infections have rarely been described, since virtually all are mild and self-limiting; however, the pattern of giant cell pneumonia has been reported in several cases.[468] Roentgenographic changes are relatively nonspecific, consisting of diffuse or local accentuation of lung markings in the lower lobes caused by peribronchial and peribronchiolar inflammation.[469]

In children the symptoms are those of croup, sometimes with intermittent rales suggesting bronchiolitis; the commonest manifestation in adults is acute pharyngitis and tonsillitis. The white blood cell count usually is normal but may increase to 15,000 cells per mL. The organism may be isolated by the culture of sputum on monkey tissue; growth requires 3 to 21 days. As in influenza infections, an immu-

nofluorescence test is useful in identifying the virus in nasopharyngeal secretions.[470] Serologic diagnosis may be achieved by agglutinin neutralization and complement-fixation tests and by hemadsorption with guinea pig erythrocytes.

Respiratory Syncytial Virus

The respiratory syncytial virus (RSV) is responsible for a small number of cases of coryza in children and adults and is a major cause of severe bronchiolitis and bronchopneumonia in infants and small children. Although often sporadic, epidemic outbreaks have been described.[471] Infants and children younger than 2 years of age (boys outnumber girls by approximately two to one) are particularly susceptible; the lower respiratory tract is affected in one third to one half of patients.[472] Adult infection is usually mild, presumably reflecting immunity as a result of childhood infection; however, in the elderly and chronically ill[473] and in the immunosuppressed,[474] it may be more virulent. Infections occur predominantly during the winter months and early spring; the incubation period is 3 to 5 days.

The pathogenesis of RSV bronchiolitis and pneumonia is not certain. Although it may be related to direct airway and alveolar epithelial damage by the virus,[475] there is also evidence that it may represent a hypersensitivity reaction. According to this hypothesis, disease is mediated by complexes of RSV and maternal IgG antibodies in infants who have no local IgA antibody of their own to intercept the virus and prevent its combination with IgG deeper in the bronchial wall. This hypothesis could explain the disastrous effects in some infants in whom infection due to RSV develops after they receive killed RSV parenteral vaccines.[456]

Histologically, RSV infection may be confined mainly to the alveolar interstitium in the form of a mononuclear infiltrate or giant cell pneumonia.[476] When airway involvement predominates, the most severe changes occur in bronchioles and consist of epithelial necrosis and a variably intense peribronchial mononuclear inflammatory infiltrate. Eosinophilic cytoplasmic viral inclusions occasionally may be seen in the degenerating epithelial cells.

In one radiographic study of 65 patients, the dominant findings in 60 cases were bronchial wall thickening, peribronchial shadowing, and perihilar linearity (sic).[477] Findings suggestive of sublobular or lobular consolidation were present in 39 cases, whereas more homogeneous shadowing was present in 10; multiple areas of involvement were common. Air trapping was evident in 41 cases.

Symptoms associated with rhinitis, pharyngitis, and conjunctivitis are frequent. In the presence of bronchiolitis or pneumonia, cough, wheezing, dyspnea, cyanosis, and retraction of the rib cage may be present in addition to signs of parenchymal consolidation. Infection appears to confer excellent immunity, since adults who are challenged with the virus manifest no symptoms or signs or exhibit, at most, symptoms of a mild common cold. The disease may be detected by complement-fixation and neutralization tests, and the diagnosis established early with immunofluorescence antibody methods.

Although the disease is usually mild, it has been estimated to be fatal in 2 to 6 per cent of children.[456] The long-term effects in those who survive are controversial; in some follow-up studies of infants and children, many have been found to have episodes of wheezing, persistent reduction in maximal expiratory flow, and greater bronchial lability than control subjects.[478] By contrast, in one study of twenty-five 8- to 12-year-old children who had suffered mild bronchiolitis, pulmonary function was normal.[479]

Measles Virus

Measles (rubeola) is a highly contagious systemic viral disease that occurs predominantly in the late winter and early spring. Transmission is believed to occur by droplet inhalation from person to person. The incubation period averages 11 days. Before measles vaccine was available, serologic evidence of infection was present in the vast majority of individuals before adolescence. However, since the introduction of active immunization programs in 1963, there has been a remarkable reduction in the number of

reported cases.[480] In its natural form, the disease is found principally in small children. In societies with active immunization programs, however, there is evidence that increasing numbers of older persons are contracting the illness.[481]

In the typical case, prodromal symptoms such as fever, malaise, myalgia, headache, conjunctivitis, sneezing, coughing, and nasal discharge are present for 2 to 4 days before the characteristic blotchy erythematous rash appears. In the United States, it has been estimated that 1 in 15 patients suffers an additional complication, of which respiratory tract involvement is the commonest (38 per 1000 cases).[480]

Pulmonary disease as a consequence of measles takes one of three forms: (1) primary measles virus pneumonia; (2) secondary bacterial pneumonia (the commonest form, usually caused by S. pneumoniae, S. aureus, H. influenzae, or N. meningitidis); or (3) atypical measles pneumonia (see later).[480] Although most cases of pneumonia occur in children, adults (particularly Armed Forces recruits) are also susceptible. The risk of primary measles pneumonia appears to be much greater in patients who are immunocompromised as a result of congenital immunodeficiency syndromes, malignancy (usually lymphoma or leukemia), or immunosuppressive therapy.[482] Such patients frequently have a clinical course different from the usual one, characterized chiefly by a lack of rash and, in some cases, by prolonged illness.

An entirely different form of disease occurs in children in whom measles develops or who receive live measles virus vaccine after having been immunized with killed or live attenuated measles vaccine. In this "altered measles syndrome" ("atypical measles"),[483] there is a maculopapular rash that appears first on the extremities and spreads centrifugally, with limb edema in many cases and moderate eosinophilia in some. Although the precise mechanisms by which these abnormalities occur are unknown, the roentgenographic appearance of the chest (see later) and rapid resolution suggest an immune response.

Pathologic Characteristics. The pathologic characteristics of fatal cases of typical measles pneumonia without bacterial superinfection are those of so-called giant cell pneumonia.[482] Histologically, alveolar airspaces and interstitium contain fluid, fibrin, and a mononuclear cellular infiltrate; hyaline membranes may be present (Fig. 6–54). Characteristically, giant cells containing numerous nuclei and eosinophilic nuclear and cytoplasmic viral inclusions are also present. Although this histologic reaction is caused most often by measles, an identical appearance can occur in RSV and parainfluenza virus infections. To our knowledge, there have been no pathologic descriptions of the lung in atypical measles syndrome.

Roentgenographic Manifestations. Primary pneumonia caused by the measles virus produces a reticular and patchy airspace pattern throughout the lungs. In children, hilar lymph node enlargement is usual. In contrast, roentgenographic evidence of lymph node enlargement in adults tends to occur only with atypical measles syndrome.[484] In addition to the interstitial pneumonitis, segmental pneumonia and atelectasis caused by bacterial superinfection develop in many cases. In view of the fact that viral and bacterial pneumonias cause fairly distinctive reticulonodular and segmental opacities, respectively, it is surprising that the pneumonia that complicates measles in adults almost

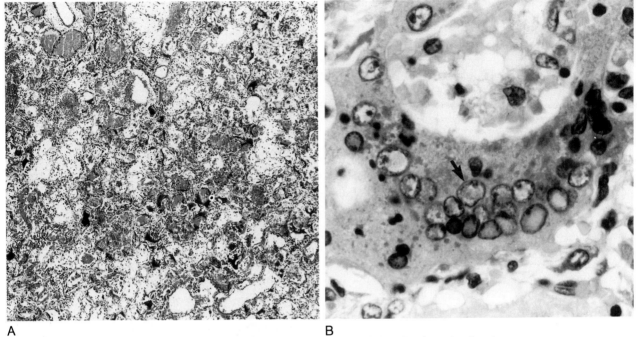

A   B

Figure 6–54. Measles (Giant Cell) Pneumonia. *A,* Low-power view showing extensive airspace consolidation by proteinaceous debris, macrophages, and red blood cells. Irregular or sickle-cell–shaped giant cells are clearly visible. *B,* Magnified view of giant cell showing numerous nuclei, some of which contain lightly stained but well-defined viral inclusions *(arrow).* (*A* × 40; *B* × 800.)

invariably is associated with an interstitial pattern regardless of whether cultures are positive or negative for "pathogenic bacteria."[482]

The chest roentgenogram in the atypical measles syndrome is sufficiently characteristic to suggest the diagnosis when the clinical findings are taken into consideration.[485] Consolidation is generally lobar or segmental in distribution. Pleural effusion and hilar lymph node enlargement are common. In contrast with the pneumonia of typical measles, the consolidation tends to resolve, and the effusions absorb very rapidly; however, residual nodules may persist for years and may even calcify.

Clinical Manifestations. Primary measles pneumonia characteristically develops before or coincident with the peak of the measles exanthem. Liver function abnormalities and evidence of infection in the paranasal sinuses and middle ear are common accompaniments in adults.[484] Superimposed bacterial pneumonia usually develops several days after the rash, when the patient's condition has begun to improve. It should be suspected when cough, purulent expectoration, tachycardia, rise in temperature, and sometimes pleural pain develop during early convalescence.

The diagnosis of atypical measles syndrome should be suspected when a child or adolescent who has previously received killed or live attenuated measles virus vaccine and who has a hemorrhagic vesicular rash on peripheral limb areas develops prodromal symptoms of measles, nonproductive cough, and pleuritic pain. It may be confirmed by the demonstration of a fourfold increase in serum antibody titer to measles antigen.

The white blood cell count in primary pneumonia usually is normal but may be low; in the presence of secondary bacterial pneumonia, polymorphonuclear leukocytosis commonly develops. The virus may be isolated on tissue cultures of throat washings or blood.

Picornaviruses

The picornaviruses are a group of small, ribonucleic acid (RNA) viruses that include two subgroups pathogenic for humans: the enteroviruses and the rhinoviruses. The latter are responsible for more than 50 per cent of cases of coryza. Lower respiratory tract infections, including bronchitis, croup, bronchiolitis, and bronchopneumonia, are very uncommon but have been described in children and occasionally adults. The roentgenographic and clinical findings are identical to those of other nonbacterial pneumonias.[486]

The enteroviruses include the coxsackieviruses, echoviruses, and polioviruses. Respiratory infection caused by the first two is usually limited to the upper tract and tends to be mild; pneumonia is rare. Pleurodynia (Bornholm's disease) is most often caused by coxsackievirus B. It is characterized by gripping chest pain, with remission and exacerbations that may last several weeks, usually accompanied by difficulty in breathing and by fever. We have seen several cases with persistent widespread bilateral pleural friction rubs. The effects of the polioviruses on the thorax are indirect only; paralysis of the muscles of respiration results in alveolar hypoventilation and respiratory failure.

Adenovirus

Adenoviruses are a group of nonenveloped, DNA-containing organisms, of which approximately 40 serotypes have been identified. The majority of sporadic infections are caused by types 1, 2, and 5[487]; epidemics are more frequently associated with types 3, 4, and 7, and the majority of fatalities are associated with types 3 and 7. Epidemics occur especially in military populations recently removed from civilian life. All types have a common complement-fixing antibody and may be differentiated by serum neutralization tests. They grow readily in tissue culture of human and simian cells, producing a distinctive cytopathologic appearance.

Adenovirus infection forms a small but significant proportion of respiratory disease. In one study of more than 18,000 infants and children followed for 10 years,[487] a minimum of 7 per cent of respiratory infections were estimated to be caused by the virus, although other studies[488] have reported a lower incidence. Infection occurs most often in healthy individuals; however, immunocompromised patients appear to be at increased risk. Disease may occur as pharyngitis, pharyngoconjunctivitis, or a nonspecific "acute respiratory syndrome," with or without clinically significant pulmonary involvement; it has also been suggested that chronic infection may by related to the development of bronchiectasis.[489]

Pathologic Characteristics. The lungs of patients who have died of acute adenovirus pneumonia characteristically show necrotizing bronchitis and bronchiolitis most prominent in the smaller airways, frequently associated with occlusion of the lumina by necrotic material and inflammatory exudate. The parenchyma shows similar necrotic changes. Viral nuclear inclusions ("smudge cells") are most prominent in alveolar lining cells but may be seen in airway epithelium. Bronchiectasis and bronchiolitis obliterans have been described as morphologic sequelae of the acute infection.[490]

Roentgenographic Manifestations. The typical roentgenographic findings, as described in one 5-year study of 69 patients (most younger than 1 year of age), were diffuse bilateral "bronchopneumonia" and severe overinflation.[491] Lobar collapse was a frequent complication, in the right upper lobe in 20 instances and the left lower lobe in six, and re-expansion did not occur in 10 (*see* Fig. 4–17, page 179). In uncomplicated cases, the roentgenographic changes resolved within 2 weeks, but of particular importance was the incidence of subsequent chronic pulmonary disease. Of the 58 children adequately followed up, 21 (36 per cent) had some form of chronic pulmonary disease. Roentgenographic evidence of unilateral hyperlucent lung (Swyer-James or Macleod's syndrome) may be apparent.

Clinical Manifestations. The adenoviruses are perhaps the commonest cause of "acute respiratory disease," a somewhat ill-defined syndrome of fever (which tends to persist for 4 to 5 days), pharyngitis, cough, hoarseness, chest pain, and conjunctivitis. Occasionally, infection presents clinically as whooping cough that is indistinguishable from pertussis.[492] When pneumonia occurs, it usually is mild and always is associated with typical upper respiratory symptoms. Physical findings include pharyngitis, which frequently is exudative and closely resembles that produced by streptococcal infection, and diffuse rales and rhonchi indicative of bronchiolitis; in some cases there are definite signs of consolidation. The white blood cell count usually is normal but may be slightly increased and, in very ill patients, may exceed 30,000 cells per mL.

Herpes Simplex

Herpes simplex virus is composed of two antigenically similar types, type I (HSV-I) and type II (HSV-II), which differ considerably in their clinical and epidemiologic char-

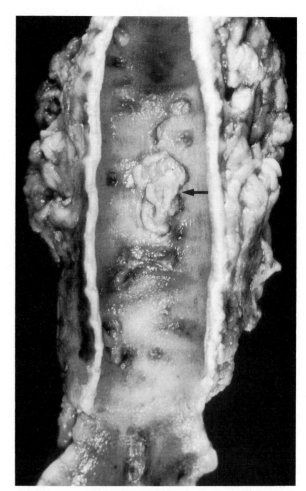

Figure 6–55. Herpes Simplex Tracheitis. The trachea of this 40-year-old burn patient has been opened posteriorly and reveals multiple foci of ulceration, some covered with a pyogenic membrane *(arrow)*.

acteristics. HSV-I is transmitted in situations of close personal contact through saliva or, possibly, by droplet inhalation and is most commonly associated with oral disease. Pneumonia, which may have a focal or diffuse interstitial pattern, is almost always associated with mucocutaneous involvement and frequently with tracheobronchitis (Fig. 6–55).[493] Disseminated disease may or may not affect the lungs and usually occurs in immunocompromised patients.[494] HSV-II is best known as the cause of herpes genitalis, a sexually transmitted disease characterized by recurrent genital ulcers. Neonatal infection is usually acquired during passage of the baby through an infected birth canal[494]; pneumonia may occur as part of the systemic disease.

Clinically, HSV-I pneumonia occurs most frequently in patients with severe burns and in those whose immune status is compromised.[495] HSV-II infection occurs most frequently in neonates during the first 2 weeks of life[495]; disease is usually disseminated and is associated with cutaneous or conjunctival vesicles, fever, jaundice, seizures, and signs of pneumonia.

The diagnosis may be made by the cytologic identification of eosinophilic intranuclear inclusions in pulmonary epithelial cells; confirmation may be obtained by viral cultures or by immunofluorescence or immunoperoxidase techniques. Bronchoscopy is valuable for identifying ulcerations or pseudomembranes in the respiratory tract and for improving the sensitivity and specificity of the cytologic diagnosis.[496]

Herpes Varicellae

Herpes varicellae (varicella-zoster virus) infection is seen in two clinical forms:[497] chickenpox (varicella), representing primary disease in previously uninfected individuals, and zoster (shingles), usually considered to represent reactivation of latent virus.

The overall incidence of pneumonia in patients with chickenpox appears to be about 15 per cent,[498] although in adults admitted to the hospital it may be as high as 50 per cent. About 90 per cent of affected patients are aged 20 years or older, a relatively high incidence of pneumonia in sharp contrast with the low incidence of varicella itself in this age group—50 per cent of cases occur in children younger than 6 years of age, and only 20 per cent occur in adults.[499] In both adults and children, pre-existing neoplastic disease, particularly leukemia and lymphoma, and corticosteroid and broad-spectrum antibiotic therapy predispose to pneumonia. In addition, the incidence of both pneumonia and mortality from it are much higher in pregnant women.

Zoster is usually a localized disease that is seen most frequently and is most severe in patients with lymphoreticular neoplasms (particularly Hodgkin's disease) or in those receiving immunosuppressive therapy or having recently received irradiation. It is in these persons that systemic dissemination is particularly likely to occur, in some cases with pneumonia. Zoster also may be complicated by unilateral diaphragmatic paralysis, presumably as a result of extension of the latent infection from the dorsal root ganglia to the adjacent spinal cord; it may occur in the absence of a cutaneous lesion.[500]

Pathologic Characteristics. Histologic features of pneumonitis in chickenpox and zoster are similar and consist of an interstitial mononuclear inflammatory infiltrate, associated with intra-alveolar proteinaceous exudate, hyaline membrane formation, and type 2 cell hyperplasia (diffuse alveolar damage). Intranuclear inclusions indistinguishable from those of herpes simplex may be seen in type 2 cells and airway epithelial cells. Vesicles similar to those on the skin and mucous membranes also may be present in the trachea and larger bronchi and on the pleural surface.[501]

Pathologic features of remote chickenpox infection consist of spherical nodules scattered randomly throughout the lung parenchyma.[502] Histologically, they are composed of an outer, often lamellated fibrous capsule frequently enclosing areas of hyalinized collagen or necrotic tissue.

Roentgenographic Manifestations. The characteristic roentgenographic pattern of acute varicella pneumonia is patchy, diffuse, airspace consolidation manifested by a multitude of acinar shadows (Fig. 6–56).[501] Hilar lymph node enlargement may be present but may be difficult to appreciate because of contiguity of the consolidation in the parahilar parenchyma. Pleural effusion is very uncommon and never large. Roentgenographic clearing may take from 9 days to several months.

An unusual manifestation of chickenpox pneumonia consists of tiny widespread foci of calcification throughout both lungs in persons who had the disease many years before in adulthood (Fig. 6–57).[503] The calcifications vary in size and number but seldom exceed 2 to 3 mm in diameter; they predominate in the lower half of the lungs. Hilar lymph nodes do not calcify.

Clinical Manifestations. In most cases of chickenpox, there is a history of contact with an affected child 3 to 21 days before the development of disease. The onset often is marked by high fever, which may precede the rash by 2 to 3 days. The latter may be scarlatiniform in its early stages but rapidly becomes maculopapular, vesicular, and pustular. Symptoms and signs of pneumonia develop a few days after the rash appears and consist of cough, dyspnea, hemoptysis, tachypnea, pleuritic chest pain, and cyanosis, with temperature as high as 40°C. Expectoration is not purulent. When pneumonia develops, the rash tends to be unusually severe and often extends onto the mucosa of the mouth and pharynx.[501]

In approximately one third of cases the white blood cell count exceeds 10,000 cells per mL and is associated with polymorphonuclear leukocytosis. Complement-fixing, neutralizing, and fluorescent antibodies are found in both varicella and herpes zoster infections, from about the fifth day of illness. Clinical improvement usually antedates roentgenographic clearing by several weeks. Although it is probable that many cases of varicella pneumonia are mild and are overlooked, a mortality as high as 11 per cent has been reported, and patients with acute pneumonia may die suddenly without warning.[501]

Cytomegalovirus

Cytomegalovirus (CMV) is the cause of a variety of illnesses whose manifestations depend largely on the age and immunologic status of the host. Infection may be congenital or acquired, the former usually occurring by transplacental spread of organisms from an asymptomatic mother. In neonates and infants, infection usually is acquired during passage through an infected birth canal or from maternal milk; in older individuals it is derived from direct interpersonal contact through saliva or genitourinary secretions. The virus also may be transmitted through contaminated blood and from infected cells in organ transplants.

Most persons who acquire the disease are asymptomatic; occasionally, there are clinical findings suggesting infectious mononucleosis. When more serious disease occurs, it usually represents reactivation of latent virus acquired earlier in life[504] and thus is seen almost exclusively in patients with immunodeficiency or lymphoreticular malignancy or who are receiving immunosuppressive therapy. Organ transplant recipients[505] and patients with AIDS (*see* page 298) are at particular risk.

Both humoral and cell-mediated immunity appear to be important in the defense against CMV infection. Patients who have CMV-specific antibodies before institution of immunosuppressive drug therapy or who respond to CMV infection with an increase in antibody production usually shed virus asymptomatically rather than develop clinically significant disease.[506] By contrast, patients who die from CMV infection typically fail to mount a significant complement-fixing antibody response.[507] Despite these observations, patients at risk are primarily deficient in cell-mediated immunity.[508]

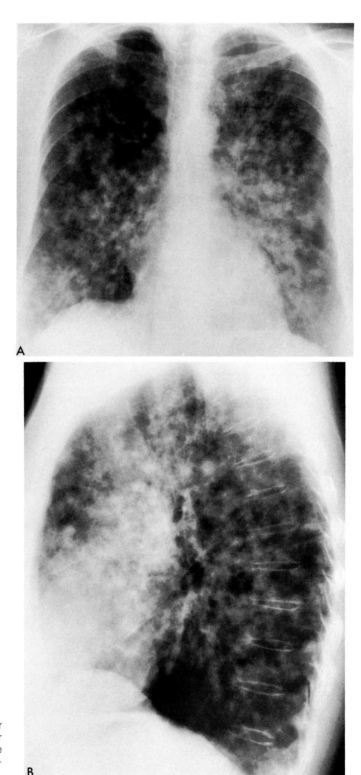

Figure 6–56. Acute Varicella-Zoster Pneumonia. Posteroanterior *(A)* and lateral *(B)* roentgenograms reveal widespread acinar shadows possessing a pattern characteristic of patchy airspace consolidation. A 42-year-old woman with non-Hodgkin's lymphoma treated with antineoplastic agents.

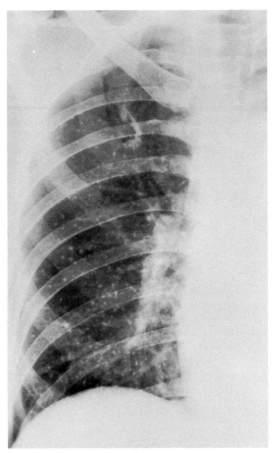

Figure 6–57. Healed Varicella-Zoster (Chickenpox) Pneumonia. A posteroanterior roentgenogram demonstrates a multitude of tiny calcific shadows measuring 1 to 2 mm in diameter scattered widely and uniformly throughout the right lung (the left lung was similarly affected). This 42-year-old asymptomatic man had had florid chickenpox 15 years previously; the presence of acute pneumonia was recognized at the time. (Courtesy of Dr. Romeo Ethier, Montreal Neurological Hospital.)

Pathogenesis and Pathologic Characteristics. It is likely that CMV is of little or no pathogenetic importance in many patients in whom it is cultured or identified pathologically. Thus, viral inclusions may be identified diffusely throughout the lung parenchyma without evidence of lung damage or inflammation. In addition, isolation of the organism from blood or BAL fluid may be unassociated with clinical evidence of disease[509] or an increased risk of death.[42] When the organism is associated with disease, the precise pathogenesis is unclear; although it may be related to viral toxicity, there is also evidence that immunologic mechanisms may be important.[510]

Two morphologic patterns have been described in CMV pneumonia,[511] the first and commonest consisting of small, relatively well-defined, hemorrhagic nodules scattered randomly throughout the parenchyma. Histologically, these are composed of intra-alveolar hemorrhage, edema, and necrotic debris; a mononuclear cell interstitial infiltrate of variable severity is usually present. Characteristic nuclear and cytoplasmic inclusions (Fig. 6–58) may be identified in the abnormal areas, both singly and in small clusters. The second pattern affects most of the parenchyma, with histologic features of either diffuse alveolar damage or chronic interstitial pneumonitis.

Roentgenographic Manifestations. The usual manifestation of CMV lung infection consists of a diffuse reticulonodular pattern that is particularly prominent in the outer one third of the lungs (Fig. 6–59).[512] Airspace consolidation may be evident as acinar shadows, but not as prominently as in *Pneumocystis carinii* pneumonia, one of the main conditions to be differentiated. Small unilateral or bilateral pleural effusions are common.

Clinical Manifestations. Symptoms and signs of pulmonary infection are nonspecific. Some patients present with disease that resembles infectious mononucleosis, consisting of fever, malaise, hepatosplenomegaly, lymph node enlargement, jaundice, atypical lymphocytosis, and, occasionally, pneumonia.[513] This may occur following extracorporeal circulation and multiple blood transfusions but also may develop spontaneously in otherwise healthy persons.

CMV may be isolated from blood and many body secretions, including sputum and BAL fluid. The organism may be cultured in human fibroblasts, in which it produces characteristic cytopathogenic cell rounding and enlargement; however, BAL with centrifugation culture is a more rapid method whose sensitivity and specificity closely approximate the results of viral tissue culture.[514] Testing for CMV antigen has been proposed as a useful way of diagnosing pneumonia when associated with lymphopenia in BAL fluid.[515]

Epstein-Barr Virus

Intrathoracic disease in infectious mononucleosis is uncommon. In one series of 59 cases,[516] hilar lymph node enlargement was identified in eight patients (13 per cent) and a diffuse reticular pattern in three (5 per cent); pleural effusion also was found in three individuals. The commonest roentgenologic finding was splenomegaly, observed in 28 patients (47 per cent), and the authors suggested that

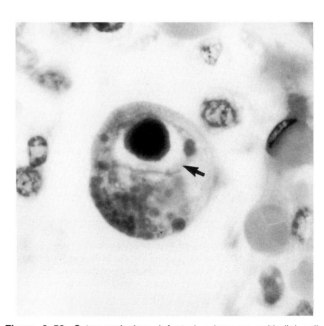

Figure 6–58. Cytomegalovirus. Infected pulmonary epithelial cell, showing a deeply basophilic round nuclear inclusion that is surrounded by a clear halo (the nuclear membrane is indicated by an *arrow*). Numerous discrete intracytoplasmic inclusions are also present. (× 1500.)

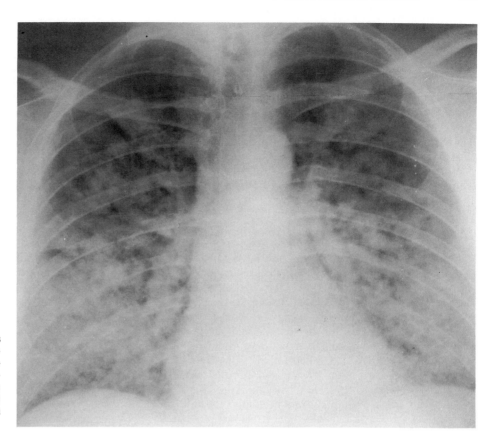

Figure 6–59. Acute Cytomegalovirus Pneumonia in a Renal Transplant Patient. A posteroanterior chest roentgenogram reveals widespread patchy airspace consolidation, more marked in the lower lobes. At autopsy several days later, severe CMV pneumonia was found.

this finding, in association with one or more of the thoracic abnormalities, should alert the radiologist to the possibility of infectious mononucleosis.

Patients complain of pharyngitis and, with pulmonary involvement, cough productive of small amounts of tenacious sputum. Fatigue and fever are frequent, and physical examination may show lymph node enlargement and hepatosplenomegaly. The diagnosis may be confirmed by the characteristic findings in peripheral blood lymphocytes.

The Epstein-Barr virus has also been associated with the development of lymphocytic interstitial pneumonia, particularly in patients with the acquired immunodeficiency syndrome.[517]

Papillomaviruses

Papillomaviruses have been shown to be present in laryngeal papillomas and are undoubtedly responsible for similar lesions in the lower respiratory tract.[518] There is also evidence that the viruses are associated with the occasional development of pulmonary carcinoma in patients with tracheobronchial papillomatosis (*see* page 491).

Chlamydiae

Chlamydiae are small, obligate intracellular organisms that are properly classified as bacteria. They differ from the latter (including intracellular forms such as rickettsiae) chiefly by their unique mode of reproduction and by their inability to synthesize high-energy compounds, such as adenosine triphosphate (ATP) and guanosine triphosphate (GTP).[519] The organisms exist in an extracellular form as

"elementary bodies." These attach to and are phagocytosed by susceptible cells, within which they convert to "reticulate bodies" that undergo division to form intracellular colonies. This process occurs within the host phagosomes, which remain intact as the colonies develop. The reticulate bodies themselves are noninfectious and eventually undergo conversion into elementary bodies, at which point the phagosome membrane disrupts, the cell dies, and the elementary bodies are released.

Three species—*Chlamydia pneumoniae*, *C. trachomatis*, and *C. psittaci*—can cause pulmonary disease in humans.

Chlamydia Pneumoniae

This organism was originally believed to be a strain of *C. psittaci* (TWAR); however, recent studies have shown it to be a separate species that is frequently the cause of minor epidemics in confined groups.[520] Pneumonia caused by this organism appears to be relatively mild compared with mycoplasmal or viral pneumonias, and there is reason to believe that healthy individuals act as chronic carriers.[521]

Chlamydia Trachomatis

It has been estimated that 2 to 13 per cent of women in city hospitals in the United States are infected with *C. trachomatis* and that infants born to such mothers have a 50 per cent chance of acquiring inclusion conjunctivitis and a 10 to 20 per cent risk of developing pneumonia.[522] The latter invariably occurs before the age of 6 months (usually from 2 to 14 weeks) and is said to account for about 30 per cent of all pneumonias in hospitalized infants during this neonatal period.[523] The chest roentgenogram has been described as showing bilateral diffuse interstitial and alveolar disease associated with overinflated lungs and areas of atelectasis.[524] Affected infants have a staccato cough and tachypnea.

Chlamydia trachomatis also has been shown to cause pneumonia in both immunocompromised[525] and immunocompetent[526] adults. Clinically, such infection ranges from acute bronchitis to severe diffuse interstitial pneumonia. A sensitive enzyme-linked fluorescence immunoassay has been described in which reticulate and elementary bodies from *C. trachomatis* are employed as antigens to detect IgM antibody.[527]

Chlamydia Psittaci

Chlamydia psittaci is a common pathogen of many birds and mammals. Most cases of human disease in which a history of animal exposure can be obtained appear to be acquired from birds, particularly parakeets, pigeons, budgerigars, and poultry.* The organisms are excreted in the feces and urine of infected birds, especially at breeding time in crowded and unsanitary conditions. They are resistant to drying and remain viable for at least a month at ambient temperature. Although the bird or birds responsible may have been obviously ill or may have died from the disease, this is not by any means invariable. In addition, infection may be acquired from a bird recently purchased from a dealer, who, having acquired immunity, remains healthy. A history of avian exposure may not always be obtained; for example, only about 15 per cent of the patients in sporadic cases in England in 1980 had known contact with birds.[528] The mode of infection in such cases is possibly person-to-person transmission.[529]

The reported incidence of disease is low. Despite this, it is probable that the disease is underdiagnosed and that some cases labeled as "primary atypical" or viral pneumonia could be proved to be ornithosis with careful history-taking and serologic testing. Disease may occur sporadically or in epidemics, the latter usually among poultry workers.[530] It may be acquired any time of the year, but the incidence is increased slightly during the cold months and early spring. The incubation period ranges from 6 to 20 days.

The microscopic appearance is variable and nonspecific, consisting of intra-alveolar edema, hemorrhage, and a mononuclear inflammatory infiltrate. Hyaline membranes may be present. Intracytoplasmic inclusions may be identified, but usually with difficulty.

The chest roentgenogram has been described as consisting of a homogeneous ground-glass opacity (sometimes containing small areas of radiolucency),[529] a patchy reticular pattern radiating out from the hilar areas or involving the lung bases, and segmental or lobar consolidation with or without atelectasis. Enlargement of hilar lymph nodes may occur. Roentgenographic resolution often is delayed for many weeks after clinical cure has occurred; one report indicated a return to normal in 6 weeks by 50 per cent of patients and in 12 weeks by 75 per cent.[528]

Clinically, ornithosis varies in intensity from a mild febrile episode to severe disease simulating typhoid, including the presence of bradycardia and even "rose spots." Headaches, fever, and chills are almost invariable. Respiratory symptoms and signs may or may not be present.[531] Cough usually is dry but may produce nonpurulent mucoid material; hemoptysis occurs in a few cases. Pleuritic pain is uncommon. Dyspnea may be severe in cases of overwhelming infection. The systemic symptoms include malaise, anorexia, nausea and vomiting, polyarthritis, myalgia, abdominal pain, and delirium. The physical signs of pulmonary disease may consist only of basal crepitations, although signs of frank parenchymal consolidation and a friction rub may be present. Hepatosplenomegaly, superficial lymph node enlargement, and erythema nodosum may occur.

The white blood cell count ranges from normal to moderately increased, with or without eosinophilia. Hemolytic anemia and proteinuria may occur, and liver function may be disturbed. Electrocardiographic abnormalities are frequent. The organism may be recovered from the blood during the first 4 days and from the sputum during the first 2 weeks of illness. It may be isolated by culture of spleen or liver tissue in the intraperitoneal cavity of mice, in chicken embryos, and on tissue; growth occurs in 5 to 30 days. Complement-fixation antibodies appear in the second to fourth week of the disease.

Rickettsiae

Rickettsiae are small, obligate intracellular organisms that are properly classified as bacteria but that are discussed at this point because of the similarity between pneumonia caused by them and by viruses. Four groups cause disease in humans, of which the major organism responsible for respiratory disease is *Coxiella burnetii*.

Coxiella Burnetii

Coxiella burnetii, the causative agent of Q fever, is distinguished from other rickettsiae by its gram-positivity, lack of pathogenicity for mice, and a variety of antigenic and metabolic characteristics. It is exceptionally resistant to drying and to destruction by chemical agents and can survive for many months in a hostile extracellular environment. It may be isolated by inoculation of infected material into the peritoneal cavity of guinea pigs and may be cultured in chick embryos, growth occurring in 4 to 14 days.

Its natural reservoir appears to be ticks, from which it is often transmitted to other hosts by bites. In the United States, the infection is widely prevalent among livestock, particularly sheep, cattle, and goats. The usual mode of transmission to humans is by inhalation from laboratory cultures,[532] from dust in sheep and cattle sheds,[533] or directly from infected animals used in research or slaughtered in abattoirs. Animals are especially contagious after parturition. As might be expected, there is a strong occupational association, farmers, abattoir and stockyard workers, and veterinary and medical laboratory personnel being particularly susceptible. The incubation period ranges from 1 to 6 weeks, averaging about 14 days. As with viral pulmonary infection, many cases of Q fever are probably misdiagnosed.[533a]

---

*Since the disease in humans was initially associated with birds of the order Psittaciformes, it has been widely known as "psittacosis," although the presence of disease in many other birds suggests that the term "ornithosis" is more appropriate.

The few reports documenting pathologic changes have described extensive parenchymal consolidation caused by a combination of airspace hemorrhage, edema, and a mononuclear inflammatory cell infiltrate; necrosis may be present. Airways contain similar exudate, and their walls may show focal areas of epithelial ulceration. Organisms may be identified in some cases by Macchiavello's stain.

In one review of 32 patients with serologically confirmed Q fever (of whom 28 manifested pulmonary abnormalities), there were multiple round areas of consolidation measuring 5 to 20 cm in diameter that were of ground-glass density and were usually situated in the lower lobes.[534] Some patients manifest lobar or sublobar consolidation associated with loss of volume (Fig. 6–60). Resolution tends to be slow, ranging from 10 days to as long as 6 months.[534a]

Onset of the disease is usually insidious, with malaise for several days followed by headaches (which may be severe), chills, myalgia, and arthralgia. Myocarditis, endocarditis, hepatitis, or phlebitis also may occur. Involvement of the upper respiratory tract is frequent and causes a troublesome dry cough. Physical examination of the lungs commonly reveals little abnormality despite fairly extensive parenchymal disease visible on roentgenographic examination. Fever is frequently remittent. The organism may be isolated from the urine, blood, sputum, or pleural fluid. Complement-fixing and agglutinating antibodies appear within 2 to 3 weeks, and the titer is maximal approximately 30 days after onset of clinical symptoms.

The illness may relapse and recur in some cases.[532] It is usually self-limited, however, and the mortality is probably less than 1 per cent.

Rickettsia Rickettsii

This organism is the cause of Rocky Mountain spotted fever, an acute and often fulminant disease found exclusively in North and South America. Despite its name, the disease is most prevalent in the eastern United States. Humans are infected by the bite of several species of tick, so that the majority of cases occur during the warm months. From the initial site of inoculation, the organisms disseminate via the bloodstream and invade capillary endothelial cells, in which they multiply and eventually cause endothelial necrosis, vasculitis, and thrombosis. The result is widespread areas of tissue necrosis and hemorrhage. Typically, the skin, subcutaneous tissues, and central nervous system are most severely affected.

Although pathologic abnormalities in the lungs have been found in a high proportion of patients at autopsy,[535] roentgenologic manifestations are seen less often and are quite variable. Of the 13 patients with abnormal chest roentgenograms in one series,[536] the predominant abnormalities were local or diffuse airspace consolidation, diffuse interstitial disease, and/or pleural effusion. Clinically, patients present with fever, rash, headache, and myalgia. Cough, rales, and evidence of impaired gas exchange are common.[537]

PARASITIC INFESTATION

Protozoa

Entamoeba Histolytica (Amebiasis)

Although human infestation is sometimes caused by other amebae, the term "amebiasis" is reserved for that caused by *Entamoeba histolytica*, a species usually associated with colonic disease (amebic dysentery). The latter is of worldwide distribution, with areas of high endemicity in regions where hygiene and therapeutic measures are inadequate. Cysts are passed in the feces of affected individuals (who are frequently asymptomatic) and are usually ingested in contaminated water or food. Person-to-person transmission also occurs and has been said to be the commonest mode of spread in the United States.[538] Whereas amebic dysentery shows no age or sex predominance, for unknown reasons pleuropulmonary involvement develops most frequently between the ages of 20 and 40 years and is 10 to 15 times commoner in men.[539] Such involvement has been estimated to occur in approximately 1 in 1000 patients with amebic dysentery; however, when the liver is involved, the incidence is 15 to 20 per cent.[540]

Pathogenesis and Pathologic Characteristics. The cysts of *Entamoeba histolytica* are acid-resistant and are able to travel through the stomach to the small intestine, where trophozoites excyst. These move on to the colon, where they multiply and pass through the epithelium into the submucosa. Penetration of the mucosa is associated with necrosis and ulceration and the characteristic symptoms of amebic dysentery. Organisms may subsequently spread to the liver, with the development of microabscesses and, eventually, macroabscesses.

Pleuropulmonary disease can occur by several mechanisms, the most frequent of which is extension of disease from a hepatic abscess, usually located in the right lobe. Such abscesses may extend into the subphrenic space and form a separate subdiaphragmatic abscess, in which circumstance intrathoracic complications such as pleural effusion and basal pulmonary disease result from the subphrenic inflammation rather than from direct invasion by the parasite. In other instances, empyema or basal pulmonary disease results from direct transdiaphragmatic extension of infection, either in association with a hepatic abscess alone or with combined hepatic and subphrenic abscesses.

Sections of the lung infected by *E. histolytica* show poorly defined areas of necrosis that are frequently soft to semifluid in consistency and possess a characteristic mucinous, hemorrhagic appearance likened to anchovy paste or chocolate sauce. Histologically, there is a variable degree of necrosis, fibrosis, and mononuclear inflammatory infiltrate. Trophozoites may be identified at the margins of the necrotic areas contiguous with normal lung.

Roentgenographic Manifestations. Right-sided pleural effusion combined with basal pulmonary disease constitutes the usual picture of pleuropulmonary amebic infestation. In one study of 88 cases of amebic empyema, the chest roentgenograms showed total or nearly total opacification of the right hemithorax and marked mediastinal shift to the left.[541] Pulmonary parenchymal involvement usually consists of ill-defined homogeneous consolidation of the right lower or middle lobe, without clear-cut segmental distribution. Some of these areas of consolidation progress to abscess formation and, later, cavitation. Ultrasonography, occasionally with percutaneous fine-needle aspiration,[542] and MRI[543] can be very useful in evaluating both liver and lung abscesses.

Clinical Manifestations. The possibility of pleuropulmonary amebiasis should be considered in a patient who is or has been a resident of an endemic area and complains of right upper quadrant abdominal pain and a dry cough,

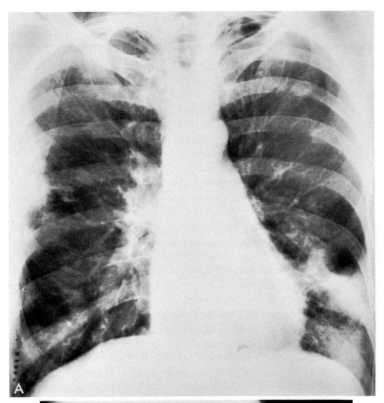

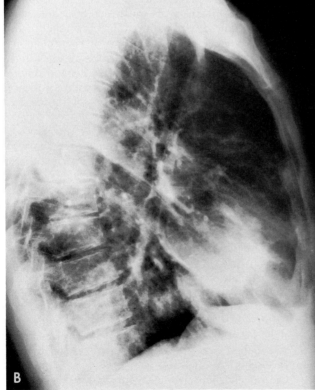

Figure 6–60. Q Fever Pneumonia. Posteroanterior *(A)* and lateral *(B)* roentgenograms reveal local areas of homogeneous consolidation in the right upper and lower lobes, the lingula, and the left lower lobe. Four serum samples showed a rising titer of complement-fixing antibodies to *Coxiella burnetii* during the 4 weeks following these roentgenograms. (Courtesy of Sherbrooke Hospital, Sherbrooke, Quebec.)

particularly if there is a history of diarrhea. The dry cough characterizes the early stages of pleuropulmonary involvement; later it may become productive of "chocolate-sauce" material and may be accompanied by severe cachexia. Expectoration of bile (biloptysis) also may occur, most often as a result of a bronchohepatic or, less often, bronchobiliary fistula.[544] Physical examination may reveal a palpable, tender liver, lower intercostal tenderness, or both.

Leukocytosis is usually moderate and may be associated with eosinophilia and anemia. A positive diagnosis can be made by the demonstration of trophozoites in the sputum, pleural exudate, or material obtained by needle aspiration; however, recovery of the organism from these sources is exceedingly difficult in most patients. A presumptive diagnosis can be made if stool contains trophozoites or cysts. Results of serologic tests for amebiasis are positive in almost all cases.[540]

The overall mortality rate associated with thoracic amebiasis has been estimated to be about 10 to 15 per cent.[539]

Toxoplasma Gondii (Toxoplasmosis)

Toxoplasmosis is caused by *Toxoplasma gondii,* an obligate intracellular protozoan that causes widespread infestation that is rarely manifested clinically. The organism is found in many wild and domestic animals throughout the world. Humans usually acquire infection by ingestion of material contaminated by oocyst-infected stool or of poorly cooked, cyst-containing meat, particularly lamb.[545]

On ingestion, the oocysts are disrupted by digestive enzymes and release trophozoites that enter the intestinal mucosa and disseminate via the bloodstream. In immunologically competent persons the disease is usually limited, intracellular infestation and cell death occurring predominantly in cardiac and skeletal muscle and the brain. The organisms encyst in these organs and occasionally other sites, where they remain viable and can serve as a source of disease in individuals who subsequently lose their immunologic competence.

Disease occurs in several clinicopathologic forms.[546] Lymph node enlargement, with or without symptoms similar to infectious mononucleosis, is the commonest clinically recognized form of the disease in adults; a variety of lymph node groups, including those in the mediastinum, may be affected. Generalized disease in adults usually occurs in immunocompromised hosts.

In disseminated disease, the lungs show interstitial pneumonitis and a largely mononuclear inflammatory infiltrate; in severe cases, an alveolar exudate and necrosis ensue. Trophozoites may be identified lying free in tissue, and cysts are found in macrophages and in alveolar epithelial and capillary endothelial cells. Roentgenographically, pulmonary disease is usually manifested by a focal reticular pattern resembling acute viral pneumonia; in some cases, there is airspace consolidation. Hilar lymph node enlargement is common.

Clinically, toxoplasmosis in adults commonly resembles infectious mononucleosis.[546] Patients may be asymptomatic or may manifest low-grade fever and lymph node enlargement, with or without a rash, over a period of several weeks or months. Anemia and lymphocytosis are common. Disseminated disease is characterized by fever, disorientation,

confusion, and headache, in addition to the clinical manifestations of myocarditis. Pneumonia is associated with nonproductive cough, tachypnea, dyspnea, and cyanosis. An IgM titer of 1:160 or greater is the best indicator of an infestation acquired during the previous 2 to 4 months.[547]

Pneumocystis Carinii

Pneumocystis carinii is an organism of uncertain taxonomic status, being considered a protozoan by most authors but recently having been shown to possess biochemical and genetic features more suggestive of a fungus.[29] *In vivo,* it exists in two forms:[548] (1) thick-walled, round or crescent-shaped cysts measuring 3 to 6 μm in diameter that may contain as many as eight intracystic bodies, believed to represent developing trophozoites (sporozoites); and (2) extracystic trophozoites, most of which range in diameter from 1 to 5 μm and are pleomorphic in shape. Routine laboratory culture methods are not available.

Organisms that are morphologically identical to *P. carinii* are found in the lungs of many animals, including the rat, mouse, rabbit, and dog; other natural habitats have not been identified. Although some of these organisms have been shown to be antigenically distinct,[29] the possibility that a single agent infects both an animal species and humans, the former serving as a reservoir for human infection, has not been excluded. If the organism is truly a fungus, it is also possible that an environmental source, such as water and soil, may eventually be identified.[29]

Because of the universal presence of the organism within the lungs, the mode of transmission is assumed to be by inhalation. Although occasional clusters of human cases have suggested direct person-to-person transmission,[549] it is probable that most cases of clinical disease result from reactivation of latent infection acquired during the early life of a patient who has subsequently become immunocompromised.

Although *P. carinii* infection is common—as evidenced by the presence of antibodies to the organism in a high proportion of healthy individuals at an early age[550]—and may cause subclinical pneumonitis in apparently healthy individuals,[550a] it causes clinically significant pneumonia only in persons with underlying disease. It occurs in two clinicopathologic forms: (1) an "endemic infantile type" that was described in Europe during and immediately after World War II as a disease limited to marasmic infants between the ages of 2 and 5 months; and (2) a sporadic disease in children and adults whose immune status is compromised.

Pathogenesis. The factors involved in the transformation from a state of apparent symbiosis to one of active disease and the mechanisms by which *P. carinii* produces tissue damage and clinical disease are not well understood. As indicated, it is clear that immunosuppression is one of the most important factors associated with the development of disease. This effect might be related to an abnormality in macrophage function; both trophozoites and cysts may be seen within alveolar macrophages by electron microscopy,[548] and it is conceivable that a decrease in ordinary surveillance by these cells might be sufficient to allow endogenously inactive organisms to multiply. Support for this hypothesis comes from the finding of a paucity of alveolar

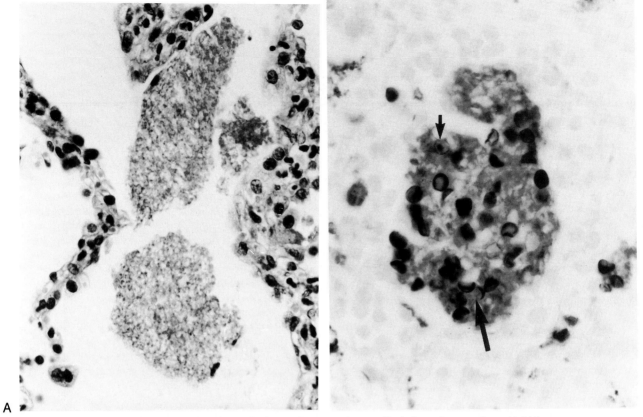

A   B

Figure 6–61. *Pneumocystis Carinii* Pneumonia. *A,* A magnified view of a transbronchial biopsy specimen from a 42-year-old man with AIDS shows mild interstitial thickening due to edema and a mononuclear inflammatory cell infiltrate; two clusters of finely vacuolated proteinaceous material are present within alveolar airspaces. *B,* Silver stain of one of these clusters shows it to contain multiple more or less round or sickle-shaped *(long arrow)* cysts. (*A* × 440; *B* Grocott silver methenamine, × 1000.)

macrophages in bronchoalveolar washings of immunocompromised patients with *P. carinii* pneumonia.[551]

The trophozoites produce no known toxins. They are found predominantly within alveolar airspaces and seldom in the alveolar interstitium or elsewhere in the body,[552] indicating a limited capacity to invade tissue. Experiments with rats—that consistently develop *P. carinii* pneumonia after several weeks of corticosteroid treatment—have shown close apposition and apparent attachment of trophozoites to type I alveolar epithelial cells,[553] which subsequently undergo degeneration and necrosis.[554] However, the mechanism by which this damage occurs is not known. There is evidence that the development of a host inflammatory reaction (particularly involving polymorphonuclear leukocytes) may be important in determining both the severity of clinical manifestations and the prognosis.[32] It has been speculated that a deficiency in surfactant phospholipid may underlie abnormalities in pulmonary function.[555]

Pathologic Characteristics. In the typical case of *P. carinii* pneumonia seen at autopsy, infection is diffuse, all lobes possessing a firm, rubbery consistency. Occasionally (usually in patients with AIDS), it is focal and limited predominantly to one lobe in either a diffuse or a nodular fashion. Histologically, there is a variable degree of edema and infiltration of the alveolar interstitium by lymphocytes and plasma cells, and a characteristic foamy, eosinophilic intra-alveolar exudate containing scattered macrophages

(Fig. 6–61). Other histologic changes that may occur either alone or in association with the typical features include interstitial and intra-alveolar granulomatous inflammation, vasculitis, and diffuse alveolar damage with hyaline membranes.[556]

The cysts are seen to best advantage with silver stain, with which they appear as clusters of round, oval, or crescent-shaped structures within the foamy exudate (*see* Fig. 6–61). Trophozoites may also be identified with special stains but, because of their small size, with less ease and reliability than cysts. Although cysts may disappear rapidly following therapy, resolution may be very slow, particularly in patients with AIDS.[557] Organizing pneumonia and interstitial fibrosis may be seen in some cases of healing or apparently healed disease.

Roentgenographic Manifestations. In the early stages of disease, a granular or reticulogranular pattern is apparent, particularly in perihilar areas.[558] In later stages the pattern progresses to airspace consolidation, patchy areas of homogeneous consolidation being interspersed with foci of atelectasis and overinflation, particularly in peripheral zones (Fig. 6–62). The changes are diffuse and may resemble those of pulmonary edema. Terminally, the lungs may be massively consolidated, to a point of almost complete airlessness. The hilar lymph nodes do not enlarge. Although pleural effusion is very uncommon, its presence does not necessarily exclude the diagnosis.[559]

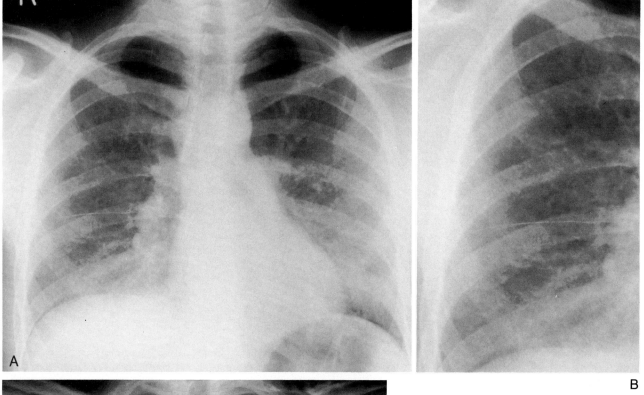

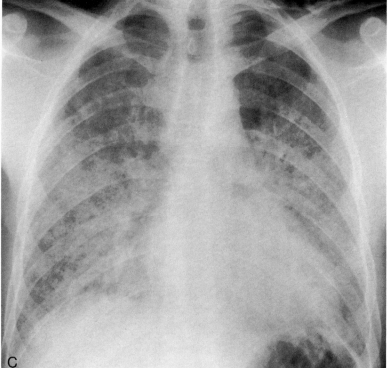

Figure 6–62. *Pneumocystis Carinii* Pneumonia in a Man with AIDS. A posteroanterior chest roentgenogram *(A)* and a close-up view of the right lung *(B)* show a diffuse, medium reticular pattern throughout both lungs, worse in the lower lobes; normal lung markings are effaced. The appearance is characteristic of a predominantly interstitial abnormality and, in this clinical setting, is suggestive of early *P. carinii* pneumonia. Several days later *(C)*, the disease had progressed and now exhibited an extensive airspace component; the previous interstitial pattern has been obscured.

Although the constellation of findings previously described is characteristic of *Pneumocystis* pneumonia, it may be seen in other conditions, especially viral pneumonia. In addition, variations in the typical pattern are common, particularly in patients with AIDS (*see* page 297); atypical findings include marked unilateral predominance, lobar or segmental consolidation in addition to diffuse involvement, a pseudonodular pattern simulating metastases, basal atelectasis, and cavity formation. In fact, in some series a "classic" roentgenographic presentation is seen in fewer than half of all patients.[560]

Despite the fact that many other pulmonary diseases can cause an increased uptake of gallium-67, the value of a positive scan in supporting a clinical diagnosis of *P. carinii* pneumonia has been convincingly demonstrated.[561]

Clinical Manifestations. The onset of clinical disease is variable. In patients with AIDS, there is often a prodrome of fever, lymph node enlargement, weight loss, and malaise over a 2- to 3-week period, followed by an abrupt onset of dyspnea, hypoxemia, and increased A-a oxygen gradient. In patients without AIDS, the disease is likely to present more acutely with fever and hypoxemia.[562] A dry, hacking cough may be present, but pleural pain and hemoptysis do not occur. Some patients are afebrile. Physical signs are minimal and include a few scattered rales or rhonchi. The clinical course of the disease lasts for 6 to 8 weeks, but roentgenographic changes may persist much longer.

Laboratory Findings. In most patients, the white blood cell count is slightly to moderately increased, with polymorphonuclear leukocytes predominating. Leukopenia is seen particularly in patients with AIDS[562] and is a bad prognostic sign. Lymphopenia is found in approximately 50 per cent of patients.[563] Serum lactate dehydrogenase is elevated in *P. carinii* pneumonia much more often than in other pneumonias, and its measurement has been advocated as a useful test in differential diagnosis.[564] Impairment of gas transfer may be considerable, even in the presence of a normal chest roentgenogram.[565]

Although the disease may be strongly suspected from the combination of roentgenologic and clinical findings in an immunocompromised individual, definitive diagnosis requires demonstration of the organism. In the majority of cases, this can readily be accomplished by BAL and pathologic examination of the resulting fluid, the sensitivity being about 90 to 95 per cent. In addition to standard BAL, studies of patients with AIDS have supported the efficacy of less invasive procedures (e.g., control-tipped catheterization without bronchoscopy to induce BAL, a procedure that possesses a sensitivity of 85 to 90 per cent[566]) or noninvasive procedures (e.g., sputum induction with 3 per cent saline, which has a sensitivity of 75 to 80 per cent[567]). This surprisingly high yield undoubtedly reflects the overwhelming *P. carinii* infection that is so common in patients with AIDS. Although data are sparse, such results are not seen in patients with other underlying conditions, such as organ transplant recipients[558]; in these individuals, transbronchial and sometimes open lung biopsy may be necessary for diagnosis.

Prognosis. Although *P. carinii* pneumonia constitutes a potentially life-threatening complication of diseases associated with immune suppression, aggressive therapy in the intensive care unit results in reversal of the disease in a substantial number of individuals.[568] However, a small but important number—particularly those with AIDS—succumb to the acute infection.[568a] Follow-up studies of patients who have survived the infestation have shown that children tend to be free from morphologic or functional defects,[569] whereas physiologic and pathologic abnormalities tend to persist in adults. Although these abnormalities are usually not severe, residual restrictive disease may occur.[570]

Nemathelminths (Roundworms)

Ascaris Lumbricoides (Ascariasis)

In the great majority of cases, human ascariasis is caused by *Ascaris lumbricoides*. The adult female worm lives in the small intestine, where it produces up to 250,000 eggs per day. These are passed in the feces to the external environment, where they are resistant to drying and freezing and can remain viable for many years. When ingested, the ovum hatches in the small intestine, and the larvae enter the portal veins or intestinal lymphatics. From there they pass by way of the right heart to the lungs, where they are trapped by the alveolar capillaries and exit into the airspaces. At this point they molt and develop into third stage larvae. These then migrate up the airways to the larynx, where they are swallowed, and complete their odyssey by developing into mature worms in the small intestine.

Pulmonary disease usually is caused as larvae pass through the lungs. Roentgenographically, there are patchy areas of homogeneous consolidation; in many cases, these are transient and without clear-cut segmental distribution in the characteristic pattern of Löffler's syndrome (*see* page 428). The shadows may be several centimeters in diameter and, in cases of moderate severity, tend to be rather discrete and concentrated in the perihilar regions; with more severe involvement, they tend to coalesce and assume a lobular pattern.[571]

Pulmonary symptoms consist of nonproductive cough, retrosternal chest pain, and, in more severe cases, hemoptysis and dyspnea. A transient, intensely pruritic skin eruption may appear within 4 or 5 days after the onset of respiratory symptoms.[571] Low-grade fever may be present, and scattered rhonchi and rales may be heard over the lungs. Leukocytosis of 20,000 to 25,000 cells per mL is common, with an eosinophilia of 30 to 70 per cent. The diagnosis is made by the discovery of larvae in the sputum or gastric aspirate; the identification of adult worms or ova in the stools strongly supports the diagnosis.

Strongyloides Stercoralis (Strongyloidiasis)

The great majority of cases of strongyloidiasis are caused by the nematode *Strongyloides stercoralis,* a parasite prevalent in tropical and temperate climates throughout the world. The life cycle of the organism is complex. Free-living filariform larvae penetrate the undamaged skin and pass via the bloodstream to the lung, where they migrate from the capillaries into the alveoli, and thence up the airways to the larynx and down the esophagus to the gut. Within the small intestine, they develop into adult females

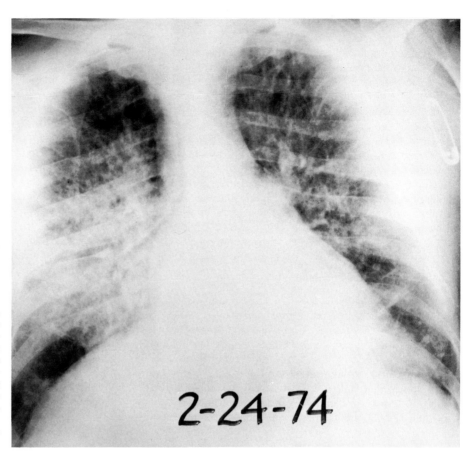

Figure 6–63. Pulmonary Strongyloidiasis. An anteroposterior roentgenogram exposed with the patient in the supine position reveals widespread disease of both lungs in a pattern suggesting extensive involvement of both interstitium and airspaces. Confluent airspace consolidation is particularly evident in the right lung. The larvae of *Strongyloides stercoralis* were identified in both the sputum and the stool. (Courtesy of the General Hospital, Wayne County, Missouri.)

that take up residence and lay eggs in the mucosal crypts. In their subsequent passage through the gut, the eggs develop into noninfectious rhabditiform larvae; these in turn may be passed in the stool and develop directly into filariform larvae in the soil or may transform directly into the filariform larvae within the gut, leading to autoinfection through direct penetration of the intestinal mucosa or perianal skin. This ability of the organism to migrate through the lungs without a soil cycle permits persistence of chronic and recurrent infestation for years, long after residence in an endemic area has terminated.

The disease is endemic in rural tropical areas where the climate is warm and the soil moist (including the southern United States); in these regions, infestation has been estimated to affect up to 35 per cent of the population.[572] Since the larvae parasitize humans through penetration of the skin, the disease is seen most frequently in areas where people walk barefoot on soil contaminated by feces. In the majority of cases, infestation is accompanied by mild or no clinical symptoms. In recent years, however, severe disease (so-called hyperinfection) has been recognized with increasing frequency in immunocompromised hosts[573] and in patients with asthma or chronic obstructive pulmonary disease receiving corticosteroid therapy.[574]

Roentgenographically, infestation can appear as nonsegmental, patchy areas of consolidation (Fig. 6–63), presumably caused by an allergic reaction to the migration of the filariform larvae through the lungs. Various patterns have been described with hyperinfection, including airspace consolidation and diffuse nodular or reticulonodular disease.

In most cases, pulmonary symptoms are mild or absent; in more severe disease, there may be dyspnea, hemoptysis, and bronchospasm. Abdominal pain and diarrhea, or diarrhea alternating with constipation, are common.[575] IgE and total blood eosinophil levels are usually increased.

The diagnosis is made by finding larvae in the sputum, gastric washings, or BAL fluid[576]; a presumptive diagnosis can be based on their detection in stool. An ELISA employing antigen extracted from third stage larvae has been found to be positive for antibody in approximately 80 per cent of patients in whom infestation has been proved; in immunocompromised patients, however, this test is of limited value.[577]

Trichinella Spiralis (Trichinosis)

Trichinosis results from the ingestion of larvae of the round worm *Trichinella spiralis*. It is worldwide in distribution and is found wherever contaminated meat, particularly pork, is eaten raw or undercooked. Live encysted larvae in the meat reach the small intestine, where they mature, mate, and produce eggs. When the eggs hatch, the larvae penetrate the duodenal wall and are carried to the lungs, from which they pass via the pulmonary circulation into the systemic circulation and are distributed to striated muscles throughout the body. Although any muscle may be parasitized, the diaphragm is perhaps the most frequently involved. Within muscle, the coiled *Trichinella* larvae encyst and become surrounded by a thick refractile hyaline layer that frequently calcifies 6 to 18 months after infestation.

Roentgenographically, there are no abnormalities related to the lungs, since the larvae produce minimal reaction in their passage through the pulmonary circulation. Calcified walls of larval cysts within the respiratory muscles may be visible as oval opacities 1.0 cm in their longest diameter.

Clinically, no symptoms result from passage of the parasite through the lungs. Diarrhea develops 2 to 4 days after the ingestion of contaminated meat; fever, muscular pains, facial edema, and central nervous system symptoms may develop by the seventh day. Deposition of the larvae in the skeletal muscles occurs by the tenth day and may result in dyspnea and tachypnea.[578] Leukocytosis with some degree of eosinophilia is common. The skin test and serologic test results become positive 3 weeks after infestation.

Tropical (Filarial) Eosinophilia

As the name suggests, this is a disease confined largely to the tropics and is characterized clinically by asthma associated with moderate to severe leukocytosis and eosinophilia. The etiologic agents have not been precisely identified but are believed to be parasitic microfilariae. The organisms most strongly implicated are *Wuchereria bancrofti* and *Brugia malayi*, best known as the causes of Bancroft's and Malayan filariasis.[579] It has been speculated that in tropical eosinophilia adult worms somewhere in the body release into the bloodstream microfilariae that are trapped largely in the lungs, where they cause a local inflammatory reaction[579]; this would explain the prominence of respiratory symptoms and the relative absence of circulating systemic microfilariae (in contrast with the typical forms of filariasis). The reason that the pathogenesis of tropical eosinophilia differs from that of classic Bancroft's or Malayan filariasis is not understood.

Tropical eosinophilia is confined to regions in which appropriate mosquito vectors live—the Indian subcontinent, Malaysia, southern Asia, northern Africa, and certain areas of South America. Most patients are adult men between the ages of 20 and 40 years.

Pathologic findings consist of a prominent eosinophilic leukocyte infiltrate located within the alveolar interstitium and airspaces and around bronchovascular structures.[580] Roentgenographically, lung involvement is diffuse and symmetric and is characterized by a reticulonodular pattern, the nodules sometimes measuring 2 to 5 mm in diameter; middle and lower lung zones are predominantly affected (Fig. 6–64). Hilar lymph node enlargement occurs in some cases.[581] Pleural effusion is rare. The chest roentgenogram may show complete clearing with appropriate therapy, but the changes may be permanent.

The main symptom is cough, usually productive of small amounts of mucoid or mucopurulent material. It tends to be particularly bothersome at night when it occurs in paroxysms, sometimes with the production of blood-streaked

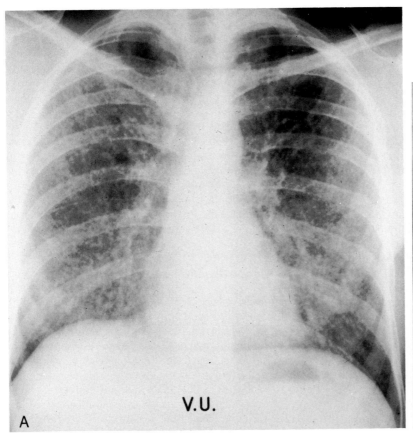

V.U.

A

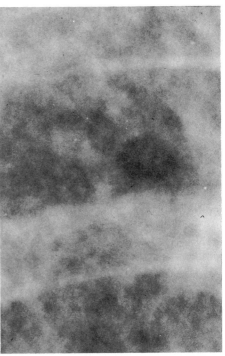

B

Figure 6–64. Tropical Eosinophilia. A posteroanterior chest roentgenogram *(A)* and a magnified view of the right upper lobe *(B)* reveal a diffuse reticulonodular pattern throughout both lungs. There is no evidence of hilar or mediastinal lymph node enlargement. The patient was a young man from East India who presented with nocturnal cough, fever, and high blood eosinophilia.

sputum. Attacks of coughing and dyspnea may be so severe as to suggest status asthmaticus. Weight loss, fatigue, low-grade fever, and slight enlargement of the liver and spleen are frequent.[581] There may be physical signs of broncho-spasm.

Leukocytosis is usually severe—60,000 white blood cells per mL is not unusual—with eosinophilia, sometimes as high as 60 per cent. Very high levels of serum and BAL fluid IgE and filarial-specific antibodies are also found in acute disease.[582] Confirmation of the diagnosis may be provided by complement-fixation and skin tests using *Dirofilaria immitis* antigen. Pulmonary function test results show either a restrictive pattern or a combined restrictive and obstructive pattern. Occasionally, such aberrations become irreversible[583]; affected patients have chronic hypoxemia, although PCO_2 and pulmonary arterial pressures remain within normal limits.

Dirofilaria Immitis (Dirofilariasis)

Pulmonary disease caused by *Dirofilaria immitis* has been recognized with increasing frequency since its original description in 1961.[584] The organism is a natural parasite of dogs and, less commonly, cats and a variety of wild carnivores. In these animals, it is initially present in the subcutaneous tissue; from there, it migrates to the right heart chambers and main pulmonary artery, where one or several worms take up residence and release microfilariae into the blood. Mosquitos subsequently transmit filariae both to the definitive host and to humans. Since humans are not a natural host, the organism does not complete its life cycle and dies before reaching sexual maturity; it is then carried into the pulmonary circulation, where it lodges in a peripheral vessel and causes necrosis of surrounding tissue.

The lesions are usually located in the periphery of the lung in the form of circumscribed, more or less spherical nodules. Histologically, there is a central region of coagulative necrosis surrounded by a variable amount of fibrous tissue and inflammatory infiltrate. One or occasionally several worms may be identified within a pulmonary artery in the central portion of the nodule. This pathologic appearance likely results from an inflammatory reaction to antigen released by the degenerating worm rather than vascular occlusion and ischemia.

Roentgenographically, the typical manifestation is a solitary, spherical or wedge-shaped, well-defined nodule, 1 to 2 cm in diameter.[585] Multiple nodules occur in about 10 per cent of cases.[584] A pneumonic pattern has also been described, evolving eventually to a solitary nodule.

Most cases of human disease have been in adults from the southeastern United States (particularly Florida and Texas).[584] The majority of patients are asymptomatic, the diagnosis being made after pulmonary resection because of suspicion of pulmonary carcinoma. Systemic eosinophilia is uncommon. Serologic tests may be helpful in diagnosis in some patients.[586] However, antibody levels may decrease substantially after the organism dies and there is cross-reaction with other parasites.[584]

Pulmonary Larva Migrans

Pulmonary larva migrans results from infestation by larvae of the dog and cat roundworms *Toxocara canis* and *T.*

cati. It occurs predominantly in children who swallow soil containing eggs passed in the feces of dogs or cats. The eggs develop into larvae in the intestine, pass into the bloodstream, and are carried to many organs and tissues, including the lungs. Since humans are not the definitive host, the larvae cannot complete their life cycle; they become trapped within small blood vessels, penetrate their walls, and migrate into contiguous tissue. Here they may either remain dormant or die, provoking an intense inflammatory (typically granulomatous) reaction. Roentgenographically, approximately 50 per cent of patients with pulmonary symptoms have transient local or diffuse patchy areas of ill-defined consolidation.[540]

Children with this disease may be asymptomatic or may complain of cough, wheezing, dyspnea, cyanosis, abdominal pain, and neurologic symptoms. Hepatosplenomegaly is usual. Leukocytosis of 40,000 cells per mL or more is common, usually with eosinophilia of at least 30 per cent. The diagnosis may be made by the identification of granulomas containing larvae on liver biopsy. A skin test and immunofluorescent antibody test are considered practical and reliable.[587] Using larval antigens or their metabolic products, an ELISA has been reported to have a sensitivity of about 80 per cent and a specificity of 90 per cent.[588]

Platyhelminths (Flatworms)

Echinococcus Granulosus (Echinococcosis)

Echinococcosis (hydatid disease) is caused by larvae of the class Cestoda, of which *E. granulosus* is responsible for the vast majority of human pulmonary infestations. The adult worm consists of four segments: a head (scolex) that is composed of four suckers and a rostellum that contains a double row of hooklets for attachment to the intestinal mucosa, and three proglottids, the last of which is the egg-laying organ.

Disease occurs in two forms. The *pastoral variety* is the commoner and, as the name implies, occurs in rural settings in which sheep, cows, or pigs are the intermediate hosts, and dogs the usual definitive hosts. Humans usually acquire the disease by direct contact with infested dogs or by ingestion of egg-contaminated water, food, or soil; humans thus become accidental intermediate hosts. The disease is particularly common in the sheep-raising Mediterranean regions and in Russia, Argentina, Chile, Uruguay, Australasia, and portions of Africa. The *sylvatic variety* is very likely caused by a different strain of the tapeworm, the definitive hosts being species of the Canidae family, including the dog, wolf, arctic fox, and coyote. A variety of herbivores, including moose, deer, reindeer, elk, caribou, and bison, serve as intermediate hosts. The disease is seen primarily in Alaska and northern Canada. It is acquired by the same mechanism as the pastoral variety.

Pathogenesis and Pathologic Characteristics

The mature adult worms live in the small intestine of the definitive host. Eggs are passed in the feces to grazing land or water, and are ingested by the intermediate hosts. In these, larvae develop in the duodenum, penetrate the wall, and pass in the portal bloodstream to the liver, where the majority are trapped in hepatic sinusoids. Of those that escape, most are trapped in the alveolar capillary sieve. The majority of entrapped larvae are killed by natural host defenses, but the few that survive develop into solitary or multiple cysts that produce brood capsules containing immature worms. The life cycle of the parasite is completed when the definitive host feeds on the remains of an intermediate host that harbors the cystic stage of the disease, with subsequent intraintestinal development of adult worms.

The ability of the hepatic and pulmonary capillary sieves to contain the larvae is largely responsible for the preponderance of disease in these organs. In the pastoral variety, approximately 65 to 70 per cent of cysts occur in the liver, and 15 to 30 per cent in the lungs. For reasons that are unclear, however, lung cysts show a clear preponderance over liver cysts in sylvatic disease.[589]

Within the lung, hydatid cysts typically are spherical or oval in shape (Fig. 6–65) and are surrounded by a layer of fibrous tissue containing a nonspecific chronic inflammatory infiltrate (the pericyst). The cyst itself is composed of two layers: (1) a laminated, outer chitinous membrane (the exocyst) that serves to protect the developing organisms from the host; and (2) a thin, inner layer formed by a syncytium of cells (the endocyst) that constitutes the germinal layer.

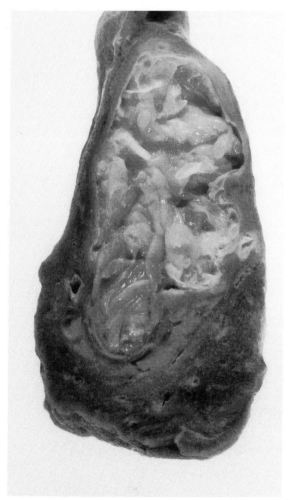

Figure 6–65. *Echinococcus Granulosus* Infestation. Wedge resection of lung showing multiple daughter cysts (mostly collapsed due to loss of fluid from sectioning) surrounded by a well-developed fibrous capsule (pericyst).

The latter produces the intracystic fluid and gives origin to numerous brood capsules (daughter cysts) within which develop larval scolices.

Although intrapulmonary hydatid cysts may cause symptoms by direct compression of surrounding structures, the disease most often becomes clinically evident as a result of rupture into contiguous bronchi. This may occur in two ways:

1. Through pericyst, exocyst, and endocyst, the contents being expelled into the airway and replaced by air. This variety is commonly followed by secondary bacterial infection.

2. Through the pericyst only, establishing communication between the bronchial tree and the potential space between exocyst and pericyst. When this occurs, air accumulates around the exocyst so that the germinal layer tends to collapse.

A cyst may also rupture directly into lung parenchyma, resulting in pneumonitis, or into the pleural cavity, producing pyopneumothorax. Rupture is said to occur more frequently in the pastoral than in the sylvatic type.[589]

Roentgenographic Manifestations

Pulmonary echinococcosis characteristically presents as a sharply circumscribed, spherical or oval mass of unit density surrounded by normal lung.[590] Cysts are multiple in 20 to 30 per cent of patients (Fig. 6–66). Their size ranges from 1 cm to over 20 cm in diameter; the larger cysts usually are of the pastoral type, the sylvatic variety rarely exceeding 10 cm.[589] The majority are located in the lower lobes, more often posteriorly than anteriorly, and somewhat more commonly on the right. Occasionally they have a bizarre, irregular shape, possibly because as the cyst grows, it impinges on relatively rigid structures such as bronchovascular bundles, becoming indented and lobulated.[591] Similarly, a cyst that is near the diaphragm, chest wall, or mediastinum tends to flatten against it. Calcification is rare.[590]

Most cysts appear as homogeneous masses indistinguishable from other solitary masses such as pulmonary carcinoma, in which case the diagnosis becomes evident only when communication develops between some portion of the cyst and the bronchial tree. When this occurs between the pericyst and the exocyst, air enters between these layers, producing the appearance of a thin crescent of air around the periphery of the cyst—variously termed the "meniscus sign," the "double-arch sign," the "moon sign," or the "crescent sign." Despite the emphasis that has been placed on this sign in the literature, some investigators have observed it in only 5 per cent of their patients[592]; it is a particularly rare manifestation of the sylvatic type of infestation.[589] When bronchial communication occurs directly with the endocyst (Fig. 6–67), the expulsion of cyst contents produces an air-fluid level; cyst fluid that is "aspirated" into surrounding parenchyma results in pneumonic consolidation.

After the cyst has ruptured into the bronchial tree, its membrane may float on the fluid within the cyst, giving rise to the classic "water-lily sign" or "sign of the camalote."[593] This sign also may be seen in pleural fluid when rupture of the cyst into the pleural space has resulted in hydropneu-

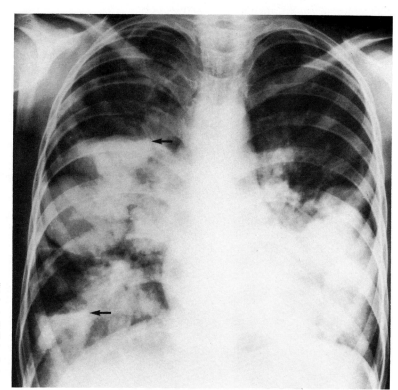

Figure 6–66. Multiple Hydatid Cysts. A multitude of sharply defined masses ranging from 1 to 7 cm in diameter are scattered widely throughout both lungs. The majority are intact, but at least four have ruptured into the tracheobronchial tree and show prominent fluid levels (two of these are indicated by *arrows*); note the irregular configuration of the air-fluid interface due to floating membranes (the water-lily sign or sign of the camalote). (Courtesy of Dr. Hassan Fateh, Teheran, Iran.)

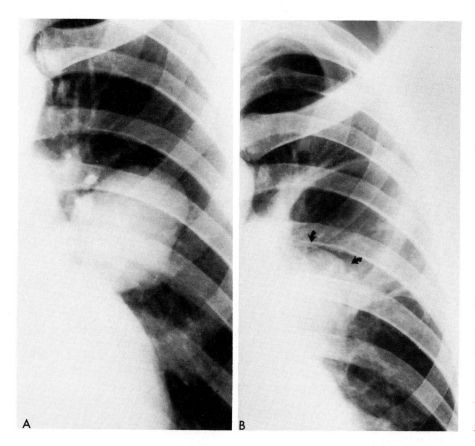

Figure 6–67. Hydatid Cyst with Rupture. In *A*, a sharply circumscribed homogeneous mass is visible in the left midlung, possessing a smooth but somewhat lobulated contour. Four years later *(B)*, the cyst has expelled all of its liquid contents into the tracheobronchial tree and is now air-containing; an irregular mass is present at the bottom of the cyst *(arrows)*, representing collapsed membranes. (Courtesy of Alfred Hospital, Melbourne, Australia.)

mothorax or pyopneumothorax.[594] Again, this sign is very uncommon in the sylvatic form of the disease.[589]

Although CT is not as useful in the diagnosis of pulmonary echinococcal disease as it is for that in the liver, it may distinguish cystic from solid lesions and may be of some use in identifying features in ruptured or complicated hydatid cysts, such as detached or collapsed endocyst membranes, collapsed daughter cyst membranes, and intact daughter cysts.[595, 596]

Clinical Manifestations

The majority of intact pulmonary hydatid cysts—particularly those of the sylvatic form—cause no symptoms. Occasionally an unruptured cyst may cause nonproductive cough and minimal hemoptysis.[591] When a cyst ruptures, there is often an abrupt onset of cough, expectoration, and fever; an acute hypersensitivity reaction may develop, with urticaria, pruritus, and, in some cases, hypotension. The patient may complain of chest pain, and the sputum may become purulent and contain fragments of hydatid membrane.

Unlike its occurrence in many other parasitic diseases, eosinophilia is relatively uncommon in echinococcosis, its incidence ranging from 25 to 50 per cent. Severe eosinophilia is usually a feature of anaphylaxis following cyst rupture. The use of skin and serologic tests is limited by cross-reactions with other parasitic antigens[597] and by antigenic similarity of the cysts with pulmonary carcinoma.[598] Specimens of pleural fluid or sputum may reveal scolices or hooklets, confirming the diagnosis.

Paragonimus Westermani (Paragonimiasis)

Paragonimiasis is caused by flukes of the genus Paragonimus, of which P. westermani is the best-known and the most frequent etiologic agent. It is seen most frequently in Southeast Asia, and migration of refugees from this region has resulted in an increased incidence of the disease in the western world.[599] Humans acquire the disease by ingesting raw or undercooked crabs or crayfish or by drinking water contaminated by them. As a result, the disease tends to occur in families, reflecting the common dietary exposure.

Pathogenesis and Pathologic Characteristics

The life cycle of P. westermani is one of the most fascinating of all parasites. Within the lungs of humans or animals, the larval forms develop into adult flukes that possess oral and ventral suckers for attachement to adjacent tissue. Eggs are deposited in burrows in lung parenchyma and are coughed up or swallowed and excreted in the feces. Under suitable moist conditions, they develop into ciliated miracidia, which infest freshwater snails. Within the snail, further larval forms develop and, after about 2 months, are liberated as cercariae. These are actively motile parasites that penetrate the soft periarticular tissues of certain species of crayfish and crabs. When ingested by the definitive host, metacercariae are liberated in the jejunum, from which they penetrate the wall of the small bowel into the peritoneal cavity, burrow through the diaphragm into the pleural space, and finally invade the lung. The mature parasite lives for many years in the lung, producing ova continuously.

Pathologic examination of the lungs shows single or multiple, 1 to 3 cm cystic spaces containing reddish brown mucinous fluid and usually a single adult parasite. The cysts are frequently located near larger bronchioles or bronchi. Microscopically, the parasites are surrounded by an infiltrate composed largely of eosinophils. Fibrosis eventually develops. When erosion occurs into a draining airway, the contents of the cyst may spread to other portions of the lung, resulting in bronchopneumonia.

Roentgenographic Manifestations

The chest roentgenogram is normal in 20 per cent of patients in whom Paragonimus eggs are identified in the sputum.[600] When the roentgenogram is abnormal, several patterns may be recognized:[600] (1) a poorly defined, somewhat hazy, inhomogeneous shadow, present in approximately one third of the patients; (2) shadows of homogeneous density and with better defined margins, occurring with about equal frequency; (3) one to four smoothly outlined cystic areas, 4 to 20 mm in diameter, within the shadows, observed in about 10 per cent; and (4) a similar type of shadow as described in (1) and (2) but containing "linear streaks"; and (5) ring shadows or thin-walled cysts 6 mm to 4 or 5 cm in diameter, often with a crescent-shaped opacity along one aspect of the inner lining (Fig. 6–68).[601] A characteristic feature of the last-named is the presence of irregular tracks or burrows joining two cysts, with a lumen measuring up to 5 mm in diameter (compared with the expected bronchial diameter of 2 to 3 mm).

From studies of immigrants to the United States who have resided in various endemic areas,[599] an additional and somewhat different pattern has become evident. In this, the opacities tend to mimic postprimary tuberculosis, particularly in the upper lobes, and it is probable that many of these immigrant patients have been treated erroneously for that disease. This error in diagnosis perhaps applies mostly to patients who have pleural effusion in addition to parenchymal disease, a manifestation formerly thought to be rare in paragonimiasis but now recognized as being common and sometimes massive.[602]

Clinical Manifestations

Symptoms do not develop for 1 year or longer after the presumed time of the infestation. Although hemoptysis has been considered to be an almost invariable symptom, it was noted in only 64 per cent of one series of 25 patients.[599] It tends to occur sporadically for months or even years in the absence of other signs of illness. There may be dyspnea, low-grade fever, anorexia, and weight loss; if pleural effusion or pneumothorax develops, there may be pleural pain.

Neither leukocytosis nor blood eosinophilia is usual. Some patients are anemic. Pleural fluid has been reported to show eosinophilia, a low glucose level and pH, and high protein and lactate dehydrogenase levels.[603] The diagnosis may be made readily in most patients by identifying the eggs in the sputum, stools, or pleural fluid. When considered in association with the clinical and roentgenographic findings, the complement-fixation test is a justified method of diagnosis.[599]

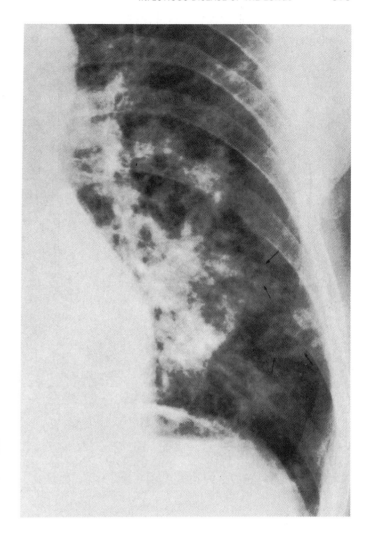

Figure 6–68. Paragonimiasis. A view of the lower two thirds of the left hemithorax from a posteroanterior roentgenogram reveals extensive parenchymal disease, of which the most characteristic change consists of irregular cystic spaces possessing walls of moderate thickness *(arrows).* In the medial portion of the lobe, consolidation of lung parenchyma is more confluent. Fluid obtained from the left lower lobe by aspiration needle biopsy contained *Paragonimus westermani.* (Courtesy of Montreal Chest Hospital Center.)

Schistosoma Species (Schistosomiasis)

Schistosomiasis is caused by flukes of the class Trematoda, of which three (*S. mansoni, S. japonicum,* and *S. haematobium*) are traditionally regarded as the most important in human infestation. *S. mekongi* also has recently been identified as an important etiologic agent in parts of Southeast Asia.[604] Acquisition of disease is limited to areas inhabited by the intermediate host, the snail. With increasing development of agriculture and associated irrigation projects in these regions, these hosts have been able to proliferate, and the prevalence of disease is increasing.[605]

The geographic distribution of schistosomiasis varies considerably with the specific organism. Both *S. mansoni* and *S. haematobium* are endemic in the Middle East (especially Egypt and parts of Saudi Arabia) and in large areas of central and southern Africa; *S. mansoni* is also found in the Caribbean islands and in South America, particularly Brazil. *Schistosoma japonicum* is predominant in China, Japan, and the Philippines, and *S. mekongi* in Laos, Kampuchea, and Thailand. The great majority of patients with schistosomiasis seen in the United States are Puerto Ricans infested with *S. mansoni.* Although infestation may occur at any age, pulmonary disease usually appears between the ages of 12 and 35 years.

Pathogenesis and Pathologic Characteristics

Humans acquire the infestation by drinking, swimming, working, or washing in fresh water containing the infective cercariae. The larvae penetrate the skin or, less commonly, the mucosa of the mouth or pharynx and travel as schistosomula via the venous circulation to the pulmonary capillaries. They pass through the pulmonary capillary sieve to the systemic circulation and traverse the mesenteric vessels into the intrahepatic portion of the portal system. There they develop into adolescent worms, which migrate against the portal blood flow to the superior mesenteric (*S. japonicum* and *S. mekongi*), inferior mesenteric (*S. mansoni*), and vesical (*S. haematobium*) venules. The adult male and female worms copulate in these venules, and the females then migrate to smaller venous channels in the submucosa and mucosa of the bowel or bladder and lay their eggs. Many of these eggs are extruded into the lumen of the bowel or urinary bladder and are passed in the feces or urine; those that reach fresh water develop into larvae, which enter snails. Several transformations take place within the snail, with infective cercariae eventually emerging. Penetration of the skin of a person in contact with the contaminated water completes the odyssey.

Tissue damage results from the release into host tissues

of various enzymes and antigens derived from the egg, with consequent inflammation and fibrosis.[605] These effects may occur during the extrusion of eggs into the lumen of the bowel or bladder, damage thus remaining localized to the gastrointestinal or vesical mucosa. However, some eggs also are released directly into venous blood. In the case of *S. mansoni, S. japonicum,* and *S. mekongi,* this usually occurs into the portal system with deposition in the liver; with *S. haematobium,* release is into the inferior vena cava with direct embolization to the lungs. Eggs of the former three species may also reach the lungs once the liver has become cirrhotic as a result of schistosomal fibrosis, the development of anastomotic channels permitting passage of the ova between the portal and the systemic venous systems.

Once they reach the lungs, most embolized eggs become impacted in small pulmonary arteries and arterioles, following which they are extruded into the surrounding perivascular tissue. The presence of the eggs causes an inflammatory reaction and fibrosis that, when widespread, can result in vascular sclerosis and pulmonary hypertension. Less often, pulmonary disease is recognized during the passage of cercariae through the pulmonary capillaries (Löffler's syndrome) or following embolization of adult worms.

Roentgenographic Manifestations

The appearance of the chest roentgenogram varies considerably, depending on the number of eggs that reach the lung and the time of roentgenography following extrusion of the eggs. Some cases, perhaps the majority, show a diffuse miliary or reticulonodular pattern presumably caused by inflammatory and fibrotic reactions to the ova after they have migrated through vessel walls.[606] Areas of pneumonic consolidation may develop around dead adult worms and occluded arteries. Pleural effusion does not occur, although focal pleural thickening may develop. Pulmonary arterial hypertension is indistinguishable from that due to any other cause, there being a marked degree of dilatation of the main pulmonary artery and its branches with rapid tapering toward the periphery.

Clinical Manifestations

These occur in three very distinct time intervals following parasitization. Migration of the schistosomula from the skin through the pulmonary circulation to the intrahepatic portal veins is associated with an acute syndrome consisting of fever, cough, diarrhea, arthralgia, anorexia, malaise, and hives; leukocytosis and eosinophilia are almost invariable. It is at this stage that transitory opacities may be seen on the chest roentgenogram. This acute form of schistosomiasis is seldom seen in inhabitants of endemic areas but is characteristic of the reaction to infestation that develops in visitors.[607]

Somewhat later, following deposition of eggs in the intestinal and bladder venules, cough, dyspnea, hypoxemia, and pulmonary edema may develop acutely, findings that are believed to constitute an allergic reaction to the sudden mobilization of many eggs to the lungs.[608] A similar syndrome may be observed when chemotherapy is instituted in patients with schistosomiasis.[609]

In the third and most important group, clinical manifes-

tations are those of pulmonary hypertension, usually after years of persistent disease. Evidence of cirrhosis (in cases of *S. mansoni* and *S. japonicum* infestation) or dysuria and terminal hematuria (*S. haematobium*) may be present. Moderate leukocytosis and eosinophilia are usual, the latter to as high as 33 per cent.

In patients with suspected schistosomiasis, concentrated specimens of stool and urine should be examined repeatedly for ova. Infestation also may be demonstrated in many cases by the finding of eggs in biopsy specimens of the rectal and bladder mucosa; however, examination of the sputum seldom reveals ova, and lung biopsy may be necessary to establish the presence of pulmonary involvement. Specific IgE against soluble egg antigen is found in high titer during the acute, but not the chronic stages. Levels of IgM and IgG antibody to cercarial antigen are increased in acute disease, and levels of IgG to the adult worm are increased in chronic schistosomiasis.[610] Specific skin tests and precipitin tests are available for individual species.[606]

References

1. Putnam JS, Tuazon CU: Symposium on infectious lung diseases: Foreword. Med Clin North Am 64: 317, 1980.
2. George WL, Finegold SM: Today's practice of cardiopulmonary medicine. Chest 81: 4, 1982.
3. Pääkkö P, Särkioja T, Hirvonen J, et al: Postmortem radiographic, histological, and bacteriological studies of terminal respiratory infections and other pulmonary lesions in hospital and non-hospital necropsies. J Clin Pathol 37: 1282, 1984.
4. Chretien J, Holland W, Macklem P, et al: Acute respiratory infections in children: A global public health problem. N Engl J Med 310: 982, 1984.
5. Transmission of tuberculosis by flexible fiberbronchoscopes. Am Rev Respir Dis 127: 97, 1983.
6. Riley RL: Indoor spread of respiratory infection by recirculation of air. Bull Eur Physiopathol Resp 15: 699, 1979.
7. Johanson WG Jr, Harris GD: Aspiration pneumonia, anaerobic infections and lung abscess. Med Clin North Am 64: 385, 1980.
8. Huxley EJ, Viroslav J, Gray WRT, et al: Pharyngeal aspiration in normal adults and patients with depressed consciousness. Am J Med 64: 546, 1978.
9. Fang GD, Fine M, Orloff J, et al: New and emerging etiologies for community-acquired pneumonia with implications for therapy: A prospective multicenter study of 359 cases. Medicine 69: 307, 1990.
9a. The British Thoracic Society Research Committee and the Public Health Laboratory Service: The aetiology, management, and outcome of severe community-acquired pneumonia on the intensive care unit. Respir Med 86(1): 7, 1992.
10. Boonsawat W, Boonma P, Tangdajahiran T, et al: Community-acquired pneumonia in adults at Scrinagarind Hospital. J Med Assoc Thai 73: 345, 1990.
11. White RJ, Blainey AD, Harrison KJ, et al: Causes of pneumonia presenting to a district general hospital. Thorax 36: 566, 1981.
12. Woodhead MA, Radvan J, Macfarlane JT: Adult community-acquired staphylococcal pneumonia in the antibiotic era: A review of 61 cases. Q J Med 64: 783, 1987.
13. Adebonojo SA, Grillo IA, Osinowo O, et al: Suppurative diseases of the lung and pleura: A continuing challenge in developing countries. Ann Thorac Surg 33: 40, 1982.
14. Winterbauer RH, Bedon GA, Ball WC Jr: Recurrent pneumonia: Predisposing illness and clinical patterns in 158 patients. Ann Intern Med 70: 689, 1969.
15. Eickhoff TC: Nosocomial infections. N Engl J Med 306: 1545, 1982.
16. A'Court C, Garrard CS: Nosocomial pneumonia in the intensive care unit: Mechanisms and significance. Thorax 47: 465, 1992.
17. Stevens GP, Jacobson JA, Burke JP: Changing patterns of hospital infections and antibiotic use: Prevalence surveys in a community hospital. Arch Intern Med 141: 587, 1981.
18. Rello J, Quintana E, Ausina V, et al: Risk factors for *Staphylococcus*

aureus nosocomial pneumonia in critically ill patients. Am Rev Respir Dis 142: 1320, 1990.

19. Heiner DC, Myers A, Beck CS: Deficiency of IgG4: A disorder associated with frequent infections and bronchiectasis may be familial. Clin Rev Allergy 1: 259, 1983.

20. Chipps BE, Talamo RL, Windelstern JA: IgA deficiency, recurrent pneumonias and bronchiectasis. Chest 73: 519, 1978.

21. Knowles GK, Stanhope R, Green M: Bronchiectasis complicating chronic lymphatic leukaemia with hypogammaglobulinaemia. Thorax 35: 217, 1980.

22. Ferguson A: Hazards of hyposplenism. Br Med J 285: 1375, 1982.

23. Murray JF: Personal communication.

24. Schnittman SM, Greenhouse JJ, Psallidopoulos MC, et al: Increasing viral burden in CD4+ T cells from patients with progressive immunosuppression and clinical disease. Ann Intern Med 113: 438, 1990.

25. Masur H, Ognibene FP, Yarchoan R, et al: CD4 counts as predictors of opportunistic pneumonias in human immunodeficiency virus (HIV) infection. Ann Intern Med 111: 223, 1989.

26. Dean NC, Golden JA, Evans LA, et al: Human immunodeficiency virus recovery from bronchoalveolar lavage fluid in patients with AIDS. Chest 93: 1176, 1988.

27. Goedert JJ: Testing for human immunodeficiency virus. Ann Intern Med 105: 609, 1986.

28. Murray JF, Mills J: State of the art: Pulmonary infectious complications of human immunodeficiency virus infection. Part I. Am Rev Respir Dis 141: 1356, 1990.

29. Murray JF, Mills J: State of the art: Pulmonary infectious complications of human immunodeficiency virus infection. Part II. Am Rev Respir Dis 141: 1582, 1990.

30. White DA, Matthay RA: State of the art: Noninfectious pulmonary complications of infection with the human immunodeficiency virus. Am Rev Respir Dis 140: 1763, 1989.

31. Kuhlman JE, Fishman EK, Hruban RH, et al: Diseases of the chest in AIDS: CT diagnosis. Radiographics 9: 827, 1989.

32. Limper AH, Offord KP, Smith TF, et al: *Pneumocystis carinii* pneumonia: Differences in lung parasite number and inflammation in patients with and without AIDS. Am Rev Respir Dis 140: 1204, 1989.

33. Travis WD, Pittaluga S, Lipschik GY, et al: Atypical pathologic manifestations of *Pneumocystis carinii* pneumonia in the acquired immune deficiency syndrome: Review of 123 lung biopsies from 76 patients with emphasis on cysts, vascular invasion, vasculitis, and granulomas. Am J Surg Pathol 14: 615, 1990.

34. Chaffey MH, Klein JS, Gamsu G, et al: Radiographic distribution of *Pneumocystis carinii* pneumonia in patients with AIDS treated with prophylactic inhaled pentamidine. Radiology 175: 715, 1990.

35. Panicek DM: Cystic pulmonary lesions in patients with AIDS. Radiology 173: 12, 1989.

36. Newsome GS, Ward DJ, Pierce PF: Spontaneous pneumothorax in patients with acquired immunodeficiency syndrome treated with prophylactic aerosolized pentamidine. Arch Intern Med 150: 2167, 1990.

37. Groskin SA, Massi AF, Randall PA: Calcified hilar and mediastinal lymph nodes in an AIDS patient with *Pneumocystis carinii* infection. Radiology 175: 345, 1990.

38. Miller WT Jr, Edelman JM, Miller WT: Cryptococcal pulmonary infection in patients with AIDS: Radiographic appearance. Radiology 175: 725, 1990.

39. Johnson PC, Hamil RJ, Sarosi GA: Clinical review: Progressive disseminated histoplasmosis in the AIDS patient. Semin Respir Infect 4: 139, 1989.

40. Fish DG, Ampel NM, Galgiani JN, et al: Coccidioidomycosis during human immunodeficiency virus infection: A review of 77 patients. Medicine 69: 384, 1990.

41. Denning DW, Follansbee SE, Scolaro M, et al: Pulmonary aspergillosis in the acquired immunodeficiency syndrome. N Engl J Med 324: 654, 1991.

42. Millar AB, Patou G, Miller RF, et al: Cytomegalovirus in the lungs of patients with AIDS: Respiratory pathogen or passenger? Am Rev Respir Dis 141: 1474, 1990.

43. Long R, Scalcini M, Manfreda J, et al: Impact of human immunodeficiency virus type 1 on tuberculosis in rural Haiti. Am Rev Respir Dis 143: 69, 1991.

44. Shafer RW, Goldberg R, Sierra M, et al: Frequency of *Mycobacterium tuberculosis* bacteremia in patients with tuberculosis in an area endemic for AIDS. Am Rev Respir Dis 140: 1611, 1989.

45. Bishburg E, Sunderam G, Reichman LB, et al: Central nervous system tuberculosis with the acquired immunodeficiency syndrome and its related complex. Ann Intern Med 105: 210, 1986.

46. Long R, Maycher B, Scalcini M, et al: The chest roentgenogram in pulmonary tuberculosis patients seropositive for human immunodeficiency virus type 1. Chest 99: 123, 1991.

47. Schlamm HT, Yancovitz SR: *Haemophilus influenzae* pneumonia in young adults with AIDS, ARC, or risk of AIDS. Am J Med 86: 11, 1989.

48. Redd SC, Rutherford GW III, Sande MA, et al: The role of human immunodeficiency virus infection in pneumococcal bacteremia in San Francisco residents. J Infect Dis 162: 1012, 1990.

49. O'Brien RF, Cohn DL: Serosanguineous pleural effusions in AIDS-associated Kaposi's sarcoma. Chest 96: 460, 1989.

50. Teirstein AS, Rosen MJ: Lymphocytic interstitial pneumonia. Clin Chest Med 9: 467, 1988.

51. Itescu S, Brancato LJ, Buxbaum J, et al: A diffuse infiltrative CD8 lymphocytosis syndrome in human immunodeficiency virus (HIV) infection: A host immune response associated with HLA-DR5. Ann Intern Med 112: 3, 1990.

52. Simmons JT, Suffredini AF, Lack EE, et al: Nonspecific interstitial pneumonitis in patients with AIDS: Radiologic features. Am J Roentgenol 149: 265, 1987.

53. Oldham SA, Castillo M, Jacobson FL, et al: HIV-associated lymphocytic interstitial pneumonia: Radiologic manifestations and pathologic correlation. Radiology 170: (1 Pt 1): 83, 1989.

54. Pluda JM, Yarchoan R, Jaffe ES, et al: Development of non-Hodgkin's lymphoma in a cohort of patients with severe human immunodeficiency virus (HIV) infection on long-term antiretroviral therapy. Ann Intern Med 113: 276, 1990.

55. Stern RG, Gamsu G, Golden JA, et al: Intrathoracic adenopathy: Differential feature of AIDS and diffuse lymphadenopathy syndrome. Am J Roentgenol 142: 689, 1984.

56. Spencer RC, Philp JR: Effect of previous antimicrobial therapy on bacteriological findings in patients with primary pneumonia. Lancet 2: 349, 1973.

57. Winterbauer RH, Hutchinson JF, Reinhardt GN, et al: The use of quantitative cultures and antibody coating of bacteria to diagnose bacterial pneumonia by fiberoptic bronchoscopy. Am Rev Respir Dis 128: 98, 1983.

58. Fekety FR Jr, Caldwell J, Gump D, et al: Bacteria, viruses, and mycoplasmas in acute pneumonia in adults. Am Rev Respir Dis 104: 499, 1971.

59. Mostow SR: Pneumonias acquired outside the hospital—recognition and treatment. Med Clin North Am 58: 555, 1974.

60. Gerrard CS, Levandowski RA, Gerrity TR, et al: The effects of acute respiratory virus infection upon tracheal mucous transport. Arch Environ Health 40: 322, 1985.

61. Jakab GJ: Immune impairment of alveolar macrophage phagocytosis during influenza virus pneumonia. Am Rev Respir Dis 126: 778, 1982.

62. Plotkowski M-C, Puchelle E, Beck G, et al: Adherence of Type I *Streptococcus pneumoniae* to tracheal epithelium of mice infected with influenza A/PR8 virus. Am Rev Respir Dis 134: 1040, 1986.

63. George WL, Finegold SM: Bacterial infections of the lung. Chest 81: 502, 1982.

64. Mufson MA, Kruss DM, Wasil RE, et al: Capsular types and outcome of bacteremic pneumococcal disease in the antibiotic era. Arch Intern Med 134: 505, 1974.

65. Foy HM, Wentworth B, Kenny GE, et al: Pneumococcal isolations from patients with pneumonia and control subjects in a prepaid medical care group. Am Rev Respir Dis 111: 595, 1975.

66. Bisno AL, Freeman JC: The syndrome of asplenia, pneumococcal sepsis, and disseminated intravascular coagulation. Ann Intern Med 72: 389, 1970.

67. Powers D, Overturf G, Weiss J, et al: Pneumococcal septicemia in children with sickle cell anemia: Changing trend of survival. JAMA 245: 1839, 1981.

68. Moss JM: Pneumococcus infection in diabetes mellitus. JAMA 243: 2301, 1980.

69. Winklestein JA, Tomasz A: Activation of the alternative pathway by pneumococcal cell walls. J Immunol 118: 451, 1977.

70. Reed WP, Davidson MS, Williams RC Jr: Complement system in pneumococcal infections. Infect Immun 13: 1120, 1976.

71. Lonky SA, Marsh J, Steele R, et al: Protease and antiprotease responses in lung and peripheral blood in experimental canine pneumococcal pneumonia. Am Rev Respir Dis 121: 685, 1980.

72. Rhodes GC, Lykke AW, Tapsall JW, et al: Abnormal alveolar epithelial repair associated with failure of resolution in experimental streptococcal pneumonia. J Pathol 159: 245, 1989.

73. Leatherman JW, Iber C, Davies SF: Cavitation in bacteremic pneumococcal pneumonia: Causal role of mixed infection with anaerobic bacteria. Am Rev Respir Dis 129: 317, 1984.

74. Goodman LR, Goren RA, Teplick SK: The radiographic evaluation of pulmonary infection. Med Clin North Am 64: 553, 1980.

75. Kalin M, Lindberg AA: Diagnosis of pneumococcal pneumonia: A comparison between microscopic examination of expectorate, antigen detection and cultural procedures. Scand J Infect Dis 15: 247, 1983.

76. Barrett-Connor E: The nonvalue of sputum culture in the diagnosis of pneumococcal pneumonia. Am Rev Respir Dis 103: 845, 1971.

77. Gong H Jr, Soffer MJ, Ertie AR, et al: Diagnostic efficacy of nasotracheal protected specimen brush in patients with suspected bacterial pneumonia. Diagn Microbiol Infect Dis 11: 87, 1988.

78. Conces DJ Jr, Clark SA, Tarver RD, et al: Transthoracic aspiration needle biopsy: Value in the diagnosis of pulmonary infections. Am J Roentgenol 152: 31, 1989.

79. Ortqvist A, Kalin M: Bacteremic pneumococcal pneumonia in Stockholm, Sweden, in 1984. Scand J Infect Dis 20: 451, 1988.

79a. Kuikka A, Syrjänen J, Renkonen OV, Valtonen VV: Pneumococcal bacteraemia during a recent decade. J Infect 24(2): 157, 1992.

80. Brummitt CF, Crossley KB, Falken M, et al: Penicillin-resistant *Streptococcus pneumoniae*: Report of a case and results of a clinical laboratory proficiency survey in Minnesota. Am J Clin Pathol 89: 238, 1988.

81. Fedson DS, Harward MP, Reid RA, et al: Hospital-based pneumococcal immunization: Epidemiologic rationale from the Shenandoah study. JAMA 264: 1117, 1990.

82. Gerber GJ, Farmer WC, Fulkerson LL: Beta-hemolytic streptococcal pneumonia following influenza. JAMA 240: 242, 1978.

83. Kevy SV, Lowe BA: Streptococcal pneumonia and empyema in childhood. N Engl J Med 264: 738, 1961.

84. Anthony BF: Carriage of group-B streptococci during pregnancy. J Infect Dis 145: 789, 1982.

85. Bayer AS, Chow AW, Anthony BF, et al: Serious infections in adults due to group B streptococci. Am J Med 61: 498, 1976.

86. Kasian GF, Bingham WT, Steinberg J, et al: Bacterial tracheitis in children. Can Med Assoc J 140: 46, 1989.

87. Jackson JR, Gibbons RJ, Magner D: The effects of staphylococcal toxin on the lungs of rabbits. Am J Pathol 34: 1051, 1958.

88. Dines DE: Diagnostic significance of pneumatocele of the lung. JAMA 204: 1169, 1968.

89. Wiita RM, Cartwright RR, Davis JG: Staphylococcal pneumonia in adults: A review of 102 cases. Am J Roentgenol 86: 1083, 1961.

90. Dalldorf FG, Kaufmann AF, Brachman PS: Woolsorters' disease: An experimental model. Arch Pathol 92: 418, 1971.

91. Ananthraman A, Israel RH, Magnussen CR: Pleural-pulmonary aspects of *Listeria monocytogenes* infection. Respiration 44: 153, 1983.

92. Dobie RA, Tobey DN: Clinical features of diphtheria in the respiratory tract. JAMA 242: 2197, 1979.

93. Dorff GJ, Rytel MW, Farmer SG, et al: Etiologies and characteristic features of pneumonias in a municipal hospital. Am J Med Sci 266: 349, 1973.

94. Pierce AK, Sanford JP: Aerobic gram-negative bacillary pneumonias. Am Rev Respir Dis 110: 647, 1974.

95. Flynn DM, Weinstein RA, Kabins SA: Infections with gram-negative bacilli in a cardiac surgery intensive care unit: The relative role of *Enterobacter*. J Hosp Infect 11(Suppl A): 367, 1988.

96. Meltz DJ, Grieco MH: Characteristics of *Serratia marcescens* pneumonia. Arch Intern Med 132: 359, 1973.

97. Reed WP: Indolent pulmonary abscess associated with *Klebsiella* and *Enterobacter*. Am Rev Respir Dis 107: 1055, 1973.

98. Karnad A, Alvarez S, Berk SL: *Enterobacter* pneumonia. South Med J 80: 601, 1987.

99. Jonas M, Cunha BA: Bacteremic *Escherichia coli* pneumonia. Arch Intern Med 142: 2157, 1982.

100. Aguado JM, Obeso G, Cabanillas JJ, et al: Pleuropulmonary infections due to nontyphoid strains of *Salmonella*. Arch Intern Med 150: 54, 1990.

101. Han T, Sokal JE, Neter E: Salmonellosis in disseminated malignant disease: A seven-year review (1959–1965). N Engl J Med 276: 1045, 1967.

102. Tillotson JR, Lerner AM: Characteristics of pneumonias caused by Bacillus Proteus. Ann Intern Med 68: 287, 1968.

103. Leads from the MMWR: Plague pneumonia: California. JAMA 252: 1399, 1984.

104. Barnes AM, Poland JD: Plague in the United States, 1983. MMWR 33: 15SS, 21SS, 1984.

105. Alsofrom DJ, Mettler FA, Mann JM: Radiographic manifestations of plague in New Mexico, 1975–1980: A review of 42 proved cases. Radiology 139: 561, 1981.

106. Sites VR, Poland JD: Mediastinal lymphadenopathy in bubonic plague. Am J Roentgenol 116: 567, 1972.

107. Holloway WJ, Scott EG, Adams YB: *Pasteurella multocida* infection in man: Report of 21 cases. Am J Clin Pathol 51: 705, 1969.

108. Steyer BJ, Sobonya RE: *Pasteurella multocida* lung abscess: A case report and review of the literature. Arch Intern Med 144: 1081, 1984.

109. Slater LN, Guarnaccia J, Makintubee S, et al: Bacteremic disease due to *Haemophilus influenzae* capsular type f in adults: Report of five cases and review. Rev Infect Dis 12: 628, 1990.

110. Bates JH: The role of infection during exacerbations of chronic bronchitis. Ann Intern Med 97: 130, 1982.

111. Musher DM, Kubitschek KR, Crennan J, et al: Pneumonia and acute febrile tracheobronchitis due to *Haemophilus influenzae*. Ann Intern Med 99: 444, 1983.

112. Trollfors B, Claesson B, Lagergard T, et al: Incidence, predisposing factors and manifestations of invasive *Haemophilus influenzae* infections in adults. Eur J Clin Microbiol 3: 180, 1984.

113. Goldstein E, Daly AK, Seamans C: *Haemophilus influenzae* as a cause of adult pneumonia. Ann Intern Med 66: 35, 1967.

114. Takala AK, Eskola J, van Alphen L: Spectrum of invasive *Haemophilus influenzae* type b disease in adults. Arch Intern Med 150: 2573, 1990.

115. Sturm AW, Mostert R, Rouing PJ, et al: Outbreak of multiresistant non-encapsulated *Haemophilus influenzae* infections in a pulmonary rehabilitation centre. Lancet 335: 214, 1990.

116. Leading article: *Pseudomonas* infection in hospital. Br Med J 4: 309, 1967.

117. Tillotson JR, Lerner AM: Characteristics of nonbacteremic *Pseudomonas* pneumonia. Ann Intern Med 68: 295, 1968.

118. Freeman R, McPeake PK: Acquisition, spread, and control of *Pseudomonas aeruginosa* in a cardiothoracic intensive care unit. Thorax 37: 732, 1982.

119. Lead article: Cystic fibrosis and *Pseudomonas* infection. Lancet 1: 257, 1983.

119a. Pollack M: *Pseudomonas aeruginosa* exotoxin A. N Engl J Med 302: 1360, 1980.

120. Pedersen SS, Hiby N, Espersen F, et al: Role of alginate in infection with *Pseudomonas aeruginosa* in cystic fibrosis. Thorax 47: 6, 1992.

121. McHenry MC, Baggentoss AH, Martin WJ: Bacteremia due to gram-negative bacilli: Clinical and autopsy findings in 33 cases. Am J Clin Pathol 50: 160, 1968.

122. Iannini PB, Claffey T, Quintiliani R: Bacteremic *Pseudomonas* pneumonia. JAMA 230: 558, 1974.

123. Simmonds EJ, Conway SP, Ghoneim AT, et al: *Pseudomonas cepacia*: A new pathogen in patients with cystic fibrosis referred to a large centre in the United Kingdom. Arch Dis Child 65: 874, 1990.

124. Conly JM, Klass L, Larson L, et al: *Pseudomonas cepacia* colonization and infection in intensive care units. Can Med Assoc J 134: 363, 1986.

125. Koponen MA, Zlock D, Palmer DL, et al: Melioidosis: Forgotten, but not gone! Arch Intern Med 151: 605, 1991.

126. Guard RW, Khafagi FA, Brigden MC, et al: Melioidosis in far North Queensland: A clinical and epidemiological review of 20 cases. Am J Trop Med Hyg 33: 467, 1984.

127. Poe RH, Vassallo CL, Domm BM: Melioidosis: The remarkable imitator (case reports). Am Rev Respir Dis 104: 427, 1971.

128. Pigott JA, Hochholzer L: Human melioidosis. Arch Pathol 90: 101, 1970.

129. Dhiensiri T, Puapairoj S, Susaengrat W: Pulmonary melioidosis: Clinical-radiologic correlation in 183 cases in northeastern Thailand. Radiology 166: 711, 1988.

130. Sweet RS, Wilson ES Jr, Chandler BF: Melioidosis manifested by cavitary lung disease. Am J Roentgenol 103: 543, 1968.

131. Everett ED, Nelson RA: Pulmonary melioidosis: Observations in thirty-nine cases. Am Rev Respir Dis 112: 331, 1975.

132. Lindquist DS, Nygaard G, Thacker WL, et al: Thirteenth serogroup of *Legionella pneumophila* isolated from patients with pneumonia. J Clin Microbiol 26: 586, 1988.

133. Edelstein PH, Meyer RD, Finegold SM: Laboratory diagnosis of Legionnaires' disease. Am Rev Respir Dis 121: 317, 1980.

134. Foy HM, Broome CV, Hayes PS, et al: Legionnaires' disease in a prepaid medical-care group in Seattle 1963–75. Lancet 1: 767, 1979.

135. Bartlett JG: New developments in infectious diseases for the critical care physician. Crit Care Med 11: 563, 1983.

136. Yu VL, Kroboth FJ, Shonnard J, et al: Legionnaires' disease: New clinical perspective from a prospective pneumonia study. Am J Med 73: 357, 1982.

137. Friis-Moller A, Rechnitzer C, Black FT, et al: Prevalence of Legionnaires' disease in pneumonia patients admitted to a Danish department of infectious diseases. Scand J Infect Dis 18: 321, 1986.

138. Poshni IA, Millian SJ: Seroepidemiology of Legionella pneumophila serogroup 1 in healthy residents of New York City. NY State J Med 85: 10, 1985.

139. Stout J, Yu VL, Vickers RM, et al: Potable water supply as the hospital reservoir for Pittsburgh pneumonia agent. Lancet 1: 471, 1982.

140. Addiss DG, Davis JP, LaVenture M, et al: Community-acquired Legionnaires' disease associated with a cooling tower: Evidence for longer-distance transport of Legionella pneumophila. Am J Epidemiol 130: 557, 1989.

141. Aubertin J, Dabis F, Fleurette J, et al: Prevalence of legionellosis among adults: A study of community-acquired pneumonia in France. Infection 15: 328, 1987.

142. Cordonnier C, Farcet J-P, Desforges L, et al: Legionnaires' disease and hairy-cell leukemia: An unfortuitous association? Arch Intern Med 144: 2373, 1984.

143. Helms CM, Viner JP, Weisenburger DD, et al: Sporadic Legionnaires' disease: Clinical observations on 87 nosocomial and community-acquired cases. Am J Med Sci 288: 2, 1984.

144. Wong KH, Moss CW, Hochstein DH, et al: "Endotoxicity" of the Legionnaires' disease bacterium. Ann Intern Med 90: 624, 1979.

145. Williams A, Baskerville A, Dowsett AB, et al: Immunocytochemical demonstration of the association between Legionella pneumophila, its tissue-destructive protease, and pulmonary lesions in experimental legionnaires' disease. J Pathol 153: 257, 1987.

146. Winn WC, Myerowitz RL: The pathology of the Legionella pneumonias. Hum Pathol 12: 401, 1981.

147. Theaker JM, Tobin JO, Jones SEC, et al: Immunohistological detection of Legionella pneumophila in lung sections. J Clin Pathol 40: 143, 1987.

148. Kroboth FJ, Yu VL, Reddy SC, et al: Clinicoradiographic correlation with the extent of Legionnaires' disease. Am J Roentgenol 141: 263, 1983.

149. Kirby BD, Snyder KM, Meyer RD, et al: Legionnaires' disease: Report of sixty-five nosocomially acquired cases and review of the literature. Medicine 59: 188, 1980.

150. Fairbank JT, Mamourian AC, Dietrich PA, et al: The chest radiograph in Legionnaires' disease. Radiology 147: 30, 1983.

151. Evans AF, Oakley RH, Whitehouse GH: Analysis of the chest radiograph in Legionnaires' disease. Clin Radiol 32: 361, 1981.

152. Van Arsdall JA II, Wunderlich HF, Melo JC, et al: The protean manifestations of Legionnaires' disease. J Infect 7: 51, 1983.

153. Davis GS, Winn WC Jr, Beaty HN: Legionnaires' disease: Infections caused by Legionella pneumophila and Legionella-like organisms. Clin Chest Med 2: 145, 1981.

154. Storch G, Hayes PS, Meyers JD, et al: Legionnaires' disease bacterium: Prevalence of antibody reacting with the organism in patients suspected of having infection with Pneumocystis carinii. Am Rev Respir Dis 121: 483, 1980.

155. Harrison TG, Dournon E, Taylor AG: Evaluation of sensitivity of two serological tests for diagnosing pneumonia caused by Legionella pneumophila serogroup 1. J Clin Pathol 40: 77, 1987.

156. Sathapatayavongs B, Kohler RB, Wheat LJ, et al: Rapid diagnosis of Legionnaires' disease by urinary antigen detection: Comparison of ELISA and radioimmunoassay. Am J Med 72: 576, 1982.

157. Gea J, Rodriguez-Roisin R, Torres A, et al: Lung function changes following Legionnaires' disease. Eur Respir J 1: 109, 1988.

158. Irwin RS, Woelk WK, Coudon WL III: Primary meningococcal pneumonia. Ann Intern Med 82: 493, 1975.

159. Harrison LH, Armstrong CW, Jenkins SR, et al: A cluster of meningococcal disease on a school bus following epidemic influenza. Arch Intern Med 151: 1005, 1991.

160. McLeod DT, Ahmad F, Capewell S, et al: Increase in bronchopulmonary infection due to Branhamella catarrhalis. Br Med J 292: 1103, 1986.

161. Diamond LA, Lorber B: Branhamella catarrhalis pneumonia and immunoglobulin abnormalities: A new association. Am Rev Respir Dis 129: 876, 1984.

162. Wright PW, Wallace RJ Jr, Shepherd JR: A descriptive study of 42 cases of Branhamella catarrhalis pneumonia. Am J Med 88(5A): 2S, 1990.

163. Buxton AE, Anderson RL, Werdegar D, et al: Nosocomial respiratory tract infection and colonization with Acinetobacter calcoaceticus: Epidemiologic characteristics. Am J Med 65: 507, 1978.

164. Rudin ML, Michael JR, Huxley EJ: Community-acquired Acinetobacter pneumonia. Am J Med 67: 39, 1979.

165. Edwards KM: Diphtheria, tetanus, and pertussis immunizations in adults. Infect Dis Clin North Am 4: 85, 1990.

166. Herwaldt LA: Pertussis in adults: What physicians need to know. Arch Intern Med 151: 1510, 1991.

167. Fawcitt J, Parry HE: Lung changes in pertussis and measles in childhood: A review of 1894 cases with a follow-up study of the pulmonary complications. Br J Radiol 30: 76, 1957.

168. Grob PR, Crowder MJ, Robbins JF: Effect of vaccination on severity and dissemination of whooping cough. Br Med J 282: 1925, 1981.

169. Mertsola J, Ruuskanen O, Kuronen T, et al: Serologic diagnosis of pertussis: Evaluation of pertussis toxin and other antigens in enzyme-linked immunosorbent assay. J Infect Dis 161: 966, 1990.

170. Respiratory sequelae of whooping cough: Swansea Research Unit of the Royal College of General Practitioners. Br Med J 290: 1937, 1985.

171. Krantz I, Bjure J, Claesson I, et al: Respiratory sequelae and lung function after whooping cough in infancy. Arch Dis Child 65: 569, 1990.

172. Leading article: Granulomatous pleuritis caused by Francisella tularensis: Possible confusion with tuberculous pleuritis. Am Rev Respir Dis 128: 314, 1983.

173. Rubin SA: Radiographic spectrum of pleuropulmonary tularemia. Am J Roentgenol 131: 277, 1978.

173a. Scofield RH, Lopez EJ, McNabb SJ: Tularemia pneumonia in Oklahoma, 1982–1987. J Okla State Med Assoc 85(4): 165, 1992.

174. Buchanan TM, Brooks GF, Brachman PS: The tularemia skin test: Three hundred twenty-five skin tests in 210 persons: Serologic correlation and review of the literature. Ann Intern Med 74: 336, 1971.

175. Felgin RD, Lobes LA Jr, Anderson D, et al: Human leptospirosis from immunized dogs. Ann Intern Med 79: 777, 1973.

176. Lee REJ, Terry SI, Walker TM, et al: The chest radiograph in leptospirosis in Jamaica. Br J Radiol 54: 939, 1981.

177. Im JG, Yeon KM, Han MC, et al: Leptospirosis of the lung: Radiographic findings in 58 patients. Am J Roentgenol 152: 955, 1989.

178. Bodner SJ, Koenig MG, Goodman JS: Bacteremic Bacteroides infections. Ann Intern Med 73: 537, 1970.

179. Editorial: Chronic destructive pneumonia. Lancet 2: 350, 1980.

180. Finegold SM: Pathogenic anaerobes. Arch Intern Med 142: 1988, 1982.

181. Felner JM, Dowell VR Jr: "Bacteroides" bacteremia. Am J Med 50: 787, 1971.

182. Patel SB, Mahler R: Clostridial pleuropulmonary infections: Case report and review of the literature. J Infect 21: 81, 1990.

183. Bartlett JG, Gorbach SL, Thadepalli H, et al: Bacteriology of empyema. Lancet 1: 338, 1974.

184. Landay MJ, Christensen EE, Bynum LJ, et al: Anaerobic pleural and pulmonary infections. Am J Roentgenol 134: 233, 1980.

185. Rohlfing BM, White EA, Webb WR, et al: Hilar and mediastinal adenopathy caused by bacterial abscess of the lung. Radiology 128: 289, 1978.

186. Tillotson JR, Lerner AM: Bacteroides pneumonias: Characteristics of cases with empyema. Ann Intern Med 68: 308, 1968.

187. Raff MJ, Johnson JD, Nagar D, et al: Spontaneous clostridial empyema and pyopneumothorax. Rev Infect Dis 61: 715, 1984.

188. Gopalakrishna KV, Lerner PI: Primary lung abscess: Analysis of 66 cases. Cleve Clin Q 42: 3, 1975.

189. Sudenfeld SM, Sutker WL, Luby JP: Fusobacterium necrophorum septicemia following oropharyngeal infection. JAMA 248: 1348, 1982.

190. Guidol F, Manresa F, Pallares R, et al: Clindamycin vs. penicillin for anaerobic lung infections: High rate of penicillin failures associated with penicillin-resistant Bacteroides melaninogenicus. Arch Intern Med 150: 2525, 1990.

191. Goodwin RA, Des Prez RM: Apical localization of pulmonary tuberculosis, chronic pulmonary histoplasmosis, and progressive massive fibrosis of the lung. Chest 83: 801, 1983.

192. Fanning A, Edwards S: Mycobacterium bovis infection in human beings in contact with elk (Cervus elaphus) in Alberta, Canada. Lancet 338: 1253, 1991.

193. Wilkins EG, Griffiths RJ, Roberts C: Pulmonary tuberculosis due to Mycobacterium bovis. Thorax 41: 685, 1986.

194. Sparks FC: Hazards and complications of BCG immunotherapy. Med Clin North Am 60: 499, 1976.

195. Au FC, Webber B, Rosenberg SA: Pulmonary granulomas induced by BCG. Cancer 41: 2209, 1978.

196. Grzybowski S: Tuberculosis: A look at the world situation. Chest 84: 756, 1983.

197. Comstock GW: Epidemiology of tuberculosis. Am Rev Respir Dis 125: 8, 1982.

198. Warren CPW, Enarson DN, Chaisson RE, et al: Symposium: Tuberculosis: Trends in Canada. Ann R Coll Phys Surg Can 22: 455, 1989.

199. McAdam JM, Brickner PW, Scharer LL, et al: The spectrum of tuberculosis in a New York City men's shelter clinic (1982–1988). Chest 97: 798, 1990.

200. Frew AJ, Mayon-White RT, Benson MK: An outbreak of tuberculosis in an Oxfordshire school. Br J Dis Chest 81: 293, 1987.

201. Stead WW, Lofgren JP, Warren E, et al: Tuberculosis as an endemic and nosocomial infection among the elderly in nursing homes. N Engl J Med 312: 1483, 1985.

202. Minh V-D, Prendergast TJ, Engle P: Tuberculosis in refugees from Southeast Asia. Chest 82: 133, 1982.

203. Yeager H Jr, Lacy J, Smith LR, et al: Quantitative studies of mycobacterial populations in sputum and saliva. Am Rev Respir Dis 95: 998, 1967.

204. Davies BH: Infectivity of tuberculosis. Thorax 35: 481, 1980.

205. Stead WW, Dutt AK: What's new in tuberculosis? Am J Med 71: 1, 1981.

206. Glassroth J, Robbins AG, Snider DE Jr: Tuberculosis in the 1980s. N Engl J Med 302: 1441, 1980.

207. Friedman LN, Sullivan GM, Bevilaqua RP, et al: Tuberculosis screening in alcoholics and drug addicts. Am Rev Respir Dis 136: 1188, 1987.

208. Nagami P, Yoshikawa TT: Aging and tuberculosis. Gerontology 30: 308, 1984.

209. Bobrowitz ID: Active tuberculosis undiagnosed until autopsy. Am J Med 72: 650, 1982.

210. Lurie MB, Dannenberg AM Jr: Macrophage function in infectious disease with inbred rabbits. Bacteriol Rev 29: 466, 1965.

211. Comstock GW: Tuberculosis in twins: A re-analysis of the Prophit survey. Am Rev Respir Dis 117: 621, 1978.

212. Singh SPN, Mehra NK, Dingley HB, et al: Human leukocyte antigen (HLA)–linked control of susceptibility to pulmonary tuberculosis and association with HLA-DR types. J Infect Dis 148: 676, 1983.

213. Morgan EJ: Silicosis and tuberculosis. Chest 75: 202, 1979.

214. Holden HM, Hiltz JE: The tuberculous diabetic. Can Med Assoc J 87: 797, 1962.

215. Andrew OT, Schoenfeld PY, Hopewell PC, et al: Tuberculosis in patients with end-stage renal disease. Am J Med 68: 59, 1980.

216. Shachor Y, Schindler D, Siegal A, et al: Increased incidence of pulmonary tuberculosis in chronic interstitial lung disease. Thorax 44: 151, 1989.

217. Reyes JM, Putong PB: Association of pulmonary alveolar lipoproteinosis with mycobacterial infection. Am J Clin Pathol 74: 478, 1980.

218. Leff A, Geppert EF: Public health and preventive aspects of pulmonary tuberculosis: Infectiousness, epidemiology, risk factors, classification, and preventive therapy. Arch Intern Med 139: 1405, 1979.

219. Snider DE: Jejunoileal bypass for obesity: A risk factor for tuberculosis. Chest 81: 531, 1982.

220. Snider GL, Placik B: The relationship between pulmonary tuberculosis and bronchogenic carcinoma: A topographic study. Am Rev Respir Dis 99: 229, 1969.

221. Haroutunian LM, Fisher AM, Smith EW: Tuberculosis and sarcoidosis. Bull Johns Hopkins 115: 1, 1964.

222. Millar JW, Horne NW: Tuberculosis in immunosuppressed patients. Lancet 1: 1176, 1979.

222a. Fischl MA, Uttamchandani RB, Daikos GL, et al: An outbreak of tuberculosis caused by multiple drug–resistant tubercle bacilli among patients with HIV infection. Ann Intern Med 117(3): 177, 1992.

223. Goren MB: Immunoreactive substances of mycobacteria. Am Rev Respir Dis 125: 50, 1982.

224. Diaz GA, Wayne LG: Isolation and characterization of catalase produced by *Mycobacterium tuberculosis*. Am Rev Respir Dis 110: 312, 1974.

225. Stead WW, Bates JH: Evidence of a "silent" bacillemia in primary tuberculosis. Ann Intern Med 74: 559, 1971.

226. Stead WW, Kerby GR, Schlueter DP, et al: The clinical spectrum of primary tuberculosis in adults: Confusion with reinfection in the pathogenesis of chronic tuberculosis. Ann Intern Med 68: 731, 1968.

227. Weber AL, Bird KT, Janower ML: Primary tuberculosis in childhood with particular emphasis on changes affecting the tracheobronchial tree. Am J Roentgenol 103: 123, 1968.

228. Choyke PL, Sostman HD, Curtis AM, et al: Adult-onset pulmonary tuberculosis. Radiology 148: 357, 1983.

229. Solomon A, Rabinowitz L: Primary cavitating tuberculosis in childhood. Clin Radiol 23: 483, 1972.

230. Dhand S, Fisher M, Fewell JW: Intrathoracic tuberculous lymphadenopathy in adults. JAMA 241: 505, 1979.

231. Matthews JI, Matarese SL, Carpenter JL: Endobronchial tuberculosis simulating lung cancer. Chest 86: 642, 1984.

232. Enarson DA, Dorken E, Gryzbowski S: Tuberculous pleurisy. Can Med Assoc J 126: 493, 1982.

233. West JB: Localization of disease: Pulmonary tuberculosis. *In* Regional Differences in the Lung. New York, Academic Press, 1977, p 236.

234. Slavin RE, Walsh TJ, Pollack AD: Late generalized tuberculosis: A clinical pathologic analysis and comparison of 100 cases in the preantibiotic and antibiotic eras. Medicine 59: 352, 1980.

235. Ip MSM, So SY, Lam WK, et al: Endobronchial tuberculosis revisited. Chest 89: 727, 1986.

236. Plessinger VA, Jolly PN: Rasmussen's aneurysms and fatal hemorrhage in pulmonary tuberculosis. Am Rev Tuberc 60: 589, 1949.

237. Jacobson HG, Shapiro JH: Pulmonary tuberculosis. Radiol Clin North Am 1: 411, 1963.

238. Berger HW, Granada MG: Lower lung field tuberculosis. Chest 65: 522, 1974.

239. Kuhlman JE, Deutsch JA, Fishman EK, et al: CT features of thoracic mycobacterial disease. Radiographics 10: 413, 1990.

240. Woodring JH, Vandivere HM, Fried AM, et al: Update: The radiographic features of pulmonary tuberculosis. Am J Roentgenol 146: 497, 1986.

241. Bobrowitz ID: Reversible roentgenographic progression in the initial treatment of pulmonary tuberculosis. Am Rev Respir Dis 121: 735, 1980.

242. Woodring JH, Vandivere HM, Lee C: Intrathoracic lymphadenopathy in postprimary tuberculosis. South Med J 81: 992, 1988.

243. Hadlock FP, Park SK, Awe RJ, et al: Unusual radiographic findings in adult pulmonary tuberculosis. Am J Roentgenol 134: 1015, 1980.

244. Massaro D, Katz S: Rapid clearing in hematogenous pulmonary tuberculosis. Arch Intern Med 113: 573, 1964.

245. Biehl JP: Miliary tuberculosis. A review of sixty-eight adult patients admitted to a municipal general hospital. Am Rev Tuberc 77: 605, 1958.

246. Dee P, Teja K, Korzeniowski O, et al: Miliary tuberculosis resulting in adult respiratory distress syndrome: A surviving case. Am J Roentgenol 134: 569, 1980.

247. Stinghe RV, Mangiulea VG: Hemoptysis of bronchial origin occurring in patients with arrested tuberculosis. Am Rev Respir Dis 101: 84, 1970.

248. Van den Brande PM, Van de Mierop F, Verbeken EK, et al: Clinical spectrum of endobronchial tuberculosis in elderly patients. Arch Intern Med 150: 2105, 1990.

249. Choe KO, Jeong HJ, Sohn HY: Tuberculous bronchial stenosis: CT findings in 28 cases. Am J Roentgenol 155: 971, 1990.

250. Sochocky S: Tuberculoma of the lung. Am Rev Tuberc 78: 403, 1958.

251. Antoniskis D, Amin K, Barnes PF: Pleuritis as a manifestation of reactivation tuberculosis. Am J Med 89: 447, 1990.

252. Donath J, Khan FA: Tuberculosis and posttuberculous fistula: Ten-year clinical experience. Chest 86: 697, 1984.

253. Byram D, Hatton P, Williams S, et al: The form and presentation of tuberculosis over a 10-year interval in Leeds. Br J Dis Chest 79: 152, 1985.

254. Myers JA, Bearman JE, Botkins AC: The natural history of tuberculosis in the human body: X. Prognosis among students with tuberculin reaction conversion before, during, and after school of nursing. Dis Chest 53: 687, 1968.

255. Styblo K, van Geuns HA, Meijer J: The yield of active case-finding in persons with inactive pulmonary tuberculosis of fibrotic lesions: A 5-year study in tuberculosis clinics in Amsterdam, Rotterdam, and Utrecht. Tubercle 65: 237, 1984.

256. Barnes PF, Chan LS, Wong SF: The course of fever during treatment of pulmonary tuberculosis. Tubercle 68: 255, 1987.

257. LeRoux BT: Unusual presentations of tuberculosis. Thorax 26: 343, 1971.

258. Munt PW: Miliary tuberculosis in the chemotherapy era: With a clinical review in 69 American adults. Medicine 51: 139, 1972.

259. Heffner JE, Strange C, Sahn SA: The impact of respiratory failure on the diagnosis of tuberculosis. Arch Intern Med 148: 1103, 1988.

260. McCulloch DK, Malone DNS: Presentation of tuberculosis in an acute medical unit. Lancet 1: 702, 1980.

261. Levenson MJ, Ingerman M, Grimes C, et al: Laryngeal tuberculosis: Review of twenty cases. Laryngoscope 94: 1094, 1984.

262. Pettengell KE, Larsen C, Garb M, et al: Gastrointestinal tuberculosis in patients with pulmonary tuberculosis. Q J Med 74: 303, 1990.

263. Bowry S, Chan CH, Weiss H, et al: Hepatic involvement in pulmonary tuberculosis: Histologic and functional characteristics. Am Rev Respir Dis 101: 941, 1970.

264. Kim TC, Blackman RS, Heatole KM, et al: Acid-fast bacilli in sputum smears of patients with pulmonary tuberculosis: Prevalence and significance of negative smears pretreatment and positive smears post-treatment. Am Rev Respir Dis 129: 264, 1984.

265. Chan HS, Sun AJ, Hoheisel GB: Bronchoscopic aspiration and bronchoalveolar lavage in the diagnosis of sputum-negative pulmonary tuberculosis. Lung 168: 215, 1990.

266. Wallace JM, Deutsch AL, Harrell JH, et al: Bronchoscopy and transbronchial biopsy in evaluation of patients with suspected active tuberculosis. Am J Med 70: 1189, 1981.

267. Dahlgren SE, Ekström P: Aspiration cytology in the diagnosis of pulmonary tuberculosis. Scand J Respir Dis 53: 196, 1972.

268. Morris CD, Bird AR, Nell H: The haematological and biochemical changes in severe pulmonary tuberculosis. Q J Med 73: 1151, 1989.

269. Fuss M, Karmali R, Pepersack T, et al: Are tuberculous patients at a great risk from hypercalcemia? Q J Med 69: 869, 1988.

270. Hill AR, Uribarri J, Mann J, et al: Altered water metabolism in tuberculosis: Role of vasopressin. Am J Med 88: 357, 1990.

271. Bothamley GH, Rudd R, Festenstein F, et al: Clinical value of the measurement of *Mycobacterium tuberculosis*–specific antibody in pulmonary tuberculosis. Thorax 47: 270, 1992.

272. Levy H, Feldman C, Wadee AA, et al: Differentiation of sarcoidosis from tuberculosis using an enzyme-linked immunosorbent assay for the detection of antibodies against *Mycobacterium tuberculosis*. Chest 94: 1254, 1988.

273. de Lassence A, Lecossier D, Pierre C, et al: Detection of mycobacterial DNA in pleural fluid from patients with tuberculous pleurisy by means of the polymerase chain reaction: Comparison of two protocols. Thorax 47: 265, 1992.

274. Simpson DG, Kuschner M, McClement J: Respiratory function in pulmonary tuberculosis. Am Rev Respir Dis 87: 1, 1963.

275. Williams MH Jr, Yoo OH, Kane C: Pulmonary function in miliary tuberculosis. Am Rev Respir Dis 107: 858, 1973.

276. Bates JH: Ambulatory treatment of tuberculosis–an idea whose time is come. Am Rev Respir Dis 109: 317, 1974.

277. Leading article: Drug-resistant tuberculosis. Br Med J 283: 336, 1981.

278. Carpenter JL, Obnibene AJ, Gorby EW, et al: Antituberculosis drug resistance in south Texas. Am Rev Respir Dis 128: 1055, 1983.

279. Davis CE Jr, Carpenter JL, McAllister CK, et al: Tuberculosis: Cause of death in antibiotic era. Chest 88: 726, 1985.

280. Wolinsky E: Nontuberculous mycobacteria and associated disease. Am Rev Respir Dis 119: 107, 1979.

281. Robakiewicz M, Grzybowski S: Epidemiologic aspects of nontuberculous mycobacterial disease and of tuberculosis in British Columbia. Am Rev Respir Dis 109: 613, 1974.

282. Penny ME, Cole RB, Gray J: Two cases of *Mycobacterium kansasii* infection occurring in the same household. Tubercle 63: 129, 1982.

283. Hutchins GM, Boitnott JK: Atypical mycobacterial infection complicating mineral oil pneumonia. JAMA 240: 539, 1978.

284. Weinstein RA, Golomb HM, Grumet G, et al: Hairy-cell leukemia: Association with disseminated atypical mycobacterial infection. Cancer 48: 380, 1981.

285. Good RC, Snider DE Jr: Isolation of nontuberculous mycobacteria in the United States, 1980. J Infect Dis 146: 829, 1983.

286. Tellis CJ, Putnam JS: Pulmonary disease caused by nontuberculosis mycobacteria. Med Clin North Am 64: 433, 1980.

286a. Kilby JM, Gilligan PH, Yankaskas JR, et al: Nontuberculous mycobacteria in adult patients with cystic fibrosis. Chest 102(1): 70, 1992.

287. Lillo M, Orengo S, Cernoch P, et al: Pulmonary and disseminated infection due to *Mycobacterium kansasii*: A decade of experience. Rev Infect Dis 12: 760, 1990.

288. Ahn CH, Lowell JR, Onstad GD, et al: Elimination of *Mycobacterium intracellulare* from sputum after bronchial hygiene. Chest 76: 480, 1979.

289. Dutt AK, Stead WW: Long-term results of medical treatment in *Mycobacterium intracellulare* infection. Am J Med 67: 449, 1979.

290. Marchevsky A, Damsker B, Gribetz A, et al: The spectrum of pathology of nontuberculous mycobacterial infections in open-lung biopsy specimens. Am J Clin Pathol 78: 695, 1982.

291. Woodring JH, Vandivere M, Melvin IG, et al: Roentgenographic features of pulmonary disease caused by atypical mycobacteria. South Med J 80: 1488, 1987.

292. Christensen EE, Dietz GW, Ahn CH, et al: Radiographic manifestations of pulmonary *Mycobacterium kansasii* infections. Am J Roentgenol 131: 985, 1978.

293. Christiansen EE, Dietz GW, Ahn CH, et al: Pulmonary manifestations of *Mycobacterium intracellulare*. Am J Roentgenol 133: 59, 1979.

294. Albelda SM, Kern JA, Marinelli DL, et al: Expanding spectrum of pulmonary disease caused by nontuberculous mycobacteria. Radiology 157: 289, 1985.

295. Zvetina JR, Demps TC, Maliwan N, et al: Pulmonary cavitations in *Mycobacterium kansasii*: Distinctions from *M. tuberculosis*. Am J Roentgenol 143: 127, 1984.

296. Saito H, Tasaka H, Osasa S, et al: Disseminated *Mycobacterium intracellulare* infection. Am Rev Respir Dis 109: 572, 1974.

297. The Tuberculin Skin Test. Supplement to Diagnostic Standards and Classification of Tuberculosis and Other Mycobacterial Diseases. New York, American Lung Association, 1974.

298. Francis PB, Jay SJ, Johanson WG Jr: The course of untreated *Mycobacterium kansasii* disease. Am Rev Respir Dis 111: 477, 1975.

299. Ahn CH, Lowell JR, Ahn SS, et al: Short-course chemotherapy for pulmonary disease caused by *Mycobacterium kansasii*. Am Rev Respir Dis 128: 1048, 1983.

300. Reich JM, Johnson RE: *Mycobacterium avium* complex pulmonary disease: Incidence, presentation, and response to therapy in a community setting. Am Rev Respir Dis 143: 1381, 1991.

301. Goodwin RA Jr, Des Prez RM: Histoplasmosis. Am Rev Respir Dis 117: 929, 1978.

302. Furcolow ML: Environmental aspects of histoplasmosis. Arch Environ Health 10: 4, 1965.

303. Baker RD: Histoplasmosis in routine autopsies. Am J Clin Pathol 41: 457, 1964.

304. Storch G, Burford JG, George RB, et al: Acute histoplasmosis: Description of an outbreak in northern Louisiana. Chest 77: 38, 1980.

305. Defaveri J, Graybill JR: Immunohistopathology of murine pulmonary histoplasmosis during normal and hypersensitive conditions. Am Rev Respir Dis 144: 1366, 1991.

306. Goodwin RA Jr, Loyd JE, Des Prez RM: Histoplasmosis in normal hosts. Medicine 60: 231, 1981.

307. Medeiros AA, Marty SD, Tosh FE, et al: Erythema nodosum and erythema multiforme as clinical manifestations of histoplasmosis in a community outbreak. N Engl J Med 27: 415, 1966.

308. Riggs W Jr, Nelson P: The roentgenographic findings in infantile and childhood histoplasmosis. Am J Roentgenol 97: 181, 1966.

309. Babbitt DP, Waisbren BA: Epidemic pulmonary histoplasmosis: Roentgenographic findings. Am J Roentgenol 83: 236, 1960.

310. Wynne JW, Olsen GN: Acute histoplasmosis presenting as the adult respiratory distress syndrome. Chest 66: 158, 1974.

311. Connell JV Jr, Muhm JR: Radiographic manifestations of pulmonary histoplasmosis: A 10-year review. Radiology 121: 281, 1976.

312. Palayew MJ, Frank H: Benign progressive multinodular pulmonary histoplasmosis: A radiological and clinical entity. Radiology 111: 311, 1974.

313. Prager RL, Burney DP, Waterhouse G, et al: Pulmonary, mediastinal, and cardiac presentations of histoplasmosis. Ann Thorac Surg 30: 385, 1980.

314. Baum GL: Cavitation in histoplasmosis: Some further comments. Chest 67: 625, 1975.

315. Landay MJ, Rollins NK: Mediastinal histoplasmosis granuloma: Evaluation with CT. Radiology 172: 657, 1989.

316. Goodwin RA Jr, Shapiro JL, Thurman GH, et al: Disseminated histoplasmosis: Clinical and pathologic correlations. Medicine 59: 1, 1980.

317. Wheat J, French MLV, Kohler RB, et al: The diagnostic laboratory tests for histoplasmosis: Analysis of experience in a large urban outbreak. Ann Intern Med 97: 680, 1982.

318. Jacobson ES, Straus SE: Reevaluation of diagnostic *Histoplasma* serologies. Am J Med Sci 281: 143, 1981.

319. Richert JH, Campbell CC: The significance of skin and serologic tests in the diagnosis of pulmonary residuals of histoplasmosis: A review of 123 cases. Am Rev Respir Dis 86: 381, 1962.

320. Sarosi GA, Voth DW, Dahl BA, et al: Disseminated histoplasmosis: Results of long-term follow-up: A Centers for Disease Control cooperative mycoses study. Ann Intern Med 75: 511, 1971.

321. Drutz DJ, Catanzaro A: Coccidioidomycosis. Part I. Am Rev Respir Dis 117: 559, 1978.

322. Drutz DJ, Catanzaro A: Coccidioidomycosis. Part II. Am Rev Respir Dis 117: 727, 1978.

323. Greendyke WH, Resnik DL, Harvy WC: The varied roentgen manifestations of primary coccidioidomycosis. Am J Roentgenol 109: 491, 1970.

324. Werner SB, Pappagianis D, Heindl L, et al: An epidemic of coccidioidomycosis among archeology students in northern California. N Engl J Med 286: 507, 1972.

325. Klein EW, Griffin JP: Coccidioidomycosis (diagnosis outside the Sonoran Zone): The roentgen features of acute multiple pulmonary cavities. Am J Roentgenol 94: 653, 1965.

326. Spivey CG Jr, Jones FL, Bopp RK: Cavitary coccidioidomycosis: Experience in a tuberculosis hospital outside the endemic area. Dis Chest 56: 13, 1969.

327. Bayer AS, Yoshikawa TT, Guze LB: Chronic progressive coccidioidal pneumonitis: Report of six cases with clinical, roentgenographic, serologic, and therapeutic features. Arch Intern Med 139: 536, 1979.

328. Baker EJ, Hawkins JA, Waskow EA: Surgery for coccidioidomycosis in 52 diabetic patients with special reference to related immunologic factors. J Thorac Cardiovasc Surg 75: 680, 1978.

329. Goldstein E: Miliary and disseminated coccidioidomycosis. Ann Intern Med 89: 365, 1978.

330. Wallace JM, Catanzaro A, Moser KM, et al: Flexible fiberoptic bronchoscopy for diagnosing pulmonary coccidioidomycosis. Am Rev Respir Dis 123: 286, 1981.

331. Bayer AS: Fungal pneumonias: Pulmonary coccidioidal syndromes: Part I. Primary and progressive primary coccidioidal pneumonias—diagnostic, therapeutic, and prognostic considerations. Chest 79: 575, 1981.

332. Levine HB, Gonzalez-Ochoa A, TenEyck DR: Dermal sensitivity to *Coccidioides immitis*: A comparison of responses elicited in man by spherulin and coccidioidin. Am Rev Respir Dis 107: 379, 1973.

333. Sarosi GA, Davies SF: Blastomycosis. Am Rev Respir Dis 120: 911, 1979.

334. Furcolow ML, Chick EW, Busey JF, et al: Prevalence and incidence studies of human and canine blastomycosis: I. Cases in the United States, 1885–1968. Am Rev Respir Dis 102: 60, 1970.

335. Kravitz GR, Davies SF, Eckman MR, et al: Chronic blastomycotic meningitis. Am J Med 71: 501, 1981.

336. Recht LD, Davies SF, Eckman MR, et al: Blastomycosis in immunosuppressed patients. Am Rev Respir Dis 125: 359, 1982.

337. Schwarz J, Salfelder K: Blastomycosis: A review of 152 cases. Curr Top Pathol 65: 166, 1977.

338. Halvorsen RA, Duncan JD, Merten DF, et al: Pulmonary blastomycosis: Radiologic manifestations. Radiology 150: 1, 1984.

339. Sheflin JR, Campbell JA, Thompson GP: Pulmonary blastomycosis: Findings on chest radiographs in 63 patients. Am J Roentgenol 154: 1177, 1990.

340. Kinasewitz GT, Penn RL, George RB: The spectrum and significance of pleural disease in blastomycosis. Chest 86: 580, 1984.

341. Stelling CB, Woodring JH, Rehm SR, et al: Miliary pulmonary blastomycosis. Radiology 150: 7, 1984.

342. Skillrud DM, Douglas WW: Survival in adult respiratory distress syndrome caused by blastomycosis infection. Mayo Clin Proc 60: 266, 1985.

342a. Winer-Muram HT, Beals DH, Cole FH Jr: Blastomycosis of the lung: CT features. Radiology 182(3): 829, 1992.

343. Klein BS, Vergeront JM, Weeks RJ, et al: Isolation of *Blastomyces dermatitidis* in soil associated with a large outbreak of blastomycosis in Wisconsin. N Engl J Med 314: 529, 1986.

344. Williams JE, Murphy R, Standard PG, et al: Serologic response in blastomycosis: Diagnostic value of double immunodiffusion assay. Am Rev Respir Dis 123: 209, 1981.

345. Klein BS, Kuritsky JN, Chappell WA, et al: Comparison of the enzyme immunoassay, immunodiffusion, and complement fixation tests in detecting antibody in human serum to the A antigen of *Blastomyces dermatitidis*. Am Rev Respir Dis 133: 144, 1986.

346. Sutliff WD, Cruthirds TP: *Blastomyces dermatitidis* in cytologic preparations. Am Rev Respir Dis 108: 149, 1973.

347. Bouza E, Winston DJ, Rhodes J, et al: Paracoccidiodomycosis (South American blastomycosis) in the United States. Chest 72: 100, 1977.

348. Murray HW, Littman ML, Roberts RB: Disseminated paracoccidioidomycosis (South American blastomycosis) in the United States. Am J Med 56: 209, 1974.

349. Restrepo A, Robledo M, Gutierrez F, et al: Paracoccidioidomycosis (South American blastomycosis): A study of 39 cases observed in Medellin, Colombia. Am J Trop Med Hyg 19: 68, 1970.

350. Severo LC, Porto NS, Camargo JJ, et al: Multiple paracoccidioidomas simulating Wegener's granulomatosis. Mycopathologia 91: 117, 1985.

351. Londero AT, Ramos CD, Lopes JOS: Progressive pulmonary paracoccidioidomycosis: A study of 34 cases observed in Rio Grande do Sul (Brazil). Mycopathologia 63: 53, 1978.

352. Restrepo A, Cano LE, Tabares AM: A comparison of mycelial filtrate and yeast lysate–paracoccidioidin in patients with paracoccidioidomycosis. Mycopathologia 84: 49, 1983.

353. Londero AT, Ramos CD: Paracoccidioidomycosis: A clinical and mycologic study of forty-one cases observed in Santa Maria, RS, Brazil. Am J Med 52: 771, 1972.

354. Farhi F, Bulmer GS, Tacker JR: *Cryptococcus neoformans*: IV. The not-so-encapsulated yeast. Infect Immun 1: 526, 1970.

355. Bulmer GS, Sans MD: *Cryptococcus neoformans*: III. Inhibition of phagocytosis. J Bacteriol 95: 5, 1968.

356. Harding SA, Scheld WM, Feldman PS, et al: Pulmonary infection with capsule-deficient *Cryptococcus neoformans*. Virchows Arch 382: 113, 1979.

357. McDonnell JM, Hutchins GM: Pulmonary cryptococcosis. Hum Pathol 16: 121, 1985.

358. Gordonson J, Birnbaum W, Jacobson G, et al: Pulmonary cryptococcosis. Radiology 112: 557, 1974.

359. Feigin DS: Pulmonary cryptococcosis: Radiologic-pathologic correlates of its three forms. Am J Roentgenol 141: 1263, 1983.

360. Khoury MB, Godwin JD, Ravin CE, et al: Thoracic cryptococcosis: Immunologic competence and radiologic appearance. Am J Roentgenol 142: 893, 1984.

361. Hammerman KJ, Powell KE, Christianson CS, et al: Pulmonary cryptococcosis: Clinical forms and treatment. A Centers for Disease Control cooperative mycoses study. Am Rev Respir Dis 108: 1116, 1973.

362. Walter JE, Jones RD: Serodiagnosis of clinical cryptococcosis. Am Rev Respir Dis 97: 275, 1968.

363. Atkinson AJ, Bennett JE: Experience with a new skin test antigen prepared from *Cryptococcus neoformans*. Am Rev Respir Dis 97: 637, 1968.

364. Meunier-Carpentier F, Kiehn TE, Armstrong D: Fungemia in the immunocompromised host: Changing patterns, antigenemia, high mortality. Am J Med 71: 363, 1981.

365. Dubois PJ, Myerowitz RL, Allen CM: Pathoradiologic correlation of pulmonary candidiasis in immunosuppressed patients. Cancer 40: 1026, 1977.

366. Buff SJ, McLelland R, Gallis HA, et al: *Candida albicans* pneumonia: Radiographic appearance. Am J Roentgenol 138: 645, 1982.

367. Watanakunakorn C: Acute pulmonary mycetoma due to *Candida albicans* with complete resolution. J Infect Dis 148: 1131, 1983.

368. Guinan ME, Portas MR, Hill HR: The *Candida* precipitin test in an immunosuppressed population. Cancer 43: 299, 1979.

369. Bardana EJ Jr: The clinical spectrum of aspergillosis: Part I. Epidemiology, pathogenicity, infection in animals, and immunology of *Aspergillus*. CRC Crit Rev Clin Lab Sci, November 1980, p 21.

370. Beaumont F, Kauffmann HF, Sluiter HJ, et al: Environmental aerobiological studies in allergic bronchopulmonary aspergillosis. Allergy 39: 183, 1984.

371. Kothary MH, Chase T Jr, MacMillan JD: Correlation of elastase production by some strains of *Aspergillus fumigatus* with ability to cause pulmonary invasive aspergillosis in mice. Infect Immun 43: 320, 1984.

372. Waldorf AR, Levitz SM, Diamond RD: In vivo bronchoalveolar macrophage defense against *Rhizopus orzae* and *Aspergillus fumigatus*. J Infect Dis 150: 752, 1984.

373. Robertson MD, Seaton A, Milne LJR, et al: Resistance of spores of *Aspergillus fumigatus* to ingestion by phagocytic cells. Thorax 42: 466, 1987.

374. Robertson MD, Seaton A, Milne LJR, et al: Suppression of host defences by *Aspergillus fumigatus*. Thorax 42: 19, 1987.

374a. Fraser RS: Pulmonary aspergillosis: Pathologic and pathogenetic features. Pathol Annu 28: 231, 1993.

375. Bardana EJ Jr: The clinical spectrum of aspergillosis: Part 2. Classification and description of saprophytic, allergic, and invasive variants of human disease. CRC Crit Rev Clin Lab Sci 13: 85, 1980.
376. Wollschlager C, Khan F: Aspergillomas complicating sarcoidosis: A prospective study in 100 patients. Chest 86: 585, 1984.
377. Le Hegarat R, Vie A, Allain YM, et al: L'épaississement des parois, signe précoce et peu connu dans l'aspergillome pulmonaire: (Thickening of the walls, early and little-known sign of pulmonary aspergilloma.) J Radiol Electrol Med Nucl 47: 535, 1966.
378. Roberts CM, Citron KM, Strickland B: Intrathoracic aspergilloma: Role of CT in diagnosis and treatment. Radiology 165: 123, 1987.
379. Pennington JE: *Aspergillus* lung disease. Med Clin North Am 64: 475, 1980.
380. Research Committee of the British Thoracic and Tuberculosis Association: Aspergilloma and residual tuberculous cavities—the results of a resurvey. Tubercle 51: 227, 1970.
381. Schwartz HJ, Greenberger PA: The prevalence of allergic bronchopulmonary aspergillosis in patients with asthma, determined by serologic and radiologic criteria in patients at risk. J Lab Clin Med 117: 138, 1991.
382. Nicolai T, Arleth S, Spaeth A, et al: Correlation of IgE antibody titer to *Aspergillus fumigatus* with decreased lung function in cystic fibrosis. Pediatr Pulmonol 8: 12, 1990.
383. Katzenstein A-L, Liebow AA, Friedman PJ: Bronchocentric granulomatosis, mucoid impaction, and hypersensitivity reactions to fungi. Am Rev Respir Dis 111: 497, 1975.
384. Henderson AH: Allergic aspergillosis: Review of 32 cases. Thorax 23: 501, 1968.
385. Mintzer RA, Rogers LF, Kruglik GD, et al: The spectrum of radiologic findings in allergic bronchopulmonary aspergillosis. Radiology 127: 301, 1978.
386. Shah A, Khan ZU, Chaturvedi S, et al: Allergic bronchopulmonary aspergillosis with coexistent aspergilloma: A long-term follow-up. J Asthma 26: 109, 1989.
387. Breslin AB, Jenkins CR: Experience with allergic bronchopulmonary aspergillosis: Some unusual features. Clin Allergy 14: 21, 1984.
388. Malo J-L, Hawkins R, Pepys J: Studies in chronic allergic bronchopulmonary aspergillosis: 1. Clinical and physiological findings. Thorax 32: 254, 1977.
389. Patterson R, Greenberger PA, Radin RC, et al: Allergic bronchopulmonary aspergillosis: Staging as an aid to management. Ann Intern Med 96: 286, 1982.
390. Imbeau SA, Nichols D, Flaherty D, et al: Relationships between prednisone therapy, disease activity, and the total serum IgE in allergic bronchopulmonary aspergillosis. J Allergy Clin Immunol 62: 91, 1978.
391. Wang JLF, Patterson R, Roberts M, et al: The management of allergic bronchopulmonary aspergillosis. Am Rev Respir Dis 120: 87, 1979.
392. Lee TM, Greenberger PA, Patterson R, et al: Stage V (fibrotic) allergic bronchopulmonary aspergillosis: A review of 17 cases followed from diagnosis. Arch Intern Med 147: 319, 1987.
393. Young RC, Bennett JE, Vogel CL, et al: Aspergillosis: The spectrum of the disease in 98 patients. Medicine 49: 147, 1970.
394. Albeda SM, Talbot GH, Gerson SL, et al: Pulmonary cavitation and massive hemoptysis in invasive pulmonary aspergillosis: Influence of bone marrow recovery in patients with acute leukemia. Am Rev Respir Dis 131: 115, 1985.
395. Clarke A, Skelton J, Fraser RS: Fungal tracheobronchitis: Report of 9 cases and review of the literature. Medicine 70: 1, 1991.
396. Orr DP, Myerowitz RL, Dubois PJ: Pathoradiologic correlation of invasive pulmonary aspergillosis in the compromised host. Cancer 41: 2028, 1978.
397. Herbert PA, Bayer AS: Fungal pneumonia: Part 4. Invasive pulmonary aspergillosis. Chest 80: 220, 1981.
398. Curtis AM, Smith GJW, Ravin CE: Air crescent sign of invasive aspergillosis. Radiology 133: 17, 1979.
399. Young RC, Vogel CL, Devita VT: *Aspergillus* lobar pneumonia. JAMA 208: 1156, 1969.
400. Kuhlman JE, Fishman EK, Burch PA, et al: CT of invasive pulmonary aspergillosis. Am J Roentgenol 150: 1015, 1988.
401. Herold CJ, Kramer J, Sertl K, et al: Invasive pulmonary aspergillosis: Evaluation with MR imaging. Radiology 173: 717, 1989.
402. Binder RE, Faling LJ, Pugatch RD, et al: Chronic necrotizing pulmonary aspergillosis: A discrete clinical entity. Medicine 61: 109, 1982.
403. Yu VL, Muder RR, Poorsattar A: Significance of isolation of *Aspergillus* from the respiratory tract in diagnosis of invasive pulmonary aspergillosis: Results from a three-year prospective study. Am J Med 81: 249, 1986.
404. Kahn FW, Jones JM, England DM: The role of bronchoalveolar lavage in the diagnosis of invasive pulmonary aspergillosis. Am J Clin Pathol 86: 518, 1986.
405. Matsushima T, Soejima R, Nakashima T: Solitary pulmonary nodule caused by phycomycosis in a patient without obvious predisposing factors. Thorax 35: 877, 1980.
406. Zagoria RJ, Choplin RH, Karstaedt N: Pulmonary gangrene as a complication of mucormycosis. Am J Roentgenol 144: 1195, 1985.
407. Ross JD, Reid KDG, Speirs CF: Bronchopulmonary geotrichosis with severe asthma. Br Med J 1: 1400, 1966.
408. Fishbach RS, White ML, Finegold SM: Bronchopulmonary geotrichosis. Am Rev Respir Dis 108: 1388, 1973.
409. England DM, Hochholzer L: Primary pulmonary sporotrichosis: Report of eight cases with clinicopathologic review. Am J Surg Pathol 9: 193, 1985.
410. Lowenstein M, Markowitz SM, Nottebart HC, et al: Existence of *Sporothrix schenckii* as a pulmonary saprophyte. Chest 73: 419, 1978.
411. Trevathan RD, Phillips S: Primary pulmonary sporotrichosis: Case Report. JAMA 195: 965, 1966.
412. England DM, Hochholzer L: *Sporothrix* infection of the lung without cutaneous disease. Arch Pathol Lab Med 111: 298, 1987.
413. Schneidau JD, Lamar LM, Hairston MA: Cutaneous hypersensitivity to sporotrichin in Louisiana. JAMA 188: 371, 1964.
414. Kathuria SK, Rippon J: Non-*Aspergillus* aspergilloma. Am J Clin Pathol 78: 870, 1982.
415. Travis LB, Roberts GD, Wilson WR: Clinical significance of *Pseudallescheria boydii*: Review of 10 years' experience. Mayo Clin Proc 60: 531, 1985.
416. McCarthy DS, Longbottom JL, Riddell RW, et al: Pulmonary mycetoma due to *Allescheria boydii*. Am Rev Respir Dis 100: 213, 1969.
417. Smith DL, Lockwood WR: Disseminated actinomycosis. Chest 67: 242, 1975.
418. Behbehani MJ, Heely JD, Jordan HV: Comparative histopathology of lesions produced by *Actinomyces israelii*, *Actinomyces naeslundii*, and *Actinomyces viscosus* in mice. Am J Pathol 110: 267, 1983.
419. Brown JR: Human actinomycosis: A study of 181 subjects. Hum Pathol 4: 319, 1973.
420. Kwong JS, Müller NL, Godwin JD, et al: Thoracic actinomycosis: CT findings in eight patients. Radiology 183: 189, 1992.
421. Balikian JP, Cheng TH, Costello P, et al: Pulmonary actinomycosis: A report of three cases. Radiology 128: 613, 1978.
422. Schwarz J, Baum GL: Actinomycosis. Semin Roentgenol 5: 58, 1970.
423. Harrison RN, Thomas DJB: Acute actinomycotic empyema. Thorax 34: 406, 1979.
424. Curry WA: Human nocardiosis: A clinical review with selected case reports. Arch Intern Med 140: 818, 1980.
425. Lovett IS, Houang ET, Burge S, et al: An outbreak of *Nocardia asteroides* infection in a renal transplant unit. Q J Med 50: 123, 1981.
426. Frazier AR, Rosenow EC III, Roberts GD: Nocardiosis: A review of 25 cases occurring during 24 months. Mayo Clin Proc 50: 657, 1975.
427. Rosett W, Hodges GR: Recent experiences with nocardial infections. Am J Med Sci 276: 279, 1978.
428. Baily GG, Neill P, Robertson VJ: Nocardiosis: A neglected chronic lung disease in Africa? Thorax 43: 905, 1988.
429. Andriole VT, Ballas M, Wilson GL: The association of nocardiosis and pulmonary alveolar proteinosis: A case study. Ann Intern Med 60: 266, 1964.
430. Gorevic PD, Katler EI, Agus B: Pulmonary nocardiosis: Occurrence in men with systemic lupus erythematosus. Arch Intern Med 140: 361, 1980.
431. Neu HC, Silva M, Hazen E, et al: Necrotizing nocardial pneumonitis. Ann Intern Med 66: 274, 1967.
432. Habermehl KO: Rapid diagnosis of respiratory virus infections in patients with acute respiratory disease. Diagn Microbiol Infect Dis 4(3 Suppl): 17S, 1986.
433. Collier AM, Clyde WA Jr: Appearance of *Mycoplasma pneumoniae* in lungs of experimentally infected hamsters and sputum from patients with natural disease. Am Rev Respir Dis 110: 765, 1974.
434. Embree JE, Embil JA: Mycoplasmas in diseases of humans. Can Med Assoc J 123: 105, 1980.
435. Foy HM, Loop J, Clarke ER, et al: Radiographic study of *Mycoplasma pneumoniae* pneumonia. Am Rev Respir Dis 108: 469, 1973.

436. Purcell RH, Chanock RM: Role of mycoplasmas in human respiratory disease. Med Clin North Am 51: 791, 1967.

436a. Khatib R, Schnarr D: Point-source outbreak of *Mycoplasma pneumoniae* infection in a family unit. J Infect Dis 151: 186, 1985.

437. Noah ND: *Mycoplasma pneumoniae* infection in the United Kingdom, 1967–73. Br Med J 2: 544, 1974.

438. Murphy GF, Brody AR, Craighead JE: Exfoliation of respiratory epithelium in hamster tracheal organ cultures infected with *Mycoplasma pneumoniae*. Virchows Arch 389: 93, 1980.

439. Kist M, Koester H, Bredt W: *Mycoplasma pneumoniae* induces cytotoxic activity in guinea pig bronchoalveolar cells. Am Rev Respir Dis 131: 669, 1985.

440. Cassell GH, Cole BC: Mycoplasmas as agents of human disease. N Engl J Med 304: 80, 1981.

441. Cameron DC, Borthwick RN, Philp T: The radiographic patterns of acute *Mycoplasma* pneumonitis. Clin Radiol 28: 173, 1977.

442. George RB, Ziskind MM, Rasch JR, et al: *Mycoplasma* and adenovirus pneumonias: Comparison with other atypical pneumonias in a military population. Ann Intern Med 65: 931, 1966.

443. Putman CE, Curtis AM, Simeone JF, et al: *Mycoplasma* pneumonia: Clinical and roentgenographic patterns. Am J Roentgenol 124: 417, 1975.

444. Ali NJ, Sillis M, Andrews BE, et al: The clinical spectrum and diagnosis of *Mycoplasma pneumoniae*. Q J Med 58: 241, 1986.

445. Shulman ST, Bartlett J, Clyde WA Jr, et al: The unusual severity of mycoplasmal pneumonia in children with sickle-cell disease. N Engl J Med 287: 164, 1972.

446. Lind K: Manifestations and complications of *Mycoplasma pneumoniae* disease: A review. Yale J Biol Med 56: 461, 1983.

447. Murray HW, Tuazon C: Atypical pneumonias. Med Clin North Am 64: 507, 1980.

448. Jones MC: Arthritis and arthralgia in infection with *Mycoplasma pneumoniae*. Thorax 25: 748, 1970.

449. Sands MJ Jr, Satz JE, Turner WE Jr, et al: Pericarditis and perimyocarditis associated with active *Mycoplasma pneumoniae* infection. Ann Intern Med 86: 544, 1977.

450. Tablan OC, Reyes MP: Chronic interstitial pulmonary fibrosis following *Mycoplasma pneumoniae* pneumonia. Am J Med 79: 268, 1985.

451. Sabato AR, Martin AJ, Marmion BP, et al: *Mycoplasma pneumoniae*: Acute illness, antibiotics, and subsequent pulmonary function. Arch Dis Child 59: 1034, 1984.

452. Lehtomäki K: Rapid etiological diagnosis of pneumonia in young men. Scand J Infect Dis Suppl 54: 1, 1988.

453. Vikerfors T, Brodin G, Grandien M, et al: Detection of specific IgM antibodies for the diagnosis of *Mycoplasma pneumoniae* infections: A clinical evaluation. Scand J Infect Dis 20: 601, 1988.

454. Madsen RD, Weiner LB, McMillan JA, et al: Direct detection of *Mycoplasma pneumoniae* antigen in clinical specimens by a monoclonal antibody immunoblot assay. Am J Clin Pathol 89: 95, 1988.

455. Wells DL, Hopfensperger DJ, Arden NH, et al: Swine influenza virus infections: Transmission from ill pigs to humans at a Wisconsin agricultural fair and subsequent probable person-to-person transmission. JAMA 265: 478, 1991.

455a. Chapman LE, Tipple MA, Schmeltz LM, et al: Influenza—United States, 1989–90 and 1990–91 seasons. MMWR 41(3): 35, 1992.

456. Hobson D: Acute respiratory virus infections. Br Med J 2: 229, 1973.

457. Glezen WP, Keitel WA, Taber LH, et al: Age distribution of patients with medically attended illnesses caused by sequential variants of influenza A/H1N1: Comparison to age-specific infection rates, 1978–1989. Am J Epidemiol 133: 296, 1991.

458. Schwarzmann SW, Adler JL, Sullivan RJ Jr, et al: Bacterial pneumonia during the Hong Kong influenza epidemic of 1968–1969: Experience in a city-county hospital. Arch Intern Med 127: 1037, 1971.

459. Ershler WB, Moore AL, Socinski MA: Influenza and aging: Age-related changes and the effects of thymosin on the antibody response to influenza vaccine. J Clin Immunol 4: 445, 1984.

460. Feldman PS, Cohan MA, Hierholzer WJ Jr: Fatal Hong Kong influenza: A clinical microbiological and pathological analysis of nine cases. Yale J Biol Med 45: 49, 1972.

461. McQuillin J, Gardner PS, McGuckin R: Rapid diagnosis of influenza by immunofluorescent techniques. Lancet 2: 690, 1970.

462. Galloway RW, Miller RS: Lung changes in the recent influenza epidemic. Br J Radiol 32: 28, 1959.

463. Monto AS, Koopman JS, Longini IM Jr: Tecumseh study of illness: XIII. Influenza infection and disease, 1976–1981. Am J Epidemiol 121: 811, 1985.

464. Louria DB, Blumenfeld HL, Ellis JT, et al: Studies on influenza in the pandemic of 1957–1958: II. Pulmonary complications of influenza. J Clin Invest 38: 213, 1959.

465. Doller PC, Doller G, Gerth HJ: Immunofluorescence test with antigen-loaded erythrocytes: Detection of influenza virus–specific IgG, IgA, and IgM antibodies. Med Microbiol Immunol 173: 291, 1985.

466. Rosenzweig DY, Dwyer DJ, Ferstenfeld JE, et al: Changes in small airway function after live attenuated influenza vaccination. Am Rev Respir Dis 111: 399, 1975.

467. Reichman RC, Dolin R: Viral pneumonias. Med Clin North Am 64: 491, 1980.

468. Akizuki S, Masu N, Setoguchi M, et al: Parainfluenza virus pneumonitis in an adult. Arch Pathol Lab Med 115: 824, 1991.

469. Wenzel RP, McCormick DP, Beam WE Jr: Parainfluenza pneumonia in adults. JAMA 221: 294, 1972.

470. Gardner PS, McQuillin J, McGuckin R, et al: Observations on clinical and immunofluorescent diagnosis of parainfluenza virus infections. Br Med J 2: 7, 1971.

471. Agius G, Dindinaud G, Biggar RJ, et al: An epidemic of respiratory syncytial virus in elderly people: Clinical and serological findings. J Med Virol 30: 117, 1990.

472. McLelland L, Hilleman MR, Hamparain VV, et al: Studies of acute respiratory illnesses caused by respiratory syncytial virus: 2. Epidemiology and assessment of importance. N Engl J Med 264: 1169, 1961.

473. Mathur U, Bentley DW, Hall CB: Concurrent respiratory syncytial virus and influenza A infections in the institutionalized elderly and chronically ill: Part I. Ann Intern Med 93: 49, 1980.

474. Englund JA, Sullivan CJ, Jordan MC, et al: Respiratory syncytial virus infection in immunocompromised adults. Ann Intern Med 109: 203, 1988.

475. Gardner PS, McQuillin J, Court SDM: Speculation on pathogenesis of death from respiratory syncytial virus infection. Br Med J 1: 327, 1970.

476. Aherne W, Bird T, Court SDM, et al: Pathological changes in virus infections of the lower respiratory tract in children. J Clin Pathol 23: 7, 1970.

477. Osborne D: Radiologic appearance of viral disease of the lower respiratory tract in infants and children. Am J Roentgenol 130: 29, 1978.

478. Pullan CR, Hey EN: Wheezing, asthma, and pulmonary dysfunction 10 years after infection with respiratory syncytial virus in infancy. Br Med J 284: 1665, 1982.

479. McConnochie KM, Mark JD, McBride JT, et al: Normal pulmonary function measurements and airway reactivity in childhood after mild bronchiolitis. J Pediatr 107: 54, 1985.

480. Barkin RM: Measles mortality: Analysis of the primary cause of death. Am J Dis Child 129: 307, 1975.

481. Weiner LB, Corwin RM, Nieburg PI, et al: A measles outbreak among adolescents. J Pediatr 90: 17, 1977.

482. Becroft DMO, Osborne DRS: The lungs in fatal measles infection in childhood: Pathological, radiological and immunological correlations. Histopathology 4: 401, 1980.

483. Henderson JAM, Hammond DI: Delayed diagnosis in atypical measles syndrome. Can Med Assoc J 133: 211, 1985.

484. Gremillion DH, Crawford GE: Measles pneumonia in young adults: An analysis of 106 cases. Am J Med 71: 539, 1981.

485. Young LW, Smith DI, Glasgow LA: Pneumonia of atypical measles: Residual nodular lesions. Am J Roentgenol 110: 439, 1970.

486. George RB, Mogabgab WJ: Atypical pneumonia in young men with rhinovirus infections. Ann Intern Med 71: 1073, 1969.

487. Brandt CD, Kim HW, Vargosko AJ, et al: Infections in 18,000 infants and children in a controlled study of respiratory tract disease: I. Adenovirus pathogenicity in relation to serologic type and illness syndrome. Am J Epidemiol 90: 484, 1969.

488. Glezen WP, Denny FW: Epidemiology of acute lower respiratory disease in children. N Engl J Med 288: 498, 1973.

489. Hogg JC, Irving WL, Porter H, et al: In situ hybridization studies of adenoviral infections of the lung and their relationship to follicular bronchiectasis. Am Rev Respir Dis 139: 1531, 1989.

490. Becroft DMO: Bronchiolitis obliterans, bronchiectasis, and other sequelae of adenovirus type 21 infection in young children. J Clin Pathol 24: 72, 1971.

491. Gold R, Wilt JC, Adhikari PK, et al: Adenoviral pneumonia and its complications in infancy and childhood. J Can Assoc Radiol 20: 218, 1969.

492. Connor JD: Evidence for an etiologic role of adenoviral infection in pertussis syndrome. N Engl J Med 283: 390, 1970.

493. Sherry MK, Klainer AS, Wolff M, et al: Herpetic tracheobronchitis. Ann Intern Med 109: 229, 1988.

494. Nahmias AJ, Roizman B: Infection with herpes-simplex viruses 1 and 2. (Third of three parts.) N Engl J Med 289: 781, 1973.

495. Nash G, Foley FD: Herpetic infection of the middle and lower respiratory tract. Am J Clin Pathol 54: 857, 1970.

496. Graham BS, Snell JD Jr: Herpes simplex virus infection of the adult lower respiratory tract. Medicine 62: 384, 1983.

497. Feldman S, Stokes DC: Varicella zoster and herpes simplex virus pneumonias. Semin Respir Infect 2: 84, 1987.

498. Weber DM, Pellecchia JA: Varicella pneumonia: Study of prevalence in adult men. JAMA 192: 572, 1965.

499. Guess HA, Broughton DD, Melton LJ III: Chickenpox hospitalizations among residents of Olmsted County, Minnesota, 1962 through 1981: A population-based study. Am J Dis Child 138: 1055, 1984.

500. Leading article: Paralyzed hemidiaphragm and shingles. Br Med J 1: 382, 1970.

501. Sargent EN, Carson MJ, Reilly ED: Roentgenographic manifestations of varicella pneumonia with postmortem correlation. Am J Roentgenol 98: 305, 1966.

502. Knyvett AF: The pulmonary lesions of chicken pox. Q J Med (New Series 35) 39: 313, 1966.

503. Brunton FJ, Moore ME: A survey of pulmonary calcification following adult chicken-pox. Br J Radiol 42: 256, 1969.

504. Meyers JD, Flournoy N, Thomas ED: Risk factors for cytomegalovirus infection after human marrow transplantation. J Infect Dis 153: 478, 1986.

505. Schulman LL, Reison DS, Austin JH, et al: Cytomegalovirus pneumonitis after cardiac transplantation. Arch Intern Med 151: 1118, 1991.

506. Rasmussen L, Kelsall D, Nelson R, et al: Virus-specific IgG and IgM antibodies in normal and immunocompromised subjects infected with cytomegalovirus. J Infect Dis 145: 191, 1982.

507. Skinhoj P, Anderson HK, Moller J, et al: Cytomegalovirus infection after bone marrow transplantation: Relation of pneumonia to postgrafting immunosuppressive treatment. J Med Virol 14: 91, 1984.

508. Quinnan V Jr, Kirmani N, Rook AH, et al: Cytotoxic T cells in cytomegalovirus infection: HLA-restricted T-lymphocyte and non–T-lymphocyte cytotoxic responses correlate with recovery from cytomegalovirus infection in bone-marrow transplant recipients. N Engl J Med 307: 7, 1982.

509. Ruutu P, Ruutu T, Volin L, et al: Cytomegalovirus is frequently isolated in bronchoalveolar lavage fluid of bone marrow transplant recipients without pneumonia. Ann Intern Med 112: 913, 1990.

510. Shanley JD, Pesanti EL, Nugent KM: The pathogenesis of pneumonitis due to murine cytomegalovirus. J Infect Dis 146: 388, 1982.

511. Beschorner WE, Hutchins GM, Burns WH, et al: Cytomegalovirus pneumonia in bone marrow transplant recipients: Miliary and diffuse patterns. Am Rev Respir Dis 122: 107, 1980.

512. Goodman N, Daves ML, Rifkind D: Pulmonary roentgen findings following renal transplantations. Radiology 89: 621, 1967.

513. Idell S, Johnson M, Beauregard L, et al: Pneumonia associated with rising cytomegalovirus antibody titres in a healthy adult. Thorax 38: 957, 1983.

514. Crawford SW, Bowden RA, Hackman RC, et al: Rapid detection of cytomegalovirus pulmonary infection by bronchoalveolar lavage and centrifugation culture. Ann Intern Med 108: 180, 1988.

515. Woods GL, Thompson AB, Rennard SL, et al: Detection of cytomegalovirus in bronchoalveolar lavage specimens: Spin amplification and staining with a monoclonal antibody to the early nuclear antigen for diagnosis of cytomegalovirus pneumonia. Chest 98: 568, 1990.

516. Lander P, Palayew MJ: Infectious mononucleuosis–a review of chest roentgenographic manifestations. J Can Assoc Radiol 25: 303, 1974.

517. Barberà JA, Hayashi S, Hegele RG, et al: Detection of Epstein-Barr virus in lymphocytic interstitial pneumonitis by in situ hybridization. Am Rev Respir Dis 145: 940, 1992.

518. Byrne JC, Tsao MS, Fraser RS, et al: Human papillomavirus-11 DNA in a patient with chronic laryngotracheobronchial papillomatosis and metastatic squamous-cell carcinoma of the lung. N Engl J Med 317: 873, 1987.

519. Ward JK: Chlamydial classification, development, and structure. Br Med Bull 39: 109, 1983.

520. Thom DH, Grayston JT, Wang SP, et al: *Chlamydia pneumoniae* strain TWAR, *Mycoplasma pneumoniae*, and viral infections in acute respiratory disease in a university student health clinic population. Am J Epidemiol 132: 248, 1990.

521. Chirgwin K, Roblin PM, Gelling M, et al: Infection with *Chlamydia pneumoniae* in Brooklyn. J Infect Dis 163: 757, 1991.

522. Schachter J: Chlamydial infections (three parts). N Engl J Med 298: 428, 490, 540, 1978.

523. Hammerschlag MR: Chlamydial pneumonia in infants [editorial]. N Engl J Med 298: 1083, 1978.

524. Radkowski MA, Kranzler JK, Beem MO, et al: *Chlamydia* pneumonia in infants: Radiography in 125 cases. Am J Roentgenol 137: 703, 1981.

525. Meyers JD, Hackman RC, Stamm WE: *Chlamydia trachomatis* infection as a cause of pneumonia after human marrow transplantation. Transplantation 36: 130, 1983.

526. Sundkvist R, Mardh PA: Serological evidence of *Chlamydia trachomatis* infection in non-immunocompromised adults with pneumonia. J Infect 9: 143, 1984.

527. Numazaki K, Chiba S, Yamanaka T, et al: Detection of IgM antibodies against *Chlamydia trachomatis* by enzyme-linked fluorescence immunoassay. J Clin Pathol 38: 733, 1985.

528. MacFarlane JT, MacRae AD: Psittacosis. Br Med Bull 39: 163, 1983.

529. Barrett PKM, Greenberg MJ: Outbreak of ornithosis. Br Med J 2: 206, 1966.

530. Andrews BE, Major R, Palmer SR: Ornithosis in poultry workers. Lancet 1: 632, 1981.

531. Kuritsky JN, Schmid GP, Potter ME, et al: Psittacosis: A diagnostic challenge. J Occup Med 26: 731, 1984.

532. Johnson JE, Kadull PJ: Laboratory-acquired Q fever: A report of 50 cases. Am J Med 41: 391, 1966.

533. Brown GL: Q fever. Br Med J 2: 43, 1973.

533a. Tissot Dupont H, Raoult D, Brouqui P, et al: Epidemiologic features and clinical presentation of acute Q fever in hospitalized patients. 323 French cases. Am J Med 93(4): 427, 1992.

534. Millar JK: The chest film findings in "Q" fever–a series of 35 cases. Clin Radiol 29: 371, 1978.

534a. Smith DL, Wellings R, Walker C, et al: The chest X-ray in Q fever: A report on 69 cases from the 1989 West Midlands outbreak. Br J Radiol 64(768): 1101, 1991.

535. Roggli VL, Keener S, Bradford WD, et al: Pulmonary pathology of Rocky Mountain spotted fever (RMSF) in children. Pediatr Pathol 4: 47, 1985.

536. Martin W III, Choplin RH, Shertzer ME: The chest radiograph in Rocky Mountain spotted fever. Am J Roentgenol 139: 889, 1982.

537. Donohue JF: Lower respiratory tract involvement in Rocky Mountain spotted fever. Arch Intern Med 140: 223, 1980.

538. Krogstad DJ, Spencer HC Jr, Healy GR: Current concepts in parasitology. N Engl J Med 298: 262, 1978.

539. Ibarra-Perez C: Thoracic complications of amebic abscesses of the liver: Report of 501 cases. Chest 79: 672, 1981.

540. Barrett-Connor E: Parasitic pulmonary disease. Am Rev Respir Dis 126: 558, 1982.

541. Ibarra-Perez C, Selman-Lama M: Diagnosis and treatment of amebic "empyema": Report of 88 cases. Am J Surg 134: 283, 1977.

542. Ralls PW, Barnes PF, Johnson MB, et al: Medical treatment of hepatic amebic abscess: Rare need for percutaneous drainage. Radiology 165: 805, 1987.

543. Elizondo G, Weissleder R, Stark DD, et al: Amebic liver abscess: Diagnosis and treatment evaluation with MR imaging. Radiology 165: 795, 1987.

544. Roy DC, Ravindran P, Padmanabhan R: Bronchobiliary fistula secondary to amebic liver abscess. Chest 62: 523, 1972.

545. Leading article: Toxoplasmosis. Br Med J 282: 249, 1981.

546. Quinn EL, Fisher EJ, Cox F Jr, et al: The clinical spectrum of toxoplasmosis in the adult. Cleve Clin Q 42: 71, 1975.

547. Welsch PC, Masur H, Jones TC, et al: Serologic diagnosis of acute lymphadenopathic toxoplasmosis. J Infect Dis 142: 256, 1980.

548. Hasleton PS, Curry A, Rankin EM: *Pneumocystis carinii* pneumonia: A light microscopical and ultrastructural study. J Clin Pathol 34: 1138, 1981.

549. Singer C, Armstrong D, Rosen PP, et al: *Pneumocystis carinii* pneumonia: A cluster of eleven cases. Ann Intern Med 82: 772, 1975.

550. Tauber MI, Beckers ML, Sieben M: Parasitologic and serologic observations of infection with *Pneumocystis* in humans. J Infect Dis 136: 43, 1977.

550a. Stiller RA, Paradis IL, Dauber JH: Subclinical pneumonitis due to *Pneumocystis carinii* in a young adult with elevated antibody titers to Epstein-Barr virus. J Infect Dis 166(4): 926, 1992.

551. Fleury J, Escudier E, Pocholle M-J, et al: Cell population obtained by bronchoalveolar lavage in *Pneumocystis carinii* pneumonitis. Acta Cytol 29: 721, 1985.

552. Dembinski AS, Smith DM, Goldsmith JC, et al: Widespread dissemination of *Pneumocystis carinii* infection in a patient with acquired immune deficiency syndrome receiving long-term treatment with aerosolized pentamidine. Am J Clin Pathol 95: 96, 1991.

553. Long EG, Smith JS, Meier JL: Attachment of *Pneumocystis carinii* to rat pneumocytes. Lab Invest 54: 609, 1986.

554. Yoneda K, Walzer PD: Mechanism of pulmonary alveolar injury in experimental *Pneumocystis carinii* pneumonia in the rat. Br J Exp Pathol 62: 339, 1981.

555. Sheehan PM, Stokes DC, Yeh Y-Y, et al: Surfactant phospholipids and lavage phospholipase A_2 in experimental *Pneumocystis carinii* pneumonia. Am Rev Respir Dis 134: 526, 1986.

556. Weber WR, Asken FB, Dehner LP: Lung biopsy in *Pneumocystis carinii* pneumonia: A histopathologic study of typical and atypical features. Am J Clin Pathol 67: 11, 1977.

557. DeLorenzo LJ, Maguire GP, Wormser GP, et al: Persistence of *Pneumocystis carinii* pneumonia in the acquired immunodeficiency syndrome. Chest 88: 79, 1985.

558. Peters SG, Prakash UB: *Pneumocystis carinii* pneumonia: Review of 53 cases. Am J Med 82: 73, 1987.

559. Forrest JV: Radiographic findings in *Pneumocystis carinii* pneumonia. Radiology 103: 539, 1972.

560. Doppman JL, Geelhoed GW, DeVita VT: Atypical radiographic features in *Pneumocystis carinii* pneumonia. Radiology 114: 39, 1975.

561. Fineman DS, Palestro CJ, Kim CK, et al: Detection of abnormalities in febrile AIDS patients with In-111–labeled leukocyte and Ga-67 scintigraphy. Radiology 170(3 Pt 1): 677, 1989.

562. Sterling RP, Bradley BB, Khalil KG, et al: Comparison of biopsy-proven *Pneumocystis carinii* pneumonia in acquired immune deficiency syndrome patients and renal allograft recipients. Ann Thorac Surg 38: 494, 1984.

563. Bradshaw M, Myerowitz RL, Schneerson R, et al: *Pneumocystis carinii* pneumonitis. Ann Intern Med 73: 775, 1970.

564. Kagawa FT, Kirsch CM, Yenokida GG, et al: Serum lactate dehydrogenase activity in patients with AIDS and *Pneumocystis carinii* pneumonia: An adjunct to diagnosis. Chest 94: 1031, 1988.

565. Barron TF, Birnbaum NS, Shane LB, et al: *Pneumocystis carinii* pneumonia studied by gallium-67 scanning. Radiology 154: 791, 1985.

566. Caughey G, Wong H, Gamsu G, et al: Nonbronchoscopic bronchoalveolar lavage for the diagnosis of *Pneumocystis* pneumonia in the acquired immunodeficiency syndrome. Chest 88: 659, 1985.

567. Zaman MK, Wooten OJ, Suprahmanya B, et al: Rapid noninvasive diagnosis of *Pneumocystis carinii* from induced liquefied sputum. Ann Intern Med 109: 7, 1988.

568. Friedman Y, Franklin C, Freels S, et al: Long-term survival of patients with AIDS, *Pneumocystis carinii* pneumonia, and respiratory failure. JAMA 266: 89, 1991.

568a. Speich R, Opravil M, Weber R, et al: Prospective evaluation of a prognostic score for *Pneumocystis carinii* pneumonia in HIV-infected patients. Chest 102(4): 1045, 1992.

569. Sanyai SK, Mariencheck WC, Hughes WT, et al: Course of pulmonary dysfunction in children surviving *Pneumocystis carinii* pneumonitis: A prospective study. Am Rev Respir Dis 124: 161, 1981.

570. Suffredini AF, Owens GR, Tobin MJ, et al: Long-term prognosis of survivors of *Pneumocystis carinii* pneumonia: Structural and functional correlates. Chest 89: 229, 1986.

571. Gelpi AP, Mustafa A: *Ascaris* pneumonia. Am J Med 44: 377, 1968.

572. Humphreys K, Hieger LR: *Strongyloides stercoralis* in routine Papanicolaou-stained sputum smears. Acta Cytol 23: 471, 1979.

573. Stone WJ, Schaffner W: *Strongyloides* infections in transplant recipients. Semin Respir Infect 5: 58, 1990.

574. Chu E, Whitlock WL, Dietrich RA: Pulmonary hyperinfection syndrome with *Strongyloides stercoralis*. Chest 97: 1475, 1990.

575. Grove DI: Strongyloidiasis in Allied ex-prisoners of war in Southeast Asia. Br Med J 280: 598, 1980.

576. Williams J, Nunley D, Dralle W, et al: Diagnosis of pulmonary strongyloides by bronchoalveolar lavage. Chest 94: 643, 1988.

577. Neva FA, Gam AA, Burke J: Comparison of larval antigens in an enzyme-linked immunosorbent assay for strongyloidiasis in humans. J Infect Dis 144: 427, 1981.

578. Robin ED, Crump CH, Wagman RJ: Low sedimentation rate, hypofibrinogenemia, and restrictive pseudo-obstructive pulmonary disease associated with trichinosis. N Engl J Med 262: 758, 1960.

579. Udwadia FE: Pulmonary eosinophilia, Chapter III: Tropical eosinophilia, *in* Herzog H (ed): Progress in Respiration Research. Vol. 7, New York, 1975.

580. Udwadia FE, Joshi VV: A study of tropical eosinophilia. Thorax 19: 548, 1964.

581. Khoo FY, Danaraj TJ: The roentgenographic appearance of eosinophilic lung (tropical eosinophilia). Am J Roentgenol 83: 251, 1960.

582. Nutman TB, Vijayan VK, Pinsdton P, et al: Tropical pulmonary eosinophilia: An analysis of antifilarial antibody localized to the lung. J Infect Dis 160: 1042, 1989.

583. Rom WN, Vijayan VK, Cornelius MJ, et al: Persistent lower respiratory tract inflammation associated with interstitial lung disease in patients with tropical pulmonary eosinophilia following conventional treatment with diethylcarbamazine. Am Rev Respir Dis 142: 1088, 1990.

584. Ro JY, Tsakalakis PJ, White VA, et al: Pulmonary dirofilariasis: The great imitator of primary or metastatic lung tumor: A clinicopathologic analysis of seven cases and a review of the literature. Hum Pathol 20: 69, 1989.

585. Levinson ED, Ziter FMH Jr, Westcott JL: Pulmonary lesions due to *Dirofilaria immitis* (dog-heartworm): Report of 4 cases with radiologic findings. Radiology 131: 305, 1979.

586. Larrieu AJ, Wiener I, Gomez LG, et al: Human pulmonary dirofilariasis presenting as a solitary pulmonary nodule. Chest 75: 511, 1979.

587. Woodruff AW: Toxocariasis. Br Med J 3: 663, 1970.

588. Fanning M, Hill A, Langer HM, et al: Visceral larva migrans (toxocariasis) in Toronto. Can Med Assoc J 124: 21, 1981.

589. Wilson JF, Diddams AC, Rausch RL: Cystic hydatid disease in Alaska: A review of 101 autochthonous cases of *Echinococcus granulosus* infection. Am Rev Respir Dis 98: 1, 1968.

590. Beggs I: The radiology of hydatid disease. Am J Roentgenol 145: 639, 1985.

591. Sadrich M, Dutz W, Navabpoor MS: Review of 150 cases of hydatid cyst of the lung. Dis Chest 52: 662, 1967.

592. McPhail JL, Arora TS: Intrathoracic hydatid disease. Dis Chest 52: 772, 1967.

593. Bloomfield JA: Protean radiological manifestations of hydatid infestation. Aust Radiol 10: 330, 1966.

594. Rakower J, Milwidsky H: Hydatid pleural disease. Am Rev Respir Dis 90: 623, 1964.

595. von Sinner WN: New diagnostic signs in hydatid disease; radiography, ultrasound, CT and MRI correlated to pathology. Eur J Radiol 12: 150, 1991.

596. von Sinner WN, Rifal A, te Strake L, et al: Magnetic resonance imaging of thoracic hydatid disease: Correlation with clinical findings, radiography, ultrasonography, CT, and pathology. Acta Radiol 31: 59, 1990.

597. Iacona A, Pini C, Vicari G: Enzyme-linked immunosorbent assay (ELISA) in the serodiagnosis of hydatid disease. Am J Trop Med Hyg 29: 95, 1980.

598. van Knapen F: *Echinococcus granulosus* infection and malignancy. Br Med J 281: 195, 1980.

599. Johnson RJ, Johnson JR: Paragonimiasis in Indochinese refugees: Roentgenographic findings with clinical correlations. Am Rev Respir Dis 128: 534, 1983.

600. Ogakwu M, Mwokolo C: Radiological findings in pulmonary paragonimiasis as seen in Nigeria: A review based on one hundred cases. Br J Radiol 46: 699, 1973.

601. Suwanik R, Harinsuta C: Pulmonary paragonimiasis: An evaluation of roentgen findings in 38 positive sputum patients in an endemic area in Thailand. Am J Roentgenol 81: 236, 1959.

602. Minh V-D, Engle P, Greenwood JR, et al: Pleural paragonimiasis in a Southeast Asian refugee. Am Rev Respir Dis 124: 186, 1981.

603. Romeo DP, Pollock JJ: Pulmonary paragonimiasis: Diagnostic value of pleural fluid analysis. South Med J 79: 241, 1986.

604. Hofstetter M, Nash TE, Cheever AW, et al: Infection with *Schistosoma mekongi* in Southeast Asian refugees. J Infect Dis 144: 420, 1981.

605. Mahmoud AA: Medical intelligence: Current concepts in schistosomiasis. N Engl J Med 297: 1329, 1977.

606. Kagan IG, Rairigh DW, Kaiser RL: A clinical, parasitologic, and immunologic study of schistosomiasis in 103 Puerto Rican males residing in the United States. Ann Intern Med 56: 457, 1962.

607. Nash TE, Cheever AW, Ottesen EA, et al: Schistosome infections in humans: Perspectives and recent findings. Ann Intern Med 97: 740, 1982.

608. Wessell HU, Sommers HM, Cugell DW, et al: Variants of cardio-

pulmonary manifestations of Manson's schistosomiasis: Report of two cases. Ann Intern Med 62: 757, 1965.

609. Davidson BL, el-Kassimi F, Uz-Zaman A, et al: The "lung shift" in treated schistosomiasis: Bronchoalveolar lavage evidence of eosinophilic pneumonia. Chest 89: 455, 1986.

610. Lunde MN, Ottesen EA: Enzyme-linked immunosorbent assay (ELISA) for detecting IgM and IgE antibodies in human schistosomiasis. Am J Trop Med Hyg 29: 82, 1980.

611. Rose HD, Dorff GJ, Lauwasser M, et al: Pulmonary and disseminated *Mycobacterium simiae* infection in humans. Am Rev Respir Dis 126: 110, 1982.

612. Maloney JM, Gregg CR, Stephens DS, et al: Infections caused by *Mycobacterium szulgai* in humans. Rev Infect Dis 9: 1120, 1987.

613. Clague H, Hopkins CA, Roberts C, et al: Pulmonary infection with *Mycobacterium gordonae* in the presence of bronchial carcinoma. Tubercle 66: 61, 1985.

614. Tenholder MF, Moser RJ 3rd, Tellis CJ: Mycobacteria other than tuberculosis: Pulmonary involvement in patients with acquired immunodeficiency syndrome. Arch Intern Med 148: 953, 1988.

615. Prince DS, Peterson DD, Steiner RM, et al: Infection with *Mycobacterium avium* complex in patients without predisposing conditions. N Engl J Med 321: 863, 1989.

616. Contreras MA, Cheung OT, Sanders DE, et al: Pulmonary infection with nontuberculous mycobacteria. Am Rev Respir Dis 137: 149. 1988.

617. Tsukamura M, Kita N, Otsuka W, et al: A study of taxonomy of the *Mycobacterium nonchromogenicum* complex and report of six cases of lung infection due to *Mycobacterium nonchromogenicum*. Microbiol Immunol 27: 219, 1983.

618. Banks J, Jenkins PA, Smith AP: Pulmonary infection with *Mycobacterium malmoense*: A review of treatment and response. Tubercle 66: 197, 1985.

619. Pacht E: *Mycobacterium fortuitum* lung abscess: Resolution with prolonged trimethoprim-sulfamethoxazole therapy. Am Rev Respir Dis 141: 1599, 1990.

620. Wallace RJ Jr, Swenson JM, Silcox VA, et al: Spectrum of disease due to rapidly growing mycobacteria. Rev Infect Dis 5: 657, 1983.

621. Rolston KV, Jones PG, Fainstein V, et al: Pulmonary disease caused by rapidly growing mycobacteria in patients with cancer. Chest 87: 503, 1985.

622. Taylor LQ, Williams AJ, Santiago S: Pulmonary disease caused by *Mycobacterium asiaticum*. Tubercle 71: 303, 1990.

623. Liu F, Andrews D, Wright DN: *Mycobacterium thermoresistible* infection in an immunocompromised host. J Clin Microbiol 19: 546, 1984.

7

DISEASES OF ALTERED IMMUNOLOGIC ACTIVITY

CONNECTIVE TISSUE DISEASES

The autoimmune connective tissue diseases are a group of disorders whose common denominator is immune-mediated damage to components of connective tissue at a variety of sites in the body. Although a consideration of clinical, laboratory, roentgenologic, and pathologic information leads to a definitive diagnosis of a specific entity in most cases, in some patients precise classification is not possible.[1] This has led to the description of several "mixed" or "overlap" forms of disease, some of which are sufficiently characteristic to suggest that they may represent discrete clinicopathologic entities (e.g., mixed connective tissue disease). In addition, some conditions with symptoms and signs characteristic of autoimmune disease are impossible to categorize precisely, either as known entities or overlap syndromes. Such conditions should be left unclassified until follow-up reveals additional features that permit a more precise diagnosis. Although it might reasonably be argued that the vasculitides also are part of the connective tissue disease group—in fact, several such entities occasionally manifest this process—for purposes of discussion we have grouped them separately.

Systemic Lupus Erythematosus

The lungs and pleura are involved more frequently in systemic lupus erythematosus (SLE) than in any other connective tissue disease, the prevalence ranging from 30 to 70 per cent in different series.

Etiology and Pathogenesis

Research from a number of sources indicates that SLE is a clinically heterogeneous disease of multifactorial origin, the heterogeneity being related in part to the types of autoantibodies found in the serum (see later). The recognized etiologic and pathogenetic factors are genetic, immunologic, environmental, and endocrine.

Genetic Factors. Heredity is clearly an important determinant: estimates of the incidence of SLE in close relatives of patients with the disease range from 5 to 10 per cent.[2] Moreover, whereas dizygotic twins have no more risk than first-degree relatives, monozygotic twins have 69 per cent disease concordance. (The lack of concordance in the remaining 31 per cent has been postulated to be related to either incomplete penetrance or the effect of environmental factors.[3]) An association with the DR2 and DR3 genes of the major histocompatibility complex also has been described.[3]

Environmental Factors. Environmental agents such as ultraviolet light are well known to induce a flare-up of SLE in susceptible individuals. There is also circumstantial evidence suggesting that viral infection may act in the same way.[4] In addition, the SLE syndrome, including the presence of antinuclear antibodies (ANA) and a positive LE cell test, can be induced by certain drugs, such as hydralazine, isoniazid, phenytoin and other similar antiepileptics, quinidine, methyldopa, and the beta-adrenoreceptor–blocking agents such as propranolol. Affected patients are commonly found to be HLA-DR4 positive, in contrast to the predominance of DR3 or DR2 in idiopathic disease.[3] In addition,

they are almost invariably slow acetylators of the responsible medication; a dose-related factor is reflected in the few affected patients who are fast acetylators but are receiving large doses of the drug.[5]

Endocrine Factors. The susceptibility of females to SLE raises the possibility of an endocrine component in the pathogenesis of the disease. There is a good deal of evidence to support this hypothesis, most of it based on variations in incidence following the administration of hormones or male castration in the murine model.[3]

Immune Factors. There is general agreement that immunoregulation is distinctly abnormal in SLE. The mechanisms are multiple and complex and are likely at least partly responsible for the variations in the clinical presentation of the disease.[6] As a rule, T lymphocytes (particularly suppressor cells[2]) are reduced in number and B cells are hyperreactive.[7] An exception to this is drug-induced SLE, in which abnormal immunoregulation appears to be related to enhanced helper T cell activity rather than impaired suppressor T cell function.[8]

Whatever the form of deranged immunoregulation, the result is the production of a variety of autoantibodies (see later). These are likely responsible for the majority of disease, either directly by cytotoxicity or indirectly via the formation of immune complexes. There is also evidence that defects in response to and in impaired production of interleukin-1 and interleukin-2 and disturbances in the activity of interferon may play pathogenetic roles.[3]

Pathologic Characteristics

Pathologic changes in the lungs and pleura are common in patients with SLE at autopsy. However, because of the frequent involvement of other organs and tissues, it is not always clear in an individual case which of these changes is related to a direct effect of SLE and which to an effect of therapy or of complicating disease in the lungs or other sites. In many instances, it is undoubtedly the indirect effects that are important. Pathologic findings that have been proposed as being caused by SLE itself include pleuritis and pleural fibrosis (the most common abnormalities[9]), interstitial pneumonitis and fibrosis, vasculitis, and changes indicative of pulmonary arterial hypertension.

Diffuse interstitial lung disease similar to that of rheumatoid disease or progressive systemic sclerosis (PSS) is uncommon in SLE; for example, in one series of 120 patients, only five such cases were identified.[10] In the few cases we have seen and in those reported in the literature,[11] histologic findings have been those of fibrosing alveolitis. Immunopathologic studies of biopsy specimens in one study showed granular deposition of immunoglobulin G (IgG), C3, and DNA in alveolar walls, and electron microscopy revealed electron-dense deposits in a similar location, suggesting that immune complex deposition may be responsible.[11]

"Acute lupus pneumonitis" refers to an uncommon manifestation of SLE characterized by fever, dyspnea, hypoxemia, and patchy, diffuse roentgenographic opacities; the term should be restricted to patients with these clinical and roentgenographic features who respond to corticosteroid and azathioprine therapy but not to antibiotics.[12] Pathologic features in these patients are variable. Some cases show diffuse alveolar damage (intra-alveolar proteinaceous exudate with hyaline membranes, interstitial edema, and an interstitial mononuclear inflammatory infiltrate),[13] and others leukocytoclastic vasculitis (patchy but more or less diffuse alveolar septal infiltrate by polymorphonuclear leukocytes associated with intracapillary fibrin thrombi and airspace hemorrhage [*see* page 417]).[14, 15] Granular immunofluorescent deposits of DNA, anti-DNA antibody, IgG, and C3 as well as subendothelial electron-dense deposits can be identified within the lungs of many of these latter patients,[14, 15] again suggesting the possibility of immune complex–mediated damage.

Disease of the larger pulmonary vessels is also uncommon. Occasional cases of necrotizing vasculitis involving small pulmonary arteries and arterioles have been reported,[16] and some patients develop isolated pulmonary hypertension, characterized pathologically by intimal fibrosis, medial hypertrophy, and sometimes plexiform lesions[17]; in most of these, there is a history of concomitant Raynaud's phenomenon.

Roentgenographic Manifestations

Roentgenologic abnormalities may be seen in the lungs, pleura, and cardiovascular system, alone or in combination. Pleural effusion, which is probably the most common manifestation, is frequently bilateral and usually small. Of 57 cases in one series,[18] it occurred in 42; in three of these, pleuritis appeared as an isolated first sign, and in 16 others it was associated with only minor antecedent symptoms. The importance of distinguishing pleural effusion due to direct involvement of the pleura by SLE from that associated with lupus nephritis has been emphasized[19]; the former characteristically is accompanied by pain and splinting, whereas the serous effusions of nephritis are painless.

Roentgenographic changes in the lungs usually are nonspecific, consisting of rather poorly defined patchy opacities (Fig. 7–1), usually in the lung bases and situated peripherally. These changes often are acute and may represent "lupus pneumonitis," edema, or infection. Frequently, only the response to various therapeutic agents provides a definitive answer as to etiology, although diffuse pulmonary hemorrhage can be readily detected by magnetic resonance imaging (MRI).[20] Horizontal line shadows, usually in both bases and sometimes migratory, are probably attributable to discoid atelectasis. In some cases, sequential roentgenologic studies show progressive loss of lung volume,[12] "shrinkage" that may be associated with an elevated, sluggish diaphragm.

Cardiovascular changes frequently occur in association with other abnormalities. Increase in the size of the cardiopericardial silhouette is generally the result of pericardial effusion, which usually is relatively small but may be massive. The roentgenographic manifestations of drug-induced SLE are no different from those of the idiopathic form.

Clinical Manifestations

As its name implies, SLE is a multisystem disease that most commonly involves extrapulmonary structures. The classic clinical picture is that of a young adult woman presenting with fever, arthralgias, facial rash, nephritis, and pleural effusion; however, clinical manifestations vary widely from patient to patient. Diagnosis may be difficult in the early stages of the disease if only one organ system is affected; however, suspicion should be aroused when progression of the disease through several exacerbations indicates widespread tissue and organ involvement.

Symptoms referable to the respiratory tract include cough (with or without mucoid sputum), dyspnea (sometimes caused by interstitial pneumonitis and fibrosis[21] and sometimes by diaphragmatic dysfunction[22]), and hoarseness. Hemoptysis is rare[15] but may be massive; this is particularly the case in children, in whom the pulmonary hemorrhage may occur long before SLE is suspected and can appear identical to idiopathic pulmonary hemorrhage.[23] Pleuritis occurs in 35 to 40 per cent of patients and may be associated with fever and pleural pain, either unilateral or bilateral.

Although clinically evident pulmonary hypertension is believed to be rare (only 46 patients were reported by 1986[17]), there is evidence that mild hypertension may not be uncommon.[24] Most often, it presents in patients with known SLE as rapidly progressive dyspnea and cardiac failure; death within 2 years is the rule. Raynaud's phenomenon is present in 75 per cent of cases, and many patients have positive reactions for ribonucleoprotein (RNP), rheumatoid factor, and lupus anticoagulants.

Symptoms and signs of disease affecting organs or tissues other than the lungs and pleura are almost always present. Arthritis and arthralgia are the most common, being observed in 95 per cent of patients; they tend to be nonerosive and nondeforming[25] and may be associated with the periarticular subcutaneous nodules usually considered characteristic of rheumatoid disease. Cutaneous manifestations are also frequent and include the "butterfly" rash (seen in 50 per cent of patients)[25] and discoid lupus, alopecia, and photosensitivity (seen in 20 per cent). Patients rarely, if ever, present initially with neuropsychiatric complaints, although seizures or psychotic episodes develop eventually in 50 to 70 per cent.[26] A similar percentage show evidence of renal disease. Other less common but still appreciable manifestations include pericarditis, hepatosplenomegaly, and Raynaud's phenomenon. Muscle weakness usually develops after institution of corticosteroid therapy and is most marked in the proximal limb muscles; however, we have seen several patients whose dyspnea could be explained only by diaphragmatic myopathy.

The clinical manifestations of drug-induced lupus do not appear until months or years after the initiation of therapy. In most cases, onset is insidious, usually heralded by prolonged discomfort in the joints.[27] In addition to arthralgia, common findings include pleuritis, pericarditis, fever, and skin rash; renal, central nervous system (CNS), and pulmonary involvement are rare.[28] Clinical manifestations disappear within days to weeks of cessation of drug therapy, whereas serologic abnormalities may continue for months.

Laboratory Findings

The detection of antibodies against specific nuclear and cytoplasmic antigens is used not only for diagnostic purposes but also to establish prognosis. The screening test most commonly used when SLE is suspected is a search

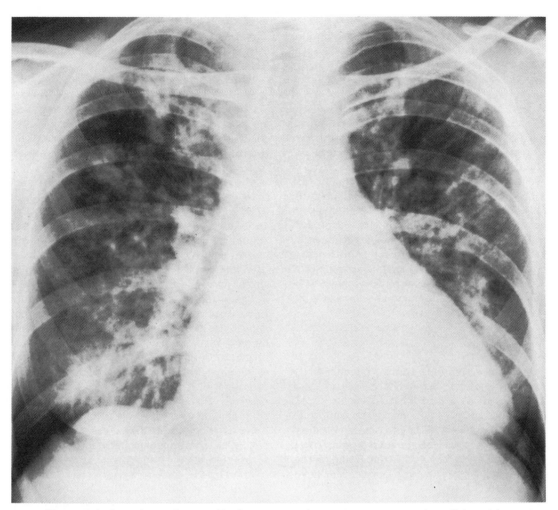

Figure 7–1. Acute Lupus Pneumonitis. A posteroanterior roentgenogram reveals multiple patchy shadows of homogeneous density distributed widely throughout both lungs; the cardiopericardial silhouette is moderately enlarged and possesses a contour consistent with pericardial effusion. Although the shadows could conceivably represent either infection or edema, institution of corticosteroid therapy resulted in complete roentgenographic resolution in 1 week, despite persistence of the cardiac enlargement.

for ANAs. Four patterns of antinuclear reaction have been described by immunofluorescence: (1) *speckled,* the most frequent pattern, is present in sera containing antibodies to such well-defined nuclear antigens as nRNP and Sm (a non-nucleic glycoprotein macromolecule), two antigens present in the saline-soluble extractable nuclear antigen (ENA); (2) *rim,* a pattern that is highly specific for SLE and is associated with antibodies in the serum against native DNA (nDNA); (3) *nucleolar,* which is present in 50 per cent of patients with PSS but seldom in those who have SLE; and (4) *homogeneous,* the pattern seen in patients with antibodies against nucleoprotein. Any individual patient can exhibit several patterns of ANA reaction.

Some of the 5 to 10 per cent of patients with SLE who are ANA negative have high titers of antibody to single-stranded (denatured) DNA (anti-ssDNA Ab).[29] These include the anti-Ro Ab and the anti-La Ab, both of which are commonly found in patients with Sjögren's syndrome (hence the designations SSA and SSB); in SLE, they are seen most often in the elderly and have been associated particularly with the presence of interstitial pneumonitis.[30]

Antibodies to native DNA (anti-nDNA Ab) are present in patients who are at greater risk for developing renal disease and are often associated with a positive response to direct immunofluorescence examination of clinically normal skin (the lupus band test).[29] In contrast to patients who manifest a positive reaction to anti-nDNA Ab only and whose disease pattern is confined largely to the kidneys, those with anti-nDNA Ab and anti-Sm Ab have a much wider distribution of lesions in skin, lungs, and heart.[31]

Patients with drug-induced SLE rarely have antibodies to native DNA but may show antibodies to denatured DNA; ANAs are common, but hypocomplementemia is rare.

The majority of patients eventually have anemia, usually caused by impaired erythropoiesis but occasionally by increased hemolysis. Leukopenia and elevated levels of serum gamma globulins are almost invariable, and thrombocytopenia, antiplatelet antibody, and platelet functional disorders can occur. Antibodies against factors VIII, IX, and XII can cause significant coagulation abnormalities.[25]

In most cases, pleural effusions are exudates that contain

LE cells and are characterized by a high ANA titer (greater than or equal to 1:160), low complement component, and a pleura-serum ANA ratio of at least 1:1 (*see* page 873).

Pulmonary Function Tests

Pulmonary function studies typically reveal decreases in lung volume, diffusing capacity, and arterial oxygen saturation with low or normal PCO_2, compensated respiratory alkalosis, and reduced lung compliance.[32] Evidence of airway obstruction is present in a minority of patients[33]; in some, it is severe and of recent onset, resembling that described with obliterative bronchiolitis in patients with rheumatoid disease. A characteristic of the function values in SLE is impairment so profound that it is out of proportion to the rather mild changes usually apparent clinically and roentgenographically. In some cases, this discrepancy can be explained by impaired diaphragmatic function[34]; weakness of both expiratory and inspiratory muscles of breathing, unrelated to steroid therapy, also has been described.[22]

Prognosis

SLE commonly has a chronic course, punctuated by acute exacerbations, some of which may be drug induced. Death occurs after many years from renal failure, CNS involvement, or myocardial infarction. Pleuropulmonary disease, although sometimes a cause of considerable morbidity, rarely is fatal. It should be remembered, however, that patients who are receiving corticosteroid and immunosuppressive therapy are at risk for opportunistic infection, particularly of the lungs.

Hypocomplementemic Urticarial Vasculitis

The term "hypocomplementemic urticarial vasculitis" has been used to refer to a syndrome characterized by persistent urticaria, leukocytoclastic vasculitis, and hypocomplementemia. A variety of other presumably immune-mediated effects also may be present, including arthritis and arthralgias, glomerulonephritis, episcleritis, uveitis, and CNS abnormalities. Although the syndrome shares many features with SLE, the paucity of serum autoantibodies as well as the characteristic cutaneous findings suggest that it may be a distinct entity.[35, 36]

Obstructive lung disease has been described in a number of patients; although many have been smokers, it has been suggested that the severity of disease and age of onset cannot be adequately explained by cigarette smoking alone. Pulmonary vasculitis has not been documented.

Rheumatoid Disease

The incidence of pleuropulmonary abnormalties in patients with rheumatoid disease varies considerably in reported series, depending at least partly on the criteria for diagnosis. For example, in one study of 54 patients with rheumatoid arthritis (RA) who had positive agglutination tests, roentgenographic changes in the lungs or pleura consistent with "rheumatoid disease" were present in 29 (54 per cent)[37]; however, in another review of 180 patients, only nine (5 per cent) had demonstrable thoracic disease.[38]

The majority of patients with pleuropulmonary disease have clinical evidence of RA, and in about 70 to 80 per cent of cases[25] serologic tests are positive for rheumatoid factor. In some cases, however, arthritis may not be clinically evident when the pleuropulmonary abnormality becomes manifest; in such circumstances the diagnosis may be suggested by positive serologic test results alone or may not be suspected until the arthritis is manifested later.[39] In contrast to the female sex predominance characteristic of RA, extra-articular manifestations of rheumatoid disease are more common in males.

Most patients with rheumatoid disease also have high titers of antiglobulin antibody (rheumatoid factor), and 15 to 30 per cent have ANAs; in some, LE cell preparations are positive.[25] Although low titers of antinuclear and rheumatoid factors may be found in approximately 5 per cent of normal control subjects and in some patients with pulmonary interstitial fibrosis of various causes, high titers are almost invariably associated with rheumatoid disease.

The pathogenesis of rheumatoid pleuropulmonary disease is poorly understood. In contrast to synovitis (which appears to result from a disturbance in cell-mediated immunity), pleuropulmonary abnormalities seem to be closely related to dysfunction of humoral immunity. For example, in rheumatoid pleural and pericardial effusions, immune complexes are virtually always present and levels of rheumatoid factor are high, and those of complement low. In addition, immunofluorescence examination of lung tissue in some cases reveals a striking deposition of IgM and rheumatoid factor in pulmonary arterioles and alveolar walls and in parenchyma adjacent to cavitary rheumatoid lung nodules.[40] Despite these observations, it is likely that some abnormality of cell-mediated immunity is also important in the pathogenesis, in at least some manifestations.[41]

The pleuropulmonary manifestations of rheumatoid disease can be considered under seven headings: (1) diffuse interstitial pneumonitis and fibrosis, (2) upper lobe fibrobullous disease, (3) pleural disease, (4) the necrobiotic nodule, (5) Caplan's syndrome, (6) pulmonary vascular disease, and (7) bronchiolitis. Although these abnormalities may be present in any combination, each is sufficiently distinctive clinically, pathologically, and roentgenographically to warrant separate consideration.

Diffuse Interstitial Pneumonitis and Fibrosis

This form of disease has been estimated to occur in 10 to 50 per cent of patients with rheumatoid disease (albeit in a severe form in fewer than 5 per cent).[42] If lymphocytosis in bronchoalveolar lavage (BAL) fluid is accepted as evidence of disease, the incidence probably is even greater.[43] It is generally accepted that its presence is related to the duration or severity of arthritis and that it is more prone to occur in males and in the presence of subcutaneous rheumatoid nodules.[44]

Histologic changes in the early stages of the disease consist of an interstitial infiltrate of lymphocytes, plasma cells, and histiocytes; focal nodular aggregates of lymphocytes, sometimes with germinal centers, can be prominent. With progression of the disease, the infiltrate decreases in severity and is replaced by mature fibrous tissue, which in the advanced stage has the appearance of honeycomb lung.

These changes are entirely nonspecific and cannot by themselves confirm a diagnosis of rheumatoid disease.

The roentgenographic pattern in early disease has been described as punctate or nodular[37]; when small, it bears some resemblance to miliary tuberculosis and when larger it is similar to the pattern of sarcoidosis or asbestosis. In the later stages, the pattern changes to one of medium to coarse reticulation, often more prominent in the bases than elsewhere and virtually indistinguishable from that seen in advanced PSS or idiopathic fibrosing alveolitis (Fig. 7–2); a "honeycomb" pattern is fairly common in advanced disease. High-resolution computed tomography (CT) scans have

been reported to reveal a predominantly peripheral pattern and have been shown to be more sensitive than conventional radiography in detecting abnormalities.[45] Serial roentgenographic studies may reveal progressive loss of lung volume.

The most common symptom is dyspnea on effort, sometimes associated with cough and pleuritic pain. Finger clubbing may be present and is not uncommonly associated with cor pulmonale. Anemia and slight lymphocytosis develop in some advanced cases. Pulmonary function tests show a restrictive ventilatory defect. In addition, the diffusing capacity is commonly reduced, even in patients with

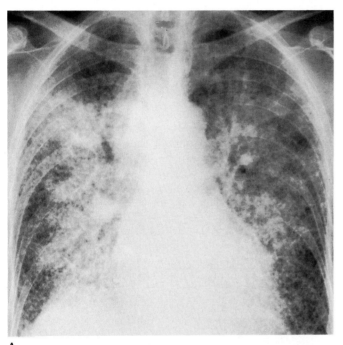

A

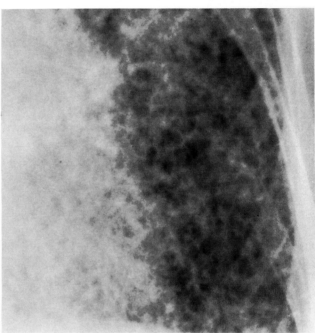

B

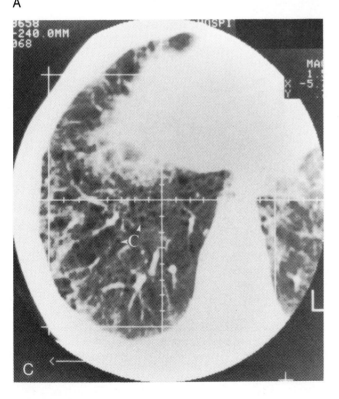

C

Figure 7–2. Rheumatoid Disease: Diffuse Interstitial Fibrosis. A coarse reticular pattern involves virtually all portions of both lungs, more severely on the right *(A* and *B).* In lower lung zones, the pattern is honeycomb in type. *C,* A transverse CT scan through the right lower lobe reveals the reticulation to possess considerable peripheral predominance; cystic spaces (C) measuring 3 to 5 mm in diameter are numerous. (*C* from Genereux GP: Med Radiogr Photogr 61: 2–31, 1985, with permission of the Eastman Kodak Co.)

normal chest roentgenograms. This has been shown by one group of investigators to be caused primarily by a reduction in pulmonary capillary blood volume rather than by any change in the membrane component.[46]

In our experience, roentgenographically demonstrable interstitial lung disease associated with rheumatoid disease is not reversible. Though stabilization can occur spontaneously, it has also been ascribed to immunosuppressive therapy.[47]

Upper Lobe Fibrobullous Disease

Although rare, the number of reports of fibrosis and bullous or cavitary disease confined to the upper lobes has been sufficient to justify inclusion of this form of parenchymal abnormality as a separate manifestation of rheumatoid disease.[48, 49] The pathogenesis of the condition is unknown; however, an important negative observation is that searches for acid-fast organisms have been consistently fruitless. Chest roentgenograms reveal patchy upper lobe fibrosis and cystic spaces consistent with either cavities or bullae. The pattern closely resembles that observed with advanced ankylosing spondylitis (Fig. 7–3).

Pleural Disease

Pleural effusion is probably the most frequent manifestation of rheumatoid disease in the thorax. Its only unique radiologic characteristic is a tendency to remain relatively unchanged for many months or even years.[50] It is unilateral and bilateral in roughly equal proportions and, in the great majority of cases, is the sole abnormality roentgenographi-

cally apparent in the thorax. In fact, it has been suggested that the presence of associated parenchymal disease should suggest a nonrheumatoid etiology.[50] Pleural thickening without effusion is seen in some cases. Details of clinical and laboratory features are discussed on page 873.

The Necrobiotic Nodule

A necrobiotic (rheumatoid) nodule is a well-circumscribed "tumor" found most commonly in the subcutaneous tissues. It is a relatively rare manifestation of pleuropulmonary rheumatoid disease and typically is associated with advanced RA and multiple subcutaneous nodules on the elbows or elsewhere.[51] Grossly, the nodules are usually well circumscribed and situated peripherally in relation to the pleura. Histologically, the central portion is composed of necrotic material and is surrounded by a layer of palisaded epithelioid histiocytes (Fig. 7–4); the adjacent tissue shows fibrosis and a variably intense plasma cell and lymphocyte infiltrate.

Typically, the nodules present roentgenographically as well-defined opacities ranging from 5 mm to 5 cm in diameter and situated in the periphery of the lung (Fig. 7–5).[52] They may be very numerous and resemble metastases (Fig. 7–6). Cavitation is common, the walls being of moderate thickness and possessing a smooth inner lining. The nodules may wax and wane in concert with the subcutaneous nodules and in proportion to the activity of the RA.[53] During remission of the arthritis, the cavities may become thin-walled and gradually disappear, and during exacerbations they may fill again and become opacified.

Necrobiotic nodules usually do not occasion symptoms;

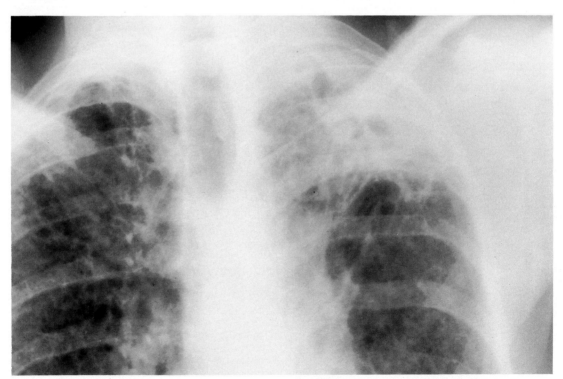

Figure 7–3. Rheumatoid Disease: Upper Lobe Fibrobullous Disease. A magnified view of both upper lungs reveals inhomogeneous consolidation in the apical portion of the left upper lobe; the left hilum is elevated. A coarse reticular pattern is present in the right upper lobe, and a fine reticulation elsewhere in both lungs.

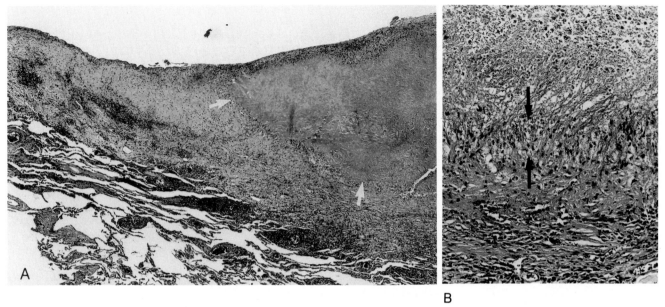

Figure 7–4. Rheumatoid Nodule. *A*, Fibrous tissue and chronic inflammatory cells are present in a subpleural location and surround a well-defined zone of necrosis *(arrows)*. *B*, Magnified view showing layer of palisaded epithelioid histiocytes *(between arrows)* adjacent to necrotic debris. (*A* × 25; *B* × 100.) (Courtesy of Dr. S. Sahai, Reddy Memorial Hospital, Montreal.)

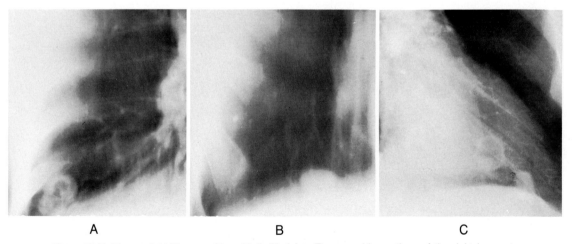

Figure 7–5. Rheumatoid Disease: Necrobiotic Nodules. Tomographic sections of the right base at different levels *(A* and *B)* show at least two nodules just above the costophrenic angle (one of which is cavitated) and a third nodule of homogeneous density more posteriorly situated. Six years later, an oblique roentgenogram of the lower portion of the left lung *(C)* reveals two nodules, one of which presents as a ring shadow, and the other as a nodule of homogeneous density.

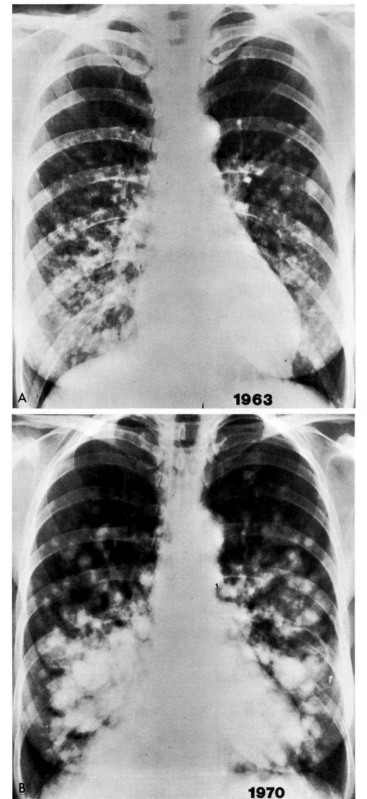

Figure 7–6. Rheumatoid Disease: Necrobiotic Nodules. *A,* Multiple, small, discrete nodules ranging in size from barely visible to approximately 1 cm are scattered throughout both lungs, with some midzonal and basal predominance. Seven years later *(B),* the nodules had increased markedly in size, some reaching a diameter of 3 cm; none showed evidence of cavitation. The patient manifested no symptoms or signs referable to her chest, although she had had clinical evidence of rheumatoid arthritis for many years. Biopsy of a left-sided nodule revealed a typical necrobiotic nodule.

occasionally, they cause hemoptysis, or sudden pain or dyspnea when pneumothorax results from rupture into the pleural cavity. Although most often seen in patients with typical features of rheumatoid disease, they may develop in patients without rheumatoid factor and in the absence of symptomatic arthritis.[51] The possibility of pulmonary carcinoma must be carefully excluded before accepting this diagnosis for a solitary nodule.[54]

Caplan's Syndrome

This uncommon manifestation of rheumatoid disease is characterized roentgenographically by single or multiple well-defined spherical opacities in the lungs of individuals exposed to inorganic particles such as silica[55] or coal dust.[56] The lesions usually develop rapidly, tend to appear in "crops," and range from 0.5 to 5.0 cm in diameter. In many cases, the background of simple pneumoconiosis is slight or even absent. An indication of the incidence of Caplan's syndrome may be obtained from one report of 26 patients with combined pneumoconiosis and RA, 30 per cent of whom were found to have typical nodules in the lungs.[57] Although the pathogenesis of the nodules is unknown, the evidence supports the hypothesis that these lesions represent a hypersensitivity reaction to irritating dust particles in the lungs.[58]

Pathologically, the lesions appear as well-delimited nodules that characteristically show alternating concentric rings of light and dark tissue. Histologically, the central portion of the nodule is composed of necrotic collagen that is surrounded by zones of macrophages and polymorphonuclear leukocytes, some of which contain dust particles. It is thought that when these cells die the dust remains behind, forming the characteristic darkened ring that distinguishes the Caplan's nodule from the necrobiotic nodule of uncomplicated rheumatoid disease.[59]

Roentgenographically, there is little to distinguish the nodular lesions of Caplan's syndrome from the necrobiotic nodules of rheumatoid disease without pneumoconiosis. The nodules tend to develop rapidly and appear in crops. They may increase in number, remain unchanged, or calcify. Cavitation may occur and may be followed by fibrosis or disappearance of the lesion.[56] The opacities may appear before, coincident with, or after the clinical onset of arthritis, and there is no apparent relationship between the severity of the arthritis and the extent and type of roentgenographically apparent change in the lungs.

Pulmonary Vascular Disease

In rheumatoid disease, pulmonary arterial hypertension occurs most frequently in association with diffuse interstitial fibrosis.[60] Its pathogenesis, pathologic characteristics, and roentgenographic manifestations in this situation differ in no way from those associated with fibrosis of other etiologies. Pulmonary hypertension also has been reported in the absence of parenchymal disease, in which case it is associated with Raynaud's phenomenon (Fig. 7–7).[61] Although vasculitis affecting the systemic circulation is not uncommon in rheumatoid disease, its occurrence in the pulmonary circulation is extremely rare.[62]

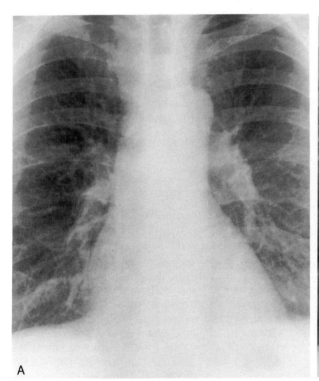
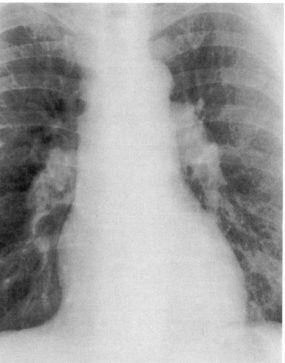

A   B

Figure 7–7. Rheumatoid Disease: Precapillary Pulmonary Hypertension Unassociated with Interstitial Pulmonary Fibrosis. The initial posteroanterior *(A)* chest roentgenogram of this 51-year-old man is normal. Three years later *(B)*, there had developed enlargement of both hila compatible with pulmonary arterial dilatation. Cardiac size is unchanged. Note that the lungs show no evidence of interstitial lung disease. The patient presented with Raynaud's phenomenon.

Bronchiolitis

Two clinicopathologic forms of bronchiolitis have been recognized as complications of rheumatoid disease: bronchiolitis obliterans and follicular bronchiolitis. The former shows a strong association with the presence of an HLA-DQw1 allotype[63] and is characterized functionally by the rapid development of obstructive airway disease.[64] Pathologically, there is an inflammatory infiltrate of lymphocytes and plasma cells in and around the walls of bronchioles associated with a variable degree of intraluminal fibrosis. Typically, the surrounding parenchyma and pulmonary vasculature are unremarkable; however, in some cases an organizing pneumonia can be found (bronchiolitis obliterans with organizing pneumonia [BOOP]).[65]

The chest roentgenogram has usually been reported to show only hyperinflation[64]; occasionally, however, a fine nodularity or ill-defined airspace disease has been described. Clinically, patients have shortness of breath that worsens rapidly, at a rate that is rarely seen in chronic obstructive pulmonary disease.[66] A midinspiratory squeak is often present on physical examination. Arthritic deformity is usually evident.

Follicular bronchiolitis is a rare manifestation of pulmonary rheumatoid disease characterized histologically by the presence of abundant lymphoid tissue, frequently with prominent germinal centers, situated about bronchioles and, to a lesser extent, bronchi.[67] The abnormality is not specific and can be found in association with other connective tissue diseases and a variety of other conditions. Despite the name, it is not clear whether it represents active inflammation of the bronchioles (i.e., a true bronchiolitis) or simply hyperplasia of the lymphoid tissue that normally occurs in this region.

The chest roentgenogram characteristically shows a diffuse reticulonodular pattern.[67] The most common clinical finding is progressive shortness of breath; cough, fever, and recurrent pneumonia are occasionally present. For unknown reasons, follicular bronchiolitis is more common in adolescents who have clinical features of juvenile rheumatoid arthritis (JRA) than in adults. Although the roentgenographic pattern suggests restrictive lung disease, pulmonary function studies reveal evidence of airway obstruction.[68]

Juvenile Rheumatoid Arthritis

JRA is a disease characterized by chronic synovitis and a variety of visceral abnormalities that, by definition, appear before age 16 years. Pleuropulmonary manifestations are uncommon: in one report of 191 patients with active disease, only eight (4 per cent) were found to be so affected; review of the literature to 1980 revealed only eight other cases.[69] Pleuritis, pleural effusion, and follicular bronchiolitis are the most common manifestations. Most affected patients have systemic signs and symptoms such as fever, rash, lymph node enlargement, and hepatosplenomegaly.

Progressive Systemic Sclerosis

PSS is a generalized fibrotic disorder of connective tissue often accompanied by vasculopathy. The majority of patients are affected in the fourth, fifth, or sixth decade of life. There is a three-to-one female predominance.[70]

Pulmonary disease is common: morphologic evidence of pulmonary fibrosis has been documented in as many as 90 per cent of patients[71] and alveolitis (inferred from the results of BAL) in about half[72]; in addition, pulmonary function is also almost invariably abnormal.[73] Despite these observations, clinical findings and abnormalties detected by standard roentgenography are relatively uncommon; in one review of 800 patients,[73] roentgenologic changes in the lungs were found in only 25 per cent and pulmonary symptoms in only 16 per cent. It should be remembered, however, that high-resolution CT findings may be abnormal in many patients who have a normal roentgenogram.[74]

Pathogenesis

Although the pathogenesis of PSS is poorly understood, some derangement of immune function is likely. The disease is clearly associated with other readily accepted disorders of immune function such as SLE and Sjögren's syndrome. In addition, autoantibodies, such as ANAs and rheumatoid factor as well as circulating immune complexes, are present in many individuals (see later).

The mechanism of pulmonary fibrosis is unknown. Studies in which BAL and lung biopsies have been correlated suggest that it is preceded by alveolitis, and it has been postulated that abnormal collagen production is caused at least partly by the release of fibronectin and growth factors from alveolar macrophages.[75] It also has been suggested that occult aspiration related to esophageal sclerosis and gastroesophageal reflux may be a factor in some cases.[76]

The pathogenesis of pulmonary arterial hypertension unassociated with interstitial fibrosis is also unclear. However, the frequent association of this abnormality with Raynaud's phenomenon (sometimes as part of PSS and sometimes as an isolated condition[77]), the observation that the digital arteries in patients with Raynaud's phenomenon show similar histologic changes to those in the lung,[78] and the finding that exposing the hand of some patients with PSS to cold can cause a decrease in pulmonary blood-flow[79] all suggest the presence of a more or less diffuse vascular abnormality or of a blood-borne substance affecting multiple vessels.

Pathologic Characteristics

Pleural fibrosis is observed at autopsy in 25 to 50 per cent of patients[80] and may be either local or diffuse. Some degree of parenchymal interstitial fibrosis also is common, although in many cases it is only focal. The more severely diseased lungs show bilateral interstitial thickening that is most marked in the subpleural regions of the lower lobes and is grossly and microscopically indistinguishable from idiopathic fibrosing alveolitis.[81]

Although pathologic evidence of pulmonary arterial hypertension is seen most often in association with diffuse interstitial fibrosis, vascular changes also can be present in areas of lung uninvolved by the latter process and, occasionally, can occur when there is no interstitial disease.[82] In these latter cases, the intima is moderately to severely thickened by fibroblastic connective tissue that, in later stages, is transformed into mature collagen (Fig. 7–8). The media usually shows some degree of hypertrophy.

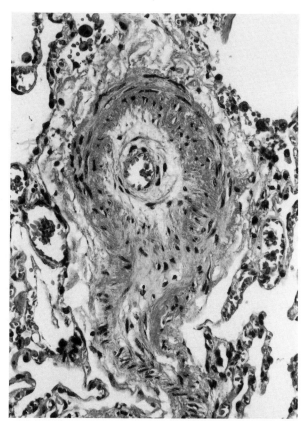

Figure 7–8. Overlap Syndrome (SLE with CREST) and Pulmonary Arterial Hypertension. A 26-year-old woman with long-standing celiac disease presented with findings consistent with SLE according to ARA criteria. She subsequently developed the CREST syndrome and evidence of pulmonary hypertension; she died 1 month later. Autopsy showed normal lung parenchyma and extensive narrowing of small pulmonary arteries and arterioles caused by muscle hypertrophy and proliferation of loose subendothelial connective tissue. (× 250.)

Roentgenographic Manifestations

In the early stages, the roentgenographic pattern of pulmonary disease is typically a fine reticulation (Fig. 7–9). With progression of disease, the reticulation tends to become coarser and may possess a nodular component attributable to projection of the coarse interstitial strands on end rather than *en face*. As with idiopathic fibrosing alveolitis, there is a tendency for predominant involvement of the lower lung zones.[83] High-resolution CT has been shown to be much more sensitive than conventional roentgenography in revealing evidence of interstitial disease[84] and may yield information that helps discriminate between areas that are predominantly fibrotic and areas that have an important inflammatory cellular component.[84a] Serial roentgenograms over a period of 2 to 3 years may show progressive and uniform loss of lung volume in addition to worsening of the interstitial disease, a finding of considerable value in diagnosis; we have been impressed repeatedly by the tendency for both PSS and idiopathic pulmonary fibrosis to show this progressive loss of volume, in contrast to other causes of diffuse interstitial fibrosis. Despite pathologic observations, roentgenographic evidence of pleural fibrosis is uncommon. Changes of pulmonary arterial hypertension and cor pulmonale may be present, with or without evidence of interstitial disease.

The esophagus is reported to be involved clinically and roentgenologically in more than 50 per cent of cases of PSS, a feature typically manifested by dilatation and aperistalsis. Whereas the presence or absence of esophageal aperistalsis must be assessed by fluoroscopic study and barium swallow, the atrophy and atony may be manifested on plain roentgenograms as an air esophagogram. In fact, the presence of a lot of gas in the esophagus on a lateral roentgenogram of the chest is a useful sign of PSS, especially if

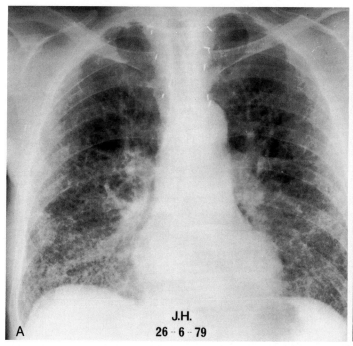
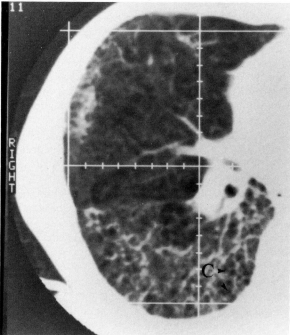

Figure 7–9. Progressive Systemic Sclerosis: Interstitial Fibrosis. A posteroanterior chest roentgenogram *(A)* reveals a medium reticular pattern in the lower lung zones and a coarser reticulation in the upper zones. *B*, A CT scan of the right lower zone also shows medium reticulation, the pattern being indistinguishable from that of rheumatoid lung disease. Centimeter scale is depicted. (*B* from Genereux GP: Med Radiogr Photogr 61: 2–31, 1985; with permission of the Eastman Kodak Co.)

it is not associated with an air-fluid level and if gas is present in the gastric fundus.[85] (The latter two qualifications are important, since an esophageal air-fluid level and a gasless stomach are characteristic features of achalasia, the chief differential diagnostic possibility.) When associated with reticular or reticulondular pulmonary disease, an air-containing esophagus is virtually pathognomonic of PSS.

Clinical Manifestations

Like SLE and rheumatoid disease, PSS is a systemic process affecting multiple organs and tissues. The skin is characteristically thickened, inelastic, and waxy in appearance, particularly about the face and extremities; it is frequently bronzed and sometimes contains calcium deposits. As seen by widefield microscopy, the nailfold capillary beds are abnormal in most patients, a finding that is highly suggestive of the disease.[86] Esophageal involvement can be suspected if the patient complains of difficulty in swallowing, but esophageal dilatation and disturbed motility can be detected in some patients by manometry and fluoroscopic examination before dysphagia becomes clinically manifest. Hiatus hernia also is a frequent complication of the esophageal fibrosis and atrophy, and the resulting gastroesophageal reflux may give rise to esophagitis. Arthralgia, particularly of the hands, is common, appearing in 50 to 80 per cent of patients at some stage in the course of the disease.[87] Clinical evidence of renal involvement occurs in approximately 25 per cent. In addition to the symptoms and signs referable to these specific organs and tissues, patients may manifest weight loss and low-grade fever.

Pulmonary involvement may cause a slightly productive cough and progressive dyspnea; it is usually a late feature of widespread systemic disease but occasionally is the initial mode of presentation.[88] Basilar rales are reported to occur in approximately 50 per cent of cases.[89]

Cardiovascular disease is also common. Raynaud's phenomenon occurs in the majority of cases of PSS (and in fact is considered by some to be a variant of the disease). It usually precedes skin changes and may antedate or occur simultaneously with clinical or function test evidence of pulmonary parenchymal involvement. Cardiac decompensation may develop as a result of pulmonary hypertension and cor pulmonale, cardiac fibrosis, or a combination of the two.

Some patients with PSS have symptoms and signs of other connective tissue diseases, placing them in a category commonly referred to as an *overlap syndrome*. For example, a scleroderma-like syndrome with skin, joint, and pulmonary manifestations has been described in children with insulin-dependent diabetes mellitus,[90] and a combined clinical presentation of myxedema, systemic sclerosis, and circulating antithyroid antibodies has been recognized.[91] Another complex that some authorities regard as a variant of PSS is diffuse fasciitis with eosinophilia (eosinophilic fasciitis), a syndrome that has distinctive features, including sparing of the skin of the hands and feet, blood eosinophilia, increased serum levels of eosinophilic chemotactic factor, and sometimes polyarthritis.[92] As the name implies, the inflammatory process involves fascia; although the lungs are spared, the chest wall may be involved, resulting in a restrictive defect.[93]

Laboratory Findings

Positive serologic test results for syphilis and rheumatoid factor have been reported in 5 and 35 per cent of patients, respectively.[94] The prevalence of ANAs ranges from 30 to 80 per cent in different series,[94] the predominant pattern of fluorescence being speckled.[95] One specific ANA, termed Scl-70, has been found in as many as 70 per cent of patients and has been hypothesized to be relatively specific for the condition. LE cell tests are positive in 2 to 5 per cent of patients judged clinically to have the disease, but most of these patients have clinical features of both PSS and SLE.[96] Protein electrophoresis reveals an increase in gamma globulin in about 50 per cent of patients.

Pulmonary Function Tests

As indicated previously, pulmonary function is almost invariably disturbed, even when the chest roentgenogram is normal. Aberrations usually consist of a restrictive insufficiency with diminished vital capacity and residual volume.[97] In the past, the finding of a predominant obstructive pattern has been ascribed to cigarette smoking, but more recent studies indicate that obstruction may be present in the absence of a smoking history[98]; in fact, one group of workers has found that a majority of patients with PSS show normal FEV_1/FVC ratios and increased residual volume, an association suggestive of small airway disease.[99] Both diffusing capacity and lung compliance are almost invariably reduced.[98] Diaphragmatic muscle dysfunction can result in ventilatory failure.[100]

Prognosis

The prognosis of PSS is unfavorable: approximately one third of patients die within 5 years of the onset of disease,[101] and in 15 to 20 per cent the course is rapidly progressive.[102] The outlook is poorer for males and blacks than for females and whites,[103] and the survival time of older patients is decreased, even after allowance has been made for the natural increase in mortality with age.[101] The cause of death may be cardiovascular, pulmonary, or renal.

Involvement of the lungs is not necessarily a bad prognostic sign; in one series, the interval from the onset of clinically evident pulmonary disease to death ranged from 2 months to 37 years.[89] However, in one follow-up study of 71 patients with PSS, lowered diffusing capacity for carbon monoxide was associated with a poor prognosis, particularly if the overall pattern was obstructive and the patient was male.[104] Although there is controversy, most observers believe that patients with PSS are at increased risk for pulmonary carcinoma.[105]

The CREST Syndrome

The CREST syndrome (subcutaneous *c*alcification, *R*aynaud's phenomenon, *e*sophageal dysfunction, *s*clerodactyly, and *t*elangiectasia) possesses certain clinical and laboratory features that differ from those of PSS, and it is generally regarded as a variant of this disorder. The most distinctive serologic abnormality is the presence of an anticentromere antibody, which has been found in the sera of 50 to 95 per cent of patients judged on clinical grounds to have the CREST syndrome, in fewer than 10 per cent of those with PSS, and rarely in patients with other connective tissue diseases.[106] Clinically, patients with CREST syndrome have an appreciably lower incidence of arthralgia and arthritis than those with PSS,[107] and their skin involvement is limited to the distal portions of the extremities.[106]

The varieties of pulmonary disease in the CREST syndrome are identical to those in PSS, but they occur with different frequency.[108] Particularly noteworthy in this regard is pulmonary hypertension, which tends to occur as an isolated finding without evidence of other significant pulmonary disease. In one study of 331 patients with the syndrome, 30 (9 per cent) were so affected[109]; in contrast, none of 342 patients with PSS and no CREST features had pulmonary hypertension. Pathologic and roentgenographic findings in these cases are similar to those in hypertension associated with other connective tissue diseases or primary (idiopathic) pulmonary hypertension. The combination of a low diffusing capacity and a relatively high vital capacity should suggest the possibility of this complication. The prognosis is poor; in the series previously cited, the rate of 2-year survival was only 40 per cent.[109]

Dermatomyositis and Polymyositis

The terms "dermatomyositis" and "polymyositis" (DM/ PM) refer to a group of disorders generally considered to be autoimmune that are characterized by weakness, and sometimes pain, in the proximal limb muscles and occasionally in the muscles of the neck. In about half the reported cases, a characteristic violaceous skin rash is associated (in which case the appropriate term is dermatomyositis), and in a minority of cases neoplastic disease. Although the clinical picture differs considerably from case to case, the common denominator is muscle weakness.

The disease is worldwide in distribution and occurs twice as often in women as in men; it shows two age peaks, the first during the first decade and the second in the fifth and sixth decades. It has been classified clinically into five groups:[110] (1) primary idiopathic polymyositis, (2) primary idiopathic dermatomyositis, (3) dermatomyositis or polymyositis associated with neoplasia, (4) dermatomyositis or polymyositis developing in childhood and associated with vasculitis, and (5) dermatomyositis or polymyositis associated with other connective tissue diseases.

The thorax is commonly affected at some point in the disease, generally in one or more of three forms: (1) hypoventilation and respiratory failure as a result of direct involvement of the respiratory muscles; (2) interstitial pneumonitis and fibrosis, bronchiolitis obliterans with organizing pneumonia, or diffuse alveolar damage; and (3) aspiration pneumonia secondary to pharyngeal muscle paralysis.

Pathogenesis

Most studies suggest an abnormality of cell-mediated immunity. Human muscle homogenates have been shown to cause blastogenesis when incubated with lymphocytes of patients with polymyositis but not with those of controls.[111] Peripheral lymphocytes of patients with active polymyositis have been found to be cytotoxic to human fetal muscle cell cultures[112] and to produce lymphotoxin when incubated with autologous muscle.[113] Immunosuppression results in a return to normal of lymphocyte-mediated myotoxicity values[112] and has been reported in some studies[114] to bring about significant clinical improvement in patients with corticosteroid-resistant polymyositis.

Pathologic Characteristics

Histologic examination of muscle biopsy specimens from patients with polymyositis may reveal both degenerative and regenerative muscle changes, a mononuclear inflammatory infiltrate, and interstitial fibrosis. Identical changes can be seen in the diaphragm and intercostal muscles at autopsy. Pathologic changes of interstitial pneumonitis are indistinguishable from those of idiopathic fibrosing alveolitis.[115, 116] In contrast to DM/PM of childhood, in which necrotizing vasculitis may be widespread, histologic evidence of vascular involvement is rare in adult disease.[117] Bronchiolitis with organizing pneumonia or diffuse alveolar damage is seen in some patients.[118]

Roentgenographic Manifestations

Many patients have normal chest roentgenograms. Several abnormal patterns are possible, depending on the presence and nature of an associated connective tissue disease and on what muscle groups are affected. In approximately 5 to 15 per cent of cases,[119, 119a] a diffuse reticular or reticulonodular pattern is seen, involving predominantly the lung bases; such cases may have the clinical features of PSS or rheumatoid disease and characteristically respond dramatically to corticosteroid therapy.[119] When disease involves the muscles of respiration, diaphragmatic elevation and small volume lungs may be apparent, often in conjunction with basal linear opacities. Pharyngeal muscle paralysis can lead to unilateral or bilateral segmental pneumonia as a result of aspiration.

Clinical Manifestations

Patients usually present with symmetric weakness of the neck and proximal limb muscles. This tends to progress rapidly over a period of weeks or months rather than years, as is characteristic of the muscular dystrophies.[110] Sometimes, manifestations of other connective tissue diseases overshadow those of muscle weakness, and the latter may be overlooked. The prevalence of coexistent carcinoma is about 5 to 25 per cent[119a, 120]; a variety of primary sites have been documented, including the stomach, prostate, pancreas, and ovary.

Only a minority of patients manifest symptoms and signs referable to the respiratory system; in one study, respiratory muscle weakness was severe enough to cause respiratory embarrassment in only six of 89 patients.[121] When present, however, such weakness can result in extreme dyspnea, cyanosis, and ineffective cough. Interstitial pulmonary disease sometimes causes dyspnea, and this may be the major presenting symptom. More often, however, extensive disease is unassociated with symptoms and is discovered on a screening chest roentgenogram.[119] Some patients present with only minor skin involvement and Raynaud's phenomenon; in this group, esophageal dysperistalsis frequently leads to dysphagia and, sometimes, to aspiration pneumonia.[122]

In one study of 124 patients followed over a period of 2½ years,[123] the overall mortality rate from the time of first hospitalization was 36 per cent; death usually was caused by aspiration pneumonia. The prognosis is considerably poorer for adults than for children and for patients with pulmonary fibrosis.[124]

Laboratory Findings

Measurement of enzyme levels is useful in establishing the diagnosis, although values may be within normal limits even in patients with active myositis and muscle atrophy resulting from severe, long-standing disease. Muscle biopsy results are reported to be normal in 10 to 50 per cent of cases[125]; in one series, positive electromyographic changes were observed in 56 of the 61 patients in whom this procedure was performed.[121]

Antibodies to one or more of three aminoacyl-tRNA synthetases (histadyl-tRNA synthetase [anti-JO-1], alanyl-tRNA synthetase [anti-PL-12], or threonyl-tRNA synthetase [anti-PL7]) have been shown to be fairly specific for the combination of interstitial lung disease and polymyositis.[126] Affected patients commonly have arthritis, keratoconjunctivitis sicca, sclerodactyly, Raynaud's phenomenon, hepatitis, or subcutaneous calcinosis.[127]

Pulmonary Function Tests

Pulmonary function tests show no abnormality in most patients; in those who have developed interstitial fibrosis, findings are identical to those of PSS.[128] When the diaphragm is affected in the absence of other muscle involvement, the vital capacity is decreased, flow rates and the transdiaphragmatic pressure are reduced, and hypoxemia develops, with or without a rise in P_{CO_2}.[129]

Sjögren's Syndrome

Sjögren's syndrome is a chronic autoimmune disorder involving principally the glands of the oral cavity, nose, and eyes and characterized clinically by keratoconjunctivitis sicca, xerostomia, and recurrent swelling of the parotid gland. It can occur as an isolated disorder (primary Sjögren's syndrome, sicca syndrome), but more often is associated with other well-defined connective tissue diseases (secondary Sjögren's syndrome). Rheumatoid disease is probably the most common of such associated disorders; it has also been documented in PSS, primary biliary cirrhosis, Hashimoto's thyroiditis, pernicious anemia, and primary hypothyroidism. The syndrome has also been identified in individuals with immune system abnormalities that are not usually considered as part of the spectrum of connective tissue diseases. These include recipients of bone marrow transplants (in whom the pathogenesis may be related to graft-versus-host disease)[130] and individuals infected with human immunodeficiency virus (HIV).[131]

Etiology and Pathogenesis

The etiology of Sjögren's syndrome is unknown. In view of the occurrence of the disease in families, genetic factors have been implicated[132]; these appear to be expressed as depression of immune surveillance, permitting increased antibody responses and the development of both benign and malignant lymphocyte proliferations. As in SLE, it is possible that antigenic alteration and resultant autoantibody production are related to viral infection, in this instance originating in the salivary gland. The human leukocyte antigens HLA-Dw2 and Dw3 are commonly present in patients with Sjögren's syndrome, including both primary disease and the secondary form associated with SLE, whereas HLA-Dw4 is characteristic of Sjögren's syndrome associated with rheumatoid disease. HLA-B8 is found in 55 per cent of cases of primary Sjögren's syndrome but does not occur in secondary Sjögren's syndrome associated with rheumatoid disease or SLE.[133]

Evidence of an autoimmune pathogenesis in Sjögren's syndrome is as strong as in SLE. As in the latter condition, many features of Sjögren's syndrome are reflected in the spontaneous disease of NZB/W mice, which develop lymphoid infiltrates in the salivary glands that are remarkably similar to those observed in naturally occurring Sjögren's syndrome in humans.[134] A variety of autoantibodies can also be detected in this disorder. The presence of lymphocytes within salivary glands and other affected glands, in association with fibrosis and glandular atrophy, has also suggested a lymphocyte-mediated autoimmune process. Unexplained findings that suggest an immune-mediated or allergic pathogenetic component in Sjögren's syndrome are blood eosinophilia and a remarkable hypersensitivity to drugs, both of which have been reported in 20 to 50 per cent of patients.[135]

Pathologic Characteristics

Pulmonary disease in Sjögren's syndrome can occur in the airways or (more commonly) the parenchymal interstitium. Atrophy of tracheobronchial mucous glands associated with a lymphoplasmacytic cellular infiltrate has been reported in occasional cases.[136] These findings are believed to be analogous to salivary gland involvement and to be responsible for the chronic cough observed clinically. Fibrosis and mononuclear cell infiltration of small airways have also been reported in patients who manifest evidence of obstructive airway disease.[137]

Pulmonary parenchymal disease may take several forms, the most common of which is a diffuse, usually bilateral, interstitial lymphoplasmacytic infiltrate (lymphocytic interstitial pneumonitis [see page 509]).[138] This infiltrate is usually most dense in relation to bronchioles and their accompanying vessels but also extends into the alveolar interstitium itself, where fibrosis may develop. The pathologic differentiation from lymphoma can be difficult.

Roentgenographic Manifestations

In one study of 42 chest roentgenograms of patients with Sjögren's syndrome,[139] 14 (33 per cent) showed a reticulo-nodular pattern similar to that of other connective tissue

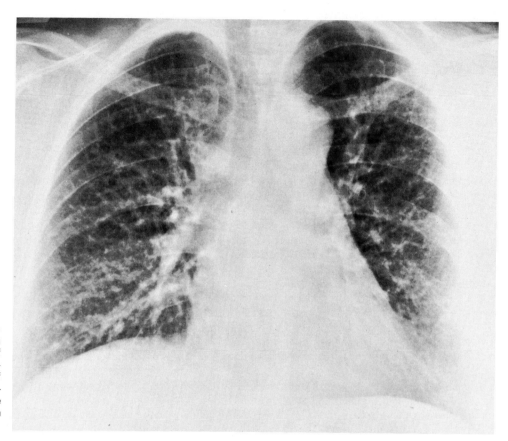

Figure 7–10. Sjögren's Syndrome. This 45-year-old woman presented with the classic triad of keratoconjunctivitis sicca, xerostomia, and recurrent swelling of the parotid glands. Her roentgenogram reveals a diffuse, coarse reticular pattern throughout both lungs.

diseases (Fig. 7–10). Pneumonitis and atelectasis are two additional complications that are commonly seen.[139]

Clinical Manifestations

The chief symptoms of Sjögren's syndrome are grittiness or burning sensation of the eyes and dryness of the mouth, nose, and skin. Lacrimal or salivary gland enlargement occurs in 25 to 50 per cent of patients.[140] With the exception of the parotid gland, such enlargement is usually bilateral. Involvement of the larynx and tracheobronchial mucous glands may result in hoarseness and a persistent cough productive of thick, tenacious sputum. Interstitial cellular infiltration and fibrosis of the lungs may be associated with dyspnea. Physical signs of pulmonary involvement include those of complicating pneumonia and, in some patients with diffuse interstitial disease, crepitations at the lung bases. Approximately one half to two thirds of patients manifest symptoms and signs of an associated connective tissue disease.

Patients with Sjögren's syndrome, either primary or secondary, are at increased risk for the development of non-Hodgkin's lymphoma, often with pulmonary involvement.[141] Those who develop this complication generally manifest a severe sicca syndrome associated with parotid swelling; there is often lymph node enlargement, splenomegaly, leukopenia, vasculitis, neuropathy, Raynaud's phenomenon, and/or hyperglobulinemia.

Laboratory Findings and Pulmonary Function Tests

Although the diagnosis of Sjögren's syndrome usually is based on characteristic clinical manifestations, it may be substantiated by tests of glandular secretory function, by biopsy of minor salivary glands, and by the detection of various serum antibodies. The first-named include Schirmer's test for the measurement of tear formation and slit lamp examination of the eyes for identification of superficial corneal scarring due to inadequate lacrimal gland secretion.

A variety of autoantibodies, including rheumatoid factor and ANAs, may be found; though they occur in both primary and secondary disease, they are much more common in the latter. Antibodies to ribonucleoproteins (termed SS-A(Ro) and SS-B(La)) are common in Sjögren's syndrome; the latter particularly has been found to be useful in arriving at a precise diagnosis.[142] A high percentage of patients have circulating immune complexes, the binding of complement being caused largely by IgG.[143] Bronchoalveolar lavage specimens show a greater number of cells and an increased proportion of lymphocytes in patients with primary Sjögren's syndrome than in normal controls;[144] in addition, patients with evidence of more severe alveolitis tend to have more frequent clinical and roentgenographic manifestations and poorer lung function.

As is to be expected in a disease that can involve the pulmonary interstitium or bronchial glands exclusively or both areas simultaneously, pulmonary function test results may be restrictive, obstructive, or mixed.[145] They may appear early in the course of the disease and progress over a relatively short time.[146]

Mixed Connective Tissue Disease

In 1972, Sharp and associates[147] described a symptom complex that included features of a variety of connective tissue disorders that they and others[148] were prepared to accept as a distinct entity. Patients with this mixed connective tissue disease (MCTD) manifest clinical features of SLE, DM/PM, and PSS. Antinuclear antibodies to native DNA and high titers of antibody to an extractable nuclear antigen consisting mainly of ribonucleoprotein (anti-nRNP Ab) differentiate this syndrome from SLE. Despite this, acceptable clinical cases of MCTD account for only 5 to 10 per cent of patients with "pure" anti-nRNP Ab, and in some patients who manifest the clinical criteria of MCTD the results of this antibody determination are negative.

Pulmonary abnormalities in mixed connective tissue disease have been described infrequently. There have been several reports of interstitial pneumonitis and fibrosis and of pulmonary hypertension unassociated with parenchymal disease.[149] Pathologic features in these latter cases have included plexogenic pulmonary arteriopathy and recurrent small vessel thromboemboli.

As might be expected, the clinical and radiologic manifestations of MCTD are quite variable and can include any of the features seen with SLE, DM/PM, or PSS. Follow-up of the original 25 patients reported by Sharp and coworkers showed that, with time, the arthritis, serositis, fever, and myositis became less severe and responded to corticosteroids and the clinical picture evolved to resemble PSS; renal disease remained relatively infrequent.[150] On the other hand, a prospective analysis of 34 patients in whom a diagnosis of MCTD was eventually made and who were followed for a mean period of more than 6 years indicated that some who presented with rather limited disease and were diagnosed as having SLE or PSS may progress to a clinical picture more compatible with MCTD.[151]

MCTD has been considered to be a relatively benign form of connective tissue disease; however, some studies indicate that patients may develop the more ominous features of connective tissue diseases that respond poorly to corticosteroid therapy, including encephalitis and glomerulonephritis.[25] Fatal diffuse interstitial lung disease and pulmonary arterial hypertension also have been decribed.[149]

Relapsing Polychondritis

Relapsing polychondritis is characterized principally by inflammation and destruction of cartilage at several sites, including the ribs, tracheobronchial tree, earlobes, nose, and axial and peripheral joints; involvement of the eye, ear, and systemic vessels is seen occasionally. There is no sex predominance, and the disease occurs at all ages (peak incidence at age 40 to 60 years).

The etiology and pathogenesis are unknown. An associated autoimmune disorder has been found in 20 to 25 per cent of cases,[152] suggesting that the disease may have an immunologic basis. In support of this hypothesis are studies documenting the presence of anticartilage antibodies in some patients.[153] In addition, it has been shown that exposure of peripheral blood lymphocytes to cartilage antigen in vitro results in increased blastogenesis[154] and the production of macrophage migration–inhibiting factor.[155] Whatever the pathogenesis, damage to cartilage causes local areas of tracheomalacia or bronchomalacia, which in turn leads to expiratory airway obstruction and increased risk of pulmonary infection.

The gross appearance of the trachea and major bronchi at autopsy has been described infrequently, but in a few cases severe narrowing has been observed.[156] Microscopically, affected cartilage shows fragmentation and fibrosis. In clinically active disease, an inflammatory infiltrate composed of lymphocytes, plasma cells, and occasional neutrophils is often present at the fibrocartilaginous interface.

Roentgenographic manifestations include articular cartilage destruction, calcification of the earlobes, and narrowing of the tracheal and major bronchial air columns (Fig. 7–11).[157] Computed tomography of the airways or tracheobronchography at different lung volumes is necessary to identify the site of the obstruction. High-resolution CT can reveal considerable deformity of peripheral as well as central airways.

As the name indicates, the disease is typically relapsing and remitting and usually has a prolonged course. The most common clinical manifestations are swelling, erythema, and pain of the ears and arthralgia.[152] Nasal chondritis is also frequent and may result in a saddle deformity. The larynx and trachea are involved in about 50 per cent of cases, and in 15 per cent are responsible for the presenting signs and symptoms.[152] Tracheobronchial disease is manifested by dyspnea and portends a poor prognosis; in fact, respiratory complications are responsible for many of the reported deaths. In one series of 112 patients, the 5- and 10-year probabilities of survival after diagnosis were 74 and 55 per cent, respectively.[158]

The predominant mechanism of expiratory airway obstruction in relapsing polychondritis is the airway abnormality itself and not a loss of elastic recoil forces of the lung.[159] The site of airway obstruction is usually fixed, as assessed by maximal inspiratory and expiratory flow-volume loops.[160] If it is variable and intrathoracic,[161] the expiratory flow-volume loop is markedly flattened.

PULMONARY VASCULITIS

Here we describe a variety of conditions whose sole or predominant histologic feature is inflammation of pulmonary vessels. Discussion is limited to those disorders in which the inflammatory reaction is directed *primarily* against the vessel wall and is of proved or presumed immunologic origin. When assessing such inflammatory processes, it is important to remember that a number of conditions, particularly infections, can result in vasculitis simply by extension of pulmonary parenchymal disease into the vessel wall. These conditions are best considered secondary vasculitides, since the primary pathogenetic mechanism is not related to vascular damage. This process is fairly common, and in order to be confident of a diagnosis of primary vasculitis, it is important that appropriate cultures be performed on biopsy material and that tissue be thoroughly

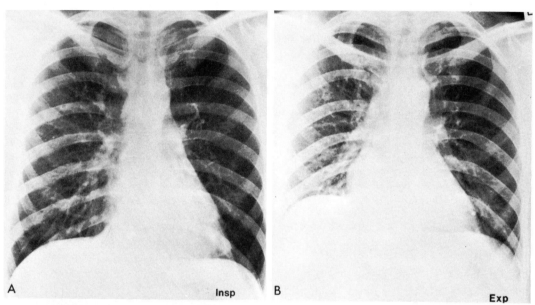

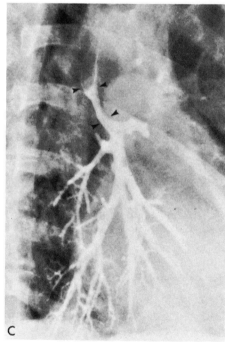

Figure 7–11. Relapsing Polychondritis. The major symptom of this 25-year-old man was polyarthralgia. In addition, he manifested a saddle deformity of his nose and an ulcer on the pinna of one ear. He had no symptoms referable to his chest. Postero-anterior roentgenograms at inspiration *(A)* and expiration *(B)* reveal a moderate degree of oligemia of the whole of the left lung, although the left hilum is only slightly smaller than the right. The volume of the left lung on inspiration is roughly normal, although it shows a severe degree of air trapping on expiration *(B)*. These plain roentgenographic findings are consistent with a diagnosis of Swyer-James syndrome. A left bronchogram was performed *(C)* and demonstrated a severe degree of narrowing of the whole length of the left main bronchus *(arrowheads)*; the lower lobe bronchi were otherwise normal. (Courtesy of Dr. John Henderson, Ottawa General Hospital.)

examined histologically to exclude an infectious etiology, particularly when disease is relatively localized.

Clinical and roentgenographic manifestations of pulmonary vasculitis can be related to the vascular inflammation itself or to the pneumonitis that accompanies some of the disorders. During the acute stages, the effects of vasculitis include alveolar hemorrhage and vascular thrombosis, with or without parenchymal necrosis. With more prolonged disease, weakening of the vessel wall can result in aneurysm formation, and obliteration of the vessel lumina can cause pulmonary hypertension. Because of the frequent occurrence of concomitant extrapulmonary vasculitis and the occasional presence of glomerulonephritis, signs and symptoms of extrathoracic disease may overshadow the pulmonary manifestations.

In addition to the specific disease entities to be described in the following sections, there exist a number of rare cases associated with pulmonary vasculitis that defy precise clinicopathologic classification. Some of these may simply represent *formes frustes* of the better-characterized vasculitides and have been termed "polyangiitis overlap syndrome" by Leavitt and Fauci.[162] These authors have listed combinations of diseases such as Takayasu's arteritis plus PAN, allergic granulomatosis plus PAN, giant cell arteritis plus Wegener's granulomatosis, and so on. Although the precise nature of these cases is even less clear than that of their better-defined "relatives," there is no question that they occasionally occur and can cause considerable diagnostic difficulty. In this regard, it is important to remember that the possibility of pulmonary vasculitis should not be discounted simply because of a lack of clinicopathologic features that make precise classification possible.

Wegener's Granulomatosis

In its classic form, Wegener's granulomatosis is a multisystem disease characterized pathologically by necrotizing granulomatous inflammation of the upper and lower respiratory tract, glomerulonephritis, and necrotizing vasculitis of the lungs and of a variety of systemic organs and tissues. Four diagnostic criteria have been proposed by the American College of Rheumatology:[163] abnormal urinary sediment (red cell casts or more than 5 red cells per high-power field); nodular cavities or fixed "infiltrates" *(sic)* on chest roentgenograms; oral ulcers or nasal discharge; and granulomatous inflammation on tissue biopsy. In one series of 807 patients with vasculitis, the presence of two or more of these criteria was associated with diagnostic sensitivity and specificity rates of 88 and 92 per cent, respectively.[163]

The disease also may be manifested primarily or solely in the respiratory tract, in which case it is referred to as "limited" Wegener's granulomatosis.[164] It is important to emphasize that in many such cases the qualifier "limited" refers chiefly to the clinical manifestations, especially in relation to an absence of renal and other visceral disease; concomitant involvement of the upper respiratory tract and skin is not uncommon, and a number of patients with apparently limited disease have been found at autopsy or biopsy to have histologic evidence of glomerulonephritis or systemic vasculitis and granulomatous inflammation.[164] Thus, from a pathogenetic point of view, it may be appropriate to consider these cases as part of a spectrum of disease rather than as separate entities. The diagnosis of limited Wegener's granulomatosis, especially when disease is manifested by a solitary pulmonary nodule or mass, should be made only after extensive investigations have excluded the possibility of an infectious etiology.

Etiology and Pathogenesis

The prominent involvement of the upper and lower respiratory tract, as well as the occurrence of occasional cases predominantly limited to these sites, strongly suggests that the etiology of Wegener's granulomatosis is related to an inhaled substance; however, what substance this might be is entirely unknown. Lung and BAL cultures are typically sterile, and no organisms have been identified by light or electron microscopic examination.[165] An inflammatory reaction closely resembling that of Wegener's granulomatosis has been induced in previously sensitized rabbits following inhalation of an aerosol consisting of bovine serum albumin and the T cell mitogen concanavalin A, suggesting that inhalation of naturally occurring concanavalin A or other plant lectins might be a causal factor.[166] Although familial cases do occur,[167] there is little evidence of a hereditary influence.[168]

Although the pathogenesis of Wegener's granulomatosis is also poorly understood, both immunologic and pathologic manifestations implicate an autoimmune process,[169] a concept supported by the dramatic therapeutic response to immunosuppresive and cytotoxic drugs in many cases. Available evidence suggests a possible role for both immune complex and cell-mediated immune reactions. Circulating immune complexes have been demonstrated in some patients with active disease and, in one case,[170] were found to disappear during remission induced by immunosuppressive therapy. On the other hand, immunohistochemical and ultrastructural examination of pulmonary tissue has led to mostly negative results: although some studies have reported deposition of immunoglobulin and C3 in the walls of alveoli and blood vessels,[171] most have found no evidence of immune complex deposition.[172] The frequent presence of granulomatous inflammation in active lesions, both in relation to vessels and to extravascular tissue, implies a cell-mediated component in the pathogenesis. In support of this, immunohistochemical studies demonstrate that the majority of inflammatory cells in the parenchyma and vascular infiltrates are T cells and monocytes.[172]

Pathologic Characteristics

Pathologic features of Wegener's granulomatosis are variable but overall quite characteristic of the disease.[173, 174] Although virtually any organ or tissue can be involved, changes are seen most often in the lungs, upper respiratory tract, kidneys, and spleen; the heart, gastrointestinal tract, skin, and nervous system are less frequently affected.

Grossly, pulmonary involvement is characterized by well-circumscribed nodules or masses ranging in diameter from 1 to 10 cm, often with central necrosis; occasionally, there is a more or less diffuse hemorrhagic consolidation.[173] Microscopically, the nodules are composed of variable amounts of inflammatory and necrotic tissue. In early le-

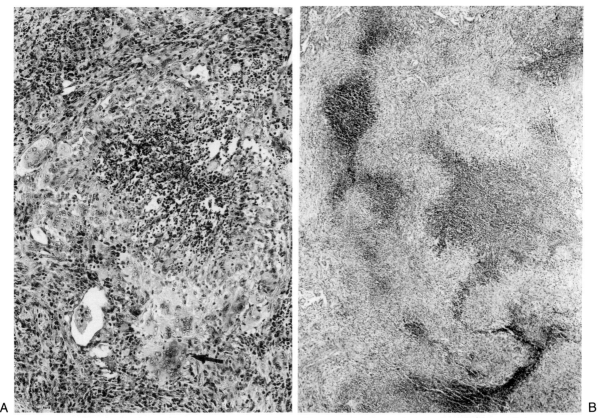

A   B

Figure 7–12. Wegener's Granulomatosis. *A,* Magnified view of a focus of parenchymal inflammation shows necrotic tissue surrounded by epithelioid histiocytes and multinucleated giant cells *(arrow). B,* Enlargement and coalescence of such necrotic areas result in an irregular (serpiginous) outline. (*A* × 120; *B* × 40.)

sions, the latter tend to be minute and multifocal; as the disease progresses, however, individual necrotic areas enlarge and coalesce, producing a rather characteristic serpiginous outline (Fig. 7–12). The necrotic tissue is often bordered by a layer of palisaded epithelioid histiocytes, which, in turn, is surrounded by a polymorphic inflammatory infiltrate. The inflammation is most prominent in the parenchyma, but involvement of the tracheobronchial tree is also fairly common, either by direct extension from a parenchymal focus or independently.

Pulmonary arteries and veins of small to medium size typically manifest one or more of three patterns of inflammation: (1) fibrinoid "necrosis" of the media, with or without a polymorphonuclear leukocyte infiltrate; (2) focal or diffuse infiltration of all vascular layers by a polymorphic infiltrate (Fig. 7–13); or (3) well-defined granulomas or numerous multinucleated giant cells. In the presence of diffuse hemorrhagic consolidation, vasculitis predominates in arterioles, capillaries, and venules and is best described as leukocytoclastic vasculitis (*see* page 417).[175]

By definition, classic Wegener's granulomatosis is always associated with disease in extrapulmonary sites. In the upper respiratory tract, involvement of the mucous membranes of the paranasal sinuses results in thickening in the early stages and, in some cases, eventuates in destruction of bone and cartilage. The middle ear and orbital cavity may also be involved. The inflammatory and necrotic components are similar to those seen in the lung parenchyma,

although evidence of granulomatous inflammation and vasculitis are often absent, especially in small biopsy specimens.[176] Characteristically, the kidneys show focal and segmental necrotizing glomerulonephritis. Vasculitis in systemic vessels is similar to that seen in polyarteritis nodosa; as in this disease, the bronchial arteries are occasionally affected.

Roentgenographic Manifestations

The typical roentgenographic pattern in the lungs is that of rounded opacities, usually sharply defined, ranging from a few millimeters to 10 cm in diameter (Fig. 7–14). They are commonly multiple, bilateral, and widely distributed, with no predilection for any zone.[177] Cavitation occurs eventually in one third to one half of cases. The cavities are thick-walled and tend to have an irregular, rather shaggy inner lining; the thickness of the walls may diminish gradually until the cavities become thin-walled cystic spaces similar to those seen in coccidioidomycosis.[178] After appropriate therapy—and rarely even without treatment—cavities may disappear altogether. Distinct "feeding" vessels related to the nodules and abnormalities suggestive of infarcts may be seen with CT.[178a]

Endotracheal or endobronchial masses can cause airway narrowing with resultant peripheral oligemia and sometimes lobar and total lung atelectasis.[179] Widespread airspace opacities can be caused by diffuse pulmonary hemor-

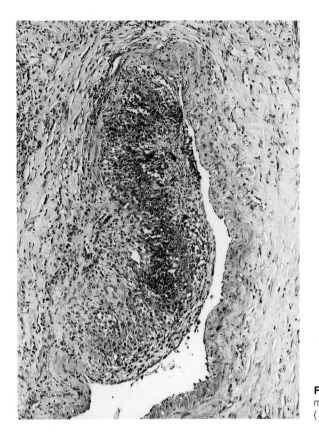

Figure 7–13. Wegener's Granulomatosis: Vasculitis. A pulmonary artery of medium size shows focal acute inflammation and necrosis within its media. (× 80.)

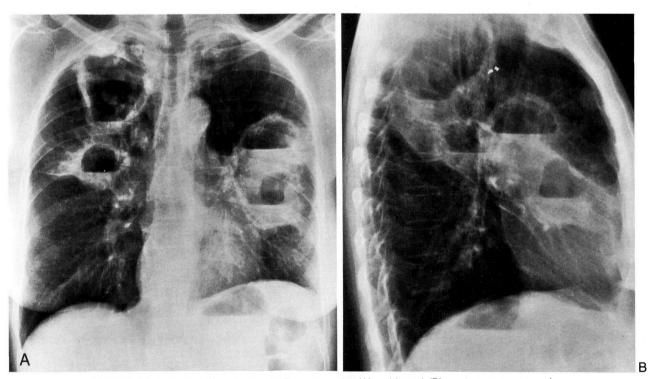

Figure 7–14. Wegener's Granulomatosis. Posteroanterior *(A)* and lateral *(B)* roentgenograms reveal multiple, large, thick-walled cavities situated in both upper lobes. Although poorly seen on these reproductions, the left upper lung zone was markedly oligemic, suggesting the possibility of involvement of the left upper lobe bronchus and resulting hypoxic vasoconstriction.

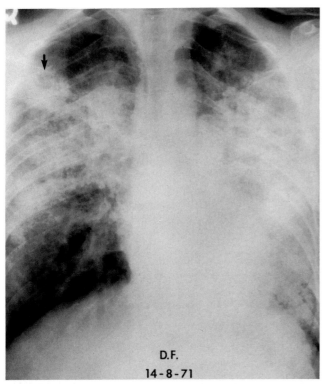

Figure 7–15. Wegener's Granulomatosis: Diffuse Pulmonary Hemorrhage. A posteroanterior chest roentgenogram demonstrates extensive consolidation in both lungs, the left worse than the right. A small cavity is present in a more focal opacity in the right upper lobe (*arrow*). The patient was a 41-year-old man with hemoptysis, sinusitis, and necrotizing glomerulonephritis confirmed at autopsy to be Wegener's granulomatosis.

rhage (Fig. 7–15).[180] Pleural effusion has been reported in about 50 per cent of cases.[181] With cytotoxic drug therapy, there is usually dramatic resolution of the pulmonary lesions. Despite this, intrathoracic relapse is common (18 of 19 patients in one series)[182]; in a third of these patients, roentgenographic abnormalities differed from those at initial presentation. No distinctive radiologic features distinguish the "limited" from the classic form of the disease.

Clinical Manifestations

Wegener's granulomatosis typically affects adults in their fifth decade, men slightly more often than women.[183] The onset can be acute and its course fulminating, but it is more commonly insidious. Although initially the disease may be associated with such nonspecific symptoms as fever, malaise, weight loss, and fatigue, the majority of patients present with complaints referable to the nose, paranasal sinuses, or chest. A few present with symptoms and signs of widespread disease, including exophthalmos, hematuria, and vesicular and hemorrhagic cutaneous lesions. Although renal manifestations occur in the majority of patients at some time in the course of the disease, only rarely are they the presenting clinical features.

Virtually any organ or tissue can be affected in Wegener's granulomatosis. Nasal disease is manifested by rhinitis, sinusitis, and epistaxis. Joint involvement is common and usually takes the form of arthralgia or a nondeforming arthritis. Myalgias are also not infrequent. Neurologic manifestations may be central or peripheral, the latter presenting as mononeuritis multiplex or polyneuritis. Cardiac manifestations include conduction abnormalities and pericarditis. Thoracic symptoms consist of intractable cough, often with hemoptysis, dyspnea, and pleuritic pain. Hemoptysis is occasionally massive, the clinical presentation mimicking idiopathic pulmonary hemorrhage or Goodpasture's syndrome.

Laboratory Findings

Laboratory findings include anemia (sometimes hemolytic), thrombocytosis, and leukocytosis, occasionally with eosinophilia. Rheumatoid factor may be detected in the serum, usually in low titer, and some patients have elevated levels of IgE.[184] Pulmonary function tests may show restrictive or obstructive disease, the latter generally resulting from involvement of large airways.

The discovery of the relationship between antineutrophil cytoplasmic antibodies (ANCAs) and Wegener's granulomatosis has been one of the most important recent events with respect to both diagnosis and therapy of the disease. These antibodies can be detected in serum and BAL specimens[165] by indirect immunofluorescence or enzyme-linked immunosorbent assay (ELISA) techniques and appear to be related to several lysosomal enzymes; specific antibodies may develop in different vasculitides.[185] They are elevated in a large percentage of patients with Wegener's granulomatosis, although they also have been reported in individuals with microscopic polyarteritis, idiopathic (crescentic) glomerulonephritis,[186, 187] and allergic granulomatosis.[185] The antibodies also have been found to vary in titer with activity of disease[186, 188] and to correlate with active renal disease,[189] suggesting that it might be possible to monitor and treat the disease by sequential antibody measurements. In fact, in one study in which 20 patients were randomly assigned to therapy or control groups on the basis of an increase in titer, the treated group experienced no clinical relapse[190]; by contrast, the 9 of 11 control patients relapsed within 6 months.

Prognosis

Until fairly recently, the prognosis for classic Wegener's granulomatosis was poor: death occurred within 6 months, from uremia or less often from respiratory failure or coronary vasculitis and pancarditis.[191] In recent years, however, combined corticosteroid and cytotoxic drug therapy, primarily with cyclophosphamide, not only has resulted in clinical remissions of the disease but also has led to apparent cures; despite this, morbidity related to therapy or the disease itself may be profound.[191a] In patients who develop irreversible renal failure despite control of active disease with immunosuppressive therapy, renal transplantation has proved successful and has not been associated with evidence of recurrent glomerulonephritis.[192] The prognosis for patients with the limited form of disease is better than for those with classic Wegener's granulomatosis,[164] presumably because of the absence of serious renal involvement.

Allergic Granulomatosis

Allergic granulomatosis (Churg-Strauss syndrome) is an uncommon and somewhat controversial clinicopathologic abnormality. The American College of Rheumatology has proposed six criteria for its diagnosis[193]: asthma, eosinophilia greater than 10 per cent on differential white blood cell count, mononeuropathy or polyneuropathy, non-fixed pulmonary "infiltrates" (sic) on roentgenography, paranasal sinus abnormalities, and biopsy containing a blood vessel showing vasculitis and extravascular eosinophils. In their investigation of 807 patients with vasculitis, the presence of four or more of these criteria was found to yield a sensitivity and specificity for diagnosis of 85 and 97 per cent, respectively.[193]

Despite these observations, it is necessary to note that the existence of allergic granulomatosis as a distinct entity has been questioned.[194, 195] For example, it has been suggested that it may simply represent a variant of Wegener's granulomatosis, with the prominent tissue eosinophilia representing a coincidental reactive process in asthmatic patients. In addition, Leavitt and Fauci[162] have pointed out that a number of cases of otherwise typical PAN possess features of allergic granulomatosis and that, in some instances, it may be difficult to classify a disease into one or the other of these two entities with conviction. They have proposed the term "overlap syndrome" for these cases, thus suggesting the existence of a spectrum of disease. These arguments possess some merit, and undoubtedly there are cases in which a clinical and pathologic distinction between Wegener's granulomatosis, PAN, and allergic granulomatosis is difficult to make. However, we believe that in most instances strict attention to clinical, pathologic, and serologic features provides a basis for choosing one of the subtypes. We thus prefer to regard these conditions separately until our knowledge of etiology and pathogenesis is sufficient to specify possible interrelationships more precisely.

The etiology and pathogenesis of allergic granulomatosis are unknown. The association with asthma and rhinitis, the presence of elevated levels of serum IgE, the response to corticosteroids, and the pathologic findings all suggest a hypersensitivity reaction to an unidentified antigen or antigens. Some investigators have found an association with a history of vaccination or desensitization therapy.[196]

Allergic granulomatosis is a multisystem disease with predilection for involvement of the lungs, skin, and nervous system; the lower urinary tract, spleen, gastrointestinal tract, and heart are less commonly affected,[162, 197] and virtually any organ or tissue is involved occasionally. Although renal disease, manifested by necrotizing glomerulonephritis or vasculitis, was common in Churg and Strauss's initial series,[198] others have found the kidneys to be infrequently affected.[197]

The characteristic microscopic findings are a combination of vasculitis and necrotizing, extravascular granulomatous inflammation.[199] The former occurs predominantly in small to medium-sized arteries and veins and consists of a transmural infiltrate of lymphocytes, plasma cells, histiocytes, multinucleated giant cells, and relatively numerous eosinophils. Extravascular granulomatous inflammation typically consists of a central focus of necrotic material, frequently with admixed eosinophils, surrounded by palisaded epithelioid histiocytes and multinucleated giant cells.

The chest roentgenogram is abnormal in approximately 75 per cent of cases,[200] the pattern consisting of either nonsegmental airspace consolidation in a peripheral distribution similar to eosinophilic pneumonia (Fig. 7–16) or multinodular disease, almost invariably without cavitation. Diffuse interstitial disease, sometimes with a miliary pattern, and hilar lymph node enlargement occur occasionally. Pleural effusions may develop and usually contain large numbers of eosinophils.

The disease usually occurs in middle age and has an insidious onset. Asthma and peripheral blood eosinophilia are present in almost all patients; allergic rhinitis, often complicated by nasal polyposis and sinusitis, occurs in many. This clinical picture of allergy may precede the other components of the disease by months or years, and, strangely, the asthma may diminish in severity when the clinical manifestations of vasculitis become apparent.[197] Other relatively common clinical findings include peripheral neuropathy, usually in the form of mononeuritis multiplex, and skin rash, frequently consisting of palpable nodules or purpura.[197] Severe renal disease is uncommon. Both peripheral blood and BAL fluid[201] typically reveal abundant eosinophils.

The abnormality usually responds to corticosteroid therapy, although some patients may require cyclophosphamide.

Polyarteritis Nodosa

PAN is a relatively common condition characterized by necrotizing vasculitis that affects predominantly small to medium-sized muscular arteries of the systemic circulation. Renal disease—vasculitis, glomerulonephritis, or both—is common. Although involvement of the bronchial arteries as part of the systemic vasculitis can occur, the incidence of vasculitis in the pulmonary circulation is very low, if it occurs at all. Some cases exist that possess clinicopathologic features common to both allergic granulomatosis and PAN, and the precise classification of these into one category or the other can be difficult.

Pathologically, the lesions of PAN are patchy in distribution and are often located at arterial branch points of the systemic circulation; histologic features range from acute inflammation with necrosis of the vessel wall to healing and fully healed stages. Extravascular granulomatous inflammation and tissue eosinophilia are not found.

Although roentgenographic abnormalities in the thorax may be present in classic PAN, it is probable that the majority are coincidental and not related to involvement of the lungs by the primary disease process. For example, in one review of the roentgenographic findings in 14 children with PAN, chest abnormalities were identified in eight, but all were consistent with the effects of chronic renal disease, hypertension, or cardiac decompensation.[202] Despite the foregoing, occasional cases of parenchymal hemorrhage may be caused by bronchial arteritis.

The predominant symptoms in PAN are related to the gastrointestinal tract, the kidneys, and the nervous system. Renal involvement is said to occur in 80 per cent of cases,[203] and systemic hypertension is a common clinical manifestation. As indicated previously, symptoms of pleuropulmonary disease are probably caused in most cases by compli-

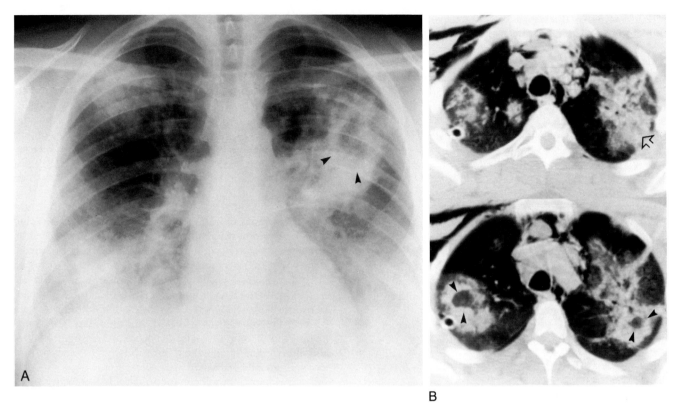

Figure 7–16. Allergic Granulomatosis. A conventional posteroanterior *(A)* chest roentgenogram discloses diffuse airspace disease throughout both lungs with moderate lower zonal predominance. The consolidation on the left contains a large central lucency *(arrowheads)*, suggesting cavitation. Small, bilateral pleural effusions were documented by decubitus views *(not shown)*. Several days later, transverse CT scans through the upper lobes *(B)* reveal broad zones of airspace consolidation *(open arrows)*; both upper lobes contain lucencies *(small arrowheads)* consistent with cavitation. Open lung biopsy confirmed allergic granulomatosis.

cating infection or by renal or cardiac failure; they include cough, wheezing, pleuritic pain, and occasionally hemoptysis.

Necrotizing Sarcoid Granulomatosis

Necrotizing sarcoid granulomatosis (NSG) is a rare disorder characterized pathologically by confluent granulomas associated with a variable amount of necrosis and prominent, focally destructive vasculitis.[204] The etiology and pathogenesis are unknown, and it is not certain if the histologic appearance represents a disease entity or simply an unusual reaction to one of a variety of inciting agents. The vascular involvement, granulomatous inflammation, and apparently good response to corticosteroid therapy have suggested a hypersensitivity reaction; however, the putative antigen is unknown. Non-necrotizing granulomatous inflammation of vessel walls is common in otherwise classic sarcoidosis,[205] although it is usually less marked in extent and severity than in NSG. This observation, in addition to the occasional presence of granulomatous disease in hilar lymph nodes and extrapulmonary sites,[206] suggests that some cases of NSG might be variants of classic sarcoidosis, possibly representing the histologic counterpart of the large nodular form of the disease observed roentgenographically.

Roentgenographically, the condition presents as multiple well-defined nodules or ill-defined opacities[207]; occasionally, a solitary mass resembling carcinoma may be present. Small

or large nodules may cavitate, and pleural effusion may develop.[204] The incidence of hilar lymph node enlargement is quite variable in different series, ranging from 8 per cent[204] to 50 per cent.[206]

Most patients are middle-aged adults, and there is a distinct female predominance.[206] Clinically, patients may be asymptomatic or have cough, fever, sweats, malaise, dyspnea, hemoptysis, or pleuritic pain. Extrapulmonary findings are usually absent. Culture and thorough examination of tissue with special stains must always be performed to exclude the possibility of infection; we and others[206] have observed cases simulating NSG in which these studies have provided proof of an infectious etiology.

The course of NSG is typically benign. Roentgenographic evidence of disease diminishes with corticosteroid therapy or, occasionally, spontaneously; however, relapse has occurred after cessation of therapy.[204]

Takayasu's Arteritis

Takayasu's arteritis (pulseless disease) is an uncommon vasculitis that occurs predominantly in women in the second or third decade of life. It is worldwide in distribution, although most affected individuals have been Japanese. Although the arteritis is often confined to the aorta and its major branches, pulmonary artery involvement also is present in an appreciable number of cases; for example, in one autopsy review, the main pulmonary artery was found to be affected in 34 of 76 cases and the intrapulmonary arterial branches in 21 cases.[208] In fact, the main pulmonary artery can be the initial site of involvement.[209]

The etiology and pathogenesis are, again, unknown. A majority of patients have evidence of active or remote tuberculosis.[210] This observation, together with the fact that in some cases granulomas are found in arterial walls, has suggested an infectious etiology; however, since the pathologic appearance and clinical course are generally unlike those of tuberculosis and since organisms have not been identified within the vascular lesions,[210] it seems unlikely that the vascular changes are the result of direct infection. The possibility that the condition represents an unusual form of hypersensitivity reaction to *Mycobacterium* organisms has been suggested.[210] A variety of serologic abnormalities and an association with connective tissue disease[211] also have been reported, raising the possibility that the pathogenesis is related to an immune mechanism.

Pathologically, most changes are limited to the larger, elastic vessels and consist of adventitial fibrosis and a mixed, largely mononuclear, inflammatory cellular infiltrate, intimal fibrosis, and, in active lesions, necrotizing or non-necrotizing granulomatous inflammation of the media.

The vascular fibrosis is responsible for appreciable stenosis, resulting in the pulmonary artery hypertension that is the principal manifestation of the disease in the lungs. In one study of the pulmonary circulation of 11 patients, pulmonary hypertension was found to be moderate in degree and to result from stenosis of the main pulmonary artery and its major branches down to subsegmental levels.[210] The angiographic pattern was similar to that commonly observed in pulmonary thromboembolism. In addition to the changes anticipated in the lungs from pulmonary arterial hypertension, the chest roentgenogram may reveal abnormalities of the aorta, including prominence of the ascending arch, irregularity of contour of the entire thoracic aorta, and intimal calcification.[212]

Clinical manifestations consist of both nonspecific constitutional symptoms and a variety of specific symptoms related to localized vascular insufficiency. These include angina pectoris, headaches, syncope, impaired vision, and claudication in upper or lower extremities. Localized pain over the affected arteries may be present, and arterial pulses may be absent. In some cases, a midsystolic murmur in the pulmonic area may suggest pulmonary artery involvement, particularly when an early systolic click is absent.[210]

Temporal (Giant Cell) Arteritis

Temporal arteritis is a relatively common systemic arteritis that affects predominantly older individuals. Vasculitis, as seen both pathologically and symptomatically, is most frequent in the larger vessels of the head and neck; involvement of both large elastic and medium-sized muscular pulmonary arteries also has been documented but is rare.[213]

Symptoms usually consist of headache, jaw claudication, and blindness; occasionally there may be high fever, anemia, and polymyalgia rheumatica. One report has stressed the importance of respiratory tract symptoms and signs as initial findings[214]; these included sore throat, hoarseness, choking sensation, tenderness of cervical structures, and glossitis and were presumably caused by either ischemia of

affected tissues or a reaction to the inflammation in the arteries supplying the laryngeal and pharyngeal tissue.

Behçet's Disease

Behçet's disease is an uncommon systemic disorder characterized principally by recurrent aphthous stomatitis, genital ulcers, skin lesions, and uveitis. Pulmonary manifestations are generally considered to be rare: only 28 examples had been documented in world literature by 1986.[215] However, in a more recent report of 72 patients, seven (10 per cent) were considered to have pulmonary vascular involvement.[216]

The basic pathogenesis is believed to be vasculitis, probably on the basis of immune complex deposition. Focal and segmental glomerulonephritis have been documented in some cases[217] and have been associated with subendothelial electron-dense deposits and immunofluorescence evidence of IgG and C3 deposition. In addition, several studies of affected patients have found circulating immune complexes whose levels have shown some correlation with disease activity.[218] The etiology is unknown, but there has been speculation that it may be a virus.[219] Several investigators have also noted that attacks were precipitated by a variety of foods, especially walnuts.[220]

The principal pathologic abnormality is a transmural inflammatory infiltrate (predominantly lymphocytic) that can affect any or all pulmonary vessels from arteries to alveolar capillaries to large veins.[215, 219] The inflammatory process can be so marked as to result in aneurysmal dilatation and can extend into adjacent airways with bronchial artery erosion and resultant massive hemoptysis. Recent or organized thrombi and parenchymal infarcts may be present and may be related to either local vasculitis and thrombosis or thromboembolism secondary to systemic thrombophlebitis.[215]

Roentgenographic manifestations are varied and consist of focal or diffuse airspace opacities, reflecting infarction or hemorrhage. Proximal pulmonary arteries may be prominent; in one study, aneurysms were identified in 7 of 13 patients examined by angiography.[216]

Clinically, Behçet's disease is a systemic abnormality characterized by recurrent exacerbations and remissions.[221] Men are affected more often than women, and patients are generally 20 to 30 years old at diagnosis. The incidence is highest in the Middle East and Japan. In addition to the characteristic triad of uveitis and oral and genital ulcers, systemic disease can result in an assortment of skin lesions (including erythema nodosum), arthritis, thrombophlebitis, and various neurologic syndromes.

Pulmonary manifestations usually appear 3 to 4 years after the onset of systemic disease and are related to both thromboembolism and pulmonary vasculitis. Typically, they consist of recurrent episodes of hemoptysis, chest pain, dyspnea, and cough.[216] Obstructive airway disease, which sometimes is responsive to bronchodilator therapy, also has been noted.[222]

Essential Mixed Cryoglobulinemia

Essential mixed cryoglobulinemia is an uncommon disease characterized by purpura, arthralgia, glomerulonephritis, and the presence in the serum of globulins that precipitate on exposure to cold (cryoglobulins). Pulmonary involvement has been described in several clinicopathologic reports[223, 224] and in one series of 23 patients whose lung function was studied.[225] In that series, roentgenographic evidence of diffuse interstitial pulmonary disease was present in 18. Symptoms related to the chest, however, were unusual: one patient presented with hemoptysis, another with pleural pain, and a third with a clinical picture of asthma. Pulmonary function test results indicated small airway obstruction and an increase in the alveolar-arterial gradient for oxygen. Pathologic features have rarely been documented and appear to be variable.

Henoch-Schönlein Purpura

Henoch-Schönlein purpura is characterized by purpura, abdominal pain, gastrointestinal hemorrhage, arthritis or arthralgia, and glomerulonephritis. Although the disease appears most often during childhood or adolescence, it can occur at any age.[226] Many patients give a history of antecedent infection or drug ingestion, but no single factor has emerged as a likely etiology. Circulating and tissue-related immune complexes, most often containing IgA, have been identified in a number of cases, and it has been speculated that the disease results from activation of complement by IgA via the alternate pathway.[194]

Involvement of the respiratory tract is rare; in one review of 77 adults with the condition, only four patients were identified with evidence of pulmonary disease, and in none of these was a biopsy performed.[226] In the occasional fatal case in which the histologic appearance has been described, there has been leukocytoclastic vasculitis and intra-alveolar hemorrhage.[227]

Roentgenographic manifestations are typically those of bilateral airspace disease, reflecting intra-alveolar hemorrhage; however, the pattern may be predominantly interstitial in some cases.[228] Clinically, the disease is characterized by episodes of remission and relapse, typically ending with complete spontaneous resolution. Pulmonary involvement is manifested by hemoptysis.[227]

Leukocytoclastic Vasculitis

Leukocytoclastic vasculitis (microangiitis, hypersensitivity vasculitis, necrotizing alveolitis) is an uncommon pathologic reaction in the lung that is characterized by alveolar hemorrhage associated with inflammation and necrosis of small parenchymal vessels. It is important to recognize that the abnormality represents an unusual histologic reaction rather than a specific disease entity; some patients manifest features of the better-characterized vasculitides such as Wegener's granulomatosis[175] or Henoch-Schönlein purpura[229]; others have evidence of a connective tissue disease (usually SLE[15]) or drug hypersensitivity.[229]

There is a variety of evidence suggesting that the underlying pathogenetic mechanism is related to immune complex deposition. A histologic appearance similar to that of human disease has been produced experimentally in rats by intratracheal instillation of preformed immune complexes[230] and of horseradish peroxidase (in animals with circulating autologous anti–horseradish peroxidase antibodies).[231] In

addition, occasional patients have glomerulonephritis, some with electron microscopic and immunofluorescence evidence of immune complex deposition[232] and others with documented systemic necrotizing vasculitis.[229] Finally, in some patients, granular deposition of IgG and subepithelial electron-dense deposits consistent with immune complexes have been identified on the alveolar wall.[232] The reason for the localization of the tissue reaction in alveolar capillaries and adjacent interstitium with minimal involvement of larger vessels is not clear; presumably it relates to differences in antigen or in immunologic characteristics of the host.

Histologically, the lungs show extensive intra-alveolar hemorrhage and a neutrophilic infiltrate associated with edema, necrosis, and fibrin thrombi in the alveolar septa (Fig. 7–17). Arterioles and venules may be affected, but larger vessels typically are normal.

Roentgenographic features consist of patchy, bilateral airspace opacities caused by alveolar hemorrhage (see Fig. 7–15, page 413). Hemoptysis is common, and cough, chest pain, and shortness of breath may be present.[229] Other clinical and laboratory findings are quite variable, depending on the extent and nature of associated renal and systemic vascular involvement.

BRONCHOPULMONARY HYPERSENSITIVITY

A variety of inhaled organic particles can cause bronchopulmonary disease by inciting hypersensitivity reactions. The particular form of disease depends on the size and chemical nature of the inhaled particles as well as the immunoreactivity of the individual. The diseases produced include asthma (see page 635), allergic bronchopulmonary aspergillosis (see page 345), bronchocentric granulomatosis (BCG), byssinosis, and extrinsic allergic alveolitis.

Bronchocentric Granulomatosis

Bronchocentric granulomatosis is a descriptive term coined by Liebow in 1973 to refer to an uncommon histologic reaction involving chiefly small bronchi and bronchioles.[233] From a conceptual point of view, it is important to realize that it does not refer to a specific disease entity "but rather identifies a distinctive pathologic process [that] does not necessarily imply a uniform pathogenesis."[234] Some cases clearly represent active infection, usually by fungi or mycobacteria. In others, however, there is evidence that the histologic appearance represents an unusual hypersensitivity reaction to one of a variety of antigens; because of this, the condition is discussed at this point.

The characteristic and most prominent histologic feature is necrotizing granulomatous inflammation centered about the small airways (Fig. 7–18).[234] Early in the course of the disease, residual bronchiolar epithelium can often be identified on one portion of the airway wall, clearly establishing the bronchiolocentric nature of the process; in later stages, both the lining and underlying lamina propria are destroyed and replaced by a layer of palisaded epithelioid histiocytes that surrounds necrotic intraluminal debris. An infiltrate of plasma cells, lymphocytes, histiocytes, and eosinophils surrounds the layer of palisaded histiocytes.

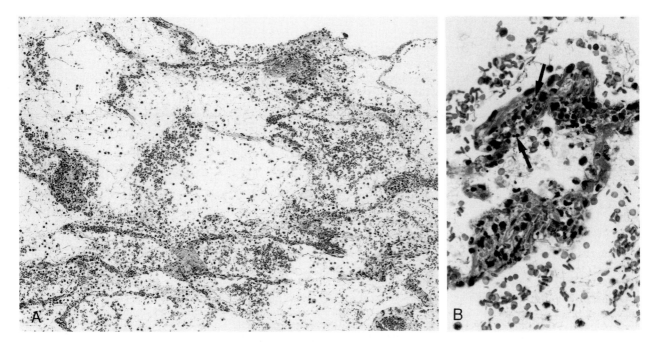

Figure 7–17. Pulmonary Leukocytoclastic Vasculitis. *A,* Section of lung parenchyma from a patient with hemoptysis and patchy, bilateral airspace opacities. Airspaces contain red blood cells and fibrin; an inflammatory cellular infiltrate is located predominantly around the alveolar septa. *B,* Magnified view showing intact and fragmented *(arrows)* leukocytes in the alveolar wall. (*A* × 100; *B* × 325.)

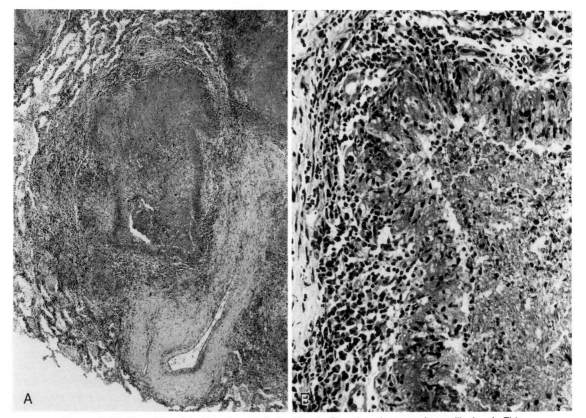

Figure 7–18. Bronchocentric Granulomatosis in Allergic Bronchopulmonary Aspergillosis. *A,* This specimen from an open lung biopsy from a 27-year-old asthmatic patient with ill-defined bilateral upper lobe opacification shows a large focus of necrotic material situated adjacent to a thick-walled pulmonary artery; no residual airway structure is apparent. *B,* Magnified view shows palisaded epithelioid histiocytes adjacent to the necrotic material and surrounded by abundant mononuclear inflammatory cells. Small fragments of degenerated fungal hyphae consistent with *Aspergillus* sp. were present within the necrotic material. (*A* × 40; *B* × 250.)

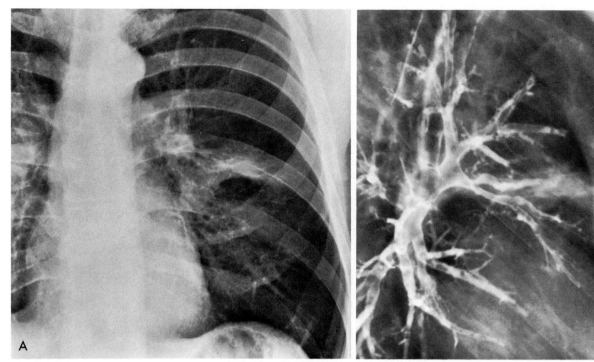

Figure 7–19. Bronchocentric Granulomatosis. A view of the left hemithorax from a posteroanterior roentgenogram *(A)* reveals a rather poorly defined opacity extending horizontally outward from the left hilum. At bronchography *(B)*, contrast medium fills a slightly dilated, irregular superior segmental bronchus of the lingula, the dilated airway being in the central portion of the opacity. In view of the uncertain nature of the lesion, thoracotomy was performed. Histologic examination of the resected specimen revealed occlusive granulomatous disease of the distal bronchi and bronchioles. (Courtesy of Dr. D. J. Willans and Dr. Archie MacPherson, Edmonton General Hospital, Edmonton, Alberta.)

The etiology of BCG is variable. Katzenstein and colleagues[234] delineated two groups of patients, one made up of young persons with prominent tissue and blood eosinophilia and a history of asthma and the other of patients without these features. In the asthmatic group, a hypersensitivity reaction was suggested in several cases by the finding of noninvasive fungal hyphae in the necrotic bronchiolar material and by the presence of serum precipitins to *Aspergillus* species and *Candida albicans*. In fact, many patients show the typical roentgenographic, clinical, and laboratory features of allergic bronchopulmonary aspergillosis (*see* page 345), and BCG is best regarded as one histologic manifestation of that condition.

Although the etiologic factors in the nonasthmatic group were less clear to Katzenstein and her colleagues, they speculated that a hypersensitivity reaction to an unidentified antigen might be responsible in these cases as well.[234] In support of this hypothesis is the observation that histologically typical BCG can occur with *Echinococcus* infestation, the reaction possibly being related to spillage of cystic contents into the airways.[235] Associations of BCG with rheumatoid disease,[236] ankylosing spondylitis,[237] glomerulonephritis,[238] and tuberculosis[239] also have been reported.

Roentgenographically, the manifestations of BCG are similar to those of bronchopulmonary aspergillosis and mucoid impaction, consisting of lobar and segmental consolidation and atelectasis, irregular masses, linear opacities, and shadows due to abnormal bronchi (Fig. 7–19).

Clinical findings are variable: of the 23 patients reported by Katzenstein and colleagues,[234] 10 were asthmatic and

their average age was 22 years; by contrast, the 13 nonasthmatics noted the onset of symptoms much later, at an average age of 50 years. Symptoms were present in the majority of patients and included dyspnea, cough, hemoptysis, malaise, and fever.

Byssinosis

Byssinosis is an unusual condition that occurs in workers engaged in the initial processing of cotton, flax, soft hemp, and sisal fibers[240] and is defined clinically by the presence of dyspnea, wheezing, and cough on return to work after a brief absence. Although traditionally considered a distinct entity, there is evidence that the condition should be considered a form of occupational asthma.[240a] By far the most important setting for exposure is cotton processing; the incidence of the disease in this industry is highest in cardroom and blowroom workers, who are exposed to the highest concentration of cotton dust and for whom the prevalence is between 5 per cent[241] and 15 per cent.[242] The disease also can develop in workers employed in spinning rooms,[242] in weavers who manufacture heavy cotton from unsized yarn,[243] and in cotton mill workers who process raw cotton into crude, thick lint.[244]

Other vegetable fiber dusts, including jute, Manila sisal, and several varieties of hard hemp, can cause pulmonary disease characterized by tightness in the chest and decreased flow rates during the day but without the typical clinical history of byssinosis.[245] The relationship of the abnormalities caused by these fibers to those of byssinosis is not clear.

Pathogenesis

The mechanism by which bronchoconstriction develops in byssinosis is not fully understood. Three substances have been suspected of inducing the symptoms.

The first is an uncharacterized chemical contained in water-soluble extract from cotton plant bracts. For more than a decade it has been recognized that inhalation of such an extract can cause reversible bronchoconstriction in non-byssinotic subjects as well as in patients with the disease.[246] The decrease in expiratory flow rates that characteristically follows exposure can be prevented by administration of either a bronchodilator or an antihistamine, and it can be reduced by beclomethasone dipropionate or sodium cromoglycate.[247] The fact that this substance is water-soluble explains the absence of the disease in workers who handle medical cotton that has been pretreated with alkali.

Contamination of the cotton plant with gram-negative bacteria and their endotoxin is a second potential mechanism. Support for this hypothesis is provided by the considerable variation in the prevalence of the disease in different mills[248] and by the fact that the decrease in FEV observed in affected workers correlates better with the number of cultured gram-negative bacteria[249] and with the endotoxin concentration[250] than with dust levels in the mills. Similar contamination of flax and soft hemp could explain the respiratory tract symptoms experienced by workers exposed to these vegetable fibers and the characteristic febrile reaction observed in some workers following initial heavy exposure to cotton ("mill fever").

The third incriminated substance is a polyphenol compound extracted from cotton dust whose action has been postulated to be mediated by an antigen-antibody reaction. The original proposal that this might be the etiologic agent was based partly on the reproduction of characteristic symptoms following inhalation challenge with this substance by patients with byssinosis and the absence of such symptoms in controls[251]; however, more recent attempts to confirm these findings have been unsuccessful.[252]

Pathologic Characteristics

Pathologic changes in the lungs of individuals with a history of long-standing byssinosis are those of chronic obstructive pulmonary disease. However, several reports in which autopsy findings have been compared in textile workers and unexposed controls have emphasized the absence of a significant excess of emphysema or bronchial abnormalities in persons exposed to cotton dust.[253, 254] "Byssinosis bodies," consisting of roughly spherical particles measuring up to 10 μm in diameter and possessing a central black spot and a peripheral clear halo, can be identified in a minority of cases; their nature and significance are unclear. Cotton fibers themselves are not found.

Roentgenographic Manifestations

Changes in the chest roentgenogram are negligible during reversible stages of the disease, as evidenced by one study in which the chest roentgenograms of symptomatic patients were indistinguishable from those of control subjects.[255] In advanced disease the findings are those of chronic bronchitis and emphysema; nothing specifically suggests the diagnosis of byssinosis.

Clinical Manifestations

The clinical history of patients with byssinosis is characterized by the gradual onset of dyspnea during the first day at work after an absence (usually a Monday) and is accompanied by cough, tightness in the chest, and general malaise. The Monday morning dyspnea correlates well with a decrease in the FEV_1; in fact, in some persons, exposure to the dust can result in a drop in FEV_1 without the development of symptoms.[256, 257] Physical findings are of limited value, although wheezing heard after a work shift may be helpful in suggesting the diagnosis.

In addition to these reversible functional abnormalities, physiologic evidence of chronic obstructive lung disease, usually mild, is present in some patients.[258] Some prefer to ascribe these findings to cigarette smoking while accepting a higher incidence of simple bronchitis[259]; others believe that retired workers have an increased incidence of irreversible obstructive disease[260] and that individuals with long-standing respiratory complaints associated with exposure to dust are considerably more responsive to provocation tests with cotton dust.[261]

Extrinsic Allergic Alveolitis

The term "extrinsic allergic alveolitis" (EAA, hypersensitivity pneumonitis, alveolar hypersensitivity) denotes a group of pulmonary diseases characterized by an inflammatory reaction to specific antigens contained in a variety of organic dusts. (An exception is disease caused by compounds of the inorganic chemical *di-isocyante*, which appears to be identical to that of organic dust EAA).[262] The condition occurs in two clinical forms: (1) an acute illness characterized by fever, dyspnea, cough, and malaise that resolves spontaneously following cessation of antigen exposure; and (2) an insidious, relatively asymptomatic disease that is usually recognized at a stage of irreversible interstitial fibrosis. Of these two forms, the first is by far the more common.

The list of causative antigens and corresponding "diseases" associated with EAA has increased steadily since "farmer's lung" was first clearly described in 1924[263] and now contains a multitude of conditions ranging from this entity, which is probably the most common and the most widely recognized, to such unusual conditions as pituitary snuff-taker's lung and hen-litter hypersensitivity (Table 7-1). Regardless of the name of the disease and the specific exposure involved, striking similarities exist among the clinical, pathologic, and roentgenologic features of all these diseases, suggesting that they share a common pathogenesis. Although many cases of EAA are associated with a specific occupational setting, inciting causes also can be found within the home or office.[264]

The exact criteria required to make the diagnosis of EAA are by no means clearly defined. The following list includes findings that, if all were observed, would definitely justify

Table 7–1. **VARIETIES OF EXTRINSIC ALLERGIC ALVEOLITIS**

Disease	Principal Responsible Antigen(s)	Exposure Source	Additional Feature(s)	Selected Reference(s)
Farmer's lung	Thermophilic bacteria *Micropolyspora faeni* *Thermoactinomyces* spp.	Moldy hay	Affects males aged 40–50 yr. Peak incidence during season when stored hay is used for cattle feeding. Acute illness in 1/3 of patients; insidious in remainder. Prevalence among farmers in different communities 1–10%	391, 392
Bagassosis	*Thermoactinomyces sacchari*	Moldy sugar cane residue (bagasse)		393–395
Mushroom-worker's lung	*Micropolyspora faeni* *Micromonospora vulgaris*	Compost used for mushroom culture	Steam pasturization during culture of mushroom encourages rapid growth of thermophylic actinomycetes	396
Humidifier lung	Bacteria: *Thermoactinomyces* spp. Fungi: *Penicillium* spp., *Cladosporium* Amebae: *Sphaeropsidales* spp., *Acanthamoeba castellani*, *Naegleria gruberi*	Air conditioners, humidifiers, damp floors or walls, hot tubs	May be difficult to diagnose because of obscurity of exposure history. Symptoms may develop in the evening of the first day back at work after a long weekend	397–400
Maple bark disease	*Cryptostroma corticale*	Tree bark	Affects sawmill workers	401
Malt-worker's lung	*Aspergillus clavatus*	Moldy malt		402
Japanese summer-type allergic alveolitis	*Trichosporum cutaneum*	House dust	Principal form of EAA in Japan; occurs in summer months and subsides in autumn	403
Domestic allergic alveolitis	Various fungi: (*Serpula*, *Paecilomyces*, *Aspergillus*, *Leucogyrophana*)	Decayed wood, damp walls	Prevalent in Australia	404
Suberosis	*Penicillium frequentans*, toluene di-isocyanate (?)	Moldy cork	Occurs principally in cork workers in Portugal. Evidence exists that the disease may coexist with asthma related to toluene di-isocyanate	405, 406
Wood pulp–worker's disease	*Alternaria* spp.	Wood pulp		407
Cheese-washer's lung	*Penicillium* spp.	Moldy cheese		408
Sequoiosis	*Aureobasidium pullulans* (?), *Graphium* spp. (?)	Moldy redwood sawdust		409
Oyster mushroom–worker's lung	*Pleurotus ostreatus*	Spores released during mushroom harvesting		410
New Guinea lung	*Streptomyces viridis* (?)	Thatched roofs		411
Detergent-worker's lung	*Bacillus subtilis*	Exposure occurs during manufacture of proteolytic enzyme by *B. subtilis* for use in detergents		412
Bird-fancier's (pigeon-breeder's) lung	Avian proteins contained in serum, excreta, or feathers	Pigeons, budgerigars, canaries, parakeets, chickens, ducks, turkeys, geese	With farmer's lung, the most common form of EAA	413–416
Pituitary snuff-taker's lung	Pig or ox pituitary extract	Extract used for treatment of diabetes insipidus		417
Prawn-worker's lung	Shellfish protein (?)	Forced air used to blow meat out of tails		418
Fishmeal-worker's lung	Fish protein (?)	Preparation of meat		419
Coffee-worker's lung	?	Coffee bean roasting		420

inclusion of a condition in the group of extrinsic allergic alveolitides; confidence in the diagnosis diminishes as the number of these findings decreases, particularly with respect to the first seven.

1. A history of exposure to an organic dust of sufficiently small particle size to penetrate into the lung parenchyma

2. Episodes of dyspnea, frequently accompanied by a dry cough, fever, and malaise, occurring some hours after exposure to the relevant antigen

3. Roentgenologic findings of a diffuse reticulonodular or nodular pattern, commonly associated in the acute stage with an airspace component

4. Pulmonary function tests revealing a reduction in vital capacity, carbon monoxide diffusing capacity, arterial oxygen pressure (PO_2), and static compliance

5. The development, some hours after aerosol provocation by the specific antigen, of appropriate symptoms, with or without impairment of pulmonary function and the appearance of abnormalities on the chest roentgenogram

6. The presence on lung biopsy of bronchiolitis and interstitial pneumonitis with granuloma formation

7. Resolution of the episodic systemic and respiratory symptoms after cessation of exposure to the antigen

8. Crepitations heard by auscultation over the lung bases bilaterally

9. A "late" (Arthus) or delayed hypersensitivity reaction after intracutaneous injection of the appropriate antigen

10. The presence in the serum of precipitins against the suspected antigen and their disappearance after cessation of exposure

11. The demonstration *in vitro* of blastogenesis and the production of migration inhibitory factor on stimulation of lymphocytes with specific antigens

12. The finding in fluid obtained on BAL of an increased number of T lymphocytes, predominantly of the suppressor type, and an increased level of immunoglobulins

Pathogenesis

The development of EAA depends on the size, immunogenicity, and number of inhaled organic particles and on the immune response of the affected host. Although precise figures are not available for many antigens, a large amount of inhaled particles is probably necessary to provide a strong stimulus for a hyperimmune response, particularly in the acute form of disease. Investigations of situations known to lead to EAA have shown this to be the case; for example, it has been estimated that there are as many as 500 million fungal spores per gram of moldy bagasse![265]

Most investigations of host immune response in EAA have focused on type III (immune complex) and type IV (cell-mediated) mechanisms. Immune complex disease has been suggested by a variety of clinical and experimental observations, including (1) the typical onset of disease 4 to 6 hours after exposure; (2) the occasional demonstration by immunofluorescence studies of the presence of antigen and antibodies in the bronchioles or pulmonary vessels[266] of acutely ill patients; (3) the association of late-onset skin reactions with complement consumption[267] and with skin biopsy–proven vasculitis and immunoglobulin and complement deposition[268]; (4) the ability to passively transfer Ar-

thus skin reactivity to laboratory animals with serum from affected patients[265]; and (5) the observation that animals depleted of complement by cobra venom factor prior to antigen challenge have a significant reduction in the number of histologic lesions characteristic of EAA.[269]

Specific IgG, IgA, and IgM antibodies can be detected by immunoprecipitation or by ELISA[270] in many patients with EAA. Titers of these antibodies are generally higher in symptomatic than asymptomatic persons and decrease with clinical improvement[271] and following removal from the source of antigen.[272] There is also a relationship between the presence of a positive precipitation reaction and the rapidity of clinical presentation, a positive reaction being detected in virtually all patients with acute disease but in only about half of those with more chronic disease.[273]

Although these observations suggest a specific role for precipitating antibodies in the pathogenesis of EAA, it is clear that they cannot be the sole factor, since it is now well recognized that the majority of patients who have been exposed to organic dust and whose serum contains precipitins are asymptomatic.[274] In fact, in the population at large there is a high prevalence of antibodies to ubiquitous organic materials such as house dust, human dandruff, and thermophilic actinomycetes[275]; individuals with precipitins to such organic antigens are no more likely to have symptoms of EAA than those who are seronegative. In addition, epidemiologic studies have shown that a change in precipitin status, from either positive to negative or vice versa, is not associated with the development or amelioration of symptoms.[276] These observations have led some authorities to conclude that precipitins do not play a pathogenic role in this disease.[277]

The results of a variety of experimental animal and clinical studies have also suggested that a type IV delayed hypersensitivity reaction is involved in the pathogenesis of EAA. For example, acute pneumonitis has been produced in several animals in response to the inhalation of aerosolized antigens implicated in human EAA, including bagasse and *Micropolyspora faeni*.[278] Such disease is characterized by abnormalities of cell-mediated immunity, including proliferation of macrophages and the presence of macrophage inhibition factor in BAL fluid. Also supporting this hypothesis is the typical presence of granulomatous inflammation in human biopsy specimens.

Although a type IV mechanism thus seems likely to be involved in EAA, the details of the process are undoubtably complex. For example, repeated intratracheal injection of *M. faeni* into rabbits results in a diminution in both pulmonary histologic abnormalities and the amount of serum antibody directed toward *M. faeni*, findings that are not associated with a reduction in lymphocyte reactivity to antigen or in local specific antibody levels.[278] This unexpected observation may be at least partly explained by the results of studies of BAL fluid in human EAA. In this situation, antigen challenge results in an alveolitis that is initially neutrophilic but then becomes lymphocytic.[279] Both patients with active EAA and asymptomatic individuals simply exposed to the implicated antigen manifest a striking increase in the number of lymphocytes in BAL fluid compared with normal subjects; these cells are predominantly T8+ suppressor cells. With avoidance of further antigen exposure, the number of suppressor cells decreases and the number of helper cells increases. Furthermore, in one study in which symptomatic and asymptomatic bird breeders with equal lymphocyte proliferation of BAL T8+ cells were compared, there was a distinct difference between the two groups with respect to the results of their *in vitro* BAL lymphocyte tests of cell-mediated immunity, indicating a discrepancy between the phenotype and function of immunoregulatory T cell subsets.[280] Different forms of cytotoxic lymphocytes may also be related to these differences.[281]

The number of mast cells in BAL fluid is much greater in patients with acute EAA than in controls; on the basis of this observation, it has been suggested that mast cell degranulation may play a role in regulating the number of immune and inflammatory cells in the lung[282] or in fibroblastic activation.[283]

A highly significant positive correlation has been reported between lack of cigarette smoking and both the development of active EAA[284] and specific serum antibodies.[285] Although these observations are unexplained, they could be due to a protective factor in smoker's cough that cleanses the airways of antigen, or, perhaps more likely, to a depressant action of inhaled tobacco ingredients on alveolar macrophages that makes smokers less immunocompetent.

The precise reasons why some individuals develop acute, symptomatic EAA and others manifest insidious, relatively asymptomatic disease are not clear. Presumably they are related to variations in the concentration of antigen to which a person is exposed, the frequency of antigen exposure, and individual immune responses. Although the effect of variable dust exposure is difficult to ascertain in many cases, it appears to be clear in others. For example, pigeon breeders usually suffer acute symptoms that develop 4 to 6 hours after exposure to the antigen,[286] whereas budgerigar fanciers, whose exposure to antigen in the home tends to be continuous and in lower concentrations than those to which pigeon breeders are exposed, tend to develop the insidious form of the disease.[287]

Pathologic Characteristics

The histologic features of the different varieties of EAA are strikingly similar and, with few exceptions (such as suberosis, in which cork dust may be identified[289]), do not permit identification of the etiologic agent. During the acute stage of disease, the histologic appearance consists of a combination of bronchiolitis and alveolitis with granuloma formation.[290, 291] The alveolitis is manifested by both interstitial and intra-alveolar components. Within the interstitium, there is an inflammatory infiltrate that consists predominantly of lymphocytes (Fig. 7–20); it is usually patchy in distribution, with a tendency to more severe involvement

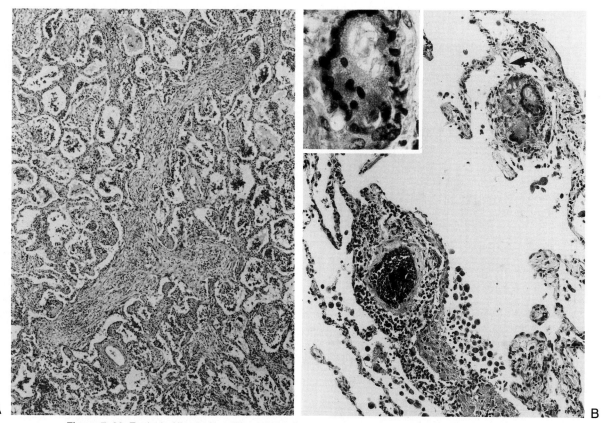

Figure 7–20. **Extrinsic Allergic Alveolitis.** *A,* Magnified view of an open lung biopsy shows a moderate degree of interstitial pneumonitis and a branching plug of fibroblastic tissue occluding the lumen of several transitional airways (bronchiolitis obliterans). No granulomata are evident. *B,* Section from a less severely affected patient shows that a perivascular lymphocytic infiltrate surrounds a small vessel and extends into the adjacent alveolar interstitium. A single granuloma is present *(arrow).* Note the foreign material present within the multinucleated giant cells, seen to better advantage in the magnified inset. (*A* × 50; *B* × 100; *inset* × 480.)

of peribronchiolar regions. Within alveolar airspaces, a similar cellular infiltrate is frequently present; foamy macrophages also are prominent in some cases, probably as a consequence of airway obstruction secondary to bronchiolitis obliterans. Evidence of alveolar epithelial and capillary endothelial damage, consisting either of intra-alveolar proteinaceous material or of loose intra-alveolar fibroblastic tissue, is seen in about two thirds of cases.

Granulomas composed of epithelioid cells or clusters of multinucleated giant cells are present in 65 to 75 per cent of cases. Unlike the granulomas typical of sarcoidosis, those of EAA are often somewhat irregular in shape and poorly defined at their periphery, without surrounding fibrosis. Birefringent foreign material is frequently present within the granulomas or in isolated multinucleated giant cells (see Fig. 7–20). Bronchiolitis is also a common finding, being observed in half of the 60 cases of farmer's lung in one review,[290] and showing an overall prevalence ranging from 25 to 100 per cent in different series. The usual pattern consists of an organizing exudate or mass of loose connective tissue adjacent to a focus of epithelial ulceration (bronchiolitis obliterans).

Depending on the severity and frequency of the individual episodes of lung damage, interstitial fibrosis may supervene. As in the acute inflammatory stage, the fibrosis is at first mild and patchy in distribution at the microscopic level, but eventually it progresses into grossly visible scars.[290] These also can be patchy and irregular in shape, with prominence in peribronchial or periseptal areas, or

may be diffuse and relatively uniform, resembling advanced idiopathic interstitial fibrosis with honeycombing.

Roentgenographic Manifestations

As with the pathologic manifestations, the roentgenographic changes vary with the stage of EAA. Early in the course of acute disease, the chest roentgenogram may show no discernible abnormality.[292] Once they are visible, abnormalities usually parallel the severity of the clinical symptoms,[293] the impairment of pulmonary function, and the cellular composition of BAL fluid.[294] (Despite this, it is important to remember that roentgenographic changes consistent with the diagnosis occasionally are present in the absence of clinical symptoms.[295])

The most common roentgenographic abnormality consists of a reticular or reticulonodular pattern involving both lungs diffusely without zonal predominance. When present, nodules range from less than 1 mm to several mm in diameter and are sometimes so numerous as to create a ground-glass opacity (Fig. 7–21). The reticulonodular pattern is characteristic of the subacute stage of the disease, usually seen between acute episodes. In the acute stage (shortly after heavy exposure to the appropriate antigen), acinar shadows are commonly present, particularly in the lower lung zones (Fig. 7–22). Such airspace consolidation may be quite extensive and may obscure the reticular or nodular pattern characteristic of the subacute stage. Within a few days after removal from the source of antigen expo-

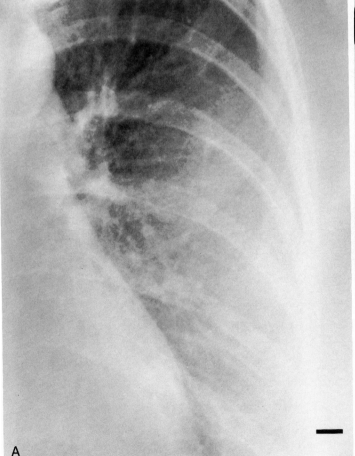

A

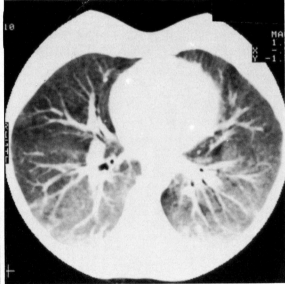

B

Figure 7–21. Extrinsic Allergic Alveolitis (Farmer's Lung). A detail view of the left lung from a posteroanterior chest roentgenogram *(A)* reveals a ground-glass opacity or fine reticulation that shows considerable lower zonal predominance. Identical features were seen in the right lung *(not shown)*. (Bar = 1 cm.) *B,* A CT scan through the lower zone demonstrates a ground-glass increase in CT density involving both the cortex and the medulla, more marked in the latter. The patient is a young woman who presented with progressive dyspnea following an unusually heavy exposure to moldy hay.

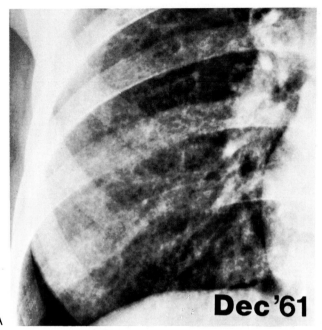 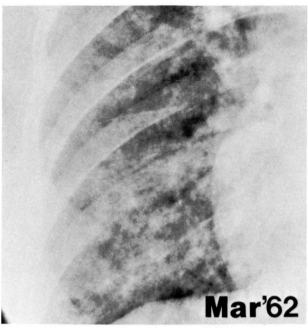

Figure 7–22. Extrinsic Allergic Alveolitis (Farmer's Lung). This 25-year-old woman, the wife of a farmer, was admitted to the hospital with a 2-week history of moderate dyspnea, mildly productive cough, and daily temperature rise to 103° F. A detail view of the lower half of the right lung *(A)* reveals a coarse reticulonodular pattern. She was placed on antibiotic therapy, and over the next 5 or 6 days her temperature gradually returned to normal. Three months after her original acute episode, she was admitted for a second time following the acute onset of dyspnea, cough, and high fever. The chest roentgenogram at this time *(B)* revealed definite extension of the disease, an acinar pattern being superimposed on the reticulonodular pattern seen earlier.

sure, the acinar pattern resolves, once again permitting identification of the reticulonodular pattern. This sequence of roentgenologic changes should strongly suggest the diagnosis of EAA. The absence of hilar lymph node enlargement is an important feature that distinguishes this disease from others with which it can be confused roentgenographically, particularly sarcoidosis.[296] CT examination of patients in both acute and subacute stages reveals airspace and interstitial patterns similar to those seen on conventional roentgenograms.[297]

The subsequent course of the roentgenographic changes depends on whether exposure to the antigen continues. If the patient is removed from antigen exposure, the chest roentgenogram may return to normal in 10 days to several weeks. If exposure is continued or repeated or if the initial exposure is especially severe, the diffuse nodular pattern characteristic of the acute and subacute stages may be replaced by changes characteristic of diffuse interstitial fibrosis—a medium to coarse reticular pattern, loss of lung volume, a honeycomb pattern, and sometimes compensatory overinflation of lung zones that are least affected. The loss of lung volume tends to show a striking upper zone predominance (Fig. 7–23).[298]

Clinical Manifestations

Intermittent exposure of susceptible individuals to high concentrations of antigen is accompanied by recurrent episodes of fever, chills, dry cough, and dyspnea, whereas continuous exposure to lower concentrations characteristically results in gradually progressive dyspnea in the absence of detectable systemic symptoms.[299] In a small number of patients, usually those with a history of allergy, the clinical presentation may suggest asthma.[300] Chronic bronchitis has been documented in 25 per cent of patients and occasionally is the sole clinical manifestation of disease.[301]

There are no physical findings that aid in the diagnosis. Auscultatory examination of the chest may or may not reveal crackles or a peculiar inspiratory "squawk,"[302] findings that are attributable to the opening up of airways of various sizes and which are common to many interstitial and bronchiolar diseases. Clubbing of fingers has been noted in as many as 50 per cent of patients in some studies and has been considered to be an unfavorable prognostic sign.[303]

Perhaps the most important step in diagnosis of EAA is meticulous history-taking in an attempt to uncover a possible source of environmental dust exposure coincident with the development of acute respiratory symptoms. This is usually fairly straightforward in patients with EAA related to specific occupations, such as farming; however, in disease caused by exposure to antigen in the home or office building, identification of dust exposure may be quite difficult. In these cases, the antigenic material (usually molds) may originate in air conditioners, humidifiers, or even on the walls of the building.[264] Undoubtedly, many patients with such exposure are misdiagnosed as having mycoplasmal or viral disease, and it is only when it is recognized that the attacks are intermittent and repeated and occur on returning home from the hospital or on starting work each Monday morning that the correct diagnosis is suspected. The diagnosis is supported by subsidence of the disease on removal of the patient from the presumed source of expo-

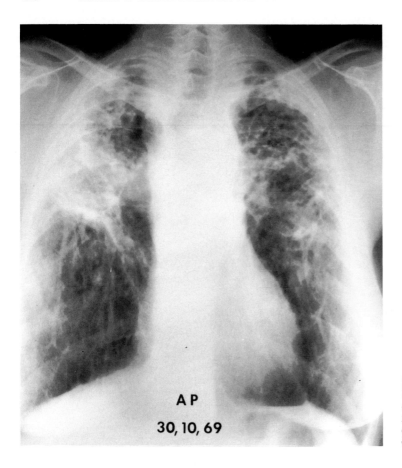

AP

30, 10, 69

Figure 7–23. Extrinsic Allergic Alveolitis (Bird-Fancier's Lung). A posteroanterior chest roentgenogram reveals a coarse reticulation that shows marked upper and middle zonal predominance. Emphysematous changes are present in the lower lobes. The patient is a 61-year-old woman with a long history of exposure to household birds.

sure; however, confirmation may necessitate inhalation challenge testing with the suspected material (*see* later on).

Although the pathologic manifestations of EAA are confined to the lungs, an association has been noted between the abnormality and celiac disease. For example, in one study,[304] jejunal biopsies were performed on 14 patients with bird-fancier's lung because of symptoms and results of special investigations that suggested malabsorption; villous atrophy was found in five. The pathogenetic basis of this association is uncertain; however, it is possible that malabsorption in patients with celiac disease results in pulmonary alveolar sensitization by permitting increased entrance of an antigen through the gastrointestinal tract.

Laboratory Findings

A useful diagnostic procedure considered to reflect both type I and type III immune reactions is the allergen inhalation (provocation) test, or challenge test. Reactions to aerosolized extracts of the appropriate antigen or directly to the suspected source of antigen (e.g., from a pet bird brought into the laboratory[305]) may be immediate, late, or dual in terms of their time of appearance. *Immediate reactions* are classically seen in atopic individuals exposed to specific antigens to which they have become sensitized[306]; they develop within minutes of the inhalation challenge and resolve spontaneously within 1 to 3 hours. In asthmatic patients the immediate response consists of bronchospasm without associated systemic features such as fever and leukocytosis. *Late reactions* become manifest 4 to 6 hours after inhalation, progress to maximal intensity more slowly, and

usually resolve within 24 to 48 hours; they may be associated with some degree of bronchospasm but the pulmonary function pattern is usually restrictive rather than obstructive. Systemic symptoms include fever, chills, malaise, and anorexia. Provocation tests are positive not only in patients with a history of recurrent acute attacks but also in those with the more insidious form of the disease. Immediate reactions can be inhibited by beta-receptor stimulants and by disodium cromoglycate administered before the allergen challenge, but not by corticosteroids. The latter drugs do inhibit late reactions. In *dual reactions*, the immediate response resolves before the appearance of symptoms associated with the late reaction. In patients with EAA, a dual reaction is less common than a late reaction alone. Almost all patients who manifest either dual or late reactions to inhalation challenge have serum precipitins to the appropriate antigen. In addition, positive responses correlate closely with results of skin testing.[306]

Generally speaking, other laboratory tests are not particularly useful in confirming a diagnosis of EAA. Neutrophilia with a shift to the left may be seen in acute-onset cases or following provocation antigen testing. In two studies of patients with farmer's[307] and pigeon breeder's lung,[308] serum angiotensin-converting enzyme levels were found to be normal. Nonspecific delayed cutaneous hypersensitivity is commonly impaired.[309]

Pulmonary Function Tests

The overall pattern of pulmonary function tests in the acute stage is one of restrictive disease, reflecting the interstitial thickening seen pathologically.[310] Typically, there is a slight to moderate reduction in FEV_1 that is proportional to a decrease in vital capacity and a reduction in static compliance and diffusing capacity.[311] In addition, some patients show evidence of small airway obstruction, as reflected by the air trapping demonstrated by a comparison of gas dilution and plethysmographic methods of measuring lung volume.[312] Such changes presumably are related to the presence of bronchiolitis. Removal of patients from their hazardous environment frequently results in restoration of pulmonary function to normal, but in some cases it continues to be impaired even after the chest roentgenogram has returned to normal.

Prognosis

The prognosis is generally good for patients whose disease is recognized in its early stages and who are removed from exposure to antigen[313] (although there is some evidence that this may not be the case in older individuals[304]). In patients who do well, most of the clinical improvement occurs during the first few months, and very little after 6 months.[314] In the more insidious cases, considerable fibrosis can develop before the cause is detected, and the patient may have incurred some degree of permanent pulmonary insufficiency.

The natural history of the disease in individuals who are recognized as having EAA and who continue to be exposed to the culpable antigen is not as clear. In some studies,[315] a progressive decline in pulmonary function has been demonstrated, whereas in others[316] clinical symptoms and pulmonary function have been found to remain stable or even improve.

EOSINOPHILIC LUNG DISEASE

Pulmonary disease affecting the major airways or parenchyma (or both) associated with either blood or tissue eosinophilia (or both) comprises a group of conditions so diverse as to render logical classification exceedingly difficult. Despite this, Crofton and associates[317] formulated a classification of these diseases in 1952 based on clinical characteristics; more recently, this was modified by Citro and colleagues,[318] who used as their basis combined clinical and roentgenologic features. These authors employed the term "eosinophilic lung disease" to categorize these entities, and we feel that this term obviates some of the problems of nomenclature.

The classification we have employed (Table 7–2) is a modification and extension of the one formulated by Citro and associates and includes three groups of conditions whose etiologic, clinical, roentgenologic, and pathologic features differ.

1. Conditions of unknown etiology that are characterized roentgenographically by foci of local, nonsegmental, usually peripheral parenchymal consolidation, sometimes transient and sometimes prolonged, associated with blood eosinophilia. These conditions range from the relatively benign Löffler's syndrome through the more severe acute and chronic eosinophilic pneumonias to the systemic and potentially fatal entity known as hypereosinophilic syndrome
2. Conditions in which a specific endogenous or exogenous etiology, including drugs, parasites, and fungi, can be recognized
3. Conditions associated with the systemic connective tissue diseases or vasculitis

Table 7–2. **EOSINOPHILIC LUNG DISEASE**

Main Classification	Subclassification	Disease or Specific Agent	Selected References
Idiopathic eosinophilic lung disease		Idiopathic Löffler's syndrome	319, 320
		Acute eosinophilic pneumonia	322
		Chronic eosinophilic pneumonia	325, 326
		Hypereosinophilic syndrome	331
Eosinophilic lung disease of specific etiology	Drug-induced	Nitrofurantoin	421
		Penicillin	422
		Sulfonamides	423
		Mecamylamine	425
		Nonsteroidal anti-inflammatory agents	426
		Aminosalicylic acid	427
		Para-aminosalicylic acid	428
		Imipramine	429
		Trimipramine	430
		Hydrochlorothiazide	431
		Cromolyn sodium	432
	Parasite-induced	Ascariasis	433
		Paragonomiasis	434
		Strongyloidiasis	See page 372
		Tropical eosinophilia	See page 374
		Pulmonary larva migrans	435
		Schistosomiasis	436
		Ancylostomiasis	437
	Fungus-induced	Allergic bronchopulmonary aspergillosis	See page 345
		Allergic bronchopulmonary disease caused by other fungi	438, 439
Eosinophilic lung disease with connective tissue disease and/or vasculitis		Rheumatoid disease	
		Wegener's granulomatosis	
		Allergic granulomatosis	
		Polyarteritis nodosa	

We emphasize that this section does not include all pulmonary diseases associated with eosinophilia, only those whose pathogenesis appears to be predominantly allergic or immune-mediated. Similarly, we do not wish to imply that all the eosinophilic lung diseases can be fitted into specific slots as listed in the classification; as in many other disorders of immunoreactivity, considerable overlap occurs among entities and one must exercise caution in attempting to apply a specific label to a clinical and roentgenologic presentation that may defy precise categorization.

Löffler's Syndrome

Löffler's syndrome is an uncommon abnormality in which local nonsegmental areas of parenchymal consolidation, usually transient, are associated with blood eosinophilia. Although the diagnosis can be made only on the basis of positive roentgenologic findings, it should be suspected whenever blood eosinophilia develops in a patient with a background of atopy. The syndrome may occur without any inciting extrinsic factor, or its onset may be related to fungal infection, parasitic infestation, drug therapy, or any of a variety of miscellaneous causes. In all these circumstances, we prefer to use the more precise etiologic designations listed in Table 7–2.

Because of its benign and transient nature, the pathology of the parenchymal consolidation has been documented only rarely; in the few cases in which biopsy has been reported, there was interstitial and alveolar edema admixed with a large number of eosinophilic leukocytes.[319]

Roentgenographically, areas of consolidation may be single or multiple and are typically homogeneous in density, ill-defined, and nonsegmental in distribution in the lung periphery (Fig. 7–24). The transient and shifting nature of the consolidation is a characteristic feature, but the term "fleeting" perhaps exaggerates the rapidity with which change may occur. We have observed several cases in which very little change was seen over several days. Even a slight decrease in the size of one area of parenchymal consolidation over a 24-hour period, if associated with a new area of consolidation elsewhere, is highly suggestive of the diagnosis in the appropriate clinical background.

In some cases the syndrome is not associated with symptoms, and it may be detected only when the patient is referred for roentgenographic examination for investigation of asthma. Conversely, symptoms may be severe, with high fever and dyspnea requiring immediate corticosteroid therapy for relief.[320] A dry or mildly productive cough is often noted, but it may be due to underlying asthma.

Leukocytosis is common, to a total white cell count of more than 20,000 cells per mL; an increase in eosinophils is responsible for most of this elevation. When pulmonary parenchymal involvement is extensive, results of function tests usually indicate restrictive insufficiency, with arterial oxygen desaturation and a decrease in diffusing capacity.[321]

Acute Eosinophilic Pneumonia

Acute eosinophilic pneumonia is a recently described condition that differs from the chronic form of disease in its abrupt onset, rapid development of respiratory distress associated with severe hypoxemia, diffuse interstitial and airspace disease on chest roentgenography, and a rapid and apparently complete response to corticosteroid therapy.[322,323] The etiology and pathogenesis are unknown, although a hypersensitivity reaction to one or more inciting agents has been hypothesized. Occasional cases have been identified in immunocompromised patients.[324] Transbronchial biopsy specimens have shown alveolar interstitial and airspace inflammation with prominent eosinophils. Bronchoalveolar lavage also reveals abundant eosinophils (20 to 50 per cent) and has been recommended as a method of diagnosis. Blood eosinophilia may or may not be present.

Chronic Eosinophilic Pneumonia

This is an uncommon disorder that has a more protracted clinical and roentgenologic course than either acute eosinophilic pneumonia or Löffler's syndrome. Approximately 120 cases had been reported by 1988.[325] As in Löffler's syndrome, an atopic background (particularly asthma) is common. Females are affected more than twice as often as males; about half of the cases occur between 30 and 50 years of age.

Although the precise etiology and pathogenesis are unknown, an autoimmune or hypersensitivity reaction has been strongly implicated. In our experience and that of others,[326] there appears to be an association with therapeutic desensitization to a variety of allergens; however, no consistent agent has been identified. It has been speculated that tissue damage may be related to the release of substances within eosinophil granules, possibly in response to locally deposited immune complexes.[327] High levels of circulating IgE have been reported during peak disease activity, which return to normal during remissions,[328] with or without treatment, suggesting that the abnormality may be reagin-mediated.

The most characteristic pathologic feature is massive infiltration of alveolar airspaces by a mixed inflammatory infiltrate containing a large proportion of eosinophils.[326] Although necrosis of lung parenchyma is unusual, eosinophilic "abscesses," consisting of aggregates of necrotic eosinophils surrounded by a rim of palisaded histiocytes, are often seen. Small airway epithelium may be ulcerated and associated with bronchiolitis obliterans, a finding possibly related to the development of obstructive airway disease in some cases.

Roentgenologically, the typical pattern is identical to that of Löffler's syndrome, consisting of nonsegmental homogeneous consolidation in the lung periphery (Fig. 7–25). Compared with the transitory and migratory character of the consolidation in Löffler's syndrome, however, the lesions of chronic eosinophilic pneumonia tend to persist unchanged for many days or even weeks unless corticosteroid therapy is instituted. Although this appearance is highly suggestive of the diagnosis, it should be remembered that it occurs in fewer than half the patients.[325] In fact, in many patients, peripheral predominance is not identified, the consolidation being most marked in the middle and upper lung zones.[329]

Clinically, the majority of patients are only mildly affected or are completely asymptomatic; however, some have severe symptoms, including high fever, malaise, weight loss, cough, and dyspnea.

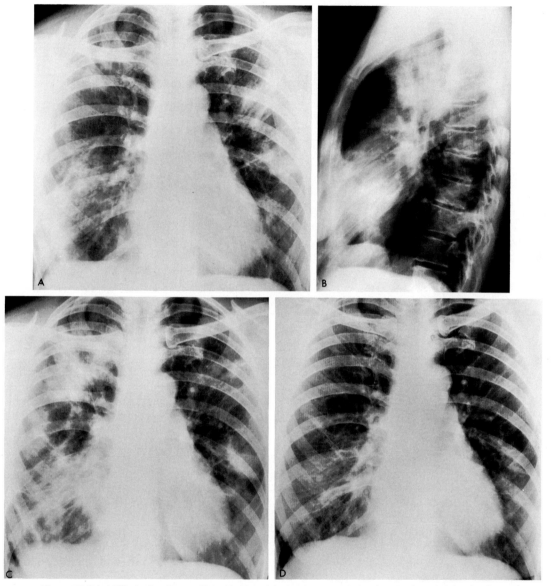

Figure 7–24. Löffler's Syndrome. This 61-year-old woman was admitted to the hospital for the first time with a 2-month history of anorexia, a 10-pound weight loss, afternoon fever, and mild cough productive of greenish phlegm occasionally flecked with blood; there was no history of allergies. On admission, posteroanterior (A) and lateral (B) roentgenograms revealed numerous shadows of homogeneous density in both lungs, occupying no precise segmental distribution; note particularly the broad shadow of increased density along the lower axillary zone of the right lung. At this time her total white cell count was 11,000 per mL with 1700 (15 per cent) eosinophils. One week later (C), the anatomic distribution of the shadows had changed considerably, being more extensive in the right upper and both lower lobes and less extensive in the left upper lobe; at this time the total white cell count was 14,000 per mL with 20 per cent eosinophils. A diagnosis of Löffler's syndrome was made, and the institution of ACTH therapy resulted in prompt remission of symptoms. One week later the white cell count had returned to normal levels, the eosinophilia had disappeared, and the roentgenographic abnormalities had completely resolved (D).

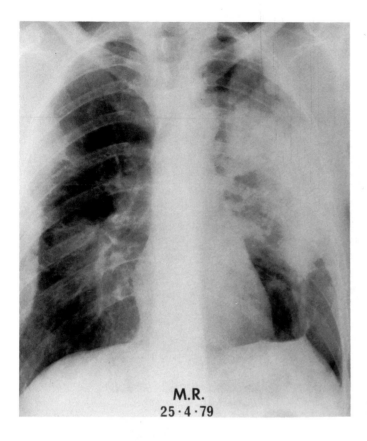

M.R.
25·4·79

Figure 7–25. Chronic Eosinophilic Pneumonia. A posteroanterior chest roentgenogram reveals peripherally located subpleural airspace consolidation in both lungs, more marked on the left.

Laboratory investigation reveals blood eosinophilia greater than 6 per cent in about 90 per cent of patients; however, the absence of eosinophilia should not exclude the diagnosis when clinical and roentgenographic findings are compatible.[326] In the appropriate clinical and roentgenologic setting, the diagnosis can be confirmed by demonstration of numerous eosinophils in BAL fluid.[201] Pulmonary function tests show a restrictive pattern with reduced diffusing capacity and impaired gas exchange, accompanied in some cases during the acute phase by severe hypoxemia; following remission, there may be evidence of small airway obstruction or residual reduction in diffusion.[327]

Response to corticosteroid therapy is often dramatic, with rapid roentgenographic resolution and clinical improvement. However, many patients require prolonged therapy lasting for months or even years; similarly, exacerbations are common when corticosteroids are reduced or stopped.[330] Despite these features, there is little evidence that the disease results in chronic pulmonary insufficiency.[325]

Hypereosinophilic Syndrome

Hypereosinophilic syndrome (HES) is an uncommon and poorly understood condition characterized by prolonged blood eosinophilia and multiple organ dysfunction.[331] The etiology usually is unknown (idiopathic HES) and is probably multifactorial. In one series of 50 patients, 35 (70 per cent) noted the onset of disease between the ages of 20 and 50 years (mean, 33 years).[331] Although the sex incidence was not revealed in this series, other authors have noted a male predominance.[332]

The principal organs affected in HES are the heart (manifested by valvular fibrosis with regurgitation) and nervous system (with meningitis, peripheral neuropathies, and behavioral or cognitive abnormalities). Direct involvement of the respiratory system is relatively uncommon but can take several forms, including vascular infiltration by eosinophils and interstitial fibrosis.

Chest roentgenograms may reveal transient airspace opacities that can resolve spontaneously and are sometimes associated with bronchospasm. At a stage when other organs are involved, an interstitial pattern has been described, presumably caused by perivascular eosinophilic infiltration or fibrosis.[331, 333] Cardiac decompensation is manifested by cardiomegaly, pulmonary edema, and pleural effusion.

Initial symptoms are nonspecific, and the diagnosis is often considered only when leukocytosis and eosinophilia are detected. Cough and dyspnea may reflect either pulmonary or cardiac involvement (or both).

MISCELLANEOUS CONDITIONS OF ALTERED IMMUNOLOGIC ACTIVITY

Goodpasture's Syndrome and Idiopathic Pulmonary Hemorrhage

Both of these diseases are characterized by repeated episodes of pulmonary hemorrhage, iron-deficiency anemia, and, in long-standing cases, pulmonary insufficiency; Goodpasture's syndrome includes glomerulonephritis as well as the pulmonary manifestations. In addition to this important clinical distinction, the epidemiology of the two conditions also differs: idiopathic pulmonary hemorrhage (IPH) occurs most commonly in children, usually those younger than 10 years of age, and shows no sex predominance; by contrast, Goodpasture's syndrome is a disease of young adults and shows a striking male predominance.[334]

A short discussion of terminology is appropriate before considering the specific manifestations of these entities in greater detail. The term "Goodpasture's syndrome" is still used by some to include disease in any patient in whom hemoptysis is associated with hematuria.[335] However, since this combination can be seen in several other disease entities, most authorities agree that this practice inevitably results in confusion and that the eponym should be reserved for disease characterized by the presence of anti–basement membrane antibodies and evidence of pulmonary hemorrhage. Since hemorrhage is the primary abnormality in IPH and since hemosiderosis is only part of the pathologic consequences of the disease (and sometimes only a very minor part) we prefer *idiopathic pulmonary hemorrhage* to the more traditional "hemosiderosis."

Etiology and Pathogenesis

There is abundant evidence that the pathogenesis of both renal and pulmonary lesions in Goodpasture's syndrome is related to an antibody that cross-reacts with alveolar basement membrane (ABM) and glomerular basement membrane (GBM). Circulating antibodies against both basement membranes have been found repeatedly, and immunofluorescence studies have demonstated the presence of IgG (and frequently complement) in a linear pattern in renal glomeruli and pulmonary alveoli (Fig. 7–26).[336] Moreover, acid elution of the kidneys of patients with Goodpasture's syndrome has been shown to yield an IgG antibody that binds to the basement membrane of glomeruli and alveoli *in vitro*.[337] Finally, both acute and chronic pulmonary and renal lesions closely resembling those in Goodpasture's syndrome have been produced in animals by injection of antilung serum[338] or heterologous antilung antibody.[339]

Although the likelihood that an antibody is involved in the pathogenesis of Goodpasture's syndrome thus seems well established, details of the mechanism by which it causes disease are far from certain. For example, it is not clear whether the lung or the kidney is primarily affected. Because of the relatively greater affinity of glomeruli for anti–basement membrane antibodies, it is often assumed that the primary target organ is the kidney. This is supported by the observation that bilateral nephrectomy usually results in cessation of further episodes of pulmonary hemorrhage.[340] However, in some patients pulmonary symptoms are associated with minimal evidence of renal disease,[341] and in others the illness appears to follow an upper respiratory tract viral infection (*see* later). Both of these observations favor the concept that the primary damage is in the lungs.

The precise nature of the inciting antigen is not known; however, there is evidence that it is related to a specific portion—the globular domain—of basement membrane collagen IV.[342] The reasons for the renal-pulmonary association without clinical evidence of involvement of other basement membranes are not clear. Normal human ABM and GBM exhibit cross-reacting antigenicity,[343] and it is possible that the association is related to an alteration of ABM by inhaled material[342] with subsequent reaction of an anti-ABM antibody with GBM. The occasional association

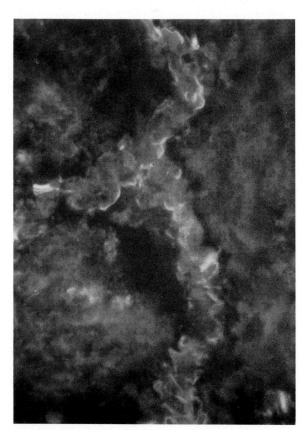

Figure 7–26. Goodpasture's Syndrome. A section of lung incubated with anti-IgG from a 43-year-old woman who presented with hemoptysis shows linear fluorescence corresponding to the site of the alveolar basement membrane. Adjacent airspaces contain blood.

of Goodpasture's syndrome with influenza infection[344] or inhalation of volatile hydrocarbons[345] may reflect such a mechanism. However, basement membranes at a number of other sites, including liver, adrenal, breast, and thyroid, also have been shown to contain the same antigen as that in lung and kidney[346]; why these tissues are not affected is a mystery.

The pathogenesis of the pulmonary hemorrhage in Goodpasture's syndrome is also uncertain. In the kidney, it is generally accepted that complement activation and inflammatory cell infiltration are responsible for glomerular damage. In the lung, however, an inflammatory reaction is typically absent, implying that other factors are involved at this site. One such factor may be cigarette smoking, which has been associated with pulmonary hemorrhage in a number of cases[347]; however, the mechanism behind this is obscure.

The etiology and pathogenesis of IPH are also unknown. Although the clinical and pathologic similarities to Goodpasture's syndrome suggest an autoimmune disease, serologic evidence for this is lacking in most cases.[348] In addition, immunologic and ultrastructural studies of lung tissue invariably have failed to reveal evidence of deposition of immunoglobulin or complement components.[349, 350] On the other hand, the recent discovery of an association between IPH and celiac disease[351] suggests that some immunologic abnormality may be important.

Pathologic Characteristics

The gross and light microscopic features of the lungs in Goodpasture's syndrome and IPH are identical. Airspace hemorrhage is confined largely to the alveoli and smaller airways; in fact, massive blood loss can occur into the lungs without associated hemoptysis, and the trachea and major bronchi may contain little or no blood. Other histologic changes depend on the duration and severity of the disease at the time of examination, but they usually include the presence of hemosiderin-laden macrophages in alveolar airspaces and interstitial tissue, mild to moderate interstitial fibrosis, and type II cell hyperplasia. Necrosis, vasculitis, and an inflammatory exudate are absent.

Electron microscopic studies of alveolar walls in both Goodpasture's syndrome and IPH have shown variable results: some investigators have found no abnormality, and others have found thickening, splitting, discontinuity, or smudging of the basement membrane.[350] Whether these findings are primary and related pathogenetically to the alveolar hemorrhage or are simply a reflection of nonspecific alveolar wall damage has not been determined. Electron-dense deposits suggestive of immune complexes have not been demonstrated.[349]

Immunofluorescence studies of fresh lung tissue obtained from patients with Goodpasture's syndrome by either open lung or transbronchial biopsy typically show diffuse linear staining along the alveolar wall (see Fig. 7–26).[336] IgG is the usual antibody detected, although IgA and IgM are occasionally present as well; C3 is variably present. In distinct contrast to the positive immunofluorescence studies in Goodpasture's syndrome, the results in IPH are negative.

Roentgenographic Manifestations

The changes apparent in the chest roentgenogram in Goodpasture's syndrome and IPH also are identical and depend in large measure on the number of hemorrhagic episodes that have occurred in the past. In the early stages of disease, the pattern is one of patchy airspace consolidation scattered fairly evenly throughout the lungs (Fig. 7–27). The opacities are confluent in many areas, but individual acinar shadows may be apparent. An air bronchogram should be identifiable in areas of major airspace consolidation. Distribution usually is widespread but may be more prominent in the perihilar areas and in the middle and lower lung zones.

Serial roentgenograms obtained in the first weeks after an acute episode usually reveal a highly predictable progressive change in the pattern (see Fig. 7–27). The opacities characteristic of acinar consolidation disappear within 2 to 3 days and are replaced by a reticular pattern whose distribution is identical to that of the airspace disease.[352] This transition presumably represents a stage in which intra-alveolar blood is being transported by macrophages up the mucociliary escalator and into the interstitial space and lymphatics. This reticular pattern gradually diminishes during the next several days, and the appearance of the chest roentgenogram usually returns to normal in about 10 to 12 days after the original episode. With repeated episodes, increasing amounts of hemosiderin are deposited within the interstitial tissue and there is progressive interstitial fibrosis. Once these irreversible changes have developed, fresh episodes of pulmonary hemorrhage usually cause the typical pattern of airspace consolidation to be superimposed upon the diffuse interstitial disease.[353]

Hilar lymph nodes may be enlarged, especially during the acute stage. However, pleural effusion is rare, and its presence usually indicates cardiac decompensation or superimposed acute pneumonia.

As with other interstitial diseases, CT—particularly high-resolution—may reveal evidence of disease in patients with normal chest roentgenograms. The presence of indistinct nodules in a centrilobular location has been found to be suggestive of the disease.[353a, 353b]

Clinical Manifestations

The onset of IPH is usually insidious, with anemia, pallor, weakness, lethargy, and sometimes a dry cough; occasionally, the onset is acute, with fever and hemoptysis. It is important to note that the typical features of airspace hemorrhage may be apparent roentgenographically without a clear-cut episode of hemoptysis. Physical examination during the stage of active pulmonary hemorrhage may reveal fine rales and dullness to percussion over the affected areas of lung. In more chronic cases, the liver, spleen, and lymph nodes are palpably enlarged in 20 to 25 per cent of patients and finger clubbing may be seen.

Iron-deficiency anemia usually develops, but it may not be detectable when intrapulmonary hemorrhage is small and does not severely deplete bone marrow iron stores.[354] Discrepancy between the degree of hemoptysis or extent of radiographic disease and the severity of the anemia can

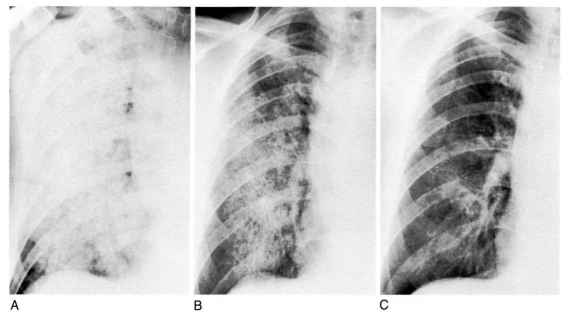

A   B   C

Figure 7–27. Goodpasture's Syndrome. A view of the right lung from a posteroanterior roentgenogram *(A)* reveals massive consolidation of virtually the whole lung (the left was also involved but somewhat less severely). A well-defined air bronchogram is visualized. Seven days later *(B)*, the pattern has become distinctly reticular. Six days later *(C)*, only a fine reticular pattern remains in an anatomic distribution identical to the original involvement.

be explained in some cases by unrecognized malabsorption caused by celiac disease.[355] Although bilirubinemia, predominantly indirect, and the excretion of excessive amounts of urobilinogen are often present and suggest a hemolytic process, the serum iron values and the iron-binding capacity are characteristic of severe iron-deficiency anemia, and it is generally agreed that hemolysis is rare.

In Goodpasture's syndrome, hemoptysis commonly precedes the clinical manifestations of renal disease by several months.[334] It is seldom as copious as in IPH and may occur late in the course of the disease or be absent altogether. Other presenting symptoms include dyspnea, fatigue, weakness, lassitude, pallor, and cough. Physical findings are similar to those of IPH. Although the initial urinalysis may be normal, proteinuria, hematuria, and cellular and granular casts almost invariably develop at some stage. In the occasional patient whose urinary sediment is normal, the presence of renal involvement can be established only by biopsy.[356] Anemia and leukocytosis (with a shift to the left) are common.

There are few reports that describe pulmonary function in patients with either IPH or Goodpasture's syndrome. Some patients tested during remission have had a predominantly restrictive pattern, with decreased diffusing capacity and sometimes a fall in resting PaO_2.[357] Such a pattern has been said to persist in both diseases after the chest roentgenogram has returned to normal.[358] A greater than normal uptake of carbon monoxide is a useful sign that the airspace opacities observed roentgenographically are caused by hemorrhage.[359]

The diagnosis of Goodpasture's syndrome can be confirmed by the demonstration of circulating or tissue-bound anti–basement membrane antibodies by immunofluorescent examination. Most other disorders characterized by hemoptysis and renal dysfunction, including Wegener's granulomatosis and SLE, can be recognized by associated clinical and laboratory manifestations of immune-complex disease[360] or by the observation of a granular pattern of deposition of immunoglobulin and complement in a kidney biopsy specimen. Several authors have stressed the feasibility of making the diagnosis of Goodpasture's syndrome based on examination of a transbronchial biopsy specimen[336]; however, a negative result does not exclude the diagnosis, since anti-GBM antibody may not be identified in pulmonary tissue even when it is present in glomeruli.[361]

It should be evident that the lack of specific morphologic or other findings in patients with IPH make this diagnosis largely one of exclusion, particularly in adults and in patients who do not manifest iron-deficiency anemia. The condition that is most likely to mimic it is aspiration of blood from the nose, esophagus, or stomach. The criteria for the diagnosis of IPH should thus consist of laboratory or clinical evidence of episodes of pulmonary hemorrhage, airspace abnormalities on a chest roentgenogram, a histologically normal renal biopsy specimen showing negative fluorescence, and the absence of a detectable cause for bleeding in the lung or elsewhere.

Prognosis

The prognosis in IPH varies considerably. In one series, the average interval from onset of symptoms until death was only 2½ years[362]; however, individual patients are known to have survived for as long as 40 years.[363] The prognosis appears to be better when the disease is acquired in adulthood than in childhood.[364]

In contrast to IPH, for which there is no convincing evidence that any form of therapy alters the course of the disease, several therapeutic measures clearly affect the prognosis of Goodpasture's syndrome. Perhaps the most important of these are plasmapheresis and immuno-suppression,[365] the response to the combination of these two forms of therapy generally being a reduction in circulating anti-GBM antibodies and cessation of pulmonary hemorrhage. Although renal failure progresses in some cases, the renal component of the disease has also been noted to improve.

Pulmonary Disease in Bone Marrow Transplantation

Pulmonary disease is common in patients receiving bone marrow transplants, whatever their genetic relationship to the donor.[366] Infection is by far the most frequent complication, and is usually caused by cytomegalovirus (CMV), *Aspergillus* species, or a variety of bacterial pathogens. Interstitial pneumonitis, acute airspace disease, and bronchiolitis are also important complications.

Interstitial pneumonitis occurs in 40 to 50 per cent of all patients; approximately 60 per cent of them die.[367] Many cases are caused by infection, particularly by CMV; pneumonitis caused by *herpes simplex, herpes zoster,* or *Pneumocystis carinii* also occurs with some frequency. In 10 to 20 per cent of patients with interstitial pneumonitis, no organism can be identified by either histologic examination or tissue culture.[368] The pathogenesis of disease in these cases has not been definitively established, but it has been attributed to pretransplant chemotherapy and irradiation, post-transplant immunosuppressive therapy, and graft-versus-host disease (GVHD).[369] Alteration of the helper-suppressor T-cell ratio in BAL fluid,[370] as well as histologic findings in experimental animals, has provided support for the last hypothesis. However, the roughly equal prevalence of idiopathic interstitial pneumonitis in patients with allogeneic and syngeneic transplants has implied that the influence of GVHD is small.[371] Most cases of idiopathic interstitial pneumonitis occur in the first 2 months after transplantation. Symptoms are nonspecific and include cough and increasing dyspnea. A reduction of diffusing capacity is usually the first indication of pulmonary dysfunction.

Acute, often diffuse airspace disease also develops in a substantial number of patients in the first 2 months after transplantation. Again, the etiology may be infectious (most often gram-negative bacteria or fungi[373]) or unknown. In one study, pathologic findings in the latter situation were those of diffuse alveolar damage associated with alveolar hemorrhage.[368] Experimental studies in animals suggest that this pattern of disease may also be related to a graft-versus-host reaction. The clinical course is characterized by progressive dyspnea, cough, and hypoxia.

Obstructive airway disease, characterized pathologically by bronchiolitis obliterans (Fig. 7–28), is a relatively uncommon complication of bone marrow transplantation. Most patients have manifestations of chronic GVHD elsewhere in the body, and it has been suggested that the bronchiolitis may represent a primary manifestation of this process in the lungs.[374] However, other mechanisms (e.g., CMV infection and the action of cytotoxic drugs) also have been proposed.[375] The abnormality usually develops within 18 months of transplantation. Roentgenograms are often normal but may show evidence of hyperinflation. Recurrent pneumothorax and pneumomediastinum have been described in several patients.[366] Pulmonary symptoms include cough, wheezing, and exertional dyspnea. Findings of

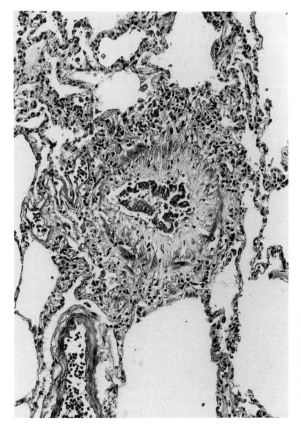

Figure 7–28. Bronchiolitis Obliterans Following Bone Marrow Transplantation. Section from a 37-year-old woman with acute myelogenous leukemia who had a partially matched bone marrow transplant. Six months later she was admitted to the hospital with evidence of chronic graft-versus-host disease and a 1-month history of dry, nonproductive cough and increasing dyspnea. A chest roentgenogram taken 3 days before death was normal. At autopsy many small bronchioles showed partial or complete luminal obliteration by fibroblastic tissue with mild peribronchiolar lymphocytic inflammation. The parenchyma was normal. (× 150.)

chronic GVHD, such as scleroderma, dryness of the eyes and mouth, dysphagia, serositis, and hepatic disease, are often present. The serum immunoglobulin level frequently is decreased, and pulmonary function studies show an obstructive pattern.[376]

Lung Transplantation

In recent years, there has been increased interest in lung and heart-lung transplantation for the treatment of some forms of advanced (end-stage) pulmonary disease, particularly cystic fibrosis, emphysema due to alpha$_1$-antiprotease deficiency, idiopathic fibrosing alveolitis, and arterial hypertension. Although this therapy has been enthusiastically supported by many physicians as a ray of hope for otherwise incurable patients, it is itself associated with substantial morbidity and mortality. Complications are associated predominantly with technical problems related to surgery, infection and pulmonary rejection.

There are three major technical problems in lung and heart-lung transplantation. The first is intraoperative hemorrhage from systemic vessels within fibrotic pleura; as discussed previously (see page 280), such vessels can be numerous in chronic inflammatory abnormalities such as cystic fibrosis and postviral bronchiectasis, and the resulting hemorrhage during recipient lung excision can be fatal. A temporary (and usually reversible) alteration in pulmonary function and gas exchange frequently occurs in the first few days after transplantation. Variably termed the "reimplantation response" or "reperfusion injury," this may be caused in part by bronchial arterial and lymphatic interruption, although ischemia to the donor lung prior to transplantation is likely a more important factor.[377] Roentgenographic manifestations are those of pulmonary edema, and pathologic examination shows diffuse alveolar damage. This complication usually resolves in a matter of days; in severe cases, however, significant pulmonary fibrosis may ensue. Ischemic necrosis at the site of tracheal or bronchial anastomosis is also an important complication of surgery, particuarly in isolated lung transplants. In the first weeks after transplantation, such necrosis can result in anastomotic dehiscence with bronchopleural or bronchomediastinal fistula or, if associated with necrosis of the adjacent pulmonary artery wall, in massive hemorrhage. In the long term, bronchomalacia or fibrotic stricture may result in significant functional or anatomic airway obstruction.

As might be predicted, infection is an important cause of morbidity and mortality, particularly during the first 6 months after transplantation. The causative organisms include *Staphylococcus aureus* and the usual gram-negative organisms seen in a hospital environment[378] as well as opportunists such as CMV, herpes viruses, *Aspergillus*, and *P. carinii*.[379]

Host-mediated pulmonary rejection is also a major problem that occurs in the majority of patients at some time after transplantation, despite the use of potent immunosupressant agents such as cyclosporine. From both clinical and pathologic points of view, it is appropriate to consider such rejection as occurring in acute and chronic forms.

Acute Rejection. The majority of cases develop in the first 3 months after transplantation; in most of these, the first episode is seen in the second or third week. Histologi-cally, the characteristic finding is the presence of a perivascular infiltrate of mononuclear inflammatory cells; similar inflammatory cells often are present in airway mucosa. In relatively mild disease, the infiltrate is found solely in relation to airways and vessels; in more severe forms, it extends into alveolar interstitial tissue and is associated with parenchymal necrosis.

The principal roentgenographic findings seen in acute rejection are ill-defined, symmetrical, parahilar opacities, not uncommonly associated with pleural effusion.[380, 381] Nodular opacities, which may progress to involve a substantial portion of lung parenchyma, also may be apparent in the lower lung zones.

Clinical findings include dyspnea, leukocytosis, and fever. As such observations may also reflect infection, definitive diagnosis based on these alone is difficult, if not impossible. As a result, some investigators advocate the use of ancillary techniques such as transbronchial biopsy to confirm the diagnosis.[382]

By increasing immunosuppressant therapy most episodes of acute rejection can be effectively controlled. However, there is evidence that the complication may be related to the development of bronchiolitis obliterans, particularly if it is severe and repeated. In addition, the effect of increased immunotherapy itself cannot be discounted, since it increases the risk of infection and, possibly, of a post-transplant lymphoproliferative disorder.[382a]

Chronic Rejection. In addition to clearly defined episodes of acute rejection, it has become clear that there are a variety of pulmonary abnormalities that develop insidiously in long-term lung transplant survivors, many of which are believed to represent a manifestation of chronic rejection. Perhaps the most distressing of such complications is bronchiolitis obliterans, which has been estimated to develop in as many as 50 per cent of patients who leave the hospital with normal cardiopulmonary function.[383] Pathologically, the process is similar to that of bronchiolitis obliterans in bone marrow transplantation, consisting of fibroblastic connective tissue located eccentrically or concentrically within the bronchiolar lumen, causing partial or complete airway obstruction (see Fig. 7–28). Roentgenographs of affected patients may be normal or show evidence of hyperinflation. Symptoms consist of cough, with or without sputum production, and progressive dyspnea. Many patients have a history of episodes of acute rejection.[384] The diagnosis can be confirmed by pulmonary function tests (which reveal air flow obstruction) and transbronchial biopsy (which is positive in many affected patients).[385] Although there is evidence that increased immunosuppression may be beneficial,[386] in most cases the progression to respiratory failure is inexorable.

Other long-term sequelae of lung transplantation that may be related to chronic rejection include bronchitis, bronchiectasis (sometimes severe), and arterial and venous intimal fibrosis.[387]

As might be expected from this rather lengthy list of complications, the prognosis for patients with either isolated lung or heart-lung transplants is guarded. Although some individuals fare remarkably well and are able to return to nearly normal daily activities, many experience significant morbidity. In addition, the mortality rate is high: in 1989, it was estimated that the worldwide death rate for

255 heart-lung transplant recipients was 40 per cent at 1 year and 80 per cent at 5 years[378]; patients undergoing heart-lung[387a] or bilateral lung[387b] transplantation for cystic fibrosis have a mortality rate of about 50 per cent at 3 years. Death is usually due to complications of surgery or infection.

Pulmonary Abnormalities Associated with Inflammatory Bowel Disease

Pulmonary function abnormalities, consisting of a decrease in the diffusing capacity of the lungs for carbon monoxide[388] and an increase in functional residual capacity,[389] have been recorded in a number of patients with ulcerative colitis and Crohn's disease. The anatomic basis of these abnormalities is poorly described, although some patients have evidence of fibrosing alveolitis.[388] In several patients, biliary cirrhosis has been described in association with the sicca syndrome, pulmonary interstitial or obstructive disease, and abnormal pulmonary function.[390]

References

1. Taormina VJ, Miller WT, Gefter WB, et al: Progressive systemic sclerosis subgroups: Variable pulmonary features. Am J Roentgenol 137: 277, 1981.
2. Decker JL, Steinberg AD, Reinertsen JL, et al: Systemic lupus erythematosus: Evolving concepts. Ann Intern Med 91: 587, 1979.
3. Steinberg AD, Raveche ES, Laskin CA, et al: Systemic lupus erythematosus: Insights from animal models. Ann Intern Med 100: 714, 1984.
4. Rich S: Human lupus inclusions and interferon. Science 213: 772, 1981.
5. Harland SJ, Facchini V, Timbrell JA: Hydralazine-induced lupus erythematosus–like syndrome in a patient of the rapid acetylator phenotype. Br Med J 281: 273, 1980.
6. Smolen JS, Chused TM, Leiserson WM, et al: Heterogeneity of immunoregulatory T-cell subsets in systemic lupus erythematosus: Correlation with clinical features. Am J Med 72: 783, 1982.
7. Blaese RM, Grayson J, Steinberg AD: Increased immunoglobulin-secreting cells in the blood of patients with active systemic lupus erythematosus. Am J Med 69: 345, 1980.
8. Miller KB, Salem D: Immune regulatory abnormalities produced by procainamide. Am J Med 73: 487, 1982.
9. Miller LR, Greenberg SD, McLarty JW: Lupus lung. Chest 88: 265, 1985.
10. Haupt HM, Moore GW, Hutchins GM: The lung in systemic lupus erythematosus. Analysis of the pathologic changes in 120 patients. Am J Med 71: 791, 1981.
11. Inque T, Kanayama Y, Ohe A, et al: Immunopathologic studies of pneumonitis in systemic lupus erythematosus. Ann Intern Med 91: 30, 1979.
12. Hoffbrand BI, Beck ER: "Unexplained" dyspnoea and shrinking lungs in systemic lupus erythematosus. Br Med J 1: 1273, 1965.
13. Matthay RA, Schwartz MI, Petty TL, et al: Pulmonary manifestations of systemic lupus erythematosus. Review of twelve cases of acute lupus pneumonitis. Medicine 54: 397, 1975.
14. Churg A, Franklin W, Chan KL, et al: Pulmonary hemorrhage and immune-complex deposition in the lung. Complications in a patient with systemic lupus erythematosus. Arch Pathol Lab Med 104: 388, 1980.
15. Myers JL, Katzenstein A-LA: Microangitis in lupus-induced pulmonary hemorrhage. Am J Clin Pathol 85: 552, 1986.
16. Gross M, Esterly JR, Earle RH: Pulmonary alterations in systemic lupus erythematosus. Am Rev Resp Dis 105: 572, 1972.
17. Pulmonary hypertension and systemic lupus erythematosus [Editorial]. J Rheumatol 13: 1, 1986.
18. Winslow WA, Ploss LN, Loitman B: Pleuritis in systemic lupus erythematosus: Its importance as an early manifestation in diagnosis. Ann Intern Med 49: 70, 1958.
19. Levin DC: Proper interpretation of pulmonary roentgen changes in systemic lupus erythematosus. Am J Roentgenol 111: 510, 1971.
20. Hsu BY, Edwards DK III, Trambert MA: Pulmonary hemorrhage complicating systemic lupus erythematosus: Role of MR imaging in diagnosis. AJR 158: 519, 1992.
21. Weinrib L, Sharma OP, Quismorio FP Jr: A long-term study of interstitial lung disease in systemic lupus erythematosus. Semin Arthritis Rheum 20: 48, 1990.
22. Martens J, Demedts M, Vanmeenen MT, et al: Respiratory muscle dysfunction in systemic lupus erythematosus. Chest 84: 170, 1983.
23. Ramirez RE, Glasier C, Kirks D, et al: Pulmonary hemorrhage associated with systemic lupus erythematosus in children. Radiology 152: 409, 1984.
24. Simonson JS, Schiller NB, Petri M, et al: Pulmonary hypertension in systemic lupus erythematosus. J Rheumatol 16: 918, 1989.
25. Kohler PF, Vaughan J: The autoimmune diseases. JAMA 248: 2646, 1982.
26. Abel T, Gladman DD, Urowitz MB: Neuropsychiatric lupus. J Rheumatol 7: 325, 1980.
27. Hughes GRV: Hypotensive agents, beta-blockers, and drug-induced lupus. Br Med J 284: 1358, 1982.
28. Bass BH: Hydralazine lung. Thorax 36: 695, 1981.
29. Synkowski DR, Mogavero HS Jr, Provost TT: Lupus erythematosus: Laboratory testing and clinical subsets in the evaluation of patients. Med Clin North Am 64: 921, 1980.
30. Hedgpeth MT, Boulware DW: Interstitial pneumonitis in antibody-negative systemic lupus erythematosus: A new clinical manifestation and possible association with anti-Ro (SS-A) antibodies. Arthritis Rheum 31: 545, 1988.
31. Beaufils M, Kouki F, Mignon F, et al: Clinical significance of anti-Sm antibodies in systemic lupus erythematosus. Am J Med 74: 201, 1983.
32. Huang CT, Lyons HA: Comparison of pulmonary function in patients with systemic lupus erythematosus, scleroderma, and rheumatoid arthritis. Am Rev Respir Dis 93: 865, 1966.
33. Kinney WW, Angelillo VA: Bronchiolitis in systemic lupus erythematosus. Chest 82: 646, 1982.
34. Jacobelli S, Moreno R, Massardo L, et al: Inspiratory muscle dysfunction and unexplained dyspnea in systemic lupus erythematosus. Arthritis Rheum 28: 781, 1985.
35. Zeiss CR, Burch FX, Marder RJ, et al: A hypocomplementemic vasculitic urticarial syndrome: Report of four new cases and definition of the disease. Am J Med 68: 867, 1980.
36. Schwartz HR, McDuffie FC, Black LF, et al: Hypocomplementemic urticarial vasculitis: Association with chronic obstructive pulmonary disease. Mayo Clin Proc 57: 231, 1982.
37. Locke CB: Rheumatoid lung. Clin Radiol 14: 43, 1963.
38. Horler AR, Thompson M: The pleural and pulmonary complications of rheumatoid arthritis. Ann Intern Med 51: 1179, 1959.
39. Nusslein HG, Rodl W, Giedel J, et al: Multiple peripheral pulmonary nodules preceding rheumatoid arthritis. Rheumatology 7: 89, 1987.
40. DeHoratius RJ, Abruzzo JL, Williams RC Jr: Immunofluorescent and immunologic studies of rheumatoid lung. Arch Intern Med 129: 441, 1972.
41. Balbi B, Cosulich E, Risso A, et al: The interstitial lung disease associated with rheumatoid arthritis: Evidence for imbalance of helper T-lymphocyte subpopulations at sites of disease activity. Bull Eur Physiopathol Respir 23: 241, 1987.
42. Gilligan DM, O'Connor CM, Ward K, et al: Bronchoalveolar lavage in patients with mild and severe rheumatoid lung disease. Thorax 45: 591, 1990.
43. Popp W, Ritschka L, Scherak O, et al: Bronchoalveolar lavage in rheumatoid arthritis and secondary Sjögren's syndrome. Lung 168: 221, 1990.
44. Hakala M, Ruuska P, Hameenkorpi R, et al: Diffuse interstitial lung disease in rheumatoid arthritis: Views on immunological and HLA findings. Scand J Rheumatol 15: 3268, 1986.
45. Fewins HE, McGowan I, Whitehouse GH, et al: High-definition computed tomography in rheumatoid arthritis associated with pulmonary disease. Br J Rheumatol 30: 214, 1991.
46. Hills EA, Geary M: Membrane diffusing capacity and pulmonary capillary volume in rheumatoid disease. Thorax 35: 851, 1980.
47. Cohen JM, Miller A, Spiera H: Interstitial pneumonitis complicating rheumatoid arthritis: Sustained remission with azathioprine therapy. Chest 72: 521, 1977.

48. Petrie GR, Bloomfield P, Grant IWB, et al: Upper lobe fibrosis and cavitation in rheumatoid disease. Br J Dis Chest 74: 263, 1980.
49. McCann BG, Hart GJ, Stokes TC, et al: Obliterative bronchiolitis and upper-zone pulmonary consolidation in rheumatoid arthritis. Thorax 38: 73, 1983.
50. Carr DT, Mayne JG: Pleurisy with effusion in rheumatoid arthritis, with reference to the low concentration of glucose in pleural fluid. Am Rev Resp Dis 85: 345, 1962.
51. Walters MN, Ojeda VJ: Pleuropulmonary necrobiotic rheumatoid nodules: A review and clinicopathological study of six patients. Med J Aust 144: 648, 1986.
52. Rubin EH, Gordon M, Thelmo WL: Nodular pleuropulmonary rheumatoid disease. Report of two cases and review of the literature. Am J Med 42: 567, 1967.
53. Morgan WKC, Wolfel DA: The lungs and pleura in rheumatoid arthritis. Am J Roentgenol 98: 334, 1966.
54. Jolles H, Moseley PL, Peterson MW: Nodular pulmonary opacities in patients with rheumatoid arthritis. A diagnostic dilemma. Chest 96: 1022, 1989.
55. Caplan A, Cowen EDH, Gough J: Rheumatoid pneumoconiosis in a foundry worker. Thorax 13: 181, 1958.
56. Caplan A: Certain unusual radiological appearances in the chest of coal miners suffering from rheumatoid arthritis. Thorax 8: 29, 1953.
57. Fritze E, Dickmans H; Pneumoconiosis causing a round infiltrate. Radiology 2: 270, 1964.
58. Benedek TG: Rheumatoid pneumoconiosis. Documentation of onset and pathogenic considerations. Am J Med 55: 515, 1973.
59. Gough J, Rivers D, Seal RME: Pathological studies of modified pneumoconiosis in coal-miners with rheumatoid arthritis (Caplan's syndrome). Thorax 10: 9, 1955.
60. Heath D, Gillund TD, Kay JM, et al: Pulmonary vascular disease in honeycomb lung. J Pathol Bacteriol 95: 423, 1968.
61. Walker WC, Wright V: Pulmonary lesions and rheumatoid arthritis. Medicine 47: 501, 1968.
62. Armstrong JG, Steele RH: Localised pulmonary arteritis in rheumatoid disease. Thorax 37: 313, 1982.
63. Wise RA, Wigley FM, Scott TE, et al: DQ$_W$ alloantigens and pulmonary dysfunction in rheumatoid arthritis. Chest 94: 609, 1988.
64. Geddes DM, Corrin B, Brewerton DA, et al: Progressive airway obliteration in adults and its association with rheumatoid disease. Q J Med 46: 427, 1977.
65. Yousem SA, Cobly TV, Carrington CB: Lung biopsy in rheumatoid arthritis. Am Rev Respir Dis 131: 770, 1985.
66. Begin R, Masse S, Cantin A, et al: Airway disease in a subset of nonsmoking rheumatoid patients. Characterization of the disease and evidence for an autoimmune pathogenesis. Am J Med 72: 743, 1982.
67. Yousem SA, Colby TV, Carrington CB: Follicular bronchitis/bronchiolitis. Hum Pathol 16: 700, 1985.
68. Fortoul TI, Cano-Valle F, Oliva E, et al: Follicular bronchiolitis in association with connective tissue diseases. Lung 163: 305, 1985.
69. Athreya BH, Doughty RA, Bookspan M, et al: Pulmonary manifestations of juvenile rheumatoid arthritis. Clin Chest Med 1: 361, 1980.
70. Medsger TA Jr, Masi AT: Epidemiology of systemic sclerosis (scleroderma). Ann Intern Med 74: 714, 1971.
71. Piper WN, Helwig EB: Progressive systemic sclerosis. Visceral manifestations of generalized scleroderma. Arch Dermatol 72: 535, 1955.
72. Silver RM, Miller KS, Kinsella MB, et al: Evaluation and management of scleroderma lung disease using bronchoalveolar lavage. Am J Med 88: 470, 1990.
73. Bianchi FA, Bistue AR, Wendt VE, et al: Analysis of twenty-seven cases of progressive systemic sclerosis (including two with combined systemic lupus erythematosus) and a review of the literature. J Chron Dis 19: 953, 1966.
74. Harrison NK, Glanville AR, Strickland B, et al: Pulmonary involvement in systemic sclerosis: The detection of early changes by thin section CT scan, bronchoalveolar lavage and ^{99m}Tc-DTPA clearance. Respir Med 83: 403, 1989.
75. Rossi GA, Bitterman PB, Rennard SI, et al: Evidence for chronic inflammation as a component of the interstitial lung disease associated with progressive systemic sclerosis. Am Rev Respir Dis 131: 612, 1985.
76. Johnson DA, Drane WE, Curran J, et al: Pulmonary disease in progressive systemic sclerosis. A complication of gastroesophageal reflux and occult aspiration? Arch Intern Med 149: 589, 1989.
77. Winters WJ Jr, Joseph RR: "Primary" pulmonary hypertension and Raynaud's phenomenon. Case report and review of the literature. Arch Intern Med 114: 821, 1964.
78. Rodnan GP, Myerowitz RL, Justh GO: Morphologic changes in the digital arteries of patients with progressive systemic sclerosis (scleroderma) and Raynaud phenomenon. Medicine 59: 393, 1980.
79. Yamauchi K, Arimori S: Alteration in pulmonary blood flow induced by cold exposure to the hand in progressive systemic sclerosis. Jpn J Med 28: 506, 1989.
80. D'Angelo WA, Fries JF, Masi AT, et al: Pathologic observations in systemic sclerosis (scleroderma): A study of fifty-eight autopsy cases and fifty-eight matched controls. Am J Med 46: 428, 1969.
81. Harrison NK, Myers AR, Corrin B, et al: Structural features of interstitial lung disease in systemic sclerosis. Am Rev Respir Dis 144: 706, 1991.
82. Young RH, Mark GJ: Pulmonary vascular changes in scleroderma. Am J Med 64: 998, 1978.
83. Divertie MB: Lung involvement in the connective-tissue disorders. Med Clin North Am 48: 1015, 1964.
84. Schurawitzki H, Stiglbauer R, Graninger W, et al: Interstitial lung disease in progressive systemic sclerosis: High-resolution CT versus radiography. Radiology 176: 755, 1990.
84a. Wells AU, Hansell DM, Corrin B, et al: High-resolution computed tomography as a predictor of lung histology in systemic sclerosis. Thorax 47: 508, 1992.
85. Martinez LO: Air in the esophagus as a sign of scleroderma (differential diagnosis with some other entities). J Can Assoc Radiol 25: 234, 1974.
86. Harper FE, Maricq HR, Turner RE, et al: A prospective study of Raynaud phenomenon and early connective tissue disease: A 5-year report. Am J Med 72: 883, 1982.
87. Clark JA, Winkelmann RK, McDuffie FC, et al: Synovial tissue changes and rheumatic factor in scleroderma. Mayo Clin Proc 46: 97, 1971.
88. Lomeo RM, Cornella RJ, Schabel SI, et al: Progressive systemic sclerosis sine scleroderma presenting as pulmonary interstitial fibrosis. Am J Med 87: 525, 1989.
89. Weaver AL, Divertie MB, Titus JL: Pulmonary scleroderma. Dis Chest 54: 490, 1968.
90. Buckingham BA, Uitto J, Sandborg C, et al: Scleroderma-like changes in insulin-dependent diabetes mellitus: Clinical and biochemical studies. Diabetes Care 7: 163, 1984.
91. Gordon MB, Klein I, Dekker A, et al: Thyroid disease in progressive systemic sclerosis: Increased frequency of glandular fibrosis and hypothyroidism. Ann Intern Med 95: 431, 1981.
92. Kent LT, Cramer SF, Moskowitz RW, et al: Eosinophilic fasciitis: Clinical, laboratory, and microscopic consideration. Arthritis Rheum 24: 677, 1981.
93. Wood SH, Cantrell BB, Shulman LE: Eosinophilic fasciitis. Johns Hopkins Med J 148: 81, 1981.
94. Clark JA, Winkelmann RK, Ward LE: Serologic alterations in scleroderma and sclerodermatomyositis. Mayo Clin Proc 46: 104, 1971.
95. Jordon RE, DeHeer D, Schroeter A, et al: Antinuclear antibodies: Their significance in scleroderma. Mayo Clin Proc 46:111, 1971.
96. Dubois EL, Chandor S, Friou GJ, et al: Progressive systemic sclerosis (PSS) and localized scleroderma (morphea) with positive LE cell test and unusual systemic manifestations compatible with systemic lupus erythematosus (SLE). Medicine 50: 199, 1971.
97. Schneider PD, Wise RA, Hochberg MC, et al: Serial pulmonary function in systemic sclerosis. Am J Med 73: 385, 1982.
98. Blom-Bulow B, Jonson B, Brauer K: Lung function in progressive systemic sclerosis is dominated by poorly compliant lungs and stiff airways. Eur J Respir Dis 66: 1, 1985.
99. Guttadauria M, Ellman H, Emmanuel G, et al: Pulmonary function in scleroderma. Arthritis Rheum 20: 1071, 1977.
100. Chausow AM, Kane T, Levinson D, et al: Reversible hypercapnic respiratory insufficiency in scleroderma caused by respiratory muscle weakness. Am Rev Respir Dis 130: 142, 1984.
101. Medsger TA Jr, Masi AT, Rodnan GP, et al: Survival with systemic sclerosis (scleroderma). Life-table analysis of clinical and demographic factors in 309 patients. Ann Intern Med 75: 369, 1971.
102. Lally EV, Jimenez SA, Kaplan SR: Progressive systemic sclerosis: Mode of presentation, rapidly progressive disease course, and mortality based on an analysis of 91 patients. Semin Arthritis Rheum 18: 1, 1988.
103. Masi AT, D'Angelo WA: Epidemiology of fatal systemic sclerosis

(diffuse scleroderma). A 15-year survey in Baltimore. Ann Intern Med 66: 870, 1967.

104. Peters-Golden M, Wise RA, Hochberg MC, et al: Carbon monoxide diffusing capacity as predictor of outcome in systemic sclerosis. Am J Med 77: 1027, 1984.

105. Peters-Golden M, Wise RA, Hochberg M, et al: Incidence of lung cancer in systemic sclerosis. J Rheumatol 12: 1136, 1985.

106. Steen VD, Ziegler GL, Rodnan GP, et al: Clinical and laboratory associations of anticentromere antibody in patients with progressive systemic sclerosis. Arthritis Rheum 27: 125, 1984.

107. Velayos EE, Masi AT, Stevens MB, et al: The "CREST" syndrome: A distinct serologic entity with anticentromere antibodies. Am J Med 69: 520, 1980.

108. Yousem SA: The pulmonary pathologic manifestations of the CREST syndrome. Hum Pathol 21: 467, 1990.

109. Stupi AM, Steen VD, Owens GR, et al: Pulmonary hypertension in the CREST syndrome variant of systemic sclerosis. Arthritis Rheum 29: 515, 1986.

110. Bohan A, Peter JB: Polymyositis and dermatomyositis (first of two parts). N Engl J Med 292: 344, 1975.

111. Currie S, Saunders M, Knowles M, et al: Immunological aspects of polymyositis: The in vitro activity of lymphocytes on incubation with muscle antigen and with muscle cultures. Q J Med 40: 63, 1971.

112. Dawkins RL, Mastaglia FL: Cell-mediated cytotoxicity to muscle in polymyositis: Effects of immunosuppression. N Engl J Med 288: 434, 1973.

113. Johnson RI, Fink CW, Ziff M: Lymphotoxin formation by lymphocytes and muscle in polymyositis. J Clin Invest 51: 2435, 1972.

114. Rowen AJ, Reichel J: Dermatomyositis with lung involvement successfully treated with azathioprine. Respiration 44: 143, 1983.

115. Schwarz MI, Matthay RA, Sahn SA, et al: Interstitial lung disease in polymyositis and dermatomyositis: Analysis of six cases and review of the literature. Medicine 55: 89, 1976.

116. Thomson PL, MacKay IR: Fibrosing alveolitis and polymyositis. Thorax 25: 504, 1970.

117. Salmeron G, Greenberg SD, Lidsky MD: Polymyositis and diffuse interstitial lung disease. A review of the pulmonary histopathologic findings. Arch Intern Med 141: 1005, 1981.

118. Tazelaar HD, Viggiano RW, Pickersgill J, et al: Interstitial lung disease in polymyositis and dermatomyositis. Clinical features and prognosis as correlated with histologic findings. Am Rev Respir Dis 141: 727, 1990.

119. Frazier AR, Miller RD: Interstitial pneumonitis in association with polymyositis and dermatomyositis. Chest 65: 403, 1974.

119a. Hidano A, Torikai S, Uemura T, Shimizu S: Malignancy and interstitial pneumonitis as fatal complications in dermatomyositis. J Dermatol 19: 153, 1992.

120. Benbassat J, Gefel D, Larholdt K, et al: Prognostic factors in polymyositis/dermatomyositis: A computer-assisted analysis of ninety-two cases. Arthritis Rheum 28: 249, 1985.

121. Rose AL, Walton JN: Polymyositis: A survey of 89 cases with particular reference to treatment and prognosis. Brain 89: 747, 1966.

122. Hepper NGG, Ferguson RH, Howard FM Jr: Three types of pulmonary involvement in polymyositis. Med Clin North Am 28: 1031, 1964.

123. Medsger TA Jr, Robinson H, Masi AT: Factors affecting survivorship in polymyositis. A life-table study of 124 patients. Arthritis Rheum 14: 249, 1971.

124. Arsura EL, Greenberg AS: Adverse impact of interstitial pulmonary fibrosis on prognosis in polymyositis and dermatomyositis. Semin Arthritis Rheum 18: 29, 1988.

125. Bohan A, Peter JB: Polymyositis and dermatomyositis (second of two parts). N Engl J Med 292: 403, 1975.

126. Targoff IN, Arnett FC: Clinical manifestations in patients with antibody to PL-12 antigen (alanyl-tRNA synthetase). Am J Med 88: 241, 1990.

127. Marguerie C, Bunn CC, Beynon HL, et al: Polymyositis, pulmonary fibrosis and autoantibodies to aminoacyl-tRNA synthetase enzymes. Q J Med 77: 1019, 1990.

128. Pace WR Jr, Decker JL, Martin CJ: Polymyositis: Report of two cases with pulmonary function studies suggestive of progressive systemic sclerosis. Am J Med Sci 245: 322, 1963.

129. Schiavi EA, Roncoroni AJ, Puy RJM: Isolated bilateral diaphragmatic paresis with interstitial lung disease: An unusual presentation of dermatomyositis. Am Rev Respir Dis 129: 337, 1984.

130. Gratwhol AA, Moutsopoulos HM, Chused TM, et al: Sjögren-type

131. Itescu S, Brancato IJ, Buxbaum J, et al: A diffuse infiltrative CD8 lymphocytosis syndrome in human immunodeficiency virus (HIV) infection: A host immune response associated with HLA-DR5. Ann Intern Med 112: 3, 1990.

132. Reveille JD, Wilson RW, Provost TT, et al: Primary Sjögren's syndrome and other autoimmune diseases in families: Prevalence and immunogenetic studies in six kindreds. Ann Intern Med 101: 748, 1984.

133. Manthorpe R, Frost-Larsen K, Isager H, et al: Sjögren's syndrome: A review with emphasis on immunological features. Allergy 36: 129, 1981.

134. Kessler HS: A laboratory model for Sjögren's syndrome. Am J Pathol 52: 671, 1968.

135. Whaley K, Webb J, McEvoy BA, et al: Sjögren's syndrome: 2. Clinical associations and immunological phenomena. Q J Med 42: 513, 1973.

136. Bucher UG, Reid L: Sjögren's syndrome. Report of a fatal case with pulmonary and renal lesions. Br J Dis Chest 53: 237, 1959.

137. Newball HH, Brahim SA: Chronic obstructive airway disease in patients with Sjögren's syndrome. Am Rev Respir Dis 115: 295, 1977.

138. Liebow AA, Carrington CB: Diffuse pulmonary lymphoreticular infiltrations associated with dysproteinemia. Med Clin North Am 57: 809, 1973.

139. Silbiger ML, Peterson CC Jr: Sjögren's syndrome. Its roentgenographic features. Am J Roentgenol 100: 554, 1967.

140. Shearn MA: Sjögren's syndrome. Med Clin North Am 61: 271, 1977.

141. Hansen LA, Prakash UB, Colby TV: Pulmonary lymphoma in Sjögren's syndrome. Mayo Clin Proc 64: 920, 1989.

142. Isenberg DA, Hammond L, Fisher C, et al: Predictive value of SS-B precipitating antibodies in Sjögren's syndrome. Br Med J 284: 1738, 1982.

143. Moutsopoulos HM, Chused TM, Mann DL, et al: Sjögren's syndrome (sicca syndrome): Current issues. Ann Intern Med 92: 212, 1980.

144. Dalavanga YA, Constantopoulos SH, Galanopoulou V, et al: Alveolitis correlates with clinical pulmonary involvement in primary Sjögren's syndrome. Chest 99: 1394, 1991.

145. Papathanasiou MP, Constantopoulos SH, Tsampoulas C, et al: Reappraisal of respiratory abnormalities in primary and secondary Sjögren's syndrome: A controlled study. Chest 90: 370, 1986.

146. Kelly C, Gardiner P, Pal B, et al: Lung function in primary Sjögren's syndrome: A cross-sectional and longitudinal study. Thorax 46: 180, 1991.

147. Sharp GC, Irvin WS, TAn EM, et al: Mixed connective tissue disease—apparently distinct rheumatic disease syndrome associated with a specific antibody to an expractable nuclear antigen (ENA). Am J Med 52: 148, 1972.

148. Silver TM, Farber SJ, Bole GG, et al: Radiological features of mixed connective tissue disease and scleroderma–systemic lupus erythematosus overlap. Radiology 120: 269, 1976.

149. Weiner-Kronish JP, Solinger AM, Warnock ML, et al: Severe pulmonary involvement in mixed connective tissue disease. Am Rev Respir Dis 124: 499, 1981.

150. Nimelstein SH, Brody S, McShane D, et al: Mixed connective tissue disease: A subsequent evaluation of the original 25 patients. Medicine 59: 239, 1980.

151. Sullivan WD, Hurst DJ, Harmon CE, et al: A prospective evaluation emphasizing pulmonary involvement in patients with connective tissue disease. Medicine 63: 92, 1984.

152. McAdam LP, O'Hanlan MA, Bluestone R, et al: Relapsing polychondritis: Prospective study of 23 patients and a review of the literature. Medicine 55: 193, 1976.

153. Homma S, Matsumoto T, Abe H, et al: Relapsing polychondritis: Pathological and immunological findings in an autopsy case. Acta Pathol Jpn 34: 1137, 1984.

154. Herman JH, Dennis MV: Immunopathologic studies in relapsing polychondritis. J Clin Invest 52: 549, 1973.

155. Rajapakse DA, Bywaters EGL: Cell-mediated immunity to cartilage proteoglycan in relapsing polychondritis. Clin Exp Immunol 16: 497, 1974.

156. Kindblom L-G, Dalen P, Edmar G, et al: Relapsing polychondritis. A clinical, pathologic-anatomic and histochemical study of 2 cases. Acta Pathol Microbiol Scand 85: 656, 1977.

157. Dolan DL, Lemmon GB Jr, Teitelbaum SL: Relapsing polychondri-

tis. Analytical literature review and studies on pathogenesis. Am J Med 41: 285, 1966.

158. Michet CJ Jr, McKenna CH, Luthra HS, et al: Relapsing polychondritis: Survival and predictive role of early disease manifestations. Ann Intern Med 104: 74, 1986.

159. Krell WS, Staats BA, Hyatt RE: Pulmonary function in relapsing polychondritis. Am Rev Respir Dis 133: 1120, 1986.

160. Mohsenifar Z, Tashkin DP, Carson SA, et al: Pulmonary function in patients with relapsing polychondritis. Chest 81: 711, 1982.

161. Gibson GJ, Davis P: Respiratory complications of relapsing polychondritis. Thorax 29: 726, 1974.

162. Leavitt RY, Fauci AS: Pulmonary vasculitis. Am Rev Respir Dis 134: 149, 1986.

163. Leavitt RY, Fauci AS, Bloch DA, et al: The American College of Rheumatology 1990 criteria for the classification of Wegener's granulomatosis. Arthritis Rheum 33: 1101, 1990.

164. Carrington CB, Liebow AA: Limited forms of angiitis and granulomatosis of Wegener's type. Am J Med 41: 497, 1966.

165. Hoffman GS, Sechler JM, Gallin JI, et al: Bronchoalveolar lavage analysis in Wegener's granulomatosis. A method to study disease pathogenesis. Am Rev Respir Dis 1431: 401, 1991.

166. Willoughby WF, Barbaras JE, Wheelis R: Immunologic mechanisms in experimental interstitial pneumonitis. Chest 69: 290, 1976.

167. Hay EM, Beaman M, Ralston AJ, et al: Wegener's granulomatosis occurring in siblings. Br J Rheumatol 30: 144, 1991.

168. Murty GE, Mains BT, Middleton D, et al: HLA antigen frequencies and Wegener's granulomatosis. Clin Otolaryngol 16: 448, 1991.

169. Fauci AS, Balow JE, Brown R, et al: Successful renal transplantation in Wegener's granulomatosis. Am J Med 60: 437, 1976.

170. Howell SB, Epstein WV: Circulating immunoglobulin complexes in Wegener's granulomatosis. Am J Med 60: 259, 1976.

171. Shasby DM, Schwarz MI, Forstot JZ, et al: Pulmonary immune complex deposition in Wegener's granulomatosis. Chest 81: 3, 1982.

172. Gephardt GN, Shah LF, Tubbs RR, et al: Wegener's granulomatosis. Immunomicroscopic and ultrastructural study of four cases. Arch Pathol Lab Med 114: 961, 1990.

173. Yoshikawa Y, Watanabe T: Pulmonary lesions in Wegener's granulomatosis: A clinicopathologic study of 22 autopsy cases. Hum Pathol 17: 401, 1986.

174. Mark EJ, Matsubara O, Tan-Liu NS, et al: The pulmonary biopsy in the early diagnosis of Wegener's (pathergic) granulomatosis: A study based on 35 open lung biopsies. Hum Pathol 19: 1065, 1988.

175. Myers JL, Katzenstein AA: Wegener's granulomatosis presenting with massive pulmonary hemorrhage and capillaritis. Am J Surg Pathol 11: 895, 1987.

176. Devaney KO, Travis WD, Hoffman G, et al: Interpretation of head and neck biopsies in Wegener's granulomatosis. A pathologic study of 126 biopsies in 70 patients. Am J Surg Pathol 14: 555, 1990.

177. Gohel VK, Dalinka MK, Israel HL, et al: The radiological manifestations of Wegener's granulomatosis. Br J Radiol 46: 427, 1973.

178. Israel HL, Patchefsky AS: Wegener's granulomatosis of lung: Diagnosis and treatment, experience with 12 cases. Ann Intern Med 74: 881, 1971.

178a. Kuhlman JE, Hruban RH, Fishman EK: Wegener granulomatosis: CT features of parenchymal lung disease. J Comput Assist Tomogr 15: 948, 1991.

179. Maguire R, Fauci AS, Doppman JL, et al: Unusual radiographic features of Wegener's granulomatosis. AJR 130: 233, 1978.

180. Travis WD, Carpenter HA, Lie JT: Diffuse pulmonary hemorrhage: An uncommon manifestation of Wegener's granulomatosis. Am J Surg Pathol 11: 702, 1987.

181. Pinching AJ, Lockwood CM, Pussell BA, et al: Wegener's granulomatosis: Observations on 18 patients with severe renal disease. Q J Med 52: 435, 1983.

182. Aberle DR, Gamsu G, Lynch D: Thoracic manifestations of Wegener's granulomatosis: Diagnosis and course. Radiology 174: 703, 1990.

183. Littlejohn GO, Ryan PJ, Holdsworth SR: Wegener's granulomatosis: Clinical features and outcome in seventeen patients. Aust NZ J Med 15: 241, 1985.

184. Brandwein S, Esdaile J, Danoff D, et al: Wegener's granulomatosis: Clinical features and outcome in 13 patients. Arch Intern Med 143: 476, 1983.

185. Tervaert JW, Limburg PC, Elema JD, et al: Detection of autoantibodies against myeloid lysosomal enzymes: A useful adjunct to classification of patients with biopsy-proven necrotizing arteritis. Am J Med 91: 59, 1991.

186. Specks U, Wheatley CL, McDonald TJ, et al: Anticytoplasmic autoantibodies in the diagnosis and follow-up of Wegener's granulomatosis. Mayo Clin Proc 64: 28, 1989.

187. Cohen Tervaert JW, Goldschmeding R, Elema JD, et al: Autoantibodies against myeloid lysosomal enzymes in crescentic glomerulonephritis. Kidney Int 37: 799, 1990.

188. Egner W, Chapel HM: Titration of antibodies against neutrophil cytoplasmic antigens is useful in monitoring disease activity in systemic vasculitides. Clin Exp Immunol 82: 244, 1990.

189. Mustonen J, Soppi E, Pasternack A, et al: Clinical significance of autoantibodies against neutrophil cytoplasmic components in patients with renal disease. Am J Nephrol 1016: 482, 1990.

190. Cohen Tervaert JW, Hultema MG, Hené RJ et al: Prevention of relapses in Wegener's granulomatosis by treatment based on antineutrophil cytoplasmic antibody titre. Lancet 336: 709, 1990.

191. Fauci AS, Wolff SM: Wegener's granulomatosis: Studies in eighteen patients and a review of the literature. Medicine 52: 535, 1973.

191a. Hoffman GS, Kerr GS, Leavitt RY, et al: Wegener granulomatosis: An analysis of 158 patients. Ann Intern Med 116: 488, 1992.

192. Chandran PKG, First MR, Weiss MA, et al: Wegener's granulomatosis: Prolonged patient survival after pneumonectomy and renal transplantation. Am J Nephrol 2: 325, 1982.

193. Masi AT, Hunder GG, Lie JT, et al: The American College of Rheumatology 1990 criteria for the classification of Churg-Strauss syndrome (allergic granulomatosis and angiitis). Arthritis Rheum 33: 1094, 1990.

194. Fauci AS, Haynes BF, Katz P: The spectrum of vasculitis. Clinical, pathologic, immunologic, and therapeutic considerations. Ann Intern Med 89: 660, 1978.

195. Fienberg R: Allergic granulomatosis. Am J Surg Pathol 6: 189, 1982.

196. Guillevin L, Guittard T, Bletry O, et al: Systemic necrotizing angiitis with asthma: Causes and precipitating factors in 43 cases. Lung 165: 165, 1987.

197. Chumbley LC, Harrison EG Jr, DeRemee RA: Allergic granulomatosis and angiitis (Churg-Strauss syndrome) report and analysis of 30 cases. Mayo Clin Proc 52: 477, 1977.

198. Churg J, Strauss L: Allergic granulomatosis, allergic angiitis, and periarteritis nodosa. Am J Pathol 27: 277, 1951.

199. Koss MN, Antonovych T, Hochholzer L: Allergic granulomatosis (Churg-Strauss syndrome) pulmonary and renal morphologic findings. Am J Surg Pathol 5: 21, 1981.

200. Hunninghake GW, Fauci AS: Pulmonary involvement in the collagen vascular diseases. Am Rev Respir Dis 119: 471, 1979.

201. Olivieri D, Pesci A, Bertorelli G: Eosinophilic alveolitis in immunologic interstitial lung disorders. Lung 168: 964, 1990.

202. Fujioka M, Bender T, Young LW, et al: Polyarteritis nodosa in children: Radiological aspects and diagnostic correlation. Radiology 136: 359, 1980.

203. Hinshaw HC, Garland LH: Diseases of the Chest. 3rd ed. Philadelphia, WB Saunders, 1969.

204. Koss MN, Hochholzer L, Feigin DS, et al: Necrotizing sarcoid-like granulomatosis: Clinical, pathologic, and immunopathologic findings. Hum Pathol 11: 510, 1980.

205. Rosen Y, Moon S, Huang C-T, et al: Granulomatous pulmonary angiitis in sarcoidosis. Arch Pathol Lab Med 101: 170, 1977.

206. Churg A, Carrington CB, Gupta R: Necrotizing sarcoid granulomatosis. Chest 76: 706, 1979.

207. Fisher MR, Christ ML, Bernstein JR: Necrotizing sarcoid-like granulomatosis: radiologic-pathologic correlation. J Can Assoc Radiol 35: 313, 1984.

208. Nasu T: Takayasu's truncoarteritis in Japan. A statistical observation of 76 autopsy cases. Pathol Microbiol 43: 140, 1975.

209. Hayashi K, Nagasaki M, Matsunaga N, et al: Initial pulmonary artery involvement in Takayasu arteritis. Radiology 159: 401, 1986.

210. Lupi HE, Sanchez TG, Horwitz S, et al: Pulmonary artery involvement in Takayasu's arteritis. Chest 67: 69, 1967.

211. Lupi-Herrera E, Sanchez-Torres G, Marcushamer J, et al: Takayasu's arteritis. Clinical study of 107 cases. Am Heart J 93: 94, 1977.

212. Berkmen YM, Lande A: Chest roentgenography as a window to the diagnosis of Takayasu's arteritis. Am J Roentgenol 125: 842, 1975.

213. Ladanyi M, Fraser RS: Pulmonary involvement in giant cell arteritis. Arch Pathol Lab Med 111: 1178, 1987.

214. Larson TS, Hall S, Hepper NGG, et al: Respiratory tract symptoms as a clue to giant cell arteritis. Ann Intern Med 101: 594, 1984.

215. Efthimiou J, Johnston C, Spiro SG, et al: Pulmonary disease in Behçet's syndrome. Q J Med 58: 259, 1986.

216. Raz I, Okon E, Chajek-Shaul T: Pulmonary manifestations in Behçet's syndrome. Chest 95: 585, 1989.

217. Herreman G, Beaufils H, Godeau P, et al: Behçet's syndrome and renal involvement: A histological and immunofluorescent study of 11 renal biopsies. Am J Med Sci 284: 10, 1982.

218. Gupta RC, O'Duffy JD, McDuffie FC, et al: Circulating immune complexes in active Behçet's disease. Clin Exp Immunol 34: 213, 1978.

219. Slavin RE, de Groot WJ: Pathology of the lung in Behçet's disease. Case report and review of the literature. Am J Surg Pathol 5: 779, 1981.

220. Petty TL, Scoggin CH, Good GT: Recurrent pneumonia in Behçet's syndrome: Roentgenographic documentation during 13 years. JAMA 238: 2529, 1977.

221. Chajek T, Fainaru M: Behçet's disease: Report of 41 cases and a review of the literature. Medicine 54: 179, 1975.

222. Ahonen AV, Stenius-Aarniala BS, Viljanen BC, et al: Obstructive lung disease in Behçet's syndrome. Scand J Respir Dis 59: 44, 1978.

223. Cryer PE, Kissane J: Mixed cryoimmunoglobulinemia. Am J Med 61: 95, 1976.

224. Chejfec G, Lichtenberg L, Lertratanakul Y, et al: Quarterly case. Respiratory insufficiency in a patient with mixed cryoglobulinemia. Ultrastruct Pathol 2: 295, 1981.

225. Bombardieri S, Paoletti P, Ferri C, et al: Lung involvement in essential mixed cryoglobulinemia. Am J Med 66: 748, 1979.

226. Cream JJ, Gumpel JM, Peachey RDG: Schönlein-Henoch purpura in the adult. A study of 77 adults with anaphylactoid or Schönlein-Henoch purpura. Q J Med New Series 39: 461, 1970.

227. Kathuria S, Cheifec G: Fatal pulmonary Henoch-Schönlein syndrome. Chest 182: 654, 1982.

228. Fulmer JD, Kaltreider HB: The pulmonary Vasculitides. Chest 82: 615, 1982.

229. Mark EJ, Ramirez JR: Pulmonary capillaritis and hemorrhage in patients with systemic vasculitis. Arch Pathol Lab Med 109: 413, 1985.

230. Scherzer H, Ward PA: Lung and dermal vascular injury produced by preformed immune complexes. Am Rev Respir Dis 117: 551, 1978.

231. Bellon B, Bernaudin J-F, Mandet C, et al: Immune complex–mediated lung injury produced by horseradish peroxidase (HRP) and anti-HRP antibodies in rats. Am J Pathol 107: 16, 1982.

232. Fukuda Y, Yamanaka N, Ishizaki M, et al: Immune complex–mediated glomerulonephritis and interstitial pneumonia simulating Goodpasture's syndrome. Acta Pathol Jpn 32: 361, 1982.

233. Liebow AA: Pulmonary angiitis and granulomatosis. Am Rev Respir Dis 108: 1, 1973.

234. Katzenstein AL, Liebow AA, Friedman PJ: Bronchocentric granulomatosis, mucoid impaction, and hypersensitivity reactions to fungi. Am Rev Respir Dis 111: 497, 1975.

235. Hertog RWD, Wagenaar SS, Westermar CJJ: Bronchocentric granulomatosis and pulmonary echinococcosis. Case reports. Am Rev Respir Dis 126: 344, 1982.

236. Bonafede RP, Benatar SR: Bronchocentric granulomatosis and rheumatoid arthritis. Br J Dis Chest 81: 197, 1987.

237. Rohatgi PK, Turrisi BC: Bronchocentric granulomatosis and ankylosing spondylitis. Thorax 39: 317, 1984.

238. Warren J, Pitchenik AE, Saldana MJ: Bronchocentric granulomatosis with glomerulonephritis. Chest 87: 832, 1985.

239. Maguire GP, Lee M, Rosen Y, et al: Pulmonary tuberculosis and bronchocentric granulomatosis. Chest 89: 606, 1986.

240. Schilling R: Worldwide problems of byssinosis. Chest 79: 3S, 1981.

240a. Fishwick D, Pickering CAC: Byssinosis—a form of occupational asthma? Thorax 47: 401, 1992.

241. Ong SG, Lam TH, Wong CM, et al: Byssinosis and other respiratory problems in the cotton industry of Hong Kong. Am J Ind Med 12: 773, 1987.

242. Lammers B, Schilling RSF, Walford I: A study of byssinosis, chronic respiratory symptoms, and ventilatory capacity in English and Dutch cotton workers, with special reference to atmospheric pollution. Br J Ind Med 21: 124, 1964.

243. Bouhuys A: Byssinosis in a cotton weaving mill. Arch Environ Health 6: 465, 1963.

244. Arnoldsson H, Bouhuys A, Lindsell SE: Byssinosis: Differential diagnosis from bronchial asthma and chronic bronchitis. Acta Med Scand 173: 761, 1963.

245. Munt DF, Gauvain S, Walford J, et al: Study of respiratory symptoms and ventilatory capacities among rope workers. Br J Ind Med 22: 196, 1965.

246. Hamilton JD, Halprin GM, Kilburn KH, et al: Differential aerosol challenge studies in byssinosis. Arch Environ Health 26: 120, 1973.

247. Buck MG, Bouhuys A: Byssinosis: Airway constrictor response to cotton bracts. Lung 158: 25, 1980.

248. Jones RN, Diem JE, Glindmeyer H, et al: Mill effect and dose-response relationships in byssinosis: Br J Ind Med 36: 305, 1979.

249. Rylander R, Imbus HR, Suh MW: Bacterial contamination of cotton as an indicator of respiratory effects among card room workers. Br J Ind Med 36: 299, 1979.

250. Castellan RM, Olenchock SA, Kinsley KB, et al: Inhaled endotoxin and decreased spirometric values: An exposure-response relation for cotton dust. N Engl J Med 317: 605, 1987.

251. Taylor G, Massoud A, Lucas F: Studies on the etiology of byssinosis. Br J Ind Med 28: 143, 1971.

252. Edwards JH, AlZubaidy TS, Altikriti R, et al: Byssinosis: Inhalation challenge with polyphenol. Chest 85: 215, 1984.

253. Edwards C, Carlile A, Rooke G: The larger bronchi in byssinosis: A morphometric study. J Clin Pathol 37: 20, 1984.

254. Moran TJ: Emphysema and other chronic lung disease in textile workers: An 18-year autopsy study. Arch Environ Health 38: 267, 1983.

255. Mair A, Smith DH, Wilson WA, et al: Dust diseases in Dundee textile workers. An investigation into chronic respiratory disease in jute and flax industries. Br J Industr Med 17: 272, 1960.

256. Bouhuys A, van Duyn J, van Lennep HJ: Byssinosis in flax workers. Arch Environ Health 3: 499, 1961.

257. Zuskin E, Valic F: Respiratory changes in two groups of flax workers with different exposure pattern. Thorax 28: 579, 1973.

258. Schachter EN, Kapp MC, Maunder LR, et al: Smoking and cotton dust effects in cotton textile workers: An analysis of the shape of the maximum expiratory flow volume curve. Environ Health Perspect 66: 145, 1986.

259. Morgan WKC, Vesterlund J, Burrell R, et al: Byssinosis: Some unanswered questions. Am Rev Respir Dis 126: 354, 1982.

260. Beck GJ, Schachter EN, Maunder LR, et al: The relation of lung function to subsequent employment status and mortality in cotton textile workers. Chest 79: 26S, 1981.

261. Battigelli MC, Berni RJ, Sasser PE, et al: The relationship of acute respiratory response and chronic respiratory symptoms in byssinosis. Chest 79: 86S, 1981.

262. Yoshizawa Y, Ohtsuka M, Noguchi K, et al: Hypersensitivity pneumonitis induced by toluene diisocyanate: Sequelae of continuous exposure. Ann Intern Med 110: 31, 1989.

263. Cadhan FT: Asthma due to grain rusts. JAMA 82: 27, 1924.

264. Saltos N, Saunders NA, Bhagwandeen SB, et al: Hypersensitivity pneumonitis in a mouldy house. Med J Aust 2: 244, 1982.

265. Salvaggio JE: Hypersensitivity pneumonitis: Pandora's box. N Engl J Med 283: 314, 1970.

266. Braun O, Zwick H, Rauscher H, et al: Detection of antigen-specific antibodies on lung tissue in a patient with hypersensitivity pneumonitis. Virchows Arch [A] 413: 223, 1988.

267. Warren CPW, Cherniack RM, Tse KS: Extrinsic allergic alveolitis from bird exposure: Studies on the immediate hypersensitivity reaction. Clin Allergy 7: 303, 1977.

268. Edwards JH, Davies BH: Inhalation challenge and skin testing in farmer's lung. J Allergy Clin Immunol 68: 58, 1981.

269. Wilson MR, Schuyler MR, Cashner F, et al: The effect of complement depletion on hypersensitivity pneumonitis lesions induced by *Micropolyspora faeni* antigen. Clin Allergy 11: 131, 1981.

270. Konishi K, Murakami S, Kokubu K, et al: Determination by enzyme-linked immunosorbent assay (ELISA) of specific IgG antibody activities for diagnosis of farmer's lung disease. Tohoku J Exp Med 147: 135, 1985.

271. Patterson R, Schatz M, Fink JN, et al: Pigeon-breeders' disease. 1. Serum immunoglobulin concentrations; IgG, IgM, IgA, and IgE antibodies against pigeon serum. Am J Med 60: 144, 1976.

272. Lee TH, Wraith DG, Bennett CO, et al: Budgerigar fanciers' lung: The persistence of budgerigar precipitins and the recovery of lung function after cessation of avian exposure. Clin Allergy 13: 197, 1983.

273. Hapke EJ, Seal RME, Thomas GO, et al: Farmer's lung. A clinical, radiographic, functional, and serological correlation of acute and chronic stages. Thorax 23: 451, 1968.

274. Hargreave FE: Review article: Extrinsic allergic alveolitis. Can Med Assoc J 108: 1150, 1973.

275. Banaszak EF, Barboriak J, Fink JN, et al: Epidemiologic studies relating thermophilic fungi and hypersensitivity lung syndromes. Am Rev Resp Dis 110: 585, 1974.

276. Cormier Y, Bélanger J: The fluctant nature of precipitating antibodies in dairy farmers. Thorax 44: 469, 1989.

277. Burrell R, Rylander R: A critical review of the role of precipitins in hypersensitivity pneumonitis. Eur J Respir Dis 62: 332, 1981.

278. Schuyler MR, Schmitt D: Experimental hypersensitivity pneumonitis: Lack of tolerance. Am Rev Respir Dis 130: 772, 1984.

279. van den Bosch JM, Heyc C, Wagenaar SS, et al: Bronchoalveolar lavage in extrinsic allergic alveolitis. Respiration 49: 45, 1986.

280. Keller RH, Swartz S, Schlueter DP, et al: Immunoregulation in hypersensitivity pneumonitis: Phenotypic and functional studies of bronchoalveolar lavage lymphocytes. Am Rev Respir Dis 130: 766, 1984.

281. Trentin L, Zambello R, Agostini C, et al: Different types of cytotoxic lymphocytes recovered from the lungs of patients with hypersensitivity pneumonitis. Am Rev Respir Dis 137: 70, 1988.

282. Soler P, Nioche S, Valeyre D, et al: Role of mast cells in the pathogenesis of hypersensitivity pneumonitis. Thorax 42: 565, 1987.

283. Bjermer L, Engström-Laurent A, Lundgren R, et al: Bronchoalveolar mastocytosis in farmer's lung is related to the disease activity. Arch Intern Med 148: 1362, 1988.

284. Warren CPW: Extrinsic allergic alveolitis: A disease commoner in nonsmokers. Thorax 32: 567, 1977.

285. Andersen P, Christensen KM: Serum antibodies to pigeon antigens in smokers and nonsmokers. Acta Med Scand 213: 191, 1983.

286. Riley DJ, Saldana M: Pigeon breeders' lung: Subacute course and the importance of indirect exposure. Am Rev Resp Dis 107: 456, 1973.

287. Warren WP: Hypersensitivity pneumonitis due to exposure to budgerigars. Chest 62: 170, 1972.

288. Larsson K, Malmberg P, Eklund A, et al: Exposure to microorganisms, airway inflammatory changes and immune reactions in asymptomatic dairy farmers. Bronchoalveolar lavage evidence of macrophage activation and permeability changes in the airways. Int Arch Allergy Appl Immunol 87: 127, 1988.

289. Pimentel JC, Alvila R: Respiratory disease in cork workers (suberosis). Thorax 28: 409, 1973.

290. Reyes CN, Wenzel JF, Lawton BR, et al: The pulmonary pathology of farmers' lung disease. Chest 81: 142, 1982.

291. Coleman A, Colby TV: Histologic diagnosis of extrinsic allergic alveolitis. Am J Surg Pathol 12: 514, 1988.

292. Stoltz JL, Arger PH, Benson JM: Mushroom worker's lung disease. Radiology 119: 61, 1976.

293. Fraser RG, Paré JAP: Extrinsic allergic alveolitis. Semin Roentgenol 10: 1, 1975.

294. Cormier Y, Belanger J, Tardif A, et al: Relationships between radiographic change, pulmonary function, and bronchoalveolar lavage fluid lymphocytes in farmer's lung disease. Thorax 41: 28, 1986.

295. Fink JN, Schlueter DP, Sosman AJ, et al: Clinical survey of pigeon breeders. Chest 62: 277, 1972.

296. Frank RC: Farmer's lung—a form of pneumoconiosis due to organic dusts. Am J Roentgenol 79: 189, 1958.

297. Silver SF, Müller NL, Miller RR, et al: Hypersensitivity pneumonitis: Evaluation with CT. Radiology 173: 441, 1989.

298. Hargreave F, Hinson KF, Reid L, et al: The radiological appearances of allergic alveolitis due to bird sensitivity (bird fancier's lung). Clin Radiol 23: 1, 1972.

299. Pepys J: Pulmonary hypersensitivity disease due to inhaled organic antigens. Ann Intern Med 64: 943, 1966.

300. Pepys J, Jenkins PA: Precipitin (FLH) test in famer's lung. Thorax 20: 21, 1965.

301. Bourke S, Anderson K, Lynch P, et al: Chronic simple bronchitis in pigeon fanciers. Relationship of cough with expectoration to avain exposure and pigeon breeders' disease. Chest 95: 598, 1989.

302. Earis JE, Marsh K, Pearson MG, et al: The inspiratory "squawk" in extrinsic allergic and other pulmonary fibroses. Thorax 37: 923, 1982.

303. Sansores R, Salas J, Chapela R, et al: Clubbing in hypersensitivity pneumonitis: Its prevalence and possible prognostic role. Arch Intern Med 150: 1849, 1990.

304. A national survey of bird fancier's lung including its possible association with jejunal villous atrophy. (A report to the Research Committee of the British Thoracic Society.) Br J Dis Chest 78:75, 1984.

305. Harries MG, Heard B, Geddes D: Extrinsic allergic bronchiolitis in a bird fancier. Br J Ind Med 41: 220, 1984.

306. Hargreave FE, Pepys J: Allergic respiratory reactions in bird fanciers provoked by allergen inhalation provocation test. J Allergy Clin Immunol 50: 157, 1972.

307. Tewksbury DA, Marx JJ Jr, Roberts RC, et al: Angiotensin-converting enzyme in farmer's lung. Chest 79: 102, 1981.

308. McCormick JR, Thrall RS, Ward PA, et al: Serum angiotensin-converting enzyme levels in patients with pigeon-breeder's disease. Chest 80: 431, 1981.

309. Orriols R, Morell F, Curull V, et al: Impaired non-specific delayed cutaneous hypersensitivity in bird fancier's lung. Thorax 44: 132, 1989.

310. Monkare S: Clinical aspects of farmer's lung: Airway reactivity, treatment and prognosis. Eur J Respir Dis 137(Suppl): 1, 1984.

311. Warren CPW, Tse KS, Cherniack RM: Mechanical properties of the lung in extrinsic allergic alveolitis. Thorax 33: 315, 1987.

312. Sovijarvi ARA, Kuusisto P, Muittari A, et al: Trapped air in extrinsic allergic alveolitis. Respiration 40: 57, 1980.

313. Grammer LC, Roberts M, Lerner C, et al: Clinical and serologic follow-up of four children and five adults with bird fancier's lung. J Allergy Clin Immunol 85: 655, 1990.

314. Monkare S, Haahtela T: Farmer's lung: A 5-year follow-up of eighty-six patients. Clin Allergy 17: 143, 1987.

315. Schmidt CD, Jensen RL, Christensen LT, et al: Longitudinal pulmonary function changes in pigeon breeders. Chest 93: 359, 1988.

316. Bourke SJ, Banham SW, Carter R, et al: Longitudinal course of extrinsic allergic alveolitis in pigeon breeders. Thorax 44: 415, 1989.

317. Crofton JW, Livingstone JL, Oswald NC, et al: Pulmonary eosinophilia. Thorax 7: 1, 1952.

318. Citro LA, Gordon ME, Miller WT: Eosinophilic lung disease (or how to slice PIE). Am J Roentgenol 117: 787, 1973.

319. Ford RM: Transient pulmonary eosinophilia and asthma. A review of 20 cases occurring in 5,702 asthma sufferers. Am Rev Respir Dis 93: 797, 1966.

320. Incaprera FP: Pulmonary eosinophilia. Am Rev Respir Dis 84: 730, 1981.

321. Morrissey JF, Gibbs GM: Pulmonary infiltration with eosinophilia occurring postpartum. Arch Intern Med 107: 95, 1961.

322. Badesch DB, King TE Jr, Schwarz MI: Acute eosinophilic pneumonia: A hypersensitivity phenomenon? Am Rev Respir Dis 139: 249, 1989.

323. Allen JN, Pacht ER, Gadek JE, et al: Acute eosinophilic pneumonia as a reversible cause of noninfectious respiratory failure. N Engl J Med 321: 569, 1989.

324. Davis WB, Wilson HE, Wall RL: Eosinophilic alveolitis in acute respiratory failure. A clinical marker for a non-infectious etiology. Chest 90: 7, 1986.

325. Jederlinic PJ, Sicilian L, Gaensler E: Chronic eosinophilic pneumonia. A report of 19 cases and a review of the literature. Medicine 67: 154, 1988.

326. Carrington CB, Addington WW, Goff AM, et al: Chronic eosinophilic pneumonia. N Engl J Med 280: 787, 1969.

327. Fox B, Seed WA: Chronic eosinophilic pneumonia. Thorax 35: 570, 1980.

328. Gonzalez EB, Hayes D, Weedn NW: Chronic eosinophilic pneumonia (Carrington's) with increased serum IgE levels. A distinct subset? Arch Intern Med 148: 2622, 1988.

329. Mayo JR, Müller NL, Road J, et al: Chronic eosinophilic pneumonia: CT findings in six cases. Am J Roentgenol 153: 727, 1989.

330. Pearson DJ, Rosenow EC III: Chronic eosinophilic pneumonia (Carrington's). A follow-up study. Mayo Clin Proc 53: 73, 1978.

331. Fauci AS, Harley JB, Roberts WC, et al: The idiopathic hypereosinophilic syndrome. Ann Intern Med 97: 78, 1982.

332. Clinicopathologic conference: Hypereosinophilic syndrome with pulmonary hypertension. Am J Med 60: 239, 1976.

333. Hill R, Wang NS, Berry G: Hypereosinophilic syndrome with pulmonary vascular involvement. Angiology 35: 238, 1984.

334. Proskey AJ, Weatherbee L, Easterling RE, et al: Goodpasture's syndrome: A report of five cases and review of the literature. Am J Med 48: 162, 1970.

335. Holdsworth S, Boyce N, Thomson NM, et al: The clinical spectrum of acute glomerulonephritis and lung haemorrhage (Goodpasture's syndrome). Q J Med 55: 75, 1985.

336. Beechler CR, Enquist RW, Hunt KK, et al: Immunofluorescence of transbronchial biopsies in Goodpasture's syndrome. Am Rev Respir Dis 121: 869, 1980.

337. McPhaul JJ Jr, Dixon JF: Characterization of immunoglobulin G antiglomerular basement membrane antibodies eluted from kidneys of patients with glomerulonephritis. II. IgG subtypes and in vitro complement fixation. J Immunol 107: 678, 1971.

338. Hagadorn JE, Vasquez JJ, Kinney TR: Immunopathologic study on

an experimental model resembling Goodpasture's syndrome. Am J Pathol 57: 17, 1969.

339. Willoughby WF, Dixon FJ: Experimental hemorrhagic pneumonitis produced by heterologous anti-lung antibody. J Immunol 104: 28, 1970.

340. Silverman M, Hawkins D, Ackman CFD: Bilateral nephrectomy for massive pulmonary hemorrhage in Goodpasture's syndrome. Can Med Assoc J 108: 336, 1973.

341. Carre P, Lloveras JJ, Didier A, et al: Goodpasture's syndrome with normal renal function. Eur Respir J 2: 911, 1989.

342. Meyer zum Büschenfelde KH, Köhler H: Immunological properties of the human Goodpasture target antigen. Clin Exp Immunol 74: 289, 1988.

343. Pusey CD, Dash A, Kershaw MJ, et al: A single autoantigen in Goodpasture's syndrome identified by a monoclonal antibody to human glomerular basement membrane. Lab Invest 56: 23, 1987.

344. Ligler FS, Westby GR, Hertz BC, et al: Immunoregulatory cell subsets in Goodpasture's syndrome: Evidence for selective T suppressor-cell depletion during active autoimmune disease. J Clin Immunol 3: 368, 1983.

345. Bombassei GJ, Kaplan AA: The association between hydrocarbon exposure and anti–glomerular basement membrane antibody-mediated disease (Goodpasture's syndrome). Am J Ind Med 21: 141, 1992.

346. Pusey CD, Evans JD: Extraglomerular distribution of immunoreactive Goodpasture antigen. J Pathol 155: 61, 1988.

347. Donaghy M, Rees AJ: Cigarette smoking and lung hemorrhage in glomerulonephritis caused by autoantibodies to glomerular basement membrane. Lancet 2: 1390, 1983.

348. Hyatt RW, Adelstein ER, Halazun JF, et al: Ultrastructure of the lung in idiopathic pulmonary hemosiderosis. Am J Med 52: 822, 1972.

349. Donlon CJ, Srodes CH, Duffy FD: Idiopathic pulmonary hemosiderosis. Electron microscopic, immunofluorescent, and iron kinetic studies. Chest 68: 577, 1975.

350. Corrin B, Jagusch M, Devar A, et al: Fine structural changes in idiopathic pulmonary haemosiderosis. J Pathol 153: 249, 1987.

351. Wright PH, Menzies IS, Pounder RE, et al: Adult idiopathic pulmonary haemosiderosis and coeliac disease. Q J Med 50: 95, 1981.

352. Theros EG, Reeder MM, Eckert JF: An exercise in radiologic-pathologic correlation. Radiology 90: 784, 1968.

353. Brannan HM, McCaughey WTE, Good CA: The roentgenographic appearance of pulmonary hemorrhage associated with glomerulonephritis. Am J Roentgenol 90: 83, 1963.

353a. Buschman DL, Gamsu G, Waldron JA Jr, et al: Chronic hypersensitivity pneumonitis: Use of CT in diagnosis. Am J Roentgenol 159: 957, 1992.

353b. Lynch DA, Rose CS, Way D, King TE Jr: Hypersensitivity pneumonitis: Sensitivity of high-resolution CT in a population-based study. Am J Roentgenol 159: 469, 1992.

354. Ditto WR, Ognibene AJ: Idiopathic pulmonary hemosiderosis without anemia. Report of two cases. Arch Intern Med 114: 490, 1964.

355. Lane DJ, Hamilton WS: Idiopathic steatorrhoea and idiopathic pulmonary haemosiderosis. Br Med J 2: 89, 1971.

356. Mathew TH, Hobbs JB, Kalowski S, et al: Goodpasture's syndrome: Normal renal diagnostic findings. Ann Intern Med 82: 215, 1979.

357. Allue X, Wise MB, Beaudry PH: Pulmonary function studies in idiopathic hemosiderosis in children. Am Rev Respir Dis 107: 410, 1973.

358. Donald KJ, Edwarda RL, McEvoy JDS: Alveolar capillary basement membrane lesions in Goodpasture's syndrome and idiopathic pulmonary hemosiderosis. Am J Med 59: 642, 1975.

359. Addleman M, Logan AS, Grossman RF: Monitoring intrapulmonary hemorrhage in Goodpasture's syndrome. Chest 87: 119, 1985.

360. Vanhille P, Raviart B, Morel-Maroger L, et al: Circulating immune complexes appearing in Goodpasture's syndrome. Br Med J 280: 1166, 1980.

361. Kurki P, Helve T, von Bonsdorff M, et al: Transformation of membranous glomerulonephritis into crescentic glomerulonephritis with glomerular basement membrane antibodies. Nephron 38: 134, 1984.

362. Soergel H, Sommers SC: Idiopathic pulmonary hemosiderosis and related syndromes. Am J Med 32: 499, 1962.

363. Bronson SM: Idiopathic pulmonary hemosiderosis in adults. Report of a case and review of the literature. Am J Roentgenol 83: 260, 1960.

364. Chryssanthopoulos C, Cassimos C, Panagiotidou C: Prognostic criteria in idiopathic pulmonary hemosiderosis in children. Eur J Pediatr 140: 123, 1983.

365. Walker RG, Scheinkestel C, Becker GJ, et al: Clinical and morphological aspects of the management of crescentic anti–glomerular basement antibody (anti-GBM) nephritis/Goodpasture's syndrome. Q J Med 54: 75, 1985.

366. Krowka MJ, Rosenow EC, Hoagland HC: Pulmonary complications of bone marrow transplantation. Chest 87: 237, 1985.

367. Wingard JR, Santos GW, Saral R: Late-onset interstitial pneumonia following allogeneic bone marrow transplantation. Transplantation 39: 21, 1985.

368. Robbins RA, Linder J, Stahl MG, et al: Diffuse alveolar hemorrhage in autologous bone marrow transplant recipients. Am J Med 87: 511, 1989.

369. Bortin MM, Kay HEM, Gale RP, et al: Factors associated with interstitial pneumonitis after bone marrow transplantation for acute leukemia. Lancet 1: 437, 1982.

370. Perrault C, Cousineau S, D'Angelo G, et al: Lymphoid interstitial pneumonia after allogeneic bone marrow transplantation: A possible manifestation of chronic graft-versus-host disease. Cancer 55: 1, 1985.

371. Appelbaum FR, Myers JD, Fefer A, et al: Nonbacterial nonfungal pneumonia following marrow transplantation in 100 identical twins. Transplantation 33: 265, 1982.

372. Baker SB, Robinson DR: Unusual renal manifestations of Wegener's granulomatosis: Report of two cases. Am J Med 64: 883, 1978.

373. Wise RH, Shin MS, Gockerman JP, et al: Pneumonia in bone marrow transplant patients. Am J Roentgenol 143: 707, 1984.

374. Chan CK, Hyland RH, Hutcheon MA, et al: Small-airways disease in recipients of allogeneic bone marrow transplants: An analysis of 11 cases and a review of the literature. Medicine 66: 327, 1987.

375. St. John RC, Gadek JE, Tutschka PJ, et al: Analysis of airflow obstruction by bronchoalveolar lavage following bone marrow transplantation. Implications for pathogenesis and treatment. Chest 98: 600, 1990.

376. Clark JG, Crawford SW, Madtes DK, et al: Obstructive lung disease after allogeneic marrow transplantation. Clinical presentation and course. Ann Intern Med 111: 368, 1989.

377. Jamieson SW, Baldwin J, Stinson EB, et al: Clinical heart-lung transplantation. Transplantation 37: 81, 1984.

378. Cagle PT, Truong LD, Holland VA, et al: Factors contributing to mortality in lung transplant recipients: An autopsy study. Mod Pathol 2: 85, 1989.

379. Penketh ARL, Higenbottam TW, Hutter J, et al: Clinical experience in the management of pulmonary opportunist infection and rejection in recipients of heart-lung transplants. Thorax 43: 762, 1988.

380. Herman SJ, Weisbrod GL, Weisbrod L, et al: Chest radiographic findings after bilateral lung transplantation. AJR 153: 1181, 1989.

381. Herman SJ, Rappaport DC, Weisbrod GL, et al: Single-lung transplantation: Imaging features. Radiology 170: 89, 1989.

382. Higenbottom TW, Stewart S, Penketh A, et al: Transbronchial lung biopsy for the diagnosis of rejection in heart-lung transplant patients. Transplantation 46: 532, 1988.

382a. Yousem SA, Randhawa P, Locker J, et al: Posttransplant lymphoproliferative disorders in heart-lung transplant recipients: Primary presentation in the allograft. Hum Pathol 20: 361, 1989.

383. Burke CM, Glanville AR, Theodore J, et al: Lung immunogenicity, rejection, and obliterative bronchiolitis. Chest 92: 547, 1987.

384. Yousem SA, Dauber JA, Keenan R, et al: Does histologic acute rejection in lung allografts predict the development of bronchiolitis obliterans? Transplantation 47: 893, 1989.

385. Khoury GF, Klandorf H, Brems J, et al: Efficacy of transbronchial lung biopsy in the diagnosis of bronchiolitis obliterans in heart-lung transplant recipients. Transplantation 47: 893, 1989.

386. Glanville AR, Baldwin JC, Burke CM, et al: Obliterative bronchiolitis after heart-lung transplantation: Apparent arrest by augmented immunosuppression. Ann Intern Med 107: 300, 1987.

387. Tazelaar HD, Yousem SA: The pathology of combined heart-lung transplantation: An autopsy study. Hum Pathol 19: 1403, 1988.

387a. Madden BP, Hodson ME, Tsang V, et al: Intermediate-term results of heart-lung transplantation for cystic fibrosis. Lancet 339: 1583, 1992.

387b. Ramirez JC, Patterson GA, Winton TL, et al: Bilateral lung transplantation for cystic fibrosis, the Toronto Lung Transplant Group. J Thorac Cardiovasc Surg 103: 287, 1992.

388. Heatley RV, Thomas P, Prokipchuk EJ: Pulmonary function abnormalities in patients with inflammatory bowel disease. Q J Med 51: 241, 1982.

389. Pasquis P, Colin R, Denis P, et al: Transient pulmonary impairment during attacks of Crohn's disease. Respiration 41: 56, 1981.

390. Rodriguez-Roisin R, Pares A, Bruguera M, et al: Pulmonary involvement in primary biliary cirrhosis. Thorax 36: 208, 1981.

391. Smyth JT, Adkins GE, Lloyd M, et al: Farmer's lung in Devon. Thorax 30: 197, 1975.

392. Gump DW, Babbott FL, Holly C, et al: Farmer's lung disease in Vermont. Respiration 37: 52, 1979.

393. Salvaggio JE, Buechner HA, Seabury JH, et al: Bagassosis: I. Precipitins against extracts of crude bagasse in the serum of patients. Ann Intern Med 64: 748, 1966.

394. Salvaggio JE, Seabury JH, Buechner HA, et al: Bagassosis: Demonstration of precipitins against extracts of thermophilic actinomycetes in the sera of affected individuals. J Allergy 39: 106, 1967.

395. Salvaggio JE, Arquembourg P, Seabury J, et al: Bagassosis. IV. Precipitins against extracts of thermophilic actinomycetes in patients with bagassosis. Am J Med 46: 538, 544, 1969.

396. Chan-Yeung M, Grzybowski S, Schonell ME: Mushroom worker's lung. Am Rev Respir Dis 105: 819, 1972.

397. Cockroft A, Edwards J, Campbell I: Investigation of an outbreak of humidifier fever in a hospital operating theatre. Br J Dis Chest 74: 317, 1980.

398. Fergusson RJ, Milne LJR, Crompton G: *Penicillium*-allergic alveolitis: Faulty installation of central heating. Thorax 39: 294, 1984.

399. Edwards JH, Griffiths AJ, Mullins J: Protozoa as sources of antigen in "humidifier fever." Nature 264: 438, 1976.

400. Jacobs RL, Thorner RE, Holcomb JR, et al: Hypersensitivity pneumonitis caused by *Cladosporium* in an enclosed hot-tub area. Ann Intern Med 105: 204, 1986.

401. Emanuel DA, Wenzel FJ, Lawton BR: Pneumonia due to *Cryptostroma corticale* maple-bark disease. N Engl J Med 274: 1413, 1966.

402. Grant IWB, Blackadder ES, Greenberg M, et al: Extrinsic allergic alveolitis in Scottish maltworkers. Br Med J 1: 490, 1976.

403. Kawai T, Tamura M, Murao M: Summer-type hypersensitivity pneumonitis: A unique disease in Japan. Chest 85: 311, 1984.

404. Bryant DH, Rogers P: Allergic alveolitis due to wood-rot fungi. Allergy Proc 12: 89, 1991.

405. Avila R, Villar TG: Suberosis: Respiratory disease in cork workers. Lancet 1: 620, 1968.

406. Alegre J, Morell F, Cobo E: Respiratory symptoms and pulmonary function of workers exposed to cork dust, toluene diisocyanate, and conidia. Scand J Work Environ Health 16: 175, 1990.

407. Schlueter DP, Fink JN, Hensley GT: Wood-pulp worker's disease: A hypersensitivity pneumonitis caused by *Alternaria*. Ann Intern Med 77: 907, 1972.

408. Campbell JA, Kryda MJ, Truehaft MW, et al: Cheese worker's hypersensitivity penumonitis. Am Rev Respir Dis 127: 495, 1983.

409. Cohen HI, Merigan TC, Kosek JC, et al: Sequoiosis: A granulomatous pneumonitis associated with redwood sawdust inhalation. Am J Med 43: 785, 1967.

410. Cox A, Folgering HT, van Griensven LJ: Extrinsic allergic alveolitis caused by spores of the oyster mushroom *Pleurotus ostreatus*. Eur Respir J 1: 466, 1988.

411. Blackburn CRB, Green W: Precipitins against extracts of thatched roofs in the sera of New Guinea natives with chronic lung disease. Lancet 2: 1396, 1966.

412. Flood DF, Blofeld RE, Bruce CF, et al: Lung function, atopy, specific hypersensitivity, and smoking of workers in the enzyme detergent industry over 11 years. Br J Ind Med 42: 43, 1985.

413. Hendrick DJ, Faux JA, Marshall R: Budgerigar fancier's lung: The commonest variety of allergic alveolitis in Britain. Br Med J 2: 81, 1978.

414. Boyer RS, Klock LE, Schmidt CD, et al: Hypersensitivity lung disease in the turkey raising industry. Am Rev Respir Dis 109: 630, 1974.

415. Warren CPW, Tse KS: Extrinsic allergic alveolitis owing to hypersensitivity to chickens: Significance of sputum precipitins. Am Rev Respir Dis 109: 672, 1974.

416. Sutton PP, Pearson A, DuBois RM: Canary fancier's lung. Clin Allergy 14: 429, 1984.

417. Harper LO, Burrell RG, Lapp NL, et al: Allergic alveolitis due to pituitary snuff. Ann Intern Med 73: 581, 1970.

418. Gaddie J, Legge JS, Friend JAR: Pulmonary hypersensitivity in prawn workers. Lancet 2: 1350, 1980.

419. Avila R: Extrinsic allergic alveolitis in workers exposed to fish meal and poultry. Clin Allergy 1: 343, 1971.

420. van Toorn DW: Coffee worker's lung: A new example of extrinsic allergic alveolitis. Thorax 25: 399, 1970.

421. Penn RG, Griffin JP: Adverse reactions to nitrofurantoin in the United Kingdom, Sweden, and Holland. Br Med J 284: 1440, 1982.

422. Reichlin S, Loveless MH, Kane EG: Loeffler's syndrome following penicillin therapy. Ann Intern Med 38: 113, 1953.

423. Fiengenberg DS, Weiss H, Kirshman H: Migratory pneumonia with eosinophilia associated with sulfonamide administration. Arch Intern Med 120: 85, 1967.

424. Donlan CJ, Scutero JV: Transient eosinophilic pneumonia secondary to use of a vaginal cream. Chest 67: 232, 1975.

425. Rokseth R, Storstein O: Pulmonary complications during mecamylamine therapy. Acta Med Scand 167: 23, 1960.

426. Goodwin DD, Glenny RW: Nonsteroidal anti-inflammatory drug–associated pulmonary infiltrates with eosinophila. Arch Intern Med 152: 1521, 1992.

427. Warring FC Jr, Howlett KS Jr: Allergic reactions to para-aminosalicylic acid: Report of seven cases, including one of Löffler's syndrome. Annu Rev Tuberc 65: 235, 1952.

428. Wold DE, Zahn DW: Allergic (Löffler's) pneumonia occurring during antituberculous chemotherapy: Report of three cases. Annu Rev Tuberc 74: 445, 1956.

429. Wilson IC, Gambill JM, Sandifer MG: Löffler's syndrome occurring during imipramine therapy. Am J Psychiatry 119: 892, 1963.

430. Paré JAPP: Unpublished data, 1975.

431. Beaudry C, Laplante L: Severe allergic pneumonitis from hydrochlorothiazide. Ann Intern Med 78: 251, 1973.

432. Burgher LW, Kass I, Schenken JR: Pulmonary allergic granulomatosis: A possible drug reaction in a patient receiving cromolyn sodium. Chest 66: 84, 1974.

433. Phills JA, Harrold AJ, Whiteman GV, et al: Pulmonary infiltrates, asthma, and eosinophilia due to *Ascaris suum* infestation in man. N Engl J Med 286: 965, 1972.

434. Bahk YW: Pulmonary paragonimiasis as a cause of Löffler's syndrome. Radiology 78: 598, 1962.

435. Fanning M, Hill A, Langer HM, et al: Visceral larva migrans (toxocariasis) in Toronto. Can Med Assoc J 124: 21, 1981.

436. deLeon EP, Pardo de Tavera M: Pulmonary schistosomiasis in the Philippines. Dis Chest 53: 154, 1968.

437. Butland RJA, Coulson IH: Pulmonary eosinophilia associated with cutaneous larva migrans. Thorax 40: 76, 1985.

438. McAleer R, Kroenert DB, Elder JL, et al: Allergic bronchopulmonary disease caused by *Curvularia lunata* and *Drechslera hawaiiensis*. Thorax 36: 338, 1981.

439. Benatar SR, Allan B, Hewitson RP, et al: Allergic bronchopulmonary stemphyliosis. Thorax 35: 515, 1980.

8

NEOPLASTIC DISEASE OF THE LUNGS

Pulmonary neoplasms are among the commonest abnormalities encountered in respiratory medicine and enter into the differential diagnosis of many lesions seen on chest roentgenograms. Because of the presence of numerous cell types in the normal lung, a great number of histogenetic possibilities exist for these tumors, and a profusion of histologically defined types of neoplasm can be recognized. As a result, a variety of classification schemes are possible. That proposed by the World Health Organization (WHO) in 1981 (Table 8–1) is probably the best known and most widely used and, with minor modifications, is the one followed in this chapter.

CARCINOMA OF AIRWAY AND ALVEOLAR EPITHELIUM

Carcinoma of the airway and alveolar epithelium is by far the most important pulmonary neoplasm in terms of both frequency and clinical significance. In the United States, it is the commonest fatal malignancy in men and, in women, is second to breast carcinoma by only a small percentage. In 1989, the estimated percentage of lung cancer cases relative to all other cancers (excluding nonmelanoma skin cancer and carcinoma *in situ*) was 20 per cent in men and 11 per cent in women; during the same year, estimated lung cancer death rates were 35 per cent in men and 21 per cent in women.[1] The overall 5-year survival rates for all stages is only about 15 per cent.

The age-adjusted lung cancer death rate increased dramatically, from about 5 per 100,000 people in 1930 to 70 per 100,000 in 1980.[1] In the early 1980s, however, the rate in individuals younger than 45 years of age began to decline, suggesting that the overall mortality rate itself will begin to decrease in the 1990s or the early part of the next century.[2] This decreased mortality rate is particularly evident in men; in fact, it has been predicted by some investigators that the rate in females will continue to increase until the end of the century.[3] The reason for this gender discrepancy is probably related to two factors. First, women did not smoke heavily until the early 1930s, whereas heavy cigarette consumption by men began after World War I. Second, since the 1970s, the smoking rate in men has decreased much more than that in women. The difference in mortality rates is also reflected in the relative incidence of lung cancer in men and women, which had changed from

Table 8–1. HISTOLOGICAL CLASSIFICATION OF LUNG TUMOURS

I. EPITHELIAL TUMOURS

A. *Benign*
1. Papillomas
   a. Squamous cell papilloma
   b. "Transitional" papilloma
2. Adenomas
   a. Pleomorphic adenoma ["mixed" tumour]
   b. Monomorphic adenoma
   c. Others
B. *Dysplasia*
   Carcinoma *in situ*
C. *Malignant*
1. Squamous cell carcinoma [epidermoid carcinoma]
   Variant:
   a. Spindle cell (squamous) carcinoma
2. Small cell carcinoma
   a. Oat cell carcinoma
   b. Intermediate cell type
   c. Combined oat cell carcinoma
3. Adenocarcinoma
   a. Acinar adenocarcinoma
   b. Papillary adenocarcinoma
   c. Bronchioloalveolar carcinoma
   d. Solid carcinoma with mucus formation
4. Large cell carcinoma
   Variants:
   a. Giant cell carcinoma
   b. Clear cell carcinoma
5. Adenosquamous carcinoma
6. Carcinoid tumour
7. Bronchial gland carcinomas
   a. Adenoid cystic carcinoma
   b. Mucoepidermoid carcinoma
   c. Others
8. Others

II. SOFT TISSUE TUMOURS
III. MESOTHELIAL TUMOURS

A. *Benign Mesothelioma*
B. *Malignant Mesothelioma*
1. Epithelial
2. Fibrous [spindle-cell]
3. Biphasic

IV. MISCELLANEOUS TUMOURS

A. *Benign*
B. *Malignant*
1. Carcinosarcoma
2. Pulmonary blastoma
3. Malignant melanoma
4. Malignant lymphomas
5. Others

V. SECONDARY TUMOURS
VI. UNCLASSIFIED TUMOURS
VII. TUMOUR-LIKE LESIONS

A. *Hamartoma*
B. *Lymphoproliferative lesions*
C. *Tumourlet*
D. *Eosinophilic granuloma*
E. *"Sclerosing haemangioma"*
F. *Inflammatory pseudotumour*
G. *Others*

Reproduced, by permission, from: Histological typing of lung tumours, 2nd ed., Geneva, World Health Organization, 1981 (International Histological Classification of Tumours, No. 1), pp. 19–20.

a distinct male predominance prior to 1960 to a slight predominance in 1980.[4]

The figures just cited relate particularly to North America, and it is important to remember that mortality statistics vary considerably from country to country. Among men in the year 1982, the highest mortality rate was 106 per 100,000 people in Singapore, and the lowest 2.5 per 100,000 in El Salvador.[1] There is also variation among different populations in the same country; for example, in the United States, both the incidence and the mortality rate of lung cancer are greater in blacks than in whites. It is likely that at least part of these variations may be explained by regional differences in tobacco consumption; occupational and socioeconomic factors also may be important.[5]

Etiology

Because the primary function of the lungs involves their intimate exposure to air, it is inevitable that they must also be exposed to the numerous pollutants the air frequently contains. As a consequence, much investigation of the etiology of pulmonary carcinoma has focused on inhaled substances that possess potential carcinogenic activity. Undoubtedly, the most important single agent in this respect is tobacco smoke, the evidence incriminating it now being overwhelming. Despite this, the incidence of lung cancer has been increasing in nonsmokers,[6] suggesting that factors other than tobacco smoke may be assuming greater significance. Especially important in this regard are a variety of particulate and chemical substances inhaled in the workplace, particularly asbestos. Although many of these substances may have an intrinsic carcinogenic potential of their own, in most cases this potential is augmented substantially by concomitant exposure to tobacco smoke. Other etiologic factors, such as radiation, pulmonary fibrosis, and viral infection, are likely of less importance than tobacco smoke or particulate substances; however, in occasional cases they play an important role.

Tobacco Smoke. By far the most important causative agent of pulmonary carcinoma is tobacco smoke, the great majority of which emanates from cigarettes. Although squamous cell and small cell carcinoma are the most frequently associated histologic types, it is now clear that adenocarcinoma—including bronchioloalveolar carcinoma[6a]—also is related to the habit.[7] The evidence supporting these conclusions may be summarized under four headings.

Epidemiologic Studies Showing a Greater Incidence of Carcinoma in Smokers than in Nonsmokers. Many studies show that pulmonary carcinoma is commoner in cigarette smokers than in nonsmokers; for example, in one follow-up study of 6071 men aged 45 years or more, lung cancer developed in 4 per cent of those who had smoked for 40 years or more but in none of 805 nonsmokers.[8] Overall estimates suggest an incidence 4 to 10 times higher in cigarette smokers than in nonsmokers. The risk for cigar and pipe smokers, particularly those who do not inhale, is considerably less but is still greater than that in those who never smoked.[9] There is also strong evidence of an association between passive (environmental) smoking—particularly spousal—and the development of lung carcinoma[10, 10a]; in fact, it has been estimated that as many as 17 per cent of lung cancers among nonsmokers can be attributed to passive smoking during childhood and adolescence.[11]

Epidemiologic Studies Showing a Relationship Between the Incidence of Lung Cancer and the Number and Type of Cigarettes Smoked. Many studies have shown that the risk of lung cancer increases in direct proportion to the number of cigarettes smoked.[12] Similarly, it has been well established that stopping the habit or appreciably reducing the number of cigarettes smoked results in a decreased risk of developing the disease, although it may take as many as 20 years for such a decrease to be appreciated.[12] Although there are conflicting data, some studies have suggested that low-tar or filter cigarettes are associated with a lower incidence of lung carcinoma,[13] possibly because the amount of carcinogenic material inhaled is less than that from nonfilter and high-tar varieties.

Chemical and Experimental Demonstration of Potent Carcinogens in Tobacco Smoke. Numerous gaseous and particulate carcinogens and cocarcinogens have been identified in tobacco smoke,[14] including benzo[*a*]pyrene and other polycyclic aromatic hydrocarbons, nitrosamines, phenols, polonium-210, and arsenic. Although the precise agent or agents responsible for the development of neoplasia have not been identified, it is clear from experiments in several animal species that both epithelial atypia and invasive cancer can develop either from inhalation of tobacco smoke or from direct intrapulmonary inoculation of tobacco condensates.[15]

Cytologic and Histologic Demonstration of Bronchial and Epithelial Atypia in Smokers. Pathologic studies have shown that loss of normal bronchial epithelial morphology accompanied by cytologic atypia is common in cigarette smokers.[16] Furthermore, the degree of atypia as well as its extent throughout the bronchial tree is greater in those who smoke more heavily[16] and decreases in individuals who have stopped smoking.[17]

Other Inhaled Particulate and Chemical Substances. Exposure to a variety of inorganic particulate materials and organic chemicals undoubtedly results in an increased risk of developing pulmonary carcinoma (Table 8–2). The greatest risk lies in specific work environments where exposure may occur over long periods of time and the concentration of noxious materials may reach dangerous levels. Despite the undoubted association between cancer and some occupations, however, it is not always clear in a particular instance which specific substance is the sole or primary carcinogenic agent; in fact, it is possible that multiple agents are involved in some cases. In addition, it is

likely that in many patients in whom carcinoma develops, there is a synergistic effect of cigarette smoke.

The most important inhaled particulate agent in the development of pulmonary carcinoma is undoubtedly asbestos. Mortality studies based on death certificates have consistently demonstrated an excessive risk of lung cancer in asbestos-exposed individuals. In addition, several investigations have shown a dose-response relationship between the degree of asbestos exposure and the development of lung carcinoma,[18] and it is now accepted by most authorities that this substance is important in the pathogenesis of many occupationally associated pulmonary tumors.

The association between asbestos and lung carcinoma has been documented in both smokers and nonsmokers, the relative risk in the latter individuals having been estimated to be 4 or 5 times that in nonsmokers not exposed to the mineral.[19] However, the influence of asbestos is much greater when it is affiliated with tobacco smoke, with which it appears to have a synergistic effect.[20] Thus, asbestos exposure is associated with a relative risk of 20 to 1 for the development of lung cancer in heavy smokers compared with nonsmokers, and a risk as great as 50 to 1 for heavy smokers compared with nonsmokers not exposed to asbestos.

Although these epidemiologic findings implicate asbestos in the pathogenesis of lung carcinoma, the precise mechanisms involved are uncertain, and it has been debated whether asbestos truly is a carcinogen in its own right or is simply a promoter of carcinogenesis. Part of this uncertainty is related to the observation that nonsmoking, asbestos-exposed individuals only rarely develop carcinoma. In addition, experimental evidence suggests that tumorigenesis requires some substance in addition to asbestos (e.g., a polycyclic aromatic hydrocarbon).[21]

The risk of developing pulmonary carcinoma after asbestos exposure depends on several factors. The type of fiber to which an individual is exposed may be important. For example, moderate exposure to chrysotile does not necessarily result in an increased risk of pulmonary cancer, whereas exposure to amphibole fibers (crocidolite, amosite, and anthophyllite) is associated with a significantly increased tumor incidence. The duration of exposure is also

Table 8–2. SUBSTANCES IMPLICATED IN PULMONARY CARCINOGENESIS

Substance	Exposure	Selected References
Asbestos	Mining, processing, use in other occupations	*See* text
Nickel	Refining of ore	24
Chromium	Processing into dichromates; arc welding	25
Arsenic	Mining and smelting of copper, lead, zinc, etc.	26
	Production and use of pesticides	27
Chloromethyl ether	Preparation of ion-exchange resins	28
Silica	Mining, sand blasting, etc.	29
Coal dust	Mining	30
Mustard gas	Production of poison gas	31
Hydrocarbons	Work in printing, rubber industry, roofing, asphalt, coke industry, etc.	32, 33
Vinyl and polyvinyl chloride	Chemical processing	34
Synthetic mineral fibers	Rockwool and slagwool plants	35
Cadmium		36
Chlorinated chemicals		37
Beryllium		38
Formaldehyde		39

important; in most series in which an increased incidence of pulmonary carcinoma has been demonstrated,[18] workers have been exposed for at least 20 years. Most patients with asbestos-related pulmonary carcinoma also have radiologic or pathologic evidence of asbestosis[22]; despite this, some studies have found an increased incidence of carcinoma in the absence of pulmonary fibrosis.[23]

The association between asbestos and pulmonary carcinoma relates both to primary exposure in mining and milling and to secondary exposure of workers in a variety of occupations,[20] including the manufacture of asbestos friction products and textiles, the manufacture or use of insulation material in the construction industry, the production of asbestos-cement, and shipbuilding. The risk of developing carcinoma in these and other industries depends greatly on the state of the asbestos fibers during the period of exposure. For the mineral to have a pathogenic effect, it must be present in the ambient air as a free fiber; once it is incorporated into manufactured products, the fiber is well bound and is unlikely to cause harm (unless the product undergoes degradation).

Radiation. There can be little doubt that radiation is an etiologic factor in a small proportion of patients with lung carcinoma. Exposure may result from an external source or from inhalation of radioactive material. The former is a relatively uncommon cause, but it does appear to be a factor in some patients with Hodgkin's disease[40] or testicular carcinoma[41] who have been treated with supradiaphragmatic radiation or combined-modality therapy.

Exposure to inhaled radioactive material as a result of decay of radium-226, a substance normally present in the earth's crust, has long been recognized as an occupational hazard in miners[42]; recently it also has come under suspicion as a possible carcinogen in homes. However, epidemiologic studies investigating this problem have yielded conflicting results,[42a] and the relative importance of such nonoccupational exposure awaits the results of several ongoing studies.

Polonium-210, a radioactive alpha emitter, has been shown to be present in cigarette smoke, where it becomes attached to lead present in tobacco and is deposited at the bifurcation of bronchi.[43] Its concentration within the lungs has been found to be substantially higher in smokers than in nonsmokers; as a consequence, it has been proposed as a potential carcinogenic agent.

Viral Infection. Laryngotracheobronchial papillomas are known to be associated with papillomavirus infection, and it is likely that the occasional cases of pulmonary squamous cell carcinoma that develop in association with papillomas are caused by this virus (*see* page 489).[44] There is also evidence that papillomavirus[45] and, possibly, Epstein-Barr virus[46] infections may rarely be related to the development of carcinoma in the absence of classic papillomas or other pulmonary disease.

Pulmonary Fibrosis. The term "scar carcinoma" refers to a pulmonary carcinoma that is intimately related to a localized area of parenchymal fibrosis. Early investigators who studied this association postulated that the scars were related pathogenetically to the development of the carcinoma,[47] and the term has since come to encompass this connotation. The etiology of the fibrosis is varied and includes tuberculosis, infarction, chronic abscess, and organ-

ized pneumonia. The precise properties of the fibrosis that hypothetically lead to the development of carcinoma are unknown. One suggestion is that the scarring causes lymphatic obstruction that, in turn, results in a local increase in potentially carcinogenic particulate material.[47] The epithelial metaplasia and hyperplasia that are frequently present at the junction of the fibrotic and unscarred lung also may be important.

Despite the frequent association between fibrosis and carcinoma, the validity of a causal relationship has been questioned, and many observers now believe that the cancer induces the fibrosis rather than the other way around. There are several mechanisms by which this might occur. For example, it is well known that carcinomas originating in other tissues, such as breast, can induce a fibrous reaction, and there is no reason why a similar process should not occur in the lung. In support of this interpretation are immunohistochemical and biochemical investigations of peripheral "scar carcinomas" that have found evidence that the collagen is being actively produced.[48] It is also possible that other cancer-associated processes, such as vascular occlusion and lung infarction, may be responsible for focal fibrosis.

An association between diffuse interstitial pulmonary fibrosis and carcinoma also has been documented. The commonest etiology of the fibrosis is progressive systemic sclerosis[49]; however, it has also been reported in association with the diffuse fibrosis of rheumatoid disease, neurofibromatosis, sarcoidosis, dermatomyositis, and fibrosing alveolitis. In all these diseases, it is usually possible to be fairly certain on clinical and roentgenologic grounds that the fibrosis truly preceded the development of carcinoma and that there thus exists a true pathogenetic relationship between the two. The basis for this relationship is unclear, but may relate to the epithelial metaplasia and hyperplasia that are invariably present in these diffusely fibrotic lungs.

Other Concomitant Lung Diseases. The association of tuberculosis and carcinoma in the same area of the lung has been reported with sufficient frequency to suggest that the combination may be more than coincidental. In occasional cases, the malignancy appears to originate in tuberculosis scars, suggesting that the tumors represent true "scar carcinomas"; alternatively, it has been suggested that carcinoma may reactivate tuberculosis by eroding encapsulated necrotic foci.[50] Perhaps more likely than either of these explanations is the effect of the cachexia and debilitation produced by the carcinoma in reactivating dormant infection.

There is evidence that chronic airflow obstruction itself may be related to the development of pulmonary carcinoma.[51]

Dietary Factors. Most studies support an association between pulmonary carcinoma (particularly squamous cell carcinoma) and low consumption of the antioxidants vitamins A, C, and E and carotene.[52] Presumably by increasing the intake of these substances, the consumption of fruit appears to protect against the development of carcinoma.[53] Other potential dietary factors have been less thoroughly investigated; however, a significant association between total dietary fat or cholesterol intake and lung cancer has been documented in some studies.[54, 55]

Genetic Factors. The role of a hereditary factor in the

pathogenesis of pulmonary carcinoma is difficult to establish because of its relative lack of importance compared with cigarette smoking and environmental dust exposure. Nevertheless, there is epidemiologic evidence that suggests an increased risk of lung cancer in patients with a familial history of lung cancer, even after the confounding effects of cigarette smoking and occupation have been controlled.[56] Occasional reports of clustering of carcinoma within a family support this hypothesis.[57] The basis of this inherited contribution to carcinogenesis is unknown, but it has been hypothesized to be related to intracellular enzymes (e.g., cytochrome P-450[58]) that promote or activate environmental carcinogens.

Immunologic Factors. Many immunologic abnormalities have been identified in patients with lung carcinoma. Most have been described in individuals in whom the tumor has already developed, in which case these abnormalities may represent a reaction to the carcinoma rather than a factor in the pathogenesis of the neoplasm. Other abnormalities, however, have been identified in patients at risk for pulmonary carcinoma, suggesting a possible pathogenetic role. For example, there is evidence that the ratio of helper to suppressor lymphocytes is decreased in those who smoke heavily[59] and that lymphocyte cytotoxicity is deficient in patients with asbestosis.[60] There is also an increased incidence of lung cancer in patients with lymphoreticular neoplasms[61] and, possibly, individuals seropositive for the human immunodeficiency virus.[62]

Pathologic Characteristics

Of the several classifications of pulmonary carcinoma proposed in the past 30 years, that put forward by the WHO review committee in 1981 (*see* Table 8–1)[63] is probably the most widely used and, with minor changes, is the one that, in the authors' opinion, gives the most practical description of the current understanding of the clinicopathologic features of carcinoma of the lung. Most studies of interobserver and intraobserver agreement have shown a high degree of reproducibility. For example, in one investigation of 93 cases of small cell carcinoma, there was unanimity of diagnosis among three observers in 94 per cent of cases.[64] Concordance for well-differentiated forms of squamous cell and adenocarcinoma is also good[65]; however, that for poorly differentiated forms and for large cell carcinoma is considerably worse, ranging from 20 to 40 per cent in some studies.[66]

The WHO classification subdivides pulmonary carcinoma into seven major categories; the first five account for at least 95 per cent of all epithelial tumors and consist of squamous cell carcinoma (approximately 30 to 35 per cent of cases), small cell carcinoma (15 per cent), adenocarcinoma (35 to 40 per cent), large cell carcinoma (10 per cent), and adenosquamous carcinoma (1 to 2 per cent). The last two categories (carcinoid tumor and tracheobronchial gland tumors) differ substantially from the others and are considered separately.

Squamous Cell Carcinoma

Squamous cell carcinoma arises most frequently in a segmental or lobar bronchus.[67] Early lesions, consisting of *in*

situ or minimally invasive carcinoma, often can be recognized grossly as white plaques or a fine granularity of the bronchial mucosa associated with loss of normal airway markings.[68] More advanced carcinomas characteristically appear as polypoid or papillary tumors within the bronchial lumen. Because of this, airway obstruction is almost invariable, and distal atelectasis and obstructive pneumonitis are present to some degree in most cases at presentation (Fig. 8–1). In large tumors, central necrosis is frequent and may be extensive; drainage of necrotic material leads to cavitation in many cases (Fig. 8–2).

Histologically, the earliest form of squamous cell cancer is carcinoma *in situ*, in which malignant cells replace the respiratory epithelium and extend into bronchial glands without actual tissue invasion. Larger, clearly invasive neoplasms are recognized by the presence of intercellular bridges or keratinization (or both). They range from well-differentiated forms, with obvious and abundant keratinization, to poorly differentiated forms that may be difficult to distinguish from small or large cell carcinoma.

Small Cell Carcinoma

Small cell carcinoma is typically located in proximal airways, particularly lobar and mainstem bronchi (Fig. 8–3). In the early stages, it forms a poorly delimited tumor that spreads in the submucosa and peribronchovascular connective tissue. As it grows, its submucosal location becomes

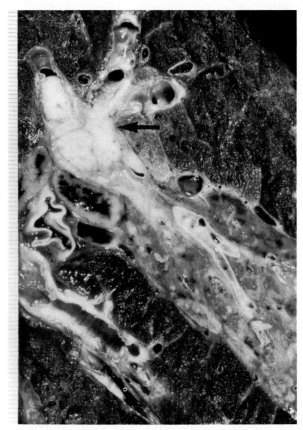

Figure 8–1. Squamous Cell Carcinoma. The upper lobe segmental bronchi are occluded by tumor that has extended locally into adjacent interstitial connective tissue *(arrow)*. The anterior segment shows obstructive pneumonitis.

classification, histologic studies have shown a continuum in nuclear and cell size rather than two distinct cell populations, and the two types have similar gross and ultrastructural features, natural histories, and prognoses.[70] For practical purposes, therefore, most pathologists now regard the two types as similar and refer to both of them as small cell carcinoma (classic or pure).[70a]

Focal areas of apparent glandular or squamous differentiation occasionally may be identified in otherwise typical small cell carcinoma, features that by themselves do not alter the diagnosis. In rare instances, however, these foci of cellular differentiation are extensive, in which case the tumors are designated "combined" small cell carcinoma. Some carcinomas also contain admixed cells that individually resemble those of large cell carcinoma. There is some evidence that this subgroup, which has been termed "small cell–large cell" carcinoma, may have a worse prognosis than that for other small cell tumors.[71]

Electron microscopic examination of small cell carcinomas reveals scanty cytoplasm, usually with few organelles. Neurosecretory granules are found in many cases and are highly suggestive of the diagnosis. They are generally fewer in number and smaller in size than those in carcinoid tumors and are frequently identified in only a small proportion of cells in any particular tumor. The presence of these granules as well as the demonstration of a variety of polypeptide and other hormones in the serum of affected patients has suggested that immunohistochemistry may also be useful in the diagnosis of small cell carcinoma. A variety of such substances have been identified, including most commonly gastrin releasing peptide, vasoactive intestinal polypeptide (VIP), serotonin, and adrenocorticotropic hormone (ACTH)[72]; in many cases, several peptides may be identified in the same tumor.

The histogenesis of small cell carcinoma has been debated. The ultrastructural demonstration of neurosecretory granules, the immunohistochemical evidence of cytoplasmic neuropeptides, and clinical and experimental evidence of the presence and secretion of polypeptide hormones all indicate a strong relationship between pulmonary neuroendocrine cells and small cell carcinoma. Although this connection has suggested that the tumor might be derived directly from the normal neuroendocrine cell, in fact several observations[73] indicate that it more likely originates from an undifferentiated bronchial epithelial cell that has the capacity for neuroendocrine differentiation.

Adenocarcinoma

Adenocarcinoma of the lung is divided into four histologic subgroups in the WHO classification—acinar carcinoma, papillary carcinoma, solid carcinoma with mucus formation, and bronchioloalveolar carcinoma. Although the histologic patterns corresponding to these subgroups are usually easily identifiable, a mixture of two or more is common in many tumors, and the distinctiveness of the subgroups themselves is open to question. In the authors' experience, the more diffuse form of bronchioloalveolar carcinoma is often histologically pure (i.e., unaccompanied by other histologic types) and shows characteristic gross pathologic, roentgenographic, and clinical features; thus, the authors favor retention of the term for such tumors and

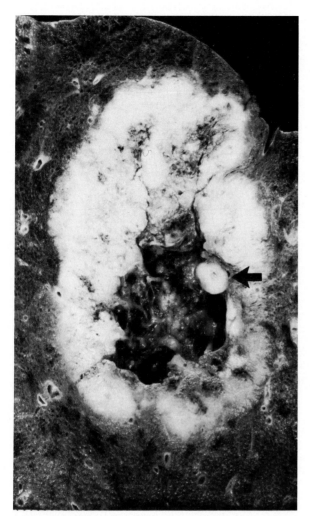

Figure 8–2. Cavitation in Squamous Cell Carcinoma. A large neoplasm arising in an upper lobe possesses prominent central cavitation. Note the shaggy appearance of the cavity wall, caused by the patchy nature of the necrosis and by nodules of viable neoplasm growing into the cavity itself *(arrow)*.

less well defined, and it appears as a poorly circumscribed mass that obliterates underlying airways and vessels. The endobronchial extension that is characteristic of squamous cell carcinoma is uncommon; when airway obstruction does occur, it is usually caused by compression by the expanding tumor rather than by intraluminal obstruction.

Histologically, four subtypes have been defined—oat cell, intermediate cell, mixed, and combined.[69] The oat cell variant consists of more or less round cells approximately one and a half to two times the size of a mature lymphocyte (Fig. 8–4). The cytoplasm is quite scanty, resulting in prominent molding of adjacent cell nuclei, which are characteristically hyperchromatic. Cells of the intermediate cell variant are somewhat larger than those of the oat cell type (two to four times the size of a lymphocyte) and may be round, polygonal, or fusiform in shape. The cytoplasm is more abundant than that in the oat cell type but is still small in amount compared with the typical squamous cell carcinoma or adenocarcinoma. Despite the distinction between oat cell and intermediate cell types in the WHO

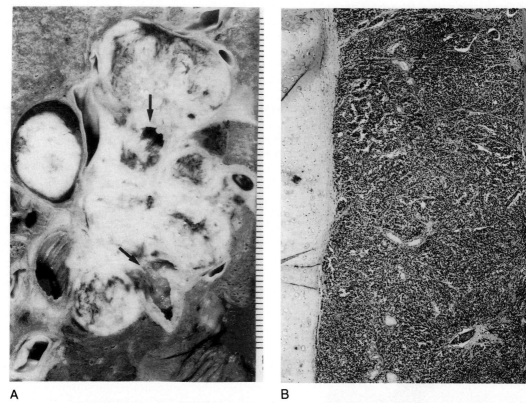

Figure 8–3. Small Cell Carcinoma. *A,* A centrally located tumor involves lymph nodes and adjacent interstitial tissue; airways *(arrows)* are surrounded and compressed by the tumor but lack the intraluminal growth typical of squamous cell carcinoma. *B,* A histologic section reveals extensive infiltration of the submucosa by a uniform population of small cells with hyperchromatic nuclei. Note that the surface respiratory epithelium is intact, and that the bronchial lumen is compressed to a minute slit *(arrow).* (× 40.)

for the uncommon solitary nodule that also shows a pure growth pattern. For practical purposes, however, the authors regard the other histologic subtypes as essentially equivalent.

The histogenesis of pulmonary adenocarcinoma is varied. Because of its typical peripheral location and lack of obvious association with major airways, many investigators believe that the tumor arises from bronchiolar or alveolar epithelium; a variety of ultrastructural,[74] histochemical,[75] and immunohistochemical[76] studies suggest that this is indeed the case. The commonest feature of cellular differentiation is mucin secretion. Since bronchiolar epithelium has the ability to undergo goblet cell metaplasia in response to a variety of noxious stimuli, it is not surprising that this inherent ability is expressed in neoplasms arising in this region. Clara cell differentiation, as evidenced by the presence of characteristic secretory granules, is present in many tumors,[74] constituting additional evidence of an origin from bronchiolar epithelium. Type II cell differentiation, demonstrated by the presence of surfactant production, is present in some tumors,[76] although undoubtedly less often than either mucus-secreting or Clara cell forms.

The great majority of pulmonary adenocarcinomas are located in the periphery of the lung, frequently in a subpleural location (Fig. 8–5). Focal fibrosis often is present in the portion of the tumor adjacent to the pleura, resulting in a puckered appearance (Fig. 8–6). Pure adenocarcinoma arising in a major airway is uncommon; when it does occur in this location, however, it is grossly indistinguishable from squamous cell carcinoma. Tumors with a pure bronchioloalveolar pattern histologically can often be recognized grossly by their characteristic nondestructive growth (Fig. 8–7), underlying structures such as airways and interlobular septa being readily identified despite being surrounded by tumor.

The histologic pattern of non–bronchioloalveolar cell carcinoma consists of acini or tubules (with or without intraluminal mucin formation), papillary projections, or solid carcinoma without structural evidence of glandular differentiation. The last-named can be distinguished from large cell carcinoma only by the presence of intracellular mucin in a large proportion of tumor cells. Frequently, more than one pattern is evident in a single tumor.

The growth pattern of bronchioloalveolar carcinoma is characterized by the presence of tumor cells spreading along the framework of normal lung parenchyma without destroying it (Fig. 8–8). Tumor cells usually form a single layer, although local proliferation may result in crowding into the airspace, resulting in a papillary appearance. Intraalveolar tumor secretion, consisting of either proteinaceous material or mucin, may be present in abundance, filling airspaces and small airways sometimes for a considerable distance from the tumor itself. Psammoma bodies also may be present, usually in association with a papillary compo-

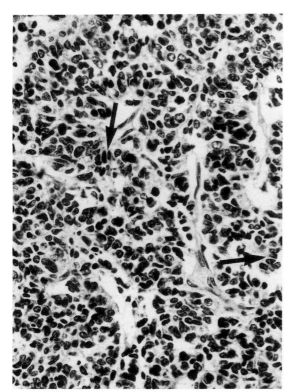

Figure 8–4. Small Cell Carcinoma. Histologic section shows cells with markedly hyperchromatic nuclei and minimal cytoplasm, the latter indicated by focal nuclear molding *(arrows)*. (× 350.)

nent,[77] and occasionally are sufficent in number to be visible roentgenographically as foci of calcification within the tumor.

Large Cell Carcinoma

This is essentially a diagnosis of exclusion and is applied to tumors that do not possess the typical appearance of small cell carcinoma and in which there is no evidence of either squamous or glandular differentiation. Although in many cases these distinctions are straightforward, differentiation of large cell carcinoma from a poorly differentiated adenocarcinoma or squamous cell carcinoma or from the intermediate form of small cell carcinoma can sometimes be difficult.

The incidence of large cell carcinoma varies substantially, depending on the amount of tissue available for examination and the techniques used to study it. Ultrastructural features of glandular, neuroendocrine, and squamous cell differentiation can be identified fairly frequently, provided that enough tissue is examined, even when they cannot be appreciated at the light microscopic level. Thus, when electron microscopic evidence of cytologic differentiation is used in classification, the incidence of large cell carcinoma is substantially decreased.[78] Since ultrastructural results are not employed in the WHO classification, however, these are not a practical consideration when using this schema. The frequency of large cell carcinoma also tends to diminish as the amount of tissue examined increases. In many cases of squamous cell carcinoma or adenocarcinoma, particularly those that are more poorly differentiated, the tumors contain areas that do not exhibit specific cellular dif-

ferentiation. If a diagnosis is made on small fragments of tissue, such as those obtained by endoscopic biopsy or transthoracic needle aspiration (TTNA), it may be impossible to identify the glandular or squamous features with confidence, and a "false diagnosis" of large cell carcinoma may result.

Grossly, large cell carcinomas tend to be bulky peripheral tumors (Fig. 8–9) with multiple foci of necrosis.[78] Histologically, they consist of sheets of cells that usually contain abundant cytoplasm and vesicular nuclei (Fig. 8–10). By definition, intercellular bridges, keratinization, and acinar or papillary structures are absent or are extremely uncommon. Mucin stains show no evidence of intracellular or extracellular secretion.

The WHO classification of large cell carcinoma includes two rare histologic subtypes—giant cell and clear cell. The former is a poorly differentiated neoplasm that contains a considerable number of very large, multinucleated tumor cells.[78a] Although its separation into a specific histologic category is somewhat arbitrary, preservation of the term may be of some value because of the almost uniformly dismal prognosis, rather distinctive histologic appearance and, possibly, an increased likelihood of gastrointestinal metastases.[78a] The clear cell variant consists of sheets of large cells with ample, lightly foamy or clear cytoplasm. As with giant cell tumors, it seems reasonable to regard these tumors as representing one end of a spectrum of histologic change in squamous cell carcinoma or adenocarcinoma, rather than a distinct entity[79]; their main significance lies in distinguishing them from metastatic clear cell carcinoma of the kidney.

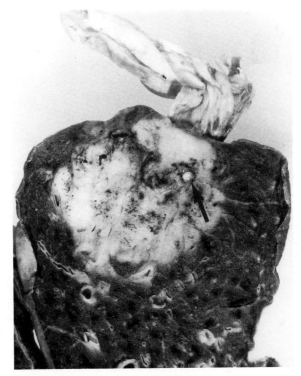

Figure 8–5. Adenocarcinoma. A well-delimited tumor is present in the apex of the upper lobe immediately adjacent to the pleura. Although it has not extended through the pleura, an inflammatory reaction has caused adhesions. Note the small focus of remote granulomatous inflammation incorporated into the tumor mass *(arrow)*.

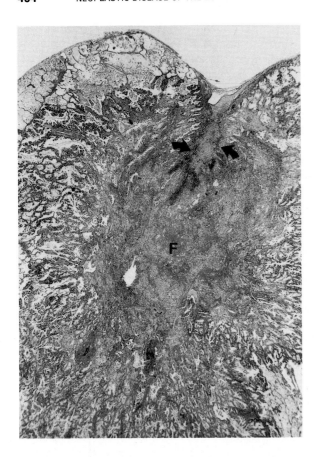

Figure 8–6. Adenocarcinoma with Central Scar and Pleural Puckering. A large focus of fibrous tissue (F) is surrounded by columnar tumor cells growing along the parenchymal framework (bronchioloalveolar cell carcinoma). The pleura *(arrows)* is focally fibrotic and has been drawn into the central portion of the scar. (× 10.)

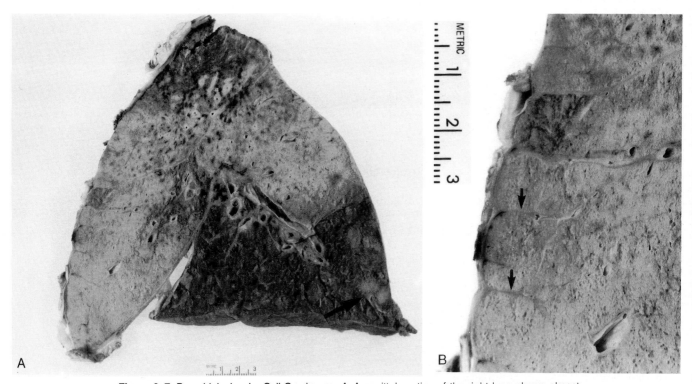

Figure 8–7. Bronchioloalveolar Cell Carcinoma. *A,* A sagittal section of the right lung shows almost complete "consolidation" of the upper and middle lobes and the superior segment of the lower lobe; several small nodular foci of early disease are present in the base of the lower lobe *(arrow). B,* On a magnified view, vessels and interlobular septa *(arrows)* are clearly visible within the tumor mass, demonstrating that the carcinoma spreads without destroying the underlying lung.

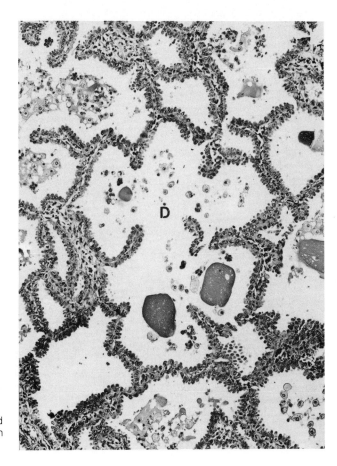

Figure 8–8. Bronchioloalveolar Carcinoma. An alveolar duct (D) and surrounding alveoli are lined by cuboidal tumor cells; airspaces contain macrophages and a small amount of proteinaceous material. (× 100.)

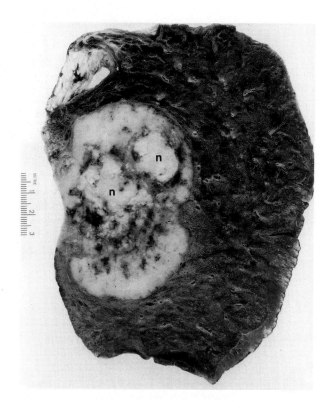

Figure 8–9. Large Cell Carcinoma. A resected upper lobe contains a large, well-defined subpleural tumor with multifocal areas of necrosis (n). Although characteristic of a large cell carcinoma, a lesion with this appearance cannot be reliably distinguished from adenocarcinoma.

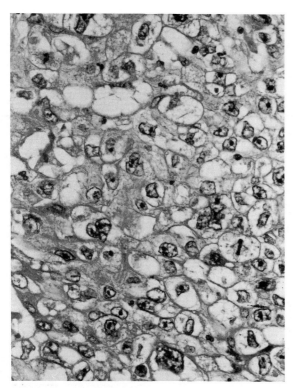

Figure 8–10. Large Cell Carcinoma. A magnified view shows cells with abundant cytoplasm, vesicular nuclei with prominent nucleoli, and occasional mitotic figures. (× 350.)

Adenosquamous Carcinoma

The incidence of adenosquamous carcinoma varies greatly, depending on the histologic criteria used for diagnosis and whether electron microscopy is employed for classification. If ultrastructural findings are used in typing, the incidence in some series is as high as 46 per cent of all lung carcinomas.[80] If only light microscopy is utilized, however, the number of cases is substantially less, ranging from 0.4 to 4.0 per cent.[81] As might be expected, the lower figures are associated with more rigid criteria for determining cellular differentiation. Most such rigidly defined tumors arise in the periphery of the lung and are grossly indistinguishable from large cell carcinoma or adenocarcinoma. In addition to areas of clear-cut glandular and squamous differentiation, many show regions of undifferentiated carcinoma, usually of the large cell type. Clinical and radiologic features are similar to those of patients with other forms of non–small cell carcinoma.[82]

Roentgenographic Manifestations

General Considerations

The roentgenographic manifestations of pulmonary carcinoma are related both to the size of the lesion and, more important, to its anatomic location, particularly with respect to its relationship to an airway. Thus, a tumor located in lung parenchyma unassociated with a relatively large airway generally appears as a solitary nodule or mass, with or without cavitation. By contrast, a carcinoma that arises in a proximal subsegmental or larger airway often is manifested by not only the tumor itself but also the consequences of obstruction of the airway in which the tumor is situated. Such consequences include obstructive pneumonitis and atelectasis, alteration of regional lung volume or blood flow, and mucoid impaction. Before considering these and other roentgenographic features of pulmonary carcinoma, a brief discussion of the general aspects of anatomic location is warranted.

It is more difficult than might be anticipated to determine the site of origin of a pulmonary carcinoma by roentgenography. The reasons for this difficulty include the large size of some cancers at the time of presentation, the tendency for some tumors (particularly squamous cell carcinoma) to extend proximally within an airway to occupy a lobar or main bronchus by the time the patient is first examined, and the problem in some cases of distinguishing the cancer itself from the obstructive pneumonitis that it induces. Despite these difficulties, some valid generalizations can be made about anatomic location.

Carcinoma occurs with a relative frequency of 3 to 2 in both the right versus the left lung and the upper versus the lower lobe. In the upper lobes, the anterior segment is most often affected. Both squamous cell and small cell carcinomas occur predominantly in a central location; by contrast, adenocarcinoma usually develops in the lung periphery. Within the bronchial tree, the site of origin of carcinoma shows a striking predominance (60 to 80 per cent) for the segmental bronchi; most of the remaining tumors arise in main and lobar bronchi. Carcinoma originating in the trachea is rare, amounting to no more than 1 per cent of cases. Approximately 4 per cent of tumors arise in the extreme apex of the upper lobes—superior sulcus (Pancoast) carcinomas.

Atelectasis and Obstructive Pneumonitis

The most frequent effect of airway obstruction is a combination of atelectasis and obstructive pneumonitis. Although to some physicians the latter term is synonymous with infection, in fact the changes seen roentgenographically are usually related solely or predominantly to the physical (and perhaps chemical) effects of airway blockage rather than to inflammation caused by infection (see page 173).[83] Despite this observation, in some patients infection may cause an acute bronchopneumonia, resulting in signs and symptoms that may be the first clinical manifestation of the malignancy. Antibiotic therapy may result in partial resolution of roentgenographic abnormalities, in which case the disease may be misdiagnosed as a slowly resolving pneumonia. As a consequence, in patients who have an increased risk of cancer, any pneumonia should be followed roentgenographically to complete resolution.

The atelectasis associated with pulmonary carcinoma is most often segmental but may affect a lobe or, occasionally, a whole lung (Fig. 8–11). Since airway obstruction is complete in most cases, air cannot pass distally, and an air bronchogram is thus absent. This sign is virtually pathognomonic of an endobronchial obstructing lesion and is of utmost importance in diagnosis. Although bronchi distal to the obstruction are frequently dilated and filled with mucus or pus, parenchymal consolidation caused by obstructive pnemonitis usually renders them invisible. Sometimes,

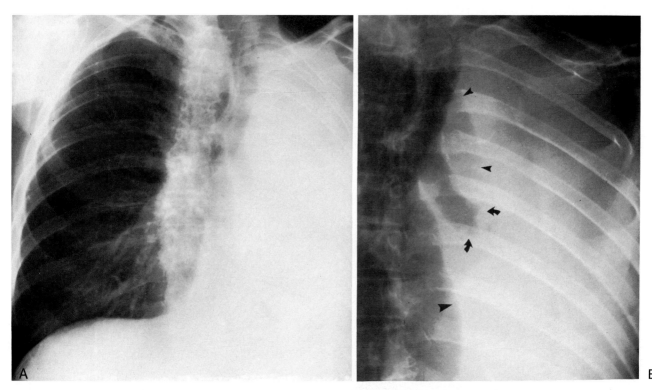

Figure 8–11. Atelectasis and Obstructive Pneumonitis of the Left Lung. A conventional posteroanterior roentgenogram *(A)* and an overpenetrated anteroposterior view *(B)* of the mediastinum show typical signs of consolidation and atelectasis of the left lung: small left hemithorax, mediastinal displacement to the left, and overinflation of the right lung manifested by displacement into the left hemithorax of the anterior *(small arrowheads)* and posterior *(large arrowhead)* mediastinal compartments. The left main bronchus is occluded *(arrows)* by an intraluminal squamous cell carcinoma.

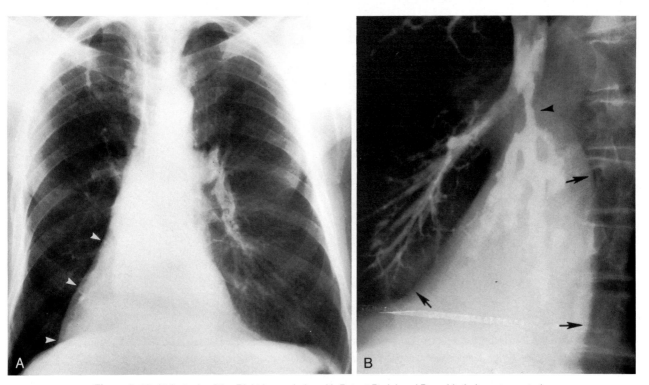

Figure 8–12. Atelectasis of the Right Lower Lobe with Patent Peripheral Bronchi. *A,* A posteroanterior chest roentgenogram shows a typical pattern of right lower lobe atelectasis *(arrowheads)*. *B,* A selective bronchogram in right posterior oblique projection reveals circumferential narrowing of the lower lobe bronchus *(arrowhead)* by a biopsy-proven squamous cell carcinoma; contrast medium has entered the dilated lower lobe bronchi, an unusual occurrence since such bronchi either are usually completely obstructed or are distended with mucus or pus. The triangular opacity *(arrows)* distal to the bronchial occlusion represents the consolidated and collapsed lower lobe.

however, obstruction is incomplete, allowing air to pass distally, in which circumstance an air bronchogram may be visible (Fig. 8–12). These statements apply only to conventional roentgenograms; it is remarkable how often an air bronchogram is visible on a computed tomography (CT) scan and yet may be inapparent on a plain chest film.

Similarly, mucoid impaction within dilated bronchi in an atelectatic segment or lobe cannot be identified on conventional roentgenograms yet should be clearly visible on contrast-enhanced CT images as relatively low-attenuation branching structures.[84] Occasionally, the tumor can be identified as a bulge deforming the apex of the triangular

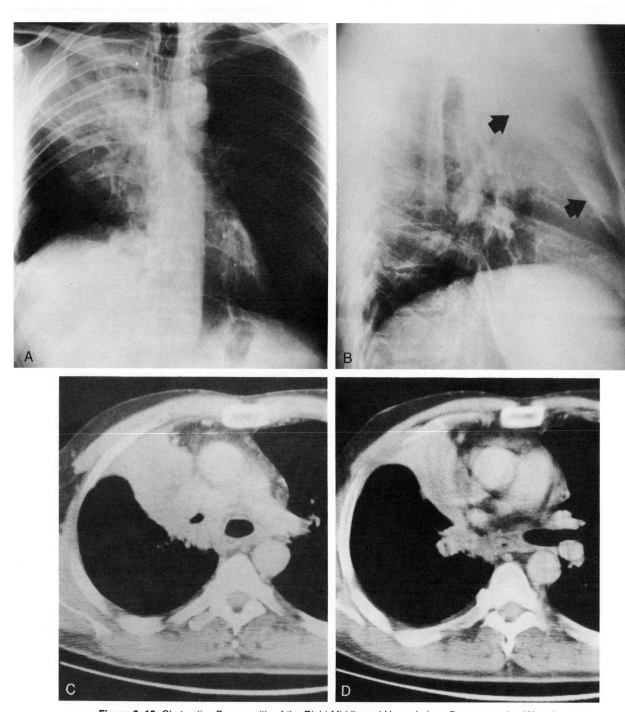

Figure 8–13. Obstructive Pneumonitis of the Right Middle and Upper Lobes. Posteroanterior *(A)* and lateral *(B)* roentgenograms of the chest reveal a homogeneous opacity occupying the upper half of the right lung and extending inferiorly to obscure the right border of the heart. The right hemidiaphragm is moderately elevated. In lateral projection, note the marked anterior displacement of the right major fissure *(arrows)*. An air bronchogram is not visible. CT scans at a level just distal to the carina *(C)* and approximately 2 cm caudad *(D)* reveal a roughly triangle-shaped homogeneous opacity extending anterolaterally to abut the pleura. In *C*, note the marked narrowing of the right main bronchus, which is surrounded by tissue of homogeneous density that possesses no clear interface with the mediastinum medially. In *D*, the bronchus intermedius has been virtually completely obliterated by neoplasm. Squamous cell carcinoma.

opacity of the atelectatic segment or lobe; obviously the part of the neoplasm that is within the opacity will not be visible, at least on conventional roentgenograms (Fig. 8–13). However, both rapid-sequence CT[85] and magnetic resonance imaging (MRI)[86] have been shown to be capable of distinguishing a central carcinoma from its associated atelectasis.

Alteration of Regional Lung Volume and Blood Volume

Although overinflation of lung distal to a partly obstructing endobronchial lesion is frequently cited as an important sign in the early diagnosis of bronchogenic carcinoma, it is in fact a rare manifestation. Instead, the volume of lung behind a partly obstructing endobronchial lesion is almost invariably *reduced* at full inspiration (Fig. 8–14). Despite this smaller volume, the density of affected parenchyma typically is less than that of the opposite lung, rather than greater as might be anticipated, an effect caused by reduction in perfusion (oligemia) resulting from hypoxic vasoconstriction in response to hypoventilation. On the other hand, *air trapping* during expiration is a dynamic event resulting from airflow obstruction as the bronchial caliber reduces to embrace the endobronchial lesion (Fig. 8–15).

Mucoid Impaction

Mucoid impaction of segmental and subsegmental bronchi is an occasional roentgenographic manifestation of an obstructing endobronchial carcinoma. The appearance is no different from that associated with allergic bronchopulmonary aspergillosis (*see* page 345) except that the impaction is localized to one specific segment (*see* Fig. 8–12). Depending on the extent of the impaction, the resultant opac-

ity may be linear or branched in a **V** or **Y** configuration. The affected bronchi are almost invariably dilated, sometimes to a marked degree (Fig. 8–16).

In order for mucoid impaction to be identified roentgenographically, the accumulation of mucus within dilated airways must be unassociated with parenchymal disease, such as obstructive pneumonitis (except on contrast-enhanced CT images, as mentioned previously). The reasons why this occasionally occurs are unclear. In addition to an absence of obstructive pneumonitis, it is necessary for collateral air drift to be sufficient to prevent atelectasis. In fact, collateral air drift effectively reduces ventilation, resulting in local hypoxia and reflex vasoconstriction; the resultant oligemia can create a zone of radiolucency that provides additional evidence of airway obstruction.

Bronchial Wall Thickening

Visualization of lobar or segmental bronchi may permit the detection of carcinoma prior to the onset of the more familiar and obvious roentgenographic signs described above.[87] This finding, which has been designated the bronchial cuff sign, consists of two components: (1) an increase in the thickness of the soft tissue compartment surrounding an end-on bronchus, often with concomitant partial or complete loss of the normal curvilinear demarcation of the bronchial wall; and (2) partial or complete envelopment of the adjacent pulmonary artery. The sign has been demonstrated in several anatomic sites (Fig. 8–17).[88]

Solitary Pulmonary Nodule

In published reports there is substantial variation in the criteria for designating a roentgenographic shadow a soli-

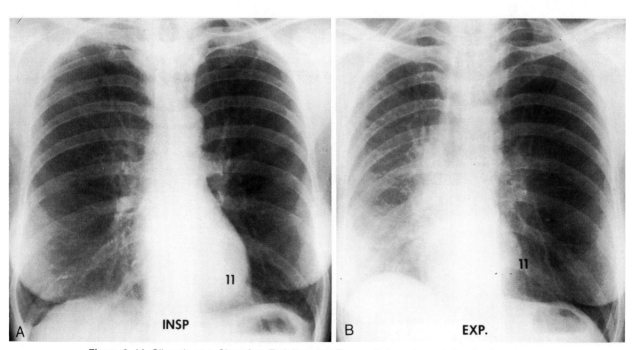

Figure 8–14. Oligemia as a Sign of an Endobronchial Tumor. *A,* A posteroanterior chest roentgenogram at full inspiration reveals small, barely visible vessels throughout the left lung, reflecting oligemia resulting from hypoxic vasoconstriction. Although the volume of the left lung is slightly reduced, the reduction in blood flow has caused hypertranslucency. *B,* A roentgenogram exposed at full expiration demonstrates air trapping in the left lung. Squamous cell carcinoma, left main bronchus.

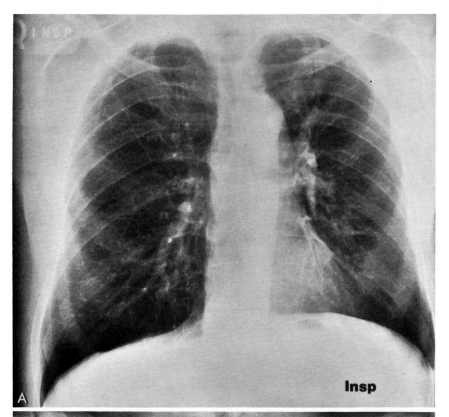

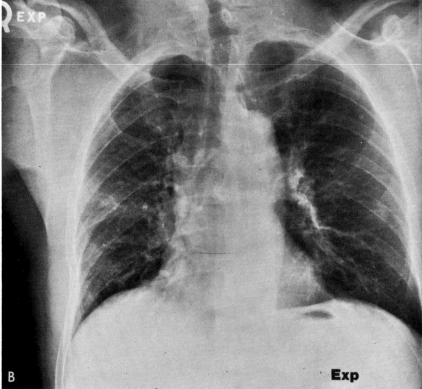

Figure 8–15. Small Cell Carcinoma, Left Main Bronchus, with Expiratory Air Trapping. A posteroanterior roentgenogram exposed at full inspiration (A) reveals considerable smallness of the left lung compared with the right; the left hemidiaphragm is moderately elevated, and the mediastinum is shifted to the left. Left lower lobe vessels are obviously smaller than corresponding vessels on the right, indicating reduced perfusion. A roentgenogram exposed at maximal expiration (B) reveals little change in the volume of the left lung from inspiration, indicating air trapping; by contrast, the right hemidiaphragm has elevated considerably, and the mediastinum has swung to the right, indicating good air flow from the right lung.

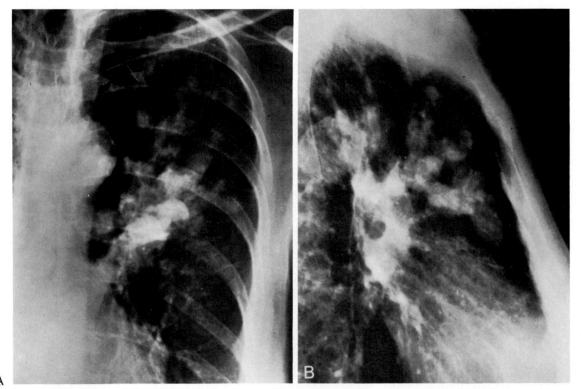

A

B

Figure 8–16. Squamous Cell Carcinoma with Mucoid Impaction. Detail views of the left lung from posteroanterior *(A)* and lateral *(B)* chest roentgenograms reveal broad, fingerlike opacities projecting into the anterior segment of the upper lobe. Although these airways are completely obstructed, the peripheral parenchyma is air-containing because of collateral air drift. At bronchoscopy, a squamous cell carcinoma was identified occluding the anterior segmental bronchus. (Courtesy of Dr. Ken Thomson, Melbourne, Australia.)

tary nodule, with resultant differences in case selection, roentgenographic findings, patient survival, and so on. The margin of the lesion is perhaps the most important criterion, most authors requiring that the lesion be "circumscribed" (i.e., surrounded by air-containing lung). The authors do not regard sharpness of definition as being important and will accept an opacity that is ill defined within this category. Nowadays, it is customary to restrict the maximum diameter to 3 cm, the term "mass" being reserved for lesions whose width is greater than that.

A great variety of conditions may result in the development of a solitary pulmonary nodule.[89] The percentage of cases of pulmonary carcinoma varies considerably from series to series, depending not only on how the solitary pulmonary nodule is defined but also on whether the lesions are discovered by mass roentgenographic survey or by hospital screening roentgenograms and whether the series includes cases referred for resection. Solitary nodules discovered in roentgenographic surveys of the general population prove to be cancer in fewer than 5 per cent of cases, whether the nodule is surgically removed at the time or the patient is followed for 5 years.[90] By contrast, patients referred for tumor resection have a malignant nodule in approximately 40 per cent of cases; of the remainder, approximately 40 per cent have a granuloma,[91] and 20 per cent benign lesions of various etiologies.[92] In any series of solitary nodules in which surgical resection is performed, malignant lesions are found in approximately 50 per cent of males older than 50 years of age.[90, 91] Even in patients with

a known extrathoracic malignancy, a solitary pulmonary nodule is much more likely to represent a second primary tumor than a single metastasis.[93]

The differentiation between a benign and a malignant solitary pulmonary nodule relies on a subjective weighing of multiple roentgenographic signs and clinical features. Although some of these signs are unquestionably of much greater significance than others, no single one or combination has proved to be invariable in this distinction. Bearing this important caveat in mind, it is still possible to make a shrewd determination as to the nature of a particular solitary pulmonary nodule. Experience has shown that it is best to divide the solitary nodule into two broad categories for the purposes of differential diagnosis: (1) lesions that are clearly benign, as determined by rigidly defined roentgenographic criteria; and (2) indeterminate nodules, comprising all other lesions. Thus, a "benign-indeterminate" categorization replaces the more traditional "benign-malignant" distinction; the main reason for this separation is simply that the stringent criteria of benignity are more certain than are the roentgenographic signs of malignancy.

The four radiologic features of greatest value in differential diagnosis are absolute size, the presence or absence of calcification, the character of the tumor-lung interface, and change in size with time.[94]

Absolute Size. Although this is an important factor in the assessment of a pulmonary mass, it is less useful for the solitary nodule. In one series, more than 80 per cent of 118 benign nodules measured 1 cm or less, and only 1 of 36

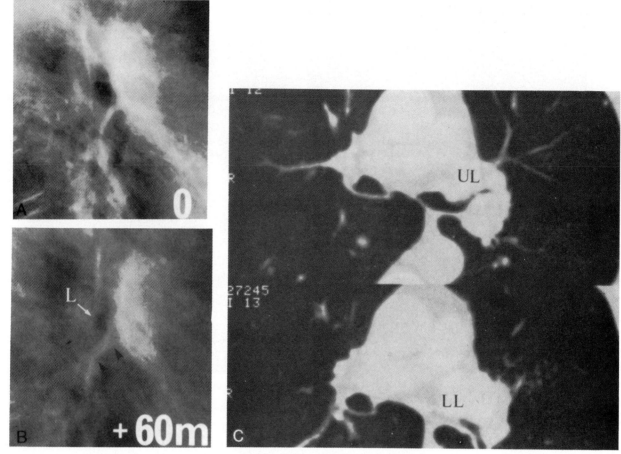

Figure 8–17. Thickened Bronchial Wall as a Sign of Pulmonary Carcinoma. *A,* A detail view of the hila from a lateral chest roentgenogram shows the left main lower lobe bronchial continuum to be normal. *B,* Five years later, slight thickening of the anterior walls of these airways *(arrowheads)* and a decrease in the size of the end-on upper lobe bronchial lumen *(arrows,* L) have occurred. These signs suggest a malignant lesion involving the upper and lower lobe central bronchi. *C,* CT scans through the carina show tumor-induced narrowing of the upper lobe (UL) and lower lobe (LL) bronchi.

"nodules" larger than 3 cm in diameter was benign[95]; by contrast, the diameters of malignant nodules were nearly uniformly distributed in the range of 1 to 6 cm. In this same series, slightly more than 50 per cent of the malignant nodules were larger than 2 cm in diameter; however, a substantital number (17.5 per cent) were 1 cm or less. Thus, it must be concluded that a 2-cm size criterion cannot be relied on by itself to indicate the nature of a solitary pulmonary nodule. However, if this value is increased to 3 cm, greater discrimination is possible, in that fewer than 5 per cent of benign solitary pulmonary nodules are larger.

Calcification. The presence or absence of calcium is undoubtedly the most important roentgenologic feature that distinguishes benign from malignant nodules. Its presence is almost certain evidence of benignity; the exceptions are the rare cases in which there is dystrophic calcification or ossification of necrotic tumor or stroma[96] or in which a calcified granuloma is engulfed by carcinoma (in which situation the calcification usually is eccentric).

Although conventional chest roentgenograms sometimes reveal convincing evidence of calcification, particularly when this is laminated or "target" in type, often it is necessary or desirable to perform conventional tomography or CT. For example, in one investigation of 384 solitary pul-

monary nodules considered not to be calcified by conventional methods, 118 (30 per cent) proved to be benign[95]; of these, 65 revealed unsuspected calcification, in 28 by direct inspection of thin-section CT scans at narrow windows and in the remaining 37 by use of a calibration phantom. Benign lesions have relatively high CT numbers (164 H or greater in one study[97]), presumably because of diffuse calcification, whereas malignant lesions have comparatively low numbers (mean CT number of 92 H, with a standard deviation of 18 H). It appears probable that digital radiography, particularly with dual-energy subtraction,[98] may prove even more successful in the benign-malignant distinction, by quantifying the calcium content of nodules (*see* Fig. 4–56, page 217).

Character of the Lung-Nodule Interface. While none of the following signs is of absolute value in distinguishing benign from malignant nodules, each is of sufficient worth to lend weight to one or the other possibility. Lobulation of outline constitutes suggestive evidence of malignancy; in fact, it has been stated that a lobulated character correctly predicts the malignancy of a lesion in more than 80 per cent of cases.[99] Shagginess of contour also supports the diagnosis of cancer and, logically, also relates to invasion of contiguous parenchyma by the neoplasm. By contrast, a

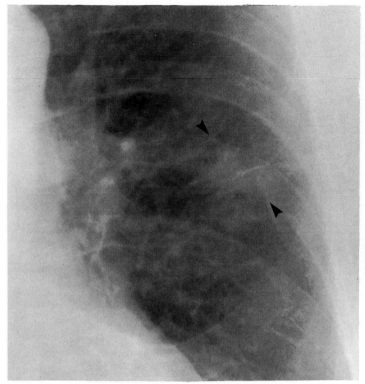
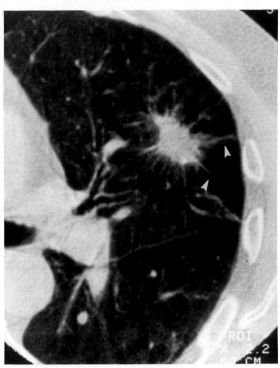

A   B

Figure 8–18. Corona Radiata. A detail view of the left lung from a posteroanterior roentgenogram *(A)* reveals a 2-cm opacity *(arrowheads)* with poorly defined margins. *B,* A CT scan through the center of the opacity shows multiple spicules *(arrowheads)* radiating from the lesion into surrounding parenchyma.

sharply defined nodule with a smooth interface provides suggestive (but by no means conclusive) evidence of a benign lesion. The shaggy margins of a malignant neoplasm are related, at least in part, to the so-called corona radiata. This sign consists of a number of fine, linear striations that extend perpendicularly outward from the periphery of a nodule for a distance of 4 or 5 mm, traversing a radiolucent halo (Fig. 8–18). While the corona radiata is not diagnostic of malignancy—for example, the authors have seen it in lipid pneumonia—it constitutes a highly suggestive sign. Although the initial studies documenting the findings described above were performed with conventional roentgenograms, high-resolution CT scans also have been reported to show a spiculated contour, lobulation, and inhomogeneous attenuation significantly more often in malignant lesions than in benign ones.[100]

The "tail sign" consists of a linear opacity that extends from a peripheral nodule or mass to the visceral pleura (Fig. 8–19). It appears to be caused by inward retraction and apposition of thickened visceral pleura. According to this hypothesis, as the visceral pleura invaginates, a small amount of pleural fluid is drawn into the area, creating the soft tissue opacity; the thin, sharp line between the apex of the pyramid and the mass represents the pleural apposition. The significance of the tail sign is contentious. For example, it has been regarded by some investigators as a fairly reliable sign of the malignant nature of a lesion, specifically indicating bronchioloalveolar carcinoma; in fact, in some series it has been observed in 25 per cent[101] of tumors of

this cell type. However, in one extensive study, it was concluded that the tail sign is an entirely nonspecific feature of peripherally located pulmonary lesions and that it cannot be used to distinguish a benign from a malignant lesion.[102]

High-resolution CT evidence of a patent bronchus leading directly to a peripheral nodular opacity—the "bronchus sign"—has been shown to be associated most often with adenocarcinoma.[103] The sign has also been advocated as being useful in predicting the success of transbronchial biopsy or brushing in providing tissue suitable for pathologic diagnosis.[104] An additional sign that may prove helpful in suggesting malignancy consists of involvement of pulmonary veins, as revealed on axial multiplanar reconstruction CT scans. In one series, such involvement was found in all 15 patients with pulmonary carcinoma but in only 1 patient of 8 with non-neoplastic lesions.[105]

Satellite lesions may be present in association with both benign and malignant nodules, although they are found much more frequently with the former. Their presence with malignant nodules usually indicates that the cancer has developed in relation to a pre-existing scar or that the carcinoma has spread by lymphatics or, possibly, pulmonary arteries to form discontinuous "skip" lesions.[106]

Change in Size with Time. Comparison of a current chest roentgenogram with previous ones is of fundamental importance in determining the benignity or malignancy of a solitary nodule. In many cases, a previous film may show an identical lesion, perhaps overlooked because of the roentgenographic technique employed or because it was

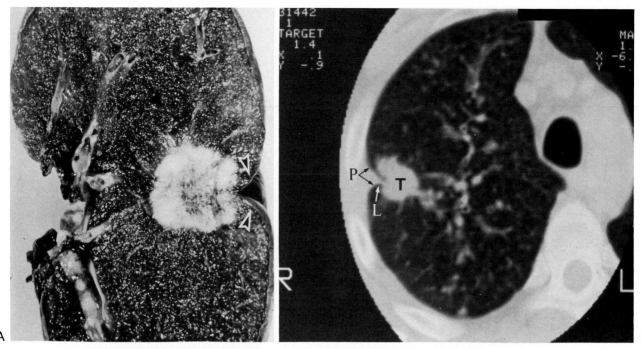

Figure 8–19. The Pyramidal Pleural Opacity (Tail Sign). *A,* Gross section of an excised upper lobe shows a peripheral carcinoma. The adjacent visceral pleura *(arrowheads)* is inverted toward the nodule, forming a triangle-shaped "defect" in the normally smooth pleural contour. *B,* In another patient, a CT scan through a right upper lobe adenocarcinoma (T) displays similar features: A pyramidal pleural opacity (P) is connected to the nodule by a short line (L).

obscured by a rib shadow. In such cases it is reasonable to withhold surgery and to follow up with periodic roentgenographic examination.

In individuals in whom a nodule has enlarged, use of doubling time* to estimate the growth rate may be of value in differentiating between benign and malignant nodules. This exercise requires at least two serial chest roentgenograms showing a roughly spherical lesion whose diameter can be averaged from measurements in at least two planes. Such measurements can be plotted against time, resulting in a curve that can be extrapolated to give an estimate of the time of onset of the cancer. According to one model,[107] 75 per cent of a cancer's lifetime occurs before the lesion is roentgenologically detectable. Calculation based on a range of doubling times from 30 to 300 days indicates that the time required for a malignant pulmonary nodule to reach 1 cm in diameter ranges from about 2.5 to more than 25 years.[107]

One problem with the radiologic estimation of doubling times is that many pulmonary carcinomas are not spherical, a fact that can lead to considerable overestimation of volume, especially of larger tumors. Another is sudden hemorrhage into the center of a malignant nodule, a process that can increase its volume dramatically and put the doubling time well within the range usually accepted as denoting benignity. Despite these and other limitations, the doubling time concept may be of use in diagnosis. In particular, it provides a more accurate assessment of the nature of a solitary nodule than does simple increase in size. Since benign lesions such as hamartomas and histoplasmomas may grow slowly, increase in size by itself should not be the sole consideration governing the therapeutic approach to a pulmonary nodule.

Although precise figures are not possible, several studies have provided data that allow reasonable generalizations about doubling time and diagnosis. For example, in two studies, the reported range of doubling times of carcinomas was 30 to 490 days (median, 120 days)[107] and 1 to 14 months.[108] In another investigation, virtually all pulmonary nodules whose doubling time was 7 days or less were benign[109]; if metastatic gestational choriocarcinoma, testicular neoplasms, and osteogenic sarcoma can be eliminated (usually relatively simple by the time pulmonary metastases appear), the doubling time for benign lesions can be confidently increased to 11 days. Similarly, nodules whose volume doubles in 460 days (the average of 14 months and 490 days) or more are almost always benign. Of the primary lung carcinomas, adenocarcinoma grows most slowly, and undifferentiated and squamous cell cancers most rapidly. Giant cell carcinoma is characterized by extremely rapid growth.

Solitary Pulmonary Mass

The rather arbitrary division of solitary opacities within the lung into two categories, nodules (measuring 3 cm or less in diameter) and masses (measuring more than 3 cm in diameter), serves only one useful purpose—a mass is much

---

*"Doubling" refers to volume, not diameter. If a nodule is spherical, multiplying its diameter by 1.25 gives the diameter of a sphere whose volume is double; for example, the volume of a nodule 2 cm in diameter is doubled by the time its diameter reaches 2.5 cm.

more likely to be malignant than is a nodule. Calcification is seldom a feature of a solitary mass. However, even when it is present, it does not argue as much against malignancy as it does in the case of a solitary nodule. Although the interface between a mass and contiguous lung may be sharply defined and smooth (e.g., a solitary "cannonball" metastasis), it is much more often ill defined, a feature that strengthens the suspicion of cancer. As with the solitary pulmonary nodule, assessment of doubling time can be important in the evaluation of a solitary mass.

Cavitation

The incidence of cavitation in patients with pulmonary carcinoma ranges from about 2 to 15 per cent.[110] In one study of 100 cases, cavity formation was of three different types:[110] (1) central necrosis of the neoplasm (77 cases); (2)

a lung abscess distal to an obstructing neoplasm (17 cases); and (3) cavitary abscesses elsewhere in the lungs, possibly resulting from "spillover" of purulent material from segmental pneumonitis and abscess formation elsewhere (6 cases). Of the 77 cases in which the neoplasm was cavitated, the commonest locations were the posterior segments of the upper lobes and the superior segments of the lower lobes. The majority of cases of cavitary carcinoma are squamous cell in type, an observation probably explained in part by the almost invariable intraluminal growth of these tumors in proximal bronchi, permitting relatively easy drainage of necrotic material.

Most cavities are thick-walled and resemble acute lung abscesses (Fig. 8–20); in fact, the vast majority of cavities whose maximum wall thickness is 4 mm or less are benign, whereas those with a maximum wall thickness of 16 mm or more are malignant.[112]

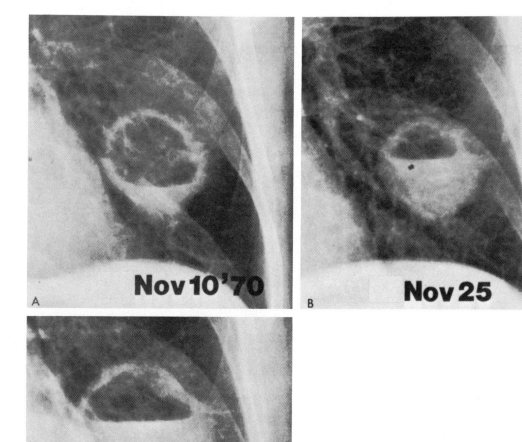

Figure 8–20. Cavitation in Primary Squamous Cell Carcinoma. The original roentgenogram of this 64-year-old asymptomatic man *(A)* reveals a 4.5-cm cavity in the left lower lobe, possessing a wall thickness of about 3 mm, and a small accumulation of fluid within it. Seven months later *(C)*, the transverse diameter of the mass had increased to 6.5 cm, which represents a tripling in volume. Note that wall thickness is essentially unchanged from the original examination.

The inner surface is usually irregular as a result of variably sized nodules of neoplastic tissue projecting into the cavity and of the patchy nature of the necrosis (*see* Fig. 8–2, page 451). Chunks of necrotic cancer sometimes become detached and lie free within the cavity, in which case differentiation from fungus ball may be difficult.

Airspace (Acinar) Pattern

This pattern of disease is almost unique to bronchioloalveolar carcinoma. The changes may be local or widely disseminated, the former predominating in 60 to 90 per cent of cases.[113] In the authors' experience, many examples of the local form of disease behave in a fashion similar to that of other histologic variants of pulmonary adenocarcinoma, often with dissemination of tumor to regional lymph nodes and extrathoracic viscera. Sometimes, however, a solitary nodule precedes the appearance of diffuse lung disease by a matter of several months, suggesting local (intrapulmonary) dissemination of tumor. In fact, it has been suggested that some patients in whom the disease appears to be local when first seen may, in fact, have deposits elsewhere in the lungs that are not demonstrable on conventional roentgenograms.[114]

Local. The commonest manifestation is a rather well-defined peripheral, homogeneous opacity ranging in size from a small nodule to a large mass occupying most of a lobe.[115] Many tumors grow very slowly, changing little for months or even years. Very occasionally, minute calcific deposits can be identified within the lesion, particularly on CT scans; these are usually caused by a multitude of psammoma bodies.[116]

An air bronchogram or bronchiologram is a common roentgenographic feature (Fig. 8–21) and is analogous to the bronchus sign previously described; it is of major importance in differential diagnosis. The explanation for its frequent presence is provided by considering the histologic appearance of the tumor; as discussed previously, the neoplastic cells grow within alveoli without destroying them, resulting in consolidation of parenchyma surrounding conducting airways. In fact, the consolidation may be caused as much by mucus or other secretion of the tumor cells as by neoplastic tissue itself. On CT, the sign is seen as stretching, spreading, and uniform narrowing of the involved airways, with or without obstruction.[117] In addition to bronchioloalveolar carcinoma, such air-containing airways may be visible in a peripheral lymphoma and inflammatory "pseudotumor"; however, they are rarely identified in other conditions.

As discussed previously (*see* page 463), the "tail sign" (consisting of a linear strand extending from the nodule to the pleural surface) has been documented in 25 per cent of

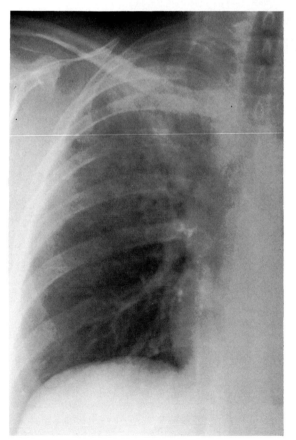

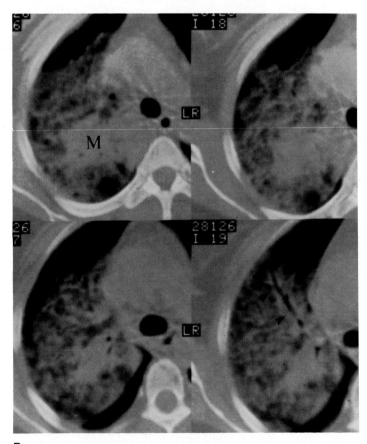

A   B

Figure 8–21. Bronchioloalveolar Carcinoma with Lobar Involvement. *A,* A view of the right lung from a posteroanterior chest roentgenogram reveals airspace consolidation occupying most of the upper lobe. An air bronchogram is present within the consolidated lung. *B,* A sequence of contiguous CT scans through the right upper lobe reveals a dominant mass superiorly (M); the air bronchogram is more clearly seen throughout the lobar consolidation.

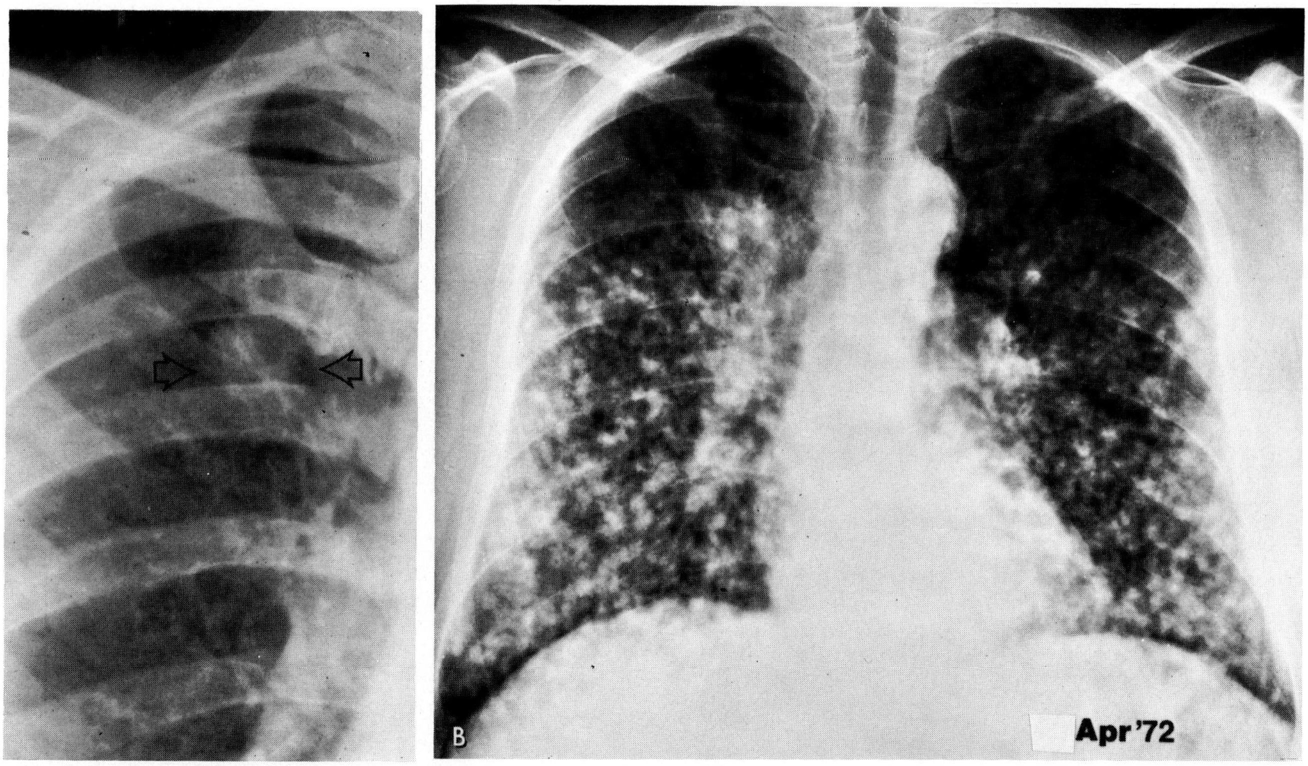

A

Figure 8–22. **Bronchioloalveolar Carcinoma Beginning as a Solitary Nodule with Subsequent Widespread Pulmonary Involvement.** A screening roentgenogram *(A)* of this 43-year-old asymptomatic man reveals a poorly defined solitary nodule 2 cm in diameter in the upper lobe *(arrows).* Nine months later *(B),* there has occurred widespread involvement of both lungs by small discrete and confluent opacities characteristic of acinar shadows. The original right upper lobe mass has undergone considerable growth.

bronchioloalveolar carcinomas.[101] Although it may also occur in granulomatous disease and other abnormalities, its association with a lesion containing an air bronchogram or bronchiologram is suggestive of this neoplasm.

Diffuse. The roentgenographic pattern of widely disseminated bronchioloalveolar carcinoma may be fairly uniform throughout both lungs (Fig. 8–22) or may vary regionally. The basic manifestation is the acinar shadow, indicating peripheral airspace consolidation. Such shadows may be discrete and readily identifiable as typical rosettes in one area of the lung, or they may be more or less confluent—sometimes to the extent of homogeneous consolidation—in other areas. Prominent line shadows extending along the bronchovascular bundles toward the hila usually represent lymphangitic carcinomatosis.

Hilar Enlargement

Unilateral hilar enlargement may be an early roentgenographic manifestation of pulmonary carcinoma, probably occurring in about 5 to 10 per cent of cases.[118] The enlargement may represent a primary carcinoma that has arisen in a mainstem or lobar bronchus (Fig. 8–23) or bronchopulmonary or hilar lymph nodes that are the site of metastases from a small primary lesion in adjacent or peripheral parenchyma. The latter process is particularly characteristic of small cell carcinoma. Even when a carcinoma is too small to enlarge the hilum, it may reveal itself by altering hilar density. The importance of CT and MRI in the evaluation of this sign cannot be overestimated.

Mediastinal Involvement

The mediastinum may be involved in patients with pulmonary carcinoma in one or both of two ways: by metastases to lymph nodes (undoubtedly the commonest mechanism) (Fig. 8–24) or by direct invasion from a contiguous neoplasm (Fig. 8–25). In most cases, there is an obvious intrapulmonary or hilar abnormality that indicates the source of the tumor. Occasionally, however, enlargement of mediastinal lymph nodes may be the main or sole abnormality seen roentgenographically,[118] a finding almost always indicating spread from a small cell carcinoma. The chief roentgenographic sign is mediastinal widening, usually with an undulating or lobular contour.

Evaluation of the presence of mediastinal lymph node involvement by metastatic pulmonary carcinoma can be best accomplished by either CT or MRI. Although there is now convincing evidence that there is no significant difference in the capability of the two techniques in demonstrating nodal metastases,[119] it is likely that MRI is superior to CT in the evaluation of the presence or absence of mediastinal invasion.[120]

Clinical manifestations of mediastinal involvement also are sometimes evident at presentation. These include signs of pericardial tamponade (corresponding roentgenographi-

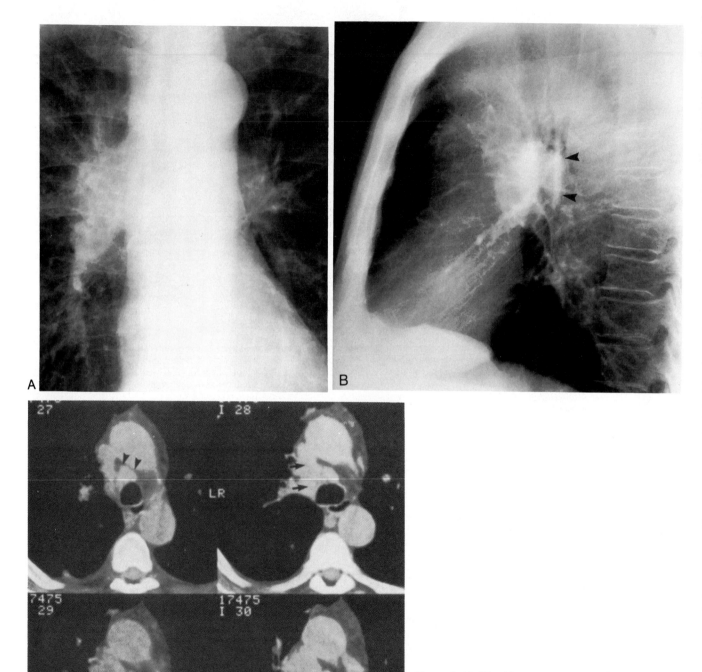

Figure 8–23. Hilar Mass without Airway Obstruction. Posteroanterior *(A)* and lateral *(B)* chest roentgenograms reveal marked asymmetry in the density and size of the hila, the right being more opaque, larger, and less well defined. Note the abnormally thick intermediate stem line *(arrowheads)* on the lateral view. *C,* Sequential CT scans disclose a right hilar mass that encircles the vasculature and major airways; several of the bronchi are narrowed. There is evidence of involvement of the mediastinum by both continuous *(arrows)* and metastatic *(arrowheads)* spread.

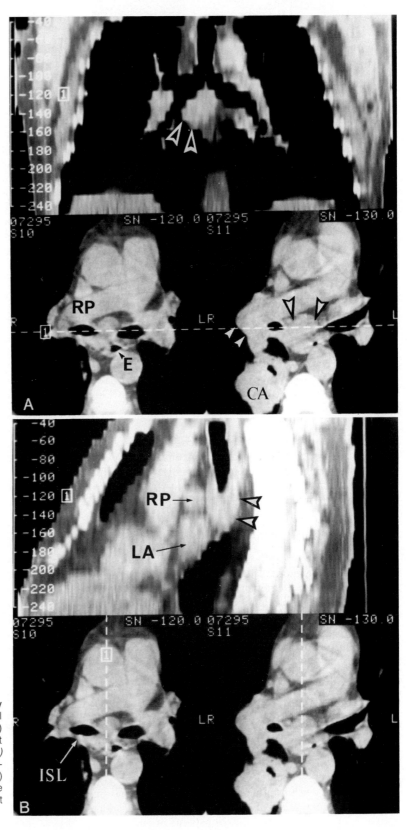

Figure 8–24. Mediastinal Involvement in Pulmonary Carcinoma: CT Manifestation. Coronal *(A)* and sagittal *(B)* re-formations (with appropriate transverse images) reveal a carcinoma in the superior segment of the right lower lobe (CA) as well as right hilar *(small arrowheads)* and subcarinal *(large arrowheads)* lymph node enlargement. Note the thickened intermediate stem line (ISL) and the relationship of the mediastinal nodes to the esophagus (E), right pulmonary artery (RP), and left atrium (LA).

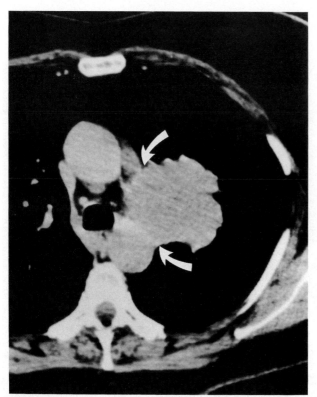

Figure 8–25. Pulmonary Carcinoma with Invasion of the Mediastinum. CT scan at the level of the aortopulmonary window shows a tumor 5 cm in diameter infiltrating the mediastinum *(curved arrows)* immediately anterior to the descending aorta.

cally to an increase in the cardiopericardial silhouette) and dysphagia caused by esophageal compression. Involvement of the subcarinal (bifurcation) or posterior mediastinal nodes also may displace the esophagus in the absence of dysphagia, a feature best revealed by CT.

Apical Pulmonary Neoplasms

Neoplasms that arise in this location have been termed Pancoast's tumor, thoracic inlet tumor, or superior pulmonary sulcus tumor (although the last-named is clearly a misnomer, since no definite sulcus exists in the extreme lung apex[121]). Although the original syndrome as described by Pancoast was characterized by pain, Horner's syndrome, destruction of bone, and atrophy of hand muscles, it has become apparent that the majority of patients with an apical neoplasm fail to fulfill all four criteria. As a result, it is now fairly well accepted that the term "Pancoast's syndrome" can be applied to any situation in which a neoplasm in the apex of a lung is accompanied by shoulder or arm pain. The symptoms or signs described are caused by direct neoplastic invasion of brachial vessels, the brachial nerve plexus, the rib cage, or the cervicothoracic sympathetic chain.

The tumors constitute about 2 to 5 per cent of all pulmonary carcinomas; squamous cell carcinoma and adenocarcinoma predominate. Of the 29 patients in one study,[121] conventional roentgenographic findings consisted of the following: an ipsilateral "apical cap" that measured more than 5 mm in thickness or a 5-mm asymmetry of apical caps on

the two sides (55 per cent); an apical mass (45 per cent); and bone destruction (34 per cent) (Figs. 8–26 and 8–27). Although these findings can confidently identify the tumors in some cases, in many other cases CT[122] or MRI[123] is necessary to confirm the diagnosis. The latter is the preferred technique for depicting the anatomic relationship of the tumor to contiguous extrathoracic structures.[120]

Pleural Involvement

Pleural involvement in primary pulmonary carcinoma is frequent and can take several forms. The commonest is probably effusion, which occurs in 5 to 15 per cent of cases at presentation. It may result from direct pleural invasion by carcinoma or from lymphatic obstruction, usually in association with metastases to hilar and mediastinal lymph nodes. Diffuse pleural thickening involving the entire surface of the lung, including the interlobar fissures, occurs occasionally, usually in association with a peripheral tumor.

Spontaneous pneumothorax is an uncommon manifestation of pulmonary carcinoma. The pathogenesis is variable and includes direct transgression of the visceral pleural surface by neoplastic cells, perforation into the pleural space by an abscess related to bronchial obstruction, and rupture of a bulla or bleb that developed as a result of the carcinoma or was present coincidentally.

Bone and Chest Wall Involvement

The skeleton may be involved in pulmonary carcinoma either by direct extension to the ribs or vertebrae (Fig. 8–28) or by metastasis via the bloodstream to remote sites. Except for Pancoast's tumor, the former can be difficult to detect, even with CT.[124] However, it is now fairly well conceded that MRI can be quite helpful.[120] An additional method that appears to hold some promise when MRI is not available is to combine CT with artificial pneumothorax.[125]

A 1973 roentgenographic analysis of the skeleton in 110 consecutive patients with pulmonary carcinoma reported bone involvement in 38 (35 per cent).[126] In 10 cases it was local and manifested by destruction of contiguous ribs or spine (mostly by squamous cell and large cell carcinoma); in 8 cases, there were distant metastases. In 9 of the 38 patients, the metastases were predominantly osteoblastic; in all of these, the cell type was either small cell carcinoma or adenocarcinoma, and there was concomitant extensive bone marrow involvement. None of the 67 patients with squamous cell or large cell carcinoma showed osteoblastic metastatic deposits.

Miscellaneous Signs

Other roentgenographic signs of pulmonary carcinoma include unilateral diaphragmatic paralysis resulting from phrenic nerve involvement (which should be differentiated from hemidiaphragmatic elevation compensatory to atelectasis and from pseudoelevation of a hemidiaphragm caused by a large infrapulmonary pleural effusion); bilateral parenchymal nodules resulting from contralateral hematogenous metastases; and a diffuse or local reticulonodular or linear pattern caused by lymphangitic carcinomatosis.

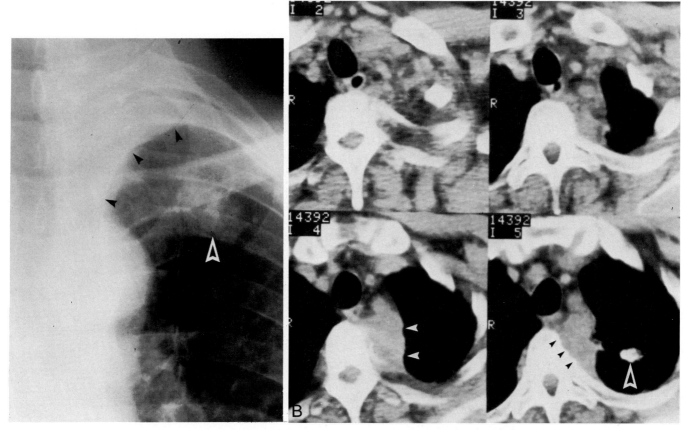

A

Figure 8–26. Role of CT in the Evaluation of Apical Pulmonary Carcinoma (Pancoast Tumor). *A,* A detail view of the left upper hemithorax from a posteroanterior chest roentgenogram shows a broad, curvilinear opacity *(arrowheads)* over the apex of the left upper lobe. A 2-cm nodule *(large arrowhead),* overlapped by the anterior end of the first and the posterior portion of the fifth ribs, is visible inferiorly; no definite calcification can be identified within the lesion. The trachea is displaced slightly to the right; there is no evidence of bone destruction. *B,* Sequential 10-mm CT scans through the left apex reveal a plaque of soft tissue superomedially *(arrowheads)* that hugs the pleural surface at the level of the second and third vertebral bodies. There is minimal bone erosion *(small arrowheads)* in the lateral part of the third vertebral body. The nodule *(large arrowhead)* in the upper lobe is a calcified granuloma (compare the CT density of the lesion with that of the adjacent bones).

Clinical Manifestations

About 10 per cent of patients with pulmonary carcinoma are asymptomatic when first seen, the diagnosis being suspected initially from an abnormal chest roentgenogram or, rarely, cytologic examination of sputum. Of the remainder, most have symptoms referable to the lungs or adjacent thoracic tissues. Occasionally, patients present with signs and symptoms related to extrathoracic metastases or a paraneoplastic disorder.

Bronchopulmonary Manifestations

The commonest symptom referable to the respiratory tract is cough, which occurs in about 75 per cent of patients.[127] Since the majority are heavy smokers and have chronic bronchitis, cough itself may not be recognized as a new symptom; a change in the character or frequency of the cough, however, has much greater significance. Hemoptysis occurs in about 50 per cent of cases and may be the only clue to the diagnosis in the patient whose chest roentgenogram is normal.[129] Increased shortness of breath

or symptoms of acute infection in a region of obstructive pneumonitis are occasionally present. In 20 to 25 per cent of cases of bronchioloalveolar carcinoma, cough is associated with abundant mucoid expectoration (bronchorrhea), a feature that is highly suggestive of the disease. Such voluminous expectoration usually indicates extensive lung involvement[128] and may result in severe hypovolemia and electrolyte depletion.

Physical examination often reveals no abnormality, although there may be a decrease in breath sounds or dullness to percussion related to airway obstruction or obstructive pneumonitis. Occasionally, a local wheeze is present.

Extrapulmonary Intrathoracic Manifestations

Complicating or presenting symptoms and signs may result from extension of the carcinoma beyond the primary site to the pleura, mediastinum, or thoracic inlet.

Pleura. Infiltration of the pleura by carcinoma may occasion pain on breathing and is frequently accompanied by effusion and its attendant signs. If the effusion is large

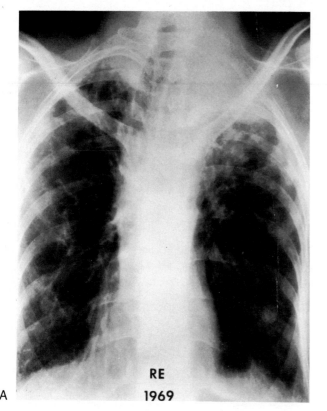

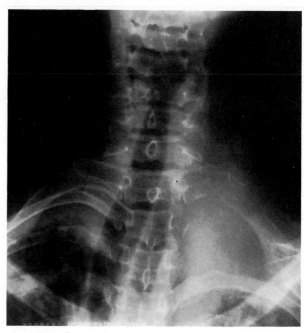

Figure 8–27. Pancoast Tumor. *A,* A posteroanterior chest roentgenogram reveals a large homogeneous soft tissue opacity over the apex of the left upper lobe. There is evidence of bone destruction in several ribs and vertebrae, seen to better advantage on an overpenetrated view of the thoracic inlet *(B).* The findings are typical of an apical or Pancoast neoplasm. Proven adenocarcinoma.

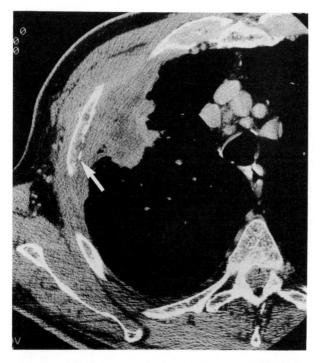

Figure 8–28. Pulmonary Carcinoma with Invasion of the Chest Wall. High-resolution CT (= 1.5-mm collimation reconstructed using a high-frequency resolution algorithm) targeted to the right lung at the level of the right upper lobe demonstrates a peripheral lung tumor 4 × 5 cm in diameter. Irregularity of the medial surface of the adjoining rib *(arrow)* is noted, indicating chest wall invasion with involvement of the rib.

enough, dyspnea may develop. Effusion also may be caused by metastases to hilar and mediastinal lymph nodes, with consequent lymphatic obstruction.

Mediastinum. Mediastinal disease in association with pulmonary carcinoma usually is caused by the neoplasm itself, either by direct extension from the primary lesion or by lymph node metastases. Nodal enlargement also may be caused by hyperplasia, representing a reaction to either infection in an obstructed region of lung or the cancer itself. The presence *per se* of enlarged nodes or neoplasm in the mediastinum seldom gives rise to symptoms; of far greater significance are the effects on the various structures that reside within the mediastinum, of which the most important are the heart, esophagus, major vessels of the venous and arterial circulation, and nerves.

Cardiac involvement is commoner than is generally realized. Pericardial infiltration is the most frequent form of disease and is usually caused by retrograde extension along lymphatics from lymph node metastases.[130] Effusion may cause cardiac tamponade; in many cases the etiology of the tamponade can be recognized by cytologic examination of pericardial fluid.

Dysphagia resulting from esophageal involvement is an uncommon symptom of pulmonary carcinoma, being observed in only 9 (2 per cent) of 405 cases in one series.[131] This low incidence is probably related to the fact that enlarged nodes usually only displace the esophagus and are unlikely to compromise function unless very large. Obstruction is most likely when the esophageal wall is invaded by neoplasm, in which case the primary site is commonly the left mainstem bronchus.

The superior vena cava syndrome—edema of the face, neck, and upper extremities, distended neck and arm veins, and sometimes headache and dizziness—is most often caused by pulmonary carcinoma.[132] In the authors' experience, this syndrome does not require emergency treatment[133]; however, compression of the trachea often coexists and is a complication that may require urgent measures to restore adequate ventilation. Occasionally, the axillary or subclavian veins alone are involved by tumor, resulting in the appropriate signs in the distribution of the affected venous drainage.[134]

Invasion or compression of the recurrent laryngeal nerve may cause hoarseness, and involvement of the vagus nerve may cause dyspnea, particularly in patients with chronic bronchitis (as is so often the case). Although involvement of the phrenic nerve causes hemidiaphragmatic paresis or paralysis, this usually does not lead to symptoms in the presence of normal respiratory reserve.

Thoracic Inlet. An apical pulmonary carcinoma invading the thoracic inlet (Pancoast's tumor) may involve one or several structures in that region, resulting in highly variable signs and symptoms, including pain and weakness of the shoulder and arm, swelling of the arm, and Horner's syndrome (*see* page 470).

Extrathoracic Metastatic Manifestations

Extrathoracic metastases of pulmonary carcinoma usually are associated with a previously diagnosed or obvious synchronous tumor. Occasionally, they may be responsible for the initial clinical manifestations, sometimes in the absence of a roentgenographically detectable primary lesion.[135]

At autopsy, metastases are almost invariable: in one necropsy review of 662 patients with lung cancer, they were identified in 96.3 per cent, the incidence being highest with small cell carcinoma and lowest with squamous cell carcinoma.[136] Although metastases can occur in virtually any organ or tissue, the most frequent sites outside the thorax are the lymph nodes, liver, adrenal glands, bone, kidneys, and brain.

Lymph Nodes. Metastases are common in the scalene group of lymph nodes; contrary to the generally accepted belief, such dissemination is chiefly ipsilateral from all parts of each lung.[137] When the carcinoma is advanced, especially in patients with extensive mediastinal lymph node involvement, spread into periaortic, mesenteric, and other intra-abdominal lymph node groups is also frequent; however, signs and symptoms caused by such invasion usually are absent.

Brain and Spinal Cord. Cerebral metastases are found at necropsy in as many as 50 per cent of cases of pulmonary carcinoma[136]; about one third are solitary. They are particularly common in patients with adenocarcinoma[138] and small cell carcinoma.[139] Now that survival is relatively prolonged in patients with treated small cell carcinoma, meningeal carcinomatosis has become a relatively common complication in this subtype.[140] An emergency situation may develop when there are metastases to the spinal cord[141]; CT and MRI are particularly useful for diagnostic purposes in this area.

Bone. Metastatic spread to bone occurs in 10 to 35 per cent of cases at some time during the course of the disease.[126] More than 20 per cent of patients have bone pain on initial evaluation; radionuclide bone scans may be abnormal in as many as 40 per cent of patients at this time. In addition, bone involvement may be manifested by features of hypercalcemia,[142] a situation that should be distinguished from a paraneoplastic syndrome (*see* later).

Abdominal Viscera. Metastatic involvement of the liver, adrenal glands, pancreas, and kidneys may cause symptoms and signs that confuse diagnosis. Small cell carcinoma, in particular, may cause extensive liver metastases, with resultant epigastric pain and jaundice and a rapid downhill course that simulates hepatitis. Jaundice may also be caused by extrahepatic biliary obstruction from pancreatic metastases.[143] Metastases to the adrenal glands are particularly common and can usually be identified by CT and confirmed (if necessary) by needle aspiration. Even though such metastases may replace much of the gland, clinical manifestations of adrenal insufficiency are very uncommon.[144] Gastrointestinal metastases have been documented in 10 to 15 per cent of cases; perforation, ulceration, and obstruction can occur at any level.[145]

Extrathoracic Nonmetastatic Manifestations

Constitutional symptoms such as malaise, weakness, lassitude, fever, and weight loss may be present in the absence of clinical evidence of extrathoracic metastases, but in most cases are manifestations of distant tumor spread. In addition to these relatively nonspecific features, some patients, particularly those with small cell carcinoma, have symptoms and signs of systemic disease not directly related to neoplastic infiltration itself. Such paraneoplastic syndromes may occur in the absence of bronchopulmonary symptoms and can be discussed under several headings.

Neuromuscular Manifestations. Neurologic abnormalities develop in about 5 per cent of cases of pulmonary carcinoma, even in the absence of central nervous system metastases.[146] Signs and symptoms typically occur only when disease is advanced and are usually progressive; in some cases, they are alleviated by removal of the primary neoplasm. The detection of antibodies to various nerve tissue components and the response to immunosuppressive therapy suggest an autoimmune pathogenesis for at least some of these disorders.[147] Small cell carcinoma is the commonest responsible primary tumor.

Myopathy. Two myopathic syndromes are seen with pulmonary carcinoma, one simulating myasthenia (the Lambert-Eaton syndrome) and the other polymyositis (*see* page 405). The Lambert-Eaton syndrome is rare and is associated with the development of immunoglobulin G (IgG) antibodies to nerve terminals. It differs from true myasthenia gravis in several respects, involved muscle groups in the extremities being proximal rather than distal and muscles being weak at the beginning of contraction and sometimes reaching normal strength with repeated or sustained effort.

Peripheral Neuropathy. In most cases, this is both motor and sensory,[146] although only pain and paresthesia may be noted in the early stages, with sensory loss, muscle weakness, and wasting occurring later. Autonomic neuropathy also has been identified in patients with pulmonary carcinoma, particularly of the small cell type.[148] Patients often present with intestinal "pseudo-obstruction" (manifested as obstipation or constipation); neurogenic bladder and abnormalities of esophageal peristalsis also may be present.

Cerebellar Dysfunction. This abnormality is a relatively common form of paraneoplastic syndrome.[149] The clinical picture varies from one of subtle signs identifiable only by examination to full-blown subacute cerebellar degeneration, with rapidly progressive ataxia, incoordination, vertigo, nystagmus, and dysarthria.

Hypertrophic Pulmonary Osteoarthropathy. This is a distinctive manifestation of pulmonary carcinoma that is found in about 3 per cent of patients,[150] most often with squamous and large cell carcinoma. The pathogenesis, roentgenographic features, and clinical manifestations are discussed on page 147. Relief of pain invariably follows resection of the primary neoplasm and is common after simple vagotomy without pulmonary resection; other features of the syndrome also may be alleviated but usually not to the same extent as pain.

Endocrine and Metabolic Manifestations

Cushing's Syndrome. Immunoreactive ACTH is commonly present in the serum of patients with small cell carcinoma. Despite this, probably no more than 1 to 2 per cent of patients develop clinical features of Cushing's syndrome. The explanation for this discrepancy is probably a combination of the short survival time of patients with small cell tumors and the observation that in many cases the immunoreactive ACTH appears to be biologically inactive.[151]

In contrast with the usual picture of Cushing's syndrome, the paraneoplastic syndrome associated with pulmonary carcinoma tends to be more acute, with a rapid, downhill course. Classic clinical and laboratory features are seldom seen, the patient presenting with progressive weakness, muscle wasting, facial edema, hyperglycemia, personality disorder, hyperpigmentation, polyuria, and hypokalemic hypochloremic alkalosis. The last-named is related to the mineralocorticoid effect of high levels of corticosteroids and is present in the majority of patients, including those with occult tumors.[152]

Hyperparathyroidlike Picture. The incidence of hypercalcemia in patients with pulmonary carcinoma depends, in large measure, on the range of values accepted as being normal. It is likely, however, that the condition is common. For example, in one study of 280 cases of early lung cancer, the serum calcium level exceeded 11.5 mg per 100 mL on two or more occasions in 19 (6.8 per cent).[150] In about 50 per cent of cases, hypercalcemia is associated with skeletal metastases. In the absence of such metastases, systemic humoral mechanisms must be responsible, and a variety of tumor-produced substances have been implicated, including a parathormonelike substance,[153] prostaglandin E_2,[154] and osteoclast activating factor. In the great majority of patients in whom the hypercalcemia is a paraneoplastic manifestation, the neoplasm is squamous cell in type.[155] In contrast with many other paraneoplastic manifestations, hypercalcemia occurs rarely, if at all, with clinically occult carcinoma.[156]

Inappropriate Secretion of Antidiuretic Hormone (ADH). This syndrome has been reported in 1 to 2 per cent of patients with pulmonary carcinoma,[150] mostly of the small cell type. It is believed to be caused by production of arginine vasopressin directly by the tumor. This leads to increased reabsorption of free water by the renal tubules under the influence of ADH. Because plasma sodium is diluted and the circulating volume is increased, hyponatremia in turn results in decreased aldosterone secretion. With the decrease in aldosterone secretion, the amount of sodium excreted in the urine is inappropriate to the low plasma sodium concentration, so the hyponatremia is both depletive and diluting.

When the serum sodium level drops below 120 mEq per L, symptoms of irritability, confusion, irresponsibility, and weakness appear, all considered to be caused by the hyponatremia. Usually, the chest roentgenogram is unequivocally abnormal.

Gonadotropin Secretion. All types of pulmonary carcinoma are capable of producing gonadotropic hormones,[157] although large cell carcinoma appears to be implicated most often. Affected patients may present with testicular atrophy and a high-pitched voice in addition to gynecomastia. Many patients have high serum levels of placental alkaline phosphatase in addition to circulating beta subunits of human chorionic gonadotropin (HCG) and estrogens.[158]

Calcitonin Secretion. The commonest polypeptide hormone produced by pulmonary neoplasms may be calcitonin.[159] Such elevation does not cause symptoms; however, levels can serve as useful markers of response to therapy or recurrence of neoplasm.

Vascular and Hematologic Manifestations

Migratory Thrombophlebitis. Although this complication much more frequently accompanies carcinoma of the pancreas, it has been well documented in cases of primary lung neoplasms. The thrombophlebitis is migratory in type, occurs in unusual sites, and tends to be resistant to anticoagulant therapy. It is associated most often with adenocarcinoma.

Leukocytosis. A leukemoid reaction (white blood cell count of 50,000 cells per mL or more) tends to be a late phenomenon, usually becoming manifest shortly before death. One review suggested an especially frequent association with large cell carcinoma.[160] Peripheral eosinophilia is present occasionally, usually in association with squamous cell and large cell carcinomas; extracts of the tumors have been shown to contain eosinophilic chemotactic factor or eosinophil colony stimulating factor.[161]

Renal Manifestations. There is evidence that both proteinuria and hematuria have an increased incidence in pulmonary carcinoma.[162] Glomerulonephritis, possibly related to immune complex formation associated with tumor antigens, is clearly present in some cases. In most of these cases, the disease is membranous in type.

Investigation of the Patient with Pulmonary Carcinoma

The patient in whom there is roentgenographic or clinical evidence suggestive of pulmonary carcinoma requires two quite distinct lines of investigation. First, it is necessary to establish the diagnosis, including a determination of the specific cell type involved. Second, since surgical excision is currently the best method of curative treatment, it is necessary to establish resectability or unresectability by a process of staging.

Since considerable variability exists in the natural history of the different histologic types of pulmonary carcinoma and in the extent of disease when the patient is first seen, the investigative protocol should ideally be tailored to the specific presentation of each patient. Nevertheless, the authors have found it desirable to develop an approach to the diagnostic and staging work-up that is organized along fairly precise lines. It is clear that such investigational protocols will vary somewhat from institution to institution, depending on the expertise of available physicians and the diagnostic equipment available, but the ones that the authors present here are those that they have personally found successful and that appear valid on the strength of information gleaned from many reports in the literature.

Clinical and Laboratory Methods of Diagnosis

Flexible fiberoptic bronchoscopy is indicated in all patients with centrally located, potentially malignant lesions. It can also be employed in peripherally located tumors, in the hope of obtaining positive cytology, although in such cases the yield is likely to be just as high with spontaneous or induced sputum specimens. Intravenous fluorescent dyes, such as a hematoporphyrin derivative and 10 per cent sodium fluoresceinate, have been administered to patients for the purpose of detecting occult pulmonary carcinomas with bronchoscopes that have been modified to permit recognition of sites of fluorescence.[163] There is no doubt that neoplastic cells can be located with this method, but because areas of inflammation and metaplasia can also fluoresce and because of the complications of skin photosensitivity the procedure has gained little popularity. Future modifications, however, may make this procedure more attractive.

A number of tumor markers, such as carcinoembryonic antigen (CEA),[164] angiotensin converting enzyme,[165] and various tumor antigens,[166] have been advocated as diagnostic aids in pulmonary carcinoma. These can be measured in serum, bronchoalveolar lavage fluid, or pleural fluid, the sensitivity and specificity of the results being manipulated by adjusting cut-off levels for positivity and negativity between control subjects and patients with carcinoma. At the time of writing, the authors believe that these methods are probably of limited diagnostic value. With increased study, however, especially in the case of new or multiple markers, these methods may prove to be useful.

Biopsy techniques used in the diagnosis of pulmonary carcinoma and a consideration of the general features of cytologic and histologic diagnosis are discussed in Chapter 2.

Roentgenographic Methods of Diagnosis

Conventional Chest Roentgenography. The presence of a potentially malignant lesion is almost invariably identified on conventional chest roentgenograms in posteroanterior and lateral projections (the exception being the rare instance in which sputum cytology is positive for malignant cells and the chest roentgenogram is normal). The importance of obtaining previous films for comparison cannot be overemphasized, particularly in the evaluation of the solitary pulmonary nodule but also in the assessment of possible lymph node enlargement in such anatomic structures as the hila and aortopulmonary window.

Conventional Tomography. Even though the morphology of a lesion may be somewhat better appreciated with conventional tomography, this modality is seldom able to establish a definitive diagnosis. In the authors' view, therefore, there are only two indications for this procedure in the evaluation of the patient with possible pulmonary carcinoma: (1) the identification of calcium within a solitary pulmonary nodule, a finding that virtually excludes the possibility of malignancy; and (2) the occasional clarification of a narrowing of the tracheal lumen in which anteroposterior and lateral tomograms may show the extent and location of a lesion to better advantage than CT.

CT and MRI. Both CT and MRI can be of inestimable value in the assessment of the patient with pulmonary carcinoma. Such benefit lies chiefly in staging (*see* later). In the authors' opinion, the only indications for CT in the *diagnosis* of primary pulmonary carcinoma are the estimation of the calcium content of a solitary pulmonary nodule (*see* page 462) and, occasionally, the confirmation of the presence of a lesion suspected on posteroanterior and lateral roentgenograms or the identification of its precise anatomic location.

Bronchography and Arteriography. In the authors' view, neither of these techniques is indicated in the investigation of a patient with suspected pulmonary carcinoma, their use having been supplanted by bronchoscopy and contrast-enhanced CT, respectively.

Scintigraphy. With the exception of the evaluation of

Table 8–3. TNM STAGING SYSTEMS

T—Primary Tumor	**N—Regional Lymph Nodes**
T0 No evidence of primary tumor.	
Tx Tumor proved by the presence of malignant cells in bronchopulmonary secretions but not visualized roentgenographically or bronchoscopically, or any tumor that cannot be assessed as in a retreatment staging.	
Tis Carcinoma in situ	
T1 A tumor that is 3.0 cm or less in greatest dimension, surrounded by lung or visceral pleura, and without evidence of invasion proximal to a lobar bronchus at bronchoscopy. (The uncommon superficial tumor of any size with its invasive component limited to the bronchial wall, which may extend proximal to the main bronchus, is classified as T1.)	

T2 A tumor more than 3.0 cm in greatest dimension, or a tumor of any size that either invades the visceral pleura or has associated atelectasis or obstructive pneumonitis extending to the hilar region. At bronchoscopy the proximal extent of demonstrable tumor must be within a lobar bronchus or at least 2.0 cm distal to the carina. Any associated atelectasis or obstructive pneumonitis must involve less than an entire lung.

T3 A tumor of any size with direct extension into the chest wall (including superior sulcus tumors), diaphragm, or the mediastinal pleura or pericardium without involving the heart, great vessels, trachea, esophagus or vertebral body, or a tumor in the main bronchus within 2 cm of the carina without involving the carina.

T4 A tumor of any size with invasion of the mediastinum or involving heart, great vessels, trachea, esophagus, vertebral body or carina or presence of malignant pleural effusion. (Most pleural effusions associated with lung cancer are due to tumor. There are, however, some few patients in whom cytopathologic examination of pleural fluid (on more than one specimen) is negative for tumor, the fluid is nonbloody and is not an exudate. In such cases, where these elements and clinical judgment dictate the effusion is not related to the tumor, the patient should be staged T1, T2, or T3, excluding effusion as a staging element.)

N—Regional Lymph Nodes

N0 No demonstrable metastasis to regional lymph nodes.

N1 Metastasis to lymph nodes in the peribronchial or the ipsilateral hilar region, or both (including direct extension).

N2 Metastasis to ipsilateral mediastinal lymph nodes and subcarinal lymph nodes.

N3 Metastasis to contralateral mediastinal lymph nodes, contralateral hilar lymph nodes, ipsilateral or contralateral scalene or supraclavicular lymph nodes.

M—Distant Metastases

N0 No (known) distant metastasis.

M1 Distant metastasis present—specify site(s).

Adapted from Mountain CF: A new international staging system for lung cancer. Chest 89: 2255, 1986.

patients for distant metastases, isotopic techniques play a limited role in the investigation of pulmonary carcinoma. Attempts to identify lung neoplasms by selective uptake of various isotopes (e.g., ^{67}GA citrate) have been disappointing,[167] partly because not all neoplasms take up the isotope, but mainly because certain infectious processes also result in positive scans.

Schemes for Staging

The most widely used scheme for staging non–small cell carcinoma of the lung is the TNM classification outlined in 1986 by the International Union Against Cancer (UICC), the American Joint Committee for Cancer Staging and End Results Reporting, and the Japanese Cancer Committee (Table 8–3).[168] According to this system, *T* designates the primary tumor, *N* represents regional lymph node involvement, and *M* specifies metastases. Various combinations of T, N, and M define different stages (Table 8–4). A more detailed discussion of stage in relation to prognosis is given on page 480.

Patients with small cell carcinoma are frequently staged in a more simple fashion into two groups: those with limited disease (defined as carcinoma confined to one hemithorax, including regional mediastinal and supraclavicular lymph nodes) and those with extensive disease. The increasing tendency to employ a surgical therapeutic approach to the occasional patient who presents with small cell carcinoma confined to the lung, with or without ipsilateral hilar and bronchopulmonary node involvement, has also suggested

that designation of another category of "very limited" disease may be necessary.

Methods of Staging

As with diagnosis, the approach to staging varies with the individual patient and the particular carcinoma and should be tailored to the presenting clinical, roentgenographic, and bronchoscopic findings.

T (The Primary Tumor). Most of the criteria that define the T categories are established during the initial diagnostic work-up. For example, conventional roentgenograms will reveal the size of the lesion in patients in whom it is

Table 8–4. STAGE GROUPING OF TNM SUBSETS

Occult Carcinoma	Tx	N0	M0
Stage 0	Tis	N0	M0
Stage I	T1	N0	M0
	T2	N0	M0
Stage II	T1	N1	M0
	T2	N1	M0
Stage IIIa	T3	N0	M0
	T3	N1	M0
	T1–3	N2	M0
Stage IIIb	Any T	N3	M0
	T4	Any N	M0
Stage IV	Any T	Any N	M1

circumscribed and the degree of associated atelectasis or obstructive pneumonitis in those in whom there is airway obstruction. In the latter event, bronchoscopy documents the proximal extent of the neoplasm. The chest roentgenogram also establishes the presence or absence of pleural effusion, the exception being the situation in which atelectasis or obstructive pneumonitis of a lower lobe obscures the presence of effusion. In such circumstances, lateral decubitus roentgenography or ultrasound examination may be helpful.

In some cases, extrapulmonary spread may also be evident without the results of special investigations. For example, direct extension of a neoplasm into the chest wall may be established by roentgenographic evidence of destruction of ribs or vertebrae or a clinically palpable mass. Evidence of invasion of the mediastinum may be suggested by elevation of a hemidiaphragm or by clinical signs of superior vena cava syndrome or laryngeal paralysis. Paramediastinal lesions sometimes displace or narrow the tracheal air column, thereby providing convincing roentgenographic evidence of mediastinal invasion. In the absence of these signs, however, conventional roentgenography is generally unreliable in detecting invasion of the chest wall, diaphragm, or mediastinum, and it is necessary to resort to CT or MRI (preferably the latter[120]) for such evaluation.

CT can correctly predict invasion of the diaphragm, chest wall, or mediastinum, provided that there is interdigitation of the carcinoma with fat or muscle or, in the case of the mediastinum, provided that major mediastinal vessels or bronchi are surrounded.[169] By contrast, a tumor that abuts but does not obviously invade mediastinal fat cannot be considered noninvasive and must be classified as indeterminate; likewise, even when the fat plane between the mediastinum and the tumor mass is obliterated, it cannot be concluded absolutely that mediastinal invasion has occurred. A similar caveat regarding tissue invasion must be made in relation to the chest wall and diaphragm:[170] when a tumor directly abuts a pleural surface or when pleural thickening is noted immediately adjacent to a tumor mass, CT findings must be interpreted as indeterminate or merely as suspicious for pleural and chest wall invasion.[169] Only when tumor obliterates fat planes between parietal pleura and chest wall muscles or when there is associated bone destruction can chest wall invasion be diagnosed with conviction.

N (Regional Lymph Nodes). Since the demonstration of mediastinal lymph node metastases may be a contraindication to definitive surgery, evaluation of these structures becomes an important part of the investigation of any patient with proven pulmonary carcinoma. Again, the investigative protocol employs both biopsy and roentgenographic techniques. The former consists of mediastinoscopy (see page 134) and, less commonly, transbronchial needle aspiration (see page 132).

With respect to roentgenographic techniques, it should be emphasized that there are no definitive criteria for determining the presence or absence of mediastinal or hilar lymph node metastases. The principal criterion on which roentgenographic evidence of metastases is based is nodal enlargement. That this approach necessarily entails a degree of inaccuracy, however, is demonstrated by two incontrovertible facts: (1) lymph nodes that are customarily considered normal in size can be the site of metastatic disease; and (2) nodes that are reasonably considered enlarged may be simply hyperplastic and may contain no malignant cells.[171, 171a] Thus, it seems reasonable to conclude that the best that current roentgenographic imaging techniques can do in assessing the presence or absence of nodal metastases is to provide an estimate of the *likelihood* that these exist.[172] In this regard, the following guidelines seem reasonable: lymph nodes whose diameter is 1 cm or less can be considered normal; those with a diameter of 1.5 cm or more should be considered pathologic and likely to contain metastases; and those of a size between these extremes should be considered indeterminate.[169] (Further discussion of the use and limitations of CT in assessing mediastinal lymph node enlargement is given on page 66.)

Comparative studies of CT and MRI in the assessment of mediastinal lymph node metastases have not convincingly demonstrated the superiority of one over the other, as long as nodal size remains the sole criterion on which the presence of metastases is based.[173] However, the situation is somewhat different when only hilar abnormality is considered; for example, in one study of 12 patients with unilateral or bilateral hilar masses, investigators were able to differentiate the mass from hilar vasculature more easily with MRI than with contrast-enhanced CT.[174] Comparison of MR and CT imaging in the investigation of hilar and mediastinal abnormalities is discussed further on page 72.

M (Distant Metastases). Imaging techniques are of vital importance in the investigation of patients with possible extrathoracic metastases, partly to confirm a clinical suspicion but more often to demonstrate occult disease. The most widely employed are radionuclide scans (used to identify potential liver, brain, or skeletal metastases) and CT and ultrasonography of the abdomen (utilized to demonstrate metastases to the adrenal glands and liver).

There is little doubt regarding the advisability of including the upper abdomen in the investigation of all patients with pulmonary carcinoma whose thorax is being examined by CT preoperatively. This is particularly useful in patients with small cell carcinoma, in whom metastases to the liver or adrenal glands have been identified in as many as 25 per cent.[175]

The use of radionuclide scanning of the liver, bone, and brain for the purpose of discovering distant metastases is controversial. Some authorities believe that in the absence of organ-specific symptoms, physical signs, or biochemical abnormalities, these procedures are of limited value.[176] Others, however, suggest that organ-specific scanning can be advantageous even in asymptomatic patients.[177] Of the three organ-specific scans, there is little doubt that the one with the highest yield is bone; in fact, bone scanning is considerably more sensitive than conventional roentgenography in the detection of metastases.[178]

Investigation of Specific Roentgenographic Patterns

Protocols for investigating the patient with pulmonary carcinoma, particularly with respect to the presence or absence of mediastinal lymph node metastases, depend in large measure on the initial roentgenologic appearance— the solitary pulmonary nodule or mass, the obstructing endobronchial lesion, or the central nonobstructing lesion.

Two algorithms are presented (Tables 8–5 and 8–6) that the authors believe represent a reasonable approach to such investigations. Clearly, these are meant to provide general guidelines only; specific circumstances and individual preferences may alter the lineage.

Solitary Pulmonary Nodule or Mass. As indicated previously, comparison of current roentgenograms with previous films is an essential first step in establishing whether a lesion is new or has grown or not grown over time. The second step is to assess the presence or absence of calcification, a determination that can sometimes be made with confidence from the conventional roentgenograms; if not, CT (or dual-energy digital radiography) is the logical next step. In the absence of calcification or other mitigating influences (e.g., age less than 35 years), the lesion must be assumed to be malignant. The presence of pleural effusion on conventional roentgenograms may already have suggested a T4 category, which can be confirmed in many cases by pleural biopsy or cytologic examination of pleural fluid. Similarly, direct chest wall or mediastinal invasion (as demonstrated by conventional procedures or CT) may establish T3 categorization. If none of these roentgenographic features is apparent, two courses of action are then possible, depending on whether conventional roentgenograms have revealed an abnormality in the hilum or mediastinum.

Mediastinum and Ipsilateral Hilum Are Roentgenographically Normal. In the absence of mitigating circumstances (e.g., signs or symptoms suggesting metastatic tumor), it is reasonable in the majority of cases to proceed directly to thoracotomy and resection. Further roentgenographic investigation is not often indicated, nor is mediastinoscopy. Hilar and mediastinal lymph nodes can be sampled at the time of surgery for staging purposes. Some would perform TTNA before thoracotomy to exclude a possible infectious etiology or small cell carcinoma.

Ipsilateral Hilum or Mediastinum is Definitely or Questionably Abnormal. Here we are dealing with the possibility of metastases in lymph nodes situated in the hilum alone, in the mediastinum alone, or in both the hilum and the mediastinum. For two reasons the authors favor CT or MRI in the evaluation of the questionably abnormal hilum. First, in recent years, CT anatomy of the hila has been described in intimate detail, and any deviation from the normal configuration should constitute convincing evidence of hilar pathology. Should confusion arise in distinguishing vascular structure from enlarged nodes, bolus contrast enhancement should provide ready differentiation. Second, since metastatic involvement of hilar nodes may be associated with proximal spread to mediastinal lymph nodes and since CT and MRI are universally regarded as more efficient methods of evaluating mediastinal nodes than con-

Table 8–5. **INVESTIGATIVE ALGORITHM BASED FIRST ON CONVENTIONAL ROENTGENOGRAMS IN POSTEROANTERIOR AND LATERAL PROJECTIONS**

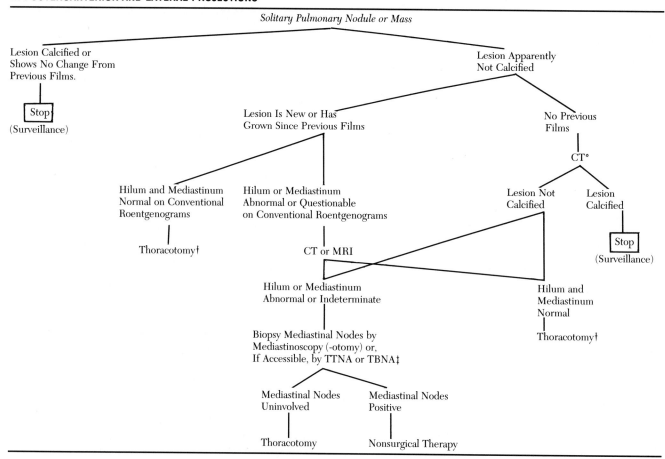

°Dual-energy digital radiography can establish the presence or absence of calcification with conviction, obviating CT.
†Some would perform TTNA before thoracotomy to reveal a possible infectious etiology or to exclude small cell carcinoma.
‡TTNA = transthoracic needle aspiration, TBNA = transbronchial needle aspiration.

Table 8–6. INVESTIGATIVE ALGORITHM BASED FIRST ON CONVENTIONAL ROENTGENOGRAMS IN POSTEROANTERIOR AND LATERAL PROJECTIONS

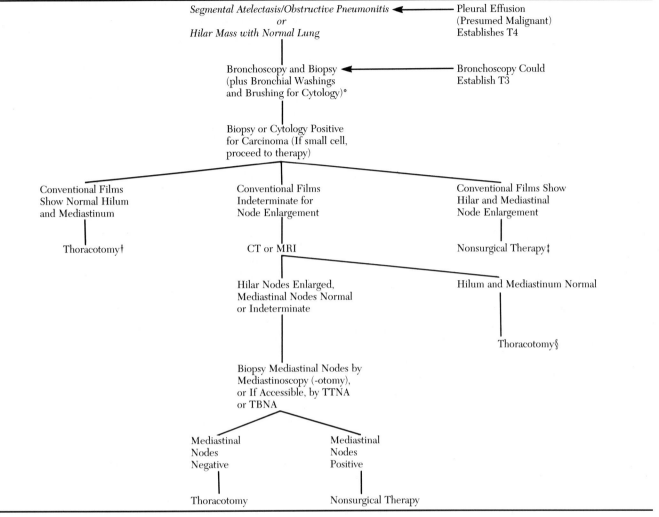

*In the presence of a hilar mass with normal lungs, if bronchoscopic biopsy and cytology are unrevealing, do TTNA.
†Some would perform CT with or without mediastinoscopy before thoracotomy.
‡Some would perform CT for radiation therapy guidance and/or lymph node biopsy or both for confirmation of metastases.
§Some would perform mediastinoscopy before thoracotomy.
   Note: All CT and MRI scans should include the upper abdomen to check for possible liver or adrenal metastases.
        For all small cell cancers, do CT or MRI of the brain and bone scintigraphy.

ventional tomography, it is logical that one of these should be the preferable method of examination in the first instance.

Should the mediastinum and ipsilateral hilum prove normal on CT or MRI, it can reasonably be assumed that the solitary nodule or mass is resectable. Should there be evidence of either hilar or mediastinal node enlargement, it becomes necessary to biopsy the mediastinal nodes. Usually, this is accomplished by mediastinoscopy; in selected cases, transbronchial needle aspiration may be employed during bronchoscopy. The decision as to which of these procedures is preferable can be aided by the anatomic distribution of abnormal nodes observed on CT or MRI.

Lobar or Segmental Atelectasis or a Hilar Mass with Normal Lungs. As with the solitary nodule or mass, the presence of pleural effusion on conventional roentgenograms may already have suggested a T4 category, which should then be confirmed pathologically. Similarly, direct mediastinal invasion or atelectasis of an entire lung may

already have established T3 categorization. If none of these roentgenographic features is apparent, one should proceed directly to bronchoscopy, which may then prove classification as T3 (proximal growth demonstrably less than 2.0 cm distal to the carina). In all these situations, the tumor is probably unresectable; however, it may still be desirable to carry out CT or MRI to establish the extent of mediastinal disease. Should bronchoscopy be inconclusive regarding the establishment of a T3 classification, it is probable that CT or MRI will provide the answer.

If the conventional roentgenograms or bronchoscopy (or a combination of the two) establish the lesion as T1 or T2, it then becomes necessary to determine the presence or absence of hilar or mediastinal lymph node enlargement. Should conventional roentgenograms reveal no abnormality of the mediastinum or ipsilateral hilum, it is reasonable to proceed directly to thoracotomy, although some physicians may wish to carry out CT and mediastinal lymph node biopsy prior to surgery. If bronchoscopic biopsy or cytology has established the cell type as small cell, it can be assumed that the lesion is unresectable, at least in the great majority of patients.

Should the hilum and mediastinum be questionable on conventional roentgenograms, it is necessary to proceed to CT or MRI, which again should establish one of two possible situations.

1. No enlarged lymph nodes are identifiable in either the hilum or the mediastinum, in which circumstance it is appropriate to proceed directly to thoracotomy (although some would perform mediastinoscopy before thoracotomy).

2. Enlarged nodes are identified in the hilum or in the hilum and mediastinum, or mediastinal nodes are indeterminate; biopsy specimens of mediastinal nodes should then be obtained. Should mediastinal nodes be negative for metastases, it is appropriate to proceed to thoracotomy.

Prognosis and Natural History

The survival of patients with pulmonary carcinoma depends on a variety of factors, some so closely inter-related that it is virtually impossible to assess their relative importance. Many can be divided into factors inherent to the host and those attributable to the neoplasm itself. The latter can be further subdivided into anatomic and clinical considerations, particularly as related to the influence of cell type and of stage. Finally, since treatment obviously affects survival, the influence of various forms of therapy must also be taken into consideration. Although these factors are discussed individually, it must be borne in mind that the complexity of their inter-relationships necessitates their overall consideration with respect to every patient.

Influence of Host Factors

The influence of race in survival from lung cancer has been evaluated infrequently. In one study, it was not found to be a factor[179]; in another, however, there was evidence for a significant role, with whites faring worse than others, at least with respect to small cell carcinoma.[180] Most studies have shown an improved survival for women.[181] In some investigations, the prognosis has been found to be poorer in patients younger than 40 years of age and in the elderly[182]; in the latter group, this appears to be because of co-morbid disease rather than inherent properties of the tumor itself.[183]

Concomitant disease, particularly chronic obstructive lung disease,[184] can play a major role in prognosis, acting as a contraindication to potentially curative surgery or as a factor that increases operative and postoperative mortality rates. Survival also may be influenced by a decision to stop smoking; in one study of patients with small cell carcinoma followed from the time of diagnosis, survival was significantly longer in those who quit than in those who did not.[185]

Influence of Cell Type

Although there can be little doubt that cell type is correlated with both natural history and prognosis in patients with carcinoma of the lung, the degree of correlation and its significance relative to other factors are difficult to determine precisely. In fact, in some studies once the effect of stage is accounted for, cell type has been found to exert no statistically significant independent influence on prognosis.[186] Despite these reservations, several general statements are applicable.

1. Small cell carcinoma is characteristically a fast-growing malignancy, and in most cases, spread has occurred beyond the thorax at the time of diagnosis. Although many tumors show a response to chemotherapy, this is often incomplete and of short duration. The overall median survival is no more than 6 to 10 months, and 5-year survival rates range from 1 to 5 per cent.[187, 188] As might be expected, a better prognosis is associated with limited as opposed to extensive disease,[70a] with demonstrable response to chemotherapy, and with surgical excision of a solitary pulmonary nodule in the absence of hilar or mediastinal node involvement.[189] Those patients with prolonged survival are at increased risk for developing acute leukemia[190] or a second pulmonary carcinoma[191] and may have significant neurologic impairment as a result of cranial irradiation.

2. Squamous cell carcinoma tends to remain localized to the thorax longer than other cell types[192] and thus causes death more frequently by local complications. Most investigators find a better prognosis, stage for stage, for squamous cell carcinoma than for adenocarcinoma or large cell carcinoma.[193] As might be expected, patients with in situ or minimally invasive carcinoma have a relatively good prognosis.[194]

3. Although in some series the prognoses for adenocarcinoma and large cell carcinoma are similar,[193] in other series that for adenocarcinoma is more favorable.[195] This latter finding may result from the inclusion of peripheral bronchioloalveolar carcinoma, a subtype with a relatively good 5-year survival when it is resected at the solitary nodule stage and that has a better prognosis than other forms of pulmonary carcinoma.[196] (Despite this, when it has metastasized, the prognosis appears to be no different from other forms of adenocarcinoma.[196a])

4. The prognosis of large cell carcinoma is generally considered to be poor.[197]

Influence of Stage

The single most important factor in the prognosis of patients with pulmonary carcinoma is the stage of disease at the time of presentation. This can be appreciated by examining data relating to individual T, N, and M subgroups (Fig. 8–29)[193] and to stage as a whole (Fig. 8–30).[168] According to the latter data, approximate overall 5-year survival rates for non–small cell carcinoma are as follows: stage I, 50 per cent; stage II, 30 per cent; stage III, 15 per cent; and stage IV, virtually zero.

The prognosis of patients in the various TNM groups previously described relates only to the histologic variants of squamous cell carcinoma, large cell carcinoma, and adenocarcinoma. Patients with small cell carcinoma are, instead, usually divided simply into those with limited disease and those with extensive disease; as might be expected, the former typically survive longer. Particularly bad prognostic indicators in these individuals are brain,[198] liver,[199] and bone marrow[200] metastases. On the other hand, in patients in whom spread occurs to supraclavicular nodes only or who develop ipsilateral pleural effusion and regional lymph node

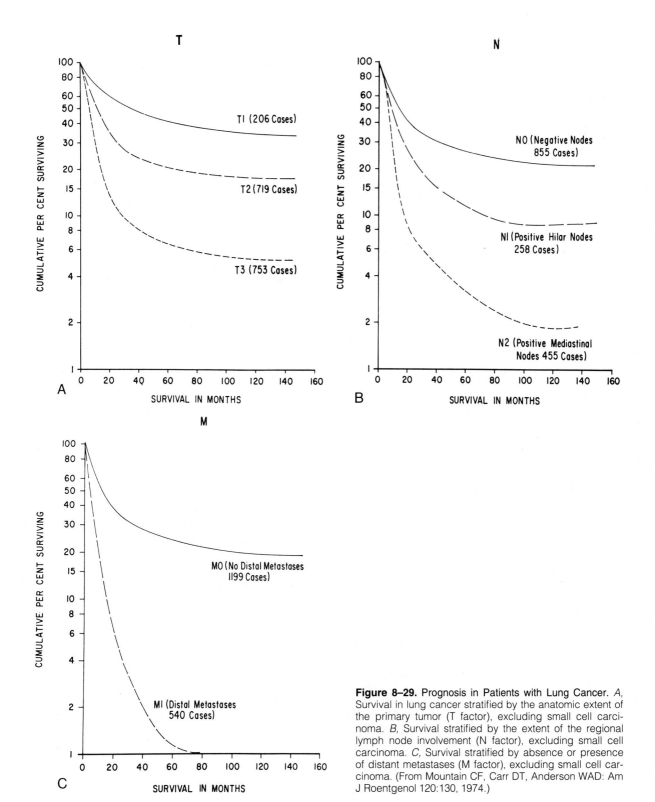

Figure 8–29. Prognosis in Patients with Lung Cancer. *A,* Survival in lung cancer stratified by the anatomic extent of the primary tumor (T factor), excluding small cell carcinoma. *B,* Survival stratified by the extent of the regional lymph node involvement (N factor), excluding small cell carcinoma. *C,* Survival stratified by absence or presence of distant metastases (M factor), excluding small cell carcinoma. (From Mountain CF, Carr DT, Anderson WAD: Am J Roentgenol 120:130, 1974.)

STAGE

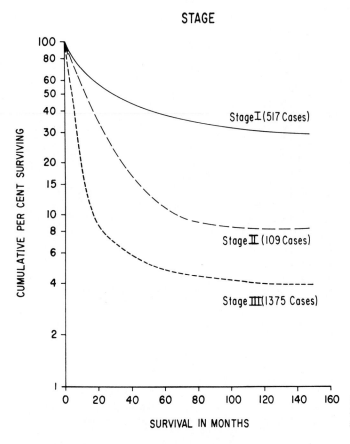

Figure 8–30. Prognosis in Patients with Lung Cancer: Influence of Stage. Cumulative proportion of patients surviving 5 years by clinical stage of disease. (From Mountain CF: Chest 89(Suppl): 225S, 1986.)

enlargement, the prognosis is just as good as that in patients without extrathoracic metastatic manifestations.[201]

Influence of Clinical and Laboratory Factors

There appears to be general agreement that asymptomatic patients survive longer than those who present with symptoms; this is most evident in the short term[202] but also applies to 5-year follow-up. In addition, the prognosis of patients with local symptoms, such as pain, hemoptysis, and cough, is better than that of patients with systemic symptoms, whether or not these are related to distant metastases. Similarly, patients who have symptoms related to the thorax for more than 6 months without accompanying systemic or metastatic symptoms have a better prognosis than those whose symptoms are of more recent onset.

In addition to their use in diagnosis, the presence of serum tumor antigens (e.g., CA125[203]) and elevated enzymes (e.g., lactate dehydrogenase [LDH][204]) have been found in some studies to be predictive of a relatively poor outcome.

Influence of Therapy

Since virtually all patients who survive 5 years or longer after diagnosis have been treated, it is clear that therapy, both surgical and to a lesser extent radiation and chemotherapy, influences survival. Since the therapeutic approach to small cell and non–small cell carcinoma differs substantially, these are best discussed separately.

Non–Small Cell Carcinoma. Few patients with lesions deemed inoperable or considered unresectable at thoracotomy live longer than 1 year, and most die within 6 months. In addition, irradiation or chemotherapy (or both) probably do not prolong life to an appreciable extent in most patients. As a result, surgical excision of the primary neoplasm and, in some instances, nodal metastases is the only practical hope of cure or significant prolongation of life. However, despite improvements in surgical techniques and in methods of establishing the diagnosis at a relatively early stage, only about 20 per cent of patients have resectable tumors; of these patients, 15 to 20 per cent will be alive after 10 years. In actual numbers, this means that only three or four patients of every 100 with pulmonary carcinoma can be considered cured.

As might be expected, the criteria by which a patient's tumor is judged to be resectable are not standard. Although chest wall invasion used to be a contraindication to curative surgery, there is now evidence that in patients with direct extension into the parietal pleura, pericardium, diaphragm, or chest wall, without accompanying regional node involvement (T3, N0, M0), 5-year survival rates between 20 and 50 per cent can be expected following resection.[205, 206] In the presence of lymph node metastases, however, there is a considerable fall-off in long-term survival. It should be stressed that this relatively favorable outcome for T3 lesions is very different from that in patients with T3 tumors that are central or are associated with pleural metastases (usually accompanied by effusion), in whom the 5-year survival is virtually nil.[207] The survival rate is not much better for stage III tumors that are associated with extensive mediastinal invasion.[208]

Although many authorities regard involvement of mediastinal lymph nodes as a contraindication to definitive surgery, a small but significant number of 5-year survivors have been reported after resection of the primary and affected lymph nodes.[209] The prognosis in such patients is related, at least in part, to the amount of tumor—those with microscopic deposits or intranodal tumor fare better than those with grossly evident disease or extranodal extension.[210]

In some situations, such as older age or poor respiratory function, operative interference is considered to be contraindicated. Although this is clearly appropriate for some patients, in others the increased risk is probably justified.[211] Even in the presence of considerable reduction in pulmonary function, morbidity and mortality can be minimal in stage I peripheral lesions; if surgery is confined to wedge resection, the 5-year survival can match that of patients subjected to lobectomy.[212]

In the vast majority of cases, nothing can be done to alter the ultimate prognosis of non–small cell carcinoma in the presence of extrathoracic spread. The exception is a solitary brain metastasis, usually adenocarcinoma, that occurs at or shortly after diagnosis of the primary lung tumor. In this situation, 5-year survival has been reported when "curative" resection of both lung and brain lesions is accomplished.[213]

Small Cell Carcinoma. The prognosis for individuals with small cell carcinoma is particularly poor, the median survival of untreated patients being measured in weeks and months. Despite this, significant prolongation of life can be attained in some patients with chemotherapy and radiotherapy; however, as indicated previously, even in this situation, the prognosis is not good, 2-year survival occurring in only about 5 to 15 per cent[188, 214] and 5-year survival in 1 to 5 per cent.[187, 188]

In an attempt to improve prognosis even further, surgical treatment of limited-stage disease has been advocated and appears to hold promise. For example, in one study of 25 patients with mediastinal metastases treated with radical surgery, chemotherapy, and radiotherapy, survival at 2 years was 38 per cent.[215] Despite the results of this and other investigations, the tendency to develop a second, often lethal malignancy and the sequelae of therapy (particularly cranial irradiation) severely limit the long-term prognosis of these individuals.[191]

Multiple Primary Carcinomas of the Lung

The criteria used to make a diagnosis of independent carcinoma, as opposed to recurrence of or metastasis from the initial neoplasm, are highly variable and can be quite complex.[216] Most authors stipulate that the tumors should be clearly situated in different parts of the lung, but there is some disagreement as to the requirement for features such as different histology and a demonstrable origin in bronchial mucosa. The development of flow cytometry is an advance that may aid the distinction.[217] In some cases, however, it may be impossible to determine with certainty the true nature of an apparent second primary lesion.

Depending on the criteria and the techniques used to establish the diagnosis, the incidence of multiple primary carcinomas probably is between 1 and 2 per cent.[216] It is important to realize, however, that these figures refer chiefly to cases in which the additional tumor becomes clinically or roentgenologically apparent during the patient's life. If incidental tumors discovered by pathologic examination are considered, there is little doubt that the true incidence is much higher.[218] This discrepancy is undoubtedly attributable to the poor prognosis associated with most lung cancers: many patients die before the second tumor has grown sufficiently to produce clinical or roentgenographic manifestations.

Multiple primary carcinomas of the lung can develop synchronously (usually defined as the presence of two tumors at the time of, or closely following, initial diagnosis) or metachronously (the second cancer appearing after an interval, usually 12 months or more). The latter constitute at least two thirds of multiple pulmonary neoplasms and, on average, are recognized 4 years after the first primary.[219] Squamous cell is the commonest histologic type, the most frequent combination being squamous-squamous, followed by squamous–small cell and squamous-adenocarcinoma. Survival after resection of the second tumor has been reported to be 30 per cent or more after 5 years and 20 per cent or more after 10 years.[220]

NEOPLASMS OF PULMONARY NEUROENDOCRINE CELLS

Several types of pulmonary neoplasm show ultrastructural and immunohistochemical features of neuroendocrine differentiation. Although some may originate directly from normal neuroendocrine cells, it is likely that others are derived from a primitive "stem" cell that, for unknown reasons, undergoes neuroendocrine differentiation.[221] Whatever their histogenesis, the vast majority of these tumors have characteristic morphologic features and can be conveniently discussed together. Although some authors consider small cell carcinoma to be one of these tumors,[222] believing it to represent the most undifferentiated end of a spectrum of neuroendocrine neoplasia, the authors prefer to consider it separately because of its closer resemblance etiologically, clinically, and prognostically to the other commoner forms of pulmonary carcinoma.

Carcinoid Tumor

Pulmonary carcinoid tumor is a low-grade malignant neoplasm that constitutes about 0.5 to 2.5 per cent of all pulmonary neoplasms. There appears to be a slight female predominance, and the incidence is distinctly higher in whites than in blacks.[223] The mean age at diagnosis is about 50 years, centrally placed carcinoids tending to become manifest some 10 years earlier than those in the periphery. There is no link with cigarette smoking or with most other agents known to be associated etiologically with pulmonary carcinoma. It should be noted that since these tumors are neither benign nor glandular, use of the term "bronchial adenoma" should be avoided.

Pathologic Characteristics

Depending on their location, there are two fairly distinct clinicopathologic subtypes of pulmonary carcinoid tumor:

central and peripheral (or "spindle-cell"). In addition, a small number of tumors in both central and peripheral locations show histologic and cytologic features suggestive of a more aggressive neoplasm. These latter variants probably represent a continuum from the so-called typical form to a clearly high-grade malignant neoplasm, and different authors have designated them "atypical carcinoid tumor"[224] or "well-differentiated (low-grade) neuroendocrine carcinoma."[221]

Central Carcinoid Tumor. About 80 per cent of pulmonary carcinoid tumors arise in a lobar, segmental, or large subsegmental bronchus. Most measure from 2 to 4 cm in diameter and extend both within the airway lumen and outside the bronchial wall (Fig. 8–31). The overlying epithelium is often intact, explaining the low incidence of diagnosis by cytologic examination of sputum or brushing or washing specimens.

Histologically, the tumors are well defined and consist of uniform cells arranged in sheets, trabeculae, or small gland-like formations (Fig. 8–32). The cytoplasm of individual cells is usually moderate in amount, and nuclei are oval or round with only mild pleomorphism; mitotic figures are scarce or absent. Cellular sheets or trabeculae are separated by a fibrovascular stroma that is usually quite thin but may be thick and hyalinized. Foci of bone formation, either in the stroma itself or in adjacent cartilage plates, are common and may be quite extensive.

Ultrastructurally, carcinoid tumors are composed of uniform cells in which neurosecretory granules—membrane-bound granules 150 to 300 μm in diameter with an electron-dense core surrounded by a clear halo—are usually abundant (*see* Fig. 8–32).[225] Immunohistochemical studies

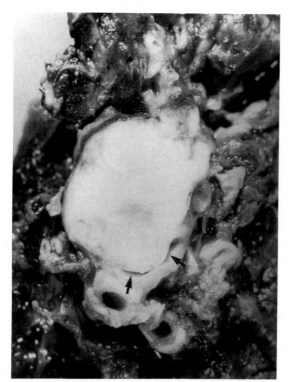

Figure 8–31. Central Carcinoid Tumor. A well-defined tumor fills the lumen of a segmental bronchus *(arrows)* and expands into the surrounding parenchyma, resulting in an "iceberg" appearance.

are also diagnostically helpful, frequently revealing intracytoplasmic, immunoreactive neuroendocrine products[225]; serotonin, gastrin releasing peptide, pancreatic polypeptide, vasoactive intestinal polypeptide, and leu-enkephalin have been most frequently identified. Most tumors display reactivity for more than one hormone, typically in a heterogeneous fashion.

The histologic diagnosis of typical central carcinoid tumor in resected specimens should present no problem; however, small tissue samples obtained by bronchoscopic or transthoracic needle biopsy may be difficult to distinguish from other tumors, especially small cell carcinoma. Because of this, it seems reasonable for both pathologist and clinician to question the diagnosis of undifferentiated or small cell carcinoma in any individual younger than 45 years of age, particularly in the absence of a history of smoking and evidence of metastasis. Similarly, the diagnosis of small cell carcinoma should be reconsidered in any patient with prolonged survival in whom the roentgenographic or clinical features are atypical.[226]

Peripheral Carcinoid Tumor. Most peripheral carcinoid tumors are situated several centimeters from the pleura, are well defined, and measure 2 to 5 cm in diameter. A remarkably high incidence in the middle lobe (10 of 29 cases) has been documented in one series.[227]

Histologically, the tumors are usually well defined and situated in close proximity to a small bronchus or bronchiole. Typically, the neoplastic cells have a whorled or spindled appearance and are separated by a loose fibrovascular stroma. As with central carcinoid tumors, diagnosis can be difficult, particularly with small tissue samples; the whorled architecture can be mistaken for that of a mesenchymal neoplasm, such as hemangiopericytoma and leiomyoma. In addition, the organoid architecture can be indistinct, resulting in a superficial resemblance to an undifferentiated pulmonary carcinoma. Electron microscopic examination usually shows evidence of intracytoplasmic neurosecretory granules.

Atypical Carcinoid Tumor. About 10 per cent of pulmonary carcinoid tumors show histologic and cytologic features suggestive of an aggressive nature. As defined by Arrigoni and colleagues,[224] this diagnostic label should be applied to a pulmonary neoplasm with the overall appearance of carcinoid tumor in which one or more of the following features are present: (1) increased mitotic activity; (2) nuclear pleomorphism and hyperchromatism associated with prominent nucleoli and an increased nucleus-to-cytoplasm ratio; (3) areas of increased cellularity associated with loss of typical architecture; and (4) necrosis. Ultrastructural study shows neurosecretory granules, although usually fewer in number and of smaller size than in typical carcinoid tumors.[225]

Roentgenographic Manifestations

Roentgenographic manifestations depend largely on the location of the carcinoid tumor. Since 80 per cent are situated centrally in major or segmental bronchi, evidence of bronchial obstruction is the commonest roentgenographic finding. When a lesion only partly occludes a bronchus, the reduction in ventilation of affected parenchyma can result in hypoxic vasoconstriction and reduction in volume. The oligemia can constitute a subtle but highly suggestive sign

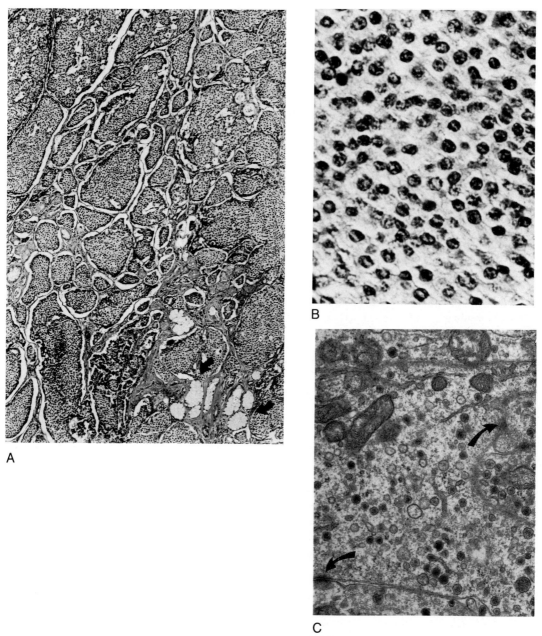

Figure 8–32. Carcinoid Tumor. *A,* Low-power view of a typical carcinoid tumor shows nests of uniform cells separated by a prominent but delicate vascular stroma. Note the remnants of bronchial gland surrounded by neoplasm *(arrows),* revealing its local infiltrative properties. *B,* A magnified view shows cells with uniform, round-to-oval nuclei, small nucleoli, ample cytoplasm, and absence of mitotic figures. *C,* Ultrastructural appearance of tumor cells, showing intercellular junctions *(arrows)* and numerous neurosecretory granules. *(A* × 60; *B* × 600; *C* × 38,300.)

of the presence of an endobronchial lesion and should lead to a recommendation for bronchoscopy (Fig. 8–33). However, in most cases, obstruction is complete, with peripheral atelectasis and obstructive pneumonitis. Thus, the characteristic roentgenographic pattern consists of a homogeneous opacity confined precisely to a lobe or to one or more segments, usually with loss of volume (Fig. 8–34).

Peripheral carcinoid tumors do not cause significant bronchial obstruction and appear roentgenographically as solitary nodules. They are usually homogeneous in density, sharply defined, round or oval, and, in many cases, slightly lobulated. They average about 4 cm in diameter (range, 1 to 10 cm) and occur most often in the right upper and middle lobes and the lingula.

Despite the fairly common demonstration of bone pathologically, evidence of calcification or ossification is rare on conventional roentgenograms, being observed in only 1 of 81 cases in one series.[228] However, in one CT study of 31 patients,[229] intratumoral calcification was indentified in 8 (26 per cent); seven of the calcified tumors were central, and one peripheral.

Computed tomography also may be of value in some cases in assessing the presence and extent of local invasion, particularly when histologic examination of biopsy specimens has revealed atypical features.[230] Magnetic resonance imaging may be useful in cases in which a CT study is nondiagnostic or equivocal.[231] Although bronchial carcinoids are very vascular, pulmonary arteriography seldom produces distinctive findings, and only injection of the bronchial arteries opacifies these tumors.[228]

Osseous metastases, which may be revealed by a roentgenographic skeletal survey, develop in few cases. Although it has been emphasized that they are frequently osteoblastic, in one series of 99 patients only 8 had osseous metastases, and all were lytic.[232]

Clinical Manifestations

Most central tumors give rise to symptoms as a result of bronchial irritation or obstruction, including cough, expectoration, fever, chest pain, and wheezing (sometimes simulating asthma[233]). Hemoptysis occurs in at least 50 per cent of patients, reflecting the highly vascular nature of these neoplasms.[234] Physical signs depend on the degree of obstruction, the size of the bronchus obstructed, and whether peripheral infection has developed.

Clinical signs and symptoms related to neuroendocrine function are distinctly uncommon. In most cases, extensive metastatic disease is necessary before they appear, possibly reflecting the need for adequate tumor bulk in order to produce sufficient amounts of active hormone. As might be expected, several clinical syndromes can occur.

Despite the name of the tumor, carcinoid syndrome is detected in fewer than 3 per cent of patients.[235] The symptoms and signs consist of flushing, fever, nausea and vomiting, diarrhea, hypotension, wheezing, and respiratory distress. Heart murmurs, which develop in a few cases, may be restricted to the left side of the heart owing to endocardial damage caused by polypeptides (principally 5-hydroxytryptamine) entering the pulmonary veins from the lungs. Cases associated with hepatic metastases show the effects of right-sided cardiac involvement. Other paraneoplastic syndromes associated with carcinoid tumor include Cushing's syndrome[236] and acromegaly.[237]

Prognosis

The overall prognosis of carcinoid tumors is good, adequate surgical excision resulting in cure in the vast majority of cases. In a National Cancer Institute review of carcinoid tumors unselected for histologic atypicality, the overall 5-year survival rate was 87 per cent (the number of patients who died with or from the neoplasm is not stated in the report).[223] If cases are selected for histologically favorable features, the survival rates are even higher.[222] Even when carcinoid tumors are metastatic, they can grow very slowly, permitting prolonged survival for many years. There are no well-documented morphologic criteria by which the "typical" tumors that will metastasize can be distinguished from those that will not.

In contrast with the typical form of pulmonary carcinoid tumor, those with atypical histologic features have a significantly worse prognosis. Evidence of distant spread is found frequently at initial presentation; in many patients it is followed by a progressive downhill course and death.[222] For example, in one series of 23 patients with atypical tumors,[224] metastases developed in 16 (70 per cent); seven (30 per cent) were considered to have died as a result of their neoplasm within an average of 27 months following resection.

Pulmonary Tumorlets

The term "pulmonary tumorlet" refers to a minute (3 mm or less) proliferation of neuroendocrine cells that usually is discovered incidentally at autopsy or in a surgical specimen excised for an independent lesion. Although they may be identified in otherwise normal lung, evidence of prior pulmonary disease, particularly bronchiectasis, is frequent.

The fundamental nature of these unusual tumors is controversial. Their multiplicity, small size, and frequent association with pulmonary fibrosis and bronchiectasis suggest that they represent a hyperplastic response to nonspecific airway injury. On the other hand, the occasional presence of tumorlets in otherwise normal lung, the rare reports of regional lymph node deposits[238] and roentgenographic evidence of increase in size over time,[239] and the morphologic resemblance to and occasional association with carcinoid tumor have suggested that they are neoplastic and, in fact, represent minute carcinoid tumors.[240] Resolution of this debate in favor of either viewpoint may be impossible; in fact, it is probably most appropriate to consider tumorlets as representing two histologically similar groups—one hyperplastic and associated with pulmonary injury and the other truly neoplastic.

The lesions are usually found in older individuals and often in females. Typically, there are no clinical manifestations. Because of their minute size, they are usually not roentgenographically apparent; however, several cases have been reported in which numerous bilateral tumorlets increased sufficiently in size to be roentgenographically visible as a nodular pattern.[239]

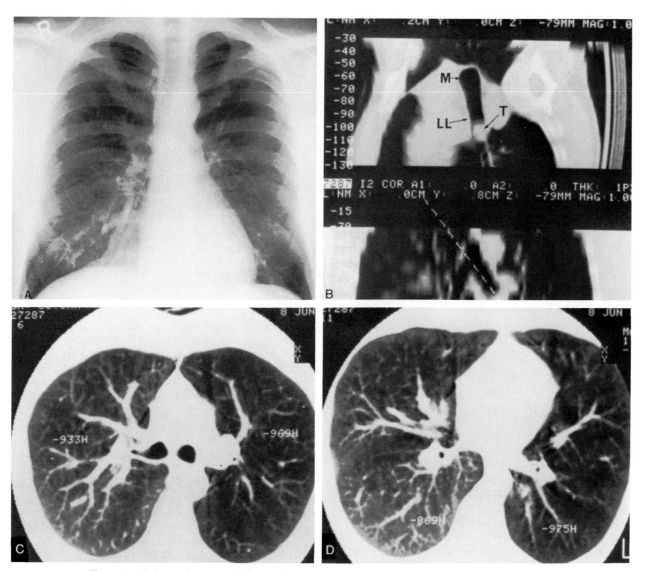

Figure 8–33. Partly Obstructing Central Carcinoid Tumor Associated with Hypoxic Vasoconstriction. *A,* A posteroanterior chest roentgenogram reveals diffuse oligemia of the left lung; volume of the lung is normal or slightly reduced. *B,* An oblique CT re-formation along the course of the left main (M) and lower lobe (LL) bronchi demonstrates the intrabronchial carcinoid tumor (T). *C* and *D,* CT scans through the upper and lower lobes reveal a unilaterally diminished CT density on the left (compare the CT attenuation values in the lungs). Note that the vessels are diffusely narrowed throughout the left lung.

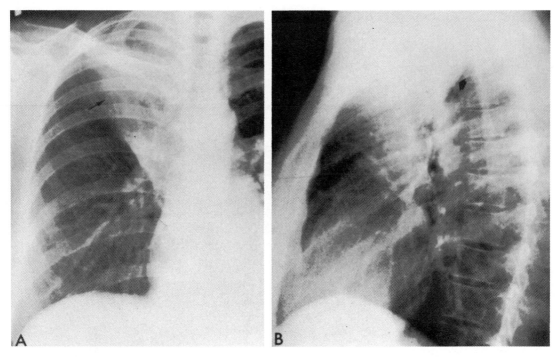

Figure 8–34. Carcinoid Tumor. Views of the right hemithorax from posteroanterior *(A)* and lateral *(B)* roentgenograms demonstrate a roughly triangular shadow of homogeneous density occupying the superomedial portion of the right lung. The inferolateral border of the shadow is formed by the upward displaced minor fissure *(arrow* in *A),* and the posterior border by the anteriorly displaced major fissure *(arrow* in *B).* This shadow represents combined consolidation and atelectasis of the right upper lobe due to an endobronchial obstructing lesion (obstructive pneumonitis).

Miscellaneous Tumors Showing Neuroendocrine Differentiation

In order to maintain some semantic benefit, the term "atypical carcinoid" should be restricted to those tumors that possess a histologic appearance at least focally recognizable as carcinoid tumor but also display necrosis or cytologic atypia. In addition to these neoplasms, however, there are a small number of tumors that lack histologic features characteristic of carcinoid tumor but still show immunochemical and ultrastructural evidence of neuroendocrine differentiation. These have been termed "large cell neuroendocrine tumors"[241] or "atypical endocrine tumors"[242] and have been considered to be intermediate between small cell carcinoma and carcinoid tumor. In general, their biologic behavior is similar to that of poorly differentiated non–small cell carcinoma.[241]

NEOPLASMS OF TRACHEOBRONCHIAL GLANDS

The development, morphology, and, to some extent, function of the tracheobronchial mucous glands are similar to those of the oropharyngeal salivary glands. These observations, in conjunction with the finding that neoplasms with an identical histologic appearance have been described in both locations, have led to the belief that a group of pulmonary tumors are histogenetically related to the airway glandular epithelium. These tumors characteristically grow intraluminally in central airways, are unassociated with cig-

arette smoking, and have a much better prognosis than that of neoplasms of surface airway epithelium. As a group, they have been estimated to account for fewer than 0.5 per cent of all lung neoplasms.[243] The vast majority are either adenoid cystic or mucoepidermoid carcinoma, the other varieties being exceptionally rare.

The diagnosis of a tracheobronchial gland tumor should be considered in anyone with roentgenographic or endoscopic evidence of a polypoid intraluminal mass in the trachea or major bronchi. Unfortunately, the tracheal air column constitutes a "blind area" for many radiologists, and the presence of these tumors on standard posteroanterior and lateral chest roentgenograms is all too frequently overlooked. The reason for this is often roentgenographic underpenetration[244]; the high-kilovoltage technique, which obviates this technical deficiency, is strongly recommended as standard technique (*see* page 118).

Although clinical features are not specific, a history of adult-onset "asthma" that has increased in severity despite adequate therapy should alert one to the possibility of a central obstructing lesion. Since the intrathoracic portion of the trachea dilates on inspiration and narrows on expiration, a lesion arising in this segment will be characterized clinically by expiratory airway obstruction and roentgenographically by expiratory air trapping. Conversely, the cervical portion of the trachea narrows on inspiration and dilates on expiration, so symptoms and signs of expiratory airway obstruction are lacking. A further indicator is the timing of a wheeze; with an intrathoracic tumor this occurs on expiration, and with a cervical one on inspiration. Because of these differences, clinical awareness of a lesion in the cervical location develops much later, enhancing the potential for local extension of the neoplasm.

Adenoid Cystic Carcinoma

Although precise figures are difficult to obtain, this tumor is clearly the commonest subtype of tracheobronchial gland tumor, probably accounting for 75 to 80 per cent of reported cases. Approximately 80 per cent arise with about equal frequency in the trachea and mainstem bronchi; most of the remainder occur in lobar bronchi. Although it forms an extremely small proportion of primary neoplasms arising in lobar bronchi, its relative incidence in the trachea is much higher, constituting about 20 to 30 per cent of primary malignant tumors at this site.[245]

Adenoid cystic carcinoma characteristically grows into the airway lumen, forming a smooth-surfaced, somewhat polypoid tumor; submucosal extension, sometimes to a considerable distance from the main tumor, is common.[243] Histologically, the tumor consists of rather uniform cells arranged in well-defined nests or trabeculae, frequently with a cribriform pattern. Mitotic activity and necrosis are seldom observed.

The conventional roentgenographic features consist of an endotracheal or endobronchial, lobulated, hemispheric mass that encroaches on the airway lumen to a variable degree. Conventional tomography in anteroposterior and lateral projections may be useful in evaluation, particularly for intratracheal tumors, although CT is clearly the preferred technique for assessing the presence or absence of mediastinal extension.[246]

Most tumors are discovered in patients aged 40 to 45 years, with no sex predominance.[247] Clinical features consist of cough, hemoptysis, dyspnea, wheeze, "asthma," and recurrent pneumonitis. Although approximately 50 per cent of patients described in the older literature either died of the neoplasm or developed recurrent disease, the more sophisticated surgical and diagnostic techniques available nowadays may be expected to result in cure in a greater proportion of cases. In some patients, however, local recurrence still develops and is complicated by direct extension into the mediastinum or lung parenchyma. Metastases are uncommon and typically appear late in the course of the disease; death is usually the result of local intrathoracic complications.[247]

Mucoepidermoid Carcinoma

Mucoepidermoid carcinoma is an uncommon tracheobronchial neoplasm whose incidence has been estimated at between 2 to 5 per 1000 primary bronchial neoplasms.[248] The lesion is considered to occur in two forms: (1) a tumor of relatively low-grade malignancy with distinctive, rather bland histologic features; and (2) a neoplasm showing histologic features of high-grade malignancy and an aggressive course.

The majority of tumors present as a polypoid mass in the lumen of a main or lobar bronchus.[249] The tumor is usually confined to the bronchial wall, although the high-grade form may extend into the peribronchial interstitium or adjacent lung parenchyma. Histologically, the low-grade form is composed of relatively uniform cells containing cyto-

plasm that is either mucus-containing or "epidermoid" in appearance. The high-grade form has a similar overall pattern but, in addition, shows areas of cytologic atypia, relatively frequent mitoses, and foci of necrosis.

Roentgenographic manifestations in 58 cases reviewed by the Armed Forces Institute of Pathology (AFIP) consisted of a solitary nodule or mass in 41 and "pneumonic consolidation" in 16.[249] Occasionally, the appearance is that of an endobronchial or endotracheal tumor similar to that of adenoid cystic carcinoma (Fig. 8–35). The low-grade and high-grade forms cannot be distinguished except by identifying extrabronchial extension using CT.

In the AFIP series, the average age of individuals with low-grade tumors was 35 years, and that of persons with high-grade forms 45 years. Symptoms are related to intraluminal growth and include cough, hemoptysis, wheeze, and recurrent pneumonia. Low-grade mucoepidermoid tumors grow slowly. Provided that they are surgically resectable, the prognosis is usually excellent, without recurrence or the development of metastases.[249] Behavior of the high-grade form, although worse than that of low-grade tumors, appears to be better than that of the commoner forms of pulmonary carcinoma.[249]

MISCELLANEOUS EPITHELIAL TUMORS

Tracheobronchial Papillomas

A papilloma can be defined as a branching or coarsely lobulated tumor composed of epithelium-lined fibrovascular stalks arising from and projecting above an epithelial surface. Although such tumors can be classified histologically into several types, depending largely on the nature of the surface lining,[250] from clinical, roentgenographic, and possibly etiologic points of view, they are best considered under the headings multiple and solitary.

Multiple Papillomas. Multiple papillomas of the respiratory tract occur most commonly in the larynx of children between 18 months and 3 years of age and are considered to be caused by human papillomavirus.[251] In the majority of cases, multiple papillomas remain localized to this site and eventually disappear spontaneously. In about 2 per cent, however, they also arise in the lower respiratory tract,[252] where they can cause local or diffuse airway obstruction. Most such cases are limited to the trachea, although extension into the bronchi, bronchioles, and even alveolar airspaces has occasionally been documented.[252] Disease can also occur in adults, usually in those who have a history of childhood papillomatosis, but occasionally in those who do not.[253]

Pathologically, the lesions consist of sessile or broadly stalked papillary growths lined by a flattened squamous epithelium. Involvement of distal airways or alveolar airspaces may be microscopic or may result in solid or cavitated masses measuring several centimeters in diameter.

Roentgenographically, papillomas located in proximal bronchi are manifested by atelectasis and obstructive pneumonitis. Involvement of distal airways and the lung parenchyma can result in multiple nodular opacities which are usually small and homogeneously opaque when first discovered. Cavitation is frequent and superficially resembles cys-

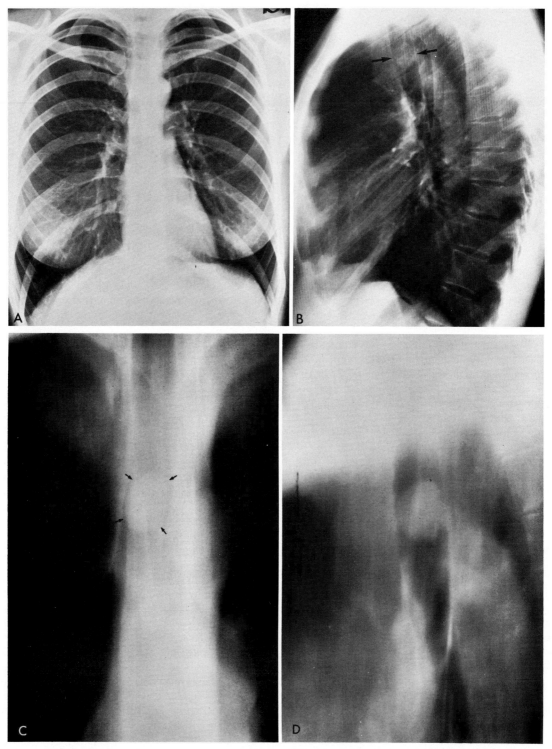

Figure 8–35. Mucoepidermoid Carcinoma. At the time of the roentgenogram illustrated in *A,* this 32-year-old woman presented with a 4-year history of sporadic attacks of acute shortness of breath that had been diagnosed and treated by her family physician as spasmodic asthma. A number of roentgenographic examinations of the chest during this period had been interpreted as normal. This posteroanterior roentgenogram reveals mild to moderate overinflation of both lungs, consistent with a diagnosis of asthma. However, note that the mediastinum is intolerably underpenetrated, to the point at which the tracheal air column is not visible. In lateral projection *(B),* a smooth, sharply demarcated mass can be identified in the plane of the tracheal air column *(arrows).* Tomographic sections of the mediastinum in anteroposterior *(C)* and lateral *(D)* projections show the mass to lie within the trachea approximately 3 cm proximal to the carina *(arrows in C).* The mass is almost completely occluding the tracheal air column. This case illustrates graphically the often repeated observation that the tracheal air column tends to be a "blind area" for many radiologists. (Courtesy of Dr. Michael Lefcoe, Victoria Hospital, London, Ontario.)

tic bronchiectasis, although CT studies reveal an absence of dilatation of airways leading to the cavities.[254] On CT, the cavity wall may be 2 to 3 mm thick; fluid levels can sometimes be identified.

Clinically, the diagnosis should be suspected in any patient with a history of laryngeal papillomas who develops cough, hemoptysis, asthmalike symptoms, recurrent pneumonia, or atelectasis. Bronchoscopy and biopsy of the lesions are usually confirmatory.

The prognosis is poor in patients with extensive tracheal and pulmonary involvement,[254] recurrent papillomas often requiring repeated excision and sometimes resulting in progressive lung destruction. In addition, there is increasing evidence that an appreciable number of lesions become frankly malignant, usually as squamous cell carcinoma.[44] Although patients who have received prior radiotherapy are probably at increased risk for this complication, it can also occur in individuals who have not had this therapy.[255]

Solitary Papilloma. Solitary papillomas of the tracheobronchial tree are less common than the multiple form. They occur almost invariably in adults, often middle-aged or older and usually male.[250] Although the etiology of most solitary papillomas is unclear, their solitary nature and their occurrence in this age group suggest that they represent an entity different from papillomatosis of childhood and adolescence.

The papillomas are usually located in lobar or segmental bronchi and measure 0.5 to 1.5 cm in diameter (Fig. 8–36). Most are histologically identical to multiple papillomas, consisting of mature squamous epithelium lining thin, fibrovascular cores. Cytologic atypia and carcinoma *in situ*

develop occasionally, either in the papillary tumor itself or in the adjacent airway epithelium.

Since most of these tumors are small and solitary, they are usually not visible roentgenographically and are manifested by atelectasis, obstructive pneumonitis, or bronchiectasis. A history of repeated or unresolved pneumonia or hemoptysis may be obtained. Surgical excision usually results in complete cure; it is important, however, to ensure that those tumors with cytologic atypia are not associated with an adjacent squamous cell carcinoma.

Pulmonary Adenoma

True adenomas of pulmonary epithelium are rare. Some are derived from tracheobronchial mucous glands. In addition, occasional tumors located in the lung periphery show pathologic features suggestive of a benign glandular neoplasm and have been termed alveolar or papillary adenomas.[256] Although the clinical history and roentgenologic findings in some cases also suggest a benign process,[250] precise pathologic criteria for distinguishing these tumors from well-differentiated adenocarcinoma are not available. In fact, some of them can be identified as small nodules separate from a clear-cut adenocarcinoma, suggesting that they may represent premalignant growths.[257]

Malignant Melanoma

Primary tracheobronchial melanoma is rare. One review documented only 20 cases in the literature by 1989,[258] and in many of these the possibility that the pulmonary tumor represented a metastasis cannot be definitely excluded. Confident diagnosis can be very difficult: there must be no history of excision of any pigmented skin lesion, no matter how remote, unless pathologic review clearly indicates a benign lesion. In addition, primary sites other than the skin, such as the eyes and the mucosa of the anal canal, vagina, and esophagus, must also be carefully excluded.

The tumors likely to represent primary tracheobronchial melanoma usually arise in proximal bronchi and grow as polypoid intraluminal lesions. Clinical and roentgenographic signs and symptoms are related to airway obstruction.

LYMPHORETICULAR NEOPLASMS AND LEUKEMIA

Hodgkin's Disease

Intrathoracic involvement in Hodgkin's disease is common, occurring most often in the form of mediastinal and hilar lymph node enlargement. In one review of 659 patients who had been staged both clinically and pathologically, the former was present at the time of diagnosis in 405 (61 per cent), and the latter in 193 (29 per cent).[259] Such involvement is usually associated with evidence of disease elsewhere in the body, primary mediastinal involvement without superficial or retroperitoneal node enlargement occurring in only 3[260] to 10 per cent[261] of cases.

Pleuropulmonary involvement is present at the time of diagnosis in 10 to 15 per cent of patients,[259] usually in

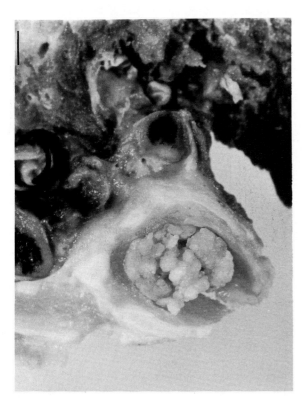

Figure 8–36. Solitary Bronchial Papilloma. A lower lobe bronchus is almost completely occluded by a coarsely lobulated tumor confined to the airway lumen. (Bar = 4 mm.)

association with mediastinal disease. Primary pulmonary Hodgkin's disease (unassociated with evidence of disease in mediastinal, hilar, or other lymph nodes) is rare.[262] Since the advent of multiagent chemotherapy, the incidence of thoracic disease at autopsy has decreased. Nevertheless, in one review of 80 patients who died between 1972 and 1977, residual disease was present in the lung and in the intrathoracic lymph nodes in 39 per cent and 59 per cent of cases, respectively.[263]

Pathologic Characteristics

Pulmonary involvement in Hodgkin's disease probably occurs most often by direct extension from affected hilar or bronchopulmonary lymph nodes; thus, the commonest pathologic appearance is thickened peribronchovascular interstitial tissue. The Hodgkin's infiltrate may extend from this location into adjacent bronchial mucosa, resulting in a plaquelike elevation or (less commonly) an endobronchial polypoid mass, both of which may cause airway narrowing with distal atelectasis and obstructive pneumonitis. The peribronchovascular interstitial infiltrate also may extend into adjacent lung parenchyma; enlargement and coalescence of such foci undoubtedly account for most of the localized nodules or masses seen grossly. Interlobular septa and pleura, with or without their adjacent parenchyma, also may be infiltrated.

Microscopically, the infiltrate is identical to that seen in affected lymph nodes, the pattern varying with the different histologic subtypes of Hodgkin's disease. By far the commonest of these is nodular sclerosis; in the review of 659 patients cited previously,[259] 77 (87 per cent) of the 89 with lung involvement had this histologic variant.

Roentgenographic Manifestations

Mediastinal Lymph Node Enlargement. This is the commonest intrathoracic roentgenographic manifestation of Hodgkin's disease. In the majority of cases, the enlarged nodes protrude into the right and left hemithoraces in an asymmetric fashion (Fig. 8–37). Unilateral node enlargement is unusual.

Although any nodal group may be affected, some observations regarding several specific groups are worthy of note. *Anterior mediastinal involvement* is common and of major importance in the differential diagnosis from sarcoidosis, which seldom produces conventional roentgenographic evidence of node enlargement at this site. By contrast, *posterior mediastinal lymph node enlargement* is uncommon. Although it can be detected by deformity of the barium-filled esophagus or paraspinal lines, usually it is necessary to confirm the presence of suspected lymph node involvement by CT, since fat accumulation cannot be distinguished from plaquelike deposits of lymphomatous tissue by conventional examination methods (Fig. 8–38). Involvement of the *diaphragmatic group* of parietal lymph nodes, particularly the anterior or prepericardiac group and the middle or lateral pericardiac (juxtaphrenic) nodes, also can simulate benign conditions such as pericardial cyst and mediastinal fat (Fig. 8–39). As with posterior disease, CT can be of great assistance in differential diagnosis.

Calcification develops in lymph nodes in some cases after radiation directed at the mediastinum (Fig. 8–40)[264] and occasionally following chemotherapy without accompanying radiation. The time interval between irradiation and the appearance of calcification may be as short as 1 year or as long as 9 years. Its development appears to indicate a favorable clinical course.

As with carcinoma, Hodgkin's disease can extend outside affected lymph nodes into mediastinal tissues and invade such structures as the esophagus, superior vena cava, and pericardium, with appropriate roentgenologic manifestations. An exception is diaphragmatic paralysis secondary to invasion of the phrenic nerve; in contrast to pulmonary carcinoma, Hodgkin's disease rarely results in this complication.[265] Involvement of the anterior mediastinal and retrosternal nodes may be associated with invasion of the sternum or the parasternal soft tissues, either unilaterally or bilaterally.[266]

Occasionally, mediastinal Hodgkin's disease presents as a relatively well-defined anterior mediastinal mass, in which case it is usually caused by primary involvement of the thymus gland rather than by enlarged lymph nodes.[267] When CT reveals the thymic mass to be cystic, differentiation is required from cystic degeneration in a thymoma or teratoma.

Pleuropulmonary Involvement. Involvement of peribronchovascular interstitial tissue by Hodgkin's disease is reflected roentgenographically by a coarse reticulonodular and linear pattern that extends outward from the hila (Fig. 8–41). Similar involvement of the interlobular septa may result in Kerley B lines.[265] Bronchopulmonary lymph nodes at the bifurcation of proximal airways also may be affected.

Consolidation of lung parenchyma remote from the mediastinum also is common in Hodgkin's disease.[268] It can occur either in the center of the lung as nodular opacities or airspace consolidation, or beneath the visceral pleura as plaquelike masses reminiscent of asbestos-related pleural disease. The size of such masses ranges widely and may vary with time; individual foci may coalesce to form a large, homogeneous, nonsegmental mass, sometimes involving a whole lobe. This type of parenchymal consolidation is purely space-occupying (Fig. 8–42) and is unassociated with loss of volume. Its borders may be shaggy and ill defined or sharply marginated. Since the airways are unaffected, an air bronchogram may be visible. Such masses may undergo necrosis and form cavities that may be thin- or thick-walled (Fig. 8–43); they are multiple in many cases and are usually situated in the lower lobes.[269]

Bronchial occlusion may result in lobar or segmental atelectasis and obstructive pneumonitis. Such occlusion is almost always caused by tumor within the airway lumen or wall[265] and seldom by airway compression by enlarged lymph nodes. In some cases, it is associated with bronchoscopic evidence of nodular endobronchial lesions elsewhere in the tracheobronchial tree that are of insufficient size to cause airway occlusion.

Pleural effusion is fairly common, occurring in approximately 30 per cent of cases, most often in association with other intrathoracic manifestations. The fluid may be serous, chylous, pseudochylous, or, rarely, serosanguineous. The incidence of pneumothorax is increased, in one series being 10 times higher than expected.[270]

Text continued on page 498

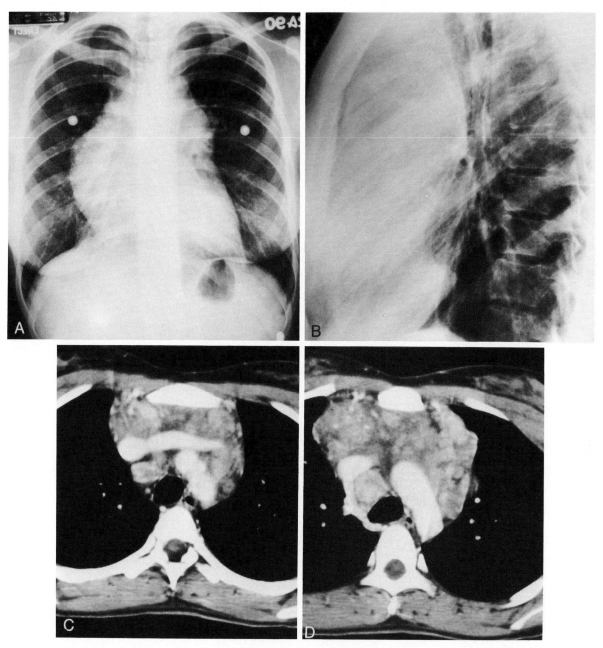

Figure 8–37. Nodular Sclerosing Hodgkin's Disease. Posteroanterior *(A)* and lateral *(B)* chest roentgenograms of this 18-year-old woman reveal a large mediastinal mass presenting to both sides of the midline but predominantly to the right. The mass extends inferiorly to obliterate most of the right heart border. In lateral projection, note the posterior displacement of the tracheal air column. CT scans at the level of the left brachiocephalic vein *(C)* and the aortic arch *(D)* show the mass to be composed of a multitude of discrete and confluent enlarged lymph nodes. In *(D)*, note the extension of the nodes lateral to the aortic arch and the large pretracheal retrocaval lymph node just medial to the azygos vein.

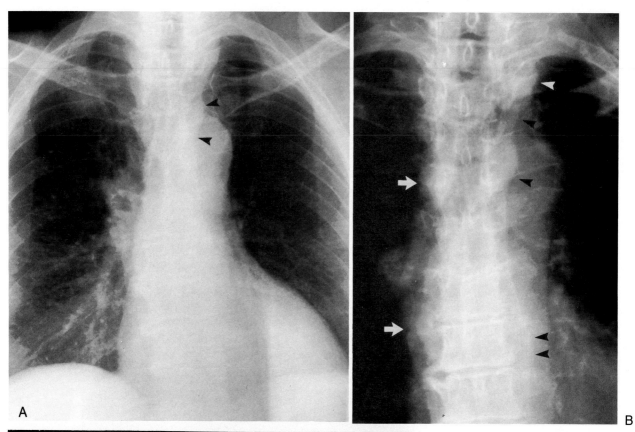

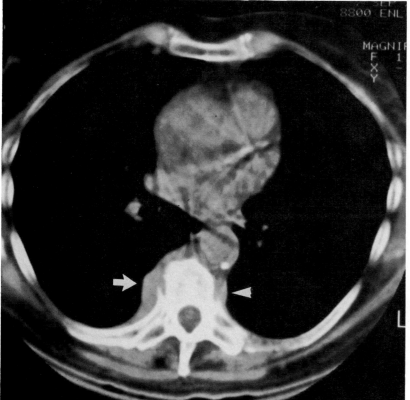

Figure 8–38. Posterior Mediastinal Lymph Node Enlargement in Hodgkin's Disease. A posteroanterior chest roentgenogram *(A)* and an anteroposterior view *(B)* of the thoracic spine reveal a lobulated contour of the right *(arrows)* and left *(arrowheads)* paraspinal lines. *C*, A transverse CT scan through the lower thorax confirms the presence of right *(arrows)* and left *(arrowheads)* paraspinal soft tissue masses consistent with lymphomatous involvement of the posterior parietal lymph nodes.

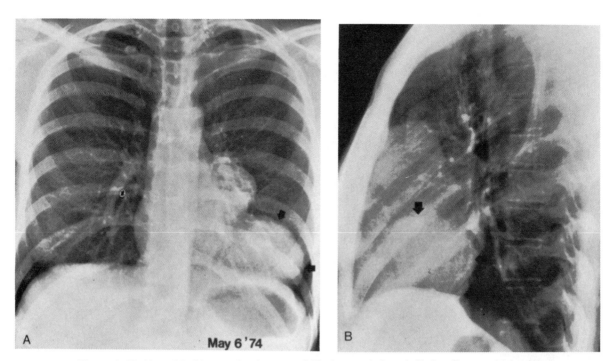

Figure 8–39. Hodgkin's Disease: Involvement of Diaphragmatic Lymph Nodes. Posteroanterior *(A)* and lateral *(B)* roentgenograms reveal large masses of lymph nodes adjacent to the apex of the heart *(arrows)* and the main pulmonary artery.

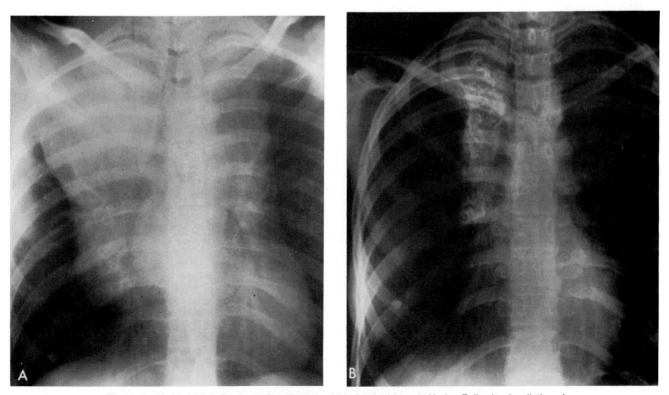

Figure 8–40. Hodgkin's Disease: Calcification of Mediastinal Lymph Nodes Following Irradiation. A posteroanterior roentgenogram *(A)* reveals marked enlargement of mediastinal lymph nodes, particularly on the right. Three years later *(B)*, the enlargement had largely disappeared, but the nodes had undergone extensive calcification. (Courtesy of Montreal Children's Hospital.)

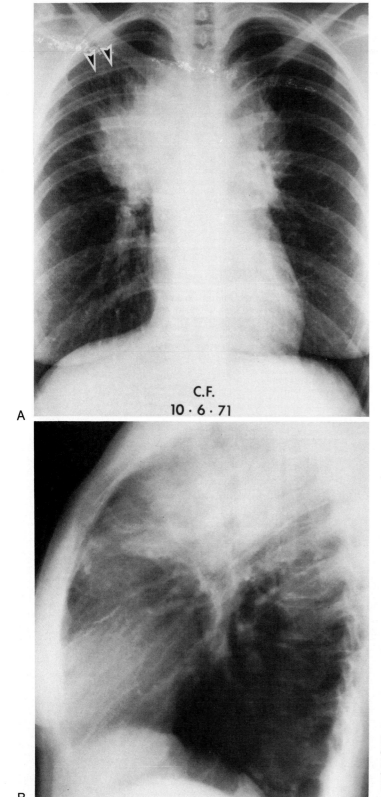

C.F.
10 · 6 · 71

A

B

Figure 8–41. Hodgkin's Disease: Invasion of Lung Paren-chyma from Mediastinal Lymph Nodes. Posteroanterior *(A)* and lateral *(B)* roentgenograms demonstrate strands *(arrowheads)* that extend from an anterosuperior mediastinal mass into the lung, representing tumor infiltration within the peribronchovas-cular interstitium.

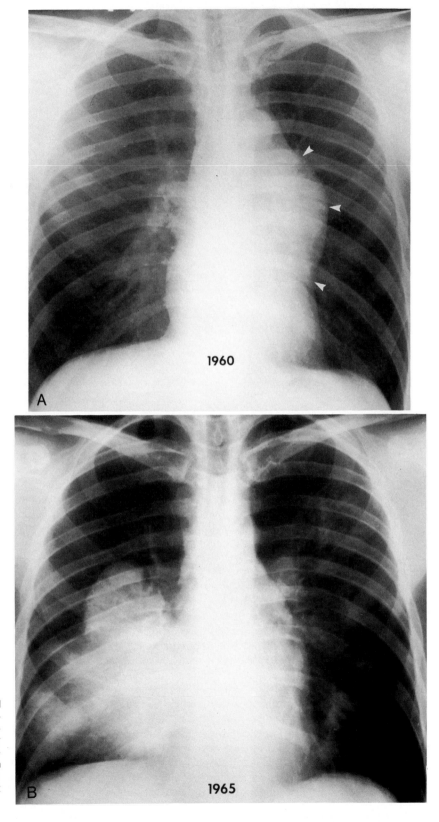

Figure 8–42. Hodgkin's Disease: Parenchymal Consolidation. *A,* A posteroanterior chest roentgenogram reveals a smoothly contoured left anterior mediastinal mass *(arrowheads)* caused by Hodgkin's involvement of lymph nodes. *B,* Five years later, a posteroanterior roentgenogram shows regression of the mediastinal lesion, but in the interim massive consolidation of the right middle and lower lobes had developed.

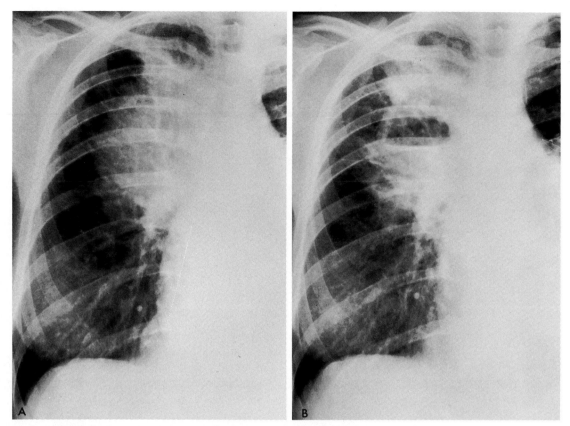

Figure 8–43. Hodgkin's Disease: Cavitation. A view of the right hemithorax from a posteroanterior roentgenogram *(A)* reveals a poorly defined mass of homogeneous density situated within the right upper lobe contiguous with the mediastinum. Three weeks later *(B)*, a large cavity had formed within the mass; the cavity possesses a thick, irregular wall and contains a prominent air-fluid level.

Chest Wall and Other Skeletal Involvement. Approximately 15 per cent of patients manifest bone involvement radiographically.[271] The thoracic skeleton is usually affected by direct extension of tumor from the mediastinum or lungs; in such cases, destruction of ribs, vertebrae, or the sternum typically results in focal lytic areas. By comparison, vertebral involvement other than by direct extension is often purely osteoblastic, resulting in an appearance sometimes referred to as "ivory" vertebra (Fig. 8–44). Involvement of the nonthoracic skeleton (most commonly the spine or pelvis) usually results in mixed lytic and blastic lesions.

Signs of Recurrent Disease. In one series of 21 patients with relapse of Hodgkin's disease, the recurrence was primarily nodal in 12, usually in the upper half of the mediastinum and sometimes in the hilar or diaphragmatic areas.[272] In only 2 of the 12 patients was there simultaneous involvement of lung parenchyma, one by direct extension from hilar nodes and the other as a discontinuous mass. Predominantly pulmonary parenchymal relapses developed in 10 of the 21 patients, in 7 of whom the lung was the only site of recurrence. In only 1 of the 10 was there associated mediastinal lymph node enlargement. Parenchymal involvement consisted of nodular masses ranging in diameter from 1 to 5 cm and usually not contiguous with the mediastinum.

Clinical Manifestations

Most patients seek the advice of a physician when they notice enlarged peripheral lymph nodes, particularly in the cervical area, an initial manifestation that occurs in roughly 90 per cent of cases. The spleen and liver are enlarged in about 50 per cent of cases. Systemic symptoms such as fever, night sweats, pruritus, weight loss, weakness, and fatigue are usually late manifestations.

Intrathoracic Hodgkin's disease is seldom asymptomatic.[273] Mediastinal lymph node enlargement may result in retrosternal pain; pulmonary involvement may be accompanied by cough, dyspnea, and pleural pain. In its later stages, especially when the patient is receiving corticosteroids or chemotherapeutic agents, Hodgkin's disease is frequently complicated by infection. The lungs are often affected, leading sometimes to difficulty in roentgenologic interpretation. Tuberculosis, formerly a common complication, now has a lower incidence than opportunistic infections.

In a minority of cases, the diagnosis of pulmonary Hodgkin's disease can be suggested by cytologic examination of sputum, transthoracic needle aspirates, or bronchoalveolar lavage fluid.[274] Investigation of the blood usually reveals a slight leukocytosis with neutrophilia; eosinophilia and lymphopenia are present in some instances. Normocytic normochromic anemia may develop early but more often is a late manifestation. A rise in the serum level of alkaline phosphatase may reflect osteoblastic bone lesions or liver disease but can also occur in their absence.[275]

Primary Non-Hodgkin's Lymphoma

The criteria for designating a lymphoma as primary in the lung are variable. Perhaps the most widely accepted are those of Saltzstein,[276] who considered lymphoma to be pri-

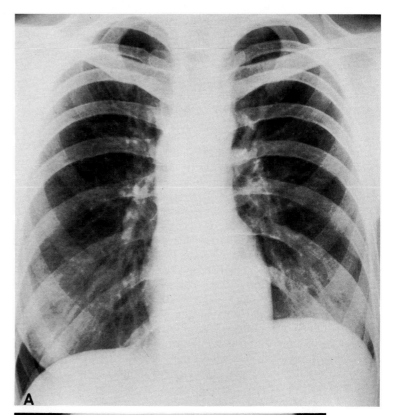

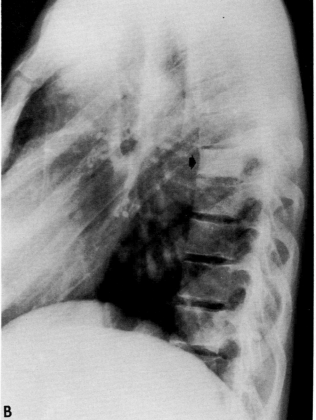

Figure 8–44. Hodgkin's Disease: Combined Splenomegaly and Bone Involvement. Posteroanterior *(A)* and lateral *(B)* roentgenograms demonstrate elevation of the left hemidiaphragm due to a markedly enlarged spleen. The lungs are clear, and there is no evidence of hilar or mediastinal node enlargement. In lateral projection, the seventh thoracic vertebral body (arrow) can be seen to be slightly compressed and to be uniformly dense ("ivory vertebra").

mary if it affected the lung (with or without involvement of regional lymph nodes) and showed no evidence of extrathoracic dissemination for at least 3 months after the initial diagnosis. While many authors abide by these criteria or minor modifications thereof, some are more liberal and others more restrictive. Because of this variability and because of the difficulty in histologic diagnosis in some cases (*see* later), the true incidence of primary pulmonary lymphoma is difficult to determine precisely. Nevertheless, it is clearly an uncommon form of disease. For example, in one review of 5030 cases of lymphoma, only 0.4 per cent were deemed to be primary in the lung.[277]

One of the major controversies concerning primary pulmonary lymphoma has been its distinction from focal areas of lymphoid hyperplasia, commonly known as "pseudolymphoma." The hypothesis that many localized intrapulmonary aggregates of lymphoid cells represent a benign, reactive process was proposed by Saltzstein in 1963.[276] However, more recent investigations have shown that many so-called "pseudolymphomas" are in fact associated with serologic or immunohistochemical evidence of a monoclonal B cell proliferation, implying neoplasia.[278] Since patients in whom such monoclonality has been identified are otherwise identical clinically, roentgenologically, and pathologically to patients in whom there is no monoclonality, it has been suggested that the majority of such tumors represent a malignant process.[279] The authors concur with this viewpoint and, in the discussion that follows, lump together those tumors that have corroborative immunologic evidence of malignancy with those that do not. It should be pointed out, however, that some tumors do seem to be both clinically and pathologically benign,[279a] and in the absence of confirmatory proof of lymphoma, some pathologists prefer to be less dogmatic and refer to these lesions in such noncommittal terms as "small (well-differentiated) lymphocytic proliferation."[280]

The origin of primary pulmonary lymphoma is not clear in the majority of cases. Presumably, many tumors arise from foci of bronchus-associated lymphoid tissue (BALT) normally present throughout the airways.[281] It is also possible that some develop within intrapulmonary lymph nodes or by extension from affected hilar nodes.

Pathologic Characteristics

Grossly, primary pulmonary lymphomas vary from well-defined nodules to more or less diffuse infiltrates in all or part of a lobe. The tumors can be conveniently divided histologically into those composed predominantly of small lymphocytes with minimal cytologic abnormality (small cell, or "well-differentiated," lymphoma) and those with clear-cut cytologic atypia (most often large cell, "histiocytic," lymphoma). The former constitute the most frequent type; for example, in one review of 131 patients, 92 per cent were small cell lymphoma.[282]

In the small lymphocyte subtype, malignant cells are found predominantly within interstitial tissue, a feature seen most clearly at the periphery of tumor nodules in relation to bronchovascular bundles and interlobular septa (Fig. 8–45). In the central portions of larger masses, expansion and confluence of the interstitial infiltrate and extension into airspaces frequently result in a more or less solid appearance. The tumor cells consist of small lymphocyte-like cells with round (less commonly cleaved) uniform nu-

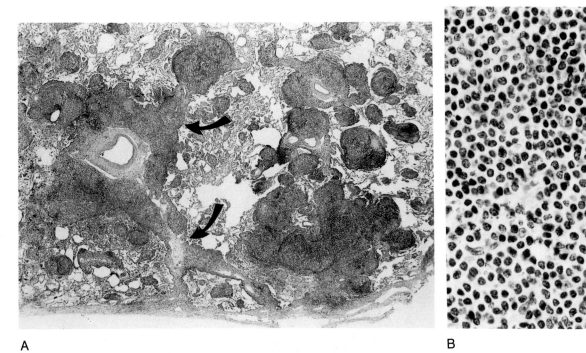

A   B

Figure 8–45. Primary Pulmonary Lymphoma. *A,* A section from the periphery of an area of poorly defined parenchymal consolidation shows abundant lymphoid cells within the interstitial tissue of an interlobular septum *(arrows).* The nodular infiltrate in the centrilobular region to the right is centered predominantly about transitional airways, although focal extension into alveolar interstitium is also present. *B,* A magnified view shows a monomorphic population of small lymphoid cells with mild nuclear atypia. (*A* × 14; *B* × 400.)

clei, small nucleoli, and rare mitotic figures. Other cells such as mature plasma cells, immunoblasts, and macrophages are usually sparse. When their numbers are considerable, the possibility of a reactive process is more likely.

The presence of monoclonality of the lymphoid cells is usually accepted as a reliable indicator of malignancy; by corollary, a polyclonal proliferation is evidence for benignity. Monoclonality reflects B cell proliferation in the majority of patients. It is important to note, however, that some lesions with a polyclonal immunohistochemical profile have subsequently progressed to clear-cut lymphoma associated with a change to a monoclonal pattern.[283]

The diagnosis of primary large cell lymphoma usually is easily made when cytologic atypia, mitotic activity, and relatively extensive necrosis are present. In contrast with the small lymphocytic lymphoma, these tumors tend to show a less prominent interstitial growth pattern.[280]

Roentgenographic Manifestations

The roentgenographic manifestations of the large cell ("histiocytic") and small cell lymphocytic forms of non-Hodgkin's lymphoma differ somewhat, the former being characterized predominantly by mediastinal and hilar lymph node enlargement, and the latter more commonly by pulmonary disease. Pulmonary disease, in turn, may occur in four roentgenographic patterns[283, 284]: (1) diffuse reticulonodular; (2) nodular; (3) parenchymal consolidation simulating pneumonia; and (4) miliary.

Reticulonodular. This is the commonest manifestation, the pattern simulating lymphangitic carcinomatosis. In most cases, there is concomitant hilar lymph node enlargement.

Nodular. These lesions are usually homogeneous in density and poorly defined and much more often multiple than solitary. They tend to be rather large when first detected and, in many cases, are better designated masses than nodules. They may be located peripherally or centrally. In the former location, they tend to assume an elongated, flattened configuration along the visceral pleura, simulating the plaques of asbestos-related disease. As in the latter condition, such lesions may be difficult to identify when viewed *en face* and may require oblique roentgenography for adequate identification. When masses are centrally located, they tend to possess smooth, fairly sharply defined margins. Cavitation is uncommon.

Parenchymal Consolidation. This pattern simulates acute airspace pneumonia and may vary in extent from a segmental opacity (Fig. 8–46) to involvement of a whole lobe or even an entire lung. One or several lobes may be involved. A characteristic of this form of disease is that it seldom obstructs the bronchial tree by either intraluminal invasion or extrabronchial compression; as a result, an air bronchogram is common. A distinctive feature of some cases of large cell lymphoma is the rapid roentgenographic progression of extensive parenchymal consolidation at some time during the course of the illness. The extreme rapidity of the process invariably leads to a suspicion of acute pneumonia, and lung biopsy is usually necessary to establish the true nature of the disease.[286]

Miliary. This form of disease is characterized by a widespread nodular or micronodular pattern resembling that of infection and is presumably caused by hematogenous dissemination.

Other Manifestations. Primary non-Hodgkin's lymphoma shows a propensity to transgress interlobar fissures and the pleura over the convexity of the lung. Pleural effusion occurs in fewer than a third of patients and is usually a late manifestation of the disease.[284]

In one study of the role of thoracic CT in the management of patients with non-Hodgkin's lymphoma,[287] it was

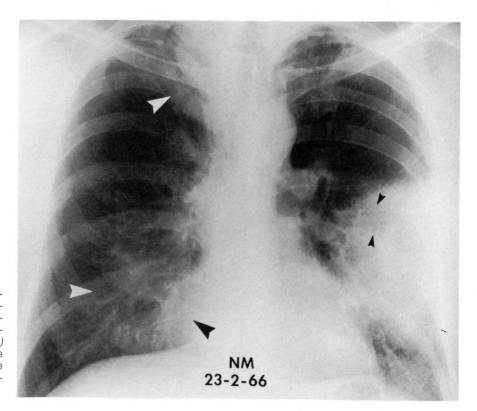

Figure 8–46. Multifocal Primary Non-Hodgkin's Lymphoma of the Lung. A posteroanterior roentgenogram reveals multifocal areas of airspace and interstitial disease in both lungs *(large arrowheads)* caused by small cell lymphoma. Note the faint air bronchogram *(arrowheads)* in the left lung, typical of a lymphomatous process.

concluded that this technique is most helpful in untreated patients with stage I or II disease unassociated with definite conventional roentgenographic abnormalities, or in those patients with abnormal conventional chest roentgenograms but no evidence of extrathoracic involvement.

Clinical Manifestations

The majority of patients with primary pulmonary lymphoma are asymptomatic when first seen, their disease being discovered on a screening chest roentgenogram. The mean age of onset is about 55 to 60 years, and men and women are equally affected.[279, 282] When present, pulmonary symptoms include cough, dyspnea, and sometimes chest pain and hemoptysis. Evidence of extrathoracic disease and systemic symptoms, such as fever and weight loss, are usually absent; their presence obviously increases the possibility of extrathoracic lymphoma.

Laboratory Findings

The presence of pulmonary lymphoma may be suspected (and occasionally diagnosed) by transbronchial biopsy or by cytologic examination of a bronchial washing or TTNA specimen or bronchoalveolar lavage fluid. However, in most cases lymph node or open lung biopsy is necessary for definitive diagnosis. The use of bronchoalveolar lavage combined with monoclonal antibodies can be particularly valuable in patients with known lymphoma when the clinical situation suggests the possibility of drug-induced or infectious interstitial disease and biopsy is considered risky because of coagulopathy.[288]

Pleural effusion in patients with non-Hodgkin's lymphoma is usually an exudate and is positive on cytologic examination in many cases.[289] When diagnosis is difficult, immunocytochemical techniques may help differentiate between benign and malignant etiologies. In the former, lymphocytes are predominantly T cells, whereas in the latter monoclonal B cells typically predominate.[290]

In a minority of patients, serum immunoelectrophoresis shows a monoclonal gammopathy, typically IgM. Free light chains, including Bence-Jones proteins, may be found in the urine of affected patients, most often with tumors that show prominent plasmacytoid differentiation.[282] The blood leukocyte count is usually within normal limits.

Prognosis

Patients with small cell lymphoma originating in the lung, with or without concomitant involvement of regional lymph nodes, generally have a good prognosis.[279, 281] For example, in one series of 32 patients with "small lymphocytic proliferation," the majority were alive without evidence of active disease after a follow-up period of 14 to 217 months.[280] Seven (22 per cent) were known to have died, and only three of these had evidence of lymphoma at autopsy. There is evidence that the prognosis of large cell lymphoma confined to the lung and regional lymph nodes is somewhat worse than that of the small cell form.[277, 280] As might be expected, pulmonary lymphoma associated with extrathoracic involvement has a worse prognosis than that of either subtype of isolated pulmonary disease.[280]

Secondary Non-Hodgkin's Lymphoma

Pleuropulmonary involvement by lymphoma in patients known to have disease outside of the thorax is much more common than primary pulmonary lymphoma. Any histologic subtype may be responsible, and since the gross pathologic, roentgenologic, and clinical manifestations tend to be similar, the following discussion applies to all. Specific features of some of the more distinctive disorders, such as mycosis fungoides and malignant histiocytosis, are discussed separately.

Pathologic Characteristics

Grossly, secondary lymphoma can possess a variety of patterns, including solitary or multiple parenchymal nodules, diffuse segmental or lobar consolidation (Fig. 8–47), and focal or extensive interstitial thickening resembling lymphangitic carcinomatosis. Although the interstitial variety may occur as an isolated finding, more commonly it is a manifestation of spread of tumor from affected hilar or bronchopulmonary lymph nodes. In this situation, marked peribronchial proliferation or endobronchial extension of tumor may cause airway compression or occlusion.

Roentgenographic Manifestations

The commonest intrathoracic manifestation of secondary pulmonary lymphoma is mediastinal or hilar lymph node enlargement. When the lungs are affected, the typical roentgenographic pattern is solitary or multiple nodules or masses 1 to 7 cm in diameter (Fig. 8–48). Multiple lesions are more frequent in the lower lobes. The nodules are round, ovoid, or polyhedral and usually possess poorly defined margins, sometimes with linear strands extending into adjacent lung parenchyma; when contiguous with the pleura, they can resemble infarcts. In cases of untreated lymphoma or in cases refractory to therapy, the nodules tend to coalesce, producing a mass that can occupy an entire lobe. Cavitation is uncommon and certainly less frequent than in Hodgkin's disease. Unlike primary pulmonary lymphoma, the secondary variety tends to affect the larger airways, resulting in atelectasis and obstructive pneumonitis. A diffuse reticulonodular pattern resembling lymphangitic carcinomatosis sometimes occurs (Fig. 8–49).

Roentgenographic evidence of involvement of the skeleton in non-Hodgkin's lymphoma is fairly common, being observed at some stage of the illness in about 15 per cent of patients. Occasionally, it is the presenting feature.[291] The lesions are characteristically osteolytic. Pleural effusion occurs in about one third of all cases.

Clinical Manifestations

As might be expected, extrathoracic manifestations often predominate in patients with secondary pulmonary lymphoma. The most frequent presenting symptoms are fever, anorexia, weight loss, and weakness, a combination that can be rapidly progressive and can suggest complicating infection.[292] As in primary pulmonary lymphoma, intrathoracic disease frequently causes no symptoms. However, cough—sometimes with hemoptysis—chest pain, and dyspnea are

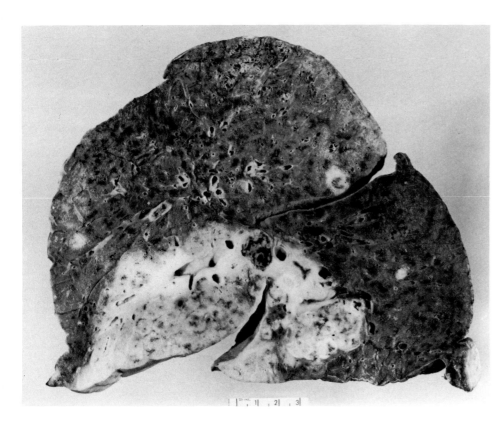

Figure 8–47. Secondary Pulmonary Lymphoma. A section of right lung removed at autopsy reveals three small parenchymal nodules and diffuse consolidation of most of the middle lobe and the anterior basal segment of the lower lobe. Disseminated large cell lymphoma. Note the patent bronchi in the middle lobe.

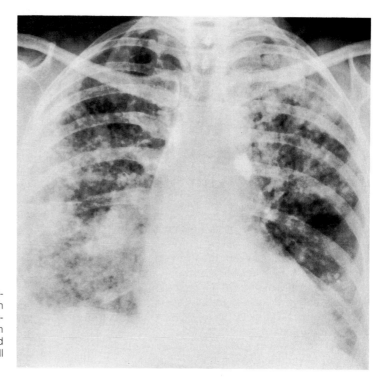

Figure 8–48. Secondary Pulmonary Lymphoma. A posteroanterior roentgenogram reveals extensive involvement of both lungs by a multitude of nodular and patchy shadows of homogeneous density. Individual shadows range from 2 to 10 mm in diameter and in some areas are confluent. Gross hilar and paratracheal lymph node enlargement is present. Large cell lymphoma.

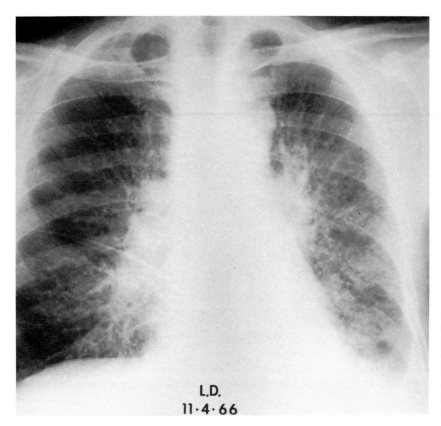

L.D.
11·4·66

Figure 8–49. Large Cell Lymphoma: Diffuse Interstitial ("Lymphangitic") Disease. A posteroanterior chest roentgenogram reveals features highly suggestive of "lymphangitic carcinomatosis"—bilateral hilar lymph node enlargement, thickening and loss of definition of the bronchovascular bundles, Kerley A lines, and small nodules. The superior mediastinum is widened as a result of lymph node enlargement.

occasionally present, particularly in patients with extensive disease. Enlarged mediastinal lymph nodes may cause obstruction of the superior vena cava and esophagus and may be associated with invasion of the recurrent laryngeal nerve, with resultant vocal cord paralysis.

Laboratory Findings

The total and differential leukocyte counts are usually within normal limits, although some patients with secondary hypersplenism have hemolytic anemia, leukopenia, or thrombocytopenia. In later stages of the disease, bone marrow replacement by lymphoma may be associated with large numbers of immature cells in the peripheral blood, resulting in a leukemic picture. Most pleural effusions are serous or serosanguineous; a few are chylous or pseudochylous.

Malignant Histiocytosis

Malignant histiocytosis is an uncommon lymphoproliferative disorder characterized by the proliferation of atypical histiocytes predominantly in the liver, spleen, lymph nodes, and bone marrow. Evidence of intrathoracic involvement is found during life in 30 to 40 per cent of patients[293] and may be the initial manifestation of the disease.[294] The pathologic diagnosis may be difficult to make, especially in those tumors with minimal cytologic atypia.

The most frequent roentgenographic manifestations are hilar and mediastinal lymph node enlargement, a reticular or reticulonodular interstitial pattern, and pleural effusion. Respiratory symptoms are usually overshadowed by systemic effects of the disease, particularly fever, weight loss,

and generalized lymph node enlargement. Cough and dyspnea may be present, and extensive pulmonary disease may occasionally cause respiratory failure. Inappropriate ADH secretion has been noted in a number of patients.

Mycosis Fungoides

Although primarily a disease of the skin, mycosis fungoides often involves the viscera late in the course of the disease, particularly lymph nodes, liver, and lungs. Roentgenographic manifestations are nonspecific and include parenchymal nodules, patchy areas of consolidation, pleural effusion, lymph node enlargement, and a diffuse reticulonodular pattern.[295] As in some cases of large cell lymphoma, airspace consolidation may develop very rapidly and may simulate acute pneumonia.[296] Dyspnea on exertion and a nonproductive cough are the usual presenting symptoms when the lungs are affected.[297] In this situation, there is usually little response to therapy, and the prognosis is dismal.

Leukemia

Necropsy studies show that thoracic involvement is a common finding in leukemia of all types. Mediastinal and hilar lymph node infiltration is the most frequent abnormality, being present in as many as 50 per cent of cases in some series[298]; pleuropulmonary infiltration is seen in about 20 to 35 per cent. Despite these figures, the incidence of clinical and roentgenographic abnormalities that may be attributed to leukemic infiltration alone is low,[299] most abnormalities being caused by pneumonia, hemorrhage, or heart failure.[300]

Pathologic Characteristics

The most frequent histologic finding is infiltration of pleural, parenchymal, or peribronchovascular interstitial tissue by leukemic cells. Although usually only microscopic in extent, infiltration in each of these areas may be severe enough to result in roentgenographic or clinical manifestations. For example, involvement of the alveolar interstitium may cause restrictive functional impairment. Similarly, a peribronchovascular infiltrate may extend into the airway mucosa and result in airway stenosis and obstructive pneumonitis.[301] Bronchiolocentric lymphocytic infiltration with relative sparing of the rest of the lung parenchyma has been reported in chronic lymphocytic leukemia and may lead to severe dyspnea.[302] Extension from any of these interstitial locations into adjacent alveolar airspaces is very uncommon.

Pulmonary leukostasis is a distinctive complication of leukemia that occurs in the absence of tissue invasion by leukemic cells. It may develop during the course of the leukemia or, less commonly, as a presenting feature; in some cases, it appears to be related directly to the institution of chemotherapy.[303] The complication invariably occurs in patients with acute leukemia or with chronic myeloid leukemia in blast crisis. The total white blood cell count is usually greater than 100,000 cells per mL, with a predominance of immature forms. Histologically, pulmonary capillaries, arterioles, and small arteries are distended and packed with blast cells. Interstitial and airspace edema, sometimes associated with a fibrinous exudate suggesting tissue damage,[304] may be present.

Roentgenographic Manifestations

The commonest roentgenographic sign of leukemia within the thorax is mediastinal and hilar lymph node enlargement (Fig. 8–50), an abnormality that occurs in about

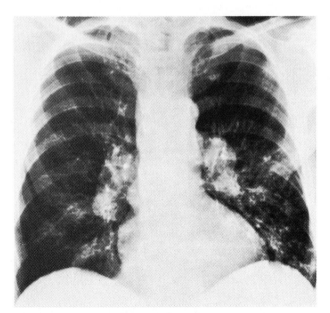

Figure 8–50. Chronic Lymphatic Leukemia: Hilar Lymph Node Enlargement. A posteroanterior roentgenogram reveals markedly enlarged lymph nodes in both hila and probably slight enlargement of the nodes in the paratracheal chain bilaterally. There is no evidence of significant pulmonary or pleural disease (the left lower lobe opacities represent resolving bronchopneumonia).

25 per cent of patients.[298] It is present much more often in the lymphatic form than in the myelogenous one. An anterior mediastinal mass, representing either thymic or lymph node enlargement and sometimes associated with pleural effusion, may be the initial roentgenographic sign of acute lymphoblastic leukemia; it is also frequently present in younger patients with lymphoblastic lymphoma who develop a leukemic phase.[305]

Pleural effusion, usually unilateral, is the second most frequent manifestation. Although it can be identified in as many as 25 per cent of patients, it is probably caused by actual leukemic infiltration in no more than 5 per cent; more probable causes are obstructed lymphatics, cardiac failure, or infection.

The commonest pulmonary abnormality is localized or diffuse airspace consolidation. As indicated previously, such disease is much more often caused by conditions other than leukemic cell infiltration. For example, in one autopsy review of 60 patients who died of acute or chronic myelogenous or lymphocytic leukemia,[300] roentgenographically demonstrable disease was related to hemorrhage in 74 per cent, to infection in 67 per cent, to edema or congestion in 57 per cent, and to leukemic infiltration in only 26 per cent. The usual pattern of pulmonary parenchymal involvement caused by leukemic cell infiltration or intravascular leukostasis consists of a diffuse bilateral reticulation or linearity that resembles interstitial edema or lymphangitic carcinomatosis.

Clinical Manifestations

Typically, acute leukemia has an abrupt onset, with major symptoms and signs related to bleeding or infection. Lymph nodes are enlarged at the onset in more than one third of cases, most frequently in lymphocytic leukemia. The spleen and liver are usually enlarged; bleeding, oral infection, and retinal hemorrhages are frequent manifestations. Fever is almost invariable, as is pallor resulting from hemolysis or hemorrhage. By contrast, chronic leukemia usually develops insidiously, revealing itself by painless lymph node enlargement or hepatosplenomegaly. Generalized weakness and loss of weight and appetite develop as the disease progresses. Anemia and hemorrhage due to thrombocytopenia occur late. Skin lesions develop in many cases, particularly in lymphocytic leukemia.

Pulmonary symptoms include cough, expectoration, and hemoptysis; as indicated previously, they are usually the result of infection, hemorrhage, or heart failure rather than leukemic infiltration. However, alveolar or bronchiolar interstitial infiltration by leukemic cells or extensive leukostasis may cause dyspnea and a reduction in diffusing capacity. Neurologic manifestations, such as confusion, somnolence, and personality disturbances, are found in some patients and have been attributed to central nervous system leukostasis, which commonly coexists with pulmonary leukostasis.

The results of pulmonary function tests are nonspecific. It is worth noting, however, that they may be abnormal in long-term survivors who, presumably, are cured of the leukemia itself. Although few of these patients are symptomatic, total lung capacity (TLC), vital capacity (VC), and diffusing capacity of carbon monoxide (DCO) may be decreased, possibly as a result of therapy or, in younger patients, a disturbance in lung growth.[306]

Multiple Myeloma

Thoracic involvement in multiple myeloma is common. In one review of 958 patients,[307] 443 (46 per cent) showed evidence of skeletal or pleuropulmonary abnormality at some time during the course of the disease; roentgenographic abnormalities were present in 25 per cent at the time of diagnosis. The pathogenesis of these abnormalities is multifactorial and may be related either to a direct effect of the neoplastic plasma cells themselves or to indirect effects caused by disease in other organs.

Neoplastic infiltration of the skeleton is undoubtedly the commonest manifestation, being identified as an isolated finding (without adjacent chest wall invasion) in 257 (28 per cent) of the cases in the series just cited; in 15 per cent, it was seen at presentation. The ribs are most frequently affected, although involvement of the vertebrae and sternum, either alone or in combination with the ribs, is also fairly common. The usual roentgenographic appearance consists of one or more well-defined, osteolytic lesions; diffuse osteoporosis, fracture, or a combination of lesions also may be seen. Extension and proliferation of tumor cells outside the ribs in the adjacent chest wall is a frequent complication and results in a rather typical roentgenographic appearance of a smooth, homogeneous soft tissue mass protruding into the thorax and compressing the lung; the mass typically is at an obtuse angle with the contiguous chest wall (Fig. 8–51).

Infiltration of the lungs or pleura by neoplastic cells is much less common than that of the skeleton, occurring in only 1 to 2 per cent of patients.[307] In fact, as with leukemia, pleuropulmonary disease is most often caused by other conditions, such as heart failure, infection, and thromboembolism. When neoplastic infiltation does occur, it may take the form of pleural effusion, a localized parenchymal mass, diffuse parenchymal infiltration, or an endobronchial or endotracheal tumor.

Thoracic signs and symptoms are uncommon and depend on the location of the lesion. Skeletal involvement may cause local tenderness and pain on respiration, and pleuropulmonary disease may be manifested by cough, chest pain, and dyspnea. Extrathoracic abnormalities are much commoner than those due to thoracic disease and include anemia, renal insufficiency, hypercalcemia, palpable liver and spleen, and proteinuria.

Plasmacytoma

A plasmacytoma can be defined as a more or less well-delimited neoplastic proliferation of plasma cells in the absence of a generalized plasma cell disorder. As such, it excludes the far commoner situation in which a localized plasma cell tumor is a manifestation of multiple myeloma. These tumors can consist of an isolated osteolytic lesion of bone or a visceral or soft tissue mass, the latter often termed "extramedullary plasmacytoma." The majority of the latter tumors are located in the pharynx; about 5 per cent occur in the lungs or trachea.

Pulmonary parenchymal tumors present roentgeno-

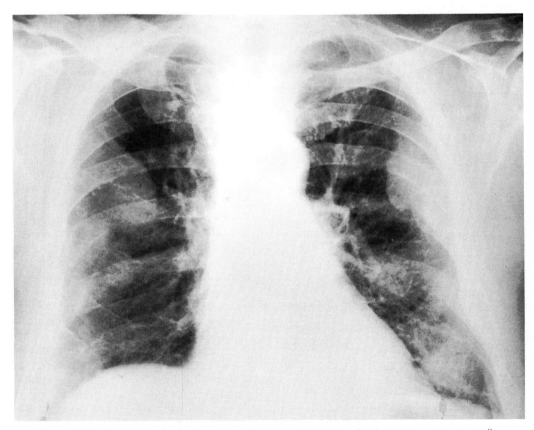

Figure 8–51. Multiple Myeloma. A posteroanterior roentgenogram demonstrates numerous, well-defined soft tissue masses of homogeneous density protruding into the thorax from the chest wall bilaterally. Each of the masses is related to a destructive lesion in an adjacent rib.

graphically as a nodule or somewhat lobulated mass indistinguishable from pulmonary carcinoma. Endobronchial tumors may cause atelectasis or obstructive pneumonitis.[308] Ossification may occasionally be identified.[309] Skeletal plasmacytomas have an appearance identical to that of skeletal tumors in multiple myeloma.

Clinical symptoms depend on the location of the lesion. Parenchymal and endobronchial tumors either cause no symptoms or are accompanied by hemoptysis, cough, dyspnea, or chest pain. Tracheal involvement may cause dyspnea, wheezing, and, in some cases, purulent expectoration. The majority of pulmonary plasmacytomas are not associated with abnormal levels of serum or urine immunoglobulins; occasionally, however, M protein may be detected, usually with very large tumors.[310]

Both localized extramedullary plasmacytomas and isolated osteolytic tumors of bone can eventually become generalized and exhibit all the clinical features of multiple myeloma. However, the survival of some patients is prolonged, without the development of other plasma cell tumors or overt multiple myeloma.

Lymphomatoid Granulomatosis

Lymphomatoid granulomatosis is an uncommon pulmonary condition characterized pathologically by a polymorphic but cytologically atypical infiltrate of lymphoreticular cells associated with necrosis and prominent vascular infiltration.[311] Recent histologic[312] and gene rearrangement[313] studies have strongly suggested that the condition represents part of a histologic spectrum of neoplastic lymphoproliferative disease. However, because of somewhat different clinical features and apparent cure in some patients who have received no therapy,[314] we describe the condition separately from pulmonary lymphoma, recognizing that a precise histologic dividing line between the two is difficult, if not impossible, to define.

Pathologically, pulmonary involvement in lymphomatoid granulomatosis is typically characterized by multiple nodules. Histologically, affected lung parenchyma is replaced by a diffuse proliferation of lymphocytes, plasma cells, histiocytes, and a variable number of cytologically atypical lymphoreticular cells (Fig. 8–52).[315] In order for the condition to be categorized as lymphomatoid granulomatosis, the last-named should be few in number and clearly admixed with benign lymphoid cells. Infiltration of the walls of vessels of small to medium size is prominent, and focal necrosis is common.

The roentgenographic manifestations are variable, depending on the acuteness of the process. In three patients the authors have seen personally who experienced acute onset of respiratory symptoms, conventional roentgeno-

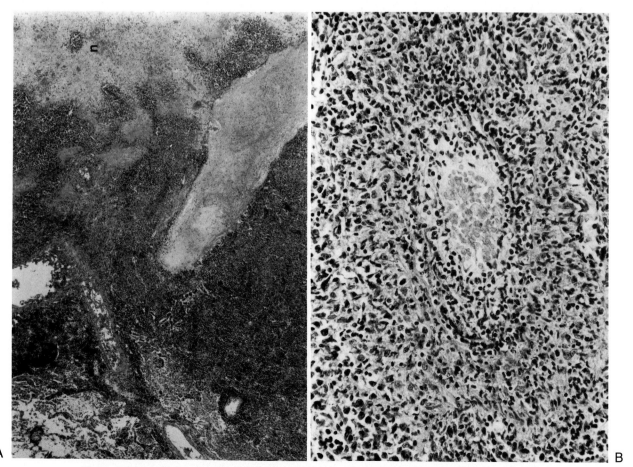

Figure 8–52. Malignant Lymphoma Simulating Lymphomatoid Granulomatosis. *A,* A histologic section of a poorly defined lung nodule shows a diffuse lymphoreticular infiltrate effacing normal lung architecture. There is prominent necrosis at the top *(n)*. *B,* The limits of the wall of a small pulmonary artery are hardly recognizable as a result of marked cellular infiltration. (*A* × 50; *B* × 100.)

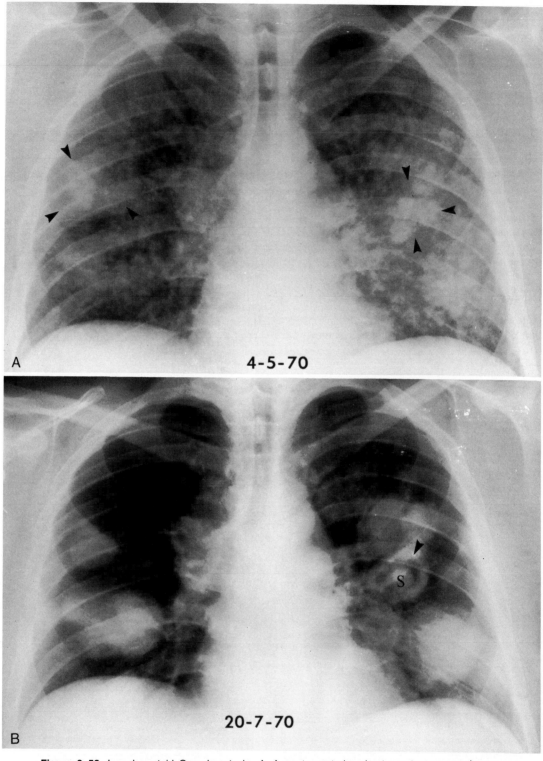

Figure 8–53. Lymphomatoid Granulomatosis. *A,* A posteroanterior chest roentgenogram demonstrates bilateral confluent and isolated nodular opacities; some of the larger opacities *(arrowheads)* possess features of airspace consolidation. Bilateral hilar lymph node enlargement is present, and the aortopulmonary window is prominent, suggesting mediastinal node involvement. *B,* Two months later, a repeat chest roentgenogram shows that the diffuse disease has resolved but has been replaced by large cavitary and noncavitary nodules. One cavitary lesion on the left *(arrowhead)* contains a central loose body (S) that could represent necrotic tissue or a blood clot.

grams revealed extensive bilateral, poorly defined opacities that displayed a striking similarity to airspace consolidation caused by infection. During the following days, however, this appearance changed to one of multiple, well-defined nodules that were close to or abutted a pleural surface, reminiscent of pulmonary infarcts (Fig. 8–53). Unlike the latter, however, several of the nodules possessed thick-walled cavities. Of the 40 cases described by Liebow and colleagues,[311] cavitation was present in 12 (30 per cent). In most cases, nodules show a distinct lower lobe predominance.[311, 315] Sequential films may show that the nodules increase or decrease in size, occasionally with complete disappearance.[315] Hilar node enlargement is uncommon. Pleural effusion occurs in about one third of patients.

The mean age at presentation is about 50 years, and there is a slight male-to-female predominance.[316] Thoracic symptoms (cough, dyspnea, chest pain) and systemic complaints (fever, weight loss, malaise) are present in most patients at the time of diagnosis. Manifestations of central nervous system involvement, cranial and peripheral neuropathies, and cutaneous disease (either an erythematous rash or skin nodules) are present in about one third of patients. Lymph node enlargement, hepatosplenomegaly, and laboratory evidence of bone marrow involvement are relatively uncommon.

The prognosis of lymphomatoid granulomatosis is guarded. In one series, approximately two thirds of patients died, with a median survival time of only 14 months.[317] A more recent review, however, documented a median survival of 72 months.[316] Progression to frank lymphoma (as defined by the presence of lymph node involvement by the atypical infiltrate) has been reported in 10 to 50 per cent of cases.[311, 316] In most instances, death is related to progressive pulmonary or central nervous system disease.

Lymphocytic Interstitial Pneumonia

Lymphocytic interstitial pneumonia (LIP) is an uncommon condition characterized pathologically by more or less diffuse expansion of the pulmonary interstitium by an infiltrate of mature lymphocytes, plasma cells, and histiocytes (Fig. 8–54).[317a] As with pseudolymphoma, differentiation from frank lymphoma can be difficult, and for this reason the condition is discussed at this point. The etiology and pathogenesis may be multifactorial. In some cases, it appears to be related to infection by Epstein-Barr virus[318]; however, its association with a variety of immunologic abnormalities in other cases suggests that some derangement of immune function is involved.

The roentgenographic features are nonspecific and, depending on the severity of involvement and acuteness of onset, can easily be confused with airspace pneumonia or lymphangitic carcinomatosis. The most frequently reported pattern is that of a bilateral reticulation or reticulonodulation,[317] variably described as coarse or finely nodular. Branching and linear opacities in the periphery of the lungs early in the course of the disease, consistent with septal lines and distended bronchovascular bundles, have also been described (Fig. 8–55).[319] As the process worsens, expansion of the interstitium may encroach on the alveolar spaces, creating an airspace pattern that may include a prominent air bronchogram. Multiple, poorly defined nodules have also been described.[317] In some patients, the

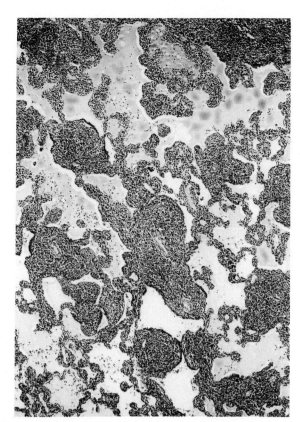

Figure 8–54. Lymphoid Interstitial Pneumonitis. A histologic section reveals diffuse infiltration, focally nodular, of lung parenchyma by mature lymphocytes. (× 40.)

process can eventuate in an "end-stage" (honeycomb) lung.[319] Hilar or mediastinal lymph node enlargement and pleural effusion are rarely observed.

Clinically, most patients are adults, a mean age of 52 years being found in the 18 patients reviewed in one series.[317a] A 2-to-1 female predominance has been noted.[317] Dyspnea and cough are the major pulmonary complaints. Most cases are associated with other conditions, particularly those in which there are abnormalities of immune function, such as Sjögren's syndrome, hypergammaglobulinemia, and AIDS (*see* page 299).

The prognosis of LIP is variable and difficult to predict. Many patients show roentgenographic improvement or stability (occasionally with no therapy). Some, however, die as a result of progression of lung disease or the development of frank lymphoma.[317]

Angioimmunoblastic Lymphadenopathy

Angioimmunoblastic lymphadenopathy (immunoblastic lymphadenopathy) is a disease of poorly defined etiology and pathogenesis that commonly affects mediastinal lymph nodes and occasionally involves the lungs and pleura.[320] It manifests several serologic abnormalities suggestive of an autoimmune or hyperimmune disorder. In fact, many patients associate the onset of symptoms with recent drug ingestion,[320] suggesting that the condition may represent an unusual hypersensitivity reaction to a foreign antigen.

The pathologic changes are best observed in lymph nodes and consist of effacement of normal architecture by

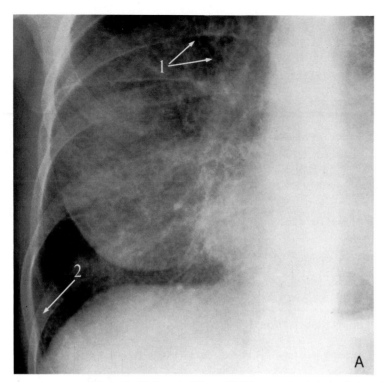 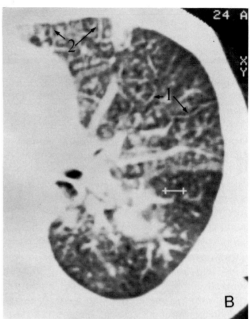

Figure 8–55. Lymphoid Interstitial Pneumonia. *A,* A detail view of the right lung from a posteroanterior chest roentgenogram reveals an admixture of small nodules, coarsened bronchovascular bundles, and Kerley A (1) and B (2) lines. Identical features were present in the left lung. *B,* A CT scan through the lower hilum of the left lung confirms the findings described previously. The bronchovascular bundles are particularly thickened in the lower lobe. Kerley A (1) and B (2) lines are visible in the upper lobe.

a polymorphous infiltrate of lymphocytes, plasma cells, and immunoblasts. In addition, there is a striking proliferation of small blood vessels, usually accompanied by deposition of eosinophilic hyaline material in the perivascular space.

Thoracic disease is most commonly manifested roentgenographically by mediastinal (particularly paratracheal) and hilar lymph node enlargement. Pulmonary disease is also fairly common. Although some cases probably represent pneumonia, others are undoubtedly caused by infiltration of peribronchovascular, interlobular, or alveolar septal interstitial tissue by an immunoblastic-plasmacytic infiltrate identical to that seen in lymph nodes, resulting in a linear or reticulonodular pattern.[321] Confluence of the interstitial disease may result in an airspace pattern that simulates pneumonia or edema or in multiple confluent nodules. Pleural effusion has been identified in approximately 15 per cent of patients.[321]

Clinically, the disease is commonest in patients older than 40 years of age; there is no sex predominance. Constitutional symptoms, including fever, weight loss, sweats, and fatigue, are present in most patients at the outset. Lymph node enlargement, usually generalized, is almost invariable. A maculopapular rash is also frequent. Laboratory abnormalities, such as polyclonal gammopathy, anemia (often Coombs'-positive), and lymphopenia, are present in most patients.

Although spontaneous remission and apparent response to corticosteroid therapy can occur, the course of the disease usually is progressive, most patients dying of infection (septicemia or pneumonia). Approximately 20 per cent develop clear-cut lymphoma.[322]

NEOPLASMS OF SOFT TISSUE, BONE, AND CARTILAGE

Neoplasms of Muscle

Leiomyoma and Leiomyosarcoma

Neoplasms of smooth muscle are among the commonest primary soft tissue tumors of the lung. Since smooth muscle is normally found throughout the conducting and transitional airways and the pulmonary vessels, tumors derived from this tissue can occur in any of these sites and can be conveniently discussed under the headings parenchymal, tracheobronchial, and vascular.

Parenchymal Leiomyoma and Leiomyosarcoma. The commonest location of pulmonary leiomyosarcoma is in the parenchyma itself; leiomyomas are equally distributed between parenchymal and endobronchial locations. Both tumors occur most commonly in adults. Malignant forms tend to be more frequent in men, and benign tumors commoner in women.[323, 324]

Pathologically, parenchymal tumors are lobulated, well-defined nodules or masses that are usually located in the periphery of the lung. In the malignant forms, necrosis and hemorrhage are frequent. Microscopically, the majority of tumors consist of interlacing fascicles of spindle cells with varying degrees of nuclear atypia.

Roentgenographically, these tumors are sharply defined, smooth or lobulated in contour, and homogeneous in density; cavitation occurs occasionally.[324] Calcification may be present and presumably occurs in areas of ischemic tissue damage. More than 90 per cent of pulmonary parenchymal leiomyomas are incidental findings on chest roentgenograms. Leiomyosarcoma may be associated with cough, chest pain, or hemoptysis.

As in smooth muscle tumors in other locations, the pathologic distinction between benignity and malignancy can be difficult. The features that seem to best predict behavior are size and mitotic activity.[324] The possibility that a parenchymal smooth muscle neoplasm represents a metastasis should always be considered, particularly in patients with multiple tumors and in women with uterine leiomyomas or a history of hysterectomy (*see* page 529).

Tracheobronchial Leiomyoma and Leiomyosarcoma. Endobronchial and endotracheal smooth muscle tumors are rare.[324, 325] Pathologically, bronchial tumors are typically located in a main or lobar airway and are fleshy, pedunculated masses more or less completely filling the airway lumen. Roentgenographic findings consist of atelectasis and obstructive pneumonitis. Defects in the air column of the trachea or bronchi may be apparent, even when the lesions are not obstructive. CT and, occasionally, conventional tomography may be useful in assessment.

As might be expected, the majority of patients are symptomatic, complaining of cough, hemoptysis, or dyspnea.

Provided that the tumors can be adequately excised surgically, the prognosis is excellent. Both local recurrence and metastases are exceptional.[324]

Vascular Leiomyosarcoma. Because of a similar clinical and roentgenologic appearance and prognosis, discussions of sarcomas arising in the pulmonary artery often include tumors with a variety of pathologic subtypes.[326] Despite this, since most neoplasms appear to be most appropriately classified as leiomyosarcoma, the authors include all histologic varieties in the following discussion.

In virtually all cases, the tumors develop in a main or proximal pulmonary artery branch or on the pulmonary valve. They tend to spread along the vascular lumen and, in about half the cases, remain entirely confined to this site.[327] In other cases, there is direct transmural extension to adjacent lymph nodes, bronchial wall, and lung parenchyma (Fig. 8–56). Metastases to the lungs are common, but only seldom do they occur systemically.[326] Pulmonary infarcts, also frequent, are caused either by tumor emboli themselves or by thromboemboli induced by the neoplasm.

Roentgenographically, the most characteristic sign is a lobulated parahilar mass corresponding to the distribution of bronchovascular bundles.[327] Such a mass represents neoplastic distention of the pulmonary artery, in some cases

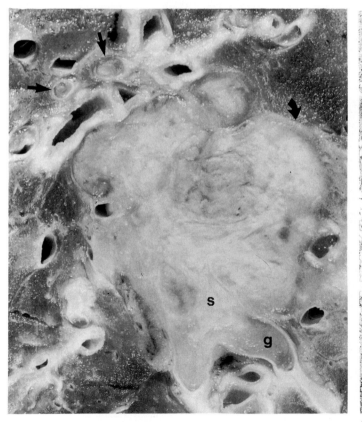

A

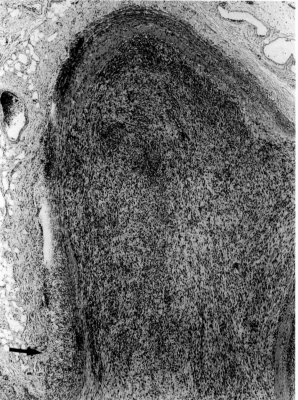

B

Figure 8–56. Pulmonary Artery Leiomyosarcoma. *A,* A magnified view of resected right lung reveals occlusion of segmental and subsegmental branches of the pulmonary artery by gelatinous (g) and more solid white tissue (s), consisting (respectively) of thrombus and sarcoma. Superiorly, the tumor has spread outside the vessel wall, forming a solid mass and invading parenchyma *(curved arrow).* A few smaller vessels, separate from the mass itself, also contain tumor *(straight arrows).* (Straight arrow = 5 mm.) *B,* A histologic section of a branch of a segmental pulmonary artery shows it to be completely filled by spindle cell sarcoma. Although most of the tumor is confined to the vessel lumen, extramural extension is present focally *(arrow).*

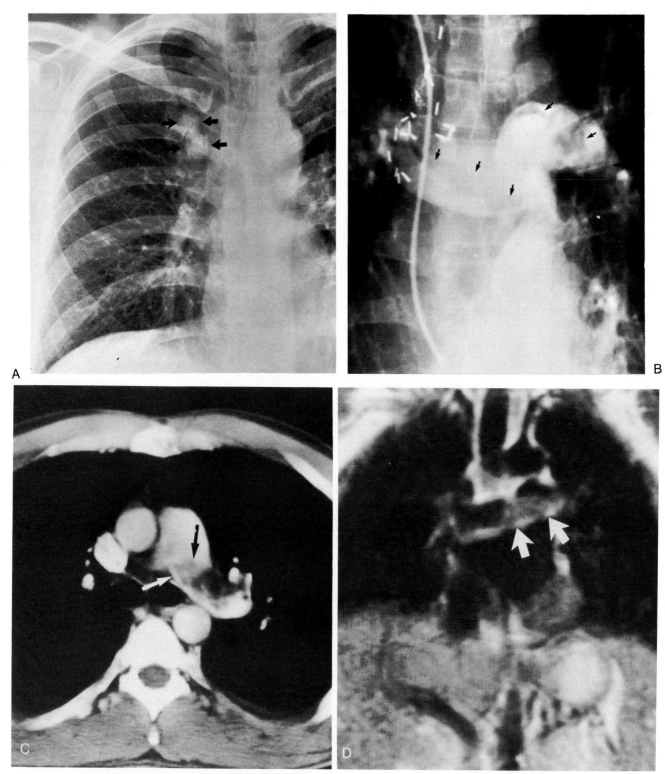

Figure 8–57. Pulmonary Artery Sarcoma. The initial chest roentgenogram *(A)* of this 41-year-old man revealed a poorly defined, somewhat lobulated mass projected just above the right hilum *(arrows)*. At thoracotomy, the right upper lobe was resected. Pathologically, the mass was situated within vascular channels in the right upper lobe and was identified histologically as leiomyosarcoma. Approximately 1 year later, a pulmonary arteriogram *(B)* revealed a multitude of filling defects within the right and left main pulmonary arteries *(arrows)* presumed to represent recurrent sarcomatous masses. *C,* A CT scan from another patient at the level of the carina reveals a filling defect in the main pulmonary artery *(arrows)*; cuts at other levels showed similar defects in the right and left pulmonary arteries. A coronal MR image at the plane of the right and left pulmonary arteries *(D)* shows a large, well-defined filling defect situated chiefly in the left pulmonary artery extending to the point of division into upper and lower branches *(arrows)*. The mass was isointense on T_1 and very hyperintense on T_2, favoring the presence of tumor rather than clot. At autopsy, a poorly differentiated sarcoma was identified arising just distal to the pulmonic valve. (Courtesy of Dr. M. Burke.)

combined with transmural extension into contiguous structures (Fig. 8–57). In the absence of a mass, both the clinical and roentgenographic presentation may be identical to that of pulmonary thromboembolism, with or without infarction.[328] Pulmonary angiography is the investigative procedure of choice for confirming the diagnosis, revealing multiple intravascular defects extending anywhere from the pulmonary valve distally. MRI also can be beneficial in some cases.

Early clinical manifestations include chest pain and dyspnea; cough, hemoptysis, fever, and palpitations also occur in roughly a third of patients.[326] Late manifestations are chiefly those of right heart failure. A heart murmur is identified in about 50 per cent of cases. The prognosis is poor, with almost all patients dying of heart failure within 2 years of diagnosis.[326]

Neoplasms of Vascular Tissue

Hemangiopericytoma

As the name indicates, these neoplasms are believed to be derived from the vascular pericyte. They occur most often as solitary, well-defined masses unrelated to major airways or vessels.[331] Microscopically, they consist of numerous vascular spaces of variable size and shape separated by aggregates of tightly packed oval to spindle-shaped cells.

The roentgenographic appearance is that of a well-demarcated nodule or mass, occasionally with calcification.[331] Most reported cases have occurred in adults, about equally in men and women. Approximately half the patients are asymptomatic when the tumor is discovered; sometimes, there is cough and hemoptysis. Although some tumors behave in a benign fashion, many invade the chest wall or mediastinum at the time of diagnosis or recur following removal and metastasize and cause death.

Kaposi's Sarcoma

Kaposi's sarcoma is believed to be derived from primitive vasoformative mesenchyme or from endothelial or pericytic cells of small vessels. Several epidemiologic and experimental observations suggest an association with viral infection, especially cytomegalovirus. The tumors occur in two clinical settings: (1) as an aggressive neoplasm involving mucosal surfaces, viscera, and lymph nodes in children and young adults, especially Africans and individuals with AIDS; and (2) as a relatively indolent tumor confined predominantly to the skin in non-African individuals of advanced age. Pulmonary involvement usually occurs in the former setting, the incidence in patients with AIDS having been estimated to be as high as 50 per cent at autopsy (*see* page 299).

Pulmonary tumors are usually multiple and are located primarily in peribronchovascular or subpleural interstitial connective tissue (Fig. 8–58). When they are present in airway mucosa, they appear as red or purplish, plaquelike elevations.[332] Expansion and coalescence of several tumor foci can result in parenchymal disease, often with a nodular appearance. Histologically, the tumors are composed of fascicles of cytologically atypical spindle cells between which are numerous, slitlike vascular spaces containing hemosiderin-laden macrophages and red blood cells.

Roentgenographic features of pulmonary Kaposi's sarcoma take two predominant forms: bilateral ill-defined nod-

ular opacities and a rather coarse linear or reticulonodular pattern (Fig. 8–59).[333] Involvement is diffuse in the majority of patients. Hilar node enlargement is present in about 20 per cent, and pleural effusion in a third.[334] Sometimes, the pattern is obscured by pneumonia, in the majority of cases by *Pneumocystis carinii*, or by hemorrhage from the tumor itself. Mediastinal lymph node enlargement occurs in some patients, either with or without concomitant pulmonary disease.

Clinically, pulmonary involvement usually causes few symptoms or signs; however, hoarseness, cough, dyspnea, stridor, and hemoptysis (rarely fatal) may occur.[335]

Intravascular Bronchioloalveolar Tumor (Epithelioid Hemangioendothelioma)

This is a rare, usually multifocal pulmonary tumor initially believed to represent an unusual form of bronchioloalveolar neoplasia characterized by extensive intravascular spread (hence the rather cumbersome designation of intravascular bronchioloalveolar tumor, or IVBAT).[336] However, more recent electron microscopic and immunohistochemical evidence has suggested an origin from (or differentiation toward) endothelial cells, and the tumor is now sometimes termed "epithelioid hemangioendothelioma."

The usual pathologic finding is multiple well-demarcated parenchymal nodules ranging in diameter from 0.3 to 3.0 cm. Light microscopic appearances are characteristic: a relatively acellular sclerotic central portion is surrounded by a somewhat nodular, more cellular periphery composed of intra-alveolar collections of oval to spindle-shaped cells separated by myxomatous interstitial tissue. In the cellular zones, tumor frequently extends into lymphatics and blood vessels.

Roentgenographic manifestations simulate metastases or infarcts (Fig. 8–60) and consist of multiple well- or ill-defined nodules.[336] Sometimes, these show little or no growth on serial roentgenograms; however, they can also enlarge slowly and eventually cause respiratory insufficiency.[337] There is usually no evidence of hilar or mediastinal lymph node enlargement. Pleural effusion is uncommon.

Clinically, these neoplasms predominate in young women, an association that may be linked to the presence of estrogen within the cytoplasm of tumor cells.[338] Most patients are initially asymptomatic, the lesions being discovered as an incidental finding on a screening roentgenogram. Occasionally, there is a history of cough, chest pain, increasing dyspnea, malaise, and weight loss.

The tumors are probably best considered low-grade sarcomas, intrathoracic spread and systemic metastases having been well documented.[336] They are relatively slow-growing, and survival may be prolonged even with widespread pulmonary involvement. Despite this, approximately 40 per cent of patients for whom follow-up information has been recorded have died, usually as a result of respiratory failure.

Neoplasms of Bone and Cartilage

Chondroma

Solitary tumors composed of pure cartilage can arise in two locations and are probably pathogenetically distinct. Some grow predominantly within the airway lumen and

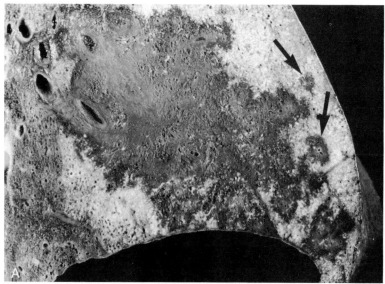

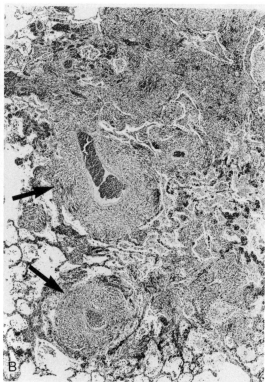

Figure 8–58. Kaposi's Sarcoma. *A,* The basal portion of a lower lobe shows extensive consolidation by an ill-defined hemorrhagic mass. At its periphery, the tumor is clearly related to small blood vessels *(arrows).* A histologic section *(B)* shows the tumor to be located in perivascular interstitial tissue *(arrows)* as well as adjacent parenchyma. (× 25.)

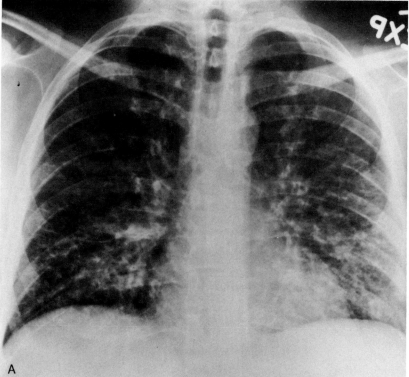

Figure 8–59. Kaposi's Sarcoma: Conventional Radiographic and CT Manifestations. A posteroanterior roentgenogram *(A)* reveals a coarse reticular and linear pattern throughout both lungs, not unlike that produced by lymphangitic carcinomatosis. *B,* A CT scan confirms the presence of nodularity and a marked increase in the volume of vascular bundles extending from the hila peripherally, in some areas as far as the visceral pleura.

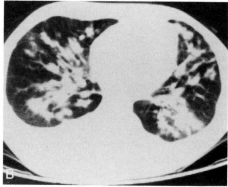

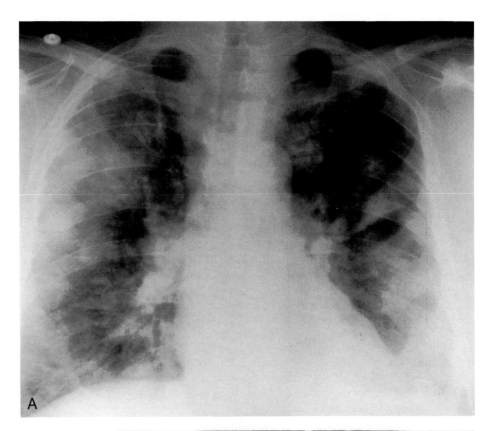

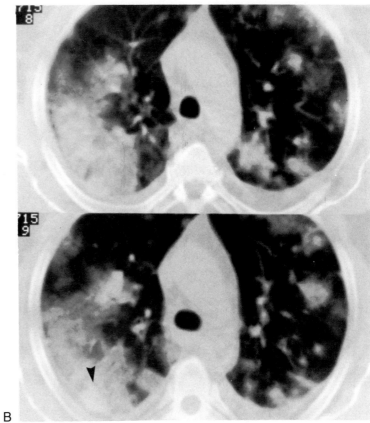

Figure 8–60. Intravascular Bronchioloalveolar Tumor (IVBAT). *A,* A posteroanterior chest roentgenogram reveals nodular and airspace opacities throughout both lungs, the right being more severely involved. The hila are slightly enlarged, suggesting node enlargement. *B,* CT scans through the apices disclose a predominantly airspace pattern with peripheral rather than central predilection. In most areas, the opacities are confluent and involve several contiguous segments. Isolated, nodular opacities *(arrowhead)* are visible in some areas.

appear to develop directly from tracheobronchial cartilage in a fashion analogous to enchondroma of bone.[339] Others (undoubtedly the majority) are situated within the lung parenchyma itself. As discussed elsewhere (see page 518), it is probable that these represent one-sided development of neoplasms derived from a bronchial mesenchymal cell and that they are analogous to so-called hamartomas.

Multiple chondromas themselves may have a separate pathogenesis. These are seen most often in *Carney's triad,* an unusual syndrome consisting of pulmonary chondromas, gastric epithelioid leiomyosarcoma (leiomyoblastoma), and extra-adrenal paraganglioma.[340] The condition is usually seen between the ages of 10 and 30 years, and almost all patients are female. The tumors are frequently multiple and can develop synchronously or metachronously. Although commonly referred to as Carney's triad, in approximately two thirds of cases only two of the three types of tumor have been documented.[341]

As might be expected, roentgenographic manifestations of Carney's triad consist of multiple nodules, with or without evidence of calcification. Pulmonary symptoms are usually absent, the chondromas being discovered on a screening roentgenogram or as part of a work-up for a previously diagnosed gastric leiomyosarcoma. Extra-adrenal paragangliomas can arise in any of the usual sites but are commonest within the thorax; paroxysmal headaches, hypertension, and tachycardia are frequent findings.

Although in most cases the follow-up period has not been long, this condition appears to have a better prognosis than the multiplicity of neoplasms might suggest.[342]

Chondrosarcoma and Osteosarcoma

Primary pulmonary chondrosarcomas are rare tumors that, in most cases, are believed to be derived from normal tracheobronchial cartilage.[343] The roentgenographic manifestations are those of either an intrapulmonary mass (that may or may not be calcified) or atelectasis and obstructive pneumonitis secondary to airway obstruction. The usual presenting symptom is cough, chest pain, or dyspnea. Adequate surgical excision is probably curative in most cases.

Primary osteosarcoma is even rarer than chondrosarcoma. The roentgenographic and clinical features are nonspecific. It is somewhat surprising that neither calcification nor ossification has been demonstrated on conventional roentgenograms or tomograms, although CT has been reported to show both quite clearly.[344]

The diagnosis of both these tumors should never be accepted unless the possibility of a metastasis from a skeletal primary tumor has been carefully excluded.

Neoplasms of Neural Tissue

Neurofibroma, Schwannoma, and Neurogenic Sarcoma

Although relatively common in the mediastinum, primary neurogenic neoplasms rarely occur in the lungs.[345] Patients with neurofibromatosis (von Recklinghausen's disease) are at increased risk. Most lesions have been classified as neurofibromas. Schwannoma (neurilemmoma) is second in frequency, and 20 to 25 per cent have been reported as neurogenic sarcoma.[345] The tumors are usually manifested roentgenographically as a solitary nodule; less commonly,

atelectasis or obstructive pneumonitis is present as a result of bronchial obstruction. Most patients are asymptomatic.

Granular Cell Tumor

Granular cell tumors are fairly common neoplasms that are most often found in the tongue, skin, subcutaneous tissue, or breast. Their presence in the lungs has been documented in about 5 per cent of cases.[346] They are somewhat more frequent in males, and two thirds of cases occur between the ages of 30 and 49 years. Most recent studies suggest an origin from either the neural sheath or, more likely, Schwann cells.

The majority of respiratory tract tumors arise in the larynx or main bronchi, in the latter often at or near their bifurcations. Multicentric tumors occur in 10 to 15 per cent of patients. The neoplasms are usually small (1 to 2 cm) and appear as white, plaquelike thickenings of the bronchial wall or as polypoid projections into the airway lumen. Microscopically, they consist of nests of polygonal cells containing abundant diastase-resistant granular cytoplasm that is positive for periodic acid–Schiff (PAS) stain.

Roentgenographically, granular cell tumor presents as a solitary nodule or as atelectasis and obstructive pneumonitis when there is sufficient bronchial occlusion.[347] The major symptoms are hemoptysis and productive cough caused by recurrent pneumonia. The prognosis is usually excellent, although neoplasms excised bronchoscopically may recur.

Neoplasms of Adipose Tissue

Lipoma

Lipomas occur only very occasionally in the lungs, usually in the tracheobronchial wall and infrequently in lung parenchyma itself.[348] In fact, many benign fatty tumors of the lung do not consist purely of adipose cells but rather contain a mixture of myxomatous, fibroblastic, chondroid, or smooth muscle elements. For this reason, it has been argued that these tumors should probably be considered as neoplasms derived from bronchial mesenchymal cells that exhibit multifaceted differentiation and that they are analogous to the commoner chondromatous hamartoma (see page 518).[339] Roentgenographically, the tumor presents most commonly as atelectasis and obstructive pneumonitis. When symptoms and signs are present, they are related to recurrent pneumonia.

Neoplasms of Fibrohistiocytic Tissue

Fibroma

Like lipomas and chondromas, many so-called pulmonary fibromas may simply represent a one-sided histologic expression of a hamartoma. It is also possible that some represent a predominantly fibrous form of benign fibrous histiocytoma (see later) or a neoplasm analogous to the localized fibrous tumor of pleura (see page 884).[349] Pathologically, the lesions are well defined and consist of spindle-shaped fibroblastlike cells embedded in a variable amount of intercellular collagen.

The roentgenographic and clinical manifestations are similar to those of other benign pulmonary neoplasms.

Those in an endobronchial or endotracheal location can cause atelectasis or obstructive pneumonitis or can simulate asthma. Parenchymal lesions usually present as an asymptomatic solitary nodule. Neoplasms that recur are best regarded as fibrosarcomas. Thorough sampling and mitotic counts of cellular tumors should enable prediction of such behavior in the majority of cases.

Fibrosarcoma

Fibrosarcoma is probably the second commonest soft tissue sarcoma of the lung (the commonest being leiomyosarcoma). Like the latter tumor, it can arise in the bronchial wall, lung parenchyma, or pulmonary artery. Histologically, the neoplasms are similar at all sites and are composed of fascicles of spindle-shaped cells with cytologically atypical nuclei. Mitotic figures are usually evident and may be numerous.

The majority of cases of endobronchial fibrosarcoma occur in children and young adults. They usually arise in lobar or mainstem bronchi, protruding into the lumen and causing variable degrees of obstruction.[324] Almost all patients are symptomatic, usually presenting with cough, hemoptysis, or chest pain. Roentgenographic findings are those of atelectasis or obstructive pneumonitis. Intrapulmonary tumors tend to arise in middle-aged or elderly adults and often do not cause symptoms.[324] Roentgenographically, they present as a smooth or lobulated mass indistinguishable from other solitary tumors. The clinical and roentgenographic features of fibrosarcoma of the pulmonary artery are identical to those of leiomyosarcoma and other sarcomas of that site (see page 511).

Endobronchial tumors are often amenable to local surgical excision, following which long-term survival is the rule.[350] By contrast, intrapulmonary lesions often behave in a highly malignant fashion, death occurring within 2½ years. Pulmonary artery tumors are invariably fatal, usually within a short time of presentation.

Malignant Fibrous Histiocytoma

Intrathoracic malignant fibrous histiocytoma most commonly originates from the chest wall; despite this, an appreciable number of pulmonary cases have been reported.[351] Most occur in older adults. Although there is no sex predominance, there appears to be a significant predilection for whites over blacks.[351]

Pathologically, these tumors typically consist of well-defined, smooth or lobulated masses, usually without an obvious site of origin. The histologic appearance is quite variable, the commonest consisting of fascicles of spindle-shaped cells arranged in a cartwheel pattern, interspersed between which are large, polygonal (histiocytelike) cells possessing highly pleomorphic nuclei.

Roentgenographically, most tumors present as nonspecific, smooth or lobulated nodules or masses within lung parenchyma.[351] Many patients are asymptomatic, although cough, dyspnea, hemoptysis, and chest pain may be present. When the neoplasm is confined to the lung, the prognosis is difficult to predict. Apparent cure after surgical excision has been noted in some cases,[352] whereas in others survival is measured in months. Extension into the chest

wall or mediastinum is a poor prognostic sign, and extrathoracic metastases invariably herald death.[351]

MISCELLANEOUS NEOPLASMS OF UNCERTAIN HISTOGENESIS

Benign Clear Cell Tumor

This is a rare pulmonary neoplasm whose histogenesis is uncertain, electron microscopic and immunohistochemical studies having been variably interpreted as providing evidence for a neuroectodermal, bronchiolar (Clara cell), smooth muscle, or pericytic origin.[353] Pathologically, the tumors are well-delimited but nonencapsulated nodules usually measuring 2 cm or less in diameter. Microscopically, they consist of sheets of polygonal cells with minimal nuclear pleomorphism and abundant, clear or finely vacuolated cytoplasm. Special stains reveal abundant glycogen.

Most reported patients have been adults, and there is a 2-to-1 female predominance. The majority are asymptomatic, the lesion being discovered as a peripheral, well-defined nodule on a screening roentgenogram. Almost all cases have behaved in a benign fashion, unassociated with recurrence or metastases. It is obviously necessary to differentiate them from primary or metastatic clear cell carcinoma.

Paraganglioma (Chemodectoma)

Paragangliomas (chemodectomas) are uncommon neoplasms that arise from the extra-adrenal paraganglia of the autonomic nervous system. Within the thorax, they are most frequently found near the ascending or transverse portion of the aortic arch or in the posterior mediastinum (see page 924). Occasional tumors interpreted as paragangliomas also have been reported in the trachea[353a] and in the lung itself.[353b]

Roentgenographic features are nonspecific, usually consisting of a solitary nodule. The tumors occur in adults who are usually asymptomatic; although some patients have had systemic hypertension, biochemical determinations of catecholamine levels were not performed to confirm a relationship with the tumor. Most tumors appear to behave in a benign fashion.

Sclerosing Hemangioma

The fundamental nature and histogenesis of sclerosing hemangioma are controversial. Although this tumor was originally hypothesized to be a vascular neoplasm, more recent ultrastructural and immunohistochemical investigations have suggested that the tumor cells are derived from epithelium, specifically from alveolar pneumocytes or terminal bronchiolar cells.[354, 355] The alternative designation "sclerosing pneumocytoma" has been proposed to emphasize this origin.

The tumor typically consists of a solitary well-defined nodule 1 to 4 cm in diameter; most arise in the peripheral parenchyma, commonly in a subpleural location. Microscopically, the tumor is variable in appearance, usually consisting of a combination of solid or papillary areas, relatively acellular sclerotic regions, and dilated blood-filled spaces.

Roentgenographically, sclerosing hemangioma characteristically presents as a well-defined, homogeneous nodule or mass without preference for any lobe. Calcification is unusual, and cavitation does not occur. Slow growth is the rule; in 14 of 51 patients reviewed in one series,[356] the lesions had been apparent roentgenographically from 1 to 14 years (average 5 years) before definitive surgery.

Approximately 80 per cent of patients are women in their fourth and fifth decades.[356] The majority are asymptomatic, the abnormality being discovered on a screening chest roentgenogram. Occasionally, a history of cough or of recent or remote hemoptysis is obtained. The tumors usually behave in a benign fashion.

Carcinosarcoma

A carcinosarcoma can be defined as a neoplasm composed of an admixture of histologically malignant epithelial and mesenchymal tissues. Pathologically, it may present as either a polypoid intrabronchial tumor with or without extension into contiguous parenchyma or a bulky peripheral mass without obvious association with an airway. Histologically, the epithelial component is most often squamous cell carcinoma. The sarcoma is usually composed of spindle cells without obvious differentiation.[357] Less often, malignant cartilaginous, muscular, or osteoid tissue may be identified. Metastases may be sarcomatous, epithelial, or a combination of both.

In one review of 44 patients,[358] the mean age was 64 years, and there was a male-to-female predominance of 4 to 1. Roentgenographic findings are nonspecific and reflect the location of the tumor, those with intrabronchial growth causing atelectasis or obstructive pneumonitis and those in the parenchyma presenting as a nodule or mass. Symptoms, including cough, hemoptysis, and chest pain, tend to occur predominantly in patients with intrabronchial lesions.

As might be expected, endobronchial tumors, especially when they are unassociated with parenchymal extension, appear to have a better prognosis than do predominantly intraparenchymal tumors. Despite this, the 1-year survival rate of 23 cases reviewed in the literature between 1951 and 1977 was only 36 per cent.[359] Both endobronchial tumors accompanied by parenchymal invasion and peripheral parenchymal lesions tend to behave in an aggressive fashion, with local invasion of contiguous structures, widespread metastases, and rapid death.

Pulmonary Blastoma

Pulmonary blastoma is a malignant tumor of uncertain histogenesis that histologically and immunohistochemically recapitulates the pseudoglandular period of early fetal life. Despite this resemblance, the appropriateness of the term "blastoma" has been questioned,[360] and some authors consider this neoplasm to represent a variant of carcinosarcoma. Usually, the tumors are large, well-defined masses located in the periphery of the lung.[361] Microscopically, they consist of primitive-appearing epithelium surrounded by polygonal or spindle-shaped stromal cells.

The peak incidence in an AFIP review of 52 cases was in the fourth decade.[361] Although many patients are asymptomatic, hemoptysis, cough, and chest pain are not infrequent

complaints. There are no specific roentgenographic features that help distinguish this neoplasm from any other peripheral pulmonary mass.

The prognosis is difficult to determine in a particular individual, but is generally not good. In one series of 39 patients,[360] 17 (44 per cent) developed metastases, and only 2 of these survived longer than 2 years. Despite this, occasional patients show exceptionally long survival, even in the presence of metastatic disease.

Pulmonary Germ Cell Neoplasms

Occasional examples of both teratoma[362] and choriocarcinoma[363] have been reported in the lung. The former usually consists of a well-defined, cystic parenchymal mass filled with sebaceous material. The roentgenographic presentation is as a peripheral mass, nonspecific in appearance except for the occasional presence of calcification or a tooth. CT scans may reveal areas of radiolucency indicating the presence of lipid—additional support for the diagnosis. Most patients come to clinical attention during the third or fourth decade. The presenting clinical features include hemoptysis and, rarely, expectoration of hair (trichoptysis). The majority behave in a benign fashion.

Pulmonary Thymoma

The presence of tumors histologically resembling thymoma but situated entirely within the lung parenchyma or in the lung and adjacent hilum has been reported occasionally.[364] The pathologic appearance, clinical manifestations and behavior are similar to those of the commoner mediastinal tumor.

MISCELLANEOUS TUMORS OF NON-NEOPLASTIC OR UNCERTAIN NATURE

Hamartoma

A hamartoma may be defined as a developmental malformation composed of tissues that normally constitute the organ in which the tumor occurs, but in which the tissue elements, although mature, are disorganized. In the lung, the term traditionally refers to a well-defined tumor consisting predominantly of cartilage and adipose tissue. It can occur within the lung parenchyma or in an endobronchial location. The parenchymal form is somewhat lobulated in contour and contains peripheral clefts lined by respiratory-type epithelium. Although tumors with this appearance are commonly designated hamartoma, it has been proposed that they are better regarded as benign neoplasms, probably derived from a bronchial wall mesenchymal cell.[365] Evidence in support of this hypothesis includes the following:

1. The tumors appear to have an onset in adult life. The peak age incidence is in the sixth decade, and they are identified uncommonly in individuals younger than 30 years of age.[366]

2. Serial roentgenograms sometimes reveal slow (and occasionally rapid) growth.[367]

3. Histologic studies suggest that the peripheral epithelium-lined clefts represent passive entrapment of adjacent

bronchial epithelium within an expanding mesenchymal proliferation, rather than separate elements of a hamartomatous process.[365]

On the strength of these observations, it appears that the diagnostic label "hamartoma" is pathogenetically incorrect and that these tumors are described more appropriately by a term such as "mesenchymoma."[366] Because of the widespread use of the designation "hamartoma," however, the authors retain this nomenclature, recognizing that the true nature of the tumor may be other than its name implies.

In addition to the controversy surrounding the fundamental nature of pulmonary hamartomas, there is also uncertainty regarding their relationship to other benign pulmonary tumors, such as fibromas, chondromas, and lipomas. The tissue composing each of these tumors occurs in varying proportion in the typical hamartoma, and it is conceivable that the former tumors might represent simply a one-sided expression of mesenchymal differentiation in a hamartoma.

Hamartomas are relatively common pulmonary tumors, representing about 5 per cent of solitary lung nodules.[368] They occur most often in males, the gender predominance being 2 or 3 to 1.

Pathologic Characteristics. Approximately 90 per cent of pulmonary hamartomas are located within the parenchyma, usually in a peripheral location. At this site, they are well-circumscribed tumors that, on cut section, consist of lobules of white, cartilaginous-appearing tissue (Fig. 8–61). Histologically, the lobules are often composed of a central area of more or less well-developed cartilage surrounded by loose myxomatous or fibroblastic tissue (Fig. 8–61). Adipose tissue, smooth muscle, seromucinous bronchial glands, and chronic inflammatory cells also may be seen in variable proportions. Thin, slitlike spaces or clefts lined by ciliated columnar or cuboidal epithelium are frequently present between the lobules, most prominently at the periphery of the tumor.

Although endobronchial hamartomas may be morphologically identical to the parenchymal variety, more frequently they appear as fleshy, polypoid tumors attached to the bronchial wall by a narrow stalk. Histologically, they often lack epithelial clefts and possess a central portion composed of a core of adipose tissue surrounded by somewhat compressed fibrous tissue. Cartilage is usually absent or present in small amounts.[369]

Roentgenographic Manifestations. Pulmonary hamartomas typically are well-defined, solitary nodules without lobar predilection.[368] The majority are smaller than 4 cm in diameter, although some occasionally grow to a very large size. Approximately one third have a smooth outline, which may aid in differentiating them from the almost invariably lobulated pulmonary carcinoma. Although some studies have reported an incidence of calcification as high as 25 to 30 per cent,[368] others have identified it far less often.[370] When calcification is present, however, the roentgeno-

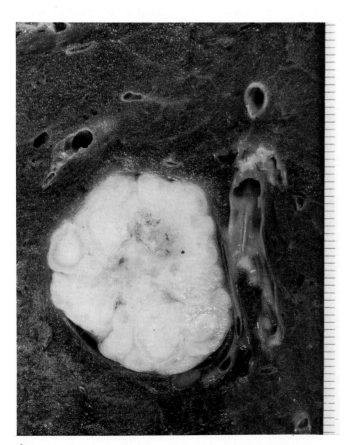

A

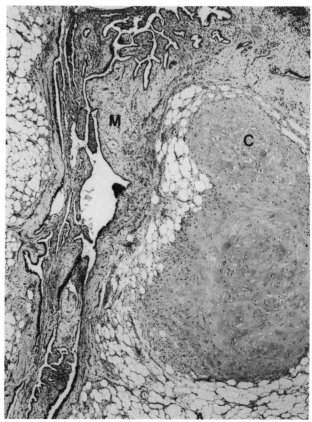

B

Figure 8–61. Pulmonary Hamartoma. *A,* A magnified view of a lower lobe reveals a well-circumscribed peribronchial tumor that consists of lobules of white tissue resembling cartilage. *B,* A histologic section demonstrates mature cartilage *(C),* adipose tissue, undifferentiated mesenchymal tissue *(M),* and multiple epithelium-lined clefts. (*B* × 40.)

graphic pattern most often resembles popcorn, a finding that is almost diagnostic (*see* Fig. 4–55, page 216). The presence of fat and calcium make the CT diagnosis exquisitely accurate (Fig. 8–62).[371] Serial films may reveal slow or (exceptionally) rapid growth of these lesions,[367] increasing the difficulty in differentiating them from pulmonary carcinoma.

Endobronchial hamartomas lead to airway obstruction, with atelectasis, obstructive pneumonitis, and progressive peripheral lung destruction.

Clinical Manifestations. Because of their predominantly peripheral location, most hamartomas do not cause symptoms. When symptoms are present, hemoptysis is the commonest. An association with multiple hamartomas of ectodermal, mesodermal, and endodermal origin (Cowden's syndrome) has been noted by some authors.[372] In the few cases in which the lesion obstructs a bronchus, there may be fever, cough, expectoration, and chest pain.

In the absence of the characteristic "popcorn" pattern of calcification, the differential diagnosis includes all other solitary pulmonary nodules, particularly carcinoma. Although thoracotomy may be required for definitive diagnosis, TTNA can provide adequate tissue for diagnosis in many instances.[373] Bronchoscopy and biopsy usually reveal the diagnosis in the endobronchial forms. Hamartomas are benign, and surgical excision should result in cure.

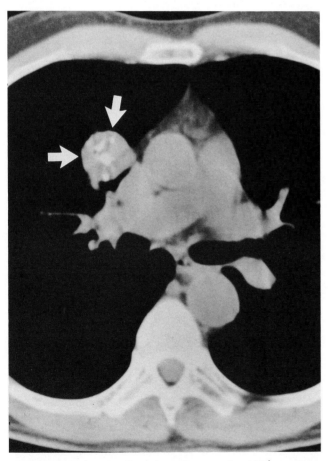

Figure 8–62. Pulmonary Hamartoma. A conventional CT scan (5-mm collimation) demonstrates a nodule 2.5 cm in diameter *(arrows)* abutting the mediastinum. Popcorn calcification is present within the nodule.

Inflammatory Tracheobronchial Polyps

Several pathogenetic mechanisms have been proposed for inflammatory tracheobronchial polyps. In some cases, a history of chronic bronchitis or bronchiectasis has suggested that they represent an exaggerated but localized inflammatory reaction to chronic airway irritation.[374] In others, aspirated foreign material[375] or thermal injury[376] has resulted in the formation of exuberant granulation tissue that constitutes the polypoid mass. Despite these examples, in most cases there is no history of concomitant pulmonary abnormality to explain polyp formation.

The polyps are usually solitary and may be pedunculated or attached to the airway wall by a broad base. Histologically, the surface epithelium often shows squamous metaplasia and may be ulcerated. The underlying stroma has a variable appearance, depending on the number of blood vessels, the maturity of connective tissue, and the severity of inflammatory cellular infiltrate.

The roentgenographic manifestations are those of airway obstruction and include bronchiectasis, atelectasis, and obstructive pneumonitis. Most patients are between 30 and 60 years of age. The clinical findings include hemoptysis, cough (frequently with sputum production), and dyspnea; wheezing may simulate asthma. A history of recurrent pneumonia is common.

Plasma Cell Granuloma and Fibrous Histiocytoma

These two terms refer to a group of pulmonary tumors characterized histologically by a mixture of fibroblasts, histiocytes, lymphocytes, and plasma cells. Since the proportion of these elements varies considerably from tumor to tumor, a variety of terms has been employed to describe them and a dual concept of their pathogenesis has arisen. Those with a predominance of plasma cells have been considered to represent an unusual chronic inflammatory reaction to an unidentified agent and have been termed "plasma cell granuloma" or "postinflammatory pseudotumor."[377, 378] By contrast, those with a relative absence of these inflammatory cells and an abundance of fibroblasts and macrophages have been interpreted by some as being neoplastic and as representing the pulmonary counterpart of benign fibrous histiocytomas that arise elsewhere in the body. To further confuse matters, there is evidence that the two groups of tumors may not be as pathogenetically distinct as this discussion suggests; for example, in one series of 27 lesions, there was considerable histologic overlap.[377]

Pathologically, the tumors are usually well defined and may be situated in parenchymal, endobronchial, or endotracheal locations. Roentgenographic manifestations consist of either a solitary pulmonary nodule or a homogeneous area of consolidation.[379] Calcification is present occasionally, and cavitation rarely. Endobronchial tumors may cause atelectasis and obstructive pneumonitis.

The tumors can develop at any age, although a relatively high proportion occur in children and adolescents.[378] Many patients are asymptomatic, the lesion being discovered on a screening chest roentgenogram. When symptoms are present, they include cough, hemoptysis, and chest pain; signs and symptoms of bronchial or tracheal obstruction may be present in some patients.

In general, neither recurrence nor metastases are detected following surgical excision. In fact, in some patients in whom the diagnosis has been established by biopsy only, the lesions have been seen to regress.[380] Despite these observations, in some cases there is evidence of locally aggressive behavior, with "invasion" of contiguous chest wall or mediastinum.[378]

Hyalinizing Granuloma

The term "hyalinizing granuloma" refers to an unusual pulmonary tumor characterized histologically by numerous regularly arranged lamellae of hyalinized fibrous tissue. The pathogenesis of the nodules is unclear. Some authors have speculated that they represent an exaggerated or abnormal host reaction to one of a number of unidentified agents.[381] Of some interest in this respect is the presence in some patients of immunologic abnormalities such as circulating immune complexes and autoantibodies.[382]

Pathologically, the tumors are well demarcated and consist of numerous lamellae of homogeneous, hyalinized connective tissue. Plasma cells and lymphocytes often are present in small numbers between the lamellae and in relation to blood vessels.

Roentgenographically, the nodules are usually multiple, round, homogeneous, and well defined. Most range from 2 to 4 cm in diameter. Cavitation[381] and calcification[382] have been noted occasionally. Serial roentgenograms may reveal slow growth, a feature that can lead to a false diagnosis of metastases.

Clinically, many patients are asymptomatic; however, cough, dyspnea, chest pain, and hemoptysis may occur. The condition is benign, and the prognosis usually very good. Increasing dyspnea associated with enlarging nodules, however, was noted in 6 of 19 cases in one series.[382] Concomitant retroperitoneal or mediastinal fibrosis, or both, have also been reported as complications in several patients.[382]

Endometriosis

Several mechanisms have been proposed to explain the presence of endometrial tissue within the thorax.[383]

1. Trauma to the endometrium results in embolization of minute tissue fragments from the uterus to the lungs via the pulmonary arteries. Support for this mechanism was provided by one review of 65 cases of pleural and parenchymal endometriosis in which all patients with evidence of pulmonary parenchymal involvement had a history of at least one spontaneous vaginal delivery or gynecologic operation.[384]

2. Endometrial tissue is regurgitated through the fallopian tubes or is released into the peritoneal cavity from foci of peritoneal endometriosis and subsequently migrates to the pleura through diaphragmatic fenestrations. Such fenestrations measure up to several millimeters in diameter and have been identified in approximately 33 per cent of patients with pleural endometriosis.[385]

3. Pleural mesothelium and submesothelial connective tissue develop directly into endometrial tissue by a process of metaplasia.[383]

Grossly, pleural endometriosis typically appears as multiple bluish-purple nodules ranging from 1 mm to several centimeters in diameter. The right pleural cavity is affected in more than 90 per cent of cases. Involvement of lung parenchyma may occur by direct extension from a focus in the pleura or as an entirely separate nodule.

The roentgenographic appearance in the few reported cases of parenchymal endometriosis is that of a solitary nodule measuring up to 4 cm in diameter[386]; cystic change may occur. Occasionally, nodules can be seen to increase and decrease in size with the menstrual cycle. In clinically suspected cases, CT may be of value in identifying lesions that are not apparent on conventional roentgenograms.[387] In pleural endometriosis, the usual roentgenographic manifestations are those of pneumothorax or hemothorax.

Most women with thoracic endometriosis are between 20 and 40 years of age. Individuals with pulmonary parenchymal involvement usually present with a history of recurrent episodes of hemoptysis. Pleural endometriosis usually manifests itself as catamenial pneumothorax or hemothorax, the main symptoms being shoulder or chest pain and dyspnea. Symptoms appear within 72 hours of the onset of menses and are typically recurrent.

Hemangioma (Pulmonary Arteriovenous Malformation)

Most, if not all, pulmonary tumors designated "hemangioma" represent either a developmental or an acquired vascular malformation rather than a true neoplasm. In the former instance, the tumor has been more appropriately termed "arteriovenous malformation" when large, and "telangiectasia" when small, although it is unclear whether there are pathogenetic differences between the two (see page 277). Acquired fistulas, more appropriately termed shunts, may be seen in a variety of circumstances and are discussed in relation to specific disease entities.

SECONDARY NEOPLASMS

The entire output of the right side of the heart as well as virtually all lymphatic fluid produced by body tissues flows through the pulmonary vascular system. It is not surprising, therefore, that secondary neoplastic involvement of the lungs is extremely common: in autopsy series of extrapulmonary cancer, the incidence of pulmonary metastases ranges from 30 to 50 per cent. The condition is thus one of great importance, because of both its serious prognostic implications and its frequency.

Pathogenesis

Secondary neoplastic involvement of the lungs, pleura, and trachea may occur by two mechanisms: (1) direct extension of tumor situated in the mediastinum, chest wall, or subphrenic space; and (2) true metastasis, usually via the pulmonary arteries, less commonly via the bronchial arteries or pulmonary lymphatics or across the pleural cavity, and rarely via the airways. Although there is overlap, each of these mechanisms and routes of spread is associated with characteristic pathologic, roentgenologic, and clinical features.

Direct Neoplastic Extension

Secondary involvement of the lung or trachea by direct extension is much less common than by metastasis. It occurs most often by invasion from a primary neoplasm in a contiguous organ or tissue, the commonest of which are thyroid[388] and esophageal carcinoma, mediastinal neoplasms such as thymoma, and chest wall sarcomas. In addition, any neoplasm metastatic to ribs or mediastinal lymph nodes can extend into the adjacent trachea or lung. Although the secondary nature of the pulmonary involvement is usually evident in these cases, the extrapulmonary source of neoplasm is occasionally inapparent. This is particularly so in the paramediastinal region, in which encroachment or invasion of the pulmonary parenchyma can simulate primary pulmonary carcinoma extending into the mediastinum.

Metastasis

Metastasis refers to the transport of viable tumor cells from one site in the body to another. Although many consider the term to include evidence of autonomous extravascular growth as well, for purposes of this discussion the authors include strictly intravascular tumor emboli as constituting true metastases. With respect to the lungs and pleura, such metastases can occur by four routes.

Spread via the Pulmonary Arteries. In this situation, tumor cells are carried to the lungs in blood of the inferior or superior vena cava or in the lymph draining from the main or right thoracic ducts. The details of the pathogenesis of metastases in these circumstances are incompletely understood and quite complex. The initial event clearly must be vascular invasion at the site of the primary neoplasm. In the case of venous invasion, individual cells or fragments of tumor (with or without admixed thrombus) are then dislodged and carried as tumor emboli to the lungs,[389] where they lodge chiefly within small pulmonary arteries or arterioles.

The fate of the emboli depends on several factors, including host inflammatory and immunologic reactions, the extent and rapidity of organization of any associated thrombus, the viability of tumor cells in their new environment, and the effects on the tumor cells of physical trauma resulting from embolization.[389, 390] In the majority of cases, it is probable that conditions are unsuitable for survival of malignant cells. Occasionally, however, there is proliferation within the vascular lumen and invasion of the adjacent wall. The location of this proliferation, perhaps in addition to as yet undefined properties of the tumor cells themselves,[391] determines the subsequent morphologic appearance of the metastasis. In most cases, there is extension of the newly formed tumor into the surrounding lung parenchyma, forming a relatively well-defined nodule. Less often, tumor cells remain confined largely to the perivascular interstitium, spreading along it and within its lymphatic channels. These are the two major morphologic manifestations of metastatic cancer in the lung and are discussed in greater detail later on.

Spread via the Pulmonary and Pleural Lymphatics. Metastatic spread within the lungs and pleura via lymphatic channels may occur in two ways. As discussed earlier, the first is by hematogenous dissemination to small pulmonary arteries and arterioles, followed by invasion of the adjacent interstitial space and lymphatics and spread along these pathways toward the hilum or periphery of the lung. That

this is the pathogenetic mechanism in most cases of pulmonary lymphangitic spread is suggested by the high frequency of concurrent intravascular cancer or thrombosis, or both, and by the frequent absence of neoplasm in bronchopulmonary and hilar lymph nodes.[392]

The second mechanism is by retrograde extension along lymphatic channels. In the usual course of events, tumor first spreads from an extrathoracic site to mediastinal lymph nodes. This is followed by retrograde extension to hilar and bronchopulmonary nodes and then by spread within pleural and pulmonary lymphatics. Communicating lymphatic channels between the basal pulmonary and diaphragmatic pleura and upper abdominal lymph nodes[393] and the peritoneal cavity[394] also may provide a direct route for lymphatic spread of intra-abdominal malignancy.

Spread via the Pleural Space. Such spread occurs when individual tumor cells or small tumor fragments are liberated into the pleural space and are carried within pleural fluid to another site. The precise mechanisms of tumor adherence and invasion at the secondary foci are not clear. In one histologic study of peritoneal metastases of ovarian carcinoma,[395] tumor cells were associated with focal mesothelial damage and an underlying inflammatory reaction. The tumor appeared to proliferate in the resulting exudate as it organized, eventually forming a well-developed metastatic nodule. Similar mechanisms presumably prevail in transpleural metastases.

Spread via the Airways. This method of tumor dissemination has been proposed for both extrapulmonary and primary pulmonary tumors (especially bronchioloalveolar carcinoma); however, except for the latter condition, its existence is probably rare and, in an individual patient, difficult to prove.

Patterns of Secondary Neoplastic Disease

Although metastasis by each of the routes just described frequently results in characteristic pathologic and roentgenologic manifestations, overlap is common. For example, tumor that metastasizes via the pulmonary artery can result in either a nodular parenchymal or an interstitial pattern of growth or both. Because of this, it is useful to discuss the clinicopathologic and roentgenologic features of pulmonary metastases in terms of patterns of disease, of which five can be recognized: parenchymal nodules, lymphatic and interstitial spread, tumor emboli, endobronchial tumor, and pleural effusion (the last-named being discussed in Chapter 18).

Parenchymal Nodules

This is the commonest manifestation of metastatic disease to the lungs. The nodules are multiple in 75 per cent of cases (Fig. 8–63) and tend to be most numerous in the basal portions of the lungs, reflecting gravity-induced preferential blood flow.[396] They range in size from barely visible to huge growths that occupy virtually the entire volume of one lung. Although most often discrete, individual deposits may enlarge and become confluent, resulting in multinodular masses. Rarely, nodular deposits are so numerous and of such minute size as to suggest miliary tuberculosis (Fig. 8–64).

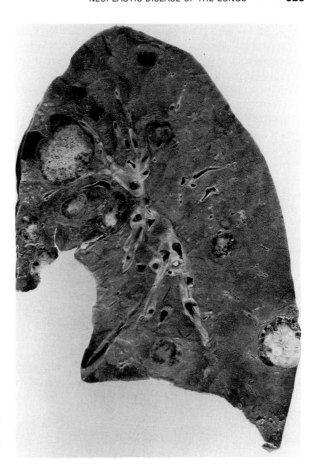

Figure 8–63. Metastatic Choriocarcinoma: Multiple Parenchymal Nodules. A slice of right lung obtained at autopsy of a young man with testicular chorio-carcinoma reveals multiple, variably sized, well-circumscribed nodules in the lung parenchyma.

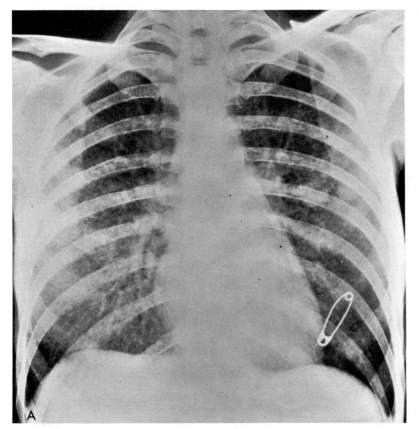

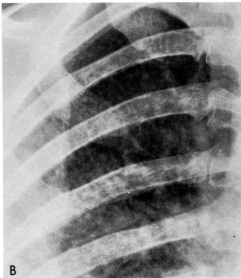

Figure 8–64. Diffuse Micronodular Metastases: Cho-riocarcinoma. An anteroposterior roentgenogram *(A)* reveals widespread nodular deposits distributed evenly throughout both lungs. In some areas, the nodules are sharply defined, but in others they are indistinct and partly coalescent, as revealed to bet-ter advantage in the magnified view of the right up-per zone *(B)*.

When nodules are multiple, the probability that they represent metastases is obviously increased. Conversely, although a solitary nodule can be a metastasis, the possibility that it represents a primary carcinoma is greater. From a diagnostic viewpoint, therefore, nodular metastases are best discussed under the headings solitary and multiple.

Solitary Nodules. Metastatic neoplasms that present as solitary parenchymal nodules are distinctly uncommon; in the all-male Veterans' Administration series of 887 asymptomatic patients with solitary pulmonary "nodules" 7 cm or less in diameter, only 3 per cent were metastases.[91] The vast majority occurred in patients aged 50 years or more, in whom the incidence was 5 per cent. Although identification of a primary neoplasm elsewhere or a history of resection of a primary neoplasm greatly increases the likelihood of a lesion being metastatic, it must be remembered that even in these situations, this is not invariable. For example, in one study of 50 patients previously treated for a malignancy and without evidence of metastases elsewhere, 18 had single intrathoracic lesions that proved to be unrelated pulmonary or mediastinal tumors.[397]

Certain neoplasms are more likely than others to produce solitary metastases. These include carcinoma of the colon (particularly of the rectosigmoid area, which accounts for 30 to 40 per cent of all cases); sarcomas (particularly those originating in bone); carcinoma of the kidney, testicle, and breast; and melanoma.[91]

In those situations with known extrathoracic malignancy, TTNA may be helpful in determining the primary or metastatic nature of the pulmonary nodule. By demonstrating other pulmonary nodules not visible on plain roentgenograms, CT scanning can also aid in distinguishing primary from metastatic tumors.

Multiple Nodules. The roentgenographic pattern of multiple pulmonary nodules varies from diffuse micronodular shadows resembling miliary disease to multiple, large, well-defined masses—the "cannonball" type of metastases (Fig. 8–65). The lesions may be of uniform size, indicating a simultaneous origin in one shower of emboli, or may differ, suggesting embolic inoculations of different ages. This latter pattern is rare in cases of benign diffuse nodular pulmonary disease. Most individual shadows are fairly sharply defined. Occasionally, some are rather indistinct, with fuzzy margins; when these reach 5 to 6 mm in diameter, they can simulate the rosette pattern of acinar filling diseases.

Cavitation of metastatic parenchymal nodules is not as common as with primary lung carcinoma. As with the latter, cavitation occurs most often in squamous cell carcinoma and is commoner in the upper than in the lower lobes. The site of the primary neoplasm is most frequently in the head and neck or cervix. Calcification of metastatic lesions is rare and almost invariably indicates that the primary neoplasm is osteogenic sarcoma, chondrosarcoma, or synovial sarcoma.[398] Mediastinal and hilar nodes are usually not enlarged.

The great majority of patients have a previously diagnosed extrathoracic neoplasm or clinical findings directly referable to a synchronous primary tumor. The signs and symptoms related to parenchymal nodules themselves are very uncommon but can be identical to those of primary pulmonary tumors. Extension of tumor into an adjacent

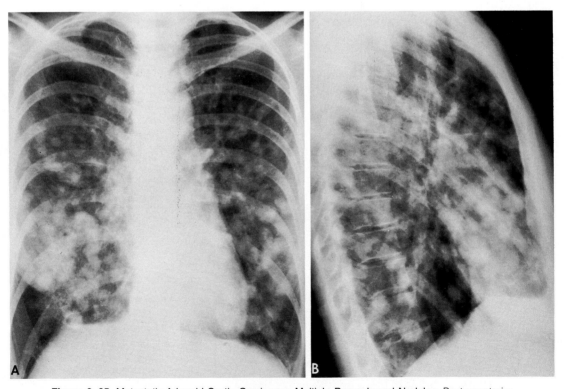

Figure 8–65. Metastatic Adenoid Cystic Carcinoma: Multiple Parenchymal Nodules. Posteroanterior *(A)* and lateral *(B)* roentgenograms reveal multiple nodules of homogeneous density ranging in size from 5 mm to 2 cm, distributed widely throughout both lungs. The apices and bases are relatively less affected than the midzones. There is no evidence of cavitation.

bronchial wall may result in cough, hemoptysis, or wheezing, and invasion of the apical chest wall may result in Pancoast's syndrome. When tumor volume is substantial, dyspnea may result. The occurrence of hypertrophic pulmonary osteoarthropathy[399] or spontaneous pneumothorax[400] should suggest sarcoma as the primary neoplasm.

Lymphatic and Interstitial Infiltration (Lymphangitic Carcinomatosis)

These terms refer to tumor growth in lymphatic channels and in the peribronchovascular and interlobular connective tissue that surrounds them (Fig. 8–66). Although any metastatic neoplasm can have this pattern, the commonest are those found in the breast, stomach, pancreas, and prostate.[392]

Roentgenographic evidence of lymphangitic carcinomatosis is much less common than is found pathologically.[396] The pattern consists of coarsened bronchovascular markings of irregular contour, sometimes indistinctly defined, simulating interstitial pulmonary edema (Fig. 8–67). Septal lines (Kerley B lines) are present in most cases (Fig. 8–68). In the majority of patients, the pattern is uniform throughout both lungs, although it is more obvious in the lower zones. In some cases, however, the disease is unilateral. The linear accentuation is sometimes associated with a nodular component, resulting from intraparenchymal extension of tumor, thus creating a very coarse reticulonodular pattern. Hilar and mediastinal lymph node enlargement or pleural effusion are present in some cases.

CT findings in lymphangitic carcinomatosis include thickening of the pulmonary interstitium, an increase in the number of peripheral lines (1 to 2 cm in length), a diffuse increase in linear and curvilinear structures toward the center of the lung, polygonal structures 1 to 2 cm in diameter (not seen at all in normal subjects), and thickening of interlobar fissures.[401]

The commonest clinical manifestation is dyspnea; it is typically insidious in onset but progresses rapidly and within a few weeks can cause severe disability. In fact, in the authors' experience, patients who present with rapidly progressive dyspnea and a coarse linear or reticulonodular pattern on chest roentgenograms have almost invariably been shown to have lymphangitic carcinomatosis, even in the absence of a clinically recognized primary site. The exception is the patient with acute interstitial edema secondary to cardiac failure.

Tumor Emboli

Intravascular neoplasm in metastatic carcinoma to the lungs is common at autopsy. It is seen most often with adenocarcinoma,[402] especially of the breast or stomach. As might be expected, the frequency and extent of vascular involvement is higher in cases with concomitant liver metastases.[403] Probably for the same reason, an unusually high frequency of this form of metastisis is seen in hepatoma, out of proportion to the incidence of the neoplasm.[402] Usually, tumor is identified only histologically, in small to medium-sized muscular arteries and arterioles. Occasionally, emboli occur in segmental and larger arteries and may result in infarction or sudden death.[403]

Although intravascular tumor emboli are usually accompanied by evidence of another pattern of pulmonary involvement (most often lymphangitic carcinomatosis), they may be the sole manifestation of metastatic pulmonary disease. In such cases, the chest roentgenogram may be entirely normal or may show dilatation of central pulmonary arteries and the right ventricle, reflecting pulmonary hypertension.[404] Radionuclide perfusion lung scans may show mismatched ventilation-perfusion defects that are virtually indistinguishable from pulmonary thromboembolic disease.

Clinical symptoms caused by tumor emboli alone are usually absent, and the condition is not regarded as a common cause of death.[403] When present, the commonest complaint is dyspnea; signs of cor pulmonale of relatively recent onset are often present. Occasionally, pleuritic chest pain and hemoptysis indicate infarction. A past history of carcinoma or evidence of a coexisting extrathoracic primary is usually evident.

Bronchial and Tracheal Metastases

Neoplastic infiltration of a bronchial wall is usually caused by direct extension from a parenchymal tumor or an involved lymph node or by more or less diffuse mucosal infiltration as part of lymphangitic carcinomatosis. The majority of cases are incidental microscopic findings seen by the pathologist at autopsy; even those grossly visible are usually of such small size that they do not manifest themselves either roentgenographically or clinically. Occasionally, however, involvement of a bronchial wall may be relatively well localized. Considerable intraluminal growth may then occur in the absence of other recognizable pulmonary metastases or primary neoplasm, leading to an erroneous diagnosis of primary bronchogenic carcinoma. The commonest neoplasms to present in this way are breast, colorectum, kidney, and melanoma.

The usual roentgenologic findings are those of bronchial obstruction, either partial (causing oligemia and expiratory air trapping) or complete (with atelectasis and obstructive pneumonitis). In most cases, the primary site is clinically apparent before symptoms related to endobronchial metastases develop.[405] When they occur, symptoms consist of wheeze, hemoptysis, and persistent cough; the last-named may result in expectoration of diagnostic tumor fragments.

Specific Primary Sites and Tumors

Lung. Autopsy studies have shown the presence of lung metastases from primary pulmonary carcinoma in 7 to 50 per cent of cases.[406, 407] The high incidence in these series reflects a thorough pathologic search for tumor deposits, many of which are undetectable on conventional chest roentgenograms. As might be expected, poorly or undifferentiated carcinomas are most commonly implicated.

Roentgenographic detection of lung metastases from primary pulmonary carcinoma at the time of presentation is very uncommon, with two exceptions: (1) small cell carcinoma, in which metastases to the opposite lung have been found at the time of diagnosis in as many as 8 per cent of patients in some studies[408]; and (2) the diffuse form of bronchioloalveolar cell carcinoma, in which bilateral and sometimes extensive lung involvement is common. With

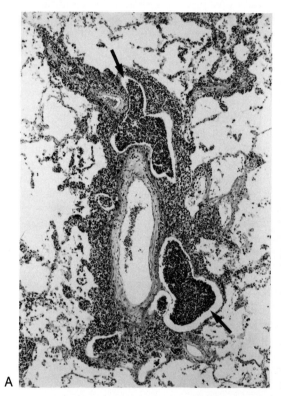

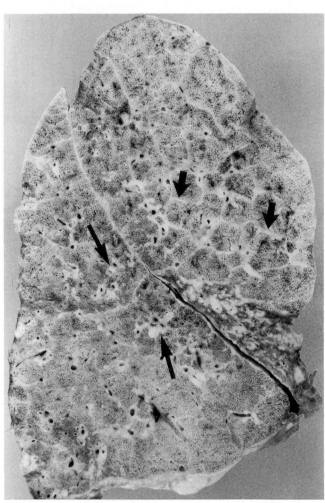

Figure 8–66. Metastatic Carcinoma: Lymphangitic Spread. *A,* Histologic appearance, showing the tissue surrounding a pulmonary vein to be thickened by a combination of intralymphatic tumor plugs *(arrows)* and interstitial tumor infiltration by small cell lung carcinoma. *B,* Gross appearance manifested in a section of left lung showing extensive infiltration of interlobular septa *(short arrows)* and peribronchovascular tissue *(long arrows)* by breast carcinoma. *(A × 52.)*

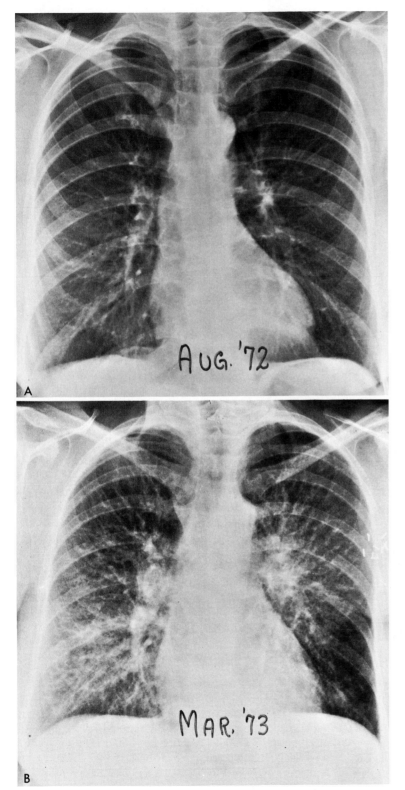

Figure 8–67. Lymphangitic Spread: Carcinoma of the Breast. At the time of the normal roentgenogram illustrated in *A*, this 50-year-old woman was discovered to have a carcinoma of the left breast, and a modified radical mastectomy was carried out. Seven months later, at which time she was complaining of progressively increasing dyspnea, a roentgenogram *(B)* revealed extensive involvement of both lungs by a coarse linear and reticular pattern associated with bilateral hilar lymph node enlargement. Note the loss of lung volume that has occurred in this interval as a result of reduced compliance.

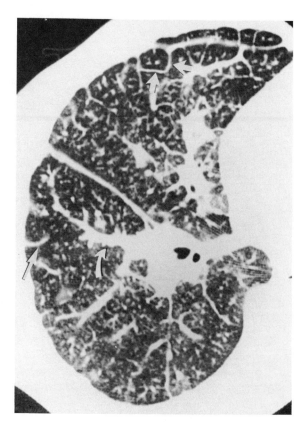

Figure 8–68. Lymphangitic Spread: CT Manifestations. High-resolution CT scan of the right lung shows irregular nodular thickening of the bronchovascular bundles *(curved arrow)* and interlobular septa *(straight arrows)*. Although these findings are characteristic of lymphangitic carcinomatosis, a similar appearance can also be seen in lymphoma, Kaposi's sarcoma, and pulmonary edema. (From Mathieson JR, Mayo JR, Staples CA, Müller NL: Chronic diffuse infiltrative lung disease: Comparison of diagnostic accuracy of CT and chest radiography. Radiology 171: 111–116, 1989.)

other forms of carcinoma, the presence of metastases can be identified with certainty only in the presence of multiple nodules. When only two tumor masses are seen, it is more likely that they represent separate primary tumors rather than a primary tumor with a solitary metastasis.

Kidney. Since approximately 30 per cent of all cases of renal cell carcinoma have distant metastases when first seen and since as many as 30 to 40 per cent of patients with pulmonary metastases have no symptoms referable to the kidney,[409] differentiation of a solitary metastasis from a primary pulmonary carcinoma can be a problem, especially if the metastasis is predominantly endobronchial. This difficulty is compounded by the histologic variability of the tumor: although most metastases have the classic clear cell appearance of renal cell carcinoma, occasionally the presence of a sarcomatous or other histologic pattern can cause considerable diagnostic problems for the pathologist.

The commonest intrathoracic roentgenologic presentation of metastatic renal cell carcinoma is as a solitary or multiple pulmonary nodules. Occasionally, these grow very slowly. Metastases are also fairly frequently endobronchial, in which circumstance they may be associated with roentgenographic evidence of partial or complete airway obstruction. Occasionally, hilar node enlargement without associated pulmonary disease is the sole manifestation.[410]

Except in the occasional patient with an endobronchial metastasis, in whom there may be cough and hemoptysis, symptoms are usually absent. A history of previous renal cell carcinoma or evidence of a synchronous tumor is often apparent; however, as noted previously, many patients have no renal symptomatology when the carcinoma is discov-

ered. It is important to remember that there may be a considerable time interval between the initial discovery of the renal tumor and the identification of metastasis; presentation up to 50 years after excision of the primary tumor has been documented.[411]

Colorectum. Metastases to the lung in colorectal carcinoma are second in frequency only to those to the liver, the overall frequency probably being 15 to 20 per cent.[412] Although metastases are usually multiple, a solitary metastasis is not infrequent. In fact, the tumor accounts for 30 to 40 per cent of all solitary metastatic neoplasms to the lung[91] and is much more likely than other primary tumors to be the cause of such a nodule. Despite this, in a patient with a solitary nodule and known colonic carcinoma, the metastatic nature of the nodule is not at all certain.[413]

Liver. Pulmonary metastases in hepatocellular carcinoma have been recorded in almost two thirds of cases in some series.[414] As might be expected, their presence is closely related to intrahepatic vascular invasion. Tumor emboli, particularly those grossly visible, are especially common.[402]

Breast. Although metastases from breast carcinoma can occur both hematogenously and by lymphatic and interstitial spread, it is probable that the latter is the commoner mechanism.[415] Detailed examination of mediastinal lymph nodes suggests that the mechanism of spread in many cases is metastasis from the breast to mediastinal lymph nodes, and thence to the pleura and lung. Clinically significant endobronchial tumor also occurs relatively frequently. Although an uncommon presenting feature, it may be the first indication of recurrence of a previously resected tumor.[416] Pleural effusion tends to be a late manifestation; most effusions are unilateral and located on the same side as the affected breast.

Thyroid. In patients with anaplastic thyroid carcinoma, direct extension of tumor into the trachea is a common occurrence,[388] in which case it is often an important factor in causing death; pulmonary metastases are also frequent. By contrast, pulmonary metastases are rather uncommon in papillary and follicular carcinomas, occurring in only 5 to 10 per cent of patients.[417] Roentgenographically, the former tends to have a micronodular pattern (resembling miliary tuberculosis) or a reticulonodular pattern (simulating interstitial fibrosis). It is often associated with cervical lymph node metastases but not with systemic spread. By contrast, metastases from follicular carcinoma tend to develop into larger parenchymal nodules and are frequently associated with concomitant skeletal metastases.

Oral Cavity and Larynx. Patients with pulmonary carcinoma are at increased risk for the development of carcinoma elsewhere, especially in the oral cavity and larynx.[418] In many of these patients, the pulmonary tumor is detected after that in the head and neck region, raising the possibility that it is, in fact, a metastasis. In the authors' experience, however, this is an uncommon occurrence and usually is associated with cervical lymph node enlargement.

Testis. Pulmonary metastases occur with considerable frequency with any of the histologic variants of malignant testicular neoplasms and usually take the form of solitary or, more commonly, multiple parenchymal nodules. CT scans reveal enlarged, low-density abdominal and pelvic lymph nodes in almost 50 per cent of patients. This low-density characteristic can also be present in metastases, and it has been suggested that when a low-attenuation pulmonary or mediastinal mass is discovered in a patient of appropriate age, search for a primary testicular neoplasm should be initiated.[419]

Clinical signs and symptoms are seldom apparent; occasionally, choriocarcinoma causes pulmonary hemorrhage and hemoptysis. A history of a previous testicular tumor can usually be obtained.

Melanoma. Pulmonary metastases from melanoma were documented in 12 per cent of patients in one large series.[420] Although many occur early in the course of disease, a substantial number are identified 10 years or more after the appearance of the skin tumor. Solitary or multiple nodules are the typical roentgenographic appearance.

Endometrium. Endometrial adenocarcinoma metastasizes to the lungs infrequently. In one series of 470 patients, only 11 (2.3 per cent) developed the complication within the follow-up period of 2 to 12 years.[421] Most have concomitant disease in other viscera or lymph nodes.

Uterine Cervix. The incidence of pulmonary metastases in patients with invasive cervical carcinoma has been estimated to be about 10 per cent.[422] The likelihood of pulmonary involvement correlates with the stage of the disease and the cell type. Metastases seldom develop in patients with squamous cell carcinoma diagnosed in its early stages, whereas in patients with adenocarcinoma, metastases tend to occur regardless of the stage at diagnosis.[423] Multiple nodules are the usual manifestation.

Ovary. Thoracic metastases in ovarian carcinoma have

been detected in about 50 per cent of patients at autopsy.[424] Pleural effusion is the commonest manifestation, a finding undoubtedly related to the high incidence of visceral and parietal pleural disease caused by direct spread from the peritoneal cavity via diaphragmatic lymphatics.[394] In most cases, pulmonary parenchymal tumor is contiguous with pleural metastases and probably represents direct extension from these sites rather than independent hematogenous deposits.

Prostate. Roentgenographically detectable lesions are present in about 5 to 15 per cent of cases of prostatic carcinoma.[425] Osteoblastic metastases to the thoracic skeleton may be present and are a clue to the diagnosis.

Choriocarcinoma. Pulmonary metastases in gestationally related choriocarcinoma are extremely common.[426] They are invariably hematogenous and are usually manifested roentgenographically by multiple parenchymal nodules (see Fig. 8–63, page 523). Less often, there are numerous tiny opacities simulating miliary tuberculosis. Therapy usually results in complete regression of the nodules, although fibrosis (with or without dystrophic calcification) is sometimes evident at the site of previous disease. Symptoms are usually absent, although dyspnea may develop and progress to respiratory failure,[427] and hemoptysis can occur as a result of intrapulmonary hemorrhage.[426]

Leiomyosarcoma. Metastatic leiomyosarcoma to the lungs may be clearly malignant histologically and clinically, in which circumstance there is usually a well-documented history of an extrathoracic primary tumor (most often of the uterus), and the diagnosis is straightforward. Sometimes, however, diagnostic difficulties arise when an excised pulmonary nodule of apparent smooth muscle origin possesses a bland histologic appearance, and there is no clear-cut evidence of an extrathoracic malignancy. Several interpretations have been given for these tumors.

1. Some tumors are presumed to represent primary pulmonary smooth muscle neoplasms.

2. Others have been referred to as "pulmonary fibroleiomyomas" and have been hypothesized to represent an unusual form of hamartoma.

3. Still others are associated with known uterine "leiomyomas" and have been considered to represent metastases from this site (so-called benign metastasizing leiomyomas). For a variety of reasons, it is now clear that tumors in the last two groups in fact represent metastatic well-differentiated leiomyosarcoma.[428]

Roentgenographically, these uncommon tumors are usually multiple and bilateral and range from 0.5 to 5.0 cm in diameter.[428] They can increase both in size and in number,[429] or new nodules may appear while others shrink and actually disappear. Such regression has been reported following termination of pregnancy, suggesting a hormonal effect on tumor growth.[430] Calcification is usually not evident.

Because the uterus is by far the commonest primary tumor site, these neoplasms occur almost exclusively in women. The pulmonary lesions can be present at the same time the uterine neoplasm is recognized, but more often they appear after hysterectomy, sometimes after an interval of 20 to 30 years. Metastases usually do not produce symptoms and are discovered incidentally on a screening chest roentgenogram. The prognosis is variable and difficult to predict. One review documented an excellent prognosis in patients with only a few nodules; however, even with extensive pulmonary involvement, both long-term and short-term survivors were found.[431]

Other Soft Tissue Sarcomas. The lung is the commonest site of metastasis for a variety of other soft tissue sarcomas.[432] In most cases, a primary source is clearly evident, and the diagnosis of metastasis is easily established on plain roentgenograms. Rarely, one or more lung nodules are evident before the clinical appearance of the primary sarcoma, notably in relation to alveolar soft part sarcoma.[433]

Sarcoma of Bone. Metastases to the lungs from sarcomas of bone are frequent, especially from osteosarcoma. The typical roentgenographic appearance is of multiple nodules, usually bilateral and, in cases of osteogenic sarcoma, calcified or ossified. A history of synchronous or previous primary bone neoplasm is almost invariable.[434] The majority of metastases do not produce symptoms; however, they can be so numerous as to cause respiratory insufficiency. Spontaneous pneumothorax is a well-recognized complication of osteogenic sarcoma.[400]

Laboratory Findings

Cytology

Malignant cells can be detected in sputum or bronchial washings in 35 to 50 per cent of patients with metastatic cancer to the lungs.[435] Cytologic examination of pleural fluid of malignant origin gives a somewhat higher yield, most series obtaining an accuracy of about 50 per cent.[436] Of greater importance in the diagnosis of metastatic disease is TTNA; with this technique, experienced practitioners can prove the malignant nature of a lesion in 85 to 90 per cent of cases. In fact, when the site of the extrathoracic primary tumor is known, a definitive cytologic diagnosis of metastatic cancer is frequently possible.

Bronchoscopy

Bronchoscopic examination is not as productive in the diagnosis of pulmonary metastases as in primary lung cancer. In one study of patients with lung metastases who underwent bronchoscopy, the incidence of a positive diagnosis was highest in colorectal (79 per cent) and breast cancers (57 per cent), and lowest in genitourinary cancer (33 per cent).[437] As might be expected, a positive yield is highest in tumors with endobronchial extension.

Pulmonary Function Tests

During the early stages of disease, the great majority of patients with pulmonary metastases have normal pulmonary function. In fact, metastases may be widespread before patients note the onset of dyspnea. Both diffusing capacity and lung compliance are uniformly reduced in patients with lymphangitic carcinomatosis. In those with hematogenous metastases, however, they are reduced only if the nodules are exceptionally numerous.[438]

References

1. Silverberg E, Lubera JA: Cancer Statistics, 1989. CA 39: 3, 1989.
2. Devesa SS, Blot WJ, Fraumeni JF Jr: Declining lung cancer rates among young men and women in the United States: A cohort analysis. J Natl Cancer Inst 81: 1568, 1989.
3. Brancker A: Lung cancer and smoking prevalence in Canada. Health Rep 2: 67, 1990.
4. Andrews JL Jr, Bloom S, Balogh K, et al: Lung cancer in women: Lahey Clinic experience, 1957–1980. Cancer 55: 2894, 1985.
5. Sterling TD, Weinkam JJ: Comparison of smoking-related risk factors among black and white males. Am J Ind Med 15: 319, 1989.
6. Enstrom J: Rising lung cancer mortality among nonsmokers. J Natl Cancer Inst 62: 755, 1979.
6a. Morabia A, Wynder EL: Relation of bronchioloalveolar carcinoma to tobacco. Br Med J 304: 541, 1992.
7. Brownson RC, Reif JS, Keefe TJ, et al: Risk factors for adenocarcinoma of the lung. Am J Epidemiol 125: 25, 1987.
8. Boucot KR, Cooper DA, Weiss W, et al: Cigarettes, cough, and cancer of the lung. JAMA 196: 985, 1966.
9. Higgins IT, Mahan CM, Wynder EL: Lung cancer among cigar and pipe smokers. Prev Med 17: 116, 1988.
10. Spitzer WO, Lawrence V, Dales R, et al: Links between passive smoking and disease: A best-evidence synthesis. A report of the Working Group on Passive Smoking. Clin Invest Med 13: 17, 1990.
10a. Trichopoulos D, Mollo F, Tomatis L, et al: Active and passive smoking and pathological indicators of lung cancer risk in an autopsy study. JAMA 268: 1697, 1992.
11. Janerich DT, Thompson WD, Varela LR, et al: Lung cancer and exposure to tobacco smoke in the household. N Engl J Med 323: 632, 1990.
12. Ockene JK, Kuller LH, Svendsen KH, et al: The relationship of smoking cessation to coronary heart disease and lung cancer in the Multiple Risk Factor Intervention Trial (MRFIT). Am J Public Health 80: 954, 1990.
13. Kaufman DW, Palmer JR, Rosenberg L, et al: Tar content of cigarettes in relation to lung cancer. Am J Epidemiol 129: 703, 1989.
14. Wynder EL, Hoffman D: Tobacco and health: A societal challenge. N Engl J Med 300: 894, 1979.
15. Stanton MF, Miller E, Wrench C, et al: Experimental induction of epidermoid carcinoma in the lungs of rats by cigarette smoke condensate. J Natl Cancer Inst 49: 867, 1972.
16. Auerbach O, Stout AP, Hammond EC, et al: Changes in bronchial epithelium in relation to cigarette smoking and in relation to lung cancer. N Engl J Med 265: 253, 1961.
17. Auerbach O, Stout AP, Hammond EC, et al: Bronchial epithelium in former smokers. N Engl J Med 267: 119, 1962.
18. Finkelstein MM: Mortality among employees of an Ontario asbestos-cement factory. Am Rev Respir Dis 129: 754, 1984.
19. Enterline FE: Attributability in the face of uncertainty. Chest 78: 377, 1980.
20. Becklake MR: Asbestos-related diseases of the lung and other organs: Their epidemiology and implications for clinical practice. Am Rev Respir Dis 14: 187, 1976.
21. Mossman BT, Eastman A, Bresnick E: Asbestos and benzo[a]pyrene act synergistically to induce squamous metaplasia and incorporation of (^{3}H)thymidine in hamster tracheal epithelium. Carcinogenesis 5: 1401, 1984.
22. Hughes JM, Weill H: Asbestosis as a precursor of asbestos-related lung cancer: Results of a prospective mortality study. Br J Ind Med 48: 229, 1991.
23. Warnock ML, Isenberg W: Asbestos burden and the pathology of lung cancer. Chest 89: 20, 1986.
24. Chovil A, Sutherland RB, Halliday M: Respiratory cancer in a cohort of nickel sinter plant workers. Br J Ind Med 38: 327, 1981.
25. Davies JM, Easton DF, Bidstrup PL: Mortality from respiratory cancer and other causes in United Kingdom chromate production workers. Br J Ind Med 48: 299, 1991.
26. Welch K, Higgins L, Oh M, et al: Arsenic exposure, smoking, and respiratory cancer in copper smelter workers. Arch Environ Health 37: 325, 1982.
27. Ott MG, Holder BB, Gordon HL: Respiratory cancer and occupational exposure to arsenicals. Arch Environ Health 29: 250, 1974.
28. McCallum RI, Woolley V, Petrie A: Lung cancer associated with

chloromethyl methyl ether manufacture: An investigation at two factories in the United Kingdom. Br J Ind Med 40: 384, 1983.

29. Infante-Rivard C, Armstrong B, Petitclerc M, et al: Lung cancer mortality and silicosis in Québec, 1938–85. Lancet 2: 1504, 1989.

30. Meijers JM, Swaen GM, Slangen JJ, et al: Long-term mortality in miners with coal workers' pneumoconiosis in The Netherlands: A pilot study. Am J Ind Med 19: 43, 1991.

31. Wada S, Miyanishi M, Nishimoto Y, et al: Mustard gas as a cause of respiratory neoplasia in man. Lancet 1: 1161, 1968.

32. Parkes HG, Vevs CA, Waterhouse JAH, et al: Cancer mortality in the British rubber industry. Br J Ind Med 39: 209, 1982.

33. Bertrand JP, Chau N, Patris A, et al: Mortality due to respiratory cancers in the coke oven plants of the Lorraine coal-mining industry (Houilleres du Bassin de Lorraine). Br J Ind Med 44: 559, 1987.

34. Hagmar L, Akesson B, Nielsen J, et al: Mortality and cancer morbidity in workers exposed to low levels of vinyl chloride monomer at a polyvinyl chloride processing plant. Am J Ind Med 17: 553, 1990.

35. Simonato L, Fletcher AC, Cherrie J, et al: Updating lung cancer mortality among a cohort of man-made mineral fibre production workers in seven European countries. Cancer Lett 30: 18, 1986.

36. Kazantizis G, Lam TH, Sullivan KR: Mortality of cadmium-exposed workers: A five-year update. Scand J Work Environ Health 14: 220, 1988.

37. Wong O: A cohort mortality study of employees exposed to chlorinated chemicals. Am J Ind Med 14: 417, 1988.

38. Steenland K, Ward E: Lung cancer incidence among patients with beryllium disease: A cohort mortality study. J Natl Cancer Inst 83: 1380, 1991.

39. Sterling TD, Weinkam JJ: Reanalysis of lung cancer mortality in a National Cancer Institute study on mortality among industrial workers exposed to formaldehyde. J Occup Med 30: 895, 1988.

40. List AF, Doll DC, Greco FA: Lung cancer in Hodgkin's disease: Association with previous radiotherapy. J Clin Oncol 3: 215, 1985.

41. Fosså SD, Langmark F, Aass N, et al: Second non–germ cell malignancies after radiotherapy of testicular cancer with or without chemotherapy. Br J Cancer 61: 639, 1990.

42. Harley NH, Harley JH: Potential lung cancer risk from indoor radon exposure. CA 40: 265, 1990.

42a. Neuberger JS: Residential radon exposure and lung cancer: An overview of published studies. Cancer Detect Prev 15: 435, 1991.

43. Little JB, Radford EP Jr, McCombs HL, et al: Distribution of polonium-210 in pulmonary tissues of cigarette smokers. N Engl J Med 273: 1343, 1965.

44. Byrne JC, Tsao M, Fraser RS, et al: Human papillomavirus-11 DNA in a patient with chronic laryngotracheobronchial papillomatosis and metastatic squamous-cell carcinoma of the lung. N Engl J Med 317: 873, 1987.

45. Béjui-Thivolet F, Liagre N, Chignol MC, et al: Detection of human papillomavirus DNA in squamous bronchial metaplasia and squamous cell carcinoma of the lung by in situ hybridization using biotinylated probes in paraffin-embedded specimens. Hum Pathol 21: 111, 1990.

46. Butler AE, Colby TV, Weiss L, et al: Lymphoepithelioma-like carcinoma of the lung. Am J Surg Pathol 13: 632, 1989.

47. Auerbach O, Garfinkel L, Parks VR: Scar cancer of the lung: Increase over a 21-year period. Cancer 43: 636, 1979.

48. El-Torky M, Giltman LI, Dabbous M: Collagens in scar carcinoma of the lung. Am J Pathol 121: 322, 1985.

49. Roumm AD, Medsger TA Jr: Cancer and systemic sclerosis: An epidemiologic study. Arthritis Rheum 28: 1336, 1985.

50. Snider GL, Placik B: The relationship between pulmonary tuberculosis and bronchogenic carcinoma: A topographic study. Am Rev Respir Dis 99: 229, 1969.

51. Nomura A, Stemmermann GN, Chyou PH, et al: Prospective study of pulmonary function and lung cancer. Am Rev Respir Dis 144: 307, 1991.

52. Menkes MS, Comstock GW, Vuilleumier JP, et al: Serum beta-carotene, vitamins A and E, selenium, and the risk of lung cancer. N Engl J Med 315: 1250, 1986.

53. Fraser DE, Beeson WL, Phillips RL: Diet and lung cancer in California Seventh-day Adventists. Am J Epidemiol 133: 683, 1991.

54. Wynder EL, Hebert JR, Kabat GC: Association of dietary fat and lung cancer. J Natl Cancer Inst 79: 631, 1987.

55. Shekelle RB, Rossof AH, Stamler J: Dietary cholesterol and incidence of lung cancer: The Western Electric Study. Am J Epidemiol 134: 480, 1991.

56. Howowitz RI, Smaldone LF, Viscoli CM: An ecogenetic hypothesis for lung cancer in women. Arch Intern Med 148: 2609, 1988.

57. Paul SM, Bacharach B, Goepp C: A genetic influence on alveolar cell carcinoma. J Surg Oncol 36: 249, 1987.

58. Nakachi K, Imai K, Hayashi S, et al: Genetic susceptibility to squamous cell carcinoma of the lung in relation to cigarette smoking dose. Cancer Res 51: 5177, 1991.

59. Ginns LC, Goldenheim PD, Miller LG, et al: T-lymphocyte subsets in smoking and lung cancer: Analysis by monoclonal antibodies and flow cytometry. Am Rev Respir Dis 126: 265, 1982.

60. Kubota M, Kagamimori S, Yokoyama K, et al: Reduced killer cell activity of lymphocytes from patients with asbestosis. Br J Ind Med 42: 276, 1985.

61. Van Leeuwen FE, Somers R, Taal BG, et al: Increased risk of lung cancer, non-Hodgkin's lymphoma, and leukemia following Hodgkin's disease. J Clin Oncol 7: 1046, 1989.

62. Braun MA, Killam DA, Remick SC, et al: Lung cancer in patients seropositive for human immunodeficiency virus. Radiology 175: 341, 1990.

63. Kreyberg L: International histological classification of tumours. In Histological Typing of Lung Tumours. Geneva, World Health Organization, 1981.

64. Hirsch FR, Matthews MJ, Yesner R: Histopathologic classification of small cell carcinoma of the lung. Cancer 50: 1360, 1982.

65. Haratake J, Horie A, Tokudome S, et al: Inter- and intra-pathologist variability in histologic diagnoses of lung cancer. Acta Pathol Jpn 37: 1053, 1987.

66. Feinstein AR, Gelfman NA, Yesner R, et al: Observer variability in the histopathologic diagnosis of lung cancer. Am Rev Respir Dis 101: 671, 1970.

67. Lisa JR, Trinidad S, Rosenblatt MB: Site of origin, histogenesis, and cytostructure of bronchogenic carcinoma. Am J Clin Pathol 44: 375, 1965.

68. Nagamoto N, Saito Y, Suda H, et al: Relationship between length of longitudinal extension and maximal depth of transmural invasion in roentgenographically occult squamous cell carcinoma of the bronchus (nonpolypoid type). Am J Surg Pathol 13: 11, 1989.

69. Carter D: Small-cell carcinoma of the lung. Am J Surg Pathol 7: 787, 1983.

70. Nomori H, Shimosato Y, Kodama T, et al: Subtypes of small cell carcinoma of the lung: Morphometric, ultrastructural, and immunohistochemical analyses. Hum Pathol 17: 604, 1986.

70a. Fraire AE, Johnson EH, Yesner R, et al: Prognostic significance of histopathologic subtype and stage in small cell lung cancer. Hum Pathol 23: 520, 1992.

71. Radice PA, Matthews MJ, Ihde DC, et al: The clinical behavior of "mixed" small cell–large cell bronchogenic carcinoma compared to "pure" small cell subtypes. Cancer 50: 2894, 1982.

72. Gould VE, Warren WH, Memoli VA: Neuroendocrine neoplasms of the lung. In Becker KL, Gazdar AF (eds): The Endocrine Lung in Health and Disease. Philadelphia, WB Saunders, 1984, p 406.

73. Said JW, Vimadalal S, Nash G, et al: Immunoreactive neuron-specific enolase, bombesin, and chromogranin as markers for neuroendocrine lung tumors. Hum Pathol 16: 236, 1985.

74. Ogata O, Endo K: Clara cell granules of peripheral lung cancers. Cancer 54: 1635, 1984.

75. Kimula Y: A histochemical and ultrastructural study of adenocarcinoma of the lung. Am J Surg Pathol 2: 253, 1978.

76. Singh G, Katyal SL, Torikata C: Carcinoma of type II pneumocytes. Am J Pathol 102: 195, 1981.

77. Unterman DH, Reingold IM: The occurrence of psammoma bodies in papillary adenocarcinoma of the lung. Am J Clin Pathol 57: 297, 1972.

78. Yesner R: Large cell carcinoma of the lung. Semin Diagn Pathol 2: 255, 1985.

78a. Ginsberg SS, Buzaid AC, Stern H, Carter D: Giant cell carcinoma of the lung. Cancer 70: 606, 1992.

79. Katzenstein AL, Prioleau PG, Askin FB: The histologic spectrum and significance of clear-cell change in lung carcinoma. Cancer 45: 943, 1980.

80. McDowell EM, McLaughlin JS, Merenyl DK, et al: The respiratory epithelium: V. Histogenesis of lung carcinomas in the human. J Natl Cancer Inst 61: 587, 1978.

81. Fitzgibbons PL, Kern WH: Adenosquamous carcinoma of the lung: A clinical and pathologic study of seven cases. Hum Pathol 16: 463, 1985.

82. Sridhar KS, Bounassi MJ, Raub W Jr, et al: Clinical features of adenosquamous lung carcinoma in 127 patients. Am Rev Respir Dis 142: 19, 1990.

83. Burke M, Fraser RS: Obstructive pneumonitis: A pathologic and pathogenetic reappraisal. Radiology 166: 699, 1988.

84. Glazer HS, Anderson DJ, Sagel SS: Bronchial impaction in lobar collapse: CT demonstration and pathologic correlation. Am J Roentgenol 153: 485, 1989.

85. Onitsuka H, Tsukuda M, Araki A, et al: Differentiation of central lung tumor from postobstructive lobar collapse by rapid-sequence computed tomography. J Thorac Imaging 6: 28, 1991.

86. Bourgouin PM, McLoud TC, Fitzgibbon JF, et al: Differentiation of bronchogenic carcinoma from postobstructive pneumonitis by magnetic resonance imaging: Histopathologic correlation. J Thorac Imaging 6: 22, 1991.

87. Genereux GP: Unusual intrathoracic manifestations of bronchogenic carcinoma. In Margulis AR, Gooding CA (eds): Diagnostic Radiology 1977. San Francisco, University of California, 1977, pp 553–584.

88. Spizarny DL, Cavanaugh B: The anterior bronchus sign: A new clue to hilar abnormality. Am J Roentgenol 145: 265, 1986.

89. Godwin JD: The solitary pulmonary nodule. Radiol Clin North Am 21: 709, 1983.

90. Holin SM, Dwork RE, Glaser S, et al: Solitary pulmonary nodules found in a community-wide chest roentgenogram survey: A five-year follow-up study. Am Rev Tuberc 79: 427, 1959.

91. Steele JD: The solitary pulmonary nodule: Report of a cooperative study of resected asymptomatic solitary pulmonary nodules in males. J Thorac Cardiovasc Surg 46: 21, 1963.

92. Steele J, Kleitsch W, Dunn J, et al: Survival in males with bronchogenic carcinoma resected as asymptomatic solitary pulmonary nodules. Ann Thorac Cardiovasc Surg 2: 368, 1966.

93. Cahan WG, Shah JP, Castro EB: Benign solitary lung lesions in patients with cancer. Ann Surg 187: 241, 1978.

94. Webb WR: Radiologic evaluation of the solitary pulmonary nodule. Am J Roentgenol 154: 701, 1990.

95. Zerhouni EA, Stitik FP, Siegelman SS, et al: CT of the pulmonary nodule—a cooperative study. Radiology 160: 319, 1986.

96. Mahoney MC, Shipley RT, Corcoran HL, et al: CT demonstration of calcification in carcinoma of the lung. Am J Roentgenol 154: 255, 1990.

97. Siegelman SS, Zerhouni EA, Leo FP, et al: CT of the solitary pulmonary nodule. Am J Roentgenol 135: 1, 1980.

98. Fraser RG, Barnes GT, Hickey N, et al: Potential value of digital radiography: Preliminary observations on the use of dual-energy subtraction in the evaluation of pulmonary nodules. Chest (Suppl) 89: 249S, 1986.

99. Nordenstrom B: New trends and technics of roentgen diagnosis of bronchial carcinoma. In Simon M, Potchen EG, LeMay M (eds): Frontiers of Pulmonary Radiology. New York, Grune & Stratton, 1969.

100. Zwirewich CV, Vedal S, Miller RR, et al: Solitary pulmonary nodule: High-resolution CT and radiologic-pathologic correlation. Radiology 179: 469, 1991.

101. Schraufnagel DE, Peloquin A, Paré JAP, et al: Differentiating bronchioloalveolar carcinoma from adenocarcinoma. Am Rev Respir Dis 125: 74, 1982.

102. Hill CA: "Tail" signs associated with pulmonary lesions: Critical reappraisal. Am J Roentgenol 139: 311, 1982.

103. Kuriyama K, Tateishi R, Doi O, et al: Prevalence of air bronchograms in small peripheral carcinomas of the lung on thin-section CT: Comparison with benign tumors. Am J Roentgenol 156: 921, 1991.

104. Gaeta M, Pandolfo I, Volta S, et al: Bronchus sign on CT in peripheral carcinoma of the lung: Value in predicting results of transbronchial biopsy. Am J Roentgenol 157: 1181, 1991.

105. Mori K, Saitou Y, Tominaga K, et al: Small nodular lesions in the lung periphery: New approach to diagnosis with CT. Radiology 177: 843, 1990.

106. Heitzman ER, Markarian B, Raasch BN, et al: Pathways of tumor spread through the lung: Radiologic correlations with anatomy and pathology. Radiology 144: 3, 1982.

107. Steele JD, Buell P: Asymptomatic solitary pulmonary nodules, host survival, tumor size, and growth rate. J Thorac Cardiovasc Surg 65: 140, 1973.

108. Weiss W: Peripheral measurable bronchogenic carcinoma: Growth rate and period of risk after therapy. Am Rev Respir Dis 103: 198, 1971.

109. Nathan MH, Collins VP, Adams RA: Differentiation of benign and malignant pulmonary nodules by growth rate. Radiology 79: 221, 1962.

110. Chaudhuri MR: Primary pulmonary cavitating carcinomas. Thorax 28: 354, 1973.

111. Sagel SS, Ablow RC: Hamartoma: On occasion a rapidly growing tumor of the lung. Radiology 91: 971, 1968.

112. Woodring JH, Fried AM: Significance of wall thickness in solitary cavities of the lung: A follow-up study. Am J Roentgenol 140: 473, 1983.

113. Schraufnagel DE, Peloquin A, Paré JAP, et al: Radiographic differences between two subtypes of bronchioloalveolar carcinoma. J Can Assoc Radiol 36: 244, 1985.

114. Huang D, Weisbrod GL, Chamberlin DW: Unusual radiologic presentations of bronchioloalveolar carcinoma. J Can Assoc Radiol 37: 94, 1986.

115. Epstein DM, Grefter WB, Miller WT: Lobar bronchioloalveolar cell carcinoma. Am J Roentgenol 139: 463, 1982.

116. Mallens WMC, Mijuis-Heddes JMA, Bakker W: Calcified lymph node metastases in bronchioloalveolar carcinoma. Radiology 161: 103, 1986.

117. Hill CA: Bronchioloalveolar carcinoma: A review. Radiology 150: 15, 1984.

118. Cohen S, Hossain Md Saha-Adat: Primary carcinoma of the lung: A review of 417 histologically proved cases. Dis Chest 49: 67, 1966.

119. Webb WR, Gatsonis C, Zerhouni EA, et al: CT and MR imaging in staging non–small cell bronchogenic carcinoma: Report of the Radiologic Diagnostic Oncology Group. Radiology 178: 705, 1991.

120. Webb WR, Sostman HD: MR imaging of thoracic disease: Clinical uses. Radiology 182: 621, 1992.

121. O'Connell RS, McLoud TC, Wilkins EW: Superior sulcus tumor: Radiographic diagnosis and workup. Am J Roentgenol 140: 25, 1983.

122. Bilbey JH, Müller NL, Connell DG, et al: Thoracic outlet syndrome: Evaluation with CT. Radiology 171: 381, 1989.

123. Heelan RT, Demas BE, Caravelli JF, et al: Superior sulcus tumors: CT and MR imaging. Radiology 170: 637, 1989.

124. Glazer HS, Duncan-Meyer J, Aronberg DJ, et al: Pleural and chest wall invasion in bronchogenic carcinoma: CT evaluation. Radiology 157: 191, 1985.

125. Yokoi K, Mori K, Miyazawa N, et al: Tumor invasion of the chest wall and mediastinum in lung cancer: Evaluation with pneumothorax CT. Radiology 181: 147, 1991.

126. Napoli LD, Hansen HH, et al: The incidence of osseous involvement in lung cancer, with special reference to the development of osteoblastic changes. Radiology 108: 17, 1973.

127. Chute CG, Greenberg ER, Baron J, et al: Presenting conditions of 1539 population-based lung cancer patients by cell type and stage in New Hampshire and Vermont. Cancer 56: 2107, 1985.

128. Marcq M, Galy P: Bronchioloalveolar carcinoma: Clinicopathologic relationships, natural history, and prognosis in 29 cases. Am Rev Respir Dis 107: 621, 1973.

129. Santiago SM, Lehrman S, Williams AJ: Bronchoscopy in patients with haemoptysis and normal chest roentgenograms. Br J Dis Chest 81: 186, 1987.

130. Fraser RS, Viloria JB, Wang N-S: Cardiac tamponade as presentation of extracardiac malignancy. Cancer 45: 1697, 1980.

131. Stankey RM, Roshe J, Sogocio RM: Carcinoma of the lung and dysphagia. Dis Chest 55: 13, 1969.

132. Parish JM, Marschke RF Jr, Dines DE, et al: Etiologic considerations in superior vena cava syndrome. Mayo Clin Proc 56: 407, 1981.

133. Schraufnagel DE, Hill R, Leech JA, et al: Superior vena caval obstruction: Is it a medical emergency? Am J Med 70: 1169, 1981.

134. Mason BA: Axillary-subclavian vein occlusion in patients with lung neoplasms. Cancer 48: 1886, 1981.

135. Clary CF, Michel RP, Wang N-S, et al: Metastatic carcinoma. Cancer 51: 362, 1983.

136. Auerbach O, Garfinkel L, Parks VR: Histologic type of lung cancer in relation to smoking habits, year of diagnosis and sites of metastases. Chest 67: 382, 1975.

137. Baird JA: The pathways of lymphatic spread of carcinoma of the lung. Br J Surg 52: 868, 1965.

138. Sorensen JB, Hansen HH, Hansen M, et al: Brain metastases in

adenocarcinoma of the lung: Fequency, risk, groups, and prognosis. J Clin Oncol 6: 1474, 1988.

139. Hirsch FR, Paulson OB, Hansen HH, et al: Intracranial metastases in small cell carcinoma of the lung: Correlation of clinical and autopsy findings. Cancer 50: 2433, 1982.

140. Rosen ST, Aisner J, Makuch RW, et al: Carcinomatous leptomeningitis in small cell lung cancer: A clinicopathologic review of the National Cancer Institute experience. Medicine 61: 45, 1982.

141. Murphy KC, Feld R, Evans WK, et al: Intramedullary spinal cord metastases from small cell carcinoma of the lung. J Clin Oncol 1: 99, 1983.

142. Campbell JH, Ralston S, Boyle IT, et al: Symptomatic hypercalcaemia in lung cancer. Respir Med 85: 223, 1991.

143. Johnson DH, Hainsworth JD, Greco FA: Extrahepatic biliary obstruction caused by small-cell lung cancer. Ann Intern Med 102: 487, 1985.

144. Seidenwurm DJ, Elmer EB, Kaplan LM, et al: Metastases to the adrenal glands and the development of Addison's disease. Cancer 54: 552, 1984.

145. Antler AS, Ough Y, Pitchumoni CS, et al: Gastrointestinal metastases from malignant tumors of the lung. Cancer 49: 170, 1982.

146. Morton DL, Itabashi HH, Grimes DF: Nonmetastatic neurological complications of bronchogenic carcinoma: The carcinomatous neuromyopathies. J Thorac Cardiovasc Surg 51: 14, 1966.

147. Popp W, Drlicek M, Grisold W, et al: Circulating antineuronal antibodies in small cell lung cancer. Lung 166: 243, 1988.

148. Chinn JS, Schuffler MD: Paraneoplastic visceral neuropathy as a cause of severe gastrointestinal motor dysfunction. Gastroenterology 95: 1279, 1988.

149. Wessel K, Diener HC, Dichgans J, et al: Cerebellar dysfunction in patients with bronchogenic carcinoma: Clinical and posturographic findings. J Neurol 235: 290, 1988.

150. Rassam JW, Anderson G: Incidence of paramalignant disorders in bronchogenic carcinoma. Thorax 30: 86, 1975.

151. Ayvazian LF, Schneider B, Gewirtz G, et al: Ectopic production of big ACTH in carcinoma of the lung: Its clinical usefulness as a biologic marker. Am Rev Respir Dis 111: 279, 1975.

152. Findling JW, Tyrell JB: Occult ectopic secretion of corticotropin. Arch Intern Med 146: 929, 1986.

153. Hardi CF, Faro JC: Localization of parathyroid hormone–like substance in squamous cell carcinomas: An immunoperoxidase study with ultrastructural correlation. Arch Pathol Lab Med 109: 752, 1985.

154. Robertson RP: Prostaglandins and hypercalcemia of cancer. Med Clin North Am 65: 845, 1981.

155. Bender RA, Hansen H: Hypercalcemia in bronchogenic carcinoma, a prospective study of 200 patients. Ann Intern Med 80: 205, 1974.

156. Coggeshall J, Merrill W, Hande K, et al: Implications of hypercalcemia with respect to diagnosis and treatment of lung cancer. Am J Med 80: 325, 1986.

157. Fusco FD, Rosen SW: Gonadotropin-producing anaplastic large-cell carcinomas of the lung. N Engl J Med 275: 507, 1966.

158. Braunstein GD, Vaitukaitis JL, Carbone PP, et al: Ectopic production of human chorionic gonadotropin by neoplasms. Ann Intern Med 78: 39, 1973.

159. Krauss S, Macy S, Ichiki AT: A study of immunoreactive calcitonin (CT), adrenocorticotropic hormone (ACTH), and carcinoembryonic antigen (CEA) in lung cancer and other malignancies. Cancer 47: 2485, 1981.

160. Ascensao JL, Oken MM, Ewing SL, et al: Leukocytosis and large cell lung cancer: A frequent association. Cancer 60: 903, 1987.

161. Kodama T, Takada K, Kameya T, et al: Large cell carcinoma of the lung associated with marked eosinophilia. Cancer 54: 2313, 1984.

162. Puolijoki H, Mustonen J, Pettersson E, et al: Proteinuria and haematuria are frequently present in patients with lung cancer. Nephrol Dial Transplant 4: 947, 1989.

163. Lam S, Palcic B, McLean D, et al: Detection of early lung cancer using low-dose Photofrin II. Chest 97: 333, 1990.

164. Ogushi F, Fukuoka M, Takada M, et al: Carcinoembryonic antigen (CEA) levels in pleural effusions and sera of lung cancer patients. Jpn J Clin Oncol 14: 321, 1984.

165. Schweisfurth H, Heinrich J, Brugger E, et al: The value of angiotensin-1-converting enzyme determinations in malignant and other diseases. Clin Physiol Biochem 3: 184, 1985.

166. Margolis ML, Desal B, Gracely E, et al: Frequency and clinical implications of monoclonal antibody detection of tumor-associated antigens in serum of patients with lung cancer. Am Rev Respir Dis 142: 1059, 1990.

167. Ito Y, Okuyama S, Awano T, et al: Diagnostic evaluation of ^{67}Ga scanning of lung cancer and other diseases. Radiology 101: 355, 1971.

168. Mountain CF: A new international staging system for lung cancer. Chest 89: 225S, 1986.

169. Baron RL, Levitt RG, Sagel SS, et al: Computed tomography in the preoperative evaluation of bronchogenic carcinoma. Radiology 145: 727, 1982.

170. Scott IR, Müller NL, Miller RR, et al: Resectable stage III lung cancer: CT, surgical, and pathologic correlation. Radiology 166: 75, 1988.

171. Kerr KM, Lamb D, Wathen CG, et al: Pathological assessment of mediastinal lymph nodes in lung cancer: Implications for non-invasive mediastinal staging. Thorax 47: 337, 1992.

171a. McLoud TC, Bourgouin PM, Greenberg RW, et al: Bronchogenic carcinoma: Analysis of staging in the mediastinum with CT by correlative lymph node mapping and sampling. Radiology 182: 319, 1992.

172. Staples CA, Müller NL, Miller RR, et al: Mediastinal nodes in bronchogenic carcinoma: Comparison between CT and mediastinoscopy. Radiology 167: 367, 1988.

173. McLoud TC, Bourgouin PM, Greenberg RW, et al: Bronchogenic carcinoma: Analysis of staging in the mediastinum with CT by correlative lymph node mapping and sampling. Radiology 182: 319, 1992.

174. Webb WR, Gamsu G, Stat DD, et al: Magnetic resonance imaging of the normal and abnormal pulmonary hila. Radiology 152: 89, 1984.

175. Hirleman MT, Yiu-Chiu VS, Chiu LC, et al: The resectability of primary lung carcinoma: A diagnostic staging review. CT 4: 146, 1980.

176. White DM, McMahon LJ, Denny WF: Usefulness outcome in evaluating the utility of nuclear scans of the bone, brain, and liver in bronchogenic carcinoma patients. Am J Med Sci 283: 114, 1982.

177. Turner P, Haggith JW: Preoperative radionuclide scanning in bronchogenic carcinoma. Br J Dis Chest 75: 291, 1981.

178. Donato AT, Ammerman EG, Sullesta O: Bone scanning in the evaluation of patients with lung cancer. Ann Thorac Surg 27: 300, 1979.

179. Lipford EH III, Eggleston JC, Lillemoe KD, et al: Prognostic factors in surgically resected limited-stage, non–small cell carcinoma of the lung. Am J Surg Pathol 8: 357, 1984.

180. Nomura A, Kolonel L, Rellahan W, et al: Racial survival patterns for lung cancer in Hawaii. Cancer 48: 1265, 1981.

181. Ferguson MK, Skosey C, Hoffman PC, et al: Sex-associated differences in presentation and survival in patients with lung cancer. J Clin Oncol 8: 1402, 1990.

182. Antkowiak JG, Regal AM, Takita H: Bronchogenic carcinoma in patients under age 40. Ann Thorac Surg 47: 391, 1989.

183. O'Rourke MA, Feussner JR, Feigl P, et al: Age trends of lung cancer stage at diagnosis: Implications for lung cancer screening in the elderly. JAMA 258: 921, 1987.

184. Boushy SF, Helgason AH, Billig DM, et al: Clinical, physiologic, and morphologic examination of the lung in patients with bronchogenic carcinoma and the relation of the findings to postoperative deaths. Am Rev Respir Dis 101: 685, 1970.

185. Johnston-Early A, Cohen MH, Minna JD, et al: Smoking abstinence and small cell lung cancer survival: An association. JAMA 244: 2175, 1980.

186. Fraire AE, Roggli VL, Vollmer RT, et al: Lung cancer heterogeneity: Prognostic implications. Cancer 60: 370, 1987.

187. Nou E, Brodin O, Bergh J: A randomized study of radiation treatment in small cell bronchial carcinoma treated with two types of four-drug chemotherapy regimens. Cancer 15: 1079, 1988.

188. Johnson BE, Grayson J, Makuch RW, et al: Ten-year survival of patients with small-cell lung cancer treated with combination chemotherapy with or without irradiation. J Clin Oncol 8: 396, 1990.

189. Albain KS, Crowley JJ, Livingston RB: Long-term survival and toxicity in small cell lung cancer. Chest 99: 1425, 1991.

190. Chak LY, Sikic BI, Tucker MA, et al: Increased incidence of acute nonlymphocytic leukemia following therapy in patients with small cell carcinoma of the lung. J Clin Oncol 2: 385, 1984.

191. Armstrong J, Shank B, Scher H, et al: Limited small-cell lung cancer: Do favorable short-term results predict ultimate outcome? Am J Clin Oncol 14: 285, 1991.

192. Stanley K, Cox JD, Petrovich Z, et al: Patterns of failure in patients with inoperable carcinoma of the lung. Cancer 47: 2725, 1981.
193. Mountain CF, Carr DT, Anderson WAD: A system for the clinical staging of lung cancer. Am J Roentgenol 120: 130, 1974.
194. Cortese DA, Pairolero PC, Bergstralh EJ, et al: Roentgenographically occult lung cancer: A ten-year experience. J Thorac Cardiovasc Surg 86: 373, 1983.
195. Gail MH, Eagan RT, Feld R, et al: Prognostic factors in patients with resected stage 1 non–small cell lung cancer. Cancer 54: 1802, 1984.
196. Daly RC, Trastek VF, Pairolero PC, et al: Bronchoalveolar carcinoma: Factors affecting survival. Ann Thorac Surg 51: 368, 1991.
196a. Feldman ER, Eagan RT, Schaid DJ: Metastatic bronchioloalveolar carcinoma and metastatic adenocarcinoma of the lung: Comparison of clinical manifestations, chemotherapeutic responses, and prognosis. Mayo Clin Proc 67: 27, 1992.
197. Downey RS, Sewell CW, Mansour KA: Large cell carcinoma of the lung: A highly aggressive tumor with dismal prognosis. Ann Thorac Surg 47: 806, 1989.
198. Hirsch FR, Paulson OB, Hansen HH, et al: Intracranial metastases in small cell carcinoma of the lung: Prognostic aspects. Cancer 51: 529, 1983.
199. Mulshine JL, Makuch RW, Johnston-Early A, et al: Diagnosis and significance of liver metastases in small cell carcinoma of the lung. J Clin Oncol 2: 733, 1984.
200. Hirsch FR, Hansen HH: Bone marrow involvement in small cell anaplastic carcinoma of the lung: Prognostic and therapeutic aspects. Cancer 46: 206, 1980.
201. Livingston RB, McCracken JD, Trauth CJ, et al: Isolated pleural effusion in small cell lung carcinoma—favorable prognosis: A review of Southwest-Oncology Group experience. Chest 81: 208, 1982.
202. Hyde L, Wolf J, McCracken S, et al: Natural course of inoperable lung cancer. Chest 64: 309, 1973.
203. Kimura Y, Fujii T, Hamamoto K, et al: Serum CA125 level is a good prognostic indicator in lung cancer. Br J Cancer 62: 676, 1990.
204. Sagman U, Feld R, Evans WK, et al: The prognostic significance of pretreatment serum lactate dehydrogenase in patients with small-cell lung cancer. J Clin Oncol 9: 954, 1991.
205. McCaughan BC, Martini N, Bains MS, et al: Chest wall invasion in carcinoma of the lung: Therapeutic and prognostic implications. J Thorac Cardiovasc Surg 89: 836, 1985.
206. Ricci C, Rendina EA, Venuta F: En bloc resection for T3 bronchogenic carcinoma with chest wall invasion. Eur J Cardiothorac Surg 1: 23, 1987.
207. Albain KS, Hoffman PC, Little AG, et al: Pleural involvement in stage IIIM0 non–small cell bronchogenic carcinoma: A need to differentiate subtypes. Am J Clin Oncol 9: 255, 1986.
208. Burt ME, Pomerantz AH, Bains MS, et al: Results of surgical treatment of stage III lung cancer invading the mediastinum. Surg Clin North Am 67: 987, 1987.
209. Martini N, Flehinger BJ: The role of surgery in N2 lung cancer. Surg Clin North Am 67: 1037, 1987.
210. Ishida T, Tateishi M, Kaneko S, et al: Surgical treatment of patients with nonsmall-cell lung cancer and mediastinal lymph node involvement. J Surg Oncol 43: 161, 1990.
211. Ebner H, Sudkamp N, Wex P, et al: Selection and preoperative treatment of over-seventy-year-old patients undergoing thoracotomy. Thorac Cardiovasc Surg 33: 268, 1985.
212. Read RC, Yoder G, Schaeffer RC: Survival after conservative resection for T1 N0 M0 non–small cell lung cancer. Ann Thorac Surg 49: 391, 1990.
213. Mandell L, Hilaris B, Sullivan M, et al: The treatment of single brain metastasis from non–oat cell lung carcinoma: Surgery and radiation versus radiation therapy alone. Cancer 58: 641, 1986.
214. Watkin SW, Hayhurst GK, Green JA: Time trends in the outcome of lung cancer management: A study of 9,090 cases diagnosed in the Mersey region, 1974–86. Br J Cancer 61: 590, 1990.
215. Salzer GM, Müller LC, Huber H, et al: Operation for N2 small cell carcinoma. Ann Thorac Surg 49: 759, 1990.
216. Bewtra C: Multiple primary bronchogenic carcinomas, with a review of the literature. J Surg Oncol 25: 207, 1984.
217. Ichinose Y, Hara N, Ohta M: Synchronous lung cancers defined by deoxyribonucleic acid flow cytometry. J Thorac Cardiovasc Surg 102: 418, 1991.
218. Auerbach O, Saccomanno G, Kuschner M, et al: Histologic findings in the tracheobronchial tree of uranium miners and non-miners with lung cancer. Cancer 42: 483, 1979.
219. Rosengart TK, Martini N, Ghosn P, et al: Multiple primary lung carcinomas: Prognosis and treatment. Ann Thorac Surg 52: 773, 1991.
220. Mathisen DJ, Jensik R, Faber LP, et al: Survival following resection for second and third primary lung cancers. J Thorac Cardiovasc Surg 88: 502, 1984.
221. Gould VE, Linnoila I, Memoli VA, et al: Biology of disease. Neuroendocrine components of the bronchopulmonary tract: Hyperplasias, dysplasias, and neoplasms. Lab Invest 49: 519, 1983.
222. Paladugu RR, Benfield JR, Pak HY, et al: Bronchopulmonary Kulchitsky cell carcinomas. Cancer 55: 1303, 1985.
223. Godwin JD II: Carcinoid tumors: An analysis of 2837 cases. Cancer 36: 560, 1975.
224. Arrigoni MG, Woolner LB, Bernatz PE: Atypical carcinoid tumors of the lung. J Cardiovasc Surg 64: 413, 1972.
225. Gould VE, Linnoila RI, Memoli VA, et al: Neuroendocrine cells and neuroendocrine neoplasms of the lung. Pathol Ann 18: 287, 1983.
226. Warren WH, Memoli VA, Jordan AG, et al: Reevaluation of pulmonary neoplasms resected as small cell carcinomas: Significance of distinguishing between well-differentiated and small cell neuroendocrine carcinomas. Cancer 65: 1003, 1990.
227. Ranchod M, Levine GD: Spindle-cell carcinoid tumors of the lung: A clinicopathologic study of 35 cases. Am J Surg Pathol 4: 315, 1980.
228. Leriche H, Catach D, Levasseur P, et al: Artériographie bronchique selective et tumeur carcinoide. (Selective bronchial arteriography in carcinoid tumor of the lung.) Ann Radiol 16: 629, 1973.
229. Zweibel BR, Austin JHM, Grimes MM: Bronchial carcinoid tumors: Assessment with CT location and intratumoral calcification in 31 patients. Radiology 179: 483, 1991.
230. Magid D, Siegelman SS, Eggleston JC, et al: Pulmonary carcinoid tumors: CT assessment. J Comput Assist Tomogr 13: 244, 1989.
231. Doppman JL, Pass HI, Nieman LK, et al: Detection of ACTH-producing bronchial carcinoid tumors: MR imaging vs CT. Am J Roentgenol 156: 39, 1991.
232. Giustra PE, Stassa G: The multiple presentations of bronchial adenomas. Radiology 93: 1013, 1969.
233. Wynn SR, O'Connell EJ, Frigas E, et al: Exercise-induced "asthma" as a presentation of bronchial carcinoid. Ann Allergy 57: 139, 1986.
234. Todd TR, Cooper JD, Weissberg D, et al: Bronchial carcinoid tumors: 20 years' experience. J Thorac Cardiovasc Surg 79: 532, 1980.
235. Hurt R, Bates M: Carcinoid tumours of the bronchus: A 33-year experience. Thorax 39: 617, 1984.
236. Leinung MC, Young WF Jr, Whitaker MD, et al: Diagnosis of corticotropin-producing bronchial carcinoid tumors causing Cushing's syndrome. Mayo Clin Proc 65: 1314, 1990.
237. Scheithauer BW, Carpenter PC, Bloch B, et al: Ectopic secretion of a growth hormone–releasing factor: Report of a case of acromegaly with bronchial carcinoid tumor. Am J Med 76: 605, 1984.
238. D'Agati VD, Perzin KH: Carcinoid tumorlets of the lung with metastasis to a peribronchial lymph node: Report of a case and review of the literature. Cancer 55: 2472, 1985.
239. Rodgers-Sullivan RF, Weiland LH, Palumbo PJ, et al: Pulmonary tumorlets associated with Cushing's syndrome. Am Rev Respir Dis 117: 799, 1978.
240. Bonikos DS, Archibald R, Bensch KG: On the origin of the so-called tumorlets of the lung. Hum Pathol 17: 461, 1976.
241. Hammond ME, Sause WT: Large cell neuroendocrine tumors of the lung. Cancer 56: 1624, 1985.
242. Neal MH, Kosinski R, Cohen P, et al: Atypical endocrine tumors of the lung: A histologic, ultrastructural, and clinical study of 19 cases. Hum Pathol 17: 1264, 1986.
243. Spencer H: Bronchial mucous gland tumors. Virchows Arch [Pathol Anat Histol] 383: 101, 1979.
244. Janower ML, Grillo HC, MacMillan AS Jr, et al: The radiological appearance of carcinoma of the trachea. Radiology 96: 39, 1970.
245. Olmedo G, Rosenberg M, Fonseca R: Primary tumors of the trachea: Clinicopathologic features and surgical results. Chest 81: 701, 1982.
246. Spizarny DL, Shepard JA, McLoud TC, et al: CT of adenoid cystic carcinoma of the trachea. Am J Roentgenol 146: 1129, 1986.
247. Hajdu SI, Huvos AG, Goodner JT, et al: Carcinoma of the trachea: Clinicopathologic study of 41 cases. Cancer 25: 1448, 1970.

248. Klacsmann PG, Olson JL, Eggleston JC: Mucoepidermoid carcinoma of the bronchus: An electron microscopic study of the low-grade and the high-grade variants. Cancer 43: 1720, 1979.
249. Yousem SA, Hochholzer L: Mucoepidermoid tumors of the lung. Cancer 60: 1346, 1987.
250. Spencer H, Dail DH, Arneaud J: Non-invasive bronchial epithelial papillary tumors. Cancer 45: 1486, 1980.
251. Levi JE, Delcelo R, Alberti VN, et al: Human papilloma-virus DNA in respiratory papillomatosis detected by in situ hybridization and the polymerase chain reaction. Am J Pathol 135: 1179, 1989.
252. Singer DB, Greenberg SD, Harrison GM: Papillomatosis of the lung. Am Rev Respir Dis 94: 777, 1966.
253. Nikolaidis ET, Trost DC, Buchholz CL, et al: The relationship of histologic and clinical factors in laryngeal papillomatosis. Arch Pathol Lab Med 109: 24, 1985.
254. Kramer SS, Wehunt WD, Stocker JT, et al: Pulmonary manifestations of juvenile laryngotracheal papillomatosis. Am J Roentgenol 144: 687, 1985.
255. Lindeberg H, Elbrønd O: Malignant tumours in patients with a history of multiple laryngeal papillomas: The significance of irradiation. Clin Otolaryngol 16: 149, 1991.
256. Yousem SA, Hochholzer L: Alveolar adenoma. Hum Pathol 17: 1066, 1986.
257. Miller RR: Bronchioloalveolar cell adenomas. Am J Surg Pathol 14: 904, 1990.
258. Bagwell SP, Flynn SD, Cox PM, et al: Primary malignant melanoma of the lung. Am Rev Respir Dis 139: 1543, 1989.
259. Colby TV, Hoppe RT, Warnke RA: Hodgkin's disease: A clinicopathologic study of 659 cases. Cancer 49: 1848, 1981.
260. Johnson DW, Hoppe RT, Cox RS, et al: Hodgkin's disease limited to intrathoracic sites. Cancer 52: 8, 1983.
261. Ultmann JE, Moran EH: Clinical course and complications in Hodgkin's disease. Arch Intern Med 131: 332, 1973.
262. Radin AI: Primary pulmonary Hodgkin's disease. Cancer 65: 550, 1990.
263. Colby TV, Hoppe RT, Warnke RA: Hodgkin's disease at autopsy: 1972–1977. Cancer 47: 1852, 1981.
264. Brereton HD, Johnson RE: Calcification in mediastinal lymph nodes after radiation therapy of Hodgkin's disease. Radiology 112: 705, 1974.
265. Martin JJ: The Nisbet Symposium: Hodgkin's disease: Radiological aspects of the disease. Australas Radiol 11: 206, 1967.
266. Press GA, Glazer HS, Wasserman TH, et al: Thoracic wall involvement by Hodgkin disease and non-Hodgkin lymphoma: CT evaluation. Radiology 157: 195, 1985.
267. Heron CW, Husband JE, Williams MP: Hodgkin disease: CT of the thymus. Radiology 167: 647, 1988.
268. Lewis ER, Caskey CI, Fishman EK: Lymphoma of the lung: CT findings in 31 patients. Am J Roentgenol 156: 711, 1991.
269. Madewell JE, Daroca PJ, Reed JC: Pulmonary parenchymal Hodgkin's disease. RPC from the AFIP. Radiology 117: 555, 1975.
270. Yellin A, Benfield JR: Pneumothorax associated with lymphoma. Am Rev Respir Dis 134: 590, 1986.
271. Beachley MC, Lau BP, King ER: Bone involvement in Hodgkin's disease. Am J Roentgenol 114: 559, 1972.
272. Costello P, Mauch P: Radiologic features of recurrent intrathoracic Hodgkin's disease following radiation therapy. Am J Roentgenol 133: 201, 1979.
273. Winterbauer RH, Belic N, Moores KD: A clinical interpretation of bilateral hilar adenopathy. Ann Intern Med 78: 65, 1973.
274. Morales FM, Matthews JI: Diagnosis of parenchymal Hodgkin's disease using bronchoalveolar lavage. Chest 91: 785, 1987.
275. Aisenberg AC: Malignant lymphoma. N Engl J Med 288: 883, 1973.
276. Saltzstein SL: Pulmonary malignant lymphomas and pseudolymphomas: Classification, therapy, and prognosis. Cancer 16: 928, 1963.
277. L'Hoste RJ, Filippa DA, Lieberman PH, et al: Primary pulmonary lymphoma. Cancer 54: 1397, 1984.
278. Chee YC, Yap CH, Poh SC: Pulmonary lymphoma or pseudolymphoma: A diagnostic dilemma. Ann Acad Med Singapore 15: 113, 1986.
279. Turner RR, Colby TV, Doggett RS: Well-differentiated lymphocytic lymphoma. Cancer 54: 2088, 1984.
279a. Holland EA, Ghahremani GG, Fry WA, Victor TA: Evolution of pulmonary pseudolymphomas: Clinical and radiologic manifestations. J Thorac Imaging 6: 74, 1991.
280. Kennedy JL, Nathwani BN, Burke JS, et al: Pulmonary lymphomas and other pulmonary lymphoid lesions: A clinicopathologic and immunologic study of 64 patients. Cancer 56: 539, 1985.
281. Li G, Hansmann ML, Zwingers T, et al: Primary lymphomas of the lung: Morphological, immunohistochemical and clinical features. Histopathology 16: 519, 1990.
282. Koss, MN, Hochholzer L, Nichols PW, et al: Primary non-Hodgkin's lymphoma and pseudolymphoma of lung: A study of 161 patients. Hum Pathol 14: 1024, 1983.
283. Evans HL: Extranodal small lymphocytic proliferation: A clinicopathologic and immunocytochemical study. Cancer 49: 84, 1982.
284. Burgener FA, Hamlin DJ: Intrathoracic histiocytic lymphoma of the lungs. Radiology 132: 569, 1979.
285. Balikian JP, Herman PG: Non-Hodgkin lymphoma of the lungs. Radiology 132: 569, 1979.
286. Dunnick NR, Parker BR, Castellino RA: Rapid onset of pulmonary infiltration due to histiocytic lymphoma. Radiology 118: 281, 1976.
287. Khoury MB, Goodwin JD, Halvorsen R, et al: Role of chest CT in non-Hodgkin lymphoma. Radiology 158: 659, 1986.
288. Costabel U, Bross KJ, Matthys H: Diagnosis by bronchoalveolar lavage of cause of pulmonary infiltrates in haematological malignancies. Br Med J 290: 1041, 1985.
289. Xaubet A, Diumenjo MC, Marin A, et al: Characteristics and prognostic value of pleural effusions in non-Hodgkin's lymphomas. Eur J Respir Dis 66: 135, 1985.
290. Das DK, Gupta SK, Ayyagari S, et al: Pleural effusions in non-Hodgkin's lymphoma: Cytomorphologic, cytochemical and immunologic study. Acta Cytol 31: 119, 1987.
291. Ngan H, Preston BJ: Non-Hodgkin's lymphoma presenting with osseous lesions. Clin Radiol 26: 351, 1975.
292. Kennedy P, Buck M, Joshua DE, et al: Rapidly progressive fatal pulmonary infiltration by lymphoma. Aust NZ J Med 15: 62, 1985.
293. Ducatman BS, Wick MR, Morgan TW, et al: Malignant histiocytosis: A clinical, histologic, and immunohistochemical study of 20 cases. Hum Pathol 15: 368, 1984.
294. Colby TV, Carrington CB, Mark GJ: Pulmonary involvement in malignant histiocytosis. Am J Surg Pathol 5: 61, 1981.
295. Marglin SI, Soulen RI, Blank N, et al: Mycosis fungoides: Radiographic manifestations of extracutaneous intrathoracic involvement. Radiology 130: 35, 1979.
296. Foster GH, Eichenhorn MS, Van Slyck EJ: The Sézary syndrome with rapid pulmonary dissemination. Cancer 56: 1197, 1985.
297. Stokar LM, Vonderheid EC, Abell E, et al: Clinical manifestations of intrathoracic cutaneous T-cell lymphoma. Cancer 56: 649, 1985.
298. Klatte EC, Yardley J, Smith EB, et al: The pulmonary manifestations and complications of leukemia. Am J Roentgenol 89: 598, 1963.
299. Marsh WL Jr, Bylund DJ, Heath VC, et al: Osteoarticular and pulmonary manifestations of acute leukemia: Case report and review of the literature. Cancer 57: 385, 1986.
300. Maile CW, Moore AV, Ulreich S, et al: Chest radiographic-pathologic correlation in adult leukemia patients. Invest Radiol 18: 495, 1983.
301. Chernoff A, Rymuza J, Lippman ML: Endobronchial lymphocytic infiltration. Am J Med 77: 755, 1984.
302. Palosaari DE, Colby TV: Bronchiolocentric chronic lymphocytic leukemia. Cancer 58: 1695, 1986.
303. Myers TJ, Cole SR, Klatsky AU, et al: Respiratory failure due to pulmonary leukostasis following chemotherapy of acute nonlymphocytic leukemia. Cancer 51: 1808, 1983.
304. Tryka AF, Godleski JJ, Fanta CH: Leukemic cell lysis pneumonopathy. Cancer 50: 2763, 1982.
305. Nathwani BN, Diamond LW, Winberg CD, et al: Lymphoblastic lymphoma: A clinicopathologic study of 95 patients. Cancer 48: 2347, 1981.
306. Shaw NJ, Tweeddale PM, Eden OB: Pulmonary function in childhood leukaemia survivors. Med Pediatr Oncol 17: 149, 1989.
307. Kintzer JS, Rosenow EC, Kyle RA: Thoracic and pulmonary abnormalities in multiple myeloma. Arch Intern Med 138: 727, 1978.
308. Tenholder MF, Scialla SJ, Weisbaum G: Endobronchial metastatic plasmacytoma. Cancer 49: 1465, 1982.
309. Morinaga S, Watanabe H, Gemma A, et al: Plasmacytoma of the lung associated with nodular deposits of immunoglobulin. Am J Surg Pathol 11: 989, 1987.
310. Baroni CD, Mineo TC, Ricci C, et al: Solitary secretory plasmacytoma of the lung in a 14-year-old boy. Cancer 40: 2329, 1977.

311. Liebow AA, Carrington CRB, Friedman PJ: Lymphomatoid granulomatosis. Hum Pathol 3: 457, 1972.

312. Colby TV, Carrington CB: Pulmonary lymphomas simulating lymphomatoid granulomatosis. Am J Surg Pathol 6: 19, 1982.

313. Gaulard P, Henni T, Marolleau J-P, et al: Lethal midline granuloma (polymorphic reticulosis) and lymphomatoid granulomatosis: Evidence for monoclonal T-cell lymphoproliferative disorder. Cancer 62: 705, 1988.

314. Leavitt RY, Fauci AS: Pulmonary vasculitis. Am Rev Respir Dis 134: 149, 1986.

315. Koss MN, Hochholzer L, Langloss JM, et al: Lymphomatoid granulomatosis: A clinicopathologic study of 42 patients. Pathology 18: 283, 1986.

316. Pisani RJ, DeRemee RA: Clinical implication of the histopathologic diagnosis of pulmonary lymphomatoid granulomatosis. Mayo Clin Proc 65: 151, 1990.

317. Katzenstein AL, Carrington CB, Liebow AA: Lymphomatoid granulomatosis. Cancer 43: 360, 1979.

317a. Koss MN, Hochholzer L, Langloss JM, et al: Lymphoid interstitial pneumonia: Clincopathological and immunopathological findings in 18 cases. Pathology 19: 178, 1987.

318. Barberà JA, Hayashi S, Hegele RG, et al: Detection of Epstein-Barr virus in lymphocytic interstitial pneumonitis by in situ hybridization. Am Rev Respir Dis 145: 940, 1992.

319. Liebow AA, Carrington CB: The interstitial pneumonias. In Simon M, Potchen EJ, Le May M (eds): Frontiers of Pulmonary Radiology. New York, Grune & Stratton, 1969, p 102.

320. Lukes RJ, Tindle BH: Immunoblastic lymphadenopathy: A hyperimmune entity resembling Hodgkin's disease. N Engl J Med 292: 1, 1975.

321. Limpert J, MacMahon H, Variakojis D: Angioimmunoblastic lymphadenopathy: Clinical and radiological features. Radiology 152: 27, 1984.

322. Pangalis GA, Moran EM, Nathwani BN, et al: Angioimmunoblastic lymphadenopathy. Cancer 52: 318, 1983.

323. Vera-Roman JM, Sobonya RE, Gomez-Garcia JL, et al: Leiomyoma of the lung: Literature review and case report. Cancer 52: 936, 1983.

324. Guccion JG, Rosen SH: Bronchopulmonary leiomyosarcoma and fibrosarcoma: A study of 32 cases and review of the literature. Cancer 30: 836, 1972.

325. Yellin A, Rosenman Y, Lieberman Y: Review of smooth muscle tumours of the lower respiratory tract. Br J Dis Chest 78: 337, 1984.

326. Baker PB, Goodwin RA: Pulmonary artery sarcomas: A review and report of a case. Arch Pathol Lab Med 109: 35, 1985.

327. Moffat RE, Chang CHJ, Slaven JE: Roentgen considerations in primary pulmonary artery sarcoma. Radiology 104: 283, 1972.

328. Olsson HE, Spitzer RM, Erston WF: Primary and secondary pulmonary artery neoplasia mimicking acute pulmonary embolism. Radiology 118: 49, 1976.

329. Liew S-H, Leong AS-Y, Tang HM: Tracheal paraganglioma: A case report with review of the literature. Cancer 47: 1387, 1981.

330. Hangartner JRW, Loosemore TM, Burke M, et al: Malignant primary pulmonary paraganglioma. Thorax 44: 154, 1989.

331. Yousem SA, Hochholzer L: Primary pulmonary hemangiopericytoma. Cancer 59: 549, 1987.

332. Fouret PJ, Pauboul JL, Mayaud CM, et al: Pulmonary Kaposi's sarcoma in patients with acquired immune deficiency syndrome: A clinicopathological study. Thorax 42: 262, 1987.

333. Naidich DP, Tarras M, Garay SM, et al: Kaposi's sarcoma. CT-radiographic correlation. Chest 96: 723, 1989.

334. Sivit CJ, Schwartz AM, Rockoff SD: Kaposi's sarcoma of the lung in AIDS: Radiologic-pathologic analysis. Am J Roentgenol 148: 25, 1987.

335. Medur GU, Stover DE, Lee M, et al: Pulmonary Kaposi's sarcoma in the acquired immune deficiency syndrome. Am J Med 81: 11, 1986.

336. Dail DH, Liebow AA, Gmelich JT, et al: Intravascular, bronchiolar, and alveolar tumor of the lung (IVBAT): An analysis of twenty cases of a peculiar sclerosing endothelial tumor. Cancer 51: 452, 1983.

337. Sicilian L, Warson F, Carrington CB, et al: Intravascular bronchioloalveolar tumor (IV-BAT). Respiration 44: 387, 1983.

338. Nakatani Y, Aoki I, Misugi K: Immunohistochemical and ultrastructural study of early lesions of intravascular bronchioloalveolar tumor with liver involvement. Acta Pathol Jpn 35: 1453, 1985.

339. Tomashefski JF Jr: Benign endobronchial mesenchymal tumors: Their relationship to parenchymal pulmonary hamartomas. Am J Surg Pathol 6: 531, 1982.

340. Keyhani-Rofagha S, O'Dorisio TM, Lucas JG, et al: Extra-adrenal paraganglioma and pulmonary chondroma: A case report and review of the literature. J Surg Oncol 35: 89, 1987.

341. Mishkin FS, Vasinrapee P, Vore L, et al: Carney's triad: Radiographic diagnosis, natural history and importance of pulmonary chondromas. J Can Assoc Radiol 38: 264, 1985.

342. Tisell L-E, Angervall L, Dahl I, et al: Recurrent and metastasizing gastric leiomyoblastoma (epithelioid leiomyosarcoma) associated with multiple pulmonary chondro-hamartomas: Long survival of a patient treated with repeated operations. Cancer 41: 259, 1978.

343. Yellin A, Schwartz L, Hersho E, et al: Chondrosarcoma of the bronchus: Report of a case with resection and review of the literature. Chest 84: 224, 1983.

344. Stark P, Smith DC, Watkins GE, et al: Primary intrathoracic extraosseous osteogenic sarcoma: Report of three cases. Radiology 174: 725, 1990.

345. Roviaro G, Montorsi M, Varoli F, et al: Primary pulmonary tumours of neurogenic origin. Thorax 38: 942, 1983.

346. Oparah SS, Subramanian VA: Granular cell myoblastoma of the bronchus: Report of 2 cases and review of the literature. Ann Thorac Surg 22: 199, 1976.

347. Korompai FL, Awe RJ, Beall AC, et al: Granular cell myoblastoma of the bronchus: A new case, 12-year followup report, and review of the literature. Chest 66: 578, 1974.

348. Hirata T, Reshad K, Itoi K, et al: Lipomas of the peripheral lung—a case report and review of the literature. Thorac Cardiovasc Surg 37: 385, 1989.

349. Yousem SA, Flynn SD: Intrapulmonary localized fibrous tumor: Intraparenchymal so-called localized fibrous mesothelioma. Am J Clin Pathol 89: 365, 1988.

350. Tan-Liu NS, Matsubara O, Grillo HC, et al: Invasive fibrous tumor of the tracheobronchial tree: Clinical and pathologic study of seven cases. Hum Pathol 20: 180, 1989.

351. Yousem SA, Hochholzer L: Malignant fibrous histiocytoma of the lung. Cancer 60: 2532, 1987.

352. Lee JT, Shelburne JD, Linder J: Primary malignant fibrous histiocytoma of the lung: A clinicopathologic and ultrastructural study of five cases. Cancer 53: 1124, 1984.

353. Gaffey MJ, Mills SE, Askin FB, et al: Clear cell tumor of the lung: A clinicopathologic, immunohistochemical, and ultrastructural study of eight cases. Am J Surg Pathol 14: 248, 1990.

353a. Liew S-H, Leong AS-Y, Tang HM: Tracheal paraganglioma: A case report with review of the literature. Cancer 47: 1387, 1981.

353b. Singh G, Lee RE, Brooks DH: Primary pulmonary paraganglioma: Report of a case and review of the literature. Cancer 40: 2286, 1977.

354. Satoh Y, Tsuchiya E, Weng SY, et al: Pulmonary sclerosing hemangioma of the lung: A type II pneumocytoma by immunohistochemical and immunoelectron microscopic studies. Cancer 64: 1310, 1989.

355. Yousem SA, Wick MR, Singh G, et al: So-called sclerosing hemangiomas of the lung: An immunohistochemical study supporting a respiratory epithelial origin. Am J Surg Pathol 12: 582, 1988.

356. Katzenstein AL, Gmelich JT, Carrington CB: Sclerosing hemangioma of the lung. Am J Surg Pathol 4: 343, 1980.

357. Humphrey PA, Scroggs MW, Roggli VL, et al: Pulmonary carcinomas with a sarcomatoid element: An immunocytochemical and ultrastructural analysis. Hum Pathol 19: 155, 1988.

358. Roth JA, Elguezabal A: Pulmonary blastoma evolving into carcinosarcoma: A case study. Am J Surg Pathol 2: 407, 1978.

359. Ludwigsen E: Endobronchial carcinosarcoma: A case with osteosarcoma of pulmonary invasive part, and a review with respect to prognosis. Virchows Arch [Pathol Anat Histol] 373: 293, 1977.

360. Fung CH, Lo JW, Yonan TN, et al: Pulmonary blastoma: An ultrastructural study with a brief review of literature and a discussion of pathogenesis. Cancer 39: 153, 1977.

361. Koss MN, Hochholzer L, O'Leary T: Pulmonary blastomas. Cancer 67: 2368, 1991.

362. Prauer HW, Mack D, Babic R: Intrapulmonary teratoma 10 years after removal of a mediastinal teratoma in a young man. Thorax 38: 632, 1983.

363. Pushchak MJ, Farhi DC: Primary choriocarcinoma of the lung. Arch Pathol Lab Med 111: 477, 1987.

364. Kung ITM, Loke SL, So SY, et al: Intrapulmonary thymoma: Report of two cases. Thorax 40: 471, 1985.

365. Bateson EM: Histogenesis of intrapulmonary and endobronchial hamartomas and chondromas (cartilage-containing tumours): A hypothesis. J Pathol 101: 77, 1970.

366. Van Den Bosch JMM, Wagenaar SS, Corrin B, et al: Mesenchymoma of the lung (so-called hamartoma): A review of 154 parenchymal and endobronchial cases. Thorax 42: 790, 1987.

367. Sagel SS, Ablow RC: Hamartoma: On occasion a rapidly growing tumor of the lung. Radiology 91: 971, 1968.

368. Bateson EM: An analysis of 155 solitary lung lesions illustrating the differential diagnosis of mixed tumours of the lung. Clin Radiol 16: 51, 1965.

369. Bateson EM: Relationship between intrapulmonary and endobronchial cartilage-containing tumors (so-called hamartomata). Thorax 20: 447, 1965.

370. Poirier TJ, Van Ordstrand HS: Pulmonary chondromatous hamartomas: Report of seventeen cases and review of the literature. Chest 59: 50, 1971.

371. Siegelman SS, Khouri NF, Scott WW, et al: Pulmonary hamartoma: CT findings. Radiology 160: 313, 1986.

372. Gabrail NY, Zara B: Pulmonary hamartoma syndrome. Chest 97: 962, 1990.

373. Hamper UM, Khouri NF, Stitik FP, et al: Pulmonary hamartoma: Diagnosis by transthoracic needle aspiration biopsy. Radiology 155: 15, 1985.

374. Ashley DJB, Danino EA, Davies HD: Bronchial polyps. Thorax 18: 45, 1963.

375. Berman DE, Wright ES, Edstrom HW: Endobronchial inflammatory polyp associated with a foreign body. Chest 86: 483, 1984.

376. Adams C, Moisan T, Chandrasekhar AJ, et al: Endobronchial polyposis secondary to thermal inhalational injury. Chest 75: 643, 1979.

377. Spencer H: The pulmonary plasma cell–histiocytoma complex. Histopathology 8: 903, 1984.

378. Bahadori M, Liebow AA: Plasma cell granulomas of the lung. Cancer 31: 191, 1973.

379. Schwartz EE, Katz SM, Mandell GA: Postinflammatory pseudotumors of the lung: Fibrous histiocytoma and related lesions. Radiology 136: 609, 1980.

380. Mandelbaum I, Brashear RE, Hull MT: Surgical treatment and course of pulmonary pseudotumor (plasma cell granuloma). J Thorac Cardiovasc Surg 82: 77, 1981.

381. Engleman P, Liebow AA, Gemlich J, et al: Pulmonary hyalinizing granuloma. Am Rev Respir Dis 115: 997, 1977.

382. Yousem SA, Hochholzer L: Pulmonary hyalinizing granuloma. Am J Clin Pathol 87: 1, 1987.

383. Karpel JP, Appel D, Merav A: Pulmonary endometriosis. Lung 163: 151, 1985.

384. Foster DC, Stern JL, Buscema J, et al: Pleural and parenchymal pulmonary endometriosis. Obstet Gynecol 58: 552, 1981.

385. Slasky BS, Siewers RD, Lecky JW, et al: Catamenial pneumothorax: The roles of diaphragmatic defects and endometriosis. Am J Roentgenol 138: 639, 1982.

386. Jelihovsky T, Grant AF: Endometriosis of the lung: A case report and brief review of the literature. Thorax 23: 434, 1968.

387. Hertzanu Y, Heimer D, Hirsch M: Computed tomography of pulmonary endometriosis. Comput Radiol 11: 81, 1987.

388. Tsumori T, Nakao K, Miyata M, et al: Clinicopathologic study of thyroid carcinoma infiltrating the trachea. Cancer 56: 2843, 1985.

389. Wallace AC, Chew E-C, Jones DS: Arrest and extravasation of cancer cells in the lung. In Weiss L, Gilbert HA (eds): Pulmonary Metastasis. Boston, GK Hall, 1978, p 26.

390. Weiss L: Factors leading to the arrest of cancer cells in the lungs. In Weiss L, Gilbert HA (eds): Pulmonary Metastasis. Boston, GK Hall, 1978, p 5.

391. Kim U: Pathogenesis of lung metastases. In Weiss L, Gilbert HA (eds): Pulmonary Metastases. Boston, GK Hall, 1978, p 76.

392. Janower ML, Blennerhassett JB: Lymphangitic spread of metastatic cancer to the lung: A radiologic-pathologic classification. Radiology 101: 267, 1971.

393. Meyer KK: Direct lymphatic connections from the lower lobes of the lung to the abdomen. J Thorac Surg 35: 726, 1958.

394. Feldman GB, Knapp RG: Lymphatic drainage of the peritoneal cavity and its significance in ovarian cancer. Am J Obstet Gynecol 119: 991, 1974.

395. Sampson JA: Implantation peritoneal carcinomatosis of ovarian origin. Am J Pathol 7: 423, 1931.

396. Crow J, Slavin G, Kreel L: Pulmonary metastasis: A pathologic and radiologic study. Cancer 47: 2595, 1981.

397. Adkins PC, Wesselhoeft CW Jr, Newman W, et al: Thoracotomy on the patient with previous malignancy: Metastasis or new primary? J Thorac Cardiovasc Surg 56: 351, 1968.

398. Zollikofer C, Castaneda-Zuniga W, Stenlund R, et al: Lung metastases from synovial sarcoma simulating granulomas. Am J Roentgenol 135: 161, 1980.

399. Firooznia H, Seliger G, Genieser NB, et al: Hypertrophic pulmonary osteoarthropathy in pulmonary metastases. Radiology 115: 269, 1975.

400. Dines DE, Cortese DA, Brennan MD, et al: Malignant pulmonary neoplasms predisposing to spontaneous pneumothorax. Mayo Clin Proc 48: 541, 1973.

401. Stein MG, Mayo J, Müller N, et al: Pulmonary lymphangitic spread of carcinoma: Appearance on CT scans. Radiology 162: 371, 1987.

402. Kane RD, Hawkins HK, Miller JA, et al: Microscopic pulmonary tumor emboli associated with dyspnea. Cancer 36: 1473, 1975.

403. Winterbauer RH, Elfenbein IB, Ball WC Jr: Incidence and clinical significance of tumor embolization to the lungs. Am J Med 45: 271, 1968.

404. Altemus LR, Lee RE: Carcinomatosis of the lung with pulmonary hypertension: Pathoradiologic spectrum. Arch Intern Med 119: 32, 1967.

405. Braman SS, Whitcomb ME: Endobronchial metastasis. Arch Intern Med 135: 543, 1975.

406. Gonzalez-Vitale JC, Garcia-Bunuel R: Pulmonary tumor emboli and cor pulmonale in primary carcinoma of the lung. Cancer 38: 2105, 1976.

407. Onuigbo WIB: Contralateral pulmonary metastases in lung cancer. Thorax 29: 132, 1974.

408. Hirsch FR: Histopathologic Classification and Metastatic Pattern of Small Cell Carcinoma of the Lung. Copenhagen, Munksgaard, 1983.

409. Latour A, Shulman HS: Thoracic manifestations of renal cell carcinoma. Radiology 121: 43, 1976.

410. Merine D, Fishman EK: Mediastinal adenopathy and endobronchial involvement in metastatic renal cell carcinoma. J Comput Tomogr 12: 216, 1988.

411. Katzenstein A-L, Purvis R Jr, Gmelich J, et al: Pulmonary resection for metastatic renal adenocarcinoma. Cancer 41: 712, 1978.

412. August DA, Ottow RT, Sugarbaker PH: Clinical perspective of human colorectal cancer metastasis. Cancer Metastasis Rev 3: 303, 1984.

413. Cahan WG, Castro EB, Hajdu SI: The significance of a solitary lung shadow in patients with colon carcinoma. Cancer 33: 414, 1974.

414. Sawabe M, Nakamura T, Kanno J, et al: Analysis of morphological factors of hepatocellular carcinoma in 98 autopsy cases with respect to pulmonary metastasis. Acta Pathol Jpn 37: 1389, 1987.

415. Thomas JM, Redding WH, Sloane JP: The spread of breast cancer: Importance of the intrathoracic lymphatic route and its relevance to treatment. Br J Cancer 40: 540, 1979.

416. Ettensohn DB, Bennett JM, Hyde RW: Endobronchial metastases from carcinoma of the breast. Med Pediatr Oncol 13: 9, 1985.

417. Massin J-P, Savoie J-C, Garnier H, et al: Pulmonary metastases in differentiated thyroid carcinoma. Cancer 53: 982, 1984.

418. Shibuya H, Hisamitsu S, Shiori S, et al: Multiple primary cancer risk in patients with squamous cell carcinoma in the oral cavity. Cancer 60: 3038, 1987.

419. Yousem DM, Scatarige JC, Fishman EK, et al: Low-attenuation thoracic metastases in testicular malignancy. Am J Roentgenol 146: 291, 1986.

420. Harpole DH Jr, Johnson CM, Wolfe WG, et al: Analysis of 945 cases of pulmonary metastatic melanoma. J Thorac Cardiovasc Surg 103:743, 1992.

421. Ballon SC, Donaldson RC, Growdon WA, et al: Pulmonary metastases in endometrial carcinoma. In Weiss L, Gilbert HA (eds): Pulmonary Metastasis. Boston, GK Hall, 1978, p 182.

422. Tellis CJ, Beechler CR: Pulmonary metastasis of carcinoma of the cervix: A retrospective study. Cancer 49: 1705, 1982.

423. Sostman HD, Matthay RA: Thoracic metastases from cervical carcinoma: Current status. Invest Radiol 15: 113, 1980.

424. Kerr VE, Cadman E: Pulmonary metastases in ovarian cancer: Analysis of 357 patients. Cancer 56: 1209, 1985.

425. Apple JS, Paulson DF, Baber CB, et al: Advanced prostatic carcinoma: Pulmonary manifestations. Radiology 154: 601, 1985.

426. Bagshawe KD, Noble MIM: Cardiorespiratory aspects of trophoblastic tumours. Q J Med 35: 39, 1966.

427. Kelly MP, Rustin GJ, Ivory C, et al: Respiratory failure due to choriocarcinoma: A study of 103 dyspneic patients. Gynecol Oncol 38: 149, 1990.

428. Wolff M, Gordon K, Silva F: Pulmonary metastases (with admixed epithelial elements) from smooth muscle neoplasms. Am J Surg Pathol 3: 325, 1979.

429. Sargent EN, Barnes RA, Schwinn CP: Multiple pulmonary fibroleiomyomatous hamartomas: Report of a case and review of the literature. Am J Roentgenol 110: 694, 1970.

430. Horstmann JP, Pietra GG, Harman JA, et al: Spontaneous regression of pulmonary leiomyomas during pregnancy. Cancer 39: 314, 1977.

431. Bachman D, Wolff M: Pulmonary metastases from benign-appearing smooth muscle tumors of the uterus. Am J Roentgenol 127: 441, 1976.

432. Vezeridis MP, Moore R, Karakousis CP: Metastatic patterns in soft-tissue sarcomas. Arch Surg 118: 915, 1983.

433. Cordier JF, Bailly C, Tabone E, et al: Alveolar soft part sarcoma presenting as asymptomatic pulmonary nodules: Report of a case with ultrastructural diagnosis. Thorax 40: 203, 1985.

434. McKenna RJ, McKenna RJ Jr: Patterns of pulmonary metastases—an orthopedic hospital experience. *In* Weiss L, Gilbert HA (eds): Pulmonary Metastasis. Boston, GK Hall, 1978, p 168.

435. Rosenberg F, Spjut HJ, Gedney MM: Exfoliative cytology in metastatic cancer of the lung. N Engl J Med 261: 226, 1959.

436. Light RW, Erozan YS, Ball WC Jr: Cells in pleural fluid: Their value in differential diagnosis. Arch Intern Med 132: 854, 1973.

437. Poe RH, Ortiz C, Israel RH: Sensitivity, specificity, and predictive values of bronchoscopy in neoplasm metastatic to lung. Chest 88: 84, 1985.

438. Emirgil C, Zsoldos S, Heinemann H: Effect of metastatic carcinoma to the lung on pulmonary function in man. Am J Med 36: 382, 1964.

9

EMBOLIC AND THROMBOTIC DISEASES OF THE LUNGS

PULMONARY THROMBOSIS

Although embolization is undoubtedly the most frequent mechanism invoked to explain the presence of intrapulmonary thrombus, *in situ* thrombosis of pulmonary vessels is probably more common than is generally appreciated. Its pathogenesis and effects are related to some extent to the site of thrombosis.

Pulmonary Arteries. Probably the most common cause of *in situ* arterial thrombosis is infection, particularly abscesses and foci of active granulomatous inflammation. Thrombosis related to primary or metastatic neoplasm is also relatively common, as a result of either vascular invasion or compression by expanding tumor. Less common causes include immune-mediated vasculitis,[1] trauma,[2] aneurysms,[3] indwelling catheters,[4] congenital heart anomalies associated with decreased pulmonary blood flow such as tetralogy of Fallot,[5] and sickle cell trait or disease.[6]

Pathologically, *in situ* arterial thrombosis should be suspected if there is adjacent parenchymal disease or if there is an associated vascular abnormality known to cause thrombosis (e.g., vasculitis or tumor). Despite these diagnostic clues, the distinction between *in situ* thrombosis and embolism can be difficult and, in some cases, impossible.

Since thrombosis occurs most often in small elastic or muscular arteries supplying lung that is already involved by disease, the role of the thrombus in determining roentgenographic or clinical manifestations is probably limited in most cases. An exception is the necrosis and cavitation that develop in some cases of pneumonia (lung "gangrene") or vasculitis, the pathogenesis being related at least in part to the thrombosis and resulting ischemia.

Pulmonary Arterioles and Capillaries. Thrombosis of small pulmonary vessels occurs frequently in immune-mediated leukocytoclastic vasculitis (*see* page 417); in this situation, it is usually associated with other evidence of vascular damage, particularly parenchymal hemorrhage. Fibrin thrombi, believed to be the product of an acute hypercoagulability state, also are found in the lungs of patients who have died of shock or disseminated intravascular coagulation[7] related to such conditions as septicemia and amniotic fluid embolism. *In situ* thrombosis of small as well as large pulmonary vessels can occur in sickle cell disease.[6]

Pulmonary Veins. As in the arterial circulation, pulmonary venous thrombosis commonly develops secondary to an infectious process or neoplasm. Other related conditions include those in which there is decreased blood flow, such as tetralogy of Fallot,[5] sclerosing mediastinitis,[8] and venoocclusive disease.

PULMONARY THROMBOEMBOLISM

Bland thrombi are by far the most common clinically significant emboli to the lungs, and the majority of this section is concerned with their features. The occasional case in which the thrombus is associated with infection (septic thromboembolism) is considered separately (*see* page 557).

Epidemiology

Estimates of the incidence of pulmonary thromboemboli vary considerably in different series, largely as a result of differences in the character of the population under study and the techniques and criteria used in diagnosis. In general, however, they are an infrequent cause of both hospital admission and a *diagnosed* complication of hospitalization. Despite this, it is well recognized that the true incidence of thromboembolism is much greater than clinical studies suggest, a belief that is based on three observations: (1) Signs and symptoms of thromboembolism are lacking in as many as 80 per cent of patients[9]; (2) even in the presence of symptoms and signs[10] and even when the embolism is of

major degree,[11] a definitive diagnosis can be difficult to make during life; and (3) thromboemboli are frequently identified at autopsy. In retrospective necropsy studies, the prevalence in most series ranges from 5 to 30 per cent,[12–14] and if lungs are examined in detail prospectively, the incidence is as high as 64 per cent.[15]

An accurate estimate of the frequency of pulmonary thromboembolism as a major or significant contributory cause of death also is difficult to establish because of the subjectivity involved in such estimates. Nevertheless, the condition is clearly of great importance; for example, it has been hypothesized that it is responsible for 50,000 deaths per year in the United States.[16] According to information derived from death certificates, the age-standardized death rate increased by 50 to 100 per cent in several countries (including Canada, Sweden and the United States) between the early 1960s and the mid 1970s[17]; since then, there has been a 20 to 30 per cent decrease. The death rate is slightly greater in men than in women and almost twice as great in blacks as in whites. It shows a progressive and significant increase with age; for example, between 1985 and 1987, the death rates per 100,000 Canadian men were 0.94 between ages 40 and 44 years, 2.48 between 50 and 54, 8.30 between 60 and 64, and 24.90 between 70 and 74.[17]

Etiology and Pathogenesis

The pathogenesis of pulmonary thromboembolism can be considered under two headings: (1) the development of venous and cardiac thrombosis, and (2) the effects on the lungs of the thromboemboli themselves.

Venous and Cardiac Thrombosis

Since pulmonary thromboembolism, by definition, is characterized by the transport to and impaction within the lung of a fragment of thrombus, the process must be preceded by the development of thrombus elsewhere in the circulatory system. In the great majority of cases, this occurs in the veins of the legs, particularly the thighs. Other relatively common sites are the pelvic veins (including the periprostatic veins in men), the inferior vena cava, and the right atrium. The right ventricle,[18] right-sided heart valves, superior vena cava,[19] and the veins of the neck and arms[20] are infrequent sources. It should be emphasized that the source of thrombus is not found during life in as many as 50 per cent of cases of fatal embolism and may not be identifiable even at autopsy. In addition, foci of peripheral thrombosis are sometimes multiple, making detection of the precise source of an embolus difficult.

The pathogenesis of cardiac and venous thrombosis is complex and is related to one or more of three major factors: (1) alteration in blood flow, (2) endothelial damage, and (3) a change in the coagulability of blood. It is important to realize that in many clinical conditions, two and, sometimes, all three of these are involved and that assessment of the relative importance of each can be difficult.

Altered Blood Flow. The rate of blood flow through the systemic veins to the heart depends on the input from the arterial side of the circulation, the resistance to venous flow, the milking action of the local musculature, and, in those veins in which they are present, intraluminal valves.

An alteration in any of these can lead to a decrease in blood flow that may predispose to thrombus formation. Many of the clinical conditions associated with venous thrombosis, particularly in the legs, are in turn associated with an abnormality of one or more of these factors. Such conditions include left-sided heart failure and shock (decreased arterial input); obesity, pregnancy, intra-abdominal tumors, right-sided heart failure, external pressure from leg casts or bandages (increased resistance to flow); strokes and the postsurgical or paraplegic state (immobility with loss or decrease of muscle activity); and varicose veins (valvular abnormalities).

Because of the effect of gravity and the relatively high frequency of immobility, the legs are the most vulnerable site for an alteration in venous blood flow and, thus, for the development of thrombosis. In fact, isotopic scanning and radiographic phlebography have shown deep venous thrombosis in the legs of as many as 60 per cent of patients with strokes,[21] and about 35 per cent of patients with myocardial infarction.[22] In the legs, most thrombi appear to be initiated by local fibrin–platelet–red blood cell aggregates, often in the region of a valve pocket.[23] Although many initially form in the calf, it is clear from postmortem anatomic studies[23] and *in vivo* phlebographic investigations[24] that a substantial proportion arise in the veins of the thigh. It is widely believed that it is from this site rather than the calf that the majority of clinically significant pulmonary thromboemboli arise.

In addition to stasis, localized areas of blood turbulence may be a factor in the development of thrombosis, particularly with respect to foreign objects such as indwelling Swan-Ganz arterial catheters,[25] pacing catheters,[26] and cerebrospinal fluid shunt[27] or inferior vena cava plication[28] devices.

Endothelial Injury. Venous thrombosis secondary to injury or inflammation of the vessel wall (thrombophlebitis) is uncommon compared to the typical bland thrombosis unassociated with these events. Despite this, endothelial injury may be a significant factor in some situations, such as total hip replacement.[24] It is likely that it is also important in the thrombosis associated with bacterial endocarditis and immune-mediated vasculitis. Paradoxically, the contrast medium used to detect venous thrombosis can itself initiate thrombosis, possibly as a result of endothelial damage.[29]

Coagulation Abnormalities. Most instances of venous thrombosis and pulmonary thromboembolism are associated with medical, surgical, or obstetric conditions that have well-defined risk factors,[30] but some patients who develop peripheral venous thrombosis, with or without associated embolization, are otherwise healthy. In many such cases, questioning reveals other potential pathogenetic factors for the thrombosis, such as sitting for long periods in a cramped position while traveling[31] or prolonged standing at work in occupations such as nursing.[32] In such circumstances and when no other pathogenetic factors are evident, the possibility of a hypercoagulable state should be considered. Several of these are possible. For example, a familial deficiency of antithrombin III, an alpha$_2$-globulin capable of inactivating thrombin and factor Xa, is associated with a substantially increased incidence of deep venous thrombosis.[33] Similarly, a deficiency of either of the coagulation inhibition proteins, C or S,[34, 35] or the presence of lupus

anticoagulant[36] is associated with recurrent venous thrombosis and pulmonary thromboembolism.

Two other factors that predispose to thrombus formation—neoplasms and oral contraceptives—deserve specific mention. Patients with certain neoplasms, particularly those of the lung and gastrointestinal tract, show a propensity for the development of venous thrombosis, and such patients have an increased incidence (approximately fourfold) of pulmonary thromboembolism. The pathogenesis is unclear but probably is multifactorial. In some cases, the thrombus has been intimately associated with intravascular mucus, suggesting that this might be the initiator of the thrombosis; in others, the normal levels of coagulation factors such as fibrinogen, antithrombin, and thromboplastin are altered.[37] A substance has been identified in the blood of some patients with cancer that is capable of causing thrombosis experimentally, but its precise nature is not known.[38]

In the late 1960s it became evident that there is an increased risk of venous thrombosis and pulmonary thromboembolism in women taking oral contraceptives.[39] Although more recent analysis of the results of epidemiologic studies investigating this association has revealed a number of methodologic flaws,[40] overall the evidence still suggests a positive relationship. The culpable ingredient in the hormone pill is thought to be estrogen, which both augments clotting and impairs fibrinolysis[41]; in fact, there is evidence that the use of relatively low-dose estrogen contraceptives is associated with a decreased risk of thrombosis.[41a] In the 1960s, it was estimated that healthy women between ages 20 and 34 years who took oral contraceptives ran a risk of death from pulmonary or cerebral embolism seven to eight times that in nonusers.[42] Stated another way, one of every 2000 women taking oral contraceptives required inpatient treatment for venous thrombosis, in contrast to only one of 20,000 who did not take these drugs.[43]

Thromboembolism

A fragment of embolized thrombus lodged within a pulmonary artery has two possible immediate consequences—an increase in pressure proximal to the thrombus and a decrease or cessation of flow distal to it. The effects of thromboemboli are largely a result of these two consequences, the final clinical, roentgenographic, and pathologic manifestations being modified by a number of factors, including the size of the embolus, the presence of bacteria within the thrombus (septic embolism), the presence and extent of underlying lung abnormality (including previous thromboemboli), and the presence of extrapulmonary disease, particularly of the cardiovascular system. These manifestations can be discussed under four headings: (1) hemorrhage and infarction, (2) atelectasis, (3) hypertension, and (4) edema.

Hemorrhage and Infarction. Excluding septic embolism, parenchymal consolidation secondary to occlusion of a pulmonary artery is due to either hemorrhage alone or hemorrhage with necrosis of lung parenchyma (infarction). Both processes are a direct consequence of a deficiency of pulmonary arterial blood flow and may represent, at least in part, different manifestations of the severity of the vascular occlusion. It should be noted that because clinical and roentgenographic findings seldom permit reliable differentiation between hemorrhage and infarction, at least in their early stages, the two are usually referred to by the single term "infarction." Apart from pathologic examination, the true nature of the abnormality can be determined only by observing its roentgenologic evolution: should follow-up examinations show rapid clearing, it is reasonable to consider a lesion to be caused by hemorrhage alone; should the opacity clear slowly over several weeks, the inference can be made that the vascular insult resulted in tissue death.

Although the precise pathogenesis of pulmonary hemorrhage following thromboembolism has not been clearly established, the probable mechanism is ischemic damage to endothelial and alveolar epithelial cells, permitting the passage of red blood cells and edema into the airspaces. The hemorrhage has been considered to be derived from the bronchial arteries via bronchopulmonary anastomoses[44] but, theoretically, may also come from the pulmonary artery itself when the vessel is only partly occluded or after clot retraction or fibrinolysis has partly reopened the vessel.

It is unclear why some thromboemboli have no effect on the lung parenchyma or result in hemorrhage alone, whereas others cause infarction. However, it is known that pulmonary vascular occlusion usually results in no permanent tissue damage unless other factors coexist[45]; in fact, some necropsy reviews have suggested that the incidence of infarction is as low as 10 to 15 per cent of all cases of thromboemboli.[15] The most common underlying condition that predisposes to infarction is congestive heart failure, an association believed to be explained by increased pulmonary venous pressure and resulting decreased bronchial artery blood flow. Other conditions associated with an increased likelihood of infarction include shock, malignancy (especially of the lung in one series[46]), multiple emboli, the number of lobes containing emboli, and the presence of peripheral (as opposed to central) emboli.[13]

Atelectasis. The pathophysiologic consequences of sudden occlusion of a pulmonary vessel include local decrease in compliance and in ventilation, caused at least partly by bronchoconstriction. This may result from decreased PCO_2 within the bronchus supplying the occluded segment[47] or from the release of vasoactive and bronchoconstrictive substances such as serotonin, prostaglandins, and histamine. Although such bronchoconstriction may be in part a cause of loss of lung volume, it is likely that this is attributable mostly to surfactant depletion. This manifestation of pulmonary embolism is a common roentgenographic finding and is usually more striking when accompanied by infarction.[48]

Hypertension. Occlusion of a major portion of the pulmonary vascular tree almost inevitably results in acute pulmonary hypertension and right-sided heart failure. However, even if there are multiple pulmonary emboli, hypertension is not sustained until at least 50 per cent (probably closer to 70 per cent) of the pulmonary vascular tree is occluded.[49] Despite this, transient pulmonary hypertension may result from vasoconstriction, particularly when smaller vessels are occluded[49]; this may depend on a reflex or humoral mechanism.[50]

When an increase in pulmonary artery pressure is discovered in patients with recent pulmonary embolism, it is usually necessary to exclude previous embolic occlusions or underlying disease as being responsible. In patients with chronic obstructive pulmonary disease (COPD), measurement of the FEV_1 as an indicator of the severity of disease may be useful in distinguishing underlying disease from embolic disease as the cause of the rise in pulmonary artery pressure.[51]

Pulmonary Edema. Diffuse pulmonary edema sometimes develops after pulmonary embolism.[52] Many patients are in heart failure at the time of the embolic episode, in which case the edema is readily explained on this basis alone. Another possible pathogenetic mechanism, applicable in patients manifesting focal edema, is the pulmonary arterial hypertension that sometimes accompanies obstruction of a large cross-section of the pulmonary vascular bed. Since right ventricular output must pass through a markedly reduced vascular bed, the pulmonary hypertension that inevitably ensues can conceivably cause high capillary hydrostatic pressures with resultant edema localized to the regions of the lung not directly affected by emboli.[53]

Pathologic Characteristics

Most thromboemboli occur in the lower lobes, probably as a result of relatively greater blood flow to these regions due to the effect of gravity. The right lung is involved more frequently than the left and the posterior basal segment is particularly affected.

In the majority of instances, lung parenchyma distal to a pulmonary thromboembolus is either normal or shows only mild atelectasis and minimal intra-alveolar hemorrhage. When changes are more marked, they consist of either hemorrhage alone or a combination of hemorrhage and necrosis. In the early stages, the two may be difficult to distinguish grossly, each appearing as a more or less wedge-shaped area of red consolidation whose base abuts the pleura. In the absence of tissue death, parenchymal hemorrhage usually disappears fairly rapidly, and its residue may not be grossly detectable if the lung is examined a week or more after the embolic episode. Within 1 or 2 days of the thromboembolic event, however, an infarct becomes recognizable as a distinctly firm area of hemorrhagic consolidation (Fig. 9–1). Although it is usually well demarcated, patchy areas of parenchymal hemorrhage may be present adjacent to it, a feature that probably explains the poor definition of infarcts roentgenographically. With time, the necrotic parenchyma becomes clearly demarcated from adjacent lung by a zone of organization tissue and, eventually, is completely replaced by fibrous tissue, resulting in a contracted, somewhat elongated scar associated with pleural puckering (see Fig. 9–1).

Cavitation within an infarct usually but not invariably[54] indicates the presence of superimposed infection. It is typically associated with a prominent leukocytic infiltrate, the enzymes from the latter presumably causing liquefaction of necrotic tissue as a precursor to drainage and cavity formation.

Histologically, infarcted lung parenchyma shows coagulative necrosis and extensive airspace hemorrhage. Organization by granulation tissue is identifiable at the periphery after several days. Reactive type 2 pneumocytes are often present at the margin of the infarct at this time; when expectorated, these cells occasionally give rise to a false-positive cytologic diagnosis of malignancy.[55] Long-standing

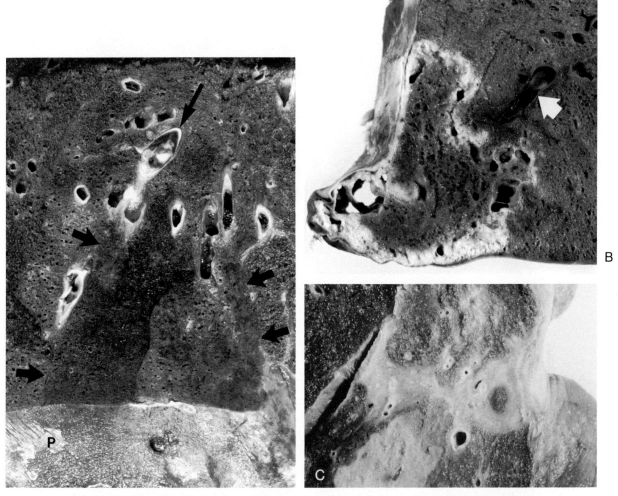

Figure 9–1. Pulmonary Infarcts: Gross Appearance. *A,* Recent infarct consisting of a wedge-shaped focus of hemorrhagic and necrotic lung parenchyma adjacent to the pleura *(small arrows).* Note the thrombus in the feeding pulmonary artery *(large arrow)* and the fibrinous pleuritis (P). *B,* An organizing infarct in the basal aspect of the lower lobe shows a distinct zone of white tissue at the junction of necrotic and viable parenchyma, representing an acute inflammatory reaction. In relation to this, there is focal cavitation. Note again the pulmonary artery thrombus *(arrow)* and the residual pleuritis. *C,* Organized infarct in a superior segment of a lower lobe consisting of a roughly linear band of fibrous tissue associated with pleural puckering. (*C* from Fraser RS: Pathologic characteristics of venous thromboembolism. *In* Leclerc JR [ed]: Venous Thromboembolic Disorders. Philadelphia, Lea & Febiger, 1991. Reproduced with permission.)

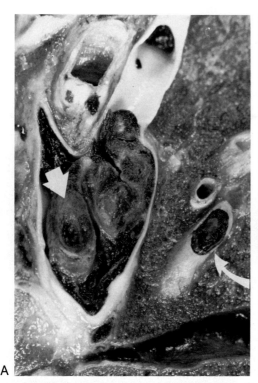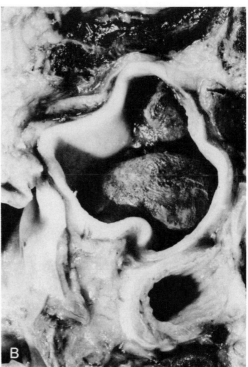

Figure 9–2. Recent Thromboemboli. Section through a lobar pulmonary artery *(A)* shows a recent thromboembolus, focally laminated *(short arrow)*. Occlusion of a small segmental branch is also apparent *(curved arrow)*. A slice at the origin of the right interlobar artery *(B)* from another patient shows complete occlusion by a smooth-surfaced, coiled thrombus. (*B* from Fraser RS: Pathologic characteristics of venous thromboembolism. *In* Leclerc JR [ed]: Venous Thromboembolic Disorders. Philadelphia, Lea & Febiger, 1991. Reproduced by permission.)

infarcts show dense parenchymal fibrosis; the adjacent pleura in the vicinity of the infarct typically shows a prominent increase in vascularity as well as fibrosis and retraction into the lung itself.

The fate of thromboemboli depends on multiple factors, including the status of the patient's fibrinolytic system, the degree of organization of the thrombus before its embolization, and the amount of new thrombus added *in situ.* However, the vast majority are largely degraded in several days to several weeks by one or more of three mechanisms—lysis, fragmentation and peripheral embolization, and organization and recanalization.

Roentgenographic and perfusion scanning studies in both humans[56] and animals[57] have established that, in many cases, flow through obstructed arteries returns relatively rapidly in the first few days after embolization, suggesting the effect of fibrinolysis. This phenomenon also may be important in preventing or decreasing the amount of thrombus added to the embolus within the pulmonary artery. Despite the angiographic evidence of rapid dissolution in some cases, many recent thromboemboli remain intact and can be recognized grossly at necropsy by one or more of three characteristics: (1) the presence of distinct laminations (Fig. 9–2) (corresponding to alternating bands of platelet-fibrin deposition during the initial stages of venous thrombosis); (2) adherence to the vessel wall (indicating organization); or (3) in larger vessels, the presence of a coiled appearance, due to imperfect fit and folding of the thrombus as it lodges in the artery (*see* Fig. 9–2).

In some experimental studies,[57] clots appear to fragment into multiple small pieces, which embolize farther toward the periphery of the lung; this phenomenon is observed somewhat later than lysis and is most prominent after the first week following embolization. The mechanism of this fragmentation may be related to splitting of the thrombus into smaller and smaller pieces as a result of ingrowth of endothelial cells and macrophages from the vessel wall.[58] Such ingrowth can also result in organization of the thrombus and its eventual conversion into fibrous tissue. Histologically, this can take the form of an eccentric plaque adjacent to the vessel wall or multiple variously thick bands traversing the lumen (recanalization) (Fig. 9–3). Although the lumina of such embolized vessels are inevitably diminished in cross-sectional area, these processes undoubtedly result in much greater flow than would have been possible without organization.

Experimental investigations in dogs and observations on humans with protracted pulmonary artery occlusion reveal a gradual increase in the bronchial circulation, which anastomoses freely with pulmonary vessels until the normal pulmonary arterial blood flow is equaled.[59] Systemic-pulmonary arterial anastomoses are usually inapparent on postmortem aortography 3 to 7 days after embolization but are well formed by 3 to 4 weeks; these anastomoses presumably play a major role in the lung's response to later emboli.[60]

Roentgenographic Manifestations

Consideration of the manifestations of pulmonary thromboembolic disease should be prefaced by a further re-

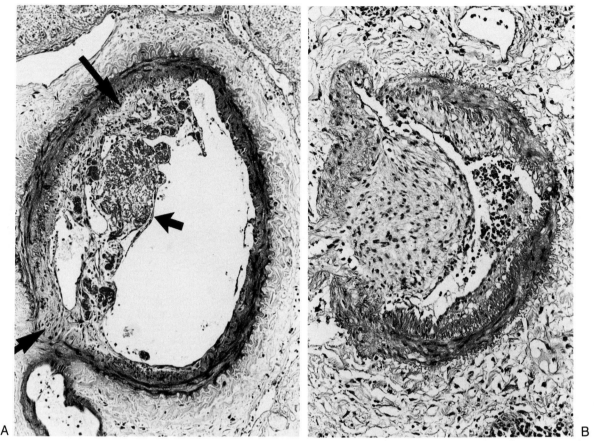

Figure 9–3. Organizing Thromboemboli. A histologic section of a muscular artery of medium size *(A)* shows a small amount of thrombus *(short arrow)* covered by endothelial cells; the thrombus has been partly replaced by fibrous tissue *(long arrows)*, which is firmly attached to the intima. A section of another vessel *(B)* shows a more advanced stage of organization, the thrombus being completely replaced by an eccentric plaque of fibrous tissue.

minder that most episodes are asymptomatic and produce no detectable changes on plain chest roentgenograms. Even if the diagnosis is suspected clinically and confirmed angiographically, in many cases no abnormalities are seen on plain films.[61] Roentgenologically apparent changes usually occur only when a fairly large segmental artery is occluded or when obstruction of many small vessels has impaired pulmonary hemodynamics.[62] The statement made by Figley and associates[63] in discussing life-threatening embolism is appropriate: "The principal evidence of embolism on the chest roentgenogram is often the paucity of abnormalities for a patient in such dire straits."

Those cases in which the roentgenographic manifestations are apparent can be divided into those with and without increased roentgenographic density—that is, with and without "infarction."

Thromboembolism Without Infarction

Four abnormalities can be appreciated in this group: oligemia, change in vessel size, alteration in size and configuration of the heart, and loss of lung volume.

Oligemia. Oligemia may be local, in which case it is caused by occlusion of a fairly large lobar or segmental pulmonary artery (Fig. 9–4), or general, due to the result of widespread small vessel thromboembolism. It is more often detected when a whole lung or a major part of it is deprived of its pulmonary artery circulation, the unilateral oligemia contrasting markedly with the pleonemia of the other lung.

Despite the previous statements about the lack of roentgenographic abnormalities in thromboembolism, oligemia is a relatively common finding, at least in association with massive pulmonary embolism. For example, in one study of 25 patients with this complication in whom plain film and angiographic abnormalities were correlated,[48] *local oligemia* (Westermark's sign) was observed in *all*. In fact, 79 per cent of such zones apparent on the arteriogram were recognizable on the plain roentgenogram.

There is evidence that computed tomography (CT) also may be able to detect oligemia with a high degree of accuracy; for example, in one experimental study carried out on dogs following balloon occlusion of a major lower lobe artery, lung parenchyma distal to the occluded vessel revealed an appreciable reduction in Hounsfield units compared to identical anatomic zones of the contralateral lung, reflecting oligemia.[64] Assuming that the results of such animal experimentation can be extrapolated to humans, it appears that CT possesses considerable promise for identification of oligemia in acute pulmonary embolism in humans

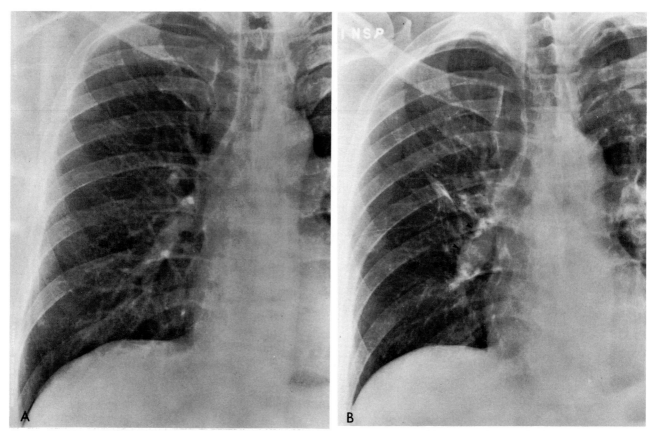

Figure 9–4. Pulmonary Embolism Without Infarction: The Westermark Sign. On admission of a 52-year-old man to the hospital, a posteroanterior roentgenogram *(A)* revealed no significant abnormalities. Several days following abdominal surgery, he experienced abrupt onset of right chest pain and dyspnea. *B*, A roentgenogram at this time showed an obvious increase in diameter and a change in configuration of the right interlobar artery *(arrowheads);* also, the distal end of this artery appeared "knuckled," and the vessels peripheral to it diminutive. The overall density of the right lower zone was considerably less than that of the left, indicating diminished perfusion (the Westermark sign).

(Fig. 9–5); however, since prompt radionuclide scanning can be expected to yield similar information at much lower cost, routine use of CT in this clinical setting is unlikely.

General pulmonary oligemia in thromboembolic disease is almost invariably the result of widespread occlusion of smaller arteries and is nearly always accompanied by signs of pulmonary artery hypertension—enlargement of the central pulmonary arteries, cor pulmonale, cardiac decompensation, and dilatation of the superior vena cava and azygos vein (Fig. 9–6).[65] Absence of overinflation differentiates diffuse thromboembolism from diffuse emphysema.

Changes in the Pulmonary Artery. Enlargement of a major pulmonary artery is an important sign of pulmonary embolism.[66] The normal maximal diameter of the right interlobar artery at total lung capacity is 16 mm in men and 15 mm in women; that of the left interlobar artery is approximately 18 mm. When these values are exceeded, it may be reasonably concluded that a vessel is enlarged.[67] Of greater reliability than these absolute measurements, however, is increase in size of the affected vessel in serial examinations, an observation that is strong evidence of thromboembolism, especially if peripheral oligemia is present (*see* Fig. 9–4). Widening of the pulmonary artery usually diminishes rapidly, and the artery reverts to normal size within a few days after lysis and fragmentation of the thrombus.[63]

It is almost certain that the increase in size of these arteries is the result of distention of the vessel by the thrombus itself, *not* of increased vascular pressure. This is because the increase in resistance due to local embolization causes redistribution of blood flow to areas of normal vascular resistance throughout both lungs; in fact, this redistribution of blood flow may itself be evidenced on plain roentgenograms by an increase in the size of the vessels (*see* Fig. 9–5). Only when there is widespread involvement in both lungs (70 per cent or more of the cross-sectional area of the vascular bed) does the increased resistance result in dilatation of the hilar artery; such an increase in size is bilateral and symmetric.

Of diagnostic importance equal to the increase in size of an interlobar artery is abrupt diminution in caliber of the occluded vessel distally owing to a lack of blood flow; the vessel may taper gradually or terminate completely, creating the so-called knuckle sign (Fig. 9–7).[68] Occluded vessels also may be more sharply delineated than normal, a sign probably attributable to diminished amplitude of pulsation.

Cardiac Changes (Cor Pulmonale). Cor pulmonale is an uncommon roentgenologic accompaniment of thromboembolism and occurs most often with multiple peripheral emboli; when a large enough area of the arterial system is occluded, it can also be seen with massive central embolization (*see* Fig. 4–77, page 238). The signs are those of

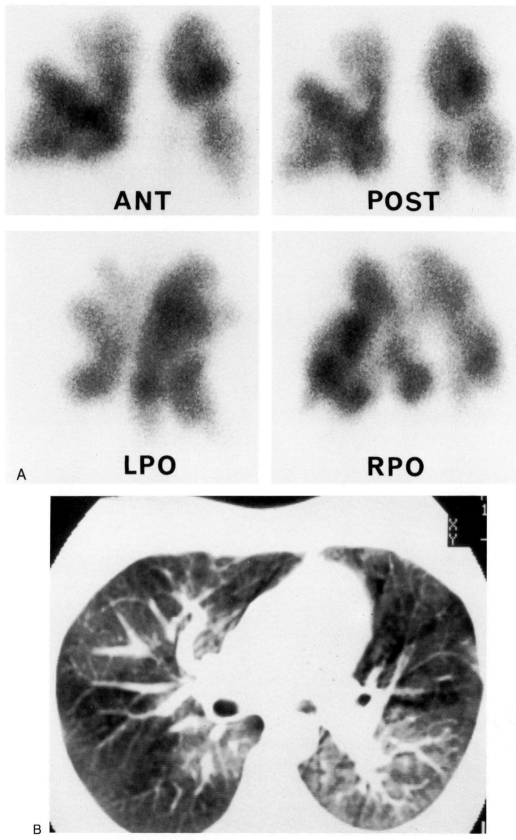

Figure 9–5. CT Depiction of Chronic Thromboembolism. A perfusion lung scintigram *(A)* in anterior (ANT), posterior (POST), right posterior oblique (RPO), and left posterior oblique (LPO) projections shows multiple segmental deficits in both lungs. A ventilation scan (not shown) was normal. The combined scintigraphic findings are highly suggestive of thromboembolic disease. A CT scan through the lower lobes *(B)* reveals sharply contrasting, contiguous areas of high and low CT attenuation that represent zones of increased perfusion and oligemia, respectively. In those areas with increased perfusion, the vessels are larger than normal, contrasting with the smaller size of those in the hyperlucent lung.

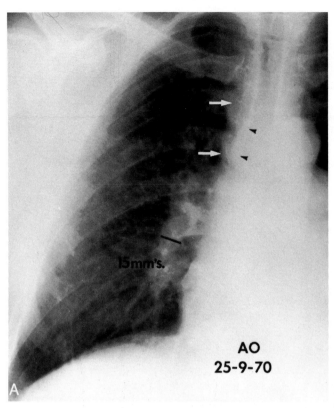
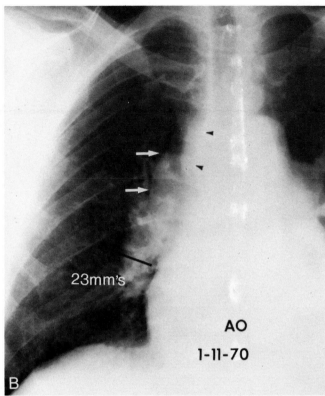

Figure 9–6. Acute Cor Pulmonale and Systemic Venous Hypertension Caused by Massive Pulmonary Thromboembolism. A detail view of the right lung *(A)* is normal; note the appearance of the superior vena cava *(arrows)*, azygos vein *(arrowheads)*, and right interlobar artery (measuring 15 mm in transverse diameter). Two months later, this elderly man suffered the sudden onset of retrosternal pain and dyspnea 10 days after prostatic surgery; a repeat chest roentgenogram *(B)* discloses marked enlargement of the vena cava *(arrows)* and azygos vein *(arrowheads)*; the hilar arterial vasculature is distinctly dilated, the right interlobar artery now measuring 23 mm. The combined features are highly suggestive, if not diagnostic, of cor pulmonale associated with massive thromboembolism. A perfusion lung scan *(not shown)* disclosed an absence of perfusion in the right lung and large deficits in the left middle and lower lung zones.

cardiac enlargement due to dilatation of the right ventricle, increase in size of the main pulmonary artery, and, usually, increase in size and rapidity of tapering of the hilar pulmonary vessels.[68]

Loss of Lung Volume. Loss of volume of a lower lobe in pulmonary embolism without infarction may be manifested roentgenographically by elevation of the hemidiaphragm, or downward displacement of the major fissure, or both.

Thromboembolism with Infarction

The roentgenologic changes in embolism with and without infarction are basically the same, except that in the former instance the oligemia is replaced by parenchymal opacification. Increased size and abrupt tapering of the feeder artery occur with equal frequency in both conditions, but loss of lung volume is seen more often and is more severe with infarction (Fig. 9–8). In fact, it has been stated that elevation of the hemidiaphragm is the single most useful roentgenographic sign of infarction.[69] It is usually most evident during the first 24 hours following embolization.[70]

The roentgenographic patterns of pulmonary infarction are specific only insofar as the shadows are segmental in distribution and homogeneous in density. In the early stages particularly, any increase in density is ill defined; it is most common in the base of the right lower lobe, often nestled in the costophrenic sinus. The majority of cases involve one or perhaps two bronchopulmonary segments, thus affecting a relatively small volume of lung parenchyma. The oft-repeated observation that infarction invariably relates to a visceral pleural surface is of little value in differential diagnosis, since the majority of pneumonias do also. The interval between the embolic episode and any increase in roentgenographic density ranges from 10 to 12 hours to several days after occlusion.[71]

The "classic" configuration of a pulmonary infarct consists of a zone of homogeneous wedge-shaped consolidation in the lung periphery, with its base contiguous to a visceral pleural surface and its rounded, convex apex toward the hilum (Figs. 9–9 and 9–10).[71] Originally described by Hampton and Castleman[72] in 1940, this configuration is fairly common and has come to bear the euphonious eponym of "Hampton's hump"; it is highly suggestive of pulmonary infarction. The size of the consolidated area varies from patient to patient and, in the case of multiple infarcts, from one area to another. They are usually 3 to 5 cm in

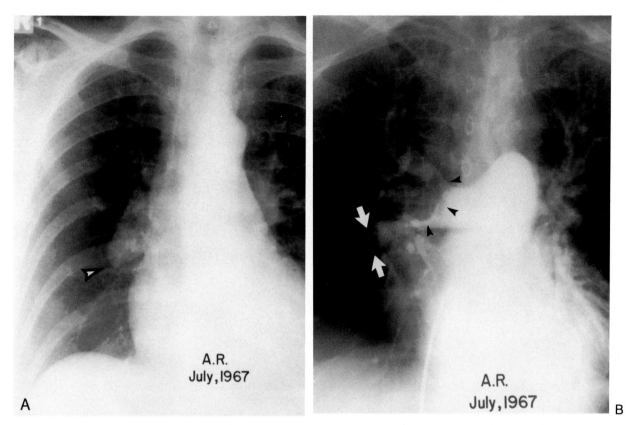

Figure 9–7. Dilatation and Amputation of the Right Interlobar Artery (Knuckle Sign) as Evidence of Pulmonary Thromboembolism. A detail view of the right lung *(A)* reveals dilatation and abrupt termination of the right interlobar artery, constituting a positive knuckle sign *(arrowhead)*. B, A pulmonary angiogram in anteroposterior projection discloses a large saddle embolus *(arrowheads)* partly obstructing the bifurcation of the ascending and descending branches of the right pulmonary artery. The right interlobar artery is completely occluded *(arrows)*, accounting for the features illustrated in *A.*

Figure 9–8. Pulmonary "Infarction" with Rapid Resolution. A view of the right lung from a conventional posteroanterior chest roentgenogram *(A)* reveals a homogeneous opacity occupying the lower half of the right lower lobe. The right hemidiaphragm is moderately elevated, and the right interlobar artery is plump. The findings are highly suggestive of pulmonary infarction. Eight days later *(B)*, the lower-lobe consolidation has resolved, and the hemidiaphragm has descended to a position consistent with emphysema. The rapidity of resolution is compatible with pulmonary hemorrhage secondary to thromboembolism.

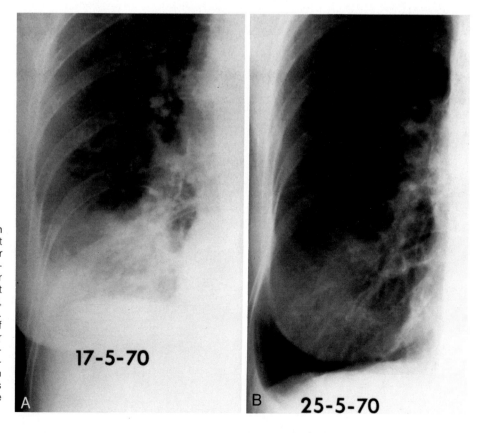

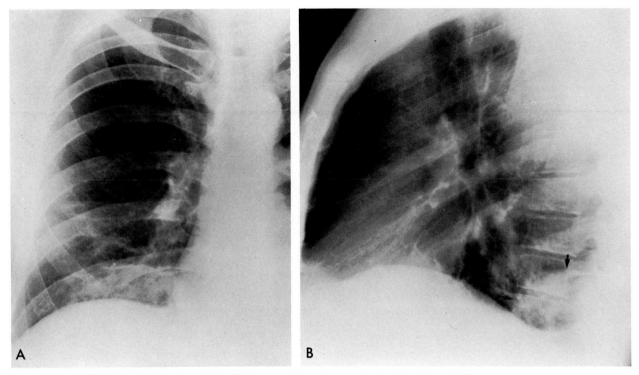

Figure 9–9. Pulmonary Infarct, Right Lower Lobe. Posteroanterior *(A)* and lateral *(B)* roentgenograms reveal a fairly well defined shadow of homogeneous density occupying the posterior basal segment of the right lower lobe. In lateral projection, the shadow has the shape of a truncated cone with its apex directed toward the hilum (Hampton's hump) *(arrows)*. A small effusion can be identified in lateral projection. This combination of changes is highly suggestive of pulmonary infarction.

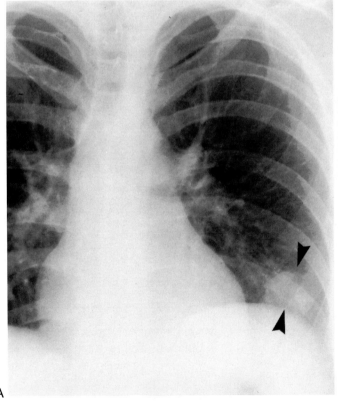

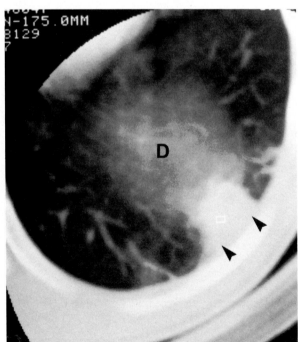

Figure 9–10. CT Depiction of Acute Pulmonary Thromboembolism and Infarction (Hampton's Hump). A conventional posteroanterior chest roentgenogram *(A)* discloses a round, homogeneous opacity *(arrowheads)* in the left lower lobe; the left hemidiaphragm is slightly elevated. *B,* A detail view of the left lower lobe from a transverse CT scan shows a pleural-based, truncated opacity *(arrowheads)* in the posterolateral costophrenic recess. The blunted medial contour is typical of a Hampton's hump. The top of the left hemidiaphragm (D) can be identified anterior to the infarct.

diameter. An air bronchogram is rarely seen[73]; absence of this finding, combined with peripheral homogeneous consolidation, should strongly suggest infarction rather than acute airspace pneumonia. Cavitation is rare[68] and usually indicates septic embolism.

Just as CT appears to be capable of revealing zones of oligemia with greater accuracy than conventional roentgenography, it is likely that it is able to demonstrate pulmonary infarcts with greater precision.[74, 75] Similarly, magnetic resonance imaging (MRI) appears to hold considerable promise in the study of pulmonary thromboembolism, both in the experimental animal[76] and in humans.[77, 77a] Again, it is clear that since radionuclide scans detect lobar or segmental defects with as much accuracy as CT or MRI, and since scintigraphy costs much less, it appears unlikely that these techniques will gain much support as cost-effective procedures.

The time course of resolution of the opacity distal to a thromboembolus is a reliable indicator of the nature of the consolidative process. If embolism results only in parenchymal hemorrhage and edema, clearing may occur within 4 to 7 days, often without residua; when it leads to necrosis, however, resolution averages 20 days[63] and may take as long as 5 weeks.[78]

The pattern of resolution can also be a valuable clue in differentiating pulmonary infarction from acute pneumonia.[79] The shadow of acute pneumonia appears to break up, rendering an originally homogeneous opacity inhomogeneous as scattered areas of radiolucency appear within it; by contrast, the shadow of a pulmonary infarct gradually diminishes but maintains its homogeneity and, roughly, its original shape (the "melting icecube" sign). However, these observations are applicable only in the resolving stages of either lesion and, therefore, have no value at a time when the institution of appropriate therapy is vital.

The outcome of pulmonary infarction includes complete resolution in approximately half the patients, residual pleural scarring in a quarter,[80] and linear opacities caused by parenchymal fibrosis in the remainder.

As a roentgenographic manifestation of thromboembolic disease, pleural effusion is as common as, if not more common than, parenchymal consolidation[66]; it nearly always indicates infarction. The parenchymal shadow may be diminutive or hidden by the fluid, so confusing the diagnostic possibilities that an embolic episode will be suggested only if the physician has a high index of suspicion. The amount of pleural fluid is frequently small but may be abundant. It is more often unilateral. When predominantly infrapulmonary, it may be mistaken for hemidiaphragmatic elevation.[71] Fluid usually develops and absorbs synchronously with the infarct, but sometimes it appears later and clears sooner.[63]

The Accuracy of Chest Roentgenography in the Diagnosis of Pulmonary Thromboembolism

Possibly the most definitive study to date that has been carried out to test the accuracy of the chest roentgenogram in the diagnosis of pulmonary embolism was carried out by Greenspan and colleagues[81] and published in 1982. These authors garnered the chest roentgenograms of 152 patients, all of whom were suspected at one time of having pulmonary embolism but in whom only 108 proved to have em-

bolism on the basis of a positive pulmonary angiogram (the remaining 44 patients were assumed not to have embolism on the basis of either a normal perfusion scintiscan or a pulmonary angiogram). The roentgenograms were randomized and presented for interpretation to nine readers (seven of whom were radiologists specializing in pulmonary disease). The question "Does this patient have pulmonary embolism?" required a "yes," "no," or "don't know" answer. The results were dismal: the predictive index, reflecting the overall accuracy of diagnosis, was 0.40 (range 0.17 to 0.57) for the entire group.

On the basis of this study, the authors concluded that although the chest roentgenogram may provide additional information in the evaluation of patients suspected of having pulmonary embolism, it cannot be considered a definitive examination, in and of itself. Its major importance lies in the exclusion of other disease processes that can mimic acute pulmonary embolism and in providing correlation with V̇/Q̇ lung scans.

Special Investigative Techniques

Because of the unreliability of standard chest roentgenography in the diagnosis of pulmonary thromboembolism, additional investigations are frequently required to confirm or exclude the diagnosis. The most useful of these are angiography and scintigraphy.

Pulmonary Angiography

Pulmonary arteriography is the single most useful technique for investigating suspected pulmonary thromboembolic disease.[82, 83] Best results are obtained if the contrast medium is injected through a catheter whose tip is in the right or left pulmonary artery (Fig. 9–11). This permits not only a clear view of the ipsilateral pulmonary arterial tree but also the measurement of pulmonary artery pressure. The study may reveal partial or complete occlusion of lobar or segmental vessels but is seldom useful when the obstructed vessels are subsegmental or smaller. In such cases, it may be necessary to perform subsegmental arteriography, first in anteroposterior (AP) projection[84] and then in other projections if the AP study is inconclusive.

Digital subtraction angiography (DSA) has been shown in some investigations of both animals[85] and humans[86] to have considerable potential benefit in the diagnosis of pulmonary embolism. For example, in one study of 33 patients with suspected embolism, the overall diagnostic accuracy was about 90 per cent.[86] However, not all studies have had the same success[87] and although there is little argument that DSA is less expensive and safer, faster, and easier to perform than conventional pulmonary arteriography, there is some doubt regarding its reliability as an acceptable substitute. For the demonstration of central pulmonary emboli, cine-gradient-refocused MRI has been shown to be an accurate method of investigation in some patients.[88]

The angiographic criteria reported for the diagnosis of pulmonary embolism are listed in Table 9–1. Although the importance of secondary signs has been stressed, it should be remembered that they reflect nothing more than diminished pulmonary arterial perfusion, a common manifesta-

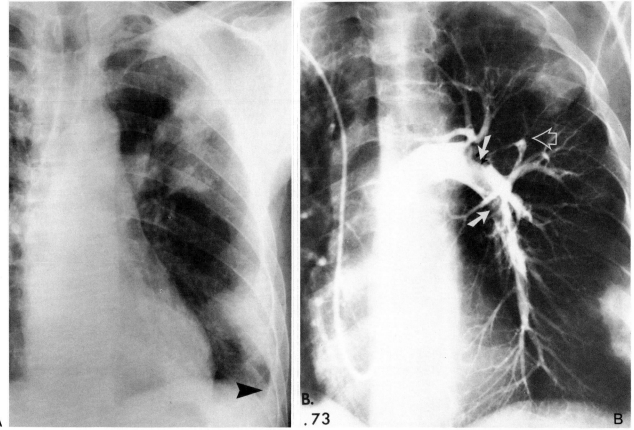

Figure 9–11. Value of Oblique Arteriography in the Demonstration of Pulmonary Thromboembolism. A conventional posteroanterior chest roentgenogram *(A)* shows multiple well-defined and poorly defined homogeneous opacities in the left lung. The lesions relate intimately to visceral pleura and are associated with a small pleural effusion *(arrowhead)*. Cardiac size and configuration are normal. *B,* A selective left pulmonary arteriogram in left anterior oblique projection reveals multiple intraluminal filling defects *(arrows)*. A segmental artery *(open arrow)* in the upper lobe is amputated.

tion of several pulmonary and cardiac diseases from which pulmonary embolism must be differentiated (Table 9–2). In fact, there is only one established angiographic criterion for the definitive diagnosis of pulmonary embolism—direct observation of an intraluminal filling defect.[66] Despite this, the secondary signs listed in Table 9–1 may be useful by

Table 9–1. ANGIOGRAPHIC CRITERIA FOR THE DIAGNOSIS OF PULMONARY EMBOLISM

Primary Sign
A. Filling defect
   1. Persistent intraluminal radiolucency, central or marginal, without complete obstruction of blood flow
   2. Trailing edge of an intraluminal radiolucency when there is complete obstruction of distal blood flow

Secondary Signs
A. Abrupt occlusion ("cutoff") of a pulmonary artery without visualization of an intraluminal filling defect
B. Perfusion defect (asymmetric filling)
   1. Areas of oligemia or avascularity
   2. Focal areas in which the arterial phase is prolonged (especially when localized to the lower lung fields); this is usually accompanied by slow filling and emptying of the pulmonary veins
   3. Tortuous, abruptly tapering peripheral vessels, with a paucity of branching vessels ("pruning")

With permission from Sagel SS, Greenspan RH: Nonuniform pulmonary arterial perfusion: Pulmonary embolism? Radiology 99: 541, 1971.

directing attention to areas where manifestations of embolism may be subtle; in such cases, segmental or wedge arteriography, especially with magnification, may reveal intraluminal defects in smaller vessels.

Care must be taken not to misinterpret an opacified artery seen end-on as a blunt obstruction. Tapering of vessels usually denotes circumferential organization and recanalization and, therefore, an old thromboembolic episode.[89] In follow-up angiographic studies,[90] weblike deformities of vessels identified *in vivo* at the precise sites of intra-arterial filling defects previously shown angiographically have been assumed to be remnants of emboli.

Measurement of the right ventricular and pulmonary arterial pressures is often very helpful in the evaluation of patients with thromboembolic disease,[91] and these pressures should always be carefully recorded before pulmonary angiography. Even if the angiogram reveals no evidence of major vessel occlusion, the pulmonary arterial pressure may be raised, suggesting the presence of multiple small emboli throughout the lungs. However, some investigators believe that this combination of findings is more characteristic of primary pulmonary hypertension,[92] since the hypertension that accompanies multiple pulmonary emboli almost invariably results from embolization of vessels large enough to be seen angiographically. The pressure probably is raised in most patients with positive angiographic findings, and

Table 9–2. CONDITIONS ASSOCIATED WITH NONUNIFORM PULMONARY ARTERIAL PERFUSION

I. *Emphysema (focal or diffuse)*
II. *Inflammatory diseases*
 Pneumonia (including tuberculosis)
 Lung abscess
 Bronchiectasis
 Pulmonary fibrosis:
  Interstitial fibrosis
  Fibrothorax
III. *Congenital*
 Absence or hypoplasia of a pulmonary artery
 Peripheral pulmonary artery stenosis
 Bronchopulmonary sequestration
IV. *Extrinsic obstruction of a pulmonary artery or vein by compression or actual invasion*
 Neoplasms:
  Benign
  Malignant
 Inflammatory:
  Fibrosing mediastinitis
 Aortic aneurysms
V. *Intrinsic obstruction of a pulmonary artery*
 Thromboembolic disease:
  Blood clot
  Tumor
  Fat
 The Eisenmenger reaction: superimposed obliterative arteriolitis develops in large left-to-right intracardiac and extracardiac shunts
 Arteritis
VI. *Postcapillary pulmonary (venous) hypertension*
 Left ventricular failure
 Mitral valvular disease
 Pulmonary veno-occlusive disease
VII. *Focal hypoventilation (frequently associated with atelectasis or air trapping)*
 Bronchial obstruction:
  Inflammatory process
  Neoplasm
  Reflex bronchoconstriction
   Asthma
   Pulmonary embolism
 Splinting from pleural irritation:
  Inflammation ("pleuritis")
  Rib fractures

With permission from Sagel SS, Greenspan RH: Nonuniform pulmonary arterial perfusion: Pulmonary embolism? Radiology 99: 541, 1971.

those with a mean right ventricular pressure exceeding 22 mm Hg are likely to die.[93]

Scintigraphy

Although it is well recognized that pulmonary angiography is the definitive method of establishing the diagnosis of embolism and of demonstrating its extent, it is expensive and time-consuming and has the potential for significant morbidity and mortality. As a result, it is now well accepted that ventilation-perfusion scintigraphy is the technique of choice as the initial screening procedure in the diagnosis of pulmonary embolism.[94]

Pulmonary emboli are rarely, if ever, identified angiographically in patients with normal perfusion images, so when scintigraphy is normal, arteriography is not indicated.[95] Similarly, when $\dot{V}/\dot{Q}$ studies demonstrate perfusion defects that correspond in size and location to zones of decreased ventilation ($\dot{V}/\dot{Q}$ match), embolism is unlikely and no further evaluation is usually required.[96] By contrast, when $\dot{V}/\dot{Q}$ studies demonstrate sizable perfusion defects in

the absence of ventilatory impairment ($\dot{V}/\dot{Q}$ mismatch) or of associated roentgenographic abnormalities, the probability of embolism is high (*see* Fig. 9–5).

In addition to these relatively straightforward situations, there are certain instances in which abnormalities observed on conventional roentgenograms and $\dot{V}/\dot{Q}$ scans are such that a conclusive statement regarding the presence or absence of embolism cannot be made: the findings are indeterminate.[96] The most frequent of these is one in which the scintigraphic abnormalities correspond in anatomic distribution to opacities identified on chest roentgenograms. The three combinations of perfusion patterns and roentgenographic abnormalities that can be seen in this situation are associated with different probabilities of embolism: (1) when the perfusion defect is substantially smaller than the corresponding roentgenographic abnormality, pulmonary embolism is present infrequently; (2) when the perfusion defect is substantially larger than the corresponding roentgenographic opacity, pulmonary embolism is present in a large percentage of patients; and (3) when the perfusion defect and radiographic opacity are of about equal size, the frequency of pulmonary embolism is approximately 25 per cent.

On the basis of these and the foregoing observations, a scheme for the interpretation of $\dot{V}/\dot{Q}$ images has been proposed by Biello and associates (Table 9–3).[97] For comparison purposes, another set of criteria selected by the multiinstitutional committee involved in the prospective National Institutes of Health–sponsored PIOPED trial (Prospective Investigation of Pulmonary Embolism Diagnosis) is also listed. Not included are the criteria established by McNeil[98] and more recently by Biello,[99] although a recent study suggests that the latter scheme represents the best compromise of the three sets of criteria (including PIOPED).[100]

Patients with COPD who are suspected of having acute pulmonary embolism are a problematic diagnostic group. These persons often have ventilation and perfusion abnormalities caused by the underlying COPD that make the interpretation of $\dot{V}/\dot{Q}$ scans very difficult. Because of this, ventilation imaging probably is not warranted in patients with roentgenographic or clinical evidence of severe disease[101] (although some investigators have found no significant difference in the diagnostic utility of $\dot{V}/\dot{Q}$ scans in patients with and without prior cardiac or pulmonary disease[101a]). However, when an attempt is made to distinguish $\dot{V}/\dot{Q}$ matching that is compatible with pulmonary embolism from that caused by COPD, a computation of the actual $\dot{V}/\dot{Q}$ ratio may be useful; in one study[102] in which a $\dot{V}/\dot{Q}$ ratio of 1.25 or higher was used to define an area of mismatch, the percentage of patients classified correctly as having either pulmonary embolism or COPD increased from 56 to 88 per cent, based simply on a consideration of the matched or mismatched character of perfusion.

Comparison of Angiography and Isotopic Scanning

Pulmonary scintigraphy and angiography have been correlated in the evaluation of patients with pulmonary embolism in several studies.[103, 104] By and large, all agree on two basic principles: (1) pulmonary $\dot{V}/\dot{Q}$ scans and angiograms are complementary, not competitive, techniques for the evaluation of pulmonary embolic disease; and (2) each method has diagnostic limitations. For example, in one

Table 9–3. **TWO SCHEMES FOR INTERPRETATION OF V̇/Q̇ IMAGES**

Probability of Pulmonary Embolism	A*	B†
None	Normal perfusion	Normal perfusion
Low	Small V̇/Q̇ mismatches	Small Q̇ defects regardless of number, ventilation or chest X-ray findings
		Q̇ defect substantially smaller than chest roentgenogram
	Focal V̇/Q̇ matches with no corresponding radiographic abnormalities	
	Perfusion defects substantially smaller than radiographic abnormalities	V̇/Q̇ match in 50% of one lung or 75% of one lung zone; chest roentgenogram normal or nearly normal
		Single moderate Q̇ defect with normal chest roentgenogram (V̇ irrelevant)
		Nonsegmental Q̇ defects
Intermediate	Diffuse, severe airway obstruction	Abnormality that is not defined by either "high" or "low"
	Matched perfusion defects and radiographic abnormalities	
	Single moderate V̇/Q̇ mismatch without corresponding radiographic abnormality	
High	Perfusion defects substantially larger than radiographic abnormalities	Two or more large Q̇ defects; V̇ and chest roentgenogram normal
	One or more large or two or more moderate-sized V̇/Q̇ mismatches with no corresponding radiographic abnormalities	Two or more large Q̇ defects in which Q̇ is substantially larger than either matching V̇ or chest roentgenogram
		Two or more moderate Q̇ and one large Q̇; V̇ and chest roentgenogram normal
		Four or more moderate Q̇; V̇ and chest roentgenogram normal

*Proposed by Biello et al[96] (slightly modified).
†Proposed by PIOPED. Wellman.[96a]

study of 14 patients with pulmonary embolism established by both lung scanning and selective pulmonary angiography, the findings with both correlated reasonably well overall in the assessment of embolic involvement[105]; however, the lung scan better depicted capillary flow and the angiogram better detected embolic material in large vessels. When embolization involved less than 40 per cent of the lung, it was better demonstrated by the perfusion scan, whereas more extensive involvement was more reliably detected by angiography. In another study of 71 patients with findings indicative of pulmonary embolism who underwent lung scanning and then pulmonary angiography,[106] the scan predicted specific arteriographic evidence of pulmonary embolism in 75 per cent of those whose scan defects were characteristic of embolism (i.e., the perfusion defects corresponded to specific anatomic segments and the chest roentgenograms were normal or suggested pulmonary embolism). Although scanning is not as reliable as angiography in assessing oligemia at the lung bases, all correlative studies have shown that it has the theoretical advantage of depicting the circulation in the lung periphery, an area poorly visualized by angiography.[82]

Because of the lower cost, relative ease of performance, and lower morbidity and mortality rates, it seems reasonable to utilize V̇/Q̇ scintigraphy as the initial screening procedure in patients suspected of having acute pulmonary embolism. If the findings are abnormal but inconclusive and if the suspicion of embolism is high based on clinical and roentgenographic findings, angiography should be performed. We are in general agreement with the requirement for angiography before the institution of thrombolytic therapy or any form of surgery but do not favor its routine use before starting anticoagulant therapy. If a pulmonary scan is positive and there is strong clinical evidence of an acute embolic episode but the chest roentgenogram is normal, we feel that anticoagulant therapy should be started without further diagnostic intervention. In fact, if the chest roentgenogram reveals an abnormality consistent with embolism and infarction and the patient has symptoms and signs of peripheral venous thrombosis, there seems to be little indication for a scan. In such cases, the results of this procedure should not influence the decision to institute anticoagulant therapy.

Computed Tomography and Magnetic Resonance Imaging

In patients in whom pulmonary arteriography is contraindicated, MRI[77, 77a, 107] and CT[108, 108a] are noninvasive alternatives in certain circumstances (Fig. 9–12). For example, the results of one experimental study suggested that CT with contrast enhancement may permit identification of emboli in both lobar and segmental arteries.[108] MRI has been shown to hold some promise for the identification of central pulmonary emboli.[88]

Methods of Diagnosis of Deep Vein Thrombosis

Knowledge of the presence or absence of deep venous thrombosis can be helpful in assessing the likelihood of pulmonary embolism; for example, in one prospective study, 70 per cent of patients with pulmonary embolism proven by angiography showed clinical evidence of thrombosis of the deep veins of the legs.[109] However, since clinical features are notoriously inaccurate for suggesting the diagnosis, special investigative techniques, of which there are several, must be performed in most cases.

Phlebography (Venography). This technique is used to outline the deep veins extending from the calf to the inferior vena cava, to determine the presence and site of

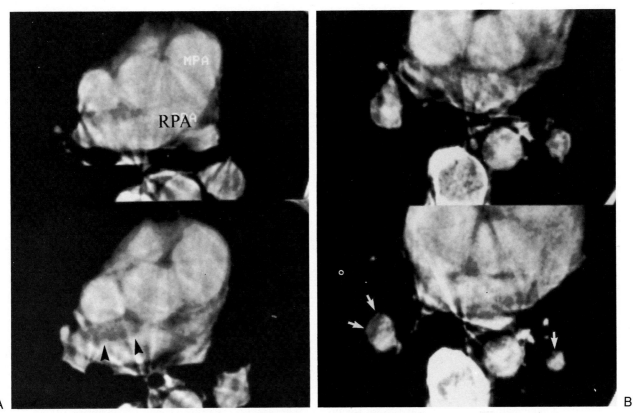

Figure 9–12. Chronic Pulmonary Thromboembolism: CT Manifestations. Contrast-enhanced CT scans through the right pulmonary artery (RPA) *(A)* and its descending branches *(B)* reveal an elongated filling defect *(arrowheads)* adjacent to the anterior wall of the right pulmonary artery, and a number of smaller, eccentric defects on the anterior parts of the descending arteries *(arrows)*.

thrombus formation. Usually, the veins are opacified by injecting contrast medium into a foot vein; however, with this method, the external and common iliac veins are inadequately opacified in as many as 15 to 20 per cent of patients. Visualization of these veins in these patients is more difficult and requires direct femoral vein or intraosseous injection.[110] Venography has at least two other disadvantages: it is painful and it can itself induce thrombosis in 3 to 4 per cent of patients. Despite this, the procedure is recommended for patients with recurrent pulmonary embolism when thrombectomy and venous ligation are being contemplated,[111] particularly if anticoagulant therapy has apparently been unsuccessful.

Scintigraphy. This method is performed by intravenously injecting ^{125}I-labeled fibrinogen into a patient who has taken daily oral doses of iodine. This is followed by scanning of the legs, with or without an ultrasound flow detector test or impedance plethysmography. The technique can be used to monitor deep vein thrombosis postoperatively, to detect extension of thrombosis from the leg into the thigh, and to decide whether anticoagulant therapy is needed[111]; however, it is inaccurate in assessing thrombosis of the veins of the upper thigh and pelvis.

It has been shown in both animals[112] and humans[113] that ^{111}In-labeled autologous platelets can adhere to venous thrombi, target-to-background ratios being sufficient to permit external "hot spot" imaging with a scintillation camera. The correlation between venography and scintigraphy in the diagnosis of deep venous thrombosis is excellent.[114]

Whereas ^{125}I-labeled fibrinogen has been found to be useful in the detection of calf vein thrombosis as it forms, ^{111}In-labeled platelets reveal established thrombi high in the iliofemoral segment.[115]

Ultrasonography. A noninvasive procedure that shows a high degree of accuracy in the detection of fresh thrombi in popliteal and proximal veins is the Doppler ultrasound flow detection method.[116] Normal venous sound is recognized by its cyclic nature, coincident with the respiratory cycle, and by its modification with the Valsalva and Mueller maneuvers. Thrombosis in the iliofemoral veins is readily recognizable by alteration in audible sounds or flow-velocity patterns recorded over the common femoral vein. This method is said to correlate well with iliac phlebography[117] and has been recommended for screening high-risk patients; phlebography is reserved to confirm the diagnosis before starting therapy. However, some investigators[118] have reported a small percentage of positive findings in patients with pulmonary emboli; as a result, this method of assessing flow variation has largely been replaced by impedance plethysmography.

Impedance Plethysmography. This technique is based on variations in blood flow measured by a change in electrical resistance between electrodes fastened to the calf.[119] Since blood is an excellent conductor of electricity, the change in limb venous blood volume when a thigh cuff is inflated normally results in decreased resistance; when the cuff pressure is released, a prompt increase in resistance follows. Constant dilatation of the deep venous system caused by thrombotic occlusion results in little or no change in resistance with this maneuver. The technique appears to be a safe and reliable non-invasive method of determining deep vein patency, especially when combined with fibrinogen scanning.

Thermography. Liquid crystal contact color thermography is a relatively new technique based on the fact that cholesteric crystals possess the property of changing colors in consistent, predictable patterns in response to local temperature changes.[120] The technique consists of embedding liquid crystals in elastic, flexible sheets, which are then inflated and adapted to the contour of extremities of various sizes and shapes. Preliminary results have shown excellent correlation with ascending phlebography, the two methods being in agreement in 90 per cent of cases.

Magnetic Resonance Imaging. In one study of 16 patients in which limited flip-angle, gradient-refocused MRI was compared with venography in the detection of deep venous thrombosis, MRI allowed accurate detection and localization of the thrombi that had been identified by venography in 16 of 17 extremities.[121] Although these results suggest a use for MRI in this situation, because of expense and time involved in this technique it is unlikely to be useful routinely.

Clinical Manifestations

The clinical manifestations of pulmonary thromboembolic disease depend on a combination of several factors, including (1) the presence or absence of underlying cardiopulmonary disease; (2) the size, number, and location of emboli; (3) whether vessel occlusion is complete or partial; and (4) when embolic episodes are multiple, the time interval between them.

Many thromboemboli produce no symptoms or cause such minimal distress that they may be recognized only in retrospect. However, in a patient with underlying disease, particularly of the lungs or heart, they are much more likely to lead to complications such as pulmonary infarction, cardiac arrhythmia, systemic hypotension, and death. Symptoms and signs also are often absent during individual episodes of multiple pulmonary emboli that are of sufficient severity to cause chronic cor pulmonale.[122] It should be emphasized that a major clue to the diagnosis of pulmonary thromboembolism is the presence of a well-defined predisposing condition. In addition, in about 50 per cent of cases, close questioning elicits a history of one or more transitory episodes of dyspnea in the past, harbingers of later, more distressing embolism and infarction.[123]

As a generalization, clinical features of pulmonary thromboembolic disease are related to one of four processes: (1) sudden occlusion of a small portion of the vascular bed (undoubtedly the most common situation, in which there may be no more than a transient episode of dyspnea or tachypnea[123a] associated with a normal chest roentgenogram); (2) sudden occlusion of a relatively large portion of the vascular bed (massive pulmonary embolism); (3) pulmonary infarction; and (4) multiple, often undetected episodes of thromboembolism resulting in pulmonary hypertension.

Massive pulmonary embolism results when a thrombus lodges in one or more proximal pulmonary arteries, ob-

structing at least 50 per cent of the pulmonary vascular bed. As a result of acute right ventricular strain, central venous pressure rises and cardiac output falls. Peripheral venous vasoconstriction may prevent systemic hypotension, but with very high resistance in the lesser circulation the blood pressure falls, and the clinical presentation is that of circulatory collapse.[124] Patients complain of severe dyspnea and retrosternal pain similar to that of angina pectoris; tachycardia, tachypnea, and, occasionally, cyanosis develop. Auscultation may reveal bronchial breathing but rarely rales or a friction rub. The jugular veins are distended, and a gallop rhythm is invariably audible. There may be a diffuse systolic lift at the left sternal edge, with accentuation of the pulmonic component of the second heart sound.

When there is pulmonary infarction, the patient may complain of dyspnea of acute onset, pain on breathing, and hemoptysis (the last-named in 20 to 33 per cent of cases[30]). Tachycardia and fever are often present; the latter is usually low grade (37.2 to 37.7°C) and occurs in about 20 to 50 per cent of cases.[66, 125] Physical findings include locally decreased breath sounds, rales, rhonchi, friction rub, and signs of pleural effusion. The differential diagnosis includes pneumonia, atelectasis, and primary pleural effusion. It may be particularly difficult to rule out atelectasis, since both complications are common postoperatively. However, pneumonia usually causes higher fever and purulent expectoration and the onset is more insidious. The pleural effusion of pulmonary infarction is usually grossly bloody unless it is diluted with the transudate of heart failure.

Occasionally, multiple thromboemboli, often of small to intermediate size, occur repeatedly without acute symptoms or signs. If only a small cross-section of the vascular bed is occluded, most patients remain asymptomatic. However, if more than 50 per cent is affected, progressive dyspnea on exertion and, in some patients, right ventricular failure develop. Some complain of episodic transient dyspnea, presumably a result of intermittent microembolism (see page 584).

The presence of signs and symptoms of deep venous thrombosis, particularly in the legs, is supportive evidence of pulmonary thromboembolism and must be carefully assessed in all patients in whom the latter diagnosis is entertained. Localized pain or tenderness in the calf, popliteal fossa, or thigh, especially if associated with a discrepancy in the diameter of the legs, suggests venous thrombosis. In some cases, pain may be elicited by dorsiflexion of the foot (Homans' sign). Although these findings are helpful when present, their absence does not in any way militate against a diagnosis of thromboembolism: approximately 50 per cent of patients who suffer a fatal embolism show no clinical evidence of deep vein thrombosis.[126]

Laboratory Findings

Measurement of levels of serum enzymes such as lactate dehydrogenase (LDH) and serum glutamic oxaloacetic transaminase (SGOT) is of little value in the diagnosis of thromboembolic disease. Wacker's triad—an increased level of LDH, a normal level of SGOT, and a slightly increased level of serum bilirubin—occurs in approximately 10 per cent of cases and has not been found to be useful in distinguishing embolism from myocardial infarction or pneumonia.[70] However, an elevation of creatine phosphokinase suggests myocardial infarction rather than massive pulmonary embolism.[127]

The leukocyte count may be elevated, but it seldom exceeds 15,000 cells per mL³. Such an increase is usually associated with fever and symptoms and signs of pulmonary infarction.

Pulmonary function studies reveal restrictive disease: the resting lung volume is decreased, airway resistance is increased, and lung compliance and diffusing capacity are reduced. Arterial blood gas analysis typically reveals hypoxemia and respiratory alkalosis. The hypoxemia cannot always be corrected by breathing 100 per cent oxygen, suggesting intrapulmonary venous shunting that may be due to pulmonary edema[128]; in most cases, however, it is probably caused chiefly by $\dot{V}/\dot{Q}$ abnormality. Despite the foregoing, alterations in arterial blood gases, dead space measurement, and arterial–end tidal carbon dioxide gradient are neither sufficiently sensitive nor specific to be of great use in differential diagnosis.[129]

Electrocardiographic changes appear early and are often transient; they are caused by acute pulmonary hypertension and hypoxemia and therefore are most common after massive pulmonary embolism.[130] Nonspecific ST segment and T wave changes are probably the most common[123a]; however, certain patterns are highly suggestive of the diagnosis, including an S wave in lead I and an inverted Q wave or T wave, or both, in lead III, with inversion of the T waves recorded over the right side of the heart. Other less reliable changes are those of right axis deviation and a pattern of right bundle branch block or right ventricular hypertrophy. Atrial arrhythmias are frequent, particularly in patients with established heart disease.[70] Early and frequent tracings may be necessary to detect these changes.

Prognosis

As discussed previously, most thromboembolic episodes go unrecognized clinically; careful search of the pulmonary vascular tree at necropsy reveals recent or organized thrombi in more than 50 per cent of unselected patients, most of whom have neither a clinical history suggestive of thromboembolic episodes nor pathologic evidence that the emboli have caused morbidity or mortality.[15] It thus must be concluded that the prognosis for the majority of thromboembolic events is good.

In most of these cases, however, the emboli are small and lodge in subsegmental or segmental vessels. The outcome in cases with larger thromboemboli (affecting the pulmonary trunk or large portions of one or both main pulmonary arteries) is substantially less favorable, and it is probable that many patients so affected die within minutes to hours.[50] The prognosis for patients who are symptomatic with smaller emboli is variable: in some, the course is similar to that of massive pulmonary embolus; others survive the acute event but develop complications such as pulmonary infarction. With appropriate anticoagulation therapy, few patients die from subsequent thromboemboli[130a]; however, mortality related to underlying predisposing factors such as cancer or congestive heart failure is substantial.[130a]

In patients with clinical manifestations who survive the acute event, partial or complete resolution of the thrombo-

embolism is the rule; in nearly all, this is complete or almost complete roentgenographically, angiographically and hemodynamically within 4 to 6 weeks of the acute event.[131]

SEPTIC THROMBOEMBOLISM

Although secondary bacterial infection of initially sterile infarcts can occur (Fig. 9–13), many cases of pulmonary infection associated with thromboembolism are the result of the presence of organisms in the thrombus itself (septic emboli). Such emboli can originate from the heart (in association with bacterial endocarditis of the tricuspid valve or a ventricular septal defect) or the peripheral veins (in which case there is invariably infectious thrombophlebitis). The source of the thrombophlebitis in these latter cases includes the pharynx (infection extending to the parapharyngeal space and internal jugular venous system),[132] arm veins in patients with a history of intravenous drug abuse, pelvic veins in association with pelvic inflammatory disease,[133] bones in individuals with osteomyelitis (particularly staphylococcal[134]), and veins near infected indwelling catheters and arteriovenous shunts such as those used for hemodialysis.[135]

The organisms most often grown on blood cultures are *Staphylococcus aureus* and streptococci.[136] Oral anaerobes,

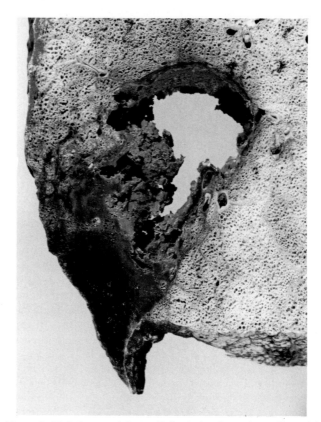

Figure 9–13. Pulmonary Infarct with Cavitation Secondary to Bacterial Superinfection. A magnified view of a slice of left lower lobe shows a well-defined, recent infarct with proximal cavitation. Note the focus of shaggy necrotic lung projecting into the cavity. The patient had multiple foci of bronchopneumonia and bland infarction but no evidence of extrathoracic infection. Thus, the cavitation was considered to represent secondary infection of a previously sterile infarct rather than septic embolization.

particularly *Bacteroides* and *Fusobacterium* species, are the most common pathogens when there is associated pharyngeal infection. When host defenses are impaired, opportunistic infections must be considered, and blood samples should be cultured for fungi as well as bacteria.

Pulmonary disease secondary to septic emboli is usually manifested by multiple, rather ill-defined, round or wedge-shaped opacities in the periphery of the lungs. They may be uniform in size or vary widely, reflecting recurrent showers of emboli. Cavitation is frequent (Fig. 9–14) and may occur rapidly; the cavities are usually thin-walled, and may have no fluid level. Occasionally, a central loose body develops within one or more cavities, resulting in an appearance sometimes termed the "target sign."[137] These bodies represent pieces of necrotic lung that have detached from the adjacent parenchyma and roentgenographically simulate the intracavitary loose bodies that develop in some patients with invasive aspergillosis. Hilar and mediastinal lymph node enlargement can occur.[138] CT has been shown to be complementary to other imaging techniques in the recognition of septic emboli,[139] even in the presence of a normal chest roentgenogram.[140]

Septic pulmonary embolism is seen most often in people younger than 40 years of age.[136] A predisposing factor is nearly always present, most often drug addiction, alcoholism, immune deficiency (particularly lymphoma), congenital heart disease, or an intravenous catheter. Some patients present with a sore throat, although the initial pharyngitis may have cleared by the time the infection reaches the retropharyngeal space.[141]

Fever, cough (with or without expectoration of purulent material), and hemoptysis (sometimes massive) are the most common symptoms. Infection originating in a right heart valve may give rise to a murmur, but in many cases this is soft and atypically located and its significance may be overlooked.

EMBOLI OF EXTRAVASCULAR TISSUES AND SECRETIONS

Fragments of virtually any organ, normal tissue, or body secretion can theoretically gain access to the systemic circulation and be transported to the lungs. Some, such as megakaryocytes and trophoblast cells, do this with such frequency that the process can be considered a normal phenomenon. Other fragments are found only in pathologic conditions, in which circumstances tissue disruption with venous laceration is a necessary precondition; thus, the underlying pathogenesis is frequently trauma, most often associated with labor, accidental or battlefield injuries, or procedures such as venipuncture or surgery. As a result of their inherent invasive properties, neoplastic cells can gain access to the systemic circulation without the aid of trauma; although in these circumstances emboli are usually microscopic and of no consequence from a vascular point of view, occasionally, large fragments or numerous small ones can cause significant vascular obstruction.

With the exception of neoplastic tissue, amniotic fluid, and possibly fat, the vast majority of these emboli are discovered incidentally at autopsy and are of minimal or no clinical or roentgenographic importance.

Fat Embolism

Although intact fragments of adipose tissue occasionally are found in the pulmonary arteries following severe trauma, the term "fat embolism" traditionally refers to the presence of globules of free fat within the vasculature. Exogenous fatty material, such as ethiodized oil used as a roentgenographic contrast medium, is also usually excluded from the definition and is discussed farther on (*see* page 568).

Pathogenesis and Pathologic Characteristics

By far the most common source of fat emboli is the bone marrow.[142] Additional potential origins include fatty liver (induced by a variety of drugs such as steroids[143] and alcohol and by poisons), intravenously infused lipid emulsions utilized in long-term hyperalimentation,[144] and deposits of normal extraosseous adipose tissue (following liposuction[145] and, possibly, crush injury without bone fracture[146]).

Fat emboli can be identified in many cases of accidental or battlefield trauma; in fact, such trauma probably is the most common antecedent of embolism. Autopsy series on patients who have died after injury show an incidence ranging from 67 to almost 100 per cent.[147, 148] In addition to trauma, any condition or procedure that disrupts the marrow has the potential of causing embolization. Examples include sickle cell disease with bone marrow infarction, intraosseous venography,[149] epilepsy,[150] replacement arthroplasty,[151] acute osteomyelitis,[152] and external cardiac massage. The widespread use of the last-named procedure probably makes it the most common cause of fat embolism after accidental fractures; in one necropsy study of 57 patients who had had external cardiac massage, emboli were identified in 46 (80 per cent).[153] Pulmonary fat embolism also has been associated occasionally with a variety of nontraumatic conditions such as diabetes mellitus,[142] pancreatitis,[154] and severe burns.

Although it is well accepted that the vast majority of fat emboli to the lungs and systemic organs are derived from traumatized bone marrow, the effects of the fat and the possible pathogenetic mechanisms of these effects are controversial. The presence of roentgenographic changes and of signs and symptoms of pulmonary disease shortly after trauma has led, understandably, to the belief that the intravascular fat itself is responsible. However, in some autopsy studies,[155] little correlation has been found between the presence of intravascular fat and clinical manifestations, leaving the pathogenetic relationship of the two open to question. In fact, it has been argued that pulmonary fat emboli are unlikely to be of clinical significance in previously healthy individuals and that pulmonary manifestations are more likely to be secondary to the complications of systemic emboli, particularly to the brain, or to conditions such as the adult respiratory distress syndrome that result from the initial injury or its nonembolic complications.[142]

Even if fat emboli are accepted as an important cause of pulmonary disease, the pathogenetic mechanisms are unclear. Fat appears to be transported to the lungs as neutral triglycerides,[156] and it has been proposed[157] that these are converted by intrapulmonary lipases into free fatty acids that can exert a direct toxic effect on the pulmonary endothelium. Supporting this hypothesis are experimental stud-

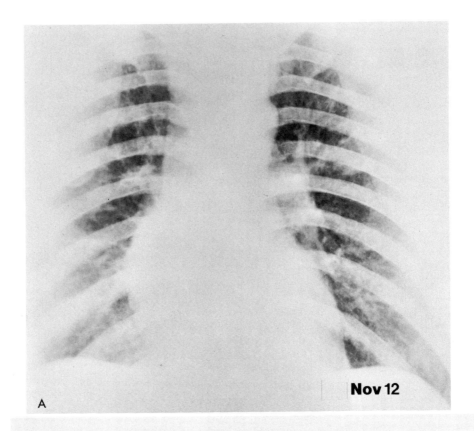

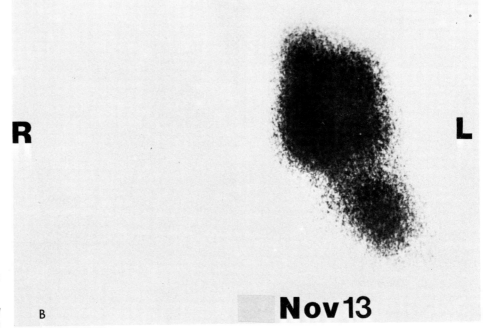

Figure 9–14. Massive Septic Embolism. Shortly before the roentgenogram illustrated in *A,* a 31-year-old man suffered a massive right pulmonary embolism related to severe thrombophlebitis of one leg. This film reveals relatively clear lungs, a normal left hilum, and an almost absent right hilum. A lung scan performed shortly thereafter *(B)* reveals a total lack of perfusion of the right lung and a segmental defect in the midportion of the left lung.

Illustration continued on following page

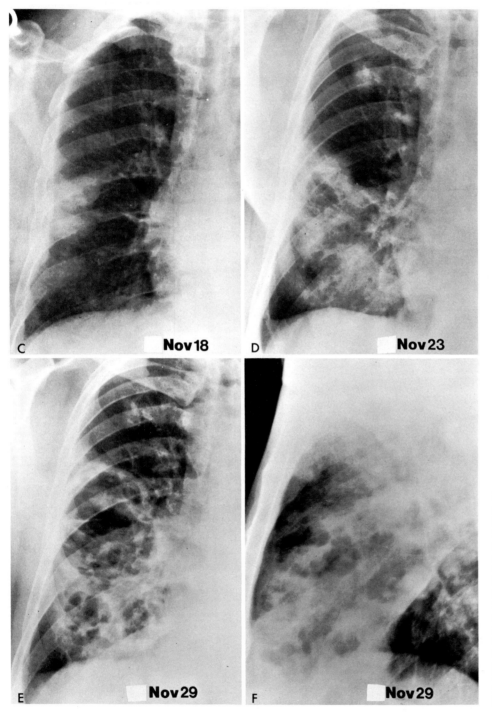

Figure 9–14 *Continued* Five days after the acute episode *(C)*, a poorly defined opacity has appeared in the axillary portion of the right lung in a configuration compatible with a pulmonary infarct. Five days later *(D)*, much of the lower half of the right lung has become consolidated, several areas of radiolucency scattered throughout the consolidated lobe suggesting cavitation. After another 5 days *(E* and *F)*, numerous shaggy cavities have appeared in the consolidation, representing multiple abscesses as a result of septic infarction. The disease is situated predominantly in the middle and upper lobes.

ies in which severe pulmonary edema and hemorrhage have resulted from the injection of free fatty acids into the pulmonary arteries.[158] However, other investigations in which neutral fat has been injected have not found evidence for conversion to free fatty acids.[159] It is also possible that fat emboli, if sufficient in number, can cause vascular obstruction; however, in most cases the typical 1- to 3-day delay of symptoms and the usual absence of acute right-side heart failure suggest that this is not an important mechanism of disease.

Pathologically,[160] the lungs of patients who have died with fat emboli are frequently heavy and show patchy areas of hemorrhage and edema. Fat is best identified in frozen sections with fat-soluble dyes.

Roentgenographic Manifestations

Pulmonary fat embolism is unrecognized in many cases, partly because symptoms are mild or absent but especially because the chest roentgenogram is often normal.[161] When present, roentgenographic appearances in the lungs are those of adult respiratory distress syndrome, consisting of widespread airspace consolidation often with discrete aci-

nar shadows (Fig. 9–15). The distribution is predominantly peripheral rather than central,[162] usually involving the basal regions to a greater degree than does pulmonary edema of cardiac origin. Further differentiation from cardiogenic edema is provided by the absence of cardiac enlargement and of signs of pulmonary venous hypertension.

Since trauma is responsible for most cases of fat embolism, the possibility of lung contusion must also be considered in differential diagnosis. In traumatic lung contusion, however, the roentgenographic opacity invariably appears immediately after injury and usually clears rapidly (in 24 to 26 hours); by contrast, in fat embolism, there is typically a time lapse of 1 or 2 days between trauma and roentgenographic signs,[162] and resolution takes 1 to 4 weeks.[163] Further differentiation lies in the extent of lung involvement: lung contusion seldom affects both lungs diffusely and symmetrically; when both lungs are involved, the roentgenographic changes are usually more severe in the lung deep to the site of maximal trauma.

Clinical Manifestations

The clinical manifestations of fat embolism can be divided into those arising from the lungs and those originat-

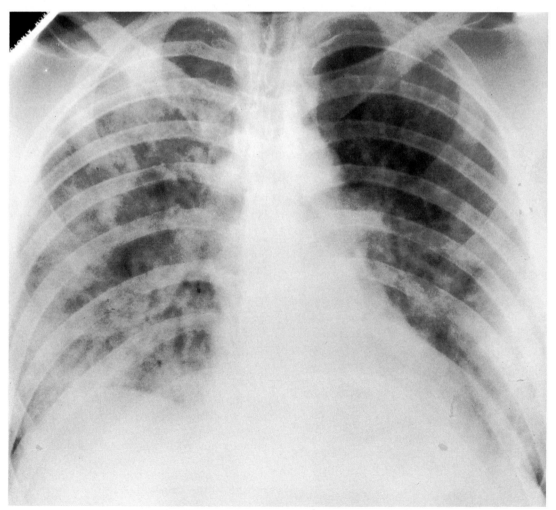

Figure 9–15. Traumatic Fat Embolism. An anteroposterior roentgenogram of a 21-year-old man 3 days after a severe automobile accident reveals extensive involvement of both lungs by patchy shadows of unit density. In many areas the shadows are confluent. For unknown reason, the left upper lung is less severely involved. Complete roentgenographic resolution occurred 7 days later.

ing in other viscera. Symptoms of pulmonary involvement usually appear 1 to 2 days after injury and include cough, dyspnea, hemoptysis, and pleural pain; signs include pyrexia, tachypnea, tachycardia, rales, rhonchi, and friction rub. Acute cor pulmonale with cardiac failure, cyanosis, and circulatory shock may occur.[164]

Manifestations of fat embolism elsewhere are chiefly caused by involvement of the central nervous system and skin; they include confusion, restlessness, stupor, delirium, and coma (the last signifying a poor prognosis). Petechiae are common,[164] particularly along the anterior axillary folds and in the conjunctiva and retina, a distribution that has been attributed to fat floating on the bloodstream and thus affecting vessels that are uppermost.[165]

Laboratory findings are mostly nonspecific. Hypocalcemia usually develops because of the affinity of calcium ions for free fatty acids released by the hydrolysis of fat emboli, and it may have prognostic value.[164] Fat droplets may be detected in alveolar macrophages in sputum or bronchoalveolar lavage fluid.[166] Pulmonary function tests reveal decreased compliance, a diffusion defect, increase in the alveolar-arterial oxygen gradient, and $\dot{V}/\dot{Q}$ inequality. Severe hypoxemia may persist despite inhalation of 100 per cent oxygen.[167]

Bone Marrow Embolism

Pulmonary bone marrow emboli are seen commonly at necropsy in individuals who have sustained accidental fractures or been subjected to external cardiac massage.[168] As in fat embolism, in the vast majority of cases the pathogenesis is related to traumatic fragmentation of marrow and its entry under pressure into disrupted marrow sinusoids or veins. Free fat emboli are probably also present in the majority of cases.[169] The embolized fragments usually are identified histologically within small muscular arteries or arterioles. Infarction of lung parenchyma has not been documented.

The vast majority of these emboli are of no clinical significance, being discovered incidentally at autopsy or in surgically excised lungs. Although they have been implicated as a major or contributory cause of death in some patients,[170] a true pathogenetic relationship is questionable; in these cases, clinical effects are more likely related to associated free fat embolism or to other systemic disease. Despite this, experimental studies in rabbits have suggested the possibility of the development of chronic hypertension.[171]

Amniotic Fluid Embolism

Amniotic fluid embolism is a rare but highly lethal complication of pregnancy in which amniotic fluid enters the bloodstream through tears in the uterine veins and is carried to the lungs. The incidence of the condition is uncertain. It has been estimated that it results in a maternal mortality rate of one in 20,000 to 30,000 deliveries and accounts for 5 to 10 per cent of maternal deaths.[172, 173] However, because of the difficulty in making the diagnosis at autopsy and because of the undoubted presence of nonlethal but unsubstantiated disease in an unspecified number of women,[174] the true incidence is likely to be somewhat higher.

Pathogenesis

Amniotic fluid is composed of fetal urine, secretions from the amniotic membrane, and a variety of particulate material derived from the fetus, including squames and lanugo hairs from the skin, fat from the vernix caseosa, and mucin and bile from the meconium. It is these particulates that are believed to be responsible for the clinical and pathologic manifestations of disease, meconium being particularly important in this regard.[175]

Virtually no amniotic fluid escapes into the maternal circulation during normal pregnancy, labor, or delivery.[176] Only when there is disruption of the uterine wall in association with rupture of the placental membranes can embolization take place. Such disruption can develop in three regions:

1. The veins of the endocervix or lower uterine segment; tears at this site can occur during normal labor but are of no significance if covered by the fetal membranes. If these have separated, however, uterine contractions against a head impacted in the birth canal can repeatedly pump amniotic fluid into the maternal circulation.

2. The placental implantation site, usually in cases of uterine rupture, placenta previa, premature separation, or cesarean section when the incision involves the placental implantation site.

3. Less commonly, elsewhere in the uterine wall in association with some form of myometrial trauma.

The pathophysiologic consequences of intravascular amniotic fluid are related to three mechanisms.

1. Once amniotic fluid enters the maternal circulation, particulate matter is quickly filtered out in the pulmonary vascular bed. Pulmonary artery pressure rises abruptly as a result of mechanical obstruction and (probably) reflex vasoconstriction, resulting in acute right ventricular failure.[175] Blood flow to the left side of the heart decreases and cardiac output falls, followed by systemic hypotension and peripheral vascular collapse. Permeability pulmonary edema develops rapidly.

2. Some cases of amniotic fluid embolism are associated with prolonged rupture of membranes and the presence of infected amniotic fluid.[175] In this circumstance, systemic hypotension may be related in part to endotoxemia. In the appropriate clinical setting, the presence of positive blood cultures and histologic evidence of chorioamnionitis should suggest this mechanism.

3. Amniotic fluid is a powerful coagulant: 1 mL of a thrombokinase-like constituent in it is capable of coagulating 10 L of blood.[177] Because of this property and because the fluid constitutes a volume equivalent to one quarter of the total maternal blood volume at term, its introduction into the systemic circulation can cause profound disturbances in blood coagulation. Such disturbances occur in as many as 40 per cent of patients who survive the first hour after the initial embolic event[178] and are probably related chiefly to a decrease in circulating fibrinogen. This results in severe fibrin depletion and the clinical and pathologic picture of disseminated intravascular coagulation.[179]

Pathologic Characteristics

Grossly, the lungs are frequently unremarkable,[175] although they may be edematous and show focal areas of hemorrhage. The most striking histologic finding is the presence of foreign material within medium-sized to small pulmonary arteries and arterioles. This consists of squames, fragments of hair, and somewhat amorphous basophilic material that is considered to represent mucin and bile derived from meconium. Although much of this material can be recognized with hematoxylin and eosin stain, it is more easily demonstrated with special techniques, the most useful being those that demonstrate acid mucopolysaccharides.[180]

Roentgenographic Manifestations

Roentgenographic changes in the lungs are poorly documented; in most cases, the condition is so rapidly fatal that roentgenograms are not obtained. The major roentgenologic sign is airspace pulmonary edema, which is indistinguishable from acute pulmonary edema of other cause. The differential diagnosis includes massive pulmonary hemorrhage and aspiration of liquid gastric contents (Mendelson's syndrome).

Clinical Manifestations

Predisposing factors to amniotic fluid embolism include tumultuous labor, uterine stimulants, meconium in the amniotic fluid, intrauterine fetal distress and death, older age of the mother, premature placental separation, and multiparity. The first two are important because of the attendant increase in uterine pressure, but it is important to recognize that they are not absolute prerequisites for embolization.[181]

Typically, the clinical manifestations are abrupt in onset and rapidly progressive, consisting of dyspnea and cyanosis, sudden profound shock disproportionate to the blood loss, and signs of central nervous system irritability such as convulsions and hyper-reflexia. Most patients die as a direct result of the embolic episode, almost all within 6 hours of the clinical onset. However, the disease is occasionally nonfatal,[175] the diagnosis being made in some cases by cytologic examination of blood aspirated from a Swan-Ganz catheter.[182]

Embolic Manifestations of Parasitic Infestation

Immature forms of many human metazoan parasites travel through the systemic circulation to the lungs, where they lodge within pulmonary arterioles and capillaries. Although strictly speaking, this represents embolization, in most cases the clinical and pathologic effects are not related to vascular obstruction or damage; instead, pulmonary disease typically occurs in the adjacent lung parenchyma and represents a host reaction to the migrating organism during part of its life cycle. Examples of parasites that cause this form of disease include *Ascaris lumbricoides*, *Strongyloides stercoralis*, *Ancylostoma duodenale*, *Necator americanus*, *Toxicara canis* and *T. cati*, *Paragonimus* species, and probably *Wuchereria bancrofti* and *Brugia malayi*.

In some instances, however, parasites cause disease that is related directly to pulmonary vascular obstruction. Undoubtedly, the most important of these organisms are *Schistosoma* species, whose eggs released into the systemic or portal venous circulation lodge within pulmonary arteries and arterioles and cause endarteritis obliterans and

pulmonary arterial hypertension. Occasionally, whole mature organisms can be transported to the lung and become lodged within larger pulmonary vessels; the most common of these is *Dirofilaria immitis*,[183] which is typically associated with adjacent parenchymal necrosis that is roentgenographically manifested by a solitary pulmonary nodule. A more thorough discussion of these parasites and the diseases they cause is given in Chapter 6.

Embolism of Neoplastic Tissue

Since all cases of hematogenous pulmonary metastases must be derived from tumor fragments lodged within pulmonary vessels, it is evident that these are one of the most common forms of emboli. Because of the small size of most tumor fragments, however, effects related to vascular obstruction are seldom apparent. When tumor emboli are of sufficient size or number to mimic thromboemboli, the clinical, pathologic, and roentgenographic manifestations can be identical, including pulmonary infarction, acute cor pulmonale and sudden death, or progressive dyspnea and pulmonary hypertension.[183a] The subject is considered in greater detail on page 525.

Miscellaneous Tissue Emboli

Pulmonary embolism of *trophoblast cells* is virtually a normal finding in pregnancy[184]; in the vast majority of patients, their presence is of no clinical or pathologic significance, and they disappear mostly by *in situ* degeneration shortly after they appear in the lungs.[185] *Megakaryocytes* are so frequently identified within pulmonary vessels at autopsy and in surgically excised lung tissue that their presence can be considered normal. In fact, it has been suggested that a substantial proportion of platelet production occurs within the lungs.[186]

In addition to these relatively common substances, virtually any normal body tissue or secretion can occasionally serve as a source of emboli to the lungs. These include skin (possibly derived from venipuncture[187]), liver (secondary to massive hepatic necrosis or trauma[188]), bone (following bone marrow transplantation[189]), myocardium (after cardiovascular surgery[190]), neural tissue (secondary to severe trauma during birth or accidental or battlefield injury[191]), and bile (usually in patients with a combination of biliary tract obstruction and liver trauma, the latter secondary to accidental injury, percutaneous cholangiography, or needle biopsy[192]).

EMBOLI OF FOREIGN MATERIAL

Air Embolism

Air may gain access to the vascular system via two routes: in the first (pulmonary, or venous, air embolism), it enters the systemic venous circulation and passes to the right side of the heart and then to the lungs; in the second (systemic, or arterial, air embolism), air enters the pulmonary venous circulation and passes to the left side of the heart and then to the systemic arterial network. Just as these routes are different, so are the pathologic and clinical manifestations of the emboli. In pulmonary air embolism, the effects derive from obstruction of the pulmonary circulation and thus are felt *by* the lungs; in systemic air embolism, the effects derive from an abnormality *within* the lung and are felt chiefly by the two vital organs, the heart and the brain.

Pathogenesis

Systemic Air Embolism. The most frequent site of air entry in systemic air embolism is the pulmonary veins. This can occur only when there is disruption of the wall of a vessel exposed to air and when the pressure of the air exceeds the pressure in the vessel. These two criteria are met in a variety of circumstances, the most common of which is probably penetrating thoracic trauma occasioned by stabbing, missile injury, bronchoscopy,[193] or the insertion of a needle into the thoracic cavity for thoracocentesis or aspiration biopsy.[194]

Embolism can also occur in several situations in which the thorax is intact. One of the most common is scuba diving, in which the pathogenesis may be related to poor ventilation of a bulla because of partial or complete obstruction of its feeding airway. The volume of air in a space distal to a partly or completely occluded bronchus doubles with every 33 feet of a diver's ascent,[195] producing sufficient distention to explode the airspace. Similar circumstances are possible during assisted positive-pressure breathing[196] and in severe asthma[197] and some forms of diffuse lung disease, such as hyaline membrane disease of the newborn.[198] In all these situations, the sequence of events probably consists of alveolar rupture, interstitial emphysema, and tracking of air into the adjacent vascular lumen.

Pulmonary Air Embolism. Pulmonary air embolism is usually iatrogenic and occurs most often in a surgical setting. Any procedure that involves an incision above the level of the heart—for example, craniotomy with the patient in the sitting (Fowler's) position[199]—places the patient at risk for this complication. Air also can enter systemic veins and pass to the pulmonary circulation through an intravenous apparatus, during diagnostic or therapeutic air insufflation into joints, urinary bladder, vagina, fallopian tubes, uterus, or the peritoneal or retroperitoneal space, after gunshot or accidental trauma,[200] and during operative obstetrics or at delivery of patients with placenta previa.[201] In the case of infusion catheters, the usual mode of entry is direct injection,[202] a potential hazard particularly of centrally placed catheters for recording central venous pressure and for hyperalimentation.

The pathogenesis of pulmonary disease in air embolism cannot be attributed solely to vascular obstruction by air bubbles.[203] In fact, when blood and air are whipped together in the chambers of the right heart, blood is altered and liberates fibrin (probably as a result of platelet damage, since a significant decrease in platelets in the peripheral blood is usual with this condition). Contraction of the right ventricle forces the altered blood into the pulmonary circulation, where the fibrin mesh becomes impacted in terminal branches of the pulmonary arteries, blocking the passage of air bubbles caught in the mesh behind them and arresting the pulmonary circulation. Although this description refers specifically to pulmonary air embolism, cerebral and cardiac effects of systemic air embolism are probably of the same nature. However, it is important to note that a much smaller quantity of air is needed to cause death when air originates in the lesser circulation and goes to the heart and brain than when air enters the systemic venous system and is trapped in the lungs.

Pathologic Characteristics

The gross morphologic changes in those who die from pulmonary air embolism are well documented, both in humans[204] and experimental animals.[203] Bloody froth, formed by the whipping action of the right atrium and ventricle, fills these chambers and extends into the central and peripheral branches of the pulmonary artery, and sometimes the superior and inferior vena cava. The pulmonary veins are virtually empty of blood; so also are the left atrium and left ventricle, which are contracted upon themselves and contain only a very small quantity of very dark blood. The systemic arterial system contains no air bubbles.

Roentgenographic Manifestations

The principal roentgenographic sign is visible gas in an abnormal location.[202, 205] In pulmonary air embolism, it is present in right heart chambers and central pulmonary arteries; in systemic air embolism, it can be identified in the left heart chambers, aorta, or more peripheral branches of the systemic arterial tree such as the neck, shoulder girdles, or upper abdomen. Other features that have been observed include pulmonary edema, focal oligemia, enlarged central pulmonary arteries, and atelectasis.[206]

Clinical Manifestations

In most instances, air embolism is a benign occurrence not recognized by any clinical findings; however, if the amount of air entering the lung is considerable, there may be pulmonary edema[207] or systemic hypotension. A precordial murmur resembling the sound of a "mill wheel" has been described in some patients.[208]

Embolism of Talc, Starch, and Cellulose

Emboli of talc, starch, and cellulose are seen in individuals who have repeatedly abused intravenous drugs. In most instances, the complication occurs with medications intended solely for oral use; pills are crushed in a spoon or bottle top, water is added, and the mixture is heated, drawn into a syringe, and injected. The habit is usually a result of a shortage of available heroin, although some addicts use the drugs in this manner to counteract the sedative effect of the narcotic drugs themselves. Oral medication misused in this way includes amphetamines[209] and closely related drugs such as methylphenidate hydrochloride (Ritalin) and tripelennamine, methadone hydrochloride, hydromorphone hydrochloride (Dilaudid), phenyltoloxamine, propoxyphene (Darvon), secobarbital, pentazocine (Talwin), meperidine, and propylhexedrine.

All these oral medications have in common an insoluble filler added to bind the medicinal particles together and to act as a lubricant to prevent the tablets from sticking to punches and dies during manufacture.[210] The most widely used filler is talc; cornstarch and microcrystalline cellulose are also present in relatively large amounts in some drugs.

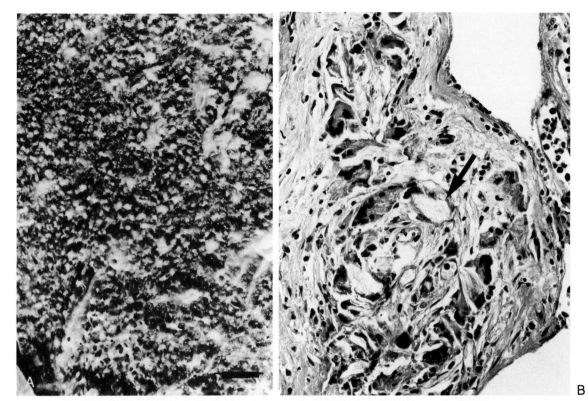

Figure 9–16. Pulmonary Talcosis Associated with Intravenous Drug Abuse. *A,* Magnified view of a slice of upper lobe from a previous heroin and methadone addict shows a myriad of minute nodules throughout the lung parenchyma. (Bar = 1 cm.) *B,* A histologic section through one nodule reveals loose aggregates of multinucleated foreign body giant cells, scattered mononuclear inflammatory cells, and fibrous tissue; finely fibrillar talc crystals are indicated by arrow. (*B* × 250.) (*B* from Paré JAP, Coté G, Fraser RS: Am Rev Respir Dis 139: 233, 1989.)

When injected intravenously, the fillers become trapped within pulmonary arterioles and capillaries. Although initially they cause vascular occlusion, sometimes associated with thrombosis, in time they migrate through the vessel wall and come to lie in the adjacent perivascular and parenchymal interstitial tissue

Pathologic Characteristics

In the early stages of disease, the lungs show variable numbers of more or less discrete parenchymal nodules measuring up to 1 mm in diameter (Fig. 9–16). In long-standing disease, there is a tendency for the nodules to become confluent, especially in the upper lobes, producing large areas of consolidation resembling the progressive massive fibrosis seen in the pneumoconioses.[211] Panacinar emphysema, sometimes with bulla formation, is often evident.

Histologically, the small nodules are mostly present in the parenchymal interstitium and consist of loosely formed granulomas containing many large multinucleated giant cells (*see* Fig. 9–16). Sections of the large foci of upper lobe consolidation seen in long-standing disease show sheets of multinucleated giant cells, usually not organized in discrete granulomas; a variable degree of fibrosis is also present. Foreign material is readily identifiable within the giant cells and is particularly well seen in polarized light.

Roentgenographic Manifestations

The earliest finding is widespread micronodulation, the diameter of individual nodules ranging from barely visible to about 1 mm (Fig. 9–17); the pattern does not have a reticular component, the opacities being distinct and "pinpoint" in character, simulating alveolar microlithiasis.[212] Although some authors have described a midzonal predominance of these micronodules,[213] the distribution we have observed has been diffuse and uniform throughout the lungs. In some patients, the widespread nodularity is associated with loss of volume, which occasionally is severe.

In the later stages of the disease, the opacities in the upper lobes may coalesce to form an almost homogeneous opacity that closely resembles the progressive massive fibrosis of silicosis or coal-worker's pneumoconiosis, except for the presence of an air bronchogram (Fig. 9–18).[211] Signs of pulmonary arterial hypertension and cor pulmonale may develop. In the very late stages of the disease, increasing disability and deteriorating function are associated with roentgenographic evidence of emphysema and bullae.

Clinical Manifestations

Most addicts who inject oral medications are asymptomatic; granulomas are found incidentally at necropsy in those who die from other causes. Symptoms usually de-

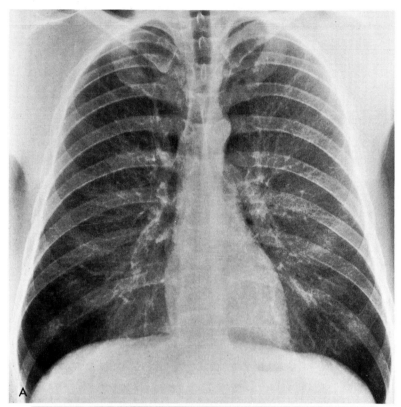

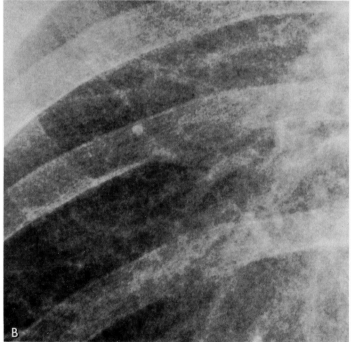

Figure 9–17. Pulmonary Talcosis Associated with Intravenous Drug Abuse. This asymptomatic 22-year-old man had been "shooting" heroin and methadone for 4 years at the time these roentgenograms were obtained. There is widespread involvement of both lungs by tiny micronodular opacities *(A)*, seen to better advantage on a roentgenographically magnified image (2:1) of the right lower zone *(B)*. There is no anatomic predominance.

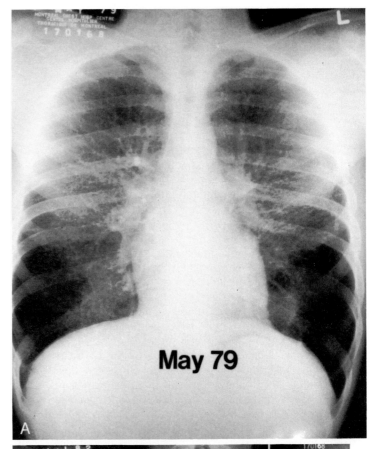

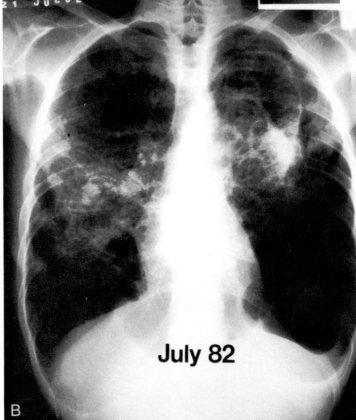

Figure 9–18. Progressive Massive Fibrosis As a Long-Term Effect of Talcosis of Drug Abuse. A conventional chest roentgenogram *(A)* reveals a diffuse micronodular pattern throughout both lungs with considerable upper and midzonal predominance. Three years later *(B)*, large irregular opacities have appeared in both midlung zones, simulating the progressive massive fibrosis seen in silicosis. A pneumothorax is present on the left.

velop in very heavy users and consist of dyspnea and occasionally persistent cough; disability increases after cessation of exposure.[212] Cor pulmonale may be manifest as a result of extensive vascular and parenchymal disease. Glistening particles can be seen in the fundi, principally at the posterior pole surrounding the foveal area. These may be the earliest clue to illicit use of such drugs, since they have been detected in addicts whose chest roentgenograms and pulmonary function are normal.[212]

In the early stages, pulmonary function tests show significant impairment of gas transfer accompanied by a strange combination of obstructive and restrictive insufficiency but little or no hyperinflation or air trapping. In advanced disease, however, both are apparent and are accompanied by a severe reduction of flow rates and diffusion.[211]

Iodized Oil Embolism

Iatrogenic pulmonary oil embolism is almost invariably a complication of lymphangiography with ethiodized poppyseed oil (Ethiodol). Most affected patients have pelvic or abdominal lymphatic obstruction.[214] It is postulated that such obstruction permits uptake of the contrast medium by systemic veins, so that the oil arrives in the lungs earlier and in greater concentration than it would otherwise.

In one study, lung biopsy performed within 12 hours after the lymphatic injection of ethiodized oil showed lipid droplets widely distributed throughout the pulmonary capillary bed, corresponding to fine granular stippling observed throughout both lungs roentgenologically[215]; biopsy specimens obtained the next day revealed that much lipid had passed into the bronchovascular interstitial tissue. At this

stage, roentgenography usually shows a fine reticular pattern, which may persist as long as 11 days.[216]

Few patients have symptoms, the only evidence of disease being the development of fever within 48 hours of lymphangiography. However, in some patients (particularly those known to have had pulmonary insufficiency previously[217]), lymphangiography provokes severe reactions and even death.

Pulmonary function tests may reveal decreased diffusing capacity after lymphangiography.[218] This is maximal at 24 to 48 hours, with an early fall in gas transfer being attributed to reduced pulmonary capillary blood flow and a later drop to interference with the membrane component of diffusion when the oil moves into the interstitial tissue.

Metallic Mercury Embolism

Pulmonary embolization of mercury may be accidental or intentional—accidental from injury from a broken thermometer or from venous blood sampling with a mercury-sealed syringe, and intentional from injection by drug abusers or patients attempting suicide.[219] Pathologically, the inflammatory reaction in the lungs is relatively mild.[220] The mercury may remain within the pulmonary arteries, eventually becoming encased in thrombus, or may migrate into the adjacent interstitium and alveolar airspaces, where it causes a foreign body giant cell reaction.

Roentgenographically, the appearance is distinctive because of the very high density of mercury and takes the form of small spherules or short tubular structures representing mercury-filled arterial segments (Fig. 9–19). The distribution is usually bilateral and fairly symmetric. A local

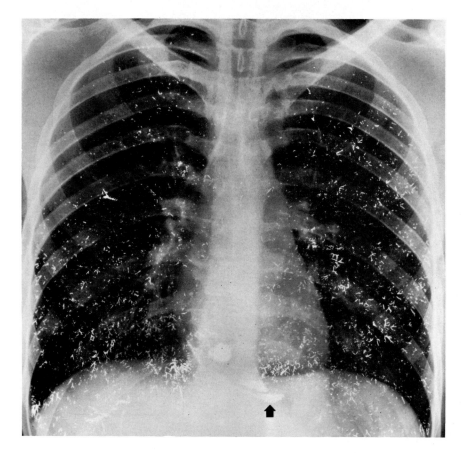

Figure 9–19. Metallic Mercury Embolization. A posteroanterior roentgenogram reveals a multitude of short linear and branching opacities of metallic density distributed widely throughout both lungs. It would be difficult to be certain whether this metallic mercury was within the vascular or airway system of the lungs if it were not for the presence of a pool of mercury lying in the inferior aspect of the right ventricular chamber *(arrow)*. This young male drug addict injected metallic mercury into an antecubital vein for a special ''kick.'' (Courtesy of Dr. William Beamish, University Hospital, Edmonton, Alberta.)

collection of mercury may be apparent in the heart, usually near the apex of the right ventricle.

Clinically, the body's reaction to pulmonary mercury embolism varies but appears to be predominantly systemic. Toxicity is manifested by a metallic taste, excessive salivation, gingivitis, stomatitis, diarrhea, nephrosis, tremor (hatter's shakes), and erethism.[220]

Metallic mercury also can enter the lungs by aspiration; since to the best of our knowledge, this does not cause mercurialism, it should be distinguished from embolization whenever possible. Roentgenographically, this can be difficult, since the appearance of intrabronchial and intravascular mercury are virtually identical, especially when the metal is in the lung periphery. However, its presence within the heart chambers (see Fig. 9–19) proves its vascular location. Aspiration usually occurs after accidental breakage of a thermometer or indwelling intestinal tube[221] or during a suicide attempt.[222]

Barium Embolism

Barium embolization to the lungs has been observed as a rare complication of routine barium enema[223] and of barium enema inadvertently administered via the vagina.[224] Mucosal lacerations can usually be identified that afford entry of injected barium into the venous system. The condition is serious: the majority of reported patients have died either immediately or within 24 hours of the event.

Miscellaneous Foreign Body Embolism

Macroscopic Foreign Bodies

Bullets or bullet fragments can enter the extrathoracic systemic veins or the right side of the heart and be carried to the lungs to lodge within pulmonary arteries.[225] Both clinical observations and experimental studies[226] have shown that they can remain within the pulmonary vasculature for prolonged periods without producing untoward effects.

Radiopaque foreign material, such as wire loops, balloons filled with contrast medium, and silicone-tantalum mixtures, are used therapeutically in both the pulmonary and the systemic circulation to obliterate arteriovenous malformations or to control intractable hemorrhage.[227, 228] In the systemic circulation, escape of material to the venous side can result in opacities of metallic density within the lungs.

Plastic intravenous catheters, whole or in fragments, may be carried in the systemic venous circulation to the right heart chambers and pulmonary circulation, a complication that usually occurs when a polyethylene catheter is cut by the sharp bevel of the needle it encloses. The catheter may break or be cut during dressing changes or may be detached from the connector.[229] Occasionally, the catheter fractures spontaneously.[230]

Microscopic Foreign Bodies

A variety of particulate materials, including glass, rubber, plastic, and cellulose, have been found in fluid destined for intravenous injection[231]; some are undoubtedly retained within the lungs after infusion. Although there are no known clinical or roentgenographic manifestations of these emboli, the granulomatous reaction that may develop in relation to some of the foreign material may be a source of confusion in the interpretation of biopsy specimens. Pulmonary granulomas and isolated interstitial giant cells containing foreign material also have been detected in patients on long-term hemodialysis.[232] Although the nature of the foreign material has not been identified in all cases, in some it has been shown to be silicone, apparently derived from the dialysis tubing.

BRONCHIAL ARTERY EMBOLISM

The vast majority of bronchial artery emboli consist of foreign material introduced therapeutically in an attempt to control recurrent or massive hemoptysis.[233] The embolic material is varied and includes absorbable gelatinous sponge (Gelfoam), polyvinyl alcohol (Ivalon), isobutyl-2-cyanoacrylate (Bucrylate), and Gianturco coils.[234] Such substances either can completely obstruct the lumen of the vessel following injection or can partly obstruct it and induce thrombosis that causes complete luminal obliteration. Although we have seen focal bronchial wall necrosis, resulting clinical and roentgenographic effects appear to be minimal.

Roentgenographically, the appearances are as might be anticipated (*see* Fig. 2–5, page 126): Initial opacification of the bronchial artery and its peripheral arborization usually reveals a markedly dilated, hypertrophic vascular tree. Following embolization, the artery can be seen to be completely blocked at a variable distance from its origin, peripheral flow being nonexistent.

References

1. Slavin RE, de Groot WJ: Pathology of the lung in Behçet's disease. Am J Surg Pathol 5: 779, 1981.
2. Dimond EG, Jones TR: Pulmonary artery thrombosis simulating pulmonic valve stenosis with patent foramen ovale. Am Heart J 47: 105, 1954.
3. Chiu B, Magil A: Idiopathic pulmonary arterial trunk aneurysm presenting as cor pulmonale: Report of a case. Hum Pathol 16: 947, 1985.
4. Connors AF, Castele RJ, Farhat NZ, et al: Complications of right heart catheterization. Chest 88: 567, 1985.
5. Ferencz C: The pulmonary vascular bed in tetralogy of Fallot. I. Changes associated with pulmonic stenosis. Bull Johns Hopkins Hosp 106: 81, 1960.
6. Haupt HM, Moore GW, Bauer TW, et al: The lung in sickle cell disease. Chest 81: 332, 1982.
7. Robboy SJ, Colman RW, Minna JD: Pathology of disseminated intravascular coagulation. Hum Pathol 3: 327, 1972.
8. Berry DF, Buccigrossi D, Peabody J, et al: Pulmonary vascular occlusion and fibrosing mediastinitis. Chest 89: 296, 1986.
9. Spittell JA Jr: Pulmonary thromboembolism—some editorial comments. Dis Chest 54: 401, 1968.
10. Mercer J, Talbot IC: Clinical diagnosis: A post-mortem assessment of accuracy in the 1980s. Postgrad Med J 61: 713, 1985.
11. Goldhaber SZ, Hennekens CH, Evans DA, et al: Factors associated with correct antemortem diagnosis of major pulmonary embolism. Am J Med 73: 822, 1982.
12. Diebold J, Löhrs U: Venous thrombosis and pulmonary embolism. A study of 5039 autopsies. Path Res Pract 187: 260, 1991.
13. Tsao M, Schraufnagel D, Wang N: Pathogenesis of pulmonary infarction. Am J Med 72: 599, 1982.
14. Beckering RE Jr, Titus JL: Femoral-popliteal venous thrombosis and pulmonary embolism. Am J Clin Pathol 52: 530, 1969.

15. Freiman DG, Suyemoto J, Wessler S: Frequency of pulmonary thromboembolism in man. N Engl J Med 272: 1278, 1965.
16. Moser KM: Venous thromboembolism. Am Rev Respir Dis 141: 235, 1990.
17. Soskolne CL, Wong AW, Lilienfeld DE: Trends in pulmonary embolism death rates for Canada and the United States, 1962-87. Can Med Assoc J 142: 321, 1990.
18. Waller BF, Dean PJ, Mann O, et al: Right ventricular outflow obstruction from thrombus with small peripheral pulmonary emboli. Chest 79: 224, 1981.
19. Goldstein MF, Nestico P, Olshan AR, et al: Superior vena cava thrombosis and pulmonary embolus: Association with right atrial mural thrombus. Arch Intern Med 142: 1726, 1982.
20. Coon WW, Willis PW III: Thrombosis of axillary and subclavian veins. Arch Surg 94: 657, 1967.
21. Warlow C, Ogston D, Douglas AS: Venous thrombosis following strokes. Lancet 1: 1305, 1972.
22. Maurer BJ, Wray R, Shillingford JP: Frequency of venous thrombosis after myocardial infarction. Lancet 2: 1385, 1971.
23. Sevitt S: The structure and growth of valve-pocket thrombi in femoral veins. J Clin Pathol 27: 517, 1974.
24. Stamatakis D, Kakkar VV, Sagar S, et al: Femoral vein thrombosis and total hip replacement. Br Med J 2: 223, 1977.
25. Yorra FH, Oblath R, Jaffe H, et al: Massive thrombosis associated with use of the Swan-Ganz catheter. Chest 65: 682, 1974.
26. Prozan GB, Shipley RE, Madding GF, et al: Pulmonary thromboembolism in the presence of an endocardiac pacing catheter. JAMA 206: 1564, 1968.
27. Gibney RTN, Donovan F, Fitzgerald MX: Recurrent symptomatic pulmonary embolism caused by an infected Pudenz cerebrospinal fluid shunt device. Thorax 33: 662, 1978.
28. Braun TI, Goldberg SK: An unusual thromboembolic complication of a Greenfield vena caval filter. Chest 87: 127, 1985.
29. Winter JH, Fenech A, Bennett B, et al: Thrombosis after venography in familial antithrombin III deficiency. Br Med J 283: 1436, 1981.
30. Wenger NK, Stein PD, Willis PW III: Massive acute pulmonary embolism: the deceivingly nonspecific manifestations. JAMA 220: 843, 1972.
31. Pulmonary embolism in active-duty servicemen [Editorial]: JAMA 196: 360, 1966.
32. Ramsay LE, MacLeod MA: Incidence of idiopathic venous thromboembolism in nurses. Br Med J 4: 446, 1973.
33. Marciniak E, Farley CH, DeSimone PA: Familial thrombosis due to antithrombin III deficiency. Blood 43: 219, 1974.
34. Comp PC, Esmon CT: Recurrent venous thromboembolism in patients with a partial deficiency of proteins. N Engl J Med 311: 1525, 1984.
35. Griffin JH, Evatt B, Zimmerman TS, et al: Deficiency of protein C in congenital thrombotic disease. J Clin Invest 68: 1370, 1981.
36. Espinoza LR, Hartman RC: Significance of the lupus anticoagulant. Am J Hematol 22: 331, 1986.
37. Min K-W, Gyorkey F, Sato C: Mucin-producing adenocarcinomas and nonbacterial thrombotic endocarditis. Pathogenetic role of tumor mucin. Cancer 45: 2374, 1980.
38. Maruyama M, Yagawa K, Hayashi S, et al: Presence of thrombosis-inducing activity in plasma from patients with lung cancer. Am Rev Respir Dis 140: 778, 1989.
39. Inman WHW, Vessey MP, Westerholm B, et al: Thromboembolic disease and the steroidal content of oral contraceptives. A report to the Committee on safety of drugs. Br Med J 2: 203, 1970.
40. Realini JP, Goldzieher JW: Oral contraceptives and cardiovascular disease: A critique of epidemiologic studies. Am J Obstet Gynecol 152: 729, 1985.
41. Blood clotting and the pill. Br Med J 4: 378, 1972.
41a. Vessey M, Mant D, Smith A, et al: Oral contraceptives and venous thromboembolism: Findings in a large prospective study. Br Med J 292: 526, 1986.
42. Inman WHW, Vessey MP: Investigation of deaths from pulmonary, coronary, and cerebral thrombosis and embolism in women of childbearing age. Br Med J 2: 193, 1968.
43. Vessey MP, Doll R: Investigation of relation between use of oral contraceptives and thromboembolic disease. Br Med J 2: 199, 1968.
44. Dalen JE, Haffajee CI, Alpert JS, et al: Pulmonary embolism, pulmonary hemorrhage and pulmonary infarction. N Engl J Med 296: 1431, 1977.

45. Parker BM, Smith JR: Pulmonary embolism and infarction. A review of the physiologic consequences of pulmonary arterial obstruction. Am J Med 24: 402, 1958.
46. Schraufnagel DE, Tsao M, Yao YT, et al: Factors associated with pulmonary infarction. Am J Clin Pathol 84: 15, 1985.
47. Comroe JH Jr: Pulmonary arterial blood flow: Effects of brief and permanent arrest. Am Rev Respir Dis 85: 179, 1962.
48. Kerr IH, Simon G, Sutton GC: The value of the plain radiograph in acute massive pulmonary embolism. Br J Radiol 44: 751, 1971.
49. Dexter L, Smith GT: Quantitative studies of pulmonary embolism. Am J Med Sci 247: 641, 1964.
50. Gorham LW: A study of pulmonary embolism: Part II. The mechanism of death; based on a clinicopathological investigation of 100 cases of massive and 285 cases of minor embolism of the pulmonary artery. Arch Intern Med 108: 189, 1961.
51. Fanta CH, Wright TC, McFadden ER: Differentiation of recurrent pulmonary emboli from chronic obstructive lung disease as a cause of cor pulmonale. Chest 79: 92, 1981.
52. Dombert MC, Rouby JJ, Smiejan JM, et al: Pulmonary oedema during pulmonary embolism. Br J Dis Chest 81: 407, 1987.
53. Hyers TM, Fowler AA, Wicks AB: Focal pulmonary edema after massive pulmonary embolism. Am Rev Respir Dis 123: 232, 1981.
54. Redline S, Tomashefski JF Jr, Altose MD: Cavitating lung infarction after bland pulmonary thromboembolism in patients with the adult respiratory distress syndrome. Thorax 40: 915, 1985.
55. Bewtra C, Dewan N, O'Donahue WJ Jr: Exfoliative sputum cytology in pulmonary embolism. Acta Cytol 27: 489, 1983.
56. Dalen JE, Banas JS Jr, Brooks HL, et al: Resolution rate of acute pulmonary embolism in man. N Engl J Med 280: 1194, 1969.
57. Austin JHM, Wilner GD, Dominguez C: Natural history of pulmonary thromboemboli in dogs: Serial radiographic observation of clots labeled with powdered tantalum. Radiology 116: 519, 1975.
58. Sevitt S: Organic fragmentation in pulmonary thromboemboli. J Pathol 122: 95, 1977.
59. Gahagan T, Manzor A, Isaac B, Mathur AN: Reestablishment of pulmonary-artery flow after prolonged complete occlusion: Studies in dogs. JAMA 198: 639, 1966.
60. Smith GT, Dexter L, Dammin GJ: Postmortem quantitative studies in pulmonary embolism. In Sasahara AA, Stein M (eds): Pulmonary Embolic Disease. New York, Grune & Stratton, 1965, pp 120–130.
61. Kakkar VV, Howe CT, Flanc C, et al: Natural history of postoperative deep-vein thrombosis. Lancet 2: 230, 1969.
62. Torrance DJ Jr: Roentgenographic signs of pulmonary artery occlusion. Am J Med Sci 237: 651, 1959.
63. Figley MM, Gerdes AJ, Ricketts HJ: Radiographic aspects of pulmonary embolism. Semin Roentgenol 2: 389, 1967.
64. Grossman D, Ritter CA, Tarner RJ, et al: Successful identification of oligemic lung by transmission computed tomography after experimentally produced acute pulmonary arterial occlusion in the dog. Invest Radiol 16: 275, 1981.
65. Fleischner FG: Recurrent pulmonary embolism and cor pulmonale. N Engl J Med 276: 1213, 1967.
66. Wiener SN, Edelstein J, Charms BL: Observations on pulmonary embolism and the pulmonary angiogram. Am J Roentgenol 98: 859, 1966.
67. Chang CH, Davis WC: A roentgen sign of pulmonary infarction. Clin Radiol 16: 141, 1965.
68. Williams JR, Wilcox WC: Pulmonary embolism: Roentgenographic and angiographic considerations. Am J Roentgenol 89: 333, 1963.
69. Talbot S, Worthington BS, Roebuck EJ: Radiographic signs of pulmonary embolism and pulmonary infarction. Thorax 28: 198, 1973.
70. Szucs MM Jr, Brooks HL, Grossman W, et al: Diagnostic sensitivity of laboratory findings in acute pulmonary embolism. Ann Intern Med 74: 161: 1971.
71. Fleischner FG: Roentgenology of the pulmonary infarct. Semin Roentgenol 2: 61, 1967.
72. Hampton AO, Castleman B: Correlation of postmortem chest teleroentgenograms with autopsy findings. With special reference to pulmonary embolism and infarction. Am J Roentgenol 43: 305, 1940.
73. Bachynski JE: Absence of the air bronchogram sign: A reliable finding in pulmonary embolism with infarction or hemorrhage. Radiology 100: 547, 1971.
74. Lourie GL, Pizzo SV, Ravin C, et al: Experimental pulmonary infarction in dogs: A comparison of chest radiography and computed tomography. Invest Radiol 17: 224, 1982.

75. Sinner WN: Computed tomographic patterns of pulmonary thromboembolism and infarction. J Comput Assist Tomogr 2: 395, 1978.
76. Pope CF, Sostman D, Carbo P, et al: The detection of pulmonary emboli by magnetic resonance imaging. Evaluation of imaging parameters. Invest Radiol 22: 937, 1987.
77. White RD, Winkler ML, Higgins CB: MR imaging of pulmonary arterial hypertension and pulmonary emboli. Am J Roentgenol 149: 15, 1987.
77a. Kessler R, Fraisse P, Krause D, et al. Magnetic resonance imaging in the diagnosis of pulmonary infarction. Chest 99: 298, 1991.
78. Fleischner FG: Observations on the radiologic changes in pulmonary embolism. *In* Sasahara AA, Stein M (eds): Pulmonary Embolic Disease, New York, Grune & Stratton, 1965, pp 206-213.
79. Woesner ME, Sanders I, White GW: The melting sign in resolving transient pulmonary infarction. Am J Roentgenol 111: 782, 1971.
80. McGoldrick PJ, Rudd TG, Figley MM, et al: What becomes of pulmonary infarcts? Am J Roentgenol 133: 1039, 1979.
81. Greenspan RH, Ravin CE, Polansky SM, et al: Accuracy of the chest radiograph in diagnosis of pulmonary embolism. Invest Radiol 17: 539, 1982.
82. Weidner W, Swanson L, Wilson G: Roentgen techniques in the diagnosis of pulmonary thromboembolism. Am J Roentgenol 100: 397, 1967.
83. Sagel SS, Greenspan RH: Nonuniform pulmonary arterial perfusion: Pulmonary embolism? Radiology 99: 541, 1971.
84. Bookstein JJ: Segmental arteriography in pulmonary embolism. Radiology 93: 1007, 1969.
85. Reilley RF, Smith CW, Price RR, et al: Digital subtraction angiography: Limitations for the detection of pulmonary embolism. Radiology 149: 379, 1983.
86. Pond GD, Ovitt TW, Capp MP: Comparison of conventional pulmonary angiography with intravenous digital subtraction angiography for pulmonary embolic disease. Radiology 147: 345, 1983.
87. Musset D, Rosso J, Peitpretz P, et al: Acute pulmonary embolism: Diagnostic value of digital subtraction angiography. Radiology 166: 455, 1988.
88. Posteraro RH, Sostman HD, Spritzer CE, et al: Cine-gradient–refocused MR imaging of central pulmonary emboli. Am J Roentgenol 152: 465, 1989.
89. Williams JR, Wilcox WC: Pulmonary embolism: Roentgenographic and angiographic considerations. Am J Roentgenol 89: 333, 1963.
90. Peterson KL, Fred HL, Alexander JK: Pulmonary arterial webs. A new angiographic sign of previous thromboembolism. N Engl J Med 277: 33, 1967.
91. MacLean LD, Shibata HR, McLean APH, et al: Pulmonary embolism: The value of bedside scanning, angiography and pulmonary embolectomy. Can Med Assoc J 97: 991, 1967.
92. Haegelin HF, Murray JF: Means of distinguishing pulmonary emboli and other causes of pulmonary hypertension. Dis Chest 53: 138, 1968.
93. Del Guercio LRM, Cohn JD, Feins NR, et al: Pulmonary embolism shock: Physiologic basis of a bedside screening test. JAMA 196: 751, 1966.
94. Alderson PO, Martin EC: Pulmonary embolism: Diagnosis with multiple imaging modalities. Radiology 164: 297, 1987.
95. Kipper MS, Moser KM, Kortman KE, et al: Long-term follow-up of patients with suspected pulmonary embolism and a normal lung scan. Chest 82: 411, 1982.
96. Biello DR, Mattar AG, Osei-Wusu A, et al: Interpretation of indeterminate lung scintigrams. Radiology 133: 189, 1979.
96a. Wellman HM: Pulmonary thromboembolism: Current status report on the role of nuclear medicine. Semin Nucl Med 16: 236, 1986.
97. Biello DR, Mattar AG, McKnight RC, et al: Ventilation-perfusion studies in suspected pulmonary embolism. Am J Roentgenol 133: 1033, 1979.
98. McNeil BJ: Ventilation-perfusion studies and the diagnosis of pulmonary embolism: Concise communication. J Nucl Med 21: 319, 1980.
99. Biello DR: Radiological (scintigraphic) evaluation of patients with suspected pulmonary embolism. JAMA 257(23): 3257, 1987.
100. Webber MM, Gomes AS, Roe D, et al: Comparison of Biello, McNeil and PIOPED criteria for the diagnosis of pulmonary emboli on lung scans. Am J Roentgenol 154: 975, 1990.
101. Smith R, Ellis K, Alderson PO: Role of chest radiography in predicting the extent of airway disease in patients with suspected pulmonary embolism. Radiology 159: 391, 1986.
101a. Stein PD, Coleman RE, Gottschalk A: Diagnostic utility of ventilation/perfusion lung scans in acute pulmonary embolism is not diminished by pre-existing cardiac or pulmonary disease. Chest 100: 604, 1991.
102. Meignan M, Simonneau G, Oliveira L, et al: Computation of ventilation-perfusion ratio with Kr-81m in pulmonary embolism. J Nucl Med 25: 149, 1984.
103. Spies WG, Burstein SP, Dillehay GL, et al: Ventilation-perfusion scintigraphy in suspected pulmonary embolism: Correlation with pulmonary angiography and refinement of criteria for interpretation. Radiology 159: 383, 1986.
104. Braun SD, Newman GE, Ford K, et al: Ventilation-perfusion scanning and pulmonary angiography: Correlation in clinical high-probability pulmonary embolism. Am J Roentgenol 143: 977, 1984.
105. McIntyre KM, Sasahara AA: Correlation of pulmonary photoscan and angiogram as measures of the severity of pulmonary embolic involvement. J Nucl Med 12: 732, 1971.
106. Poulose KP, Reba RC, Gilday DL, et al: Diagnosis of pulmonary embolism: A correlative study of the clinical, scan, and angiographic findings. Br Med J 3: 67, 1970.
107. Fisher MR, Higgins CB: Central thrombi in pulmonary arterial hypertension detected by MR imaging. Radiology 158: 223, 1986.
108. Ovenfors C-O, Goodwin JD, Brito AC: Diagnosis of peripheral pulmonary emboli by computed tomography in the living dog. Radiology 141: 519, 1981.
108a. Remy-Jardin M, Remy J, Wattinne L, et al: Central pulmonary thromboembolism: Diagnosis with spiral volumetric CT with the single-breath-hold technique—comparison with pulmonary angiography. Radiology 185: 381, 1992.
109. Hull RD, Hirsh J, Carter CJ, et al: Pulmonary angiography, ventilation lung scanning, and venography for clinically suspected pulmonary embolism with abnormal perfusion lung scan. Ann Intern Med 98: 891, 1983.
110. Management of pulmonary embolism. Br Med J 4: 133, 1968.
111. Browse NL: Prophylaxis of pulmonary embolism. Br Med J 2: 780, 1970.
112. Sostman HD, Neumann RD, Zoghbi SS, et al: Experimental studies with [111]Indium-labeled platelets in pulmonary embolism. Invest Radiol 17: 367, 1982.
113. Sostman HD, Newmann RD, Loke J, et al: Detection of pulmonary embolism in man with ^{111}In-labeled autologous platelets. Am J Roentgenol 138: 945, 1982.
114. Fenech A, Hussey JK, Smith FW, et al: Diagnosis of deep vein thrombosis using autologous indium-111–labeled platelets. Br Med J 282: 1020, 1981.
115. Fenech A, Dendy PP, Hussey JK, et al: Indium-111–labeled platelets in diagnosis of leg-vein thrombosis: Preliminary findings. Br Med J 280: 1571, 1980.
116. Little JM, Binns M: Spontaneous change in frequency of deep-vein thrombosis detected by ultrasound. Lancet 2: 1229, 1972.
117. Yao ST, Gourmos C, Hobbs JT: Detection of proximal-vein thrombosis by Doppler ultrasound flow-detection method. Lancet 1: 1, 1972.
118. Cheely R, McCartney WH, Perry JR, et al: The role of noninvasive tests versus pulmonary angiography in the diagnosis of pulmonary embolism. Am J Med 70: 17, 1981.
119. Hull R, Hirsh J, Sackett DL, et al: Replacement of venography in suspected venous thrombosis by impedance plethysmography and ^{125}I-fibrogen leg scanning: A less invasive approach. Ann Intern Med 94: 12, 1981.
120. Pochaczevsky R, Pillari G, Feldman F: Liquid crystal contact thermography of deep venous thrombosis. Am J Roentgenol 138: 717, 1982.
121. Spritzer CE, Sussman SK, Blinder RA, et al: Deep venous thrombosis evaluation with limited flip-angle, gradient-refocused MR imaging: Preliminary experience. Radiology 166: 371, 1988.
122. Moser KM, Spragg RG, Utley J, et al: Chronic thrombotic obstruction of major pulmonary arteries: Results of thromboendarterectomy in 15 patients. Ann Intern Med 99: 299, 1983.
123. Prevention of pulmonary embolism. Br Med J 2: 1, 1973.
123a. Stein PD, Terrin ML, Hales CA, et al: Clinical, laboratory, roentgenographic, and electrocardiographic findings in patients with acute pulmonary embolism and no pre-existing cardiac or pulmonary disease. Chest 100: 598, 1991.
124. Oakley CM: Diagnosis of pulmonary embolism. Br Med J 2: 773, 1970.

125. Sasahara AA: Clinical studies in pulmonary thromboembolism. *In* Sasahara AA, Stein M (eds): Pulmonary Embolic Disease. New York, Grune & Stratton, 1965, pp 256–264.

126. Sevitt S: Venous thrombosis and pulmonary embolism. Their prevention by oral anticoagulation. Am J Med 33: 703, 1962.

127. Coodley EL: Enzyme profiles in the evaluation of pulmonary infarction. JAMA 207: 1307, 1969.

128. Dexter L: Cardiovascular responses to experimental pulmonary embolism. *In* Sasahara AA, Stein M (eds): Pulmonary Embolic Disease. New York, Grune & Stratton, 1965, pp 101–109.

129. Dantzker DR, Bower JS: Alterations in gas exchange following pulmonary thromboembolism. Chest 81: 495, 1982.

130. Winsor T: Electrocardiogram and pulmonary infarction (acute cor pulmonale). JAMA 204: 807, 1971.

130a. Carson JL, Kelley MA, Duff A, et al: The clinical course of pulmonary embolism. N Engl J Med 326: 1240, 1992.

131. Riedel M, Stanek V, Widimsky J, et al: Long-term follow-up of patients with pulmonary thromboembolism: Late prognosis and evolution of hemodynamic and respiratory data. Chest 81: 151, 1982.

132. Hadlock FP, Wallace RJ, Rivera M: Pulmonary septic emboli secondary to parapharyngeal abscess: Postanginal sepsis. Radiology 130: 29, 1979.

133. Fred HL, Harle TS: Septic pulmonary embolism. Dis Chest 55: 483, 1969.

134. Felman AH, Shulman ST: Staphylococcal osteomyelitis, sepsis, and pulmonary disease: Observations of 10 patients with combined osseous and pulmonary infections. Radiology 117: 649, 1975.

135. Levi J, Robson M, Rosenfeld JB: Septicaemia and pulmonary embolism complicating use of arteriovenous fistula in maintenance haemodialysis. Lancet 2: 288, 1970.

136. Jaffe RB, Koschmann EB: Septic pulmonary emboli. Radiology 96: 527, 1970.

137. Zelefsky MN, Lutzker LG: The target sign: A new radiologic sign of septic pulmonary emboli. Am J Roentgenol 129: 453, 1977.

138. Gumbs RV, McCauley DI: Hilar and mediastinal adenopathy in septic pulmonary embolic disease. Radiology 142: 313, 1982.

139. Huang R-M, Naidich DP, Lubat E, et al: Septic pulmonary emboli: CT-radiographic correlation. AJR 153: 41, 1989.

140. Kuhlman JE, Fishman EK, Teigen C: Pulmonary septic emboli: Diagnosis with CT. Radiology 174: 211, 1990.

141. Hadlock FP, Wallace RJ Jr, Rivera M: Pulmonary septic emboli secondary to parapharyngeal abscess: Postanginal sepsis. Radiology 130:29, 1979.

142. Sevitt S: Fat Embolism. London, Butterworths, 1962.

143. Pastore L, Kessler S: Pulmonary fat embolization in the immunocompromised patient. Am J Surg Pathol 6: 315, 1982.

144. Kitchell CC, Balogh K: Pulmonary lipid emboli in association with long-term hyperalimentation. Hum Pathol 17: 83, 1986.

145. Ross RM, Johnson GW: Fat embolism after liposuction. Chest 93: 1294, 1988.

146. Lessells AM: Fatal fat embolism after minor trauma. Br Med J 282: 1586, 1981.

147. Benatar SR, Ferguson AD, Goldschmidt RB: Fat embolism—some clinical observations and a review of controversial aspects. Q J Med 41: 85, 1972.

148. Sevitt S: The significance and classification of fat embolism. Lancet 2: 825, 1960.

149. Thomas ML, Tighe JR: Death from fat embolism as a complication of intraosseous phlebography. Lancet 2: 1415, 1973.

150. Kaufman HD, Finn R, Bourdillon RE: Fat embolism following an epileptic seizure. Br Med J 1: 1089, 1966.

151. Gresham GA, Kuczynski A, Rosborough D: Fatal fat embolism following replacement arthroplasty for transcervical fractures of femur. Br Med J 2: 617, 1971.

152. Broder G, Ruzumna L: Systemic fat embolism following acute primary osteomyelitis. JAMA 199: 1004, 1967.

153. Jackson CT, Greendyke RM: Pulmonary and cerebral fat embolism after closed-chest cardiac massage. Surg Gynecol Obstet 120: 25, 1965.

154. Guardia SN, Bilbao JM, Murray D, et al: Fat embolism in acute pancreatitis. Arch Pathol Lab Med 113: 498, 1989.

155. Dines DE, Burgher LW, Okazaki H: The clinical and pathologic correlation of fat embolism syndrome. Mayo Clin Proc 50: 407, 1975.

156. Hallgren B, Kerstall J, Rudenstam C-M, et al: A method for the isolation and chemical analysis of pulmonary fat embolism. Acta Chir Scand 132: 613, 1966.

157. Peltier LF: Fat embolism. III. The toxic properties of neutral fat and free fatty acids. Surgery 40: 665, 1956.

158. Derks CM, Jacobovitz-Derks D: Embolic pneumopathy induced by oleic acid. Am J Pathol 87: 143, 1977.

159. Jones JG, Minty BD, Beeley JM, et al: Pulmonary epithelial permeability is immediately increased after embolisation with oleic acid but not with neutral fat. Thorax 37: 169, 1982.

160. Scully RE: Fat embolism in Korean battle casualties: Its incidence, clinical significance, and pathologic aspects. Am J Pathol 32: 379, 1956.

161. Glas WW, Grekin TD, Musselman MM: Fat embolism. Am J Surg 85: 363, 1953.

162. Berrigan TJ Jr, Carsky EW, Heitzman ER: Fat embolism. Roentgenographic pathologic correlation in 3 cases. Am J Roentgenol 96: 967, 1966.

163. Williams JR, Bonte FJ: Pulmonary damage in nonpenetrating chest injuries. Radiol Clin North Am 1: 439, 1963.

164. Burgher LW, Dines DE, Linscheid RL: Fat embolism and the adult respiratory distress syndrome. Mayo Clin Proc 49: 107, 1974.

165. Tachakra SS: Distribution of skin petechiae in fat embolism rash. Lancet 1: 284, 1976.

166. Chastre J, Fagon JY, Soler P, et al: Bronchoalveolar lavage for rapid diagnosis of the fat embolism syndrome in trauma patients. Ann Intern Med 113: 583, 1990.

167. Wiener L, Forsyth D: Pulmonary pathophysiology of fat embolism. Am Rev Respir Dis 92: 113, 1965.

168. Carstens PHB: Pulmonary bone marrow embolism following external cardiac massage. Acta Pathol Microbiol Scand 76: 510, 1969.

169. Bierre AR, Koelmeyer TD: Pulmonary fat and bone marrow embolism in aircraft accident victims. Pathology 15: 131, 1983.

170. Pyun KS, Katzenstein RE: Widespread bone marrow embolism with myocardial involvement. Arch Pathol 89: 378, 1970.

171. Yamamoto M: Pathology of experimental pulmonary bone marrow embolism. II. Post-embolic pulmonary arteriosclerosis and pulmonary hypertension in rabbits receiving an intravenous infusion of allogeneic bone marrow. Acta Pathol Jpn 37(5): 705, 1987.

172. Courtney LD: Amniotic fluid embolism. Obstet Gynecol Surv 29: 169, 1974.

173. Philip RS: Amniotic fluid embolism. NY State J Med 67: 2085, 1967.

174. Masson RG, Ruggieri J, Siddiqui MM: Amniotic fluid embolism: Definitive diagnosis in a survivor. Am Rev Respir Dis 120: 187, 1979.

175. Attwood HD: Amniotic fluid embolism. Pathol Annu 7: 145, 1972.

176. Sparr RA, Pritchard JA: Studies to detect the escape of amniotic fluid into the maternal circulation during parturition. Surg Gynecol Obstet 107: 560, 1958.

177. Weiner AE, Reid DE, Roby CC: The hemostatic activity of amniotic fluid. Science 110: 190, 1949.

178. Aguillon A, Andjus T, Grayson A, Race GJ: Amniotic fluid embolism: A review. Obstet Gynecol Surv 17: 619, 1962.

179. Woodfield DG, Galloway RK, Smart GE: Coagulation defect associated with presumed amniotic fluid embolism in the mid-trimester of pregnancy. J Obstet Gynaecol Br Comm 78: 423, 1971.

180. Roche WD Jr, Norris HJ: Detection and significance of maternal pulmonary amniotic fluid embolism. Obstet Gynecol 43: 729, 1974.

181. Morgan M: Amniotic fluid embolism. Anaesthesia 34: 20, 1979.

182. Lee KR, Catalano PM, Ortiz-Giroux S: Cytologic diagnosis of amniotic fluid embolism. Report of a case with a unique cytologic feature and emphasis on the difficulty of eliminating squamous contamination. Acta Cytol 30: 177, 1986.

183. Neafie RC, Piggott J: Human pulmonary dirofilariasis. Arch Pathol 92: 342, 1971.

183a. Schriner RW, Ryu JH, Edwards WD: Microscopic pulmonary embolism causing subacute cor pulmonale: A difficult antemortem diagnosis. Mayo Clin Proc 66: 143, 1991.

184. Attwood HD, Park WW: Embolism to the lungs by trophoblast. J Obstet Gynaecol Br Comm 68: 611, 1961.

185. Park WW: Experimental trophoblastic embolism of the lungs. J Pathol Bacteriol 75: 257, 1958.

186. Aabo K, Hansen KB: Megakaryocytes in pulmonary blood vessels. I: Incidence at autopsy: Clinicopathological relations especially to disseminated intravascular coagulation. Acta Pathol Microbiol Scand 86: 285, 1978.

187. Nosanchuk JS, Littler ER: Skin embolus to lung. Arch Pathol 87: 542, 1969.

188. Straus R: Pulmonary embolism caused by liver tissue. Arch Pathol 33: 69, 1942.

189. Abrahams C, Catchatourian R: Bone fragment emboli in the lungs of patients undergoing bone marrow transplantation. Am J Clin Pathol 79: 360, 1983.

190. Lie JT: Myocardium as emboli in the systemic and pulmonary circulation. Arch Pathol Lab Med 111: 261, 1987.

191. Bohm N, Keller KM, Kloke WD: Pulmonary and systemic cerebellar tissue embolism due to birth injury. Virchows Arch 398: 229, 1982.

192. Balogh K: Pulmonary bile emboli: Sequelae of iatrogenic trauma. Arch Pathol Lab Med 108: 814, 1984.

193. Peachey T, Eason J, Moxham J, et al: Systemic air embolism during laser bronchoscopy. Anaesthesia 43: 872, 1988.

194. Tolly TL, Feldmeier JE, Czarnecki D: Air embolism complicating percutaneous lung biopsy. AJR 150: 555, 1988.

195. Smith FR: Air embolism as a cause of death in scuba diving in the Pacific Northwest. Dis Chest 52: 15, 1967.

196. Kogutt MS: Systemic air embolism secondary to respiratory therapy in the neonate: Six cases including one survivor. Am J Roentgenol 131: 425, 1978.

197. Segal AJ, Wasserman M: Arterial air embolism: A cause of sudden death in status asthmaticus. Radiology 99: 271, 1971.

198. Siegle RL, Eyal FG, Rabinowitz JG: Air embolus following pulmonary interstitial emphysema in hyaline membrane disease. Clin Radiol 27: 77, 1976.

199. Campkin TV, Perks JS: Venous air embolism. Lancet 1: 235, 1973.

200. Adams VI, Hirsch CS: Venous air embolism from head and neck wounds. Arch Pathol Lab Med 113: 498, 1989.

201. O'Quin RJ, Lakshminarayan S: Venous air embolism. Arch Intern Med 142: 2173, 1982.

202. Tuddenham WJ, Paskin DL: Radiographic demonstration of air embolism. Med Radiogr Photogr 50: 16, 1974.

203. Hartveit F, Lystad H, Minken A: The pathology of venous air embolism. Br J Exp Pathol 49: 81, 1968.

204. Gottlieb JD, Ericsson JA, Sweet RB: Venous air embolism: A review. Anesth Analg 44: 773, 1965.

205. Faer JM, Messerschmidt GL: Nonfatal pulmonary air embolism: Radiographic demonstration. Am J Roentgenol 131: 705, 1978.

206. Kizer KW, Goodman PC: Radiographic manifestations of venous air embolism. Radiology 144: 35, 1982.

207. Clark MC, Flick MR: Permeability pulmonary edema caused by venous air embolism. Am Rev Respir Dis 129: 633, 1984.

208. Ericsson JA, Gottlieb JD, Sweet RB: Closed-chest cardiac massage in the treatment of venous air embolism. N Engl J Med 270: 1353, 1964.

209. Kalant H, Kalant OJ: Death in amphetamine users: Causes and rates. Can Med Assoc J 112: 299, 1975.

210. Hopkins GB: Pulmonary angiothrombotic granulomatosis in drug offenders. JAMA 221: 909, 1972.

211. Paré JAP, Cote G, Fraser RS: Long-term follow-up of drug abusers with intravenous talcosis. Am Rev Respir Dis 139: 233, 1989.

212. Paré JAP, Fraser RG, Hogg JC, et al: Pulmonary "mainline" granulomatosis: Talcosis of intravenous methadone abuse. Medicine 58: 229, 1979.

213. Douglas FG, Kafilmout KJ, Patt NL: Foreign particle embolism in drug addicts: Respiratory pathophysiology. Ann Intern Med 75: 865, 1971.

214. Bron Klaus M, Baum S, Abrams HL: Oil embolism in lymphangiography: Incidence, manifestations, and mechanism. Radiology 80: 194, 1963.

215. Fraimow W, Wallace S, Lewis P, et al: Changes in pulmonary function due to lymphangiography. Radiology 85: 231, 1965.

216. Gough JH, Gough MH, Thomas ML: Pulmonary complications following lymphography with a note on technique. Br J Radiol 37: 416, 1964.

217. Weg JG, Harkleroad LE: Aberrations in pulmonary function due to lymphangiography. Dis Chest 53: 534, 1968.

218. White RJ, Webb JAW, Tucker AK, et al: Pulmonary function after lymphography. Br Med J 4: 775, 1973.

219. Hill DM: Self-administration of mercury by subcutaneous injection. Br Med J 1: 342, 1967.

220. Naidich TP, Bartelt D, Wheeler PS, et al: Metallic mercury emboli. Am J Roentgenol 117: 886, 1973.

221. Tsuji HK, Tyler GC, Reddington JV, et al: Intrabronchial metallic mercury. Chest 57: 322, 1970.

222. Schulze W: Röntgenologische Studien nach Aspiration von metallischen Quecksilber. (Roentgenographic studies of metallic mercury aspiration.) Fortschr Roentgenstr 89: 24, 1958.

223. Truemner KM, White S, Vanlandingham H: Fatal embolization of pulmonary capillaries. JAMA 173: 119, 1960.

224. David R, Berezesky IK, Bohlman M, et al: Fatal barium embolization due to incorrect vaginal rather than colonic insertion. Arch Pathol Lab Med 107: 548, 1983.

225. Hafez A, Dartevelle P, Lafont D, et al: Pulmonary arterial embolus by an unusual wandering bullet. Thorac Cardiovasc Surg 31: 392, 1983.

226. Brewer LA III, Bai AF, King EL, et al: The pathologic effects of metallic foreign bodies in the pulmonary circulation. J Thorac Cardiovasc Surg 38: 670, 1959.

227. Terry PB, Barth KH, Kaufman SL, et al: Balloon embolization for treatment of pulmonary arteriovenous fistulas. N Engl J Med 302: 1189, 1980.

228. Leitman BS, McCauley DI, Firooznia H: Multiple metallic pulmonary densities after therapeutic embolization. JAMA 248: 2155, 1982.

229. Bernhardt LC, Wegner GP, Mendenhall JT: Intravenous catheter embolization to the pulmonary artery. Chest 57: 329, 1970.

230. Prager D, Hertzberg RW: Spontaneous intravenous catheter fracture and embolization from an implanted venous access port and analysis by scanning electron microscopy. Cancer 60: 270, 1987.

231. Turco SJ, Davis NM: Detrimental effects of particulate matter on the pulmonary circulation. JAMA 217: 81, 1971.

232. Krempien B, Bommer J, Ritz E: Foreign body giant cell reaction in lungs, liver and spleen. Virchows Arch [A] 392: 73, 1981.

233. Uflacker R, Kaemmerer A, Picon PD, et al: Bronchial artery embolization in the management of hemoptysis: Technical aspects and long-term results. Radiology 157: 637, 1985.

234. Tomashefski JF Jr, Cohen AM, Doershuk CF: Long-term histopathologic follow-up of bronchial arteries after therapeutic embolization with polyvinyl alcohol (Ivalon) in patients with cystic fibrosis. Hum Pathol 19: 555, 1988.

10

PULMONARY HYPERTENSION AND EDEMA

GENERAL CONSIDERATIONS OF PULMONARY BLOOD FLOW AND PRESSURE

The anatomy and physiology of the normal pulmonary circulation are discussed in detail in Chapter 1, and only a few points relevant to an understanding of altered pulmonary hemodynamics are reviewed here. Unlike the case in the tracheobronchial tree, in which most of the resistance to airflow occurs in the large airways, in the pulmonary arterial tree most of the resistance is in the smaller blood

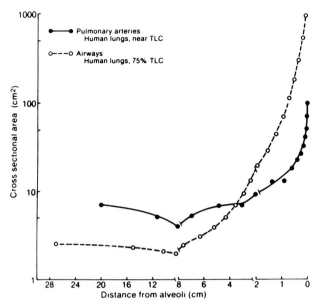

Figure 10–1. Pulmonary Arterial and Airway Cross-Sectional Area. The total cross-sectional area of the tracheobronchial tree and the pulmonary vascular tree increases greatly as they branch toward the gas-exchanging portion of the lung. These data show that the total area occupied by small airways exceeds that occupied by small pulmonary vessels. (Reproduced, with permission, from Culver BH, Butler J: Mechanical influences on the pulmonary microcirculation. Annual Review of Physiology 40:187, 1980. © 1980 by Annual Reviews Inc.)

vessels (muscular arteries and arterioles). As shown in Figure 10–1,[1] it is apparent that the tracheobronchial and pulmonary arterial trees begin with similar-sized "trunks" but that the total cross-sectional area of the airways greatly exceeds that of the blood vessels in the periphery of the lung. These small vessels are also the site of the majority of vascular smooth muscle, and it is the modulation of their caliber that causes the best match of ventilation and perfusion.

The pulmonary vascular circuit is a low-pressure system, the mean arterial pressure being only about one sixth of the systemic arterial pressure. It has a remarkable capacity to compensate for a large physiologic increase in blood flow (e.g., during exercise) without a corresponding increase in pressure. This reduction in vascular resistance is achieved mainly by "recruiting" pulmonary vessels that are not perfused at rest. This ability to recruit vessels with minor increases in pressure results in a pulmonary vascular pressure-flow curve, as illustrated in Figure 10–2. When the cardiac output is low (A), pulmonary vascular resistance is given by the slope A-X or

16 mm Hg/5 L/minute = 3.2 mm Hg/L/minute

If the cardiac output is increased to 15 L per minute (B), pulmonary artery pressure increases only slightly, to 18 mm Hg, and now pulmonary vascular resistance is given by the slope B-X or

18 mm Hg/15 L/minute = 1.2 mm Hg/L/minute

This substantial decrease in resistance occurs simply because of vascular recruitment and *not* because of relaxation of pulmonary vascular smooth muscle.

Pulmonary vascular resistance (PVR) is calculated by dividing the driving pressure by the cardiac output:

$$PVR = Ppa - Pla/\dot{Q}$$

where PVR = pulmonary vascular resistance, Ppa = pulmonary artery pressure, Pla = left atrial pressure, and $\dot{Q}$ = cardiac output. The driving pressure is the difference between mean pulmonary arterial and mean left atrial pressure. In practice, the pulmonary wedge pressure provides a reliable estimate of left atrial pressure in the absence of large vein obstruction. An increase in pulmonary arterial pressure can occur because of an increase in blood flow, because of increased resistance to flow through arteries, capillaries, or veins, or because of an increased left atrial pressure.

In the roentgenologic assessment of diseases of the pulmonary vascular system, signs are related to a relative change in the caliber of hilar pulmonary arteries and of lobar and segmental pulmonary arteries as they proceed distally, the size and contour of the heart, and the caliber of the pulmonary veins. Whereas severe degrees of overvascularity (pleonemia) and undervascularity (oligemia) may be readily apparent, minor degrees may be exceedingly difficult to appreciate on standard roentgenograms. Although serial roentgenography and tomography (either conventional or computed) may aid in evaluation, only angiography can provide proof of vascular abnormality in questionable cases.

PULMONARY HYPERTENSION

Pulmonary arterial hypertension may be defined as an increase in systolic pressure to 30 mm Hg or higher, an increase in mean pressure to 18 mm Hg or higher, or both.[2] Pulmonary venous hypertension is present when the pressure in the pulmonary veins measured indirectly by a catheter wedged in a pulmonary artery exceeds 12 mm Hg. Slight increases in pulmonary arterial pressure generally cause no clinical, roentgenographic, or electrocardiographic signs, even with mean pulmonary arterial pressures as high

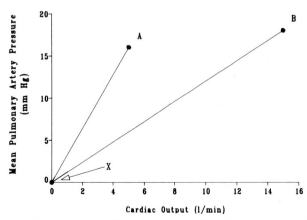

Figure 10–2. Pulmonary Vascular Pressure Flow Curves. Mean pulmonary arterial pressure is plotted against cardiac output. The slope of the line is pulmonary vascular resistance. A large increase in cardiac output is associated with only a slight increase in mean pulmonary vascular pressure. *See* text for discussion.

as 24 mm Hg.[3] As the resistance to pulmonary blood flow increases, however, the increase in right ventricular afterload produces clinical and electrocardiographic signs and, eventually, roentgenologic changes indicative of strain and resultant hypertrophy of the right ventricle. With further rises in pressure, catheterization studies may show elevation not only of pulmonary arterial and right ventricular systolic pressures but also of right ventricular diastolic pressure, indicating the onset of right ventricular failure.

Pathologic Characteristics

Many of the pathologic abnormalities that occur in the vasculature in pulmonary hypertension are similar, despite differences in etiology. In arterial hypertension of significant degree, the large elastic arteries, especially the main pulmonary artery, are often dilated, sometimes so severely that localized aneurysm formation is the result. An increase in acidic ground substance and a focal loss of elastic tissue in the media (so-called cystic medial necrosis) are sometimes present in such vessels; as in the aorta, these can be associated with dissection.[4] Although some degree of atherosclerosis is a common manifestation of aging in elastic pulmonary arteries, in the presence of pulmonary hypertension, it increases in both severity and extent.[5] Despite this, complicating features such as necrosis, calcification, and ulceration are rare.

Medial hypertrophy of muscular arteries is seen in almost all forms of pulmonary hypertension (Fig. 10–3). Although it is most often caused by a combination of muscle hypertrophy and hyperplasia, in some cases there is also an increase in intermuscular connective tissue.[6] Intimal fibrosis is frequently associated with medial hypertrophy[6a] and may be so severe as to virtually obliterate the vascular lumen (see Fig. 10–3); paradoxically, the media in such cases may be atrophic. Muscle hypertrophy also occurs in pulmonary arterioles. In some cases, this is caused by an increase in the size and number of muscle fibers already present in the arteriolar wall, but in others it represents extension of muscle into vessels that formerly contained none (so-called arterialization of pulmonary arterioles). These new muscle cells appear to be derived from pericytes and "intermediate cells" normally present in the arteriolar wall.[7]

In addition to the changes just described, several distinctive abnormalities are often present in small to medium-sized muscular arteries in cases of primary pulmonary hypertension and in hypertension associated with congenital cardiac disease, hepatic disease, and anorexic drugs. These changes include intimal cellular proliferation, plexiform lesions, "fibrinoid necrosis," and vasculitis, the combination of which characterizes "plexogenic pulmonary arteriopathy." In this abnormality, intimal thickening is caused by a proliferation of loose connective tissue containing cells that typically are elongated and arranged in more or less con-

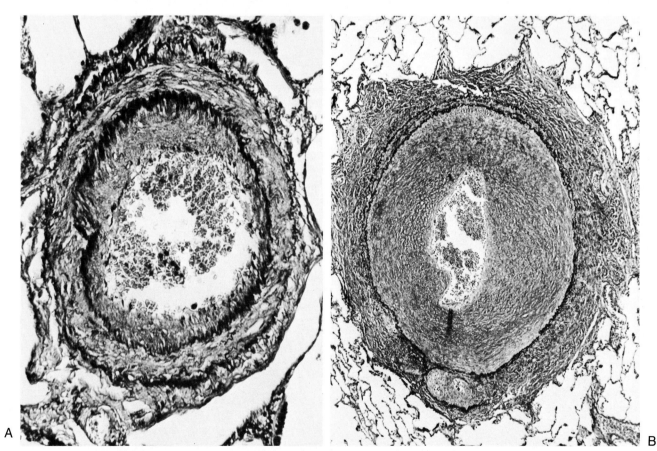

A   B

Figure 10–3. Pulmonary Hypertension: Medial and Intimal Changes. A histologic section *(A)* of a medium-sized muscular artery shows a moderate degree of medial thickening and mild intimal fibrosis. *B,* A section from another patient shows predominantly intimal fibrosis with fairly extensive medial atrophy. (Verhoeff–van Gieson; *A* × 200; *B* × 52.)

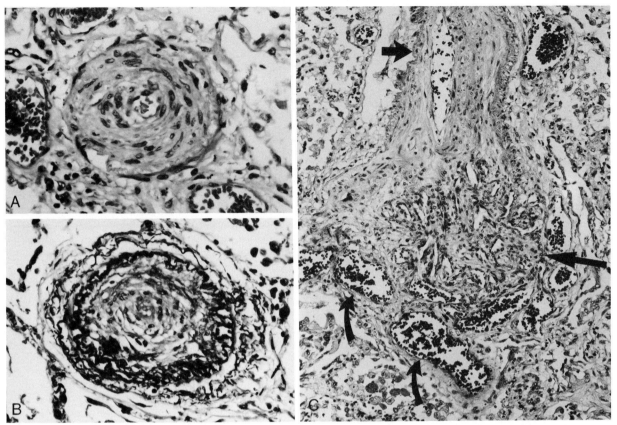

Figure 10–4. Pulmonary Hypertension: Plexogenic Arteriopathy. A histologic section of a small pulmonary artery *(A)* from a young man with an atrial septal defect shows almost complete luminal obliteration by cellular fibrous tissue with a somewhat whorled appearance. A section of the same vessel stained for elastic tissue *(B)* shows the cellular proliferation to be entirely within the intima. *C,* A section of a medium-sized pulmonary artery from a patient with cirrhosis and portal hypertension reveals moderate intimal fibrosis *(short arrow)* and a plexus of small, irregularly shaped vascular channels *(long arrow)*. The plexus itself is continuous with a dilated, relatively thin-walled vascular channel *(curved arrows)*. *(A × 160; B,* Verhoeff–van Gieson, × 160; *C × 130.)*

centric layers, creating a distinctive "onion skin" appearance (Fig. 10–4). This cellular proliferation is often out of proportion to the degree of medial hypertrophy and can result in almost complete luminal obliteration. Identification of this change in a lung biopsy is important, because there is evidence that it is associated with progressive pulmonary vascular disease despite repair of cardiovascular anomalies.[8]

A plexiform lesion refers to a distinctive abnormality of small muscular arteries that often develops just beyond the origin of the vessel from its parent branch. The lesion consists of localized vascular dilatation associated with an intraluminal plexus of numerous slitlike vascular channels (*see* Fig. 10–4). The pathogenesis of these lesions is uncertain, but they may result from organization of intraluminal thrombus, possibly secondary to inflammation of the adjacent vessel wall.

The term "fibrinoid necrosis" is used to describe the presence of homogeneous eosinophilic material in the wall of small pulmonary arteries and arterioles. Although the term is commonly used, it is incorrect, strictly speaking, because there is usually no evidence of tissue necrosis. Instead, the lesion most likely represents the accumulation of fibrin and other proteins within the media unaccompanied by true cell death. Whatever its nature, however, it is

a not uncommon finding in plexogenic arteriopathy, particularly in the presence of high pulmonary arterial pressures. Occasionally, these foci are associated with an acute inflammatory reaction, indicating true vasculitis.

Pathogenesis

Several factors determine normal pulmonary vascular pressures, and an alteration in any one can result in hypertension (Table 10–1). The pressure across any vascular bed is directly related to the blood flow through that particular bed and the blood viscosity within it; an increase in either will cause an increase in pressure for any given vascular geometry. The pressure across the vascular bed also is inversely related to the number and radii of its vessels. The total cross-sectional area of the vascular tree can decrease because of a loss of pulmonary vessels, intraluminal occlusion of a proportion of the vessels, or a decrease in vascular radius as a result of smooth muscle contraction or wall thickening. Finally, pulmonary arterial pressure can be increased as a result of an increase in the downstream or venous pressure.

Pulmonary artery vasoconstriction can be produced by hypoxemia or acidosis, either metabolic or respiratory in origin,[238, 239] and thus may be reversed, at least partly, by

Table 10–1. **CLASSIFICATION OF PULMONARY HYPERTENSION**

Precapillary Pulmonary Hypertension
Primary Vascular Disease
1. Increased flow (large left-to-right shunts)
2. Decreased flow (tetralogy of Fallot)
3. Primary pulmonary hypertension
4. Pulmonary embolic disease:
    Thrombus
    Metastatic neoplasm
    Parasites
    Miscellaneous: fat, talc, amniotic fluid
5. Immunologic abnormalities: e.g., SLE, PSS
6. High altitude
Primary Pleuropulmonary Disease
1. Emphysema
2. Diffuse interstitial or airspace disease
    Fibrosis: e.g., connective tissue disease, fibrosing
        alveolitis, sarcoidosis
    Neoplasm
    Postpulmonary resection
    Miscellaneous: alveolar microlithiasis, idiopathic hemosiderosis,
        alveolar proteinosis, cystic fibrosis, bronchiectasis
3. Pleural disease (fibrothorax)
4. Chest wall deformity
    Thoracoplasty
    Kyphoscoliosis
Alveolar Hypoventilation
1. Neuromuscular
2. Obesity
3. Chronic upper airway obstruction in children
4. Idiopathic
Postcapillary Hypertension
Cardiac
1. Left ventricular failure
2. Mitral valvular disease
3. Myxoma (or thrombus) of the left atrium
4. Cor triatriatum
Pulmonary Venous
1. Congenital stenosis of the pulmonary veins
2. Chronic sclerosing mediastinitis
3. Idiopathic veno-occlusive disease
4. Anomalous pulmonary venous return
5. Neoplasms
6. Thrombosis

Abbreviations: SLE, systemic lupus erythematosus; PSS, progressive systemic sclerosis.

the administration of oxygen or by raising the pH of the blood.[9] Vasoconstriction also can be caused by a variety of mediators of inflammation, including serotonin, histamine, angiotensin, catecholamines, prostaglandins, and leukotrienes.[10] The release of such mediators is probably the mechanism of acute pulmonary hypertension in pulmonary thromboembolic disease. The increase in pressure in the pulmonary arteries resulting from postcapillary hypertension (*see* later) also is initially vasospastic in origin, probably mediated through a vasovagal reflex originating from a rise in left atrial and pulmonary venous pressures.

It is useful conceptually to divide the causes of pulmonary hypertension into three general groups, each of which shows somewhat different clinical, physiologic, and roentgenologic characteristics (*see* Table 10–1): (1) those in which the major mechanisms of production are *precapillary* in location, (2) those in which the significant physiologic disturbance arises from disease in the *postcapillary vessels,* and (3) those in which the hypertension reflects a disturbance in vessels on both sides of the capillary bed—*com-*

bined precapillary and postcapillary hypertension. In each of these groups, the capillaries may be involved to some extent and may contribute considerably to the increase in vascular resistance.

The multiple causes of pulmonary arterial hypertension have recently been reviewed, accompanied by excellent radiologic-pathologic correlation.[11]

Precapillary Pulmonary Hypertension

Increased Flow

Included in this category are the congenital cardiovascular defects that result in a left-to-right shunt (atrial septal defect [ASD], ventricular septal defect [VSD], patent ductus arteriosus [PDA], aorticopulmonary window, and partial anomalous pulmonary venous drainage) and conditions associated with an increase in total blood volume, such as thyrotoxicosis and chronic renal failure.

The main roentgenographic sign in these conditions is an increase in caliber of all the pulmonary arteries throughout the lungs (Fig. 10–5). Since the hemodynamic change is one of increased flow, the degree of enlargement of the main and hilar pulmonary arteries usually is directly related to the degree of distention of the intrapulmonary vessels. Thus, when peripheral resistance is normal, the arteries taper gradually and proportionately distally. Vascular markings that normally are invisible in the peripheral 2 cm of the lungs may become visible. Appreciation of venous as well as arterial caliber is important in the assessment of shunt lesions. For example, with the development of increased vascular resistance and pulmonary hypertension, the shunt becomes balanced and eventually reversed (Eisenmenger's reaction) (Fig. 10–6), with resultant reduction in right ventricular output and a decrease in pulmonary venous caliber. Occasionally, large left-to-right shunts are not reflected in roentgenographically demonstrable enlargement of the pulmonary vascular bed or in cardiomegaly.[12]

It may be extremely difficult roentgenologically to recognize the presence of pulmonary arterial hypertension in cases of left-to-right shunt. It might be assumed that increased rapidity of tapering or a disparity between proximal and peripheral pulmonary vessel sizes would constitute reliable evidence for the presence of hypertension. However, it has been shown that although the small branches of the pulmonary arterial tree are narrowed in some instances, usually they are beyond the range of visibility on plain roentgenography or angiography.[13] In fact, only in very severe cases can the presence of pulmonary hypertension be determined from the chest roentgenogram. The difficulty is compounded by the fact that other signs of pulmonary arterial hypertension, such as enlargement of the main and hilar pulmonary arteries, are unreliable, since these structures may be greatly enlarged when resistance is normal. In most patients, cardiac catheterization, with or without angiocardiography, is necessary for thorough assessment of left-to-right shunts, particularly in the presence of suspected pulmonary arterial hypertension (Fig. 10–7).

Clinically, many patients with left-to-right shunts are asymptomatic. If the shunt is large, some physical underdevelopment and a tendency to respiratory infections may occur. The patient may complain of fatigue, palpitations,

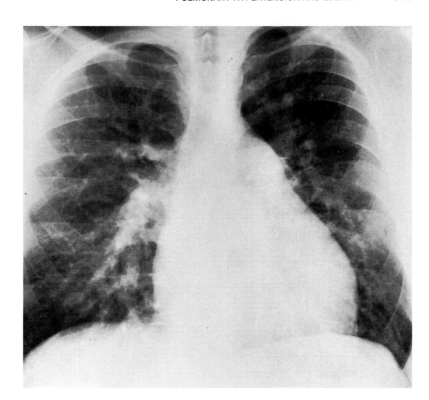

Figure 10–5. Pulmonary Pleonemia: Atrial Septal Defect. A Posteroanterior roentgenogram of an asymptomatic 19-year-old male reveals a marked increase in the caliber of the pulmonary arteries and veins throughout both lungs; the vessels taper normally. The heart is moderately enlarged, possessing a contour consistent with enlargement of the right atrium and right ventricle. An atrial septal defect was satisfactorily corrected surgically.

and dyspnea on exertion and may exhibit signs of cardiac failure. Uncomplicated ASD is characterized by an ejection murmur, an early systolic click, and a wide splitting of the second cardiac sound (0.05 seconds or more) that does not vary with respiration; cardiac enlargement and bulging of the precordial chest cage may develop. A VSD produces a pansystolic murmur maximal at the third or fourth left interspace close to the sternum; the second sound is normally split or widened but, unlike its behavior in ASD, varies with respiration. The murmur of PDA before the development of pulmonary hypertension usually is long and rumbling and occupies most of systole and diastole. It is loudest in the second left interspace near the sternum and sometimes is associated with crescendo accentuation in late systole. The second pulmonic sound is increased in amplitude but normally split and changing with respiration. A widely patent left-to-right shunt caused by PDA produces systemic peripheral vascular signs of a high pulse pressure.

The development of pulmonary hypertension in cases of left-to-right shunt gives rise to changes in the physical findings. In ASD, atrial fibrillation is a frequent occurrence and may be followed by tricuspid regurgitation and heart failure. The fixed splitting of the second heart sound becomes much narrower, and the systolic murmur may become fainter. In VSD, the systolic murmur decreases in length, and an ejection systolic murmur and click may appear. In PDA, as the pressure in the pulmonary circulation rises and the shunt decreases, the murmur is reduced in intensity, and in many cases the diastolic component disappears. Pulmonary hypertension also causes accentuation of the second pulmonic sound and an early diastolic murmur along the left sternal border as a result of pulmonary valvular insufficiency. The parasternal thrust, tricuspid insufficiency, and liver and neck pulsations are caused by cor pulmonale and failure of the right ventricle. Retrosternal pain, identi-

cal to angina pectoris, may occur when the pulmonary arterial pressure becomes very high.

Decreased Flow (Tetralogy of Fallot)

Pulmonary hypertension sometimes develops prior to any attempt at surgical correction in tetralogy of Fallot. In such cases, the hypertension may be caused by multiple foci of pulmonary arterial thrombosis resulting from slowing of the pulmonary circulation and a tendency to polycythemia.[14] Surgical creation of a left-to-right shunt with a Blalock-Taussig or Potts's anastomosis causes pulmonary hypertension in patients older than 5 years of age, but usually not in younger children.[15] When pulmonary hypertension does develop, the central pulmonary arteries dilate, cyanosis increases, the continuous murmur disappears, and a loud pulmonary valve closure sound develops.[16] Factors that may lead to irreversible pulmonary hypertension after surgical correction include failure to recognize associated anomalous pulmonary venous drainage,[17] undetected agenesis of a pulmonary artery, peripheral pulmonic stenosis (coarctation), too large a shunt from a previous Blalock (or more likely Potts's) anastomosis leading to heart failure, and obstruction of the pulmonary vascular bed associated with inadequate closure of the VSD and relief of the pulmonic stenosis.

Primary Pulmonary Hypertension

Primary pulmonary hypertension is a relatively uncommon condition,[18] the authenticity of which has been questioned by some on the basis of the demonstration at necropsy of multiple pulmonary emboli in patients considered to have had this disease during life.[19, 20] However, the dramatic response in some patients to the intravenous injection

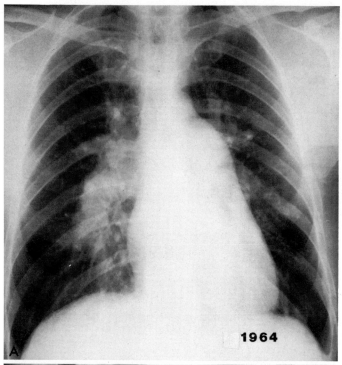

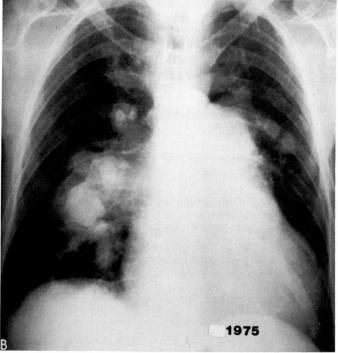

Figure 10–6. Severe Eisenmenger Syndrome Caused by Atrial Septal Defect. A roentgenogram taken in 1964 *(A)* reveals marked enlargement of the hilar pulmonary arteries, which taper rapidly as they proceed distally. The peripheral vasculature is clearly diminished, and the size and configuration of the heart are consistent with cor pulmonale. Cardiac catheterization at this time revealed a secundum-type atrial septal defect. There was a right-to-left shunt of approximately 21 per cent; pulmonary vascular resistance was equivalent to that of the systemic circulation.

B, Eleven years later the main pulmonary arteries and the heart have undergone remarkable enlargement; the peripheral oligemia is much more evident. (Courtesy of St. Boniface Hospital, Manitoba.)

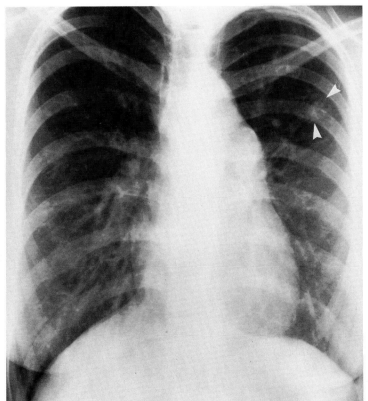
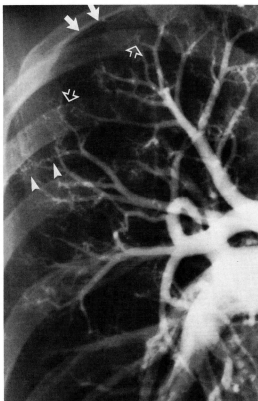

A

B

Figure 10–7. Precapillary Pulmonary Hypertension Caused by a Ventricular Septal Defect: Angiographic Features. A conventional posteroanterior chest roentgenogram *(A)* discloses a prominent main pulmonary artery segment. The hilar arteries are increased in size, and the lungs plethoric. Several poorly defined nodular opacities can be identified in the lungs, the most notable being in the left upper lobe *(arrowheads)*. A right pulmonary arteriogram *(B)* reveals multiple, small, sinuous arteries in the distal parenchyma *(arrowheads)*, amputation of arteries *(open arrows)*, and subpleural collaterals *(closed arrows)*. The nodular opacities in *A* were shown to be caused by enlarged, branchless, serpiginous segmental arteries that terminated in a bulbous structure. Cardiac catheterization disclosed pressures within the pulmonary artery that were almost the same as those in the systemic circulation.

of acetylcholine and other vasodilating agents,[21] the presence of characteristic plexogenic arteriopathy (a pathologic abnormality that is rarely associated with thromboemboli), and the tendency to familial occurrence strongly support the existence of this condition as a distinct entity. Although the majority of cases appear to occur sporadically, the disease may occur in a familial pattern generally conforming to an autosomal dominant inheritance.[22]

The pathogenesis of the disease is uncertain. The finding of a plasmin inhibitor in some patients suggests that normally occurring microemboli or foci of *in situ* thrombosis may be unable to be lysed.[23] Exogenous substances, such as those contained in *Crotalaria fulva*, a plant ingested in the West Indies as a component of bush tea, can cause pulmonary hypertension in rats[24]; however, there is no evidence that they do so in humans. A condition resembling primary pulmonary hypertension can occur in patients who have cirrhosis and portal hypertension, especially those who have a surgical portacaval shunt.[25] It has been suggested that in these patients, vasoactive substances normally metabolized by the liver reach the pulmonary circulation.[26] The frequent association of primary pulmonary hypertension with Raynaud's phenomenon, either as an isolated finding or in association with systemic lupus erythematosus (Fig. 10–8)

or the CREST syndrome (*see* pages 394 and 404), suggests the possibility that it is part of a generalized angiopathic process.[27] This hypothesis is supported by experimental studies in which immersion of a hand in cold water has been followed by evidence of pulmonary artery vasoconstriction.[28]

It is believed that the early stages of primary pulmonary hypertension are characterized by vasoconstriction of pulmonary vascular smooth muscle, a situation which is potentially reversible; however, with prolonged vasoconstriction there occurs intimal fibrosis, medial smooth muscle hyperplasia, and other changes of plexogenic pulmonary arteriopathy. Unfortunately, by the time the vast majority of patients first come to medical attention, these anatomic changes have already developed, and the hypertension is irreversible.

Roentgenographically, the lungs show evidence of diffuse oligemia, the peripheral pulmonary arteries being narrow and inconspicuous (Fig. 10–9).[29] The hilar pulmonary arteries are enlarged and taper rapidly distally; the main pulmonary artery usually is prominent and often shows increased amplitude of pulsation fluoroscopically. Evidence of right ventricular enlargement may be present. Overinflation does not occur, permitting ready differentiation from

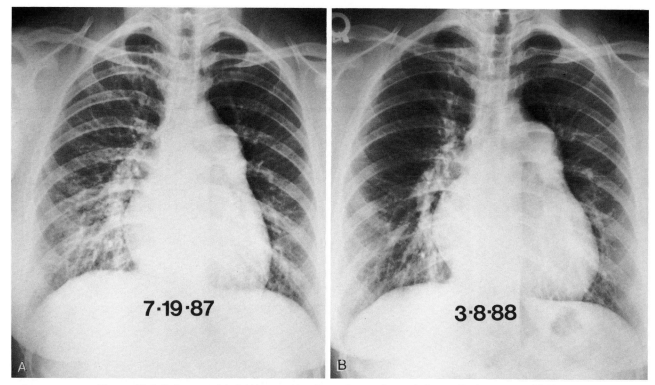

Figure 10–8. Pulmonary Arterial Hypertension Secondary to Systemic Lupus Erythematosus (SLE). The first chest roentgenogram in posteroanterior *(A)* projection on this 32-year-old woman with SLE reveals exceptional prominence of the main pulmonary artery and mild to moderate cardiomegaly consistent with right ventricular enlargement. The pulmonary vasculature looks plethoric, but the lungs are otherwise unremarkable. Eight months later, a repeat chest roentgenogram *(B)* showed an increase in the size of the heart and greater prominence of the main and hilar pulmonary arteries. However, a more remarkable change has occurred in the pulmonary vasculature, which now displays diffuse oligemia. (Courtesy Dr. M. O'Donovan, Montreal General Hospital.)

the diffuse pulmonary oligemia associated with emphysema. Lung perfusion scans are abnormal in most patients, the majority of the abnormalities on perfusion scintigraphy consisting of diffuse, patchy defects that have a low probability of representing pulmonary embolism.[30]

Measurement of the transverse diameter of the right and left interlobar arteries provides reliable evidence of the presence or absence of dilatation and thus the likelihood of the presence of pulmonary arterial hypertension (provided that conditions of increased flow, such as left-to-right shunt, have been excluded). The upper limit of the transverse diameter of the right interlobar artery from its lateral aspect to the air column of the intermediate bronchus is 16 mm in men and 15 mm in women.[31] However, since the transverse diameter of the left interlobar artery is often impossible to measure on a conventional posteroanterior roentgenogram, a useful alternative is to measure the vessel on a lateral roentgenogram from the circular lucency created by the left upper lobe bronchus viewed end-on to the posterior margin of the vessel as it loops over the bronchus, the accepted upper limits of normal for this measurement being 18 mm. Computed tomography (CT) can also allow precise noninvasive measurement of the diameter of pulmonary arteries: It has been shown that in normal subjects the upper limit of the diameter of the main pulmonary artery is 28.6 mm,[32] a diameter greater than this readily predicting the presence of pulmonary hypertension.

The mean age of the patients with primary pulmonary hypertension is 36 ± 15 years, and there is a female-to-male predominance of 1.7 to 1.[30] The mean interval from the onset of symptoms to diagnosis is 2 years, and the most frequent presenting symptoms are dyspnea (60 per cent), fatigue (20 per cent), and syncope or near-syncope (about 15 per cent). Raynaud's phenomenon is observed in 10 per cent of patients, virtually all of whom are female, and a positive antinuclear antibody test is found in about 30 per cent, 70 per cent of whom are female.

Signs of cor pulmonale and cardiac failure may be present, including giant jugular A waves, right atrial gallop (60 per cent), a loud pulmonary ejection click, an accentuated pulmonic sound (90 per cent), a palpable lift along the left sternal border, and murmurs caused by pulmonic and tricuspid insufficiency (40 per cent).[30] Cyanosis and peripheral edema occur in the later stages of the disease.

Catheterization of the right side of the heart reveals arterial hypertension, a normal pulmonary wedge pressure, high pulmonary vascular resistance, and, in patients with right ventricular failure, a low cardiac output.[29] In 187 patients studied by the National Institutes of Health (NIH),[30] the mean pulmonary arterial pressure was 60 ± 18 mm Hg, the pulmonary wedge pressure averaged 9 mm Hg, and the cardiac index was mildly reduced at 2.27 ± 0.9 L per minute per m².

Mild lung restriction and significant gas exchange impair-

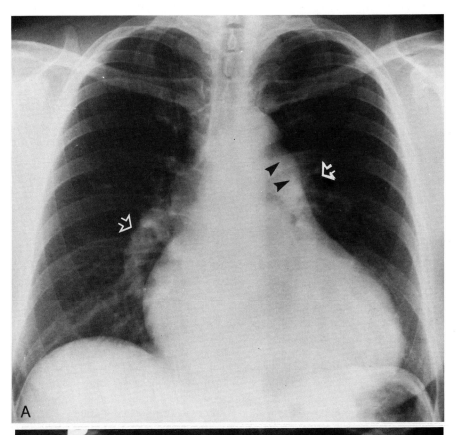

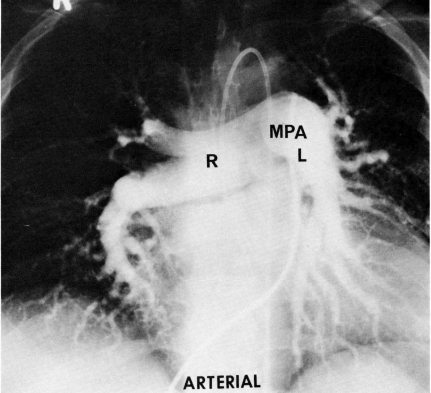

Figure 10–9. Primary Pulmonary Hypertension. A conventional posteroanterior chest roentgenogram *(A)* reveals enlargement of the right ventricle, dilatation of the main *(arrowheads)* and hilar *(open arrows)* pulmonary arteries, and increased rapidity of tapering of pulmonary arteries as they proceed distally. These findings are confirmed on a pulmonary angiogram during the arterial phase *(B)* (main pulmonary artery [MPA], right [R] and left [L] pulmonary arteries); the distal pulmonary arteries taper rapidly, displaying a sinuous ("corkscrew") appearance.

ment characterize the pulmonary function.[33] In the NIH study,[30] total lung capacity (TLC) and vital capacity (VC) were mildly decreased, and there was a moderate decrease in pulmonary diffusing capacity (68 per cent predicted), arterial partial pressure of oxygen (PaO_2 = 70 mm Hg), and arterial partial pressure of carbon dioxide ($PaCO_2$ = 30 mm Hg). Hypoxemia worsens during exercise because of a failure of cardiac output to increase and a reduction in mixed venous oxygen saturation.[34]

The majority of patients with primary pulmonary hypertension have progressive disease, and the median survival time is no more than 2 to 3 years,[18] although there are occasional patients who have prolonged survival or even improvement.[35] Raynaud's phenomenon and right ventricular hemodynamic dysfunction are associated with shortened survival.[36]

Pulmonary Embolic Disease

Multiple pulmonary thromboemboli occurring over a period of months or years is probably the most common cause of precapillary pulmonary hypertension. Less common causes of pulmonary embolic hypertension include microemboli from platelet-fibrin thrombi in patients with eclampsia,[37] tumor emboli, schistosomiasis, and talc emboli from the intravenous injection of oral medications. Rarely, pulmonary hypertension results from chronic thrombotic occlusion of the major pulmonary arteries.[38]

The major diagnostic difficulty is in distinguishing patients whose pulmonary hypertension is due to multiple small pulmonary emboli from those in whom it is primary. The chest roentgenograms can be identical in the two con-

ditions. Perfusion scintigraphy may show patchy diffuse nonsegmental perfusion defects in patients with thromboembolic disease.[39] The morphologic features of thromboembolic disease are sufficiently distinctive to suggest the cause of the hypertension in most cases.[40] Although affected patients may have a history of an acute pulmonary thromboembolic episode,[41] the majority do not.[42] In the absence of discrete episodes suggestive of acute pulmonary embolism, the symptoms and signs are identical to those of primary pulmonary hypertension.

Miscellaneous Causes

A wide variety of primary diseases of the lungs, pleura, chest wall, and respiratory control center can cause precapillary pulmonary hypertension (see Table 10–1). In most patients, the hypertension is secondary to hypoxemia and respiratory acidosis, but hypervolemia, polycythemia, pulmonary capillary bed destruction, and anastomoses between the systemic bronchial circulation and the pulmonary circulation are contributing factors.

Pulmonary hypertension in chronic obstructive pulmonary disease (COPD) appears to be caused predominantly by a combination of hypoxemia and destruction of the microvasculature. Physiologic studies have shown a close correlation between pulmonary vascular resistance, oxygen saturation, and diffusing capacity during exercise.[43] The roentgenographic manifestations of pulmonary hypertension in emphysema can be readily distinguished from primary vascular disease by the invariable presence of overinflation (Fig. 10–10). The pulmonary hypertension in patients who have diffuse interstitial or airspace disease is

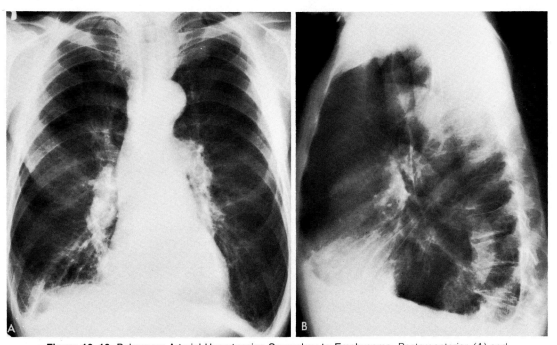

Figure 10–10. Pulmonary Arterial Hypertension Secondary to Emphysema. Posteroanterior *(A)* and lateral *(B)* roentgenograms reveal marked overinflation of both lungs, with a low flat position of the diaphragm and a marked increase in the depth of the retrosternal airspace. The lungs are diffusely oligemic, the peripheral vessels being narrow and attentuated. A discrepancy in the size of the central and peripheral pulmonary vessels is caused not only by a decrease in caliber peripherally but also by an increase in size centrally; this increase in central caliber constitutes convincing evidence of pulmonary arterial hypertension.

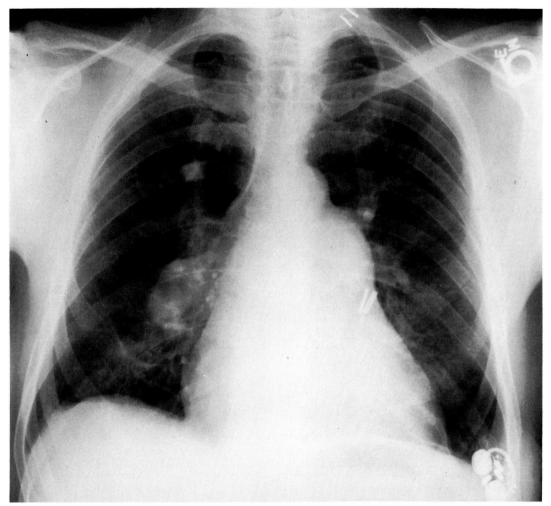

Figure 10–11. Severe Pulmonary Arterial Hypertension in Primary Alveolar Hypoventilation. A postero-anterior roentgenogram of a 55-year-old white man reveals marked dilatation of the main pulmonary artery and its hilar branches, with rapid diminution in caliber of pulmonary arteries as they proceed distally. The heart is moderately enlarged in a configuration compatible with cor pulmonale. The lungs are not overinflated and show no evidence of primary disease. (Courtesy of Dr. Richard Greenspan, Yale University, New Haven.)

caused by hypoxemia, decreased lung volumes, and structural abnormalities in the vessels. Roentgenologic changes almost invariably are dominated by the underlying pulmonary disease, and in many cases the peripheral vascular markings are obscured.[44]

Pulmonary hypertension occasionally develops in patients after pneumonectomy,[45] in patients with severe chest wall restriction or distortion such as kyphoscoliosis, in patients with acquired immunodeficiency syndrome (AIDS),[45a] and in individuals with alveolar hypoventilation from any cause (Fig. 10–11). Mediastinal or hilar lesions may sometimes compress the major pulmonary arteries and also lead to pulmonary hypertension. The causes include aortic aneurysm, dissection of the aorta[46] or pulmonary artery,[47] and fibrosing mediastinitis.[48]

Postcapillary Pulmonary Hypertension

Postcapillary pulmonary hypertension results from any condition that increases pulmonary venous pressure above a critical level. Undoubtedly, the most common of these are diseases of the left side of the heart that cause left ventricular failure, such as systemic hypertension, coronary artery disease, and mitral stenosis. Less common causes include atrial myxoma and congenital cardiac anomalies, such as cor triatriatum. Pulmonary venous obstruction from a variety of causes, including total anomalous venous drainage and primary veno-occlusive disease, results in similar functional effects.

Pathologic Characteristics

Both arteries and veins show medial hypertrophy and intimal fibrosis. In the veins, more definite internal and external elastic laminae may develop (Fig. 10–12).[49] In the lung parenchyma, patchy accumulation of hemosiderin-laden macrophages and interstitial fibrosis are common ("brown induration"), and there may be evidence of recent interstitial or airspace hemorrhage. Occasionally, small foci of connective tissue may become ossified.

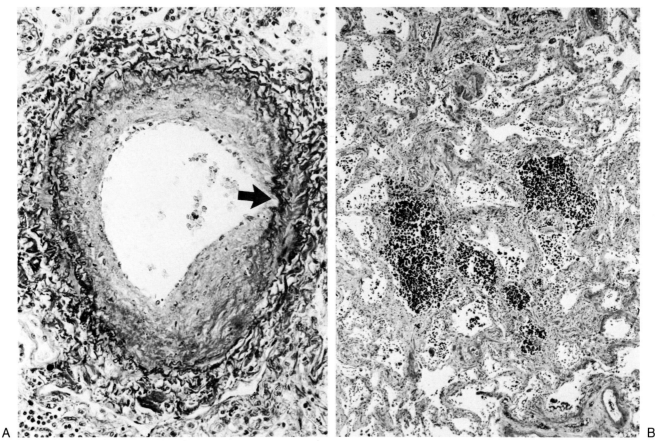

Figure 10–12. Postcapillary Hypertension in Mitral Stenosis. A histologic section of a medium-sized pulmonary vein (A) shows intimal fibrosis and focal medial hypertrophy (arrow) associated with two fairly distinct elastic laminae resembling those seen in pulmonary arteries. A section of lung parenchyma (B) shows several intra-alveolar aggregates of hemosiderin-laden macrophages and a moderate degree of interstitial fibrosis. (A, Verhoeff–van Gieson, × 200; B × 40.)

Roentgenographic Manifestations

When pulmonary vascular resistance is increased in part of the lungs and unaffected elsewhere, blood flow is redistributed from zones of high resistance to those of normal resistance. When areas of lung thus affected are sufficiently large, the discrepancy in size between normal and abnormal lung markings is readily apparent roentgenographically. This effect is observed in several primary pulmonary abnormalities, such as local obstructive emphysema (Fig. 10–13), as well as in some diseases of the cardiovascular system. The authors are concerned with the latter group here.

In erect humans, pulmonary venous pressure is higher in the lower than in the upper lobes because of a difference in hydrostatic pressure (averaging approximately 12 to 15 mm Hg in adult subjects). Therefore, peripheral vascular resistance typically rises first in the lower zones. Since resistance in the upper lobes is unchanged initially, blood is diverted to these regions, resulting in a roentgenographic picture of upper lobe pleonemia and lower lobe oligemia (Fig. 10–14). This is in striking contrast with the normal situation, in which pulmonary perfusion increases from apex to base. With continued increase in venous pressure, the reduction in venous caliber progresses upward from the lung bases and eventually involves the upper lobes, producing a pattern of diffuse alteration in the pulmonary vasculature. The inevitable result is generalized elevation of pulmonary arterial vascular resistance and pulmonary arterial hypertension.[50]

This disparity between the calibers of upper and lower lobe vessels represents one of the most useful roentgenographic signs of pulmonary venous hypertension. Although it is common to hear the term "upper lobe venous engorgement" used to describe this sign, in fact the redistribution of blood flow is *arterial* rather than venous and thus is a *flow* phenomenon caused by increased resistance to blood flow through the lower lung zones. Thus, *both* arteries and veins show distention, and it is conceptually preferable to employ the phrase "upper zone vascular distention" to indicate redistribution of blood flow. In fact, since distention of upper zone vessels occurs in five situations other than pulmonary venous hypertension (a supine position, predominantly lower zonal parenchymal disease, left-to-right shunts, hypervolemia, and pulmonary arterial hypertension), it is advisable *as a first approximation* to refer to the abnormality as "recruitment of upper zone vessels" (Fig. 10–15).

It is customary for roentgenologists to assess the caliber of upper zone vessels by comparing them with lower zone vessels. While it is clear that a disparity must exist in order for redistribution of flow to be present, the authors feel that it is often exceedingly difficult to be convinced of an

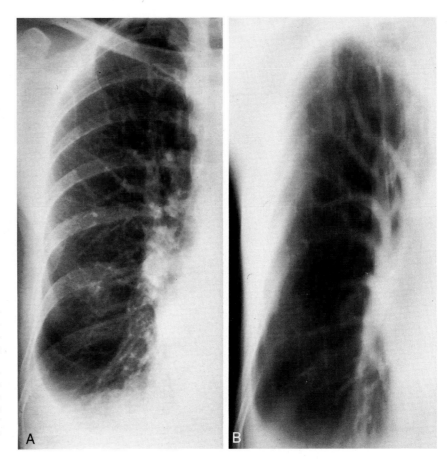

Figure 10–13. Redistribution of Blood Flow Caused by Predominantly Lower Lobe Emphysema. A view of the right lung from a conventional posteroanterior chest roentgenogram *(A)* reveals dilatation of upper lobe vessels, reduced caliber of lower-lobe vessels, and lower-zonal hyperinflation and oligemia. These findings are more clearly demonstrated on an anteroposterior linear tomogram *(B)*. The pleural thickening at the base is caused by fibrosis, which may have contributed to the reduced perfusion.

increase in upper zonal vessel caliber by such a comparison. It has been their experience that subjective assessment of the caliber of vessels in the upper zones, based on experience of what constitutes the normal, is more dependable.

It is important to recognize the fact that signs of left ventricular failure may be apparent roentgenographically without clinical evidence of decompensation. For example, of 94 patients who had chest roentgenograms obtained on admission to a coronary care unit, 31 (33 per cent) were found to have roentgenographic evidence of pulmonary venous hypertension (manifested most commonly by distention of upper zone vessels) without associated clinical signs.[51] In 23 of these, however, clinically evident failure developed subsequently. In a study of 30 patients with recent myocardial infarction,[52] the severity of roentgenographic abnormality generally correlated well with levels of pulmonary capillary wedge pressure. It was found that redistribution of blood flow was the earliest manifestation of elevated wedge pressure, followed, sequentially, by loss of the normal sharp margins of the pulmonary vessels, the development of perihilar haze, and, finally, overt airspace edema.

In addition to the typical alteration in vascular pattern observed in pulmonary venous hypertension, particularly in mitral stenosis, other pulmonary changes occur that are worthy of note. Signs of interstitial pulmonary edema frequently are visible, including septal edema (Kerley A and B lines; *see* Fig. 4–39, page 203) and perivascular edema (manifested by loss of definition of pulmonary vascular markings). Hemosiderosis, although often visible pathologically, is not readily identifiable roentgenographically unless

severe, probably because of the low density of the deposits. It is manifested by tiny punctate shadows situated mainly in the middle and lower lung zones (Fig. 10–16). Associated pulmonary fibrosis may be apparent as a rather coarse, poorly defined reticulation.

Bone formation occurs occasionally in mitral stenosis and is virtually pathognomonic of this entity.[53] Roentgenographically, it is manifested by densely calcified nodules 1 to 5 mm in diameter, mainly in the midlung zones and sometimes containing demonstrable trabeculae (Fig. 10–17). They are more numerous in the right lung[54] and range in incidence in reported series from 3 to 13 per cent.[55] Although pulmonary venous hypertension is invariably present, there is no apparent relationship between the development of the nodules and the degree of hypertension or associated hemosiderosis.[55]

Clinical Manifestations

In left ventricular failure and mitral stenosis, the symptoms and signs are predominantly those arising from acute or subacute pulmonary edema and are readily differentiated from those of precapillary hypertension. Patients typically are dyspneic and orthopneic and may be subject to paroxysmal nocturnal dyspnea. In mitral stenosis, in addition to the pink, frothy expectoration typical of acute pulmonary edema, bright-red blood also may be expectorated. Pulmonary venous hypertension caused by myxoma or thrombus that blocks the mitral valve usually is punctuated by episodes of pulmonary edema or syncope that can be

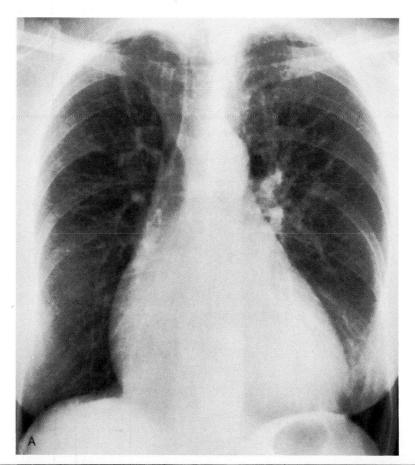

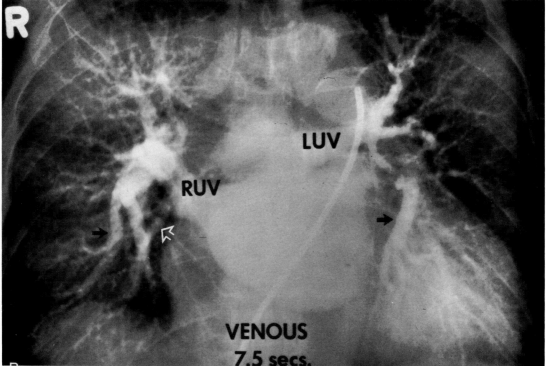

Figure 10–14. Redistribution of Blood Flow to Upper Lung Zones Caused by Pulmonary Venous Hypertension. A posteroanterior roentgenogram *(A)* reveals unusually prominent vascular markings in the upper zones and rather sparse markings in the lower zones. The patient, a 42-year-old woman, had recurrent episodes of left ventricular decompensation consequent on cardiomyopathy. During the venous phase of a pulmonary arteriogram of a different patient *(B),* the right (RUV) and left (LUV) superior veins are well opacified, whereas there is only slight filling and a narrower caliber of lower lobe veins *(open arrow).* Note the persistent opacification of the lower lobe arteries *(arrows).* The findings indicate combined precapillary and postcapillary pulmonary hypertension.

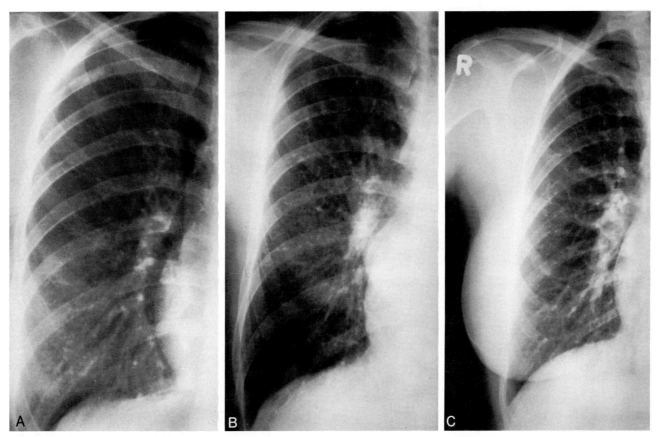

Figure 10–15. Recruitment of Upper Lobe Vessels in Postcapillary Hypertension and Left-to-Right Shunt: Roentgenographic Distinction. A view of the right lung from a conventional posteroanterior chest roentgenogram (A) is normal. Note that in the erect position, the upper-lobe arteries and veins are much smaller than those in the lower lobe, a reflection of the influence of gravity on blood flow. The vasculature is well defined throughout. Contrast this appearance with that in two patients with increased blood flow to the upper lobes, in B caused by mitral stenosis and in C by an atrial septal defect (ASD). B, Upper-lobe vessels are dilated; lower-lobe vessels are narrowed and ill defined as a result of interstitial edema. These features are typical of postcapillary hypertension. C, Upper-lobe and lower-lobe vessels are larger than normal and are sharply defined, findings indicative of a left-to-right shunt (ASD in this instance). Note that the cause of the upper-zone vessel recruitment in B and C cannot be distinguished by the appearance of the upper-lobe vessels alone.

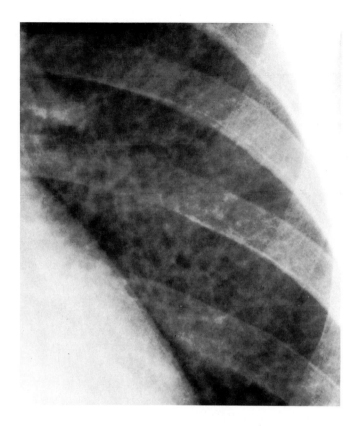

Figure 10–16. Pulmonary Hemosiderosis and Fibrosis Secondary to Recurrent Episodes of Pulmonary Edema. A magnified view of the midportion of the left lung reveals a medium reticular pattern that did not change on sequential examinations.

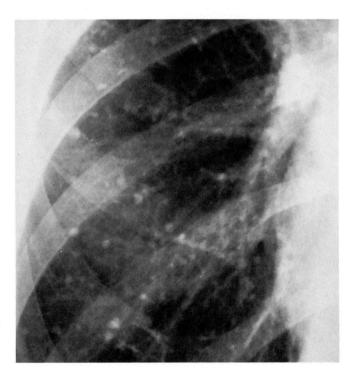

Figure 10–17. Ossific Nodules in Mitral Stenosis. A view of the right lung from a conventional posteroanterior chest roentgenogram demonstrates multiple, sharply defined 1- to 3-mm calcific (ossific) nodules.

relieved by a change in position. In some instances, left atrial myxomas give rise to systemic embolization or are associated with constitutional findings, such as fever, weight loss, raised sedimentation rate, anemia, and elevation of gamma globulin levels.[56] Patients with postcapillary pulmonary hypertension caused by increased resistance between the pulmonary capillaries and the left atrium have symptoms identical to those of mitral stenosis but without the characteristic accentuation of the first heart sound, the opening snap, or the rumbling diastolic murmur.

The electrocardiographic findings in postcapillary hypertension may be identical to those of primary pulmonary hypertension, reflecting the increase in right ventricular afterload, and in addition may show changes related to the cause of the increase in venous pressure, such as P mitrale in mitral stenosis and left ventricular hypertrophy in mitral insufficiency. Pulmonary function studies in patients who have long-standing venous hypertension show progressive lung restriction and a decrease in diffusing capacity.[57]

Pulmonary Veno-occlusive Disease

Pulmonary veno-occlusive disease is a disorder of unknown etiology characterized by progressive narrowing of small pulmonary veins and venules due to intimal cellular proliferation and fibrosis. The disease shows no sex predilection and has been reported from infancy to old age.[58] It can occur in family clusters[59] and in association with chronic active hepatitis, celiac disease,[59] Raynaud's phenomenon,[60] and the use of oral contraceptives.

Pathologically, there is narrowing or obliteration of the lumina of small pulmonary veins and venules by intimal

fibrous tissue (Fig. 10–18), usually widespread throughout both lungs. Larger pulmonary veins are usually spared. It is probable that the venous occlusions are thrombotic in origin, although the cause of the thrombosis is unknown. Histologic evidence of severe pulmonary arterial hypertension is usually present in the form of medial hypertrophy of small pulmonary arteries, with or without intimal fibrosis and thrombi. The plexiform lesions characteristic of primary pulmonary hypertension are absent.

Roentgenographically, signs of pulmonary arterial hypertension are no different from those associated with primary or thromboembolic disease, but with the important additions of normal left atrial size and signs of postcapillary hypertension, chiefly pulmonary edema (Fig. 10–19).

Clinically, affected patients typically have slowly progressive dyspnea and orthopnea punctuated by attacks of acute pulmonary edema; hemoptysis may occur. Rales may be heard over the lung bases, and the second pulmonic sound is accentuated in most cases. As the condition progresses, a right ventricular heave develops, together with murmurs indicative of pulmonic and tricuspid insufficiency. Pulmonary function tests reveal arterial oxygen desaturation and a reduction in diffusing capacity and lung compliance.[61] The pulmonary arterial wedge pressure is usually normal or low.[62] The only other condition that causes a similar constellation of findings is left atrial myxoma. Most patients die within 2 years of the onset of symptoms.[63]

Cor Pulmonale

The term "cor pulmonale" should be restricted to those instances in which an abnormality of lung structure or func-

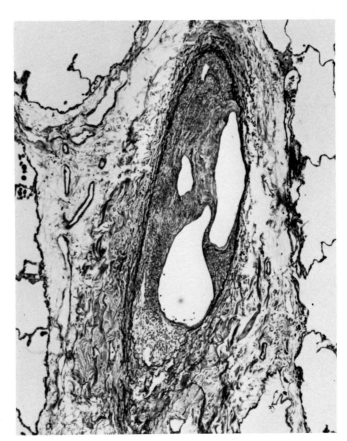

Figure 10–18. Veno-occlusive Disease. A histologic section of a medium-size pulmonary vein shows intraluminal fibrosis and multiple vascular spaces, suggesting canalized thrombus. (× 40.)

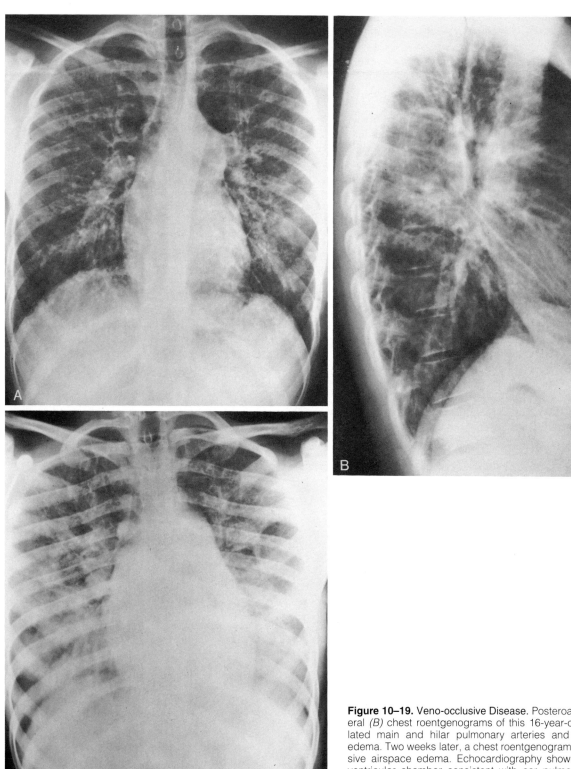

Figure 10–19. Veno-occlusive Disease. Posteroanterior *(A)* and lateral *(B)* chest roentgenograms of this 16-year-old male reveal dilated main and hilar pulmonary arteries and diffuse interstitial edema. Two weeks later, a chest roentgenogram *(C)* revealed massive airspace edema. Echocardiography showed a dilated right ventricular chamber consistent with cor pulmonale but no other structural abnormality; specifically, the mitral valve and left atrium were normal in appearance. This combination of findings is highly suggestive of veno-occlusive disease. (Courtesy of the Birmingham Children's Hospital.)

tion results in right ventricular hypertrophy. Approximately 80 per cent of cases result from COPD.[64] Although the presence of pulmonary hypertension does not necessarily imply cor pulmonale, it does indicate that there is a strain on the right ventricle that, if prolonged, will inevitably lead to the abnormality.

Roentgenologically, cardiac enlargement is not always apparent, even when right ventricular hypertrophy is evident at postmortem examination.[65] This is particularly likely to occur in the presence of pulmonary emphysema, when only serial roentgenography may reveal evidence of increased heart size.

Clinically, right ventricular thrust, usually felt along the left sternal border, also may be obscured by pulmonary overinflation in emphysema. A systolic thrust, sometimes a diastolic shock, and a systolic thrill may be felt over the pulmonary area. A loud P_2 sound with a pulmonary systolic ejection click and, in some cases, harsh systolic and diastolic murmurs may be heard over the same area. As right-sided heart failure develops, a systolic murmur that is louder during inspiration becomes audible along the left sternal border. It may be associated with a palpable pulse in the (enlarged) liver, a systolic venous pulse in the neck, and, in many cases, peripheral edema and ascites.

The electrocardiogram (ECG) may be normal, even in cases of known severe right ventricular hypertrophy.[66] The Expert Committee Report for the World Health Organization suggested the following criteria for ECG diagnosis, indicating that at least two should be present: R/S less than 1 in V_5 and V_6; predominant S wave in lead I or incomplete right bundle branch block; P waves taller than 2 mm in lead II; right axis deviation greater than 110 degrees; and inversion of T waves in V_1 to V_4 or V_2 and V_3.[67] This last finding is of less diagnostic value.[65]

Pulmonary Artery Aneurysms

Aneurysms of the pulmonary artery are uncommon, and the etiology and pathogenetic mechanisms diverse (Table 10–2).[68] The most frequent causes are probably congenital cardiovascular disease, infection, and trauma. Aneurysms may be solitary or multiple and range in size from microscopic foci to lesions 5 cm in diameter. Most occur in the pulmonary trunk or its major branches (Fig. 10–20), but presentation in a peripheral artery as a solitary nodule can

occur. Signs and symptoms are usually absent; in some cases, cough, dyspnea, and hemoptysis may be present. Physical examination may reveal a thrill or murmur over the aneurysm. Complications are uncommon, although rupture into an airway can result in massive hemorrhage. Dissecting aneurysms may present with precordial pain; as in aortic aneurysms, proximal extension with intrapericardial hemorrhage and tamponade is a frequent cause of death.[69]

Hughes-Stovin syndrome is a rare disorder characterized by aneurysms of the large and small pulmonary arteries and thrombosis of peripheral veins and dural sinuses.[70] It is possible that there are several pathogenetic mechanisms, including congenital cardiovascular defects and vasculitis (Behçet's disease). Recurrent episodes of fever, lack of response to antibiotics, hemoptysis, and respiratory symptoms resulting from recurrent pulmonary artery occlusions are prominent clinical features. A common terminal event is massive hemoptysis.

PULMONARY EDEMA

A variety of anatomic and physiologic mechanisms keep the alveoli dry or, perhaps more correctly, ideally moist. Although the absolute amount of fluid within the pulmonary interstitium and alveolar airspaces is more or less constant, there is considerable transport of water between different tissue compartments within the lung. Normally, an ultrafiltrate of plasma moves from the pulmonary microvessels through the endothelium into the interstitial tissue. The fluid is removed from this space by the pulmonary lymphatics, evaporative water loss from the alveolar surface, resorption into the pulmonary and bronchial microvasculature, and transport into the pleural space. The volume of water and protein movement are dependent on the balance of pressures across the pulmonary microvasculature (determined by the relationship between the microvascular and perimicrovascular hydrostatic pressure and the plasma and perimicrovascular osmotic pressure) and the permeability of the microvascular membrane. A disturbance of sufficient magnitude in one or both of these factors will result in an increase in the transudation or exudation of fluid from the microvessels into the interstitial tissue. Sufficient accumulation of fluid in this compartment constitutes interstitial edema; when the storage capacity of the interstitial space is

Table 10–2. ETIOLOGY AND PATHOGENESIS OF PULMONARY ARTERY ANEURYSMS

Etiology	Pathogenesis	Selected References
Congenital	Deficiency of vessel wall	240
	Postvalvular or arterial stenosis	241
Degenerative-metabolic	Marfan's syndrome	242
	"Cystic medial necrosis" (dissecting aneurysm)	4
Traumatic		243
Infectious (mycotic)	Syphilis	244
	Tuberculosis	245
	Pyogenic bacterial	246
	Others (e.g., fungi)	247
Immunologic	Behçet's disease (?Hughes-Stovin syndrome)	248
	Polyarteritis nodosa (bronchial arteries)	
Secondary to pulmonary disease	Hypertension (including dissecting aneurysms)	249
	Bronchiectasis	
Idiopathic	Hughes-Stovin syndrome	248

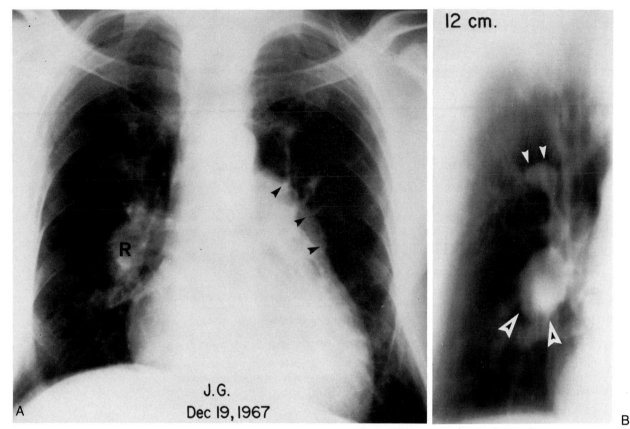

Figure 10–20. Aneurysms of the Pulmonary Arteries Secondary to Chronic Thromboembolism. A posteroanterior *(A)* chest roentgenogram shows features of severe chronic cor pulmonale—cardiomegaly with a configuration compatible with right atrial and ventricular dilatation, and marked enlargement of the main pulmonary artery *(arrowheads)* and the right (R) interlobar artery. Detail view of the right lung from a conventional full lung tomogram *(B)* reveals an aneurysm in the truncus anterior *(small arrowheads)* and marked dilatation and abrupt termination of the interlobar artery *(large arrowheads)*. At autopsy, these vessels were focally dilated (saccular aneurysms) proximal to totally occluded partially recanalized emboli.

exceeded, airspace edema develops. Excellent reviews of the topic are available.[71–73]

Anatomic Considerations

Pulmonary Circulation and Microvascular Endothelium

The alveolar septa have a thin and a thick side (*see* page 9), the former for gas exchange and the latter for structural support and fluid exchange.[74] On the thin side, the membrane is between 0.3 and 0.5 μm thick and consists of the epithelial and endothelial cell cytoplasm with a shared basement membrane and no interstitial space. On the thick side, the basement membranes of the endothelium and epithelium are separated by an interstitial compartment consisting of collagen and elastic fibers, interstitial cells, and connective tissue matrix. When excess water and protein accumulate in the alveolar septa, as in interstitial pulmonary edema, they do so exclusively or predominantly on the thick side (Fig. 10–21).[75] Although most of the fluid transport within the lungs takes place across the capillaries, there is good evidence that the larger precapillary arterioles and postcapillary venules also take part.[76]

The exact pathway for fluid and solute transport across the pulmonary microvasculature is still uncertain. Presum-ably, lipid-soluble substances can traverse the capillary endothelium by passing directly through cell membranes. By contrast, in order to cross the endothelium, water-soluble substances must be transported by pinocytosis or must pass through the "paracellular pathway" (intercellular "pores"). Selective sieving of protein molecules according to their molecular size suggests that the latter mechanism is the more important. Small molecules traverse the pulmonary capillary endothelium with ease, whereas larger molecules are excluded in direct proportion to their molecular size; very large molecules do not reach the pulmonary interstitium at all.

The anatomic counterpart of the physiologic "pores" is uncertain but may be discontinuities in the tight junctions that join the endothelial cells.[77] The junctional complexes of the capillary endothelium are much less developed than those of the alveolar epithelium, and studies have shown that there is a correlation between the number of junctional strands and the permeability of a cellular membrane.[78] It has been theorized that a rise in pulmonary microvascular pressure can increase the size of the intercellular space between endothelial cells, thus increasing protein permeability (the stretched-pore theory). This theory remains controversial; however, it is probable that within a range of

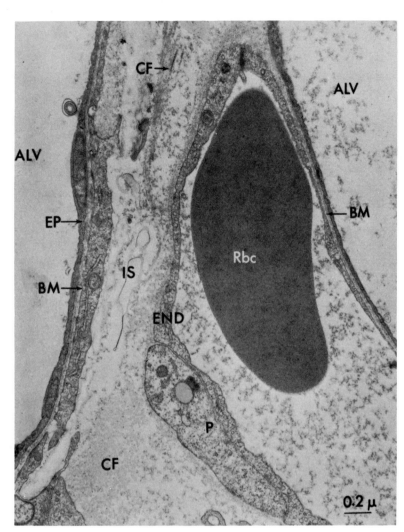

Figure 10–21. Interstitial Pulmonary Edema. The interstitial space (IS) of the thick portion of the alveolar septum has been considerably widened by fluid during hemodynamic pulmonary edema, whereas the opposite thin part, containing the fused basement membranes (BM), remains unchanged in thickness. ALV = alveolar space; EP = alveolar epithelium; BM = basement membrane; IS = interstitial space; CF = collagen fibers; END = capillary endothelium; Rbc = red blood cell. (× 12,000.) (Reprinted from Fishman A: Pulmonary edema: The water-exchanging function of the lung. Circulation 46: 389, 1972. With permission of the author and editor.)

moderately elevated microvascular pressures, lung endothelial permeability is not directly affected by pressure.[79] It should be appreciated that the "pores" through which fluid movement occurs in the pulmonary microvasculature represent a minute fraction of the total capillary surface area.[80] As a result, a doubling or tripling of the surface area occupied by pores might not be detected by conventional microscopic techniques, whereas it would markedly enhance fluid and solute transport.

Pulmonary Interstitium

As indicated, excess fluid accumulates first in the pulmonary interstitium. This can be divided into two functionally distinct compartments—an alveolar wall (parenchymal) compartment and a peribronchovascular and interlobular septal (axial) compartment. Although the former compartment constitutes a large percentage of the total interstitial space, it is very noncompliant, so fluid tends to accumulate to a much lesser extent in alveolar walls than in the peribronchovascular and interlobular septal connective tissue (*see* Fig. 4–38, page 202).[81]

The interstitial connective tissue is a gel that contains fibers and cells. The gel itself is composed of a matrix of highly polymerized mucopolysaccharides that, in combination with proteins, form proteoglycans (glycosaminoglycans). In the lung, the principal mucopolysaccharides are chondroitin sulfate and hyaluronic acid. The proteoglycan complexes are extremely hydrophilic and can bind large amounts of water. Thus, the interstitial tissue normally contains 40 per cent of the extravascular water; during the development of pulmonary edema, this volume can more than double before alveolar flooding occurs. This fluid storage capacity of the interstitial space increases with lung volume.[82] In fact, when positive end-expiratory pressure (PEEP) is used to increase lung volume, fluid can shift from alveolar airspace to the interstitial space, where it has a less detrimental effect on gas exchange.[83]

Alveolocapillary Membrane

Although the surface area of the epithelial side of the alveolocapillary membrane is approximately equal to that of the capillary endothelial surface, it is much less permeable. This is reflected in physiologic tracer studies, which show that the epithelium is restrictive to all but small molecules such as urea, sucrose, and sodium.[84] The "pore" size for the epithelium has been calculated to average 3 to 4 nm,[84] while "pores" as large as 100 nm are postulated to account for the permeability of pulmonary capillary endothelium.[85]

Lymphatic Drainage

Pulmonary lymphatic drainage is one of the important mechanisms by which interstitial fluid is removed from the lung. As discussed previously (*see* page 63), the lymphatics begin as blind-ended vessels in the region of the alveolar ducts and respiratory bronchioles and course in the interstitial connective tissue of the bronchovascular bundles and interlobular septa. Fluid that enters the lymphatics is pumped toward the hila by the passive action of respiratory motion and by active contraction of the lymphatic vessels, which in large lymphatics can generate pressures as high as 60 cm H_2O.

Physiologic Considerations

Starling Equation

The factors that govern the formation and removal of extravascular water within the lungs are described by the fluid transport equation originally proposed by Starling (Fig. 10–22).[86]

$$\dot{Q}f = Kf\,[(Pmv - Ppmv) - \sigma(\pi mv - \pi pmv)]$$

where $\dot{Q}f$ = the net transvascular fluid flow; Kf = the filtration coefficient, a measure of fluid conductance of the microvascular endothelium; Pmv = the hydrostatic pressure in the lumen of the fluid-exchanging microvessels; Ppmv = the hydrostatic pressure in the interstitial tissue surrounding the fluid-exchanging microvessels; σ = the osmotic reflection coefficient (i.e., a number between 0 and 1 that describes the effectiveness of the membrane in preventing the flow of protein compared with the flow of

water); πmv = the protein osmotic pressure in the microvascular lumen; and πpmv = the protein osmotic pressure in the interstitial fluid surrounding the microvessels.

The movement of protein across the endothelium occurs by diffusion and is related to the concentration difference between capillary lumen and interstitial space and to the size of the protein molecules relative to that of the endothelial "pores." Since the endothelial permeability is different for protein molecules of different sizes, their net flux will be inversely related to molecular weight, and the steady-state interstitial concentrations of proteins relative to their plasma concentration will also vary with molecular size. When pulmonary microvascular permeability and pressures are normal, the ratios of interstitial to plasma protein concentrations for albumin, globulin, and fibrinogen are approximately 0.8, 0.5, and 0.2, respectively.[87]

Under normal steady-state conditions, there is a continual net outward flow of fluid and protein from the pulmonary microvasculature to the interstitium; these substances are then returned to the bloodstream by the lymphatics. When this balance is disrupted, edema results. Although an increase in capillary hydrostatic pressure (Pmv) or an increase in endothelial permeability (Kf) are the most common causes of edema, it is of some value to discuss each of the factors in the Starling equation individually because all are important determinants of transvascular fluid flux.

Microvascular Hydrostatic Pressure (Pmv). The hydrostatic pressure in the fluid-exchanging vessels of the lung must be somewhere between the mean pulmonary arterial pressure (about 20 cm H_2O) and the mean left atrial pressure (about 5 cm H_2O). The actual value is dependent on the relative resistances of the vessels upstream and

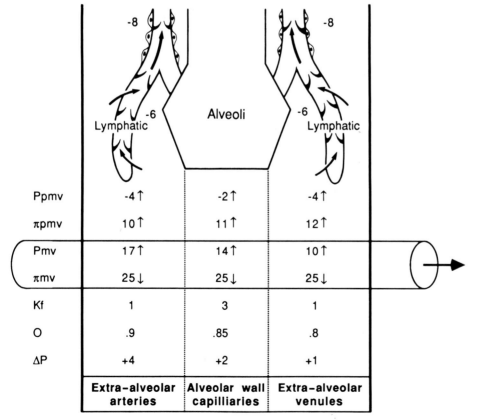

	Extra-alveolar arteries	Alveolar wall capilliaries	Extra-alveolar venules
	−8		−8
	−6 Lymphatic	Alveoli	−6 Lymphatic
Ppmv	−4 ↑	−2 ↑	−4 ↑
πpmv	10 ↑	11 ↑	12 ↑
Pmv	17 ↑	14 ↑	10 ↑
πmv	25 ↓	25 ↓	25 ↓
Kf	1	3	1
O	.9	.85	.8
ΔP	+4	+2	+1

Figure 10–22. A Three-Compartment Model of Starling Forces. The values for microvascular and perimicrovascular hydrostatic and osmotic pressures represent rough estimates and have been chosen to illustrate the longitudinal variation of the net driving pressure (Δ P) within the exchanging vessels. The arbitrary values for Kf illustrate the relative importance of the different compartments to overall lung fluid exchange, and the values for the reflection coefficient (σ) reflect the morphometric complexity of endothelial intercellular junctions on the arterial and venous side of the microcirculation. A value of 1.0 for σ would represent a membrane that was freely permeable to water but completely impermeable to protein. The driving pressure is greatest in the precapillary vessels and least in the postcapillary venules. There is a gradient in interstitial pressure that drives fluid from the pericapillary interstitial space toward the hilum. (Modified from Staub NC: Pathophysiology of pulmonary edema. *In* Staub NC, Taylor AE [eds]: Edema. New York, Raven Press, 1984, p 719.)

downstream from the fluid-exchanging vessels. If arterial resistance is high relative to venous resistance, microvascular pressure will be close to venous pressure. Conversely, if venous resistance is high relative to arterial resistance, pulmonary microvascular pressure will approach arterial pressure.

Normally, arterial resistance is slightly higher than venous resistance, resulting in an average capillary pressure of approximately 10 cm H_2O.[88] The microvascular pressure differs between the arterial and the venous ends of the fluid-exchanging vessels as a result of capillary resistance, and there may be fluid filtration at the arterial end of the capillaries and reabsorption at the venous end.[87]

Although it is usual to talk of a single microvascular pressure within the pulmonary vasculature, pulmonary arterial and venous pressures decrease or increase by 1 cm H_2O pressure for each centimeter that the vessel in question is above or below the left atrium. Since there is as much lung above as below this level, the integrated microvascular pressure over the height of the lung is not much different from that which would be calculated from the average Ppa and Pla at the level of the left atrium.[87]

Perimicrovascular Interstitial Hydrostatic Pressure (Ppmv). Just as there is no unique value for microvascular pressure, there is also no single value that describes the interstitial pressure of the lung. The pressure in the interstitial space in close proximity to the alveolar walls is about −3 cm H_2O.[89] Direct measurements of pressure in the perihilar connective tissue show values of −5 cm H_2O, decreasing to about −12 cm H_2O when the lung is inflated to TLC.[90] It is apparent that there is a gradient in pressure that drives fluid from the pericapillary to the perihilar (axial) interstitial space (see Fig. 10–22).[87] There is also a vertical gradient in interstitial pressure from the top to the bottom of the lung, the interstitial pressure being more negative at the apex of the lung.

Plasma Protein Osmotic Pressure (πmv). The pressure exerted by plasma proteins is dependent on both their concentration and the permeability of the endothelial membrane to protein. The πmv represents the maximal osmotic pressure that would be produced by that concentration of plasma protein acting across a membrane that was completely impermeable to protein.

Interstitial Protein Osmotic Pressure (πpmv). Like the osmotic pressure of the plasma, the interstitial osmotic pressure is related to the protein concentration. It is generally assumed that the protein concentration of the lung lymph represents the average protein concentration within the lung interstitium. Interstitial protein concentration decreases as fluid filtration increases, and this represents one of the safety factors that protects against the development of pulmonary edema.

Filtration Coefficient (Kf). The filtration coefficient (the units for which are mL per minute per cm H_2O per unit lung weight) is a measure of endothelial permeability to water. The more permeable the endothelium, the larger is the value for Kf (i.e., the greater the fluid flux for a given driving pressure). It is impossible to measure Kf in vivo, and even in excised lung preparations the reported values simply represent the best estimates. However, it is clear that in many forms of pulmonary edema, an increase in Kf—rather than an imbalance in hydrostatic and osmotic pressure—is responsible for edema formation.

Osmotic Reflection Coefficient (σ). The reflection coefficient is a numerical estimate of the permeability of the membrane to a solute and therefore is also an estimate of the effectiveness with which a given concentration of solute can exert osmotic pressure. A reflection coefficient of 1 means that the membrane is completely impermeable to the solute and that the osmotic pressure exerted by that solute will be equal to that measured in an osmometer. When the reflection coefficient is 0, the membrane is completely permeable to the solute, and the solute exerts no osmotic pressure.[72] Reflection coefficients for albumin, globulin, and fibrinogen are 0.85, 0.9, and 0.98.[87] In the presence of noncardiogenic pulmonary edema, the capillary endothelial permeability for water (Kf) and protein (σ) are altered; when the endothelium is severely damaged, the reflection coefficient approaches 0. In this case, plasma proteins exert no effective pressure across the endothelium, and the most powerful force preventing the formation of edema is lost.

Fluid Transport Across the Alveolar Epithelium

The principles that govern fluid and solute transport across the epithelium are the same as those that operate across the endothelium, but the fluid conductivity is at least one order of magnitude lower. The epithelium can even restrict the movement of electrolytes so that they can exert an osmotic pressure, and their concentration can be altered by active transport of electrolytes across the epithelial cells.[91] The surface tension present at the interface between alveolar liquid and air exerts a pressure that tends to suck fluid from the interstitium into the airspaces. Because surfactant lowers surface tension, this pressure is small (about 15 cm H_2O). When surfactant is deficient or inactivated, however, the increase in surface tension can play an important role in the formation of alveolar edema.[92]

Safety Factors

Normally, the alveolar airspaces remain ideally moist despite substantial changes in microvascular and interstitial pressure related to posture, gravity, variations in the state of hydration, and changes in lung volume. This homeostasis is provided by a number of safety factors that tend to minimize accumulation of fluid in the lung.[87]

Lung lymph flow is one such factor. In the presence of an acute increase in microvascular pressure or permeability, lymph flow from the lung can increase 10-fold or more before there is significant accumulation of interstial fluid.[88] The precise rate of lung lymph flow during pulmonary edema is unknown in humans, but maximal flows of 200 mL per hour are predicted from animal studies.[93] In conditions associated with repeated episodes of pulmonary edema, such as chronic left ventricular failure, lymphatic vessels proliferate and increase in caliber,[94] and their flow capacity can increase three to four times.[95]

A second safety factor that operates in hydrostatic, but not in permeability, edema is dilution of the interstitial protein. This mechanism is dependent on the relative impermeability of the microvascular endothelium to protein. As transvascular fluid movement increases as a result of elevated microvascular hydrostatic pressure, water transport outstrips protein transport. The resulting dilution of interstitial protein decreases the interstitial osmotic pressure.[96]

A third factor that tends to minimize the accumulation of edema within the lungs is the increase in tissue pressure that accompanies the swelling of the interstitium. As fluid accumulates in the interstitial space, the tightly compacted gel resists deformation, and pressure increases. Morphologic studies suggest that the pressure-volume characteristics of the peribronchovascular interstitium are such that this space may be more compliant than that of the alveolar walls because it is in this loose connective tissue that fluid first accumulates.[81] When the fluid storage capacity of the interstitium is exceeded, the high interstitial pressure disrupts the alveolar epithelium, and alveolar flooding occurs.[97] The increase in interstitial pressure associated with fluid accumulation may be an explanation for the redistribution of pulmonary blood flow evident on erect chest roentgenograms in patients with pulmonary venous hypertension; presumably, the interstitial edema accumulates predominantly in lower lung zones.

Development and Classification of Pulmonary Edema

The sequence of events that occur during the development of pulmonary edema is similar for both hydrostatic and permeability edema (*see* Fig. 4–38, page 202).[81] The earliest manifestation observed through the light micro-

scope is the appearance of fluid in the loose connective tissue around extra-alveolar vessels and conducting airways. Excess fluid widens the peribronchovascular interstitial space and interlobular septa and distends the lymphatics (Fig. 10–23). The appearance of fluid within this tissue occurs before there is evidence of alveolar flooding and when measurements of alveolar wall thickness are virtually normal.

As the amount of fluid increases, there is a progressive increase in alveolar wall thickness as fluid accumulates in the thick side of the alveolocapillary membrane. There also may be accumulation of small amounts of fluid within the airspaces confined to the alveolar "corners." When the fluid storage capacity of the interstitium is exceeded, alveolar flooding tends to occur in an all-or-nothing manner, individual alveoli being either liquid filled or air filled.[81] In both hydrostatic and permeability edema, the protein content of the fluid in the flooded alveolar airspaces is the same as that in the interstitium,[98, 99] suggesting that during alveolar flooding the epithelium loses all ability to sieve and thus permits the outpouring of pure interstitial fluid.

It is convenient to classify the multiple causes of pulmonary edema into two major categories on the basis of the underlying pathogenetic abnormality: an increase in pulmonary microvascular pressure or an increase in microvascular permeability (cardiogenic and noncardiogenic pulmonary edema) (Table 10–3). Left ventricular decom-

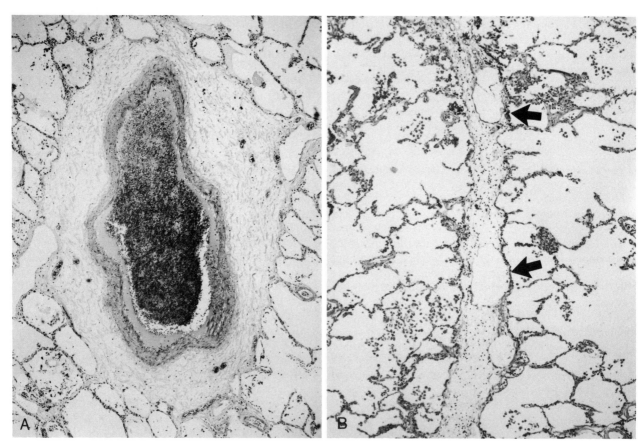

Figure 10–23. Interstitial Pulmonary Edema. *A,* A histologic section reveals widening of the perivascular interstitial tissue as a result of the presence of abundant fluid separating the connective tissue fibers. A section of an interlobular septum *(B)* shows similar widening as well as dilated lymphatic channels *(arrows).* (A × 40; B × 60.)

Table 10–3. **CLASSIFICATION OF PULMONARY EDEMA**

Elevated Microvascular Pressure
Cardiogenic
    Left ventricular failure
    Mitral valvular disease
    Left atrial myxoma or thrombus
    Cor triatriatum
Pulmonary Venous Disease
    Primary veno-occlusive disease
    Chronic sclerosing mediastinitis
    Anomalous pulmonary venous drainage
    Congenital venous stenosis or atresia
    Some forms of congenital heart disease
Neurogenic
    Head trauma
    Increased intracranial pressure
    Postictal
Normal Microvascular Pressure (Increased Capillary Permeability)
    Inhalation of noxious fumes and soluble aerosols (*see* Chapter 14)
    Aspiration of noxious fluids (*see* Chapter 13)
    High altitude
    Transient tachypnea of the newborn
    Rapid re-expansion of lung in thoracentesis
    Pancreatitis
    Severe upper airway obstruction
    Pheochromocytoma
    Diabetic ketoacidosis
    Traumatic fat embolism
    Post-traumatic (contused lung)
    Acute radiation reaction
    Circulating toxins (alloxan, snake venom)
    Circulating vasoactive substances (histamine, kinins, prostaglandins, serotonin)
    Decreased capillary oncotic pressure
    Lymphatic insufficiency
Combined Elevation of Microvascular Pressure and Increased Capillary Permeability

---

pensation is the most important cause of cardiogenic edema; others include mitral stenosis and atrial myxoma. Although many specific insults can cause noncardiogenic pulmonary edema, the resulting constellation of clinical, roentgenographic, and pathologic manifestations are remarkably similar and are called the adult respiratory distress syndrome (ARDS).[100] A combination of permeability and cardiogenic edema is common and is particularly devastating, because many of the safety factors that normally impede the accumulation of excess extravascular water are lost when the endothelium loses its selectivity for solutes.

PULMONARY EDEMA ASSOCIATED WITH ELEVATED MICROVASCULAR PRESSURE

Cardiogenic Pulmonary Edema

The most common cause of interstitial and airspace pulmonary edema is a rise in pulmonary venous pressure secondary to disease of the left side of the heart. Increased pressure within the left atrium is transmitted to the pulmonary veins as a result of back-pressure, most often from a failing left ventricle or obstruction to the left atrial outflow.

Roentgenographic Manifestations

There are two major roentgenographic patterns, related to whether edema fluid remains relatively localized in the interstitial space or whether it occupies the airspaces of the lung also.

Interstitial Edema. As discussed previously, transudation of fluid into the interstitial space of the lung inevitably constitutes the first stage of pulmonary edema. When pulmonary venous hypertension is moderate in degree or transient, fluid transudation occurs into the alveolar interstitial space, from which it flows centripetally and accumulates within the peribronchovascular and interlobular septal connective tissue. This anatomic localization produces the typical roentgenographic findings of loss of the normal sharp definition of pulmonary vascular markings and thickening of the interlobular septa (A and B lines of Kerley; Fig. 10–24). Although the presence of septal lines can be of value in confirming the diagnosis when other signs are equivocal, in the authors' experience the frequency with which they can be identified is low compared with loss of definition of vessel markings. Thus, the absence of septal lines should not be construed as evidence against the diagnosis. Similarly, the authors have not been impressed with the value of loss of definition of hilar pulmonary vessels (parahilar haze) as a sign of interstitial edema. Although it is frequently cited as a reliable sign, in the authors' opinion it should be considered a sign of airspace edema rather than interstitial edema.

Disappearance of septal lines generally parallels that of other signs of the edema, and their persistence after adequate therapy (e.g., mitral commissurotomy for mitral stenosis) usually indicates that chronic congestion and edema of the septa have led to irreversible fibrosis. Occasionally, the development of interstitial edema in patients with emphysema will make visible the walls of air sacs that cannot be seen in its absence.

In circumstances in which edema fluid accumulates in the *parenchymal* interstitial tissues (the alveolar wall phase of Staub and associates[81]) before the development of overt airspace edema, the accumulation usually is invisible or only faintly discernible roentgenographically as a "haze" that tends to be predominantly in the lower lung zones.

If evidence for interstitial pulmonary edema is equivocal as judged from the signs described, confirmatory evidence may be provided in some cases by appreciating an increased thickness of the wall of bronchi commonly seen end-on in the parahilar zones (bronchial wall "cuffing"). These bronchial walls are normally hairline in thickness, but when fluid accumulates in the loose interstitial tissue surrounding them, their shadow thickens and loses its sharp definition (Fig. 10–25).[101] In the individual patient, however, it is often difficult to exclude chronic bronchitis as the cause of the thickening, particularly in the absence of a clinical history, and the authors now regard the sign as being of questionable value.

Another sign of interstitial edema—but one that usually becomes evident only when the accumulation of excess water is severe—is thickening of the interlobar fissures (Fig. 10–26).[102] The pleural connective tissue layer is in continuity with the interlobular septa, and when sufficient fluid accumulates in the latter sites (creating Kerley B lines) it also collects in the pleural interstitium. This sign should not be misconstrued as evidence of pleural effusion within the fissures.

It has been shown that a very good correlation exists between pulmonary arterial wedge pressure and evidence

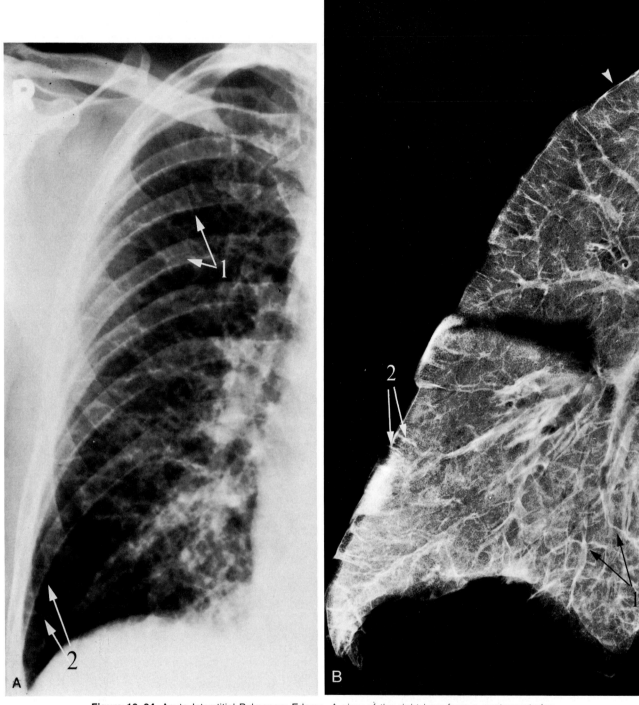

Figure 10–24. Acute Interstitial Pulmonary Edema. A view of the right lung from a posteroanterior chest roentgenogram *(A)* reveals the classic features of interstitial edema—septal A (1) and B (2) lines, and thickened and ill-defined bronchovascular bundles. A roentgenogram of a coronal slice through the right lung following an autopsy of a different patient *(B)* reveals similar features—septal A lines (1) and B lines (2) and thickened peribronchovascular interstitium. Note the thickened pleura *(arrowhead)*, indicating the presence of pleural edema. (From Genereux GP: Pattern recognition in diffuse lung disease: A review of theory and practice. Med Radiogr Photogr 61: 2, 1985.)

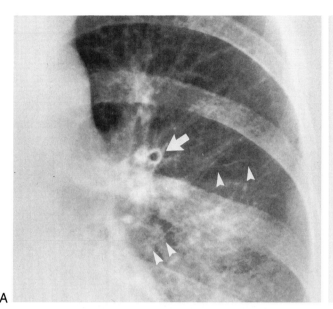
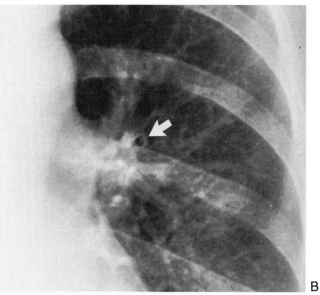

A   B

Figure 10–25. Peribronchial Cuffing in Pulmonary Edema. A detail view of the upper half of the left lung from a posteroanterior chest roentgenogram *(A)* reveals distended upper-lobe vessels, perihilar haze, septal A lines *(arrowheads)*, and a thickened bronchial wall viewed end-on *(arrow)*. A few days later, following diuretic therapy *(B)*, signs of pulmonary edema had resolved. Note the decreased thickness of the bronchial wall *(arrow)*.

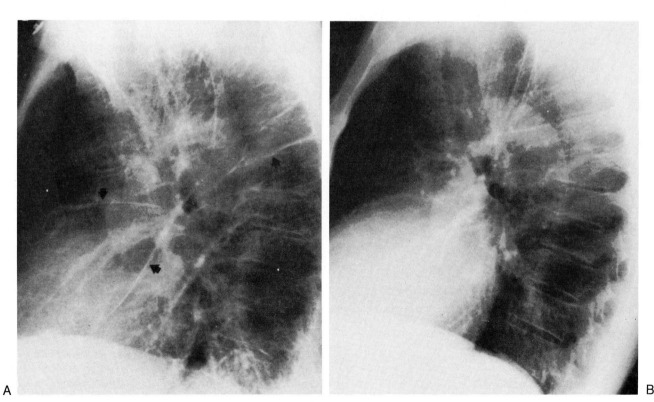

A   B

Figure 10–26. Pleural Edema. In lateral projection *(A)*, the interlobar fissures are very prominent *(arrows)* as a result of pleural edema. Twenty-four hours later *(B)*, the edema had cleared completely.

of pulmonary venous hypertension as assessed from bedside chest roentgenograms. In general, a normal chest roentgenogram is an exceptional feature of the early stages of recent myocardial infarction, since evidence for pulmonary venous hypertension presents itself immediately after mean left ventricular filling pressure rises above 10 mm Hg.[103] However, considerable phase lags have also been observed[52]; that is, pulmonary wedge pressure can rise before roentgenographic signs become apparent, and pulmonary edema can persist following successful therapy and lowering of wedge pressure to normal. Despite these phase lags, the chest roentgenogram remains a reasonably accurate subjective method of diagnosing pulmonary edema. With adequate treatment, the roentgenologic signs may disappear within a matter of hours (*see* Fig. 10–27).

Airspace Edema. The hallmark in the roentgenologic diagnosis of airspace edema is the acinar shadow (Fig. 10–27). In the majority of cases, these shadows are confluent, creating irregular, rather poorly defined, patchy opacities of unit density scattered randomly throughout the lungs. In the medial third of the lungs particularly, coalescence of acinar consolidation is common. Although the distribution varies from patient to patient, it may be surprisingly similar during different espisodes in one patient. In acute pulmonary edema resulting from left ventricular failure, patchy airspace consolidation sometimes extends to the subpleural zone or "cortex" of the lung, although the cortex may be completely spared, thus creating the "bat's-wing" or "butterfly" pattern of edema (*see* later). The effects of gravity on the distribution of edema fluid within the lungs tend to be similar to those of blood flow and ventilation. Although there are opposing forces in action, from a practical point of view, they result in maximal fluid accumulation in the lower and central lung zones.

Edema caused by cardiac disease usually is bilateral and fairly symmetric, although it may be predominantly unilateral or in other respects "inappropriate"; that is, occupying zones of one or both lungs out of keeping with the "expected" distribution of disease arising from a central influence (Fig. 10–28).[104] Unilateral pulmonary edema can oc-

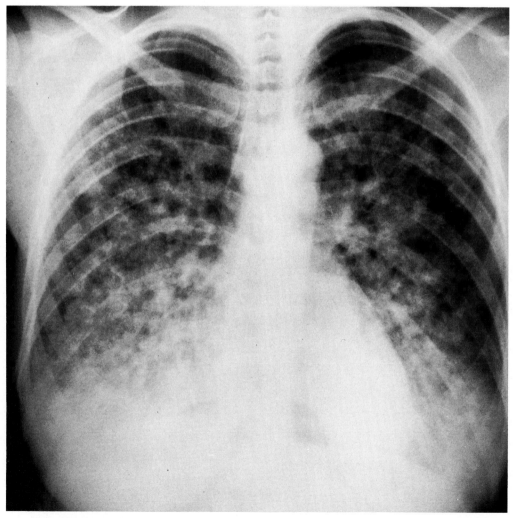

Figure 10–27. Acute Airspace Pulmonary Edema. A posteroanterior roentgenogram reveals widespread patchy airspace consolidation. Individual acinar shadows can be visualized in some areas, although generally these are coalescent, particularly in the lower lung zones. Cardiac size and configuration are normal. This 28-year-old woman had severe, periodic systemic arterial hypertension caused by a pheochromocytoma of the adrenal gland. The possibility that this represented permeability edema (ARDS) rather than cardiogenic edema was not excluded.

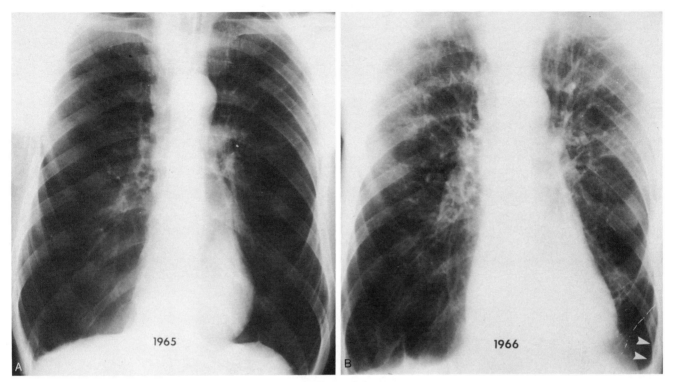

Figure 10–28. Atypical Pattern of Pulmonary Edema Associated with Predominantly Lower-Lobe Emphysema. A posteroanterior chest roentgenogram *(A)* shows pulmonary overinflation and striking lower-lobe oligemia indicative of advanced emphysema. Approximately 1 year later *(B)*, the heart had increased in size, and upper-lobe vessels had become larger and poorly defined as a result of the accumulation of interstitial edema; note that lower-lobe vessels remain inconspicuous. A small pleural effusion is present on the left *(arrowheads)*.

cur in a wide variety of conditions in which the pathogenetic mechanism exists either on the same side as the edema (ipsilateral edema) or on the opposite side (contralateral edema).[105] In patients with cardiac decompensation, unilateral edema is probably related primarily to dependency.[106]

Like interstitial pulmonary edema, airspace pulmonary edema usually clears fairly rapidly in response to adequate treatment of the underlying condition, and resolution appears complete roentgenographically in no more than 3 days in most cases. Since the presence of edema causes a reduction in the compliance of the lungs, resolution can result in a roentgenographically apparent increase in lung volume (Fig. 10–29).

The "bat's-wing" or "butterfly" pattern describes an anatomic distribution of airspace edema in which the hilum and "medulla" of the lungs are fairly uniformly consolidated and the peripheral 2 to 3 cm of lung parenchyma—the "cortex"—is relatively uninvolved (Fig. 10–30). Definition of the margin of consolidated parenchyma often is rather indistinct but may be remarkably sharp. Resolution of the edema generally begins in the periphery and spreads medially.[107] An incidence of 5 per cent in 110 cases of moderate to severe edema of varying etiology has been recorded.[108] Many theories have been propounded to explain the mechanism of this unusual anatomic distribution of edema[109–111]; however, none is completely convincing.

Although it has been said that the "bat's-wing" pattern of edema is seen commonly in association with uremia, we

and others[112] consider that there is convincing evidence that the pattern is the result of acute left ventricular failure and that it bears no specific relationship to uremia. Localization of the edema to the hilar and medullary portions of the lungs may be apparent in both posteroanterior and lateral roentgenographic projections[113] and can be identified in interstitial as well as airspace pulmonary edema, particularly on CT (Fig. 10–31). The freedom from involvement of the "cortex" usually extends along the interlobar lung fissures as well as around the convexity of the thorax, thereby creating a waistlike indentation visible in posteroanterior projection in the region of the minor fissure. Similarly, the upper and lower paramediastinal zones may be relatively free from involvement.

Clinical Manifestations

The clinical manifestations of cardiogenic pulmonary edema depend on whether the onset is acute or insidious. The acute form is dramatic: severe dyspnea develops over a short period (minutes to hours), and the patient characteristically sits bolt upright using the accessory muscles of respiration. Peripheral and central cyanosis, tachycardia, pallor, cool sweaty skin, anxiety, and an elevated blood pressure often are present. These latter findings are related to marked sympathetic stimulation. In severe cases, the patient may expectorate frothy, blood-tinged fluid; in some cases, there is frank hemoptysis. Physical examination may reveal an elevated jugular venous pressure. However, the

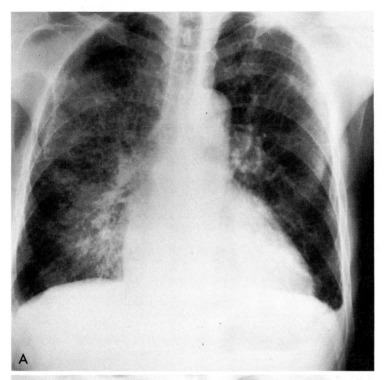

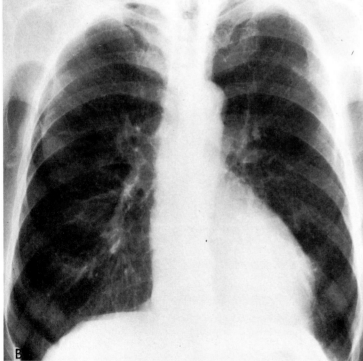

Figure 10–29. Effect on Compliance of Diffuse Interstitial Edema. A posteroanterior roentgenogram *(A)* of a 70-year-old man admitted with acute myocardial infarction reveals diffuse interstitial and patchy airspace pulmonary edema. A roentgenogram following resolution of the edema *(B)* shows a marked increase in volume of both lungs characteristic of diffuse emphysema. The diffuse edema observed in *A* had reduced pulmonary compliance to the degree where lung volume was within normal limits, obscuring the presence of emphysema.

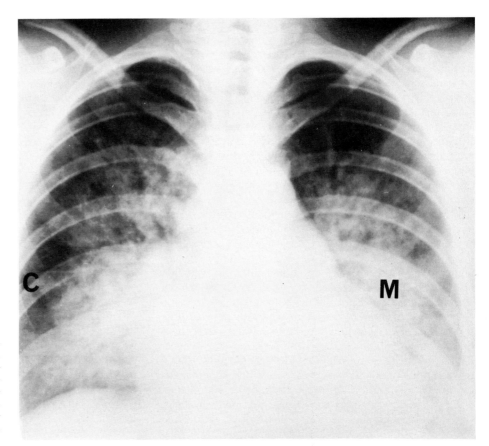

Figure 10–30. Acute Airspace Pulmonary Edema: The "Bat's-Wing" Pattern. A posteroanterior chest roentgenogram reveals a classic bat's-wing pattern of airspace consolidation consisting of a dense central core (medulla, M) surrounded by a radiolucent peripheral zone of normal lung (cortex, C).

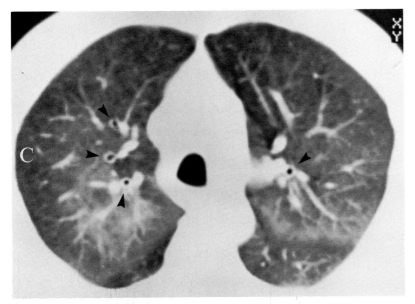

Figure 10–31. Pulmonary Edema: CT Manifestations. A CT scan through the superior aspect of the hila shows a fairly symmetric increase in CT density in the medulla of each lung; note that the cortex (C) is relatively spared. Segmental bronchi are thickened (arrowheads) as a result of interstitial edema. This CT pattern is typical of postcapillary hypertension and pulmonary edema.

jugular veins may be difficult to evaluate owing to the patient's use of the cervical accessory muscles of respiration and to the considerable swings in pleural pressure. Other signs of congestive failure, such as hepatosplenomegaly and peripheral edema, may be present. Auscultation of the thorax reveals widespread crackles and expiratory wheezes. In the terminal stage, there is a decrease in level of consciousness and circulatory collapse.

The only potentially confusing possibilities in the differential diagnosis are acute bronchoconstriction and upper airway obstruction. In patients who have acute bronchoconstriction, evidence for sympathetic hyper-reactivity is almost always lacking; examination of the chest reveals high-pitched wheezing without crackles. In acute upper airway obstruction, the chest is usually silent except for stridorous sounds confined to the central airway.

In patients in whom pulmonary edema develops less precipitously, there may be few physical findings. In fact, it is well to remember that the chest roentgenogram usually is more accurate in diagnosis than physical examination, particularly when the edema is predominantly interstitial. A history of orthopnea and paroxysmal nocturnal dyspnea is a helpful diagnostic feature, although nocturnal dyspnea and cough are also common in patients with asthma or COPD. When the edema is confined to the interstitial space, there may be no auscultatory findings, although expiratory wheezing is present in some patients. The quieter chest allows more careful auscultation of the heart, which may reveal a gallop rhythm or a murmur caused by valvular dysfunction. Another clue in diagnosis is a change in clinical findings. Cardiogenic pulmonary edema is not a static condition, and there is usually improvement or worsening during a relatively short time course.

The clinical manifestations of "butterfly" edema may be almost as unimpressive as the roentgenographic appearance is dramatic. Even when there is roentgenographic evidence of massive consolidation of the medial two thirds of the lungs, the clinical presentation may be unremarkable, and those patients who complain of increased dyspnea and orthopnea may have minimal or nonexistent physical signs— much the same as in diffuse interstitial edema.

Physiologic Manifestations

Although pulmonary vascular congestion by itself can cause a slight stiffening of the lung,[114] the development of airspace edema results in more pronounced decreases in compliance and lung volumes (TLC and VC) as a result of replacement of alveolar air and a disruption of the normal surfactant-lined air-liquid interface.[115] Airway resistance is increased in both acute and chronic pulmonary edema[116] and is probably attributable to accumulation of fluid in the peribronchial interstitial space.[116] An increase in closing volume may be an early sign of interstitial edema.[117]

As edema develops, there is a tendency for perfusion to increase to the upper lung, resulting in a more uniform pattern of blood flow.[118] It is unclear whether this change is related to perivascular interstitial edema increasing pulmonary vascular resistance at the lung base[119] or is secondary to the development of alveolar edema.[120] Despite this apparent uniformity of perfusion, patchy inhomogeneity in ventilation and perfusion causes ventilation and perfusion

mismatching and arterial hypoxemia. The $\dot{V}/\dot{Q}$ mismatch and hypoxemia are relatively mild when edema is confined to the interstitium, but the development of true intrapulmonary shunting associated with airspace edema causes more profound hypoxemia. The PCO_2 is usually normal or low,[121] although in about 10 per cent of cases of severe pulmonary edema, hypercapnea and respiratory acidosis occur.[122] Most patients who have moderate to severe pulmonary edema develop metabolic lactic acidosis as a result of hypoperfusion of peripheral tissues.[123]

Pulmonary Edema Associated with Renal Disease, Hypervolemia, or Hypoproteinemia

Both acute and chronic renal disease—with or without uremia—can be associated with acute pulmonary edema. Acute glomerulonephritis in children is frequently associated with pulmonary edema and, in fact, can be implicated in approximately 75 per cent of all possible causes of pulmonary edema in this age group.[124] A variable combination of decreased serum oncotic pressure, hypervolemia, increased capillary permeability, and left ventricular failure secondary to hypertension is responsible.[125]

The administration of a large volume of intravenous fluid has been shown to cause pulmonary edema in patients without underlying heart disease,[126] particularly during the postoperative period and in the elderly. In many of these patients, the volume loading may serve to unmask the presence of borderline left ventricular function; however, there also may be a contribution from decreased serum colloid osmotic pressure.[127]

The pulmonary edema that occasionally develops in association with blood transfusion also may be the result of overloading of the circulation. However, in some cases the pathogenesis is related to blood type incompatibility, leuko-agglutinins causing neutrophil accumulation in the lung, which results in an increase in pulmonary microvascular permeability.[128] Affected patients have an abrupt onset of chills, fever, tachycardia, nonproductive cough, and dyspnea; sometimes, they manifest blood eosinophilia.[129]

Pulmonary edema also occurs with increased frequency in patients with hepatic disease,[72] particularly acute failure.[130] Again, it is likely that a combination of increased capillary pressure, increased endothelial permeability, and decreased plasma osmotic pressure is responsible.

Neurogenic and Postictal Pulmonary Edema

Acute pulmonary edema in association with raised intracranial pressure, head trauma, and seizures is a well-known but infrequent phenomenon. Its mechanism is poorly understood.[131] Experimental studies have provided evidence for a transient, massive sympathetic discharge from the central nervous system, which results in generalized vasoconstriction, a shift of blood into the pulmonary vascular compartment, and consequent elevation of pulmonary microvascular pressure.[132] Clinical investigations have also suggested that there may be an alteration in microvascular permeability, since normal microvascular pressures have been found in association with protein-rich edema fluid in some patients.[133] It is possible that a combination of the two mechanisms is involved: an acute increase in intracranial pressure may cause sufficient sympathetic discharge to increase microvascular pressure, in turn producing baro-trauma to the endothelium and consequent increased permeability.

Of the various causes of neurogenic edema, head trauma is probably the most frequent; although it is often severe, it may be relatively mild and nonfatal.[134] Postictal pulmonary edema may develop immediately after a seizure or may be delayed for several hours. It occurs most often in young patients with idiopathic epilepsy and in those in whom seizures relate to expanding intracranial lesions.[135] Characteristically, the edema disappears within several days following surgical relief of increased intracranial pressure.

PULMONARY EDEMA ASSOCIATED WITH NORMAL MICROVASCULAR PRESSURE

Following trauma, shock, sepsis, aspiration, or a variety of other direct or indirect pulmonary insults, a number of patients develop progressive respiratory distress characterized by (1) tachypnea, dyspnea, cough, and the physical findings of airspace consolidation; (2) diffuse airspace disease on chest roentgenography; (3) severe arterial desaturation that is resistant to even high concentrations of inhaled oxygen; and (4) pulmonary function evidence of increased pulmonary vascular pressures and resistance and decreased lung compliance. This constellation of findings has come to be known as ARDS (shock lung). Although some authorities have opposed the use of the term "ARDS" on the grounds that it serves to decrease the attention devoted to the search for specific clinical and pathophysiologic features in the various causes of the syndrome,[136, 137] because of its familiarity and brevity, the designation is employed throughout this text.

Pathogenesis

Although an increase in microvascular permeability and the development of interstitial and airspace edema are perhaps the major consequences of ARDS, in most cases the injury goes far beyond a simple increase in capillary "pore" size and involves severe damage to endothelial and epithelial cells. The pathogenesis involves a complex series of inflammatory events, including participation of preformed plasma-derived inflammatory mediators and newly generated arachidonic acid mediators from both the cyclooxygenase and the lipoxygenase pathways. Activation of the complement and blood clotting systems can also be involved, in addition to recruitment of numerous inflammatory cell types. Despite the variety of precipitating events of ARDS, the pathologic characteristics are similar in all cases, suggesting that either there is one common activating factor or the lung is capable of reacting to injury in only a limited manner.[138]

Role of Shock. In experimental studies, prolonged hypotension can result in both pulmonary endothelial damage[139] and increased microvascular permeability.[80] In addition, episodes of hypotension, either brief or prolonged, are frequent in patients who subsequently develop ARDS and may be caused by either hypovolemia or a decrease in systemic vascular smooth muscle tone. Despite these obser-

vations, it is difficult to cause ARDS by shock alone,[140] and it is probable that other factors are involved in producing the complete syndrome.

Role of Polymorphonuclear Leukocytes. A large pool of marginated neutrophils normally reside in the pulmonary capillaries (see page 52).[141] Both these cells and circulating neutrophils can be activated by a variety of mechanisms, resulting in penetration of the cells through junctions between endothelial cells as well as the generation and release of oxygen free radicals, lysosomal enzymes, and arachidonate metabolites.[142] These products of activated neutrophils have the capacity to damage the capillary endothelium and the alveolar epithelium. Evidence in support of a role for leukocytes in the development of ARDS includes the following:

1. Animal models of acute lung injury that are dependent on the presence of neutrophils.[143]
2. The presence of numerous neutrophils in some biopsy and postmortem lung specimens from patients with established ARDS.[144]
3. The presence of increased numbers of neutrophils and of neutrophil-derived products such as neutrophil elastase in bronchoalveolar lavage (BAL) fluid of similarly affected patients.[145]
4. The recognition that many of the risk factors for ARDS are associated with complement activation and leukopenia secondary to sequestration of leukocytes within the lungs.[146]
5. The demonstration that severe, acute leukopenia frequently predates the onset of clinical ARDS.[147]
6. Animal models in which chemotactic agents such as C5a have been shown to attract leukocytes to the pulmonary microvasculature with resulting pulmonary microvascular injury.

Although these experimental and clinical studies provide strong support for the important contribution that neutrophils make to the pulmonary damage in ARDS, there is also convincing evidence that the syndrome can occur in the absence of circulating or tissue neutrophils.[148]

Role of Surfactant. Abnormalities of surfactant function have been demonstrated in alveolar fluid obtained from patients who have ARDS,[149] and animal studies of acute lung injury have been shown to be associated with decreased phospholipid synthesis by alveolar type II cells.[150] However, it is probable that these abnormalities are the result rather than the cause of ARDS. This is not to say that the disruption of the surfactant layer is not an important mechanism contributing to the development of alveolar edema in ARDS. In fact, disruption of surfactant by itself can increase lung water, presumably by increasing the surface tension at the alveolar fluid-air interface, resulting in the suction of water from the interstitial space.[92]

Role of Complement. A number of clinical and experimental observations suggest a role for complement in ARDS. It can both attract and activate neutrophils and may itself have a direct toxic effect on capillary endothelium and other lung cells.[151] Both trauma and infection, the most common causes of ARDS, can cause activation of the complement system. In addition, the blood and BAL fluid of patients who have ARDS have been shown to contain increased levels of activated complement components.[152] Despite these observations, some studies have shown that a large percentage of patients with sepsis and other risk factors for the development of ARDS manifest complement activation *in vivo* unaccompanied by the subsequent development of pulmonary dysfunction.[153]

Role of the Clotting System. There is considerable evidence to suggest that activation of the blood clotting system is associated with ARDS,[154, 155] particularly when it follows major trauma. For example, severely injured patients who develop the disease have lower platelet counts and levels of antithrombin III, fibrinogen, and plasminogen than those of similarly injured patients who do not develop ARDS.[156] Likewise, radiolabeled fibrinogen accumulates rapidly in the lungs of patients with established ARDS, but not in the lungs of patients who are equally ill but who do not have ARDS.[157] In addition, patients with established ARDS frequently have elevated blood levels of fibrin degradation products,[158] and in fact disseminated intravascular coagulation (DIC) occurs in as many as 25 per cent of patients.[159]

In experimental animals, activation of the clotting system is associated with increased microvascular permeability and the development of pulmonary edema.[160] Although these effects are dependent on the activation of the coagulation cascade, they also require complement and polymorphonuclear leukocytes.[161] A proposed sequence of events to account for these experimental observations is (1) the generation of fibrin from fibrinogen; (2) the activation by fibrin of the fibrinolytic system, causing the generation of plasmin; and (3) the formation by plasmin of the complement fragments C3a and C5a, which then activate neutrophils.[160]

Role of Oxygen Radicals. A variety of unstable oxygen free radicals are generated by neutrophils, by certain specific enzymes normally present within the body, and by a variety of toxic substances. These cytotoxic molecules include the superoxide radical (O_2^-), hydrogen peroxide (H_2O_2), and the hydroxyl radical (OH•). Under normal conditions, the body tissues are protected from their effects by a battery of antioxidant defense mechanisms that include specific enzymes such as (1) *superoxide dismutase,* which catalyzes the conversion of O_2^- to hydrogen peroxide (see figure below); (2) *catalase,* which catalyzes the conversion of hydrogen peroxide to oxygen and water; and (3) *glutathione peroxidase,* which converts peroxide radicals to nontoxic lipids.

Oxygen free radicals can damage the lung by denaturation of lipids associated with the plasma membrane, by inactivation of sulfhydryl-containing protein enzymes, and by depolymerization of polysaccharides. Their toxicity is enhanced by hyperoxic conditions and lessened by hypoxic conditions. Experimental studies suggest that damage caused by them may be the final common pathway in a variety of acute lung injuries, including pneumonitis caused by radiation, the herbicide paraquat, chemotherapeutic agents such as bleomycin and doxorubicin (Adriamycin),

and drugs such as alloxan and streptozotocin.[162] However, because oxygen free radicals are extremely short-lived, it is difficult to gather direct evidence that incriminates their formation in the pathogenesis of ARDS in humans. Indirect evidence for their role derives from studies that have shown an increased amount of oxidized substances such as alpha₁-proteinase inhibitor in the BAL fluid of affected patients.[163]

Role of Enzymes and Mediators. There is evidence that both the mediators of inflammation and a variety of enzymes have important roles in initiating or modifying lung injury in ARDS. The products of arachidonic acid metabolism, prostaglandins and leukotrienes, can either cause or protect against lung injury. Thromboxane causes platelet aggregation and pulmonary vascular constriction, whereas prostacyclin is a potent pulmonary arterial dilator and is capable of causing disaggregation of platelets. The leukotrienes can cause edema either directly by increasing vascular permeability or indirectly by inducing vascular smooth muscle contraction and chemotaxis of leukocytes to the site of mediator release.

Although plasma levels of prostaglandins are not increased in patients with ARDS,[164] increased levels of leukotrienes have been identified in the edema fluid of such patients but not in those with hydrostatic edema of similar severity.[165] There is also evidence for decreased pulmonary removal of certain prostaglandins, such as prostaglandin E₁, probably secondary to the diffuse endothelial injury that constitutes the basic feature of ARDS.[166]

Prekallikrein is the inactive precursor of plasma kallikrein, which is both a component of the coagulation and fibrinolytic systems and an activator of the kinin system. There is some evidence for prekallikrein activation in the blood and BAL fluid of patients with ARDS[167, 168]; in addition, in animal models of acute lung injury,[169] bradykinin generation has been demonstrated and has been accompanied by increased pulmonary vascular permeability. Greatly increased concentrations of elastase[170] and other neutrophil-derived enzymes[171] can be detected in the blood and BAL fluid of patients with ARDS. It is likely that these increased enzyme levels represent a marker of leukocyte activation, although it is possible that the enzymes themselves cause tissue injury. Increased levels of the enzyme phospholipase A₂ have been demonstrated in the blood of patients with gram-negative sepsis, the levels being particularly high in those who develop ARDS.[172] If the phospholipase gained access to the alveolar compartment, it could cause degradation of surfactant and thus contribute to the decreased lung compliance characteristic of ARDS.

Pathologic Characteristics

The pathologic changes in the lungs of patients with ARDS are virtually the same regardless of etiology and are frequently described by the term "diffuse alveolar damage." Although a continuum of histologic abnormalities exists, for

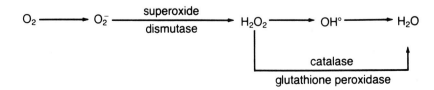

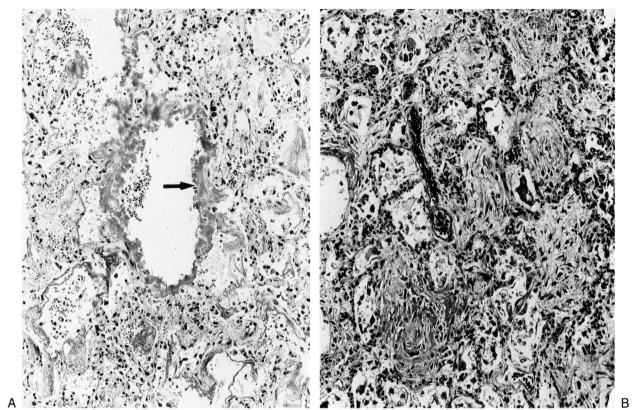

Figure 10–32. Diffuse Alveolar Damage. A histologic section of lung in the early exudative phase of diffuse alveolar damage *(A)* shows filling of alveolar airspaces by a proteinaceous exudate containing red blood cells. Inflammatory cells are few in number, and there is a mild to moderate degree of interstitial edema. A prominent hyaline membrane *(arrow)* is present. A section from another patient with more advanced disease (organizing phase) *(B)* shows almost complete consolidation by loose connective tissue. Alveolar walls are clearly recognizable and are only slightly thickened, indicating that the fibroblastic reaction is occurring within alveolar airspaces. (*A* and *B* × 120.)

purposes of discussion the changes can conveniently be described in three phases: exudative, proliferative, and fibrotic.[173]

The early exudative phase begins within hours of the onset of pulmonary damage and lasts for 2 to 3 days. It is characterized by diffuse interstitial edema, capillary congestion, and an airspace exudate composed of fluid, fibrin, and red blood cells (Fig. 10–32). In the later exudative phase (2 to 7 days), this exudate becomes more compact and eosinophilic in appearance and is transformed into hyaline membranes, particularly along the walls of alveolar ducts and distal respiratory bronchioles. Type II alveolar cell proliferation is usually a prominent feature.[174]

Changes of the proliferative phase can be identified between 1 to 4 weeks after the initial pulmonary insult and are characterized largely by proliferation of fibroblasts in the alveolar airspaces and interstitium (*see* Fig. 10–32)[175]; a mononuclear inflammatory cell infiltrate, composed predominantly of lymphocytes, may be apparent. In patients who die during this period, focal areas of bronchopneumonia caused by bacterial superinfection are common.

In some cases, the end result of the first two stages is the deposition of mature collagen, resulting in chronic interstitial fibrosis. In others, however—presumably those with relatively mild disease—much of the fibroblastic proliferation resolves without functionally significant residual fibrosis.

Roentgenographic Manifestations

Remarkably good correlation has been reported between the roentgenographic patterns observed during life and the pathologic changes observed at necropsy.[174, 176]

Up to Twelve Hours. All observers report a characteristic delay of up to 12 hours from the clinical onset of respiratory failure to the appearance of abnormalities on the chest roentgenogram. In some series,[177] evidence of interstitial pulmonary edema is remarkably infrequent; in others,[178] however, it is relatively common.

Twelve to Twenty-Four Hours. Patchy, ill-defined opacities appear throughout both lungs. The appearance is similar to that of airspace edema of cardiac origin, except that the heart size is usually normal and the edema tends to show a more peripheral distribution. Although upper zone vessels are often more prominent than normal, this sign is of no value as evidence of pulmonary venous hypertension, since the majority of patients are radiographed in the supine position.

Twenty-Four Hours to Four Days. The patchy zones of consolidation rapidly coalesce to a point of massive airspace consolidation of both lungs (Fig. 10–33). Characteristically, involvement is diffuse, affecting all lung zones from apex to base and to the extreme periphery of each lung. In the authors' experience, this widespread distribution can be of considerable value in distinguishing ARDS

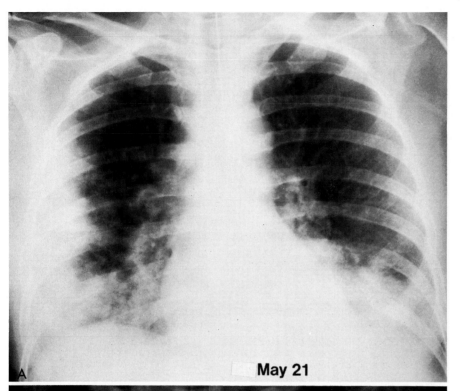

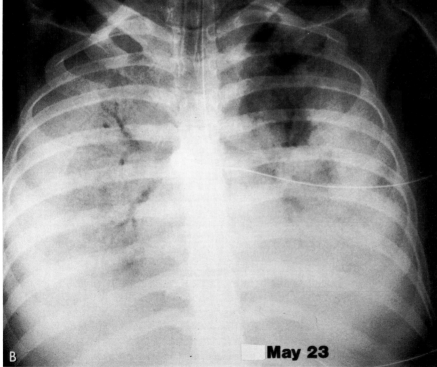

Figure 10–33. Acute Post-traumatic Respiratory Insufficiency ("Shock Lung," ARDS). This 18-year-old girl was admitted to the intensive care unit in severe shock following a motor vehicle accident. A roentgenogram the day after admission (A) revealed homogeneous consolidation of the left lower lobe and the axillary portion of the right lung. Two days later (B), both lungs were massively consolidated by pulmonary edema; note the prominent air bronchogram.

from cardiogenic pulmonary edema, whose distribution is seldom as extensive. Similarly, in contrast with cardiogenic edema, an air bronchogram is frequently visible. Pleural effusion is characteristically absent; its presence should strongly suggest a complicating acute pneumonia or pulmonary infarction.

Four to Seven Days. Characteristically, improvement in the roentgenographic picture occurs, the homogeneous consolidation becoming inhomogeneous, suggesting diminution of the amount of alveolar edema.

The institution of PEEP can result in dramatic variations in the appearance of parenchymal opacities in technically identical roentgenograms exposed over a 10- to 15-minute period.[179] In fact, patients who demonstrate roentgenographic evidence of diffuse pulmonary edema in the absence of mechanical ventilation can show an almost complete disappearance of roentgenographic abnormality within minutes of the institution of PEEP therapy. Continuous positive-pressure ventilation can also lead to diffuse interstitial emphysema that may be readily visible against the background of extensive parenchymal consolidation. It is important to recognize this development because of the frequency of complicating pneumomediastinum or pneumothorax.

More Than Seven Days. The lungs remain diffusely abnormal, but the pattern tends to become reticular[174] or "bubbly"[178] in appearance. It is likely that this pattern represents diffuse interstitial and airspace fibrosis characteristic of the proliferative and fibrotic phases of the disease (Fig. 10–34).

Differential Diagnosis

In roentgenologic differential diagnosis, the major conditions to be considered are severe cardiogenic pulmonary edema and widespread bacterial pneumonia. The latter may be impossible to differentiate from ARDS except on clinical grounds. However, the roentgenographic pattern frequently permits the distinction between cardiogenic and permeability edema with a high degree of accuracy. Milne and colleagues[180] carried out an independent two-observer study in which 216 chest roentgenograms obtained on 119 patients with pulmonary edema were reviewed with respect to the presence or absence of nine features; 61 of the patients had cardiac disease, 30 had renal failure or overhydration, and 28 had ARDS. Three principal—the first three in the list that follows—and six ancillary roentgenographic features were identified, the assessment of which

permitted the cause of the edema to be determined correctly in a high percentage of patients (Table 10–4).

Distribution of Pulmonary Blood Flow. Of the three patterns of blood flow distribution—normal, balanced, and inverted—50 per cent of patients with cardiogenic edema showed an inverted flow, and 40 per cent a balanced distribution; 80 per cent of patients with renal failure had a balanced distribution, and 20 per cent were normal; 40 per cent of those with increased capillary permeability had normal distribution, and 50 per cent a balanced distribution. Of note is the observation that in none of the patients with renal failure and in only 10 per cent of those with ARDS was pulmonary blood flow inverted.

Distribution of Pulmonary Edema. Although there were many variations in the distribution of edema, all could be grouped into three principal categories—even, central, and peripheral. Ninety per cent of patients with cardiogenic edema showed an even distribution pattern (more or less homogeneous from chest wall to heart), and in only 10 per cent was the pattern predominantly central. In these cases, the distribution of edema was clearly affected by gravity, being most marked at the lung bases. In the patients with renal failure, central edema predominated (70 per cent of cases), and in none was a peripheral pattern observed. In contrast with these two patterns, in 45 per cent of patients with ARDS a peripheral distribution was shown, and in 35 per cent it was widespread from chest wall to mediastinum. The pattern was often patchy with small intervening unaffected regions of lung parenchyma.

Width of the Vascular Pedicle. In the cardiac failure group, 60 per cent of patients showed an increased vascular pedicle width, and 40 per cent were in the normal range. In the renal-overhydration group, 85 per cent of patients showed a widened vascular pedicle, and only 15 per cent were normal. Of the patients with capillary permeability edema, 35 per cent had a normal pedicle, and 35 per cent a narrowed pedicle. Of note with respect to the ARDS group is the observation that 60 per cent of patients were radiographed in the supine position, which increased the vascular pedicle width by an average of 20 per cent.[181]

Pulmonary Blood Volume. This parameter was assessed by estimating the size of visible lung markings. A decrease in blood volume was seen in a small number of patients with ARDS on PEEP and in a few cardiac cases with very low cardiac output. In general, the pulmonary blood volume tended to be increased in patients with renal failure or overhydration (70 per cent) but in only 40 per cent of those with cardiogenic edema and 20 per cent of

Table 10–4. RADIOGRAPHIC FEATURES OF PULMONARY EDEMA

	Cardiac	Renal	Injury
Heart size	Enlarged	Enlarged	Not enlarged
Vascular pedicle	Normal or enlarged	Enlarged	Normal or reduced
Pulmonary blood flow distribution	Inverted	Balanced	Normal or balanced
Pulmonary blood volume	Normal or increased	Increased	Normal
Septal lines	Not common	Not common	Absent
Peribronchial cuffs	Very common	Very common	Not common
Air bronchogram	Not common	Not common	Very common
Lung edema, regional distribution (horizontal axis)	Even	Central	Peripheral
Pleural effusions	Very common	Very common	Not common

From Milne ENC, Pistolesi M, Miniati M, et al: The radiologic distinction of cardiogenic and noncardiogenic edema. Am J Roentgenol 144: 879, 1985.

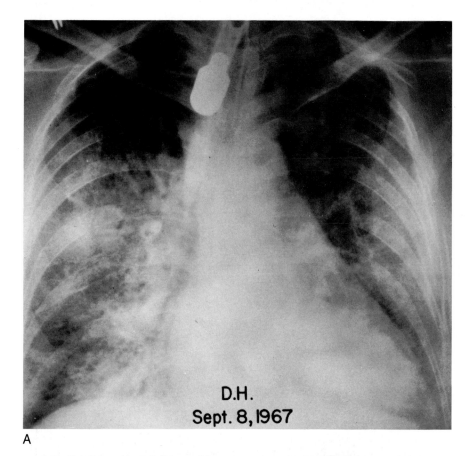

A

B

Figure 10–34. Adult Respiratory Distress Syndrome (ARDS) with a Prolonged Course and Partial Resolution. Four days after admission of a young woman with multiple bone fractures sustained in a motor vehicle accident, a roentgenogram *(A)* demonstrates severe airspace consolidation highly suggestive of ARDS. Approximately 2 months later, a predischarge roentgenogram *(B)* shows that most of the airspace component has resolved; however, there is persistent coarse reticulation that almost certainly represents residual parenchymal fibrosis. Follow-up films over the ensuing months demonstrated only modest further improvement.

those with permeability edema; it was normal in 80 per cent of patients with ARDS.

Septal Lines and Peribronchial Cuffing. Septal lines were observed in approximately 30 per cent of patients with either cardiac or renal-overhydration edema but in none of the patients with ARDS.

Air Bronchograms. This sign was identified frequently in patients with capillary permeability edema (70 per cent), but in only 20 per cent of the cardiac and renal-overhydration cases.

Pleural Effusion. Pleural effusion was identified in approximately 40 per cent of patients with cardiac edema and in 30 per cent of those with renal edema, but in only about 10 per cent of those with permeability edema.

Lung Volume. Lung volume was usually normal or slightly increased in patients with renal-overhydration edema, reduced in patients with cardiac edema (reflecting diminished compliance), and normal in patients with ARDS (except in patients on PEEP).

Heart Size. Cardiac enlargement was identified in 85 per cent of patients with renal-overhydration edema and in 72 per cent of patients with cardiogenic edema, but in only 32 per cent of those with capillary permeability edema.

In a subsequent study by this same group of investigators,[182] 119 roentgenograms of patients with pulmonary edema caused by left heart decompensation, renal failure, and microvascular injury were retrospectively analyzed to assess the value of the chest roentgenogram in distinguishing these types of pulmonary edema. Two trained observers who were unaware of the clinical diagnosis assigned chest roentgenograms to the corresponding group with an accuracy of 86 and 90 per cent, respectively. In addition, roentgenographic findings were used as input variables for discriminant analysis: when the three groups are considered together, computer-generated numerical functions identified the etiology of pulmonary edema with an accuracy of 88 per cent. When groups were compared as pairs, percentages of correct classification were 91 (group 1 versus group 2), 93 (group 1 versus group 3), and 100 (group 2 versus group 3).

Although some investigators have failed to reproduce the results previously described,[183] on the basis of personal examination of many cases and on the strength of the findings in other studies[180, 182, 184] the authors believe that it is possible to distinguish cardiogenic edema from permeability edema on the basis of these roentgenographic observations with a reasonable degree of accuracy in the majority of patients. Despite this, there is no question that the measurement of pulmonary arterial wedge pressure is almost always necessary to provide an objective criterion on which to estimate the presence or absence of increased pressure in the left atrium and pulmonary veins.

Clinical and Physiologic Manifestations

The major risk factors for the development of ARDS include sepsis, aspiration of liquid gastric contents, multiple trauma (including long bone and pelvic fractures and lung contusion), multiple blood transfusions, overwhelming pneumonia, and DIC (often associated with sepsis).[185] The likelihood of developing ARDS increases if more than one of the risk factors is present.[186]

Clinical manifestations can develop either insidiously, hours or days after the initiating event (e.g., sepsis or fat emboli), or acutely, coincident with the event (e.g., aspiration of liquid gastric contents). Typical symptoms are dyspnea, tachypnea, dry cough, retrosternal discomfort, and agitation; cyanosis may be present. The expectoration of copious blood-tinged fluid signifies the presence of the full-blown syndrome. Examination of the chest reveals coarse crackles and bronchial breath sounds. Arterial blood analysis shows severe hypoxemia and a normal or decreased $PaCO_2$. The hypoxemia is difficult or impossible to correct even with the use of very high concentrations of inspired oxygen. Clinical deterioration is usual, requiring endotracheal intubation to maintain oxygen saturation greater than 90 per cent.

As indicated previously, the measurement of pulmonary vascular pressures is an essential procedure in the diagnosis and management of many patients. Pulmonary arterial and pulmonary arterial wedge (PAW) pressures can be easily measured using a balloon-tipped, flow-directed catheter.[187] In the absence of significant pulmonary venous obstruction, PAW represents an estimate of left ventricular filling pressure. Since an elevated left ventricular filling pressure is the hallmark of cardiogenic pulmonary edema, the finding of a normal wedge pressure provides convincing evidence that the edema is the result of increased permeability.

Correct measurement of the arterial wedge pressure as an estimate of pulmonary venous pressure requires that the catheter be located in a region where zone III blood flow conditions exist (pulmonary arterial pressure > pulmonary venous pressure > pulmonary alveolar pressure). Erroneous values for PAW can occur when alveolar pressure is increased using PEEP or when pulmonary arterial pressure is decreased (as in shock). Whether or not the pulmonary artery catheter is in zone III can be determined by obtaining a lateral roentgenogram of the chest with a horizontal x-ray beam. If the mean pulmonary artery pressure (referenced to midthorax) and the alveolar pressure at end-expiration are known, the vertical level at which zone I flow conditions will begin can be calculated. In addition, some of the PEEP can be transmitted to the pleural space, increasing the pressure around the heart and causing an overestimation of ventricular filling pressure.

Besides giving an accurate estimate of left ventricular filling pressure, the pulmonary wedge pressure provides an estimate of the microvascular pressure in the exchanging vessels. As discussed previously, pulmonary capillary pressure is dependent on the relative resistance of the arterial and venous systems. During occlusion of the pulmonary artery, any pressure drop between the pulmonary microvessels and the major pulmonary veins disappears, so pulmonary wedge pressure is less than pulmonary capillary pressure. The magnitude of this difference is related directly to the pulmonary venous resistance. Since pulmonary venous resistance is relatively low and since few conditions selectively increase it, in most cases it is reasonable to use the pulmonary wedge pressure as an estimate of pulmonary microvascular pressure.

In addition to its use as a method of determining whether pulmonary edema is caused by increased microvascular pressure or increased permeability, the measurement of wedge pressure can be a very effective management tool

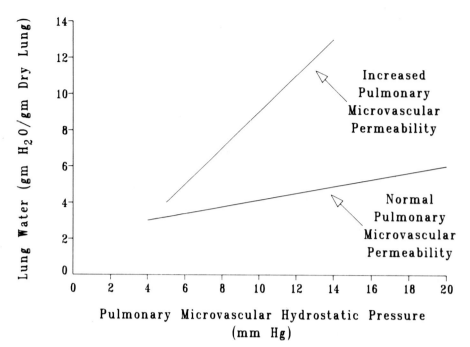

Figure 10–35. Lung Water versus Pulmonary Microvascular Pressure. Lung water, expressed as grams of water per gram of dry lung, is plotted against mean pulmonary microvascular pressure. When pulmonary microvascular permeability is normal, increased microvascular pressure causes a modest increase in lung water (hydrostatic edema); when microvascular permeability is increased, the same change in pressure causes a marked accumulation of lung water.

in testing the effectiveness of agents and therapies designed to lower intravascular pressure. In the presence of increased microvascular permeability, edema formation is critically dependent on microvascular pressure. Although an increase in microvascular pressure is not the *primary* cause of edema in such circumstances, transient or prolonged elevation of microvascular pressure can significantly exaggerate the formation of edema (Fig. 10–35).

In patients with pulmonary edema who are intubated, sampling of the edema fluid through the endotracheal tube permits measurement of the protein concentration in the fluid. The ratio of this concentration to that in serum is significantly higher in patients with permeability edema than in those with cardiogenic edema, permitting clear separation of the two entities in patients in whom the diagnosis is not obvious.[188]

The most important pathophysiologic effect of the edema in patients with ARDS is on gas exchange, profound hypoxemia rather than ventilatory failure being the major indication for intubation and mechanical ventilation. The hypoxemia is caused by intrapulmonary shunting of blood through edematous lung regions.[189] The intrapulmonary shunt in patients with ARDS increases when total pulmonary blood flow is increased,[190] an effect that is probably related to an increase in mixed venous P_{O_2} and decreased hypoxic vasoconstriction.

ARDS is often accompanied by pulmonary arterial hypertension,[191] and the resultant increase in right ventricular afterload can cause right ventricular dysfunction. There is also evidence that right ventricular dysfunction can result in left ventricular dysfunction, most likely related to a shift in the shared interventricular septum.[192] The progression or regression of pulmonary edema in ARDS can be followed using serial chest roentgenograms, serial studies of gas exchange, and estimates of pulmonary extravascular water using techniques such as the double indicator dilution technique.[193] This involves injecting a cold dye into the pulmo-

nary circulation and measuring the appearance of dye and the change in temperature in the systemic arterial system. Since the volume of distribution of the dye is the intravascular space and the change in temperature affects the entire lung water compartment, the difference in transit time of these indicators gives an estimate of total lung water.

Prognosis

The mortality rate of ARDS is invariably over 50 per cent.[194, 195] Although the lung is the primary organ affected, death is often caused by multiple organ failure rather than by respiratory failure. For example, in one study only 40 per cent of those with pulmonary insufficiency alone died, whereas patients with evidence of disease in two, three, four, and five organs showed mortality rates of 54, 72, 84, and 100 per cent, respectively.[196] Coincident renal failure is particularly important in this regard.[197] Persistent sepsis is also a frequent fatal complication of ARDS, in addition to being the most common initiator of the syndrome.[198]

Maintenance of normal arterial blood gases throughout the period of acute lung injury does not guarantee survival, because lung repair and reversal of the injury do not necessarily occur. In one study in which oxygenation was effectively maintained using extracorporeal membrane oxygenation, 82 of 90 patients died.[199] Patients who die of pulmonary insufficiency usually show a progressive decrease in lung compliance and worsening gas exchange. In the terminal stages, hypercapnia may develop despite an enormous minute ventilation. This process can occur over an extremely short time course.[200]

Patients who survive ARDS manifest surprisingly little long-term impairment of lung function.[201] They may have mild restrictive impairment and gas-exchange deficit[202] and occasionally can exhibit partly reversible airway obstruction.[203] Long-term abnormalities of function are more likely to be present in patients who have had the most severe disturbances in lung mechanics and gas exchange during their acute illness and in those treated for prolonged periods who have a fractional inspired oxygen (FIO$_2$) value greater than 0.5.[204]

Specific Forms of Permeability Edema

High-Altitude Pulmonary Edema

A small percentage of persons arriving at high altitudes develop overt pulmonary edema, which occasionally proves fatal.[205] Many more individuals develop altitude sickness, a symptom complex that includes headache, dizziness, tiredness, weakness, body aches, anorexia, nausea, vomiting, insomnia, and restlessness. Physical examination of some of these patients reveals crackles, suggesting that subclinical pulmonary edema may develop more frequently than the occurrence of symptoms.[206] The edema can develop during acute[207] or prolonged[208] exposure to high altitudes, although it is more common in the former situation. The likelihood of developing edema increases with altitude; it is rare for it to develop at altitudes less than 3350 m (11,000 feet). Physical exertion and cold weather are considered precipitating factors in some cases.[209] Individuals returning to high altitudes after a sojourn at lower elevations or who develop pulmonary edema after one exposure to high altitude are particularly susceptible. In one study, the recurrence rate following one episode of edema was an astounding 66 per cent.[210]

The pathophysiology of high-altitude pulmonary edema is unknown and may involve an increase in either vascular pressure or microvascular permeability (or both). Individuals who develop the complication have a decreased ventilatory drive to hypoxemia,[211] and the resultant more severe hypoxemia causes more severe pulmonary hypertension.[212] In addition, right-heart catheterization in susceptible individuals has shown increased pulmonary arterial pressure but normal pulmonary wedge pressure in the presence of edema.[213] However, exactly how the increased arterial pressure might cause increased transudation of fluid into the lung or damage the capillary endothelium is unclear. There also is evidence that increased permeability may be involved in the pathogenesis. For example, one study of the constituents of BAL fluid in climbers at a camp at 4400 m showed increased protein content in fluid from individuals with edema compared with fluid from nonaffected climbers.[214] The edema fluid also contains increased inflammatory cells and vasoactive mediators.

The roentgenographic appearances are typical of acute pulmonary edema, although the distribution tends to be rather irregular and patchy. Although the central pulmonary vessels may be prominent as a result of acute pulmonary hypertension, cardiac enlargement has not been noted.

Symptoms develop within 12 hours to 3 days after arrival at high altitude[215] and consist of cough, dyspnea, weakness, and hemoptysis, often associated with substernal discomfort. Common findings include cyanosis and tachycardia, and crackles may be heard throughout the lungs. Papilledema and retinal hemorrhages have been described.[213] Fever occurs in about one third of patients, and leukocytosis is common, ranging from 13,000 cells per mL to as many as 30,000 cells per mL.[207] The ECG may show nonspecific changes, such as right atrial enlargement or right axis shift, but is usually normal.[216]

Patients respond rapidly to the administration of oxygen or to a return to lower altitudes. The chest roentgenogram clears within 24 to 48 hours.[217]

Re-expansion of Lung at Thoracentesis

Pulmonary edema can occur in the ipsilateral lung when a pneumothorax or hydrothorax is removed,[216] almost certainly much more commonly than reports indicate. Such re-expansion edema is most likely to develop when the lung has been collapsed for a long time and when the pneumothorax or hydrothorax is large and rapidly drained.[218] The development of edema is often preceded by a feeling of tightness in the chest and by spasmodic coughing. When such symptoms develop, thoracentesis should be discontinued. Typically, the edema resolves spontaneously within a few days.

Re-expansion pulmonary edema is clearly associated with increased microvascular permeability, since the protein content of edema fluid is high.[219] Postulated mechanisms include the following:

1. A sudden increase in negative interstitial pressure, causing increased fluid transudation (however, this does not explain the high protein content of edema fluid or the frequent presence of alveolar edema[220]).
2. A delay in venous or lymphatic return caused by stasis in the pulmonary venules and lymphatics during prolonged collapse.[221]
3. An alteration in alveolar surface tension caused by prolonged atelectasis.[222]
4. Reperfusion injury to the pulmonary endothelium.

According to this last hypothesis, when the lung is re-expanded, there is a rapid but incomplete return of blood flow. It is this sudden reperfusion that causes endothelial damage.[223] Several experimental observations support this idea. It has been shown that reperfusion of the heart and kidneys causes damage in these organs; similarly, rapid reperfusion of lung made ischemic by pulmonary artery occlusion has been shown to cause fever, leukopenia, and pulmonary edema.[224] Although the mechanism of such perfusion injury of the lung is unknown, it may be related to the generation of oxygen radicals by tissue enzymes that were depleted of substrate and O$_2$ during ischemia and are suddenly presented with an abundance of both. It is also possible that leukocytes play a role, since rapid re-expansion of collapsed lung can be associated with the acute development of leukopenia.

It is important to be aware of this potential complication of rapid thoracentesis in pneumothorax or hydrothorax, since fatalities have been reported[225] and since it may be prevented by slow withdrawal of gas or liquid by underwater drainage.

Pulmonary Edema Associated with Severe Upper Airway Obstruction

Diffuse pulmonary edema occurs sometimes in patients with severe upper airway obstruction. It occurs exclusively in lesions affecting the extrathoracic airway from the nasopharynx to the thoracic inlet.[226] Since airway obstruction above the thoracic inlet is predominantly inspiratory, efforts to inspire are associated with an increase in negative intrathoracic pressure; it has been suggested that this exaggerated negative alveolar and interstitial pressure causes the edema.[227] However, the fact that the edema often appears only after the obstruction has been relieved—frequently after intubation in patients with severe laryngospasm[228-230]—suggests that another mechanism may be responsible, possibly "flooding" of the pulmonary circulation following prolonged hypoxic vasoconstriction. Whatever the cause, vigorous treatment usually results in prompt resolution.[231]

Miscellaneous Causes of Permeability Edema

The multiple direct and indirect pulmonary insults that have been associated with the development of ARDS are listed in Table 10–5. The clinical features, pathophysiology, and roentgenographic appearance of most of these conditions are described in the sections of this text dealing directly with these etiologic agents. Some of the causes that are not dealt with elsewhere are discussed briefly in the following sections.

ARDS develops in a small but significant proportion of patients with acute pancreatitis unassociated with other precipitating causes, such as sepsis and aspiration. The mechanisms by which this disorder causes pulmonary edema are uncertain; however, it has been proposed that the pancreatic enzymes in the blood could cause activation of the coagulation pathway, generation of kinins,[232] or activation of the complement system.[233]

ARDS frequently occurs following major trauma, particularly in the presence of multiple pelvic and long bone fractures (Fig. 10–36). As discussed in the section on pul-

Table 10–5. **CAUSES OF ADULT RESPIRATORY DISTRESS SYNDROME**

Direct Pulmonary Insults
  Inhalation or aspiration
    Smoke
    Toxic chemicals (e.g., NO_2)
    Gastric acid
    Oxygen
    Water (near-drowning)
  Drugs and chemicals (e.g., paraquat, heroin, salicylates, bleomycin)
  Infection
  Fat emboli
  Amniotic fluid emboli
  Air emboli
  Decompression sickness
  Pulmonary contusion
  Radiologic contrast media
  Thoracic irradiation
Indirect Pulmonary Insults
  Sepsis
  Anaphylaxis
  Multisystem trauma
  Multiple transfusions
  Antilymphocyte globulin therapy
  Disseminated intravascular coagulation
  Pancreatitis
  Pheochromocytoma
  Diabetic ketoacidosis
  Cardiopulmonary bypass
  High altitude
  Rapid lung re-expansion
  Neurogenic
  Sickle-cell crisis
  Hyperthermia
  Extreme physical exertion

monary fat embolism (*see* page 558), the contribution of this condition to post-traumatic ARDS remains unresolved. Patients with multiple trauma are frequently hypotensive, have massive transfusions, or develop sepsis, each of which

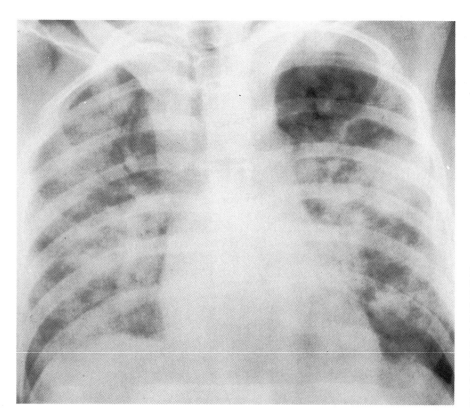

Figure 10–36. Adult Respiratory Distress Syndrome Associated with Traumatic Fat Embolism. A roentgenogram of the chest in anteroposterior projection, supine position, shows diffuse airspace consolidation with some peripheral predominance. Cardiac size is normal. The patient, a young woman with multiple leg fractures sustained in a motor vehicle accident, died shortly thereafter. At autopsy, the arterioles and capillaries were widely occluded by fat.

by itself is a risk factor for the development of ARDS, and it is not certain to what extent fat emboli themselves contribute to pulmonary damage.

Some patients with pheochromocytoma present with episodes of acute pulmonary edema. By the time they are examined, signs of left ventricular failure or elevated pulmonary microvascular pressure are usually absent, and the clinical syndrome has all the features of permeability pulmonary edema.[234]

Rarely, patients with *diabetic ketoacidosis* develop noncardiogenic pulmonary edema that does not appear to be related to other well-defined predisposing factors, such as sepsis.[235] The mechanism of edema formation is unknown.

Pulmonary edema has been described following the parenteral administration of two different forms of contrast media: (1) after injection of the oil-based medium used for lymphangiography, in which the edema develops some days after the lymphatic injection of ethiodized oil[236]; and (2) following injection of the water-based media employed in urography and arteriography, in which the edema accompanies anaphylactic shock.[237] In this situation, the onset of pulmonary edema is characteristically acute, occurring minutes to hours after the injection, and is associated with evidence of systemic hypotension and complement activation.[237]

References

1. Culver BH, Butler J: Mechanical influences on the pulmonary microcirculation. Annu Rev Physiol 42: 187, 1980.
2. Fowler Noble O, Westcott RN, Scott RC: Normal pressure in the right heart and pulmonary artery. Am Heart J 46: 264, 1953.
3. Sasamoto H, Hosono K, Katayama K, et al: Electrocardiographic findings in patients with chronic cor pulmonale. Respir Circ 9: 55, 1961.
4. Shilkin KB, Low LP, Chen BTM: Dissecting aneurysm of the pulmonary artery. J Pathol 98: 25, 1969.
5. Moore GW, Smith RRL, Hutchins GM: Pulmonary atherosclerosis: Correlation with systemic atherosclerosis and hypertensive pulmonary vascular disease. Arch Pathol Lab Med 106: 378, 1982.
6. Wagenvoort CA, Wagenvoort M: Smooth muscle content of pulmonary arterial media in pulmonary venous hypertension compared with other forms of pulmonary hypertension. Chest 81: 581, 1982.
6a. Wright JL, Petty T, Thurlbeck WM: Analysis of the structure of the muscular pulmonary arteries in patients with pulmonary hypertension and COPD: National Institutes of Health nocturnal oxygen therapy trial. Lung 170: 109, 1992.
7. Meyrick B, Reid L: Ultrastructural findings in lung biopsy material from children with congenital heart defects. Am J Pathol 101: 527, 1980.
8. Wagenvoort CA: Open lung biopsies in congenital heart disease for evaluation of pulmonary vascular disease: Predictive value with regard to corrective operability. Histopathology 9: 417, 1985.
9. Fritts HW Jr, Harris P, Clauss HH, et al: The effect of acetylcholine on the human pulmonary circulation under normal and hypoxic conditions. J Clin Invest 37: 99, 1958.
10. Rounds S, Hill NS: Pulmonary hypertensive diseases. Chest 85: 397, 1984.
11. Randall PA, Heitzman ER, Bull MJ, et al: Pulmonary arterial hypertension: A contemporary review. Radiographics 9: 905, 1989.
12. Baltaxe HA, Amplatz K: The normal chest roentgenogram in the presence of large atrial septal defects. Am J Roentgenol 107: 322, 1969.
13. Doyle AE, Goodwin JF, Harrison CV, et al: Pulmonary vascular patterns in pulmonary hypertension. Br Heart J 19: 353, 1957.
14. Ferencz C: The pulmonary vascular bed in tetralogy of Fallot. I. Changes associated with pulmonic stenosis. II. Changes following a systemic-pulmonary arterial anastomosis. Bull Johns Hopkins Hosp 106: 81, 1960.
15. von Bernuth G, Ritter DG, Schattenbert TT, et al: Severe pulmonary hypertension after Blalock-Taussig anastomosis in a patient with tetralogy of Fallot. Chest 58: 380, 1970.
16. Puyau FA, Meckstroth GR: Evaluation of pulmonary perfusion patterns in children with tetralogy of Fallot. Am J Roentgenol 122: 119, 1974.
17. Muster AJ, Paul MH, Nikaidoh H: Tetralogy of Fallot associated with total anomalous pulmonary venous drainage. Chest 64: 323, 1973.
18. Hughes JD, Rubin LJ: Primary pulmonary hypertension: An analysis of 28 cases and a review of the literature. Medicine 65: 56, 1986.
19. Shinnick JP, Cudkowicz L, Blanco G, et al: A problem in pulmonary hypertension. Part 1: The clinical course. Chest 65: 69, 1974.
20. Shinnick JP, Cudkowicz L, Saldana M, et al: A problem in pulmonary hypertension. Part 2: The final course and autopsy findings. Chest 65: 192, 1974.
21. Elkayam U: Vasodilator therapy in primary pulmonary hypertension. Chest 79: 254, 1981.
22. Thompson P, McRae C: Familial pulmonary hypertension, evidence of autosomal dominant inheritance. Br Heart J 32: 758, 1970.
23. Inglesby TV, Singer JW, Gordon DS: Abnormal fibrinolysis in familial pulmonary hypertension. Am J Med 55: 5, 1973.
24. Wagenvoort CA, Wagenvoort N, Dijk HJ: Effect of fulvine on pulmonary arteries and veins of the rat. Thorax 29: 522, 1974.
25. Lebrec D, Capron JP, Dhumeaux D, et al: Pulmonary hypertension complicating portal hypertension. Am Rev Respir Dis 120: 849, 1979.
26. Kibria G, Smith P, Heath D, et al: Observations on the rare association between portal and pulmonary hypertension. Thorax 35: 945, 1980.
27. Berliner S, Schoenfeld Y, Dean H, et al: Primary pulmonary hypertension: A facet of a diffuse angiopathic process? Respiration 43: 76, 1982.
28. Kunichiko Y, Suzuki Y, Ichikawa Y, et al: Abnormalities of pulmonary blood flow during cold exposure in systemic lupus erythematosus. Nucl Med Commun 9: 423, 1988.
29. Walcott G, Burchell HB, Brown AL Jr: Primary pulmonary hypertension. Am J Med 49: 70, 1970.
30. Rich S, Dantzker DR, Ayres SM, et al: Primary pulmonary hypertension: A national prospective study. Ann Intern Med 107: 216, 1987.
31. Chang CH: The normal roentgenographic measurement of the right descending pulmonary artery in 1,085 cases. Am J Roentgenol 87: 929, 1962.
32. Kuriyama K, Gamsu G, Stern RG, et al: CT-determined pulmonary artery diameters in predicting pulmonary hypertension. Invest Radiol 19: 16, 1984.
33. Scharf SM, Feldman NT, Graboys TB, et al: Restrictive ventilatory defect in a patient with primary pulmonary hypertension. Am Rev Respir Dis 118: 409, 1978.
34. Dantzker DR, D'Alonzo GE, Bower JS, et al: Pulmonary gas exchange during exercise in patients with chronic obliterative pulmonary hypertension. Am Rev Respir Dis 130: 412, 1984.
35. Yu N: Primary pulmonary hypertension: Report of six cases and review of the literature. Ann Intern Med 49: 1138, 1958.
36. D'Alonzo GE, Barst RJ, Ayres SM, et al: Survival in patients with primary pulmonary hypertension: Results from a national prospective registry. Ann Intern Med 115: 343, 1991.
37. Starkie CM, Harding LK, Fletcher DJ, et al (The Birmingham Eclampsia Study Group): Intravascular coagulation and abnormal lung-scans in pre-eclampsia and eclampsia. Lancet 2: 889, 1971.
38. Moser KM, Spragg RG, Utley J, et al: Chronic thrombotic obstruction of major pulmonary arteries: Results of thromboendarterectomy in 15 patients. Ann Intern Med 99: 299, 1983.
39. Rich S, Pietra GG: Primary pulmonary hypertension: Radiographic and scintigraphic patterns of histologic subtypes. Ann Intern Med 105: 499, 1986.
40. Pietra GG, Ruttner JR: Specificity of pulmonary vascular lesions in primary pulmonary hypertension: A reappraisal. Respiration 52: 81, 1987.
41. de Soyza NDB, Murphy ML: Persistent post-embolic pulmonary hypertension. Chest 62: 665, 1972.
42. Rich S, Levitsky S, Brundage BH: Pulmonary hypertension from chronic pulmonary thromboembolism. Ann Intern Med 108: 425, 1988.
43. Emirgil C, Sobol BJ, Herbert WH, et al: Routine pulmonary function studies as a key to the status of the lesser circulation in chronic obstructive pulmonary disease. Am J Med 50: 191, 1971.

44. Steckel RJ, Bein ME, Kelly PM: Pulmonary arterial hypertension in progressive systemic sclerosis. Am J Roentgenol 124: 461, 1975.

45. Fry WA, Archer FA, Adams WE: Long-term clinical-pathologic study of the pneumonectomy patient. Dis Chest 52: 720, 1967.

45a. Polos PG, Wolfe D, Harley RA, et al: Pulmonary hypertension and human immunodeficiency virus infection: Two reports and a review of the literature. Chest 101: 474, 1992.

46. Nasraliah A, Goussous Y, El-Said G, et al: Pulmonary artery compression due to acute dissecting aortic aneurysm: Clinical and angiographic diagnosis. Chest 67: 228, 1975.

47. Tikoff G, Bloom S: Complete interruption of the aortic arch in an adult associated with a dissection aneurysm of the pulmonary artery. Am J Med 48: 782, 1970.

48. Cheris DN, Dadey JL: Fibrosing mediastinitis: An unusual cause for cor pulmonale. Am J Roentgenol 100: 328, 1967.

49. Wagenvoort CA: Pathology of congestive pulmonary hypertension. Prog Respir Res (Basel) 9: 195, 1975.

50. Milne ENC: Pulmonary blood flow distribution. Invest Radiol 12: 479, 1977.

51. Chait A, Cohen HE, Meltzer LE, et al: The bedside chest radiograph in the evaluation of incipient heart failure. Radiology 105: 563, 1972.

52. McHugh TJ, Forrester JS, Adler L, et al: Pulmonary vascular congestion in acute myocardial infarction: Hemodynamic and radiologic correlations. Ann Intern Med 76: 29, 1972.

53. Legge DA, Miller WE, Ludwig J: Pulmonary findings associated with mitral stenosis. Chest 58: 403, 1970.

54. Fleming HA, Robinson CLN: Pulmonary ossification with cardiac calcification in mitral valve disease. Br Heart J 19: 532, 1957.

55. Galloway RW, Epstein EJ, Coulshed N: Pulmonary ossific nodules in mitral valve disease. Br Heart J 23: 297, 1961.

56. Symbas PN, Abbott OA, Logan WD, et al: Atrial myxomas: Special emphasis on unusual manifestations. Chest 59: 504, 1971.

57. Palmer WH, Gee JBL, Mills FC, et al: Disturbances of pulmonary function in mitral valve disease. Can Med Assoc J 89: 744, 1963.

58. Wagenvoort CA: Pulmonary veno-occlusive disease: Entity or syndrome? Chest 69: 82, 1976.

59. Hasleton PS, Ironside JW, Whittaker JS, et al: Pulmonary veno-occlusive disease: A report of four cases. Histopathology 10: 933, 1986.

60. Leinonen H, Pohjola-Sintonen S, Krogerus L: Pulmonary veno-occlusive disease. Acta Med Scand 221: 307, 1987.

61. Stovin PGI, Mitchinson MJ: Pulmonary hypertension due to obstruction of intrapulmonary veins. Thorax 20: 106, 1965.

62. Rambihar VS, Fallen EL, Cairns JA: Pulmonary veno-occlusive disease: Antemortem diagnosis from roentgenographic and hemodynamic findings. Can Med Assoc J 120: 1519, 1979.

63. Shackelford GD, Sacks EJ, Mullins JD, et al: Pulmonary veno-occlusive disease: Case report and review of the literature. Am J Roentgenol 128: 643, 1977.

64. Stevens PM, Terplan M, Knowles JH: Prognosis of cor pulmonale. N Engl J Med 269: 1289, 1963.

65. Chronic cor pulmonale: Report of an expert committee. (Reprinted from World Health Organization Technical Report Series No. 213.) Circulation 27: 594, 1963.

66. Seplveda G, Ris E, Len J, et al: Clinico-pathologic correlation in chronic cor pulmonale. Dis Chest 52: 205, 1967.

67. World Health Organization (Report of an Expert Committee): Definition and diagnosis of pulmonary diseases with special reference to chronic bronchitis and emphysema. In Chronic Cor Pulmonale, WHO Technical Report Series No. 213, 1961, pp 14–19.

68. Bartter T, Irwin RS, Nash G: Aneurysms of the pulmonary arteries. Chest 94: 1065, 1988.

69. Shilken KB, Low LP, Chen BTM: Dissecting aneurysm of the pulmonary artery. J Pathol 98: 25, 1968.

70. Teplick JG, Haskin ME, Nedwich A: The Hughes-Stovin syndrome: Case report. Radiology 113: 607, 1974.

71. Staub NC: "State of the art" review: Pathogenesis of pulmonary edema. Am Rev Respir Dis 109: 358, 1974.

72. Pritchard JS: Edema of the Lung. Springfield, IL, Charles C Thomas, 1982.

73. Effros RM: Pulmonary microcirculation and exchange. In Renkin EM, Michel CG (eds): Handbook of Physiology: The Cardiovascular System. IV. Oxford, Oxford University Press, 1984, pp 865–915.

74. Fishman AP: Pulmonary edema: The water-exchanging function of the lung. Circulation 46: 390, 1972.

75. Cottrell TS, Levine OR, Senior RM, et al: Electron microscopic alterations at the alveolar level in pulmonary edema. Circ Res 21: 783, 1967.

76. Albert RK, Lakshminarayan S, Charan NB, et al: Extra-alveolar vessel contribution to hydrostatic pulmonary edema in in situ dog lungs. J Appl Physiol 54: 1010, 1983.

77. Schneeburger EE: Barrier function of intercellular junctions in adult and foetal lungs. In Fishman AP, Renkin EM (eds): Pulmonary Edema. Baltimore, Williams & Wilkins, 1979.

78. Claude P, Goodenough DA: Fracture faces of zonulae occludentes from "tight" and "leaky" epithelium. J Cell Biol 58: 390, 1973.

79. Brigham K: Lung edema due to increased vascular permeability. In Staub NC (ed): Lung Water and Solute Exchange. New York, Marcel Dekker, Inc, 1978, p 235.

80. Todd TRJ, Baile E, Hogg JC: Pulmonary capillary permeability during hemorrhagic shock. J Appl Physiol 45: 298, 1978.

81. Staub NC, Nagano H, Pearce ML: Pulmonary edema in dogs, especially the sequence of fluid accumulation in lungs. J Appl Physiol 22: 227, 1967.

82. Gee MH, Williams DO: Effect of lung inflation on perivascular cuff fluid volume in isolated dog lung lobes. Microvasc Res 17: 192, 1979.

83. Malo J, Ali J, Duke K, et al: Effects of PEEP on lung liquid distribution and pulmonary shunt in canine oleic acid pulmonary edema. Clin Res 28: 703, 1980.

84. Egan EA: Effect of lung inflation on alveolar permeability to solutes. In Lung Liquids. Ciba Symposium (New Series) 38. New York, Excerpta Medica, 1976.

85. Harris TR, Roselli RJ: A theoretical model of protein, fluid, and small molecule transport in the lung. J Appl Physiol 50: 1, 1981.

86. Starling EH: On the absorption of fluids from the connective tissue spaces. J Physiol (Lond) 19: 312, 1896.

87. Staub NC: Pathophysiology of pulmonary edema. In Staub NC, Taylor AE (eds): Edema. New York, Raven Press, 1984, p 719.

88. Staub NC: Pulmonary edema. Physiol Rev 54: 678, 1974.

89. Bhattacharya J, Staub MC: Direct measurement of microvascular pressures in the isolated perfused dog lung. Science 210: 327, 1980.

90. Lai-Fook SJ: Perivascular interstitial fluid pressure measured by micro-pipettes in isolated dog lung. J Appl Physiol 52: 9, 1982.

91. Olver RE: Ion transport and water flow in the mammalian lung. In Lung Liquids. Ciba Symposium (New Series) 38. New York, Excerpta Medica, 1976.

92. Albert RK, Lakshminarayan S, Hildebrandt J, et al: Increased surface tension favours pulmonary edema formation in anesthetized dogs' lungs. J Clin Invest 63: 115, 1979.

93. Brigham KL, Woolverton WC, Staub NV: Increased pulmonary vascular permeability after Pseudomonas aeruginosa bacteremia in unanesthetized sheep. Fed Proc 32: 440, 1973.

94. Sampson JJ, Leeds SE, Uhley HN, et al: Studies of lymph flow and changes in pulmonary structures as indexes of circulatory changes in experimental pulmonary edema. Isr J Med Sci 5: 826, 1969.

95. Leeds SE, Uhley HN, Sampson JJ, et al: Significance of changes in the pulmonary lymph flow in acute and chronic experimental pulmonary edema. Am J Surg 114: 254, 1967.

96. Erdmann AJ, Vaughan TR, Brigham KL, et al: Effect of increased vascular pressure on lung fluid balance in unanesthetized sheep. Circ Res 37: 271, 1975.

97. Montaner JSG, Tsang J, Evans KG, et al: Alveolar epithelial damage: A critical difference between high pressure and oleic acid–induced low pressure pulmonary edema. J Clin Invest 77: 1786, 1986.

98. Vreim CE, Staub NC: Protein composition of lung fluid in acute alloxan edema in dogs. Am J Physiol 230: 376, 1976.

99. Vreim CE, Snashall PD, Staub NC: Protein composition of lung fluid in anesthetized dogs with acute cardiogenic edema. Am J Physiol 231: 1466, 1976.

100. Petty TL, Ashbaugh DG: The adult respiratory distress syndrome: Clinical features, factors influencing prognosis, and principles of management. Chest 60: 233, 1971.

101. Heitzman ER: The Lung: Radiologic-Pathologic Correlations. St. Louis, CV Mosby, 1973, pp 127, 137.

102. Meszaros WT: Cardiac Roentgenology: Plain Films and Angiocardiographic Findings. Springfield, IL, Charles C Thomas, 1969, p 103.

103. Bennett ED, Rees S: The significance of radiological changes in the lungs in acute myocardial infarction. Br J Radiol 47: 879, 1974.

104. Richman SM, Godar TJ: Unilateral pulmonary edema. N Engl J Med 264: 1148, 1961.

105. Calenoff L, Kruglik GD, Woodruff A: Unilateral pulmonary edema. Radiology 126: 19, 1978.
106. Leeming BWA: Gravitational edema of the lungs observed during assisted respiration. Chest 64: 719, 1973.
107. Herrnheiser G, Hinson KFW: An anatomical explanation of the formation of butterfly shadows. Thorax 9: 198, 1954.
108. Nessa CG, Rigler LG: The roentgenological manifestations of pulmonary edema. Radiology 37: 35, 1941.
109. Prichard MML, Daniel PM, Ardran GM: Peripheral eschaemia of the lung: Some experimental observations. Br J Radiol 27: 93, 1954.
110. Borgstrom KE, Ising U, Linder E, et al: Experimental pulmonary edema. Acta Radiol 54: 97, 1960.
111. Fleischner FG: The butterfly pattern of acute pulmonary edema. Am J Cardiol 20: 39, 1967.
112. Hodson CJ: Pulmonary oedema and the "bat's-wing" shadow. J Fac Radiol 1: 176, 1950.
113. Hughes RT: The pathology of butterfly densities in uraemia. Thorax 22: 97, 1967.
114. Cooke CD, Mead J, Schreiner GL, et al: Pulmonary mechanics during induced pulmonary edema in anesthetized dogs. J Appl Physiol 14: 17, 1969.
115. Said SI, Longacre JW, David RK, et al: Pulmonary gas exchange during induction of pulmonary edema in anesthetized dogs. J Appl Physiol 19: 403, 1964.
116. Hogg JC, Agarawal JB, Gardiner AJF, et al: Distribution of airway resistance with developing pulmonary edema in dogs. J Appl Physiol 32: 20, 1972.
117. Hales CA, Kazemi H: Small airway function in myocardial infarction. N Engl J Med 290: 761, 1974.
118. West JB, Dollery CT, Heard BE: Increased pulmonary vascular resistance in the dependent zone of the isolated dog lung caused by perivascular edema. Circ Res 17: 191, 1965.
119. West JB: Perivascular oedema: A factor in pulmonary vascular resistance. Am Heart J 70: 570, 1965.
120. Muir AL, Hall DL, Despas P, et al: Distribution of blood flow in the lungs in acute pulmonary edema in dogs. J Appl Physiol 33: 763, 1972.
121. Aberman A, Fulop M: The metabolic and respiratory acidosis of acute pulmonary edema. Ann Intern Med 76: 173, 1972.
122. Anthonisen NR, Smith HJ: Respiratory acidosis as a consequence of pulmonary edema. Ann Intern Med 62: 991, 1965.
123. Fulop M, Horowitz M, Aberman A, et al: Lactic acidosis in pulmonary edema due to left ventricular failure. Ann Intern Med 79: 180, 1973.
124. Macpherson RI, Banerjee AK: Acute glomerulonephritis: A chest film diagnosis? J Can Assoc Radiol 25: 58, 1974.
125. Gibson DG: Hemodynamic factors in the development of acute pulmonary oedema in renal failure. Lancet 2: 1217, 1966.
126. Stein L, Beraud J, Cavonilles J, et al: Pulmonary edema during fluid infusion in the absence of heart failure. JAMA 229: 65, 1974.
127. Westcott JL, Rudick MG: Cardiopulmonary effects of intravenous fluid overload: Radiologic manifestations. Radiology 129: 577, 1978.
128. Levy GJ, Shabot MM, Hart ME, et al: Transfusion-associated non-cardiogenic pulmonary edema: Report of a case and a warning regarding treatment. Transfusion 26: 278, 1986.
129. Ward HN: Pulmonary infiltration associated with leukoagglutinin transfusion reactions. Ann Intern Med 73: 688, 1970.
130. Trewby PN, Warren R, Contini S, et al: Incidence and pathophysiology of pulmonary oedema in fulminant hepatic failure. Gastroenterology 74: 859, 1978.
131. Bekemeyer WB, Pinstein ML: Neurogenic pulmonary edema: New concepts of an old disorder. South Med J 82: 380, 1989.
132. Worthen M, Argano B, Siwadiowski W, et al: Mechanisms of intracisternal veratrine pulmonary edema. Dis Chest 55: 45, 1969.
133. Melon E, Bonnet F, Lepresle F, et al: Altered capillary permeability in neurogenic pulmonary oedema. Intensive Care Med 11: 323, 1985.
134. Felman AH: Neurogenic pulmonary edema: Observations in 6 patients. Am J Roentgenol 112: 393, 1971.
135. Teplinsky K, Hall J: Post-ictal pulmonary edema: Report of a case. Arch Intern Med 146: 801, 1986.
136. Murray JF: The adult respiratory distress syndrome (may it rest in peace). Am Rev Respir Dis 111: 716, 1975.
137. Fishman AP: Shock lung: A distinctive nonentity. Circulation 47: 921, 1973.
138. Blennerhassett JB: Shock lung and diffuse alveolar damage: Pathological and pathogenetic considerations. Pathology 17: 239, 1985.
139. Connell RS, Swank RL, Webb MC: The development of pulmonary ultrastructural lesions during hemorrhage shock. J Trauma 15: 116, 1975.
140. Blaisdell FW, Schlobohm RM: The respiratory distress syndrome: A review. Surgery 74: 251, 1973.
141. Hogg JC: Neutrophil kinetics and lung injury. Physiol Rev 67: 1249, 1987.
142. Cochrane CG: The enhancement of inflammatory injury. Am Rev Respir Dis 136: 1, 1987.
143. Flick MR, Perel G, Staub NC: Leukocytes are required for increased lung microvascular permeability after microembolism in sheep. Circ Res 48: 344, 1981.
144. Elliott CG, Zimmerman GA, Orme JF, et al: Granulocyte aggregation in adult respiratory distress syndrome (ARDS): Serial histologic and physiologic observations. Am J Med Sci 289: 70, 1985.
145. Fowler AA, Hyers TM, Fisher BJ, et al: The adult respiratory distress syndrome: Cell populations and soluble mediators in the air spaces of patients at high risk. Am Rev Respir Dis 136: 1225, 1987.
146. Warshawski FJ, Sibbald WJ, Driedger AA, et al: Abnormal neutrophil-pulmonary interaction in the adult respiratory distress syndrome: Qualitative and quantitative assessment of pulmonary neutrophil kinetics in humans with in vivo [111]indium neutrophil scintigraphy. Am Rev Respir Dis 133: 797, 1986.
147. Thommasen HB: The role of the polymorphonuclear leukocyte in the pathogenesis of the adult respiratory distress syndrome. Clin Invest Med 8: 185, 1985.
148. Maunder RJ, Hackman RC, Riff E, et al: Occurrence of the adult respiratory distress syndrome in neutropenic patients. Am Rev Respir Dis 133: 313, 1986.
149. Hallman M, Spragg R, Harrell JH, et al: Evidence of lung surfactant abnormality in respiratory failure. J Clin Invest 70: 673, 1982.
150. Ryan SF, Liau DF, Bell ALL, et al: Correlation of lung compliance and quantities of surfactant phospholipids after acute alveolar injury from N-nitroso-N-methylurethane in the dog. Am Rev Respir Dis 123: 200, 1981.
151. Muller-Eberhard HJ: Complement. Annu Rev Biochem 44: 697, 1975.
152. Langlois PF, Gawryl MS: Accentuated formation of the terminal C5b-9 complement complex in patient plasma precedes development of the adult respiratory distress syndrome. Am Rev Respir Dis 138: 368, 1988.
153. Duchateau J, Haas M, Schreyen H, et al: Complement activation in patients at risk of developing the adult respiratory distress syndrome. Am Rev Respir Dis 130: 1058, 1984.
154. Malik AB: Mediators of pulmonary vascular injury and edema after thrombin. In Said SI (ed): The Pulmonary Circulation and Acute Lung Injury. Mount Kisco, NY, Futura Publishing Co, 1985, p 429.
155. El-Kassimi FA, Al-Mashhadani DCP, Abdullah AK, et al: Adult respiratory distress syndrome and disseminated intravascular coagulation complicating heat stroke. Chest 90: 571, 1986.
156. Modig J, Bagge L: Specific coagulation and fibrinolysis tests as biochemical markers in traumatic-induced adult respiratory distress syndrome. Resuscitation 13: 87, 1986.
157. Quinn DA, Carvalho AC, Geller E, et al: ^{99m}Tc-fibrinogen scanning in adult respiratory distress syndrome. Am Rev Respir Dis 135: 100, 1987.
158. Haynes AB, Hyers TM, Giclas PC, et al: Elevated fibrin(ogen) degradation products in the adult respiratory distress syndrome. Am Rev Respir Dis 122: 841, 1980.
159. Carlson RW, Schaeffer RC, Carpio M, et al: Edema fluid and coagulation changes during fulminant pulmonary edema. Chest 79: 43, 1981.
160. Malik AB: Pulmonary microembolism. Physiol Rev 63: 1114, 1983.
161. Johnson A, Blumenstock FA, Malik AB: Effect of complement depletion on lung fluid balance after thrombin. J Appl Physiol 55: 1480, 1983.
162. Frank L: Oxidant injury to pulmonary endothelium. In Said SI (ed): The Pulmonary Circulation and Acute Lung Injury. Mount Kisco, NY, Futura Publishing Co, 1985, p 283.
163. Cochrane CG, Spragg R, Revak SD: Pathogenesis of the adult respiratory distress syndrome: Evidence of oxidant activity in bronchoalveolar lavage fluid. J Clin Invest 71: 754, 1983.
164. Slotman GJ, Burchard KW, Yellin SA, et al: Prostaglandin and complement interaction in clinical acute respiratory failure. Arch Surg 121: 271, 1986.
165. Matthay MA, Eschenbacher WL, Goetzl EJ: Elevated concentrations

of leukotriene D$_4$ in pulmonary edema fluid of patients with the adult respiratory distress syndrome. J Clin Immunol 4: 479, 1984.

166. Cox JW, Andreadis NA, Bone RC, et al: Pulmonary extraction and pharmacokinetics of prostaglandin E$_1$ during continuous intravenous infusion in patients with adult respiratory distress syndrome. Am Rev Respir Dis 137: 5, 1988.

167. Schapira M, Gardaz JP, Py P, et al: Prekallikrein activation in the adult respiratory distress syndrome. Bull Eur Physiopathol Respir 21: 237, 1985.

168. Idell S, Kucich U, Fein A, et al: Neutrophil elastase-releasing factors in bronchoalveolar lavage from patients with adult respiratory distress syndrome. Am Rev Respir Dis 132: 1098, 1985.

169. O'Brodovich HM, Stalcup SA, Pang LM, et al: Bradykinin production and increased pulmonary endothelial permeability during acute respiratory failure in unanesthetized sheep. J Clin Invest 67: 514, 1981.

170. McGuire WW, Spragg RG, Cohen AB, et al: Studies on the pathogenesis of the adult respiratory distress syndrome. J Clin Invest 69: 543, 1982.

171. Johnson AR, Coalson JJ, Ashton J, et al: Neutral endopeptidase in serum samples from patients with adult respiratory distress syndrome: Comparison with angiotensin-converting enzyme. Am Rev Respir Dis 132: 1262, 1985.

172. Vadas P: Elevated plasma phospholipase A$_2$ levels: Correlation with the hemodynamic and pulmonary changes in gram-negative septic shock. J Lab Clin Med 104: 873, 1984.

173. Blennerhasset JB: Shock lung and diffuse alveolar damage: Pathological and pathogenetic considerations. Pathology 17: 239, 1985.

174. Ostendorf P, Birzle H, Vogel W, et al: Pulmonary radiographic abnormalities in shock: Roentgen clinical-pathological correlation. Radiology 115: 257, 1975.

175. Fukuda Y, Ishizaki M, Masuda Y, et al: The role of intra-alveolar fibrosis in the process of pulmonary structural remodeling in patients with diffuse alveolar damage. Am J Pathol 126: 171, 1987.

176. Greene R: Adult respiratory distress syndrome: Acute alveolar damage. Radiology 163: 57, 1987.

177. Joffe N: The adult respiratory distress syndrome. Am J Roentgenol 122: 719, 1974.

178. Dyck DR, Zylak CJ: Acute respiratory distress in adults. Radiology 106: 497, 1973.

179. Zimmerman JE, Goodman LR, Shahvari MBG: Effect of mechanical ventilation and positive end-expiratory pressure (PEEP) on chest radiograph. Am J Roentgenol 133: 811, 1979.

180. Milne ENC, Pistolesi M, Miniati M, et al: The radiologic distinction of cardiogenic and noncardiogenic edema. Am J Roentgenol 144: 879, 1985.

181. Pistolesi M, Milne EWC, Miniati M, et al: The vascular pedicle of the heart and the vena azygos. Part II: Acquired heart disease. Radiology 152: 9, 1984.

182. Miniati M, Pistolesi M, Paoletti P, et al: Objective radiographic criteria to differentiate cardiac, renal, and injury lung edema. Invest Radiol 23: 433, 1988.

183. Aberle DR, Wiener-Kronish JP, Webb WR, et al: Hydrostatic versus increased permeability pulmonary edema: Diagnosis based on radiographic criteria in critically ill patients. Radiology 168: 73, 1988.

184. Smith RC, Mann H, Greenspan RH, et al: Radiographic differentiation between different etiologies of pulmonary edema. Invest Radiol 22: 859, 1987.

185. Petty TL: Indicators of risk, course, and prognosis in adult respiratory distress syndrome (ARDS). Am Rev Respir Dis 132: 471, 1985.

186. Fowler AA, Hamman RF, Good JT, et al: Adult respiratory distress syndrome: Risk with common predisposition. Ann Intern Med 98: 593, 1983.

187. O'Quin R, Marini JJ: Pulmonary artery occlusion pressure: Clinical physiology, measurement, and interpretation. Am Rev Respir Dis 128: 319, 1983.

188. Sprung CL, Long WM, Marcial EH, et al: Distribution of proteins in pulmonary edema: The value of fractional concentrations. Am Rev Respir Dis 136: 957, 1987.

189. Ralph DD, Robertson HT, Weaver LJ, et al: Distribution of ventilation and perfusion during positive end-expiratory pressure in the adult respiratory distress syndrome. Am Rev Respir Dis 131: 54, 1985.

190. Breen PH, Schumacker PT, Hedenstierna G, et al: How does increased cardiac output increase shunt in pulmonary edema? J Appl Physiol 53: 1273, 1982.

191. Zapol WM, Snider MT: Pulmonary hypertension in severe acute respiratory failure. N Engl J Med 296: 476, 1977.

192. Sibbald WJ, Driedger AA, Cunningham DG, et al: Right and left ventricular performance in acute hypoxemic respiratory failure. Crit Care Med 14: 852, 1986.

193. Rinaldo JE, Borovetz HS, Mancini MC, et al: Assessment of lung injury in the adult respiratory distress syndrome using multiple indicator dilution curves. Am Rev Respir Dis 133: 1006, 1986.

194. Respiratory Diseases. Task Force Report on Problems, Research Approaches, Needs. National Heart and Lung Institute. DHEW Pub. No. NIH 73-432, 1972, pp 167–80.

195. Bernard GR, Brigham KL: The adult respiratory distress syndrome. Annu Rev Med 36: 195, 1985.

196. Bartlett RH, Morris AH, Fairley HB, et al: A prospective study of acute hypoxic respiratory failure. Chest 89: 684, 1986.

197. Gillispie DJ, Marsh HM, Divertie MB, et al: Clinical outcome of respiratory failure in patients requiring prolonged (greater than 24 hours) mechanical ventilation. Chest 90: 364, 1986.

198. Seidenfeld JJ, Pohl DF, Bell RC, et al: Incidence, site, and outcome of infections in patients with the adult respiratory distress syndrome. Am Rev Respir Dis 134: 12, 1986.

199. National Heart, Lung, and Blood Institute: Extracorporeal Support for Respiratory Insufficiency: Collaborative Study. Washington, DC, National Heart, Lung, and Blood Institute, December, 1979.

200. Auler JO, Calheiros DF, Brentani MM, et al: Adult respiratory distress syndrome: Evidence of early fibrogenesis and absence of glucocorticoid receptors. Eur J Respir Dis 69: 261, 1986.

201. Buchser E, Leuenberger P, Chiolero R, et al: Reduced pulmonary capillary blood volume as a long-term sequela of ARDS. Chest 87: 608, 1985.

202. Elliott CG, Morris AH, Cengiz M: Pulmonary function and exercise gas exchange in survivors of adult respiratory distress syndrome. Am Rev Respir Dis 123: 492, 1981.

203. Simpson DL, Goodman M, Spector SL, et al: Long-term follow-up and bronchial reactivity testing in survivors of the adult respiratory distress syndrome. Am Rev Respir Dis 117: 449, 1978.

204. Elliott CG, Rasmusson BY, Crapo RO, et al: Prediction of pulmonary function abnormalities after adult respiratory distress syndrome (ARDS). Am Rev Respir Dis 135: 634, 1987.

205. Hurtado A: Some clinical aspects of life at high altitudes. Ann Intern Med 53: 247, 1960.

206. Wilson R: Acute high-altitude illness in mountaineers and problems of rescue. Ann Intern Med 78: 421, 1973.

207. Kamat SR, Banerjil BC: Study of cardiopulmonary function on exposure to high altitude. I. Acute acclimatization to an altitude of 3500 to 4000 meters in relation to altitude sickness and cardiopulmonary function. Am Rev Respir Dis 106: 404, 1972.

208. Kamat SR, Rao TL, Sama BS, et al: Study of cardiopulmonary function on exposure to high altitude. II. Effects of prolonged stay at 3500 to 4000 meters and reversal on return to sea level. Am Rev Respir Dis 106: 414, 1972.

209. Fred HL, Schmidt AM, Bates T, et al: Acute pulmonary edema of altitude: Clinical and physiologic observations. Circulation 25: 929, 1962.

210. Vock P, Fretz C, Franciolli M, et al: High-altitude pulmonary edema: Findings at high-altitude chest radiography and physical examination. Radiology 170: 661, 1989.

211. Hyers TM, Scoggin CH, Will DH, et al: Accentuated hypoxemia at high altitude in subjects susceptible to high-altitude pulmonary edema. J Appl Physiol 46: 41, 1979.

212. Hackett PH, Roach RC, Schoene RB, et al: Abnormal control of ventilation in high-altitude pulmonary edema. J Appl Physiol 64: 1268, 1988.

213. Schoene RB, Swenson ER, Pizzo CJ, et al: The lung at high altitude: Bronchoalveolar lavage in acute mountain sickness and pulmonary edema. J Appl Physiol 64: 2605, 1988.

214. Schoene RB, Hackett PH, Henderson WR, et al: High-altitude pulmonary edema: Characteristics of lung lavage fluid. JAMA 256: 63, 1986.

215. Hultgren HN, Flamm MD: Pulmonary edema. Mod Concepts Cardiovasc Dis 31: 1, 1969.

216. Kleiner JP, Nelson WP: High-altitude pulmonary edema: A rare disease? JAMA 234: 491, 1975.

217. Hultgren HN, Spickard WB, Hellreigel K, et al: High-altitude pulmonary edema. Medicine 40: 289, 1961.

218. Waqaruddin M, Bernstein A: Re-expansion pulmonary oedema. Thorax 30: 54, 1975.

219. Sprung CL, Loewenherz JW, Baier H, et al: Evidence for increased permeability in re-expansion pulmonary edema. Am J Med 71: 497, 1981.
220. Humphreys RL, Berne AS: Rapid re-expansion of pneumothorax: A cause of unilateral pulmonary edema. Radiology 96: 509, 1970.
221. Rigler LG, Surprenant EL: Pulmonary edema. Semin Roentgenol 2: 33, 1967.
222. Ratliff JL, Chavez CM, Jamchuk A, et al: Re-expansion pulmonary edema. Chest 64: 654, 1973.
223. Yamazaki S, Ogawa J, Shohzu A, et al: Pulmonary blood flow to rapidly re-expanded lung in spontaneous pneumothorax. Chest 81: 1, 1982.
224. Bishop MJ, Boatman ES, Ivey TD, et al: Reperfusion of ischaemic dog lung results in fever, leukopenia, and lung edema. Am Rev Respir Dis 134: 752, 1986.
225. Mahfood S, Hix WR, Aaron BL, et al: Re-expansion pulmonary edema. Ann Thorac Surg 45: 340, 1988.
226. Lagler U, Russi E: Upper airway obstruction as a cause of pulmonary edema during late pregnancy. Am J Obstet Gynecol 156: 643, 1987.
227. Warren MF, Peterson DK, Drinker CK: The effects of heightened negative pressure in the chest, together with further experiments upon anoxia in increasing the flow of lung lymph. Am J Physiol 137: 641, 1942.
228. Szucs RA, Floyd HL: Laryngospasm-induced pulmonary edema. Radiology 170: 446, 1989.
229. Oudjhane K, Bowen A, Sang K, et al: Pulmonary edema complicating upper airway obstruction in infants and children. Can Assoc Radiol J 43: 278, 1992.
230. Willms D, Shure D: Pulmonary edema due to upper airway obstruction in adults. Chest 94: 1090, 1988.
231. Lorch DG, Sahn SA: Post-extubation pulmonary edema following anesthesia induced by upper airway obstruction: Are certain patients at increased risk? Chest 90: 802, 1986.
232. Satake K, Rozmanith JS, Appert H, et al: Hemodynamic change and bradykinin levels in plasma and lymph during experimental acute pancreatitis in dogs. Ann Surg 178: 659, 1973.
233. Minta JO, Man D, Movat HZ: Kinetic studies on the fragmentation of the third component of complement (C3) by trypsin. J Immunol 118: 2192, 1977.
234. deLeeuw PW, Waltman FL, Birkenhager WH: Noncardiogenic pulmonary edema as the sole manifestation of pheochromocytoma. Hypertension 8: 810, 1986.
235. Botha J, van Niekerk DJ, Rossouw DJ, et al: The adult respiratory distress syndrome in association with diabetic keto-acidosis: A case report. S Afr Med J 71: 535, 1987.
236. Silvestri RC, Huseby JS, Rughani I, et al: Respiratory distress syndrome from lymphangiography contrast medium. Am Rev Respir Dis 122: 543, 1980.
237. Boden WE: Anaphylactoid pulmonary edema ("shock lung") and hypotension after radiologic contrast media injection. Chest 81: 759, 1982.
238. Harvey RM, Enson Y, Ferrer MI: A reconsideration of the origins of pulmonary hypertension. Chest 59: 82, 1971.
239. Vogel JHK, Blount SG Jr: The role of hydrogen ion concentration in the regulation of pulmonary artery pressure: Observations in a patient with hypoventilation and obesity. Circulation 32: 788, 1965.
240. Plokker HWM, Wagenaar S, Bruschke AVG, et al: Aneurysm of a pulmonary artery branch: An uncommon cause of a coin lesion. Chest 68: 258, 1975.
241. Baum D, Khoury GH, Ongley PA, et al: Congenital stenosis of the pulmonary artery branches. Circulation 29: 680, 1964.
242. Tung H, Liebow AA: Marfan's syndrome. Lab Invest 1: 382, 1952.
243. Symbas PN, Scott HW Jr: Traumatic aneurysm of the pulmonary artery. J Thorac Cardiovasc Surg 45: 645, 1963.
244. Deterling RA Jr, Clagett OT: Aneurysm of the pulmonary artery: Review of the literature and report of a case. Am Heart J 34: 471, 1947.
245. Auerbach O: Pathology and pathogenesis of pulmonary arterial aneurysm in tuberculous cavities. Am Rev Tuberc 39: 99, 1939.
246. Jaffe RB, Condon VR: Mycotic aneurysms of the pulmonary artery and aorta. Radiology 116: 291, 1975.
247. Choyke PL, Edmonds PR, Markowitz RI, et al: Mycotic pulmonary artery aneurysm: Complication of *Aspergillus* endocarditis. Am J Roentgenol 138: 1172, 1982.
248. Slavin RE, deGroot WJ: Pathology of the lung in Behçet's disease. Am J Surg Pathol 5: 779, 1981.
249. Steurer J, Jenni R, Medici TC, et al: Dissecting aneurysm of the pulmonary artery with pulmonary hypertension. Am Rev Respir Dis 142: 1219, 1990.

11

DISEASES OF THE AIRWAYS

This chapter is concerned with a variety of lung diseases that are grouped together because of their common characteristic of obstruction of the airways. Such obstruction may be acute or chronic, and acute episodes may be isolated or recurrent. It can occur in either the upper* or the lower airways, and in the latter site it may be local or diffuse.

The designation "chronic obstructive pulmonary disease" (COPD) is frequently used to describe patients who have persistent diffuse lower airway obstruction. In its broadest sense, the term is applied to patients who have chronic bronchitis with airway narrowing, intractable asthma, emphysema, bronchiectasis, cystic fibrosis, or a combination of these disorders. However, it is also frequently used in a narrower sense to describe patients with largely irreversible obstruction to expiratory flow in whom a specific diagnosis cannot be made. These patients are usually heavy cigarette smokers, and the airway obstruction is related to a combination of loss of lung elasticity and narrowing of the membranous and respiratory bronchioles. For the most part, use of the term COPD in this chapter refers to this more restrictive definition.

OBSTRUCTIVE DISEASE OF THE UPPER AIRWAYS

Although the clinical manifestations of obstruction of the upper airways are usually sufficiently distinctive to permit prompt recognition, an appreciable number of cases are misdiagnosed. Since appropriate roentgenographic procedures and physiologic measurements readily distinguish upper from lower airway obstruction, these examinations should be performed in all cases of possible obstructive upper airway disease to prevent needless—and sometimes life-threatening—misdiagnosis.

Acute Upper Airway Obstruction

The disorders that cause acute upper airway obstruction occur most commonly in infants and young children because of the small intraluminal caliber and greater compliance of their upper airways. The sudden onset of dyspnea, hoarseness, and stridor are the most frequent clinical manifestations. The cause of the obstruction is often apparent from the history. For example, fever and cough are usually present with infections, and previous episodes of obstruction with angioneurotic edema. Although roentgenographic manifestations vary according to the specific etiology, the combination of relatively small lung volume plus dilatation of the airway proximal to the site of obstruction should alert the radiologist to the diagnosis.[1]

The causes of acute upper airway obstruction include faulty placement of an endotracheal tube (*see* page 805), infection, edema, hemorrhage, and foreign body aspiration.

Infection

Infection can cause severe narrowing of the upper airways, particularly in infants and young children. Acute

---

*The upper airway is defined as the portion of the conducting system from the nose or mouth to the tracheal carina.

pharyngitis and tonsillitis, which may be complicated by retropharyngeal abscess (Fig. 11–1), are caused most commonly by beta-hemolytic streptococci[2] and less often by adenoviruses[3] and coxsackieviruses.[4] Acute laryngotracheitis (croup) is caused by parainfluenza or respiratory syncytial viruses and results in a characteristic narrowing of the subglottic trachea; staphylococcal tracheitis can closely simulate it clinically.[5] Whooping cough may be associated with upper airway obstruction and is caused by *Bordetella pertussis* and adenovirus.[6]

Acute epiglottitis is caused most often by *Haemophilus influenzae* and occasionally by *Staphylococcus aureus* or *Streptococcus pneumoniae*.[7] Although it usually affects infants and young children, acute epiglottitis also occurs in adults, in whom it often goes unrecognized.[8] Roentgenographic findings include swelling of the epiglottis, aryepiglottic folds, arytenoids, uvula, and prevertebral soft tissues. The hypopharynx and oropharynx tend to be ballooned, and the valleculae obliterated. Narrowing of the subglottic trachea, simulating croup, occurs in roughly a quarter of affected children.[9] The presenting symptoms are severe sore throat, difficulty in breathing, and hoarseness; stridor may be present.

Edema

Edema of noninfective origin characteristically affects the larynx and may be caused by angioneurotic edema, trauma, or inhalation of noxious gases. The first-named is the commonest cause and can be classified as allergic, hereditary, or idiopathic.[10] The allergic form occurs in atopic individuals and is often associated with multiple pruritic and usually nonpainful swellings in the subcutaneous tissue of the face, hands, feet, and genitalia; some patients develop urticaria. A type I (immunoglobulin G [IgG]–mediated) response to foreign antigens contained in foods, inhalants, bee stings, or drugs is the mechanism for the edema in some individuals; a type III (IgG-mediated) allergic response to antiserum, certain drugs such as penicillin, or radiocontrast material may be responsible in others. Despite these observations, the responsible antigen is identified in fewer than 20 per cent of cases.

The hereditary form of angioneurotic edema usually begins in childhood and is characterized by recurrent attacks, often in association with abdominal cramps.[11] The attacks are not precipitated by allergens but may follow local trauma, such as tonsillectomy and tooth extraction, or may be associated with emotional upsets. The form of inheritance is autosomal dominant, the underlying defect being an absence of a serum alpha₂ globulin esterase inhibitor of the first component of complement. It is believed that the byproducts of the complement cascade are responsible for the release of vasoactive substances, which in turn produce angioedema. The prognosis is grave, with approximately one third of affected family members dying of suffocation.[10] Careful management and long-term prophylactic measures, however, can save a considerable number of lives.[11]

Hoarseness or singeing of nasal hairs in a patient who has been exposed to smoke indicates that mucosal damage is likely at the level of the larynx and that life-threatening airway obstruction as a result of edema, hyperemia, and ulceration may develop within hours. Inspiratory and expiratory flow-volume loops can be helpful in assessing the

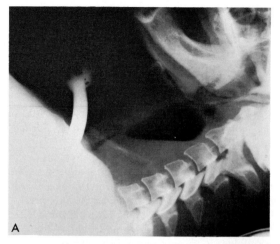

Figure 11–1. Acute Retropharyngeal and Mediastinal Abscess. A 29-year-old woman was admitted to the hospital with an 8-day history of increasing dyspnea, difficulty in swallowing, and loss of voice. An emergency tracheostomy was performed. Lateral roentgenography of the soft tissues of the neck with a horizontal x-ray beam (A) revealed a large accumulation of gas and fluid in the retropharyngeal space associated with complete obliteration of the airspace of the hypopharynx and anterior displacement of the cervical trachea. Anteroposterior (B) and lateral (C) roentgenograms of the chest showed a large mediastinal mass projecting predominantly to the right of the midline, situated mainly behind the trachea, and causing anterior displacement and narrowing of this structure.

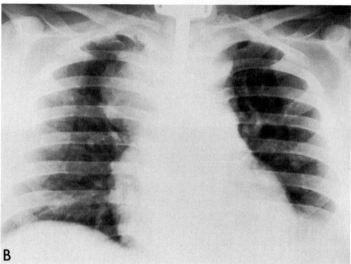

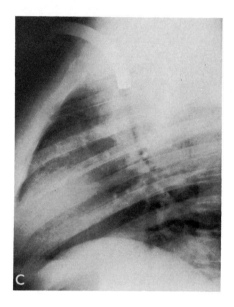

presence of upper airway involvement and the need for intubation.[12]

Retropharyngeal Hemorrhage

Acute upper airway obstruction can result from hemorrhage into the retropharyngeal space from a variety of causes, including neck surgery, external trauma, carotid angiography, transbrachial retrograde catheterization,[13] and erosion of an artery secondary to infection. Hemorrhage also can occur spontaneously in hemophiliacs or in patients with acute leukemia or those receiving anticoagulant therapy.[14]

Foreign Bodies

The aspiration of food (often partly masticated meat) and its lodgment in the larynx is the commonest cause of the "café-coronary syndrome" (Fig. 11–2) (see page 741). As might be anticipated, such obstruction occurs more often in patients with dysfunction of the pharyngeal muscles.

Chronic Upper Airway Obstruction

In contrast with acute upper airway obstruction, the cause of which is generally apparent, chronic obstructive disease of the pharynx, larynx, and trachea frequently is misdiagnosed as asthma or chronic obstructive lung disease. Dyspnea is the usual presenting complaint, often first noted on exertion and sometimes exacerbated when the patient assumes a recumbent position. The diagnosis can be confirmed by the application of standard and specialized roentgenographic procedures and by the demonstration of characteristic physiologic abnormalities on pulmonary function testing.

Physiologic Manifestations

An excellent method of portraying how physiologic determinants of flow can be affected by various obstructing lesions of the conducting system is the flow-volume loop, which combines maximal expiratory and inspiratory curves from total lung capacity (TLC) and residual volume (RV), respectively (Fig. 11–3). In normal subjects, the maximal, or peak, expiratory flow rate (PEFR) occurs early in forced expiration, and the flow ratio between expiratory and inspiratory limbs at mid–vital capacity (VC)(50 per cent) is approximately 1.[15] In asthma, COPD, and other conditions that cause diffuse lower airway obstruction, peak expiratory flow is decreased less than flow at lower lung volumes, and expiratory flow is decreased much more than inspiratory flow, so the mid-VC expiratory-inspiratory ratio is usually

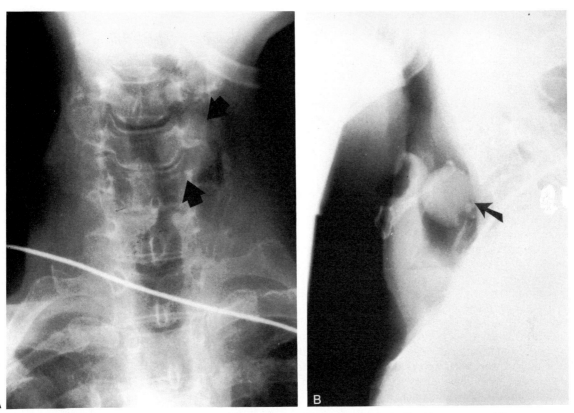

Figure 11–2. Acute Upper Airway Obstruction Caused by a Foreign Body. Roentgenograms of the neck in anteroposterior *(A)* and lateral *(B)* projections reveal a grape-size opacity *(arrows)* situated in the region of the left pyriform sinus immediately above the false vocal cords. This 71-year-old woman presented in acute respiratory distress; direct laryngoscopy revealed a grape, the removal of which resulted in prompt improvement. (Courtesy of Dr. John Fleetham, Health Sciences Centre Hospital, University of British Columbia, Vancouver.)

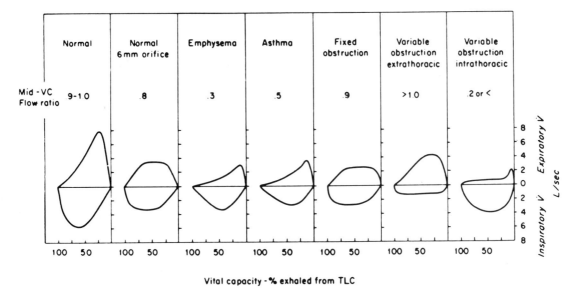

Figure 11–3. Flow-Volume Loops in Various Obstructive Conditions Compared with Normal. Volume is given as a percentage of vital capacity exhaled from total lung capacity. Representative mid–vital capacity flow ratios are given. (Reproduced from Miller RD, Hyatt RE: Obstructing lesions of the larynx and trachea: Clinical and physiologic characteristics. Mayo Clin Proc 44: 145, 1969, with permission of the authors and editor.)

less than 0.5 (*see* Fig. 11–3). By contrast, in upper airway obstruction, flow is decreased to approximately the same extent throughout the forced VC (FVC) and there tends to be a plateau in one or both segments of the flow-volume curve.

The dynamic effects of lesions of the upper airway depend in part on the extent to which the obstruction is "fixed" or "variable." In the former situation, the airway is unable to change cross-sectional area in response to transmural pressure differences, usually as a result of a circumferential benign stricture. By contrast, in "variable" obstruction—a situation that occurs most often with neoplasms that arise from the airway wall and create a crescentic lumen—the airway is able to respond to transmural pressure, thus permitting a variable cross-sectional diameter throughout the forced ventilatory cycle. Characteristic flow-volume loop patterns are produced by fixed and variable lesions (*see* Fig. 11–3). Since fixed upper airway obstruction, either intrathoracic or extrathoracic, is not influenced by transmural pressure gradients, both inspiratory and expiratory flow are proportionally lowered.

When a lesion is variable, however, its location (intrathoracic or extrathoracic) becomes important because the airway responds to transmural pressure. During inspiration, the extrathoracic airway has a transmural pressure favoring narrowing because intraluminal pressure is subatmospheric while extraluminal pressure is approximately atmospheric. During expiration, intraluminal pressure is positive relative to extraluminal pressure, thus tending to dilate the airway and obscure the presence of the lesion. Thus, a variable extrathoracic lesion tends to cause a predominant decrease in maximal inspiratory flow and has relatively little effect on maximal expiratory flow.[16]

This situation is reversed when a variable lesion is intrathoracic in location. During inspiration, extraluminal pressure (equivalent to pleural pressure) is negative relative to intraluminal pressure, so transmural pressure favors airway dilatation. By contrast, during expiration, extraluminal pressure is positive relative to intraluminal pressure, so airway narrowing occurs. Thus, a variable intrathoracic lesion results in a predominant reduction in maximal expiratory flow with relative preservation of maximal inspiratory flow (*see* Fig. 11–3).[16] In addition to these patterns that suggest anatomic upper airway obstruction, periodic flow oscillations caused by fluttering of upper airway structures, either passively or as a result of periodic muscle contraction, may be an important indicator of an abnormality of control of upper airway caliber in neuromuscular disease.[16a]

Since flow-volume loops are not routinely performed in many laboratories, it is important to examine the results of simple spirometry for clues to upper airway obstruction. The diagnosis is suggested by finding a peak expiratory flow rate that is reduced proportionately greater than forced expiratory volume in 1 second (FEV_1).[17] A comparison of FEV_1 and midexpiratory phase forced expiratory flow ($FEF_{25\%-75\%}$) also may be helpful. In the absence of airflow obstruction, the numerical values of FEV_1 and $FEF_{25\%-75\%}$ are roughly comparable, but as lower airway obstruction develops, the $FEF_{25\%-75\%}$ becomes disproportionately lowered. In upper airway obstruction, however, the FEV_1 (reflecting both effort-dependent and effort-independent flow) is decreased to the same extent as $FEF_{25\%-75\%}$, which reflects effort-independent flow only.[18]

Roentgenographic Manifestations

Although theoretically the effects on lung volume of variable intrathoracic and extrathoracic obstructing lesions should be different—the former being associated with expiratory air trapping and overinflation, whereas the latter is not—the assessment of pulmonary overinflation on standard posteroanterior and lateral roentgenograms is subject to so much individual variation that it is of questionable value. However, unequivocal evidence of pulmonary overinflation, particularly in a young patient, should immediately raise the suspicion of upper airway obstruction, especially since overinflation is such a surprisingly infrequent manifestation of spasmodic asthma.

Of much greater importance than this indirect sign of obstructive airway disease is the direct identification of airway narrowing, and it is by this that the roentgenologist can play a very useful—and sometimes vital—role. Obviously, narrowing is almost always identified first on conventional posteroanterior and lateral roentgenograms, bearing in mind the requirement for adequate penetration of the mediastinum in order to see the whole length of the tracheal air column. Once a lesion has been identified, its more precise anatomic nature can be established by tomography, either conventional or computed (CT) (Fig. 11–4). The authors have been repeatedly impressed by the superiority of linear tomography over CT in establishing the extent of tracheal narrowing in cases of postintubation stenosis. However, in patients with primary or secondary neoplasms involving the trachea, CT has been shown to be more accurate in demonstrating the intraluminal presence of tumor, the degree of airway compression, and, most important, the presence or absence of extratracheal extension.[19]

Other roentgenographic techniques that may be of value in selected cases include lateral roentgenograms of the soft tissues of the neck (particularly in infants and young children, in whom abnormalities such as hypertrophied tonsils and adenoids may be responsible for upper airway obstruction), positive contrast laryngography and tracheography, and cine CT.[20]

Two unusual roentgenographic manifestations of chronic upper airway obstruction relate to the heart and pulmonary circulation. The first is pulmonary edema, a complication that is thought to be related to heart failure caused by the very negative intrathoracic pressures acting as an afterload to ventricular ejection. The second is cardiac enlargement resulting from pulmonary arterial hypertension secondary to chronic hypoxemia and acidosis.[21] In fact, some children with certain forms of chronic upper airway obstruction, such as hypertrophied tonsils, can present for the first time in frank right ventricular failure.

Clinical Manifestations

The symptoms of chronic upper airway obstruction are dyspnea and nonproductive cough. Stridor also may be noted either at rest or during exercise, and its timing may be inspiratory, expiratory, or both. The major effect of the

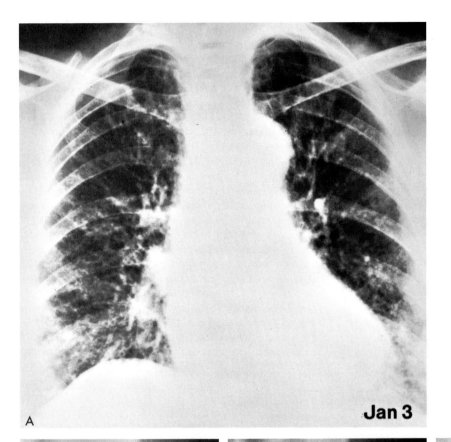

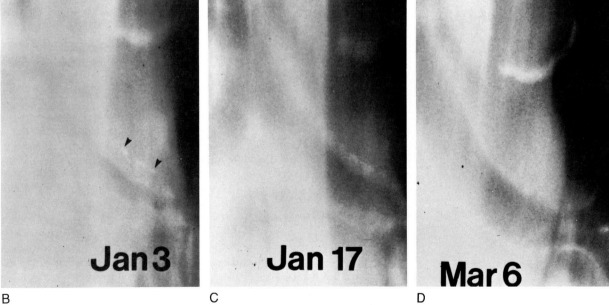

Figure 11–4. Severe Airway Obstruction Caused by Widespread Submucosal Lymphoma. This 71-year-old woman presented for the first time with a 4-month history of increasing dyspnea on mild exertion. The initial roentgenogram *(A)* revealed a rather coarse reticular pattern throughout both lungs. A tomogram of the major airways in anteroposterior projection *(B)* revealed marked narrowing of the airways of the main bronchi. The small *arrowheads* point to calcified cartilaginous rings of the bronchi, indicating marked increase in soft tissue thickness between these rings and the airways owing to thickening of the submucosa. A transbronchial biopsy revealed lymphocytic lymphoma. Antineoplastic therapy was begun immediately, and 2 weeks later the submucosal thickening had diminished considerably *(C)*. Two months after the institution of therapy, the tomogram *(D)* had returned to normal. (Courtesy of The Royal Adelaide Hospital, Adelaide, Australia, and Dr. Peter Macklem, The Royal Victoria Hospital, Montreal.)

obstruction is alveolar hypoventilation, with resultant hypoxia, hypercapnia, and pulmonary arterial hypertension and cor pulmonale.[22]

Hypertrophy of Tonsils and Adenoids

Hypertrophy of the palatine tonsils results in a characteristic roentgenographic appearance of a smooth, well-defined, elliptical mass of unit density extending downward from the soft palate into the hypopharynx (Fig. 11–5). Hypertrophy of the nasopharyngeal adenoids is commonly associated. Both should be readily apparent on lateral roentgenograms of the soft tissues of the neck.

Laryngeal Dysfunction

There are 24 sets of skeletal muscles that are involved in stabilization and closure of the upper airway, most of which are laryngeal muscles. The larynx, therefore, is the site with the greatest potential for upper airway dysfunction. The major laryngeal dilator muscle (abductor) is the posterior cricoarytenoid, and the major constrictors (adductors) are the thyroarytenoid and lateral cricoarytenoid. Paralysis of the abductors causes fixed obstruction of the upper air-

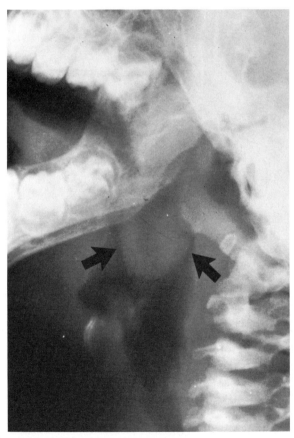

Figure 11–5. Hypertrophied Tonsils Resulting in Upper Airway Obstruction. A view of the soft tissues of the neck in lateral projection reveals a large soft tissue mass *(arrows)* protruding downward into the hypopharynx from the oropharynx. This represents huge hypertrophied tonsils. In addition, there is evidence of moderate enlargement of the nasopharyngeal adenoids. This 3-month-old girl was experiencing severe respiratory distress. (Courtesy of Dr. Bernard Epstein, University of Texas, San Antonio.)

way,[23] whereas unopposed action of adductors results in "laryngospasm." Bulbar involvement in generalized neuromuscular disease causes weakness of the upper airway muscles that may be associated with inspiratory upper airway obstruction and characteristic flow oscillations on flow-volume curves.[24]

One of the principal causes of respiratory obstruction during the neonatal period is collapse of the hypotonic larynx, caused chiefly by infolding of the arytenoid cartilages during inspiration.[25] Congenital hypoplasia of laryngeal structures and redundancy of the mucous membranes of the larynx and subglottic segment of the trachea result in dyspnea and inspiratory-expiratory stridor.

Interruption of the superior laryngeal nerves at the time of thyroidectomy is the commonest cause of bilateral vocal cord paralysis in the adult. It can also occur in rheumatoid disease or poliomyelitis, following viral infections, in association with Guillain-Barré syndrome, or for no apparent reason (idiopathic). Vocal cord paralysis predominantly affects inspiratory flow rates; in one series of 10 patients, the mean expiratory to inspiratory flow ratio at 50 per cent vital capacity was 1.65.[23] Some degree of obstruction can also be caused by unilateral vocal cord paralysis.[26]

A syndrome that mimics asthma termed "emotional laryngeal wheezing" occurs in emotionally disturbed patients and is caused by expiratory glottic narrowing.[27] Episodic, paradoxical inspiratory laryngeal narrowing and stridor result in a syndrome in adults that resembles croup.[28] It can be precipitated by respiratory tract infection and histamine inhalation and abolished by continuous positive airway pressure.

Tracheal Stenosis

One of the commonest causes of chronic upper airway obstruction is tracheal stenosis that occurs as a complication of intubation or tracheostomy. In one study of 342 patients who required prolonged endotracheal intubation,[29] 5 per cent manifested stridor following extubation, and 1.8 per cent required reintubation or tracheostomy. Although reversible laryngeal edema and inflammation were the major causes of the stridor, stricture developed as a result of fibrosis in four patients.

Plastic tubes with inflatable high-compliance balloons are now the most commonly used endotracheal and tracheostomy devices. Once the tube is in position, the cuff is inflated with sufficient air to occlude the tracheal lumen in order to provide an air-tight system at the maximum ventilatory pressure required by the patient. Since the trachea is not circular in cross-section, the circumferential cuff can attain an air-tight seal only by expanding the tracheal lumen and deforming its wall. The tracheal mucosa is easily compressed between the cuffed balloon and the nonyielding tracheal cartilage, and since the pressure may easily exceed capillary pressure, blood supply to the mucosa is compromised, resulting in ischemic necrosis. The lesion begins as a superficial tracheitis and progresses to shallow mucosal ulcerations, usually 2 days or more following the inflation of the cuff. As the tracheal mucosa becomes eroded, the cartilaginous rings are exposed and become softened, split, fragmented, and eventually completely destroyed.[30] Following deflation of the cuff and removal of the tracheostomy tube, fibrosis may occur in the damaged tracheal wall and result in stenosis. Stenosis also may occur at the level of the stoma or, rarely, where the tip of the tube impinges on the tracheal mucosa.[31]

The narrowing of the tracheal lumen typically begins 1 to 1.5 cm distal to the inferior margin of the tracheostomy stoma and involves 1.5 to 2.5 cm of tracheal wall (including two to four cartilaginous rings).[30] Three different roentgenographic appearances have been described: (1) circumferential narrowing of the tracheal lumen over a distance of approximately 2 cm; (2) a thin membrane or diaphragm (caused by granulation tissue rather than mature fibrous tissue) that projects almost at right angles from the tracheal wall; and (3) a long, thickened, eccentric opacity of soft tissue density. Adequate roentgenographic assessment can usually be made by standard films of the chest along with tomography in anteroposterior and lateral projections. Sometimes, precise delineation of the length of stenosis may require opacification. Tracheal cross-sectional areas can be evaluated from posteroanterior and lateral chest roentgenograms or from CT scans[32] and can be compared to published normal values.[33]

Occasionally, tracheomalacia rather than cicatricial stenosis occurs, usually as a result of excessive removal of cartilage at the time of tracheostomy or destruction of cartilage by pressure necrosis and infection.[34] In such circumstances, the increased compliance of the affected tracheal segment can be appreciated by fluoroscopic examination or cinefluorography.

Clinically, most patients are symptom-free for a variable period following removal of the tracheostomy tube. Eventually, however, those who develop stenosis experience increasing difficulty in raising secretions and shortness of breath on exertion. These symptoms may progress to stridor and marked dyspnea on minimal exertion.[30]

Tracheal Neoplasms

Squamous cell carcinoma constitutes 50 per cent or more of cases of primary cancer of the trachea (Fig. 11–6).[35] Adenoid cystic carcinoma is slightly less common. Patients with both neoplasms are frequently treated for asthma for considerable periods of time before the correct diagnosis is made.[36] Dyspnea, hoarseness, and cough are common symptoms. Stridor (inspiratory with extrathoracic lesions, and expiratory with intrathoracic lesions) helps distinguish these patients from those who have lower airway obstruction.

"Saber-Sheath" Trachea

Although considerable variation exists in the shape of the tracheal cartilage rings,[37] the coronal and sagittal diameters of the tracheal air column are roughly equal on posteroanterior and lateral roentgenograms. A condition called "saber-sheath" trachea is characterized by a flattening of the trachea so that the coronal diameter of the intrathoracic trachea is no more than one half of the corresponding sagittal diameter (Fig. 11–7).[38] Generally, the narrow coronal diameter extends the entire length of the intrathoracic trachea from carina to thoracic outlet, at which point the coronal diameter abruptly widens and the sagittal diameter

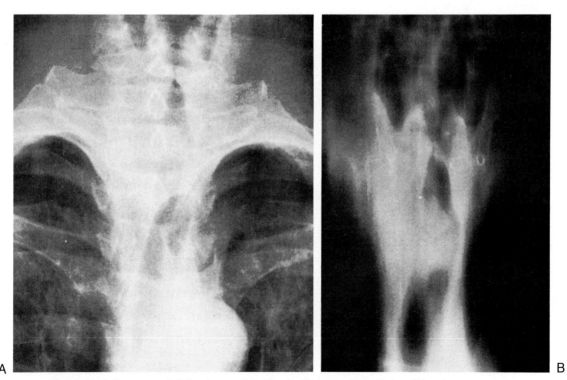

A   B

Figure 11–6. Squamous Cell Carcinoma of the Cervical Trachea. A detail view *(A)* and an anteroposterior tomogram *(B)* reveal severe narrowing of the air column approximately 2 cm distal to the larynx. A large mass can be identified arising from the right wall and extending over a distance of at least 3 cm.

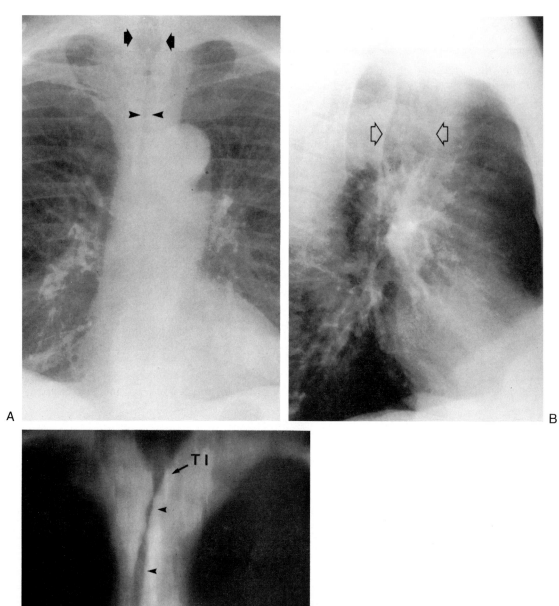

Figure 11–7. Saber-Sheath Trachea. Postero-anterior *(A)* and lateral *(B)* chest roentgeno-grams reveal severe narrowing of the intrathoracic trachea in the coronal plane *(arrowheads)* and widening in the sagittal plane *(open arrows)*, resulting in an abnormal "tracheal index" of 0.20 or less (see text). Note that the extrathoracic trachea *(arrows)* is normal, the narrowing beginning at the thoracic inlet. A linear tomogram in anteroposterior projection *(C)* confirms the narrowing and lobulation *(arrowheads)* and shows that the most severe reduction in caliber extends from the thoracic inlet (TI) to a point slightly above the aortic arch (A). Note that the diameter of the left main bronchus (LB) exceeds that of the trachea.

narrows, the air column thus assuming a normal configuration. This abrupt change in tracheal configuration from intrathoracic to extrathoracic trachea is a consistent finding and almost certainly reflects the influence of intrathoracic transmural pressures. The abnormality occurs in men who are chronic smokers and is associated with chronic obstructive lung disease.[39]

Relapsing Polychondritis

Relapsing polychondritis is an uncommon systemic autoimmune disease that affects cartilage throughout the body, including that in the tracheobronchial tree (see page 408). It can result in thickening of the central airway walls with fixed obstruction[40] or can produce increased compliance and flaccidity of the airways.[41] Either can be rapidly progressive and severe and generally represents a poor prognostic feature of the disease.

Tracheobronchomegaly

This uncommon disorder is characterized by cystic dilatation of the tracheobronchial tree that may extend all the way from the larynx to the periphery of the lung.[42] Although the etiology and pathogenesis are uncertain in all cases, it may be familial[43] and has been associated with Ehlers-Danlos syndrome in adults[44] and cutis laxa in children,[45] suggesting the presence of an underlying defect in connective tissue.

Pathologically, both the cartilaginous and the membranous portions of the trachea and mainstem bronchi show atrophic muscle and elastic tissue, abnormalities that are reflected in easy collapsibility of the airways during forced expiration and cough. This, in turn, leads to recurrent pneumonia, emphysema, bronchiectasis, and parenchymal scarring.

Roentgenologically, the diagnosis is usually apparent at a glance. The calibers of the trachea and major bronchi generally are increased, and the air columns have an irregular corrugated appearance caused by the protrusion of redundant mucosal and submucosal tissue between the cartilaginous rings (sometimes called tracheal diverticulosis). This appearance is often best visualized in lateral projection.[42] Both CT and magnetic resonance imaging (MRI) can be used to demonstrate the abnormal tracheal and bronchial dilatation.[46]

The symptoms of tracheobronchomegaly are usually indistinguishable from those of chronic bronchitis or bronchiectasis. However, the presence of prolonged cough and a loud, harsh, rasping sound on auscultation in a patient who complains of inability to expectorate secretions should arouse suspicion of the diagnosis.[47] Pulmonary function tests typically show decreased expiratory flow rates.[43]

Tracheobronchopathia Osteochondroplastica

Tracheobronchopathia osteochondroplastica (tracheoosteoma, tracheitis chronica ossificans, tracheopathia osteoplastica) is a rare condition characterized by the development of nodules or spicules of cartilage and bone in the submucosa of the trachea and bronchi.[48] It occurs almost exclusively in men older than 50 years of age. In the majority of reported cases, the condition is diagnosed only at

necropsy, having been unsuspected during life.[49] The etiology and pathogenesis are unknown.

Pathologically, the nodules are usually confined to the portions of the tracheal and bronchial walls that normally contain cartilage and can be seen as sessile and polypoid elevations that give the airways a beaded appearance. They may be composed of cartilage alone or of bone with a variable amount of marrow.

Roentgenologically, the findings are variable and are chiefly those resulting from bronchial obstruction.[49] Tomography should clearly reveal the irregular nodular appearance of the tracheal and bronchial air columns and permit identification of bone. CT reveals the tracheal deformity to excellent advantage (Fig. 11–8).[50] Coronal and sagittal MRI or dual-energy digital radiography should demonstrate the deformity even more clearly.

The majority of patients are asymptomatic, the degree of osteochondromatous proliferation being insufficient to cause clinically significant airway narrowing. Occasionally, there is dyspnea, hoarseness, cough, expectoration, wheezing, and hemoptysis.[51] The diagnosis is made most easily at bronchoscopy, the spiculelike formations of bone and cartilage producing a grating sensation as the instrument is passed.

Tracheomalacia

Rather than a specific disease entity, tracheomalacia (tracheobronchomalacia) is a descriptive term that refers to weakness of the tracheal walls and supporting cartilages with resultant easy collapsibility. It is most often acquired, usually secondary to intubation or COPD but occasionally following trauma, chronic or recurrent infection, or relapsing polychondritis.[52] It can also be seen as a primary condition, most often in children and usually associated with a deficiency of cartilage in the tracheobronchial tree.[53] As

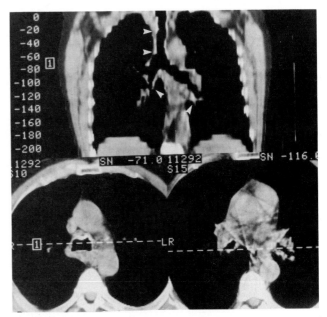

Figure 11–8. Tracheobronchopathia Osteochondroplastica. A coronal CT re-formation and appropriate transverse images through the carina demonstrate extensive tracheal and bronchial wall calcification (*arrowheads*). The tracheal lumen is irregular and slightly narrowed anteriorly and on its right lateral wall.

with tracheobronchomegaly, abnormal flaccidity causes inefficiency of the cough mechanism, resulting in the retention of mucus, recurrent pneumonitis, and bronchiectasis. The symptoms include stridor and shortness of breath.

Miscellaneous Causes of Upper Airway Obstruction

Vascular malformations of the great vessels can result in obstruction of the trachea and main bronchi, the commonest being double and right-sided aortic arch. Aberrant subclavian, innominate, or common carotid arteries[54] and aneurysms of the ascending aorta[55] are also occasional causes. Ankylosis of the cricoarytenoid joint in patients with long-standing rheumatoid arthritis can result in severe airway obstruction.[56] Sarcoidosis,[57] amyloidosis,[58] and substernal goiter[59] should also be borne in mind when evaluating a patient with chronic upper airway obstruction.

OBSTRUCTIVE SLEEP APNEA

Obstructive sleep apnea is a clinical syndrome characterized by asphyxia and sleep fragmentation caused by repeated episodes of upper airway obstruction during sleep. Its prevalence in the general population is unknown, in part because of lack of precise definition of the condition. One definition that has been suggested[60] is more than five instances of apnea per hour of sleep (an instance of apnea being defined as cessation of breathing for more than 10 seconds). If this definition is used, the incidence in the general population is more than 1 per cent.[61] However, this may overestimate the prevalence of the condition, especially in older persons.[62]

To understand the pathophysiology of obstructive sleep apnea, it is necessary to have some knowledge of the physiologic interactions of sleep and breathing. Sleep is categorized as either non–rapid eye movement (NREM) or rapid eye movement (REM) based on the electroencephalographic pattern and on the presence or absence of rapid phasic eye movements on an electro-oculogram. NREM sleep is subdivided into four stages in which there is progressively slower electroencephalographic activity. During the initial 10 to 60 minutes of sleep, frequent changes occur between wakefulness and stages 1 and 2 of NREM sleep. There is irregular breathing, and the average alveolar ventilation decreases with a slight increase in arterial partial pressure of carbon dioxide ($PaCO_2$). With the onset of stages 3 and 4 of NREM sleep, breathing becomes remarkably regular, although tidal volume (VT) and overall expired volume per unit time ($\dot{V}E$) decrease further, and $PaCO_2$ rises 2 to 7 mm Hg.[63] The decreased ventilation during NREM sleep is due primarily to an increase in upper airway resistance caused by decreased activation of upper airway dilating and stabilizing muscles.[64]

With the onset of REM sleep, breathing becomes irregular again. Tidal volume decreases concomitantly with the development of episodes of REMs, and an irregular pattern of rapid, shallow breathing is observed. There is a decrease in neural activation of intercostal respiratory muscles that is part of a generalized supraspinal inhibition of skeletal muscle and a further increase in upper airway resistance.[65] Ventilatory chemosensitivity decreases during all stages of sleep, both hypoxic and hypercapnic ventilatory responses

being depressed. In general, this depression is more pronounced during REM than during NREM sleep. The compensatory response to added external resistive loads is also diminished.[66]

Thus, sleep is a time of particular vulnerability for the respiratory system—the resistance of the system is increased and at the same time both chemical and mechanical sensors of trouble are depressed.

Diagnostic Techniques

The diagnosis of obstructive sleep apnea requires the study of breathing during sleep. The techniques of polysomnography have been reviewed.[67] For physicians interested specifically in respiration, these include sleep staging and the measurement of respiratory effort, air flow, and changes in arterial blood gas tensions. Sleep is staged by visually scoring the polysomnographic record and by categorizing short time periods (called *epochs*) into the appropriate stage based on recordings of the electroencephalogram (EEG) (usually with two electrode positions), the electro-oculogram, and the electromyogram (EMG) of a skeletal muscle (usually the submental).

Respiration is assessed by measuring airflow and respiratory movement. Respiratory effort can be determined with devices that measure rib cage and/or abdominal movement or changes in intrathoracic pressure. Chest and abdominal movements can be measured with a circumferential strain gauge, by transthoracic impedance pneumography, or, most commonly, by respiratory inductance plethysmography (Respitrace). Respiratory air flow can be assessed with a thermistor, a microphone, a pneumotachograph, or an expired carbon dioxide–sensing device. A pneumotachograph requires the use of a face mask, which can interfere with sleep and with the breathing pattern during sleep; however, only this device provides an estimate of VT.

Changes in arterial oxygen saturation can be monitored noninvasively using a pulse oximeter, and there are also devices that measure mean capillary PO_2 and PCO_2 transcutaneously. The final measurements that complete a polysomnographic record are an electrocardiogram to record cardiac dysrhythmias and an audio signal to detect snoring.

At present a complete overnight sleep study is the accepted method for definite diagnosis of obstructive sleep apnea. There is increasing interest, however, in screening for diagnosis in the home or during short-term monitoring.

Pathogenesis

Obstructive sleep apnea results from repeated obstruction of the upper airway, usually at the level of the oropharynx. It has many predisposing factors (Fig. 11–9), two of the most important being gender and obesity. The condition develops 6 to 10 times more frequently in men than in women[67]; in the latter, it usually occurs during the postmenopausal period. The influence of gender may be related to differences in hormones between the sexes. Women with obstructive sleep apnea have elevated androgen levels, and administration of androgens can induce the abnormal state in previously unaffected men and women.[68]

Although early reports suggested that obstructive sleep apnea occurs typically in very obese individuals, the diagnosis is now made more frequently in patients who are of

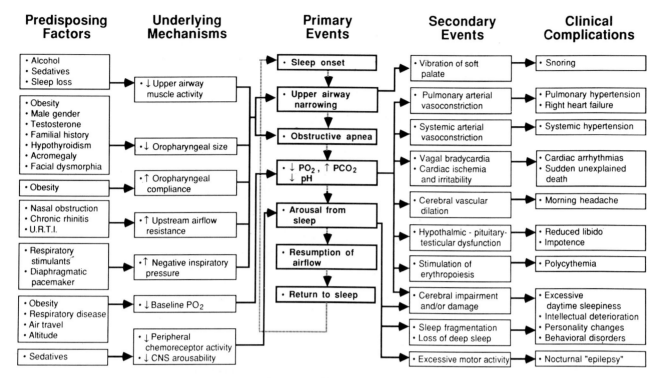

Figure 11–9. The Pathogenesis of Obstructive Sleep Apnea. (Modified from a table constructed by Dr. John Fleetham, Health Sciences Centre Hospital, University of British Columbia, Vancouver.)

normal weight or are only slightly overweight.[69] However, obesity is associated with a higher incidence and severer form of the disorder.[70] The relationship between obesity and obstructive sleep apnea is complex and incompletely understood. It is possible it may increase the risk of the condition by affecting upper airway geometry, since deposition of adipose tissue in the submucosa of the oropharynx and the soft palate can narrow the upper airway and increase its compliance. Supporting this hypothesis is the observation that the pharyngeal cross-sectional area in obese patients with obstructive sleep apnea is less than that in equally obese patients without the disorder.[71] Obesity also decreases functional residual capacity (FRC), especially when the person is in the supine posture. Should FRC fall to a level below closing capacity, nocturnal hypoxemia would result, thus contributing to severer arterial oxygen desaturation during apneic episodes.

The principal mechanisms that have been implicated in the pathogenesis of obstructive sleep apnea include an anatomically narrowed airway, an abnormally collapsible airway (increased compliance), decreased neural drive to upper airway dilating muscles, decreased chemoreceptor stimulation and load compensation of upper airway dilating muscles,[69] and uncoordinated activation of the upper airway muscles (*see* Fig. 11–9).

Structural Narrowing

Although the obstruction of sleep apnea usually occurs at the level of the oropharynx, it can be precipitated by airway narrowing upstream (e.g., in the nasal passages) by virtue of the more negative downstream inspiratory pressures that must be generated.[72] Nasal obstruction also causes mouth breathing, which in itself narrows the lumen by causing the tongue to be displaced posteriorly.

CT or MRI studies of the oropharyngeal airway sometimes show a narrowing of the airway not attributable to a specific cause (Figs. 11–10 and 11–11).[73] Because MRI is sensitive in detecting water content, it also may prove useful in determining whether significant soft tissue swelling contributes to the upper airway narrowing.[74] Snoring may cause edema of the soft palate and uvula, which can exacerbate the obstruction.[75]

Anatomic upper airway narrowing may be suggested by inspiratory-expiratory flow-volume curves that show a ratio of midexpiratory to midinspiratory flow greater than 1[76] or by a "saw-tooth" pattern of flow.[77]

Increased Compliance

The compliance of the upper airway can be measured during sleep by applying negative pressure at the airway opening and determining the negative pressure that results in airway closure.[78] In normal subjects, negative pressures lower than -25 cm H_2O can be applied before closure occurs. In patients with obstructive sleep apnea, however, closure occurs with pressures as low as -0.5 cm H_2O (mean -2.4 during REM and -4.2 cm H_2O during slow wave sleep). Although the principal site of airway narrowing in obstructive sleep apnea is the oropharynx, there is evidence that the nasopharyngeal airway is also narrower and more compliant.[79] The site of the major increase in resistance can differ from patient to patient, which may explain why a single surgical procedure is not universally successful therapy.[80]

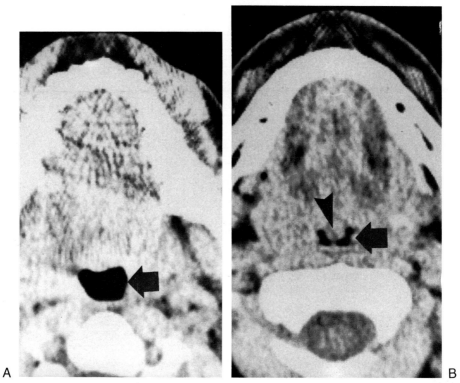

Figure 11–10. Computed Tomography (CT) of the Upper Airway in a Normal Subject and a Patient with Obstructive Sleep Apnea. A CT slice at the level of the oropharynx in a normal subject *(A)* reveals a widely patent oropharynx *(arrow)*. In a patient with obstructive sleep apnea, a CT slice at approximately the same level *(B)* shows a markedly reduced cross-sectional area of the airway *(arrowhead)* and a prominent uvula *(arrowhead)*.

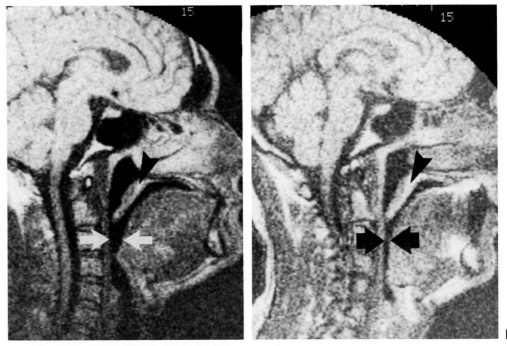

Figure 11–11. Magnetic Resonance imaging (MRI) of the Upper Airway in a Normal Subject and a Patient with Obstructive Sleep Apnea. A sagittal reconstructed magnetic resonance image of the head and neck of a normal subject *(A)* demonstrates the uvula *(arrowhead)* and hypopharyngeal airway *(arrows)*. A similar image of a patient with obstructive sleep apnea *(B)* reveals a slightly enlarged uvula *(arrowhead)* and a markedly narrowed hypopharyngeal airway *(arrows)*. These images were obtained at 8:00 A.M. following an overnight sleep study.

Neuromuscular Dysfunction

Contraction of oropharyngeal muscles during inspiration normally stiffens the walls of the oropharynx, counteracting its tendency to narrow in response to the negative intraluminal pressure that develops during inspiration. Abnormal function of these muscles, therefore, can contribute to upper airway obstruction. The activity of the oropharyngeal muscles is influenced by a number of factors, including changes in lung volume, changes in chemical drive, and input from upper airway receptors.[72] Neural activation of the upper airway dilating muscles is depressed during sleep and by alcohol and sedative drugs.[81, 82] In fact, the sleep deprivation and hypoxia that result from obstructive sleep apnea can cause depression of phasic respiratory activity in the upper airway muscles and can lead to a vicious circle of worsening obstruction and more fragmented sleep.[83]

The pathophysiologic sequence that results in obstructive sleep apnea thus can be summarized as follows. Oropharyngeal narrowing (caused by structural changes and/or a diminution of the force generated by the muscles that maintain airway patency) results in an increase in pharyngeal resistance that causes more negative intrapharyngeal inspiratory pressures and airway closure. Although airway closure increases the neural input to the pharyngeal dilator muscles, it also increases drive to the diaphragm and intercostal inspiratory muscles, thus generating more negative intra-airway pressures, which keep the oropharynx closed. The only escape from such a vicious circle is arousal accompanied by higher center activation of the upper airway dilator muscles and consequent relief of the obstruction.

It is not known which stimulus causes arousal during apneic episodes. Although hypoxemia seems to be the most obvious candidate, administration of oxygen does not invariably prolong the apneic episodes. Arousal frequently occurs when the amount of tension generated by the inspiratory muscles against the occluded upper airway approaches the amount of tension that causes muscle fatigue, suggesting that a message from inspiratory muscles may be an important stimulus.[84]

Clinical Manifestations

Snoring is an invariable sign in patients who suffer from obstructive sleep apnea. It is by no means a sensitive indicator of the disorder, however, since 40 per cent of men and 30 per cent of women are occasional or habitual snorers.[85] In patients with obstructive sleep apnea, snoring is typically interrupted by frequent periods of silent apnea, during which progressively greater inspiratory efforts are expended against a completely closed airway. The apneic periods are terminated by loud snorting and motor activity associated with arousal. With resumption of sleep, rhythmic snoring returns.

A characteristic symptom of obstructive sleep apnea is excessive daytime sleepiness that can range from mild to severe. The frequency and duration of periods of nocturnal apnea and the severity of nocturnal arterial oxygen desaturation correlate well with the severity of hypersomnolence. Patients who have mild hypersomnolence fall asleep while reading, watching television, or listening to lectures, but sleepiness does not interfere with work. As hypersomnolence worsens, patients fall asleep while driving, talking, eating, or relating a medical history and become unable to work. Thirty to 60 apneic episodes per night cause mild hypersomnolence; severe hypersomnolence results when there are more than 400.[75] The severity of hypersomnolence can be quantitated by measuring the time it takes to fall asleep (sleep latency test).[86] Sleep fragmentation caused by frequent arousals, and episodic nocturnal hypoxia probably combine to produce daytime hypersomnolence.[87, 88]

Episodic hypoxemia and profound sleep fragmentation also are the most likely causes of the changes in personality and behavior that can accompany severe obstructive sleep apnea. Confusion with a psychiatric disorder is likely if the excessive sleepiness is attributed to depression. There is a striking incidence of severe psychosocial disruption in the lives of patients with sleep apnea that affects their family, social interactions, and work situations.[89]

The arterial oxygen desaturation associated with apneic episodes causes pulmonary arterial hypertension and an increase in right ventricular afterload.[90] Since prolonged pulmonary hypertension can result in irreversible vascular narrowing, the hypertension may eventually persist during the waking hours, despite correction of hypoxemia. The almost inevitable result is cor pulmonale and, ultimately, right ventricular failure.[91]

Patients with obstructive sleep apnea also may present with systemic arterial hypertension,[92] and this diagnosis must be considered in hypertensive patients, especially when they are obese males or have symptoms of hypersomnolence and snoring.[91] The disorder also can be associated with decreased libido and impotence,[93] nocturnal bradycardia, and, rarely, serious conduction defects or dysrhythmias.[94] Nocturnal hypoxemia can also stimulate erythropoietin secretion and may cause secondary polycythemia.[95]

The prognosis of obstructive sleep apnea is variable. Moderate weight loss and a change in sleeping posture from supine to lateral decubitus can be beneficial in alleviating the symptoms, but these measures are seldom sufficient to reverse them completely.[96] In some patients, surgical removal of part of the uvula, soft palate, and pharyngeal wall (uvulopalatopharyngoplasty) causes long-term relief of symptoms; however, in others this procedure is ineffective. The variation in response is probably related to the variable site of upper airway narrowing. The prospective use of cephalometric roentgenograms, somnofluoroscopy,[97] and CT reconstruction of the upper airway[98] may prove to be beneficial in identifying the patients who will benefit from surgery and may aid in the planning of individual surgical procedures.

ASTHMA

Asthma is a disease characterized by wide variations over short periods of time in resistance to air flow in intrapulmonary airways.[99] In addition, asthmatic subjects show an increased responsiveness of the tracheobronchial tree to a variety of stimuli.[100] The airway narrowing that occurs in asthma is intermittent and variable, complete remission between attacks usually occurring spontaneously or as the result of therapy. However, some residual abnormality of function is often detectable with sensitive tests.[101] Although the reversibility of airway obstruction may be suspected from the clinical history, it should always be evaluated objectively by measurement of airway function after administration of a bronchodilator.[102]

Although asthma is a common disease,[103] there are considerable racial and geographic variations in its prevalence, estimates in children ranging from less than 1 per cent to 20 per cent in different countries.[104] It is unknown to what extent this variation is related to genetic factors, to climate, or to differences in the degree of antigen exposure.[105, 106] The lower incidence of asthma in some tropical countries is believed by some to be related to a protective effect of high serum IgE levels induced by parasitic infestation.[107] That the prevalence of asthma within a population can change is illustrated by the dramatic increase in the number of Papua New Guinea Melanesians who have acquired the disease during the past decade.[108]

Although there may be some overlap, asthma is generally characterized as falling into two major categories, extrinsic and intrinsic.

Extrinsic Asthma. This form occurs in patients who are atopic, a term used to refer to the genetic predisposition to respond to antigenic challenge with excessive IgE production. The inheritance is complex but usually incomplete, and it increases greatly if both parents are atopic. The prevalence of atopy increases until approximately age 20 years, at which point it gradually declines. Peak IgE levels occur at age 14 years; in infants and young children, atopy and asthma are twice as common in males.[109] Besides demonstrating increased blood levels of IgE, atopic individuals characteristically show immediate skin test responses to a variety of antigens and have a high incidence of eczema and rhinitis.

Although patients with extrinsic asthma are invariably atopic, it is important to realize that atopy itself is not synonymous with asthma. The former occurs in more than 30 per cent of the population, whereas the incidence of asthma is generally less than 5 per cent. In addition, although both identical twins invariably develop atopy if one is affected, the development of asthmatic symptoms and nonspecific bronchial hyper-responsiveness are discordant.[110]

Patients with extrinsic asthma are distinguished by several features, including (1) a family history of atopy; (2) onset during the first three decades of life; (3) seasonal symptoms; (4) elevated blood levels of IgE; (5) positive skin and bronchial challenge tests to specific allergens; and (6) a tendency for the disease to remit in later life.[99]

Intrinsic Asthma. Intrinsic (cryptogenic) asthma occurs in patients in whom atopy or specific external triggers of bronchoconstriction cannot be identified. Affected patients are characterized by (1) being older than patients with extrinsic disease; (2) a lack of family history of asthma or allergic disease; (3) an absence of elevated blood levels of IgE or positive skin or bronchial response to allergen challenge; (4) increased numbers of blood and sputum eosinophils; (5) an increased incidence of autoimmune disease and of autoantibodies to smooth muscle; (6) decreased responsiveness to therapy; and (7) a tendency to persistent and progressive disease resulting in fixed airflow obstruction.[99]

Pathologic Characteristics

The basic pathophysiologic abnormality that determines the functional and symptomatic status of an asthmatic pa-

tient is airway narrowing. This may occur by three main mechanisms: (1) airway smooth muscle contraction; (2) edema and congestion of the airway wall; and (3) plugging of the airway lumen by mucus and inflammatory exudate. For the most part, it is difficult, if not impossible, to determine in a given patient at a given time what proportion of obstruction is caused by each of these mechanisms. However, it may be reasonably concluded that when obstruction is rapidly reversible following inhalation of cholinergic antagonists or beta-adrenergic agonists, the pathogenesis is smooth muscle contraction. On the other hand, when obstruction responds over a period of days to steroids and other therapeutic interventions, it is probably caused predominantly by edema and mucous plugging.[111]

At autopsy, the lungs of patients who die of asthma are distended and typically project above the cut ends of the ribs and across the midline of the thorax when the chest is opened. There is evidence of subsegmental atelectasis, and the bronchi are plugged with viscid, tenacious mucus (the increased viscidity being at least partly related to an increase in mucus protein content, particularly of albumin).[112] The mucus plugs are most frequent in bronchi and larger membranous bronchioles, but they often extend to the level of respiratory bronchioles[113] and typically completely fill the airway lumen (Fig. 11–12). Scattered within them is a variable number of eosinophils and ciliated cells derived from the airway epithelium.

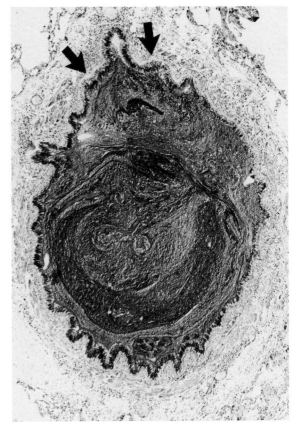

Figure 11–12. Asthma: Mucous Plugging. A histologic section of a small bronchus shows it to be completely occluded by a dense plug of mucus strongly positive for periodic acid–Schiff (PAS) stain. Thickening of the basement membrane is evident as a lightly stained subepithelial stripe *(arrows)*. Note the strong PAS positivity of the epithelium, indicating extensive goblet cell hyperplasia. (PAS × 40.)

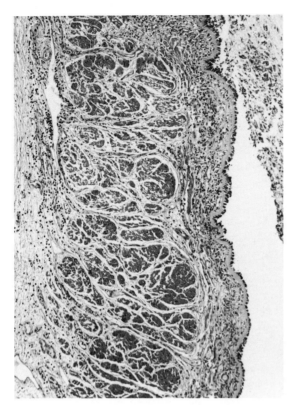

Figure 11–13. Asthma: Bronchial Wall Abnormalities. A histologic section of bronchial wall shows marked thickening of the muscularis mucosa, numerous inflammatory cells, and a uniformly thickened basement membrane. The bronchial epithelium is composed only of a row of cuboidal basal cells, the ciliated and goblet cells having been shed into the overlying mucus. (× 40.)

the mediators actually stimulate increased ciliary beat frequency.[117] Despite this, some asthmatic patients have been found to have a ciliary inhibitory compound in their sputum.[118] Prolonged therapy of asthmatic patients with corticosteroids for 4 weeks has been shown to result in improved mucociliary clearance, despite more peripheral deposition of the inhaled radiolabel.[119]

Nonspecific Bronchial Responsiveness

Nonspecific bronchial hyper-responsiveness (NSBH, bronchial hyper-reactivity, bronchial hyperexcitability) represents the exaggerated airway narrowing that occurs in response to inhalation of a variety of nonallergenic, usually pharmacologic stimuli. The authors use "nonspecific bronchial responsiveness" as the generic term for this phenomenon and "nonspecific bronchial hyper-responsiveness" for the exaggerated responsiveness seen in asthmatic patients.[120] Although all the stimuli used to demonstrate NSBH result in some degree of airway narrowing in normal subjects, it is the excessive narrowing at very much lower doses or concentrations that characterizes NSBH. This narrowing is caused predominantly by airway smooth muscle shortening, since it is rapid in onset and readily reversible with bronchodilators.[121]

NSBH renders asthmatic subjects susceptible to excessive airway narrowing in response to a wide variety of inhaled irritants. In fact, it is probable that the majority of everyday symptoms experienced by asthmatic patients are secondary to an exaggerated response to otherwise trivial inhalational exposures. The nonspecific nature of the exaggerated response has become increasingly apparent, and the list of substances to which asthmatic patients respond excessively is continually enlarging. Among the pharmacologic agents are histamine, pilocarpine, methacholine, carbachol, acetylcholine, serotonin, bradykinin, prostaglandin $F_{2\alpha}$ ($PGF_{2\alpha}$), leukotrienes C_4 and D_4, and adenosine.[121] Asthmatics also show excessive airway narrowing in response to inhalation of atmospheric pollutants, dust, hypotonic or hypertonic aerosols, and cold and dry air, and to certain respiratory maneuvers such as a deep inspiration or forced expiration to RV.[121]

It is most likely that NSBH is a consequence of asthma rather than a genetically determined factor predisposing to its development.[122] NSBH can change over time with exposure to infectious agents,[123] environmental pollutants,[124] or specific antigens or sensitizers.[125] Normal airway responsiveness has been reported in asymptomatic monozygotic twins of asthmatic patients who have airway hyper-responsiveness.[122]

NSBH is so characteristic of asthma that it is questionable whether a diagnosis can be made in its absence.[126] Rarely, patients with occupational asthma or nonoccupational extrinsic asthma do not show increased NSBH at the time of diagnosis but develop increased responsiveness with prolonged exposure.[127] Although NSBH is virtually 100 per cent sensitive in the *diagnosis* of asthma, it is far from being specific. For example, it has been demonstrated in patients with sarcoidosis,[128] extrinsic allergic alveolitis,[129] and COPD,[130] although in these conditions it appears to be related to a baseline decrease in airway caliber. In addition, about 5 to 6 per cent of otherwise normal individuals dem-

Most knowledge of the histologic features of asthma has been derived from the study of lungs obtained at autopsy. Evidence provided by bronchial biopsy, however, confirms that similar changes occur in less severe disease, although they can diminish between attacks.[113a] Such changes include goblet cell metaplasia, basement membrane thickening, edema and vascular congestion of the lamina propria, smooth muscle hyperplasia, and a more or less intense mural infiltrate of eosinophilic leukocytes (Fig. 11–13). Often, there is also histologic evidence of airway epithelial damage, particularly in patients who have died of the disease. In these individuals, the surface columnar cells are typically detached, leaving only a layer of basal cells. The pathogenesis of this damage is unknown.

Mucus and Mucociliary Clearance in Asthma

Although airway mucous plugging plays an important role in the pathogenesis of asthma, there are no specific abnormalities in the biochemical composition or viscoelastic properties of airway mucus in asthmatic subjects.[114] A long list of putative mediators of asthma are known to increase the quantity of mucus secretion, including histamine, prostaglandins, alpha-adrenergic agonists, and lipoxygenase products of arachidonic acid metabolism.[115] Radioaerosol techniques reveal impaired mucociliary clearance rates in patients with stable asthma.[116] The depressed clearance is most likely related to the excessive mucus production, since

onstrate bronchial hyper-responsiveness.[131] The methods that can be used to quantify nonspecific bronchial responsiveness are described in Chapter 3 (*see* page 160).

Pathogenesis

Many factors have been proposed to explain NSBH, including a change in the starting airway caliber, altered bronchial mucosal permeability, abnormalities of smooth muscle and neurohormonal control, decreased muscle load, and inflammation.

Starting Airway Caliber. Because airway resistance is related to the fourth power of the radius with both laminar and turbulent flow regimens, the effect of a given degree of narrowing is greater in previously narrowed airways. This observation has led to the theory that decreased starting airway caliber could be a contributor to NSBH. In addition to this geometric effect, decreased baseline airway caliber could alter the deposition pattern of inhaled aerosol particles. Since central airway resistance is an important component of total resistance, preferential central deposition could result in NSBH.

If starting airway caliber were an important contributor to NSBH, a relationship would be expected between the baseline resistance or expiratory flow rates and the responsiveness to challenge. Although such a relationship has been clearly shown in patients with COPD and other nonasthmatic diseases associated with NSBH,[132] studies in asthmatic subjects have generally failed to show such a relationship.[133] However, airway wall thickening internal to the smooth muscle layer as a result of edema or connective tissue deposition might have only a slight effect on baseline resistance but may still greatly amplify the effects of smooth muscle contraction.[134] The importance of starting airway caliber in general and airway wall thickening caused by edema and/or smooth muscle hypertrophy, in particular, awaits more quantitative studies of airway morphometry in normal and diseased airways.[134]

Increased Bronchial Mucosal Permeability. To have any effect, inhaled agonists must cross a layer of respiratory tract secretions, bronchial epithelium, and lamina propria to reach receptor sites on smooth muscle. Since the respiratory epithelium is characteristically damaged in patients with asthma, it seems reasonable to assume that a greater proportion of inhaled agonist might reach receptors on smooth muscle.[135] There is poor correlation, however, between measures of bronchial mucosal permeability and NSBH in asthmatic subjects,[136] and smokers who do have increased mucosal permeability do not necessarily demonstrate hyper-responsiveness.[137]

Abnormalities of Neurohormonal Control. Airway smooth muscle is innervated by the autonomic nervous system and is equipped with membrane receptors for a wide variety of circulating excitatory and inhibitory substances.[121] Thus, bronchial hyper-responsiveness could theoretically be caused by excessive cholinergic efferent activity, excessive afferent stimulation with resultant reflex bronchoconstriction, deficient beta-adrenergic relaxation, or deficient noncholinergic, nonadrenergic inhibitory innervation.

Although there is some evidence that the cholinergic parasympathetic system is excessively responsive in asthmatic subjects,[138] it cannot explain NSBH because it fails to

account for the nonspecificity of the exaggerated airway response. Asthmatic subjects show exaggerated responsiveness to agents that do not act via the afferent cholinergic pathway. A similar argument dictates that increased sensitivity of vagal afferents cannot explain the nonspecific nature of the hyper-responsiveness; asthmatic subjects show exaggerated airway narrowing in response to methacholine, which has little effect on vagal afferents.[139] It is possible that excessive release of inflammatory neuropeptides, such as substance P, could contribute to airway hyper-responsiveness by provoking an inflammatory response in the airway wall.

The most persistent hypothesis to explain NSBH is the theory of partial beta-adrenergic blockade.[140] There is considerable evidence that beta-adrenergic responsiveness is altered in asthma. The blood leukocytes of asthmatic subjects have decreased beta-adrenergic receptor number and function.[141] Deficient beta-adrenergic relaxation of airway smooth muscle from asthmatic subjects has been reported *in vitro*.[142] Some studies suggest that the decreased responsiveness is the result of exogenous beta-adrenergic administration, with resulting down-regulation of beta-receptor number and function.[143] Others, however, have found an increase in the density of beta-adrenergic receptors on the airway smooth muscle of asthmatic patients who have died. Further support for a role of the beta-adrenergic system in the abnormal control of airway caliber in asthma is provided by the studies that show profound bronchoconstriction following administration of beta-blocking drugs.[144] Despite this evidence, deficient beta-adrenergic responses cannot be the sole or even the major cause of NSBH, since exaggerated bronchoconstriction does not develop in normal subjects in response to nonspecific stimuli, even when profound beta-adrenergic blockade is produced by systemic or inhaled beta-blocking agents.[145]

The third component of the airway autonomic nervous system is the so-called nonadrenergic noncholinergic inhibitory system (NANCi). NANCi-induced relaxation of human airway smooth muscle can be demonstrated *in vitro*[146] and *in vivo*,[147] but there does not appear to be a deficiency of this relaxation in asthmatic airway tissue[147a] or subjects.[148] There is evidence to support vasoactive intestinal polypeptide (VIP) and/or nitric oxide (NO) as the primary mediators of the NANCi responses.[149]

Abnormalities of Smooth Muscle. Several alterations in airway smooth muscle might underlie NSBH. When smooth muscle is activated by a neurotransmitter or a mediator, calcium enters the cytosol from intracellular sequestration sites and from the extracellular space. The high levels of calcium initiate an enzymatic process that ultimately causes cross-bridge formation between actin and myosin filaments. It is these cross-bridges that generate smooth muscle tension and shortening and that cause airway narrowing.[150] Removal of free calcium from the cytosol causes smooth muscle relaxation. Thus, airway hyper-responsiveness could occur as a result of either increased calcium availability from one of its sources or decreased removal of intracellular calcium. Increased contraction of the actin-myosin chain in response to calcium release is another possible cause.[151] Alternatively, the increased smooth muscle mass that has been well documented in the airways of asthmatic subjects could be responsible for exaggerated airway narrowing.[152]

If a basic abnormality of smooth muscle contraction was at the basis of airway hyper-responsiveness, one might expect to be able to demonstrate an exaggerated response *in vitro*. However, in the few studies in which human asthmatic airway tissue has been available for pharmacologic study, the results have been disappointing.[153] Although a small number of asthmatic patients appear to have supernormal contractile responses to histamine,[154] in most the potency and efficacy of contractile agonists are the same as those in nonasthmatic subjects.

Decreased Smooth Muscle Load. Once smooth muscle is activated, it narrows the airway by shortening. The degree to which it does this in response to a given stimulus depends on the load against which the muscle must shorten. Smooth muscle acts against elastic loads that increase as shortening increases and that ultimately limit the degree of shortening.[155] In large cartilaginous airways, the muscle is loaded by the outward recoil of airway cartilage,[156] whereas in smaller intraparenchymal airways it is the elastic recoil of the lung that imparts the elastic load. As the airway narrows, local lung parenchyma becomes distorted, increasing transmural pressure and converting more of the smooth muscle activation to tension generation rather than to shortening.[134] Another load on smooth muscle is related to the folding of the basement membrane, lamina propria, and epithelium that is produced as the airway narrows.[157] Softening of airway cartilage, decrease in lung elastic recoil or increased deformability of the airway wall could contribute to the increased airway responses of asthma by decreasing the elastic load on airway smooth muscle.

Inflammation. Bronchial hyper-responsiveness develops in normal subjects following viral respiratory tract infections[158] or exposure to ozone or other atmospheric pollutants.[124] NSBH also increases with infection and pollutant exposure in asthmatic subjects and is enhanced following specific antigen challenge.[159] Occupational exposure to plicatic acid, a component in Western Red Cedar (*Thuja plicata*) dust[160] and to toluene diisocyanate (TDI) in the plastic and paint industries[161] may lead to profound NSBH in sensitive individuals, and the hyper-responsiveness may diminish or disappear following cessation of exposure.[162] A feature common to all these agents is the development of airway inflammation.[163] This is characterized by an initial exudative phase, during which mucosal and vascular permeability is increased, and is followed by a cellular phase, during which acute inflammatory cells migrate from the circulation into the airway wall, particularly the epithelium. This in turn is accompanied by sloughing of epithelial cells and by mucus hypersecretion.[124]

There are several mechanisms by which airway inflammation might result in hyper-responsiveness. As discussed previously, the increased endothelial and epithelial permeability may result in greater exposure of airway smooth muscle and irritant receptors to inhaled antigens. However, failure to demonstrate hyperpermeability in stable but hyper-responsive asthmatic patients makes this unlikely as the sole explanation for NSBH.[136] Alternatively, the increased vascular permeability caused by the inflammatory process could result in airway wall edema.[164] By the geometric factors discussed previously, the resulting thickening may enhance the airway narrowing effect of a given degree of smooth muscle shortening. Finally, the release of secondary mediators from inflammatory cells may directly alter smooth muscle responsiveness.[165]

The suggestion that chronic airway inflammation might be the underlying pathophysiologic inducer of NSBH has resulted in a number of studies designed to decrease hyper-responsiveness with chronic anti-inflammatory therapy. In these studies, prolonged (weeks to months) treatment with inhaled sodium cromoglycate[166] or inhaled[167] or oral[168] corticosteroids has generally shown some decrease in NSBH.

Clinical Usefulness

There are patients in whom the clinical history of asthma may not be clear and who demonstrate normal spirometric values at the time of examination, thus precluding assessment of bronchodilator response; in these subjects, measurement of NSBH is a very useful adjunct to diagnosis (Fig. 11–14).[169] Such measurement is particularly helpful in patients with the isolated symptom of chronic cough, in whom the demonstration of increased NSBH aids in predicting whether the patient will respond symptomatically to the inhalation of beta-adrenergic agents.[169] Tests of NSBH are less useful in patients who are already obstructed[132, 170]; in these patients, the history and response to bronchodilators are usually diagnostic.[171]

Because NSBH can be altered by treatment, it also can be used as an indicator of the effectiveness of therapy and the need for more or less intensive therapy.[172] In an occupational setting, serial measurements of NSBH also may be of particular value; the development or worsening of NSBH with occupational exposure and its gradual improvement following withdrawal of exposure constitute strong evidence that the symptoms are work related.[173]

Provoking Factors

Although asthma is a chronic disease, there are a variety of insults that provoke exacerbations of the process, result-

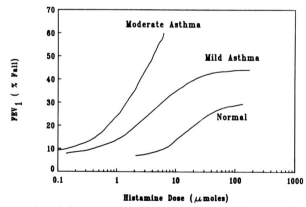

Figure 11–14. Histamine Dose-Response Curves. The percentage fall in the forced expiratory volume in 1 second (FEV_1) is plotted against the dose of inhaled histamine for a normal subject and patients with mild and moderate asthma. In the normal subject and the patient with mild asthma, a plateau is reached on the dose-response curve. In the patient with moderate asthma, there is no plateau despite a 60 per cent decrease in FEV_1. Asthma is characterized by a shift of the dose-response curve to the left and an increase in the maximal response. (Modified from Woolcock AJ, Salome CM, Yan K: The shape of the dose-response curve to histamine in asthmatic and normal subjects. Am Rev Respir Dis 130: 71, 1984.)

ing in acute episodes of dyspnea and wheezing. Some of these provoking factors contribute to the ongoing inflammatory process as well as cause acute airway narrowing. Other factors simply stimulate airway narrowing by the mechanism of NSBH.[174]

Allergens

Specific antigens can provoke asthmatic attacks in sensitized persons. Such individuals frequently suffer from other allergic manifestations, such as hay fever and eczema, and usually manifest positive prick or intradermal skin tests to a variety of allergens. Such hypersensitivity is common. Surveys of the population at large using skin tests indicate that approximately 30 per cent of individuals have a positive reaction to at least one allergen.[175] Fortunately, many of these sensitive individuals are asymptomatic, and those with allergies usually suffer from only seasonal or perennial rhinitis. Besides skin tests, specific allergy to individual antigens can be proved by using an inhalation challenge test[176] or by employing an assay of the specific IgE blood levels for various antigens—the radioallergosorbent test (RAST).[177]

Potential antigens in our environment are innumerable. Although grass and tree pollens cause positive skin reactions and inhalation challenge in many atopic asthmatic subjects, they are not thought to be common causes of asthmatic attacks. Whole ragweed pollen grains are too large to be inspired into the lower respiratory tract; however, fragmented particles are a common cause of hay fever and asthma.[178] Fungal spores are a major source of airborne allergens, usually outnumbering pollen spores by as much as 1000 to 1. The most commonly recognized forms are the imperfect fungi, which include *Alternaria, Aspergillus, Cladosporium, Mucor,* and *Penicillium* species; however, additional entire families have been relatively ignored and may be important.[179] Animal dander from a variety of household pets, including the gerbil and guinea pig in addition to the more ubiquitous cat and dog, may cause ocular and nasal symptoms as well as asthma.[179] Proteins derived from a variety of insects also are an important source of aeroallergens; the most potent and ubiquitous is that derived from the house dust mite *Dermatophagoides pteronyssinus.* This organism thrives in house dust, especially in damp environments, and is an important cause of asthma, especially in children.[180] In addition to aeroallergens, a variety of protein antigens in foods, particularly eggs, fish, nuts, spices, and chocolate, can cause allergy and asthma, again especially in children.

The pathogenesis of allergen-mediated asthma is related to binding of IgE to tissue mast cells and blood basophils. When a specific allergen is inhaled or ingested and comes in contact with antibody in the airway, it causes synthesis and release of inflammatory mediators. These mediators cause contraction of airway smooth muscle, increased bronchial vascular and airway epithelial permeability, increased airway mucus secretion, and attraction of inflammatory cells to the airway as well as their activation.

When IgE antibody and antigen interaction occurs on mast cells throughout the body, anaphylaxis occurs. Airway narrowing as a result of the local release of mediators in the airways is only a component of this generalized re-

sponse, in which hypotension and upper airway obstruction caused by edema may play a more striking role. Anaphylaxis may occur after the oral or parenteral administration of drugs,[181] of which penicillin is the most frequent culprit.[182] Other causes include bee and wasp stings[181] and parenteral administration of iodinated contrast agents.[183] The condition can be rapidly fatal, most often as a result of asphyxia due to laryngeal edema or acute bronchoconstriction. Sometimes, the clinical presentation may be one of circulatory collapse and hypovolemia.[184]

When a sensitized individual inhales antigen, mediators released from mast cells cause an immediate or early response characterized by bronchoconstriction, which reaches a maximum in 15 to 30 minutes and is followed by a return toward normal lung function even without treatment.[185] The severity of bronchoconstriction is related to the degree of allergy and the nonspecific bronchial responsiveness.[186] The former can be determined by quantitative skin testing[186] or RAST testing[187] and relates to the amounts of specific IgE and mediator released for a given antigen dose. The severity of NSBH determines the degree of bronchial narrowing that will occur when a given amount of mediator is released.

In some patients, the early response is followed by a late or delayed response that comes on between 3 and 10 hours after the initial challenge and may persist for 48 hours (Fig. 11–15). This late response may be related to the presence of inflammatory cells attracted by chemotactic factors released during the early response. In some patients, a single-antigen inhalation challenge is followed by recurrent noc-

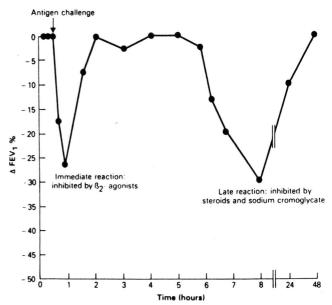

Figure 11–15. Immediate and Late Allergic Airway Response. This graph reveals the response when asthmatic patients are challenged with a specific antigen to which they are allergic: they can develop an immediate bronchoconstriction that generally wanes by 1 hour, followed by a late reaction that begins 4 to 6 hours after challenge and can last as long as 24 hours. Beta-adrenergic agonists effectively inhibit the immediate allergic reaction but have less effect on alleviating the late response. Both the immediate and the late responses can be inhibited by sodium cromoglycate, whereas steroid therapy attenuates the late response but has no influence on the immediate response.

turnal episodes of asthma.[188] Occasionally, individuals develop only a delayed response to inhaled antigen. Although it was initially believed that the late response might be mediated by IgG antibody, it is now accepted that it is a delayed result of the immediate IgE–mast cell interaction.

Besides being more prolonged, the late asthmatic response differs from the immediate response with respect to modulation by pharmacologic interventions. Beta-adrenergic agonists in sufficient concentration effectively block the immediate response but are much less effective against the delayed response; corticosteroids do not influence the immediate response but attenuate the late response; and sodium cromoglycate blocks both the immediate and the late responses.[189] The similarity of the pathology of the late phase response to that of chronic asthma suggests that the former may be the link between immediate hypersensitivity reactions and the subacute or chronic airway disease that characterizes the majority of patients with asthma. Re-

peated late responses to antigen can result in chronic structural and functional changes in the airway. A similar common final pathway of airway inflammation may explain the similarity of airway function and pathology in asthmatic patients in whom asthma is triggered by nonallergic mechanisms.[190]

Mediators and Cells

The inflammatory mediators and cells that have been implicated in the acute and chronic inflammatory reactions of asthma are summarized in Table 11–1.

Histamine. Several experimental observations suggest that this is an important mediator in asthma. Administration of histamine by aerosol can cause many of the symptoms and physiologic derangements that occur during acute attacks of asthma. The fact that oral or parenteral antihistamine administration does not significantly decrease the re-

Table 11–1. INFLAMMATORY MEDIATORS AND CELLS INVOLVED IN ASTHMA

Mediator or Cell	Source	Stimulus	Action(s)
Histamine	Mast cells and basophils present preformed in granules	Allergen-IgE interaction Exercise Distilled water aerosol Dry air hyperpnea	Smooth muscle contraction Increased vascular permeability Increased mucus secretion Stimulation of afferent nerves
Neutrophil chemotactic factor of anaphylaxis (NCFA)	Mast cells present preformed in granules	Allergen-IgE interaction Exercise Dry air hyperpnea	Chemotactic: Attracts and activates neutrophils
Eosinophil chemotactic factor of anaphylaxis (ECFA)	Mast cells present preformed in granules	Allergen-IgE interaction Exercise Dry air hyperpnea	Chemotactic: Attracts and activates eosinophils
Platelet activating factor (PAF)	Mast cells + basophils	Allergen-IgE interaction	Smooth muscle contraction Increased vascular permeability Chemotactic for inflammatory cells Smooth muscle hyperplasia or hypertrophy?
Prostaglandins (PGD_2, $PGF_{2\alpha}$, PGE_1, PGE_2)	A variety of inflammatory and tissue cells. Synthesized de novo	Allergen-IgE interaction Other nonspecific stimuli	PGD_2 + $PGF_{2\alpha}$ Smooth muscle contraction Increased vascular permeability Chemotactic for inflammatory cells PGE_1 and PGE_2 Bronchodilatation
Leukotrienes (LTC_4, LTD_4, + LTE_4, LTB_4)	A variety of inflammatory and tissue cells Synthesized de novo	Allergen-IgE interaction Other nonspecific stimuli	LTC_4, LTD_4, + LTE_4 Smooth muscle contraction Increased vascular permeability Increased mucus production LTB_4 Chemotactic for inflammatory cells
Kallikreins	Basophils	Allergen-IgE interaction Other nonspecific stimuli?	Generates kinins from plasma kininogen Smooth muscle contraction Stimulation of afferent receptors Increased vascular permeability
Neutral proteases and acid hydrolases	Mast cells present preformed in granules	Allergen-IgE interaction	Tissue injury?
Substance P and other neuropeptides	Afferent nerve fibers in the airway wall	Afferent nerve stimulation	Smooth muscle contraction Increased vascular permeability Increased mucus production
Toxic oxygen radicals	Activated inflammatory cells	Inflammatory cell activation	Smooth muscle contraction Tissue damage
Eosinophils	Circulating blood	Chemotactic factors	Enzyme release Major basic protein and eosinophil cationic protein release Tissue damage
Neutrophils	Circulating blood	Chemotactic factors	Enzyme, mediator, and toxic oxygen radical release Tissue damage

sponse to inhaled antigen could be related to an ineffective concentration of antagonist at the site of histamine release in the airways.[191] Although stimulation of H_2 receptors on the smooth muscle of various animal species results in bronchodilatation or attenuation of the H_1 constrictor response, the presence of significant H_2 receptor–induced relaxation of smooth muscle in humans remains doubtful.[192] On the other hand, H_2 receptors located on cells other than smooth muscle may be important modulators of the allergic response. For example, H_2 receptors on suppressor cell lymphocytes may allow histamine-induced modulation of IgE production.[193] Both H_1 and H_2 receptors may be present on mast cells, so histamine release can feed back to modulate subsequent mediator release.[194]

Neutrophil and Eosinophil Chemotactic Factors. Although these substances do not have any immediate effect on airway function, the cells that their release attracts to the airways may have an important role in inducing the late response to inhaled allergen and may contribute to the chronic inflammatory response in the airways of asthmatic subjects.[195]

Leukotrienes. These substances have a wide variety of proinflammatory effects on the airways. The leukotrienes that have been identified as the substances that make up slow-reacting substance of anaphylaxis (SRS-A) are potent bronchoconstrictors, and their inhibition by specific antagonists results in decreased response to allergen[196] and exercise[197] and improved symptoms after prolonged administration.[198] Although virtually all cells have the ability to generate prostaglandins, the amount and type produced are dependent on the enzyme content of the individual cell type. Prostaglandins can both contract and relax airway smooth muscle. In normal subjects, PGE_1 and PGE_2 usually cause bronchodilatation.[199] Prostaglandin F is the best known of the bronchoconstricting prostaglandins; asthmatic patients are up to 8000 times more sensitive to PGF than are healthy normal subjects.[200] Prostaglandin D_2 is released in substantial amounts after IgE challenge of human lung and is a potent bronchoconstrictor in normal and asthmatic subjects.[201]

Additional evidence implicating prostaglandins in the pathogenesis of asthma is provided by studies showing that acetylsalicylic acid (ASA), indomethacin, and other analgesics provoke asthma and anaphylaxis in some individuals. It is thought that this is related to the ability of these agents to block cyclooxygenase, the first enzyme in the pathway of prostaglandin synthesis (*see* later).[202]

Inflammatory Cells. Although it is believed that mast cells and basophils are the most important mediator-releasing cells, at least in allergic asthma, the "secondary" inflammatory cells, such as eosinophils, neutrophils, macrophages, and lymphocytes, probably play an important role in perpetuating the chronic inflammation and in damaging and altering airway tissue cells.

Exercise

Exercise-induced asthma (EIA) is present when excessive airway narrowing and reduction in maximal expiratory flow rates accompany moderate or vigorous exercise. It is not a separate form of asthma, but rather should be considered as a trigger for airway narrowing in patients *who have*

asthma. It is equally common in highly trained athletes and unfit subjects.[203]

Defined as a decrease in FEV_1 or PEFR greater than 10 per cent, EIA occurs in 70 to 80 per cent of patients with asthma who exercise at 80 to 90 per cent of their maximal work load for 6 to 8 minutes.[204] The bronchoconstriction usually peaks 5 to 12 minutes after the cessation of exercise and spontaneously remits within 30 to 60 minutes. The majority of patients are refractory to the induction of a second episode of EIA for approximately 2 hours. Late bronchoconstriction in response to exercise can also occur, particularly in children,[204] although it is extremely rare in adults.[205]

A major advance in our understanding of EIA came with the observation that airway narrowing can be completely abolished if the inspired air during exercise is warmed to body temperature and saturated with water vapor (37°C and a water content of about 46 mg per L).[206, 207] In fact, the degree of airway obstruction following identical exercise challenges can be modified by altering the inspired air conditions: the colder and drier the air breathed during exercise, the greater the subsequent response.[208] Moreover, exercise is not even necessary to produce "EIA," the airway response being reproducible by the isocapnic hyperventilation of unconditioned air.[209] With identical inspired air conditions, there is a dose-response relationship between ventilation and the severity of bronchoconstriction in patients with asthma whether the ventilation is associated with exercise or with isocapnic hyperventilation (hyperventilation-induced bronchoconstriction [HIB]). In individual patients, the degree of bronchoconstriction in response to either exercise or isocapnic hyperventilation depends on the level of nonspecific bronchial responsiveness.[210]

These observations have led to the conclusion that EIA is related to an exaggerated response to cooling and/or drying of the airways. When the temperature and water content of inspired air is less than 37°C and 100 per cent relative humidity, heat and water are lost from the respiratory tract. During resting levels of ventilation, especially during nose breathing, the inspired air is warmed and humidified prior to its reaching the glottis, and any cooling or drying is confined to the upper airway. During exercise or isocapnic hyperventilation, however, unconditioned air can reach the lung and cool and dry the tracheobronchial tree. It is still unclear whether it is the cooling of the lower airway or the drying of the surface liquid that triggers EIA and HIB.[211] However, when the temperature and water content of inspired air are varied so as to produce a range of total respiratory heat and water loss, the magnitude of bronchoconstriction correlates more closely with calculated water loss than with heat loss.[212] The hypothesis that drying, with consequent hyperosmolarity of the surface liquid, is the important stimulus has been strengthened by studies that have shown that inhalation of hyperosmolar aerosols elicit bronchoconstriction in patients with EIA.[213]

The bronchoconstriction that occurs in asthmatic patients in response to the ventilation of unconditioned air appears to result not from a defect in inspired air conditioning but rather from an abnormal response to a normal stimulus. Normal subjects do not seem to have more efficient air conditioning, because they develop equivalent airway cooling at matched levels of ventilation and inspired air conditions.[214] With identical levels of ventilation and inspired air conditions, nasal breathing results in much less airway cooling and bronchoconstriction than that noted with oral breathing.[215]

The precise mechanism by which airway cooling or drying results in airway narrowing remains uncertain, and several posibilities have been studied.

Release of Mediators from Mast Cells or Other Sources. Histamine and neutrophil chemotactic factor of anaphylaxis, both of which are believed to be released from mast cells, can be detected in the blood of asthmatic patients, but not normal subjects, during EIA or HIB.[216] Mediator release from mast cells in the airway may be triggered by the change in osmolarity accompanying evaporative water loss. Basophils and mast cells release preformed mediators *in vitro* in response to both hyperosmolar and hypo-osmolar challenges.[217, 218] In some individuals, exercise appears to produce generalized release of mast cell mediators that results in anaphylaxis, especially if the exercise follows the eating of specific foods.[219]

Stimulation of Afferent Receptors. Evidence to support this mechanism has come from studies showing that both local anesthetics—which inhibit the airway afferent nerves—and atropinelike drugs—which inhibit the efferent cholinergic nerves—attenuate EIA and HIB.[220, 221] However, the effect of inhaled local anesthetics may occur by decreasing ventilation,[222] and the effect of cholinergic bronchodilators may simply relate to altered baseline airway caliber.[223]

Direct Effect on Smooth Muscle. Cooling of human airway smooth muscle studied *in vitro* can potentiate the contractile response to some agonists,[224] and it is possible that the same mechanism ocurs *in vivo*.

Mucosal Dilatation and Edema. Although it is generally believed that airway smooth muscle contraction is the major cause of airway narrowing in EIA, it has been suggested that at least some of the effect may be secondary to bronchial vascular reactivity and edema.[225] In the nose, rapid changes in caliber can occur; since there is no encircling smooth muscle layer at this site, these changes are entirely attributable to vasomotion in the vascular bed of the nasal mucosa. Like the nose, the lower airway mucosa possesses a complex and extensive submucosal plexus of blood vessels,[226] and it is possible that vascular constriction induced by cold followed by vasodilation and mucosal edema could play a role in the airway obstruction of EIA.[225]

From 50 to 80 per cent of asthmatic subjects who develop EIA show a refractory period following challenge; during this period, similar levels of exercise produce no response or an attenuated response.[227, 228] The degree of attenuation of the second response is dependent on the intensity of the initial exercise and on time. Thirty minutes after an initial episode, EIA is considerably less; by 4 hours, however, the protective effect has completely disappeared.[228] The exact explanation for the refractory period is unknown, but there is some evidence to suggest that there is a relative depletion or attenuated release of mast cell mediators[229] as well as the release of bronchodilating prostaglandins[230] during the postexercise period.

Exercise and isocapnic hyperventilation of cold and/or dry air causes cough as well as bronchoconstriction. The time course of the cough is very similar to that of bronchoconstriction, peaking 5 minutes after exercise or hypoven-tilation and lasting for approximately 30 minutes. It correlates better with respiratory water loss than with heat loss and occurs in both normal and asthmatic subjects. Cough also occurs in response to inhaled hypertonic aerosols, suggesting that the stimulus is the change in airway fluid osmolarity attendant on evaporative water loss.

Infection

Viral infection of the respiratory tract can have important consequences for airway function. In otherwise normal adults, small but measurable transient changes in flow rates and pharmacologic responsiveness can result from respiratory syncytial viral infection, influenza A viral infection, or vaccination with live attenuated virus.[231] In asthmatic patients, heat-killed and live attenuated influenza vaccination as well as naturally occurring infection with respiratory syncytial virus, rhinovirus, and influenza A virus have been reported to cause increased NSBH.[232]

The effect of viruses in provoking bronchoconstriction appears to be more pronounced in children than in adults; in some studies, for example, viral infections have been associated with asthma exacerbations in as many as 70 per cent of episodes in children[233] but only 10 per cent in adults.[234] The mechanism by which infection precipitates these attacks is not clear. It is possible that airway wall edema and increased secretions within bronchial lumina further diminish the caliber of already narrowed airways. It is also conceivable that the mucosal inflammation associated with the infection results in airway smooth muscle contraction secondary to mediator release from inflammatory cells.

Analgesics

Acetylsalicylic acid (ASA) and several other analgesics and anti-inflammatory agents—including indomethacin, aminopyrine, acetaminophen, mefenamic acid, dextropropoxyphene, and tartrazine—are capable of provoking attacks in about 5 to 30 per cent of patients with asthma.[235] The typical ASA-sensitive patient is a nonatopic woman older than 20 years of age with a long history of perennial rhinitis and nasal polyps.[236] Long-standing asthma and rhinitis usually precede the development of the sensitivity, and the intolerance increases with age, being six times commoner after age 50 than before age 20.[237] Peripheral eosinophilia is observed in more than 50 per cent of patients, although serum IgE levels are usually normal[235] and specific IgE directed toward ASA is not detectable.[238]

Symptoms and signs develop anywhere from 20 minutes to 3 hours after ingestion. Two forms of response have been distinguished: a predominantly respiratory form and an urticarial-angioedema form. Rarely, both occur in the same individual.[235] The respiratory response is dominated by bronchoconstriction and can be severe and life-threatening; it is usually associated with rhinitis and conjunctivitis.

The most likely mechanism by which ASA and other nonsteroidal anti-inflammatory agents cause bronchoconstriction is through their ability to block metabolism of arachidonic acid via the cyclooxygenase pathway. Supporting this hypothesis is the observation that the degree of bronchoconstriction the drugs induce *in vivo* is proportional to their ability to retard prostaglandin synthesis *in vitro*.[239] It has been postulated that patients with ASA-sensitive asthma produce large amounts of the bronchodilator PGE_2 in compensation for continued bronchoconstriction; when ASA or other anti-inflammatory agents are administered, an acute drop in PGE_2 synthesis precipitates an acute asthmatic attack.[202] Alternatively, it has been suggested that blockade of the cyclooxygenase series of enzymes diverts more arachidonic acid toward the lipoxygenase metabolic pathway, resulting in excessive production of bronchoconstricting leukotrienes.

Gastroesophageal Reflux

Gastroesophageal reflux can theoretically trigger airway narrowing in susceptible individuals by stimulating esophageal vagal afferents or by direct aspiration of a small amount of esophageal contents.[240, 241] When acid is instilled into the esophagus of asthmatic patients, only those who develop symptoms of esophagitis exhibit bronchoconstriction.[242] It has been suggested that since reflux is exacerbated during sleep as a result of recumbency and decreased tone in the lower esophageal sphincter, it tends to cause nocturnal asthma and "morning dipping"—the latter term referring to the phenomenon in which the lowest values for expiratory flow are recorded in the early hours of the morning (2 to 4 A.M.).[243]

Emotion

It is difficult to evaluate the influence of psychological factors as provocative triggers of asthmatic attacks. Although some asthmatic patients are emotionally unstable and dependent, this is almost certainly a result of their disease rather than a factor predisposing to its development. Mild bronchoconstriction and bronchodilation can be produced by suggestion, presumably as a result of changes in cholinergic vagal activity.[244] Hyperventilation provoked by anxiety is common in asthmatic patients. In fact, a vicious cycle can be established because the hyperventilation itself can cause bronchoconstriction as a result of hypocapnia and airway drying, thus tending to increase the anxiety.[245] Although emotional distress can trigger an attack in a patient with asthma, it plays no role in the basic pathophysiologic process that causes the asthmatic state.

Environment

It is clear that low levels of atmospheric chemical pollutants can cause functional abnormalities in patients with hyper-reactive airways. In fact, epidemiologic studies in industrial areas have shown that asthma symptoms and admissions to hospital are increased during periods of heavy pollution.[246, 247] The major respirable atmospheric chemicals that affect lung function are ozone and the oxides of sulfur and nitrogen.

In normal subjects, inhalation of sulfur dioxide (SO_2) in concentrations of 0.5 to 1.0 ppm causes mild, transient, asymptomatic bronchoconstriction, albeit only when the subjects exercise during the exposure, thereby increasing the dose of SO_2 reaching the airways.[248] As might be expected, patients with asthma are more sensitive than nor-

mal subjects. A concentration as low as 0.25 ppm can cause detectable obstruction during mild exercise,[249] and 5 minutes of heavy exercise in 0.4 or 0.5 ppm SO_2 can cause transient symptomatic exacerbation (followed by recovery within 24 hours).[250]

In both normal and asthmatic subjects and at a concentration as low as 0.12 ppm, ozone causes a dose-dependent decrease in expiratory flow rates and volumes as well as TLC, making it the most potent irritant gas.[251, 252] As with SO_2, its effects are enhanced with exercise. Even brief ozone exposure increases subsequent nonspecific airway responsiveness in normal subjects[253]; animal models and human studies suggest that this effect is mediated by airway inflammation.[254]

The oxides of nitrogen are another component of smog and industrial pollution that in low concentrations can precipitate symptomatic episodes in hyper-responsive individuals. A transient increase in the nitrogen oxide level to more than 500 parts per billion was blamed for an acute outbreak of asthma in Barcelona, Spain, in which 44 patients were admitted to the hospital over a 2- to 3-hour period.[255] Inhalation of nitrogen dioxide (0.3 ppm) increases the severity of exercise-induced bronchoconstriction in asthmatic patients.[256] In most studies, low-level NO_2 exposure (0.1 ppm for 1 hour or 910 μg per m³ for 20 minutes) enhances nonspecific airway responsiveness in asthmatic subjects but does not in normal subjects.[257]

Deep Inspiration

Normal subjects show a transient decrease in airway resistance following a deep inspiration, a reaction believed to be caused by dilatation of the airways.[258] By contrast, asthmatic subjects show a paradoxical airway narrowing.[259] The difference between asthmatic subjects and normal individuals is also evident following pharmacologically induced bronchoconstriction: a deep breath in these circumstances has a profound bronchodilating effect on normal subjects that is absent or deficient in asthmatic subjects.[260] The reason for the abnormal response to a big breath in asthmatic subjects is not known. It is possible that the stretch on the airways stimulates irritant receptors and initiates reflex bronchoconstriction[261]; alternatively, the hypertrophied airway smooth muscle layer in the airways of asthmatic individuals may show a deficient or abnormal response to stretch.[262]

Miscellaneous Provoking Factors

Alcohol-containing beverages have been reported to precipitate attacks of bronchoconstriction in some patients with asthma.[263] Although in some cases this is caused by the preservative metabisulfite (*see* later), in others ethanol alone seems to be responsible. Patients develop rapid onset of flushing, nasal congestion, and wheeze; the response is attenuated by histamine H_1 and cyclooxygenase blockers but not by atropine.[264] Asians who have a very high incidence of acetylaldehyde dehydrogenase deficiency and who manifest vasomotor responsiveness to ethanol may be particularly sensitive to its bronchoconstricting effects.[264]

In addition to food itself, several artificial additives to food can provoke airway narrowing in sensitive individuals.

Metabisulfite salts are used as preservatives in a wide variety of foods and beverages and cause bronchoconstriction in approximately 4 per cent of asthmatic subjects.[265] Sensitivity can be documented by careful oral challenges with capsules containing increasing amounts of metabisulfite.[266] Monosodium glutamate and the food coloring additive tartrazine can also cause attacks.[267, 268]

A large number of asthmatic patients report a worsening of symptoms in the presence of certain odors, of which perfume and cologne are the most frequently mentioned sources.[269] Second-hand, or "side stream," cigarette smoke also can cause symptoms and airflow obstructions in asthmatic individuals.[270] As many as 30 per cent of women with asthma complain of increased symptoms and demonstrate decreased maximal flow rates during the premenstrual period[271]; although presumably related to a hormonal effect, the precise pathogenesis is unclear.

Occupational Asthma

Occupational asthma is a particularly important form of the disease to recognize, both because it is becoming more frequent[272] and because it is potentially completely reversible if recognized early. Depending on the pathogenesis, it can be divided into four categories: reflex, inflammatory, pharmacologic, and immunologic. The last-named can itself be subdivided into those exposures with proven allergic pathophysiology—in which high-molecular-weight substances can be implicated—and those in which an immunologic mechanism is likely but unproven—in which low-molecular-weight substances are the supposed offending agents.

Reflex (Nonspecific) Bronchoconstriction. Patients with asthma that is unrelated to a specific occupational exposure can suffer episodic exacerbation of their symptoms during exposure to a variety of irritants in the workplace. Because the reactions are no more than aggravations of pre-existing asthma, their inclusion within the definition of occupational asthma has been questioned.[272]

Inflammatory Bronchoconstriction. Acute exposure to a high concentration of certain gases, vapors, and smoke can produce severe bronchial and bronchiolar injury that causes narrowing and hyper-responsiveness of airways in the exposed worker.[272] This syndrome has been called "reactive airway dysfunction syndrome" (RADS) and develops following a single exposure to a high concentration of gases, such as hydrogen sulfide, ammonia, diethylene diamine, and chlorine; fumes from plastics; or smoke from a variety of materials.[273] Airway obstruction develops within 24 hours of exposure, and some degree of obstruction and exaggerated nonspecific airway responsiveness can persist for months, usually followed by slow resolution.

Pharmacologic Bronchoconstriction. Some occupations involve exposure to substances that are thought to cause a direct, nonidiosyncratic airway effect in a dose-dependent fashion in all exposed workers.[272] The commonest substances implicated in this category are cotton dust (byssinosis, *see* page 419) and grain dust.

Because of the complex composition of grain dust, it is not surprising that a number of different syndromes and mechanisms are associated with exposure. Although specific IgE-mediated allergic responses to some of its components can occur (*see* later), inhalation of grain dust more often causes a syndrome characterized by elevated temperature, flushing, headache, chest tightness, cough, dyspnea, an elevated white blood cell count, and a reduction in maximal expiratory flow ("grain fever").[274] Workers can also develop leukocytosis and a significant decrease in maximal expiratory flow over a working shift.[275] A similar syndrome can occur in factory workers exposed to the output from "contaminated" humidifiers.[276] Certain organophosphate insecticides have anticholinesterase activity and can produce vagally mediated airway narrowing.[272]

Proven Allergic Bronchoconstriction. Table 11–2 contains a list of some agents and occupations in which a specific IgE-induced allergic mechanism for asthma has been proved. For the most part, the antigens are high-molecular-weight proteins, polysaccharides, or glycoproteins derived from plants or animals. Sensitivity develops predominantly in workers with an atopic predisposition, and positive immediate skin test or specific IgE responses (RAST) can be demonstrated.

A small percentage of atopic grain workers develop IgE-mediated acute and delayed airway responses to specific antigens, such as grain mites and weevils, and the grains themselves.[272] Between 7 and 20 per cent of bakers eventually develop symptoms of allergy (rhinitis and asthma)[277]; however, unlike the reactions in most grain workers, specific allergy to cereal grains (wheat, rye, barley, oats, and triticale) can be detected in the vast majority by positive skin tests and RAST.

Possible Allergic Bronchoconstriction. There is an ever-increasing list of low-molecular-weight substances (<1000 daltons) that can induce asthma in exposed workers (*see* Table 11–2). Although the mechanism of sensitization to these substances is uncertain, some features are suggestive of an allergic origin: (1) only about 5 per cent of exposed individuals develop sensitivity; (2) there is a latent period between exposure and the onset of bronchoconstriction; (3) increasing exposure increases the incidence of sensitivity; and (4) exposure to minute quantities of the substances causes acute bronchoconstriction followed by a delayed response. On the other hand, classic skin test sensitivity is usually absent, and atopic individuals are not more likely to develop sensitivity.

The best studied agent in this category is plicatic acid.[278] Approximately 4 per cent of exposed workers develop sensitivity to this substance over an exposure period ranging from months to years. Nonatopic individuals are equally as prone as atopic patients to develop sensitization, and there are no clinical or historical characteristics that permit prediction of which workers will be affected. Specific IgE antibody to plicatic acid–human serum albumin conjugate is found in approximately 40 per cent of patients tested. Cough and dyspnea can be insidious in onset and predominantly nocturnal, presumably as a result of the delayed response; this makes diagnosis difficult. Symptoms and pulmonary function abnormalities increase with the duration and intensity of exposure.[279] Approximately 60 per cent of sensitive individuals have persistent symptoms for 4 years following cessation of exposure; those whose symptoms are of longer duration prior to diagnosis and whose pulmonary function is worse at diagnosis are less likely to recover completely.[280]

Table 11–2. **SELECTED CAUSES OF OCCUPATIONAL ASTHMA**

Pharmacologic			Not Proven Allergic		
Agent	**Occupation**	**Selected References**	**Agent**	**Occupation**	**Selected References**
Cotton dust (byssinosis)	Textile workers		*Diisocyanates*		
Grain dust	Grain elevator and storage workers, dock workers	662	Toluene, 1,5-naphthylene, diphenylmethane, and hexamethylene diisocyanate	Polyurethane industry, plastics manufacture, foundry, paint, rubber, and varnish workers	675
Humidifier pollution or contamination	Factory workers	276	*Anhydrides*		
Organophosphate insecticides	Farm workers	663	Phthalic, trimellitic, pyromellitic, tetrachlorophalic and hexahydrophalic anhydride	Epoxy resin and plastics manufacture and use	676
Isocyanates (also see below)	Polyurethane industry, plastics manufacture, paint and varnish use and manufacture		*Wood Dusts*		
Proven Allergic			Western Red Cedar, Eastern White Cedar, California redwood, e.g., Mahogany	Carpenters, cabinet makers, construction and sawmill workers	677
Animals and Animal Products			*Metals*		
Laboratory animals (rats, mice, rabbits, guinea pigs, and monkeys), hair, and urine	Laboratory workers, veterinarians, animal handlers	664	Platinum	Platinum refinery	
			Nickel	Metal plating; dental workers	678
Birds (pigeons, chickens, budgerigars)	Bird breeders and poultry workers		Cobalt, vanadium, and tungsten carbide	Hard metal workers, diamond polishers	679
Insects			*Fluxes*		
Poultry mites	Poultry workers	665	Aminoethyl ethanolamine	Aluminum soldering	
Grain mites, flour weevils	Grain and mill workers	666	Colophony	Electronics industry	
Cockroaches	Laboratory workers	667	*Drugs*		
Moths, butterflies	Entomologists	668	E.g., penicillin, cephalosporins, e.g., methyldopa, tetracycline	Pharmaceutical industry, chemists, nurses, brewers, poultry feed mixture	
Honeybees and honeybee pollen	Apiary workers	669			
Marine Animals			*Other Chemicals*		
Snow crabs and prawns	Crab and prawn processing	670	Persulfate salts and henna	Hairdressers	680
			Ethylene diamine	Photographers	
Plants and Plant Products			Glutaraldehyde, hexachlorophene, and formalin	Hospital staff	681
Grain dust	Grain elevator and storage workers, dock workers				
Wheat, rye, and buckwheat flour	Bakers and millers	671	Urea formaldehyde	Insulation and resin workers	
Castor bean, soybean	Oil industry, felt industry	672	Methyl methacrylate	Dental workers	682
Tobacco leaf	Tobacco handling and cigarette manufacture		Polyvinylchloride	Plastics manufacture and meat wrappers	683, 684
Curry, coriander, and mace	Spice industry	673			
Biologic Enzymes					
Trypsin, pancreatin, papain, pepsin	Plastics, pharmaceutical, and laboratory personnel	674			
Vegetables					
Gum acacia	Printers				

Isocyanates are used as hardeners in paint, varnish, molds, and plastics, and exposure to them, particularly toluene diisocyanate (TDI), is the commonest cause of occupational asthma. As many as 10 per cent of exposed workers develop airway sensitivity.[272] TDI hypersensitivity can cause prolonged asthma despite removal from occupational exposure.[281] The clinical, epidemiologic, and pathophysiologic features are similar to those of plicatic acid sensitivity, although nonspecific irritant and allergic alveolitis–type syndromes have also been reported.[282]

Diagnosis

The diagnosis of occupational asthma is aided by a high index of suspicion and requires the demonstration that the patient's symptoms are caused by asthma and are related to

the work environment. It is established by a combination of clinical history, pulmonary function tests, bronchodilator response, and tests of nonspecific and specific bronchial responsiveness. A carefully taken occupational history should be obtained from all patients with adult-onset asthma. It is especially helpful if symptoms develop during or immediately after exposure to a specific agent; however, symptoms can begin after working hours or can be solely nocturnal. Patients should be questioned concerning remission of their symptoms during weekends and holidays and exacerbation on return to work. Positive results of skin or RAST tests to known occupational allergens are very supportive of the diagnosis.

Patients with occupational asthma frequently manifest normal lung function at the time of presentation, and it may be necessary to document functional impairment related to work exposure.[283] Because of the potential for delayed responses, 24-hour records of PEFR with mini-peak flow meters may be particularly helpful in establishing the diagnosis.[284] Serial tests of NSBH also can help document that the asthma is work-related.[272] An increase in NSBH during a period of exposure and a decrease during absence from work provide strong evidence for occupational sensitivity. In addition, tests of NSBH help predict the severity of the response to a challenge with a specific sensitizing agent.[285]

Bronchial provocation testing with suspected occupational agents should not be undertaken lightly and should be performed only by experienced personnel in a hospital setting where resuscitation facilities are available.[272] However, a significant airway response to a specific challenge remains the most definitive means of establishing a causative relationship, provided that a nonspecific irritant response can be ruled out.

Roentgenographic Manifestations

The roentgenographic manifestations of asthma are more complex than customarily believed and, in certain combinations, may be highly suggestive, if not diagnostic.[286] Notwithstanding, in many patients the chest roentgenogram is normal.

In the presence of acute severe asthma or during prolonged, intractable asthmatic attacks, the most characteristic, although by no means invariable, roentgenographic signs are pulmonary overinflation and expiratory air trapping (Fig. 11–16). Atelectasis, pneumothorax, and/or pneumomediastinum are seen in a small percentage of cases.[287]

Prominence of the main pulmonary artery and its hilar branches with rapid midlung attenuation is probably indicative of transient precapillary pulmonary arterial hypertension secondary to hypoxia and occurs in approximately 10 per cent of patients.[286] "Subpleural oligemia," consisting of

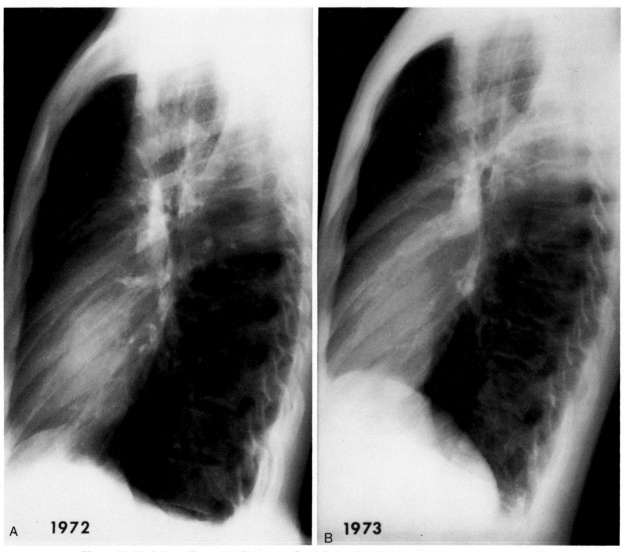

Figure 11–16. Asthma: Reversible Pulmonary Overinflation (Adult). A lateral chest roentgenogram *(A)* of an adult asthmatic during an attack of severe bronchospasm reveals a low position and flat configuration of the diaphragm, indicating severe pulmonary overinflation. Approximately 1 year later during a remission *(B)*, lung volume had returned to normal. Note that the curvature of the sternum and thoracic spine did not change, since these structures do not participate in acute hyperinflation in the adult.

a striking paucity of vessels in the outer 2 to 4 cm of the lungs (Fig. 11–17), has been identified in about one third of patients in some series.[286] It is especially evident when accompanied by an increased prominence of the hilar and midlung vessels; it is reversible with treatment. Its pathogenesis probably relates to diffuse bronchiolar mucous plugging and spasm resulting in peripheral hypoventilation and hypoxic vasoconstriction, a hypothesis that is supported by both radionuclide and CT correlative studies.

Defects in perfusion associated with ventilation inequality may cause other abnormal scintigraphic patterns.[288] One such pattern, designated the "stripe sign," is manifested by a rim of normal perfusion in the cortex alternating with contiguous zones of hypoperfusion, central to which resides a zone of medullary hypoperfusion (Fig. 11–18).[289] It has been proposed that this pattern effectively excludes thromboembolic disease as the cause of the oligemia, since thromboembolic deficits almost invariably extend to a pleural surface and hence must involve both the cortex and the medulla simultaneously.

In some patients with chronic asthma—usually those with a history of repeated episodes of infection—the bronchial walls are thickened, an abnormality that can be detected both on conventional roentgenograms and by CT.[289a] The abnormality occurs in both segmental and subsegmental bronchi and can be seen either as ring shadows when viewed end-on or as tramline opacities when viewed *en face*. Smaller bronchi measuring 3 to 5 mm in diameter, normally invisible on conventional chest roentgenograms, may be identified. These findings probably represent intramural and peribronchial thickening secondary to inflammation or fibrosis or both. In the authors' opinion, the combination of thickening of the walls of bronchi, diffuse vessel narrowing, and subpleural oligemia is highly suggestive, if not diagnostic, of bronchial asthma.

The incidence of roentgenographic abnormalities is influenced to a considerable degree by the age at onset of the asthma, its severity, and its constancy. The influence of age at onset of asthma on the presence or absence of roentgenographic changes was illustrated graphically in one study of 117 asthmatic patients older than 15 years of age.[290] In this adult group, roentgenographic abnormalities were identified in 31 per cent of the patients whose asthma had its onset before the age of 15 years but in none of those in whom it occurred after 30 years of age. The incidence of roentgenographic abnormalities also bears a relationship to the constancy or intermittent nature of symptoms. In one investigation of 218 children with asthma,[291] the most marked roentgenographic abnormalities were identified without exception in patients suffering from severe or moderately severe *constant* asthma; those with *intermittent* symptoms usually had roentgenograms that appeared normal, even during asthmatic episodes.

The chief indication for chest roentgenography in patients with bronchial asthma is to exclude other conditions that cause diffuse wheezing throughout the chest—chronic bronchitis, emphysema, bronchiectasis, and obstruction of the trachea or major bronchi. Several studies have been carried out to evaluate the usefulness of roentgenographic examination in patients with asthma.[292, 287] Although the results are not conclusive, the authors are inclined to agree with those reached by Zieverink and colleagues,[287] who con-

cluded that routine chest roentgenography is not useful in the patient with acute asthma unless the patient is unresponsive to bronchodilators or is being admitted to the hospital.

Clinical Manifestations

The diagnosis of asthma is based largely on a history of periodic paroxysms of dyspnea, when the individual is at rest as well as exercising, with intervals of complete or nearly complete remission. Some patients have a more chronic form of the disease, but periodic exacerbation and remission occur in all cases. Cough can be a prominent symptom, and nonsmoking patients with asthma can fulfill the diagnostic criteria for chronic bronchitis.[293] The diagnosis is strengthened by a history of eczema or hay fever or by a family history of allergies.

Meticulous inquiry into the circumstances that initiate attacks, although time-consuming, is a particularly important diagnostic procedure. Questioning should be directed toward the possible association with ingestion of a specific food (particularly in children) or season of the year (suggesting either pollen or insect sensitivity). Careful inquiry should be made into possible antigens in the home, especially domestic pets and feather pillows. The patient may have recognized an association between the onset of symptoms and exposure to a dusty environment at his or her place of work.

A history of drug intake should always be sought. Drug allergy most often occurs in association with intravenous or intramuscular drug administration and often is associated with acute and sometimes fatal anaphylaxis. In highly sensitive persons, however, drugs taken by mouth or administered by aerosol inhalation may produce a similar reaction, resulting in a maximum response within 5 to 30 minutes manifested by nausea, vomiting, pruritus, substernal tightness, or dyspnea.[294]

The patient should be questioned as to whether there is an association between the onset of asthmatic attacks and infections of the upper or lower respiratory tract, with particular emphasis on the occurrence of symptoms suggestive of sinusitis, such as postnasal drip and facial pain. An attempt should be made to correlate the onset of attacks with emotional disturbance; if the patient is a child, this should include interview of the parents. Finally, the patient should be questioned as to the relationship between the onset of attacks and exercise; exposure to cold air, irritating dusts, fumes, or odors; and changes in temperature and humidity.

In both atopic and nonatopic patients, particularly those who are elderly, the original asthmatic episode commonly is termed acute bronchitis, with or without fever or symptoms of upper respiratory tract disease.[295] In such patients, wheezing and paroxysmal nocturnal dyspnea often are attributed to irreversible obstructive airway disease or left ventricular failure.[296] In fact, nocturnal breathlessness is a common symptom of asthma, and careful history taking may be necessary to distinguish the disease from paroxysmal nocturnal dyspnea of cardiac origin.

In the majority of patients, the onset of an attack of asthma is heralded by an unproductive cough and wheeze; only subsequently do the sensations of suffocation and tightness in the chest develop. The onset of dyspnea is

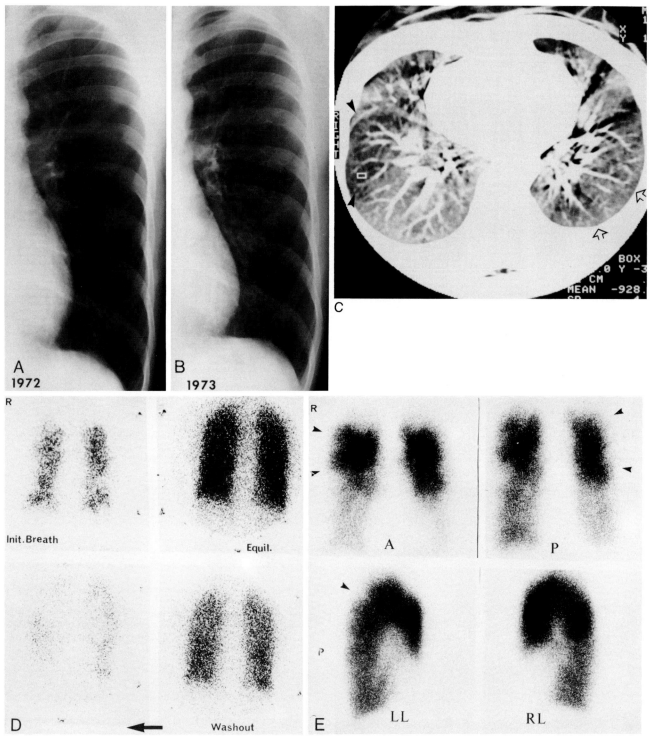

Figure 11–17. Asthma: Peripheral Oligemia. A detail view of the left lung from a posteroanterior chest roentgenogram *(A)* of a young man during an episode of acute bronchospasm reveals moderate hyperinflation. The vasculature in the outer 2 to 3 cm of lung is inconspicuous and barely visible, creating a subpleural shell of oligemic lung. A repeat study 1 year later during remission *(B)* shows less hyperinflation: the pulmonary vessels now taper normally, and most are visible well into the lung periphery. A CT scan through the lower lobes *(C)* at the time of the initial roentgenogram demonstrates low-density areas in the subpleural lung *(arrowheads)* (cursor boxes record a measurement of −928 Hounsfield units). This CT finding is indicative of decreased perfusion; however, note that cortical perfusion is normal in some areas *(open arrows)*. A ventilation lung scintigram *(D)* reveals poor filling on the initial breath, confined largely to the medulla; the end-stage of washout shows some peripheral air trapping. A perfusion scintigram *(E)* reveals poor perfusion of the lower lobes. Note the irregular subpleural shell of diminished perfusion *(arrowheads)*, corresponding with the subpleural oligemia on the conventional roentgenogram and the zone of air trapping on the ventilation scan.

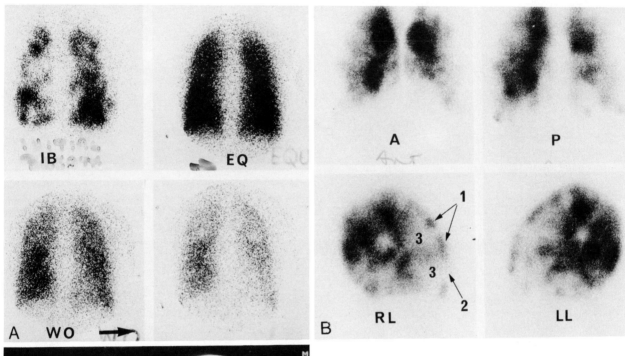

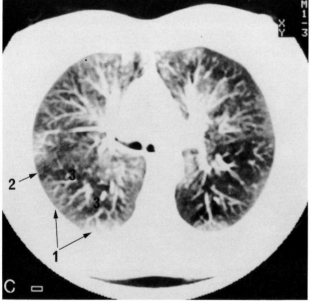

Figure 11–18. Asthma: The "Stripe Sign." A ventilation lung scinti-gram *(A)* reveals unequal deposition of the radioisotope in the cen-tral (medullary) parenchyma on the initial breath (IB), with relative sparing peripherally; equilibration (EQ) was eventually achieved centrally and peripherally, although air trapping occurred in both areas during the washout (WO) phase. A perfusion scan *(B)* in anterior (A), posterior (P), right lateral (RL), and left lateral (LL) positions demonstrates gross deficits in the perfusion pattern in the lower lobes and posterior parts of the upper lobes. Note the rim of maintained perfusion in the cortex (1) that alternates with adjacent regions of cortical hypoperfusion (2); in both instances, the proximal medulla (3) is focally underperfused. The presence of maintained perfusion adjacent to contiguous medullary hypoperfusion on a scintigram is designated the "stripe sign," effectively excluding thromboembolic disease as the cause of the oligemia. A CT scan through the carina *(C)* shows features similar to those on the perfu-sion images: Note the regions of maintained cortical perfusion (1), deficient cortical perfusion (2), and medullary hypoperfusion (3), the CT equivalent of the stripe sign.

usually gradual and seldom abrupt. Paroxysms occur most commonly at night; when they are severe, the patient may feel obliged to sit on the edge of the bed or to stagger to the window in the vain hope of obtaining more oxygen. As previously noted, the lowest values for expiratory flow are recorded in the early hours of the morning (2 to 4 A.M.) (a phenomenon known as "morning dipping").[297] The mechanism or mechanisms that cause this diurnal variation are uncertain[298]; however, the most likely is a nocturnal decrease in circulating catecholamines. Sleep itself is not a necessary factor because the obstruction develops, albeit somewhat less severely, when nocturnal sleep is prevented.[299]

Cough (with normal pulmonary function) may be the sole presenting symptom in some patients, in which case measurement of NSBH may be helpful in diagnosis.[300] Patients in whom asthma is the underlying cause of cough usually have an increase in nonspecific airway responsiveness, and the cough is alleviated by treatment of the asthma. Measurement of the total eosinophil count may be a useful screening technique to select patients for this test.[301]

Although some patients present with attacks of asthma that develop over a period of hours, most have had progressive symptoms over days to weeks, often with a more rapid deterioration during the previous 24 hours.[302] Younger atopic subjects are more likely to present with exacerbations of rapid onset.[303] Occasionally, the onset of asthma is so insidious that the diagnosis is not considered, particularly in elderly smokers, who are usually labeled as having COPD; intensive therapy in such patients may result in a dramatic reversal of obstruction.[304]

Patients with acute severe asthma may be too dyspneic or exhausted to speak and may be stuporous or even comatose as a result of hypoxemia and hypercarbia; they commonly manifest tachycardia (the heart rate is usually more than 130 beats) and exaggerated pulsus paradoxus (see later). As a result of airway obstruction and exhaustion, they usually exhibit such severe restriction of air flow that wheezing is absent, and breath sounds are barely discernible.[305] Arterial blood gas analysis is of particular value in the recognition of this state of emergency (see later).

The physical findings in asthma include hyperventilation, hyper-resonance on percussion, inspiratory and expiratory sonorous and sibilant rhonchi (low-pitched and high-pitched wheezes), decreased breath sounds, and prolonged expiration. In very severe attacks, wheezing may not be apparent, the clinical picture being one of air hunger. In this situation, there is evidence of the use of accessory muscles of respiration, diminished breath sounds without rhonchi, and often cyanosis.[306]

The correlation between physical findings suggestive of asthma, nonspecific airway responsiveness, and objective evidence of airway obstruction generally is not close, although FEV$_1$ can be roughly estimated with a combination of auscultation and palpation of the accessory muscles.[307] Of greater use is the pulsus paradoxus; correlation of clinical findings with physiologic dysfunction has indicated that its severity may be a valuable reflection of the severity of asthma.[308] On inspiration, the systolic arterial pressure of normal subjects decreases by as much as 5 mm Hg, whereas in patients with asthma the pressure may drop by

10 mm Hg or more. This is probably the result of increased negative intrathoracic pressure consequent on airway obstruction[309] and may be related to two mechanisms: (1) the increased right ventricular volume caused by the negative pressure may result in a leftward shift of the interventricular septum and interfere with left ventricular diastolic filling; and (2) because there is communication between the ventricle and the great vessels outside the thorax that are not exposed to the negative pressure, the negative intrathoracic pressure may act as an afterload on the left ventricle.[310]

Laboratory Investigation

The sputum of patients who have asthma is mucoid and characteristically contains eosinophils, although the number is not sufficiently sensitive to distinguish asthmatic patients from those who have chronic bronchitis.[311] Blood eosinophilia is also frequent and may be better able to separate these patients.[312] Skin tests may be useful in identifying specific food or aeroallergens to which patients are sensitive,[313] and confirmation of specific sensitivity may be obtained by radioallergosorbent testing.[176] It is important to remember, however, that skin application of the recommended dilutions of individual allergens may precipitate an attack. The patient must be watched carefully for reactions, and countermeasures should be at hand.[314]

Although inhalation challenge is a more reliable method of identifying specific allergens it is rarely indicated in clinical practice, since profound immediate and (more important) delayed bronchoconstriction may occur. It should be reserved for research studies in carefully controlled settings and for incriminating a specific antigen in occupational asthma.[315] Nonspecific inhalation challenge with histamine or methacholine is an important diagnostic technique in some patients and may have value in following the response to long-term therapy.

A variety of electrocardiographic changes may occur during severe episodes of asthma.[316] Sinus tachycardia is almost always present; in addition, there may be right axis deviation, clockwise rotation of the heart, right ventricular hypertrophy, right atrial P waves, and ST segment or T-wave abnormalities.

Pulmonary Function Tests

As might be expected, aberrations in pulmonary function in asthma vary, depending largely on whether the condition is in remission or exacerbation and, if the latter, on the severity of the attack. Many patients whose asthma is in remission have normal routine pulmonary function,[317] although "sensitive" tests of small airway function may demonstrate abnormalities.[318] Even when maximal expiratory flows and volumes are within the normal predicted range, inhalation of a bronchodilator may result in a greater than 15 per cent increase in FEV$_1$ or FVC. The relationship between symptoms and function depends on the patient's ability to detect airway obstruction and is quite variable. Some patients are unable to sense the presence of severe airway obstruction (FEV$_1$ less than 50 per cent predicted).[319]

Diffuse airway narrowing is the basic functional abnormality of symptomatic asthma; the resulting increase in resistance leads to decreased flow, hyperinflation, gas trapping, and, ultimately, an increase in the work of breathing.

Airway narrowing is most easily detected and quantitated by measurements of maximal expiratory flow, derived from either volume-time or flow-volume plots.[320] In addition to decreasing flow during an asthmatic attack, airway narrowing and closure[321] result in gas trapping manifested by an increase in RV and the RV-TLC ratio and by a decrease in VC.[322] The increase in airway resistance is also associated with hyperinflation, manifested by an increase in FRC[323] and, to a lesser extent, TLC.[324] Total lung capacity is significantly higher and lung elastic recoil lower in asthmatic individuals whose disease began in childhood than in those who have the adult-onset type.[325]

The hyperinflation associated with asthma has advantages and disadvantages.[326] By dilating the intraparenchymal airways, it improves the distribution of ventilation and prevents the phenomenon of tidal expiratory flow occurring on the maximal expiratory flow-volume curve.[326] On the negative side, it increases the elastic work of breathing and places inspiratory muscles on an inefficient part of their length-tension curve.

As an asthmatic episode resolves, there is improvement in expiratory flow and VC and a decrease in FRC and RV. A decrease in symptoms may accompany the return of lung volumes to normal before changes in FEV_1 are observed, presumably as a result of the reversal of hyperinflation and gas trapping.[327] Flow rates measured at low lung volumes ($FEF_{25\%-75\%}$, V_{50}, V_{25}) may take longer to improve or may never return to normal predicted values.[328]

The single-breath diffusing capacity ($DLcoSB$) is often elevated during an asthma attack.[329] The most plausible explanation for this apparent paradox is the transient increase in pulmonary capillary blood volume that occurs as the result of the more negative inspiratory intrathoracic pressure secondary to obstruction of the airways.

Most patients with asthma have some degree of hypoxemia as a result of $\dot{V}/\dot{Q}$ mismatch[330]; it is severer in patients who have the most airway obstruction.[331] Inhalation of a beta-adrenergic bronchodilator increases the perfusion to low $\dot{V}/\dot{Q}$ regions and lowers the arterial Po_2, suggesting pharmacologic reversal of hypoxic vasoconstriction in these regions.[332] Although hypoxemia is almost always observed in acute asthmatic attacks, the incidence of hypercapnia varies, being as high as 50 per cent of patients in some studies.[333] Respiratory alkalosis is the only acid-base disturbance seen during mild asthmatic attacks, but metabolic and mixed acidosis can occur during severe exacerbations.[334]

The relationship between changes in Pao_2 and FEV_1 is not clear, some investigators finding that the two vary directly,[335] and others finding a poor correlation.[336] In acute prolonged attacks, the Pao_2 generally drops to below 60 mm Hg, the FEV_1 is less than 1 L, and peak flow is less than 60 L per minute.[336] As the severity and duration of obstruction increase, patients become exhausted, their respiratory muscles fatigue, and values of $Paco_2$ rise into the hypercapnic range.[331] In asthma, unlike COPD, hypercapnia is *never* a steady-state situation. The Pco_2 generally decreases in response to therapy but can rise steeply within minutes or hours, and patients should be under constant surveillance.[337] Artificial ventilation should be considered if improvement is not prompt, the decision being influenced by the clinical state of the patient—especially the level of consciousness—and by the elapsed time on therapy.

Clinical Course and Prognosis

The complications of asthma are much commoner in children than in adults and consist of pneumonia, atelectasis, mucoid impaction and mucous plugging, pneumomediastinum, and, rarely, arterial air embolism. Roentgenographic examination of large groups of children with acute asthma demonstrate one of these complications in about 5 to 25 per cent of individuals,[338, 339] whereas similar studies in adults have shown them in as few as 1 per cent.[340]

Atelectasis is the result of mucous plugging of small airways or mucoid impaction in central airways.[338] Although the abnormality is identifiable roentgenographically only very uncommonly in adult asthmatic patients, it is probable that mucous plugging of smaller bronchi and bronchioles occurs much more frequently than is recognized, atelectasis being prevented by collateral ventilation of obstructed regions.

Pneumomediastinum is an uncommon complication that is most often identified in males. The sudden onset of chest pain should arouse suspicion of the diagnosis.[341] A precordial "click" or "crunch" synchronous with the heartbeat also should suggest the presence of pneumomediastinum, although this sign is not conclusive (*see* page 147). In infants, particularly, there is a tendency for the additional development of pneumothorax.[342] Should the pneumothorax fail to respond to chest-tube drainage and the ipsilateral lung undergo progressive loss of volume, obstruction of central airways by impacted mucus should be suspected.[343] In older children and in adults, subcutaneous "emphysema" should be easily recognizable clinically.

In addition to complications that result directly from an asthmatic attack, lower respiratory tract infection occurs more frequently among patients with asthma than in the population at large, and the clinical severity of viral infections tends to be worse in asthmatic individuals.[344] The reason for these effects is unclear.

Three issues need to be considered in determining the prognosis of patients with asthma: the determinants of recovery from an individual acute episode, the likelihood of achieving complete remission, and the chances of dying of asthma.

Recovery from Acute Asthmatic Episodes. The clinical features that have been associated with a need for hospitalization and a prolonged symptomatic and functional recovery from acute asthma include: (1) age more than 40 years; (2) nonatopic asthma; (3) a longer duration of symptoms prior to admission; (4) poor long-term control of symptoms; and (5) use of maintenance steroids.[345] The rapidity with which flow rates improve during the first 6 hours also predicts a patient's recovery time.[346] In one retrospective study, a scoring system based on pulse rate, respiratory rate, pulsus paradoxus, peak expiratory flow rate, the use of accessory muscles, and the severity of dyspnea and wheeze was 90 per cent effective in predicting the need for hospitalization and the relapse rate following discharge from the emergency room.[347]

Remission. Determination of the ultimate long-term prognosis in asthma requires a long period of follow-up.

Studies in children[348, 349] have shown that a number of factors are associated with a poor prognosis—early onset of symptoms, multiple attacks in the initial year, clinical and physiologic evidence of persisting airway obstruction, pulmonary hyperinflation, chest deformity, and impairment of growth. The prognosis in patients whose asthmatic attacks are intermittent[350] and who show evidence of lability[351] is considerably better than in those whose symptoms are continuous and whose obstruction is relatively fixed.

The likelihood of remission is much greater in childhood-onset asthma: 50 to 70 per cent of patients whose onset of disease is prior to 16 years of age experience remission in early adult life.[352, 353] The remissions experienced by adolescents and young adults may not be permanent, however. In one 14-year follow-up of 441 children, the cumulative prevalence of asthma increased until the age of 7 years, then progressively decreased until the age of 17 to 18 years, at which time 70 per cent were "cured" (no symptoms or treatment for 1 year). Subsequent "relapses" occurred, however, and at an average age of 26 years only 57 per cent were still "cured."[354] Additional relapses tend to occur with increasing age.

Although a characteristic feature of asthma is some degree of reversibility of the airflow obstruction, it is clear that long-standing asthma can lead to a relatively fixed narrowing, despite prolonged aggressive therapy with bronchodilators and corticosteroids.[355]

Mortality. Death from asthma occurs predominantly in adults between the ages of 40 and 60 years[356] and in children younger than 2 years of age. Although this outcome is unusual, there is evidence that it is increasing in frequency.[357, 358] Two largely unexplained and transient increases in asthma mortality occurred between 1959 and 1966 in the United Kingdom, New Zealand, and Australia[359] and, more recently, in New Zealand again.[360] Although excessive use of beta-adrenergic bronchodilators has been suggested as a possible cause of these "epidemics," no definitive proof of the relationship has been established. In 1980, death rates from asthma in patients aged 5 to 34 years ranged from 0.2 per 100,000 in the United States to 3 per 100,000 in New Zealand.[104]

Case-control studies have identified several factors that are linked to increased mortality, including (1) increased asthma symptoms in the week preceding death; (2) a decrease in prednisone dosage; (3) inadequate steroid and bronchodilator administration; (4) excessive theophylline dosage; (5) over-reliance on home nebulized bronchodilators; and (6) a failure to institute artificial ventilation.[361, 362] Patient education is also an important factor in preventing death. Patients who are considered to be at risk for dying should be admitted to the hospital promptly when their clinical and physiologic findings indicate a severe attack.[363] In fact, if streamlined procedures are instituted for hospital admission, death can often be prevented.[364]

CHRONIC OBSTRUCTIVE PULMONARY DISEASE

Chronic respiratory disease related to cigarette smoking has had an enormous impact on society in this century. Mortality rates for chronic obstructive respiratory diseases have increased markedly over the past 40 years,[365] and in the United States COPD now represents the fifth commonest cause of death. In addition, there is good evidence that chronic respiratory disease constitutes the most important cause of work incapacity and restricted activity in industrialized countries, such as the United States and the United Kingdom.[366]

Chronic bronchitis is a clinical diagnosis based on excessive mucous secretion. Although it was once believed that in some patients this hypersecretion was associated with airway narrowing, the classic follow-up study of Peto and associates[367] refutes any connection between coughing and sputum production and the eventual development of airflow obstruction. These investigators followed 2718 men for 20 years and showed that coughing and sputum production were not related to decline in lung function. The initial value for FEV_1 as percentage predicted and persistent smoking were the most important determinants of eventual symptomatic airflow obstruction. Despite the disassociation between airflow obstruction and chronic coughing, it is clear that chronic airflow obstruction can develop in the absence of emphysema or loss of lung elastic recoil.

What, then, are we to call the disease of patients with irreversible airflow obstruction, without proven emphysema or loss of elastic recoil? The nomenclature is in a state of transition and controversy,[368] and there are cogent arguments for and against the use of the various terms. However, for the purposes of this text, the following definitions will apply.

Chronic bronchitis refers to a clinical condition diagnosed on the basis of a history of excessive mucus expectoration on most days during at least 3 consecutive months for not less than 2 consecutive years.[369] All other causes of chronic coughing and expectoration must be eliminated before the diagnosis is accepted. It is important to remember that the definition does not include the presence of airflow obstruction[370] and does not necessarily imply the subsequent development of this complication.[367] In some cases, it may be difficult to differentiate chronic bronchitis from asthma, and the term "asthmatic bronchitis" has been used to describe patients who fulfill the diagnostic criteria for both conditions.

Emphysema is defined as abnormal permanent enlargement of airspaces distal to the terminal bronchioles, accompanied by destruction of their walls, and without obvious fibrosis.[371] Strictly speaking, the condition can be diagnosed only pathologically; however, certain clinical, pulmonary function, and roentgenographic features allow an *in vivo* estimation of its presence and severity. Although emphysema is generally accompanied by a loss of lung elastic recoil—which, in turn, is thought to cause airflow obstruction, hyperinflation, and gas trapping—loss of recoil can occur without the development of emphysema and *vice versa*.

Chronic obstructive pulmonary disease (chronic obstructive lung disease [COLD], chronic airflow obstruction [CAO], chronic airflow limitation [CAL]) is defined in functional terms as persistent, largely irreversible airway obstruction in which the underlying pathophysiology is not precisely known.[368] Thus, conditions characterized by persistent obstruction in which the mechanism of obstruction is known, such as asthma, bronchiectasis, bronchiolitis, cystic fibrosis, and alpha$_1$-protease inhibitor deficiency, are excluded. Lung function tests show that a combination of intrinsic airway narrowing and loss of lung elasticity contribute to airway narrowing in the majority of patients who have COPD.

The term "small airway disease" has been used to describe not only the pathologic abnormalities of small airways in patients with COPD but also a variant of the clinical presentation of a small number of patients with COPD.[372] The authors feel that the use of the term in the latter context should be abandoned because it only leads to confusion; disease of the small airways is one of the abnormalities that leads to airway obstruction in COPD, not a disease in its own right.

Epidemiology

A review of the sex incidence of COPD has shown a male predominance of approximately 10 to 1,[373] a difference for which cigarette consumption is a major responsible factor.[374] However, retrospective and prospective studies designed to analyze risk factors for the development of COPD show that men are at increased risk even when adjustment is made for the amount smoked.[375] Additional factors, such as genetic differences, occupational pollution, and methods of cigarette smoking, may also be responsible. Studies that have compared the disease in men and women generally agree that it is also more rapidly progressive and more severe in the former.[376] In addition, COPD is usually worse in white cigarette smokers than in nonwhite ones, a difference that cannot be explained by the amount, mechanism, or duration of cigarette smoking.[377]

Etiology

Cigarette smoking is clearly the most significant factor in the development of COPD, the condition being rare in an individual who has not smoked cigarettes. However, since only a relatively small percentage of chronic smokers develop COPD,[378] other factors must be important. Possible modifiers and amplifiers of the response to cigarette smoke include air pollution, infection, climate, socioeconomic status, altered mucus and mucociliary clearance, and genetically determined factors such as atopy, NSBH, and alpha$_1$-protease deficiency.

Cigarette Smoking. Cigarette smoking is overwhelmingly the most important etiologic agent in the development of COPD. Healthy people who are nonsmokers show a yearly decline in FEV$_1$ that is largely secondary to the age-related decrease in lung elastic recoil; smokers, however, show an exaggerated decline, the rate increasing with the intensity of cigarette smoking (Fig. 11–19).[379] A low initial value for FEV$_1$ also results in an increased rate of decline. Cigarette smoking also retards the normal increase in expiratory flow that occurs during growth in childhood or adolescence.[380] The duration and intensity of smoking are of equal importance in determining these effects.

It is not known which of the components of tobacco smoke are responsible for the changes of COPD; however, the tar content,[381] the use of filters,[382] and the development of allergy to cigarette smoke components[383] do not appear to be important. The pattern of inhalation may influence the site and intensity of lung exposure to the various particulates and gases and could be a factor leading to the variable response between individuals.[384]

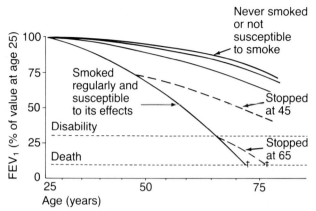

Figure 11–19. Changes in FEV$_1$ with Aging. This figure shows the percentage change of FEV$_1$ versus age for smokers and nonsmokers. Nonsmokers show a gradual decline in FEV$_1$ with age, and smokers who are not susceptible to the effects of cigarette smoke show a similar, although somewhat accelerated, decline. Individuals who are susceptible to cigarette smoke and who smoke regularly demonstrate an accelerated decline in FEV$_1$, which increases in rapidity with increasing age ("horse race effect"). Smoking cessation returns the rate of decline to that observed in the nonsmoking or nonsusceptible population. (From Peto R, Speizer FE, Cochrane AL, et al: The relevance in adults of air-flow obstruction, but not of mucus hypersecretion, to mortality from chronic lung disease: Results from 20 years of prospective observation. Am Rev Respir Dis 128: 491, 1983.)

Although personal cigarette smoking is certainly the most important risk factor in the development of COPD, passive, or side-stream, smoking may also be harmful,[385] especially in infants or children. Such individuals who live in the same household as parents or siblings who smoke have an increased incidence of respiratory illness, functional impairment, and a less than expected increase in lung function during growth.[386, 387]

Air Pollution. Air pollution may be domestic, urban, or occupational. Each may contribute to airway obstruction, although the effects are minor compared with the influence of cigarette smoking (except in heavily polluted regions and with certain industrial exposures).

Domestic exposure to pollutants is often overlooked but may be an important factor in causing disease in certain situations. For example, the use of natural gas in home cooking is associated with an increase in the incidence of childhood respiratory illness and pulmonary dysfunction that is independent of the effects of parental smoking.[388] Cooking fires are a major cause of domestic pollution worldwide, and in rural communities in developing countries prolonged exposure can lead to obstructive lung disease and cor pulmonale.[389]

Although a sudden increase in the degree of air pollution—such as occurs with smog—can result in increased morbidity and mortality in patients with established COPD,[390] there is little evidence that urban air pollution *per se* causes obstructive pulmonary disease in adult nonsmokers.[391] However, it does appear to have an effect additive to that of cigarette smoke[392] and may be partly responsible for progression of disability in patients already affected. Children with growing lungs may be particularly vulnerable to the effects of air pollution. The incidence of acute lower respiratory tract infections is higher in children who live in environments with high levels of air pollution,[393] and childhood infection is especially prone to impairing subsequent lung function.

Although some controversy exists as to the relative importance of smoking and exposure to dust in the workplace, in some occupations there is unequivocal evidence of a significant effect of dust on lung function.[394] An increased annual rate of decline in FEV_1 has been seen in workers exposed to inorganic dusts, such as coal and hard rock miners, foundry workers, and metal and chemical workers.[395, 396] Inhalation of cotton, grain, and wood dust also has been shown to contribute to chronic airway obstruction.[394, 397]

Infection. Retrospective studies have provided fairly conclusive evidence that lower respiratory tract infection in children is a significant risk factor for the subsequent development of COPD during adulthood.[398] "Childhood bronchitis," especially in children younger than 2 years of age, is associated with persistently abnormal lung function, and it is this functional impairment that later predisposes to accelerated deterioration.[399] The precise mechanism of this effect is uncertain but may be the alteration of pulmonary function, growth, or defense mechanisms. It has also been speculated that chronic latent adenovirus infection of airway epithelium may be responsible.[399a]

Respiratory infection in patients with established COPD may accelerate subsequent functional deterioration and can lead to an irreversible deficit; of importance in this regard is the possibility that established COPD itself may increase the incidence and severity of respiratory infection. However, despite a severe decline in pulmonary function during respiratory infections, most patients with COPD improve to their pre-exacerbation status after resolution of the infection.

Viral infection is responsible for the majority of clinical exacerbations in patients with COPD.[400] The rhinoviruses and myxoviruses—the latter particularly during epidemics—appear to be the commonest etiologic agents.[401] The role of bacteria in acute exacerbation is more likely that of a secondary invader following acute viral infection.

Climate. Patients with COPD often relate exacerbations of their disease to climatic factors, particularly to extreme variations in humidity and temperature. It is probable that the effect of high humidity relates not only to the water vapor but also to the high level of air pollution that often accompanies humid weather.[402] Some patients with COPD appear to be abnormally sensitive to the inhalation of cold air.[403] The degree of bronchoconstriction following cold air inhalation correlates with the magnitude of bronchodilation that occurs following inhalation of aerosol beta-adrenergic agonist[404] and with nonspecific responsiveness to methacholine.[405]

Socioeconomic Status. Epidemiologic studies have suggested an increased risk of the development of COPD in people of lower socioeconomic status. However, this effect is small and is difficult to separate from related factors, such as smoking habits, industrial exposure, passive smoking, and childhood infection.[388]

Altered Mucus and Mucociliary Clearance. The importance of alterations in the amount or characteristics of airway mucus or of the efficiency of mucociliary clearance in the pathogenesis of COPD is unclear. Cigarette smoking is associated with an increased amount of serum protein in airway mucus,[114] alterations in the viscoelastic properties of

mucus,[406] and decreased clearance of particulate matter from the airways[407]; however, patients may have significant impairment of airflow without alterations in mucociliary clearance and *vice versa*.[408] In fact, nonsmoking individuals who have primary ciliary dyskinesia and virtual absence of particulate clearance from the lung develop only mild airflow obstruction in their middle years.[409]

Heredity. First-degree relatives of patients with COPD have a likelihood of developing the disease that is 1.2 to 3 times that of the general population.[410] The observation that there is a greater concordance for indices of airway obstruction between first-degree relatives than between spouses, and between monozygotic twins than between dizygotic twins supports the influence of a genetic predisposition rather than the effects of a shared environment.

In the vast majority of cases, the underlying defect that constitutes this genetic predisposition is unknown. The exception is a deficiency of alpha$_1$-protease inhibitor (alpha$_1$PI, alpha$_1$-antitrypsin), an acute phase reactant that is synthesized in the liver and released into the blood. It is the most important circulating proteolytic enzyme inhibitor[411] and makes up the majority of the alpha$_1$ globulin peak in serum protein electrophoresis. The importance of alpha$_1$PI from a respiratory point of view is in its apparent role in maintaining normal lung structure, a deficiency of the enzyme being associated with a 30-fold increase in the incidence of emphysema.[412]

Employing immunodiffusion, values for serum concentrations of alpha$_1$PI are 200 mg per dL in normal subjects, 60 to 199 mg per dL in patients with intermediate deficiency, and less than 60 mg per dL in those with severe deficiency.[411] However, because of the well-documented overlap of serum concentrations of alpha$_1$PI, particularly between normal subjects and patients in the intermediate range, there is general agreement that protease inhibitor (Pi) phenotyping is necessary for the recognition of heterozygotes.[413]

The distribution of alpha$_1$PI levels can be explained by the presence of two genes that code for the production of alpha$_1$PI; only when both genes are defective does severe deficiency develop. Approximately 25 alleles have been described,[414] by far the commonest of which is Pi^M. A homozygous state (Pi^{MM}) is found in about 90 per cent of the general population[415] and is associated with normal quantitative determinations of alpha$_1$PI. Other alleles, designated Pi^S, Pi^F, Pi^I, Pi^X, Pi^P, Pi^Z, and so on, occur far less frequently in homozygous or heterozygous forms. In most series, the major antiprotease variants have been MS, MZ, FM, IM, SS, SZ, and ZZ, ranging from 6 per cent to less than 0.1 per cent.[416, 417]

The gene Pi^Z in the homozygous state (ZZ) is associated with the lowest serum concentration of alpha$_1$PI, the lowest total serum antiprotease activity (amounting to only 20 per cent of normal),[418] and a significant increase in the risk of developing emphysema. It has been estimated that patients with homozygous alpha$_1$PI deficiency have a 50 per cent[419] to 80 per cent[420] chance of this complication. However, they represent only about 1 per cent of individuals who have emphysema, since the homozygous state is so rare.

Pi^{ZZ} antiprotease has a lysine molecule substituted for glutamic acid at the 342 position.[421] In the normal molecule, the latter is the site of attachment of sialic acid, and it appears that the lack of sialic acid is related to defective secretions of alpha$_1$PI from hepatocytes. The accumulation of the protein in the hepatocytes results in the presence of diagnostic periodic acid–Schiff (PAS)-positive intracytoplasmic inclusion bodies; hepatitis and cirrhosis occur in some patients.

Cigarette smoking plays an important role in the production of emphysema in patients with alpha$_1$PI deficiency (*see later*). The symptoms of dyspnea and evidence of airflow obstruction bring smokers with alpha$_1$PI deficiency to medical attention in the third and fourth decades of life, whereas nonsmokers may not present until the sixth or seventh decade.[422] Pathologically, the emphysema is invariably panacinar in type and usually is more pronounced in the lower lobes.[423]

Occasionally, emphysema is described in patients showing Pi variants other than Pi^{ZZ}; the heterozygous Pi^{SZ} phenotype has been associated with alpha$_1$PI levels as low as those seen in Pi^{ZZ} patients.[424] In one study of 25 Pi^{SZ} patients, emphysema was present only in those who smoked.[425] Rare cases also have been described in which serum alpha$_1$PI has been completely absent ("null" homozygotes) accompanied by an absence of liver globules, a combination that may represent complete deletion of the gene for alpha$_1$PI synthesis.[426] Severe emphysema develops more rapidly in these patients than in those with Pi^{ZZ}. Heterozygous deficiency (PiMS) is associated with serum alpha$_1$PI levels that are approximately 60 per cent of normal, but the bulk of evidence does not support a greater incidence of COPD in heterozygotes.[427]

Nonspecific Bronchial Hyper-responsiveness (the "Dutch hypothesis"). This hypothesis proposes that patients with an atopic tendency and increased nonspecific bronchial responsiveness have an increased risk of developing irreversible airflow obstruction.[428] It is not clear exactly how these conditions might cause COPD. However, in individuals with hyper-responsive airways, it is possible that repeated episodes of acute bronchoconstriction related to smoke inhalation might by themselves cause fixed narrowing. Alternatively, an exaggerated inflammatory response to smoke in atopic individuals could be responsible.

Although a number of studies have supported a relationship between NSBH and a more rapid annual decline in FEV$_1$,[429] interpretation of some of these studies is difficult since it is possible that abnormal baseline lung function leads to airway hyper-responsiveness rather than *vice versa*.[430] Additional support for the Dutch hypothesis derives from population studies that have shown a positive relationship between decreased FEV$_1$ levels and skin test responses to allergens, blood eosinophilia, and elevated serum IgE levels.[431]

Pathogenesis

Emphysema results from the unchecked enzymatic destruction of the elastic and collagen framework of the lung.[432] The most important enzyme in this regard is elastase derived from polymorphonuclear leukocytes, although a different elastolytic enzyme in alveolar macrophages also may have a role. The lung is normally protected against excessive elastolytic damage by alpha$_1$PI. A high-molecular-weight protein, alpha$_1$-macroglobulin,[433] and low-molecular-weight antiproteases present in airway mucus[434] are less

important defenders of lung integrity. It is now accepted that an imbalance between these elastolytic and antielastolytic forces is the most important mechanism in the genesis of emphysema and loss of lung elasticity. The many factors that influence this dynamic balance are shown in Figure 11–20.

The profound effect of cigarette smoke in the pathogenesis of emphysema may be explained by its action on both elastolytic and antielastolytic factors. It decreases the level of lysyl oxidase, an enzyme involved in the repair of damaged elastin and collagen,[432] increases the number of circulating and pulmonary neutrophils,[435] delays the transit of neutrophils through the pulmonary circulation,[436] causes the release of elastase from neutrophils, and may enhance the chemotaxis of neutrophils from the vasculature to the lung interstitium.[437] The peripheral neutrophils of smokers also show a higher than normal content of myeloperoxidase—an enzyme that can oxidatively inactivate alpha$_1$PI[438]—and of neutrophil elastase.[439] Cigarette smokers also have greatly increased numbers of alveolar macrophages,[440] in which both metabolic[441] and elastolytic activity is increased.

Besides increasing the number and elastolytic capacity of inflammatory cells, smoke can tip the balance toward elastolysis by interfering with the ability of alpha$_1$PI to inhibit any elastase that is released. The active site on alpha$_1$PI is related to a methionine-serine bond that is susceptible to oxidation, and oxidant damage completely blocks the ability of alpha$_1$PI to inhibit elastase.[442] The gas phase of cigarette smoke is a rich source of oxidizing agents, and these substances have a direct effect on alpha$_1$PI.[443] Activated neutrophils and macrophages release oxygen radicals that may have a similar effect.

These hypothetical mechanisms of human emphysema are supported by many animal experiments. When administered intratracheally or by aerosol, papain,[444] pancreatic elastase,[445] and purified human neutrophil elastase[446] all are capable of causing morphologic and physiologic changes comparable to those of human emphysema. Repeated intravenous injections of endotoxin cause sequestration of neutrophils in the lungs of dogs[447] and monkeys[448] and the eventual development of emphysemalike changes; presumably, the neutrophils release proteolytic enzymes in quantities sufficient to overcome the antiproteolytic protective mechanisms. Inhibition of lysyl oxidase—the enzyme that catalyzes the cross-linking between collagen and elastin molecules—also produces emphysemalike changes in animals.[449] When inhibition is accompanied by administration of elastase, abnormalities are even more severe.[432]

Pathologic Characteristics

The majority of patients with COPD have pathologic abnormalities in the large airways, small airways, and lung parenchyma, although the changes in an individual patient may be located predominantly in one of these sites.

Large Airways

Abnormalities of the trachea and major bronchi can occur in virtually all tissues of the airway wall, including the epithelium, tracheobronchial glands, muscularis mucosa,

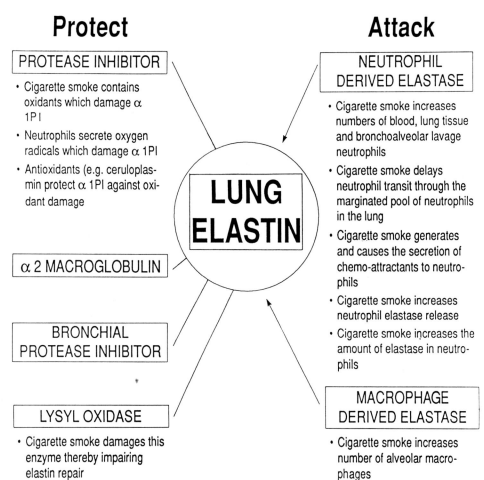

Protect

PROTEASE INHIBITOR

- Cigarette smoke contains oxidants which damage α 1PI
- Neutrophils secrete oxygen radicals which damage α 1PI
- Antioxidants (e.g. ceruloplasmin protect α 1PI against oxidant damage

α 2 MACROGLOBULIN

BRONCHIAL PROTEASE INHIBITOR

LYSYL OXIDASE

- Cigarette smoke damages this enzyme thereby impairing elastin repair

LUNG ELASTIN

Attack

NEUTROPHIL DERIVED ELASTASE

- Cigarette smoke increases numbers of blood, lung tissue and bronchoalveolar lavage neutrophils
- Cigarette smoke delays neutrophil transit through the marginated pool of neutrophils in the lung
- Cigarette smoke generates and causes the secretion of chemo-attractants to neutrophils
- Cigarette smoke increases neutrophil elastase release
- Cigarette smoke increases the amount of elastase in neutrophils

MACROPHAGE DERIVED ELASTASE

- Cigarette smoke increases number of alveolar macrophages

Figure 11–20. Pathogenesis of Emphysema. Cigarette smoke interacts with the proteolysis-antiproteolysis balance at a number of sites. The overall effect is to promote increased breakdown of elastin and to interfere with repair.

interstitial tissue, and cartilage. Hyperplasia of the tracheobronchial glands is common (Fig. 11–21) and has probably been the subject of greatest attention. Reid[450] devised an index to quantitate the hyperplasia by measuring mucous gland thickness relative to airway wall thickness and showed that an increase in the "Reid index" correlated with cough and expectoration. However, measurements of bronchial gland hyperplasia generally do not correlate with the severity of airway obstruction,[451] a lack of association that is in keeping with the failure of the clinical syndrome of chronic

bronchitis to predict the accelerated decline in expiratory flow rates that characterizes COPD.[367]

The quantity of airway cartilage, especially in the segmental and subsegmental bronchi, appears to be decreased in COPD.[452] Since cartilage provides an important contribution to the relative incompressibility of these airways, its deficiency might be expected to result in more prominent collapse. In fact, studies of the relationship between pressure and cross-sectional area of the trachea in a small number of patients with COPD[453] have shown increased "com-

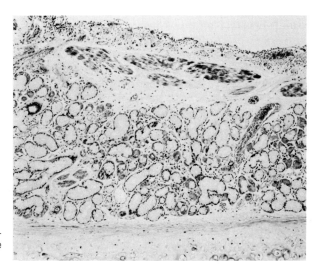

Figure 11–21. Bronchial Gland Hypertrophy in COPD. A section of segmental bronchus from a patient with chronic productive cough shows diffuse glandular hypertrophy (compare with Figure 1–9, page 7.)

pliance," suggesting that the loss of cartilage observed histologically possesses a functional counterpart.

Epithelial changes in the trachea and bronchi include hyperplasia of goblet and basal cells and squamous metaplasia, sometimes associated with dysplasia. Although such changes are not likely to contribute directly to airway obstruction, they may interfere with mucociliary clearance. Other bronchial wall abnormalities include an increase in smooth muscle (at least in some studies),[454] chronic inflammation,[455] and decreased elastic tissue.[456]

Small Airways

It is now clear that airways smaller than 2 to 3 mm in internal diameter are the major site of increased resistance to air flow in the lungs of patients with COPD.[457] Although the exact mechanism for this increase is incompletely understood, it appears to be related to a chronic inflammatory process that narrows and occasionally obliterates the membranous and respiratory bronchioles.[458] Such inflammatory changes can cause airway obstruction by several mechanisms, including (1) thickening of the airway wall by fibrous tissue and inflammatory cells; (2) plugging of the airway lumen by excessive and abnormal mucus; (3) alteration of the surface active properties of the airway liquid lining layer; and (4) disruption of the surrounding alveolar walls, which normally provide a structural support to the airways.[459]

The severity of airway narrowing can be assessed using a semiquantitative microscopic scoring system that is based on a comparison of the airways to be measured to a set of standard photomicrographs that show different degrees of cellular infiltration and fibrosis.[460] More quantitative morphometric measurements, such as the number of inflammatory cells per mm² of airway wall[461] and the thickness of the airway wall,[462] can also be used. These measurements of airway narrowing are correlated with decreased maximal expiratory flow and increased total airway resistance.[463] In addition, patients who have normal expiratory flow but abnormal test results of small airway function—such as the closing volume or the slope of phase III of the single-breath nitrogen washout test—are more likely to have pathologic abnormalities of their small airways.[464]

In many studies, an association has been found between the severity of small airway changes and the presence and degree of emphysema,[465, 466] and it is possible that the inflammation that results in narrowing of the small airways also causes destruction of alveolar walls. The two processes are not invariably associated, however; some patients with airway obstruction and pathologic abnormalities of the small airways have no morphologic emphysema.

Lung Parenchyma

The basic pathologic abnormality of the lung parenchyma in COPD is destruction of alveolar walls and the formation of enlarged airspaces (i.e., emphysema). As described in Chapter 1, the acinus consists of all tissue distal to the terminal bronchiole, comprising several generations of respiratory bronchioles, followed by alveolar ducts, alveolar sacs, and alveoli (Fig. 11–22). Selective involvement of the acinus at the level of the first and second generations of

respiratory bronchioles is termed "centrilobular emphysema," whereas diffuse and more selective terminal acinar destruction are termed "panacinar emphysema" and "distal acinar emphysema," respectively. A fourth, albeit somewhat disputed, form of emphysema is irregular, or scar, emphysema.

Centrilobular Emphysema. This form of emphysema results from destruction of parenchymal tissue in the region of the proximal respiratory bronchioles (see Fig. 11–22B). Although the term "centrilobular" is frequently used to refer to this anatomic localization, the fact that each lobule contains multiple acini means that instead of disease being found precisely in the center of the lobule, it is characteristically distributed in a multifocal fashion within it (Fig. 11–23). However, because of its widespread use, the expression "centrilobular emphysema" is used throughout this text. Of those forms of emphysema that possess clinical and functional significance, this is the commonest; it is found predominantly in cigarette smokers.

The pathology of the early stages of centrilobular emphysema and the reasons for its proximal acinar predilection have not been well established. The earliest abnormality may be fenestrae, or holes, that can be seen in the alveolar walls adjacent to small airways.[467] Theoretically, these fenestrae coalesce as they increase in size and number, so eventually the alveolar wall disappears. Morphometric studies have shown that the number of alveolar walls attached to the small airways decreases in emphysema, supporting this concept. These early morphologic abnormalities are associated with a loss of lung elasticity and decreased maximal expiratory flow and can occur in the absence of gross pathologic changes.

As the disease progresses, respiratory bronchioles dilate and the adjacent parenchymal tissue is lost, resulting in abnormal foci clearly identifiable both microscopically (Fig. 11–24) and grossly. There is usually prominent anthracotic pigment deposition in the emphysematous foci, resulting in a distinctive "checkerboard" appearance of the parenchyma (see Fig. 11–23A). With further progression, the relatively discrete foci of early disease become confluent, and eventually an entire lobule or even whole segments of lung parenchyma can be destroyed (see Fig. 11–23B).

Centrilobular emphysema shows considerable upper zone predominance, particularly affecting the apical and posterior segments of the upper lobes and the superior segment of the lower lobes.[468] The precise reasons for this are unclear but may be related to differences in zonal deposition or clearance of inhaled cigarette smoke, to differences in perfusion between upper and lower lobes (leukocyte transit time being prolonged and antielastases being less available in the relatively underperfused upper zones), or to differences in pleural pressure (the more negative pressure and resultant hyperinflation of nondependent lung regions resulting in a relatively greater mechanical stress on the alveolar walls in these regions).

Panacinar Emphysema. Panacinar (panlobular, or diffuse) emphysema has also been called "unselective" because the acinus and secondary lobules are involved diffusely rather than selectively as in proximal and distal acinar emphysema (see Fig. 11–22C). This form is characteristic of disease in alpha₁-antiprotease deficiency; however, it can also be seen in smokers and (rarely) nonsmokers without

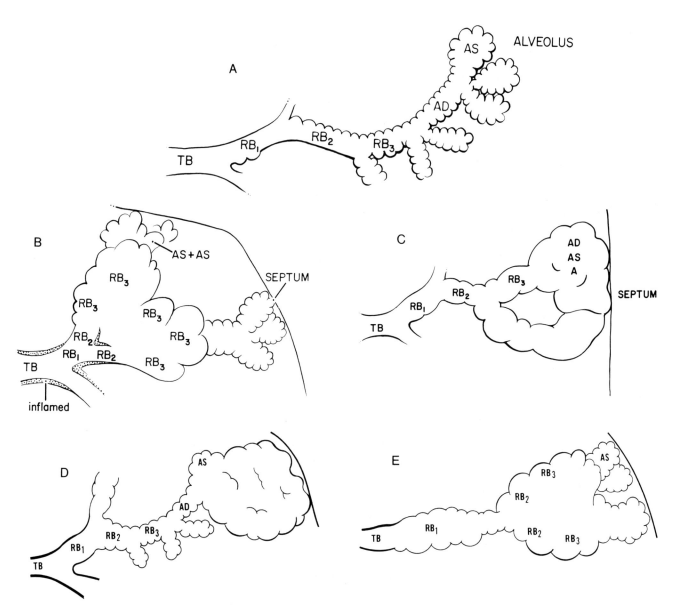

Figure 11–22. Component Parts of the Acinus. This diagrammatic representation *(A)* of the acinus shows a terminal bronchiole, respiratory bronchioles of the first (RB$_1$), second (RB$_2$), and third (RB$_3$) orders, an alveolar duct (AD), and an alveolar sac (AS). The acinus is that part of the lung distal to a terminal bronchiole, and emphysema is defined in terms of the acinus. *B,* In centrilobular (proximal acinar) emphysema, respiratory bronchioles are selectively and dominantly involved. *C,* In panacinar emphysema, the enlargement and destruction of airspaces involve the acinus more or less uniformly. *D,* In paraseptal (distal acinar) emphysema, the peripheral part of the acinus (alveolar ducts and sacs) is dominantly or selectively involved. *E,* In irregular emphysema, the acinus is irregularly involved. This form is often accompanied by scarring in the lung. *(A, D,* and *E* from Thurlbeck WM: Chronic Airflow Obstruction in Lung Disease. Philadelphia, WB Saunders Company, 1976, pp 15–17. *B,* After Leopold JG, Gough J: The centrilobular form of hypertrophic emphysema and its relation to chronic bronchitis. Thorax 12: 219, 1957; from Thurlbeck WM: Chronic obstructive lung disease. *In* Sommers SC (ed): Pathology Annual. Vol 3. New York, Appleton-Century-Crofts, 1968. *C* from Thurlbeck WM: Chronic obstructive lung disease. *In* Sommers SC (ed): Pathology Annual. Vol 3. New York, Appleton-Century-Crofts, 1968, p. 381.)

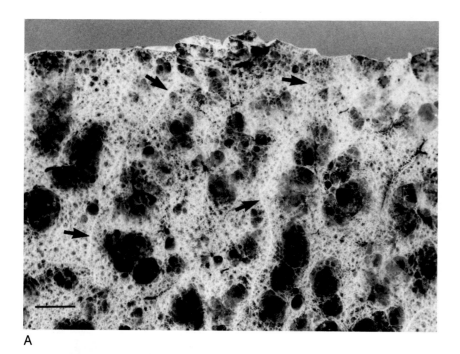

A

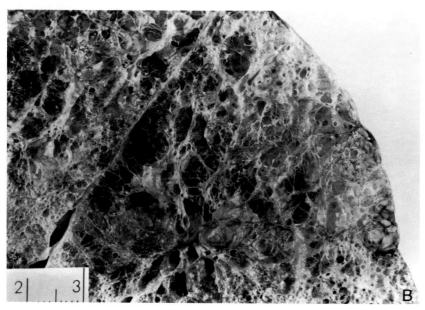

Figure 11–23. Centrilobular Emphysema: Early and Advanced. *A,* A cut section of lung parenchyma reveals multiple foci of emphysema distributed in a patchy fashion; most are associated with anthracotic pigment. The parenchyma adjacent to the interlobular septa *(arrows)* is essentially normal. The emphysematous spaces are clearly not limited to the central portion of the lobule but rather are scattered within it in a distribution corresponding approximately to the location of the proximal respiratory bronchioles. (Bar = 8 mm.) *B,* A magnified view of the superior segment of the lower lobe from another patient shows the majority of lung parenchyma to be totally destroyed and represented only by thin strands traversing emphysematous spaces.

protease deficiency.[469] As with centrilobular emphysema, the early morphologic changes have been poorly documented. However, examination of thick sections of lung reveals fenestrations in alveolar walls similar to those seen in centrilobular emphysema,[470] and it is possible that these represent the initial abnormality.

In severe disease, affected parenchyma consists of no more than large airspaces through which strands of tissue and blood vessels pass like struts—the so-called cotton-candy lung. Histologic sections show dilated airspaces with virtually no alveolar septa (*see* Fig. 11–24). The appearance in this advanced stage is indistinguishable from that in advanced centrilobular emphysema. Panacinar emphysema characteristically shows a predilection for the lower lobes and anterior lung zones, although it can occur in more or less random distribution throughout the lungs.

Distal Acinar Emphysema. Distal acinar (paraseptal) emphysema selectively involves the alveolar ducts and sacs in the peripheral portion of the acinus (*see* Fig. 11–22D). Grossly, it is usually focal and consists of a row of more or less continuous, variably sized spaces located in the periphery of the lung adjacent to the pleura or along interlobular septa (Fig. 11–25). Bullae may develop in these regions and usually are multiple; in fact, paraseptal emphysema probably represents an early form of bullous lung disease. In the vast majority of cases, this variety of emphysema is limited in extent and, with the exception of the occasional occurrence of spontaneous pneumothorax, results in no clinical disease.

Irregular Emphysema. As the name suggests, irregular (paracicatricial, or scar) emphysema shows no consistent relationship to any portion of the acinus (*see* Fig. 11–22E).

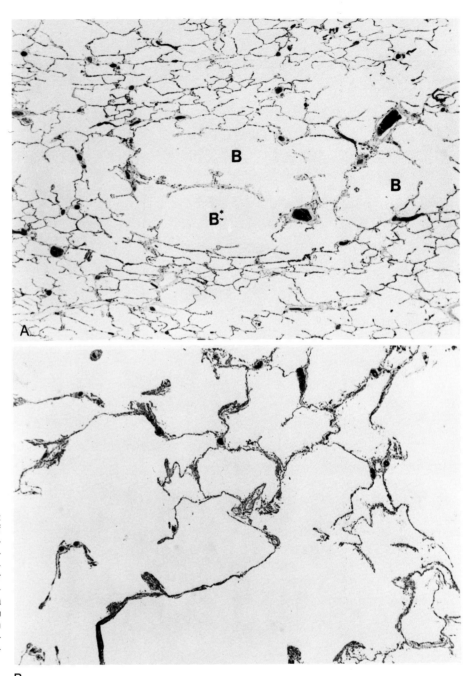

Figure 11–24. Centrilobular Emphysema: Early and Severe. A histologic section of lung parenchyma *(A)* reveals early centrilobular emphysema; note the slight dilatation of respiratory bronchioles (B) associated with blunting and loss of alveolar septa. The adjacent parenchyma is normal. *B,* A section of lung parenchyma photographed at the same magnification as *A* shows advanced emphysema, with almost no alveolar airspaces being identifiable. The appearance is similar in panacinar emphysema. (*A* and *B* × 25.)

It is always associated with fibrosis. Thus, according to the recent modification of the definition of emphysema suggested by a workshop of the National Heart, Blood, and Lung Institute, it should not even be classified as emphysema.[471] The association with fibrosis suggests a relationship with inflammation. In some instances—such as remote granulomas—this association is clearly evident (Fig. 11–26); in many others, however, it can only be assumed. Because of the frequency of pulmonary scars, irregular "emphysema" is probably the commonest form seen pathologically; typically, however, it is limited in extent and results in no functional or clinical abnormalities.

Roentgenographic Manifestations

As discussed previously, chronic bronchitis is defined clinically, emphysema pathologically, and COPD function-

ally. As a diagnostic tool that predominantly reveals morphologic abnormalities, the chest roentgenogram can demonstrate changes attributable to chronic bronchitis or emphysema but can disclose variations caused by COPD only by inference. In the following pages, therefore, only the first two of these are addressed.

Chronic Bronchitis

The roentgenographic appearances in uncomplicated chronic bronchitis are inadequately documented, mainly because no large series has been reported of an assessment of premortem roentgenograms of known bronchitic patients who have been shown to have no emphysema at necropsy. Thus, it is necessary to emphasize at the outset that although changes may be observed in the lungs *suggesting* that bronchitis may be present, it is never appropri-

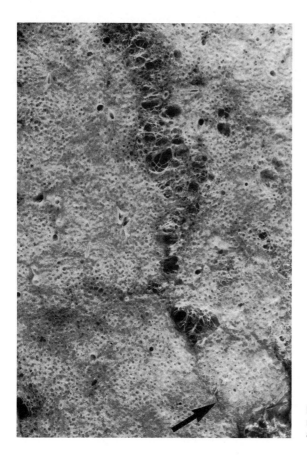

Figure 11–25. Paraseptal Emphysema. A gross specimen of lung parenchyma reveals a well-delimited zone of emphysema in a linear pattern contiguous with an interlobular septum *(arrow)*. The adjacent lung parenchyma is normal.

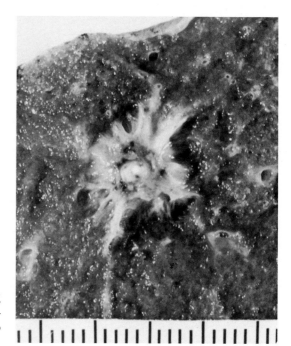

Figure 11–26. Irregular Emphysema. A slice of lung parenchyma reveals a small, round focus of necrotic material (long-standing histoplasmosis) surrounded by irregular projections of fibrous tissue and small emphysematous spaces. The latter are caused by destruction of lung tissue during the initial inflammatory reaction to *Histoplasma capsulatum.*

ate to do more than indicate that the findings are compatible with or suggestive of that diagnosis.

In reported studies of the roentgenographic features of chronic bronchitis, between 20 and 50 per cent of patients have been found to have normal examinations.[472, 473] In fact, it is probable that these figures are much too low. If one were to obtain chest roentgenograms of cigarette smokers picked at random from passers-by on the street, each of whom satisfied the clinical criteria for the diagnosis of chronic bronchitis, it is very likely that the great majority would show no changes suggesting that diagnosis.

The two roentgenographic abnormalities that are most suggestive of chronic bronchitis are thickened bronchial walls and prominent lung markings. The former can be identified in branches of the anterior or posterior segmental bronchi of the upper lobes or the superior segmental bronchi of the lower lobes. They range in diameter from approximately 3 to 7 mm and thus represent different stages in bronchial subdivision. Their accompanying arteries are nearly always identifiable but, because of slight angulation, may not be sharply defined. Thickening of these bronchial shadows viewed end-on can usually be easily identified (see Fig. 4–67, page 228).

The pattern of "prominent lung markings" (the "dirty chest") consists of a general accentuation of linear markings throughout the lungs. In one radiologic-pathologic study there was good correlation between this roentgenographic appearance and histologic evidence of interstitial edema, chronic inflammation, and mild fibrosis.[474]

Emphysema

The roentgenologic signs of emphysema include the classic triad of overinflation, oligemia, and bullae.

Overinflation. Probably the most dependable single piece of evidence of pulmonary overinflation is flattening of the diaphragmatic domes (Fig. 11–27). In fact, the authors find that if the configuration of the diaphragm is concave superiorly, the presence of emphysema is virtually certain, at least in adults. (Severe overinflation of the lungs in children—from acute bronchiolitis, for example—may result in sufficient depression of the diaphragm to show a concave configuration superiorly.) Other traditional signs of overinflation include increase in the width of the retrosternal airspace (judged by the distance from the sternum to the shadow of the ascending aorta and by the point at which the heart shadow separates from the sternum), anterior bowing of the sternum, accentuation of the thoracic kyphosis, and horizontally inclined, widely spaced ribs (see page 231).[475–477]

The development of left-sided heart failure in emphysematous patients with roentgenographic evidence of overinflation gives rise to a curious change in the chest roentgenogram: in addition to the usual evidence of interstitial pulmonary edema, the signs of overinflation may diminish or disappear altogether as a result of a drop in compliance.[478] Since roentgenologic signs of emphysema, particularly oligemia, are often more apparent in some lung zones than in others (see later), interstitial edema will be evident in those zones receiving the major blood flow; as a consequence, the edema is "inappropriately" distributed.

Alteration in Pulmonary Vasculature (Oligemia). Diminution in the caliber of the pulmonary vessels, with increased rapidity of tapering distally, is a sign of great value in differentiating emphysema from other diseases in which overinflation is an integral part, notably spasmodic asthma (Fig. 11–28). Equally important in the identification of emphysema are other vascular abnormalities, such as amputation, side branch obliteration, and curvilinear displacement, the last-named serving to indicate the presence of otherwise invisible emphysematous spaces. It is also common for blood to be diverted from more severely affected zones to those least affected, producing dilatation of segmental vessels in either upper or lower zones.

In the authors' and others'[479] experience, emphysema appears more often as local disease than is usually recognized. In one series,[479] the lower lung zones were most predominantly involved, although the authors have observed various patterns of localization to the upper lung zones, to one or two lobes of one lung, or to different lobes in the two lungs, an irregularity of distribution that has also been noted by others.[480] In a recent high-resolution CT study in which regional distribution of emphysema was correlated with pulmonary function tests in unselected smokers,[481] it was shown that predominant involvement of lower lung zones had a stronger correlation with function abnormalities than involvement of upper zones. In fact, when upper zones were predominantly affected, function tests failed to reveal the abnormality, thus representing relatively silent regions of lung destruction.

The type of emphysema associated with alpha$_1$PI deficiency usually involves the lower lobes predominantly, with relatively normal vasculature in upper lung zones (Fig. 11–29)[482] (although high-resolution CT clearly shows evidence of upper lobe involvement in many patients[482a]). However, such anatomic predilection also is found in an appreciable number of patients with normal alpha$_1$PI values.[483]

Computed tomography has been found to be an accurate method of identifying zones of oligemia in patients with emphysema (Fig. 11–30). In one study in which CT was correlated with pulmonary function tests and conventional chest roentgenograms,[484] it was found to be as sensitive as function tests and more sensitive than conventional roentgenograms in detecting emphysema. In fact, there is evidence that high-resolution CT is capable of detecting emphysema in symptomatic patients when chest roentgenograms and pulmonary function tests are nondiagnostic.[485]

Pulmonary arterial hypertension secondary to emphysema usually is easily recognizable, not by a deficiency in the peripheral vasculature alone but with the additional finding of an increase in the size of the hilar pulmonary arteries (see Fig. 11–28). In cases in which previous films are available for comparison, such increase in size should be readily apparent. When no previous films exist, a diameter of the right interlobar artery exceeding 16.0 mm should be regarded as convincing evidence of the complication.

Bullae. Bullae are local, air-containing cystic spaces within the lung, ranging from 1 cm in diameter up to the volume of a whole hemithorax. They may be single or multiple. Their walls are usually of no more than hairline thickness (Fig. 11–31), so it may be difficult to distinguish them from uninvolved parenchyma. Although they may occur in the absence of diffuse emphysema (see page 671), their identification in a patient with other roentgenographic signs of pulmonary emphysema is of diagnostic value.[486]

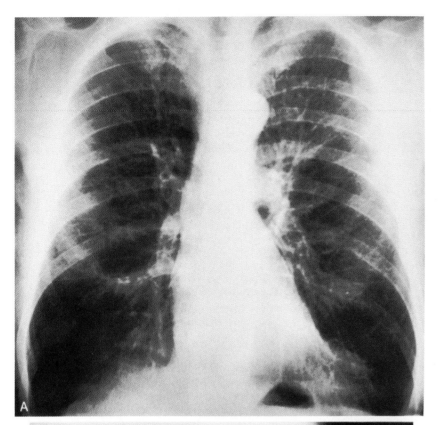

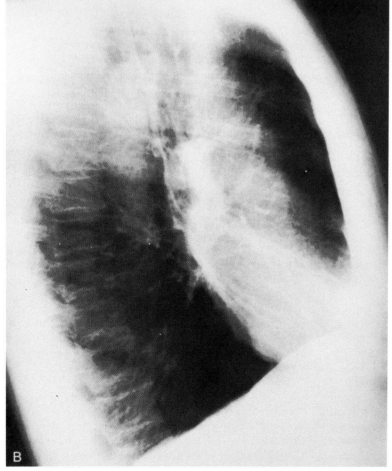

Figure 11–27. Diffuse Emphysema. Posteroanterior *(A)* and lateral *(B)* chest roentgenograms show thickened bronchial walls, marked overinflation, and bilateral lower and right upper zonal oligemia. The findings are indicative of diffuse emphysema with lower lobe predominance.

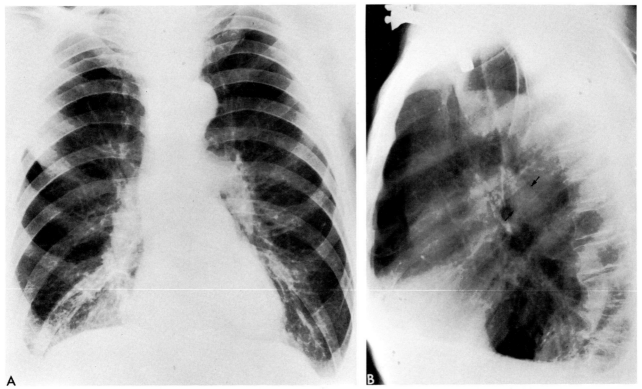

Figure 11–28. Emphysema with Pulmonary Arterial Hypertension. Posteroanterior *(A)* and lateral *(B)* roentgenograms reveal severe overinflation of both lungs as evidenced by marked flattening of the diaphragm (seen to best advantage in lateral projection). The lungs generally are oligemic, arterial deficiency being more apparent in the upper two thirds than in the bases. The hilar pulmonary arteries are moderately dilated and taper rapidly distally. In lateral projection, note the shadow of the dilated descending branch of the left pulmonary artery *(arrow)*. Despite the evidence of severe pulmonary arterial hypertension, the heart is only slightly enlarged.

The "Increased Markings" Pattern. In 1970, Thurlbeck and colleagues[487] described a series of patients with pathologically proven emphysema, in whom clinical, pulmonary function, and roentgenologic data were correlated with morphologic findings. Two different roentgenographic patterns of altered pulmonary vascularity were recognized and were designated "arterial deficiency" (AD) and "increased markings" (IM). AD represented peripheral vascular deficiency (oligemia), in most cases associated with severe overinflation. By contrast, vascular markings in the IM pattern were more prominent than normal and tended to be irregular in contour and indistinct in definition (Fig. 11–32). Thus, in contrast with the exceptionally clear lungs characteristic of "AD emphysema," the appearance was that of the "dirty chest" suggestive of some cases of chronic bronchitis. Overinflation seldom was present to the degree seen in AD disease and, in the majority of cases, was no more than slight or moderate. Pulmonary arterial hypertension (as evidenced by enlargement of the hilar pulmonary arteries) was invariable and, in many cases, was associated with cardiac enlargement; bullae were seldom seen.

Whether or not and to what extent the roentgenographic pattern of increased markings corresponds to the presence of emphysema is debatable. In fact, which label one wishes to place on this roentgenographic pattern of disease is probably more of semantic than of practical importance, although logically it should be differentiated from the classic AD pattern. However, since there is a general agreement that *all patients* with this roentgenologic pattern have severe chronic bronchitis,[487, 488] it is recommended that it be designated the "chronic bronchitic pattern with arterial hypertension."

Clinical Manifestations

Patients with COPD complain of cough, expectoration, and dyspnea. Cough can precede the onset of dyspnea by many years.[489] The majority of patients who complain of cough and expectoration have mucoid sputum, only periodically yellow or green. Hemoptysis is very uncommon, and its presence should stimulate a careful search for other causes. Most patients are heavy smokers[490]; however, in individual patients the number of years of smoking may not correlate with the amount and duration of coughing and expectoration[490] or with the degree of pulmonary dysfunction.[491]

When COPD is mild or moderate in severity, dyspnea occurs only on exertion. As the disease worsens, however, shortness of breath is precipitated by less and less effort and, in the terminal stages, is present at rest. Symptomatic airflow obstruction usually does not become apparent until after the age of 50 years[492] or until after 20 or 30 years of smoking. In patients who have severe disease, dyspnea may be influenced by posture. In some patients, it is worse when they are in the erect sitting or standing position than when they are supine or sitting leaning forward (platypnea)[493];

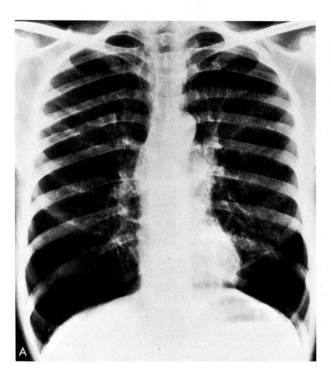

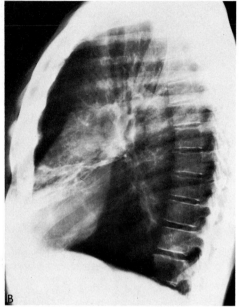

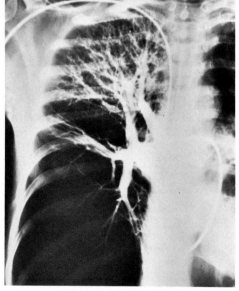

Figure 11–29. Emphysema Caused by Alpha₁-Antiprotease Deficiency. A 47-year-old woman had noted increasing shortness of breath on exertion over several years. Roentgenograms of the chest in posteroanterior *(A)* and lateral *(B)* projections reveal marked overinflation of both lungs. The lower half of both lungs shows sparse vasculature, and the vessels to the upper zones are more prominent than normal, indicating redistribution of flow. The vascular changes are particularly well seen on a pulmonary angiogram *(C)*.

C

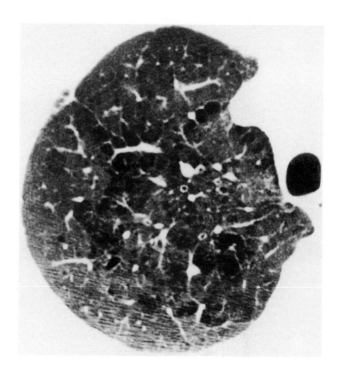

Figure 11–30. Emphysema: CT Characteristics. High-resolution CT (1.5-mm collimation reconstructed using high-frequency resolution algorithm targeted to right upper lobe) shows localized areas of abnormally low attenuation characteristic of centrilobular emphysema.

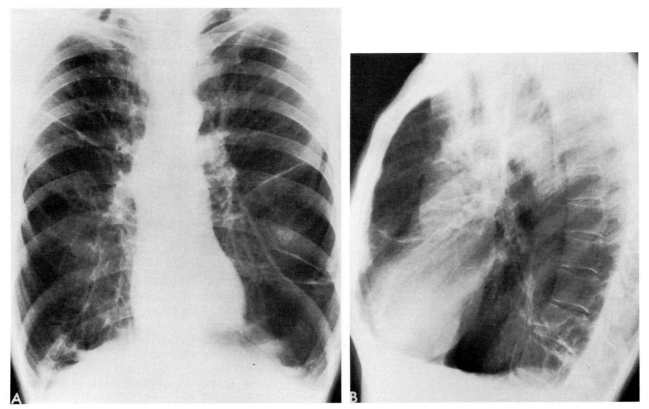

Figure 11–31. Emphysema with Bulla Formation. Posteroanterior *(A)* and lateral *(B)* roentgenograms reveal severe overinflation of both lungs. The diaphragm is low, and its superior surface concave. Note the prominent costophrenic muscle slips. The peripheral vasculature of the lungs is severely diminished, but, in contrast to the case illustrated in Figure 11–28, there is no evidence of pulmonary arterial hypertension. Several bullae are present in both lower lung zones, particularly the left.

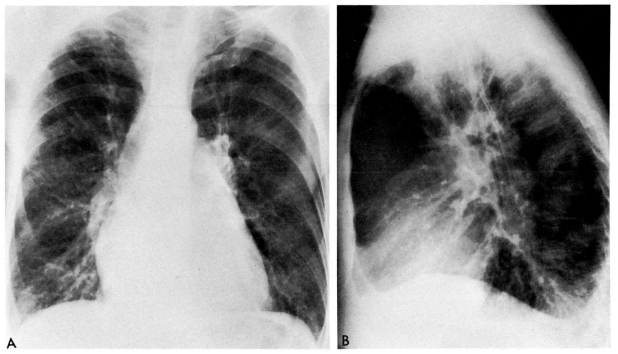

Figure 11–32. "Increased Markings" (IM) Emphysema. Roentgenograms of the chest in posteroanterior *(A)* and lateral *(B)* projections reveal only slightly increased volume (note the deep retrosternal airspace). The vascular markings throughout the lungs are prominent except in the subapical zones, where there appears to be local vascular deficiency. The heart is moderately enlarged (consistent with right ventricular enlargement), and the hilar pulmonary arteries dilated, indicating the presence of pulmonary arterial hypertension.

other patients have orthopnea. In temperate climates most patients attest to an increased frequency of respiratory infections during the winter, and such episodes also may increase the severity of dyspnea.

The dyspnea of COPD is not closely related to abnormalities of arterial blood gases, a dissociation that is highlighted by the clinical differentiation of patients with COPD into "pink puffers" and "blue bloaters."[494] A "pink puffer," or type A patient, tends to be thinner, does not have cor pulmonale or right heart failure, is relatively well oxygenated, and does not have hypercapnia but complains of severe dyspnea. A "blue bloater," or type B patient, has peripheral edema caused by right heart failure and has more severe hypoxemia and hypercapnia but less dyspnea. Although the great majority of patients with COPD cannot be placed precisely into one of these categories, the concept that there is a spectrum of clinical presentations is valuable.

The physiologic and clinical responses to a given degree of airflow obstruction differ between individuals, part of the variation probably being the result of differences in the responsiveness of the respiratory center to hypoxia and hypercapnia. It is likely that in individuals with a well-developed ventilatory responsiveness, blood gases will be preserved at the expense of increased respiratory effort. Conversely, those with relatively blunted respiratory center responsiveness may hypoventilate, thus allowing Po_2 to fall further and Pco_2 to rise higher. Genetic differences contribute to the variation in respiratory drive.[495]

In many patients with chronic cough and expectoration and mild airflow obstruction, physical examination of the chest reveals no abnormalities, at least during quiet breathing. Wheezing is usually audible during forced expiration but does not relate closely to the degree of obstruction.[496] During quiet expiration, however, it is a more reliable indicator in this regard, and symptomatic patients usually have diffuse inspiratory and expiratory wheezing. When emphysema becomes widespread it gives rise to physical signs attributable to the combination of airway obstruction, bullae, and pulmonary overinflation. The most characteristic of these additional signs is decreased intensity of breath sounds.

When lung volumes are markedly increased and the thoracic cage is fixed in an inspiratory position, the physical signs are characteristic. The chest becomes barrel shaped, the thoracic kyphosis sometimes being considerably increased, the shoulders are raised, and the chest tends to move *en bloc*, often with contraction of the accessory muscles of respiration in the neck.[497] Pulmonary overinflation may be evidenced by increased resonance of the percussion note, although this may be difficult to evaluate in obese or muscular patients. Depression of the diaphragm is believed to be responsible for a paradoxical movement of the lower thoracic costal margins during inspiration; known as Hoover's sign, it consists of an inward pulling of the costal cartilages from the flattened diaphragm.[498] Paradoxical abdominal motion at rest is a sign of inspiratory muscle fatigue or recruitment of expiratory muscles and is seen only with severe end-stage disease.

COPD is associated with several complications, the most serious of which are pulmonary arterial hypertension, right ventricular hypertrophy (cor pulmonale), and right ventricular failure. Pulmonary hypertension is caused by a combination of hypoxic vasoconstriction of the muscular pulmonary arteries, a loss of pulmonary capillary bed, a decrease of pulmonary vascular compliance, and intimal and medial hypertrophy. With mild to moderate grades of COPD (FEV_1 of 40 to 80 per cent predicted), the pulmonary artery pressure (Ppa) is usually normal at rest but increases with moderate exercise.[499] In the presence of severe COPD ($FEV_1 < 40$ per cent predicted), however, hypertension is usually present at rest (mean Ppa > 20 mm Hg) and undergoes a disproportionate increase with mild exercise[500]; its severity correlates with the degree of arterial desaturation and arterial PCO_2.[501]

Exacerbations of COPD are associated with acute worsening of pulmonary hypertension, although the Ppa usually returns to pre-exacerbation levels with treatment.[501] Ppa can also increase acutely during the episodes of hypoxemia that occur during sleep, and it has been suggested that recurrent nocturnal pulmonary hypertension can eventually result in pathologic changes in pulmonary vessels and fixed hypertension.[502] In the absence of therapy, the pulmonary hypertension in patients with COPD progresses slowly but inexorably,[503] the increase in Ppa over time correlating with decreases in FEV_1 and PaO_2.[504]

The electrocardiogram (ECG) may be perfectly normal in patients with COPD despite the development of increased pulmonary vascular resistance on exercise. As airway obstruction becomes more severe, however, signs of right axis deviation develop, with large S waves and biphasic T waves over the left precordium beyond the V_2 position. These changes correlate best with total pulmonary vascular resistance.[505] With decreasing FEV_1/FVC ratios, there is an increased frequency of P waves greater than 2.0 mm, P axis greater than $+75$ degrees, S waves greater than 5 mm in V_5 and V_6, and QRS axis greater than $+75$ degrees.[506] The most reliable indicators of right ventricular hypertrophy are S_1, Q_3 pattern, right axis deviation ($\geqq 110$), S_1, S_2, S_3 pattern, and an RS ratio in V_6 of $\leqq 1.0$.[507]

Severe COPD is associated with a significant decrease in right ventricular ejection fraction.[508] Although left ventricular function is normal in most patients who have COPD, left ventricular dysfunction may occur when cor pulmonale and right ventricular failure develop because of right ventricular dilatation, septal shift, and decreased left ventricular compliance.[509] Chronic cor pulmonale is associated with a high incidence of cardiac arrhythmias, particularly supraventricular.[510]

Secondary polycythemia develops in some hypoxemic patients with COPD, especially those who show severe nocturnal desaturation.[511] Increased carboxyhemoglobin levels can also contribute to the development of polycythemia.[512] Patients who have COPD are quite susceptible to postoperative atelectasis after upper abdominal surgery[513] and may develop marked respiratory distress after development of a spontaneous pneumothorax.[514] Air travel can be associated with significant arterial oxygen desaturation.[515]

Pulmonary Function

The most important applications of pulmonary function tests lie in detecting the presence of disease (preferably at an early stage) and in following its progression. Although

symptomatic COPD develops in only a small proportion of smokers, these individuals can be identified long before the development of symptoms because the disease follows an insidiously progressive course for years prior to clinical presentation.[516] Smoking cessation in such subjects results in some functional improvement but, more important, causes a normalization in the rate of age-related decline of lung function.[517] Thus, COPD can be prevented, but only if it is recognized at an early stage by pulmonary function testing.

Small Airway Tests. The demonstration that airways smaller than 3 mm in internal diameter were the most important site of increased resistance in the lungs of patients with established airway disease[457] led to the development of tests to detect abnormalities of small airway function.[518] It was reasoned that a test that could detect abnormal function in the airways prior to the onset of a decrease in FEV_1 would allow the identification of a small subset of smokers who had preclinical COPD and were therefore at risk for the development of symptomatic disease. Intensive smoking cessation campaigns directed at such individuals would have an important preventative effect. The so-called small airway tests that were developed include the frequency dependence of dynamic compliance (Cdyn), the single-breath nitrogen washout (Delta N_2 per L), closing volume and closing capacity, the density dependence of maximal expiratory flow, and flows at low lung volumes ($FEF_{25\%-75\%}$, $Vmax_{50}$, $Vmax_{25}$). Unfortunately, none of these tests have proved more sensitive or specific than simple spirometry in detecting "early" or mild COPD.

Maximal Expiratory Flow. A decrease in maximal expiratory flow is the diagnostic functional hallmark of COPD. Expiratory flow can be measured as peak flow (PEFR), flow in the first second of an FVC maneuver (FEV_1), average flow over the middle half of the forced expired volume ($FEF_{25\%-75\%}$, or maximal midexpiratory flow rate—MMEF), or instantaneous flow rates at different percentages of the FVC ($\dot{V}max_{50}$, $\dot{V}max_{25}$). All these measures decrease with the development of COPD. The FEV_1 has the advantage of being most reproducible in a given individual, and there is little evidence that $FEF_{25\%-75\%}$, or $\dot{V}max_{50}$, or $\dot{V}max_{25}$ is more sensitive in detecting the early stages of the disease.[519] Although there is a wide range of values within the normal population for these tests, the range can be narrowed by expressing forced expiratory flow as a percentage of FVC (FEV_1/FVC per cent). Forced expiratory flow decreases over the entire VC range, and the effort-independent portion of the curve (from 80 per cent TLC to RV) becomes more curvilinear than normal and is convex (lower toward the volume axis) (Fig. 11–33).[520]

Patients with COPD can show a substantial increase in forced expiratory flow following inhalation of a bronchodilator, 30 per cent of patients showing a greater than 20 per cent improvement in FEV_1. Patients who have asthma or COPD cannot be easily distinguished by their response to bronchodilators.[521] Some patients with COPD also show substantial improvement in function following a course of oral corticosteroid therapy[522] and, like asthmatic patients, can show substantial diurnal variation in expiratory flow.[523]

Smoking cessation results in a sustained increase in maximal expiratory flow,[524] and a normalization in the rate of decline in lung function.[525] The improvement begins as

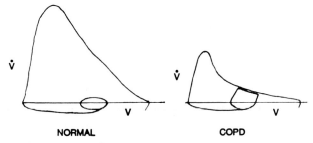

Figure 11–33. Flow-Volume Curve in a Normal Subject and a Patient with Severe Chronic Obstructive Pulmonary Disease (COPD). A normal tidal flow-volume (V̇-V) loop and a complete maximal expiratory flow-volume curve show that during tidal breathing the patient with COPD achieves maximal expiratory flow. There is considerable reserve for increased expiratory flow in the normal subject.

early as 1 week following cessation and continues for 6 to 8 months.[526]

Lung Volumes. The initial alteration in lung volumes in patients with COPD is an increase in RV.[527] This change is probably related to premature airway closure at the lung bases, as has been demonstrated in otherwise asymptomatic young smokers.[528] As RV increases further, FRC and TLC also increase, and VC decreases. Vital capacity can decrease further when patients with COPD assume the supine posture (about 10 per cent average).[529] The increase in FRC is caused by a loss of lung elastic recoil, allowing the chest wall to expand, and dynamic hyperinflation caused by the development of "auto PEEP"[530] (positive end-expiratory pressure), a phenomenon that occurs when the patient inspires prior to a reduction of alveolar pressure to zero. The resulting increased intrathoracic pressure can adversely affect venous return to the right side of the heart, and the hyperinflation puts the inspiratory muscles at a mechanical disadvantage and at a shorter length on their length-tension curve. On the positive side, the hyperinflation dilates intraparenchymal airways and decreases the resistive work of breathing.

The increase in TLC in patients who have COPD is due to a combination of a loss of lung elasticity and, possibly, an adaptive shortening of the inspiratory muscles.[531] The magnitude of the increase in TLC is controversial. Both the helium dilution technique and the body plethysmograph are subject to errors in obstructed patients. With helium, there is a tendency to underestimate TLC,[532] whereas with plethysmography thoracic gas volume may be overestimated[533] unless panting frequency is 1 Hz or less.[534]

The changes in lung distensibility that occur in COPD are reflected not only by an increase in TLC but also by an alteration in the pulmonary pressure-volume curve. The maximal elastic recoil pressure at TLC and recoil pressures at various percentages of TLC decrease with increasing age, but in smokers the decrease is accelerated.[535] The entire pressure-volume curve can be described by an exponential equation in which the constant k indicates the shape; an increased k indicates loss of recoil and correlates with the presence of emphysema in smokers.[536]

Arterial Blood Gases. Arterial blood gas tensions are commonly disturbed in patients with COPD; the more severe the disease, the more frequent the hypoxemia and hypercapnia.[487] The arterial hypoxemia is the result of al-

veolar hypoventilation and ventilation-perfusion mismatching. In COPD of mild to moderate severity, hypoxemia exists without hypercapnia. Although the V̇/Q̇ inequality impairs both the uptake of O_2 and the elimination of CO_2, the tendency for elevation of $PaCO_2$ is overcome by an increase in alveolar ventilation to well-perfused units. However, the increase in ventilation cannot correct the hypoxemia because of the nonlinear shape of the oxygen dissociation curve (*see* page 48). When COPD becomes severe, carbon dioxide retention eventually occurs as total alveolar ventilation decreases. An increase in arterial $PaCO_2$ generally does not occur until the FEV_1 is less than approximately 1.2 L, and the presence of hypercapnia in a patient with an FEV_1 greater than 1.5 L should raise the possibility of central hypoventilation.

The hypoxemia of COPD is easily corrected by increasing the concentration of inspired oxygen; however, such an increase also causes a variable increase in arterial PCO_2, especially during episodes of acute ventilatory respiratory failure.[537] The administration of supplemental oxygen causes a decrease in minute ventilation (V̇E) and a worsening of ventilation-perfusion matching, the latter as a result of the increased alveolar oxygen-attenuating hypoxic vasoconstriction.[538]

During exacerbations of COPD, blood gas tensions deteriorate. Such exacerbations are frequently associated with right-sided heart failure and fluid overload, which by themselves may impair arterial blood gas tensions. Cardiac output can influence arterial blood gases by changing the mixed venous tensions of oxygen and carbon dioxide. Given a certain disturbance of V̇/Q̇ matching and metabolic rate, mixed venous PO_2 will fall and mixed venous PCO_2 will rise as cardiac output decreases, changes that are reflected in arterial gas tensions.[539] The fluid retention associated with episodes of right-sided heart failure may also contribute to worsening gas exchange by causing mild interstitial pulmonary edema and more severe V̇/Q̇ mismatch.[540]

Sleep has profound effects on ventilatory control and arterial blood gases in patients with COPD and is frequently associated with a worsening of hypoxemia and hypercapnia.[541] Since PaO_2 values may fall onto the steep portion of the oxygen dissociation curve, the decrease in arterial saturation may be considerable. Despite the lack of frank apneas, patients with COPD may manifest episodic arterial desaturation during sleep, episodes of decreased saturation being more severe in patients categorized as blue bloaters than as pink puffers.[542] The desaturation is also more severe during REM sleep than during slow-wave sleep[543] and appears to be related to periods of hypoventilation or "hypopneas." Episodes of nocturnal desaturation are also associated with a worsening of pulmonary hypertension; although nocturnal oxygen administration does not prevent hypopnea, it does block the pulmonary vascular response.[544]

Exercise can also influence arterial blood gas tensions; in some patients, exercise induces pronounced arterial desaturation and hypercapnia, whereas in others gas exchange is improved.[545] Patients in whom desaturation occurs during exercise have significantly worse airflow obstruction, a lower diffusing capacity,[546] a higher dead space–tidal volume ratio (VD/VT), and a lower V̇T.[547] Even during maximal exercise, normal subjects do not achieve the level of ventilation of which they are capable, leaving considerable ventilatory reserve. By contrast, patients with COPD usually stop exercising when they reach their maximal achievable ventilation.

Measurement of arterial pH, hydrogen ion concentration, and bicarbonate provides important information about the acid-base status of patients with COPD. When an excess of carbon dioxide is compensated for by an increase in bicarbonate, there is clear indication that the respiratory failure is not of "acute" onset. An arterial pH within or above the normal range is unusual in uncomplicated respiratory acidosis and suggests the possibility of concomitant metabolic alkalosis, usually secondary to diuretic usage. An elevated Pco_2 associated with a normal or only slightly raised bicarbonate level indicates that the hypoventilation and respiratory acidosis are of recent onset. However, this conclusion is not justified if there is coexisting metabolic acidosis that has depressed the bicarbonate level.

Diffusing Capacity. The single-breath diffusing capacity of individuals who smoke cigarettes is lower than that of age-matched nonsmoking control subjects, even in the absence of other evidence of lung dysfunction. Part of this decrease is caused by elevated blood carboxyhemoglobin levels; however, even after correction for the back-pressure of carbon monoxide, smoking subjects have lower values of DlcoSB.[548] This decrease in DlcoSB may be a result of decreased pulmonary vascular volume in smokers.[548a]

In the presence of established COPD there is a further reduction in diffusing capacity that is related to the extent of emphysema.[487] This reduction is generally considered to be caused by both a decrease in the membrane component and $\dot{V}/\dot{Q}$ mismatch. It is probable, however, that there are other contributing factors, including reduction in capillary volume and perhaps limitation of diffusion in the gas phase of the "air pools" typical of emphysema.[549]

Prognosis

Over a period of years, most patients with COPD experience slow but inexorable worsening of symptoms and progressive impairment of pulmonary function. When the impairment results in dyspnea, progression to severe disability can be expected within 6 to 10 years.[516] In advanced disease, repeated episodes of "acute-on-chronic" respiratory failure may occur. Although 70 to 75 per cent of patients survive such crises,[550] 50 per cent die within 1 year,[551] and 70 per cent within 2 years of the initial episode.[550] Inspiratory muscle fatigue may be the final common pathway that causes ventilatory failure in these patients.

Prognosis is also significantly related to the pulmonary hemodynamic and right ventricular consequences of COPD.[552] Patients who have a pulmonary artery pressure of less than 20 mm Hg have an average 5-year survival rate of about 70 per cent compared with less than 50 per cent in those whose pressure exceeds 20 mm Hg. However, prognosis is equally well predicted by measurements of arterial PCO_2 or FEV_1.[553]

Long-term supplemental oxygen increases the survival time of patients with advanced COPD.[554] The exact mechanism by which this occurs is not clear. In one study, lung function did not show improvement in the patients who received oxygen, and pulmonary artery pressure did not decrease significantly, although the increase in pulmonary artery pressure was less than would have been expected without oxygen.[555] Prevention of severe oxygen desaturation during sleep may decrease cardiac irritability, a possible contributing factor to the beneficial effects of oxygen.[556]

Despite the foregoing, the use of *uncontrolled oxygen therapy* for respiratory failure in patients with severe COPD can cause serious complications, a high concentration of inspired alveolar oxygen causing worsening of hypercapnia by interfering with hypoxic vasoconstriction, increasing "physiologic" dead space, and depressing minute ventilation.[557] In fact, an abrupt and sometimes catastrophic rise in PCO_2 can result in coma and death.[558]

BULLOUS DISEASE OF THE LUNGS

A bulla is an air-filled, thin-walled space within the lung that is greater than 1 cm in diameter in the distended state.° Its walls are formed by pleura, connective tissue septa, or compressed lung parenchyma. Thus, the character of the wall depends to some extent on the site of the bulla.

It is useful to divide patients with bullous disease of the lungs into two groups: (1) those with COPD, in which case the bulla can be considered as a particularly large focus of otherwise typical emphysema; and (2) those judged to have normal pulmonary parenchyma between the bullae and who thus are free from airway obstruction (primary bullous disease). The pathogenesis of the latter form is unclear; however, a familial occurrence has been reported.[559] The incidence is increased in patients with Marfan's syndrome[560] and Ehlers-Danlos syndrome,[561] suggesting an underlying inherited defect in connective tissue in at least some patients.

Pathologic Characteristics

Three morphologic types of bullae have been described.[562] Type 1 bullae most commonly originate in a subpleural location in the apex of an upper lobe or along the costophrenic rim of the middle lobe and lingula. When these bullae are seen in an excised lung, they appear as variably sized, spherical sacs projecting above the pleural surface (Fig. 11–34). Of necessity, they extend into the contiguous lung *in vivo*, compressing the parenchyma and causing passive atelectasis. Each bulla characteristically has a narrow neck and usually contains no alveolar remnants or blood vessels. It is possible that this type is related to paraseptal emphysema.[563]

Type 2 bullae are also superficial in location but have a very broad neck and develop most often over the anterior edge of the upper and middle lobes and over the diaphragmatic surface. In contrast with type 1 bullae, this variety characteristically contains blood vessels and strands of partially destroyed lung. It is the most frequent of the three forms to be associated with spontaneous pneumothorax.[564]

°The term "pneumatocele" is sometimes used as a synonym for bulla; in the authors' opinion, however, use of this word should be restricted to a thin-walled, gas-filled space within the lung that develops in association with acute pneumonia, most commonly of staphylococcal etiology and almost invariably transient (*see* page 239).

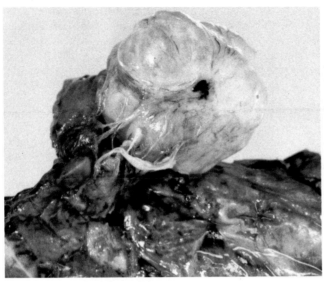
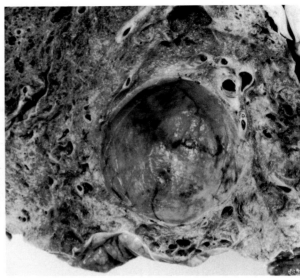

A

B

Figure 11–34. Bullae. *A,* A discrete narrow-necked bulla is present on the apical aspect of the upper lobe. *B,* The basal portion of the lower lobe from another patient shows a spherical, smooth-walled bulla within the lung parenchyma (the other half of the bulla extended to the lateral pleural surface). The remainder of the lung parenchyma shows moderate emphysema.

Type 3 bullae lie deep within the lung substance but are otherwise similar to the type 2 variety, commonly containing strands of residual lung tissue. They appear to affect both upper and lower lobes equally and usually represent an exaggerated form of generalized emphysema.

Roentgenographic Manifestations

Roentgenographically, bullae are seen much more commonly in the upper lobes than elsewhere in the lungs. The diagnosis depends on identification of local, thin-walled, sharply demarcated areas of avascularity (Fig. 11–35). The walls are characteristically apparent as hairline shadows, but since the air cysts are most often at or near the lung surface, usually only a portion of the wall is visible. Since the bullae trap air during expiration, they may be identified on roentgenograms exposed at RV and yet be barely or not at all visible on those exposed at TLC; in fact, they may undergo an increase in size during expiration. In the majority of cases, they enlarge progressively over a period of months to years (Fig. 11–36). Evidence of diffuse emphysema may be present elsewhere in the lungs (*see* Fig. 11–31, page 667).

CT can provide greatly improved visibility of a bulla already identified and may reveal bullae not suspected on plain roentgenograms (Fig. 11–37). It is particularly valuable in determining the extent of associated emphysema or parenchymal compression of adjacent lung tissue[565] and should be performed in any individual in whom surgical excision of the bulla is considered. Angiography also may be of value in preoperative assessment.[563]

Since bullous disease commonly does not produce any

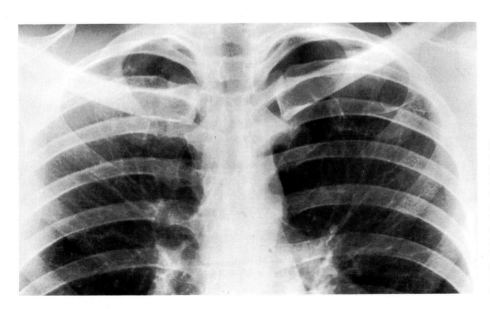

Figure 11–35. Multiple Bullae in Otherwise Normal Lung. A view of the upper half of the thorax from a posteroanterior roentgenogram reveals numerous curved hairline shadows in the upper portion of the left lung, representing the walls of multiple large bullae. A single bulla is present in the right paramediastinal area. An anteroposterior tomogram *(not illustrated)* demonstrated a normal distribution and caliber of the pulmonary vessels bilaterally, except for the avascular bullae.

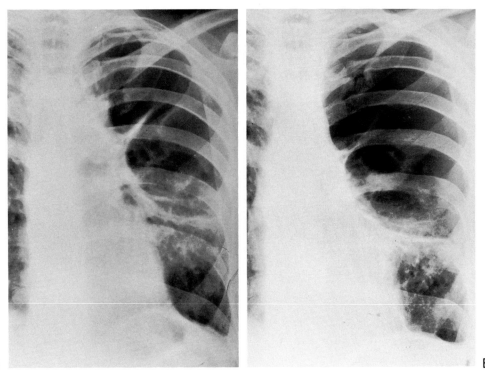

A   B

Figure 11–36. Progressive Enlargement of Bullae. A posteroanterior roentgenogram *(A)* reveals a large bulla occupying the upper half of the left lung. The parenchymal disease is due to chronic fibrocaseous tuberculosis. Approximately 1 year later *(B)*, the bulla has increased considerably in size. (Courtesy of Montreal Chest Hospital Center.)

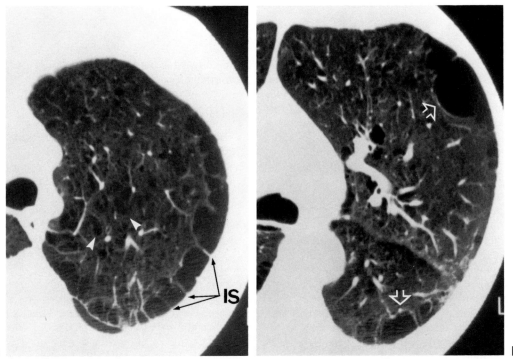

A   B

Figure 11–37. Bullae and Paraseptal Emphysema: CT Characteristics. High-resolution CT scans through the midtrachea *(A)* and carina *(B)* show multiple small cystic spaces *(arrowheads)* widely dispersed throughout the upper lobes. Additionally, there are a number of larger bullae *(open arrows)* in the subpleural parenchyma of the upper and lower lobes; interlobular septa (IS) partition the cystic areas into prominent arcades. These latter findings are characteristic of paraseptal emphysema.

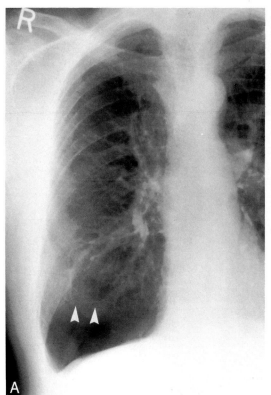 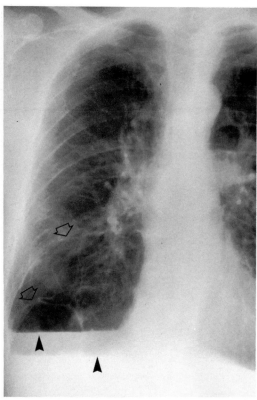

Figure 11–38. Infected Bullae. A posteroanterior chest roentgenogram *(A)* reveals typical features of diffuse emphysema. In addition, the supradiaphragmatic portion of the right lower lobe is severely oligemic, and there is displacement of vessels upwards, backwards, and laterally by one or more large bullae; a faint curvilinear opacity may represent the wall of a bulla *(arrowheads)*. Three months later *(B)*, two long fluid levels *(arrowheads)* had developed in adjacent bullae. Note that the walls of the bullae are more clearly outlined *(open arrows)*, presumably as a result of thickening of adjacent tissue by inflammatory cells, edema, and fibrovascular tissue.

symptoms, its presence may become evident only when chest roentgenography is carried out during investigation of an acute lower respiratory tract infection in which the bulla itself has become infected. In such circumstances, the roentgenographic appearance may be misinterpreted as a lung cavity secondary to abscess formation. Differentiation between the two is aided by the observations that most patients with infected bullae are much less ill than those with acute lung abscess and that most infected bullae have much thinner walls (Fig. 11–38), are surrounded by lesser degrees of pneumonitis, and usually contain much less fluid than cavitated lung abscesses. Complete clearing of fluid from infected bullae may be protracted, averaging about 6 weeks in some reports.[566]

Spontaneous pneumothorax commonly occurs in association with small bullae affecting the lung apices. Less commonly, it complicates large bullae in the lower or other lobes.[559] When pneumothorax develops in patients with peripheral lung bullae, the air sacs may be much more easily identified when the lung is collapsed than when it is fully inflated. This improved visibility results from the tendency of bullae to remain air-containing while surrounding lung collapses. Sometimes the presence of pneumothorax can be exceedingly difficult to recognize when large bullae occupy much of the volume of one lung (Fig. 11–39). In this

situation, it has been shown that CT can be of value in confirming its presence or absence.[567]

Clinical Manifestations

Primary bullous disease characteristically occasions no symptoms or signs. Typically, there is also minimal abnormality in pulmonary function. The VC usually is within normal range, although FRC and RV may be increased, especially if they are measured by body plethysmography. Flow rates and diffusing capacity are normal or nearly normal, although diffusion may be affected if adjacent lung parenchyma is severely compressed. Blood gas values usually are normal at rest but may reveal evidence of hypoxemia during exercise.[568]

Since there is no clinical disability, surgery is not indicated in the great majority of patients with primary bullous disease. However, when bullae are large, surgical removal may become necessary; in such cases, pulmonary function studies carried out before and after surgery have revealed significant improvement.[569] The rationale for bullectomy lies in the potential for healthy lung to expand and fill the space occupied by the bullae and in an increase in elastic recoil pressure that reduces the tendency for airways to collapse on expiration.[570]

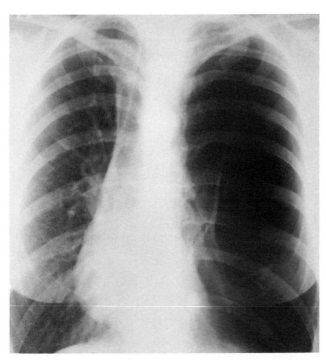

Figure 11–39. A Huge Bulla Simulating Pneumothorax. A posteroanterior chest roentgenogram demonstrates a severely overinflated and almost totally oligemic left hemithorax. A small amount of distorted and compressed left lung parenchyma is situated contiguous with the heart border. The mediastinum is displaced to the right. The vasculature of the right lung is within normal limits. The patient is an essentially asymptomatic middle-aged woman.

Patients who have bullae associated with COPD show little difference clinically or functionally from COPD without bullae.

UNILATERAL OR LOBAR EMPHYSEMA

Unilateral or lobar emphysema (unilateral hyperlucent lung, Swyer-James or Macleod's syndrome) is one of the very few conditions whose name derives entirely from the manifestations it produces roentgenographically—a state in which the density of one lung (sometimes only one lobe) is markedly less than the density of the other.

Pathogenesis and Pathologic Characteristics

The pathologic changes include bronchitis, bronchiectasis, bronchiolitis, and a variable degree of destruction of the lung parenchyma, without the anthracosis that is characteristic of centrilobular emphysema.[571] This appearance is consistent with the hypothesis that the condition begins as a viral bronchiolitis.[572] According to this interpretation, infection results in obliteration of small airways while leaving the lung parenchyma relatively unaffected, it being ventilated by collateral air drift with resulting air trapping. Although the destructive changes characteristic of emphysema ultimately occur in most cases,[573] the pathogenesis of this process is unclear. It is conceivable, however, that infection persists in the lung parenchyma, with consequent elastolysis from phagocytic cell proteases.

Roentgenographic Manifestations

The roentgenographic manifestations usually are easily recognized and are virtually pathognomonic. A posteroanterior roentgenogram of the chest exposed at TLC reveals a remarkable difference in the radiolucency of the two lungs, caused *not* by a relative increase in air in the affected lung but by decreased perfusion (Fig. 11–40). The peripheral pulmonary markings are diminutive, indicating severe narrowing and attenuation of the vessels. The ipsilateral hilum also is diminutive but is *present*, a feature of great value in the differentiation from proximal interruption of a pulmonary artery (pulmonary artery agenesis). In roentgenograms exposed at TLC, the volume of the affected lung (or lobe) either is comparable to that of the normal contralateral lung or is reduced; it is seldom, if ever, increased. The volume of the affected lung depends almost entirely on the age of the patient at the time of the infectious insult: the younger the patient, the smaller the fully developed lung, since the insult retards further maturation.[574]

One of the characteristic roentgenologic features of unilateral or lobar emphysema—in fact, a *sine qua non* for diagnosis—is the presence of air trapping during expiration (*see* Fig. 11–40). This indicates the presence of airway obstruction and is of absolute value in differentiation from other conditions that may give rise to unilateral or lobar translucency. Since the contralateral lung is normal, expiration (particularly if rapid) causes the mediastinum to swing abruptly toward the normal lung, and excursion of the hemidiaphragms is markedly asymmetric, being severely diminished on the affected side. Roentgenograms exposed at RV also accentuate the disparity in radiolucency of the two lungs, the density of the normal lung being much greater. This is not only because the normal lung contains less air but also, perhaps more important, because its blood flow is virtually the total output of the right ventricle.

Ancillary diagnostic techniques such as perfusion lung scanning or radionuclide V̇/Q̇ scans may reveal additional areas of involvement in some patients.[575] Computed tomography also has been shown to be a procedure of some value in clarifying the morphologic features of the disease.[576] Pulmonary arteriography is seldom indicated. In the majority of patients, bronchography reveals a characteristic deformity of the bronchial tree: the segmental bronchi are irregularly dilated and end abruptly in squared or tapered terminations in the vicinity of the fifth- or sixth-generation divisions. Filling of peripheral bronchioles is notable by its absence, even with repeated deep respirations.[577]

A partly obstructing lesion situated within a main bronchus can create a triad of roentgenographic signs that are indistinguishable from those of unilateral emphysema—smaller than normal lung volume, oligemia, and expiratory air trapping. As a consequence, in any patient presenting with these signs, the presence of a lesion within the ipsilateral main bronchus *must* be excluded before the diagnosis of Swyer-James syndrome is accepted. The easiest way of accomplishing this is by bronchoscopy. Other conditions that give rise to unilateral or lobar radiolucency, such as proximal interruption of a pulmonary artery, hypogenetic lung syndrome, and obstruction of a main pulmonary artery or one of its branches from thromboembolic disease, are readily differentiated by the absence of air trapping during

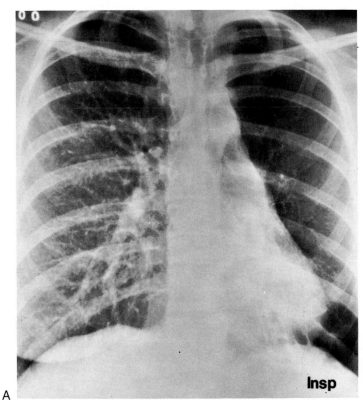

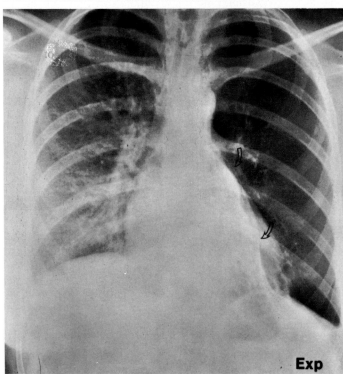

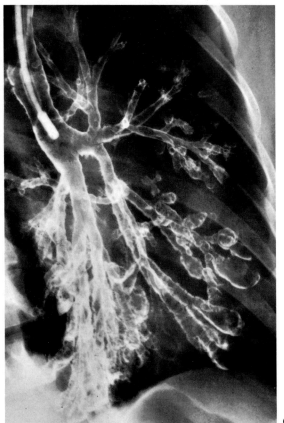

Figure 11–40. Swyer-James Syndrome Associated with Absence of the Ipsilateral Breast. Posteroanterior roentgenograms in inspiration *(A)* and expiration *(B)* reveal marked oligemia of the left lung and severe air trapping on expiration. A left breast shadow is not visualized, nor was breast tissue apparent on physical examination. The left lower lobe shows a severe degree of loss of volume *(open arrows* in *B)*, and the left hilum is diminutive. A left bronchogram *(C)* reveals bronchiectasis of all segments, those in the lower lobe being the most severely involved and thus accounting for the loss of volume. All bronchial segments terminate abruptly in a configuration characteristic of obliterative bronchiolitis. Absence of the pectoral muscles and left breast suggested the possibility of Poland's syndrome, but no other congenital anomalies were discovered. (Courtesy of Montreal Chest Hospital Center.)

expiration and by other roentgenologic signs that characterize these conditions.

Clinical Manifestations

The clinical presentation is highly variable. Some patients are completely asymptomatic,[578] some complain of dyspnea on exertion,[579] and others present with a history of repeated lower respiratory tract infections.[580] Physical examination reveals restriction of chest expansion on the affected side, associated with diminished breath sounds, relative hyperresonance, and, sometimes, scattered crackles.[581]

Blood gas concentrations usually are normal but may fall during exercise. Pulmonary function tests show a reduction in VC and expiratory flow rates as well as a decreased diffusing capacity.

BRONCHIECTASIS

General Features

Bronchiectasis is defined as irreversible abnormal dilation of the bronchial tree. As a pathologic abnormality it is common and occurs in a variety of conditions (Table 11–3). As a clinically significant affliction, however, it has decreased considerably in importance since the advent of antibiotic therapy, at least in industrialized societies.[582] It is probable that the most important cause of clinically important bronchiectasis in North America and Europe today is cystic fibrosis.[583]

Pathogenesis

One of the most important mechanisms by which bronchiectasis develops is airway infection. When bronchiectasis starts in childhood in otherwise healthy individuals, the initial infection is often measles or pertussis; when it occurs in patients with cystic fibrosis, bacteria such as *Pseudomonas* species are usually responsible. In both situations, the initial damage to the airway wall is followed by an increased susceptibility to further infectious episodes and,

Table 11–3. CLASSIFICATION OF BRONCHIECTASIS

General Category	Disease Examples
Congenital abnormality in bronchial structure	Absent or defective cartilage, intraluminal webs
Dyskinetic cilia syndrome	
Cystic fibrosis	
Deficiency in host defense	Agammaglobulinemia, chronic granulomatous disease of childhood, etc.
Immunologic abnormality	Allergic bronchopulmonary aspergillosis
Postinfectious bronchitis	Classic bronchiectasis secondary to measles or pertussis pneumonia
	Swyer-James syndrome
Post-toxic bronchitis	Ammonia inhalation, gastric acid aspiration, etc.
Acquired bronchial obstruction	Intraluminal obstruction by neoplasm, aspirated foreign body, broncholiths
	Compression by lymph nodes (neoplasms, tuberculosis, etc.)
Parenchymal fibrosis	Tuberculosis, sarcoidosis, etc.
Chronic obstructive pulmonary disease	Emphysema

in some cases, airway colonization by various microorganisms. The repetitive or continuous inflammatory reaction results in progressive bronchial wall damage and dilatation, establishing a vicious cycle of further infection and ever-increasing bronchiectasis.[584]

The bronchiectasis that develops following inhalation of various fumes or gases such as ammonia[585] or following aspiration of liquid gastric contents (especially in heroin addicts)[586] is also related to an initial damage to the airway wall followed by infection. Some of the other conditions associated with bronchiectasis, including the dyskinetic cilia syndrome and immunologic deficiency states such as agammaglobulinemia, probably act by predisposing to bronchial wall infection or colonization.

Of a somewhat different pathogenesis is the bronchiectasis that occurs in patients with chronic upper lobe tuberculosis and some interstitial lung diseases such as sarcoidosis. In these conditions, the parenchyma appears to be the primary site of disease, replacement of alveoli by fibrous tissue resulting in parenchymal retraction and secondary bronchial dilatation.

Pathologic Characteristics

The pathologic findings in bronchiectasis vary somewhat according to the severity of bronchial dilatation and the degree of distal bronchial and bronchiolar obliteration.[587] In mild disease (cylindrical bronchiectasis), the bronchi are of regular outline, their diameter remaining constant or increasing only slightly as they extend distally (Fig. 11–41). The number of subdivisions of the bronchial tree from the main bronchus to the periphery are within normal limits, but smaller bronchi and bronchioles are plugged with thick, purulent material.

In more severe disease (varicose bronchiectasis), the degree of dilatation is greater, and local constrictions cause an irregularity of outline of the bronchial wall that resembles varicose veins. The lumina of many smaller bronchi and bronchioles are obliterated by granulation or fibrous tissue. In the severest cases (saccular [cystic] bronchiectasis), bronchial dilatation increases progressively toward the periphery, resulting in cystic spaces measuring up to several centimeters in diameter (*see* Fig. 11–41). The maximum number of bronchial subdivisions that can be counted may be no more than five, and bronchioles may be entirely absent.

The intervening pulmonary parenchyma may be normal but often shows multifocal areas of organizing or organized pneumonia, reflecting the frequent bouts of infection experienced by these patients. Bronchial artery circulation typically is markedly increased[588] and is the source of hemoptysis, a frequent complication.

Roentgenographic Manifestations

Bronchiectasis is bilateral in approximately 50 per cent of patients and, in the great majority, involves the basal segments of the lower lobes. However, it often varies considerably in severity between different lobes and even between different segments in the same lobe.

The plain roentgenogram reveals changes highly suggestive of the diagnosis in the great majority of patients, the typical changes consisting of the following:

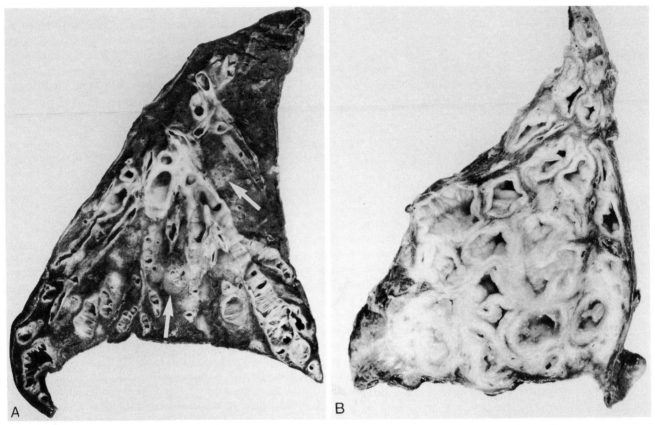

Figure 11–41. Bronchiectasis. Illustrated are the cut sections of lower lobes from two patients with bronchiectasis, that in *A* showing relatively mild ("cylindrical" and "varicose") bronchiectasis, and that in *B* severe ("saccular" or "cystic") bronchiectasis. Although much of the parenchyma in *A* is normal, focal areas of organizing or organized pneumonia are apparent *(arrows)*. This process is advanced in *B*, there being almost no residual normal parenchyma.

1. Increase in size and loss of definition of the markings in specific segmental areas of the lungs.

2. Crowded markings, indicating the almost invariable associated loss of volume.

3. Evidence of oligemia as a result of reduction in pulmonary artery perfusion (Fig. 11–42).

4. In more advanced disease, cystic spaces up to 2 cm in diameter, sometimes containing fluid levels (Fig. 11–43).

5. In very severe disease, the formation of a rather coarse "honeycomb" pattern consisting of rarefied areas that, in contrast with the cystic spaces described earlier, do not fill with contrast medium. In some cases, atelectasis may be complete and is associated with total airlessness of a lobe (Fig. 11–44).

Although the plain roentgenogram may strongly suggest the diagnosis, bronchography (Fig. 11–45) or CT (Fig. 11–46) is mandatory to establish its presence beyond question and to determine its precise extent if surgery is contemplated. Bronchography should be performed only after adequate postural drainage and antibiotic therapy have rendered the bronchial tree as free as possible from retained secretions. Only one lung should be studied at a time. Most studies have shown that CT is sensitive and accurate in the detection of bronchiectasis.[589]

The term "reversible bronchiectasis" has been used to refer to bronchial dilatation that occurs in association with acute pneumonia. Dilatation develops as a result of retained secretions and of the atelectasis that is an invariable accompaniment of resolving pneumonia. With complete resolution of the pneumonia the dilatation gradually disappears, although this may take as long as 3 or 4 months. Consequently, if surgery is contemplated it is advisable to allow 4 to 6 months to elapse after acute pneumonia before performing bronchography or CT for the assessment of the extent and severity of disease.

Clinical Manifestations

The main symptoms are cough and expectoration of purulent sputum. Although the quantity of sputum varies with the severity of the disease, most patients expectorate daily. Some patients become aware of purulent expectoration only after respiratory infections (which tend to be frequent). In cases in which the disease is a complication of measles, whooping cough, or other infection, the history commonly dates from early childhood.[590] Hemoptysis occurs in about 50 per cent of older patients, although it is relatively rare in children, and may be the presenting feature. If the disease is widespread, the patient may complain of shortness of breath.

In almost every case, persistent crackles are detectable in the area of major involvement. If the bronchiectasis is

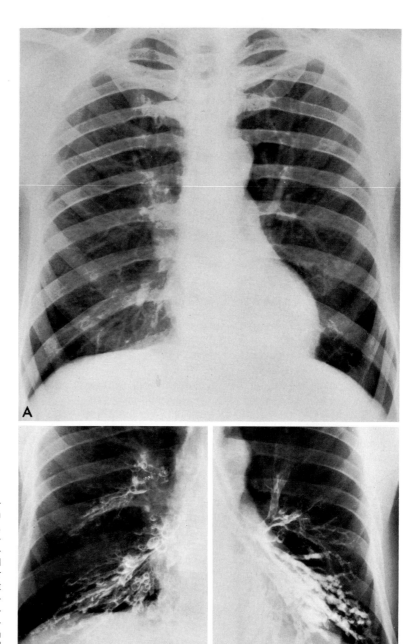

Figure 11–42. Varicose Bronchiectasis. A posteroanterior roentgenogram *(A)* shows a rather subtle change in the size of the vascular markings throughout the lungs, the upper lobe vessels being somewhat larger than normal, and the lower lobe vessels comparatively inconspicuous. Right *(B)* and left *(C)* bronchograms reveal extensive dilatation of all basal bronchi of the lower lobes and of the right middle lobe. The dilatation is not uniform but is characterized by numerous local constrictions that give the bronchi a configuration resembling varicose veins. There is a notable absence of peripheral filling. It is assumed that the alteration in vascular pattern resulted from a redistribution of blood flow from the lower lobes as a result of hypoxic vasoconstriction, bronchial artery hypertrophy, and systemic–pulmonary arterial anastomoses.

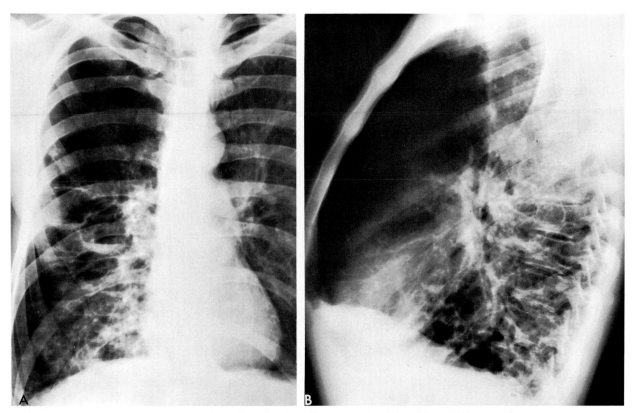

Figure 11–43. Advanced Cystic Bronchiectasis. Posteroanterior *(A)* and lateral *(B)* roentgenograms demonstrate extensive replacement of the right lower lobe by multiple thin-walled cysts, many of which contain air-fluid levels.

associated with significant airway obstruction, diffuse wheezes may be heard over both lungs. Extrathoracic manifestations include finger clubbing, seen in about one third of cases,[590] and, rarely, brain abscess and amyloidosis.

Patients who have localized bronchiectasis may have little or no functional impairment. In more generalized disease, there is a combination of restrictive and obstructive changes. The predominant functional abnormality consists of airflow obstruction unaccompanied by marked hyperinflation: FEV_1, FVC, and the ratio of FEV_1 to FVC are decreased, and RV is increased. The diffusing capacity may be mildly reduced, and there can be bronchial hyper-responsiveness and a reversible component to the obstruction.[591] A small number of patients, invariably those with diffuse disease, manifest the typical pattern of advanced COPD, including hypoxemia and carbon dioxide retention.

Prognosis

Prior to 1940, 70 per cent of patients died before the age of 40 years, about 90 per cent as a direct result of the disease.[592] With the advent of antibiotics, the prognosis has significantly improved. In 1970, the average age at death was 55 years, and in only 50 per cent of patients was death attributable to bronchiectasis itself.[593] After pulmonary resection for localized bronchiectasis, the disease commonly affects segments previously shown to be normal bronchographically.[594]

Dyskinetic Cilia Syndrome

The pathogenesis of the syndrome of situs inversus, paranasal sinusitis, and bronchiectasis (Kartagener's syndrome) was obscure until 1975, when abnormal ciliary structure and function were identified as the basic abnormalities.[595] Although the descriptive term "immotile cilia syndrome" was suggested to replace the eponymous name, it has become apparent that even the structurally abnormal cilia move, albeit in an ineffective, uncoordinated fashion.[596] As a result, the terms now accepted for these disorders are dyskinetic cilia syndrome (DCS) or primary ciliary dyskinesia. The incidence of DCS in the total white population is estimated to be 1 in 40,000.[597]

The abnormality has a strong familial association, most studies suggesting an autosomal recessive pattern of inheritance[598]; however, the variety of ultrastructural defects associated with the clinical syndrome suggests considerable genetic heterogeneity.[599] In addition, patients have been described with classic Kartagener's syndrome and abnormal airway ciliary ultrastructure but with normal spermatozoa, indicating that discordance in phenotypic presentation can occur.[600]

Ultrastructural abnormalities in each of the components of the cilium have been identified in patients with DCS (Fig. 11–47). These include a lack of outer dynein arms, absent or short radial spokes,[601] deficient central sheath, absent or defective inner dynein arms,[602] absent central microtubules, transposition of peripheral microtubules,[603]

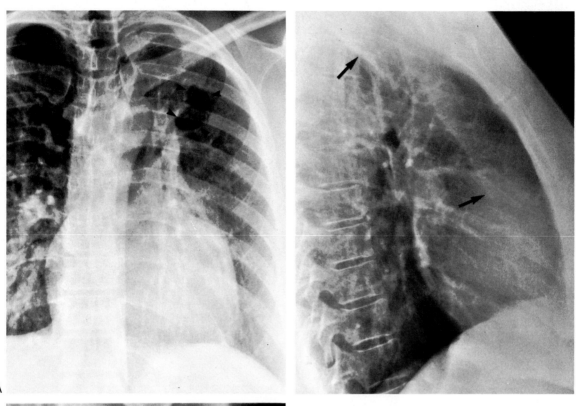

A

B

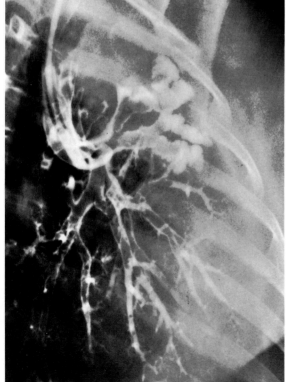

C

Figure 11–44. Severe Atelectasis of the Left Upper Lobe Associated with Bronchiectasis. Posteroanterior *(A)* and lateral *(B)* roentgenograms reveal marked loss of volume of the left upper lobe, indicated by shift of the mediastinum to the left and marked anterior displacement of the major fissure *(arrows in B)*. In lateral projection the lobe appears airless, suggesting the possibility of an endobronchial obstructing lesion, but in posteroanterior projection a broad air-containing space is visible *(arrowheads)*, which makes an endobronchial lesion most unlikely. Bronchoscopy revealed a patent left upper lobe bronchus. A left bronchogram *(C)* shows severe cystic bronchiectasis of all segments of the left upper lobe. The air-containing space in *A* represents a markedly dilated bronchus.

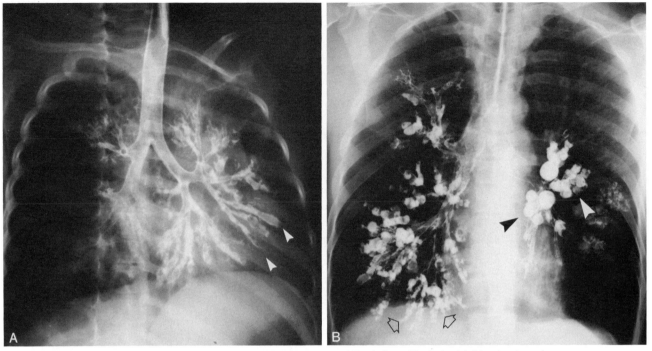

Figure 11–45. Bronchographic Features of Varicose and Cystic Bronchiectasis. A left tracheobronchogram *(A)* reveals mildly dilated and slightly irregular bronchi that terminate four to six generations of branchings from the trachea in a squared or bulbous appearance *(arrowheads)*. The findings are those of varicose bronchiectasis. In a different patient, a bilateral tracheobronchogram *(B)* demonstrates a multitude of contrast-filled cystic spaces resembling a cluster of grapes *(arrowheads)*, a characteristic feature of cystic bronchiectasis. Note that the cystic spaces appear after only two to three bronchial generations. Less severe bronchiectasis of varicose type is present in the right lower lobe *(open arrows)*.

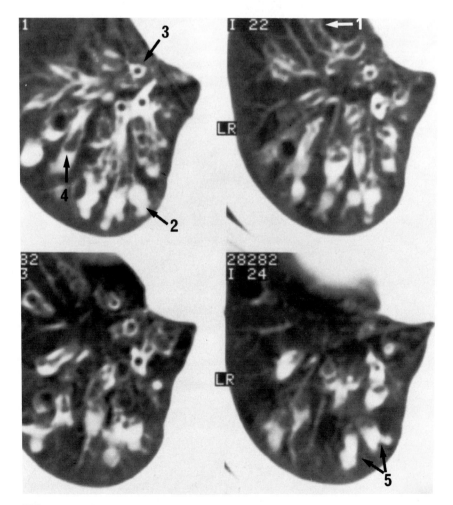

Figure 11–46. Varicose and Cystic Bronchiectasis: CT Features. A sequence of CT scans 10 mm thick, with 10-mm interspacing through the right lower lobe reveals varicose (1) and cystic (2) bronchiectasis, thickened bronchial walls (3), fluid levels (4), and mucoid impaction (5).

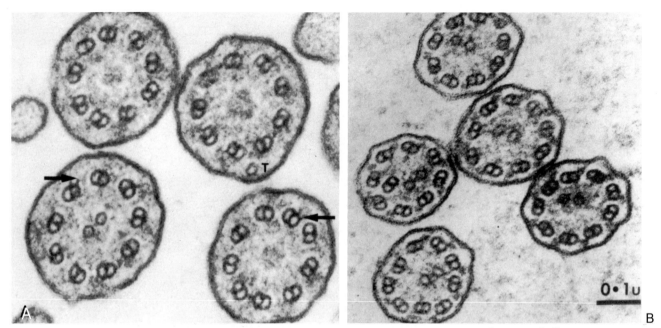

Figure 11–47. Ciliary Abnormalities in Dyskinetic Cilia Syndrome. A cross-section of a group of cilia and microvilli *(A)* shows that most of the outer ciliary doublets lack dynein arms, although occasional partial arms are present *(arrows)*. The central tubules are also absent in four of the cilia; supernumerary single tubules (T) are occasionally present. (Original magnification, × 130,000.) (From Wakefield St J, Waite D: Abnormal cilia in Polynesians with bronchiectasis. Am Rev Respir Dis 121: 1003, 1980.) A cross-section of cilia from another patient *(B)* shows the absence of inner dynein arms. (Original magnification, × 100,000.) (From Neustein HG, Nickerson B, O'Neal M: Kartagener's syndrome with absence of inner dynein arms of respiratory cilia. Am Rev Respir Dis 122: 979, 1980.)

and supernumerary microtubules[604]; the commonest of these is a lack of dynein arms. It is important to remember that structural defects of cilia can be acquired rather than congenital,[605] and it can be difficult to distinguish the two in a single biopsy specimen of nasal or bronchial mucosa.

The roentgenographic manifestations of DCS in the chest are similar to those of cystic fibrosis, although they tend to be less severe and less progressive. They include bronchial wall thickening, hyperinflation, segmental atelectasis or consolidation, and bronchiectasis.[606] In addition to these abnormalities, evidence of otitis and sinusitis and situs inversus are found in about 50 per cent of patients (Fig. 11-48).

Clinically, individuals with full-blown DCS have chronic rhinitis, sinusitis, otitis, chronic and recurrent infections of the airways, bronchiectasis, male sterility, corneal abnormalities, and a poor sense of smell. To make the diagnosis, patients should have signs of chronic bronchial infection and rhinitis from early childhood, combined with one or more of the following features: (1) situs inversus or dextrocardia in the patient or a sibling, (2) living but immotile spermatozoa of normal appearance, (3) tracheobronchial clearance that is absent or nearly so, and (4) cilia in a nasal or bronchial biopsy specimen that have ultrastructural defects characteristic of the syndrome.[607]

Patients with DCS develop mild to moderate airflow obstruction.[409] Their decrease in mucociliary clearance is profound and greater than that seen in advanced cystic fibrosis, postinfective bronchiectasis, COPD, or asthma.[608]

Cystic Fibrosis

Cystic fibrosis (CF) is a hereditary disease of autosomal recessive transmission also known as mucoviscidosis or cystic fibrosis of the pancreas. The fundamental abnormality consists of the production of abnormal secretions from a variety of exocrine glands, including the salivary and sweat glands and those of the pancreas, large bowel, and tracheobronchial tree. The major clinical manifestations are COPD (found in varying degrees of severity in almost all cases) and pancreatic insufficiency (present in 80 to 90 per cent of patients).[609]

The disease is the commonest lethal, genetically transmitted abnormality among whites, the estimated incidence in this group being approximately 1 per 2000 to 3500 live births.[610] By contrast, the disease is uncommon in nonwhites; its incidence among North American blacks is 1 in 17,000 and among North American Indians and Asians 1 in 90,000.[610] There is no sex predominance. It is chiefly a disease of infants and children, although adult cases are being recognized with greater frequency.[611] In 80 per cent of cases, the diagnosis is made before the age of 5 years; however, in 10 per cent the disease is not recognized until adolescence.[612]

Cystic fibrosis is caused by mutations in a gene that codes for a protein that functions as a transmembrane chloride channel,[613] termed cystic fibrosis transmembrane conductance regulator (CFTR).[614] In 70 per cent of cases, the defect is due to the loss of a single amino acid (phenylala-

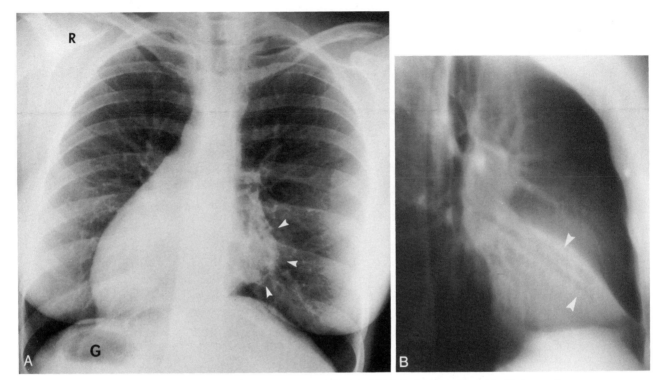

Figure 11–48. Dextrocardia, Situs Inversus, and Chronic Middle Lobe Bronchiectasis (Kartagener's Syndrome). A posteroanterior chest roentgenogram *(A)* shows dextrocardia and situs inversus; note the position of the gastric air bubble (G). The right atrial contour is effaced by an inhomogeneous triangular opacity *(arrowheads)* consistent with atelectasis. A linear tomogram through the left hilum in 55 degrees posterior oblique projection *(B)* reveals patency of the middle lobe bronchus and air-filled bronchiectatic bronchi distally *(arrowheads)*.

nine) at position 508 on the CFTR; in the other 30 per cent, there is one of a number of other mutations.

In the white population, approximately 1 in 20 individuals is heterozygous for CF. No clinical characteristics have been demonstrated that identify these people, since they do not express the disease and generally are unaware that they are carriers until they have children with CF.[615] With the identification of the specific genetic defect, however, it is now potentially possible to screen the normal population for heterozygosity. Each unaffected brother or sister of a patient with CF has a two-thirds chance of being a carrier. If a carrier of the gene marries another person who is heterozygous for the same gene, each pregnancy has a 25 per cent risk of resulting in a child with CF. If one parent has no familial history of CF and the other parent has the disease, there is a 1 in 40 chance of the child's being affected.[615]

Pathogenesis

Despite the identification of the mutant gene and its defective protein product, the precise pathogenesis of CF is still incompletely understood. CFTR functions as a chloride channel on the luminal surface of epithelial cells. When activated by cyclic adenosine monophosphate (cAMP), the channel opens and chloride is transported from the cytoplasm to the cell surface. The defective chloride transport in CF results in abnormalities in transepithelial water and sodium transport that, in turn, cause an alteration in the liquid lining layer of the airways and defec-

tive mucociliary clearance.[616] It is tempting to speculate that an increased susceptibility to infection then leads to the characteristic pulmonary changes of CF.

In fact, patients with CF clearly do have an increased susceptibility to infection, particularly with *S. aureus, Pseudomonas aeruginosa,* and *P. cepacia.*[617] However, it is difficult to explain this susceptibility purely on the basis of a defect in ion transport and mucociliary clearance, since patients who have dyskinetic ciliary syndrome and *absent* mucociliary transport do not have the same devastating and progressive pulmonary infections. Humoral immunologic host defense mechanisms are not impaired; in fact, immunoglobulin levels are often increased, presumably in response to chronic infection.

Even though there is a specific defect in a single ion channel, abnormal electrolyte secretion varies from one exocrine gland to another. For example, the concentration of sodium and chloride is slightly diminished in tracheobronchial and cervical mucus, whereas saliva from parotid, submaxillary, and sublingual glands contains normal amounts of sodium and chloride. Characteristically, the sweat of patients with CF contains elevated concentrations of sodium and chloride and, to a lesser extent, of potassium; the determination of these concentrations is a basic requirement for the diagnosis (*see* later).

In addition to pulmonary infection, there is a higher incidence of atopy and asthma among patients with CF than among the general population.[618] Many patients show type I and type III hypersensitivity reactions to a variety of antigens, including food, bacteria, and fungi.[619] Neither atopy nor allergic symptoms are associated with earlier age at onset, more severe symptoms, more rapid pulmonary function deterioration, or worse survival rates.[620] The frequency with which IgE antibodies and serum precipitins to *Aspergillus* species and *Candida albicans* have been identified also is higher in patients with CF than in those with asthma unassociated with CF.[621] The basis for these immunologic abnormalities is uncertain.

Pathologic Characteristics

Pathologic studies of neonates or infants who have died of CF show normal lungs.[622] By contrast, older patients who die of the disease invariably show pulmonary changes,[623] including airway mucous plugging, acute and organizing pneumonitis (often with abscess formation), bronchiolitis obliterans, bronchiectasis, and focal areas of atelectasis and overinflation distal to obstructed segmental bronchi (Fig. 11–49). All these changes are variable in severity and patchy in distribution; however, there is a tendency to more marked involvement of the upper lobes.[624] Focal emphysema can be present but is rarely appreciable except in patients who reach adulthood[625]; occasionally bullae and blebs are present.[623] Most adult patients who die manifest right ventricular hypertrophy at autopsy.

Roentgenographic Manifestations

Plain roentgenography reveals a pattern typical of extensive obstruction of medium-sized and small airways of the lungs; hyperinflation is almost invariable.[626] The earliest change perhaps is accentuation of the linear markings, usually generalized throughout the lungs and caused by thickening of bronchial walls (Fig. 11–50). Atelectasis may be subsegmental, segmental, or lobar (the last having been reported in 10 per cent of cases, most frequently in the right upper lobe).[627] Recurrent local pneumonitis occurs in most cases. Cylindrical and even cystic bronchiectasis may be present.

Mucoid impaction, manifested by a pattern of nodular, fingerlike shadows along the distribution of the bronchovascular bundles, occurs in some patients. In some of these, the mucus plugs contain fragments of fungal hyphae, in which case clinical and laboratory features of allergic bronchopulmonary aspergillosis are usually present. As in other diseases, CT can reveal pathologic changes not visible on conventional chest roentgenograms, particularly mucoid impaction.[628]

Clinical Manifestations

Involvement of the lungs usually is manifested clinically by recurrent chest infections associated with wheezing, dyspnea, productive cough, and hemoptysis. The organisms most often responsible for pulmonary infection are *P. aeruginosa* of the mucoid and nonmucoid types, *S. aureus*, and *H. influenzae*. The presence of *P. cepacia* is associated with the terminal stages of the disease.[617] Hemoptysis is common in advanced cases and usually occurs as a result of bron-

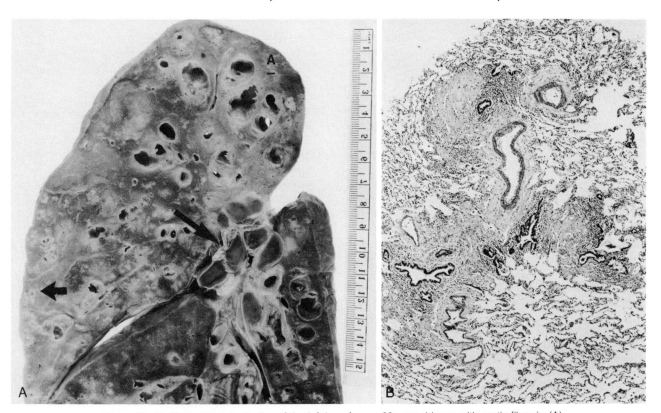

Figure 11–49. Cystic Fibrosis. A slice of the left lung from a 23-year-old man with cystic fibrosis *(A)* shows variably severe bronchiectasis, worse in the apicoposterior segment (A). Extensive organizing pneumonia in the same region and multiple foci of acute bronchopneumonia, most marked in the lingula *(short arrow)*, are present. Note the hyperplastic peribronchial lymph nodes at the junction of upper and lower lobes *(long arrow)*. A histologic section through grossly normal lung *(B)* shows severe narrowing of several bronchioles by fibrous tissue and a mild inflammatory infiltrate. (× 40.)

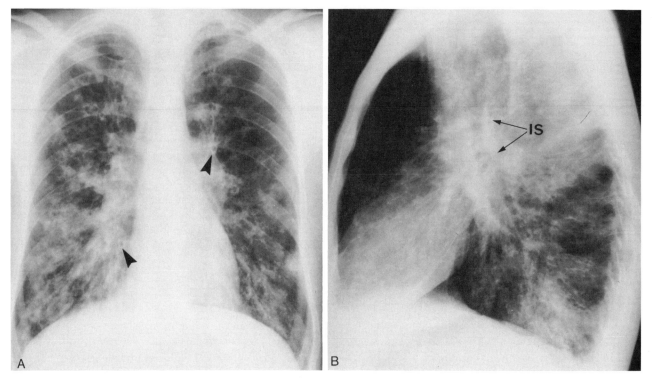

Figure 11–50. Cystic Fibrosis. Posteroanterior *(A)* and lateral *(B)* chest roentgenograms demonstrate diffuse bronchial wall thickening *(arrowheads),* diffuse small patchy opacities, and areas of inhomogeneous airspace consolidation. Note the remarkable thickening of the posterior wall of the bronchus intermedius (IS). The lungs are moderately overinflated. Both hila are enlarged, almost certainly as a result of lymph node enlargement rather than pulmonary arterial hypertension.

chiectasis; occasionally, it is massive, in which case the prognosis is poor. Pneumothorax is common and often recurrent.[629] Respiratory insufficiency and cor pulmonale develop frequently in the later stages of the disease.

The physical findings in adult patients with CF are typical of bronchiectasis and obstructive airway disease. Coarse crackles are common and often diffuse; generalized wheezing may suggest asthma. Finger clubbing is a frequent sign in patients with advanced disease, and hypertrophic pulmonary osteoarthropathy has been reported.[630]

Although gastrointestinal symptoms are minimal or absent in some patients, in many they are significant. Approximately 10 to 20 per cent of neonates develop intestinal obstruction as a result of meconium ileus; surgical therapy is usually required. Intestinal obstruction in adults usually responds to intravenous fluid administration and acetylcysteine by nasogastric tube and enema.[631] The lack of pancreatic enzymes results in poor digestion, particularly of fat, resulting in characteristic bulky, fatty stools. Malabsorption may be present, particularly in children. Malnutrition and protein depletion are also consequences of recurrent pulmonary infection, which can accelerate the course of pulmonary disease.[632] Hepatic involvement includes steatosis and focal biliary cirrhosis. Pancreatic involvement is reflected in recurrent attacks of acute pancreatitis and, in a small number of patients, diabetes mellitus.

Laboratory Features

The diagnosis of CF may be suggested by family history, or persistent respiratory disease or evidence of pancreatic insufficiency in a young individual; however, confirmation currently requires a positive sweat test (although genetic testing will likely become routinely available and capable of identifying the majority of homozygotes). The most generally accepted method is pilocarpine iontophoresis sweat collection, with chemical analysis of ionic composition.[633] Although not reliable in newborn infants, in children a chloride concentration of 60 mEq per L or higher indicates the presence of CF; a value of 50 mEq per L requires repeat testing. When this test is properly performed, it has nearly 100 per cent sensitivity and 93 per cent specificity.[634] A number of recently developed techniques (including one in which sweat osmolarity can be measured on as little as 10 μL of sweat) are promising alternatives to the gold standard.[634]

Pancreatic insufficiency can be diagnosed by measuring the trypsin and chymotrypsin content of stool, or by the determination of the bicarbonate and enzyme content of duodenal secretions obtained by intubation following stimulation with secretin and pancreozymin.[609]

Pulmonary Function Tests

Tests of small airway function are sensitive in the detection of mild pulmonary involvement.[635] As the disease progresses, VC diminishes and RV increases. FEV_1 values fall, and carbon monoxide diffusing capacity may decrease.[636] It is important to measure flow rates before and after use of a bronchodilator in order to recognize a reversible component to the obstruction; however, there is usually less response in patients with CF than in those with asthma.[637] In advanced cases, there may be some loss of elastic recoil, but this is usually minimal and consistent with the degree of emphysema observed at necropsy. Thus, the major factor that reduces expiratory flow appears to be airway obstruction.[638] Patients with advanced disease may also manifest abnormal collapse of large airways on expiration.[639]

Hypoxemia is present in some cases, and hypercapnia in a minority. The impairment in gas exchange has been shown to be caused equally by shunt and $\dot{V}/\dot{Q}$ inequality.[640] Episodes of arterial blood desaturation occur during sleep,[641] the largest decrease occurring during REM sleep. They are associated with periods of hypoventilation rather than apnea.

Prognosis

As a result of improved medical care, chiefly through antibiotic therapy, life expectancy of affected patients has increased dramatically over the last two decades.[642] Whereas the survival rate until the age of 17 years used to be approximately 5 per cent,[643] it is now closer to 50 per cent.[609] Some of the marked variability in the clinical course of CF may be related to genetic heterogeneity, although other factors must be important, since 70 per cent of patients have the same mutation and yet show marked variability in clinical progression. The prognosis varies considerably in different countries,[644] probably related to the variations in the aggressiveness of early preventative therapy. Prognosis also relates to the age at diagnosis,[645] patients diagnosed earlier by postnatal screening tending to do better.

Infants with severe pancreatic insufficiency usually die of meconium ileus, and children and young adults of progressive lung disease. In patients who live to the age of 18 years, subsequent survival is best predicted from clinical features.[646] Lung transplantation has proved life-saving in some patients with advanced disease.

Miscellaneous Causes of Bronchiectasis

Young's syndrome (obstructive azoospermia) is a condition characterized by a combination of infertility and sinopulmonary infection.[647] Patients have a decrease in mucociliary clearance and mild abnormalities of lung function.[648] The cause is unknown.

Patients with the yellow nail syndrome also have an increased incidence of chronic sinusitis, bronchiectasis, and recurrent pneumonia. The disorder begins in middle age and is characterized by the triad of yellow nails, lymphedema, and pleural effusion.[649] The pathogenesis of the bronchiectasis is not certain.[650]

Familial dysautonomia is manifested by malfunction of the autonomic nervous system with consequent hypersecretion of mucous glands and obstruction of the bronchial tree.[651] It is transmitted as an autosomal recessive trait and occurs almost exclusively in Jews. The roentgenographic manifestations resemble those of CF. Clinically, the picture is characterized by episodes of fever, cough, and shortness of breath associated with typical signs of bronchopneumonia. The prognosis is extremely poor, only a small number of patients surviving into adulthood.[652]

BRONCHOLITHIASIS

The term broncholithiasis is used to denote the presence of calcified or ossified material within the lumen of the tracheobronchial tree. The material can originate in three ways: (1) by *in situ* calcification of aspirated foreign material that has impacted within the bronchial wall; (2) by erosion of calcified or ossified bronchial cartilage plates into the airway wall and eventual extrusion into the lumen; or (3) by similar erosion and extrusion of calcified necrotic material derived from bronchopulmonary lymph nodes.[653] The last-named is by far the commonest. In North America, the most frequent etiologic agent is probably *Histoplasma capsulatum*, undoubtedly related to the high incidence of lymphadenitis in endemic areas. Elsewhere, *Mycobacterium tuberculosis* is likely commoner.

Broncholiths vary in size from less than 1 mm to the exceptional instance of one weighing 139 g.[654] They are usually quite irregular in shape and often possess multiple pointed spurs and sharp edges. Those that contain relatively little calcium may disintegrate easily, and it is presumably this type that is associated with recurrent lithoptysis. By contrast, stones that are heavily calcified or ossified have less of a tendency to break up and are more likely to cause airway occlusion, with distal obstructive effects.

Roentgenographic findings may consist only of foci of hilar or parenchymal calcification suggestive of remote granulomatous disease (*see* Fig. 4–58, page 219). Segmental or subsegmental atelectasis may be found in relation to obstruction; focal calcification near the apparent origin of the atelectasis as viewed on conventional or computed tomograms is virtually pathognomonic of the condition. Bronchography may show the intraluminal nature of the broncholith but is seldom indicated.

The most prominent symptom is cough. Although it is usually nonproductive, it is frequently associated with hemoptysis and, occasionally, with lithoptysis. Less commonly, the presence of bronchial obstruction and secondary infection causes pain, chills, and fever.

BRONCHIOLITIS

A variety of pulmonary diseases are pathologically manifested predominantly by inflammation of membranous and respiratory bronchioles. This can occur as a simple bronchiolitis, characterized by either an acute or a chronic inflammatory infiltrate within the bronchiolar wall. In addition, some cases are complicated by the development of intraluminal fibrosis, which can be severe enough to cause complete obliteration of the airway lumen (bronchiolitis obliterans). In the early stages, such fibrosis is manifested by plugs of loose connective tissue and is usually associated with epithelial destruction. Occasionally, the fibrous tissue is present between the muscularis mucosa and an intact epithelium ("constrictive" bronchiolitis) (*see* Fig. 7–28, page 434). In advanced disease, the airway lumen may be completely occluded by mature fibrous tissue. Bronchiolitis obliterans itself may be an isolated abnormality or may be associated with the presence of fibroblastic tissue within adjacent alveolar airspaces, so-called bronchiolitis obliterans with organizing pneumonia (BOOP).

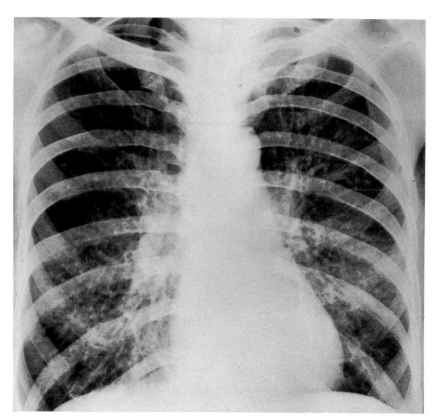

Figure 11–51. Acute Bronchiolitis in the Adult. A posteroanterior roentgenogram shows an extensive coarse reticulonodular pattern throughout both lungs associated with moderate pulmonary overinflation. This 70-year-old man was admitted to the hospital with an acute respiratory illness; pulmonary function studies revealed changes consistent with extensive obstruction of small airways. Proven *Mycoplasma* infection.

Three main roentgenographic patterns of disease are associated with bronchiolitis: (1) nodular opacities (Fig. 11–51), (2) alveolar opacities, and (3) hyperinflation (Fig. 11–52). Nodular opacities, in turn, can be considered in several categories: (a) those smaller than 5 mm in diameter (micronodular), (b) those greater than 5 mm (discrete nodular), (c) those associated with parenchymal consolidation (confluent nodular), and (d) those associated with a reticular pattern (lineonodular). These abnormalities represent a spectrum of changes seen in patients who have pure bronchiolitis, bronchiolitis obliterans, or BOOP.

The following is a brief discussion of the most important etiologies of bronchiolitis. (More information is present in appropriate sections elsewhere in the text.)

Bronchiolitis Related to Fumes and Toxic Gases. Acute exposure to smoke or to a high concentration of NO_2, SO_2, and a variety of other gases and fumes can cause bronchiolitis that is associated with severe airflow obstruction. The respiratory symptoms of cough and dyspnea appear minutes or hours following exposure and may be accompanied by the development of pulmonary edema. The pathologic changes at this stage consist mainly of necrosis of bronchiolar epithelium associated with an acute inflammatory exudate. If patients survive this acute stage, within 2 to 5 weeks there may occur a second phase characterized by increasing obstruction, cough, dyspnea, and cyanosis.[655] At this time, the pathologic findings are predominantly those of bronchiolitis obliterans (*see* Chapter 14).

Acute Infectious Bronchiolitis. Viral infection of the small airways causes severe illness most frequently in children younger than 3 years of age. The commonest etiologic agents are the respiratory syncytial virus, adenoviruses, rhi-novirus, and parainfluenza virus (especially type 3). Pathologically, disease is characterized by an acute bronchiolitis that usually completely resolves, resulting in the restoration of normal architecture. Sometimes—particularly following adenovirus infection—bronchiolitis obliterans and bronchiectasis localized to one lobe or lung remain as sequelae (unilateral or lobar emphysema) (*see* page 675). In other cases, the process is more diffuse and is manifested roentgenologically by severe, general overinflation of both lungs (*see* Fig. 11–52).

The clinical manifestations typically begin with symptoms of an upper respiratory tract infection, followed 2 to 3 days later by the abrupt onset of dyspnea, tachypnea, fever, cyanosis, and often severe prostration. The physical signs include widespread low- and high-pitched wheezes, fine and coarse crackles, and evidence of hyperinflation. The usual course of the disease consists of 2 or 3 days of severe symptoms followed by progressive recovery.

Bronchiolitis Associated with Connective Tissue Disease. Bronchiolitis, with or without bronchiolitis obliterans, is an occasional complication of a number of connective tissue diseases, particularly rheumatoid disease (*see* page 402).

Bronchiolitis Obliterans Associated with Organ Transplantation. Bronchiolitis obliterans is a particularly ominous complication of bone marrow,[656] lung, or heart-lung transplantation (*see* pages 434 and 435).[657] Clinically, the bronchiolitis is manifested months to years following successful transplantation and is associated with progressive dyspnea that may be very severe; the development of respiratory failure may indicate the need for retransplantation. The bronchiolitis is believed to be an immunologically me-

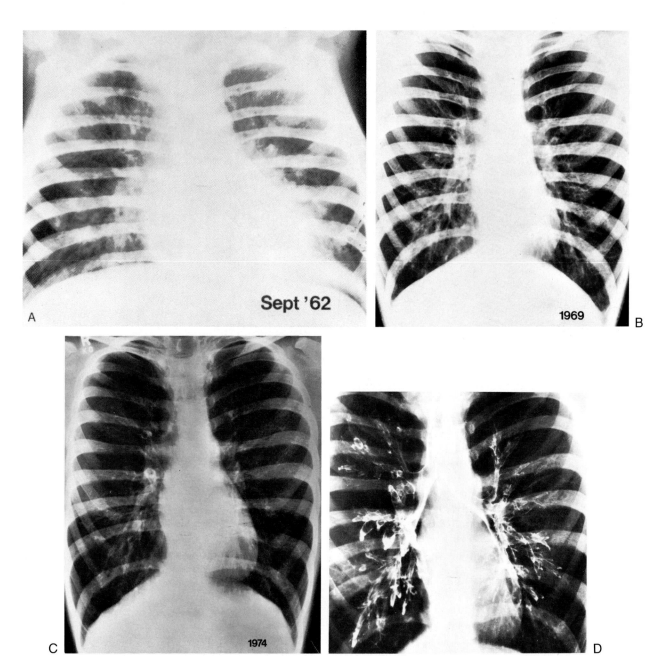

Figure 11–52. Diffuse "Emphysema" (Bronchiolitis Obliterans) in a Young Girl. This 1½-year-old girl was admitted to the hospital with an acute respiratory illness that progressed to respiratory failure. A roentgenogram on admission *(A)* reveals widespread pulmonary disease more evident in the lower lung zones and consistent with (but in no way diagnostic of) acute viral pneumonia. By the time the child was 8 years of age *(B)*, overinflation had become marked, and diffuse peripheral oligemia consistent with a diagnosis of diffuse emphysema had developed. By age 13, a roentgenogram of her chest *(C)* again revealed severe overinflation and peripheral oligemia. Pulmonary function studies showed severe airway obstruction and marked reduction in carbon monoxide diffusion. A broncho-gram *(D)* showed moderate uniform dilatation of all segmental and subsegmental bronchi of both lungs, with abrupt, conical termination of all segments distally, virtually diagnostic of widespread bronchiolitis obliterans. (Courtesy of Drs. J. S. D. McEvoy and Richard Slaughter, The Prince Charles Hospital, Brisbane, Australia.)

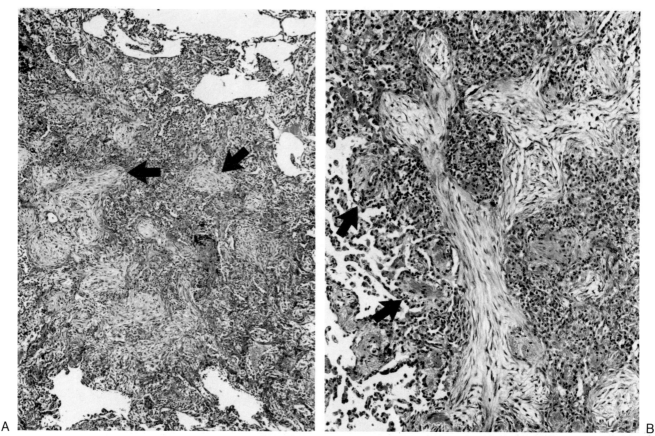

A   B

Figure 11–53. Bronchiolitis Obliterans with Organizing Pneumonia. A histologic section of lung parenchyma *(A)* shows a poorly defined focus of chronic inflammation associated with numerous small foci of loose connective tissue *(arrows)*. A magnified view of similar disease from another area *(B)* shows branching of the connective tissue plugs, implying that they are present in the lumina of alveolar ducts and respiratory bronchioles. The interstitial nature of the chronic inflammatory infiltrate is apparent at the junction with normal lung *(arrows)*. (A × 40; B × 100.)

diated manifestation of tissue incompatibility. Roentgenographic evidence of bronchiectasis has been found in a high proportion of patients in some studies of lung transplantation.[658]

Idiopathic Bronchiolitis With and Without Organizing Pneumonia. Although bronchiolitis occurs in association with a specific disease entity or possesses a specific etiology in many patients, there are also instances in which no underlying cause can be identified. Such idiopathic cases are often associated with organizing pneumonia (BOOP, cryptogenic organizing pneumonia).[659, 659a] Pathologically, this process is characteristically distributed in a patchy fashion throughout the lung. Plugs of loose fibroblastic connective tissue can be identified principally within respiratory bronchioles and alveolar ducts (Fig. 11–53). The parenchyma adjacent to the affected bronchioles shows similar fibroblastic tissue in alveolar airspaces, as well as interstitial fibrosis and chronic inflammation. Roentgenographically, BOOP is characterized by patchy areas of consolidation that are usually bilateral and peripheral (Fig. 11–54).[659b] Many cases also feature small rounded opacities that, occasionally, are the only abnormality.[660]

Clinically, BOOP usually presents as a subacute illness whose duration of symptoms prior to diagnosis ranges from 3 to 6 months.[659] The commonest symptoms are cough (90 per cent), dyspnea (80 per cent), fever (60 per cent), sputum expectoration, malaise, and weight loss (50 per cent). Crackles are audible on auscultation in 75 per cent of cases, but clubbing is not observed. The great majority of patients show restrictive disease and gas exchange impairment.[660] Some cases have been reported that show a seasonal occurrence and that are associated with intrahepatic cholestasis.[659a]

Systemic corticosteroid therapy has a salutory effect in patients with BOOP, and in many the clinical and roentgenologic signs of disease completely remit. By contrast, patients with bronchiolitis obliterans associated with the inhalation of toxic fumes, rheumatoid disease, or organ transplantation show little or no response to corticosteroid therapy.

Diffuse Panbronchiolitis. Diffuse panbronchiolitis is a disease of unknown etiology and pathogenesis characterized by chronic inflammation of respiratory bronchioles with secondary obstructive effects. It has been recognized almost exclusively in Japan; a survey in that nation between 1978 and 1980 collected more than 1000 probable cases.[661] The changes are more or less diffuse throughout the lungs, resulting in roentgenographic evidence of a disseminated nodular pattern with lower zonal predominance.[661] Evidence of hyperinflation is also present. Findings on high-

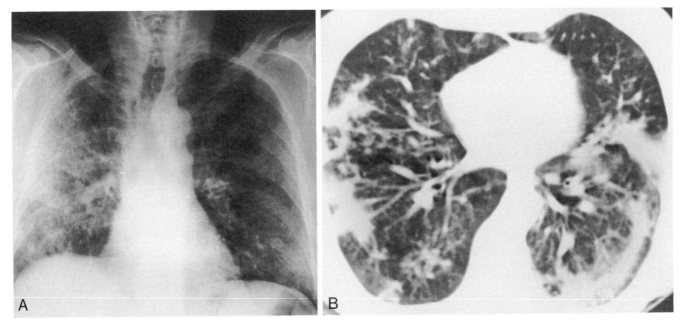

Figure 11–54. Bronchiolitis Obliterans–Organizing Pneumonia (BOOP). A posteroanterior roentgeno-gram *(A)* reveals extensive patchy opacities involving both lungs but much more marked in the right. In the axillary portions of the right upper and lower lobes, the opacities are almost homogeneous, suggesting airspace consolidation. A conventional CT scan (10-mm collimation) through the lower lung zones *(B)* shows bilateral areas of airspace consolidation involving mainly the subpleural lung regions.

resolution CT include small, rounded areas of attenuation in the central portion of pulmonary lobules and dilated airways with thick walls.[661a]

Most patients are between 30 and 60 years of age; the male to female ratio is approximately 2 to 1.[661] The chief clinical manifestations are dyspnea on exertion, productive cough, and sinusitis. Progression of disease appears to be common and is sometimes accompanied by respiratory failure.

References

1. Capitanio MA, Kirkpatrick JA: Obstructions of the upper airway in children as reflected on the chest radiograph. Radiology 107: 159, 1973.
2. Evans AS: Clinical syndromes in adults caused by respiratory infections. Med Clin North Am 51: 803, 1967.
3. Hobson D: Acute respiratory virus infections. Br Med J 2: 229, 1973.
4. Hawley HB, Morin DP, Geraghty ME, et al: Coxsackievirus B epidemic at a boys' summer camp: Isolation of a virus from swimming water. JAMA 26: 33, 1973.
5. Kasian GF, Bingham WT, Steinberg J, et al: Bacterial tracheitis in children. Can Med Assoc J 140: 46, 1989.
6. Connor JD: Evidence for an etiologic role of adenoviral infection in pertussis syndrome. N Engl J Med 283: 390, 1970.
7. Bass JW, Steele RW, Wiebe RA: Acute epiglottitis: A surgical emergency. JAMA 229: 671, 1974.
8. Ossoff RH, Wolff AP: Acute epiglottitis in adults. JAMA 244: 2639, 1980.
9. Shakelford GD, Siegel MJ, McAlister WH: Subglottic edema in acute epiglottitis in children. Am J Roentgenol 131: 603, 1978.
10. Michel RG, Hudson WR, Pope TH: Angioneurotic edema: A review of modern concepts. Arch Otolaryngol 101: 544, 1975.
11. Frank MM, Gelfand JA, Atkinson JP: Hereditary angioedema: The clinical syndrome and its management. Ann Intern Med 84: 580, 1976.
12. Haponik EF, Munster AM, Wise RA, et al: Upper airway function in burn patients: Correlation of flow-volume curves and nasopharyngoscopy. Am Rev Respir Dis 129: 251, 1984.
13. Eshagby B, Loeb HS, Miller SE, et al: Mediastinal and retropharyngeal hemorrhage: A complication of cardiac catheterization. JAMA 226: 427, 1973.
14. Duong TC, Burtch GD, Shatney CH: Upper-airway obstruction as a complication of oral anticoagulation therapy. Crit Care Med 14: 830, 1986.
15. Bass H: The flow-volume loop: Normal standards and abnormalities in chronic obstructive pulmonary disease. Chest 63: 171, 1973.
16. Miller RD, Hyatt RE: Obstructing lesions of the larynx and trachea: Clinical and physiologic characteristics. Mayo Clin Proc 44: 145, 1969.
16a. Vincken W, Dollfuss RE, Cosio MG: Upper airway dysfunction detected by respiratory flow oscillations. Eur J Respir Dis 68: 50, 1986.
17. Empey DW: Assessment of upper airways obstruction. Br Med J 3: 503, 1972.
18. Paré PD, Donevan RD, Nelems JM, et al: Clues to unrecognized upper airway obstruction: A case report. Can Med Assoc J 127: 39, 1982.
19. Kittredge RD: Computed tomography of the trachea: A review. J Comput Tomogr 5: 44, 1981.
20. Ell SR, Jolles H, Galvin JR: Cine CT demonstration of nonfixed upper airway obstruction. Am J Roentgenol 146: 669, 1986.
21. Capitanio MA, Kirkpatrick JA: Obstructions of the upper airway in children as reflected on the chest radiograph. Radiology 107: 159, 1973.
22. Djalilian M, Kern EB, Brown HA, et al: Hypoventilation secondary to chronic upper airway obstruction in childhood. Mayo Clin Proc 50: 11, 1975.
23. Cormier Y, Kashima H, Summer W, et al: Upper airways obstruction with bilateral vocal cord paralysis. Chest 75: 423, 1979.
24. Vincken W, Elleker G, Cosio MG: Detection of upper airway muscle involvement in neuromuscular disorders using the flow-volume loop. Chest 90: 52, 1986.
25. Caffey J: Pediatric X-Ray Diagnosis. 6th ed. Vol 1. Chicago, Year Book Medical Publishers, 1972, p 235.
26. Cormier Y, Kashima H, Summer W, et al: Airflow in unilateral vocal cord paralysis before and after Teflon injection. Thorax 33: 57, 1978.
27. Rodenstein DO, Francis D, Stanescu DC: Emotional laryngeal wheezing: A new syndrome. Am Rev Respir Dis 127: 354, 1983.
28. Collett PW, Brancatisano T, Engel LA: Spasmodic croup in the adult. Am Rev Respir Dis 127: 500, 1983.

29. Dixon TC, Sando MJW, Bolton JM, et al: A report of 342 cases of prolonged endotracheal intubation. Med J Aust 2: 529, 1968.

30. James AE Jr, MacMillian AS Jr, Eaton SB, et al: Roentgenology of tracheal stenosis resulting from cuffed tracheostomy tubes. Am J Roentgenol 109: 455, 1970.

31. Hemmingsson A, Lindgren PG: Roentgenologic examinations of tracheal stenosis. Acta Radiol Diagn 19: 753, 1978.

32. Griscom N, Wohl ME: Dimensions of the growing trachea related to body height, length, anteroposterior and transverse diameters, cross-sectional area, and volume in subjects younger than 20 years of age. Am Rev Respir Dis 131: 840, 1985.

33. Breatnach E, Abbott GC, Fraser RG: Dimensions of the normal human trachea. Am J Roentgenol 141: 903, 1984.

34. Harley HRS: Laryngotracheal obstruction complicating tracheostomy or endotracheal intubation with assisted respiration: A critical review. Thorax 26: 493, 1971.

35. Hadju SI, Huvos AG, Goodner JT, et al: Carcinoma of the trachea: Clinicopathologic study of 41 cases. Cancer 25: 1448, 1970.

36. Baydur A, Gottlieb LS: Adenoid cystic carcinoma (cylindroma) of the trachea masquerading as asthma. JAMA 234: 829, 1975.

37. deKock MA: Functional anatomy of the trachea and main bronchi. *In* deKock MA, Nadel JA, Lewis CM (eds): Mechanisms of Airway Obstruction in Human Respiratory Disease. Cape Town, South African Medical Research Council, 1979.

38. Greene R, Lechner GL: "Saber-sheath" trachea: A clinical and functional study of marked coronal narrowing of the intrathoracic trachea. Radiology 115: 265, 1975.

39. Greene R: "Saber-sheath" trachea: Relation to chronic obstructive pulmonary disease. Am J Roentgenol 130: 441, 1978.

40. Dolan DL, Lemmon GB Jr, Teitelbaum SL: Relapsing polychondritis: Analytical literature review and studies on pathogenesis. Am J Med 41: 285, 1966.

41. Gibson GJ, Davis P: Respiratory complications of relapsing polychondritis. Thorax 29: 726, 1973.

42. Ettman IK, Keel DT Jr: Tracheal diverticulosis. Radiology 78: 187, 1962.

43. Johnston RF, Green RA: Tracheobronchiomegaly: Report of five cases and demonstration of familial occurrence. Am Rev Respir Dis 91: 35, 1965.

44. Ayres J, Rees J, Cochrane GM, et al: Hemoptysis and non-organic upper airways obstruction in a patient with previously undiagnosed Ehlers-Danlos syndrome. Br J Dis Chest 75: 309, 1981.

45. Wonderer AA, Elliot FE, Goltz RW, et al: Tracheobronchomegaly and acquired cutis laxa in child: Physiologic and immunologic studies. Pediatrics 44: 709, 1969.

46. Rindsberg S, Friedman AC, Fiel SB, et al: MRI of tracheobronchomegaly. J Can Assoc Radiol 38: 126, 1987.

47. Al-Mallah Z, Quantock OP: Tracheobronchomegaly. Thorax 23: 230, 1968.

48. Van Nierop MA, Wagenaar SS, Van den Bosch JM, et al: Tracheobronchopathia osteochondroplastica: Report of four cases. Eur J Respir Dis 64: 129, 1983.

49. Baird RB, McCartney JW: Tracheopathia osteoplastica. Thorax 21: 321, 1966.

50. Onitsuka H, Hirose N, Watanabe K, et al: Computed tomography of tracheopathia osteoplastica. Am J Roentgenol 140: 268, 1983.

51. Lundgren R, Stjernberg NL: Tracheobronchopathia osteochondroplastica: A clinical bronchoscopic and spirometric study. Chest 80: 706, 1981.

52. Feist JH, Johnson TH, Wilson RJ: Acquired tracheomalacia, etiology and differential diagnosis. Chest 68: 340, 1975.

53. Cogbill TH, Moore FA, Accurso FJ, et al: Primary tracheomalacia. Am Thorac Surg 35: 538, 1983.

54. Maayan C, Mogle P, Tal A, et al: Prolonged wheezing and tracheal compression caused by an aberrant right subclavian artery. Thorax 36: 793, 1981.

55. MacGillivray RG: Tracheal compression caused by aneurysms of the aortic arch: Implications for the anaesthetist. Anaesthesia 40: 270, 1985.

56. Kandora TF, Gilmore IM, Sorber JA, et al: Cricoarytenoid arthritis presenting as cardiopulmonary arrest. Ann Emerg Med 14: 700, 1985.

57. Miller A, Brown LK, Teirstein AS, et al: Stenosis of main bronchi mimicking fixed upper airway obstruction in sarcoidosis. Chest 88: 244, 1985.

58. Breuer R, Simpson GT, Rubinow A, et al: Tracheobronchial amyloidosis: Treatment by carbon dioxide laser photoresection. Thorax 40: 870, 1985.

59. Karbowitz SR, Edelman LB, Nath S, et al: Spectrum of advanced upper airway obstruction due to goiters. Chest 87: 18, 1985.

60. Guilleminault C, van den Hoed J, Mitler MM: Clinical overview of the sleep apnea syndromes. *In* Guilleminault C, Dement WC (eds): Sleep Apnea Syndromes. New York, Alan R. Liss, 1978, p 1.

61. Lavie P: Sleep apnea in industrial workers. *In* Guilleminault C, Lugaresi E (eds): Sleep/Wake Disorders: Natural History, Epidemiology, and Long-Term Evolution. New York, Raven Press, 1983, p 127.

62. Ancoli-Israel S, Kripke DF, Mason W, et al: Sleep apnea and periodic movements in an aging sample. J Gerontol 40: 419, 1985.

63. Gothe B, Althose MD, Goldman MD, et al: Effect of quiet sleep on resting and CO_2-stimulated breathing in humans. J Appl Physiol 50: 724, 1981.

64. Hudgel DW, Martin RJ, Johnson B, et al: Mechanics of the respiratory system and breathing pattern during sleep in normal humans. J Appl Physiol 56: 133, 1984.

65. Krieger J: Breathing during sleep in normal subjects. Clin Chest Med 6: 577, 1985.

66. Douglas NJ: Control of ventilation during sleep. Clin Chest Med 6: 563, 1985.

67. Fletcher EC: History, techniques, and definitions in sleep-related respiratory disorders. *In* Fletcher EC (ed): Abnormalities of Respiration During Sleep. Orlando, Grune & Stratton, 1986, p 1.

68. Johnson MW, Anch AM, Remmers JE: Induction of the obstructive sleep apnea syndrome in a woman by exogenous androgen administration. Am Rev Respir Dis 129: 1023, 1984.

69. Parisi RA, Croce SA, Edelman NH, et al: Obstructive sleep apnea following bilateral carotid body resection. Chest 91: 922, 1987.

70. Wittels EH: Obesity and hormonal factors in sleep and sleep apnea. Med Clin North Am 69: 1265, 1985.

71. Hoffstein V, Zamel N, Phillipson EA: Lung volume dependence of pharyngeal cross-sectional area in patients with obstructive sleep apnea. Am Rev Respir Dis 130: 175, 1984.

72. Kuna ST, Remmers JE: Pathophysiology and mechanisms of sleep apnea. *In* Fletcher EC (ed): Abnormalities of Respiration During Sleep. Orlando, Grune & Stratton, 1986, p 63.

73. Lowe AA, Gionhaku N, Takeuchi K, et al: Three-dimensional CT reconstructions of tongue and airway in adult subjects with obstructive sleep apnea. Am J Orthod Dentofacial Orthop 90: 364, 1986.

74. Hannam A, Wood W, Fache S, et al: MR imaging and graphic reconstruction in the orofacial region. J Comput Assist Tomogr (in press).

75. Sullivan CE, Issa FG: Obstructive sleep apnea. Clin Chest Med 6: 633, 1985.

76. Sturani C, Barrot-Cortez E, Papiris S, et al: Respiratory flutter during carbon dioxide rebreathing in patients with obstructive sleep apnea syndrome. Eur J Respir Dis 69: 75, 1986.

77. Shore ET, Millman RP: Abnormalities in the flow-volume loop in obstructive sleep apnea sitting and supine. Thorax 39: 775, 1984.

78. Issa FG, Sullivan CE: Upper airway closing pressures in obstructive sleep apnea. J Appl Physiol 57: 520, 1984.

79. Suratt PM, McTier RF, Wilhoit SC: Collapsibility of the nasopharyngeal airway in obstructive sleep apnea. Am Rev Respir Dis 132: 967, 1985.

80. Hudgel DW: Variable site of airway narrowing among obstructive sleep apnea patients. J Appl Physiol 61: 1403, 1986.

81. Taasan VC, Block AJ, Boysen PG, et al: Alcohol increases sleep apnea and oxygen desaturation in asymptomatic men. Am J Med 71: 240, 1981.

82. Leiter J, Knuth S, Krol R, et al: The effect of diazepam on genioglossal muscle activity in normal human subjects. Am Rev Respir Dis 132: 216, 1985.

83. Leiter JC, Knuth SL, Bartlett D: The effect of sleep deprivation on activity of the genioglossus muscle in man. Am Rev Respir Dis 132: 1242, 1985.

84. Vincken W, Guilleminault C, Silvestri L, et al: Inspiratory muscle activity as a trigger causing the airways to open in obstructive sleep apnea. Am Rev Respir Dis 135: 372, 1987.

85. Lugaresi E, Cirignotta F, Coccagna G, et al: Some epidemiological data on snoring and cardiocirculatory disturbances. Sleep 3: 221, 1980.

86. Gyulay S, Gould D, Sawyer B, et al: Evaluation of a microprocessor-

based portable home monitoring system to measure breathing during sleep. Sleep 10: 130, 1987.

87. Orr WC, Martin RJ, Imes NK, et al: Hypersomnolent and nonhypersomnolent patients with upper airway obstruction during sleep. Chest 75: 418, 1979.

88. Sink J, Bliwise DL, Dement WC: Self-reported excessive daytime somnolence and impaired respiration in sleep. Chest 90: 177, 1986.

89. Kales A, Caldwell AB, Cadieux RJ, et al: Severe obstructive sleep apnea. II: Associated psychopathology and psychosocial consequences. J Chronic Dis 38: 427, 1985.

90. Podszus T, Bauer W, Mayer J, et al: Sleep apnea and pulmonary hypertension. Klin Wochenschr 64: 131, 1986.

91. Hudgel DW: Clinical manifestations of the sleep apnea syndrome. *In* Fletcher EC (ed): Abnormalities of Respiration During Sleep. Orlando, Grune & Stratton, 1986, pp 21–37.

92. Fletcher EC, DeBehnke RD, Lovoi MS, et al: Undiagnosed sleep apnea in patients with essential hypertension. Ann Intern Med 103: 190, 1985.

93. Santamaria JC, Prior JC, Fleetham JA: Reversible reproductive dysfunction in men with obstructive sleep apnea. Clin Endocrinol 28: 461, 1988.

94. Shephard JW Jr: Gas exchange and hemodynamics during sleep. Med Clin North Am 69: 1243, 1985.

95. Flenley DC: Sleep in chronic obstructive lung disease. *In* Kryger MH (ed): Symposium on Sleep Disorders. Philadelphia, WB Saunders, 1985.

96. McEvoy RD, Sharp DJ, Thornton AT: The effects of posture on obstructive sleep apnea. Am Rev Respir Dis 133: 662, 1986.

97. Hegstrom T, Emmons LL, Hoddes E, et al: Obstructive sleep apnea syndrome: Preoperative radiologic evaluation. Am J Roentgenol 150: 67, 1988.

98. Larsson SG, Gislason T, Lindholm CE: Computed tomography of the oropharynx in obstructive sleep apnea. Acta Radiol 29: 401, 1988.

99. Scadding JG: Definition and the clinical categories of asthma. *In* Clark TJH, Godfrey S (eds): Asthma. 2nd ed. London, Chapman & Hall, 1983, pp 1–11.

100. American Thoracic Society: Chronic bronchitis, asthma, and pulmonary emphysema. Am Rev Respir Dis 85: 762, 1962.

101. Mok JYQ, Simpson H: Pulmonary function in severe chronic asthma in children during apparent clinical remission. Eur J Respir Dis 64: 487, 1983.

102. Report of the Committee on Emphysema, American College of Chest Physicians: Criteria for the assessment of reversibility in airway obstruction. Chest 65: 552, 1974.

103. Williams E, McNicol KN: Prevalence, natural history, and relationship of wheezy bronchitis and asthma in children: An epidemiologic study. Br Med J 4: 321, 1969.

104. Woolcock AJ: Worldwide differences in asthma prevalence and mortality: Why is asthma mortality so low in the U.S.A.? Chest 90: 40S, 1986.

105. Cookson JB, Makoni G: Prevalence of asthma in Rhodesian Africans. Thorax 35: 833, 1980.

106. Ross I: Bronchial asthma in Malaysia. Br J Dis Chest 78: 369, 1984.

107. Editorial: IgE, parasites, and allergy. Lancet 1: 894, 1976.

108. Dowse GK, Smith D, Turner KJ, et al: Prevalence and features of asthma in a sample survey of urban Goroka, Papua New Guinea. Clin Allergy 15: 429, 1985.

109. Marsh G, Meyers A, Bias B: The epidemiology and genetics of atopic allergy. N Engl J Med 305: 1551, 1981.

110. Hopp RJ, Bewtra AK, Watt GD, et al: Genetic analysis of allergic disease in twins. J Allergy Clin Immunol 73: 265, 1984.

111. Hogg JC: The pathophysiology of asthma. Chest 82: 85, 1982.

112. Brogan TD, Ryley HC, Neale L, et al: Soluble proteins of bronchopulmonary secretions from patients with cystic fibrosis, asthma, and bronchitis. Thorax 30: 72, 1975.

113. Dunnill MS: The pathology of asthma, with special reference to changes in the bronchial mucosa. J Clin Pathol 13: 27, 1960.

113a. Laitinen LA, Heino M, Laitinen A, et al: Damage of the airway epithelium and bronchial reactivity in patients with asthma. Am Rev Respir Dis 131: 599, 1985.

114. Lopez-Vidriero MT, Reid L: Chemical markers of mucous and serum glycoproteins and their relation to viscosity in mucoid and purulent sputum from various hypersecretory diseases. Am Rev Respir Dis 117: 465, 1987.

115. Shelhamer J, Kaliner M: Respiratory mucus production in asthma (editorial). Clin Respir Physiol 21: 301, 1985.

116. Pavis D, Bateman JRM, Sheahan NF, et al: Tracheobronchial mucociliary clearance in asthma: Impairment during remission. Thorax 40: 171, 1985.

117. Wanner A: Allergic mucociliary dysfunction. J Allergy Clin Immunol 72: 347, 1983.

118. Dulfano MJ, Luk CK: Sputum and ciliary inhibition in asthma. Thorax 37: 646, 1982.

119. Agnew JE, Bateman JR, Sheahan NF, et al: Effect of oral corticosteroids on mucus clearance by cough and mucociliary transport in stable asthma. Bull Eur Physiopathol Respir 19: 37, 1983.

120. Dolovich J, Hargreave FE, O'Byrne P, et al: Asthma terminology: Troubles in wordland. Am Rev Respir Dis 134: 1102, 1986.

121. Boushey HA, Holtzman MJ, Shuler JR, et al: State of the art: Bronchial hyperreactivity. Am Rev Respir Dis 121: 389, 1980.

122. Zamel N, Leroux M, Vanderdoelen JL: Airway responses to inhaled methacholine in healthy nonsmoking twins. J Appl Physiol 56: 936, 1984.

123. Halperin SA, Eggleston PA, Beasley P, et al: Exacerbation of asthma in adults during experimental rhinovirus infection. Am Rev Respir Dis 132: 976, 1985.

124. Boushey HA, Holtzman MJ: Experimental airway inflammation and hyperreactivity—searching for cells and mediators. Am Rev Respir Dis 131: 312, 1985.

125. Mapp CE, Polato R, Maestrelli P, et al: Time course of the increase in airway responsiveness associated with late asthmatic reactions to toluene di-isocyanate in sensitized subjects. J Allergy Clin Immunol 75: 568, 1985.

126. Orehek J: Asthma without airway hyperreactivity: Fact or artifact? Eur J Respir Dis 63: 1, 1982.

127. Giffon E, Orehek J, Vervloet D, et al: Asthma without airway hyperresponsiveness to carbachol. Eur J Respir Dis 70: 229, 1987.

128. Olafsson M, Simonsson BG, Hansson SB: Bronchial reactivity in patients with recent pulmonary sarcoidosis. Thorax 40: 51, 1985.

129. Mönkäre S: Clinical aspects of farmer's lung: Airway reactivity, treatment, and prognosis. Eur J Respir Dis 65: 1, 1984.

130. Yan K, Salome CM, Woolcock AJ, et al: Prevalence and nature of bronchial hyperresponsiveness in subjects with chronic obstructive pulmonary disease. Am Rev Respir Dis 132: 25, 1985.

131. Woolcock AJ, Peat JK, Salome CM, et al: Prevalence of bronchial hyperresponsiveness and asthma in a rural adult population. Thorax 42: 361, 1987.

132. Bechtel JJ, Starr T, Dantzker DR, et al: Airway hyperreactivity in patients with sarcoidosis. Am Rev Respir Dis 124: 759, 1981.

133. Rubinfeld AR, Pain MCF: Relationship between bronchial reactivity, airway caliber, and severity of asthma. Am Rev Respir Dis 115: 381, 1977.

134. Moreno RH, Hogg JC, Paré PD: Mechanism of airway narrowing. Am Rev Respir Dis 133: 1171, 1986.

135. Hogg JC: Bronchial mucosal permeability and its relationship to airways hyperreactivity. J Allergy Clin Immunol 67: 421, 1981.

136. Elwood RK, Kennedy S, Belzberg A, et al: Respiratory mucosal permeability in asthma. Am Rev Respir Dis 128: 523, 1983.

137. O'Byrne PM, Dolovich M, Dirks R, et al: Lung epithelial permeability: Relation to nonspecific airway responsiveness. J Appl Physiol 57: 77, 1984.

138. Kallenbach JM, Webster T, Dowdeswell R, et al: Reflex heart rate control in asthma: Evidence of parasympathetic overactivity. Chest 87: 644, 1985.

139. Vidrukk EH, Hahn HL, Nadel JA, et al: Mechanisms by which histamine stimulates rapidly adapting receptors in dog lungs. J Appl Physiol 43: 397, 1977.

140. Szentivanyi A: The beta-adrenergic theory of the atopic abnormality in bronchial asthma. J Allergy 42: 203, 1968.

141. Kariman K: Beta-adrenergic receptor binding in lymphocytes from patients with asthma. Lung 158: 41, 1980.

142. Goldie RG, Spina D, Henry PJ, et al: *In vitro* responsiveness of human asthmatic bronchus to carbachol, histamine, beta-adrenoceptor agonists, and theophylline. Br J Clin Pharmacol 22: 669, 1986.

143. Bruynzeel PLB: Changes in the β-adrenergic system due to β-adrenergic therapy: Clinical consequences. Eur J Respir Dis 135(Suppl 65): 62, 1984.

144. Grieco MH, Pierson RN: Mechanism of bronchoconstriction due to beta-adrenergic blockade. J Allergy Clin Immunol 48: 143, 1971.

145. Kiyingi KS, Anderson SD, Temple DM, et al: Beta-adrenoceptor blockade with propranolol and bronchial responsiveness to a number

of bronchial provocation tests in non-asthmatic subjects. Eur J Respir Dis 66: 256, 1985.

146. Davis C, Kannan MS, Jones TR, et al: Control of human airway smooth muscle: In vitro studies. J Appl Physiol 53: 1080, 1982.
147. Taylor SM, Paré PD, Schellenberg R: Cholinergic and nonadrenergic mechanisms in human and guinea pig airways. J Appl Physiol 56: 958, 1984.
147a. Bai TR: Abnormalities in airway smooth muscle in fatal asthma. Am Rev Respir Dis 141: 552, 1990.
148. Michoud MC, Jeanneret-Grosjean A, Cohen A, Amyot R: Reflex decrease of histamine-induced bronchoconstriction after laryngeal stimulation in asthmatic patients. Am Rev Respir Dis 138: 1548, 1988.
149. Lei Y-H, Barnes PJ, Rogers DF: Regulation of NANC bronchoconstriction in vivo in the guinea pig: Involvement of nitric oxide, vasoactive intestinal peptide, and guanylate cyclase. Br J Pharmacol 108: 228, 1993.
150. Barnes PJ: Calcium-channel blockers and asthma. Thorax 38: 481, 1983.
151. Anderson KE: Airway hyperreactivity, smooth muscle, and calcium. Eur J Respir Dis 64(Suppl 131): 49, 1983.
152. Kaliner M, Bretz U, Holtzman MJ, et al: Bronchial obstruction: Some patho-physiological and clinical concepts. In Herzog H, Perruchoud AP (eds): Asthma and Bronchial Hyperreactivity. Basel, Karger, 1984, p 417.
153. Whicker SD, Armour CL, Black JL: Responsiveness of bronchial smooth muscle from asthmatic patients to relaxant and contractile agonists. Pulmonary Pharmacol 1: 25, 1988.
154. Schellenberg RR, Duff MJ, Foster A, et al: Asthmatic bronchial reactivity in vitro. Proc Can Soc Invest 8: A202, 1985.
155. Ishida K, Paré PD, Blogg T, et al: Effects of elastic loading on porcine trachealis muscle mechanics. J Appl Physiol 69: 1033, 1990.
156. De Kock MA: Functional anatomy of the trachea and main bronchi. In De Kock MA, Nadel JA, Lewis CM (eds): Mechanisms of Airway Obstruction in Human Respiratory Disease. Capetown, South African Medical Research Council, 1979, p 49.
157. Lambert RK: Role of basement membrane in bronchial collapse. J Appl Physiol 71: 666, 1991.
158. Walters EH: Effect of inhibition of prostaglandin synthesis on induced bronchial hyperresponsiveness. Thorax 38: 195, 1983.
159. Bar-Sela S, Schleuter DP, Kitt SR, et al: Antigen-induced enhancement of bronchial reactivity. Chest 88: 114, 1985.
160. Cartier A, L'Archeveque J, Malo JL: Exposure to a sensitizing occupational agent can cause a long-lasting increase in bronchial responsiveness to histamine in the absence of significant changes in airway caliber. J Allergy Clin Immunol 78: 1185, 1986.
161. Fabbri LM, DiGiacomo R, Dal Vecchio L, et al: Prednisone, indomethacin, and airway responsiveness in toluene diisocyanate–sensitized subjects. Bull Eur Physiopathol Respir 21: 421, 1985.
162. Lam S, Wong R, Yeung M: Nonspecific bronchial reactivity in occupational asthma. J Allergy Clin Immunol 613: 28, 1979.
163. Pauwels R: Mediators and non-specific bronchial hyperreactivity. Eur J Respir Dis 64: 95, 1983.
164. Persson CGA, Szenjö E: Airways hyperreactivity, and microvascular permeability to large molecules. Eur J Respir Dis 64(Suppl 131): 183, 1983.
165. Nadel JA: Inflammation and asthma. J Allergy Clin Immunol (Suppl) 73: 651, 1984.
166. Löwhagen O, Rak S: Modification of bronchial hyperreactivity after treatment with sodium cromoglycate during pollen season. J Allergy Clin Immunol 75: 460, 1985.
167. Ryan G, Latimer KM, Juniper EF, et al: Effect of beclomethasone dipropionate on bronchial responsiveness to histamine in controlled nonsteroid-dependent asthma. J Allergy Clin Immunol 75: 25, 1985.
168. Bhagat RG, Grunstein M: Effect of corticosteroids on bronchial responsiveness to methacholine in asthmatic children. Am Rev Respir Dis 131: 902, 1985.
169. Hargreave FE, Ramsdale H, Dolovich J: Measurement of airway responsiveness in clinical practice. In Hargreave FE, Woolcock AJ (eds): Airway Responsiveness: Measurement and Interpretation. Ontario, Astra Mississauga, 1985, p 122.
170. Freedman PM, Ault B: Bronchial hyperreactivity to methacholine in farmers' lung disease. J Allergy Clin Immunol 67: 59, 1981.
171. Woolcock AJ: Test of airway responsiveness in epidemiology. In Hargreave FE, Woolcock AJ (eds): Airway Responsiveness: Measurement and Interpretation. Ontario, Astra Mississauga, 1985, p 136.

172. Woolcock AJ, Yan K, Salome CM: Effect of therapy on bronchial hyperresponsiveness in the long-term management of asthma. Clin Allergy 18: 165, 1988.
173. Chan-Yeung M, Lam S, Tse KS: Measurement of airway responsiveness in occupational asthma. In Hargreave FE, Woolcock AJ (eds): Airway Responsiveness: Measurement and Interpretation. Ontario, Astra Mississauga, 1985, p 129.
174. Dolovich J, Hargreave F: The asthma syndrome—inciters, inducers and host characteristics. Thorax 36: 641, 1981.
175. Barbee RA, Lebowitz MD, Thompson HC, et al: Immediate skin-test reactivity in a general population sample. Ann Intern Med 84: 129, 1976.
176. Freedman SO: New perspectives in allergic asthma. Can Med Assoc J 114: 346, 1976.
177. Wide L, Bennich H, Johansson SGO: Diagnosis of allergy by an in-vitro test for allergen antibodies. Lancet 2: 1105, 1967.
178. Rosenberg GL, Rosenthal RR, Norman PS: Inhalation challenge with ragweed pollen in ragweed-sensitive asthmatics. J Allergy Clin Immunol 71: 302, 1983.
179. Salvaggio J, Aukrust L: Mold-induced asthma. J Allergy Clin Immunol 68: 327, 1981.
180. Blythe ME, Al Abaydi F, Williams JD, et al: Study of dust mites in three Birmingham hospitals. Br Med J 1: 62, 1975.
181. Barr SE: Allergy to Hymenoptera stings. JAMA 228: 718, 1974.
182. Welch H, Lewis CN, Weinstein HI, et al: Severe reactions to antibiotics: A nationwide survey. Antibiot Med Clin Ther 4: 800, 1957.
183. Austen KF: Current concepts: Systemic anaphylaxis in the human being. N Engl J Med 291: 661, 1974.
184. Hanashiro PK, Weil MH: Anaphylactic shock in man: Report of two cases with detailed hemodynamic and metabolic studies. Arch Intern Med 119: 129, 1967.
185. Wanner A, Russi E, Brodnan J, et al: Prolonged bronchial obstruction after a single antigen challenge in ragweed asthma. J Allergy Clin Immunol 76: 177, 1985.
186. Cockcroft DW, Ruffin RE, Frith PA, et al: Determinants of allergen-induced asthma: Dose of allergen, circulating IgE antibody concentration, and bronchial responsiveness to inhaled histamine. Am Rev Respir Dis 120: 1053, 1979.
187. Valenti S, Crimi E, Brusasco V: Bronchial provocation tests with RAST-standardized allergens and dosimetric technique. Respiration 48: 97, 1985.
188. Cockcroft DW, Hoeppner VH, Werner GD: Recurrent nocturnal asthma after bronchoprovocation with Western Red Cedar sawdust: Association with acute increases in nonallergic bronchial responsiveness. Clin Allergy 14: 61, 1984.
189. Kaliner M: Hypotheses on the contribution of late-phase allergic responses to the understanding and treatment of allergic disease. J Allergy Clin Immunol 73: 311, 1984.
190. Hogg JC: The pathology of asthma. Chest 87: 152S, 1985.
191. White J, Eiser NM: The role of histamine and its receptors in the pathogenesis of asthma. Br J Dis Chest 77: 215, 1983.
192. Eiser NM: Hyperreactivity: Its relationship to histamine receptors. Eur J Respir Dis 64(Suppl 131): 99, 1983.
193. Beer J, Osband E, McCaffrey P, et al: Abnormal histamine-induced suppressor-cell function in atopic subjects. N Engl J Med 306: 454, 1982.
194. Kaliner M: Human lung tissue and anaphylaxis: The effects of histamine on the immunologic release of mediators. Am Rev Respir Dis 118: 1015, 1978.
195. Wasserman SI, Center DM: The relevance of neutrophil chemotactic factors to allergic disease. J Allergy Clin Immunol 64: 231, 1979.
196. Taylor IK, O'Shaughnessy KM, Fuller RW, et al: Effect of cysteinyl-leukotriene receptor antagonist ICI204.219 on antigen-induced bronchoconstriction and airway hyperreactivity in atopic subjects. Lancet 337: 690, 1991.
197. Manning PJ, Watson RM, Margolski, et al: Inhibition of exercise-induced bronchoconstriction by MK-5, a potent leukotriene D4-receptor antagonist. N Engl J Med 323: 1736, 1990.
198. Hui KP, Barnes NC: Lung function improvement in asthma with a cysteinyl-leukotriene receptor antagonist. Lancet 337: 1062, 1991.
199. Walters EH, Davies BH: Dual effect of prostaglandin E2 on normal airways smooth muscle in vivo. Thorax 37: 918, 1982.
200. Mathé AA, Hedqvist P, Holmgren A, et al: Bronchial hyperreactivity to prostaglandin F2a and histamine in patients with asthma. Br Med J 1: 193, 1973.
201. Hardy CC, Robinson C, Tattersfield AE, et al: The bronchoconstric-

tor effect of inhaled prostaglandin D_2 in normal and asthmatic men. N Engl J Med 311: 209, 1984.

202. Parker CW: Aspirin-sensitive asthma. *In* Lichtenstein LM, Austen KF (eds): Asthma: Physiology, Immunopharmacology and Treatment. Vol II. New York, Academic Press, 1977, p 301.

203. Weiler JM, Metzger WJ, Donnelly AL, et al: Prevalence of bronchial hyperresponsiveness in highly trained athletes. Chest 90: 23, 1986.

204. Anderson SD: Exercise-induced asthma. *In* Middleton E Jr, et al (eds): Allergy: Principles and Practice. St Louis, CV Mosby, 1986.

205. Rubenstein I, Levison H, Slutsky AS, et al: Immediate and delayed bronchoconstriction after exercise in patients with asthma. N Engl J Med 317: 482, 1987.

206. Chen WY, Horton DJ: Heat and water loss from the airways and exercise-induced asthma. Respiration 34: 305, 1977.

207. Strauss RH, McFadden ER, Ingram RH: Enhancement of exercise-induced asthma by cold air. N Engl J Med 297: 743, 1977.

208. Deal EC Jr, McFadden ER Jr, Ingram RH, et al: Role of respiratory heat exchange in production of exercise-induced asthma. J Appl Physiol 46: 467, 1979.

209. Deal EC, McFadden ER, Ingram RH, et al: Hyperpnea and heat flux: Initial reaction sequence in exercise-induced asthma. J Appl Physiol 46: 476, 1979.

210. Neijens HJ, Wesselius T, Kerrebijn KF: Exercise-induced bronchoconstriction as an expression of bronchial hyperreactivity: A study of its mechanisms in children. Thorax 36: 517, 1981.

211. McFadden ER, Ingram RH: Exercise-induced airway obstruction. Annu Rev Physiol 45: 453, 1983.

212. Hahn A, Anderson SD, Norton AR, et al: A reinterpretation of the effect of temperature and water content of the inspired air in exercise-induced asthma. Am Rev Respir Dis 130: 575, 1985.

213. Schoeffel RE, Anderson SD, Altounyan RED: Bronchial hyperreactivity in response to inhalation of ultrasonically nebulized solutions of distilled water and saline. Br J Med 23: 1285, 1981.

214. Deal EC, McFadden ER, Ingram RH Jr, et al: Esophageal temperature during exercise in asthmatic and nonasthmatic subjects. J Appl Physiol 46: 484, 1979.

215. Griffin MP, McFadden ER, Ingram RH: Airway cooling in asthmatic and nonasthmatic subjects during nasal and oral breathing. J Allergy Clin Immunol 69: 354, 1982.

216. Lee TH, Nagakura T, Cromwell O, et al: Neutrophil chemotactic activity and histamine in atopic and nonatopic subjects after exercise-induced asthma. Am Rev Respir Dis 129: 409, 1984.

217. Findlay SR, Dvorak AM, Kagey-Sobotka A, et al: Hyperosmolar triggering of histamine release from human basophils. J Clin Invest 67: 1604, 1981.

218. Rimmer J, Bryant DH: Effect of hypo- and hyper-osmolarity on basophil histamine release. Clin Allergy 16: 221, 1986.

219. Kidd JM, Cohen SH, Sosman AJ, et al: Food-dependent exercise-induced anaphylaxis. J Allergy Clin Immunol 71: 407, 1983.

220. Enright PL, McNally JF, Souhrada JF: Effect of lidocaine on the ventilatory and airway responses to exercise in asthmatics. Am Rev Respir Dis 122: 823, 1980.

221. O'Byrne PM, Thomson NC, Morris M, et al: The protective effect of inhaled chlorpheniramine and atropine on bronchoconstriction stimulated by airway cooling. Am Rev Respir Dis 128: 611, 1983.

222. Griffin MP, McFadden ER, Ingram RH, et al: Controlled-analysis of the effects of inhaled lignocaine in exercise-induced asthma. Thorax 37: 741, 1982.

223. O'Byrne PM, Thomson NC, Morris M, et al: The protective effect of inhaled chlorpheniramine and atropine on bronchoconstriction stimulated by airway cooling. Am Rev Respir Dis 128: 611, 1983.

224. Black JL, Armour CL, Shaw J: The effect of alteration in temperature on contractile responses in human airways in vitro. Respir Physiol 57: 269, 1984.

225. McFadden ER, Lemmer KAM, Strohl KP: Post-exertion at airway rewarming and thermally induced asthma: New insights into pathophysiology and possible pathogenesis. J Clin Invest 78: 18, 1986.

226. Miller WS: The Lung. Springfield, IL, Charles C Thomas, 1947, p 69.

227. Lee TH, Anderson SD: Heterogeneity of mechanisms in exercise-induced asthma (editorial). Thorax 40: 481, 1985.

228. Edmunds AT, Tooley W, Godfrey S: The refractory period after exercise-induced asthma: Its duration and relation to the severity of exercise. Am Rev Respir Dis 117: 247, 1978.

229. Weiler-Ravell D, Godfrey S: Do exercise-induced and antigen-induced asthma utilize the same pathways: Antigen provocation in

230. O'Byrne PM, Jones GL: The effect of indomethacin on exercise-induced bronchoconstriction and refractoriness after exercise. Am Rev Respir Dis 134: 69, 1986.

231. O'Connor SA, Jones DP, Collinsa JV, et al: Changes in pulmonary function after naturally acquired respiratory infection in normal persons. Am Rev Respir Dis 120: 1087, 1979.

232. Jenkins CR, Breslin ABX: Upper respiratory tract infections and airway reactivity in normal and asthmatic subjects. Am Rev Respir Dis 130: 879, 1984.

233. Minor TE, Dick EC, DeMeo AN, et al: Viruses as precipitants of asthma attacks in children. JAMA 227: 292, 1974.

234. Clarke CW: Relationship of bacterial and viral infections to exacerbations of asthma. Thorax 34: 344, 1979.

235. Slepian IK, Mathews KP, McLean JA: Aspirin-sensitive asthma. Chest 87: 386, 1985.

236. Ogino S, Harada T, Okawachi I, et al: Aspirin-induced asthma and nasal polyps. Acta Otolaryngol [Suppl] (Stockh) 430: 21, 1986.

237. Settipane GA, Chafee FH, Klein DK: Aspirin intolerance. 2. A prospective study of an atopic and normal population. J Allergy Clin Immunol 53: 200, 1974.

238. Weltman JK, Szaro RP, Settipane GA: An analysis of the role of IgE in intolerance to aspirin and tartrazine. Allergy 33: 273, 1978.

239. Szczeklik A, Grylglewski RJ, Czerniawska-Mysik G: Relationship of inhibition of prostaglandin biosynthesis by analgesics to asthma attacks in aspirin-sensitive patients. Br Med J 1: 67, 1975.

240. Boyle JT, Tuchman DN, Altschuler SM, et al: Mechanisms for the association of gastroesophageal reflux and bronchospasm. Am Rev Respir Dis 131: S16, 1985.

241. Ducoloné A, Vandevenne A, Jouin H, et al: Gastroesophageal reflux in patients with asthma and chronic bronchitis. Am Rev Respir Dis 135: 327, 1987.

242. Andersen LI, Schmidt A, Bundgaard A: Pulmonary function and acid application in the esophagus. Chest 90: 358, 1986.

243. Allen CJ, Newhouse MT: Gastroesophageal reflux and chronic respiratory disease. Am Rev Respir Dis 129: 645, 1984.

244. Horton DJ, Suda WL, Kinsman RA, et al: Bronchoconstrictive suggestion in asthma: A role for airways hyperreactivity and emotions. Am Rev Respir Dis 117: 1029, 1978.

245. Demeter SL, Cordasco EM: Hyperventilation syndrome and asthma. Am J Med 81: 989, 1986.

246. Bates DV, Sizto R: A study of hospital admissions and air pollutants in Southern Ontario. *In* Lee SD, Schneider T, Grant LD, et al (eds): Aerosols. Chelsea, MI, Lewis Publishers, 1986.

247. Weill H, Ziskind MM, Dickerson RC, et al: Epidemic asthma in New Orleans. JAMA 190: 811, 1964.

248. Folinsbee LJ, Bedi JF, Horvath SM: Pulmonary response to threshold levels of sulfur dioxide (1.0 ppm) and ozone (0.3 ppm). J Appl Physiol 58: 1783, 1985.

249. Roger LJ, Kehrl HR, Hazucha M, et al: Bronchoconstriction in asthmatics exposed to sulfur dioxide during repeated exercise. J Appl Physiol 59: 784, 1985.

250. Linn WS, Venet TG, Shamoo DA, et al: Respiratory effects of sulfur dioxide in heavily exercising asthmatics: A dose-response study. Am Rev Respir Dis 127: 278, 1983.

251. Kulle TJ, Sauder LR, Hebel JR, et al: Ozone response relationships in healthy nonsmokers. Am Rev Respir Dis 132: 36, 1985.

252. McDonnell W, Chapman R, Leigh M, et al: Respiratory responses of vigorously exercising children to 0.12 ppm ozone exposure. Am Rev Respir Dis 132: 875, 1985.

253. Holtzman MJ, Cunningham JH, Sheller JR, et al: Effect of ozone on bronchial reactivity in atopic and nonatopic subjects. Am Rev Respir Dis 120: 1059, 1979.

254. Holtzman MJ, Fabbri LM, O'Byrne PM, et al: Importance of airway inflammation for hyperresponsiveness induced by ozone. Am Rev Respir Dis 127: 686, 1983.

255. Ussetti P, Roca J, Agusti AGN, et al: Another asthma outbreak in Barcelona: Role of oxides of nitrogen. Lancet 1: 156, 1984.

256. Bauer MA, Utell MJ, Morrow PE, et al: Inhalation of 0.30 ppm nitrogen dioxide potentiates exercise-induced bronchospasm in asthmatics. Am Rev Respir Dis 134: 1203, 1986.

257. Bylin G, Lindvall T, Rehn T, et al: Effects of short-term exposure to ambient nitrogen dioxide concentrations on human bronchial reactivity and lung function. Eur J Respir Dis 66: 205, 1985.

258. Parham WM, Shepard RH, Norman PS, et al: Analysis of time course

and magnitude of lung inflation effects on airway tone: Relation to airway reactivity. Am Rev Respir Dis 128: 240, 1983.

259. Liu Y, Sasaki H, Ishii M, et al: Effect of circadian rhythm on bronchomotor tone after deep inspiration in normal and in asthmatic subjects. Am Rev Respir Dis 132: 278, 1985.

260. Beaupré A, Badier M, Delpierre S, et al: Airways response of asthmatics to carbachol and to deep inspiration. Eur J Respir Dis 64: 108, 1983.

261. Hida W, Arai M, Shindoh C, et al: Effect of inspiratory flow rate on bronchomotor tone in normal and asthmatic subjects. Thorax 39: 86, 1984.

262. Burns CB, Taylor WR, Ingram RH Jr: Effects of deep inhalation in asthma: Relative airway and parenchymal hysteresis. J Appl Physiol 59: 1590, 1985.

263. Ayres JG, Clark TJH: Alcoholic drinks and asthma: A survey. Br J Dis Chest 77: 370, 1983.

264. Gong H, Tashkin DP, Calvarese BM: Alcohol-induced bronchospasm in an asthmatic patient: Pharmacologic evaluation of the mechanism. Chest 80: 167, 1981.

265. Bush RK, Taylor SL, Holden K, et al: Prevalence of sensitivity to sulfiting agents in asthmatic patients. Am J Med 81: 816, 1986.

266. Stevenson DD, Simon RA: Sensitivity to ingested metabisulfites in asthmatic subjects. J Allergy Clin Immunol 68: 26, 1981.

267. Genton C, Frei PC, Pécoud A: Value of oral provocation tests to aspirin and food additives in the routine investigation of asthma and chronic urticaria. J Allergy Clin Immunol 76: 40, 1985.

268. Allen DH, Delohery J, Baker G: Monosodium L-glutamate–induced asthma. J Allergy Clin Immunol 80: 530, 1987.

269. Shim C, Williams MH Jr: Effect of odors in asthma. Am J Med 80: 18, 1986.

270. Dahms TE, Bolin JF, Slavin RG: Passive smoking: Effects on bronchial asthma. Chest 80: 530, 1981.

271. Eliasson O, Scherzer HH, DeGraff AC Jr: Morbidity in asthma in relation to the menstrual cycle. J Allergy Clin Immunol 77: 87, 1986.

272. Chan-Yeung M, Lam S: Occupational asthma. Am Rev Respir Dis 133: 686, 1986.

273. Brooks SM, Weiss MA, Bernstein IL: Reactive airways dysfunction syndrome (RADS): Persistent asthma syndrome after high-level irritant exposures. Chest 88: 376, 1985.

274. Cockcroft AE, McDermott M, Edwards JH, et al: Grain exposure symptoms and lung function. Eur J Respir Dis 64: 189, 1983.

275. doPico GA, Reddan W, Anderson S, et al: Acute effects of grain dust exposure during a work shift. Am Rev Respir Dis 128: 399, 1983.

276. Burge PS, Finnegan M, Horsfield N, et al: Occupational asthma in a factory with a contaminated humidifier. Thorax 40: 248, 1985.

277. Theil H, Ulmer WNT: Baker's asthma: Development and possibility of treatment. Chest 78: S400, 1980.

278. Chan-Yeung M, Vedal S, Kus J, et al: Symptoms, pulmonary function, and bronchial hyperreactivity in Western Red Cedar workers compared to those in office workers. Am Rev Respir Dis 130: 1038, 1984.

279. Vedal S, Chan-Yeung M, Enarson D, et al: Symptoms and pulmonary function in Western Red Cedar workers related to duration of employment and dust exposure. Arch Environ Health 41: 179, 1986.

280. Chan-Yeung M, MacLean L, Paggiaro PL: Follow-up study of 232 patients with occupational asthma caused by Western Red Cedar (Thuja plicata). J Allergy Clin Immunol 79: 792, 1987.

281. Moller DR, McKay RT, Bernstein IL, et al: Persistent airways disease caused by toluene diisocyanate. Am Rev Respir Dis 134: 175, 1986.

282. Zeiss CR, Kanellakes TM, Bellone JD, et al: Immunoglobulin E–mediated asthma and hypersensitivity pneumonitis with precipitating anti-hapten antibodies due to diphenylmethane diisocyanate (Mdi) exposure. J Allergy Clin Immunol 65: 346, 1980.

283. Burge SP, O'Brien IM, Harries MG: Peak flow rate records in the diagnosis of occupational asthma due to isocyanates. Thorax 34: 317, 1979.

284. Burge SP, O'Brien IM, Harries MG: Peak flow rate records in the diagnosis of occupational asthma due to colophony. Thorax 34: 308, 1979.

285. Lam S, Tan F, Chan H, et al: Relationship between types of asthmatic reaction, non-specific bronchial reactivity, and specific IgE antibodies in patients with Red Cedar asthma. J Allergy Clin Immunol 72: 134, 1983.

286. Genereux GP: Radiology and pulmonary immunopathologic lung dis-

ease. In Steiner RE (ed): Recent Advances in Radiology and Medical Imaging. New York, Churchill Livingstone, 1983, pp 213–240.

287. Zieverink SE, Harper AP, Holden RW, et al: Emergency room radiography of asthma: An efficacy study. Radiology 145: 27, 1982.

288. Blair DN, Coppage L, Shaw C: Medical imaging in asthma. J Thorac Imag 1: 23, 1986.

289. Sostman HD, Gottschalk AG: The stripe sign: A new sign for diagnosis of nonembolic defects on pulmonary perfusion scintigraphy. Radiology 142: 737, 1982.

289a. Paganin F, Trussard V, Seneterre E, et al: Chest radiography and high-resolution computed tomography of the lungs in asthma. Am Rev Respir Dis 146: 1084, 1992.

290. Hodson ME, Simon G, Batten JC: Radiology of uncomplicated asthma. Thorax 29: 296, 1974.

291. Simon G, Connolly N, Littlejohns DW, et al: Radiological abnormalities in children with asthma and their relation to the clinical findings and some respiratory function tests. Thorax 28: 115, 1973.

292. Petheram IS, Kerr IH, Collins JV: Value of chest radiographs in severe acute asthma. Clin Radiol 32: 281, 1981.

293. Simonsson BG: Chronic cough and expectoration in patients with asthma and in patients with alpha$_1$-antitrypsin deficiency. Eur J Respir Dis 118: 123, 1982.

294. Parker CW: Drug therapy: Drug allergy (third of three parts). N Engl J Med 292: 957, 1975.

295. Lee HY, Stretton TB: Asthma in the elderly. Br Med J 4: 93, 1972.

296. McFadden ER Jr: Exertional dyspnea and cough as prelude to acute attacks of bronchial asthma. N Engl J Med 292: 555, 1975.

297. Turner-Warwick M: On observing patterns of airflow obstruction in chronic asthma. Br J Dis Chest 71: 73, 1977.

298. Jönsson E, Mossberg B: Impairment of ventilatory function by supine posture in asthma. Eur J Respir Dis 65: 496, 1984.

299. Catterall JR, Rhind GB, Stewart IC, et al: Effect of sleep deprivation on overnight bronchoconstriction in nocturnal asthma. Thorax 41: 676, 1986.

300. Puolijoki H, Lahdensuo A: Chronic cough as a risk indicator of broncho-pulmonary disease. Eur J Respir Dis 71: 77, 1987.

301. Cohen RM, Grant W, Lieberman P, et al: The use of methacholine inhalation, methacholine skin testing, distilled water inhalation challenge, and eosinophil counts in the evaluation of patients presenting with cough and/or nonwheezing dyspnea. Ann Allergy 56: 308, 1986.

302. Bellamy D, Collins JV: "Acute" asthma in adults. Thorax 34: 36, 1979.

303. Arnold AG, Lane DJ, Zapata E: The speed of onset and severity of acute severe asthma. Br J Dis Chest 76: 157, 1982.

304. Stellman JL, Spicer JE, Clayton RM: Morbidity from chronic asthma. Thorax 37: 218, 1982.

305. Treatment of status asthmaticus. Br Med J 4: 563, 1972.

306. McFadden ER Jr, Kiser R, de Groot WJ: Acute bronchial asthma: Relations between clinical and physiologic manifestations. N Engl J Med 288: 221, 1973.

307. Pardee NE, Winterbauer RH, Morgan EH, et al: Combinations of 4 physical signs as indicators of ventilatory abnormality in obstructive pulmonary syndromes. Chest 77: 354, 1980.

308. Knowles GK, Clark TJH: Pulsus paradoxus as a valuable sign indicating severity of asthma. Lancet 2: 1356, 1973.

309. Galant SP, Groncy CE, Shaw KC: The value of pulsus paradoxus in assessing the child with status asthmaticus. Pediatrics 61: 46, 1978.

310. McGregor M: Current concepts: Pulsus paradoxus. N Engl J Med 301: 480, 1979.

311. O'Connell JM, Baird LI, Campbell AH: Sputum eosinophilia in chronic bronchitis and asthma. Respiration 35: 65, 1978.

312. Lowell FC: The total eosinophil count in obstructive pulmonary disease. N Engl J Med 292: 1182, 1975.

313. Hendrick DJ, Davies RJ, D'Souza MF, et al: An analysis of skin prick test reactions in 656 asthmatic patients. Thorax 30: 2, 1975.

314. Beers RF Jr: Skin tests. In Samter M, Alexander HL (eds): Immunologic Disorders. Boston, Little, Brown & Co, 1965, p 539.

315. Pepys J: Current concepts: Inhalation challenge tests in asthma. N Engl J Med 293: 758, 1975.

316. Ahonen A: Analysis of the changes in ECG during status asthmaticus. Respiration 37: 85, 1979.

317. Orzalesi MM, Cook CD, Hart MC: Pulmonary function in symptom-free asthmatic patients. Acta Paediatr Scand 53: 401, 1964.

318. McCarthy D, Milic-Emili J: Closing volume in asymptomatic asthma. Am Rev Respir Dis 107: 559, 1973.

319. Rubinfeld AR, Pain MCF: Perception of asthma. Lancet 1: 882, 1976.

320. Olive JT Jr, Hyatt RE: Maximal expiratory flow and total respiratory resistance during induced bronchoconstriction in asthmatic subjects. Am Rev Respir Dis 106: 366, 1972.

321. Pedersen OF, Thiessen B, Naeraa N, et al: Factors determining residual volume in normal and asthmatic subjects. Eur J Respir Dis 65: 99, 1984.

322. Palmer KNV, Kelman GR: A comparison of pulmonary function in extrinsic and intrinsic bronchial asthma. Am Rev Respir Dis 107: 940, 1973.

323. Woolcock AJ, Read J: Lung volumes in exacerbations of asthma. Am J Med 41: 259, 1966.

324. Shore S, Milic-Emili J, Martin JG: Reassessment of body plethysmographic technique for the measurement of thoracic gas volume in asthmatics. Am Rev Respir Dis 126: 515, 1982.

325. Greaves IA, Colebatch HJ: Large lungs after childhood asthma: A consequence of enlarged air spaces. Aust NZ J Med 15: 427, 1985.

326. Macklem PT: Hyperinflation (editorial). Am Rev Respir Dis 129: 1, 1984.

327. Woolcock AJ, Read J: Improvement in bronchial asthma not reflected in forced expiratory volume. Lancet 2: 1323, 1965.

328. Wang T-R, Levison H: Pulmonary function in children with asthma at acute attack and symptom-free status. Am Rev Respir Dis 99: 719, 1969.

329. Keens TG, Mansell A, Krastins IRB, et al: Evaluation of the single-breath diffusing capacity in asthma and cystic fibrosis. Chest 76: 41, 1979.

330. Roca J, Ramis L, Rodriguez-Roison R, et al: Serial relationships between ventilation-perfusion inequality and spirometry in acute severe asthma requiring hospitalization. Am Rev Respir Dis 137: 1055, 1988.

331. Palmer KNV, Diament ML: Dynamic and static lung volumes and blood-gas tensions in bronchial asthma. Lancet 1: 591, 1969.

332. Wagner PD, Dantzker DB, Iacovoni VE, et al: Ventilation-perfusion inequality in asymptomatic asthma. Am Rev Respir Dis 118: 511, 1978.

333. Simpson H, Forfar JO, Grubb DJ: Arterial blood gas tensions and pH in acute asthma in childhood. Br Med J 3: 460, 1968.

334. Alberts WM, Williams JH, Ramsdell JW: Metabolic acidosis as a presenting feature in acute asthma. Ann Allergy 57: 107, 1986.

335. Rees HA, Millar JS, Donald KW: A study of the clinical course and arterial blood gas tensions of patients in status asthmaticus. Q J Med 37: 541, 1968.

336. Banner AS, Shah RS, Addington WW: Rapid prediction of need for hospitalization in acute asthma. JAMA 235: 1337, 1976.

337. Mountain RD, Sahn SA: Clinical features and outcome in patients with acute asthma presenting with hypercapnia. Am Rev Respir Dis 138: 535, 1988.

338. Eggleston PA, Ward BH, Pierson WE, et al: Radiographic abnormalities in acute asthma in children. Pediatrics 54: 442, 1974.

339. Gershel JC, Goldman HS, Stein EK, et al: The usefulness of chest radiographs in first asthma attacks. N Engl J Med 309: 336, 1983.

340. Findley LF, Sahn SA: The value of chest roentgenograms in acute asthma in adults. Chest 80: 535, 1981.

341. Dattwyler RJ, Goldman MA, Bloch KJ: Pneumomediastinum as a complication of asthma in teenage and young adult patients. J Allergy Clin Immunol 63: 412, 1979.

342. Bierman CW: Pneumomediastinum and pneumothorax complicating asthma in children. Am J Dis Child 114: 42, 1967.

343. Lewis M, Kallenbach J, Zaltzman M, et al: Acute respiratory failure in a young asthmatic patient. Chest 84: 733, 1983.

344. Bendkowski B: Asian influenza (1957) in allergic patients. Br Med J 2: 1314, 1958.

345. Jenkins PF, Benfield GFA, Smith AP: Predicting recovery from acute severe asthma. Thorax 36: 835, 1981.

346. Benfield GFA, Smith AP: Predicting rapid and slow response to treatment in acute severe asthma. Br J Dis Chest 77: 249, 1983.

347. Fischl MA, Pitchenik A, Gardner LB: An index predicting relapse and need for hospitalization in patients with acute bronchial asthma. N Engl J Med 305: 783, 1981.

348. McNichol KN, Williams HE: Spectrum of asthma in children. I. Clinical and physiological components. Br Med J 4: 7, 1973.

349. McNichol KN, Williams HE: Spectrum of asthma in children. II. Allergic components. Br Med J 4: 12, 1973.

350. Ogilvie AG: Asthma: A study in prognosis of 1,000 patients. Thorax 17: 183, 1962.

351. Blackhall MI: Effect of age on fixed and labile components of airway resistance in asthma. Thorax 26: 325, 1971.

352. Rackemann FN, Edwards MC: Asthma in children: A follow-up study of 688 patients after an interval of twenty years. N Engl J Med 246: 815, 1952.

353. Rackemann FN, Edwards MC: Asthma in children: A follow-up study of 688 patients after an interval of twenty years (concluded). N Engl J Med 246: 858, 1952.

354. Cserhati E, Mezei G, Keleman J: Late prognosis of bronchial asthma in children. Respiration 46: 160, 1984.

355. Brown PJ, Greville HW, Finucane KE: Asthma and irreversible airflow obstruction. Thorax 39: 131, 1984.

356. Alexander HL: A historical account of death from asthma. J Allergy 34: 305, 1963.

357. Paulozzi LJ, Coleman JJ, Buist AS: A recent increase in asthma mortality in the northwestern United States. Ann Allergy 56: 392, 1986.

358. Jenkins MA, Hurley SF, Jolley DJ, et al: Trends in Australian mortality of asthma, 1979–1985. Med J Austral 149: 620, 1988.

359. Asthma deaths: A question answered. Br Med J 4: 443, 1972.

360. Sears MR, Rea HH, Beaglehole R, et al: Asthma mortality in New Zealand: A two-year national study. NZ Med J 98: 271, 1985.

361. Eason J, Markowe HL: Controlled investigation of deaths from asthma in hospitals in the North East Thames region. Br Med J 294: 1255, 1987.

362. Sears MR, Rea HH, Fenwick J, et al: 75 deaths in asthmatics prescribed home nebulizers. Br Med J 294: 277, 1987.

363. Crompton GK, Grant IWB: Edinburgh Emergency Asthma Admission Service. Br Med J 4: 680, 1975.

364. Crompton GK, Grant IW, Chapman BJ, et al: Edinburgh Emergency Asthma Admission Service: Report on 15 years' experience. Eur J Respir Dis 70: 266, 1987.

365. Friedman D, Dales LG, Ury HK, et al: Mortality in middle-aged smokers and non-smokers. N Engl J Med 300: 213, 1979.

366. Ferris B Jr: Chronic bronchitis and emphysema: Classification and epidemiology. Med Clin North Am 57: 637, 1973.

367. Peto R, Speizer FE, Cochrane AL, et al: The relevance in adults of air-flow obstruction, but not of mucus hypersecretion, to mortality from chronic lung disease: Results from 20 years of prospective observation. Am Rev Respir Dis 128: 491, 1983.

368. Fletcher CM, Pride NB: Definitions of emphysema, chronic bronchitis, asthma, and airflow obstruction: 25 years on from the CIBA symposium (editorial). Thorax 39: 81, 1984.

369. American Thoracic Society (Statement by Committee on Diagnostic Standards for Nontuberculous Respiratory Diseases): Definitions and classification of chronic bronchitis, asthma, and pulmonary emphysema. Am Rev Respir Dis 85: 762, 1962.

370. Report of the conclusions of a Ciba Guest Symposium: Terminology, definitions, and classification of chronic pulmonary emphysema and related conditions. Thorax 14: 286, 1959.

371. Snider GL, Kleinerman JL, Thurlbeck WM, et al: The definition of emphysema: Report of a National Heart, Lung, and Blood Institute, Division of Lung Diseases Workshop. Am Rev Respir Dis 132: 182, 1985.

372. Macklem PT, Thurlbeck WM, Fraser RG, et al: Chronic obstructive disease of small airways. Ann Intern Med 74: 167, 1971.

373. Keith TA III, Schreiner AW: *Haemophilus influenzae* in adult bronchopulmonary infection. Ann Intern Med 56: 27, 1962.

374. College of General Practitioners: Chronic bronchitis in Great Britain: A national survey carried out by the Respiratory Diseases Study Group of the College of General Practitioners. Br Med J 2: 973, 1961.

375. Higgins MW, Keller JB, Landis JR, et al: Risk of chronic obstructive pulmonary disease: Collaborative assessment of the validity of the Tecumseh Index of Risk. Am Rev Respir Dis 130: 380, 1984.

376. Webster JR Jr, Kettel LJ, Moran F, et al: Chronic obstructive pulmonary disease: A comparison between men and women. Am Rev Respir Dis 98: 1021, 1968.

377. Seltzer CC, Siegelaub AB, Friedman GD, et al: Differences in pulmonary function related to smoking habits and race. Am Rev Respir Dis 110: 598, 1974.

378. Pride NB: Which smokers develop progressive airflow obstruction. Eur J Respir Dis 64(Suppl 126): 79, 1983.

379. Clément J, Van de Woestijne KP: Rapidly decreasing forced expiratory volume in one second or vital capacity and development of chronic airflow obstruction. Am Rev Respir Dis 125: 553, 1982.

380. Tager IB, Muñoz A, Rosner B, et al: Effect of cigarette smoking on the pulmonary function of children and adolescents. Am Rev Respir Dis 131: 752, 1985.

381. Sparrow D, Stefos T, Bossé R, et al: The relationship of tar content to decline in pulmonary function in cigarette smokers. Am Rev Respir Dis 127: 56, 1983.

382. Beck GJ, Doyle CA, Schachter EN, et al: Smoking and lung function. Am Rev Respir Dis 123: 149, 1981.

383. Lehrer SB, Barbandi F, Taylor JP, et al: Tobacco smoke sensitivity: Is there an immunologic basis? J Allergy Immunol 240: 73, 1984.

384. Taylor DR, Reid WD, Paré PD, et al: Cigarette smoke inhalation patterns and bronchial reactivity. Thorax 43: 65, 1988.

385. Bake B: Does environmental tobacco smoke affect lung function? Eur J Respir Dis 65(Suppl 133): 85, 1984.

386. Burchfiel CM, Higgins MW, Keller JB, et al: Passive smoking in childhood: Respiratory conditions and pulmonary function in Tecumseh, Michigan. Am Rev Respir Dis 133: 966, 1986.

387. Tsimoyianis GV, Jacobson MS, Feldman JG: Reduction in pulmonary function and increased frequency of cough associated with passive smoking in teenage athletes. Pediatrics 80: 32, 1987.

388. Ware JH, Dockery DW, Spiro A, et al: Passive smoking, gas cooking, and respiratory health of children living in 6 cities. Am Rev Respir Dis 129: 366, 1984.

389. Pandey MR: Prevalence of chronic bronchitis in a rural community of the hill region of Nepal. Thorax 39: 331, 1984.

390. Bates DV: Air pollutants and the human lung: The James Waring Memorial Lecture. Am Rev Respir Dis 105: 1, 1972.

391. Cohen CA, Hudson AR, Clausen JL, et al: Respiratory symptoms, spirometry, and oxidant air pollution in nonsmoking adults. Am Rev Respir Dis 105: 251, 1972.

392. Lambert PM, Reid DD: Smoking, air pollution, and bronchitis in Britain. Lancet 1: 853, 1970.

393. Lunn JE, Knowelden J, Handyside AJ: Patterns of respiratory illness in Sheffield infant schoolchildren. Br J Prev Soc Med 21: 7, 1967.

394. Becklake MR: Chronic airflow limitation: Its relationship to work in dusty occupations. Chest 88: 608, 1985.

395. Diem JE, Jones RN, Hendrick DJ, et al: Five-year longitudinal study of workers employed in a new toluene diisocyanate manufacturing plant. Am Rev Respir Dis 126: 420, 1982.

396. Attfield MD: Longitudinal decline in FEV_1 in United States coalminers. Thorax 40: 132, 1985.

397. Chan-Yeung M, Wong R, MacLean L, et al: Respiratory survey of workers in a pulp and paper mill in Powell River, British Columbia. Am Rev Respir Dis 122: 249, 1980.

398. Britten N, Davies JM, Colley JR: Early respiratory experience and subsequent cough and peak expiratory flow rate in 36-year-old men and women. Br Med J 294: 1317, 1987.

399. Woolcock A, Peat J, Leeder S, et al: The development of lung function in Sydney children: Effects of respiratory illness and smoking. A ten-year study. Eur J Respir Dis 65: 1, 1985.

399a. Matsuse T, Hayashi S, Kuwano K, et al: Latent adenoviral infection in the pathogenesis of chronic airways obstruction. Am Rev Respir Dis 146: 177, 1992.

400. Gump DW, Phillips CA, Forsyth BR, et al: Role of infection in chronic bronchitis. Am Rev Respir Dis 113: 465, 1976.

401. Stern H: Virus infections in chronic bronchitis: A family study. J Clin Pathol 21(Suppl 2): 99, 1968.

402. Lawther PJ, Waller RE, Henderson M: Air pollution and exacerbations of bronchitis. Thorax 25: 525, 1970.

403. Hsieh Y-C, Frayser R, Ross JC: The effect of cold-air inhalation on ventilation in normal subjects and in patients with chronic obstructive pulmonary disease. Am Rev Respir Dis 128: 236, 1983.

404. Arnup ME, Mendella LA, Anthonisen NR, et al: Effects of cold air hyperpnea in patients with chronic obstructive lung disease. Am Rev Respir Dis 128: 326, 1983.

405. Ramsdale E, Roberts R, Morris M, et al: Differences in responsiveness to hyperventilation and methacholine in asthma and chronic bronchitis. Thorax 40: 422, 1985.

406. Puchelle E, Zahm J-M, Aug F: Viscoelasticity, protein content, and ciliary transport rate of sputum in patient with recurrent and chronic bronchitis. Biorheology 18: 659, 1981.

407. Foster WM, Langenback E, Bergorfsky E, et al: Disassociation in the mucociliary function of central and peripheral airways of asymptomatic smokers. Am Rev Respir Dis 132: 633, 1985.

408. Matthys H, Vastag E, Kohler D, et al: Mucociliary clearance in patients with chronic bronchitis and bronchial carcinoma. Respiration 44: 329, 1983.

409. Mossberg B, Camner P: Impaired mucociliary transport as a pathogenetic factor in obstructive pulmonary diseases. Chest 77: 265, 1980.

410. Tockman MS, Khoury MJ, Cohen BH: The epidemiology of COPD. In Petty TL (ed): Chronic Obstructive Disease: Lefant C (ed): Lung Biology in Health and Disease. New York, Marcel Dekker, 1985, p 43.

411. Lieberman J: Alpha₁-antitrypsin deficiency. Med Clin North Am 57: 691, 1973.

412. Ad Hoc Committee to Review Antitrypsin Methods: Statement on methods for detecting alpha₁-antitrypsin abnormalities. In Mittman C (ed): Pulmonary Emphysema and Proteolysis. New York, Academic Press, 1972, p 141.

413. Talamo RC, Langley CE, Hyslop NE Jr: A comparison of functional and immunochemical measurements of serum alpha₁-antitrypsin. In Mittman C (ed): Pulmonary Emphysema and Proteolysis. New York, Academic Press, 1972, p 167.

414. Lieberman J: Elastase, collagenase, emphysema, and alpha₁-antitrypsin deficiency. Chest 70: 62, 1976.

415. Talamo RC, Thurlbeck WM: Alpha₁-antitrypsin Pi types in postmortem blood. Am Rev Respir Dis 112: 201, 1975.

416. Pierce JA, Eradio B, Dew TA: Antitrypsin phenotypes in St. Louis. JAMA 231: 609, 1975.

417. Cole RB, Nevin NC, Blundell G, et al: Relation of alpha₁-antitrypsin phenotype to the performance of pulmonary function tests and to the prevalence of respiratory illness in a working population. Thorax 31: 149, 1976.

418. Falk GA, Briscoe WA: Alpha₁-antitrypsin deficiency in chronic obstructive pulmonary disease. Ann Intern Med 72: 430, 1970.

419. Alpha₁-antitrypsin deficiency and liver disease in childhood. Br Med J 1: 758, 1973.

420. Kueppers F, Black LF: Alpha₁-antitrypsin and its deficiency. Am Rev Respir Dis 110: 176, 1974.

421. Jeppsson JO, Larsson C, Eriksson S: Characterization of alpha₁-antitrypsin in the inclusion bodies from the liver in alpha₁-antitrypsin deficiency. N Engl J Med 293: 576, 1975.

422. Black LF, Kueppers F: Alpha₁-antitrypsin deficiency in nonsmokers. Am Rev Respir Dis 117: 421, 1978.

423. Orell SR, Mazodier P: Pathological findings in alpha₁-antitrypsin deficiency. In Mittman C (ed): Pulmonary Emphysema and Proteolysis. New York, Academic Press, 1972, p 69.

424. Fagerhol MK: The incidence of alpha₁-antitrypsin variants in chronic obstructive pulmonary disease. In Mittman C (ed): Pulmonary Emphysema and Proteolysis. New York, Academic Press, 1972, p 51.

425. Hutchison DC, Tobin MJ, Cook PJL, et al: Alpha₁-antitrypsin deficiency: Clinical and physiological feautres in heterozygotes of Pi type SZ: A survey by the British Thoracic Association. Br J Dis Chest 77: 28, 1983.

426. Morse JO: Alpha₁-antitrypsin deficiency. N Engl J Med 299: 1045, 1978.

427. Bruce RM, Cohen BH, Diamond EL, et al: Collaborative study to assess risk of lung disease in Pi^{MZ} phenotype subjects. Am Rev Respir Dis 130: 386, 1984.

428. Weiss ST, Speizer FE: Increased levels of airways responsiveness as a risk factor for development of chronic obstructive lung disease: What are the issues? Chest 86: 3, 1984.

429. Postma DS, de Vries K, Köeter GH, et al: Independent influence of reversibility of air-flow obstruction and nonspecific hyperreactivity on the long-term course of lung function in chronic air-flow obstruction. Am Rev Respir Dis 134: 276, 1986.

430. Mitchell RS: Outlook in emphysema and chronic bronchitis. N Engl J Med 280: 445, 1969.

431. Taylor RG, Gross E, Joyce H, et al: Smoking, allergy, and the differential white blood cell count. Thorax 40: 17, 1985.

432. Janoff A: Elastases and emphysema: Current assessment of the protease-antiprotease hypothesis. Am Rev Respir Dis 132: 417, 1985.

433. Gadek JE, Fells GA, Zimmerman RL, et al: Antielastases of the human alveolar structures: Implications for the protease-antiprotease theory of emphysema. J Clin Invest 68: 889, 1981.

434. Hoidal JR, Niewoehner DE: Pathogenesis of emphysema. Chest 83: 679, 1983.

435. Chan Yeung M, Dy Buncio A: Leukocyte count, smoking, and lung function. Am J Med 76: 31, 1984.

436. MacNee W, Martin BA, Tanco S, et al: Cigarette smoking delays

polymorphonuclear leukocyte (PMN) transit through the pulmonary circulation. Am Rev Respir Dis 135: A146, 1987.

437. Kew RR, Ghebrehiwet B, Janoff A, et al: Cigarette smoke can activate the alternative pathway of complement in vitro by modifying the third component of complement. J Clin Invest 75: 1000, 1985.

438. Bridges RB, Wyatt RJ, Rehm SR: Effect of smoking on peripheral blood leukocytes and serum antiproteases. Eur J Respir Dis (Suppl) 139: 24, 1985.

439. Kramps JA, Bakker W, Dijkman JH, et al: A matched-pair study of the leukocyte elastase-like activity in normal persons and in emphysematous patients with and without alpha₁-antitrypsin deficiency. Am Rev Respir Dis 121: 253, 1980.

440. Harris JO, Olsen GN, Castle JR, et al: Comparison of proteolytic enzyme activity in pulmonary alveolar macrophages and blood leukocytes in smokers and nonsmokers. Am Rev Respir Dis 111: 579, 1975.

441. Kuhn C, Senior RM: The role of elastases in the development of emphysema. Lung 155: 185, 1978.

442. Cohen AB: The effects in vivo and in vitro of oxidative damage to purified alpha₁-antitrypsin and to the enzyme-inhibiting activity of plasma. Am Rev Respir Dis 119: 953, 1979.

443. Janoff A, Dearing R: Alpha₁-proteinase inhibitor is more sensitive to inactivation by cigarette smoke than is leukocyte elastase. Am Rev Respir Dis 126: 691, 1982.

444. Snider GL, Hayes JA, Franzblau C, et al: Relationship between elastolytic activity and experimental emphysema-inducing properties of papain preparations. Am Rev Respir Dis 110: 254, 1974.

445. Karlinsky JB, Snider GL, Franzblau C, et al: In vitro effects of elastase and collagenase on mechanical properties of hamster lungs. Am Rev Respir Dis 113: 769, 1976.

446. Senior RM, Tegner H, Kuhn C, et al: The induction of pulmonary emphysema with human leukocyte elastase. Am Rev Respir Dis 116: 469, 1977.

447. Guenter CA, Coalson JJ, Jacques J, et al: Emphysema associated with intravascular leukocyte sequestration: Comparison with papain-induced emphysema. Am Rev Respir Dis 123: 79, 1981.

448. Wittels EH, Coalson JJ, Welch MH, et al: Pulmonary intravascular leukocyte sequestration. A potential mechanism of lung injury. Am Rev Respir Dis 109: 502, 1974.

449. Kida K, Thurlbeck WM: Lack of recovery of lung structure and function after the administration of beta-aminoproprionitrile in the postnatal period. Am Rev Respir Dis 122: 467, 1980.

450. Reid L: Measurement of the bronchial mucous gland layer: A diagnostic yardstick in chronic bronchitis. Thorax 15: 132, 1960.

451. Jamal K, Cooney RP, Fleetham JA, et al: Chronic bronchitis: Correlation of morphologic findings to sputum production and flow rates. Am Rev Respir Dis 129: 719, 1984.

452. Nagai A, West W, Paul J, et al: The National Institutes of Health Intermittent Positive-Pressure Breathing Trial: Pathology studies. 1. Interrelationship between morphologic lesions. Am Rev Respir Dis 132: 937, 1985.

453. Baier H, Zarzecki S, Wanner A, et al: Influence of lung inflation on the cross-sectional area of central airways in normals and in patients with lung disease. Respiration 41: 145, 1981.

454. Carlile A, Edwards C: Structural variation in the named bronchi of the left lung: A morphometric study. Br J Dis Chest 77: 344, 1983.

455. Mullen JBM, Wright JL, Wiggs BR, et al: Reassessment of inflammation of airways in chronic bronchitis. Br Med J 291: 1235, 1985.

456. Bowen JH, Woodard BH, Pratt PC: Bronchial collapse in obstructive lung disease. Chest 80: 510, 1981.

457. Hogg JC, Macklem PT, Thurlbeck WM: Site and nature of airway obstruction in chronic obstructive lung disease. N Engl J Med 278: 1355, 1968.

458. Cosio MG, Hale KA, Niewoehner DE, et al: Morphologic and morphometric effects of prolonged cigarette smoking on the small airways. Am Rev Respir Dis 122: 265, 1980.

459. Petty TL, Silvers GW, Stanford RE, et al: Radial traction and small airway disease in excised human lungs. Am Rev Respir Dis 133: 132, 1986.

460. Wright JL, Cosio M, Wiggs BJ, et al: A morphologic grading scheme for membranous and respiratory bronchioles. Arch Pathol Lab Med 109: 163, 1985.

461. Wright JL, Paré PD, Nelems JM, et al: The nature of peripheral airway inflammations in emphysema. Fed Proc 39: 332A, 1980.

462. Wright JL, Hobson J, Wiggs BR, et al: Effect of cigarette smoke on structure of the small airways. Lung 165: 91, 1987.

463. Niewoehner DE, Kleinerman J: Morphologic basis of pulmonary

464. Wright JL, Lawson LM, Paré PD, et al: The detection of small airways disease. Am Rev Respir Dis 129: 989, 1984.

465. Petty TL, Silvers GW, Stanford RE, et al: Small airway disease is associated with elastic recoil changes in excised human lungs. Am Rev Respir Dis 130: 42, 1984.

466. Hale KA, Ewing SL, Gosnell BA, et al: Lung disease in long-term cigarette smokers with and without chronic air-flow obstruction. Am Rev Respir Dis 130: 716, 1984.

467. Cosio MG, Shiner RJ, Saetta M, et al: Alveolar fenestrae in smokers: Relationship with light microscopic and functional abnormalities. Am Rev Respir Dis 133: 126, 1986.

468. Anderson AE Jr, Foraker AG: Centrilobular emphysema and panlobular emphysema: Two different diseases. Thorax 28: 547, 1973.

469. Anderson AE Jr, Furlaneto JA, Foraker AG: Bronchopulmonary derangements in nonsmokers. Am Rev Respir Dis 101: 518, 1970.

470. Boren HG: Alveolar fenestrae: Relationship to the pathology and pathogenesis of pulmonary emphysema. Am Rev Respir Dis 85: 328, 1962.

471. Snider GL, Kleinerman JL, Thurlbeck WM, et al: The definition of emphysema: Report of a National Heart, Lung, and Blood Institute, Division of Lung Diseases workshop. Am Rev Respir Dis 132: 182, 1985.

472. Bates DV, Gordon CA, Paul GI, et al: Chronic bronchitis: Report on the third and fourth stages of chronic bronchitis in the Department of Veterans Affairs, Canada. Med Serv J Can 22: 5, 1966.

473. Simon G: Chronic bronchitis and emphysema: A symposium. III. Pathological findings and radiological changes in chronic bronchitis and emphysema. (b) Radiological changes in chronic bronchitis. Br J Radiol 32: 292, 1959.

474. Feigin DS, Abraham JL: "Increased pulmonary markings": A radiologic-pathologic correlation study (abstr). Invest Radiol 15: 425, 1980.

475. Nicklaus TM, Stowell DW, Christiansen WR, et al: The accuracy of the roentgenologic diagnosis of chronic pulmonary emphysema. Am Rev Respir Dis 93: 889, 1966.

476. Burki NK: Conventional chest films can identify air flow obstruction. Chest 93: 675, 1988.

477. Reich SB, Weinshelbaum A, Yee J: Correlation of radiographic measurements and pulmonary function tests in chronic obstructive pulmonary disease. Am J Roentgenol 144: 695, 1985.

478. Milne ENC, Bass H: Roentgenologic and functional analysis of combined chronic obstructive pulmonary disease and congestive cardiac failure. Invest Radiol 4: 129, 1969.

479. Fraser RG, Bates DV: Body section roentgenography in the evaluation and differentiation of chronic hypertrophic emphysema and asthma. Am J Roentgenol 82: 39, 1959.

480. Barden RP: Glimpses through the pulmonary window: Interpretation of the radiologic evidence in disorders of the lungs. Hickey Lecture, 1966. Am J Roentgenol 98: 269, 1966.

481. Gurney JW, Jones KK, Robbins RA, et al: Regional distribution of emphysema: Correlation of high-resolution CT with pulmonary function tests in unselected smokers. Radiology 183: 457, 1992.

482. Rosen RA, Dalinka MK, Gralino BJ Jr, et al: The roentgenographic findings in alpha₁-antitrypsin deficiency (AAD). Radiology 95: 25, 1970.

482a. Guest PJ, Hansell DM: High-resolution computed tomography (HRCT) in emphysema associated with alpha₁-antitrypsin deficiency. Clin Radiol 45: 260, 1992.

483. Jones MC, Thomas GO: Alpha₁-antitrypsin deficiency and pulmonary emphysema. Thorax 26: 652, 1971.

484. Sanders C, Nath PH, Bailey WC: Detection of emphysema with computed tomography: Correlation with pulmonary function tests and chest radiography. Invest Radiol 23: 262, 1988.

485. Klein JS, Gamsu G, Webb WR, et al: High-resolution CT diagnosis of emphysema in symptomatic patients with normal chest radiographs and isolated low diffusing capacity. Radiology 182: 817, 1992.

486. Simon G: Radiology and emphysema. Clin Radiol 15: 293, 1964.

487. Thurlbeck WM, Henderson JA, Fraser RG, et al: Chronic obstructive lung disease: A comparison between clinical, roentgenologic, functional, and morphological criteria in chronic bronchitis, emphysema, asthma, and bronchiectasis. Medicine 49: 81, 1970.

488. Simon G: Complexities of emphysema. In Simon M, Potchen EJ, LeMay M (eds): Frontiers of Pulmonary Radiology. New York, Grune & Stratton, 1969, pp 142–153.

489. Burrows B, Niden AH, Barclay WR, et al: Chronic obstructive lung

resistance in the human lung and effects of aging. J Appl Physiol 36: 412, 1974.

disease. II. Relationship of clinical and physiologic findings to the severity of airways obstruction. Am Rev Respir Dis 92: 665, 1965.

490. Miller RD, Hepper NGG, Kueppers F, et al: Host factors in chronic obstructive pulmonary disease in an upper mid-west rural community: Design, case selection, and clinical characteristics in a matched-pair study. Mayo Clin Proc 51: 709, 1976.

491. Kass I, O'Brien LE, Zamel N, et al: Lack of correlation between clinical background and pulmonary function tests in patients with chronic obstructive pulmonary diseases: A retrospective study of 140 cases. Am Rev Respir Dis 107: 64, 1973.

492. Mueller RE, Keble DL, Plummer J, et al: The prevalence of chronic bronchitis, chronic airway obstruction, and respiratory symptoms in a Colorado city. Am Rev Respir Dis 103: 209, 1971.

493. Seward JB, Hayes DL, Smith HC, et al: Platypnea-orthodeoxia: Clinical profile, diagnostic workup, management, and report of seven cases. Mayo Clin Proc 59: 221, 1984.

494. Burrows B, Flatcher CM, Heard BE, et al: The emphysematous and bronchial types of chronic airways obstruction. Lancet 1: 830, 1966.

495. Kawakami Y, Irie T, Shida A, et al: Familial factors affecting arterial blood gas values and respiratory chemosensitivity in chronic obstructive pulmonary disease. Am Rev Respir Dis 125: 420, 1982.

496. Marini JJ, Pierson DJ, Hudson LD, et al: The significance of wheezing in chronic airflow obstruction. Am Rev Respir Dis 120: 1069, 1979.

497. Christie RV: Emphysema of the lungs. Br Med J 1: 105, 1944.

498. Hoover CF: Definitive percussion and inspection in estimating size and contour of heart. JAMA 75: 1626, 1920.

499. Wright JL, Lawson LM, Paré PD, et al: The structure and function of pulmonary vasculature in mild chronic obstructive pulmonary disease: The effect of oxygen and exercise. Am Rev Respir Dis 128: 702, 1983.

500. Albert RK, Muramoto A, Caldwell J, et al: Increases in intrathoracic pressure do not explain the rise in left ventricular end-diastolic pressure that occurs during exercise in patients with chronic obstructive pulmonary disease. Am Rev Respir Dis 132: 623, 1985.

501. Weitzenblum E, Hirth C, Parini JP, et al: Clinical, functional, and pulmonary hemodynamic course of patients with chronic obstructive pulmonary disease followed-up over 3 years. Respiration 36: 1, 1978.

502. Midgren B, White T, Petersson K, et al: Nocturnal hypoxaemia and cor pulmonale in severe chronic lung disease. Bull Eur Physiopathol Respir 21: 527, 1985.

503. Weitzenblum E, Jezek V: Evolution of pulmonary hypertension in chronic respiratory disease. Bull Eur Physiopathol Respir 20: 73, 1985.

504. Schrijen F, Uffholtz H, Polu JM, et al: Pulmonary and systemic hemodynamic evolution in chronic bronchitis. Am Rev Respir Dis 117: 25, 1978.

505. Taha RA, Boushy SF, Thompson HK Jr, et al: The electrocardiogram in chronic obstructive pulmonary disease. Am Rev Respir Dis 107: 1067, 1973.

506. Tandon MK: Correlations of electrocardiographic features with airway obstruction in chronic bronchitis. Chest 63: 146, 1973.

507. Murphy ML, Hutcheson F: The electrocardiographic diagnosis of right ventricular hypertrophy in chronic obstructive pulmonary disease. Chest 65: 622, 1974.

508. Macnee W, Xue QF, Hannan WJ, et al: Assessment by radionuclide angiography of right and left ventricular function in chronic bronchitis and emphysema. Thorax 38: 494, 1983.

509. Jardin F, Gueret P, Prost JF, et al: 2-dimensional echocardiographic assessment of left ventricular function in chronic obstructive pulmonary disease. Am Rev Respir Dis 129: 135, 1984.

510. Holford FD, Mithoefer JC: Cardiac arrhythmias in hospitalized patients with chronic obstructive pulmonary disease. Am Rev Respir Dis 108: 879, 1973.

511. Wedzicha JA, Cotes PM, Empey DW, et al: Serum immunoreactive erythropoietin in hypoxic lung disease with and without polycythaemia. Clin Sci 69: 413, 1985.

512. Calverley MA, Leggett RJ, McElderry L, et al: Cigarette smoking and secondary polycythemia in hypoxic cor pulmonale. Am Res Respir 125: 507, 1982.

513. Palmer KNV, Gardiner AJS: Effect of partial gastrectomy on pulmonary physiology. Br Med J 1: 347, 1964.

514. Dines DE, Clagett OT, Payne WS: Spontaneous pneumothorax in emphysema. Mayo Clin Proc 45: 481, 1970.

515. Schwartz JS, Bencowitz HZ, Moser KM, et al: Air travel hypoxemia with chronic obstructive pulmonary disease. Ann Intern Med 100: 473, 1984.

516. Burrows B, Earle RH: Course and prognosis of chronic obstructive lung disease: A prospective study of 200 patients. N Engl J Med 280: 397, 1969.

517. Camilli AE, Burrows B, Knudson RJ, et al: Longitudinal changes in forced expiratory volume in one second in adults: Effect of smoking and smoking cessation. Am Rev Respir Dis 135: 794, 1987.

518. Becklake MR, Permutt S: Evaluation of tests of lung function for "screening" for early detection of chronic obstructive lung disease. In Macklem PT, Permutt S (eds): The Lung in the Transition Between Health and Disease. New York, Marcel Dekker, 1979, p 345.

519. Marrero O, Beck GJ, Schachier EN: Discriminating power of measurements from maximum expiratory flow-volume curves. Respiration 49: 263, 1986.

520. Hyatt RE, Rodarte JR: Changes in lung mechanics. In Macklem PT, Permutt S (eds): The Lung in the Transition Between Health and Disease. New York, Marcel Dekker, 1979, p 73.

521. Anthonisen NR, Wright EC: Bronchodilator response in chronic obstructive pulmonary disease. Am Rev Respir Dis 133: 814, 1986.

522. Wardman AG, Binns V, Clayden AD, et al: The diagnosis and treatment of adults with obstructive airways disease in general practice. Br J Dis Chest 80: 19, 1986.

523. Ramsdale EH, Morris MM, Hargreave FE: Interpretation of the variability of peak flow rates in chronic bronchitis. Thorax 41: 771, 1986.

524. Buist AS, Nagy JM, Sexton GJ, et al: The effect of smoking cessation on pulmonary function: A 30-month follow-up of two smoking cessation clinics. Am Rev Respir Dis 120: 953, 1979.

525. Tashkin D, Clark V, Coulson A, et al: The UCLA population studies of chronic obstructive respiratory disease. VIII. Effects of smoking cessation on lung function—a prospective study of a free-living population. Am Rev Respir Dis 130: 707, 1984.

526. Simonsson BG, Rolf C: Bronchial reactivity to methacholine in ten non-obstructive heavy smokers before and up to one year after cessation of smoking. Eur J Respir Dis 63: 526, 1982.

527. Hogg JC, Wright JL, Paré PD, et al: Airway disease: Evolution, pathology, and recognition. Med J Aust 142: 605, 1985.

528. York EL, Jones RL: Effects of smoking on regional residual volume in young adults. Chest 79: 12, 1981.

529. Dawkins KD, Muers MF: Diurnal variation in airflow obstruction in chronic bronchitis. Thorax 36: 618, 1981.

530. Fleury B, Murciano D, Talamo C, et al: Work of breathing in patients with chronic obstructive pulmonary disease in acute respiratory failure. Am Rev Respir Dis 131: 822, 1985.

531. Farkas GA, Roussos CH: Adaptability of the hamster diaphragm to exercise and/or emphysema. J Appl Physiol 53: 1263, 1982.

532. Paré PD, Coppin CA: Errors in the measurement of total lung capacity in patients with chronic obstructive pulmonary disease. Thorax 38: 468, 1983.

533. Piquet J, Harf A, Lorino H, et al: Lung volume measurements by plethysmography in chronic obstructive pulmonary disease: Influence of the panting pattern. Bull Eur Physiopathol Respir 20: 31, 1985.

534. Bégin P, Peslin R: Influence of panting frequency on thoracic gas volume measurements in chronic obstructive pulmonary disease. Am Rev Respir Dis 130: 121, 1984.

535. Colebatch HJH, Greaves IA, Ng CKY, et al: Pulmonary distensibility and ventilatory function in smokers. Bull Eur Physiopathol Respir 21: 439, 1985.

536. Paré PD, Brooks LA, Bates J, et al: Exponential analysis of the lung pressure-volume curve as a predictor of pulmonary emphysema. Am Rev Respir Dis 126: 54, 1982.

537. Aubier M, Murciano D, Fournier M, et al: Central respiratory drive in acute respiratory failure of patients with chronic obstructive pulmonary disease. Am Rev Respir Dis 122: 191, 1980.

538. Guenard H, Merhas M, Todd-Prokopek A, et al: Effects of oxygen breathing on regional distribution of ventilation and perfusion in hypoxemic patients with chronic lung disease. Am Rev Respir Dis 125: 12, 1982.

539. Mithoefer JC, Ramirez C, Cook W, et al: The effect of mixed venous oxygenation on arterial blood in chronic obstructive pulmonary disease: The basis for a classification. Am Rev Respir Dis 117: 259, 1978.

540. Paré PD, Brooks LA, Baile EM, et al: The effect of systemic venous hypertension on pulmonary function and lung water. J Appl Physiol 51: 592, 1981.

541. Flick MR, Block AJ: Continuous in-vivo monitoring of arterial oxygenation in chronic obstructive lung disease. Ann Intern Med 86: 725, 1977.

542. Guilleminault C, Cummiskey J, Motta J, et al: Chronic obstructive airflow disease and sleep studies. Am Rev Respir Dis 122: 397, 1980.

543. Douglas NJ, Calverley PM, Leggett RJ, et al: Transient hypoxaemia during sleep in chronic bronchitis and emphysema. Lancet 1: 1, 1979.

544. Boysen PG, Block AJ, Wynne JW, et al: Nocturnal pulmonary hypertension in patients with chronic obstructive pulmonary disease. Chest 76: 536, 1979.

545. Stewart RI, Lewis CM: Arterial oxygenation and oxygen transport during exercise in patients with chronic obstructive pulmonary disease. Respiration 49: 161, 1986.

546. Owens G, Rogers R, Pennock B, et al: The diffusing capacity as a predictor of arterial oxygen desaturation during exercise in patients with chronic obstructive pulmonary disease. N Engl J Med 310: 1218, 1984.

547. Giminez M, Servera E, Candina R, et al: Hypercapnia during maximal exercise in patients with chronic airflow obstruction. Bull Eur Physiopathol Respir 20: 113, 1985.

548. Miller A, Thornton JC, Warshaw R, et al: Single breath diffusing capacity in a representative sample of the population of Michigan, a large industrial state: Predicted values, lower limits of normal, and frequencies of abnormality by smoking history. Am Rev Respir Dis 127: 270, 1983.

548a. Sansores RH, Paré PD, Abboud RT: Acute effect of cigarette smoking on the carbon monoxide diffusing capacity of the lung. Am Rev Respir Dis 146: 951, 1992.

549. Williams MH Jr, Park SS: Diffusion of gases within the lungs of patients with chronic obstructive pulmonary disease. Am Rev Respir Dis 98: 210, 1968.

550. Moser KM, Shibel EM, Beamon AJ: Acute respiratory failure in obstructive lung disease. JAMA 225: 705, 1973.

551. Burk RH, George RB: Acute respiratory failure in chronic obstructive pulmonary disease. Arch Intern Med 132: 865, 1973.

552. Bishop JM, Cross KW: Physiological variables and mortality in patients with various categories of chronic respiratory disease. Bull Eur Physiopathol Respir 20: 495, 1985.

553. Weitzenblum E, Hirth C, Ducolone A, et al: Prognostic value of pulmonary artery pressure in chronic obstructive pulmonary disease. Thorax 36: 752, 1981.

554. Medical Research Council Working Party: Long-term domiciliary oxygen therapy in chronic hypoxic cor pulmonale complicating chronic bronchitis and emphysema. Lancet 1: 681, 1981.

555. Timms RM, Khaja FU, Williams GW: The Nocturnal Oxygen Therapy Trial Group: Hemodynamic response to oxygen therapy in chronic obstructive pulmonary disease. Ann Intern Med 102: 29, 1985.

556. Flick MR, Block AJ: Nocturnal vs diurnal cardiac arrhythmias in patients with chronic obstructive pulmonary disease. Chest 75: 8, 1979.

557. Sassoon CSH, Hassell KT, Mahutte CK, et al: Hyperoxic-induced hypercapnia in stable chronic obstructive pulmonary disease. Am Rev Respir Dis 135: 907, 1987.

558. McNicol MW, Campbell EJM: Severity of respiratory failure: Arterial blood-gases in untreated patients. Lancet 1: 336, 1965.

559. Gibson GJ: Familial pneumothoraces and bullae. Thorax 32: 88, 1977.

560. Wood JR, Bellamy D, Child AH, et al: Pulmonary disease in patients with Marfan syndrome. Thorax 39: 780, 1984.

561. Ayers JG, Pope FM, Reudy JF, et al: Abnormalities of the lungs and thoracic cage in the Ehlers-Danlos syndrome. Thorax 40: 300, 1985.

562. Reid L: The Pathology of Emphysema. London, Lloyd-Luke (Medical Books) Ltd, 1967.

563. Boushy SF, Kohen R, Billig DM, et al: Bullous emphysema: Clinical, roentgenologic, and physiologic study of 49 patients. Dis Chest 54: 327, 1968.

564. Ohata M, Suzuki H: Pathogenesis of spontaneous pneumothorax with special reference to the ultrastructure of emphysematous bullae. Chest 77: 771, 1980.

565. Morgan MD, Denison DM, Strickland B, et al: Value of computed tomography for selecting patients with bullous lung disease for surgery. Thorax 41: 855, 1986.

566. Stark P, Gadziala N, Green R: Fluid accumulation in preexisting pulmonary air spaces. Am J Roentgenol 134: 701, 1980.

567. Bourgouin P, Cousineau G, Lemire P, et al: Computed tomography used to exclude pneumothorax in bullous lung disease. J Can Assoc Radiol 36: 341, 1985.

568. Viola AR, Zuffardi EA: Physiologic and clinical aspects of pulmonary bullous disease. Am Rev Respir Dis 94: 574, 1966.

569. Poe RH, Willman HN, Berke RA, et al: Perfusion-ventilation scintiphotography in bullous disease of the lung. Am Rev Respir Dis 107: 946, 1973.

570. Pride NB, Hugh-Jones P, O'Brien EN, et al: Changes in lung function following the surgical treatment of bullous emphysema. Q J Med 39: 49, 1970.

571. Rakower J, Morgan E: Unilateral hyperlucent lung (Swyer-James syndrome). Am J Med 33: 864, 1962.

572. Gold RE, Wilt JC, Adhikari TK, et al: Adenoviral pneumonia and its complications in infancy and childhood. J Can Assoc Radiol 20: 218, 1969.

573. Culiner MM: The hyperlucent lung, a problem in differential diagnosis. Dis Chest 49: 578, 1966.

574. Reid L, Simon G: Unilateral lung transradiancy. Thorax 17: 230, 1962.

575. McKenzie SA, Allison DJ, Singh MP, et al: Unilateral hyperlucent lung: The case for investigation. Thorax 35: 745, 1980.

576. Marti-Bonmati L, Perales FR, Catala F, et al: CT findings in Swyer-James syndrome. Radiology 172: 477, 1989.

577. Houk VN, Kent DC, Fosburg RG: Unilateral hyperlucent lung: A study in pathophysiology and etiology. Am J Med Sci 253: 406, 1967.

578. Prowse OM, Fuchs JE, Kaufman SA, et al: Chronic obstructive pseudoemphysema: A rare cause of unilateral hyperlucent lung. N Engl J Med 271: 127, 1964.

579. Nairn JR, Prime FJ: A physiological study of Macleod's syndrome. Thorax 22: 148, 1967.

580. Margolin HN, Rosenberg LS, Felson B, et al: Idiopathic unilateral hyperlucent lung: A roentgenographic syndrome. Am J Roentgenol 82: 63, 1959.

581. Swyer PR, James GCW: A case of unilateral pulmonary emphysema. Thorax 8: 133, 1953.

582. Glauser EM, Cook CD, Harris GBC: Bronchiectasis: A review of 187 cases in children with follow-up pulmonary function studies in 58. Acta Paediatr Scand (Suppl) 165: 1, 1966.

583. Barker AF, Bardana EJ: Bronchiectasis: Update of an orphan disease. Am Rev Respir Dis 137: 969, 1988.

584. Cole PJ: Inflammation: A two-edge sword: The model of bronchiectasis. Eur J Respir Dis 69(Suppl 147): 6, 1986.

585. Hoeffler HB, Schweppe HI, Greenberg SD: Bronchiectasis following pulmonary ammonia burn. Arch Pathol Lab Med 106: 686, 1982.

586. Banner AS, Muthuswamy P, Shah RS, et al: Bronchiectasis following heroin-induced pulmonary edema: Rapid clearing of pulmonary infiltrates. Chest 69: 552, 1976.

587. Reid L: Reduction in bronchial subdivision in bronchiectasis. Thorax 5: 233, 1950.

588. Cudkowicz L: Bronchiectasis and bronchial artery circulation. In Moser KM (ed): Pulmonary Vascular Diseases. (Lung Biology in Health and Disease Series, Vol 14.) New York, Marcel Dekker, 1979, p 165.

589. Grenier P, Maurice F, Musset D, et al: Bronchiectasis: Assessment by thin-section CT. Radiology 161: 95, 1986.

590. Clark NS: Bronchiectasis in childhood. Br Med J 1: 80, 1963.

591. Bahous J, Cartier A, Pineau L, et al: Pulmonary function tests and airway responsiveness to methacholine in chronic bronchiectasis of the adult. Bull Eur Physiopathol Respir 20: 375, 1984.

592. Perry KMA, King DS: Bronchiectasis: A study of prognosis based on a follow-up of 400 patients. Am Rev Respir Dis 41: 531, 1940.

593. Konietzko NFJ, Carton RW, Leroy EP: Causes of death in patients with bronchiectasis. Am Rev Respir Dis 100: 852, 1969.

594. Helm WH, Thompson VC: The long-term results of resection for bronchiectasis. Q J Med 27: 353, 1958.

595. Camner P, Mossberg B, Afzelius BA: Evidence for congenitally nonfunctioning cilia in the tracheobronchial tract in two subjects. Am Rev Respir Dis 112: 807, 1975.

596. Rossman CM, Forrest JB, Lee RMKW: The dyskinetic cilia syndrome: Abnormal ciliary motility in association with abnormal ciliary ultrastructure. Chest 80: 860, 1981.

597. Holmes LB, Blennerhassett JB, Austen KF: A reappraisal of Kartagener's syndrome. Am J Med Sci 255: 13, 1968.

598. Rott HD: Genetics of Kartagener's syndrome. Eur J Respir Dis 127: 1, 1983.

599. Chao J, Turner JA, Sturgess JM, et al: Genetic heterogeneity of dynein-deficiency in cilia from patients with respiratory disease. Am Rev Respir Dis 126: 302, 1982.

600. Matwijiw I, Thliveris JA, Faiman C: Aplasia of nasal cilia with situs inversus, azoospermia, and normal sperm flagella: A unique variant of the immotile cilia syndrome. J Urol 137: 522, 1987.

601. Sturgess JM, Chao J, Wong J, et al: Cilia with defective radial spokes: A cause of human respiratory disease. N Engl J Med 300: 53, 1979.

602. Wilton LJ, Teichtahl H, Temple-Smith PD, et al: Kartagener's syndrome with motile cilia and immotile spermatozoa: Axonemal ultrastructure and function. Am Rev Respir Dis 134: 1233, 1986.

603. Moreau MF, Chretien MF, Dubin J, et al: Transposed ciliary microtubules in Kartagener's syndrome: A case report with electron microscopy of bronchial and nasal brushings. Acta Cytol 29: 248, 1985.

604. Antonelli M, Modesti A, Quattrucci S, et al: Supernumerary microtubules in the cilia of two siblings causing "immotile cilia syndrome." Eur J Respir 64: 607, 1983.

605. Gonzalez S, von Bassewitz DB, Grundmann E, et al: Atypical cilia in hyperplastic, metaplastic, and dysplastic human bronchial mucosa. Ultrastruct Pathol 8: 345, 1985.

606. Nadel HR, Stringer DA, Levison H, et al: The immotile cilia syndrome: Radiological manifestations. Radiology 154: 651, 1985.

607. Afzelius BA: Immotile-cilia syndrome and ciliary abnormalities induced by infection and injury. Am Rev Respir Dis 124: 107, 1981.

608. Kollberg H, Mossberg B, Afzelius BA, et al: Cystic fibrosis compared with the immotile-cilia syndrome: A study of mucociliary clearance, ciliary ultrastructure, clinical picture, and ventilatory function. Scand J Respir Dis 59: 297, 1978.

609. Wood RE, Boat TF, Doershuk CF: Cystic fibrosis. Am Rev Respir Dis 113: 833, 1976.

610. Rosenstein BJ, Langbaum TS, Metz SJ, et al: Cystic fibrosis: Diagnostic considerations. Johns Hopkins Med J 150: 113, 1982.

611. Hunt B, Geddes DM: Newly diagnosed cystic fibrosis in middle and later life. Thorax 40: 23, 1985.

612. Fitzpatrick SB, Rosenstein BJ, Langbaum TS, et al: Diagnosis of cystic fibrosis during adolescence. J Adolesc Health Care 7: 38, 1986.

613. Riordan JR, Rommens JM, Kerem B, et al: Identification of the cystic fibrosis gene: Cloning and characterization of the complementary DNA. Science 245: 1066, 1989.

614. Collins FS: Cystic fibrosis: Molecular biology and therapeutic implications. Science 256: 774, 1992.

615. Bowman BH, Mangos JA: Current concepts in genetics: Cystic fibrosis. N Engl J Med 294: 937, 1976.

616. Cuthbert AW: Abnormalities of airway epithelial function and the implications of the discovery of the cystic fibrosis gene. Thorax 46: 124, 1991.

617. Klinger JD, Thomassen MJ: Occurrence and antimicrobial susceptibility of gram-negative nonfermentative bacilli in cystic fibrosis patients. Diagn Microbiol Infect Dis 3: 149, 1985.

618. Wönne R, Hoffmann D, Posselt HG, et al: Bronchial allergy in cystic fibrosis. Clin Allergy 15: 455, 1985.

619. McFarlane H, Holzel A, Brenchley P, et al: Immune complexes in cystic fibrosis. Br Med J 1: 423, 1975.

620. Wilmott RW, Tyson SL, Matthew DJ, et al: Cystic fibrosis survival rates: The influences of allergy and *Pseudomonas aeruginosa*. Am J Dis Child 139: 669, 1985.

621. Zeaske R, Bruns WT, Fink JN, et al: Immune responses to *Aspergillus* in cystic fibrosis. J Allergy Clin Immunol 82: 73, 1988.

622. Chow CW, Landau LI, Taussig LM, et al: Bronchial mucous glands in the newborn with cystic fibrosis. Eur J Paediatr 139: 240, 1982.

623. Tomashefski JF Jr, Bruce M, Stern RC, et al: Pulmonary air cysts in cystic fibrosis: Relation of pathologic features to radiologic findings and history of pneumothorax. Hum Pathol 16: 253, 1985.

624. Tomashefski JF, Bruce M, Goldberg HI, et al: Regional distribution of macroscopic lung disease in cystic fibrosis. Am Rev Respir Dis 133: 535, 1986.

625. Sobonya RE, Taussig LM: Quantitative aspects of lung pathology in cystic fibrosis. Am Rev Respir Dis 134: 290, 1986.

626. Polgar G, Denton R: Cystic fibrosis in adults: Studies of pulmonary function and some physical properties of bronchial mucus. Am Rev Respir Dis 85: 319, 1962.

627. Stur O: Lungenverènderungen bei Mucoviscidose. (Pulmonary changes in mucoviscidosis.) Fortschr Röntgenstr 99: 625, 1963.

628. Rezek PR, Talbert WM Jr: Kongenitale (familière) zystiche Fibrose der Lunge: Beziehungen zur Metaplasie und dem Carcinoma in situ. (Congenital cystic fibrosis of the lung: Relationship to metaplasia and carcinoma in situ.) Wien Klin Wochenschr 74: 869, 1962.

629. McLaughlin FJ, Matthews WJ, Strieder DJ, et al: Pneumothorax in cystic fibrosis: Management and outcome. J Pediatr 100: 863, 1982.

630. Matthay MA, Matthay RA, Mills DM, et al: Hypertrophic osteoarthropathy in adults with cystic fibrosis. Thorax 31: 572, 1976.

631. Hodson ME, Mearns MB, Batten JC: Meconium ileus equivalent in adults with cystic fibrosis of pancreas: A report of six cases. Br Med J 2: 790, 1976.

632. Shepherd RW, Holt TL, Thomas BJ, et al: Nutritional rehabilitation in cystic fibrosis: Controlled studies of effects on nutritional growth retardation, body protein turnover, and course of pulmonary disease. J Pediatr 109: 788, 1986.

633. Gibson LE, Cooke RE: A test for concentration of electrolytes in sweat in cystic fibrosis of the pancreas utilizing pilocarpine by iontophoresis. Pediatrics 23: 545, 1959.

634. Warwick WJ, Huang NN, Waring WW, et al: Evaluation of a cystic fibrosis screening system incorporating a miniature sweat stimulator and disposable chloride sensor. Clin Chem 32: 850, 1986.

635. Landau LI, Phelan PD: The spectrum of cystic fibrosis: A study of pulmonary mechanics in 46 patients. Am Rev Respir Dis 108: 593, 1973.

636. Featherby EA, Weng T-R, Crozier DN, et al: Dynamic and static lung volumes, blood gas tensions, and diffusing capacity in patients with cystic fibrosis. Am Rev Respir Dis 102: 737, 1970.

637. Chang N, Levison H: The effect of a nebulized bronchodilator administered with or without intermittent positive-pressure breathing on ventilatory function in children with cystic fibrosis and asthma. Am Rev Respir Dis 106: 867, 1972.

638. Mansell A, Dubrawsky C, Levison H, et al: Lung elastic recoil in cystic fibrosis. Am Rev Respir Dis 109: 190, 1974.

639. Landau LI, Taussig LM, Macklem PT, et al: Contribution of inhomogeneity of lung units to the maximal expiratory flow-volume curve in children with asthma and cystic fibrosis. Am Rev Respir Dis 111: 725, 1975.

640. Dantzker DR, Patten GA, Bower JS: Gas exchange at rest and during exercise in adults with cystic fibrosis. Am Rev Respir Dis 125: 400, 1982.

641. Tepper RS, Skatrud JB, Dempsey JA, et al: Ventilation and oxygenation changes during sleep in cystic fibrosis. Chest 84: 388, 1983.

642. Wilmott RW, Tyson SL, Dinwiddie R, et al: Survival rates in cystic fibrosis. Arch Dis Child 58: 835, 1983.

643. Shwachman H, Kulczycki LL, Khaw K-T: Studies in cystic fibrosis: A report on sixty-five patients over 17 years of age. Pediatrics 36: 689, 1965.

644. Phelan P, Hey E: Cystic fibrosis mortality in England and Wales and in Victoria, Australia, 1976–1980. Arch Dis Child 59: 71, 1984.

645. Wilcken B, Chalmers G: Reduced morbidity in patients with cystic fibrosis detected by neonatal screening. Lancet 2: 1319, 1985.

646. Huang NN, Schidlow DV, Szatrowski TH, et al: Clinical features, survival rate, and prognostic factors in young adults with cystic fibrosis. Am J Med 82: 871, 1987.

647. Handelsman DJ, Conway AJ, Boylan LM, et al: Young's syndrome: Obstructive azoospermia and chronic sinopulmonary infections. N Engl J Med 310: 3, 1984.

648. Pavia D, Agnew JE, Bateman JRM, et al: Lung mucociliary clearance in patients with Young's syndrome. Chest 80: 892, 1981.

649. Nordkild P, Kormann-Andersen H, Struve-Christensen E: Yellow nail syndrome: The triad of yellow nails, lymphedema, and pleural effusions. Acta Med Scand 219: 221, 1986.

650. Hiller E, Rosenow EC III, Olsen AM: Pulmonary manifestations of the yellow nail syndrome. Chest 61: 452, 1972.

651. Riley CM, Day RL, Greeley D, et al: Central autonomic dysfunction with defective lacrimation. I. Report of five cases. Pediatrics 3: 468, 1949.

652. Brunt PW, McKusick VA: Familial dysautonomia: A report of genetic and clinical studies, with a review of the literature. Medicine 49: 343, 1970.

653. Moersch HJ, Schmidt HW: Broncholithiasis. Ann Otol 68: 548, 1959.

654. Bhagavan BS, Rao DRG, Weinberg T: Histoplasmosis producing broncholithiasis. Arch Pathol 91: 577, 1971.

655. Jones GR, Proudfoot AT, Hall JI: Pulmonary effects of acute exposure to nitrous fumes. Thorax 28: 61, 1973.

656. Johnson FL, Stokes DC, Ruggiero M, et al: Chronic obstructive airways disease after bone marrow transplantation. J Pediatr 105: 370, 1984.

657. Burke CM, Glanville AR, Theodore J, et al: Lung immunogenicity, rejection, and obliterative bronchiolitis. Chest 92: 547, 1987.

658. Skeens JL, Fuhrman CR, Yousem SA: Bronchiolitis obliterans in heart-lung transplantation patients: Radiologic findings in 11 patients. Am J Roentgenol 153: 253, 1989.

659. Epler GR, Colby TV, McCloud TC, et al: Bronchiolitis obliterans organizing pneumonia. N Engl J Med 312: 152, 1985.

659a. Spiteri MA, Klenerman P, Sheppard MN, et al: Seasonal cryptogenic organising pneumonia with biochemical cholestasis: A new clinical entity. Lancet 340: 281, 1992.

659b. Flowers JR, Clunie G, Burke M, Constant O: Bronchiolitis obliterans organizing pneumonia: The clinical and radiological features of seven cases and a review of the literature. Clin Radiol 45: 371, 1992.

660. Guerry-Force ML, Müller NL, Wright JL, et al: A comparison of bronchiolitis obliterans with organizing pneumonia, usual interstitial pneumonia, and small airway disease. Am Rev Respir Dis 135: 705, 1987.

661. Homma H, Yamanaka A, Tanimoto S, et al: Diffuse panbronchiolitis: A disease of the transitional zone of the lung. Chest 83: 63, 1983.

661a. Nishimura K, Kitaichi M, Izumi T, Itoh H: Diffuse panbronchiolitis: Correlation of high-resolution CT and pathologic findings. Radiology 184: 779, 1992.

662. Manireda J, Holford-Strevens V, Cheang M, et al: Acute symptoms following exposure to grain dust in farming. Environ Health Perspect 66: 73, 1986.

663. Bryant DH: Asthma due to insecticide sensitivity. Aust NZ J Med 15: 66, 1985.

664. Petry RW, Voss MJ, Kroutil LA, et al: Monkey dander asthma. J Allergy Clin Immunol 75: 268, 1985.

665. Lutsky I, Teichtahl H, Bar-Sela S: Occupational asthma due to poultry mites. J Allergy Clin Immunol 73: 56, 1984.

666. Belin L: Hyperreactivity in clinical practice—induction by occupational factors. Eur J Respir Dis (Suppl 131) 64: 285, 1983.

667. Spieksma FT, Vooren PH, Kramps JA, et al: Respiratory allergy to laboratory fruit flies (*Drosophila melanogaster*). J Allergy Clin Immunol 77: 108, 1986.

668. Kaufman GL, Baldo BA, Tovey ER, et al: Inhalant allergy following occupational exposure to blowflies. Clin Allergy 16: 65, 1986.

669. Ostrom NK, Swanson MC, Agarwal MK, et al: Occupational allergy to honeybee-body dust in a honey-processing plant. J Allergy Clin Immunol 77: 736, 1986.

670. Cartier A, Malo JL, Forest F, et al: Occupational asthma in snow crab–processing workers. J Allergy Clin Immunol 74: 261, 1984.

671. Prichard MG, Ryan G, Walsh BJ, et al: Skin test and RAST responses to wheat and common allergens and respiratory disease in bakers. Clin Allergy 15: 203, 1985.

672. Topping MD, Henderson RTS, Luczynska CM, et al: Castor bean allergy among workers in the felt industry. Allergy 37: 603, 1982.

673. Van Toorenenbergen AW, Dieges PH: Immunoglobulin E antibodies against coriander and other spices. J Allergy Clin Immunol 76: 477, 1985.

674. Cartier A, Malo JL, Pineau L, et al: Occupational asthma due to pepsin. J Allergy Clin Immunol 73: 574, 1984.

675. Alexandersson R, Gustafsson P, Hedenstierna G, et al: Exposure to naphthalene-diisocyanate in a rubber plant: Symptoms and lung function. Arch Environ Health 41: 85, 1986.

676. Moller DR, Gallagher JS, Bernstein DI, et al: Detection of IgE-mediated respiratory sensitization in workers exposed to hexahydrophthalic anhydride. J Allergy Clin Immunol 75: 663, 1985.

677. Cartier A, Chan N, Malo JL, et al: Occupational asthma caused by Eastern White Cedar (*Thuja occidentalis*) with demonstration that alicatic acid is present in this wood dust and is the causal agent. J Allergy Clin Immunol 77: 639, 1984.

678. Lung disease in dental laboratory technicians. Lancet 1: 1200, 1985.

679. Gheysens B, Auwerx J, Van den Eeckhout A, et al: Cobalt-induced bronchial asthma in diamond polishers. Chest 88: 740, 1985.

680. Blainey AD, Ollier S, Cundell D, et al: Occupational asthma in a hairdressing salon. Thorax 41: 42, 1986.

681. Corrado OJ, Osman J, Davies RJ: Asthma and rhinitis after exposure to glutaraldehyde in endoscopy units. Hum Toxicol 5: 325, 1986.

682. Lozewicz S, Davison AG, Hopkirk A, et al: Occupational asthma due to methyl methacrylate and cyanoacrylates. Thorax 40: 836, 1985.

683. Krumpe PE, Finley TN, Martinez NN: The search for expiratory obstruction in meat wrappers studied on the job. Am Rev Respir Dis 119: 611, 1979.

684. Baser ME, Tockman MS, Kennedy TP: Pulmonary function and respiratory symptoms in polyvinylchloride fabrication workers. Am Rev Respir Dis 131: 203, 1985.

12

PLEUROPULMONARY DISEASE CAUSED BY INHALATION OF INORGANIC DUST (PNEUMOCONIOSIS)

The inorganic dust pneumoconioses are caused by inhalation of minerals or other inorganic particles, the accumulation of which results in one or both of two pathologic reactions:

1. Fibrosis, which can be focal and nodular (as in silicosis) or diffuse (as in asbestosis). The fibrosis is probably related to a toxic effect of the inhaled substance on pulmonary epithelial or inflammatory cells; it often results in roentgenographic abnormalities and, if extensive enough, in significant functional impairment.

2. Aggregates of particle-laden macrophages with minimal or no accompanying fibrosis. This reaction is typically seen with inert dusts such as iron, tin, and barium. Al-

though sometimes associated with roentgenographic abnormalities, it usually causes few if any functional or clinical manifestations.

The establishment of a relationship between an inhaled dust and an adverse biologic effect can be difficult. A detailed occupational history is of the utmost importance, especially since certain jobs not usually regarded as harmful can become so if carried out in proximity to other potentially hazardous occupations such as welding and sandblasting.[1] Lack of a history of occupational exposure to a potentially harmful dust, however, does not exclude the possibility of pneumoconiosis. In recent years, it has become increasingly apparent that disease can develop in individuals who live in the vicinity of industrial plants (particularly those handling asbestos or beryllium) but who do not work there. Such "paraoccupational" disease occurs especially in spouses and children of workers, who transport hazardous material on clothing from the worksite into the home.[2] It is also important to remember that significant dust exposure occasionally occurs in nonoccupational settings, as exemplified by reports of silicosis in inhabitants of a Himalayan village who endured frequent dust storms[3] and a young woman who inhaled domestic scouring powder.[4]

Even when all investigations have shown convincing evidence for the presence of a pneumoconiosis, the precise etiology may not be evident. Individuals in many forms of work are exposed to more than one type of dust, and even with a detailed occupational history and analysis of lung tissue, it is occasionally difficult to attribute pathologic changes to one specific substance. For example, shale miners sometimes develop progressive massive fibrosis similar to that seen in coal miners; their lungs have been shown to contain dust composed of a combination of kaolinite, mica, and silica,[5] each of which by itself can cause pulmonary disease.

Because of regulations governing the risk of exposure to various dusts in the workplace, the incidence and prevalence of pneumoconiosis in developed countries are undoubtedly lower now than in the first part of this century. However, such regulations are not always followed,[6] and clusters of disease still occur in these regions. In addition, there is evidence that pneumoconiosis may be increasing in developing countries as a result of the expansion of mining, construction, and industry combined with relatively poor working conditions.[7]

The reaction of the lung to inhaled inorganic dust depends on several factors. The effects of particle size and shape, rate and pattern of breathing, distribution and concentration of inhaled particles, and pulmonary clearance were considered in the discussion of pulmonary defense (*see* page 52). In addition, several factors that specifically concern pneumoconiosis deserve mention.

The great majority of cases of pneumoconiosis occur only after many years of dust exposure. Occasionally, however, severe progressive lung disease develops after relatively brief exposure. In this situation, it is probable that a very high concentration of dust and individual susceptibility are responsible. There is no doubt that different workers exposed to identical amounts of dust can have profoundly different reactions. The precise reasons for such individual variation are not clear, but presumably they relate to differences in lung structure,[8] immune status,[9] efficiency of dust clearance,[10] degree of exposure to other noxious agents

such as tobacco smoke, and the presence of other disease such as tuberculosis and emphysema.

In addition to influencing the site within the respiratory tract at which a fiber or particle is deposited, size and shape can have a direct role in determining a pathologic effect. This is particularly well exemplified by asbestos, for which there is abundant evidence that fibers with a high length-diameter ratio are those that are important in the pathogenesis of mesothelioma.[11]

INTERNATIONAL CLASSIFICATION OF RADIOGRAPHS OF THE PNEUMOCONIOSES

The chest roentgenogram is an important tool in both detecting the effects of dust particle deposition in the lungs and in measuring progression.[12] In order for it to be useful in epidemiologic studies, however, it is essential that a standardized classification of extent of involvement be followed and an acceptable nomenclature be employed. A multitude of such classifications have been developed over the years, among the first of which were those of the International Labour Office (ILO) in 1930[13] and in 1958[14] and of a committee of *l'Union Internationale Contre le Cancer* (UICC) (the International Union Against Cancer) in 1967.[15] These classification schemes were combined in 1971 and subsequently modified in 1980, resulting in the one now widely used throughout the world, the ILO 1980 International Classification of Radiographs of the Pneumoconioses. Although this classification does not define pathologic entities, it possesses the considerable advantage of providing a uniform, simple, and reproducible method of reporting the type and extent of pneumoconiosis, thus leading to international comparability of pneumoconiosis statistics.

Because the 1980 ILO classification employs roentgenologic descriptors that are somewhat different from those generally used throughout this book, a short list of terms with corresponding definitions is reproduced here. A more extensive description of the classification may be obtained from *Medical Radiography and Photography*,[16] from which publication much of the material in this section has been gleaned.

Small, Rounded Opacities. These are well-defined opacities or nodules ranging in diameter from barely visible to 10 mm in diameter. The qualifiers *p, q,* and *r* subdivide the predominant opacities into three diameter ranges—up to 1.5 mm, 1.5 to 3 mm, and 3 mm to 10 mm, respectively.

Small, Irregular Opacities. This term describes a pattern that, elsewhere in this book, has been designated "linear," "reticular," or "reticulonodular"—in other words, a netlike pattern. Although the nature of these opacities is such that the establishment of quantitative dimensions is considerably more difficult than with rounded opacities, the ILO has established three categories: *s* (width up to 1.5 mm), *t* (width exceeding 1.5 mm and up to 3 mm), and *u* (width exceeding 3 mm and up to 10 mm).

To record shape and size, two letters must be used. Thus, if the reader considers that all or virtually all opacities are one shape and size, this is noted by recording the symbol twice, separated by a virgule (e.g., q/q). If, however, another shape or size is seen, this is recorded as the second letter (e.g., q/t). The designation q/t would mean that the predominant small opacity is round and of size q, but that there are, in addition, a significant number of small irregular opacities of size t. In this way, any combination of small opacities can be recorded.

Profusion. This term denotes the number of small, rounded or small, irregular opacities per unit area or zone of lung. There are four basic categories:

Category 0. Small opacities absent or less profuse than those in category 1.
Category 1. Small opacities definitely present but few in number, the normal lung markings usually being visible.
Category 2. Numerous small opacities with the normal markings typically being partly obscured.
Category 3. Very numerous small opacities, the normal markings typically being totally obscured.

These basic categories can be further subdivided by employing a 12-point scale,[17] as follows:

0/—	0/0	0/1
1/0	1/1	1/2
2/1	2/2	2/3
3/2	3/3	3/+

Employing this scale, the roentgenogram is first classified in the usual way into one of the four categories, 0, 1, 2, or 3. If during the process the category above or below is considered as a serious alternative, this is recorded; for example, a roentgenogram in which profusion is considered to be category 2 but for which category 1 was seriously considered as an alternative would be graded 2/1. If no alternative was considered (i.e., if the profusion was definitely category 2) it would be classified 2/2.

A subdivision is also possible within categories 0 and 3. Category 0/1 means profusion is category 0, but category 1 was seriously considered as an alternative. Category 0/0 describes a radiograph in which there are no small opacities or one in which a few opacities are thought to be present but are not sufficiently definite or numerous for category 1 to be considered. If the absence of small opacities is particularly obvious, profusion should be recorded as 0/—. A radiograph that shows profusion markedly greater than that classifiable as 3/3 would be recorded as 3/+.

Large Opacities. Large opacities are those larger than 10 mm. Three categories are recognized:

Category A. An opacity whose greatest diameter is at least 1 cm and possibly as large as 5 cm, or several opacities each greater than 1 cm, the sum of whose greatest diameters does not exceed 5 cm.
Category B. One or more opacities larger or more numerous than in category A whose combined area does not exceed the equivalent of the right upper lung zone.
Category C. One or more opacities whose combined area exceeds the equivalent of the right upper lung zone.

Extent. Each lung is divided into three zones—upper, middle, and lower—by horizontal lines drawn at one third and two thirds of the vertical distance between the apex of the lung and the dome of the diaphragm. The presence of disease in each of these zones is recorded; for example, "all zones of both lungs" and "both lower zones and the middle zone of the left lung."

Roentgenologic Interpretation. Much attention has been directed toward decision-making processes and observer error in the roentgenologic diagnosis of pneumoconiosis.[18–20] Common to all reports has been an exceptionally high degree of inter-reader variability and observer error, which has been attributed to a combination of lack of experience with the classification systems employed, unfamiliarity with the roentgenologic manifestations of pneumoconiosis, and poor film quality. As a result of these deficiencies, the National Institute of Occupational Safety and Health (NIOSH) has established an examination that is administered to physicians who wish to be certified as interpreters of chest roentgenograms in pneumoconiosis programs; the examination is preceded by a weekend course administered by the American College of Radiology. Completion of the course establishes the physician as an "A reader"; successful completion of the examination results in the designation "B reader."

In assessing roentgenologic progression of pneumoconiosis in individual miners, it is recommended that all films be viewed together in known chronologic order, recording into the most detailed classification available[12, 20, 21]; side-by-side reading has been shown to lead to substantially lower observer error and variability than independent reading.

THE INORGANIC DUSTS

Silica

Silica is a ubiquitous and abundant mineral composed of regularly arranged molecules of silicon dioxide (SiO_2). It exists in three forms: (1) *crystalline*, which occurs primarily as quartz, tridymite, or cristobalite; (2) *microcrystalline*, minute crystals of quartz bonded together by amorphous silica and exemplified by flint and chert; and (3) *amorphous*, which is noncrystalline and consists of kieselguhr (composed of the skeletal remains of diatoms) and several vitreous forms (derived by heating and rapid cooling of the crystalline types). Occupational exposure to and the fibrogenic potential of these different types of silica vary, a fact that is important in understanding the development of disease in different individuals. Pure ("free") silica (composed predominantly of silicon dioxide) must be distinguished from other substances in which silicon dioxide is combined with an appreciable proportion of various cations ("combined" silica); such silicates include asbestos, talc, and mica and are associated with different clinicopathologic forms of disease.

Exposure to a concentration of silica high enough to result in roentgenologic and pathologic manifestations of silicosis can occur in many occupations,[22] the most common being mining, tunneling, quarrying, foundry work, and sandblasting; use of potter's clay and powdered flint in the ceramics industry, of diatomaceous earth in the manufacture of paints, varnishes, and insecticides, or of ochre, granite, bentonite, enamel, and silica flour is also potentially hazardous. Because of the ubiquity of silica in the earth's crust, miners and quarriers of such minerals as gold, tin, iron, copper, nickel, silver, tungsten, and uranium have a particularly high occupational risk. The mining of other minerals recognized as causes of pneumoconiosis, such as coal, can also be accompanied by silica exposure, and there is no doubt that the lung disease in some affected individuals results from the silica, at least in part.

The nature of the occupations that expose workers to silica dust limits the disease mainly to men. An exception is the pottery industry in England, in which roughly half the 20,000 employees at risk are women, many of whom have exhibited typical features of pneumoconiosis.[23]

Pathogenesis

Both clinical and pathologic observations and experimental investigations have resulted in the recognition of a variety of factors that may be important in the pathogenesis of silica-induced pulmonary disease.[22, 24] Such factors must attempt to explain the two fundamental pathologic reactions to inhaled silica: (1) the silicotic nodule, which is characterized by dense, often concentric lamellae of collagen and which, when multiple and conglomerated, is termed progressive massive fibrosis (PMF); and (2) silicoproteinosis, which typically occurs in individuals or animals exposed to very high concentrations of silica and is characterized by alveolar filling by lipoproteinaceous material similar to that seen in idiopathic alveolar proteinosis. The majority of experimental investigations have focused on the first of these reactions because it is by far the more common.

One of the most important early discoveries was that silica contained within a capsule whose membrane is permeable to silicic acid and that is placed subcutaneously in an experimental animal does not result in a significant fibrotic reaction.[25] This observation led to the conclusion that direct contact between cells and silica particles is necessary for the production of a pathologic effect. There is now abundant evidence that one of the most important of these cells is the macrophage, particularly those within the interstitium.[26]

When silica is added to a macrophage cell culture, it is rapidly ingested and incorporated within phagosomes.[27] Lysosomes subsequently fuse with, and release their enzymes into, the phagosomes. However, instead of being destroyed, the silica remains intact, and the phagosomal membrane ruptures. Silica, toxic enzymes, and inflammatory mediators are thus released into the cell cytoplasm and, upon cell death, back into the culture medium. Among the substances released from the dead macrophages is an agent that causes fibroblasts to produce collagen.[28] These experimental observations led to the concept that silica induces lung fibrosis by causing phagolysosome rupture, macrophage death, and the release of fibrogenic substances. Ingestion of the released silica by new generations of macrophages and their subsequent death would then be responsible for perpetuating tissue injury.

Although this hypothetical mechanism explains many of the features of both experimental and clinical silicosis, it has become clear that it is an oversimplification. For example, more detailed studies of the interaction between macrophages and fibroblasts have shown that macrophage-derived chemical mediators can both stimulate and inhibit the production of collagen[29]; in addition, experimental studies have shown that when quartz is injected into rats, the process of fibrosis alternates with periods of lysis of collagen.[30] Both of these observations suggest that additional factors are important in affecting whether and to what degree fibrosis occurs. There is also evidence that the time course of silica-induced macrophage injury is much more prolonged *in vivo* than in tissue culture.[24, 31]

For these and other reasons, it has been suggested that silica affects macrophages while they are still alive, by altering their function rather than by causing their death and dissolution.[24, 31] This in turn suggests that other cells or cell products might be important in the pathogenesis of disease.[32] Among the most likely of these are lymphocytes, particularly helper T cells.[33] These cells are increased in number in bronchoalveolar lavage (BAL) fluid in both experimental and clinical silicosis and clearly have an effect on the character of the inflammatory reaction.[34] There is evidence, however, that they do not influence how much collagen is finally deposited,[34] and the nature and degree of their possible effect is unclear. Whatever additional cells are ultimately implicated, it seems likely that macrophage-derived clinical mediators, such as tissue necrosis factor, interleukin-1, and leukotrienes,[35] are involved at some point.

It is also possible that immune mechanisms not directly related to macrophage dysfunction are important in the pathogenesis of silicosis. Protein adsorbed onto silicon dioxide can theoretically act as an antigen, and it has been speculated that the silicotic nodule contains antigen-antibody precipitates as well as collagen.[36] Because plasma cells are prominent in some silicotic nodules and because some nodules have been reported to contain immunoglobulins,[37] it is possible that a local immunoglobulin reaction might be important.

In contrast to the fibrosis associated with long-term exposure to relatively low doses of silica, it is perhaps surprising that brief exposure to large amounts results in little collagen deposition in both animals[38] and humans.[39] Instead, abundant intra-alveolar proteinaceous debris, virtually identical histologically and ultrastructurally to that seen in alveolar proteinosis, is typically produced.[40] The precise pathogenesis of this reaction is unclear. Experimentally, instillation of silica into the lungs has been associated with type 1 alveolar cell injury and concomitant reparative type 2 cell hyperplasia,[41] suggesting that this might be a factor. It is also possible that the silica directly stimulates type 2 cells to produce excessive alveolar lining material or disturbs the ability of macrophages to handle normally produced material.[42] The reason for the lack of fibrosis in acute silicoproteinosis is also unclear, although it has been shown that coating silica particles with alveolar lining material results in significantly less cytotoxicity for ingesting macrophages.[43]

Altered macrophage function probably underlies the greater susceptibility to tuberculosis of patients with both fibrotic silicosis and acute silicoproteinosis; *Mycobacterium tuberculosis* grows much more rapidly in cultures of macrophages exposed to sublethal doses of silica than in those not so exposed.[44]

Pathologic Characteristics

Grossly, silicotic nodules range from 1 to 10 mm in diameter (although some authorities accept 2 cm as the cutoff between a single nodule and PMF[45]) and typically are more numerous in the upper lobes and parahilar regions than elsewhere (Fig. 12–1). Cut sections show the nodules to be more or less well defined, spherical or irregularly shaped,

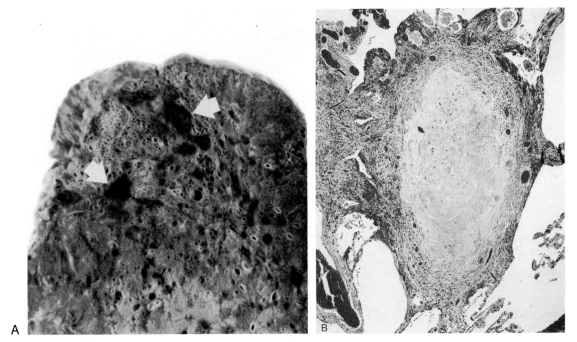

Figure 12–1. Silicosis: Silicotic Nodules. *A,* A slice of an upper lobe shows multiple, well-defined, somewhat irregularly shaped nodules within the lung parenchyma *(arrows).* The nodules are black as a result of the presence of abundant anthracotic pigment. (arrow length = 8 mm.) *B,* A histologic section shows a central zone of dense collagen and a peripheral rim of macrophages in which abundant foreign particulate material is situated. (*B* × 40.)

and firm to hard in texture. Coalescence of nodules results in larger masses that can occupy virtually an entire lobe (PMF). Such masses are usually associated with adjacent emphysema and may be cavitated as a result of ischemia, tuberculosis, or anaerobic infection.

Microscopically, the earliest lesions are located in the peribronchiolar, paraseptal, and subpleural interstitial tissue and consist predominantly of macrophages with scattered reticulin fibers. As the lesions enlarge, the central portions become relatively acellular and composed of mature collagen, often in relatively well-defined, more or less concentric lamellae; a peripheral zone of macrophages and lesser numbers of plasma cells and lymphocytes surrounds this central portion (*see* Fig. 12–1). In the cellular areas, a variable number of needle-shaped birefringent silicate crystals 1 to 3 μm in length usually can be identified. The larger conglomerate lesions are also composed of macrophages and hyalinized collagen, although the concentric lamellar appearance of the smaller nodules is frequently not as evident (Fig. 12–2). Focal necrosis is common in the central portions and is occasionally associated with granulomatous inflammation, implying tuberculous infection.

In silicoproteinosis, well-defined fibrous nodules are typically absent. Instead, there is mild interstitial fibrosis, and airspaces are more or less diffusely filled by PAS-positive, finely granular, proteinaceous material similar to that seen in alveolar proteinosis (*see* Fig. 16–1, page 816). Macrophages are present in increased numbers, and adjacent alveolar type 2 cells show a variable degree of hyperplasia. Ultrastructurally, the intra-alveolar material consists largely of membranous material resembling that seen in the normal alveolar lining layer.[40]

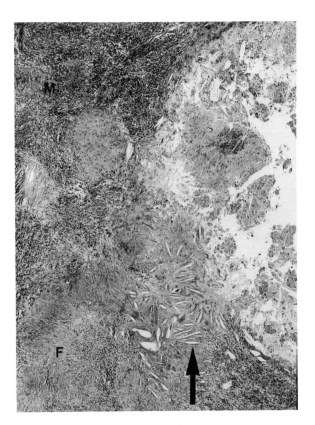

Figure 12–2. Silicosis: Progressive Massive Fibrosis. A histologic section reveals fibrosis (F), aggregates of pigment-laden macrophages (M), and multiple cholesterol clefts *(arrow).* The tissue in the right half of the illustration is necrotic and has undergone liquefaction. (× 25.)

Roentgenographic Manifestations

Ten to twenty years' exposure usually is necessary before roentgenographic abnormalities appear,[46] although the course of silicosis sometimes is rapid, particularly in patients exposed to high concentrations of dust in a relatively confined area (Fig. 12–3).[47] The classic roentgenographic pattern consists of multiple well-defined nodules of uniform density ranging from 1 to 10 mm in diameter (Fig. 12–4). Profusion can be fairly even throughout both lungs but commonly shows considerable upper zonal predominance. Calcification is uncommon.

The roentgenographic pattern of small round or irregular opacities is sometimes referred to as simple silicosis, in contrast to complicated silicosis, which is characterized by the large opacities or conglomerate shadows of PMF. These opacities appear as homogeneous areas of consolidation of nonsegmental distribution, measuring more than 1 cm in diameter and usually affecting the upper lobes. They can become very large (Fig. 12–5), some even exceeding the volume of an upper lobe, and can cavitate. The margins sometimes are irregular and somewhat ill defined, with multiple pseudopodia extending outward from their edges[48]; more commonly, however, the lateral margin is

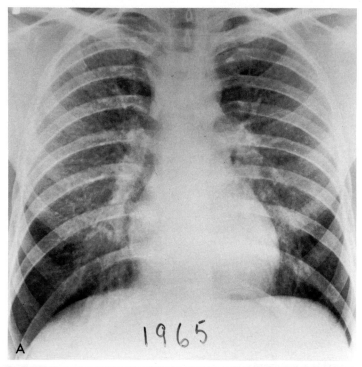

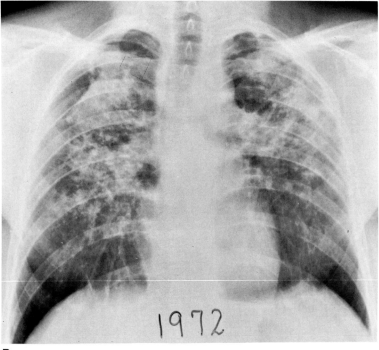

Figure 12–3. Silicosis Showing Rapid Progression. In 1965, a posteroanterior roentgenogram *(A)* reveals diffuse, predominantly irregular opacities more prominent in the upper lung zones; hilar lymph nodes are enlarged. *B,* By 1972, 7 years after the patient was originally seen, large confluent opacities have developed in both upper lobes, characteristic of progressive massive fibrosis. Note the sharply defined lateral margin of the large opacity on the right.

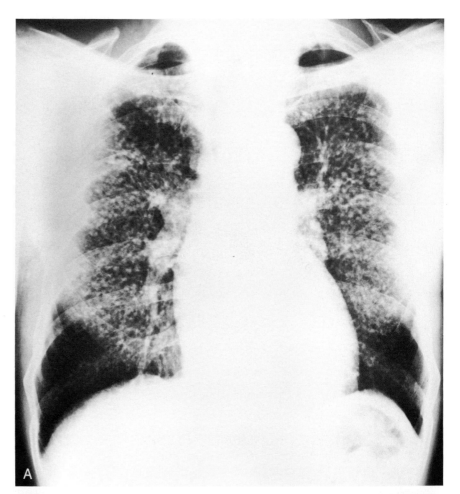

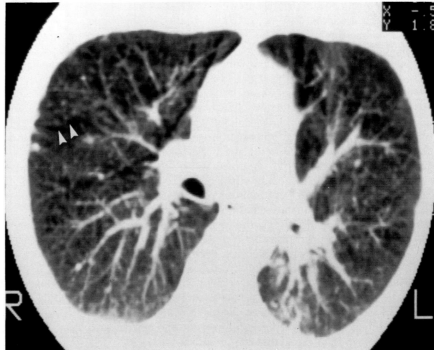

Figure 12–4. Silicosis. A posteroanterior roentgenogram *(A)* reveals a multitude of well-defined nodular opacities throughout both lungs possessing considerable mid-zonal predominance. *B,* A CT scan at the level of the hila confirms the presence of multiple nodules measuring 2 to 5 mm *(arrowheads).*

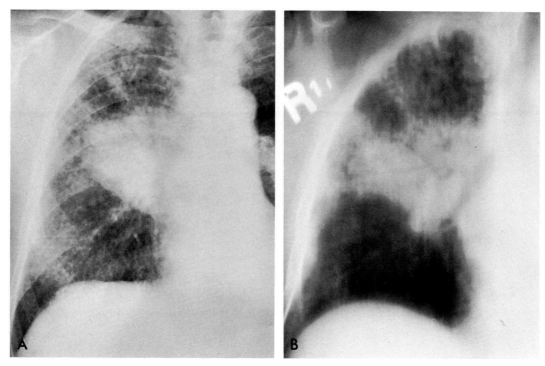

Figure 12–5. Silicosis with Progressive Massive Fibrosis. A posteroanterior roentgenogram *(A)* of a 58-year-old miner reveals combined rounded and irregular opacities throughout the right lung. A large mass of homogeneous density is situated in the parahilar area. A tomographic section *(B)* shows the homogeneity of the large parahilar mass to be disturbed by a well-defined air bronchogram; the mass is remarkably well defined.

very smooth, creating an interface that parallels the lateral chest wall. The abnormality commonly develops in the midzone or periphery of the lung and tends to "migrate" later toward the hilum, leaving overinflated emphysematous lung tissue between it and the pleural surface (Fig. 12–6).[49] The more extensive the progressive massive fibrosis, the less the apparent nodularity in the remainder of the lungs,[49] a feature presumably caused by gradual incorporation of nodular lesions into the site of massive consolidation.

Hilar lymph node enlargement is a frequent roentgenographic finding in silicosis and can occur at any stage.[49] One distinctive but uncommon feature of such enlargement is the deposition of calcium in the periphery of the nodes (so-called eggshell calcification).[50] Although this can be seen in other diseases (e.g., sarcoidosis), it is almost pathognomonic of silicosis.

Although nodularity is usually stressed as the typical roentgenographic pattern in simple silicosis, correlative studies of roentgenologic and pathologic material indicate that a linear or reticular pattern—the small irregular opacities of the ILO 1980 classification—may be present without visible nodules and may be associated with severe clinical disability.[52] This appears to be particularly characteristic of silicosis secondary to diatomaceous earth exposure.[53]

Two other variants of the classic roentgenographic changes of the disease are the acute silicosis of sandblasters and the nodular lesions of Caplan's syndrome.[54] The latter, a complication of rheumatoid disease, consists of large necrobiotic nodules superimposed on a background of simple silicosis (Fig. 12–7) *(see* page 401). Although most commonly seen in coal-worker's pneumoconiosis (CWP), the syndrome occasionally is identified in patients with silicosis.

Acute silicoproteinosis is associated with a pattern of diffuse airspace disease, identical to that of alveolar proteinosis (Fig. 12–8) *(see* page 817).[55, 56]

Roentgenographic progression of silicosis after removal from exposure is a well-accepted phenomenon; for example, in one study of 1902 workers who had no roentgenographic evidence of PMF as long as 4 years before leaving the occupation, 172 subsequently exhibited PMF on follow-up examination.[57] Despite the development of conglomerate lesions after leaving employment, this cohort of workers showed no overall progression or regression of the grades of simple pneumoconiosis.

Computed tomography (CT), particularly the high-resolution type, can be useful in the assessment of silicosis. In one study of 58 workers with long-term exposure to silica in the granite and foundry industries,[58, 59] assessment of CT and conventional chest roentgenograms yielded similar average scores for the detection (profusion) of small nodules; however, CT was able to identify large opacities in patients who, by conventional roentgenography, appeared to have only simple silicosis. Similar results were obtained in another study of 17 patients, particularly with respect to the evaluation of profusion of small opacities[60]; however, in this investigation, emphysema associated with silicosis was easily detected on CT but not on conventional roentgenograms.

Clinical Manifestations

Many patients with silicosis are totally asymptomatic when initially seen. Some may complain of shortness of breath, first noted on exertion only but becoming progressively more severe as the roentgenographic changes

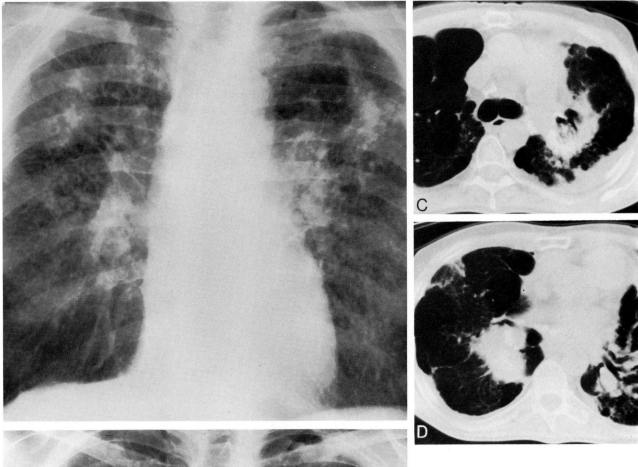

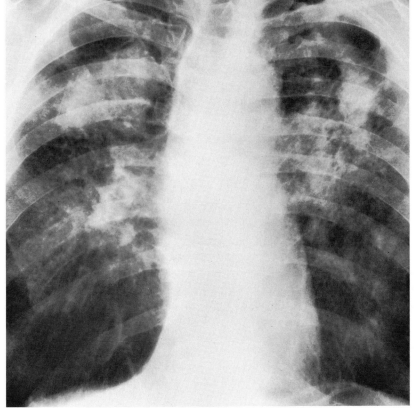

Figure 12–6. Silicosis with PMF: Progression over 4 Years and CT Appearance. A postero-anterior roentgenogram *(A)* reveals extensive irregular opacities involving predominantly the upper and middle lung zones. In the subapical regions bilaterally, poorly defined shadows of homogeneous density represent large opacities (category B). *B,* Four years later, a repeat study shows considerable enlargement of the large opacities, which are now category C. Most of the enlargement appears to have occurred hilarward, indicating medial "migration" of the lesions. The lung peripheral to the zones of PMF has shown a loss of markings, suggesting the development of emphysema; the lower lung zones also show signs of progressive emphysema. *C,* In another patient, a CT scan at the level of the carina reveals a large area of consolidation contiguous with the left hilum and mediastinum; note the central cavitation. At a slightly lower level *(D),* a similar area of consolidation is present on the right, unassociated with cavitation. In both scans, note the severe emphysema. Both of these lesions represent PMF in a patient with long-standing silicosis.

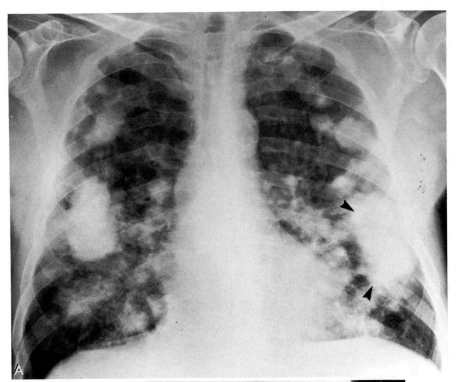

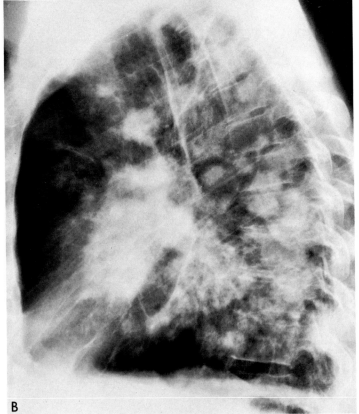

Figure 12–7. Caplan's Syndrome. Postero-anterior *(A)* and lateral *(B)* roentgenograms reveal a multitude of fairly well-defined nodules ranging in diameter from 1 to 5 cm, scattered randomly throughout both lungs with no notable anatomic predilection. No cavitation is apparent, nor is there evidence of calcification. This patient, a 56-year-old man, had been a coal miner for many years and in recent years had developed arthralgia, which proved to be due to rheumatoid arthritis. As a means of establishing the nature of the pulmonary nodules, a percutaneous needle aspiration was carried out on the large mass situated in the lower portion of the left lung *(arrowheads* in *A)*: several milliliters of inky black fluid were aspirated. The necrotic nature of this mass was thus established, as was the presence of large quantities of coal dust within it. (Courtesy of Dr. Michael O'Donovan, Montreal General Hospital.)

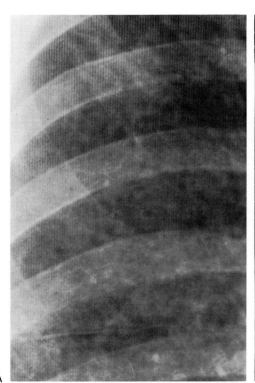
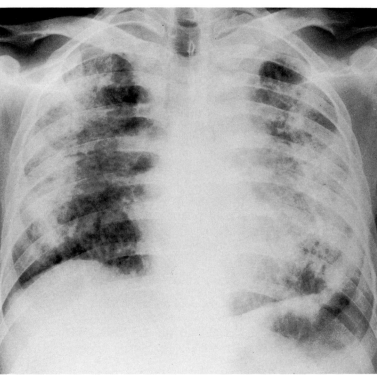

A
B

Figure 12–8. Acute Silicoproteinosis. During the previous 3 years, this 29-year-old man had been employed full time as a sandblaster inside huge, nonventilated metal tanks. On admission, a magnified view of the right upper lung *(A)* from a posteroanterior roentgenogram reveals multiple fairly well-circumscribed nodules scattered diffusely throughout the lung parenchyma. The nodules range in size from barely visible to 3 mm in diameter. The patient's subsequent course was progressively and rapidly downhill, leading to severe respiratory failure. A roentgenogram 2 years after the inital study *(B)* reveals marked loss of lung volume, much of the lung parenchyma showing a very coarse reticular pattern, which in many areas is confluent, suggesting airspace consolidation.

worsen. With progressive destruction of pulmonary tissue, pulmonary hypertension develops, resulting in cor pulmonale and, eventually, right-sided heart failure. In one series of hospitalized patients with silicosis, rales and wheezes were found to be present in the majority.[61] In our experience, however, asymptomatic ambulatory patients with silicosis usually have no adventitial signs on auscultation. This is in contrast to asbestos-exposed individuals, who often have bilateral rales despite an absence of roentgenographic abnormality in the chest.

Unlike many other inhalation dust diseases, the fibrosis and associated disability in silicosis frequently are progressive, even after removal of the patient from the dusty environment.[62, 63] Thus, it is common for patients to present with symptoms many years after leaving the occupation responsible for the dust exposure. This is an important point to remember, because only a complete occupational history, ranging over a patient's entire working life, may provide the clue to the diagnosis.

There is little question that silicosis predisposes to tuberculosis. It is customary to suspect this complication with the development of PMF, although sputum cultures of acid-fast bacilli are positive in as many patients with nodular opacities alone as in those with conglomerate shadows.[64] It must be remembered, however, that it may be extremely difficult to isolate tubercle bacilli during life in patients with PMF, despite subsequent postmortem demonstration of active tuberculous infection.[64] There is also evidence that silicosis is associated with an increased risk of pulmonary

carcinoma,[65] and a new or changing opacity should be considered with this in mind.

Silicoproteinosis (acute or accelerated silicosis) occurs in tunnelers and sandblasters[66] who are exposed to particularly high concentrations of silica. Respiratory symptoms (cough and dyspnea) develop within months to a few years; affected individuals often die in respiratory failure, not uncommonly with a complicating pneumothorax.[67]

Laboratory Findings

Silicosis may be accompanied by a rise in serum angiotensin-converting enzyme, high levels of which have been found to be associated with progression of the disease.[68] Serologic abnormalities are common and include the presence of rheumatoid factor, antinuclear antibodies, immune complexes, and a polyclonal increase in gamma globulin.[69]

Pulmonary Function Tests

Function may be normal in the early stages of disease.[70, 71] However, when dyspnea is present, impairment of function is usually evident and may be obstructive, restrictive, or a combination of both.[72] Diffusing capacity may be decreased, and the combination of this finding with hyperinflation and decrease in flow rates constitutes a pattern of functional impairment identical to that of pulmonary emphysema. In fact, because miners are usually cigarette smokers, difficulty may be encountered in assessing the specific factor responsible for pulmonary dysfunction. Further compounding this situation is the distinct possibility that symptoms of cough and dyspnea may be caused by chronic bronchitis secondary to a nonspecific effect from dust itself.[73] Although arterial oxygen saturation may be normal at rest, exercise often gives rise to hypoxemia, at least in patients with progressive massive fibrosis.[59] In the late stages of the disease, carbon dioxide retention may develop.[74]

Coal and Carbon

The inhalation and retention in the lung of dust composed predominantly of carbon (often termed "anthracosis") is seen in many individuals,[75] particularly those who smoke or live in an urban or industrial environment. Microscopically, such material is easily recognized as dense black particles, mostly 1 to 2 μm in size, within macrophages adjacent to terminal or proximal respiratory bronchioles and in the pleura. Although predominantly composed of carbon, the particles also contain traces of other substances, such as silica and iron. Nevertheless, associated fibrosis is invariably minimal or absent, and it is generally believed that the presence of such particles is of no pathologic or functional significance.

Such innocuous environmental anthracosis is caused by the inhalation of relatively small amounts of dust. It is clear, however, that inhalation of large amounts of carbon, either as coal dust or as substances derived from coal or petroleum products, can be associated with significant pulmonary disease. Because quantity is important in this effect, disease occurs almost exclusively in the workplace, where the concentration of these materials is much greater than that in nonoccupational settings. The most important occupation in terms of the number of individuals affected is coal mining, the resulting disease appropriately being called *coal-worker's pneumoconiosis* (CWP). Workers involved in the production or use of graphite,[76] carbon black,[77] and carbon electrodes[78] are affected less often. The possibility that pulmonary disease can occasionally be caused by inhalation of fly ash also has been suggested.[79]

Pathologic, roentgenographic, and clinical findings in workers exposed to large amounts of carbon, in whatever form, are similar; however, because the vast majority of such individuals are involved in coal mining, the literature reflects this fact and much of the following description relates predominantly to CWP.

Epidemiology

Coal is a sedimentary rock formed by the action of pressure, temperature, and chemical reactions on vegetable material. The percentage of pure carbon varies with the type, brown coal and lignite containing the least and anthracite the most.[80] The degree of exposure to carbon dust thus depends to some extent on the type of coal being mined, a feature that at least in part may explain the variability in incidence of CWP from colliery to colliery. Perhaps more important in this regard are local geologic variations[81]; some coal seams are very thick (up to 100 feet),[80] whereas others are much thinner and are separated by seams of siliceous rock. Mining in the latter situation can result in significant

concomitant exposure to silica and other substances, a feature that probably explains the occurrence of classic silicosis in some coal miners.[82] Specific tasks within the coal mine also influence the probability of developing disease and the form that it may take. For example, because the majority of dust is produced at the coal face, operators of cutting and loading machines are exposed to the highest concentration of pure coal dust,[80] whereas surface coal miners drilling through quartz[83] are more likely to come in contact with silica.

There is evidence that the incidence of CWP is decreasing, at least in Europe and North America. For example, epidemiologic studies carried out in the early 1970s in the Appalachian region showed approximately 10 per cent of coal miners to have pneumoconiosis and about a third of these to have PMF.[84] However, a more recent assessment of 1438 surface coal miners in the United States revealed that only 59 (4 per cent) had roentgenographic evidence of pneumoconiosis; only seven of these patients were interpreted as having opacities in category 2 or higher.[85]

Pathogenesis and Pathologic Characteristics

The two major morphologic findings in CWP are the coal macule and PMF.[86] The former is characterized by deposits of anthracotic material unassociated with fibrosis, a finding sometimes referred to as "simple" pneumoconiosis. PMF is defined as a focus of fibrosis and pigment deposition larger than 1 cm in diameter (or, according to some definitions, 2 or even 3 cm[86]) and is sometimes designated "complicated" pneumoconiosis. Despite the term, it should be understood that some lesions do not appear to be progressive, and according to the size definition, many clearly are not massive.

Grossly, coal macules are stellate or round, impalpable foci of black pigmentation that range in size from 1 to 5 mm (Fig. 12–9). They are scattered fairly uniformly throughout the lung parenchyma, although they tend to be more numerous in the upper than lower lung zones. Microscopically, the macule relates to respiratory bronchioles and consists of numerous interstitial pigment-laden macrophages; fine reticulin fibers can be identified between the macrophages, but mature collagen is minimal or absent. Bronchioles adjacent to the macrophage aggregates are frequently distended (*see* Fig. 12-9), an appearance often designated "focal emphysema." It is unclear whether the pathogenesis of this abnormality is similar to the more common centrilobular emphysema associated with cigarette smoking[75] or whether it is caused by a different mechanism related to the presence of coal dust itself.[87]

The lesions of PMF are firm in consistency and develop most often in the posterior segment of an upper lobe or superior segment of a lower lobe, a localization that is thought by some to be related to poor lymphatic drainage.[88] The lesion can extend across a fissure into an adjacent lobe. Cut section often reveals a center of necrotic dark black fluid that can be washed away, leaving a cavity. In most cases, the pathogenesis of the necrosis is probably ischemia[89]; vascular obliteration both within and adjacent to the region of PMF is a common histologic feature, and, in fact, avascular zones can be demonstrated by lung perfusion scanning.[90] Occasionally, cavitation is caused by tuberculous

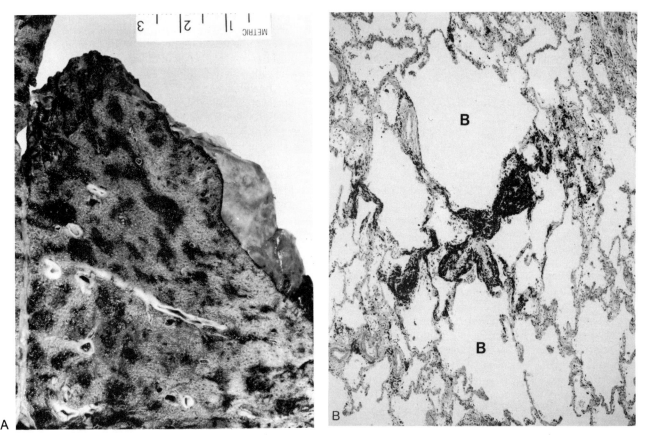

Figure 12–9. Coal-worker's Pneumoconiosis: The Coal Macule. *A,* A magnified view of the superior segment of a lower lobe shows multiple foci of dense black pigmentation that are of irregular shape but are fairly evenly spaced. Emphysema is present but is difficult to appreciate in this thick, formalin-fixed section. Note also the dense zone of subpleural pigment deposition. *B,* A histologic section shows numerous alveolar macrophages containing abundant anthracotic pigment situated in the interstitial tissue adjacent to respiratory bronchioles (B). No fibrosis is evident. The bronchioles are moderately dilated. (× 40.)

infection. Microscopically, the lesions of PMF consist of bundles of haphazardly arranged, sometimes hyalinized bands of collagen interspersed with numerous pigment-laden macrophages and abundant free pigment. Foci of degenerated and frankly necrotic tissue, cholesterol clefts, and chronic inflammatory cells often are present.

The etiology and pathogenesis of PMF are unclear, and several agents or processes, either alone or in combination, may be responsible. The lesion is more likely to occur in coal workers with heavy dust exposure and who have a large amount of dust in the lungs at autopsy, suggesting that the quantity of coal dust itself may be important.[91, 92] Because classic silicosis is associated with lesions that are similar both pathologically and radiologically to those of coal-worker's PMF, it has been suggested that contamination of coal dust by silica may be responsible.[93] However, at least three observations militate against this hypothesis. First, there is a wide variation in the amount of silica in the lungs of coal workers with PMF.[80] Second, in at least some studies, the severity of CWP is more closely related to total dust content of the lung than to the concentration of quartz.[94] Finally, as indicated previously, workers involved with carbon black or carbon electrodes who are exposed almost exclusively to carbon sometimes develop lesions similar to those that occur in underground coal workers. Despite the fore-

going observations, it is possible that silica is responsible for the development of PMF in some cases.[93]

The presence in coal miners of hypergammaglobulinemia,[95] rheumatoid factor (RF),[96] and antinuclear[97] or anti-lung antibodies,[98] as well as the characteristic association between rheumatoid disease and CWP (Caplan's syndrome),[99] have raised the possibility of an immune mechanism in the pathogenesis of CWP. Supporting this hypothesis are studies showing increasing titers of RF with increasing severity of roentgenographically determined category of disease[100] as well as the presence of tissue-bound RF and antinuclear antibodies.[96] However, despite this and other evidence suggesting a role for immune factors in the development of PMF, precise details of possible pathogenetic mechanisms are not understood.

In addition to pulmonary fibrosis, two other abnormalities are commonly found at necropsy in patients with CWP. Cor pulmonale is frequent in the complicated form of the disease and is occasionally present in those with simple pneumoconiosis.[101] In most patients in the latter group, right ventricular hypertrophy can be explained on the basis of associated chronic obstructive lung disease or silicosis, but in some the sole explanation appears to be simple pneumoconiosis itself. In several investigations, emphysema has been shown to be present more often and to be more advanced in patients with CWP than in those without it[102]; the severity correlates with the degree of exposure to coal dust[103] and has been demonstrated to be independent of age and cigarette smoking and to be positively related to the dust content of macules.[102]

Roentgenographic Manifestations

The roentgenographic appearance of simple pneumoconiosis is typically one of round opacities 1 to 5 mm in diameter (a nodular pattern).[104, 105] Occasionally, it may consist predominantly of small, irregular opacities (a reticular pattern) (Fig. 12–10).[105a] Although the nodules tend to be somewhat less well defined than those of silicosis and possess a granular density unlike the homogeneous density of silicotic nodules, it is generally agreed that the roentgenographic changes of CWP cannot be distinguished from those of silicosis with any degree of confidence.

Calcification occurs in at least a few of the nodules in as many as 10 to 20 per cent of older coal miners, particularly anthracite workers.[105a, 106] The calcification begins as a central dot, thus helping to differentiate these nodules from those of silicosis, in which the calcification tends to be diffuse. Eggshell calcification of lymph nodes is uncommon in coal-worker's pneumoconiosis, occurring in only 1.3 per cent of 1063 coal miners whose chest roentgenograms showed evidence of pneumoconiosis.[106] All had worked 20 years or more in the mines, and it is possible that the calcification was related to the effect of admixed silica.

The lesions of PMF range from a minimum of 1 cm in diameter to the volume of a whole lobe and are almost always restricted to the upper half of the lungs. They usually develop on a background of simple pneumoconiosis and are said to occur in about 30 per cent of patients with diffuse bilateral opacities[84] (although some have found a much lower prevalence[105a]); however, they have been observed in miners whose initial chest roentgenograms 4 to 5 years earlier were considered to be within normal limits.[107] The abnormality may develop after exposure to coal dust has ceased and, unlike simple pneumoconiosis, may progress in the absence of further exposure.[84, 108]

PMF typically starts near the periphery of the lung and appears as a mass with a smooth, well-defined lateral border that parallels the rib cage and projects 1 to 3 cm from it.[106] In contrast to its sharp lateral border, the medial margin of the mass is often ill defined. It tends to be thicker in one dimension than the other, appearing as a broad opacity on a posteroanterior (PA) roentgenogram and a thin shape in lateral projection, frequently paralleling the major fissure. As might be expected, this spindle-shaped configuration creates a roentgenographic opacity that is considerably less dense in one projection than in the other. The mass is usually homogeneous in density unless cavitation has developed, which occurs only occasionally.

As with the conglomerate shadows of silicosis, PMF gradually "migrates" from the lung periphery toward the hilum, leaving a zone of overinflated emphysematous lung between it and the chest wall. The presence of such a large

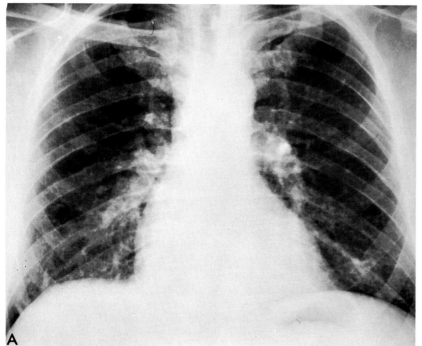
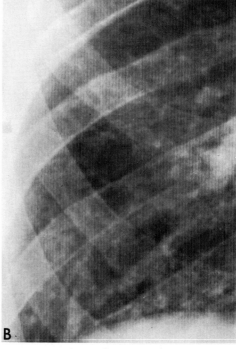

Figure 12–10. Coal-worker's Pneumoconiosis. This posteroanterior roentgenogram *(A)* and magnified view of the lower half of the right lung *(B)* reveal a coarse reticulonodular pattern throughout both lungs, affecting the upper lung zones least. Both hila are enlarged and possess a contour suggestive of lymph node enlargement. Approximately 15 years previously this 45-year-old miner had worked underground in a Belgian coal mine for 7 years and had been exposed to heavy concentrations of dust but had never worn a mask.

homogeneous mass in the parahilar area of one lung may closely simulate pulmonary carcinoma. In this situation, needless thoracotomy can be avoided if a background of pneumoconiosis is present and is recognized in the rest of the lungs. However, PMF occasionally is not associated with roentgenographic evidence of nodularity,[106] and in such cases the correct diagnosis might not be suspected in the absence of an appropriate occupational history and unless the lesions are bilateral and symmetric. Both the smooth, sharply defined lateral border and the somewhat flattened configuration characteristic of PMF can be employed to differentiate it from carcinoma, a lesion whose borders tend to be less well defined and whose configuration is typically spherical.

The pulmonary nodules described by Caplan[99] in coal workers with rheumatoid disease are more regular in contour and more peripherally located than the masses of PMF (*see* page 401). They range in size from 0.5 to 5 cm in diameter and are seen most often in workers who manifest subcutaneous rheumatoid nodules clinically and whose chest roentgenograms are classified as category 0 or 1 simple pneumoconiosis.[109]

Clinical Manifestations

Coal workers with simple pneumoconiosis suffer little clinical disability and seldom show progression of disease if they are removed from their dust-ridden environment.[110] Symptoms usually develop only when the disease becomes complicated with PMF; they include cough, mucoid expectoration, dyspnea on exertion, hemoptysis, and frequent attacks of acute purulent bronchitis. Copious amounts of black sputum and, sometimes, jet-black fluid are produced when a focus of PMF becomes necrotic and erodes into a bronchus.[111] Physical examination may reveal decreased breath sounds and a few rales. With progression of the disease, dyspnea usually worsens; cor pulmonale and right-sided heart failure may ensue.

Pulmonary Function Tests

The results of pulmonary function testing in coal workers are at variance, largely because of differences in population groups studied. For example, nonworking miners show more impairment than those who are working, an apparent paradox that presumably results from the fact that the former have left the job because of disability. An often-cited study of pulmonary function of patients with simple pneumoconiosis compared with a control group of the same age, published in 1955, showed no differences apart from minor disturbances in gas distribution.[112] More recently, however,[113] in a long-term follow-up of a group of coal miners who did not have PMF, it was found that the relationship between exposure and FEV_1 suggested that in some miners, even moderate exposure to dust can cause severe impairment of lung function. Diffusing capacity can be reduced in miners who smoke but is usually normal in nonsmoking miners with simple pneumoconiosis.[114] On the other hand, impairment of V̇/Q̇ ratio resulting in impaired gas exchange has been described in nonsmoking coal miners despite normal spirometric findings.[115]

In contrast to simple CWP, PMF is frequently associated with physiologic evidence of airway obstruction, reduced diffusing capacity, abnormal blood gases, and increased pulmonary arterial pressures.[116] In one study in which pathology and function were correlated, these changes in function were attributed not only to PMF and emphysema but also to small airway disease and interstitial fibrosis.[117]

Asbestos

Asbestos is the general term given to a group of minerals that are fibrous and are resistant to high temperatures and various chemical insults. Mineralogically they are divided into two major groups: the serpentines, of which the only member of commercial importance is chrysotile, and the amphiboles, which include amosite, crocidolite, anthophyllite, tremolite, and actinolite. Chrysotile fibers are curved or curly, whereas the amphiboles are straight (Fig. 12–11). These physical properties, as well as chemical differences, are responsible for the varying uses of asbestos and, to some extent, for their ability to cause disease. Chrysotile, amosite, crocidolite, and tremolite are responsible for the vast majority of pleuropulmonary disease.

Epidemiology

The use of asbestos in industry increased enormously during the first three quarters of this century, resulting in a dramatic increase in the number of individuals exposed to the mineral. For example, it has been estimated that in the

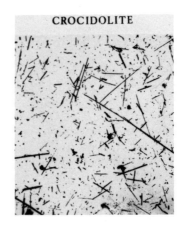

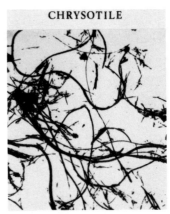

Figure 12–11. Types of Asbestos Fiber. Electron microscopic views of two different types of asbestos fiber. (Modified from Timbrell V: Physical factors as etiologic mechanisms. T.A.R.C. Scientific Publication No. 8, Lyons, 1973, p. 295.)

United States in 1983, as many as nine million people had been occupationally exposed to the mineral.[118] Although recognition of the harmful effects of asbestos exposure has resulted in better control of dust levels and, undoubtedly, an overall decrease in total exposure, the potential for the development of serious disease still exists.

There are three major sources of exposure to asbestos dust:

1. The primary occupations of asbestos mining and its processing in a mill. In such occupations, exposure occurs predominantly to only one type of fiber, although small amounts of other types may be present, even in commercially "pure" preparations.[119] By contrast, mixtures of fibers are commonly employed in construction and in the manufacture of textiles.

2. Numerous secondary occupations involving use of asbestos in a variety of industrial and commercial products. The most important uses are in the construction and automotive industries (in which asbestos is extensively incorporated in cement piping, tiles, moldings, paneling, and brake linings) and in shipbuilding and ship repair. Although risk of exposure applies during the manufacturing process, it is even greater during repair and demolition.

3. Contaminated air inhaled by individuals not directly involved in asbestos-related occupations.[120] That such exposure is common is indicated by the frequency with which asbestos bodies are found in the lungs in routine necropsies, the incidence ranging from 1 per cent in rural Italy[121] to as high as 60 per cent in New York City.[122] Although this observation indicates that asbestos exposure is almost universal, there is no evidence to date that in most individuals it represents a significant risk for the development of pleuropulmonary disease.[123] On the other hand, it is well established that individuals who live in the vicinity of a mine, mill, or factory where asbestos dust pollution is heavy have an increased incidence of pleural plaques and mesothelioma.[124] In fact, these abnormalities can develop in persons whose only exposure is the repeated handling of the clothes of asbestos workers.[125] Such disease also can occur in individuals exposed to asbestos in a nonoccupational setting; for example, a high incidence of pleural plaques and mesothelioma has been reported from the Metsovo area of northwest Greece[126] and from isolated villages in Turkey,[127] two places where the soil, which contains tremolite, is used as a whitewash for buildings. A history of such environmental or paraoccupational asbestos exposure may not be readily apparent from a cursory inquiry, because the exposure may have occurred many years prior to recognition of the disease and may have been of short duration.

Pathogenesis and Pathologic Characteristics

Pleural Manifestations
Parietal Pleural Plaques. These are almost certainly the most common form of asbestos-related pleuropulmonary disease, the incidence in consecutive routine autopsies ranging from 4 to 12 per 100 cases.[128] Pathologically, they consist of well-defined, pearly-white foci of firm, virtually acellular fibrous tissue, usually 2 to 5 mm thick and up to 10 cm in diameter.[129] They may have a smooth surface or show fine or coarse nodularity and can be round, elliptical,

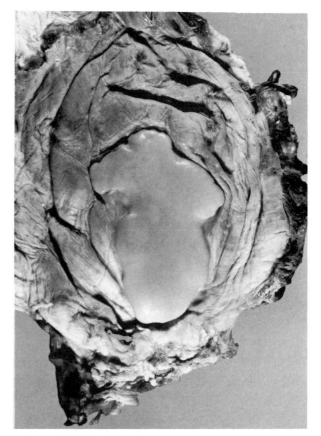

Figure 12–12. Pleural Plaque Secondary to Asbestos Exposure. A gross specimen of a hemidiaphragm reveals a smooth, well-defined focus of fibrosis on the tendinous portion. This was an incidental finding in a construction worker whose lung contained occasional asbestos bodies.

or irregularly shaped (Fig. 12–12).[130] Characteristically, plaques are located on the parietal pleura overlying the ribs and on the domes of the diaphragm. They are generally absent from the apices, costophrenic angles, and anterior chest wall and are almost always bilateral.

In most individuals with pleural plaques, there is evidence of prior asbestos exposure, as indicated by either an appropriate occupational history or the presence of a substantial number of coated or uncoated asbestos fibers in the lungs.[131] In some patients, however, these features are not evident,[131] in which case the plaques cannot be regarded as absolute evidence of asbestos-related disease. Whether such plaques are caused by trauma, infection, or inhalation of nonasbestos fibers usually cannot be established. The pathogenesis of asbestos-related pleural plaques is unclear.[127]

Focal Visceral Pleural Fibrosis. Relatively discrete foci of visceral pleural fibrosis morphologically distinct from pleural plaques are common in association with asbestos exposure (Fig. 12–13). They consist of round or elliptical areas of fibrous tissue 1 to 2 mm thick that often appear to radiate from a central focus. Unless the abnormality is associated with round atelectasis (see later) or located in a fissure, it is unlikely to be detected on conventional chest roentgenograms.

Diffuse Pleural Fibrosis. In contrast to the relatively discrete foci of visceral and parietal pleural fibrosis de-

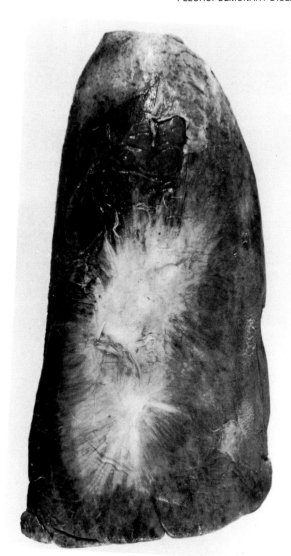

Figure 12–13. Localized Visceral Pleural Fibrosis Secondary to Asbestos Exposure. The lateral surface of this lower lobe shows a rather poorly demarcated area of fibrosis that appears to radiate out from two central foci. The fibrosis is limited to the visceral pleura, although multiple plaques were identified on the parietal pleura of the chest wall and hemidiaphragms. The underlying lung was unremarkable. The patient was a former construction worker with known asbestos exposure.

sion, in many instances without evidence of an underlying cause. Histologic examination of the pleura of these individuals has shown fibrosis and nonspecific chronic inflammation[133]; mesothelial hyperplasia also can be present and must be differentiated from mesothelioma. As with other forms of asbestos-related pleural disease, the pathogenesis of non-neoplastic effusion is unclear. It has been suggested that interaction between asbestos fibers and pleural tissue results in the release of non–complement-related chemotactic factors that cause the effusion.[134]

Mesothelioma. There is now no doubt of the association between asbestos exposure and the development of mesothelioma. The pathologic features and pathogenesis of this tumor are discussed in greater detail on page 886.

Pulmonary Manifestations

Asbestosis. Asbestosis can be defined as a pneumoconiosis characterized by more or less diffuse parenchymal interstitial fibrosis secondary to the inhalation of asbestos fibers. Grossly, the fibrosis is most prominent in the subpleural regions of the lower lobes and varies from a slightly coarse appearance of the parenchyma to obvious honeycomb change (Fig. 12–14).[130] Fibrosis of adjacent visceral pleura is common and is often accompanied by parietal pleural adhesions. As might be expected from the gross description, the microscopic appearance varies from a slight increase in interstitial collagen to complete obliteration of normal lung architecture and the formation of thick fibrous

scribed above, some patients show more diffuse pleural thickening that may be progressive and may be associated with clinical and functional abnormalities.[118] Although the fibrosis can be restricted to either the parietal or visceral pleura, it usually involves both and is accompanied by interpleural adhesions. It is not clear whether this form of disease represents an extension of one or both of the other two forms of pleural fibrosis or is a pathogenetically separate process. In one study of seven patients with diffuse pleural fibrosis, one or more episodes of pleural effusion were identified, suggesting that organization of the effusion might have been responsible for the chronic changes.[118] The presence of numerous inflammatory cells within the fibrous tissue in some cases has also raised the possibility of an immunologic pathogenesis.[132]

Pleural Effusion. Disease in some individuals with a history of asbestos exposure is manifested as pleural effu-

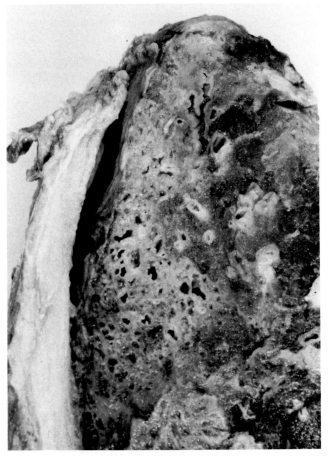

Figure 12–14. Diffuse Pleural Fibrosis and Asbestosis. A slice of a lower lobe shows severe pleural fibrosis and underlying parenchymal interstitial fibrosis with a "honeycomb" appearance.

bands and cystic spaces. Asbestos bodies are usually easily identified in tissue sections and may be present in great numbers; in fact, according to most authorities,[130] their presence is required for the histologic diagnosis. Despite this, they may be very scarce or apparently absent in some individuals.[135]

The earliest histologic change in asbestosis is considered by some investigators to consist of fibrosis in the walls of respiratory bronchioles.[130] According to this view, the process begins in the most proximal of such airways and extends to involve terminal bronchioles, more distal respiratory bronchioles and the adjacent alveolar interstitium; as the disease progresses, greater portions of lung parenchyma are affected in a centrifugal fashion. Although there is no doubt that peribronchiolar fibrosis exists in association with asbestos exposure (Fig. 12–15), there is evidence that it may represent a process pathogenetically distinct from pulmonary parenchymal fibrosis (i.e., asbestosis). For example, peribronchiolar fibrosis has been identified in patients with a history of exposure to mineral dust other than asbestos, implying that this pathologic change may be a nonspecific reaction to dust inhalation rather than a specific manifestation of asbestos toxicity.[136] Experimental studies in sheep also have demonstrated evidence for two distinct pulmonary reactions, one related to small airways and the other to the parenchymal interstitium.[137] Whatever its relationship to interstitial fibrosis, the peribronchiolar fibrosis may be related to the airflow obstruction that is observed in both patients[138] and experimental animals.[137]

The pathogenesis of asbestosis is incompletely understood. In experimental animals, inhaled asbestos fibers small enough to reach the lung parenchyma appear to be deposited preferentially at alveolar duct bifurcations.[139] Such deposition is rapidly followed by the accumulation of alveolar macrophages[140] (possibly as a result of direct activation by asbestos of a complement-dependent chemotactic factor[141]) and by proliferation of alveolar epithelial, interstitial, and endothelial cells[142] (possibly caused by the release of a diffusible growth factor.[143]) Further, there is evidence that macrophages that come in contact with asbestos fibers can release substances that stimulate growth of fibroblasts, with resulting collagen production.[144] Experiments in which human alveolar macrophages have been cultured in varying concentrations of amosite asbestos have shown significant cytotoxicity[145]; however, it is conceivable that in vivo, less severe damage results simply in abnormalities in macrophage function similar to those proposed for silicosis.

Not everyone exposed to heavy concentrations of asbestos develops asbestosis, the dose-response relationship being weaker in this condition than in other pneumoconioses such as CWP. This observation has raised the possibility that other extrinsic agents or intrinsic host factors may be important in the pathogenesis of the disease. The most extensively studied extrinsic agent is cigarette smoke. Although there is some disagreement,[146] most investigators[147, 148] have demonstrated an apparent synergistic effect of cigarette smoking on the development of roentgenographically detectable asbestosis. The pathogenetic basis for the cigarette smoke–asbestosis association is unclear. However, experimental studies in guinea pigs[149] have shown that cigarette smoking is associated with increased penetration of asbestos fibers into the walls of respiratory bronchioles, suggesting that the resulting larger interstitial fiber burden may be related to more severe fibrosis.

Intrinsic host factors that might be important in determining individual susceptibility to the harmful effects of asbestos include the efficiency of alveolar and tracheobronchial clearance,[150] underlying lung structure,[151] and immune status. The last has been studied most thoroughly, evidence for an autoimmune factor in the pathogenesis of asbestosis having been found in studies of both humoral and cellular immune function. Some asbestos workers have circulating rheumatoid factor, antinuclear antibody,[152] hypergammaglobulinemia, and immune complexes.[153] However, although such B-cell hyperactivity appears to correlate with roentgenographic progression of asbestosis,[154] there is as yet no clear-cut evidence that it is directly involved in the pathogenesis of the disease. A variety of abnormalities of cell-mediated immunity also have been documented in asbestos-exposed individuals; these include delayed skin hypersensitivity,[155] an alteration in the ratio of helper to suppressor T lymphocytes in BAL fluid,[156] and a reduction in natural killer cell activity.[157] As with abnormalities related to antibodies, however, the precise contribution of any of these to the development of asbestosis is unknown.

The Asbestos Body. The asbestos body is seen commonly in tissue sections in association with asbestos pleu-

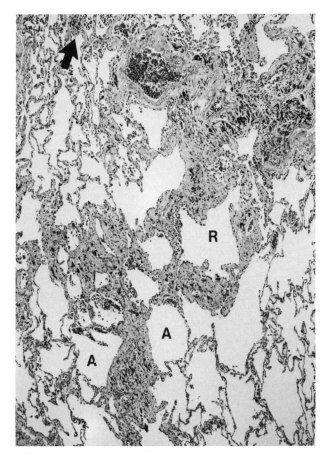

Figure 12–15. Peribronchiolar Fibrosis Associated with Asbestos Exposure. In this histologic section the wall of a respiratory bronchiole (R) and its distal divisions (A) are substantially thickened by fibrous tissue, pigmented macrophages, and a mild lymphocytic infiltrate. The adjacent parenchyma is mostly normal, although focal interstitial fibrosis is present (arrow). The patient was a 55-year-old man employed as an insulator; asbestos bodies were easily identified in lung parenchyma. (× 40.)

ropulmonary disease and consists of a core composed of a transparent asbestos fiber (usually amosite or crocidolite[158]) surrounded by a variably thick coat of iron and protein (Fig. 12–16). Most bodies measure between 2 and 5 μm in width and 20 to 50 μm in length.[158] The shape is quite variable, depending on the length of the asbestos core, the amount and pattern of deposition of the protein-iron coat, and whether the body is whole or fragmented. In tissue sections, they usually are seen within interstitial fibrous tissue or airspaces; they are rarely identified in pleural plaques. Their presence in the sputum[159] and BAL[160] and TTNA[161] specimens from individuals with occupational exposure has been well documented.

The absolute number of asbestos bodies identified in tissue sections or digested lung samples is a gross underestimation of the total number of uncoated asbestos *fibers*, as determined by electron microscopic examination of tissue samples[162]; thus, the ratio of uncoated to coated fibers in lung digests ranges from approximately 7:1 to 5000:1 in different series.[163] Since it is likely that it is the uncoated form of asbestos that exerts pathologic effects and since there are qualitative as well as quantitative differences between fibers and bodies, these distinctions are important in understanding pathogenesis.

The number of asbestos bodies and fibers per gram of digested lung tissue is roughly proportional to both the presence and severity of disease and the degree of occupational exposure. Thus, individuals with well-documented

high exposure generally have 20 to 100 times the number of fibers in the lung as those not exposed. Individuals with asbestosis or mesothelioma usually have a 100- to 1000-fold relative increase.[163]

Round Atelectasis. Pathologically, round atelectasis consists of a more or less spherical focus of collapsed parenchyma in the periphery of the lung. Although the abnormality is not related only to asbestos, the majority of cases are associated with it.[164] Grossly, the atelectatic lung is poorly defined and appears to blend imperceptibly with adjacent normal lung parenchyma (see Fig. 4–16, page 179).[165] The overlying pleura is invariably fibrotic and shows one or more invaginations, 1 mm to 3 cm in length, into the adjacent lung.

Pulmonary Carcinoma. As with mesothelioma, there is now no doubt about the relationship between asbestos exposure and pulmonary carcinoma, particularly in cigarette smokers (see page 448).

Roentgenographic Manifestations

In most reported series of asbestos-related disease, roentgenographic changes in the pleura are far more striking than those in the lung. For example, in one study of 40 patients with asbestos exposure, only five had parenchymal changes in the lung bases, pleural plaques being the sole manifestation of disease in the other 35.[166]

Pleural Manifestations

Four types of roentgenographic abnormality can be identified in the pleura: plaques, diffuse thickening, thickening of the interlobar fissure, and effusion. As a group, these are not uncommon. It has been estimated that as many as 1.3 million people in the United States may have such roentgenographically detectable abnormalities.[167]

Pleural Plaques. These may be smooth or nodular in outline and can measure up to 1 cm in thickness, although they are usually thinner (Fig. 12–17). They are most often multiple and usually occur on the posterolateral chest wall between the seventh and tenth ribs and on the lateral chest wall between the sixth and ninth ribs (Fig. 12–18)[168]; in both sites, they tend to follow the rib contours. Although plaques also occur frequently on the domes of the diaphram, their roentgenographic identification at this site can be difficult because of the absence of contrast with contiguous diaphragmatic muscle. Although it is generally thought that pleural plaques or thickening are usually bilateral and fairly symmetric, this has not been found in all studies. For example, in one review of the roentgenograms of 200 individuals with known or suspected asbestos exposure, plaques or thickening (with or without calcification) occurred solely or predominantly on the left side in 90, on the right side in 32, and equally on the two sides in only 44.[169]

Uncalcified pleural plaques may be very difficult to identify, particularly when viewed *en face*, so tangential roentgenograms in oblique projection may be necessary. In fact, the frequency with which plaques occur along the posterolateral or anterolateral portion of the thorax has suggested to some that oblique projections of the thorax should be standard in the roentgenographic investigation of patients suspected of having asbestos-related disease.[168] The validity of this approach was supported in one study of 127 asbestos

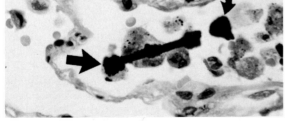

Figure 12–16. Asbestos Bodies. A histologic section *(A)* reveals a slightly curved, elongated structure with a finely beaded iron-protein coat. The asbestos fiber itself can be identified as a thin line in the center of the coat near one end of the body *(arrow)*. In another section *(B)*, other asbestos bodies show a more prominent iron-protein coat obscuring the enclosed asbestos fiber; some are fragmented *(curved arrow)*, and a characteristic drumstick form is taken by one *(straight arrow)*. (A and B × 400.)

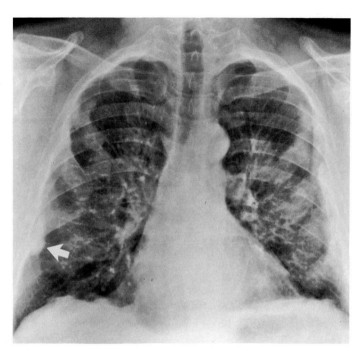

Figure 12–17. Pleural Plaques. A posteroanterior roentgenogram of the chest reveals multiple pleura-based opacities situated on all aspects of the chest wall and diaphragm. Several are viewed tangentially, the largest measuring 15 mm in width *(arrow)*, but perhaps the majority are ill defined and rather hazy, indicating their origin from the posterolateral and anterolateral chest wall. The diaphragmatic plaques have created an irregular configuration of both hemidiaphragms. The patient is a 54-year-old man with a long history of occupational asbestos exposure; he had no symptoms referable to his thorax.

workers in which the diagnostic content of three types of examination—a single PA roentgenogram, roentgenograms in four projections (PA, lateral, and both 45-degree oblique views), and CT—was evaluated.[170] It was found that the four-view roentgenograms revealed more sites of pleural plaques and the CT scans more calcified pleural plaques than could be identified on the single PA roentgenograms. It is important to realize that, depending on the criteria and techniques for diagnosis, the frequency with which plaques are recognized roentgenographically ranges from as little as 8 per cent to as much as 40 per cent of patients in whom they are demonstrated at autopsy.[128]

The greatest problem in the roentgenologic diagnosis of diffuse pleural thickening and early plaques lies in distinguishing them from the muscle and fat shadows that may be identified in as many as 75 per cent of normal PA roentgenograms along the convexity of the thorax. In fact, with standard roentgenography, it is sometimes impossible to differentiate pleural plaques from companion shadows with conviction. Several studies have documented the advantages of high-resolution CT in this situation, in comparison with both conventional roentgenograms and conventional CT.[171, 172] It is now generally agreed that scanning should be performed with the patient in the prone position, a maneuver that effectively permits distinction of structural abnormalities from gravity-related physiologic phenomena.[172]

The preceding comments relate to pleural plaques in which calcification is not apparent; when this can be identified, diagnosis clearly is greatly facilitated. The frequency of pleural plaque calcification is variable, some authors reporting calcified and noncalcified plaques in roughly equal numbers,[166] whereas others have observed calcification in only 20 per cent of cases.[173] It is possible that this variability relates to the variety of asbestos concerned; in an American survey of 261 workers exposed to asbestos in industry, pleural calcification was found in none,[174] whereas in Fin-

land (where anthophyllite is relatively abundant) it is common. Roentgenographically, calcified plaques vary from small linear or circular shadows, commonly situated over the diaphragmatic domes (*see* Fig. 12–18), to complete encirclement of the lower portion of the lungs.[175]

Diffuse Pleural Thickening. In contrast to pleural plaques, diffuse thickening is a generalized, more or less uniform increase in pleural width. Although the term is not precisely defined in the 1980 ILO classification, an acceptable definition has been provided by McLoud and colleagues: "a smooth, non-interrupted pleural density extending over at least one-fourth of the chest wall, with or without costophrenic angle obliteration."[176] In a study designed to determine the prevalence and causes of diffuse pleural thickening in an asbestos-exposed population, the chest roentgenograms of 1373 exposed individuals and 717 control subjects were evaluated.[173] Among the exposed group, plaques and diffuse thickening occurred with almost equal frequency, 16.5 and 13.5 per cent, respectively.

Thickening of the Interlobular Fissures. In one study, the incidence of interlobar fissural thickening in asbestos workers was 54 per cent, compared with 16 per cent in the unexposed control group.[177] Fissural thickening was present in 85 per cent of workers with parietal pleural plaques and in 36 per cent of those without plaques; it was particularly common (85 per cent) in patients with pulmonary fibrosis. Although the thickening in some of these patients is probably caused by plaque formation similar to that in the parietal pleura, in others it is likely due to focal fibrosis morphologically distinct from plaques (*see* page 720).

Pleural Effusion. The most comprehensive report of the prevalence and incidence of pleural effusion in an asbestos-exposed population was by Epler and colleagues,[178] who studied 1135 exposed workers and 717 control subjects. Benign asbestos effusion was defined by (1) history of exposure to asbestos; (2) confirmation by roentgenograms

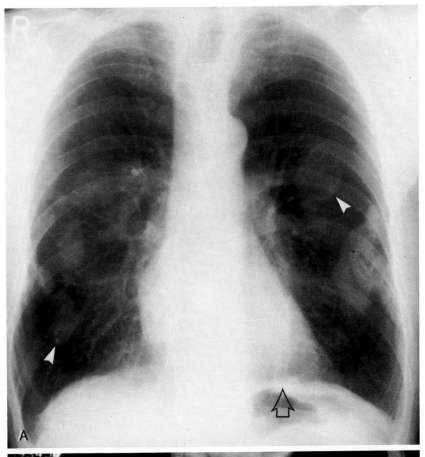

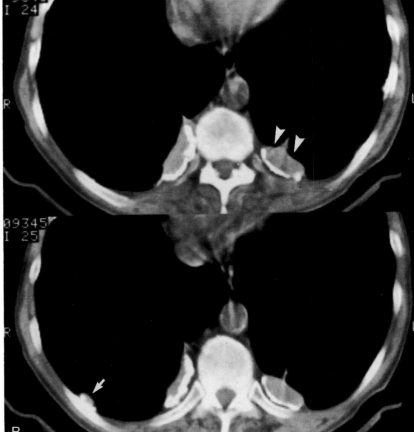

Figure 12–18. Calcified Pleural Plaques. A posteroanterior chest roentgenogram *(A)* reveals multiple round and elliptical opacities located peripherally between the sixth and tenth ribs posteriorly. Faint curvilinear and nodular calcification *(arrowheads)* can be identified in several of the lesions. There is slight irregularity on the superomedial portion of the left hemidiaphragm *(open arrow)* consistent with plaque formation. Two 10-mm-thick CT scans *(B)* through the lower lobes reveal bilateral posteromedial nodular *(arrow)* and hemispheric *(arrowheads)* opacities.

or thoracentesis or both; (3) no other disease related to pleural effusion; and (4) no malignant tumor within 3 years. These authors found 34 benign effusions among the exposed workers (3 per cent), compared with no otherwise unexplained effusions among the control subjects. The likelihood of effusion was dose related. The latency period was shorter than for other asbestos-related disorders, benign effusion being the most common abnormality during the first 20 years after exposure.

Mesothelioma. As indicated, the relationship between mesothelioma and asbestos exposure is now well recognized and is discussed further on page 886.

Pulmonary Manifestations

The roentgenographic changes of asbestosis occur in two forms, small and large opacities. The former can be round (a nodular pattern) or irregular (a reticular pattern) and may be seen in three stages:[179]

1. A fine reticulation occupying predominantly the lower lung zones and associated with a ground-glass appearance that is probably the result of combined pleural thickening[166] and early interstitial pneumonitis or fibrosis.
2. A stage in which irregular small opacities become more marked, creating a prominent reticular pattern (Fig. 12–19).
3. A late stage, in which reticulation is severe and involves all lung zones, sometimes with marked distortion of lung architecture. Hilar lymph node enlargement is seldom if ever notable on conventional roentgenograms[180]; however, mediastinal lymph nodes larger than 1.2 cm in greatest dimension are common on CT scans.[180a]

By conventional roentgenography, the small irregular opacities of asbestosis are best detected in PA projection, although shallow oblique views can sometimes demonstrate the subpleural parenchyma to better advantage by diminishing the absorptive influence of the chest wall musculature.[181] In recent years, possibly as a result of the general acceptance of the ILO 1980 International Classification, observer variability in the diagnosis of asbestosis appears to be similar to that reported in other pneumoconiosis studies.

A number of studies have shown that high-resolution CT (1- to 2-mm collimation using a high-frequency reconstruction algorithm) can demonstrate parenchymal abnormalities in patients with normal chest roentgenograms.[172, 183–188] The characteristic findings include (1) short linear opacities radiating from the subpleural parenchyma to the pleura (thickened interlobular septa); (2) nontapering linear opacities 2 to 5 cm in length extending to the pleura, usually to areas of pleural thickening ("parenchymal bands" caused by fibrous tissue in the bronchovascular sheath[189]); (3) small cystlike spaces up to 1 cm in diameter with discrete walls (honeycombing); and (4) nondependent curvilinear lines parallel to the pleura (subpleural curvilinear shadows).[190] Although these findings are characteristic of asbestosis, they may be indistinguishable from those of idiopathic pulmonary fibrosis.

Large opacities measure 1 cm or more in diameter and are an uncommon manifestation of asbestosis. They are invariably associated with prominent reticulation[191] and usually with pleural plaques. They may be well or ill de-

fined, solitary or multiple, and vary from one to several centimeters in diameter. They are typically nonsegmental in distribution. Unlike the large opacities of silicosis or CWP, the massive fibrosis of asbestosis does not appear to "migrate" toward the center of the lung, tends not to show upper lobe predominance, and has not been known to undergo roentgenographically demonstrable cavitation. The precise nature of these large opacities is unclear. In one study of affected individuals from South Africa, they were shown to consist pathologically of foci of fibrosis with or without a concentric lamellated appearance (similar to that of silicotic nodules).[191] Since South African asbestos rock has a quartz content of approximately 16 per cent, it is possible that the opacities are in fact related to inhalation of silica.

Clinical Manifestations

The great majority of patients with pleuropulmonary asbestos-related disease have no symptoms. Occasionally an acute pleural effusion is associated with pleural pain.[192] Such effusions are recurrent in 15 to 30 per cent[192, 193] of cases, are usually smaller than 500 mL, are often serosanguineous, and persist 2 weeks to 6 months. Breathlessness is almost invariably associated with interstitial fibrosis, although it can occasionally be caused partly (and, in rare cases, largely) by thickened pleura.[118] Once it begins, dyspnea is usually progressive despite discontinuation of asbestos exposure. In patients with asbestosis, shortness of breath seldom develops sooner than 20 to 30 years after initial exposure.[194] Signs and symptoms of cor pulmonale develop in some patients. Prolonged asbestos exposure also can cause cough, which can be dry or productive of mucopurulent sputum. This symptom can be present with or without dyspnea on exertion and in the absence of roentgenographic or physiologic evidence of asbestosis.[195]

Physical examination may reveal evidence of deformity of the thoracic cage caused by underlying pleural disease. Crepitations (fine rales or crackles) are common at the lung bases in workers with prolonged exposure to asbestos, particularly when there is roentgenographically demonstrable asbestosis.[196] Because their presence correlates with derangement of pulmonary function,[197] most observers would compensate a worker for asbestosis on the basis of this physical sign, even in the absence of roentgenographic abnormality, provided that the history suggests sufficiently heavy exposure and that pulmonary function tests show decreased compliance.[198]

Finger clubbing, also a frequent sign in asbestosis, has some prognostic significance. In one study,[199] patients who developed the complication were found to have lower diffusing capacity, higher mortality rate, and greater likelihood of progression of pulmonary fibrosis than patients who did not.

Pulmonary Function Tests

Patients with asbestosis usually show a restrictive pattern of pulmonary function, with decreased vital capacity, residual volume, and diffusion capacity, and preservation of relatively good ventilatory function. The decrease in vital capacity may be evident in the absence of roentgenographic abnormality.[199a] Hypoxemia may be observed on exercise,

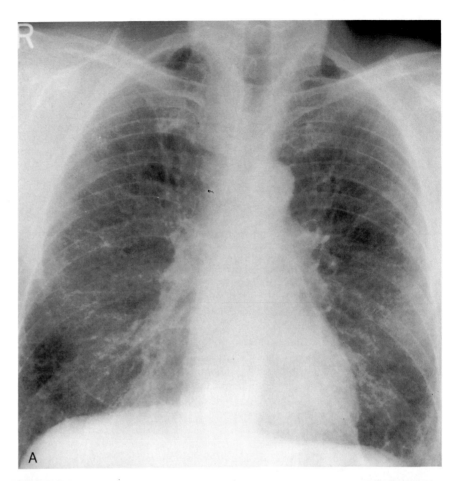

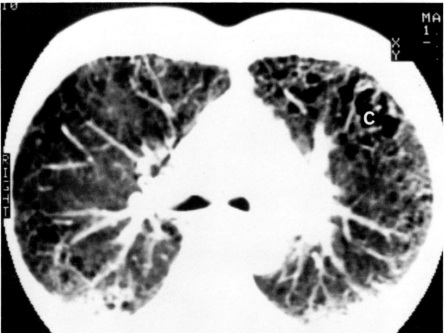

Figure 12–19. Asbestosis. A postero-anterior *(A)* chest roentgenogram discloses a diffuse medium reticular or reticulonodular pattern throughout both lungs, with some middle and lower zone predominance. No pleural abnormalities can be identified. *B,* A CT scan through the middle lung zone confirms the presence of widespread interstitial disease; cystic spaces measuring 2 to 3 cm can be identified *(C),* surrounded by thick walls.

but the Pco_2 is normal or low. Pulmonary compliance characteristically is greatly reduced.[200]

In addition to these abnormalities, tests on some asbestos workers who are smokers show an obstructive pulmonary function pattern that cannot be explained solely on the basis of cigarette consumption. Similar physiologic evidence of small airways disease also can be seen in nonsmokers.[138] As discussed previously, the anatomic basis for this obstruction may be peribronchiolar fibrosis. Because of these observations and because most individuals with asbestosis are cigarette smokers, the measurement of total lung capacity (TLC) alone is thought to be an insensitive means of assessing functional impairment.[201] However, there is evidence that measurement of the midexpiratory flow rate ($FEV_{25\%-75\%}$) may be helpful in early diagnosis.[202]

Other Silicates

Talc

Talc is a hydrated magnesium silicate that is used in the manufacture of such diverse products as leather, rubber, paper, textiles, ceramic tiles, and roofing material. It is also employed as an additive in paint, food, many pharmaceuticals, insecticides, and herbicides. Individuals in any of these occupational settings may be exposed to potentially harmful levels of dust. Others at risk include workers involved in talc mining and milling,[203] individuals who work with soapstone,[204] and people exposed to commercial talcum powder, either as an occupational hazard[205] or environmentally (the last-named usually as an obsession).[206]

Because other elements such as iron and nickel are usually incorporated in the talc crystal and because the substance is often found in association with other minerals such as quartz and asbestos, the composition of commercially available talc can differ considerably from region to region and from industry to industry.[207] As a result, the pattern of pulmonary disease associated with its inhalation is highly variable. In fact, the ability of talc in pure form to induce fibrosis has been questioned on the basis of the results of both epidemiologic and animal studies.[207] Despite this, it seems likely that true inhalational talcosis does occur, as evidenced by reported cases in which significant pulmonary disease has been caused by exposure to dust apparently uncontaminated by asbestos or silica.[204, 208]

Pathologic findings[204, 208] include pleural fibrosis (sometimes with calcification and plaque formation similar to that seen in asbestos-related pleural disease), focal nodular parenchymal fibrosis, more or less diffuse interstitial fibrosis, non-necrotizing granulomatous inflammation, and aggregates of peribronchiolar and perivascular macrophages. Multinucleated giant cells containing irregularly shaped birefringent plates or needlelike crystals, representing ingested talc, are common.

Roentgenographically, the hallmark of talc-related disease is the pleural plaque. Plaques are often diaphragmatic and bizzare in shape, and may be massive, and extend over much of the surface of both lungs.[203, 209] Parenchymal involvement is said to be similar to that in asbestosis, the roentgenographic pattern being one of general haziness, nodulation, and reticulation, with sparing of the apices and costophrenic sinuses.[203] Some cases may show confluence of lesions, creating large opacities (Fig. 12–20).[210]

Symptoms are similar to those of any other disabling pneumoconiosis and include dyspnea and productive cough. Decreased breath sounds, rales at the lung bases, limited chest expansion, and finger clubbing are found on physical examination.[211] The level of serum angiotensin-converting enzyme is increased in some patients.[212]

Decreases in vital capacity, total lung capacity, and carbon-monoxide diffusing capacity have been reported to occur in many exposed workers.[211] Diffusing capacity is said to correlate with the extent of parenchymal involvement seen roentgenographically.[211] Restrictive pulmonary function impairment has been described in patients with pleural disease only.[209]

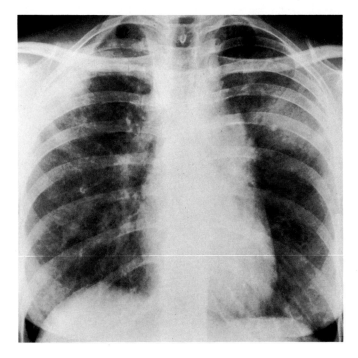

Figure 12–20. Pulmonary Talcosis. A posteroanterior roentgenogram reveals extensive involvement of both lungs by a rather coarse reticular pattern. In the upper axillary zone on the right and in the left midlung are two areas of homogeneous consolidation possessing poorly defined margins. Paratracheal lymph node enlargement is present bilaterally, more marked on the left. The patient was in the habit of spreading talcum powder liberally over her pillow and blankets at night and actually inhaled it in large amounts from her cupped hands.

Mica

Micas are complex aluminum silicates of which three forms are commercially available: (1) muscovite, which is used in the manufacture of windows for stoves and furnaces; (2) phlogopite, which is used in the electrical industry; and (3) vermiculite, whose uses relate primarily to its fire resistance, insulation, and ion-exchange properties.

Like talc, micas are often associated with other minerals, particularly the asbestos tremolite,[213] and whether they can cause disease by themselves has been questioned.[214] For example, a literature review in 1985 found 66 cases reported as mica pneumoconiosis; however, the authors concluded that the evidence that the pulmonary disease was caused by mica exposure alone was reasonably convincing in only 26.[215] In addition, animal experiments have demonstrated little or no fibrogenic activity caused by mica[37] (although the validity of these studies has been questioned[215]). Despite these uncertainties, occasional cases have been reported in which apparently pure mica exposure has been associated with pulmonary fibrosis,[214, 216] and it seems reasonable to conclude that the risk of developing pulmonary disease from mica inhalation is real but slight.

When present, roentgenographic and clinical manifestations of significant exposure to mica are virtually indistinguishable from those of exposure to asbestos or talc.

Fuller's Earth

Fuller's earth is an aluminum silicate employed in the refining of oils, as a filtering agent, as a filler in cosmetics and other products, and in the bonding of molding sands in foundry work. Prolonged exposure can result in the accumulation of dust, mainly in the upper lobes, associated with the deposition of reticulin fibers but usually little or no collagen formation or cellular reaction.[217] Roentgenographic changes are said to consist of a prominence of bronchovascular markings and, occasionally, PMF.[218]

Kaolin

The term "kaolin" (china clay) refers to a group of clays of which kaolinite, a hydrated aluminum silicate, is the most important member. This substance is used industrially as a filler in plastics, rubber, paints, and adhesives, as a coating for paper, as an absorbent, and in the making of firebricks.[219] Water is usually employed in quarrying or strip mining, to minimize the risk of dust exposure; however, subsequent drying, bagging, and transporting of kaolin can result in high concentrations of aerosolized dust. Although it seems likely that kaolinite alone can cause pulmonary disease,[219] it is probable that some cases are complicated by the inhalation of other particulates,[220] particularly silica.

The incidence of significant chest disease in reported series varies from zero[221] to as great as 23 per cent.[222] The presence and severity of abnormalities are related to the number of years of exposure.[223] In one roentgenographic survey of 1676 china clay workers from Cornwall, England, 77 per cent were judged to be normal; 18 per cent showed abnormalities in category 1, and about 4 per cent in categories 2 and 3. Nineteen workers (1 per cent) were considered to have large opacities of progressive massive fibrosis.[224]

Pathologic features are similar to those of CWP, consisting of peribronchiolar macules (composed of numerous pigment-laden macrophages and interspersed reticulin fibers) and of larger masses measuring up to 12 cm in diameter.[219] Interstitial and nodular fibrosis, the latter correlating with the pulmonary quartz content, has also been documented.[220]

The roentgenographic pattern varies widely: in some cases there is no more than a general increase in lung markings; in others (particularly those with prolonged and severe exposure), a diffuse nodular and miliary mottling is present. A late manifestation is bilateral progressive massive fibrosis identical to that seen in other pneumoconioses.[225]

Nepheline Rock Dust

Nepheline is a mineral that occurs in crystalline form in many igneous rocks. It is milled to a fine powder and used in the production of pottery glazes. Pneumoconiosis occurs rarely.[226]

Zeolites (Erionite)

Zeolites are a group of over 30 naturally occurring minerals composed of hydrated aluminum silicates that are found in deposits of volcanic ash[227] and are widely used as absorbents and for filtration. The richest deposits are in Turkey and the western United States. Most are not considered toxic, but erionite has been reported to be associated with pleural plaques, mesothelioma, pulmonary carcinoma, and interstitial pulmonary fibrosis.[227, 228]

Inert Radiopaque Dusts

Iron

Workers in many occupations are exposed to dust containing iron, usually in the form of iron oxide (Fe_2O_3). The majority are electric arc or oxyacetylene torch workers who are exposed to the substance in fumes derived from melted and boiled iron emitted during the welding process. Other individuals at risk include those involved in the mining and processing of iron ore and metallic pigments such as ocher, workers in iron and steel rolling mills, foundry workers, boiler scalers, and workers exposed to magnetite.

When inhaled in sufficient quantity in relatively pure form, iron oxide causes siderosis, a condition generally believed to be unassociated with fibrosis or functional impairment. This belief is supported by experimental studies in animals in which various iron compounds inhaled or injected intratracheally have not caused a fibrotic reaction.[229] In addition, persons exposed for many years to iron oxide in high concentration usually are not disabled and show little evidence of fibrosis at necropsy,[230] even when the iron content of their lungs is very high. Despite the relatively benign nature of pure siderosis, it is important to realize that occupations associated with iron dust or fume production frequently expose workers to other noxious materials, including asbestos and silica. As the proportion of these substances increases, the propensity for the development of pulmonary fibrosis also increases, particularly if welding or other work is carried out in inadequately ventilated areas.[230] This situation results in the clinical, roentgenographic, and pathologic features characteristic of mixed dust pneumoconiosis (siderosilicosis).

Pathologically, pulmonary siderosis is characterized by the presence of macrophages filled with iron oxide, situated predominantly in the peribronchovascular interstitium.[231] Fibrosis is typically absent or minimal. In mixed dust disease, the appearance is similar to that of silicosis and is characterized by solitary or conglomerate fibrous nodules, the latter occasionally being large enough to be designated PMF. Unlike pure silicosis, nodules are usually rather poorly defined and have stellate borders. Aggregates of iron oxide and other substances such as carbon can often be found admixed within the fibrous tissue, either free or within macrophages.

The roentgenographic pattern in pure siderosis is reticulonodular and widely disseminated (Fig. 12–21). Opacities have been shown experimentally to correlate with localized aggregates of iron oxide–laden macrophages[232] and are related to the density of the iron oxide itself.[233] The roentgenographic abnormalities can disappear partly or completely when patients are removed from dust exposure.[234] In siderosilicosis, the pattern depends on the concentration of free silica in the inhaled dust; when it is relatively low (less than 10 per cent), the appearance is similar to that of pure siderosis or CWP, but when the concentration is high, the pattern is identical to that of silicosis.[235]

Clinically, patients with siderosis are asymptomatic. However, some patients with siderosilicosis complain of cough and dyspnea. Even in the absence of roentgenographic abnormality, arc welders[236] and foundry workers[237] have been found to have a higher incidence of bronchitis than control subjects. Although some studies of pulmonary function in welders have shown values considered to be within normal limits,[231] others have found evidence of both restrictive and mixed obstructive and restrictive abnormalities.[238]

Iron and Silver

Inhalation of large amounts of iron oxide and silver can produce an unusual pneumoconiosis termed argyrosiderosis. This results from the use of jeweler's rouge (which is composed in part of iron oxide) as a polishing agent in the finishing of silver products. When the rouge is applied with a buffer, small particles of iron oxide and silver are generated that may be inhaled. Pathologic examination of lung tissue demonstrates iron within macrophages in a distribution similar to that of siderosis; in addition, the inhaled silver can be identified in connective tissue of the alveolar walls, small arteries, and veins.[239] The roentgenographic manifestation is rather characteristic, consisting of a finely stippled pattern in contrast to the reticulonodular pattern of siderosis. Patients are typically asymptomatic.

Tin

Pneumoconiosis caused by inhalation of tin (stannosis) occurs predominantly in individuals employed in the handling of the ore after it has been mined, especially in industries in which tin oxide fumes are created. Pathologically, the findings simulate the macule of CWP. Although the condition is of no clinical or functional significance,[240] the high density of tin (atomic number 50) results in a dramatic roentgenographic appearance consisting of multiple shadows of high density, about 1 mm in diameter, distributed evenly throughout the lungs[240]; larger, somewhat less numerous nodules occasionally are seen. Linear opacities may be present in the paramediastinal zone, in the vicinity of the diaphragm, and in the costophrenic angles.

Barium

Barium and its salts, particularly barium sulfate, are used as coloring or weighting agents, as fillers in numerous prod-

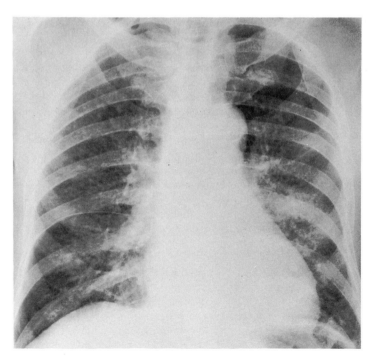

Figure 12–21. Pulmonary Siderosis. A 63-year-old man had worked as an electric arc welder for a railway company for 20 years. He was asymptomatic, this roentgenogram being part of a screening examination. The posteroanterior roentgenogram reveals a diffuse reticulonodular pattern throughout both lungs.

ucts, and in the manufacture of glass. Exposure during any of these uses, as well as in mining of the ore, can cause pulmonary disease (barytosis). The chest roentgenogram shows a variable number of discrete shadows that, because of the high radiopacity of barium (atomic number 56), are extremely dense, creating an awesome appearance.[241] The lesions may develop after only brief exposure and characteristically regress after the patient is removed from the dust-filled environment. Some affected individuals complain of chronic cough, expectoration, and asthmalike attacks[242]; however, many are asymptomatic.

Antimony

Antimony is procured mainly from the mineral stibnite and is handled either as unrefined ore or as a fine white powder.[243] It is used in cosmetics, in the manufacture of batteries, pewter, printing type, and electrodes, in the compounding of rubber, in textiles, paints, and plastics as a flame retardant, and in ceramics as an opacifier.[243] There is both pathologic[243] and experimental[244] evidence suggesting that accumulation of the mineral is accompanied by little, if any, fibrosis. The chest roentgenogram of affected individuals reveals minute dense opacites scattered widely throughout both lungs.[244] There is no evidence that the dust causes disturbances in lung function.

Rare Earths

The rare earth elements include cerium (quantitatively the most important), scandium, yttrium, lanthanum, and 14 other minerals. Although the elements have a wide variety of industrial uses, pneumoconiosis occurs chiefly in individuals working with carbon arc lamps in the graphic arts, such as photoengraving and printing.[245] Granulomatous inflammation and parenchymal fibrosis have been described in a number of cases[245]; in some, the extent and progression of disease appear to depend on the thorium content of the dust.[246] The typical roentgenographic pattern consists of widely disseminated punctate opacities of great density,[247] again related to the high atomic numbers of the inhaled dusts, which range from 51 to 71. Patients are frequently asymptomatic despite the spirometric demonstration of a restrictive impairment.

Miscellaneous Inorganic Dusts

Beryllium

The majority of cases of berylliosis reported nowadays are associated with the processing and handling of beryllium compounds in precious metal refineries,[248] in the aerospace industry, and in the manufacture of gyroscopes and nuclear reactors.[249] The disease may occur in an acute or chronic form, the latter being much more common.

Acute Berylliosis. The majority of affected patients are exposed to the dust while working in beryllium refineries. Depending on the intensity of exposure, the clinical presentation may be either fulminating or insidious. In both situations, the pathologic changes consist of bronchitis, bronchiolitis, and diffuse alveolar damage.[250] Granulomatous inflammation does not occur.

The fulminating variety develops rapidly following an overwhelming exposure. Its clinical and roentgenographic manifestations are those of acute pulmonary edema, which may be rapidly fatal. The onset is heralded by a dry cough, substernal pain, shortness of breath on exertion, anorexia, weakness, and weight loss. Auscultatory findings include rales and, in some cases, rhonchi, suggesting asthma.[251] The chest roentgenogram usually does not become abnormal until 1 to 4 weeks after the onset of symptoms. Diffuse, symmetric, bilateral "haziness" is seen in the earliest stage of the disease, with subsequent development of irregular patchy opacities scattered rather widely throughout the lungs. Subsequently, discrete or confluent mottling may be observed.[251] Complete roentgenographic clearing may take 2 to 3 months.

Pulmonary function studies in the insidious form of acute disease have shown hyperventilation, reduction in vital capacity, and normal residual volume and maximal breathing capacity. In some cases, arterial oxygen saturation is greatly decreased during exercise and even at rest, with an increase in the alveolar-arterial gradient for oxygen. Removal from exposure to the dust results in gradual return to normal function.

Chronic Berylliosis. Several clinical, pathologic, and experimental observations suggest that the pathogenesis of chronic berylliosis is immune mediated, most likely a type IV hypersensitivity reaction. Such observations include (1) the frequent delay in onset of disease from the time of exposure; (2) the poor correlation between the degree of exposure and the development of disease; (3) the common presence of granulomatous inflammation; (4) the presence of blast transformation when lymphocytes are cultured in the presence of beryllium[252]; and (5) an increased number of T lymphocytes, with an increased helper-to-suppressor ratio, in fluid obtained by BAL.[253] Although the details of the presumed immunopathogenesis are not understood, it has been proposed that the metal binds as a hapten to a tissue or blood protein, the complex then being recognized by the immune system as foreign and inducing a cellular immune response.[253]

The characteristic pathologic abnormality in chronic berylliosis is interstitial pneumonitis,[250] which varies from a more or less diffuse mononuclear cell infiltrate unassociated with granulomatous inflammation to well-formed, discrete, non-necrotizing granulomas indistinguishable from those of sarcoidosis. Interstitial fibrosis is common. In contrast to most other dusts that cause pneumoconiosis, beryllium is largely removed from the lungs with time and excreted in the urine. As a result, quantitative studies show significantly less tissue content of beryllium in chronic than in acute disease.[250]

The roentgenographic pattern is neither specific nor diagnostic.[254] When the degree of involvement is relatively minor, it has been described as a diffuse, finely granular "haziness" with a tendency to sparing of the apices and bases.[255] With more severe involvement, ill-defined round or irregular opacities of moderate size are scattered diffusely throughout the lungs, sometimes with associated lymph node enlargement.[256] Calcification of nodules occurs and, when present, permits differentiation from sarcoidosis.[257] In advanced cases, the pattern may be chiefly reticular and may be associated with a great decrease in lung volume and some conglomeration of nodular shadows. Areas of emphysema may be identified, usually in the upper lobes. Spontaneous pneumothorax occurs in slightly more than 10 per cent of cases.[257]

The majority of cases of chronic berylliosis are associated with dust exposure of more than 2 years' duration. Occasionally, patients with proven disease are asymptomatic.[258] Usually, however, symptoms develop insidiously after a latent period that may be as long as 15 years following the last exposure to dust.[251] There is some evidence that the disease can be precipitated by certain triggers, such as pregnancy, withdrawal from exposure, and even the performance of a beryllium patch test.[259] Early symptoms include cough, fatigue, weight loss, dyspnea on exertion, and, sometimes, migratory arthralgia. With progression of the disease, cyanosis may become evident, and in approximately 30 per cent of patients clubbing of the fingers and toes develops. Hypergammaglobulinemia, hypercalciuria, hypercuricemia, and polycythemia are not uncommon findings.[251]

Results of pulmonary function studies may be normal or may indicate some degree of restrictive insufficiency.[260] In many cases, the arterial oxygen tension is decreased, even at rest. Diffusing capacity may be reduced, and the alveolar-arterial oxygen difference increased, suggesting that the diffusion abnormality is caused primarily by $\dot{V}/\dot{Q}$ inequality.

The diagnosis of chronic beryllium disease may be suspected from a history of exposure to the dust and a chest roentgenogram showing diffuse nodular disease. Confirmation may be obtained by a patch test showing hypersensitivity to beryllium or by blastogenic transformation of blood[261] or alveolar[262] lymphocytes. The disease may be confused with sarcoidosis[248]; helpful points in differentiation include absence of involvement of the uveal tract, tonsils, parotid glands, and bones in berylliosis.

Aluminum

Individuals can be exposed to the potential toxic effects of aluminum in four situations: (1) the reduction of alumina to metallic aluminum during the process of smelting[263]; (2)

the preparation or use of aluminum powder[264]; (3) aluminum arc welding[265]; and (4) the grinding or polishing of aluminum products.[266] Each of these situations has been associated with pulmonary disease; however, there is often a history of concomitant exposure to other potentially toxic substances, and it is not certain that aluminum is the pathogenetic agent in every case. This pathogenetic uncertainty is underlined by several experimental and clinical studies that have shown either minimal or no pulmonary reaction to inhaled aluminum.[267, 268] Despite this, some investigators have shown a significant fibrotic reaction,[269, 270] suggesting that, at least in some cases, true toxicity is present. It has been hypothesized that host factors, perhaps mediated by immune mechanisms, may be responsible for these discrepant experimental results.[264]

Pathologic findings in the lungs of individuals exposed to aluminum are variable and include desquamative interstitial pneumonitis,[271] alveolar proteinosis,[266] interstitial fibrosis[270] (in some cases with an upper zonal predominance[269]), and granulomatous pneumonitis.[264]

Roentgenographic abnormalities may become apparent after a few months' or several years' exposure.[272] Fully developed changes consist of a fine to coarse reticular pattern widely distributed throughout the lungs (Fig. 12–22), sometimes with a nodular component.[272] Lung volume may be greatly decreased, the pleura may become thickened, and spontaneous pneumothorax may occur.

Breathlessness is the chief symptom and may be severely disabling. Chronic bronchitis[273] or asthma[263] develop in some individuals. Pulmonary function studies have shown both restrictive and obstructive disease with reduction in diffusing capacity.

Cobalt and Tungsten Carbide

The term "hard metal" is usually used to refer to an alloy of tungsten, carbon, and cobalt (occasionally small amounts of other metals are added).[274] The resulting product is ex-

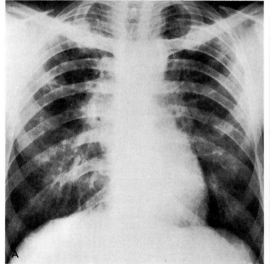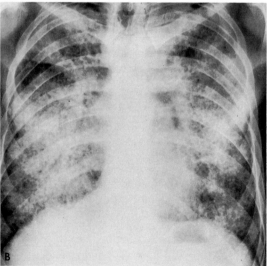

Figure 12–22. Bauxite Pneumoconiosis (Shaver's Disease). A 29-year-old man had been exposed for a number of years to bauxite in the manufacture of corundum. The first posteroanterior roentgenogram *(A)* revealed a coarse reticulonodular pattern throughout both lungs involving predominantly the upper and middle lung zones. Slightly more than 1 year later *(B)*, the disease had extended to a remarkable degree, the reticulonodular shadows being confluent in many areas. (Courtesy of Montreal Chest Hospital Center.)

tremely hard and resistant to heat and is used extensively in the drilling and polishing of other metals. Exposure to dust can occur during either the manufacture or the use of the metal.

The pathogenesis of disease is unclear. Experimental studies in animals suggest that cobalt is the etiologic agent,[274] a hypothesis supported by the finding of the disease in diamond polishers,[275] who are exposed to high concentrations of cobalt alone. However, there is evidence that the effects of cobalt are enhanced by the presence of tungsten carbide,[274] and in some autopsy studies of patients with interstitial fibrosis and a history of exposure to hard metals, cobalt has not been found in the lung tissue.[276] It has been suggested that the disease may result from a hypersensitivity reaction analogous to that seen in berylliosis.[277]

Pathologic findings are predominantly those of interstitial pneumonitis with a variable degree of fibrosis.[278] Characteristically, numerous macrophages are present in alveolar airspaces, creating a pattern simulating idiopathic desquamative interstitial pneumonitis. In many cases, multinucleated giant cells also are prominent, resulting in the pattern of giant cell interstitial pneumonitis.

Roentgenographic findings are variable[278] but characteristically consist of a diffuse micronodular and reticular pattern, sometimes with lymph node enlargement. The reticulation may be very coarse[279] and in advanced disease may be accompanied by small cystic shadows.

Symptoms include a dry cough and dyspnea on exertion; severe respiratory insufficiency sometimes develops and can prove fatal.[279] Pulmonary function tests reveal both restrictive and obstructive patterns[280] and diffusion may be reduced.

Silicon Carbide

Silicon carbide (carborundum) is produced by fusion at high temperature of high-grade sand, finely ground carbon (coke), salt, and wood dust.[281] The resulting product is extremely hard and is used as an abrasive. Although the findings in experimental studies in animals have suggested that the substance is inert,[281, 282] occasional individuals with apparently pure or predominant silicon carbide exposure have shown pathologic evidence of interstitial fibrosis and macrophage accumulation accompanied by roentgenographic and pulmonary function abnormalities.[281, 282]

Polyvinyl Chloride

In its pure form, polyvinyl chloride is a white powder that is produced by polymerization under pressure of the gas vinyl chloride[283]; it is used in the manufacture of plastics, synthetic fibers, and numerous other commercial products. There is evidence that its inhalation, during either its production or its use in the manufacture of other materials, may be associated with interstitial pneumonitis and fibrosis or the accumulation of interstitial and intra-alveolar macrophages.[283, 284] In one study of 1215 workers employed in a polyvinyl chloride production plant, 20 were considered to have roentgenographic abnormalities consistent with pneumoconiosis.[285] Some investigations have shown evidence of mild restrictive functional impairment[286] or combined restriction and obstruction.[287]

Titanium Dioxide

Titanium dioxide is derived from the ore ilmenite and is used chiefly as a pigment in paints, paper, and other products, as a mordant in dyeing, and as an alloy in some hard metals. Pathologic examination of the lungs of affected individuals has shown alveolar and interstitial accumulation of macrophages but minimal fibrosis.[288] Non-necrotizing granulomatous inflammation has been documented in a biopsy specimen from one patient[289]; because of a positive lymphocyte transformation test on exposure to titanium, the authors considered the possibility of a hypersensitivity reaction similar to that proposed for berylliosis. Roentgenographic changes considered consistent with pneumoconiosis have been reported in some workers involved in pigment production.[288, 290]

Volcanic Dust

Volcanic eruption can result in significant quantities of potentially harmful ash being liberated into the atmosphere. The best-studied eruption from the point of view of human health was at Mount Saint Helens in 1980.[291] As of 1981, 35 individuals were known to have died directly as a result of the eruption[292]; among the 25 who underwent autopsy, the majority were considered to have asphyxiated as a result of major airway plugging by mucus and inhaled volcanic ash.[293] In individuals outside the areas of most severe damage, there was a mild increase in the number of acute respiratory complaints such as cough, wheezing, and dyspnea,[291] probably secondary to airway irritation. The long-term consequences, if any, of volcanic ash inhalation are unclear.

Synthetic Mineral Fibers

Synthetic mineral fibers are amorphous silicates derived from slag, rock, or glass. Unlike natural silicates such as asbestos, synthetic fibers break transversely rather than longitudinally when traumatized, resulting in small fragments whose diameter is the same as that of their parents.[294] Because the potential for fibrous minerals to cause disease is related at least in part to a high length-diameter ratio,[294] this effect may be important in explaining the relative lack of toxicity of these substances.

Although some epidemiologic studies have suggested that inhaled synthetic mineral fibers can cause significant pulmonary damage,[295, 296] the bulk of autopsy[297] and experimental[298] evidence suggests that they have little, if any, harmful effects. In addition, other epidemiologic investigations, roentgenographic surveys, and tests of pulmonary function of workers involved with synthetic mineral fibers, have shown no differences from those of appropriate controls.[298]

Dental Technician's Pneumoconiosis

Dental technicians are exposed to a variety of inorganic materials during the process of grinding and drilling of dental prostheses, and there are several well-documented cases of lung disease related to their inhalation. Although this form of pneumoconiosis has been attributed to silicon dioxide, it is probable that other agents, such as acrylic resin,[299] are implicated as well.

Cement Dust

In one survey of 195 cement workers, many years' exposure to a high concentration of raw and mixed cement dust was associated with roentgenographic evidence of accentuation of linear markings and ill-defined micronodulation.[300] However, other epidemiologic studies have found little or no evidence of roentgenographic abnormality.[300]

References

1. Weill H: Epidemiologic methods in the investigation of occupational lung disease. Am Rev Respir Dis 112: 1, 1975.
2. Knishkowy B, Baker EL: Transmission of occupational disease to family contacts. Am J Ind Med 9: 543, 1986.
3. Norboo T, Angchuk PT, Yahya M, et al: Silicosis in a Himalayan village population: Role of environmental dust. Thorax 46: 341, 1991.
4. Dumontet C, Biron F, Vitrey D, et al: Acute silicosis due to inhalation of a domestic product. Am Rev Respir Dis 143: 880, 1991.
5. Seaton A, Lamb D, Brown WR, et al: Pneumoconiosis of shale miners. Thorax 36: 412, 1981.
6. Seaton A, Legge JS, Henderson J, et al: Accelerated silicosis in Scottish stonemasons. Lancet 337: 341, 1991.
7. van Sprundel MP: Pneumoconioses: The situation in developing countries. Exp Lung Res 16: 5, 1990.
8. Pinkerton KE, Plopper CG, Mercer RR, et al: Airway branching patterns influence asbestos fiber location and the extent of tissue injury in the pulmonary parenchyma. Lab Invest 55: 688, 1986.
9. Kreiss K, Danilovs JA, Newman LS: Histocompatibility antigens in a population based silicosis series. Br J Ind Med 46: 364, 1989.
10. Bégin R, Massé S, Sébastien P, et al: Asbestos exposure and retention as determinants of airway disease and asbestos alveolitis. Am Rev Respir Dis 134: 1176, 1986.
11. Churg A, Wiggs B: Fiber size and number in amphibole asbestos-induced mesothelioma. Am J Pathol 115: 437, 1984.
12. Amandus HE, Reger RB, Pendergrass EP, et al: The pneumoconioses: Methods of measuring progression. Chest 63: 736, 1973.
13. International Labor Office (League of Nations): Silicosis. Records of the international conference held at Johannesburg 13-27 August 1930. International Labour Office, Studies and Reports, Series F (Industrial Hygiene), No. 13, Geneva, International Labor Office, 1930, pp 86–93.
14. International Classification of Persistent Radiological Opacities in the Lung Fields Provoked by the Inhalation of Mineral Dusts. Safety Health 9: 63, 1959.
15. UICC-Cincinnati classification of the radiographic appearances of pneumoconioses. A cooperative study by the UICC committee. Chest 58: 57, 1970.
16. Russell AR (ed): Classification of radiographs of the pneumoconioses. Med Radiogr Photogr 57: 2, 1981.
17. Liddell FDK, Lindars DC: An elaboration of the I.L.O. classification of simple pneumoconiosis. Br J Ind Med 26: 89, 1969.
18. Felson B, Morgan WKC, Bristol LJ, et al: Observations on the results of multiple readings of chest films on coal miners' pneumoconiosis. Radiology 109: 19, 1973.
19. Morgan RH, Donner MW, Gayler BW, et al: Decision processes and observer error in the diagnosis of pneumoconiosis by chest roentgenography. Am J Roentgenol 117: 757, 1973.
20. Amandus HE, Pendergrass EP, Dennis JM, et al: Pneumoconiosis: Inter-reader variability in the classification of the type of small opacities in the chest roentgenogram. Am J Roentgenol 122: 740, 1974.
21. Liddell FDK: Assessment of radiological progression of simple pneumoconiosis in individual miners. Br J Ind Med 31: 185, 1974.
22. Ziskind M, Jones RN, Weill H: Silicosis. Am Rev Respir Dis 113: 643, 1976.
23. Cunningham CDB, Hugh AE: Pneumoconiosis in women. Clin Radiol 24: 491, 1973.
24. Davis GS: Pathogenesis of silicosis: Current concepts and hypotheses. Lung 164: 139, 1986.
25. Curran RC, Rowsell EV: The application of the diffusion-chamber technique to the study of silicosis. J Pathol Bacteriol 76: 561, 1958.
26. Bowden DH, Hedgecock C, Adamson IYR: Silica-induced pulmonary fibrosis involves the reaction of particles with interstitial rather than alveolar macrophages. J Path 158: 73, 1989.
27. Allison AC, Harington JS, Birbeck M: An examination of the cytotoxic effects of silica on macrophages. J Exp Med 124: 141, 1966.
28. Heppleston AG, Styles JA: Activity of a macrophage factor in collagen formation by silica. Nature 214: 521, 1967.
29. Gritter HL, Adamson IYR, King GM: Modulation of fibroblast activity by normal and silica-exposed alveolar macrophages. J Pathol 148: 263, 1986.
30. Chvapil M, Eskelson CD, Stiffel V, et al: Early changes in the chemical composition of the rat lung after silica administration. Arch Environ Health 34: 402, 1979.
31. Lowrie DB: What goes wrong with the macrophage in silicosis? Eur J Respir Dis 63: 180, 1982.
32. Schuyler MR, Ziskind MM, Salvaggio J: Function of lymphocytes and monocytes in silicosis. Chest 75: 340, 1979.
33. Struhar D, Harbeck RJ, Mason RJ: Lymphocyte populations in lung tissue, bronchoalveolar lavage fluid, and peripheral blood in rats at various times during the development of silicosis. Am Rev Respir Dis 139: 28, 1989.
34. Hubbard AK: Role for T lymphocytes in silica-induced pulmonary inflammation. Lab Invest 61: 46, 1989.
35. Dubois CM, Bissonnette E, Rola-Pleszczynski M: Asbestos fibers and silica particles stimulate rat alveolar macrophages to release tumor necrosis factor. Autoregulatory role of leukotriene B$_4$. Am Rev Respir Dis 139: 1257, 1989.
36. Vigliani EC, Pernis B: Immunological factors in the pathogenesis of the hyaline tissue of silicosis. Br J Ind Med 15: 8, 1958.
37. Parkes WR: Occupational Lung Disorders. 2nd ed. London, Butterworths, 1982.
38. Heppleston AG, Wright MA, Stewart JA: Experimental alveolar lipoproteinosis following the inhalation of silica. J Pathol 101: 293, 1970.
39. Buechner HA, Ansari A: Acute silicoproteinosis: A new pathologic variant of acute silicosis in sandblasters, characterized by histologic features resembling alveolar proteinosis. Dis Chest 55: 274, 1969.
40. Hoffman EO, Lamberty J, Pizzolato P, et al: The ultrastructure of acute silicosis. Arch Pathol 96: 104, 1973.
41. Bowden DH, Adamson IYR: The role of cell injury and the continuing inflammatory response in the generation of silicotic pulmonary fibrosis. J Pathol 144: 149, 1984.
42. Miller BE, Hook GER: Isolation and characterization of hypertrophic Type II cells from the lungs of silica-treated rats. Lab Invest 58: 565, 1988.
43. Emerson RJ, Davis GS: Effect of alveolar lining material–coated silica on rat alveolar macrophages. Environ Health Perspect 51: 81, 1983.
44. Allison AC, Hart PD: Potentiation by silica of the growth of *Mycobacterium tuberculosis* in macrophage cultures. Br J Exp Pathol 49: 465, 1968.
45. Craighead JE, Kleinerman J, Abraham JL, et al: Diseases associated with exposure to silica and nonfibrous silicate minerals. Arch Pathol Lab Med 112: 673, 1988.
46. Paterson JF: Silicosis in hardrock miners in Ontario: The problem and its prevention. Can Med Assoc J 84: 594, 1961.
47. Michel RD, Morris JF: Acute silicosis. Arch Intern Med 113: 850, 1964.
48. Greening RR, Heslep JH: The roentgenology of silicosis. Semin Roentgenol 2: 265, 1967.
49. Pendergrass EP: Caldwell Lecture 1957—Silicosis and a few of the other pneumoconioses: Observations on certain aspects of the problem, with emphasis on the role of the radiologist. Am J Roentgenol 80: 1, 1958.
50. Bellini F, Ghislandi E: "Egg-shell" calcifications at extrahilar sites in a silicotuberculotic patient. Med Lav 51: 600, 1960.
51. Jacobs LG, Gerstl B, Hollander AG, et al: Intra-abdominal egg-shell calcifications due to silicosis. Radiology 67: 527, 1956.
52. Oosthuizen SF, Theron CP: Correlation between the radiographic and pathological findings in silicosis. Med Proc 10: 337, 1964.
53. Oechsli WR, Jacobson G, Brodeur AE: Diatomite pneumoconiosis: Roentgen characteristics and classification. Am J Roentgenol 85: 263, 1961.
54. Sluis-Cremer GK, Hessel PA, Hnizdo E, et al: Relationship between silicosis and rheumatoid arthritis. Thorax 41: 596, 1986.
55. Buechner HA, Ansari A: Acute silicoproteinosis. A new pathologic variant of acute silicosis in sandblasters, characterized by histologic features resembling alveolar proteinosis. Dis Chest 55: 274, 1969.

56. Vallyathan V, Shi X, Dalal NS, et al: Generation of free radicals from freshly fractured silica dust: Potential role in acute silica-induced lung injury. Am Rev Respir Dis 138: 1213, 1988.
57. MacLaren WM, Soutar CA: Progressive massive fibrosis and simple pneumoconiosis in ex-miners. Br J Ind Med 42: 734, 1985.
58. Bégin R, Bergeron D, Samson P, et al: CT assessment of silicosis in exposed workers. Am J Roentgenol 148: 509, 1987.
59. Bégin R, Ostiguy G, Cantin A, et al: Lung function in silica-exposed workers. A relationship to disease severity assessed by CT scan. Chest 94: 539, 1988.
60. Bergin CJ, Müller NL, Vedall S, et al: CT in silicosis: Correlation with plain films and pulmonary function tests. Am J Roentgenol 146: 477, 1986.
61. Munakata M, Homma Y, Matsuzaki M, et al: Rales in silicosis. A correlative study with physiological and radiological abnormalities. Respiration 48: 140, 1985.
62. Sluis-Cremer GK, Hessel PA, Hnizdo E, et al: Relationship between silicosis and rheumatoid arthritis. Thorax 41: 596, 1986.
63. Nozaki S, Sawada Y: Progress of simple pulmonary silicosis in retired miners. Jpn J Clin Tuberc 18: 154, 1959.
64. Brink GC, Grzybowski S, Lane GB: Silicotuberculosis. Can Med Assoc J 82: 959, 1960.
65. Infante-Rivard C, Armstrong B, Peticlerc M, et al: Lung cancer mortality and silicosis in Québec, 1938–85. Lancet 2: 1504, 1989.
66. Hughes JM, Jones RN, Gilson JC, et al: Determinants of progression in sandblasters' silicosis. Ann Occup Hyg 26: 701, 1982.
67. Bailey WC, Brown M, Buechner HA, et al: Silico-mycobacterial disease in sandblasters. Am Rev Respir Dis 110: 115, 1974.
68. Nordman H, Koskinen H, Froseth B: Increased activity of angiotensin-converting enzyme in progressive silicosis. Chest 86: 203, 1984.
69. Doll NJ, Stankus RP, Hughes J, et al: Immune complexes and auto-antibodies in silicosis. J Allergy Clin Immunol 68: 281, 1981.
70. Teculescu DR, Stanescu DC: Carbon monoxide transfer factor for the lung in silicosis. Scand J Respir Dis 51: 150, 1970.
71. Renzetti AD Jr, Kobayshi T, Bigler A, et al: Regional ventilation and perfusion in silicosis and in the alveolar-capillary block syndrome. Am J Med 49: 5, 1970.
72. Becklake MR: Pneumoconioses. In Fenn WO, Rahn H (eds): Handbook of Physiology, Section III. Vol 2. Baltimore, Waverly Press, 1965, pp 1601–1614.
73. Irwiq LM, Rocks P: Lung function and respiratory symptoms in silicotic and nonsilicotic gold miners. Am Rev Respir Dis 117: 429, 1978.
74. Bates DV, Macklem PT, Christie RV: Respiratory Function in Disease: An Introduction to the Integrated Study of the Lung. 2nd ed. Philadelphia, WB Saunders, 1971.
75. Fisher ER, Watkins G, Lam NV, et al: Objective pathological diagnosis of coal workers' pneumoconiosis. JAMA 245: 1829, 1981.
76. Gaensler EA, Cadigan JB, Sasahara AA, et al: Graphite pneumoconiosis of electrotypers. Am J Med 41: 864, 1966.
77. Miller AA, Ramsden F: Carbon pneumoconiosis. Br J Ind Med 18: 103, 1961.
78. Watson AJ, Black J, Doig AT, et al: Pneumoconiosis in carbon electrode makers. Br J Ind Med 16: 274, 1959.
79. Golden EB, Varnock ML, Hulett LD Jr, et al: Fly ash lung: A new pneumoconiosis? Am Rev Respir Dis 125: 108, 1982.
80. Green FHY, Laqueur WA: Coal workers' pneumoconiosis. Pathol Annu 15: 333, 1980.
81. Naeye RL, Mahon JK, Dellinger WS: Rank of coal and coal workers' pneumoconiosis. Am Rev Respir Dis 103: 350, 1971.
82. Banks DE, Bauer MA, Castellan RM, et al: Silicosis in surface coalmine drillers. Thorax 38: 275, 1983.
83. Seaton A, Dick JA, Dodgson J, et al: Quartz and pneumoconiosis in coal miners. Lancet 2: 1272, 1981.
84. Morgan WKC: Respiratory disease in coal miners. JAMA 231: 1347, 1975.
85. Pairman RP, O'Brien RJ, Swecker S, et al: Respiratory status of surface coal miners in the United States. Arch Environ Health 32: 211, 1977.
86. Kleinerman J, Green F, Harley RA, et al: Pathology standards for coal workers' pneumoconiosis. Arch Pathol Lab Med 103: 375, 1979.
87. Duguid JB, Lambert MW: The pathogenesis of coal miners' pneumoconiosis. J Pathol Bacteriol 88: 389, 1964.
88. Goodwin RA, Des Prez RM: Apical localization of pulmonary tuberculosis, chronic plumonary histoplasmosis, and progressive massive fibrosis of the lung. Chest 83: 801, 1983.
89. Theodos PA, Cathcart RT, Fraimow W: Ischemic necrosis in anthracosilicosis. Arch Environ Health 2: 609, 1961.
90. Seaton A, Lapp NL, Chang CEJ: Lung perfusion scanning in coal workers' pneumoconiosis. Am Rev Respir Dis 103: 338, 1971.
91. Douglas AN, Robertson A, Chapman JS, et al: Dust exposure, dust recovered from the lung, and associated pathology in a group of British coalminers. Br J Ind Med 43: 795, 1986.
92. Hurley JF, Alexander WP, Hazledine DJ, et al: Exposure to respirable coalmine dust and incidence of progressive massive fibrosis. Br J Ind Med 444: 661, 1987.
93. Davis JMG, Chapman J, Collings P, et al: Variations in the histological patterns of the lesions of coal workers' pneumoconiosis in Britain and their relationship to lung dust content. Am Rev Respir Dis 128: 118, 1983.
94. Seaton A: Coalworkers' pneumoconiosis in Britain today and tomorrow. Br Med J 284: 1507, 1982.
95. Robertson MD, Boyd JE, Collins HP, et al: Serum immunoglobulin levels and humoral immune competence in coalworkers. Am J Ind Med 6: 387, 1984.
96. Wagner JC, McCormick JN: Immunological investigation of coal workers' disease. J R Coll Physicians Long 2: 49, 1967.
97. Lippman M, Eckert HL, Hahon N, et al: Circulating antinuclear and rheumatoid factors in coal miners. A prevalence study in Pennsylvania and West Virginia. Ann Intern Med 79: 807, 1973.
98. Burrell R: Immunological aspects of coal workers' pneumoconiosis. Ann NY Acad Sci 200: 94, 1972.
99. Caplan A: Certain unusual radiological appearances in the chest of coal-miners suffering from rheumatoid arthritis. Thorax 8: 29, 1953.
100. Pearson DJ, Mentnech MS, Elliot JA, et al: Serologic changes in pneumoconiosis and progressive massive fibrosis of coal workers. Am Rev Respir Dis 124: 696, 1981.
101. Fernie JM, Douglas AN, Lamb D, et al: Right ventricular hypertrophy in a group of coalworkers. Thorax 38: 436, 1983.
102. Cockcroft A, Seal RME, Wagner JC, et al: Postmortem study of emphysema in coalworkers and noncoalworkers. Lancet 2: 600, 1982.
103. Leigh J, Outhred KG, McKenzie HI, et al: Quantified pathology of emphysema, pneumoconiosis, and chronic bronchitis in coal workers. Br J Ind Med 40: 258, 1983.
104. Cockcroft AE, Wagner JC, Seal EM, et al: Irregular opacities in coalworkers' pneumoconiosis: Correlation with pulmonary function and pathology. Ann Occup Hyg 26: 767, 1982.
105. Cockcroft A, Lyons JP, Andersson N, et al: Prevalence and relation to underground exposure of radiological irregular opacities in South Wales coal workers with pneumoconiosis. Br J Ind Med 40: 169, 1983.
105a. Young RC Jr, Rachal RE, Carr PG, Press HC: Patterns of coal workers' pneumoconiosis in Appalachian former coal miners. J Natl Med Assoc 84: 41, 1992.
106. Williams JL, Moller GA: Solitary mass in the lungs of coal miners. Am J Roentgenol 117: 765, 1973.
107. Shennan DH, Washington JS, Thomas DJ, et al: Factors predisposing to the development of progressive massive fibrosis in coal miners. Br J Ind Med 38: 321, 1981.
108. Seaton A, Soutar CA, Melville AWT: Radiological changes in coalminers on leaving the industry. Br J Dis Chest 74: 310, 1980.
109. Morgan WKC, Lapp NL: Respiratory disease in coal miners. Am Rev Respir Dis 113: 531, 1976.
110. Morgan WKC, Lapp NL, Seaton A: Respiratory disability in coal miners. JAMA 243: 2401, 1980.
111. Mosquera JA: Massive melanoptysis: A serious unrecognized complication of coal worker's pneumoconiosis. Eur Respir J 1: 766, 1988.
112. Gilson J, Hugh-Jones P: Lung function in coal workers' pneumoconiosis. Medical Research Council, Special Report 290. London, HMSO, 1955.
113. Hurley JF, Soutar CA: Can exposure to coalmine dust cause a severe impairment of lung function? Br J Ind Med 43: 150, 1986.
114. Kibelstis JA: Diffusing capacity in bituminous coal miners. Chest 63: 501, 1973.
115. Susskind H, Acevedo JC, Iwai J, et al: Heterogeneous ventilation and perfusion: A sensitive indicator of lung impairment in non-smoking coalminers. Eur J Respir 1: 232, 1988.
116. Musk AW, Cotes JE, Bevan C, et al: Relationship between type of simple coal workers' pneumoconiosis and lung function. A nine-year follow-up study of subjects with small rounded opacities. Br J Ind Med 38: 313, 1981.
117. Lyons JP, Campbell H: Relation between progressive massive fibrosis, emphysema, and pulmonary dysfunction in coal workers' pneumoconiosis. Br J Ind Med 38: 125, 1981.
118. Miller A, Teirstein AS, Selikoff IJ: Ventilatory failure due to asbestos pleurisy. Am J Med 75: 911, 1983.

119. Craighead JE, Mossman BT: The pathogenesis of asbestos-associated diseases. N Engl J Med 306: 1446, 1982.

120. Young I, West S, Jackson J, et al: Prevalence of asbestos related lung disease among employees in non-asbestos industries. Med J Aust 1: 464, 1981.

121. Peacock PR, Bianciifiori C, Bucciarelli E: Examination of lung smears for asbestos bodies in 109 consecutive necropsies in Perugia. Eur J Cancer 5: 155, 1969.

122. Roberts GH: Asbestos bodies in lungs at necropsy. J Clin Pathol 20: 570, 1967.

123. Becklake MR: Asbestos-related diseases of the lung and other organs: Their epidemiology and implications for clinical practice. Am Rev Respir Dis 114: 187, 1976.

124. Parkes WR: Asbestos-related disorders. Br J Dis Chest 67: 261, 1973.

125. Vianna NJ, Polan AK: Non-occupational exposure to asbestos and malignant mesothelioma in females. Lancet 1: 1061, 1978.

126. Constantopoulos SH, Saratzis NA, Kontogiannis D, et al: Tremolite whitewashing and pleural calcifications. Chest 92: 709, 1987.

127. Yazicioglu S, Ilcayto R, Balci K, et al: Pleural calcification, pleural mesotheliomas, and bronchial cancers caused by tremolite dust. Thorax 35: 564, 1980.

128. Wain SL, Roggli VL, Foster WL Jr: Parietal pleural plaques, asbestos bodies, and neoplasia. Chest 86: 707, 1984.

129. Roberts GH: The pathology of parietal pleural plaques. J Clin Pathol 24: 348, 1971.

130. Craighead JE, Abraham JL, Churg A, et al: The pathology of asbestos-associated diseases of the lungs and pleural cavities: Diagnostic criteria and proposed grading schema. Arch Pathol Lab Med 106: 544, 1982.

131. Warnock ML, Prescott BT, Kuvahara TJ: Numbers and types of asbestos fibers in subjects with pleural plaques. Am J Pathol 109: 37, 1982.

132. O'Brien CJ, Franks AJ: Paraplegia due to massive asbestos-related pleural and mediastinal fibrosis. Histopathology 11: 541, 1987.

133. Gaensler EA, Kaplan AI: Asbestos pleural effusion. Ann Intern Med 74: 178, 1971.

134. Antony VB, Owen CL, Hadley KJ: Pleural mesothelial cells stimulated by asbestos release chemotactic activity for neutrophils in vitro. Am Rev Respir Dis 139: 199, 1989.

135. Warrock ML, Wolery G: Asbestos bodies and fibers and the diagnosis of asbestosis. Environ Res 44: 29, 1987.

136. Churg A, Wright JL: Small-airway lesions in patients exposed to non-asbestos mineral dusts. Hum Pathol 14: 688, 1983.

137. Bégin R, Massé S, Bureau MA: Morphologic features and function of the airways in early asbestosis in the sheep model. Am Rev Respir Dis 126: 870, 1982.

138. Bégin R, Cantin A, Berthiaume Y, et al: Airway function in lifetime nonsmoking older asbestos population. Am J Med 75: 631, 1983.

139. Brody AR, Roe MW: Deposition pattern of inorganic particles at the alveolar level in the lungs of rats and mice. Am Rev Respir Dis 128: 724, 1983.

140. Warheit DB, Chang LY, Hill LH, et al: Pulmonary macrophage accumulation and asbestos-induced lesions at sites of fiber deposition. Am Rev Respir Dis 129: 301, 1984.

141. Warheit DB, George G, Hill LH, et al: Inhaled asbestos activitates a complement-dependent chemoattractant for macrophages. Lab Invest 52: 505, 1985.

142. Chang L-Y, Overby LH, Brody AR, et al: Progressive lung cell reactions and extracellular matrix production after a brief exposure to asbestos. Am J Pathol 131: 156, 1988.

143. McGavran PD, Moore LB, Brody AR: Inhalation of chrysotile asbestos induces rapid cellular proliferation in small pulmonary vessels of mice and rats. Am J Pathol 136: 695, 1990.

144. Lemaire I, Beaudoin H, Massé S, et al: Alveolar macrophage stimulation of lung fibroblast growth in asbestos-induced pulmonary fibrosis. Am J Pathol 122: 205, 1986.

145. McLemore T, Corson M, Mace M, et al: Phagocytosis of asbestos fibers by human pulmonary alveolar macrophages. Cancer Lett 6: 183, 1979.

146. Hnizdo E, Sluis-Cremer GK: Effect of tobacco smoking on the presence of asbestosis at postmortem and on the reading of irregular opacities on roentgenograms in asbestos-exposed workers. Am Rev Respir Dis 138: 1207, 1988.

147. Kilburn KH, Warshaw RH: Severity of pulmonary asbestosis as classified by International Labor Organization profusion of irregular opacities in 8749 asbestos-exposed American workers. Arch Intern Med 152: 325, 1992.

148. Lilis R, Selidoff IJ, Lerman Y, et al: Asbestosis: Interstitial pulmonary fibrosis and pleural fibrosis in a cohort of asbestos workers: Influence of cigarette smoking. Am J Ind Med 10: 459, 1986.

149. McFadden D, Wright J, Wiggs B, et al: Cigarette smoke increases the penetration of asbestos fibers into airway walls. Am J Pathol 123: 95, 1986.

150. Fasske E: Pathogenesis of pulmonary fibrosis induced by chrysotile asbestos. Longitudinal light and electron microscopic studies on the rat model. Virchows Arch 408: 329, 1986.

151. Becklake MR, Toyota B, Stewart M, et al: Lung structure as a risk factor in adverse pulmonary responses to asbestos exposure. A case-referent study in Quebec chrysotile miners and millers. Am Rev Respir Dis 128: 385, 1983.

152. Turner-Warwick M, Parkes WR: Circulating rheumatoid and antinuclear factors in asbestos workers. Br Med J 1: 886, 1965.

153. Doll NJ, Diem JE, Jones RN, et al: Humoral immunologic abnormalities in workers exposed to asbestos cement dust. J Allergy Clin Immunol 72: 509, 1983.

154. Huuskonen MS, Rasanen JA, Juntunen J, et al: Immunological aspects of asbestosis: Patients' neurological signs and asbestosis progression. Am J Ind Med 5: 461, 1984.

155. Lange A, Garncarek D, Tomeczako J, et al: Outcome of asbestos exposure (lung fibrosis and antinuclear antibodies) with respect to skin reactivity: An 8-year longitudinal study. Environ Res 41: 1, 1986.

156. Sprince NL, Oliver LC, McLoud TC, et al: Asbestos exposure and asbestos-related pleural and parenchymal disease. Associations with immune imbalance. Am Rev Respir Dis 143: 822, 1991.

157. de Shazo RD, Morgan J, Bozelka B, et al: Natural killer cell activity in asbestos workers. Interactive effects of smoking and asbestos exposure. Chest 94: 482, 1988.

158. Churg AM, Warnock ML: Asbestos and other ferruginous bodies. Their formation and clinical significance. Am J Pathol 102: 447, 1981.

159. Roggli VL, Greenberg SD, McLarty JV, et al: Comparison of sputum and lung asbestos body counts in former asbestos workers. Am Rev Respir Dis 122: 941, 1980.

160. De Vuyst P, Dumortier P, Moulin E, et al: Diagnostic value of asbestos bodies in bronchoalveolar lavage fluid. Am Rev Respir Dis 136: 1219, 1987.

161. Roggli VL, Johnston WW, Kaminsky DB: Asbestos bodies in fine needle aspirates of the lung. Acta Cytol 28: 493, 1984.

162. Dodson RF, Williams MG Jr, O'Sullivan MF, et al: A comparison of the ferruginous body and uncoated fiber content in the lungs of former asbestos workers. Am Rev Respir Dis 132: 143, 1985.

163. Churg A: Fiber counting and analysis in the diagnosis of asbestos-related disease. Hum Pathol 13: 381, 1982.

164. Hillerdal G: Rounded atelectasis. Clinical experience with 74 patients. Chest 95: 836, 1989.

165. Menzies R, Fraser R: Round atelectasis. Pathologic and pathogenetic features. Am J Surg Pathol 11: 674, 1987.

166. Anton HC: Multiple pleural plaques, part II. Br J Radiol 41: 341, 1968.

167. Rogan WJ, Gladen BC, Ragan ND, et al: U.S. prevalence of occupational pleural thickening: A look at chest x-rays from the first National Health and Nutrition Examination Survey. Am J Epidemiol 126: 893, 1987.

168. Fletcher DE, Edge JR: The early radiological changes in pulmonary and pleural asbestosis. Clin Radiol 21: 355, 1970.

169. Fisher MS: Asymmetrical changes in asbestos-related disease. J Can Assoc Radiol 36: 110, 1985.

170. Bégin R, Boctor M, Bergeron D, et al: Radiologic assessment of pleuropulmonary disease in asbestos workers: Posteroanterior, four view films, and computed tomograms of the thorax. Br J Ind Med 41: 373, 1984.

171. Friedman AC, Fiel SB, Fisher MS, et al: Asbestos-related pleural disease and asbestosis: A comparison of CT and chest radiography. Am J Roentgenol 150: 269, 1988.

172. Aberle DR, Gamsu G, Ray CS, et al: Asbestos-related pleural and parenchymal fibrosis: Detection with high-resolution CT. Radiology 166: 729, 1988.

173. Freundlich IM, Greening RR: Asbestosis and associated medical problems. Radiology 89: 224, 1967.

174. Smith AR: Pleural calcification resulting from exposure to certain dusts. Am J Roentgenol 67: 375, 1952.

175. Kleinfeld M: Pleural calcification as a sign of silicatosis. Am J Med Sci 251: 215, 1966.

176. McLoud TC, Woods BO, Carrington CB, et al: Diffuse pleural thickening in an asbestos-exposed population: Prevalence and causes. Am J Roentgenol 144: 9, 1985.

177. Rockoff SD, Kagan E, Schwartz A, et al: Visceral pleural thickening

in asbestos exposure: The occurrence and implication of thickened interlobar fissures. J Thorac Imaging 2: 58, 1987.

178. Epler GR, McLoud TC, Gaensler EA: Prevalence and incidence of benign asbestos pleural effusion in working population. JAMA 247: 617, 1982.

179. Smith KW: Pulmonary disability in asbestos workers. AMA Arch Ind Health 12: 198, 1955.

180. Krige L: Asbestosis—with special reference to the radiological diagnosis. S Afr J Radiol 4: 13, 1966.

180a. Sampson C, Hansell DM: The prevalence of enlarged mediastinal lymph nodes in asbestos-exposed individuals: A CT study. Clin Radiol 45: 340, 1992.

181. Calhoun J. Personal communication.

182. Rossiter CE, Bristol LJ, Cartier PH, et al: Radiographic changes in chrysotile asbestos mine and mill workers of Quebec. Arch Environ Health 24: 388, 1972.

183. Friedman AC, Fiel SB, Fisher MS, et al: Asbestos-related pleural disease and asbestosis: A comparison of CT and chest radiography. Am J Roentgenol 150: 269, 1988.

184. Staples CA, Gamsu G, Ray CS, et al: High-resolution computed tomography and lung function in asbestos-exposed workers with normal chest radiographs. Am Rev Respir Dis 139: 1502, 1989.

185. Akira M, Yodoyama K, Yamamoto S, et al: Early asbestosis: Evaluation with high-resolution CT. Radiology 178: 409, 1991.

186. McLoud T: The use of CT in the examination of asbestos-exposed persons. Radiology 169: 862, 1988.

187. Lynch DA, Gamsu G, Aberle DR: Conventional and high resolution computed tomography in the diagnosis of asbestos-related diseases. RadioGraphics 9: 523, 1989.

188. Aberle DR, Gamsu G, Ray CS: High-resolution CT of benign asbestos-related diseases: Clinical and radiographic correlation. AJR 151: 883, 1988.

189. Akira M, Yamamoto S, Yokoyama K, et al: Asbestosis: High-resolution CT-pathologic correlation. Radiology 176: 389, 1990.

190. Yoshimura H, Hatakeyama M, Otsuji H, et al: Pulmonary asbestosis: CT study of subpleural curvilinear shadow. Radiology 158: 653, 1986.

191. Solomon A, Goldstein B, Webster I, et al: Massive fibrosis in asbestosis. Environ Res 4: 430, 1971.

192. Robinson BWS, Musk AW: Benign asbestos pleural effusion: Diagnosis and course. Thorax 36: 896, 1981.

193. Hillerdal G: Non-malignant asbestos pleural disease. Thorax 36: 669, 1981.

194. Kleinfeld M, Messite J, Shapiro J: Clinical, radiological, and physiological findings in asbestosis. Arch Intern Med 117: 813, 1966.

195. Enarson DA, Embree V, MacLean L, et al: Respiratory health in chrysotile asbestos miners in British Columbia: A longitudinal study. Br J Ind Med 45: 459, 1988.

196. Picado C, Roisin RR, Sala H, et al: Diagnosis of asbestosis: Clinical, radiological and lung function data in 42 patients. Lung 162: 325, 1984.

197. Bégin R, Cantin A, Berthiaume Y, et al: Clinical features to stage alveolitis in asbestos workers. Am J Ind Med 8: 521, 1985.

198. Johnson WM, Lemen RA, Hurst GA, et al: Respiratory morbidity among workers in an amosite asbestos insulation plant. J Occup Med 24: 994, 1982.

199. Coutts II, Gilson JC, Kerr IH, et al: Significance of finger clubbing in asbestosis. Thorax 42: 117, 1987.

199a. Miller A, Lilis R, Godbold J, et al: Relationship of pulmonary function to radiographic interstitial fibrosis in 2611 long-term asbestos insulators. Am Rev Respir Dis 145: 263, 1992.

200. Wang ML, Lu PL: Lung function studies of asbestos workers. Scand J Work Environ Health 11(Suppl 4): 34, 1985.

201. Barnhart S, Hudson LD, Mason SE, et al: Total lung capacity. An insensitive measure of impairment in patients with asbestosis and chronic obstructive pulmonary disease? Chest 93: 299, 1988.

202. Duji'c Z, Tocilj J, Saric M: Early detection of interstitial lung disease in asbestos exposed non-smoking workers by mid-expiratory flow rate and high resolution computed tomography. Br J Ind Med 48: 663, 1991.

203. Wegman DH, Peters JM, Boundy MG, et al: Evaluation of respiratory effects in miners and millers exposed to talc free of asbestos and silica. Br J Ind Med 39: 233, 1982.

204. Berner A, Gylseth B, Levy F: Talc dust pneumoconiosis. Acta Pathol Microbiol Scand (A) 89: 17, 1981.

205. Wells IP, Dubbins PA, Whimster WF: Pulmonary disease caused by the inhalation of cosmetic talcum powder. Br J Radiol 52: 586, 1979.

206. Nam K, Gracey DR: Pulmonary talcosis from cosmetic talcum powder. JAMA 221: 492, 1972.

207. Hildick-Smith GY: The biology of talc. Br J Ind Med 33: 217, 1976.

208. Vallyathan NV, Craighead JE: Pulmonary pathology in workers exposed to nonasbestiform talc. Hum Pathol 12: 28, 1981.

209. Gamble J, Greife A, Hancock J: An epidemiological–industrial hygiene study of talc workers. Ann Occup Hyg 26: 841, 1982.

210. Alivisatos GP, Pontikakis AE, Terzis B: Talcosis of unusually rapid development. Br J Ind Med 12: 43, 1955.

211. Kleinfeld M, Messite J, Shapiro J, et al: Effect of talc dust inhalation on lung function. Arch Environ Health 10: 431, 1965.

212. Tukiainen P, Nickels J, Taskinen E, et al: Pulmonary granulomatous reaction: Talc pneumoconiosis or chronic sarcoidosis? Br J Ind Med 41: 84, 1984.

213. Lockey JE, Brooks SM, Jarabek AM, et al: Pulmonary changes after exposure to vermiculite contaminated with fibrous tremolite. Am Rev Respir Dis 129: 952, 1984.

214. Davies D, Cotton R: Mica pneumoconiosis. Br J Ind Med 40: 22, 1983.

215. Skulberg KR, Gylseth B, Skaug V, et al: Mica pneumoconiosis: A literature review. Scand J Work Environ Health 11: 65, 1985.

216. Landas SK, Schwartz DA: Mica-associated pulmonary interstitial fibrosis. Am Rev Respir Dis 144: 718, 1991.

217. Sakula A: Pneumoconiosis due to fuller's earth. Thorax 16: 176, 1961.

218. McNally WD, Trostler IS: Severe pneumoconiosis caused by inhalation of fuller's earth. J Ind Hyg 23: 118, 1941.

219. Lapenas D, Gale P, Kennedy T, et al: Kaolin pneumoconiosis. Radiologic, pathologic, and mineralogic findings. Am Rev Respir Dis 130: 282, 1984.

220. Wagner JC, Pooley FD, Gibbs A, et al: Inhalation of china stone and china clay dusts: Relationship between the mineralogy of dust retained in the lungs and pathological changes. Thorax 41: 190, 1986.

221. Edenfield RW: A clinical and roentgenological study of kaolin workers. Arch Environ Health 1: 392, 1960.

222. Sheers G: Prevalence of pneumoconiosis in Cornish kaolin workers. Br J Ind Med 21: 218, 1964.

223. Altekruse EB, Chaudhary BA, Pearson MG, et al: Kaolin dust concentrations and pneumoconiosis at a kaolin mine. Thorax 39: 436, 1984.

224. Oldham PD: Pneumoconiosis in Cornish china clay workers. Br J Ind Med 40: 131, 1983.

225. Bristol LJ: Pneumoconiosis caused by asbestos and by other siliceous and non siliceous dusts. Semin Roentgenol 2: 283, 1967.

226. Olscamp G, Herman SJ, Weisbrod GL: Nepheline rock dust pneumoconiosis. A report of 2 cases. Radiology 142: 29, 1982.

227. Baris YI, Artvinli M, Sahin AA, et al: Diffuse lung fibrosis due to fibrous zeolite (erionite) exposure. Eur J Respir Dis 70: 122, 1987.

228. Casey KR, Shigeoka JW, Rom WM, et al: Zeolite exposure and associated pneumoconiosis. Chest 87: 837, 1985.

229. Stacy BD, King EJ, Harrison CV, et al: Tissue changes in rats' lungs caused by hydroxides, oxides and phosphates of aluminium and iron. J Pathol Bacteriol 77: 417, 1959.

230. Harding HE, McLaughlin AIG, Doig AT: Clinical, radiographic, and pathological studies of the lungs of electric-arc and oxacetylene welders. Lancet 2: 394, 1958.

231. Morgan WKC, Kerr HD: Pathologic and physiologic studies of welders' siderosis. Ann Intern Med 58: 293, 1963.

232. Harding HE, Grout JLA, Davies TAL: The experimental production of x-ray shadows in the lungs by inhalation of industrial dusts: I. Iron oxide. Br J Ind Med 4: 223, 1947.

233. Guidotti TL, Abraham JL, DeNee PB, et al: Arc welders' pneumoconiosis: Application of advanced scanning electron microscopy. Arch Environ Health 33: 117, 1978.

234. Sander OA: The nonfibrogenic (benign) pneumoconioses. Semin Roentgenol 2: 312, 1967.

235. McLaughlin AIG: Iron and other radiopaque dusts. In King EJ, Fletcher CM (eds): Industrial Pulmonary Diseases: A Symposium Held at the Postgraduate Medical School of London, 18–20 September 1957 and 25–27 March 1958. London, J & A Churchill, 1960, pp 146–167.

236. Antti-Poika M, Hassi J, Pyy L: Respiratory diseases in arc welders. Int Arch Occup Environ Health 40: 225, 1977.

237. Low I, Mitchell C: Respiratory disease in foundry workers. Br J Ind Med 42: 101, 1985.

238. Rastogi SK, Gupta BN, Husain T, et al: Spirometric abnormalities among welders. Environ Res 56: 15, 1991.

239. Barrie HJ, Harding HE: Argyro-siderosis of the lungs in silver finishers. Br J Ind Med 4: 225, 1947.

240. Robertson AJ, Whitaker PH: Radiological changes in pneumoconiosis due to tin oxide. J Fac Radiol 6: 224, 1955.

241. Pendergrass EP, Greening RR: Baritosis. Report of a case. AMA Arch Ind Hyg 7: 44, 1953.

242. Lévi-Valensi P, Drif M, Dat A, et al: A propos de 57 observations de barytose pulmonaire. Résultats d'une enquête systématique dans une usine de baryte. (Observations on 57 cases of barium sulfate pneumoconiosis: Results of a systematic investigation in a barium sulfate mill.) J Fr Med Chir Thorac 20: 443, 1966.

243. McCallum RI: Detection of antimony in process workers' lungs by x-radiation. Trans Soc Occup Med 17: 134, 1967.

244. Cooper DA, Pendergrass EP, Vorwald AJ, et al: Pneumoconiosis among workers in an antimony industry. Am J Roentgenol 103: 495, 1968.

245. Waring PM, Watling RJ: Rare earth deposits in a deceased movie projectionist. A new case of rare earth pneumoconiosis? Med J Aust 153: 726, 1990.

246. Cain H, Egner E, Ruska J: Ablagerungen seltener Erden in der menschlichen Lunge und in Tierexperiment. (Deposits of rare earth metals in the lungs of man, and in experimental animals). Virchows Arch 374: 249, 1977.

247. Sulotto F, Romano C, Berra A, et al: Rare-earth pneumoconiosis: A new case. Am J Ind Med 9: 567, 1986.

248. Cullen MR, Komisky JR, Rossman MD, et al: Chronic beryllium disease in a precious metal refinery. Clinical, epidemiologic, and immunologic evidence for continuing risk from exposure to low level beryllium fume. Am Rev Respir Dis 135: 201, 1987.

249. Hasan FM, Kasemi H: Chronic beryllium disease: A continuing epidemiologic hazard. Chest 65: 289, 1974.

250. Frieman DG, Hardy HL: Beryllium disease. Hum Pathol 1: 25, 1970.

251. American College of Chest Physicians Report of the Section on Nature and Prevalence Committee on Occupational Diseases of the Chest: Beryllium disease. Dis Chest 48: 550, 1965.

252. Kreiss K, Newman LS, Mroz MM, et al: Screening blood test identifies subclinical beryllium disease. J Occup Med 31: 603, 1989.

253. Daniele RP: Cell-mediated immunity in pulmonary disease. Hum Pathol 17: 154, 1986.

254. Gary JE, Schatzki R: Radiological abnormalities in chronic pulmonary disease due to beryllium. AMA Arch Ind Health 19: 117, 1959.

255. Tebrock HE: Beryllium poisoning (berylliosis). X-ray manifestations and advances in treatment. Am J Surg 90: 120, 1955.

256. Aronchick JM, Rossman MD, Miller WT: Chronic beryllium disease: Diagnosis, radiographic findings, and correlation with pulmonary function tests. Radiology 163: 677, 1987.

257. Weber AL, Stoeckle JD, Hardy HL: Roentgenologic patterns in long-standing beryllium disease. Report of 8 cases. Am J Roentgenol 93: 879, 1965.

258. Newman LS, Kreiss K, King TE Jr, et al: Pathologic and immunologic alterations in early stages of beryllium disease. Re-examination of disease definition and natural history. Am Rev Respir Dis 139: 1479, 1989.

259. Cotes JE, Gilson JC, McKerrow CB, et al: A long-term follow-up of workers exposed to beryllium. Br J Ind Med 40: 13, 1983.

260. Gaensler EA, Verstraeten JM, Weil WB, et al: Respiratory pathophysiology in chronic beryllium disease. Review of thirty cases with some observations after long-term steroid therapy. AMA Arch Ind Health 19: 32, 1959.

261. Mroz MM, Kreiss K, Lezotte DC, et al: Reexamination of the blood lymphocyte transformation test in the diagnosis of chronic beryllium disease. J Allergy Clin Immunol 88: 54, 1991.

262. Rossman MD, Kern JA, Elias JA, et al: Proliferative response of bronchoalveolar lymphocytes to beryllium: A test for chronic beryllium disease. Ann Intern Med 108: 687, 1988.

263. Abramson MJ, Wlodarczyk JH, Saunders NA, et al: Does aluminum smelting cause lung disease? Am Rev Respir Dis 139: 1042, 1989.

264. DeVuyst P, DuMortier P, Schandene L, et al: Sarcoidlike lung granulomatosis induced by aluminum dusts. Am Rev Respir Dis 135: 493, 1987.

265. Vallyathan V, Bergeron WN, Robichaux PA, et al: Pulmonary fibrosis in an aluminum arc welder. Chest 81: 372, 1982.

266. Miller R: Pulmonary alveolar proteinosis and aluminum dust exposure. Am Rev Respir Dis 130: 312, 1984.

267. Pigott GH, Gaskell BA, Ishmael J: Effects of long term inhalation of aluminum fibres in rats. Br J Exp Pathol 62: 323, 1981.

268. Musk AW, Beck BD, Greville HW, et al: Pulmonary disease from exposure to an artificial aluminum silicate: Further observations. Br J Ind Med 45: 246, 1988.

269. Gilks B, Churg A: Aluminum-induced pulmonary fibrosis: Do fibers play a role? Am Rev Respir Dis 136: 176, 1987.

270. Jederlinic PJ, Abraham JL, Churg A, et al: Pulmonary fibrosis in aluminum oxide workers. Investigation of nine workers, with pathologic examination and microanalysis in three of them. Am Rev Respir Dis 142: 1179, 1990.

271. Herbert A, Sterling G, Abraham J, et al: Desquamative interstitial pneumonia in an aluminum welder. Hum Pathol 13: 694, 1982.

272. Edling NPG: Aluminum pneumoconiosis: A roentgen diagnostic study of five cases. Acta Radiol 56: 170, 1961.

273. Nilsen AM, Mylius EA, Gullvag: Alveolar macrophages from expectorates as indicators of pulmonary irritation in primary aluminum reduction plant workers. Am J Ind Med 12: 101, 1987.

274. Rizzato G, Lo Cicero S, Barberis M, et al: Trace of metal exposure in hard metal lung disease. Chest 90: 101, 1986.

275. Demedts M: Cobalt lung in diamond polishers. Am Rev Respir Dis 130: 130, 1984.

276. Ruttner JR, Spycher MA, Stolkin I: Inorganic particulates in pneumoconiotic lungs of hard metal grinders. Br J Ind Med 44: 657, 1987.

277. Coates EO Jr, Watson JHL: Diffuse interstitial lung disease in tungsten carbide workers. Ann Intern Med 75: 709, 1971.

278. Cugell DW, Morgan WK, Perkins DG, et al: The respiratory effects of cobalt. Arch Intern Med 150: 177, 1990.

279. Forrest ME, Skerker LB, Nemirott MJ: Hard metal pneumocomiosis: Another cause of diffuse interstitial fibrosis. Radiology 128: 609, 1978.

280. Sprince NL, Chamberlin RI, Hales CA, et al: Respiratory disease in tungsten carbide production workers. Chest 86: 549, 1984.

281. Funahashi A: Pneumoconiosis in workers exposed to silicon carbide. Am Rev Respir Dis 129: 635, 1984.

282. Bégin R, Dufresne A, Cantin A, et al: Carborundum pneumoconiosis. Fibers in the mineral activate macrophages to produce fibroblast growth factors and sustain the chronic inflammatory disease. Chest 95: 842, 1989.

283. Cordasco EM, Demeter SL, Kerkay J, et al: Pulmonary manifestations of vinyl and polyvinyl chloride (interstitial lung disease). Chest 78: 6, 1980.

284. Antti-Poika M, Nordman H, Nickels J, et al: Lung disease after exposure to polyvinyl chloride dust. Thorax 41: 566, 1986.

285. Mastrangelo G, Manno M, Marcer G, et al: Polyvinyl chloride pneumocomiosis: Epidemiological study of exposed workers. J Occup Med 21: 540, 1979.

286. Boutar CA, Copland LH, Thornley PE, et al: Epidemiological study of respiratory disease in workers exposed to polyvinylchloride dust. Thorax 35: 644, 1980.

287. Ernst P, De Guire L, Armstrong B, et al: Obstructive and restrictive ventilatory impairment in polyvinylchloride fabrication workers. Am J Ind Med 14: 273, 1988.

288. Yamadori I, Ohsumi S, Taguchi K: Titanium dioxide deposition and adenocarcinoma of the lung. Acta Pathol Jpn 36: 783, 1986.

289. Redline S, Barna BP, Tomashefski JF Jr, et al: Granulomatous disease associated with pulmonary deposition of titanium. Br J Ind Med 43: 652, 1986.

290. Rode LE, Ophus EM, Gylseth B: Massive pulmonary deposition of rutile after titanium dioxide exposure. Acta Pathol Microbiol Scand (A) 89: 455, 1981.

291. Craighead JE, Adler KB, Butler GB, et al: Biology of disease. Health effects of Mount St. Helens volcanic dust. Lab Invest 48: 5, 1983.

292. Eisele JW, O'Halloran RL, Reay DT, et al: Deaths during the May 18, 1980 eruption of Mount St. Helens. Med Intelligence 305: 931, 1981.

293. Merchant JA, Baxter P, Bernstein R, et al: Health implications of the Mount St. Helens eruption: Epidemiological considerations. Ann Occup Hyg 26: 911, 1982.

294. Hill JW: Health aspects of man-made mineral fibres. A review. Ann Occup Hyg 20: 161, 1977.

295. Bayliss DL, Dement JM, Wagoner JK, et al: Mortality patterns among fibrous glass production workers. Ann NY Acad Sci 271: 324, 1976.

296. Goldsmith JR: Comparative epidemiology of men exposed to asbestos and man-made mineral fibers. Am J Ind Med 10: 543, 1986.

297. Gross P, Tuma J, deTreville RTP: Lungs of workers exposed to fiber glass. Arch Environ Health 23: 67, 1971.

298. Gross P: Man-made vitreous fibers: An overview of studies on their biologic effects. Am Ind Hyg Assoc J 47: 717, 1986.

299. Barrett TE, Pietra GG, Maycock RL, et al: Case report: Acrylic resin pneumoconiosis: Report of a case in a dental student. Am Rev Respir Dis 139: 841, 1989.

300. Sander OA: Roentgen resurvey of cement workers. AMA Arch Ind Health 17: 96, 1958.

13

PULMONARY DISEASE CAUSED BY ASPIRATION OF SOLID FOREIGN MATERIAL AND LIQUIDS

ASPIRATION OF SOLID FOREIGN BODIES

Aspiration of solid foreign bodies into the tracheobronchial tree occurs most often in small children.[1] Although a fascinating variety of objects have been described, including bone, pencils, rubber tubing, pins, needles, thermometers, plastic toys, and jewelry,[2] the most common is food, usually vegetable. In one review of 160 patients,[3] more than 85 per cent of aspirated bodies were of this type, the peanut being by far the most common.

Several specific foreign bodies deserve special comment. The flowering heads of some grasses possess inflorescences with well-developed terminal spikes. When the grass is aspirated, it projects proximally toward the larger airways, causing the spikes to be inserted farther and farther into the lung periphery, much like a lobster entering a trap. This migration may be so extensive that the grass spike traverses the pleural space and is actually extruded through the skin.[4] Broken fragments of teeth are occasionally aspirated following maxillofacial trauma, particularly by older

children,[5] and roentgenograms of the chest should be obtained as a precautionary measure whenever skull roentgenograms reveal absence or fracture of teeth following trauma. Inhaled candies can be particularly problematic when they dissolve in tracheobronchial secretions, since the resulting viscid fluid can cause significant respiratory obstruction.[6]

Pathologic Characteristics

In the early stages, the airway wall in immediate contact with the foreign body shows edema and a variable degree of inflammatory cellular infiltration or, if ulcerated, granulation tissue; these reactions themselves contribute directly to airway narrowing. Foreign bodies such as peanuts, which are high in fatty acid content, may be associated with an especially severe reaction. Occasionally, the aspirated material becomes incorporated within granulation tissue in the bronchial wall and can appear grossly as a fungating tumor simulating carcinoma.[7] In such cases, the foreign substance usually can be identified histologically in material obtained by endoscopic biopsy.[8] Chronic retention of an aspirated foreign body results in bronchial wall fibrosis and stenosis, usually accompanied by distal bronchiectasis and obstructive pneumonitis.[1, 9]

Roentgenographic Manifestations

In the majority of cases, changes in the lungs reflect the presence of partial or complete bronchial obstruction—atelectasis, with or without obstructive pneumonitis, when the obstruction is acute, and infectious pneumonia with abscess formation or bronchiectasis if it is not relieved.[10] The lower lobes are involved almost exclusively. Contrary to common belief, left-sided aspiration is almost as common as right-sided, a fact that has been attributed to the equality of the right and left bronchial angles in the majority of children up to the age of 15 years.[11]

Some investigators have reported a large number of cases of "obstructive overinflation"[3]; however, because it can be very difficult to obtain roentgenograms of the chest in infants and young children at a point of maximal inspiration, particularly if there is respiratory distress and consequent tachypnea, the authors suspect that this is a spurious observation. Instead, it is likely that in the majority of cases the affected lung is *not* overinflated at a position of full inspiration and that instead the roentgenographic appearances reflect two effects: (1) the ipsilateral lung *appears* larger because roentgenograms are exposed at a position of slight expiration, thus exhibiting air trapping; and (2) the ipsilateral lung exhibits increased radiolucency as a result of oligemia occasioned by hypoxic vasoconstriction (Fig. 13–1).

A variety of ancillary techniques are occasioinally of value in the diagnosis of foreign body aspiration. In a patient in whom a foreign body impacts in a major bronchus, a roentgenogram exposed at inspiration may reveal no abnormality if insufficient time has elapsed for much air to be absorbed. In such circumstances, a roentgenogram exposed at full expiration shows air trapping on the affected side and contralateral shift of the mediastinum. Because of the difficulty in communicating with infants and very young children and the resultant problems in obtaining good quality expiratory roentgenograms, lateral decubitus roentgenography may be particularly valuable. When a child is placed on one side, the dependent hemithorax is splinted, restricting movement of the thoracic cage on that side. As a consequence, in normal children inflation of the dependent lung tends to be less than that of the upper lung. When air trapping is present in a dependent lung, however, the affected parenchyma tends to remain hyperlucent and of large volume. Thus, the presence of an obstructing endobronchial foreign body, as well as which lung is involved, usually is established by bilateral lateral decubitus roentgenography, regardless of the degree of lung inflation at which the roentgenograms

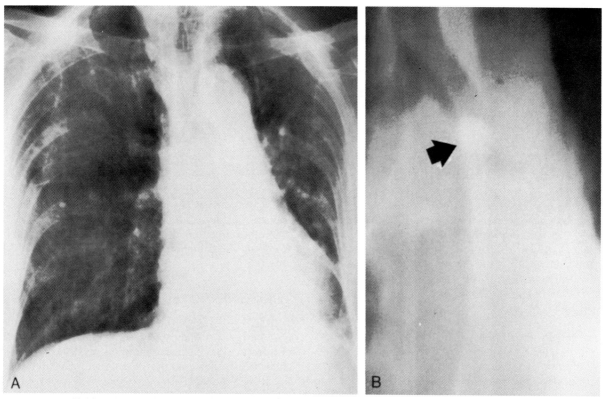

Figure 13–1. Aspiration of a Foreign Body with Impaction in a Main Bronchus. A posteroanterior roentgenogram *(A)* reveals moderate reduction in volume of the left lung accompanied by diffuse oligemia. A linear tomogram in anteroposterior projection *(B)* shows a circular opacity situated within and occupying the whole transverse diameter of the left main bronchus. A pill *(arrow)* was successfully removed bronchoscopically. (Courtesy of Dr. M. O'Donovan, Montreal General Hospital.)

are exposed. Fluoroscopic examination accomplishes the same thing, revealing mediastinal "swing" and restricted diaphragmatic excursion on the affected side on deep respiration. Both computed tomography (CT)[12] and scintiscanning[13] may be of value in selected cases.

Clinical Manifestations

As might be expected, the principal clinical manifestation of aspiration of a solid foreign body is choking, a symptom that almost all adult patients remember; in most instances, choking in children is recognized by nearby adults.[14] Occasionally, an asymptomatic interval may follow aspiration, especially when bronchi are not completely obstructed; such a latent period can extend to several months or even years if the aspirated material is bone or inorganic matter. In this circumstance, if the patient does not recall the actual event of aspiration, diagnosis is much more complicated.

Acute upper airway obstruction caused by aspiration of food (the "café coronary" syndrome[15]) results in air hunger, extreme cyanosis, venous distention, and coma. Risk factors include old age, poor dentition, alcohol consumption, sedative drugs, chronic care institutionalization, and natural diseases, particularly parkinsonism, mental retardation, and severe psychiatric disorders. The sudden onset of such a catastrophic episode can lead to a misdiagnosis of myocardial infarction, though its association with eating should suggest the true diagnosis.

ASPIRATION OF GASTRIC OR OROPHARYNGEAL SECRETIONS

Although it is often complicated by anaerobic bacterial infection, aspiration of oropharyngeal or gastric secretions, with or without admixed food particles, can occur in a pure form and can cause significant pulmonary disease. This develops most often as an isolated event in debilitated patients with a chronic disease such as cancer, in patients with oropharyngeal or airway intubation,[16] and in unconscious patients in association with general anesthesia, epileptic seizure, cardiopulmonary resuscitation,[17] electroconvulsive therapy, emergency endoscopy,[17a] trauma, alcoholic stupor, or cerebrovascular accident.

In addition to these acute, often easily recognizable forms of aspiration, more chronic insidious disease can occur in association with various abnormalities of the upper gastrointestinal tract, including hypopharyngeal (Zenker's) diverticulum, benign or malignant esophageal stricture, achalasia, congenital or acquired tracheoesophageal fistula, neuromuscular disturbances in swallowing, and gastroesophageal reflux.[18] The last-named has been extensively studied and is a well-accepted cause of respiratory disease, particularly in infants and children.[19] In addition to repeated pneumonia, there is evidence that it may cause chronic cough,[20] asthma,[21] and diffuse interstitial fibrosis.[22]

It is likely that aspiration of small amounts of oropharyngeal or gastric contents is common and is not recognized by either patient or physician. For example, of 300 unselected patients undergoing general anesthesia in whom Evans blue dye was injected into the stomach prior to anesthesia, 16 per cent showed bronchoscopic evidence of dye in the tracheobronchial tree postoperatively.[23] It is likely that such aspiration also is frequent in patients with neuromuscular disease[24] and even in normal individuals during sleep.

Pathogenesis

Because of its highly irritating character, aspirated gastric fluid unaccompanied by a significant amount of admixed particulates is usually distributed more or less diffusely throughout both lungs in an explosive fashion as a result of violent coughing and the deep inspiration that such coughing engenders. Since the aspirate is liquid, it typically passes to the most peripheral airspaces, a process that can occur within seconds.

The precise nature of the substances that cause pulmonary disease is unclear. There is no doubt that the hydrochloric acid of gastric juice can cause direct damage to the alveolar wall, with resultant increased alveolocapillary permeability. The observations of many experimental studies suggest that such damage occurs predominantly when the pH of the aspirate is less than 2.5.[25] However, several investigators have documented the development of pulmonary disease following the aspiration of fluid with a considerably higher pH. For example, aspiration of neutralized gastric liquid (pH 5.9) that has been filtered to remove food particles has been shown to result in significant but transient hypoxemia in experimental animals,[26] and pulmonary edema has been documented in patients who have aspirated fluid with a pH as high as 6.4.[27]

When the aspirated material includes an appreciable quantity of food, the pathogenesis of pulmonary damage appears to relate to both a nonspecific reaction to the liquid and a more specific inflammatory response to the various admixed particulates.[28] Gastrointestinal enzymes, such as trypsin and pepsin, are unlikely to have any pathogenetic effect by themselves.[28]

Pathologic Characteristics

Pathologic changes depend on the nature and quantity of the aspirated material and on the frequency with which bouts of aspiration occur. The reaction to aspiration of relatively pure gastric liquid of low pH is characterized by bronchitis and bronchiolitis, frequently accompanied by focal ulceration. In the early stages, the lung parenchyma shows edema and hemorrhage, followed rapidly by the appearance of necrotic debris and hyaline membranes (diffuse alveolar damage). If the patient lives long enough, the exudate undergoes organization. Aspiration of gastric liquid of pH higher than 2.5 results in less severe damage but also has been shown to cause acute pneumonitis and bronchiolitis.[26]

The pathologic reaction differs when there is a substantial amount of admixed particulate material. Edema, congestion, and hemorrhage are early findings and are rapidly followed by an influx of polymorphonuclear leukocytes, which characteristically form a mantle around the foreign material (Fig. 13–2).[29] Foreign body giant cells, often of highly irregular shape and with numerous nuclei, and well-organized granulomas subsequently develop and surround fragments of meat or vegetable material (see Fig. 13–2). Although the edema and hemorrhage of the early stage tend to be more or less diffuse throughout the parenchyma, the granulomatous inflammation often is most severe in

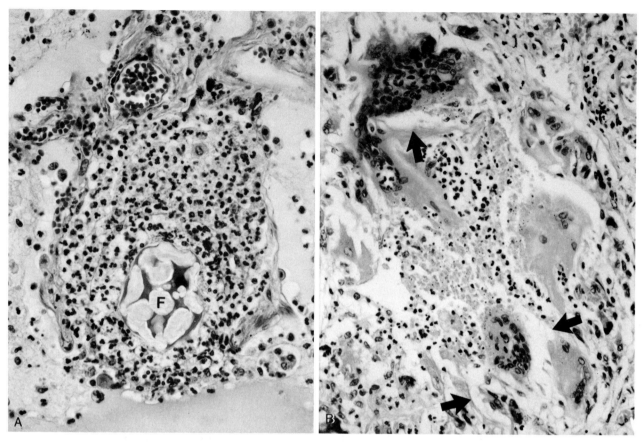

Figure 13–2. Aspiration of Gastric Contents—Inflammatory Reactions. A histologic section of lung parenchyma from a patient with recent aspiration *(A)* shows a somewhat lobulated foreign body (F) (characteristic of a leguminous vegetable) surrounded by numerous polymorphonuclear leukocytes. A section from another patient with relatively remote aspiration *(B)* shows several multinucleated giant cells surrounding necrotic material and multiple polymorphonuclear leukocytes. The vegetable fragments themselves are partly destroyed and are evident only as clear spaces within and adjacent to the giant cells *(arrows)*. (A × 300; B × 250.)

relation to membranous and respiratory bronchioles; thus, some degree of bronchiolitis obliterans is common.

Roentgenographic Manifestations

In the patient who has aspirated a large amount of relatively pure gastric secretion of low pH, the chest roentgenogram reveals generalized but patchy airspace consolidation similar to that of the adult respiratory distress syndrome (ARDS; Fig. 13–3). An anatomic distribution reflecting the influence of gravity may or may not be apparent. If the patient is lying in the prone or supine position at the time of aspiration, the highly irritative nature of the aspirate results in widespread dissemination throughout the lungs; however, predominant changes may be unilateral if the patient is lying on one side. Discrete acinar shadows may be present, but most opacities are confluent.[30] The normal size of the heart serves to distinguish the edema from that of cardiac origin. In uncomplicated cases, roentgenographic changes often worsen for several days; thereafter, resolution is relatively rapid, averaging 7 to 10 days in our experience.

In patients who aspirate oropharyngeal secretions or gastric contents with an appreciable amount of admixed food, the roentgenographic changes tend to occur in a more segmental distribution, involving one or more of the posterior segments of the upper or lower lobes (Fig. 13–4). The precise localization depends at least partly on the position of the patient at the time of aspiration.[31] Some degree of atelectasis is present in almost all cases, and the picture can be that of typical bacterial bronchopneumonia (Fig. 13–5). With repeated aspiration, serial roentgenography over a period of months or years shows much variation in the anatomic distribution of segments involved, with disease clearing rather slowly in one segment and appearing anew in another. A residuum of irregular accentuation of linear markings may remain, probably representing either peribronchial scarring or bronchiectasis.

Clinical Manifestations

Acute respiratory distress caused by aspiration of gastric contents of low pH (Mendelson's syndrome) occurs most commonly in patients in a comatose state, often following induction of anesthesia. Intubation does not necessarily protect the lungs, because aspirated material situated within the airway above an inflated cuff can flood the lungs when the cuff is deflated or when it leaks around an inflated cuff.[32] In the early stages, diffuse rales may be heard; once consolidation develops, patchy areas of bronchial breathing

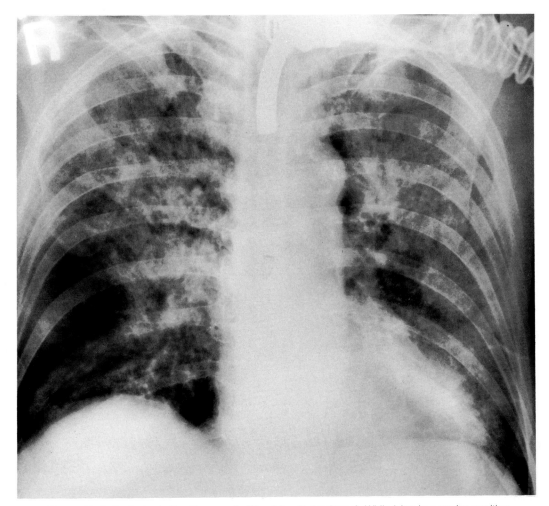

Figure 13–3. Acute Aspiration Pneumonia (Mendelson's syndrome). While lying in a supine position following anesthesia, this 68-year-old man vomited and aspirated considerable quantities of vomitus. Anteroposterior roentgenography performed within 2 hours reveals bilateral airspace consolidation typical of acute pulmonary edema. Although a few patchy shadows are present in the lower lung zones, the predominant involvement is in the upper zones, a distribution that can be explained, at least partly, by the position of the patient at the time of aspiration.

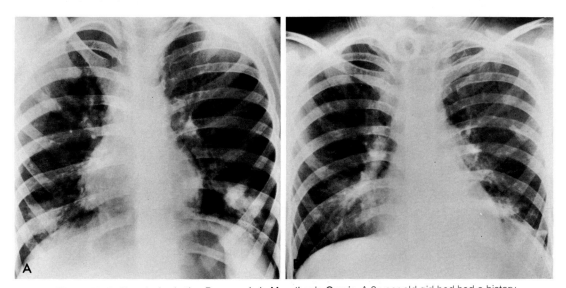

Figure 13–4. Chronic Aspiration Pneumonia in Myasthenia Gravis. A 9-year-old girl had had a history of frequent respiratory infections since infancy, complicated by bronchiolitis and bronchitis. Epilepsy and myasthenia gravis were part of the rather complicated clinical picture. The roentgenographic studies illustrated cover a period of almost 2 weeks. The first *(A)* reveals inhomogeneous segmental consolidation of both lower lobes and of the middle lobe. Approximately 2 weeks later, the disease of the right lower lobe had resolved *(B)* but the middle lobe consolidation had extended; in addition there was new disease in the left lower lobe. Approximately 6 weeks later, the pneumonia of both lower lobes had resolved completely.

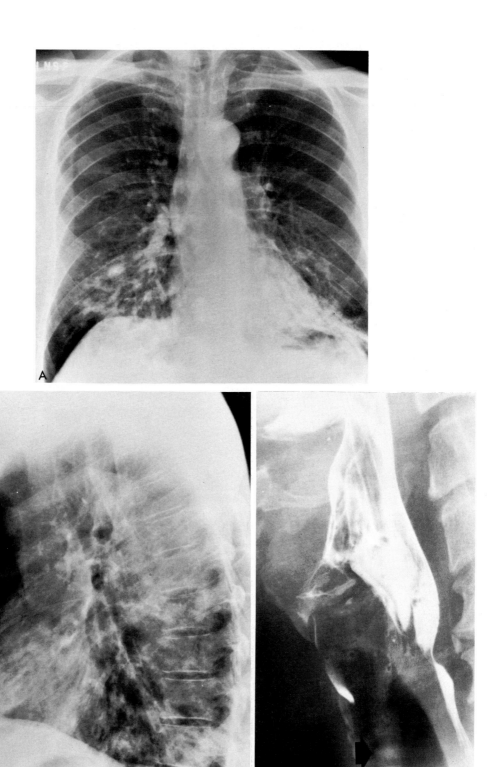

Figure 13–5. Aspiration Pneumonia (Carcinoma of the Pharynx). Chest roentgenograms in postero-anterior *(A)* and lateral *(B)* projections reveal extensive inhomogeneous, segmental consolidation of both lower lobes, the middle lobe, and the lingula. The possibility that this was caused by aspiration was considered, and a barium swallow was performed. A view of the hypopharynx and upper trachea in lateral projection *(C)* shows barium in the upper trachea *(arrow)*.

may be detected. Hypoxemia can be severe. If the patient survives the stage of acute pulmonary edema, bacterial superinfection may develop with cough productive of purulent sputum.

The presence of chronic recurrent aspiration should be suspected in any patient with an unexplained cough or a history of repeated pneumonia. Although this applies particularly to infants and children, it is also pertinent in adults, who may also complain of choking.

Although acute aspiration pneumonia was formerly a disease with substantial mortality, there is evidence that with modern intensive care therapy it has a relatively better prognosis. In the authors' experience, patients who survive usually do not show significant clinical, physiologic, or roentgenographic sequelae; however, recovery may be prolonged, and long-term follow-up has revealed persistent respiratory insufficiency in some patients.[34] During pregnancy, the morbidity appears to be particularly severe and the mortality rate increased.[35]

ASPIRATION OF LIPID

Although the term "lipid (lipoid) pneumonia" is sometimes applied to endogenous accumulation of lipid in relation to a variety of pathologic states, it is restricted here to exogenous pulmonary disease caused by the aspiration of mineral oil (the most common etiologic agent) or of the various vegetable or animal oils present in food or radiographic contrast media.

Etiology and Pathogenesis

Although a variety of cultural[36] and occupational[37] situations predispose to the aspiration of *mineral oil*, disease occurs most frequently when the oil is used medically, particularly as a lubricant in infants with feeding difficulties, in old people who are constipated, and in patients with esophageal disease. Oil-based nose drops are not used as widely now as formerly; however, cases of lipid pneumonia as a result of nasal medication containing liquid paraffin are still seen occasionally.[38] The pathogenesis of mineral oil–related fibrosis is not well understood. Chemically, the substance is a pure hydrocarbon and is believed to be inert, a feature that may explain the lack of airway-mediated cough reflex following aspiration.[39] It has been suggested that release of lysosomal enzymes by dead lipid-laden macrophages may be a factor in causing fibrosis.[39] However, it is also possible that other inflammatory or immune mediator cells may be involved.[39a]

The principal *animal oils* associated with pneumonia are those in milk or milk products. Aspiration of these substances occurs predominantly in infants and young children during feeding. In contrast to mineral oils, animal fats are hydrolyzed into fatty acids, presumably by lung lipases, and their presence in the lung can cause an acute hemorrhagic pneumonitis.[40]

Aspiration of *vegetable oils* occurs in a variety of circumstances and possesses great variability in its capacity to cause tissue damage.[40] With some oils, there is virtually no pulmonary reaction; others cause a tissue reaction similar to that associated with animal oils.[40] It is probable that these

oils are aspirated most commonly during eating or in association with vomiting of gastric contents, in which circumstances they are unlikely to be the sole offending agent. As a result, damage to the lung caused by the oil itself is difficult to assess. An exception is the aspiration of bronchographic contrast media such as Lipiodol (iodized ethyl esters of the fatty acids of poppyseed oil) and Dionosil (propyliodone in an arachis oil), which has been associated with granulomatous pneumonitis.[41]

Pathologic Characteristics

The degree and quality of tissue reaction to aspirated oil are quite variable, being related to the quantity and frequency of aspiration, to the chemical characteristics of the oil itself, and to the complicating effects of other substances that may be aspirated at the same time. The reaction to many animal oils and some vegetable oils is an acute bronchopneumonia characterized by edema, intra-alveolar hemorrhage, and a mixed polymorphonuclear and mononuclear infiltrate. By contrast, aspirated mineral oil is associated with minimal, if any, acute inflammatory reaction; instead, there is an intra-alveolar infiltrate of macrophages that rapidly phagocytose the oil. With time, these macrophages become predominantly interstitial in location and decrease in number. The oil droplets are initially small but eventually coalesce to form relatively large, round or oval droplets situated within multinucleated giant cells (Fig. 13–6). True granulomas do not develop. Fibrous tissue containing scattered collections of lymphocytes surrounds the giant cells. Grossly, the area of fibrosis can form a fairly well-circumscribed, stellate tumor ("paraffinoma") or can be more diffuse and patchy in appearance.

Roentgenographic Manifestations

The typical pattern of disease caused by mineral oil aspiration is relatively homogeneous consolidation of one or more segments, often in precise segmental distribution (Fig. 13–7). In most cases, the lower lobes are predominantly affected, although in debilitated patients in a recumbent position, involvement is likely to occur in the superior segment of a lower lobe or the posterior segment of an upper lobe.[42] The consolidated area may be several centimeters in diameter, with poorly defined or fairly sharply defined margins. Because the oil is carried from the alveoli into the interstitial space by macrophages, a predominantly interstitial pattern can develop in the later stages. Another, almost as common, manifestation is a peripheral mass, also chiefly in the dependent portions of the lung, and sometimes with poorly defined margins simulating peripheral pulmonary carcinoma (Fig. 13–8).[43] Linear shadows radiating from the periphery of such a localized mass result from the interlobular septal thickening caused by infiltration of lipid-laden macrophages and secondary fibrosis. Withdrawal of the medication may be followed by slow but progressive roentgenographic resolution (Fig. 13–9). By dint of its low attenuation, the lipid nature of a pulmonary mass can sometimes be confirmed by CT.[44]

The roentgenographic appearance of vegetable or animal oil aspiration is similar to that seen with aspirated food: segmental airspace consolidation resembling bacterial bronchopneumonia.

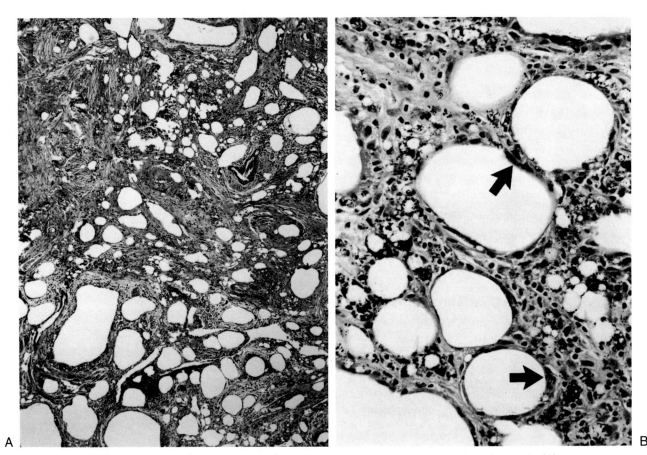

Figure 13–6. Lipid Pneumonia. A histologic section from a well-defined parenchymal nodule *(A)* shows fibrous tissue with admixed lymphocytes and numerous clear spaces of variable size and shape. At higher magnification *(B)*, many of the clear spaces can be seen to be surrounded by a thin rim of cytoplasm containing multiple, somewhat flattened nuclei *(arrows)*. The clear spaces represent foci of mineral oil within multinucleated giant cells. (*A* × 40; *B* × 250.)

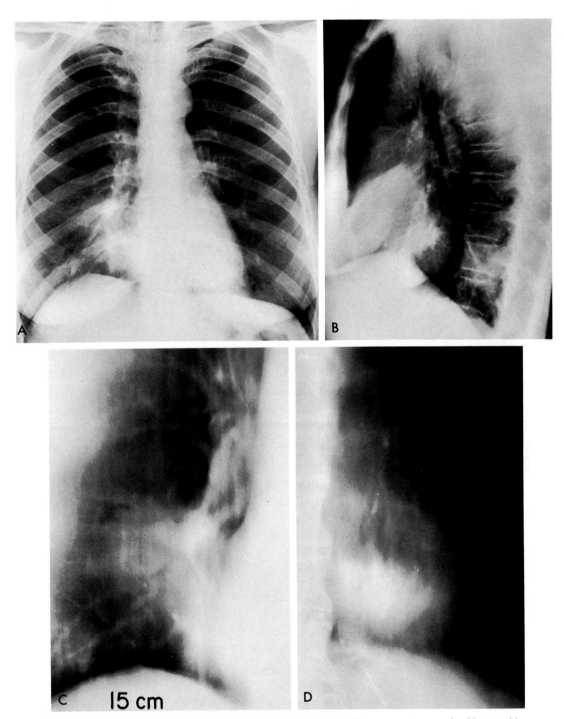

Figure 13–7. Lipid Pneumonia. Posteroanterior *(A)* and lateral *(B)* roentgenograms of a 53-year-old asymptomatic woman reveal rather poorly defined shadows of homogeneous density situated in the middle lobe, the anterior segment of the right lower lobe, and the posterior basal segment of the left lower lobe. Tomographic sections of the right and left lungs *(C* and *D)* in anteroposterior projection show the consolidation to better advantage. Necropsy revealed chronic lipid pneumonia.

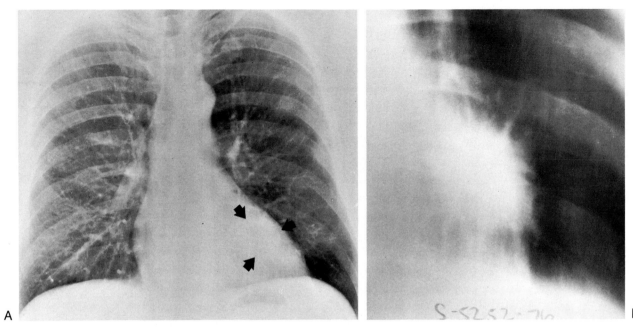

Figure 13–8. Lipid Pneumonia Simulating Carcinoma. A posteroanterior roentgenogram *(A)* reveals a poorly defined homogeneous opacity in the posterior portion of the left lower lobe *(arrows)*. A tomogram in anteroposterior projection *(B)* shows a multitude of linear strands extending outward into contiguous lung, creating an appearance usually identified with pulmonary carcinoma. The resected lobe revealed lipid pneumonia. The patient was an asymptomatic 42-year-old man who had used oily nose drops for many years.

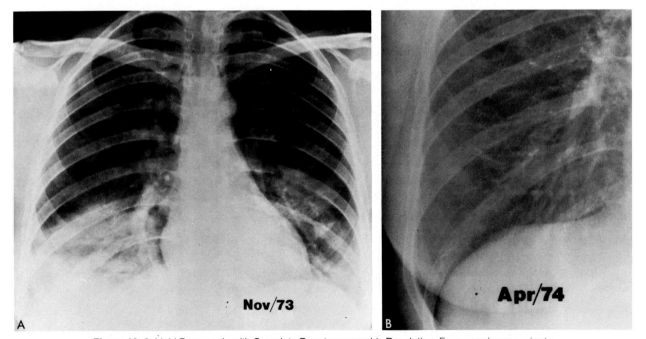

Figure 13–9. Lipid Pneumonia with Complete Roentgenographic Resolution. For several years prior to the roentgenogram illustrated in *(A)*, an asymptomatic middle-aged woman had been using oily nose drops many times a day for a stuffy nose. The roentgenogram reveals massive consolidation of both lower lung zones, the right more than the left. The consolidation is homogeneous except for a well-defined air bronchogram. No treatment was given other than a change in the nose drops to a non oily mixture. Six months later *(B)*, all signs of pulmonary disease had disappeared. (Courtesy of Queen Elizabeth Hospital, Montreal, and Montreal Chest Hospital Center.)

Clinical Manifestations

In most cases of mineral oil aspiration, the patient is asymptomatic, and the abnormality is discovered on a screening chest roentgenogram. Some patients complain of chronic cough and pleuritic pain. If sufficient oil is aspirated over a long period, diffuse pulmonary fibrosis and cor pulmonale may develop.[45]

The finding of fat droplets in macrophages in the sputum or bronchoalveolar lavage fluid[39a] adds weight to the diagnosis, although fat can sometimes be identified in the sputum of normal subjects, and its presence is not incontrovertible evidence of pulmonary disease. Quantification of the number of lipid-laden macrophages can be helpful.[46] Transthoracic needle aspiration or transbronchial biopsy can confirm the diagnosis.

ASPIRATION OF LIQUIDS

Aspiration of Water

Drowning can be defined as death caused by asphyxia as a result of submersion in liquid, provided that the victim succumbs within 24 hours of the submersion episode. *Near-drowning* occurs when an individual survives longer than this, the term still applying if the victim dies more than 24 hours after submersion. So-called *dry drowning* occurs in an individual whose laryngeal reflexes are brisk, resulting in spasm that prevents inhalation of water. If the spasm is sustained until the resulting cerebral anoxia causes paralysis of the respiratory center, the individual can lose consciousness without taking water into the lung. Because such episodes have the highest recovery rate and are reported relatively infrequently, it is difficult to estimate the number of victims who experience dry drowning. The reported prevalence ranges from 10 to 40 per cent of all cases of drowning.[47, 48]

Pathogenesis

In both drowning and near-drowning, in either seawater or fresh water, there is usually a period of apnea and struggling, which may be followed by violent inspiratory effort. Water enters the mouth, is swallowed in large quantities, and is then inhaled. The volume aspirated clearly has considerable bearing on the outcome: in one study of dogs,[49] the chance of survival was very small if the volume of seawater inhaled exceeded 10 mL per pound of body weight; the critical volume of fresh water was 20 mL per pound. These figures correspond to about 1.5 and 3 L, respectively, for a 70-kg human.[50]

The pathogenesis of the physiologic effects of aspirated water differs, depending on whether the water is fresh or salt, at least in experimental animals. Because its tonicity is greater than that of blood, when seawater enters the alveoli water is drawn out of the blood into the airspaces, and ions of sodium, magnesium, calcium, and chloride pass into the blood.[47] At the same time there is a transfer of protein into the alveoli. All of these movements result in rapid hemoconcentration and hypovolemia. There follows slowing of the pulse, a fall in blood pressure, and death within 4 to 5 minutes from hypoxemia and metabolic acidosis. When fresh water enters the alveoli, the situation is reversed. Because of the blood's greater tonicity, inhaled water is immediately absorbed into the circulation, producing marked hemodilution and hemolysis of red cells.[49] The serum potassium level rises considerably, and the serum sodium level falls. Both changes may be factors in causing ventricular fibrillation.[50]

Despite these theoretical and experimental differences between the effects of inhalation of saltwater and fresh water, where it has been possible to carry out examinations in humans, many[51] (albeit not all[51a]) studies have found no evidence of significant electrolyte transfer, hemoconcentration, or hemodilution. Similarly, no clinical differences are seen between fresh water and saltwater drowning victims.[52] Thus, although there is no conclusive evidence regarding the exact sequence of events that occur in humans, it is possible that it is not the same as the one observed in experimental animals.

As discussed on page 741 fluid entering the alveoli acts as an irritant, whatever its tonicity, and probably results in increased permeability of pulmonary capillaries. In addition to the fluid itself, aspirated water may contain debris, such as small marine organisms, sand, mud, and sewage, which can directly cause pulmonary injury and an inflammatory cellular reaction.[53] Since this reaction can take several hours to develop, deterioration in clinical status may follow initial improvement.

Roentgenographic Manifestations

There appears to be no significant difference in the roentgenographic appearances of fresh water and of seawater aspiration.[51] The basic finding is one of pulmonary edema,[54, 55] the severity of which depends, at least in part, on the amount of water inhaled. In the worst cases, there is almost complete opacification of both lungs. Opacities are generally bilateral and symmetric but, in less severe cases, can be predominantly parahilar and midzonal. It is important to note that there may be a delay in some patients before there is roentgenographic evidence of edema, sometimes as long as 24 to 48 hours.[55] In uncomplicated cases, the edema improves rather quickly over 3 to 5 days and resolves completely in 7 to 10 days.[54] In some patients, however, the roentgenographic changes persist or worsen, findings that should suggest the possibility of aspirated foreign material or secondary bacterial pneumonia, with or without ARDS (secondary near-drowning; Fig. 13–10). A few survivors manifest roentgenographic evidence of persistent fibrosis and linear opacities months after recovery.[56]

Clinical Manifestations

Depending on the volume of water aspirated and the duration of submersion, drowning victims may or may not be unconscious when they are first seen by a physician. In the more severe cases, respiratory frequency is generally increased to 30 to 40 breaths per minute during the initial 24 hours and thereafter returns to normal.[51] Fine inspiratory crackles are common, and wheezing can be noted occasionally. Metabolic acidosis is frequent and is presum-

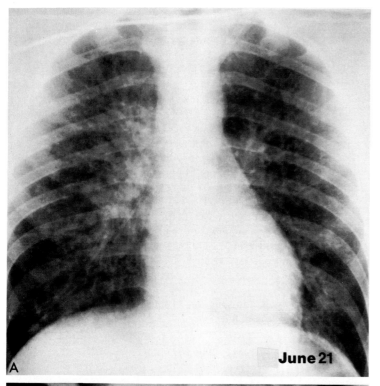

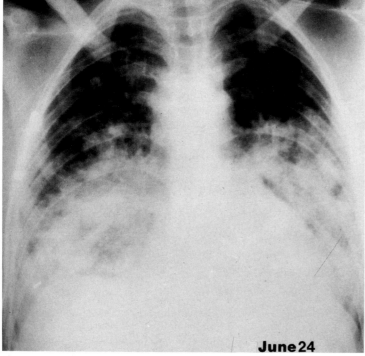

Figure 13–10. Near-Drowning in Fresh Water. A 19-year-old man was immersed in a dirty, badly polluted, fresh-water lake for a period of about 4 minutes before being rescued. The roentgenogram obtained shortly after his arrival in the emergency department *(A)* reveals widespread patchy airspace consolidation evenly distributed throughout both lungs. Heart size and configuration are normal. Three days after the acute episode *(B)*, massive airspace consolidation had developed throughout the lower two thirds of both lungs, and the patient's clinical status had deteriorated markedly, manifesting ARDS and secondary near-drowning.

ably caused by the formation of lactic acid in the hypoxic tissues of a person struggling to survive. Respiratory acidosis is usually not observed in near-drowning patients, probably because they are artificially ventilated before initial arterial blood gas samples are drawn in the hospital.[51] Serum electrolyte levels are usually within normal limits.

Prognosis

Among victims of near-drowning, those who are alert on arrival in the emergency room and those who have a normal chest roentgenogram tend to survive. However, significant hypoxemia[57] is common and the resulting cerebral hypoxia can have important aftereffects. When prolonged submersion occurs in cold water, chances of survival without residual damage are improved, possibly because the hypothermia serves to protect the brain from hypoxic injury.[58] The long-term effects on pulmonary function are variable. In one study of 10 asymptomatic children examined at a mean interval of 3.3 years after submersion accidents, only mild abnormalities of peripheral airway dysfunction were detected; however, 7 of the 10 demonstrated bronchial hyperresponsiveness to inhaled methacholine.[59]

References

1. Weissberg D, Schwarz I: Foreign bodies in the tracheobronchial tree. Chest 91: 730, 1987.
2. Jackson C: Observations on the pathology of foreign bodies in the air and food passages. Based on the analysis of 628 cases. Surg Gynecol Obstet 28: 201, 1919.
3. Brown BS, Ma H, Dunbar JS, et al: Foreign bodies in the tracheobronchial tree in childhood. J Can Assoc Radiol 14: 158, 1963.
4. Hilman BC, Kurzweg FT, McCook WW Jr, et al: Foreign body aspiration of grass inflorescences as a cause of hemoptysis. Chest 78: 306, 1980.
5. Pochaczevsky R, Leonidas JC, Feldman F, et al: Aspirated and ingested teeth in children. Clin Radiol 24: 349, 1973.
6. Mearns AJ, England RM: Dissolving foreign bodies in the trachea and bronchus. Thorax 30: 461, 1975.
7. Chopra S, Simmons DH, Cassan SM, et al: Case reports. Bronchial obstruction by incorporation of aspirated vegetable material in the bronchial wall. Am Rev Respir Dis 112: 717, 1975.
8. Ristagno RL, Kornstein MJ, Hansen-Flaschen JH: Diagnosis of occult meat aspiration by fiberoptic bronchoscopy. Am J Med 80: 154, 1986.
9. Tarkka M, Anttila S, Sutinen S: Bronchial stenosis after aspiration of an iron tablet. Chest 93: 439, 1988.
10. Kürklü EU, Williams MA, le Roux BT: Bronchiectasis consequent upon foreign body retention. Thorax 28: 601, 1973.
11. Cleveland RH: Symmetry of bronchial angles in children. Radiology 133: 89, 1979.
12. Berger PE, Kuhn JP, Kuhns LR: Computed tomography and the occult tracheobronchial foreign body. Radiology 134: 133, 1980.
13. Rudavsky AZ, Leonidas JC, Abramson AL: Lung scanning for the detection of endobronchial foreign bodies in infants and children: Clinical and experimental studies. Radiology 108: 629, 1973.
14. Laks Y, Barzilay Z: Foreign body aspiration in childhood. Pediatr Emerg Care 4: 102, 1988.
15. Mittleman RE: The fatal café coronary. JAMA 247: 1285, 1982.
16. Alessi DM, Berci G: Aspiration and nasogastric intubation. Otolaryngol Head Neck Surg 94: 486, 1986.
17. Lawes EG, Baskett PJ: Pulmonary aspiration during unsuccessful cardiopulmonary resuscitation. Intensive Care Med 13: 379, 1987.
17a. Lipper B, Simon D, Cerrone F: Pulmonary aspiration during emergency endoscopy in patients with upper gastrointestinal hemorrhage. Crit Care Med 19: 330, 1991.
18. McArthur MS: Pulmonary complications of benign esophageal disease. Am J Surg 151: 296, 1986.
19. Barish CF, Wu WC, Castell DO: Respiratory complications of gastroesophageal reflux. Arch Intern Med 145: 1882, 1985.
20. Ing AJ, Ngu MC, Breslin AB: Chronic persistent cough and gastrooesophageal reflux. Thorax 46: 479, 1991.
21. Harper PC, Bergner A, Kaye MD: Antireflux treatment for asthma. Improvement in patients with associated gastroesophageal reflux. Arch Intern Med 147: 56, 1987.
22. Mays EE, Dubois JJ, Hamilton GB: Pulmonary fibrosis associated with tracheobronchial aspiration. A study of the frequency of hiatal hernia and gastroesophageal reflux in interstitial pulmonary fibrosis of obscure etiology. Chest 69: 512, 1976.
23. Culver GA, Makel HP, Beecher HK: Frequency of aspiration of gastric contents by lungs during anesthesia and surgery. Ann Surg 133: 289, 1951.
24. Pruzanski W, Profis A: Pulmonary disease and myotonic dystrophy. Am Rev Respir Dis 91: 874, 1965.
25. Baker GL, Heublein GW: Postoperative aspiration pneumonias. Am J Roentgenol 80: 42, 1958.
26. Schwartz DJ, Wynne JW, Gibbs CP, et al: The pulmonary consequences of aspiration of gastric contents at pH values greater than 2.5. Am Rev Respir Dis 121: 119, 1980.
27. Bond VK, Stoelting RK, Gupta CD: Pulmonary aspiration syndrome after inhalation of gastric fluid containing antacids. Anesthesiology 51: 452, 1979.
28. Teabeaut JR II: Aspiration of gastric contents: An experimental study. Am J Pathol 28: 51, 1952.
29. Knoblich R: Pulmonary granulomatosis caused by vegetable particles. So-called lentil pulse pneumonia. Am Rev Respir Dis 99: 380, 1969.
30. Landay MJ, Christensen EE, Bynum LJ: Pulmonary manifestations of acute aspiration of gastric contents. Am J Roentgenol 131: 587, 1978.
31. Brock RC, Hodgkiss F, Jones HO: Bronchial embolism and posture in relation to lung abscess. Guy's Hosp Rep 91: 131, 1948.
32. MacRae W, Wallace P: Aspiration around high-volume, low-pressure endotracheal cuff. Br Med J 283: 1220, 1981.
33. Campinos L, Duval G, Couturier M, et al: The value of early fibreoptic bronchoscopy after aspiration of gastric contents. Br J Anaesth 55: 1103, 1983.
34. Sladen A, Zanca P, Hadnott WH: Aspiration pneumonitis: The sequelae. Chest 59: 448, 1971.
35. MacLennan FM: Maternal mortality from Mendelson's syndrome: An explanation? Lancet 1: 587, 1986.
36. Miller GJ, Ashcroft MT, Beadnell HMSG, et al: The lipoid pneumonia of blackfat tobacco smokers in Guyana. Q J Med 40: 457, 1971.
37. Jones JG: An investigation into the effects of exposure to an oil mist in workers in a mill for the cold reduction of steel strip. Ann Occup Hyg 3: 264, 1961.
38. Spatafora M, Bellia V, Ferrara G, et al: Diagnosis of a case of lipoid pneumonia by bronchoalveolar lavage. Respiration 52: 154, 1987.
39. Scully RE, Galdabini JJ, McNeely BU: Case 19-1977. Lipoid pneumonia. N Engl J Med 296: 1105, 1977.
39a. Lauque D, Dongay G, Levade T, et al: Bronchoalveolar lavage in liquid paraffin pneumonitis. Chest 98: 1149, 1990.
40. Pinkerton H: The reaction to oils and fats in the lung. Arch Pathol 5: 380, 1928.
41. Felton WL II: The reaction of pulmonary tissue to Lipiodol. J Thorac Surg 25: 530, 1953.
42. Sundberg RH, Kirschner KE, Brown MJ: Evaluation of lipid pneumonia. Dis Chest 36: 594, 1959.
43. Kennedy JD, Costello P, Balikian JP, et al: Exogenous lipoid pneumonia. Am J Roentgenol 136: 1145, 1981.
44. Wheeler PS, Stitik FP, Hutchins GM, et al: Diagnosis of lipoid pneumonia by computed tomography. JAMA 245: 65, 1981.
45. Casey JF: Chronic cor pulmonale associated with lipoid pneumonia. JAMA 177: 896, 1961.
46. Colombo JL, Hallberg TK: Recurrent aspiration in children: Lipid-laden alveolar macrophage quantitation. Pediatr Pulmonol 3: 86, 1987.
47. Miles S: Drowning. Br Med J 3: 597, 1968.
48. Orlowski JP: Drowning, near-drowning, and ice-water submersions. Pediatr Clin North Am 34: 75, 1987.
49. Modell JH, Moya F: Effects of volume of aspirated fluid during chlorinated fresh water drowning. Anesthesiology 27: 662, 1966.
50. Drowning. Lancet 2: 441, 1968.
51. Hasan S, Avery WG, Fabian C, et al: Near-drowning in humans: A report of 36 patients. Chest 59: 191, 1971.

51a. Cohen DS, Matthay MA, Cogan MG, et al: Pulmonary edema associated with salt water near-drowning: New insights. Am Rev Respir Dis 146: 794, 1992.

52. Bradley ME: Near-drowning: CPR is just the beginning. J Respir Dis 2: 37, 1981.

53. Noguchi M, Kimula Y, Ogata T: Muddy lung. Am J Clin Pathol 83: 240, 1985.

54. Hunter TB, Whitehouse WM: Freshwater near-drowning. Radiological aspects. Radiology 112: 51, 1974.

55. Putman CE, Tummillo AM, Myerson DA, et al: Drowning: Another plunge. Am J Roentgenol 125: 543, 1975.

56. Glauser FL, Smith WR: Pulmonary interstitial fibrosis following near-drowning and exposure to short-term high oxygen concentrations. Chest 68(Suppl): 373, 1975.

57. Modell JH, Graves SA, Ketover A: Clinical course of 91 consecutive near-drowning victims. Chest 70: 231, 1976.

58. Bolte RG, Black PG, Bowers CCP, et al: The use of extracorporeal rewarming in a child submerged for 66 minutes. JAMA 260: 377, 1988.

59. Laughlin JJ, Eigen H: Pulmonary function abnormalities in survivors of near-drowning. J Pediatr 100: 26, 1982.

14

PULMONARY DISEASE CAUSED BY DRUGS, POISONS, AND INHALED TOXIC GASES AND AEROSOLS

DRUGS

Drug reactions within the lungs can be divided into six fairly well-defined categories:[1,2] (1) bronchospasm (*see* page 643), (2) systemic lupus erythematosus–like syndrome (*see* page 393), (3) intravenous abuse of oral medications (*see* page 564), (4) Löffler's syndrome (*see* page 427), (5) interstitial or airspace pneumonitis; and (6) permeability pulmonary edema. This chapter is concerned primarily with the latter two categories; drug-induced disease of the pleura, the mediastinum, and the neuromuscular control of breathing are considered in Chapters 18, 19, and 21, respectively.

Mechanisms of drug-induced lung damage are not completely understood but appear to be either immune-mediated (usually associated with a favorable outcome) or cytotoxic (in many cases accompanied by irreparable damage and fibrosis). The toxicity of specific drugs varies, sometimes being dose related and other times not. In many cases, simultaneous use of multiple drugs, sometimes in association with irradiation, a high concentration of oxygen, or concomitant pulmonary disease can make identification of the responsible agent difficult. It is also likely that in many patients, the severity of drug-induced disease in these situations is worse than when a single drug is taken.

There are no specific clinical, functional, or roentgenographic findings in drug-induced pulmonary disease; even pathologic examination of tissue generally serves only to confirm a clinical suspicion and is not itself diagnostic. In most instances, the diagnosis is suspected because of the insidious onset of dyspnea and cough in a patient receiving a drug (or drugs) recognized as being potentially damaging to the lungs. Onset with fever is common, and diffuse rales are often audible. Drugs that initiate capillary leakage tend to be associated with a more abrupt clinical presentation, and physical examination usually reveals profuse rales. Some patients may be asymptomatic, in which case a drug reaction may be suggested by the appearance of a diffuse reticulonodular pattern on the chest roentgenogram or by a significant reduction in diffusing capacity. Since the disease process can extend from the interstitium into the alveoli, the roentgenographic pattern may be mixed or, in the case of those drugs that cause pulmonary edema, predominantly airspace. Although pulmonary dysfunction is generally restrictive and associated with a low carbon monoxide diffusing capacity, the pattern may be mixed. In fact, in some patients in whom the sensitivity to drugs has an immunologic pathogenesis, the insufficiency is predominantly obstructive.

The natural history of drug-induced pulmonary disease is quite variable, some reactions being associated with irreparable damage, disability, and even death, and others with transitory clinical and roentgenographic manifestations that eventually lead to total clinical remission. Even in the latter group, however, follow-up sometimes reveals residual derangement of pulmonary function despite the fact that patients feel well and have normal chest roentgenograms.

The mechanisms of lung injury, pathologic characteristics, roentgenographic manifestations, clinical features, and pulmonary function abnormalities of drug reactions are summarized in Table 14–1.

Chemotherapeutic Agents

Bleomycin

Bleomycin is used primarily in the treatment of lymphoma, squamous cell carcinoma, and testicular neoplasms.[3] The present therapeutic trend is to combine this agent with a variety of other cytotoxic drugs, in which case there may be some synergistic toxic effect; despite this, it is generally accepted that bleomycin is the most culpable con-

stituent. Although pulmonary disease occurs in about 3 per cent of patients in most series,[4] it is dose related and the incidence rises to 35 per cent when the cumulative dose is more than 450 units.[5] Nevertheless, disease has been reported in humans following the administration of as little as 100 units.[6] A reduction in renal function appears to be a major risk factor.[7]

In a minority of patients, pulmonary injury appears to be primarily immune-mediated and consists of reversible eosinophilic pneumonia.[8] In the majority, however, there is rapidly progressive interstitial pneumonitis that is probably related to cytotoxicity. The drug is concentrated in cells of the lung and skin, in which it has the ability to cleave deoxyribonucleic acid (DNA), possibly by generating oxygen radicals.[9] It has been speculated that the production of such radicals is responsible for cell death and, eventually, interstitial fibrosis. Since bronchoalveolar lavage (BAL) fluid from animals[10] and humans[11] receiving bleomycin has shown an excess of neutrophils, it is also possible that cell damage may be the result of oxidants or proteases released by these cells. A synergistic toxic effect is believed to occur when the drug is given simultaneously or sequentially with radiation therapy or a high concentration of oxygen. As a consequence, supplemental oxygen administered to any patient with a history of bleomycin treatment should be at the lowest possible level; in addition, when surgery is undertaken, continuous intraoperative and postoperative monitoring of arterial oxygen tension has been recommended.[12]

The earliest pathologic changes are related to endothelial cell damage and consist of interstitial and alveolar edema and hemorrhage.[13] This histologic stage may be reflected in physiologic evidence of a substantial decrease in the pulmonary capillary blood volume component of the D_{LCO}[14] and in biochemical evidence of a reduction in serum angiotensin-converting enzyme.[15] Endothelial cell damage is soon followed by injury and death of alveolar type I cells and, in severe cases, by collagen production within alveolar septa and airspaces.[13]

The principal roentgenographic abnormality consists of a reticular pattern that tends to progress to patchy or massive airspace consolidation (Fig. 14–1).[6] The lung bases are predominantly involved, most extensively in the costophrenic regions.[16] An unusual manifestation is multiple pulmonary nodules; although these can simulate metastases, they tend to disappear on drug withdrawal.[17]

Symptoms include fever, cough, and dyspnea on exertion and may develop prior to, synchronous with, or following changes in the chest roentgenogram.[1] Basilar rales may be detected. The tendency for deposition of the drug in the skin can cause hyperpigmentation and swelling of the fingers, palms, and soles of the feet. Pulmonary function tests, particularly vital capacity and diffusing capacity, may be the most sensitive method of detecting lung toxicity.

The mortality rate of pulmonary bleomycin toxicity is about 1 to 2 per cent.[19] Death usually follows a prolonged period of increasing dyspnea.

Mitomycin

Mitomycin is an alkylating antibiotic that is used in the treatment of gastrointestinal and, occasionally, breast and cervical malignancies.[1] It is usually combined with vincristine or vindesine and 5-fluorouracil, drugs not generally

Text continued on page 759

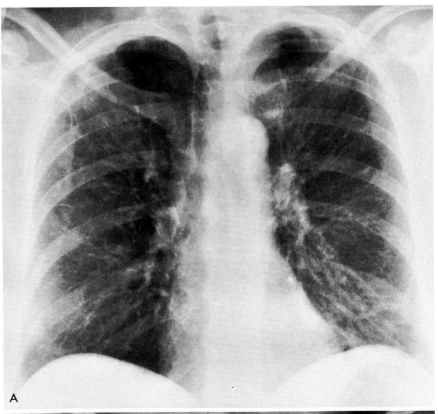

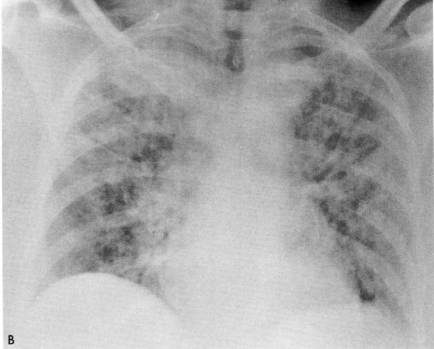

Figure 14–1. Acute Pulmonary Reaction to Bleomycin. Four months prior to the roentgenograms illustrated, large cell lymphoma was discovered in this 55-year-old woman. Shortly thereafter, chemotherapy was instituted that included bleomycin, vincristine, and prednisone. At the end of a 6-week course, she noted the onset of weakness, dry cough, and a stuffy nose. At this time, a posteroanterior roentgenogram *(A)* showed an almost normal appearance of the lungs apart from some prominence of vascular markings. Five days later *(B)* extensive disease had developed throughout both lungs, the pattern of which suggests diffuse interstitial and airspace involvement of the parenchyma. An open lung biopsy showed interstitial pneumonitis.

Table 14–1. DRUG-INDUCED DISEASE OF THE THORAX

Drug	Mechanism of Lung Injury	Pathologic Abnormalities	Roentgenographic Features	Clinical Features	Pulmonary Function Abnormalities	Selected References
Chemotherapeutic Agents						
Bleomycin	Hypersensitivity in a minority; direct toxicity in most (oxidants)	Diffuse alveolar damage; eosinophilic pneumonia in a minority	Combined coarse reticulation and airspace opacities (predominantly lower zonal)	Toxicity in 1–2%; usually progressive dyspnea, rarely acute pulmonary insufficiency; oxygen and radiation have synergistic toxicity	Reduction in vital capacity and diffusing capacity, especially capillary blood volume component	See text
Peplomycin	Same as for bleomycin	Same as for bleomycin	Same as for bleomycin	Toxicity in 5%; same as for bleomycin	Same as for bleomycin	232
Talisomycin	Same as for bleomycin	Same as for bleomycin	Same as for bleomycin	Bleomycin analogue with greater potency but less pulmonary toxicity	Same as for bleomycin	233
Mitomycin	Direct pulmonary toxicity, exact mechanism unknown	Diffuse alveolar damage in some cases	Same as for bleomycin	Toxicity in 3–5%; usually slowly progressive dyspnea and cough, rarely acute; possible synergism with other drugs	Restrictive lung disease; reduced Dlco	See text
Busulfan	Exact mechanism unknown, probably oxidants	Large, bizarre, mononuclear cells (altered type II cells); increased fibroblasts and collagen, type II cell hyperplasia	Bibasilar reticulonodular and, less frequently, airspace opacities	Toxicity in 5%; usually slowly progressive dyspnea, cough, fever, and weakness; usually long-term therapy (average 3–4 years); synergistic toxicity with other cytotoxic drugs and radiation	Restrictive lung disease; reduced Dlco	See text
Cyclophosphamide	Same as for busulfan	Similar to busulfan	Similar to busulfan	Toxicity in 1%; acute or subacute onset of dyspnea, cough, and fever at variable intervals after institution of therapy; synergistic with oxygen and radiation	Similar to busulfan	See text
Chlorambucil	Same as for busulfan	Similar to busulfan	Similar to busulfan	Rare cause of pulmonary toxicity; subacute onset of dyspnea, cough, fever, and anorexia; 50% mortality	Similar to busulfan	See text
Melphalan	Same as for busulfan	Similar to busulfan	Similar to busulfan	Rare cause of pulmonary toxicity; symptoms similar to other alkylating agents	Similar to busulfan	See text
Nitrosoureas (BCNU)	Same as for busulfan	Similar to busulfan	Similar to busulfan	Similar to other alkylating agents	Similar to busulfan	See text
Vinca alkaloids				Vinblastine or vindesine; usually used with other drugs, raising possibility of synergism		234, 235
Antimetabolites						
Methotrexate	Cellular immune response	Alveolitis ± eosinophilia ± granuloma formation; fibrosis 10%	Combined interstitial and airspace disease; rarely hilar node enlargement	Toxicity in 5%; no clear dose-response relationship; may be concurrent skin and liver involvement; 1% mortality	Restrictive; hypoxemia	See text
Azathioprine		Interstitial pneumonitis and fibrosis		High mortality in some studies		236
Cystosine arabinoside				Noncardiogenic pulmonary edema		237
Antiarrhythmics						
Amiodarone	Lysosomal storage disease (phospholipidosis); ? immune-mediated	Alveolitis and type II cell hyperplasia; lysosomal inclusions on electron microscopy	Diffuse reticular and patchy airspace disease	Toxicity in 1–5%; insidious onset of dyspnea; weakness, weight loss. Diagnosis on BAL by lysosomal inclusions in macrophages; usually reversible	Restrictive; decreased Dlco	See text
Lidocaine			ARDS picture	Rare		—
Tocainide		Interstitial pneumonitis and fibrosis	Interstitial disease	Gradual onset; reversible	Restrictive; decreased Dlco	238

Table 14–1. **DRUG-INDUCED DISEASE OF THE THORAX** *Continued*

Drug	Mechanism of Lung Injury	Pathologic Abnormalities	Roentgenographic Features	Clinical Features	Pulmonary Function Abnormalities	Selected References
Antimicrobials						
Nitrofurantoin	Acute: Immune hypersensitivity reaction	Acute: Eosinophilic pneumonia	Diffuse reticular pattern; occasionally pleural effusion	Acute: Hours to days after ingestion; blood eosinophilia + + +, fever, cough, dyspnea, chest pain, and skin rash	Restrictive; decreased DLCO	*See* text
	Chronic: Oxidant damage	Chronic: Interstitial pneumonitis and fibrosis		Chronic: Insidious course; eosinophilia +		
Furazolidone				Similar to nitrofurantoin		239
Sulfasalazine (salazosulfa-pyridine)	Immune hypersensitivity reaction	Bronchiolitis obliterans with organizing pneumonia; tissue eosinophilia and eosinophils in BAL fluid	Patchy airspace consolidation	Dry cough, fever, dyspnea; often skin rash and eosinophilia 1–6 months after starting therapy	Restrictive or obstructive pattern	239a
Sulfonamides, penicillin, para-aminosalicylic acid and tetracycline	Similar to sulfasalazine	Similar to sulfasalazine	Similar to sulfasalazine	Similar to sulfasalazine	Similar to sulfasalazine	240–242
Isoniazid						243
Minocycline		Acute eosinophilic pneumonia				244
Neomycin, streptomycin, dihydrostreptomycin, viomycin, kanamycin, and polymixin B and E	Competitive or noncompetitive blockade at neuromuscular junction		Small lungs; atelectasis	Ventilatory respiratory failure secondary to muscle weakness; patients with myasthenia and renal failure especially susceptible	Decreased lung volumes and inspiratory and expiratory pressures	
Penicillin, cephalosporins, phenylglycine acid chloride, piperazine hydrochloride, psyllium, methyldopa, spiramycin, amprolium hydrochloride, tetracycline, sulfone chloramides	Allergic or nonallergic airway narrowing		Hyperinflation	Bronchospasm in a patient with or without pre-existing asthma	Airflow obstruction	—
Anticonvulsants						
Diphenylhydantoin (phenytoin)	Immune hypersensitivity reaction	Lymphocytic alveolitis; necrotizing vasculitis	Diffuse reticulonodular pattern; mediastinal lymph node enlargement	Fever, dry cough, and dyspnea 3 to 6 weeks after starting therapy; generalized lymph node enlargement; blood eosinophilia; lymphocytes in BAL fluid; hepatitis; resolution of acute symptoms	Restriction and gas exchange impairment; residual gas exchange impairment is possible	69, 71
Carbamazepine	Similar to diphenylhydantoin	Similar to diphenylhydantoin	Similar to diphenylhydantoin	Similar to diphenylhydantoin	Similar to diphenylhydantoin	245
Analgesics						
Acetylsalicylic acid (aspirin, ASA)	Increased pulmonary microvascular permeability secondary to either increased intracranial pressure or altered prostaglandin metabolism	High-protein edema; occasionally a picture simulating desquamative interstitial pneumonia	Airspace pulmonary edema	Usually history of large-dose, long-term ASA ingestion; dyspnea, lethargy, and confusion; rapidly reversible with decreased blood ASA levels	Impairment of gas exchange	*See* text
Nonsteroidal antiinflammatory drugs (e.g., Naproxen, ibuprofen, sulindac)	? Hypersensitivity reaction	Tissue eosinophilia, sometimes with granulomas	Airspace pulmonary edema	Uncommon, but prevalence possibly underestimated; cough, fever, and blood eosinophilia; rapid resolution	Impairment of gas exchange	246, 247

Table continued on following page

Table 14–1. **DRUG-INDUCED DISEASE OF THE THORAX** *Continued*

Drug	Mechanism of Lung Injury	Pathologic Abnormalities	Roentgenographic Features	Clinical Features	Pulmonary Function Abnormalities	Selected References
Antirheumatics						
Penicillamine	Type I immune reaction for eosinophilic syndrome, type III for renal-pulmonary hemorrhage	Interrupted IgG and complement in basement membrane in renal-pulmonary hemorrhage; bronchiolitis obliterans	Three patterns: (1) Reticulonodular with some airspace opacities; (2) diffuse airspace opacity (hemorrhage); (3) hyperinflation (bronchiolitis obliterans)	Toxicity rare and dose related; at least four clinical syndromes: (1) Eosinophilic syndrome; (2) hemoptysis and hematuria (Goodpasture-like); (3) bronchiolitis obliterans (in rheumatoid arthritis); and (4) myasthenia-like	Restrictive or obstructive	*See* text
Gold	Probable hypersensitivity reaction, cell-mediated	Lymphocytic and plasma cell alveolitis ± fibrosis; type II cell hyperplasia	Diffuse interstitial and airspace opacities	Lung toxicity in 1% of patients; one third of patients have blood eosinophilia; presentation can be acute or subacute; fever, cough, and dyspnea; usually prompt resolution	Lung restriction and gas exchange impairment; may be residual impairment	*See* text
Sympathomimetics						
Terbutaline, ritodrine, isoxsuprine	? Acute increase in microvascular permeability or pressure, or both		Airspace pulmonary edema	Used for tocolytic therapy to delay preterm labor; rarely acute pulmonary edema; rapid recovery	Severe hypoxemia	90
Narcotics and Sedatives						
Heroin, methadone, Darvon, naloxone, Librium, Placidyl, paraldehyde and codeine	Increased pulmonary microvascular permeability, ? immune-mediated, ? neurologic	Pulmonary edema	Diffuse airspace pulmonary edema with normal heart size	Accompanies narcotic or sedative overdose; patients are comatose; rapid resolution	Severe hypoxemia; reversible lung restriction	*See* text
Antidepressants and Antipsychotics						
Imipramine, trimipramine, chlorpromazine	Immune hypersensitivity reaction; occasionally increased pulmonary microvascular permeability	Bronchiolitis; interstitial pneumonitis	Patchy airspace consolidation	Cough and dyspnea; acute pulmonary edema associated with the neuroleptic malignant syndrome	—	248
Miscellaneous Drugs						
Hydrochlorothiazide	Possible hypersensitivity reaction	—	Diffuse interstitial and airspace edema	Rare; rapid onset of cough, dyspnea, and cyanosis; associated dermatitis and hepatitis; rapid recovery	Severe hypoxemia	110
Beclomethasone dipropionate	Possible hypersensitivity to 10% oleic acid dispensing agent	—	Airspace consolidation	Eosinophilia and "pneumonia" on switching from oral to inhaled steroid; rapid resolution	—	249
ACE inhibitors (captopril, ramipril, enalapril)	Neutral endopeptidase inhibition; enhanced neuropeptide action	Occasionally eosinophilic pneumonia	—	Cough and bronchspasm; occasionally life-threatening angioedema	Occasionally exacerbation of airway obstruction in asthmatics; increased bronchial hyper-responsiveness	250, 251
Silicone	Increased pulmonary microvascular permeability	Diffuse alveolar damage	Interstitial and airspace pulmonary edema	Following subcutaneous injection in trans-sexual men; fever, chest pain, and dyspnea; ARDS	Gas exchange impairment	252
Cocaine	—	Diffuse alveolar damage	Airspace edema	Rarely implicated in pulmonary toxicity	Reduced diffusing capacity	111, 112
Practolol	—	Pleuropulmonary fibrosis	—	Now withdrawn from market; caused fetal respiratory failure in some cases	Lung restriction	253

Table 14–1. DRUG-INDUCED DISEASE OF THE THORAX *Continued*

Drug	Mechanism of Lung Injury	Pathologic Abnormalities	Roentgenographic Features	Clinical Features	Pulmonary Function Abnormalities	Selected References
Propranolol and other beta-blockers	Beta-adrenergic blockade removing protective effect of chronic beta stimulation in patients with asthma and COPD	Interstitial pneumonitis in some patients	Worsening hyperinflation	Worsening dyspnea, cough, and airway obstruction in patients with pre-existing asthma and COPD; pulmonary edema in patients with pheochromocytoma	Worsening airway obstruction; increased airway hyper-responsiveness	254, 255
Contrast media (ethiodized oil, sodium iothalamate and diatrizoate, meglumine [Gastrografin])	Ethiodized oil causes fatty acid embolism; water-soluble media cause damage because of hypertonicity	Alveolar inflammation and high-protein edema	Diffuse airspace edema	Acute or subacute pulmonary edema; water-soluble media predispose patients with heart disease to pulmonary edema	Hypoxemia, impaired diffusing capacity	*See text*
Disodium cromoglycate	Allergic hypersensitivity reaction	—	Patchy airspace consolidation	Rarely, pulmonary eosinophilia	Hypoxemia	—
L-Tryptophan	Eosinophilic pneumonia and vasculitis	Reticulonodular pattern		Fever, rash, myalgia, weakness and dyspnea	Reduced diffusing capacity	105, 106
Ergotomine, bromocryptine	—	Pleuropulmonary fibrosis	—	—	—	256
Nilutamide	—	? Interstitial pneumonitis	—	Antiandrogen used to treat prostatic carcinoma	Restrictive; hyoxemia	257

regarded as being toxic to the lungs[1] but perhaps capable of exerting a synergistic effect. Pulmonary toxicity is not dose related and occurs in 3 to 5 per cent of patients.[20]

The mechanism by which mitomycin induces tissue damage has not been elucidated, but since the drug possesses alkylating properties its mode of action may be comparable to that of cyclophosphamide. Pathologic characteristics are similar to those associated with other cytotoxic drugs and include endothelial damage, necrosis of type I pneumocytes, proliferation of type II cells, and collagen deposition.[20] One group of investigators has described a syndrome consisting of noncardiogenic pulmonary edema, microangiopathic hemolytic anemia, and renal failure, accompanied by immunofluorescence evidence of vascular damage.[21]

In the few descriptions of roentgenographic manifestations of mitomycin-induced pulmonary damage, the pattern has consisted of coarse reticular and airspace opacities with lower zonal predominance. It has been likened to the pattern observed in bronchiolitis obliterans and organizing pneumonia.[1, 20] Pleural effusion has been described in a number of cases and appears to be a more common feature of mitomycin toxicity than of other cytotoxic drug reactions.[1]

Mitomycin toxicity is usually suspected when the patient develops a dry cough and progressive dyspnea, symptoms that may subside with cessation of therapy.[20] Most patients remain afebrile. Other side effects include nausea, vomiting, alopecia, and renal and cardiac toxicity.[20] In a limited number of reports, pulmonary function tests have shown a restrictive defect and decreased DLCO.[1] The mortality rate is said to be about 50 per cent.[1]

Busulfan

This chemotherapeutic agent is used in the treatment of myeloproliferative disorders, particularly chronic myeloge-

nous leukemia. Although clinically recognized pulmonary toxicity occurs in only about 5 per cent of patients, some pathologic studies have revealed a much higher percentage with interstitial fibrosis.[22] Clinically apparent pulmonary toxicity tends to occur only with long-term use, ranging from months to years.[19] Prior use of other cytotoxic drugs or radiation therapy increases the risk.[23] Although toxicity does not appear to be directly dose dependent, no patient treated with a total dose less than 500 mg has developed pulmonary disease in the absence of other potentially toxic influences, such as radiation therapy and other chemotherapeutic agents.[1, 19]

The pathologic finding most characteristic of busulfan-induced pulmonary disease is the presence of large, cytologically atypical type II pneumocytes (Fig. 14–2).[22, 24] Although such pneumocytes are also found in pulmonary disease induced by other drugs, the extent and severity of atypia are generally greater with busulfan. Other pathologic manifestations include interstitial pneumonitis and fibrosis and, in the early stage, edema and hyaline membrane formation.

The chest roentgenogram usually shows a diffuse reticulonodular pattern, sometimes with lower zone predominance (Fig. 14–3). Airspace opacities also can be present and probably occur more often with busulfan than with other drugs.[1]

The onset of disease is usually insidious, the major complaints being dry cough, fever, weakness, weight loss, and dyspnea.[25] By removing an inhibitor of tyrosinase, busulfan accelerates the formation of melanin from tyrosine and thus results in hyperpigmentation of the skin. As a result, some patients resemble those with Addison's disease.[25] Once disease has become evident, lung volumes and diffusing capacity are usually reduced.[26] The mean survival time after diagnosis of pulmonary fibrosis has been reported to be only 5 months.[19]

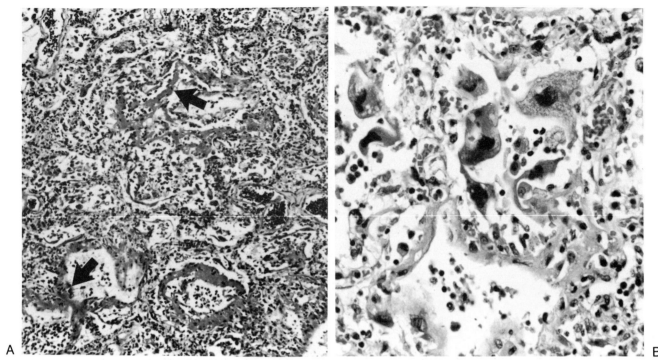

Figure 14–2. Busulfan Toxicity. A histologic section of lung parenchyma *(A)* obtained at autopsy shows a moderate degree of interstitial thickening by lymphocytes, extensive airspace filling by macrophages and other mononuclear inflammatory cells, and multifocal hyaline membranes *(arrows)*. A magnified view of three alveoli *(B)* shows type II pneumocytes to be greatly increased in size and to contain irregularly shaped, hyperchromatic nuclei. The patient was taking 3 mg of busulfan daily for therapy of acute myelogenous leukemia. *(A × 80, B × 275.)*

Cyclophosphamide

Cyclophosphamide, an alkylating cytotoxic drug, is used widely in the treatment of malignancies and autoimmune connective tissue disease. Although it is often combined with other chemotherapeutic agents, the results of both animal experimental and clinical studies indicate that the drug can cause significant pulmonary damage by itself.[27] The incidence of pulmonary toxicity is probably less than 1 per cent.[1] Irreversible pulmonary fibrosis is associated with high total doses of the drug,[28] and there appears to be a synergistic toxic effect with oxygen and probably also with irradiation.[29] The pathologic findings are said to be similar to those of busulfan toxicity.[30]

The chest roentgenogram reveals a diffuse reticulonodular pattern with basal predominance, sometimes with an airspace component (Fig. 14–4).

The clinical onset of pulmonary disease is acute or subacute more often than chronic. The interval between initiation of therapy and development of symptoms varies from months to years.[30] Cough and dyspnea are major complaints and fever occurs in more than 50 per cent of patients.[31] Pulmonary function tests show a restrictive ventilatory defect and a reduced diffusing capacity.[30]

Approximately 60 per cent of patients recover. Early cessation of cyclophosphamide therapy can be followed by resolution of the pulmonary disease, usually in association with corticosteroid administration.[32]

Chlorambucil

This alkylating agent is used chiefly in the treatment of hematologic malignancies and is a rare cause of pulmonary

toxicity.[1] There is no information in the literature to suggest a synergistic effect with other oxidants. The pathologic appearance is similar to that seen with busulfan and cyclophosphamide toxicity.[33] The chest roentgenogram reveals a diffuse, predominantly bibasilar, reticulonodular pattern.[1]

Symptoms tend to be subacute and include anorexia, weight loss, fatigue, fever, cough, and dyspnea,[33] with onset 6 months to 3 years after initiation of therapy.[1] Finger clubbing and rales have been found on physical examination. Pulmonary function tests show a restrictive pattern and a decrease in DLCO. Cessation of drug therapy and administration of steroids can result in resolution of the pulmonary disease[33]; however, about 50 per cent of reported patients have died.[1]

Melphalan

Melphalan, a phenylalanine derivative of nitrogen mustard, is used chiefly in the treatment of multiple myeloma. Since only seven documented cases of pulmonary toxicity have been reported, the incidence of toxicity is obviously very low.[1, 34] The chest roentgenogram has been reported to show a reticular pattern,[1] although a predominantly nodular pattern also has been described.[35]

Symptoms and signs tend to appear within 1 to 4 months of initiation of therapy[1] and are identical to those of chlorambucil, as are pulmonary function test abnormalities.[36] Five of the seven reported patients died of respiratory failure.[1]

Nitrosoureas

These drugs are used chiefly in the treatment of intracranial neoplasms, melanoma, gastrointestinal malignancies,

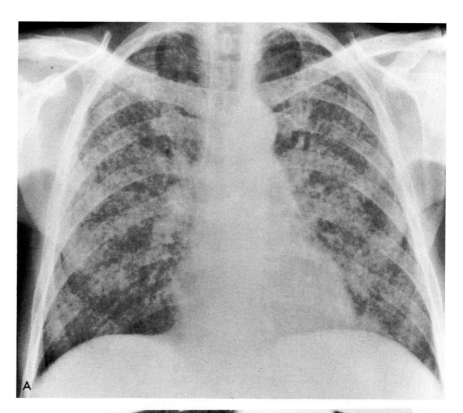

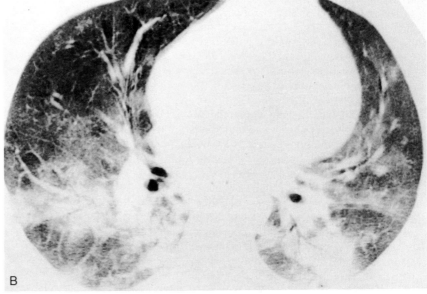

Figure 14–3. Busulfan Toxicity. This 61-year-old woman was being treated for chronic myeloid leukemia with busulfan in a dose of 2 mg three times a day. A posteroanterior roentgenogram *(A)* reveals a widespread coarse reticulonodular pattern throughout both lungs without anatomic predominance. The pattern suggests a predominant interstitial abnormality. At the time of this roentgenogram, she was complaining of severe exertional dyspnea and showed signs of congestive heart failure. *B,* A high-resolution CT (= 1.5-mm collimation reconstructed using a high-frequency resolution algorithm) through the lung bases of a different patient demonstrates bilateral areas of airspace consolidation involving predominantly the posterior lung regions.

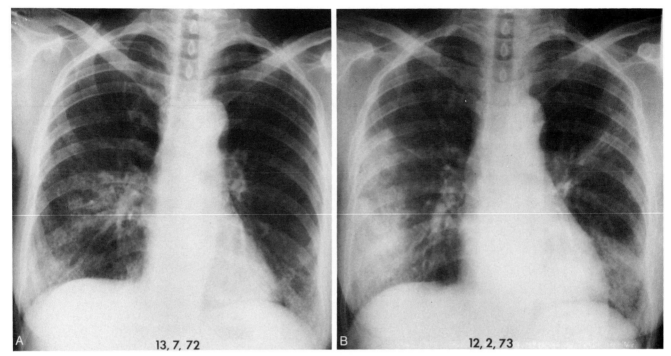

Figure 14–4. Cyclophosphamide-Induced Pulmonary Disease. A posteroanterior roentgenogram *(A)* of a middle-aged woman with lymphoma reveals ill-defined opacities in the midportion of the right lung and at both lung bases. The appearance suggests a combination of interstitial and airspace abnormality. Seven months later *(B)*, the opacities had become largely airspace in character and, on the right side at least, showed considerable peripheral dominance.

and lymphoma.[1] In a 1986 review, the number of cases of pulmonary toxicity was estimated at 70[1]; most were caused by bischloronitrosourea (carmustine, BCNU). This drug is most frequently given in combination with cyclophosphamide, and there may be a synergistic toxic effect on the lungs. Synergism with prior mediastinal irradiation also has been reported.[37] When BCNU therapy is given in a total dosage of less than 1.5 g the incidence of pulmonary toxicity is low[38]; however, more than this amount results in pulmonary fibrosis in as many as 50 per cent of cases.[39] Clinical and roentgenographic evidence of pulmonary damage usually appears some months to years after the institution of therapy.[39]

Pathologic findings include interstitial fibrosis and evidence of damage to epithelial and endothelial cells. Roentgenographic manifestations consist of a reticulonodular pattern with basal predominance. In one series, CT scans showed a pattern of upper zone fibrosis.[39]

Symptoms include dry cough, fatigue, and dyspnea.[40] One series followed 17 children treated with BCNU for brain tumors.[39] Six died of pulmonary fibrosis from 3 to 13 years after treatment, and 8 of the remaining 11 had abnormal chest roentgenograms.[39] The DLCO, arterial partial pressure of oxygen (PaO$_2$), and vital capacity are reduced.[1]

Nitrosoureas other than BCNU rarely cause pulmonary toxicity. CCNU[41] (lomustine) and methyl-CCNU[42] have been reported to induce pulmonary damage in three patients and one patient, respectively; the findings are identical to those described for BCNU.

Antimetabolites

Methotrexate

Methotrexate is used in the treatment of malignancy and a variety of nonmalignant diseases such as psoriasis, pem-

phigus, and rheumatoid arthritis. In 1986, it was estimated that more than 50 cases of pulmonary toxicity had been reported[1]; a prevalence of approximately 5 per cent is probably realistic.[43]

The drug is a folic acid analogue that inhibits cellular reproduction by causing a deficiency of folate coenzymes.[1] It is probable that the mechanism of lung damage is related to this deficiency. There is also evidence that a cellular immune response may play a role in toxicity. A clear-cut dose relationship has not been shown, and a number of reports have indicated that clinical and roentgenographic evidence of reversible interstitial disease can occur with doses as small as 5 to 15 mg per week.[44]

Biopsies of patients with reversible disease show a largely mononuclear inflammatory reaction, with or without granuloma formation and tissue eosinophilia.[19] Diffuse pulmonary edema with hyaline membrane formation also has been seen in patients who have received methotrexate intrathecally.[1]

Initially, the chest roentgenogram reveals a diffuse reticular pattern, indicating widespread interstitial disease (Fig. 14–5). This progresses rapidly to patchy acinar consolidation (Fig. 14–6), which, in time, reverts once again to an interstitial pattern followed by complete resolution.[45] Multiple nodules, hilar lymph node enlargement,[46] and pleural effusion have been described.[47]

The duration of maintenance methotrexate therapy before symptoms and signs of toxicity become clinically apparent ranges from 1 month to as long as 18 years.[48] In the majority of cases the onset is acute or subacute and is characterized by fever, cough, dyspnea, and headache. Digital clubbing has been described,[45] and skin eruptions have been noted in 15 to 20 per cent of cases.[46] Moderate blood eosinophilia is common.[1] Pulmonary function tests show a restrictive pattern,[1] often with a suprisingly low PaO$_2$.

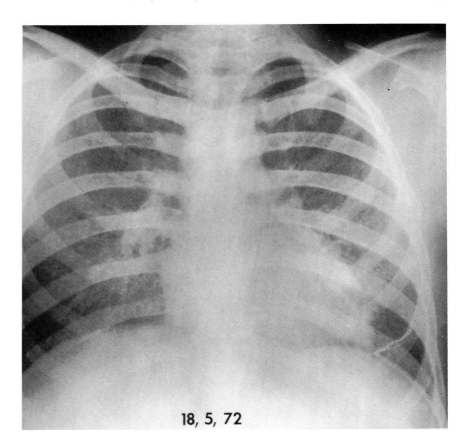

Figure 14–5. Methotrexate-Induced Pulmonary Disease. A posteroanterior roentgenogram reveals an extensive ground-glass opacity throughout both lungs, indicating diffuse interstitial lung disease. Lung volume is reduced. Middle-aged man receiving methotrexate therapy for psoriasis.

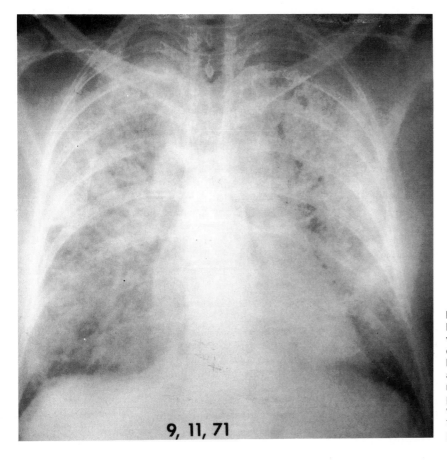

Figure 14–6. Methotrexate-Induced Pulmonary Disease. A posteroanterior roentgenogram reveals massive bilateral airspace consolidation containing a well-defined air bronchogram. The heart size is within normal limits. This appearance is highly suggestive of diffuse airspace pulmonary edema, specifically of the increased permeability type. Two weeks later, following withdrawal of methotrexate therapy for rheumatoid arthritis, the edema had cleared almost completely.

Recovery usually is rapid following withdrawal of the medication, and in some instances occurs even with continuation or reinstitution of therapy. However, in approximately 10 per cent of patients, interstitial fibrosis is either proved pathologically or is assumed to be present because of persistent roentgenographic abnormality.[49] The mortality rate has been estimated at 1 per cent.[19, 46]

Antimicrobial Agents

Nitrofurantoin

The very large number of published reports of pulmonary toxicity from this drug, used in the treatment of urinary tract infections,[2, 50] undoubtedly reflects its common use.[51]

Disease may be acute, developing hours to days after the onset of treatment, or chronic and insidious, becoming manifest after weeks to years of continuous therapy. Clinical presentation, pathologic findings and experimental studies of the former, which is much more common, support a hypersensitivity reaction: onset is abrupt, eosinophilia is found in blood and lung tissue, and resolution follows cessation of therapy. By contrast, the chronic form of disease probably represents direct tissue injury from oxidants, a conclusion based on experimental studies in animals that have shown hyperoxic enhancement and antioxidant suppression of pulmonary damage.[2] Pathologically, most cases show interstitial pneumonitis and fibrosis indistinguishable from idiopathic fibrosing alveolitis.[52]

In both the acute and chronic forms of disease, the chest roentgenogram characteristically reveals a diffuse reticular pattern with some basilar predominance. The pattern resembles interstitial pulmonary edema and, in fact, the rapid clearing that occurs when the drug is withdrawn, particularly with acute disease, suggests that edema plays a considerable role in the production of the roentgenographic opacities.[53] Pleural effusion may be present and, in the acute form, may be an isolated finding.[54]

In the acute form of the disease, fever, dyspnea and cough develop within a few days of continuous medication; a minority of patients have chest pain, skin rash, and arthralgia.[50] Symptoms develop more rapidly in patients who have received the drug previously. The chronic form of the disease has a more insidious onset, dry cough and gradually increasing shortness of breath on exertion developing after months to years of medication.[54] Rales may be heard at the lung bases. Clubbing can be found in a minority of patients. Peripheral blood eosinophilia of 5 per cent or more is present in about 85 per cent of patients with the acute form and about 40 per cent of those with chronic disease.[50] In both acute and chronic varieties, a restrictive pattern is found on physiologic assessment.[50, 54]

The prognosis is excellent in the acute variety, all evidence of disease usually disappearing within 4 to 8 weeks.[55] Death from respiratory failure is rare.[50] By contrast, the mortality rate is about 10 per cent for the chronic disease.

Sulfasalazine

Sulfasalazine is an uncommon cause of pulmonary toxicity.[56, 57] The majority of affected patients present with acute, transitory pulmonary disease accompanied by peripheral blood eosinophilia. Biopsy specimens in some cases have revealed interstitial fibrosis or bronchiolitis obliterans with organizing pneumonia.[56] Lung tissue and BAL eosinophilia also have been reported.

Descriptions of chest roentgenograms in published cases are somewhat vague. In the one patient we have seen, the chest roentgenogram showed patchy airspace opacities confined to the upper lobes; the blood eosinophilia and roentgenographic resolution following withdrawal of therapy simulated Löffler's syndrome.

The clinical presentation consists of dry cough, progressive dyspnea, and fever, often associated with a skin rash; these findings become manifest 1 to 6 months after initiation of treatment. Both restrictive and obstructive changes have been found on pulmonary function testing. Follow-up studies usually reveal a complete return to normal.[2]

Antiarrhythmics

Amiodarone

Amiodarone is an important cause of drug-induced pulmonary damage, the incidence of toxicity ranging from 1 to 6 per cent.[2, 58] The mechanism of lung damage has not been determined. Some authorities[58, 59] consider it to be analogous to a lysosomal storage disease ("phospholipidosis"), a conclusion based in part on the characteristic light and electron microscopic findings. In fact, an analysis of BAL fluid phospholipid content has been proposed as a diagnostic test.[60] Other investigators have found evidence for a disturbance of cell-mediated immunity[61] and for damage mediated by oxidants.[62]

There is strong evidence that toxicity is dose related, a concept that would explain its relatively innocuous features in Europe, where it has been used for many years in maintenance doses approximately half that used in North America. Most affected patients have received 400 mg per day or more before pulmonary disease appeared,[63] and adverse reactions are more common when serum values exceed 2.5 mg per L.[64] Lung damage has its onset months after the initiation of therapy.[2, 59] The drug is deposited throughout the body but mainly in the lungs. It is eliminated slowly, which may explain the interval of 1 month or more after the cessation of therapy before complete roentgenographic and clinical resolution occurs.

Pathologic examination typically reveals inflammation and fibrosis of the alveolar septa, hyperplasia of type II pneumocytes, and the accumulation of intra-alveolar macrophages (Fig. 14–7).[65] These macrophages—and to a lesser extent type II pneumocytes and pulmonary interstitial and endothelial cells—have a distinctive foamy cytoplasm that, by electron microscopy, can be seen to contain numerous distinctive lysosomal inclusions (see Fig. 14–7). Although the inclusion-bearing macrophages can be identified in BAL specimens, their presence is indicative only of amiodarone ingestion and does not necessarily imply drug-related tissue damage.[65]

Chest roentgenograms are almost invariably described as showing a diffuse reticular and patchy airspace pattern, the airspace opacities sometimes being predominant in the upper lobes and resembling those of eosinophilic pneumonia.[66] Pleural thickening and bilateral exudative pleural effusions also have been described.[67] CT findings of high-

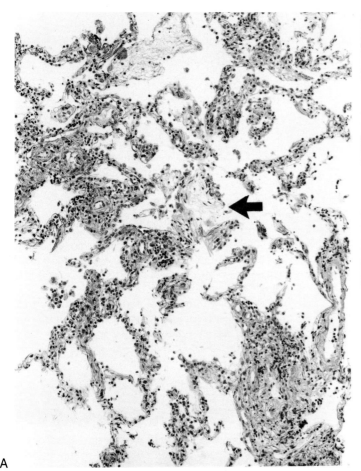

A

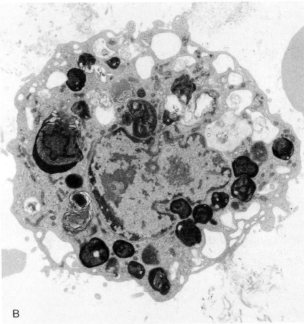

B

Figure 14–7. Amiodarone Toxicity: Interstitial Pneumonitis. A histologic section of lung parenchyma *(A)* shows a moderate degree of interstitial fibrosis and lymphocytic infiltration; focally, apparently active fibrosis is present *(arrow)*. Ultrastructural examination of an alveolar macrophage *(B)* shows the cytoplasm to contain numerous phagosomes, some of which are enlarged, and many of which contain densely osmiophilic material. Lung biopsy from a 63-year-old man who had been taking 200 mg of amiodarone daily for 2 months. *(A × 110; B × 7720.)*

attenuation parenchymal-pleural abnormalities are thought to be related to the iodinated chemistry of the drug.[68]

The clinical presentation is usually that of gradually increasing dyspnea accompanied by a dry cough, weight loss, and weakness; fever and chest pain occur rarely. Nonpulmonary complications are frequent and include blue-gray skin discoloration, photodermatitis, thyroid dysfunction (both hypo- and hyperthyroidism), corneal microdeposits, gastrointestinal symptoms, neurotoxicity (manifested by muscle weakness, peripheral neuropathy, and extrapyramidal symptoms), hepatic dysfunction, and bradycardia.[2, 59]

The white cell count is usually normal or slightly elevated. In the presence of established disease, pulmonary function tests show restrictive impairment[59] and a severe reduction in gas transfer. They are useful in assessing early pulmonary toxicity.[63]

The prognosis following withdrawal of medication and initiation of corticosteroid therapy is excellent, and very few cases of irreversible damage have been reported. Monitoring serum amiodarone concentration may be a valid means of ensuring the drug's efficacy and of avoiding toxicity.[64]

Anticonvulsants

Diphenylhydantoin

Diphenylhydantoin (phenytoin) is used principally to control seizures and is believed to act by stabilizing neuronal membranes.[2] It may produce an acute variety of pul-

monary toxicity with blood eosinophilia which resolves within 2 weeks following drug withdrawal.[69] Pathologic findings include interstitial pneumonitis[69] and necrotizing granulomatous vasculitis.[70]

Chest roentgenograms show a diffuse reticulonodular pattern, in some cases with mediastinal lymph node enlargement.[2, 71] Clinical findings include fever, dyspnea, and a nonproductive cough that appears within 3 to 6 weeks after the onset of treatment. Most patients have manifestations of systemic involvement, including generalized lymph node enlargement, dermatitis, and clinical and laboratory evidence of hepatitis. There may be severe impairment of gas exchange and reduced diffusion.[72]

Analgesics

Acetylsalicylic Acid

Acetlysalicylic acid (aspirin) toxicity occurs particularly in middle-aged and elderly individuals who become habituated as a result of ingesting large doses to alleviate pain. Fatal salicylate-induced pulmonary edema, however, can occur at any age.[73]

Animal experiments[74] and measurements of pulmonary artery wedge pressure[75] and protein content of airway fluid in humans[76] have confirmed the clinical impression that the edema results from increased capillary permeability. The mechanism of increased permeability is unknown, but two possibilities have been suggested:[2, 75] (1) increased intracranial pressure causing neurogenic pulmonary edema as a result of deposition of the drug in brain tissue; and (2) inhibition of prostaglandin production, resulting in vasodilatation and increased permeability. In some cases, hypoproteinemia also may play a role in the capillary leakage.[76] Serum salicylate levels are usually 30 mg per mL or more, but there is no clear dose relationship, since many patients with similar blood levels do not develop edema.[75]

Chest roentgenograms reveal the typical diffuse airspace pattern of pulmonary edema. Patients are dyspneic, lethargic, and confused; they tend to have proteinuria, perhaps reflecting increased capillary permeability in the renal circulation. Since the pulmonary edema responds well to measures that decrease serum salicylate levels, the prognosis is generally good.[75]

Antirheumatic Drugs

Penicillamine

Penicillamine is a chelator of lead, copper, zinc, and mercury and is used to treat heavy metal poisoning, Wilson's disease, and connective tissue diseases, particularly rheumatoid arthritis. Although uncommonly cited as a cause of lung toxicity, it is probably responsible for a greater variety of lung complications than any other drug. In addition to rare examples of lupuslike[77] and myasthenialike diseases,[78] a number of cases of presumed drug-induced alveolitis,[79] bronchiolitis obliterans,[80] and a Goodpasture's-like syndrome[81] have been reported.

Risk of toxicity is not dose related.[2] The mechanism of acute reversible pulmonary disease is very likely a type I immune reaction, whereas limited pathologic findings suggest that the pulmonary-renal syndrome is type III. Histologic findings in patients with the pulmonary-renal syndrome are identical to those of Goodpasture's syndrome; however, immunofluorescence studies with immunoglobulin G (IgG) and complement show an interrupted pattern rather than the linear reaction typical of that condition.

Roentgenographic manifestations are of three types: (1) a reticulonodular pattern, with or without limited airspace opacities, indicating the presence of interstitial disease[82]; (2) overinflation unaccompanied by parenchymal abnormality, associated with advanced bronchiolitis obliterans; and (3) diffuse opacities characteristic of airspace consolidation, typically seen in patients with the Goodpasture's-like syndrome.[2]

Patients with penicillamine-induced pulmonary disease present with insidiously developing cough and dyspnea except for those with pulmonary hemorrhage, whose symptoms come on abruptly. Other manifestations include stomatitis, dermatitis, and, rarely, cholestatic hepatitis.[79] In patients with bronchiolitis, pulmonary function tests can reveal evidence of severe obstruction, even when the chest roentgenogram is within normal limits.[2] The prognosis for patients with the acute hypersensitivity syndrome is excellent on withdrawal of medication; however, many patients with the Goodpasture's-like or bronchiolitis obliterans syndrome die.[2]

Gold

Lung toxicity has been estimated to occur in fewer than 1 per cent of patients receiving this drug.[2, 83] Although the mechanism of pulmonary damage is generally believed to be a hypersensitivity reaction, some *in vitro* studies suggest a cell-mediated immune reaction.[2, 84] Genetic susceptibility is suggested by a strong association between toxicity and the presence of certain major histocompatibility antigens.[85] Risk of toxicity does not appear to be dose related.

Pathologic findings are those of interstitial pneumonitis accompanied by a varying degree of fibrosis.[86] As with penicillamine, there are reports of patients with rheumatoid disease developing bronchiolitis obliterans while receiving gold therapy.[87] The chest roentgenogram has been described as showing diffuse interstitial and patchy airspace opacities.[88]

Unlike the interstitial pneumonitis of rheumatoid disease, that caused by gold usually presents acutely or subacutely. Patients often are febrile and complain of progressive shortness of breath on exertion and a dry cough; almost half have associated dermatitis.[2] Physical examination may reveal rales. A restrictive pattern and hypoxemia are found on physiologic assessment.[86]

The response to withdrawal of the drug is good, death being rare.[87] However, some residual restriction on pulmonary function testing or reticulonodularity on chest roentgenograms may be observed.[88]

Sympathomimetics

The tocolytic betamimetics terbutaline, ritodrine, isoxsuprine, and hexoprenaline are used in the treatment of preterm labor and have been implicated in the development of permeability pulmonary edema.[89, 90] The complication has a very low incidence, and it is probable that in some instances other factors associated with parturition may play a role. The chest roentgenogram reveals classic signs of airspace edema. Symptoms and clinical findings develop within 2 to 3 days of the initiation of therapy and can be associated with extreme hypoxemia; however, the prognosis is excellent if therapy is discontinued.[2]

Narcotics and Sedatives

Opiates and related drugs have long been recognized as causes of pulmonary edema. Compared with many other drugs, toxicity is common: at least 50 per cent of heroin addicts who have taken an overdose develop the complication.[91] Pulmonary edema also has been reported as a result of overdosage of other narcotic analgesics and benzodiazepines.[92, 93]

The mechanism of capillary leakage is uncertain; hypotheses include endothelial damage from the hypoxemia and acidosis that accompany severe respiratory center depression, an immune disorder,[94] and a neurologic abnormality[95] (which could explain the paradoxical development of edema following the administration of the opiate antagonist, naloxone[96]).

Pulmonary edema may be delayed after admission to the hospital, sometimes as long as 6 to 10 hours. The pathologic and roentgenographic manifestations of edema are indistinguishable from those of other etiologies. Roentgenographic resolution characteristically occurs in as brief a time as 24 to 48 hours.

The drug abuser with pulmonary edema is usually admitted in coma, often with frothy, pink fluid oozing from nostrils and mouth. Hypoxemia is severe and is accompanied by mixed acidosis.

Angiotensin-Converting Enzyme Inhibitors

These agents include captopril, enalapril, and ramipril and are used in the treatment of hypertension. They can cause severe coughing[97] and, occasionally, bronchospasm[98] and life-threatening angioedema.[99] Patients who develop cough have underlying bronchial hyper-reactivity.[100]

Contrast Media

Lymphangiography with ethiodized oil (see page 568) may cause a somewhat subacute form of adult respiratory distress syndrome (ARDS) that resembles fat embolism and that may have a similar pathogenesis.[101] A significant drop in diffusing capacity has been recorded that is maximal in 48 hours and returns to normal in 1 month.[102]

Water-soluble contrast media occasionally have been reported to cause pulmonary edema.[103, 104] Although this may represent an idiosyncratic reaction, it is more likely the consequence of the osmolarity of the solutions employed, particularly sodium iothalamate and diatrizoate meglumine (Gastrografin), whose osmolarity is 5 to 10 times that of plasma. In addition, some patients undergoing upper gastrointestinal examination with water-soluble contrast media develop acute pulmonary edema following aspiration of this liquid.

Miscellaneous Drugs

L-Tryptophan

L-Tryptophan is an essential amino acid that is used as a dietary supplement. It has been implicated as the cause of a myalgia-eosinophilia syndrome[105] often associated with diffuse interstitial pulmonary disease.[106, 107] The pathogenesis of toxicity is unknown; however, there is no relation between dose or duration of L-tryptophan exposure and the development of disease, suggesting an idiosyncratic reaction.

Biopsies of a number of tissues and viscera, including the lung, have revealed a largely mononuclear inflammatory infiltrate with a varying admixture of eosinophils.[105, 106] All reports have described small and medium-sized vessel vasculitis and an interstitial pneumonitis and eosinophilia. Chest roentgenograms show diffuse infiltrates (sic), which appear to have a reticulonodular pattern.

Symptoms and signs include fever, rash, severe myalgias, weakness, and shortness of breath. A few patients have had pulmonary hypertension.[106, 107] There may be severe reduction in the diffusing capacity. Respiratory failure can occur, sometimes related to muscle disease.[108] The majority of patients recover on stopping the medication, almost invariably while receiving corticosteroids.

Hydrochlorothiazide

Although hydrochlorothiazide has been implicated as a cause of permeability pulmonary edema, the incidence of such edema must be extremely low.[109] The acute onset and the association with other clinical manifestations such as

hepatitis and dermatitis suggest a hypersensitivity response.[2]

Chest roentgenograms show a combined interstitial and airspace pattern compatible with pulmonary edema; complete clearing generally occurs with cessation of therapy.[2]

One review of the literature found 90 per cent of cases to occur in women.[110] Cough, dyspnea, cyanosis, and rales at the lung bases develop within an hour after the ingestion. In most instances, complete and rapid recovery occurs on stopping the drug; however, some attacks are fatal.[110]

Cocaine

Cocaine and "crack" cocaine have been occasionally implicated as causes of pulmonary edema.[111] Inhalation of freebase cocaine also has been associated with a more prolonged pulmonary syndrome of fever, hypoxemia, hemoptysis, respiratory failure, and diffuse airspace opacities on chest roentgenography. Biopsies of some affected patients have revealed diffuse alveolar damage.[112] A patient has been reported with "crack" cocaine abuse who became ventilator dependent and whose lung on biopsy showed chronic interstitial pneumonitis and fibrosis with extensive infiltration of free silica within histiocytes.[113] Such cases may explain the persistent reduction in diffusing capacity with otherwise normal pulmonary function described in long-term inhalers.[114]

POISONS

Poison-induced pulmonary toxicity almost always occurs as a result of accidental exposure or suicidal intent. The great majority of involved toxic substances are inhaled as noxious gases or soluble aerosols, usually in an occupational setting or from environmental pollution in the vicinity of production sites or vehicular accidents during transport. A minority of poisons reach the pulmonary alveolocapillary membrane by absorption through the skin or gastrointestinal tract or directly by intravenous injection.

Insecticides and Herbicides

Organophosphates

The major examples of this group are parathion and malathion. Poisoning occurs most commonly in agricultural workers during or shortly after the spraying of crops and less often in industrial workers during manufacture and transport; it also occurs accidentally in children and in individuals committing suicide.[115]

Parathion and malathion exert their effect by inhibiting acetylcholinesterase at nerve endings.[116] Symptoms and signs are thus attributable mainly to initial stimulation, and later inhibition, of transmission at cholinergic synapses. Miosis, diaphoresis, increased salivation, bronchorrhea, bronchoconstriction, bradycardia, and hyperperistalsis develop. Muscle fasciculations, particularly of the diaphragm, are followed by fatigability and, eventually, paralysis. Pulmonary edema from increased capillary leakage may occur.[117, 118] Death can result from depression of cholinergic receptors in the central nervous system, from diaphragmatic paralysis, or from ARDS; the effects of the latter two complications are compounded by bronchoconstriction and hypersecretion of airway mucus.

Paraquat

Poisoning from this herbicide usually results from ingestion, either by mistake or for suicidal purposes. In addition, respiratory failure and death occasionally result from absorption of the poison through the skin.[119]

It is believed that paraquat acts like other oxidants (e.g., oxygen and radiation) in damaging lung tissue, a concept supported by the observation that poisoned rats administered oxygen die much more rapidly than those that breathe ambient air.[120] It has even been postulated that paraquat exerts its toxic action by sensitizing the lungs to oxygen at atmospheric pressure.[121] Pathologic features are those of diffuse alveolar damage.

Roentgenographic changes in the lungs of individuals who die within hours of paraquat ingestion show diffuse bilateral airspace consolidation. In those who survive, the chest roentgenogram reveals fine, discrete and confluent granular opacities that appear 3 to 7 days after poison ingestion. Roentgenographic changes characteristically progress rapidly to a pattern resembling severe pulmonary edema (Fig. 14–8).[122] CT scans have documented sequential changes from airspace consolidation to the fibrocystic changes of honeycomb lung.[123] Pneumomediastinum, with or without pneumothorax, frequently occurs during the course of the disease.

In most cases, a history of accidental paraquat ingestion or suicidal attempt can be obtained. Patients present with vomiting, abdominal pain, and burning of the mouth and throat. When the drug is absorbed through the skin, cutaneous lesions are common.[119]

Paraquat poisoning is a serious disease: it has been estimated that about 30 to 55 per cent of affected individuals die from pulmonary edema or renal and hepatic failure.[124] Most who survive manifest persistent radiologic changes[125] and pulmonary dysfunction.[124] Disease in individuals who absorb paraquat through the skin is less acute than that which follows ingestion, perhaps reflecting a smaller dose; however, the outcome is still often fatal.[119]

Other Insecticides

Proproxur (Baygon), a member of the carbamylester family, possesses pharmacologic action similar to that of the organophosphates (binding of acetylcholinesterase). Pulmonary edema, coma, bronchorrhea, and miosis have been described in patients who have attempted suicide with this poison.[126]

Thallium, a drug formerly recognized as a rodenticide and insecticide, is now used industrially in the production of optic lenses, low-temperature thermometers, semiconductors, pigments, and scintillation counters. It has been reported to cause ARDS.[127]

Spanish Toxic Oil Syndrome

In the summer of 1981, a previously unrecognized syndrome characterized by pneumonia, paralysis, and eosinophilia occurred in Spain in epidemic form.[128] Epidemiologic studies strongly indicated that the agent responsible for the disease was rapeseed oil that was denatured by the addition

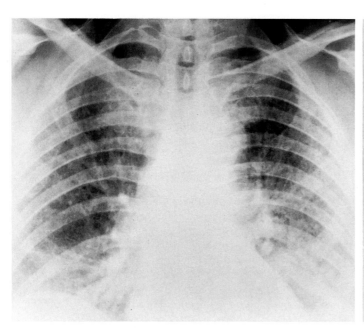
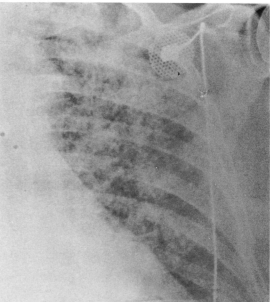

Figure 14–8. Paraquat Poisoning. During the major flood suffered by Brisbane, Australia, in 1974, this 64-year-old man added to his rum the contents of a Coke bottle that was washed up by the floods. Unfortunately, the bottle contained paraquat. On admission to the hospital, a posteroanterior roentgenogram *(A)* revealed an extensive fine granular reticulation throughout both lungs, with a suggestion of patchy airspace consolidation in both bases. Three days later *(B)*, the consolidation had extended considerably and now appeared to affect both interstitium and airspaces in a rather uniform manner. The patient died a few days later. (Courtesy of Dr. Peter Goy and Dr. Sid Moro, Royal Brisbane Hospital, Brisbane, Australia.)

of 2 per cent aniline and was illegally marketed as a cooking oil. During an 8-month period, more than 13,000 persons who had ingested this oil were hospitalized; 277 died, the mortality rate being estimated at 1 to 2 per cent.[128] The epidemic stopped when the oil was removed from the market.

To date, the specific toxin responsible has not been definitively identified. The suggestion that the poison may have been a fatty-acid anilide[129] has not been generally accepted, because oleoanilides are not regarded as sufficiently toxic to induce the high morbidity and mortality.[130] Since *Mycoplasma pneumoniae* infection appeared to be rampant at the time of the epidemic, it has been suggested that the contaminated oil may have acted synergistically with the infection to cause the disease.[131]

Pathologic changes in the early stages of the syndrome are those of pulmonary edema accompanied by a scanty, largely mononuclear, inflammatory infiltrate. Survivors of the acute event may show pulmonary vascular changes consistent with hypertension[132]; in some, lymphocytic vasculitis is also present.[133]

The initial clinical and roentgenographic presentation consisted of "atypical" pneumonia, usually accompanied by fever, rash, myalgia, and marked eosinophilia. In some patients, a period of respiratory failure terminated in death. About 20 per cent of those who survived developed a syndrome of neuromuscular disease, sicca syndrome, and scleroderma-like changes in the skin.[134] Some of these patients developed ventilatory failure as a result of respiratory muscle dysfunction. Other residual manifestations included eosinophilia (at a somewhat lower level than during the acute disease), abnormal liver function tests, and a reduced diffusing capacity suggesting persistent interstitial lung disease.[134]

Fluorocarbons and Hydrocarbons

Poisoning by these agents can take several forms, depending on the particular toxic substance involved, the mode of contamination (inhalation, ingestion, or absorption through the skin), and the dose-time relationship of exposure. Four major forms are recognized: (1) ingestion by young children of halogenated aromatic hydrocarbons (petroleum products); (2) acute inhalation by adolescents and adults of chlorinated volatile hydrocarbons; (3) long-term inhalation of aliphatic and aromatic hydrocarbons in addicts and persons exposed at work; and (4) long-term inhalation of chlorinated hydrocarbons, again in an occupational setting.

Ingestion. It has been estimated that 5 per cent of all poisonings in children are caused by ingestion of petroleum products such as kerosene, gasoline, furniture polish, lighter fluid, and cleaning fluid. In most instances, pulmonary toxicity directly follows aspiration of the poison following emesis; however, some experimental studies suggest that damage also may follow absorption from the intestinal tract followed by transport to the pulmonary endothelium.[135]

The chest roentgenogram is usually found to be abnormal within an hour of hydrocarbon ingestion. The typical pattern is one of patchy airspace consolidation characteristic of pulmonary edema, involving predominantly the basal portions of the lungs, usually bilaterally symmetrically. Res-

olution tends to be slow (up to 2 weeks) and usually lags well behind clinical improvement. In one series,[136] 134 (40 per cent) of 338 children with hydrocarbon ingestion developed acute pneumonia; of these, 14 demonstrated pneumatocele formation during resolution of the pneumonia. The pneumatoceles were often large, septate, and irregular, and some contained a fluid level.

Fortunately, most children suspected of ingesting petroleum products are not seriously affected. For example, in one series of 950 patients,[137] only 15 per cent had abnormal chest roentgenograms, and half of these remained asymptomatic. In the absence of witnesses to the incident, the diagnosis may be suspected from the odor of the offending agent on the child's breath. Vomiting follows shortly after ingestion and presumably is associated with aspiration. There is a positive correlation among the amount of hydrocarbon ingested, the severity of clinical findings, and the extent of roentgenographic abnormalities.[138] A follow-up study of 14 asymptomatic children 10 years after an episode of kerosene ingestion showed subclinical functional impairment of small airways that seemed to be related to the severity of the acute insult.[139]

Inhalation. Fluorocarbons and hydrocarbons are perhaps most commonly inhaled for "kicks" by adolescents and young adults. The hydrocarbons abused include various cements, glues, lacquers, paints, fingernail polish remover, lighter and cleaning fluids, gasoline, and antifreeze. Fluorocarbons (freons) are used as propellants in a great variety of commercial products packaged in aerosol cans and are usually inhaled from plastic bags. Occupational exposure to inhaled hydrocarbons in industries such as cable production can also cause disease.[140]

The major health hazard of inhaled hydrocarbons lies in their action on the myocardium.[141] Not only may conduction be impaired, but cardiac muscle becomes sensitive to sympathomimetic amines, resulting in arrhythmias. Since catecholamines are recognized inducers of cardiac arrhythmias, the combination of volatile hydrocarbons and bronchodilators is likely to be particularly hazardous.

In addition to arrhythmia and sudden death, inhalation of these substances can cause permeability pulmonary edema[142] and, with repeated abuse, interstitial pneumonitis[143] and fibrosis.[144] A chronic diffuse nodular pattern on chest roentgenograms also has been reported in persons who indulge in "fire breathing," a practice involving the ignition of a rapidly exhaled mouthful of a volatile hydrocarbon.[145]

Polychlorinated biphenyls (PCBs) are chlorinated aromatic hydrocarbon compounds that can exert deleterious effects on the lungs by either inhalation or absorption through the skin. Workers exposed to PCBs in power capacitor manufacturing develop cough and expectoration that correlate with blood levels of PCBs.[146] In one study of pulmonary function of 243 workers exposed to PCBs during a mean term of employment of more than 15 years, 34 workers (14 per cent) showed reduced forced vital capacity (FVC) of less than 80 per cent of predicted.[147]

INHALED TOXIC GASES AND AEROSOLS

Several gases and aerosols can cause acute (and sometimes chronic) damage to the pulmonary airways and parenchyma. Although the concentration of the gas or aerosol and the duration of exposure are the chief factors that determine the clinical presentation and pulmonary pathology, these also depend to some extent on their chemical composition. Some substances—particularly those that are highly soluble, such as sulfur dioxide, ammonia, and chlorine—are so irritating to the mucous membranes of the nose that, on exposure, individuals tend to stop breathing and try to run away, thus reducing the risk of pulmonary damage. By contrast, less soluble gases—including phosgene, nitrogen dioxide, ozone, and highly concentrated oxygen—may be inhaled deeply into the lungs before the irritating effect is perceived.

The form of pulmonary disease that results from inhalation of these toxic substances is variable. In many instances, extensive damage to the alveolocapillary membrane results in permeability pulmonary edema. In other cases, the chemical injury appears to affect predominantly the airways, resulting in bronchitis and bronchiolitis, sometimes complicated by atelectasis and bacterial pneumonia. Patients who survive the acute insult may feel relatively well for about 3 weeks and then suffer abrupt clinical deterioration, with cough, shortness of breath, and fever, a delayed development reflected pathologically by bronchiolitis obliterans. This complication also can occur in individuals with diffuse pulmonary edema. In addition to these abnormalities, it is probable that repeated exposure to a low concentration of certain gases or aerosols can cause more insidious irritation of the airways, with the development of chronic bronchitis.

Oxidants

Oxygen, ozone, and nitrogen dioxide have the potential to damage tissue by producing highly reactive metabolic products of oxygen such as hydrogen peroxide, superoxide radical, hydroxyl radical, and singlet excited oxygen.[148, 149] Although these oxygen radicals are normally present in small amounts, intracellular production increases markedly under hyperoxic conditions, resulting in peroxidation of polyunsaturated lipids situated within the cell or on the cell membrane, depolymerization of mucopolysaccharides, protein sulfhydryl oxidation and cross-linking (resulting in enzyme inactivation), and nucleic acid damage.

Animals exposed to a low concentration of ozone[150] or to one atmosphere of oxygen[151] develop a variety of histologic changes: ciliated cells become vacuolated, mitochondria become condensed, type I alveolar epithelial cells become swollen and may desquamate, and type II cells proliferate.[151] Endothelial cells and alveolar macrophages are also affected. Such abnormalities can appear in as short a time as 24 hours.[152]

Experimental animal studies also demonstrate a remarkable ability of the lung to produce a variety of antioxidant enzymes to prevent damage from cytotoxic oxygen metabolites.[148] The enzymes generally assumed to be responsible for maintaining low levels of oxygen radicals and thus protecting against oxidants include superoxide dismutase (SOD), catalase, glutathione, and the glutathione enzymes, glutathione reductase, and glucose-6-phosphate dehydrogenase (G6PD). Prior exposure to inhaled oxidants, intermittently or in low concentration, exerts a protective effect

in some species of animals, an effect that correlates with the production of these antioxidants.[148]

Oxygen

Studies directed at the assessment of clinical, physiologic, and anatomic alterations in the lungs of patients exposed to high concentrations of oxygen are complicated by the knowledge that some of the changes observed may be caused by the underlying disease, concurrent drug therapy, or artificial ventilation.[153] This dilemma is perhaps most evident in newborn infants with hyaline membrane disease, who show pathologic and roentgenographic evolution from a classic picture of infantile respiratory distress syndrome to one of inflammation and necrosis accompanied by a roentgenographic appearance of almost complete opacification of the lungs. This progresses to atelectasis, fibrosis, and emphysema, creating a "spongy" pattern roentgenographically (bronchopulmonary dysplasia). Similar pathologic changes have been described in adults with varying underlying diseases who require prolonged oxygen therapy.[153]

Although it is difficult to specify the precise level at which oxygen is inevitably toxic, there appears to be ample clinical evidence that humans can tolerate an FIO_2 of 50 per cent for prolonged periods of time without developing irreversible pulmonary damage.[154] The potential deleterious effects of a combination of oxidants should be borne in mind, however, and unless death from hypoxia appears imminent, higher concentrations of oxygen should be avoided, particularly in patients with pulmonary disease caused by other oxidants such as cytotoxic drugs, paraquat, or radiation.

Ozone

Ozone is clearly a potentially important pulmonary toxin:[155] it constitutes 90 per cent of the measured oxidants in photochemical smog,[149] and in certain urban areas its atmospheric concentration is equal to that known to cause structural and physiologic changes in animals. From a clinical point of view, it is important to note that whereas the consequences of inhaled ozone may be modest for a healthy individual, they may be more hazardous for the patient with lung disease.[156]

In experimental animal studies, the pathologic changes have been localized predominantly to respiratory bronchioles[157] or alveolar ducts[158] and consist principally of epithelial hyperplasia associated with small aggregates of macrophages in adjacent alveoli. In one study,[158] findings diminished dramatically following a 24-week "recovery period" in clean air. Functional abnormalities in the animals in this last investigation were mild but included an increase in functional residual capacity and residual volume and a decrease in DLCO; these disturbances disappeared following a 3-month recovery period.

Unlike most other toxic gases, ozone has not produced serious acute pulmonary disease in humans, to the best of the authors' knowledge. Nevertheless, a number of investigators[159, 160] have shown that acute exposure of normal volunteers to low concentrations of ozone (0.5 to 0.9 ppm) results in dry cough, chest discomfort, and impaired pulmonary function (manifested as a decrease in bronchial flow rates).[161] Considerable variation is observed among individuals in these responses, probably because of differences in airway hyper-reactivity, smoking habits, tolerance developed from prolonged exposure, and the degree of exercise attained.[159, 160] As with oxygen, there is a phenomenon of adaptation with ozone. It develops within 2 to 5 days of exposure but is relatively short-lived, lasting 4 days to 3 weeks after cessation of exposure.[162]

Nitrogen Dioxide

Nitrogen dioxide (NO_2) is a component of photochemical smog that has a biologic effect similar to that of ozone. Animal experiments have shown that short-term exposure to the gas in a concentration less than 17 ppm can result in injury to bronchopulmonary epithelial and capillary endothelial cells.[163] As with oxygen and ozone, tolerance to such damage develops with repeated exposure. Despite this, there is evidence that prolonged exposure can result in pulmonary interstitial fibrosis[164] and emphysema,[165] at least in experimental animals.

Experimental studies of the effects of low concentrations of NO_2 in humans have revealed few abnormalities[166]; however, the dangers of exposure to a high concentration are appreciable. This hazard has been recognized for many years in silo fillers and in association with industrial exposure to fuming nitric acid or the use of explosives in mining operations.[167] Silo-filler's disease is the most important condition.[168] For 3 to 10 days after a silo has been filled, the fresh silage produces nitric oxide which, on contact with air, oxidizes to form NO_2 and its polymer, dinitrogen tetroxide. These two gases are heavier than air and are apparent just above the silage as a brownish-yellow cloud. Anyone who enters the silo during this period will inhale NO_2 and will suffer bronchopulmonary irritation. Following moderate to severe exposure, the course is triphasic.

First Phase. During the first phase, there is an immediate reaction that consists of acute bronchiolitis and peribronchiolitis, sometimes accompanied by denuding of the epithelium; diffuse alveolar damage also has been documented in some patients.[168] The clinical picture is characterized by the abrupt onset of cough, dyspnea, weakness, and a choking feeling that usually persists. Pulmonary edema can develop within 4 to 24 hours.[169]

Second Phase. Symptoms abate during the second phase, which lasts 2 to 5 weeks, although cough, malaise, and shortness of breath of lesser severity may persist. Weakness may worsen. The chest roentgenogram is normal.

Third Phase. The third phase becomes manifest up to 5 weeks after the initial exposure[170, 171] and is characterized pathologically by bronchiolitis obliterans. Roentgenographically, multiple discrete nodular opacities of varying size are scattered diffusely throughout the lungs (to a point of confluence in the more severe cases). The nodules may disappear as the clinical course progresses to a stage of chronic pulmonary insufficiency, although they usually persist for a considerable time after the acute symptoms have subsided. Clinically, this stage is characterized by fever, chills, progressive shortness of breath, cough, and cyanosis. Moist rales and rhonchi may be heard on auscultation. A neutro-

philic leukocytosis develops in most cases and the $PaCO_2$ may be elevated. The patient may die of pulmonary insufficiency or may recover more or less completely during this stage. In some patients, a degree of obstructive impairment of pulmonary function remains.[172]

Nonoxidant Gases and Aerosols

Sulfur Dioxide

Sulfur dioxide (SO_2) is a highly soluble gas that, on contact with moist epithelial surfaces, is hydrated and oxidized to form sulfuric acid (H_2SO_4). It is this form that causes mucosal injury. The acid may be partly neutralized, and the damage thereby diminished, by combination with endogenous ammonia in the respiratory tract.[173]

The major source of SO_2 is atmospheric pollution, and continuous exposure to low concentrations in an urban environment may play a role in the pathogenesis of chronic obstructive pulmonary disease (see page 654). Accidental exposure to a high concentration also can result in severe acute pulmonary disease similar to that caused by NO_2. This can occur in pulp and paper factories, refrigeration plants, and oil-refining and fruit-preserving industries. H_2SO_4 itself is also used in photographic developing and is capable of causing reversible obstructive disease of small airways in photographers.[174] It is probable that inhaled SO_2 produces the same triphasic course that NO_2 does; as with other toxic gases, bronchiectasis and bronchiolitis obliterans are long-term complications of acute disease (Fig. 14–9).

Hydrogen Sulfide

Hydrogen sulfide (H_2S) produces a characteristic "rotten-egg" odor at 0.2 ppm and paralyzes the sense of smell at levels of 150 ppm. Levels of 250 ppm cause irritation of mucous membranes, with resultant keratoconjunctivitis, bronchitis, and pulmonary edema. Higher concentrations affect the central nervous system and can cause rapid death.[175] Like cyanide, sulfide ions act as direct cytotoxins, selectively binding to cytochrome oxidase within mitochondria and thereby disrupting the electron transport chain. The usual sources of exposure are petroleum and chemical industries[176] and decaying organic matter, such as liquid manure[175] and insufficiently refrigerated fish stored in an unventilated ship's hold.[177]

One review of 5 years' experience with H_2S poisoning in the Alberta oil fields revealed 221 cases of recognized exposure, with an overall mortality of 6 per cent.[176] Five per cent of victims were dead on arrival at hospital. Acute problems consisted of coma, dysequilibrium, and respiratory insufficiency as a result of pulmonary edema. Although 75 per cent of patients lost consciousness at the accident site, neurologic and respiratory sequelae were uncommon.

Ammonia

Ammonia is a toxic, highly soluble alkaline gas that may play a role along with H_2S in causing bronchopulmonary disease on exposure to decaying organic matter. However, it is better known as a cause of lung damage in industry and farming or as a result of vehicular accidents that cause leakage from tanks of concentrated ammonia.[178] Inhalation

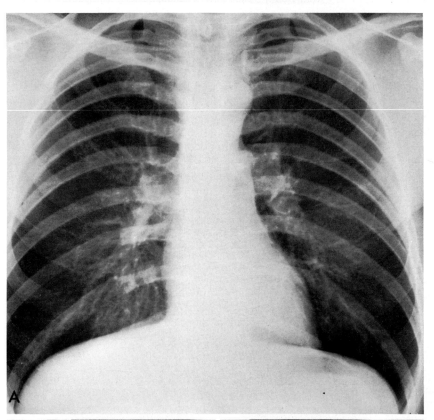

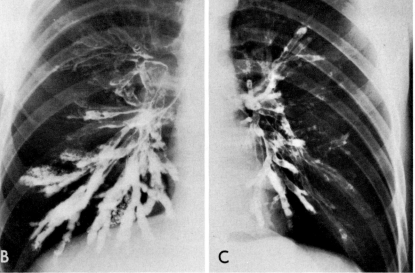

Figure 14–9. Bronchiolitis Obliterans and Bronchiectasis Secondary to Sulfur Dioxide Inhalation. Three months prior to these roentgenographic studies, this 33-year-old man was exposed to high concentrations of sulfur dioxide fumes rising from a sulfuric acid vat. Immediately following this exposure, he was said to have developed acute pulmonary edema, which gradually resolved over a period of days (this acute episode was not documented). Three months later, a posteroanterior roentgenogram *(A)* revealed numerous "tram lines" in the central and medullary portions of both lungs. The lungs were somewhat overinflated. Bilateral bronchography *(B* and *C)* demonstrated severe cylindrical and varicose bronchiectasis of all segmental bronchi of both lungs, the dilated bronchi terminating abruptly in squared or rounded extremities. There was an almost total absence of peripheral filling.

of a large quantity of the gas results in severe acute tracheobronchitis and the production of copious serosanguineous and purulent secretions. Extreme inflammation and desquamation of the mucosa of the central bronchial tree can be seen bronchoscopically.[179] Survivors may develop bronchiectasis and obliterative bronchiolitis.[180]

Chlorine

Heavy exposure to chlorine can occur in industrial accidents or when the gas escapes from broken pipes or tank containers; occupational settings at particular risk are plastic and textile industries and plants for water purification.[181] Acute exposure to a high concentration of gas results in pulmonary edema, fever, severe acute bronchitis, conjunctivitis, nausea and vomiting, stupor, shock, and hemoptysis. Less exposure results in cough and dyspnea and, sometimes, roentgenographic evidence of mild interstitial edema. Although some studies have revealed complete return to normal function in a few weeks,[182] others have shown persistent airflow impairment and, in some cases, a suspicion of chlorine induced bronchial hyper-reactivity.[183, 184]

Phosgene

Phosgene (the common name of carbon oxychloride) is known chiefly as a highly poisonous gas used in warfare, but it is also occasionally a hazard in industry.[185] Cases of poisoning have been described following accidental inhalation of carbon tetrachloride from a fire extinguisher[186] and inhalation within small, enclosed, stove-heated spaces of chemical paint removers containing methylene chloride.[187] When the gas is inhaled, it is hydrolyzed to hydrochloric acid and carbon dioxide. Probably as a result of the action of the former substance, sloughing of the bronchiolar mucosa, interstitial and alveolar edema, and patchy lobular emphysema occur.[186] As with NO_2 poisoning, there is a delay of several hours before the onset of dyspnea.

Mercury

Poisoning can occur from exposure to either the metallic (see page 568) or the vaporized form of mercury. Inhalation of the latter form usually occurs in industry when a worker is exposed in a confined space such as a tank or boiler. Accidental exposure also can occur in the home when metallic mercury is allowed to burn on a stove.[188]

Symptoms and signs tend to develop 3 to 4 hours after exposure and include gingivostomatitis, crampy abdominal pain, and diarrhea. Severe tracheitis, bronchitis, bronchiolitis, and pneumonitis may be present.[189] The condition is particularly serious in infants, in whom the bronchiolitis may be fatal. Central nervous system symptoms are very common and can develop in the absence of pulmonary disease. Other manifestations include paronychia, erosion of the nails, and a metallic taste in the mouth. Lung biopsy specimens can reveal interstitial fibrosis.[190] Pulmonary function tests performed shortly after exposure have shown a combination of obstructive and restrictive disease and a lowered diffusing capacity.[189]

Cadmium

This toxic metal is present in many foods and in tobacco. Acute exposure to a high concentration usually occurs during the heating of cadmium-coated metal with an oxyacetylene torch and results in metal fume fever (see later) or in delayed acute pulmonary edema.

Chronic exposure occurs most often in cigarette smokers, the metal being present in the smoke itself. Although the results of some studies have suggested the possibility of a pathogenetic relationship between cadmium and emphysema,[191] it seems more likely that other agents in cigarette smoke are of greater importance. Some investigators have described a restrictive dysfunction attributed to cadmium[192]; however, others have found no pulmonary defect despite exposure to a relatively high concentration (sufficient to cause renal toxicity).[193]

Trimellitic Anhydride

The culpable agent of respiratory tract disease caused by epoxy resins appears to be trimellitic anhydride (TMA), a low–molecular weight chemical widely used in the manufacture of plastics, epoxy resin coatings, and paints.[194] Four syndromes have been described following the inhalation of TMA dust or fumes:[195]

1. An immediate-type airway response (asthma-rhinitis) that is mediated by IgE antibody directed against TMA conjugated with respiratory tract proteins.
2. A late-onset respiratory syndrome, characterized by cough, wheezing, dyspnea, myalgias, and arthralgias, that develops 4 to 12 hours after exposure. In this syndrome, TMA reacts covalently with protein to form a hapten-protein complex that results in the induction of antibody, mostly IgG.
3. A TMA hemoptysis-anemia syndrome, resembling Goodpasture's syndrome, that develops following high-dose exposure to fumes when materials containing TMA are sprayed on heated metal surfaces.[196] High levels of antibodies to trimellityl human proteins and erythrocytes have been found in these patients.
4. Occupational bronchitis resulting from direct irritant properties of TMA.

Limited information indicates that removal from exposure results in rapid disappearance of symptoms and a decrease in the levels of serum antibodies. Hypoxemia, which may be severe, and a restrictive functional defect revert to normal in patients with the hemoptysis-anemia syndrome.

Fumes

Inhalation of a variety of organic and inorganic compounds in a finely dispersed form can result in an acute febrile illness commonly known as fume fever. There are three general forms.

Metal fume fever results from inhalation of minute particles of the oxides of zinc, copper, magnesium, iron, cadmium, nickel, and various other metals formed during welding or during cleaning of metal-coated tanks.[197] Inhalation of the fumes results in an acute transitory illness characterized by sudden onset of thirst, a metallic taste in the mouth, irritation of the throat, substernal tightness, malaise, headache, muscle cramps, chills, and fever. Symptoms usually appear within 12 hours of exposure and subside within 24 hours without complications or sequelae. Moist rales and rhonchi may be heard on auscultation, and there is neutrophilic leukocytosis in both peripheral blood and BAL fluid.[198] The chest roentgenogram either is normal or shows increased prominence of bronchovascular markings.

Polymer fume fever (polytetrafluoroethylene poisoning) is caused by inhalation of fumes derived by heating polytetrafluoroethylene (Fluon, Teflon) to high temperatures (above 250°C). Symptoms are similar to those of metal fume fever and include tightness in the chest, headache, shivering, fever, aching, weakness, and occasionally shortness of breath.[199] Pulmonary edema can occur.[200] In most reported cases, fume inhalation has been associated with cigarette smoking,[199, 201] the high temperatures generated by cigarette burning being sufficient to produce the toxic byproducts. Episodes of fume fever disappear after workers wash their hands thoroughly before they smoke cigarettes.

Organic dust fever is an uncommon, recently described abnormality characterized by an acute transient febrile illness after exposure to a high concentration of organic dust. By definition, there is an absence of clinical, radiologic, and immunologic features of extrinsic allergic alveolitis (with which the condition can be confused). The abnormality has occurred in such diverse settings as the unloading of moldy hay ("silo-unloader's syndrome"[202]), the handling of moldy oranges,[203] and a college fraternity party where dense airborne dust had been created from straw strewn over the floor.[204] The common feature of all of these situations seems to be contact with abundant airborne fungus (and in fact the condition has been termed "pulmonary mycotoxicosis"). The pathogenesis is unclear but appears to be related to a direct toxic effect of the fungus rather than an idiosyncratic immune reaction. The chest roentgenogram may be normal or show an airspace pattern consistent with pulmonary edema. Clinical manifestations resemble those of influenza and include chills, headache, cough, dyspnea, and fever. Precipitins to a variety of molds may or may not be found in the serum.

Formaldehyde

Increasing production and use of urea formaldehyde resins as adhesives in wood products (principally particleboard, fiberboard, and hardwood plywood) and as foam insulation in housing have made formaldehyde gas toxicity a subject of concern. Occupational exposure occurs in the manufacture of these substances, in carpentry shops,[205] and in persons exposed to formalin in pathology departments and mortician establishments. Nonoccupational exposure occurs in buildings that contain furniture treated with urea formaldehyde resins or insulated with urea formaldehyde foam insulation.[206]

It is now generally accepted that exposure to formaldehyde can cause eye irritation, rhinitis, skin rash, and upper respiratory symptoms.[206] Results of studies investigating the long-term effects of inhaled formaldehyde are variable; some suggest minor long-term pulmonary dysfunction,[207] and others no evidence of either acute or chronic impair-

ment of pulmonary function.[208, 209] Discrepancies in these results may reflect differences in the length and concentration of exposure. A possible association with pulmonary carcinoma has also been documented.[209a]

Bronchopulmonary Disease Associated with Burns

Pulmonary parenchymal and tracheobronchial disease are common and important complications of burns and can occur by three mechanisms. Assessment of the relative contribution of each can be extremely difficult in an individual patient.[210]

The inhalation of smoke and the toxic chemicals it contains is a particularly important cause of disease, especially when it occurs in confined spaces. Smoke consists of gases and a suspension of small particles in hot air. The particles are composed of carbon that is coated with combustible products such as organic acids and aldehydes. The gaseous fraction has a highly variable composition, depending on the material that is burning, although the main constituents—carbon monoxide and carbon dioxide—are always present. Toxic combustion products include cyanide (a product of fires involving material such as nylon, asphalt, wool, silk, and polyurethane that is directly related to blood carboxyhemoglobin [COHb] levels[211]) and polyvinyl chloride (PVC, a plastic solid widely used as a rubber substitute for covering electric and telephone wire and cable and in many manufactured products).[212] PVC has been implicated as a major cause of bronchopulmonary damage because hydrogen chloride gas is released when it burns. PVC degrades and releases hydrochloric acid at temperatures over 225°C. The effect of the acid in the gas phase is restricted largely to irritability and chiefly involves the upper respiratory tract; however, loosely bound hydrochloric acid can condense on soot aerosol and thereby gain access to the lung parenchyma.

Direct trauma from heat can cause severe tissue damage, particularly to the mucous membranes of the upper respiratory tract. Although such damage is most common in association with fires, it also can occur with inhalation of other hot gases, such as steam.[213]

In addition to injury caused by heat and by the inhalation of smoke, pulmonary disease can be a result of concurrent shock, sepsis, renal failure, and the consequences of therapy, including overhydration.[214]

The histopathologic findings in patients who die within 48 hours of a fire include pulmonary congestion, edema, intravascular fibrin thrombi, intra-alveolar hemorrhage, and necrosis of tracheal and proximal bronchial epithelium.[215] Although the latter abnormality is probably diffuse in most cases, it occasionally results in the formation of localized endobronchial polyps composed of granulation tissue.[216]

Pulmonary complications occur in 20 to 30 per cent of burn victims admitted to a hospital; of these, 70 to 75 per cent die.[217] The incidence correlates with the severity of the burn and with a history of being in an enclosed space. During the first 24 hours, complications result from upper airway edema caused by direct heat injury or toxic products, usually in patients with head and neck burns. After a latent period of 12 to 48 hours, symptoms and roentgenographic evidence of lower respiratory tract involvement may develop.[218] Complications that become evident at this time consist of atelectasis, pulmonary edema, and pneumonia, the last-named particularly in the presence of inhalaton injury. Atelectasis can be caused when mucus plugs large bronchi, presumably as a result of excessive smoke inhalation. Complications that arise somewhat later include pulmonary embolism and ARDS.[218]

Since transient hypoxemia in firemen overcome by smoke inhalation is a common finding,[219] it might be expected that firefighters who are repeatedly exposed to smoke would show cumulative lung damage. However, investigations of this potential problem have not produced an unequivocal answer. For example, one long-term clinical and physiologic assesment of more than 1000 Boston firefighters failed to find evidence of pulmonary disease attributable to smoke.[220] In contrast, a more recent study of 632 Baltimore city fire fighters concluded that those who were active experienced a rate of decline in FEV_1 2.5 times greater than that of a retired or resigned control group.[221] Similar conflicting results have arisen in epidemiologic surveys directed at fire-fighters' risk of dying from nonmalignant respiratory disease.[222, 223] Despite the variability of the findings of these studies, the consensus of most investigations suggests that while firefighting likely does not lead to short-term deterioration in function,[219] it may well represent a long-term risk of obstructive pulmonary disease over and above that caused by cigarette smoking.

Carbon Monoxide

Carbon monoxide (CO) is an odorless gas formed by incomplete combustion of carbon-containing matter. It is produced in high concentration in fires and inhalation of the gas is probably the most common cause of death in these circumstances. Other sources of CO include faulty heaters, automobile exhaust, tobacco smoke, mine explosions, paint removers containing methylene chloride, and "charcoal" briquets.

The deleterious effects of CO in humans are attributable to two factors: (1) tissue hypoxia resulting from the formation of carboxyhemoglobin (COHb), which reduces the oxygen transport capacity of the blood and causes a shift of the oxyhemoglobin dissociation curve to the left, thus curtailing the amount of oxygen available to the tissues; and (2) a direct cytotoxic effect.

Characteristically, clinical symptoms of acute CO poisoning develop when COHb saturation reaches 20 per cent; unconsciousness occurs at about 60 per cent, and death at about 80 per cent. Interstitial and, occasionally, airspace edema may develop. Roentgenographic manifestations include a ground-glass opacity and peribronchial or perivascular cuffing. Heart size is usually normal and clearing occurs after 3 to 5 days of hyperbaric oxygen therapy.[224] Measurement of protein content of airspace fluid in humans and experimental work in animals suggest that the pathogenesis of these abnormalities is increased permeability edema.[225] In patients who survive the acute episode, follow-up studies have demonstrated neurologic damage characterized by personality deterioration and memory impairment[226]; however, permanent respiratory damage does not occur.

Of possibly even greater clinical significance than acute CO poisoning is the morbidity associated with long-term

exposure to low concentrations of this gas. The blood COHb level of healthy nonsmokers is roughly 0.5 per cent; by contrast, the average COHb of a person who smokes one pack a day is about 6 per cent,[227] a figure that may rise to between 10 and 20 per cent with heavy smoking. The percentage of inspired CO also may be increased in heavy traffic, since car exhaust contains between 1 and 7 per cent CO. Levels of COHb can thus be obtained that result in significant hypoxia; cerebral function may be interfered with and myocardial ischemia may be increased, resulting in angina.

Thesaurosis

In its broad connotation, this term designates storage in the body of unusual amounts of normal or foreign material. However, the term has become restricted to pulmonary disease resulting from the inhalation of hairspray and characterized by a granulomatous pulmonary infiltrate resembling sarcoidosis.[228]

It is important to note that there has been some dispute about the existence of this condition. Some authors speculate that it represents simply sarcoidosis in an individual who happens to use hairspray.[229] Considering all the available evidence, it seems reasonable to conclude that hairspray-induced pulmonary disease may exist and should be considered in an individual with appropriate roentgenographic and pathologic abnormalities and a history of excessive exposure to the substance. It must be remembered, however, that sarcoidosis is a relatively common disease and that despite the widespread use of hairspray, only a small number of cases of possible thesaurosis have been reported.

Histologically, cases reported as thesaurosis have shown interstitial inflammation, predominantly in a peribronchial location but also to some extent in the lung parenchyma. The inflammatory infiltrate consists of lymphocytes and numerous multinucleated giant cells, the latter frequently containing periodic acid–Schiff (PAS)–positive material. Discrete granulomas also occur.

The roentgenographic pattern consists of a diffuse, fine micronodularity simulating the pattern seen in alveolar microlithiasis and talcosis of intravenous drug abuse.[230] Roentgenographic clearing and symptomatic improvement tend to occur fairly rapidly following discontinuance of exposure to hairspray; however, abnormalities possibly related to hairspray have been found to persist for several years in some studies of hairdressers.[231]

References

1. Cooper JAD Jr, White DA, Matthay RA: Drug-induced pulmonary disease. Part 1: Cytotoxic drugs. Am Rev Respir Dis 133: 321, 1986.
2. Cooper JAD Jr, White DA, Matthay RA: Drug-induced pulmonary disease. Part 2: Noncytotoxic drugs. Am Rev Respir Dis 133: 488, 1986.
3. Bennett JM, Reich SD: Bleomycin. Ann Intern Med 90: 945, 1979.
4. Rosenow EC III: The spectrum of drug-induced pulmonary disease. Ann Intern Med 77: 977, 1972.
5. Pascual RS, Mosher MB, Sikand RS, et al: Effects of bleomycin on pulmonary function in man. Am Rev Respir Dis 108: 211, 1973.
6. Iacovino JR, Leitner J, Abbas AK, et al: Fatal pulmonary reaction from low doses of bleomycin. An idiosyncratic tissue response. JAMA 235: 1253, 1976.
7. Van Barneveld PWC, van der Mark TW, Sleijfer DT, et al: Predictive

factors for bleomycin-induced pneumonitis. Am Rev Respir Dis 130: 1078, 1984.

8. Yousem SA, Lifson JD, Colby TV: Chemotherapy-induced eosinophilic pneumonia: Relation to bleomycin. Chest 88: 103, 1985.

9. Phan SH, Fantone JC: Inhibition of bleomycin-induced pulmonary fibrosis by lipopolysaccharide. Lab Invest 50: 587, 1984.

10. Fahey PJ, Utell MJ, Mayewski RJ, et al: Early diagnosis of bleomycin pulmonary toxicity using bronchoalveolar lavage in dogs. Am Rev Respir Dis 126: 126, 1982.

11. Akoun GM, Cadranel JL, Milleron BJ, et al: Bronchoalveolar lavage cell data in 19 patients with drug-associated pneumonitis (except amiodarone). Chest 99: 98, 1991.

12. Ingrassia TS III, Ryu JH, Trastek VF, et al: Oxygen-exacerbated bleomycin pulmonary toxicity. Mayo Clin Proc 66: 173, 1991.

13. Jones AW: Bleomycin lung damage: The pathology and nature of the lesion. Br J Dis Chest 72: 321, 1978.

14. Luursema PB, Star-Kroesen MA, van der Mark TW, et al: Bleomycin-induced changes in the carbon monoxide transfer factor of the lungs and its components. Am Rev Respir Dis 128: 880, 1983.

15. Sorensen PG, Romer FK, Cortes D: Angiotensin-converting enzyme: An indicator of bleomycin-induced pulmonary toxicity in humans. Eur J Cancer Clin Oncol 20: 1405, 1984.

16. Balikian JP, Jochelson MS, Bauer KA, et al: Pulmonary complications of chemotherapy regimens containing bleomycin. Am J Roentgenol 139: 455, 1982.

17. Glasier CM, Siegel MJ: Multiple pulmonary nodules: Unusual manifestation of bleomycin toxicity. Am J Roentgenol 137: 155, 1981.

18. Fleischman RW, Baker JR, Thompson BR, et al: Bleomycin-induced interstitial pneumonia in dogs. Thorax 26: 675, 1971.

19. Ginsberg SJ, Comis RL: The pulmonary toxicity of antineoplastic agents. Semin Oncol 9: 34, 1982.

20. Budzar AU, Legha SS, Luna MA, et al: Pulmonary toxicity of mitomycin. Cancer 45: 236, 1980.

21. Jolivet J, Giroux L, Laurin S, et al: Microangiopathic hemolytic anemia, renal failure, and noncardiogenic pulmonary edema: A chemotherapy-induced syndrome. Cancer Treat Rep 67: 429, 1983.

22. Heard BE, Cooke RA: Busulfan lung. Thorax 23: 187, 1968.

23. Soble AR, Perry H: Fatal radiation pneumonia following subclinical busulfan injury. Am J Roentgenol 128: 15, 1977.

24. Koss LG, Melamed MR, Mayer K: The effect of busulfan on human epithelia. Am J Clin Pathol 44: 385, 1965.

25. Harrold BP: Syndrome resembling Addison's disease following prolonged treatment with busulphan. Br Med J 1: 463, 1966.

26. Littler WA, Ogilvie C: Lung function in patients receiving busulphan. Br Med J 4: 530, 1970.

27. Gould VE, Miller J: Sclerosing alveolitis induced by cyclophosphamide. Ultrastructural observations on alveolar injury and repair. Am J Pathol 81: 513, 1975.

28. Maxwell I: Reversible pulmonary edema following cyclophosphamide treatment. JAMA 229: 137, 1974.

29. Trask CW, Joannides T, Harper PG, et al: Radiation-induced lung fibrosis after treatment of small cell carcinoma of the lung with very high-dose cyclophosphamide. Cancer 55: 47, 1985.

30. Batist G, Andrews JL Jr: Pulmonary toxicity of antineoplastic drugs. JAMA 246: 1449, 1981.

31. Burke DA, Stoddart JC, Ward MK, et al: Fatal pulmonary fibrosis occurring during treatment with cyclophosphamide. Br Med J 285: 696, 1982.

32. Spector JI, Zimbler H, Ross JS: Early-onset cyclophosphamide-induced interstitial pneumonitis. JAMA 242: 2852, 1979.

33. Cole SR, Myers TJ, Klatsky AU: Pulmonary disease with chlorambucil therapy. Cancer 41: 455, 1978.

34. Major PP, Laurin S, Bettez P: Pulmonary fibrosis following therapy with melphalan: Report of two cases. Can Med Assoc J 123: 197, 1980.

35. Westerfield BT, Michalski JP, McCombs C, et al: Reversible melphalan-induced lung damage. Am J Med 68: 767, 1980.

36. Goucher G, Rowland V, Hawkins J: Melphalan-induced pulmonary interstitial fibrosis. Chest 77: 805, 1980.

37. Durant JR, Norgard MJ, Murad TM, et al: Pulmonary toxicity associated with bischloroethylnitrosourea (BCNU). Ann Intern Med 90: 191, 1979.

38. Weinstein AS, Diener-West M, Nelson DF, et al: Pulmonary toxicity of carmustine in patients treated for malignant glioma. Cancer Treat Rep 70: 943, 1986.

39. O'Driscoll BR, Hasleton PS, Taylor PM, et al: Active lung fibrosis up

to 17 years after chemotherapy with carmustine (BCNU) in childhood. N Engl J Med 323: 378, 1990.

40. Ryan BR, Walters TR: Pulmonary fibrosis: A complication of 1,3-bis(2-chloroethyl)-1-nitrosourea (BCNU) therapy. Cancer 48: 909, 1981.

41. Cordonnier C, Vernant J-P, Mital P, et al: Pulmonary fibrosis subsequent to high doses of CCNU for chronic myeloid leukemia. Cancer 51: 1814, 1983.

42. Block M, Lachowiez RM, Rios C, et al: Pulmonary fibrosis associated with low-dose adjuvant methyl-CCNU. Med Pediatr Oncol 18: 256, 1990.

43. Carson CW, Cannon GW, Egger MJ, et al: Pulmonary disease during the treatment of rheumatoid arthritis with low-dose pulse methotrexate. Semin Arthritis Rheum 16: 186, 1987.

44. Ridley MG, Wolfe CS, Mathews JA: Life-threatening acute pneumonitis during low-dose methotrexate treatment for rheumatoid arthritis: A case report and review of the literature. Ann Rheum Dis 47: 784, 1988.

45. Everts CS, Westcott JL, Bragg DG: Methotrexate therapy and pulmonary disease. Radiology 107: 539, 1973.

46. Sostman HD, Matthay RA, Putman CE, et al: Methotrexate-induced pneumonitis. Medicine 55: 371, 1976.

47. Filip DJ, Logue GL, Harle TS, et al: Pulmonary and hepatic complications of methotrexate therapy of psoriasis. JAMA 216: 881, 1971.

48. Kaplan RL, Waite DH: Progressive interstitial lung disease from prolonged methotrexate therapy. Arch Dermatol 114: 1800, 1978.

49. Shapiro CL, Yeap BY, Godleski J, et al: Drug-related pulmonary toxicity in non-Hodgkin's lymphoma. Comparative results with three different treatment regimens. Cancer 68: 699, 1991.

50. Holmberg L, Boman G, Bottiger LE, et al: Adverse reactions to nitrofurantoin: Analysis of 921 reports. Am J Med 69: 733, 1980.

51. Jick SS, Jick H, Walker AM, et al: Hospitalizations for pulmonary reactions following nitrofurantoin use. Chest 96: 512, 1989.

52. Willcox PA, Maze SS, Sandler M, et al: Pulmonary fibrosis following long-term nitrofurantoin therapy. S Afr Med J 61: 714, 1982.

53. Ngan H, Millard RJ, Lant AF, et al: Nitrofurantoin lung. Br J Radiol 44: 21, 1971.

54. Hailey FJ, Glascock HW Jr, Hewitt WF: Pleuropneumonic reactions to nitrofurantoin. N Engl J Med 281: 1087, 1969.

55. Taskinen E, Tukiainen P, Sovijarvi AR: Nitrofurantoin-induced alterations in pulmonary tissue: A report on five patients with acute or subacute reactions. Acta Pathol Microbiol Scand (A) 85: 713, 1977.

56. Leino R, Liippo K, Ekfors T: Sulphasalazine-induced reversible hypersensitivity pneumonitis and fatal fibrosing alveolitis: Report of two cases. J Intern Med 229: 553, 1991.

57. Moss SF, Ind PW: Time course of recovery of lung function in sulphasalazine-induced alveolitis. Respir Med 85: 73, 1991.

58. Dean PJ, Groshart KD, Porterfield JG, et al: Amiodarone-associated pulmonary toxicity: A clinical and pathologic study of eleven cases. J Clin Pathology 87: 7, 1987.

59. Marchlinski FE, Gansler TS, Waxman HL, et al: Amiodarone pulmonary toxicity. Ann Intern Med 97: 839, 1982.

60. Nicolet-Chatelain G, Prevost MC, Escamilla R, et al: Amiodarone-induced pulmonary toxicity. Immunoallergologic tests and bronchoalveolar lavage phospholipid content. Chest 99: 363, 1991.

61. Israel-Biet D, Venet A, Caubarrere I, et al: Bronchoalveolar lavage in amiodarone pneumonitis: Cellular abnormalities and their relevance to pathogenesis. Chest 91: 214, 1987.

62. Pollak PT, Sharma AD, Carruthers SG: Relation of amiodarone hepatic and pulmonary toxicity to serum drug concentrations and superoxide dismutase activity. Am J Cardiol 65: 1185, 1990.

63. Adams PC, Gibson GJ, Morley AR, et al: Amiodarone pulmonary toxicity: Clinical and subclinical features. Q J Med 59: 449, 1986.

64. Rotmensch HH, Belhassen B, Swanson BN, et al: Steady-state serum amiodarone concentrations: Relationships with antiarrhythmic efficacy and toxicity. Ann Intern Med 101: 462, 1984.

65. Myers JL, Kennedy JI, Plumb VJ: Amiodarone lung: Pathologic findings in clinically toxic patients. Hum Pathol 18: 349, 1987.

66. Gefter WB, Epstein DM, Pietra GG, et al: Lung disease caused by amiodarone, a new antiarrhythmia agent. Radiology 147: 339, 1983.

67. Akoun GM, Milleron BJ, Madaro DM, et al: Pleural T-lymphocyte subsets in amiodarone-associated pleuropneumonitis. Chest 95: 596, 1989.

68. Kuhlman JE, Teigen C, Ren H, et al: Amiodarone pulmonary toxicity: CT findings in symptomatic patients. Radiology 177: 121, 1990.

69. Chamberlain DW, Hyland RH, Ross DJ: Diphenylhydantoin-induced lymphocytic interstitial pneumonia. Chest 90: 458, 1986.
70. Gaffey CM, Chun B, Harvey JC, et al: Phenytoin-induced systemic granulomatous vasculitis. Arch Pathol Lab Med 110: 131, 1986.
71. Heitzman ER: Lymphadenopathy related to anticonvulsant therapy: Roentgen findings simulating lymphoma. Radiology 89: 311, 1967.
72. Michael JR, Rudin ML: Acute pulmonary disease caused by phenytoin. Ann Intern Med 95: 452, 1981.
73. Fisher CJ Jr, Albertson TE, Foulke GE: Salicylate-induced pulmonary edema: Clinical characteristics in children. Am J Emerg Med 3: 33, 1985.
74. Bowers RE, Brigham KL, Owen PJ: Salicylate pulmonary edema: The mechanism in sheep and review of the clinical literature. Am Rev Respir Dis 115: 261, 1977.
75. Heffner JE, Sahn SA: Salicylate-induced pulmonary edema. Clinical features and prognosis. Ann Intern Med 95: 405, 1981.
76. Hormaechea E, Carlson RW, Rogove H, et al: Hypovolemia, pulmonary edema and protein changes in severe salicylate poisoning. Am J Med 66: 1046, 1979.
77. Chalmers A, Thompson D, Stein HE, et al: Systemic lupus erythematosus during penicillamine therapy for rheumatoid arthritis. Ann Intern Med 97: 659, 1982.
78. Bocanegra T, Espinoza LR, Vasey FB, et al: Myasthenia gravis and penicillamine therapy of rheumatoid arthritis. JAMA 244: 1822, 1980.
79. Kumar A, Bhat A, Gupta DK, et al: D-Penicillamine–induced acute hypersensitivity pneumonitis and cholestatic hepatitis in a patient with rheumatoid arthritis. Clin Exp Rheumatol 3: 337, 1985.
80. Camus P, Degat OR, Justrabo E, et al: D-Penicillamine–induced severe pneumonitis. Chest 81: 376, 1982.
81. Gibson T, Burry HV, Ogg C: Goodpasture's syndrome and D-penicillamine. Ann Intern Med 84: 100, 1976.
82. Davies D, Jones JKL: Pulmonary eosinophilia caused by penicillamine. Thorax 35: 957, 1980.
83. Cooke NT, Bamji AN: Gold and pulmonary function in rheumatoid arthritis. Br J Rheumatol 22: 18, 1983.
84. McCormick J, Cole S, Lahirir B, et al: Pneumonitis caused by gold salt therapy: Evidence for the role of cell-mediated immunity in its pathogenesis. Am Rev Respir Dis 122: 145, 1980.
85. Partanen J, van Assendelft AH, Koskimies S, et al: Patients with rheumatoid arthritis and gold-induced pneumonitis express two high-risk histocompatibility complex patterns. Chest 92: 277, 1987.
86. Geddes DM, Bristoff J: Pulmonary fibrosis associated with hypersensitivity to gold salts. Br Med J 1: 1444, 1976.
87. Holness L, Tenenbaum J, Cooter NBE, et al: Fatal bronchiolitis obliterans associated with chrysotherapy. Ann Rheum Dis 42: 593, 1983.
88. Evans RB, Ettensohn DB, Fawaz-Estrup F, et al: Gold lung: Recent developments in pathogenesis, diagnosis, and therapy. Semin Arthritis Rheum 16: 196, 1987.
89. Pisani RJ, Rosenow EC III: Pulmonary edema associated with tocolytic therapy. Ann Intern Med 110: 714, 1989.
90. van Iddekinge B, Gobetz L, Seaward PG, et al: Pulmonary oedema after hexoprenaline administration in preterm labour. A report of 4 cases. S Afr Med J 79: 620, 1991.
91. Duberstein JL, Kaufman DM: A clinical study of an epidemic of heroin intoxication and heroin-induced pulmonary edema. Am J Med 51: 704, 1971.
92. Guilleminault C: Benzodiazepines, breathing, and sleep. Am J Med 88: 255, 1990.
93. Bailey PL, Pace NL, Ashburn MA, et al: Frequent hypoxemia and apnea after sedation with midazolam and fentanyl. Anesthesiology 73: 826, 1990.
94. Smith WR, Glauser FL, Dearden LC, et al: Deposits of immunoglobulin and complement in the pulmonary tissue of patients with "heroin lung." Chest 73: 471, 1978.
95. Snyder SH: Opiate receptors in the brain. N Engl J Med 296: 266, 1977.
96. Taff RH: Pulmonary edema following naloxone administration in a patient without heart disease. Anesthesiology 59: 576, 1983.
97. Sebastian JL, McKinney WP, Kaufman J, et al: Angiotensin-converting enzyme inhibitors and cough. Prevalence in an outpatient medical clinic population. Chest 99: 36, 1991.
98. Popa V: Captopril-related (and induced?) asthma. Am Rev Respir Dis 136: 999, 1987.
99. Gianos ME, Klaustermeyer WB, Kurohara M, et al: Enalapril-induced angioedema. Am J Emerg Med 8: 124, 1990.
100. Kaufman J, Casanova JE, Riendl P, et al: Bronchial hyperreactivity and cough due to angiotensin-converting enzyme inhibitors. Chest 95: 544, 1989.
101. Silvestri RC, Huseby JS, Rughani I, et al: Respiratory distress syndrome from lymphangiography contrast medium. Am Rev Respir Dis 122: 543, 1980.
102. White RJ, Webb JAW, Tucker AK, et al: Pulmonary function after lymphography. Br Med J 4: 775, 1973.
103. Greganti MA, Flowers WM Jr: Acute pulmonary edema after the intravenous administration of contrast media. Radiology 132: 583, 1979.
104. Chamberlin WH, Stockman GD, Wray NP: Shock and noncardiogenic pulmonary edema following meglumine diatrizoate for intravenous pyelography. Am J Med 67: 684, 1979.
105. Martin RM, Duffy J, Engel AG, et al: The clinical spectrum of the eosinophilia-myalgia syndrome associated with L-tryptophan ingestion. Clinical features in 20 patients and aspects of pathophysiology. Ann Intern Med 113: 124, 1990.
106. Tazelaar HD, Myers JL, Drage CW, et al: Pulmonary disease associated with L-tryptophan–induced eosinophilic myalgia syndrome. Clinical and pathological features. Chest 97: 1032, 1990.
107. Catton CK, Elmer JC, Whitehouse AC, et al: Pulmonary involvement in the eosinophilia-myalgia syndrome. Chest 99: 327, 1991.
108. Ivey M, Eichenhorn MS, Glasberg MR, et al: Hypercapnic respiratory failure due to L-tryptophan–induced eosinophilic polymyositis. Chest 99: 756, 1991.
109. Kavaru MS, Ahmad M, Amirthalingam KN: Hydrochlorothiazide-induced acute pulmonary edema. Cleve Clin J Med 57: 181, 1990.
110. Biron P, Dessureault J, Napke E: Acute allergic interstitial pneumonitis induced by hydrochlorothiazide. Can Med Assoc J 145: 28, 1991.
111. Hoffman CK, Goodman PC: Pulmonary edema in cocaine smokers. Radiology 172: 463, 1989.
112. Forrester JM, Steele AW, Waldron JA, et al: Crack lung: An acute pulmonary syndrome with a spectrum of clinical and histopathologic findings. Am Rev Respir Dis 142: 462, 1990.
113. O'Donnell AE, Mappin FG, Sebo TJ, et al: Interstitial pneumonitis associated with "crack" cocaine abuse. Chest 100: 1155, 1991.
114. Itkonen J, Schnoll S, Glassroth J: Pulmonary dysfunction in "free base" cocaine users. Arch Intern Med 144: 2195, 1984.
115. Tsao TC, Nuang YC, Lan RS: Respiratory failure of acute organophosphate and carbamate poisoning. Chest 98: 631, 1990.
116. Neal EA: Enzymic mechanism of metabolism of the phosphorothionate insecticides. Arch Intern Med 128: 118, 1971.
117. Li C, Miller WT, Jiang J: Pulmonary edema due to ingestion of organophosphate insecticide. Am J Roentgenol 152: 265, 1989.
118. Kass R, Kocher G, Lippman M: Adult respiratory distress syndrome from organophosphate poisoning. Am J Emerg Med 9: 32, 1991.
119. Wohlfahrt DJ: Fatal paraquat poisonings after skin absorption. Med J Aust 1: 512, 1982.
120. Fisher HK, Clements JA, Wright RR: Enhancement of oxygen toxicity by the herbicide paraquat. Am Rev Respir Dis 107: 246, 1973.
121. Rebello G, Mason JK: Pulmonary histological appearances in fatal paraquat poisoning. Histopathology 2: 53, 1978.
122. Davidson JK, MacPherson P: Pulmonary changes in paraquat poisoning. Clin Radiol 23: 18, 1972.
123. Im JG, Lee KS, Han MC, et al: Paraquat poisoning findings on chest radiography and CT in 42 patients. Am J Roentgenol 157: 697, 1991.
124. Higenbottam T, Crome P, Parkinson C, et al: Further clinical observations on the pulmonary effects of paraquat ingestion. Thorax 34: 161, 1979.
125. Hudson M, Patel SB, Ewen SW, et al: Paraquat-induced pulmonary fibrosis in three survivors. Thorax 46: 201, 1991.
126. Salisburg BD, Tate CF, Davies JE: Baygon-induced pulmonary edema. Chest 65: 455, 1974.
127. Roby DS, Fein AM, Bennett RH, et al: Cardiopulmonary effects of acute thallium poisoning. Chest 85: 236, 1984.
128. Rigau-Pérez-Alvarez L, Duñas-Castro S, et al: Epidemiologic investigation of an oil-associated pneumonic paralytic eosinophilic syndrome in Spain. Am J Epidemiol 119: 250, 1984.
129. Tabuenca JM: Toxic-allergic syndrome caused by ingestion of rapeseed oil denatured with aniline. Lancet 2: 567, 1981.
130. Gordon RS: Oleoanilides and Spanish oil poisoning. Lancet 2: 1171, 1981.
131. Root-Bernstein RS, Westall FC: Mycoplasma pneumoniae and a dual etiology for Spanish oil syndrome. Nature 301: 178, 1983.
132. Gómez-Sánchez MA, Mestre de Juan MJ, Gómez-Pajuelo C, et al:

Pulmonary hypertension due to toxic oil syndrome. A clinicopathologic study. Chest 95: 325, 1989.

133. Fernández-Segoviano P, Esteban A, Martinez-Cabruja R: Pulmonary vascular lesions in the toxic oil syndrome in Spain. Thorax 38: 724, 1983.

134. Martín Escribano P, Daz de Atauri MJ, Gómez Sánchez MA: Persistence of respiratory abnormalities four years after the onset of toxic oil syndrome. Chest 100: 336, 1991.

135. Thurlbeck WM: Conference summary. Chest 66(Suppl): 40, 1974.

136. Harris VJ, Brown R: Pneumatoceles as a complication of chemical pneumonia after hydrocarbon ingestion. Am J Roentgenol 125: 531, 1975.

137. Anas N, Namasonthi V, Ginsburg CM: Criteria for hospitalizing children who have ingested products containing hydrocarbons. JAMA 246: 840, 1981.

138. Reynolds J, Bonte FJ: Kerosene pneumonitis. Tex Med 56: 34, 1960.

139. George M, Hedworth-Whitty RB: Non-fatal lung disease due to inhalation of nebulised paraquat. Br Med J 280: 902, 1980.

140. Skyberg K, Ronneberg A, Kamoy JI, et al: Pulmonary fibrosis in cable plant workers exposed to mist and vapor of petroleum distillates. Environ Res 40: 261, 1986.

141. Macdougall IC, Isles C, Oliver JS, et al: Fatal outcome following inhalation of Tipp-Ex. Scott Med J 32: 55, 1987.

142. Cane RD, Buchanan N, Miller M: Pulmonary oedema associated with hydrocarbon inhalation. Intensive Care Med 3: 31, 1977.

143. Engstrand DA, England DM, Huntington RW III: Pathology of paint sniffers' lung. Am J Forensic Med Pathol 7: 232, 1986.

144. Buchanan DR, Lamb D, Seaton A: Punk rocker's lung: Pulmonary fibrosis in a drug-snorting fire-eater. Br Med J 283: 1661, 1981.

145. Cartwright TR, Brown ED, Brashear RE: Pulmonary infiltrates following butane "fire-breathing." Arch Intern Med 143: 2007, 1983.

146. Smith AB, Schloemer J, Lowry LK, et al: Metabolic and health consequences of occupational exposure to polychlorinated biphenyls. Br J Ind Med 39: 361, 1982.

147. Warshaw R, Fischbein A, Thornton J, et al: Decrease in vital capacity in PCB-exposed workers in a capacitor manufacturing facility. Ann NY Acad Sci 320: 277, 1979.

148. Deneke SM, Fanburg BL: Normobaric oxygen toxicity of the lung. N Engl J Med 303: 76, 1980.

149. Cross CE, DeLucia AJ, Reddy AK, et al: Ozone interactions with lung tissue. Biochemical approaches. Am J Med 60: 929, 1976.

150. Boatman ES, Sato S, Frank R: Acute effects of ozone on cat lungs. II. Structural. Am Rev Respir Dis 110: 157, 1974.

151. Weibel ER: Oxygen effect on lung cells. Arch Intern Med 128: 54, 1971.

152. Currie WD, Pratt PC, Sanders AP: Hyperoxia and lung metabolism. Chest 66: 19S, 1974.

153. Gillbe CE, Salt JC, Branthwaite MA: Pulmonary function after prolonged mechanical ventilation with high concentrations of oxygen. Thorax 35: 907, 1980.

154. Jackson RM: Pulmonary oxygen toxicity. Chest 88: 900, 1985.

155. Berry M, Lioy PJ, Gelperin K, et al: Accumulated exposure to ozone and measurement of health effects in children and counselors at two summer camps. Environ Res 54: 135, 1991.

156. Bergofsky EH: The lung mucosa: A critical environmental battleground. Am J Med 91(4A): 4S, 1991.

157. Eustis SL, Schwartz LW, Kosch PC, et al: Chronic bronchiolitis in nonhuman primates after prolonged ozone exposure. Am J Pathol 105: 121, 1981.

158. Gross KB, White HJ: Functional and pathologic consequences of a 52-week exposure to 0.5 ppm ozone followed by a clean air recovery period. Lung 165: 283, 1987.

159. Kagawa J: Respiratory effects of two-hour exposure with intermittent exercise to ozone, sulfur dioxide and nitrogen dioxide alone and in combination in normal subjects. Am Ind Hyg Assoc J 44: 14, 1983.

160. Kagawa J: Exposure-effect relationship of selected pulmonary function measurements in subjects exposed to ozone. Int Arch Occup Environ Health 53: 345, 1984.

161. McDonnell WF, Kehrl HR, Abdul-Salaam S, et al: Respiratory response of humans exposed to low levels of ozone for 6.6 hours. Arch Environ Health 46: 145, 1991.

162. Horvath SM, Gliner JA, Folinsbee LJ: Adaptation to ozone: Duration of effect. Am Rev Respir Dis 123: 496, 1981.

163. Evans MJ, Stephens RJ, Freeman G: Effects of nitrogen dioxide on cell renewal in the rat lung. Arch Intern Med 128: 57, 1971.

164. Stephens RJ, Freeman G, Evans MJ: Ultrastructural changes in connective tissue in lungs of rats exposed to NO_2. Arch Intern Med 127: 873, 1971.

165. Ranga V, Kleinerman J: Lung injury and repair in the blotchy mouse: Effects of nitrogen dioxide inhalation. Am Rev Respir Dis 123: 90, 1981.

166. Folinsbee LJ, Horvath SM, Bedi JF, et al: Effect of 0.62 ppm NO_2 on cardiopulmonary function in young male nonsmokers. Environ Res 15: 199, 1978.

167. Becklake MR, Goldman HI, Bosman AR, et al: The long-term effects of exposure to nitrous fumes. Am Rev Tuberc 76: 398, 1957.

168. Douglas WW, Hepper NG, Colby TV: Silo-filler's disease. Mayo Clin Proc 64: 291, 1989.

169. Ramirez FJ: The first death from nitrogen dioxide fumes. The story of a man and his dog. JAMA 229: 1181, 1974.

170. Ramirez RJ, Dowell AR: Silo-filler's disease: Nitrogen dioxide–induced lung injury. Long-term follow-up and review of the literature. Ann Intern Med 74: 569, 1971.

171. Jones GR, Proudfoot AT, Hall JI: Pulmonary effects of acute exposure to nitrous fumes. Thorax 28: 61, 1973.

172. Fleming GM, Chester EH, Montenegro HD: Dysfunction of small airways following pulmonary injury due to nitrogen dioxide. Chest 75: 720, 1979.

173. Larson TV, Frank R, Covert DS, et al: Measurements of respiratory ammonia and the chemical neutralization of inhaled sulfuric acid aerosol in anesthetized dogs. Am Rev Respir Dis 125: 502, 1982.

174. Kipen HM, Lerman Y: Respiratory abnormalities among photographic developers: A report of three cases. Am J Ind Med 9: 341, 1986.

175. Osbern LN, Crapo RO: Dung lung: A report of toxic exposure to liquid manure. Ann Intern Med 95: 312, 1981.

176. Burnett WW, King EG, Grace M, et al: Hydrogen sulfide poisoning: Review of 5 years' experience. Can Med Assoc J 117: 1277, 1977.

177. Glass RI, Ford R, Allegra DT, et al: Deaths from asphyxia among fishermen. JAMA 244: 2193, 1980.

178. Arwood R, Hammond J, Ward GG: Ammonia inhalation. J Trauma 25: 444, 1985.

179. Flury KE, Dines DE, Rodarte JR, et al: Airway obstruction due to inhalation of ammonia. Mayo Clin Proc 58: 389, 1983.

180. Kass I, Zamel N, Dobry CA, et al: Bronchiectasis following ammonia burns of the respiratory tract. A review of two cases. Chest 62: 282, 1972.

181. Shroff CP, Khade MV, Srinivasan M: Respiratory cytopathology in chlorine gas toxicity: A study in 28 subjects. Diagn Cytopathol 4: 28, 1988.

182. Abhyankar A, Bhambure N, Kamath NN, et al: Six-month follow-up of fourteen victims with short-term exposure to chlorine gas. J Soc Occup Med 39: 131, 1989.

183. Kennedy SM, Enarson DA, Janssen RG, et al: Lung health consequences of reported accidental chlorine gas exposures among pulpmill workers. Am Rev Respir Dis 143: 74, 1991.

184. Schwartz DA, Smith DD, Lakshminarayan S: The pulmonary sequelae associated with accidental inhalation of chlorine gas. Chest 97: 820, 1990.

185. Polednak AP: Mortality among men occupationally exposed to phosgene in 1943-1945. Environ Res 22: 357, 1980.

186. Seidelin R: The inhalation of phosgene in a fire extinguisher accident. Thorax 16: 91, 1961.

187. English JM: A case of probable phosgene poisoning. Br Med J 1: 38, 1964.

188. Rowens B, Guerrero-Betancourt D, Gottlieb CA, et al: Respiratory failure and death following acute inhalation of mercury vapor. A clinical and histologic perspective. Chest 99: 185, 1991.

189. Lien DC, Todoruk DN, Rajani HR, et al: Accidental inhalation of mercury vapour: Respiratory and toxicologic consequences. Can Med Assoc J 129: 591, 1983.

190. Hallee TJ: Diffuse lung disease caused by inhalation of mercury vapor. Am Rev Respir Dis 99: 430, 1969.

191. Hirst RN, Perry HM, Cruz MG, et al: Elevated cadmium concentration in emphysematous lungs. Am Rev Respir Dis 108: 30, 1973.

192. Smith TJ, Petty TL, Reading JC, et al: Pulmonary effects of chronic exposure to airborne cadmium. Am Rev Respir Dis 114: 161, 1976.

193. Edling C, Elinder CG, Randma E: Lung function in workers using cadmium-containing solders. Br J Ind Med 43: 657, 1986.

194. Zeiss CR, Mitchell JH, Van Peenen PF, et al: A twelve-year clinical

immunologic evaluation of workers involved in the manufacture of trimellitic anhydride (TMA). Allergy Proc 11: 71, 1990.

195. Zeiss CR, Wolkonsky P, Chacon R, et al: Syndromes in workers exposed to trimellitic anhydride: A longitudinal clinical and immunologic study. Ann Intern Med 98: 8, 1983.

196. Ahmad D, Morgan WK, Patterson R, et al: Pulmonary haemorrhage and haemolytic anaemia due to trimellitic anhydride. Lancet 2: 328, 1979.

197. Vogelmeier C, Konig G, Bencze K, et al: Pulmonary involvement in zinc fume fever. Chest 92: 946, 1987.

198. Blanc P, Wong H, Berstein MS, et al: An experimental human model of metal fume fever. Ann Intern Med 114: 930, 1991.

199. Wegman DH, Peters JM: Polymer fume fever and cigarette smoking. Ann Intern Med 81: 55, 1974.

200. Evans EA: Pulmonary edema after inhalation of fumes from polytetrafluoroethylene (PTFE). J Occup Med 15: 599, 1973.

201. Williams N, Smith K: Polymer fume fever, an elusive diagnosis. JAMA 219, 1587, 1972.

202. May JJ, Stallones L, Darrow D, et al: Organic dust toxicity (pulmonary mycotoxicosis) associated with silo unloading. Thorax 41: 919, 1986.

203. Yoshida K, Ando M, Araki S: Acute pulmonary edema in a storehouse of moldy oranges: a severe case of the organic dust toxic syndrome. Arch Environ Health 44: 382, 1989.

204. Brinton WT, Vastbinder EE, Greene JW, et al: An outbreak of organic dust toxic syndrome in a college fraternity. JAMA 258: 1210, 1987.

205. Alexandersson R, Kolmodin-Hedman B, Hedenstierna G: Exposure to formaldehyde: Effects on pulmonary function. Arch Environ Health 37: 279, 1982.

206. Harris JC, Rumack BH, Aldrich FD: Toxicology of urea formaldehyde and polyurethane foam insulation. JAMA 245: 243, 1981.

207. Krzyzanowski M, Quackenboss JJ, Lebowitz MD: Chronic respiratory effects of indoor formaldehyde exposure. Environ Res 52: 117, 1990.

208. Harving H, Korsgaard J, Pedersen OF, et al: Pulmonary function and bronchial reactivity in asthmatics during low-level formaldehyde exposure. Lung 168: 15, 1990.

209. Nunn AJ, Craigen AA, Darbyshire JH, et al: Six year follow-up of lung function in men occupationally exposed to formaldehyde. Br J Ind Med 47: 747, 1990.

209a. Sterling TD, Weinkam JJ: Reanalysis of lung cancer mortality in a National Cancer Institute study on mortality among industrial workers exposed to formaldehyde. J Occup Med 30: 895, 1988.

210. Toor AH, Tomashefski JF Jr, Kleinerman J: Respiratory tract pathology in patients with severe burns. Hum Pathol 21: 1212, 1990.

211. Clark CJ, Campbell D, Reid WH: Blood carboxyhaemoglobin and cyanide levels in fire survivors. Lancet 1: 1332, 1981.

212. Dyer RF, Esch VH: Polyvinyl chloride toxicity in fires, hydrogen chloride toxicity in fire fighters. JAMA 235: 393, 1976.

213. Brinkmann B, Püschel K: Heat injuries to the respiratory system. Virchows Arch [A] 379: 299, 1978.

214. The lung in burns [editorial]. Lancet 2: 673, 1981.

215. Hasleton PS, McWilliam L, Haboubi NY: The lung parenchyma in burns. Histopathology 7: 333, 1983.

216. Williams DO, Vanecko RM, Glassroth J: Endobronchial polyposis following smoke inhalation. Chest 84: 774, 1983.

217. Teixidor HS, Novick G, Rubin E: Pulmonary complications in burn patients. J Can Assoc Radiol 34: 264, 1983.

218. Teixidor HS, Rubin E, Novick GS, et al: Smoke inhalation: Radiologic manifestations. Radiology 149: 383, 1983.

219. Tashkin DP, Genovesi MG, Chopra S, et al: Respiratory status of Los Angeles firemen: One-month follow-up after inhalation of dense smoke. Chest 71: 445, 1977.

220. Musk AW, Peters JM, Wegman DH: Lung function in fire fighters. I: A three-year follow-up of active subjects. Am J Public Health 67: 626, 1977.

221. Tepper A, Comstock GW, Levine M: A longitudinal study of pulmonary function in fire fighters. Am J Ind Med 20: 307, 1991.

222. Decoufle P, Lloyd JW, Salvin LG: Mortality by cause among stationary engineers and stationary firemen. J Occup Med 19: 679, 1977.

223. Rosenstock L, Demers P, Heyer NJ, et al: Respiratory mortality among firefighters. Br J Ind Med 47: 462, 1990.

224. Sone S, Higashihara T, Kotake T, et al: Pulmonary manifestations in acute carbon monoxide poisoning. Am J Roentgenol 120: 865, 1974.

225. Fein A, Grossman RF, Jones JG, et al: Carbon monoxide effect on alveolar epithelial permeability. Chest 78: 726, 1980.

226. Smith JS, Brandon S: Morbidity from acute carbon monoxide poisoning. A three-year follow-up. Br Med J 1: 318, 1973.

227. Goldsmith JR, Landaw SA: Carbon monoxide in human health. Science 162: 1352, 1968.

228. Bergmann M, Flance IJ, Cruz PT, et al: Thesaurosis due to inhalation of hair spray. Report of twelve new cases, including three autopsies. N Engl J Med 266: 750, 1962.

229. Herrero EU, Feigelson HH, Becker A: Sarcoidosis in a beautician. Am Rev Respir Dis 92: 280, 1965.

230. Schraufnagel DE, Paré JAP, Wang NS: Micronodular pulmonary pattern: Association with inhaled aerosol. Am J Roentgenol 137: 57, 1981.

231. Gowdy JM, Wagstaff MJ: Pulmonary infiltration due to aerosol thesaurosis: A survey of hairdressers. Arch Environ Health 25: 101, 1972.

232. Shinkai T, Saijo N, Tominaga K, et al: Pulmonary toxicity induced by pepleomycin 3-[(S)-1-phenylethylaminol propylamino-bleomycin. Jpn J Clin Oncol 13: 395, 1983.

233. Paolozzi FP, Gaver RC, Newman NB, et al: Phase I trial of tallysomycin S10b, a bleomycin analogue. Invest New Drugs 8: 171, 1990.

234. Rao SX, Ramaswamy G, Levin M, et al: Fatal acute respiratory failure after vinblastine-mitomycin therapy in lung carcinoma. Arch Intern Med 145: 1905, 1985.

235. Luedke D, McLaughlin TT, Daughaday C, et al: Mitomycin C and vindesine-associated pulmonary toxicity with variable clinical expression. Cancer 55: 542, 1985.

236. Bedrossian CWM, Sussman J, Conklin RH, et al: Azathioprine-associated interstitial pneumonitis. Am J Clin Pathol 82: 148, 1984.

237. Haupt HM, Hutchins GM, Moore GW: Ara-C lung: Noncardiogenic pulmonary edema complicating cytosine arabinoside therapy of leukemia. Am J Med 70: 256, 1981.

238. Feinberg L, Travis WD, Ferrans V, et al: Pulmonary fibrosis associated with tocainide: Report of a case with literature review. Am Rev Respir Dis 141: 505, 1990.

239. Cortez LM, Pankey GA: Acute pulmonary hypersensitivity to furazolidone. Am Rev Respir Dis 105: 823, 1972.

239a. Yamakado S, Yoshida Y, Yamada T, et al: Pulmonary infiltration and eosinophilia associated with sulfasalazine therapy for ulcerative colitis: A case report and review of literature. Intern Med 31: 108, 1992.

240. Reichlin S, Loveless MH, Kane EG: Loeffler's syndrome following penicillin therapy. Ann Intern Med 38: 113, 1953.

241. Wold DE, Zahn DW: Allergic (Löffler's) pneumonitis occurring during antituberculous chemotherapy. Report of three cases. Am Rev Tuberc 74: 445, 1956.

242. Dreis DF, Winterbauer RH, Van Norman GA, et al: Cephalosporin-induced interstitial pneumonitis. Chest 86: 138, 1979.

243. Salomaa ER, Ruokonen EL, Tevola K, et al: Pulmonary infiltrates and fever induced by isoniazid. Postgrad Med J 66: 647, 1990.

244. Yokoyama A, Mitzushima Y, Suzuki H, et al: Acute eosinophilic pneumonia induced by minocycline: Prominent Kerley B lines as a feature of positive rechallenge test. Jpn J Med 29: 195, 1990.

245. Barreiro B, Manresa F, Valldeperas J: Carbamazepine and the lung. Eur Respir J 3: 930, 1990.

246. Ogawa H, Kurashima K, Namura M, et al: Pulmonary infiltrates with eosinophilia due to naproxen. Jpn J Med 30: 32, 1991.

247. Goodwin SD, Glenny RW: Nonsteroidal anti-inflammatory drug–associated pulmonary infiltrates: Review of the literature and Food and Drug Administration Adverse Drug Reaction reports. Arch Intern Med 152: 1521, 1992.

248. Marshall A, Moore K: Pulmonary disease after amitriptyline overdosage. Br Med J 1: 716, 1973.

249. Mollura JL, Bernstein R, Fine SR, et al: Pulmonary eosinophilia in a patient receiving beclomethasone dipropionate aerosol. Ann Allergy 42: 326, 1979.

250. Barna JS, Frable MA: Life-threatening angioedema. Otolaryngol Head Neck Surg 103: 795, 1990.

251. Schatz PL, Mesologites D, Hyun J, et al: Captopril-induced hypersensitivity lung disease. An immune-complex–mediated phenomenon. Chest 95: 685, 1989.

252. Chastre J, Basset F, Viau F, et al: Acute pneumonitis after subcutaneous injections of silicone in transsexual men. N Engl J Med 308: 764, 1983.

253. Marshall AJ, Eltringham WK, Barritt DW, et al: Respiratory disease associated with practolol therapy. Lancet 2: 1254, 1977.

254. Gauthier-Rahman S, Akoun GM, Milleron BJ, et al: Leukocyte migration inhibition in propranolol-induced pneumonitis. Evidence for an immunologic cell-mediated mechanism. Chest 97: 238, 1990.

255. Sloand EM, Thompson BT: Propranolol-induced pulmonary edema and shock in a patient with pheochromocytoma. Arch Intern Med 144: 173, 1984.

256. Wiggins J, Skinner C: Bromocriptine-induced pleuropulmonary fibrosis. Thorax 41: 328, 1986.

257. Pfitzenmeyer P, Foucher P, Piard F, et al: Nilutamide pneumonitis: A report on eight patients. Thorax 47: 622, 1992.

15

DISEASES OF THE THORAX CAUSED BY EXTERNAL PHYSICAL AGENTS

Trauma to the thorax can have many effects on the chest wall, diaphragm, mediastinum, trachea, and lungs. Because the manifestations of such trauma are dissimilar in these different sites, each is considered separately. As might be anticipated, however, a great deal of overlap occurs. Also, the effects of penetrating and nonpenetrating trauma may be quite different and thus require separate consideration. *Trauma* is used here in its broad sense, to indicate all insults to the thorax resulting from external physical agents; thus, irradiation injury is included in this category. It is also appropriate to include in this chapter the consequences of surgery, both thoracic and nonthoracic, and complications caused by various diagnostic, therapeutic, and monitoring procedures involving the chest.

Although diagnosis of the majority of traumatic abnormalities of the thorax can be established with reasonable confidence by conventional roentgenographic methods, certain conditions (e.g., laceration of the aorta) require special diagnostic procedures, including computed tomography (CT) and aortography, to confirm the injury and establish its extent. CT also may provide additional information on the nature and severity of pulmonary disease.[1] For example, in one study of 85 consecutive patients with chest trauma,[2] 151 abnormalities (excluding rib fractures) were identified on roentgenograms, whereas 423 were found on CT scans.

EFFECTS ON THE LUNGS OF NONPENETRATING TRAUMA

Pulmonary Parenchymal Contusion

Pulmonary contusion consists of the exudation of edema fluid and blood into the parenchyma of the lung in both its airspace and interstitial components, in the absence of substantial tissue disruption. It is the most common pulmonary complication of blunt chest trauma, in which it occurs more often than rib fracture; in fact, rib fractures are frequently absent. The severity of the injury necessary to produce contusion varies from a trivial glancing blow to major trauma resulting from motor vehicle or aircraft accidents.

Roentgenographically, the pattern varies from irregular, patchy airspace opacities to diffuse and extensive homogeneous consolidation (Fig. 15–1). As might be expected, the distribution of the contused areas does not conform to lobes or segments.[3] The major change is usually in the lung directly deep to the traumatized areas. The time interval between the trauma and the detection of roentgenographic abnormality is important in differential diagnosis, particularly with respect to fat embolism. With contusion, changes are apparent roentgenographically soon after trauma (almost invariably within 6 hours),[3] whereas in fat embolism they usually do not become evident until at least 1 to 2 days after injury. Resolution of lung contusion typically occurs rapidly, improvement being noted within 24 to 48 hours and clearing being complete within 3 days (Fig. 15–2).[3, 4]

Clinical findings are seldom striking; in fact, symptoms may be entirely absent or may be masked by the other injuries the patient may have. Hemoptysis is said to occur in 50 per cent of cases and there may be mild fever.[3] Shortness of breath may develop in the presence of severe contusion.

Traumatic Lung Cyst and Pulmonary Hematoma

Rather uncommonly, closed chest trauma results in the development of one or more spaces within the lung that can remain air-filled (traumatic lung cyst, or pseudocyst) or that fill partly or completely with blood (pulmonary hematoma). The trauma usually is blunt and is often severe, as in automobile accidents. Children and young adults seem to be particularly vulnerable, probably because of the greater flexibility of their thoracic wall. Pulmonary hematomas indistinguishable from those caused by closed chest trauma sometimes develop following segmental or wedge resection of the lung.

The development of these cystic spaces is necessarily preceded by laceration of pulmonary parenchymal tissue which, in blunt trauma, has been hypothesized to occur by one of two mechanisms. According to the first, sudden compression of an area of lung closes off a segment of the peripheral bronchial tree and creates within it a bursting, explosive pressure that is expended in the rupture of alveolar walls.[5] In the second, the propagation of a concussion wave creates shearing stresses that tear the substance of the lung.[6]

These lesions may be apparent roentgenographically immediately after trauma, but more commonly are not seen until a few hours or even several days later. The fact that they are not identified immediately may be ascribed to two circumstances: in the absence of hemorrhage, their paper-thin margins and lack of contrast with contiguous parenchyma render them invisible; alternatively, their presence may be masked by surrounding pulmonary contusion.[7]

Roentgenographically, traumatic cysts appear as single or multiple lesions,[8] ranging from oval to spherical in shape and from 2 to 14 cm in diameter. In the majority of cases, they develop under the point of maximal injury in the periphery of the lung. Their appearance depends in large measure on whether they contain blood. Approximately half the lesions present as thin-walled, air-filled spaces, with or without a fluid level (Fig. 15–3),[9] and the remainder as homogeneous, well-defined masses of water density (Fig. 15–4). A characteristic of these lesions is their tendency to persist for a long time, frequently as long as 4 months. However, they generally decrease in size progressively; if such a lesion does not shrink within 6 weeks, the possibility must be considered that the trauma may have been purely coincidental to a solitary nodule of other etiology.

The majority of affected patients are asymptomatic. Hemoptysis occurs rarely and is probably attributable to emptying of the hematoma.[9]

Fracture of the Trachea and Bronchi

Fracture (rupture, transection) of the tracheobronchial tree is uncommon and usually results from blunt trauma to the anterior chest in vehicular accidents.[10] It has been stated that in adults particularly, the trauma is severe enough to result in concomitant fractures of the first three ribs. However, the incidence of this abnormality varies widely in different series; for example, such fractures were observed in an astonishing 91 per cent of patients in one study[11] but in only 1 of 50 patients in another.[12]

Fractures of the bronchi are more common than those of the trachea and constitute about 80 per cent of all tracheobronchial injuries.[4] They are usually parallel to the cartilage rings and involve the mainstem bronchi 1 to 2 cm distal to the carina.[4] The right side is affected more often than the left; adjacent pulmonary vessels are rarely damaged.[13] Fractures of the intrathoracic trachea are horizontal and usually occur just above the carina.[4]

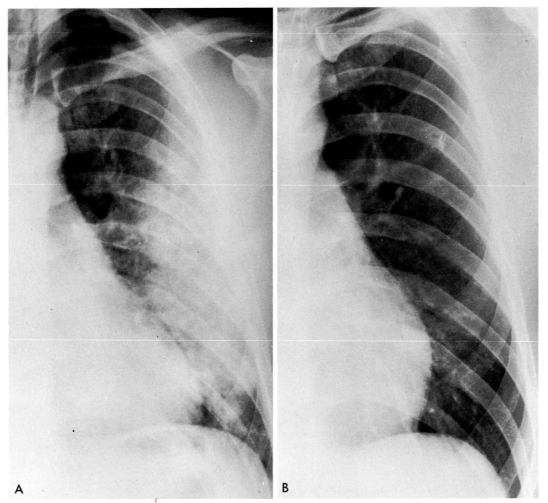

Figure 15–1. Pulmonary Contusion. Six hours before the roentgenographic examination illustrated in *(A)*, this 33-year-old man was involved in a car accident in which he suffered severe trauma to the posterior portion of his left chest. A view of the left hemithorax from an anteroposterior roentgenogram reveals homogeneous consolidation of the posterolateral portion of the left lung in nonsegmental distribution. The margins of the consolidation are very indistinctly defined, and there is no air bronchogram. No ribs were fractured. The right lung was clear. Three days later *(B)*, complete clearing had occurred.

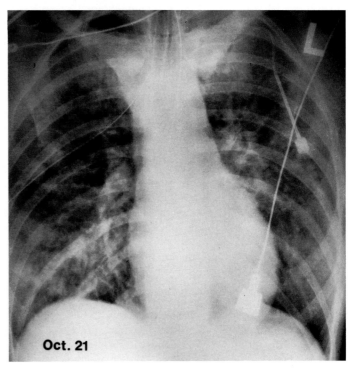

Figure 15–2. Pulmonary Contusion with Rapid Resolution. Shortly after his arrival in the emergency room following an automobile accident, this 22-year-old man showed roentgenographic evidence of poorly defined patchy airspace consolidation throughout both lungs. The appearance is one of pulmonary edema of any cause, although the history and normal cardiac size obviously favor traumatic contusion. Complete clearing had occurred 48 hours later.

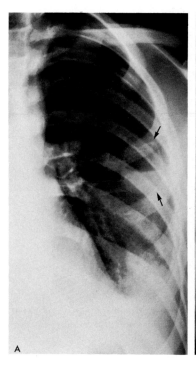
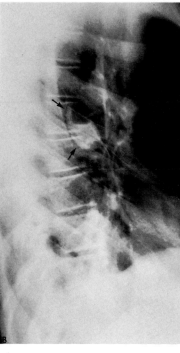

Figure 15–3. Traumatic Pulmonary Contusion, Laceration, and Hematoma. This 18-year-old man suffered a severe blow to the left side of his chest in a car accident 4 days previously. Views of the left hemithorax from posteroanterior (A) and lateral (B) roentgenograms reveal inhomogeneous, nonsegmental consolidation of the lower portion of the left lung caused by pulmonary contusion. In the midportion of the left lung is a thin-walled cystic space containing a prominent air-fluid level (*arrows* in both projections), representing a pulmonary laceration into which hemorrhage has occurred. (Courtesy of St. Paul's Hospital, Saskatoon, Saskatchewan.)

Roentgenologically, the most common finding is pneumothorax, although this may not present when fracture affects the trachea or the bronchi within the mediastinum and the mediastinal parietal pleura remains intact. In some cases, a small amount of air escapes from the airway and remains localized to the surrounding connective tissues, where it can be identified.[14] Displacement of fracture ends can result in bronchial obstruction and atelectasis of an entire lung (Fig. 15–5).[6] Perhaps more important than these individual abnormalities are certain combinations of roentgenographic findings that are considered to be highly suggestive of fracture: (1) a large pneumothorax that does not respond to chest tube drainage,[15] (2) pneumothorax and pneumomediastinum in the absence of pleural effusion, and (3) mediastinal and deep cervical emphysema in a trauma patient who is not receiving positive-pressure ventilation.[16]

In approximately 10 per cent of patients, tracheobronchial fracture is not associated with any roentgenographically demonstrable abnormality or with much in the way of symptoms or signs.[4] It is probable that in such cases the peribronchial connective tissue is preserved, preventing passage of air into the mediastinum or pleural space. Thus, the consequence of the trauma may not become evident until the patient presents with atelectasis of a lobe or lung as a result of bronchial stenosis, a condition that may not occur until weeks to months after the traumatic episode (*see* Fig. 15–5).

Symptoms and signs include cyanosis, hemoptysis, shock, cough, and sternal tenderness.[10] Air may be identifiable in the subcutaneous tissues, initially involving the neck and upper thorax and later becoming generalized.

The overall mortality rate is approximately 30 per cent, a value attributable to the severity of the trauma required to cause fracture, rather than to the fracture itself. More than half the patients succumb within 1 hour of injury, and

approximately 10 per cent who reach the hospital alive subsequently die.[11] Early diagnosis is important, since surgical repair can result in anatomic and functional restoration.[17]

Lung Torsion

Torsion occurs when a whole lung or lobe is twisted 180 degrees so that its base comes to lie at the apex of the hemithorax and its apex at the base. It has been described under three sets of circumstances:[18] (1) spontaneously (usually in association with some other pulmonary or diaphragmatic abnormality, such as pneumonia, accessory pulmonary lobe, or diaphragmatic hernia); (2) following trauma; and (3) after thoracic surgery, usually lobectomy.[19] As a complication of trauma, torsion of a whole lung occurs most commonly in children, presumably because of the easy compressibility of a child's thoracic cage. The trauma usually is severe, such as when a child is run over by a vehicle, and torsion occurs most often when the major force is applied to the compressible lower thorax.

The diagnosis should be obvious from the roentgenographic appearance of the chest. The pattern of pulmonary vascular markings is altered in a predictable manner: the interlobar artery sweeps upward toward the apex, and the lower lung vessels are comparatively diminutive. If the torsion is not relieved, the vascular supply can be compromised and the lung can become opaque as a result of exudation of edema fluid and blood into the airspaces.

Atelectasis

Post-traumatic collapse of a lobe—or very occasionally of a whole lung—is not common, but when present causes significant intrapulmonary shunting and hypoxemia at a time when a patient's clinical status may be critical. The cause of the atelectasis is not always clear, although it is probable that most cases result from bronchial obstruction from blood clots or mucus plugs. In such circumstances, bronchoscopy readily reveals the cause and permits prompt relief of the obstruction.

EFFECTS ON THE PLEURA OF NONPENETRATING TRAUMA

Hemothorax and pneumothorax are common manifestations of nonpenetrating trauma (*see* also pages 875 and 878). Although hemothorax can result from laceration of the parietal or visceral pleura by fractured ribs, it also can occur with closed chest trauma when there is no evidence of fracture. The origin of hemorrhage is important in determining the quantity of hemothorax.[14] When bleeding is from a vessel in the chest wall, diaphragm, or mediastinum, the hemothorax tends to increase despite the quantity of blood present. By contrast, when the blood comes from pulmonary vasculature, the expanding hemothorax compresses the lung, producing pulmonary vascular tamponade that may produce hemostasis.

When blood enters the pleural space it coagulates rapidly; however, presumably as a result of physical agitation produced by movement of the heart and lungs, the clot may be defibrinated and leave fluid indistinguishable roentgenologically from effusion from any other cause.[14] When a solid clot does remain, it may prove a hindrance to adequate thoracentesis, a procedure that should be carried out thoroughly to prevent later troublesome fibrothorax. As in empyema, loculation tends to occur early in hemothorax and increases still further the difficulty of achieving drainage.

Although pneumothorax most commonly develops as a consequence of pulmonary interstitial emphysema, it also may result from rib or tracheobronchial fracture or esophageal rupture. When rib fracture is present, the likely mechanism is laceration of the visceral pleura by bone fragments, and in such circumstances hemothorax may be expected as a concomitant finding. When there are no rib fractures, the likely mechanism is the same as in spontaneous pneumomediastinum: rupture of alveoli into the peribronchovascular connective tissue as a result of an abrupt increase in pressure or shear stress leads to interstitial emphysema and, by extension, pneumothorax. This explanation also provides adequate reason for the occurrence of pneumomediastinum and subcutaneous emphysema without rib fracture.

EFFECTS ON THE MEDIASTINUM OF NONPENETRATING TRAUMA

Pneumomediastinum

Like pneumothorax, pneumomediastinum can develop after closed chest trauma, in which case it is probably related to alveolar rupture and interstitial emphysema. It may also follow traumatic rupture of the esophagus or fracture of the tracheobronchial tree, in which case it may be associated with acute mediastinitis. Air may also enter the mediastinum along deep fascial planes as a result of trauma or surgical procedures to the neck or in association with zygomaticomaxillary fractures.[20] The roentgenographic signs are identical to those of pneumomediastinum from any other cause (see page 903).

Mediastinal Hemorrhage

The majority of cases of mediastinal hemorrhage result from trauma, usually following a severe automobile acci-

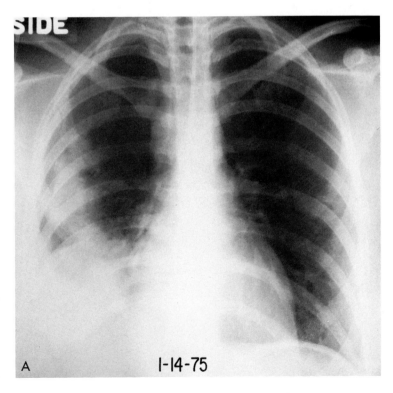

Figure 15–4. Multiple Unilateral Pulmonary Hematomas. This 17-year-old girl was involved in a two-car collision in which she sustained fractures of her right scapula and humerus. The day after admission, an anteroposterior roentgenogram *(A)* revealed extensive parenchymal consolidation in the lower two thirds of the right lung in nonsegmental distribution; the left lung was clear. There was some widening of the superior mediastinum, undoubtedly from venous hemorrhage.

Illustration continued on following page

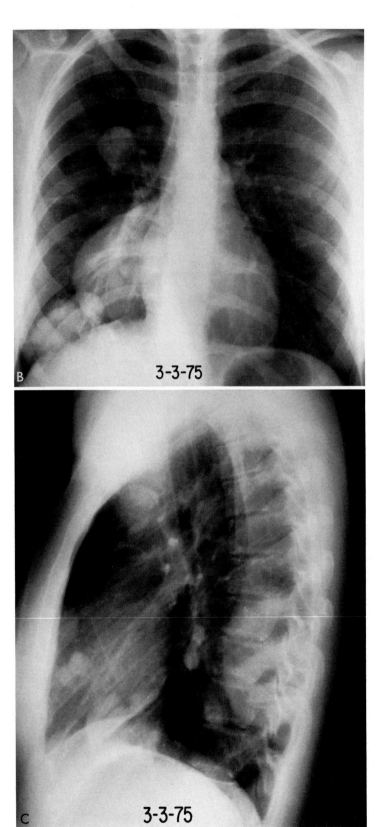

3-3-75

3-3-75

Figure 15–4 *Continued* Two months later, roentgenograms in posteroanterior *(B)* and lateral *(C)* projections revealed multiple, sharply defined, homogeneous nodules in the right lung ranging from 1 to 6 cm in diameter (12 discrete nodules can be identified). No cavitation was present, and the left lung remained clear.

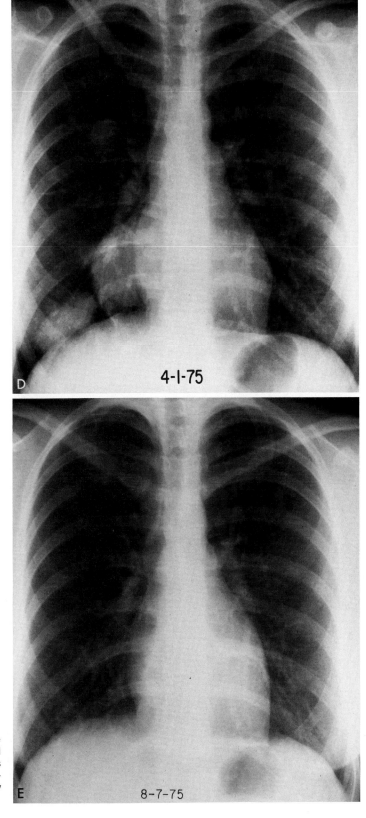

Figure 15–4 *Continued* Approximately 1 month later *(D),* the nodules had diminished considerably in size, and several had disappeared altogether. Seven months after the injury, all signs of disease had disappeared *(E).* (Courtesy of Dr. John D. Armstrong, Jr., University of Utah College of Medicine and Valley West Hospital, Salt Lake City, Utah.)

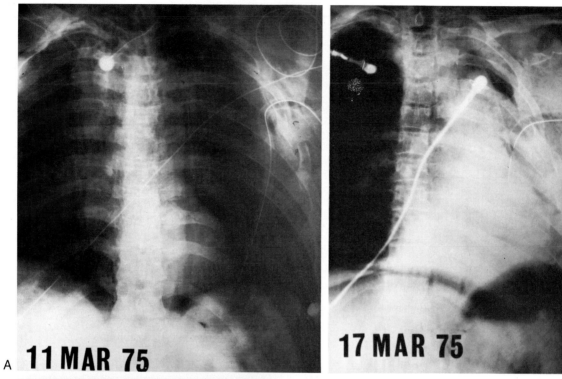

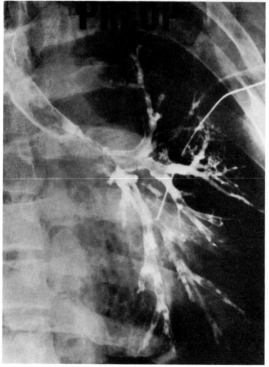

Figure 15–5. Fracture of the Left Main Bronchus. On admission to the hospital following a crushing injury to his chest, this 33-year-old man showed roentgenographic evidence *(A)* of severe subcutaneous and mediastinal emphysema and fracture of multiple left ribs, including the first, second, and third (not visible on the illustration). Bilateral pneumothorax had been treated in the emergency room by intubation. At this time, both lungs were well expanded. Six days later *(B)*, there had occurred almost total collapse of the left lung. Bronchoscopy revealed an obstruction in the midportion of the left main bronchus. The obstructing material resembled a blood clot, although in some areas the bronchoscopist thought he was looking at the edge of a cartilaginous ring. Bronchography performed shortly thereafter *(C)* revealed severe deformity and narrowing of the distal end of the left main bronchus just before its bifurcation. At thoracotomy, the left main bronchus was found to be completely disrupted just proximal to its bifurcation, and this was repaired by end-to-end anastomosis. Three months later, the left lung was well expanded, the only residual roentgenographic changes being those usually anticipated following severe trauma.

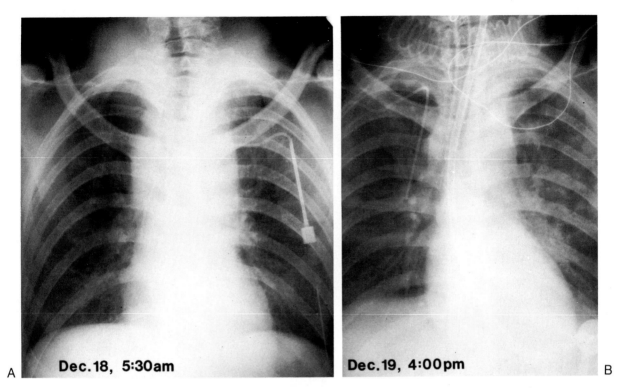

Figure 15–6. Traumatic Mediastinal Hemorrhage. A roentgenogram of the chest in anteroposterior projection, supine position *(A)* of this young man following severe closed chest trauma reveals moderate widening of the upper half of the mediastinum, roughly symmetric on both sides. The lungs are unremarkable. Approximately 36 hours later *(B)*, the widening had diminished considerably. There is now evidence of a uniform opacity over both lungs, which, in a supine view, is good evidence for bilateral pleural effusion, in this case hemothorax.

dent with chest cage compression or faulty placement of a central venous line in a subclavian vein. Less common causes include rupture of an aortic aneurysm, extension of blood from the retropharyngeal soft tissues secondary to trauma, and spontaneous hemorrhage associated with a co-agulation disorder. Undoubtedly, the majority of cases go unrecognized, the amount of bleeding being insufficient to produce symptoms and signs.

Roentgenographically, hemorrhage typically results in uniform, symmetric widening of the mediastinum in any of its compartments (Fig. 15–6). Local accumulation of blood in the form of a hematoma is manifested by a homogeneous mass that may project to one or both sides of the medias-tinum.

Rupture of the Thoracic Aorta and Its Branches

Rupture of the aorta is a well-recognized sequela of closed chest injury, particularly following severe automobile accidents.[21] Because of the variable mobility of different portions of the aorta, sudden deceleration produces shear-ing stresses, the more mobile anterior portion of the aortic arch being "whipped" on the more fixed posterior arch and paraspinal aorta.[22] Thus, approximately 95 per cent of all aortic ruptures occur in the region of the aortic isthmus at the site of the ligamentum arteriosum[22]; the remaining 5 per cent are immediately above the aortic valve. Immediate death is the usual result.

Occasionally, mediastinal hemorrhage following severe chest trauma can result from damage to one of the great vessels arising from the aortic arch. In fact, avulsion of the innominate artery from the arch has been stated to be the second most common type of aortic injury in which the patient survives long enough for diagnostic evaluation.[23] The plain roentgenographic findings are similar to those of rupture of the aorta itself, with the possible exception that the outline of the descending aorta may be preserved.

Although aortography remains the definitive method of establishing the diagnosis of aortic rupture, a variety of signs on plain roentgenograms have been described as being useful in diagnosis. It should be remembered, how-ever, that some of these—including upper mediastinal wid-ening of at least 8 cm, left apical cap, tracheal stripe wid-ened to 5 mm or more, and deviation of a nasogastric tube to the right of the T4 spinous process—are also associated with fractures of the upper thoracic spine.[24]

Widening of the Upper Half of the Mediastinum. Plain roentgenograms of the chest almost invariably reveal widening of the superior mediastinum as a result of hemor-rhage (Fig. 15–7). The extravascular blood tends to cause the pedicle to widen predominantly to the left of the mid-line while, at the same time, causing disappearance of the shadow of the tracheal stripe and the azygos vein.[25]

Loss of Contour of the Aortic Knob. The aortic knob is generally invisible, an important sign that should alert the roentgenologist to the possibility of aortic rupture (*see* Fig. 15–7). It must be emphasized, however, that in some cases the shadow of the aortic knuckle is preserved, and this finding does not rule out rupture of the vessel.

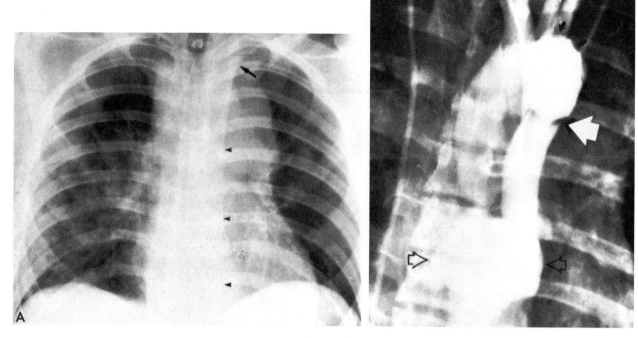

Figure 15–7. Traumatic Aneurysm and Rupture of the Thoracic Aorta. This 16-year-old boy crashed into a telephone pole in an automobile traveling at 85 mph. Shortly after his arrival in the emergency room, a chest roentgenogram in anteroposterior projection *(A)* revealed marked widening of the upper mediastinum and loss of visualization of the aortic knob. A wide paravertebral opacity *(arrow-heads)* extends up to the apex, creating an extrapleural apical cap *(arrow)*. The suspicion of aortic rupture was confirmed by aortography *(B)*. The site of primary aortic laceration is indicated by a *thick arrow*, the irregular bulge imediately above *(small arrows)* representing dissection proximally. Several centimeters distally is a large collection of contrast medium *(open arrows)*, which represents an extra-aortic hematoma from a second rupture.

Deviation of the Trachea and Left Main Bronchus. As the hematoma enlarges, the left main bronchus may be pushed anteriorly, inferiorly, and to the right, and the trachea displaced to the right. These signs are said to be present in about 75 per cent of patients.[21]

Displacement of a Nasogastric Tube. Some studies have emphasized the importance of identifying displacement of a nasogastric tube to the right. For example, one investigation found that a shift to the right of both the trachea and the nasogastric tube was associated with a 96 per cent probability of rupture.[26]

Displacement of the Right Paraspinous Interface. This sign has been found by some workers to be highly reliable in diagnosis *(see* Fig. 15–7). For example, in one retrospective review of the roentgenographic findings in 14 patients with proven acute traumatic rupture of the aorta,[27] displacement of the right paraspinous interface was identified in eight. The sign was not seen roentgenographically in any patient who did not have evidence of rupture on aortography.

Widening of the Right Tracheal Stripe. Another sign that has been suggested as a possible indicator of aortic tear is widening of the right tracheal stripe to a width greater than 5 mm *(see* Fig. 15–7). In one study of 102 patients with blunt chest trauma, all patients with a right paratracheal stripe less than 5 mm in width had a normal aortogram, whereas in those patients whose right tracheal stripe measured 5 mm or greater, aortography revealed major arterial injury in 23 per cent.[28]

The Left Apical Cap. Provided that the parietal pleura

is intact, extravasated blood from the aorta can track cephalad along the course of the left subclavian artery, between the parietal pleura and the extrapleural soft tissues. The result is a homogeneous opacity over the apex of the left hemithorax—the extrapleural apical cap *(see* Fig. 15–7). In one prospective and retrospective study that assessed the value of the left apical cap,[29] the findings suggested that *by itself* it is an unreliable sign of acute aortic rupture.

Left Hemothorax. Hemothorax complicating traumatic rupture of the aorta is common and is almost invariably left sided. It should not be attributed erroneously to left-sided rib fractures.

Fracture of the First and Second Ribs. Formerly considered a potential indicator of aortic or brachiocephalic trauma, fractures of the first and second ribs are now thought to represent unreliable signs on the strength of several well-documented studies.[12]

CT is extremely useful in diagnosing aortic rupture.[30] Findings include (1) false aneurysm; (2) linear lucency within the opacified aortic lumen caused by the torn edge of the aortic wall; (3) marginal irregularity of the opacified aortic lumen; (4) periaortic or intramural aortic hematoma; and (5) dissection. Interestingly, in some series the extent of associated mediastinal hemorrhage and the amount of blood in the pleural space have not been found to be useful indicators of aortic injury.[30] Similarly, shift of the trachea and esophagus to the right may not be discriminatory.

On the basis of the many studies that the authors have reviewed,[31–34] the following three conclusions seem to be warranted. First, when any patient suffers severe chest trauma and conventional chest roentgenograms reveal upper mediastinal widening and loss of configuration of the aortic knob, CT or aortography, or both, should be performed to establish the diagnosis and reveal the anatomic extent of the rupture. Second, patients older than 65 years probably should be examined at least with CT, whether or not there is roentgenographic evidence of mediastinal widening. Third, considered individually, it is doubtful whether the other signs described above constitute sufficient indication for aortography, but even in the absence of mediastinal widening, any combination of three of these signs should raise the index of suspicion to a high level and probably justify at least CT and, possibly, aortography.

Clinical findings that suggest the presence of traumatic rupture of the aorta include (1) a systolic murmur over the precordium or medial to the left scapula; (2) hoarseness (caused by pressure of a hematoma on the left recurrent laryngeal nerve); and (3) hypertension in the upper extremities and hypotension or weak pulses in the lower extremities.[35]

The mortality of dissecting aneurysms of nontraumatic origin is between 20 and 40 per cent.[36] Considering the additional injuries that almost inevitably occur in association with a traumatic etiology, the prognosis for this form is undoubtedly worse, many patients dying in the first week after injury. Uncommonly, aneurysms of traumatic origin go unrecognized at the time and may remain so for many years until the patient presents with chest pain and roentgenographic evidence of progressive enlargement of the aortic shadow (Fig. 15–8)[37] or until a screening chest roentgenogram of an asymptomatic patient reveals the abnormality.[38]

Perforation of the Esophagus

Rupture of the esophagus from closed chest trauma is rare.[39] Of considerably greater frequency, however, is the rupture that occurs as a complication of esophagoscopy or gastroscopy, overzealous dilation of a stricture or achalasia, or disruption of the suture line following esophageal resection and anastomosis. The usual result is acute mediastinitis (*see* page 897).

Rupture of the Thoracic Duct

Rupture of the thoracic duct may develop from surgical procedures, nonpenetrating injuries, or penetrating wounds from a bullet or knife.[14] The anatomic course of the thoracic duct and the site of damage establish the side on which the chylothorax develops. As it enters the thorax, the duct lies slightly to the right of the midline, so rupture in its lower third (an unusual site in crush injuries) leads to right-sided chylothorax. The duct crosses the midline to the left in the midthorax, so disruption above this point tends to produce left-sided chylothorax. Several days may elapse between the chest trauma and the development of roentgenographically demonstrable pleural fluid, a time lag that should strongly suggest the diagnosis.

The rupture of large quantities of chyle from the mediastinum into the pleural space may give rise to the abrupt onset of respiratory difficulty. Thoracentesis yielding milky fluid of high-fat content confirms the diagnosis, and the precise site of rupture may be established by lymphangiography.

EFFECTS ON THE DIAPHRAGM OF NONPENETRATING TRAUMA

The only abnormality of the diaphragm that occurs as a result of trauma is rupture (tear). This may be caused by direct penetrating injury or blunt nonpenetrating trauma to the abdomen or thorax; roughly equal numbers of cases are attributable to each type of trauma.[40] The most common causes are automobile accidents and falls. In some cases, herniation of abdominal contents through the site of rupture occurs at the time of the accident, but its presence is masked by injuries to other organs. In other cases, herniation may occur without associated signs or symptoms and be detected months or years later on a screening chest roentgenogram. The latter situation is probably common; it has been estimated that 9 of 10 traumatic diaphragmatic hernias are overlooked at the time of injury.[41]

Trauma accounts for only a small percentage of all diaphragmatic hernias[42]; however, 90 percent of *strangulated* diaphragmatic hernias are of traumatic origin.[4] According to the older literature, the left hemidiaphragm is affected in 90 to 95 per cent of cases,[40] a predominance hypothesized to occur because the right hemidiaphragm is protected by the liver. More recent studies, however, have documented a considerably higher incidence of right-sided hernias. For example, in one analysis of 42 cases it was found that the left hemidiaphragm was affected in 24 cases (57 per cent), the right in 15 cases (36 per cent), and both in 3 cases (7 per cent).[43] The central and posterior portions are most commonly involved. The hernia contents depend on the size and position of the rupture and can include omentum, stomach, small and large intestine, spleen, kidney, and even pancreas. As might be anticipated, there is no peritoneal sac.

Roentgenographically, the left hemidiaphragm cannot be traced, and abnormal shadows are visible in the left hemithorax (Fig. 15–9). These shadows depend on the nature of hernia contents and are commonly inhomogeneous owing to the presence of air-containing bowel, usually with fluid levels. In contrast to Bochdalek hernias, a portion of the stomach is often present. The roentgenographic appearance can simulate eventration or diaphragmatic paralysis, and differentiation may be possible only with barium examination of the gastrointestinal tract, computed tomography, or real-time sonography.[44] Of major differential importance is the fact that with hernia, afferent and efferent loops of bowel are constricted as they traverse the orifice in the diaphragm (Fig. 15–10), whereas in eventration or paralysis the loops tend to be widely separated. Unilateral pleural effusion, hemothorax, and pneumothorax are important roentgenographic signs suggesting strangulation.[45] When this complication is absent, fluid seldom collects in the affected pleural space, since any fluid that forms as a result of irritation can pass into the abdomen through the rent in the diaphragm.

When rupture occurs in the right hemidiaphragm, a portion of the liver may herniate through the rent and create a

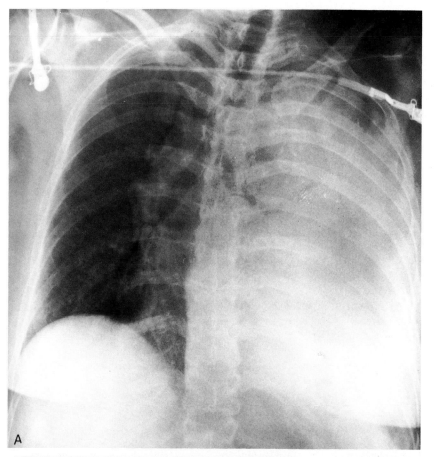

Figure 15–8. Traumatic Aneurysm of the Aorta: Delayed Rupture 20 Years After Trauma. This 53-year-old woman was admitted to the hospital approximately 24 hours after the abrupt onset of severe chest pain and worsening dyspnea. A roentgenogram of the chest in anteroposterior projection, supine position *(A)* discloses a massive left pleural effusion which, on thoracentesis, proved to be blood. A CT scan at the level of the aortic arch following a bolus injection of contrast medium *(B)* reveals a large saccular aneurysm extending off the left side of the arch *(arrows)*. An aortogram in left anterior oblique projection *(C)* demonstrates a large saccular aneurysm arising from the aorta just distal to the takeoff of the left subclavian artery. The only previous trauma that the patient could recall was an automobile accident approximately 20 years previously in which she suffered a severe injury to her thorax against a steering wheel. She had not been investigated for possible thoracic injury at that time.

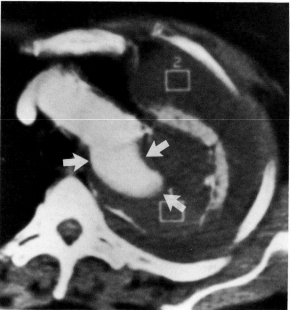

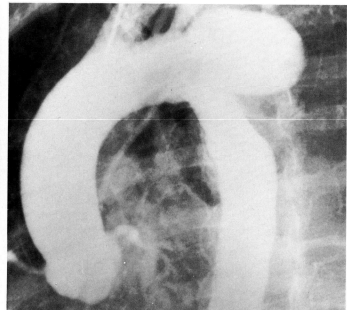

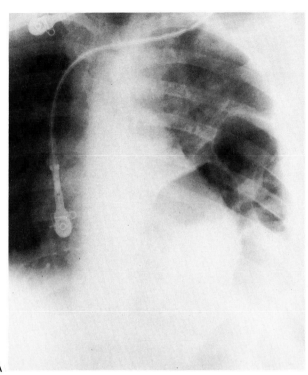
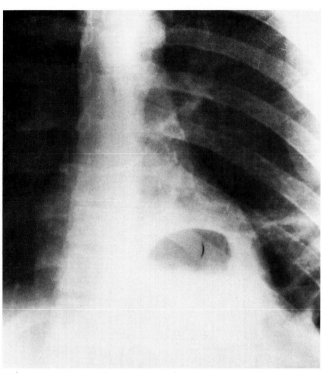

A   B

Figure 15–9. Acute Traumatic Rupture of the Left Hemidiaphragm. This 22-year-old man was involved in a car accident in which he suffered severe trauma to the left side of his chest and abdomen. An anteroposterior roentgenogram of his chest in the supine position *(A)* revealed no evidence of a left hemidiaphragm. Multiple gas-containing structures could be identified in the lower portion of the left hemithorax. Later the same day, an anteroposterior roentgenogram in the erect position *(B)* revealed a gas-containing structure in the medial portion of the left hemithorax posteriorly, showing a prominent air-fluid level—this is the stomach. In addition, there is almost total airlessness of the left lower lobe owing to atelectasis. A large left diaphragmatic laceration was satifactorily repaired.

mushroom-like mass in the right hemithorax, the herniated liver being constricted by the tear. In such circumstances, herniation may be suspected by the high position of the lower border of the liver, as indicated by the position of the hepatic flexure.[46]

Immediate symptoms consist of severe substernal pain, vomiting, shock, and dyspnea resulting from lung compression. Associated injuries are common, the most frequent being rupture of the spleen, perforation of a hollow abdominal viscus, and fractured ribs. Intestinal obstruction as a result of strangulation occurs most commonly in cases of long-standing hernia.[40]

EFFECTS ON THE CHEST WALL OF NONPENETRATING TRAUMA

Fractures of the Ribs

The possibility of complications such as hemothorax, pneumothorax, or hemopneumothorax after rib fracture renders it desirable—if not necessary—to perform chest roentgenography promptly after trauma, more for the identification of these complications than for the fractures themselves. Trauma severe enough to fracture the first and second ribs often produces serious intrathoracic damage as well, including torsion of the lung and tracheobronchial fracture.[47] Fractures of the ninth, tenth, or eleventh ribs

are apt to be associated with splenic or hepatic injury and sometimes with serious intra-abdominal hemorrhage.[35]

Cough fractures of the ribs occur more often in women than in men[48] and almost invariably involve the sixth to ninth ribs, most often the seventh and usually in the posterior axillary line.

The diagnosis of fractured ribs may be suggested clinically by the abrupt onset of chest pain after blunt trauma or a severe bout of coughing. The pain is accentuated by breathing; in some cases, a sensation of "something snapping" is noted by the patient.

Fractures of the Spine

Fractures of thoracic vertebral bodies may result in extraosseous hemorrhage and the development of unilateral or bilateral paraspinal masses. Although the fracture is usually evident roentgenographically, the major evidence of its presence may be deformity of the contiguous paraspinal soft tissues. As indicated previously (*see* page 789), some of the roentgenographic signs of a fractured upper thoracic spine are identical to those of a ruptured aorta.[24]

Post-traumatic Hernia of the Lung

Protrusion of a portion of lung through an abnormal aperture of the thoracic cage may be congenital or traumatic in origin.[49] The most common location of the latter

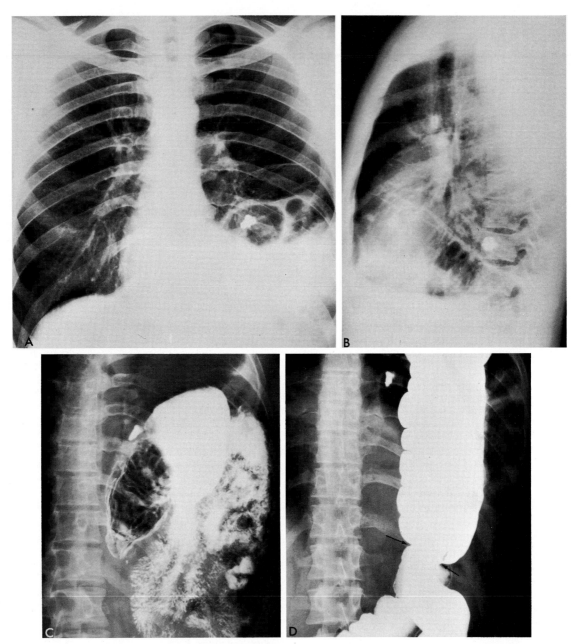

Figure 15–10. Traumatic Diaphragmatic Hernia. This 65-year-old man was admitted to the hospital with a 12-year history of discomfort in the left chest and upper abdomen, a symptom that had been present more or less continuously since he was wounded in 1944 by a piece of shrapnel that entered the left side of his chest between the eighth and ninth ribs. On admission, posteroanterior *(A)* and lateral *(B)* roentgenograms revealed numerous air-containing viscera within the lower portion of the left hemithorax. The left hemidiaphragm could not be identified clearly. The metallic foreign body was readily visualized. Barium examination of the upper gastrointestinal tract *(C)* showed much of the stomach and several loops of small bowel within the left hemithorax. Barium opacification of the colon *(D)* demonstrated a long segment of splenic flexure within the left hemithorax, the point at which the colon passed through the rent in the diaphragm being indicated by *arrows.* At thoracotomy, a large defect measuring 3 inches in diameter was found in the left hemidiaphragm; most of the stomach, part of the large bowel, and a considerable amount of small bowel were situated within the left hemithorax.

form is the parasternal region just medial to the costochondral junction, where the intercostal musculature is thinnest. The patient usually complains of a bulge appearing during coughing and straining, and, in most cases, the diagnosis is evidenced by the clinical finding of a soft, crepitant mass that develops under these conditions and disappears during expiration or rest. Chest roentgenograms reveal pulmonary parenchymal tissue herniating through an obvious defect in the rib cage or through a supraclavicular fossa. Optimal visualization requires the Valsalva maneuver, with or without tangential roentgenographic projection or CT.[50]

PULMONARY EFFECTS OF NONTHORACIC TRAUMA

A number of pleuropulmonary abnormalities occur as a consequence of trauma, but their pathogenesis is unrelated to *direct* injury to the thorax (although chest injury may have occurred as well). Some of these effects are specific to trauma, including fat embolism, air embolism, and the hypoxemia associated with severe head trauma, whereas others are nonspecific, such as pulmonary thromboembolism and adult respiratory distress syndrome. The last-named is perhaps the most common serious complication. Although the chest roentgenogram may be normal despite low values of PaO_2, it more often shows diffuse opacification. If there is reason to believe that the chest was also injured, the only other condition that need be considered in the differential diagnosis is severe pulmonary contusion. Sometimes this distinction can be difficult, although contusion tends to be less diffuse and to clear more rapidly.

EFFECTS ON THE THORAX OF PENETRATING TRAUMA

The usual roentgenographic appearance of the path of a bullet through lung parenchyma is a rather poorly defined, homogeneous shadow that, as might be expected, is more or less circular when viewed in the direction in which the bullet passed and longitudinal when viewed in perpendicular projection (Fig. 15–11). The indistinct definition is caused by hemorrhage and edema into the parenchyma surrounding the bullet track. The edema usually clears in a few days, leaving a "longitudinal" hematoma that may not resolve for several weeks or months. Resolution usually is complete and without residua, although we have seen patients in whom a longitudinal scar remained[51] and in whom a chronic abscess developed in relation to a retained shrapnel fragment (*see* Fig. 18–5, page 883).

Penetrating wounds of the thorax from a knife or bullet may induce pneumothorax, although the searing effect of a bullet as it passes through the pleura may cauterize the tissues sufficiently to prevent escape of air into the pleural space. In one series of 250 consecutive cases of gunshot wounds involving the thorax, 90 per cent presented with hemothorax or hemopneumothorax, and only 3 per cent with pneumothorax alone.[52] The incidence of other complications of penetrating injuries of the lung is low. It should be remembered, however, that associated intra-abdominal injuries are common; for example, in the series of 250 cases

cited above, 20 per cent of the patients also had injuries involving the diaphragm or one or more abdominal viscera.[52]

THE POSTOPERATIVE CHEST

Roentgenographic Manifestations

The roentgenographic abnormalities with which we are primarily concerned are those observed following thoracotomy, a subject that has been reviewed by Goodman.[53] The majority of complications occur in the immediate postoperative period (up to the tenth day), although certain manifestations may not become apparent for several weeks or even months postoperatively (e.g., following pneumonectomy).

The authors find it convenient to divide postoperative roentgenograms into three groups, depending on the nature of observed abnormalities and the requirement for early or immediate clinical attention. This rather simplified approach has proved to be of some value in determining the course to take in any given situation.

1. Changes that are ordinarily anticipated following thoracotomy, such as subcutaneous emphysema and the accumulation of a minimal amount of pleural fluid without major pulmonary abnormality. (In such cases, the authors employ the designation "satisfactory postoperative appearance" without going into any detail about the changes observed.)

2. Abnormalities that may or may not be of importance in patient care but whose nature requires that follow-up studies be performed; for example, a pneumothorax or hydrothorax of larger volume than is ordinarily anticipated, a large hematoma following wedge resection, or mediastinal widening following mediastinotomy.

3. Abnormalities that require immediate attention and are sufficiently urgent to require a telephone call to the attending physician or surgeon; for example, acute atelectasis, a large pneumothorax or hydrothorax, malposition of an endotracheal tube, and pulmonary thromboembolism.

Although roentgenographic changes observed in the lungs, thoracic cage, pleura, mediastinum, and diaphragm are in many ways interdependent and therefore should be considered together in interpretation, it serves a useful purpose to discuss them separately.

Lungs

Atelectasis is undoubtedly the most common pulmonary complication of surgical procedures, whether the surgery is thoracic or abdominal.[54] The amount of lung affected varies considerably, from a whole lobe to focal areas of discoid opacities (Fleischner's lines) to multiple small lobular units whose airlessness causes density insufficient to be appreciated roentgenologically. In the last-named circumstance, atelectasis may be evidenced only by the demonstration on pulmonary function testing of decreased lung volume, increased venous admixture, or decreased pulmonary compliance.[55]

There are several mechanisms of development of postoperative atelectasis. The most common is mucus plugging

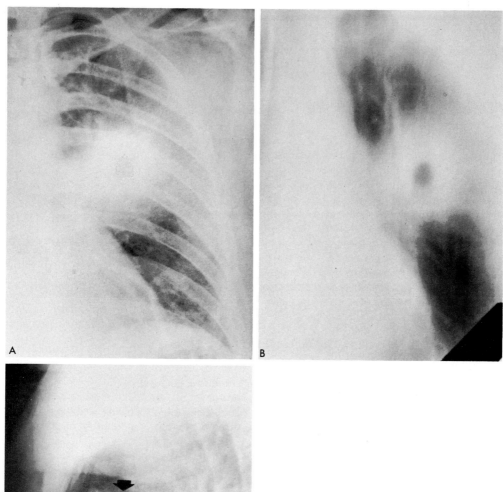

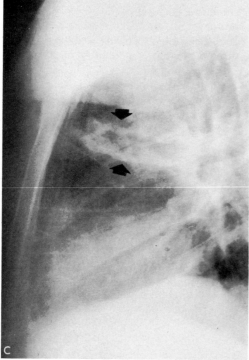

Figure 15–11. Bullet Wound of the Lung. A 36-year-old man suffered a self-inflicted bullet wound of the left chest 24 hours before the roentgenographic examination illustrated in *(A)*. This roentgenogram of the left hemithorax reveals a rather poorly defined, roughly circular shadow of increased density in the left midlung, possessing a circular radiolucency in its center. An anteroposterior tomogram performed 24 hours later *(B)* demonstrates the lesion to better effect. The major portion of this shadow is caused by traumatic pulmonary contusion. Based on an analysis of roentgenograms in frontal projection only, this could be misinterpreted as a large mass containing a central cavity (e.g., an abscess). However, subsequent lateral reontgenography *(C)* demonstrates the longitudinal nature of the central radiolucency *(arrows)*, indicating the path that the bullet took in its passage through the lung.

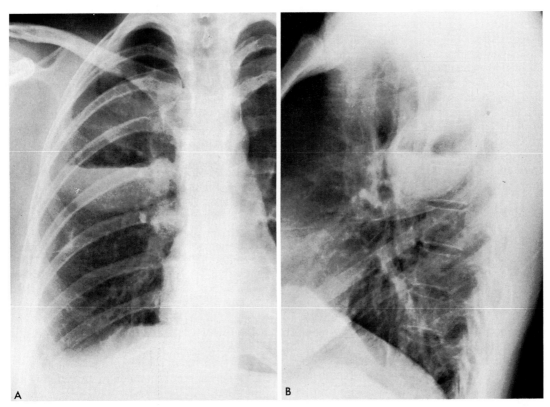

Figure 15–12. Postoperative Pulmonary Hematoma. Views of the right hemithorax from posteroanterior *(A)* and lateral *(B)* roentgenograms reveal a large, well-defined circular shadow in the upper portion of the right lung, possessing a prominent air-fluid level within it. It is very thin-walled. These roentgenograms were made approximately 3 days following wedge resection of a bulla of the right upper lobe. The shadow represents an accumulation of blood elements and gas in the bare area following resection. Over a period of 4 weeks, it underwent slow but progressive resolution and left no significant residuum.

from retained secretions, which occurs chiefly as a result of diminished diaphragmatic excursion caused by splinting as a result of pain. Disruption of mucociliary clearance[56] and surfactant deficit[57] also may be involved. The latter particularly may underlie the common though incompletely understood roentgenographic abnormality observed after cardiopulmonary bypass during open heart surgery. This appears as a relatively homogeneous opacity, usually in the left lower lobe behind the heart and often associated with an air bronchogram. Although these air-containing bronchi sometimes appear crowded, there are no other convincing signs of atelectasis; similarly, there are seldom clinical signs of pneumonia.[57] Regardless of its nature, the abnormality results in little clinical disability and is considered by some investigators to be such a frequent finding following bypass surgery that it can be regarded as an expected part of a "satisfactory postoperative appearance."

Following thoracotomy, the chest roentgenogram also may reveal changes anticipated from the nature of the surgical procedure. For example, following lobectomy the vascular markings become more widely spaced and lung density is reduced as a result of compensatory overinflation, signs that must not be confused with those resulting from atelectasis. Hematoma formation is common following wedge or segmental resection and results from hemorrhage into the potential space at the site of excision (Fig. 15–12). It must be remembered, however, that any local pulmonary

opacity identified in the postoperative period must be regarded as one of the "big four"—atelectasis, pneumonia, infarction, and edema. The manifestations of these complications are no different from those that develop in a nonsurgical setting.

Thoracic Cage

The absence of a rib, usually the fifth or sixth, is frequent following thoracotomy. Nowadays, however, the ribs often are spread rather than resected, so that an intact rib cage is quite compatible with prior thoracotomy. Ribs that have been spread may be fractured.

Median sternotomy has become the principal surgical approach to the heart and great vessels and to a variety of mediastinal abnormalities. Complications of the procedure are uncommon (less than 5 per cent) and usually become manifest between 1 and 2 weeks postoperatively. Six presentations can occur: (1) serosanguineous discharge with a stable sternum; (2) unstable sternum with or without a serosanguineous discharge; (3) sternal dehiscence without mediastinitis; (4) superficial wound infection without mediastinitis; (5) subcutaneous infection with retrosternal extension and an unstable sternum; and (6) mediastinitis with or without sternal separation. In one study, all patients in groups 1 and 2 survived with appropriate therapy, patients in groups 3 and 4 had a 24 per cent mortality rate, and for patients with deep wound infections (groups 5 and 6), the mortality rate exceeded an astonishing 70 per cent.[58] Goodman and colleagues[59] have emphasized the limited role that conventional roentgenography and tomography can play in the evaluation of these conditions and recommend CT as the investigative procedure of choice.

The so-called midsternal stripe, formerly thought to represent radiographic evidence of sternal dehiscence, can be recognized in 30 to 60 per cent of patients at some time during the postoperative period and is now known to be of no diagnostic or prognostic significance.[53] Of much greater importance in establishing sternal separation is a change in the relationship of wires to their neighbors.

Pleura

The most common roentgenographic abnormality in the thorax in the postoperative period is pleural effusion. During the 2 or 3 days after thoracotomy little or no fluid is evident, since the pleural space is effectively drained. Following removal of the drainage tube, however, a small amount of fluid often appears, only to disappear quite quickly during convalescence. Minimal residual pleural thickening may remain, particularly over the lung base.

The accumulation of fluid in larger than expected amounts may result from a variety of causes, including poor positioning of the drainage tube or hemorrhage from an intercostal vessel, particularly an artery (Fig. 15–13). In the presence of pleural adhesions, fluid may loculate in areas that are not in communication with the drainage tube, a finding that is particularly common following pleural decortication. In such circumstances, absorption of the fluid may

be prolonged, sometimes requiring several weeks. The finding is not of major importance unless the accumulation is very large or infected.

In contrast to the small amount of fluid that often accumulates, gas is seldom visible in the pleural space following removal of the drainage tube, even on roentgenograms exposed with the patient erect. A word of caution is in order regarding the assessment of possible pneumothorax: in the immediate postoperative period, roentgenograms are often exposed with the patient supine, in which position any intrapleural gas tends to be situated at the base of the hemithorax anteriorly, where it may not be in communication with the drainage tube. A pneumothorax of such small size should not cause symptoms, but when there is clinical concern, roentgenography should be performed with the patient in the lateral decubitus position to confirm or deny the presence of pneumothorax.

Postoperative pneumothorax may be due to a variety of causes. Lack of communication with the drainage tube is probably the most common, particularly if the gas is loculated or the tube is incorrectly positioned (e.g., in the major fissure). Other causes include leakage into the pleural space from a blown bronchial stump (bronchopleural fistula) or from a bare area of lung following wedge or segmental resection of lung. The incidence of bronchopleural fistula as a complication of pulmonary resection is approximately 2 per cent, and the mortality rate about 15 to 20 per cent.[60] It occurs as a result of necrosis of the bronchial stump or dehiscence of sutures and is most common after right pneumonectomy. Characteristically, it is heralded by the sudden onset of dyspnea and expectoration of bloody fluid during the first 10 days postoperatively. The chest roent-

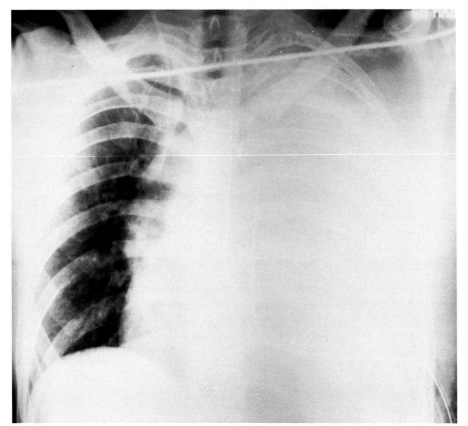

Figure 15–13. Massive Hemothorax Complicating Thoracotomy. Twenty-four hours prior to the roentgenogram illustrated, this 20-year-old man was subjected to left thoracotomy for repair of a coarctation of the aorta (minimal rib notching was apparent). The roentgenogram illustrates a massive effusion in the left pleural space with considerable shift of the mediastinum to the right. This represents a massive hemothorax caused by bleeding into the pleural space from an intercostal artery. The unusually severe hemorrhage was related to hypertrophy of the intercostal circulation secondary to coarctation.

genogram may reveal unexpected disappearance of fluid as a reflection of emptying of the pleural space by way of the tracheobronchial tree. Roentgenographic evaluation of this complication can be facilitated by CT.[61] With the introduction of a modern stapling machine to effect closure of the bronchus, fistulae are becoming much less frequent.[62]

Mediastinum

The two major roentgenographic abnormalities of the mediastinum that occur in the postoperative period are enlargement and displacement. The former results from the accumulation of either gas or fluid and should not be considered serious unless it is excessive or increasing.

Position of the mediastinum is one of the most important indicators of pulmonary abnormality during the postoperative period. Ipsilateral displacement is an expected but usually temporary finding following lobectomy or pneumonectomy; the normal midline position is regained as the remainder of the lung undergoes compensatory overinflation. Excessive displacement toward the operated side may be a sign of atelectasis in the ipsilateral lung. Mediastinal displacement away from the operated side may occur as a result of atelectasis in the contralateral lung or accumulation of excessive fluid or gas in the ipsilateral pleural space.

Within 24 hours of pneumonectomy, the ipsilateral pleural space contains air, the mediastinum is shifted slightly to the ipsilateral side, and the hemidiaphragm is slightly elevated (Fig. 15–14). The post pneumonectomy space then begins to fill with serosanguineous fluid in a progressive and normally predictable manner at a rate of approximately two rib spaces a day. The majority of cases show 80 to 90 per cent obliteration of the space at the end of 2 weeks and complete obliteration by 2 to 4 months. The process occurs not only as a result of fluid accumulation but by progressive ipsilateral displacement of the mediastinum and elevation of the hemidiaphragm. Such mediastinal displacement is an almost invariable finding and constitutes the most reliable indicator of a normal postoperative course. It generally requires 6 to 8 months to reach its maximum.

The absence of a progressive shift of the mediastinum to the operative side in the immediate postoperative period may indicate the presence of bronchopleural fistula, empyema (Fig. 15–15), hemorrhage, or occasionally chylothorax. The most sensitive indicator of late complications is return to the midline of a previously shifted mediastinum, particularly the tracheal air column. This indicates the presence within the post pneumonectomy space of an expanding process such as recurrent neoplasm (Fig. 15–16), hemorrhage, chyle, or pus. CT can be of great value in documenting tumor recurrence by demonstrating a soft tissue mass projecting into the near–water-density postpneumonectomy space.[63]

Two rare complications of pneumonectomy are herniation of the heart through a partial pericardiectomy defect[64] and the so-called right pneumonectomy syndrome.[65] The former may occur on either side and is frequently associated clinically with the abrupt onset of circulatory collapse or superior vena cava obstruction. Roentgenologically, the appearance varies with the side on which the pneumonectomy has been formed: if on the right, the heart is dextrorotated into the right hemithorax and the appearance is unmistakable; when on the left, the heart may rotate posteriorly or laterally, and herniation is usually less evident, particularly if there is a sizable accumulation of pleural fluid.

The right pneumonectomy syndrome is usually seen in children and adolescents and is manifested roentgenographically by marked rightward and posterior displacement of the mediastinum, clockwise rotation of the heart and great vessels, and marked displacement of the overinflated left lung into the anterior portion of the right hemithorax. As a result of the marked rotation of the heart and great vessels, the distal trachea and left main bronchus become compressed between the aorta and the pulmonary artery, with resulting dyspnea and recurrent left-sided pneumonia.

Diaphragm

Following pneumonectomy or lobectomy, the ipsilateral hemidiaphragm is almost invariably elevated during the first few postoperative days. In the former situation, this elevation persists along with ipsilateral mediastinal shift, despite accumulation of fluid in the pleural space. Following lobectomy, however, diaphragmatic elevation and mediastinal displacement disappear over a period of several days or weeks as the remainder of the ipsilateral lung undergoes compensatory overinflation. Marked elevation of a hemidiaphragm can result from injury to the phrenic nerve sustained during surgery. Elevation can also be caused by a number of pathologic states in the lungs, including atelectasis, bronchopneumonia, and thromboembolism.

Clinical Manifestations

Several factors determine morbidity and mortality after thoracotomy and resectional surgery.

The General Health of the Patient. This undoubtedly plays a role in the successful outcome of any operation. Both cigarette smoking and older age are risk factors for postoperative pulmonary complications.[66] There is little doubt that the prognosis can be improved with proper preparation, particularly for patients with chronic obstructive pulmonary disease (COPD) or obesity.

Preoperative Evaluation. A fundamental aspect of preoperative preparation is clinical and physiologic assessment of the patient's breathing reserve, both to determine the likelihood of survival after resection surgery and to avoid creating a respiratory cripple. An experienced physician or surgeon may feel confident in making such a judgment on the basis of history and by observing the patient as he or she walks through corridors and up stairs,[67] but most feel more comfortable with an objective determination of pulmonary function.

Pulmonary function test values that indicate a high risk of development of postoperative cardiopulmonary complications include (1) vital capacity less than 1.0 L; (2) FEV_1 less than 0.5 L; (3) maximal midexpiratory flow less than 0.6 L per second; (4) maximal voluntary ventilation less than 50 per cent of predicted; (5) PaO_2 less than 55 mm Hg; and (6) elevated preoperative PCO_2.[68] Using these values as guidelines, it is possible to adopt a prospective

Text continued on page 804

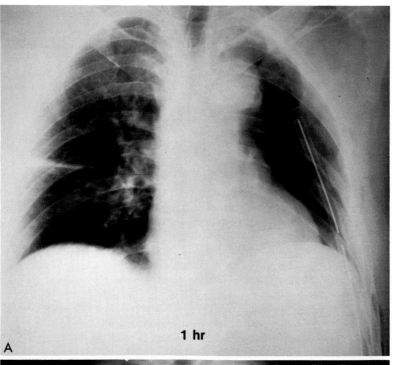

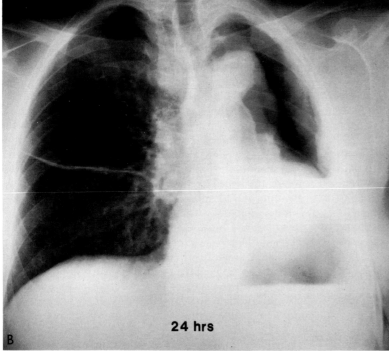

Figure 15–14. Postpneumonectomy Course, Normal. An anteroposterior roentgenogram obtained in the supine position at the bedside 1 hour following left pneumonectomy *(A)* reveals a slight reduction in the volume of the left hemithorax. The space is air-filled, and the mediastinum is in the midline. At 24 hours, a roentgenogram in the erect position *(B)* shows moderate elevation of the left hemidiaphragm (as indicated by the gastric air bubble), a moderate shift of the mediastinum to the left, and a prominent air-fluid level in the plane of the third interspace anteriorly.

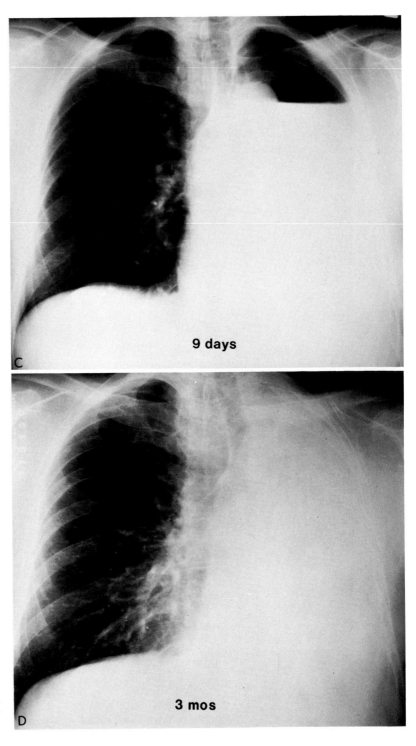

Figure 15–14 *Continued* By 9 days *(C)*, fluid had filled approximately two thirds of the cavity of the left hemithorax, but the mediastinum was still displaced to the left (note the curvature of the tracheal air column). By 3 months *(D)*, the left hemithorax had become completely airless. Note the persistent shift of the mediastinum to the left and the prominent curve of the air column of the trachea.

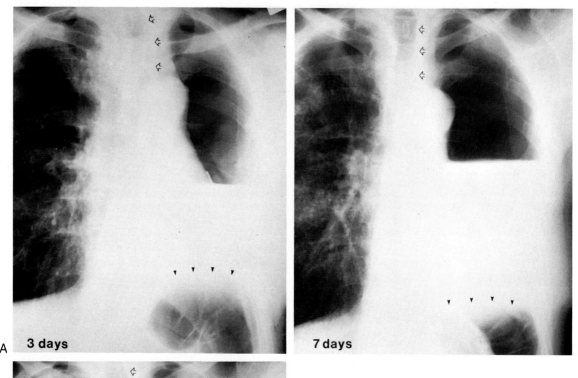

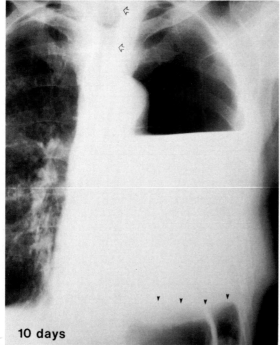

Figure 15–15. Postpneumonectomy Course Complicated by Empyema. Three days following left pneumonectomy *(A)*, the amount of fluid that has accumulated, the position of the left hemidiaphragm *(arrowheads)*, and the shift of the tracheal air column to the left *(open arrows)* all are consistent with a normal postoperative course (compare with Figure 15–14). At 7 days *(B)*, however, the left hemidiaphragm *(arrowheads)* has undergone some depression, and the tracheal air column *(open arrows)* has returned to the midline. Such a change should suggest empyema, bronchopleural fistula, pleural hemorrhage, or, conceivably, chylothorax. By 10 days *(C)*, the left hemidiaphragm *(arrowheads)* had become concave superiorly, and the mediastinum and tracheal air column *(open arrows)* had shifted further to the right. Proved left-sided empyema.

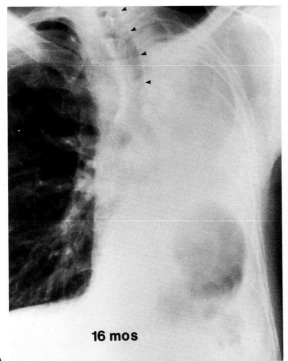

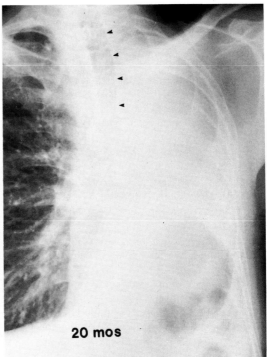

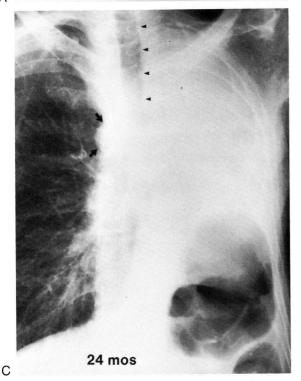

Figure 15–16. Postpneumonectomy Course: Recurrence of Neoplasm. Sixteen months following left pneumonectomy for pulmonary carcinoma, a posteroanterior roentgenogram *(A)* reveals a normal appearance (compare with Figure 15–14). The left hemidiaphragm is markedly elevated, and the heart and tracheal air column *(arrowheads)* are shifted into the left hemithorax. By 20 months *(B)*, the left side of the tracheal air column is beginning to flatten out *(arrowheads)*, suggesting the presence of an expanding process in the left hemithorax. By 24 months *(C)*, not only is the trachea in the midline *(arrowheads)*, but also there has developed a soft tissue mass in the region of the right tracheobronchial angle *(arrows)*, indicating a metastasis to the azygos lymph node. Recurrence of neoplasm in the pleural space and contralateral node metastasis were subsequently proved pathologically.

approach to the selection of patients who are capable of undergoing pneumonectomy.[69] Some groups employ ventilation-perfusion lung scans to assess the amount of functioning lung tissue preoperatively.[70] In conjunction with spirometric measurements, this procedure permits calculation of the likely functional effects of pneumonectomy.

Anesthesia Management. A variety of pulmonary function abnormalities occur during anesthesia, including decreased functional residual capacity (FRC), impaired oxygenation and CO_2 elimination, and increased venous admixture and alveolar dead space.[71] It has been shown that the development of shunt during anesthesia is related to the presence of atelectasis in dependent lung regions,[72] a conclusion that is consistent with the hypothesis that the atelectasis is caused by changes in chest wall mechanics. Serious hypoxia can result if artificial ventilation is discontinued while the respiratory center is still depressed by anesthetics or narcotics.

The Extent of the Surgery. It is probable that this exerts considerable influence on outcome. For example, the mortality rate is higher following pneumonectomy than lobectomy (although in some cases this may be simply a reflection of the area of gas exchange available to a patient whose remaining lung tissue is affected by COPD).

Pulmonary dysfunction is an invariable accompaniment of thoracic and upper abdominal surgery. A decrease occurs in all lung volumes and in compliance, and perfusion of nonventilated alveoli results in hypoxemia. These changes become maximal 48 to 72 hours after surgery and usually clear completely within 7 days, without producing symptoms or signs.[73] They probably result from persistent shallow breathing initiated by pain, narcotic drugs, and general anesthesia. Pain particularly inhibits coughing and prevents effective expectoration, in addition to reducing lung volume.[74] The major preventive measure to overcome this physiologic dysfunction is for the physician, nurse, or therapist to encourage the patient to cough and to inspire deeply in order to renew surfactant and to clear the airways. It has been shown that more effective pressure can be obtained by coughing in the sitting position and by manually assisted compression of the chest wall.[75]

Patients with pulmonary carcinoma tolerate pneumonectomy surprisingly well, considering that the majority have associated COPD.[76] Preoperatively, perfusion of the tumor-bearing lung is usually greatly reduced (to as low as 25 per cent of the total pulmonary blood flow in some cases[76]). Following pneumonectomy, PaO_2 values usually improve, presumably as a result of better matching of ventilation and perfusion.[77]

Somewhat surprisingly, the incidence of postoperative pulmonary complications has been found to be greater after abdominal than after thoracic surgery,[78] ranging from about 20 to 75 per cent depending on the criteria for diagnosing a complication and the patient population studied. (The overall incidence of complications following any form of surgery is clearly greater in patients with disturbed pulmonary function.[79]) The main risk factors are chronic airway disease, advanced age, surgery in the upper abdomen, obesity, and intra-abdominal sepsis.[79] The major thoracic complications of abdominal surgery are atelectasis, pneumonia, thromboembolism, subphrenic abscess, cardiogenic pulmonary edema, and adult respiratory distress syndrome.[80] Atelectasis is undoubtedly the most common of these and in

the majority of patients is related to mucus plugging of airways.

COMPLICATIONS OF INTUBATION AND MONITORING APPARATUS

Many complications can arise during the introduction, maintenance, and use of devices for life support and monitoring in the intensive care unit.[81]

Chest Drainage Tubes

Complications of chest drainage tubes are uncommon[82] and are usually readily apparent clinically or radiologically. Hemorrhage from a lacerated intercostal vessel can be avoided by insertion of the tube in the intercostal space as close as possible to the superior surface of a rib. Intercostal vessels may be tortuous, especially in the elderly,[83] and insertion elsewhere can be dangerous.

Malposition of the chest tube can occur within the pleural space, in which case the complication results only in inadequate drainage. Such malposition can occur in several ways. For example, a tube inserted anterolaterally and directed posteriorly will drain the posterior pleural space, but with the patient lying in a supine position it will not drain a pneumothorax situated anteriorly. Similarly, a tube in any position will not drain a loculated accumulation of fluid or gas in an area not in communication with the tube's holes. The incidence of malposition within a major fissure probably is higher than is generally believed.[84] It is important to realize that malposition often cannot be convincingly recognized on a single anteroposterior roentgenogram. Malposition of a chest tube can also occur within the chest wall or abdomen, in which case it may be associated with serious complications, such as laceration of the diaphragm, liver, stomach, or colon.[85]

Pulmonary perforation is rarely recognized *in vivo* as a complication of chest tube insertion, at least in adults,[85] and its extent is usually minimal. It is often associated with the use of a trocar to aid tube insertion. Underlying pulmonary parenchymal consolidation or interpleural fibrous adhesions probably increase the risk of perforation by decreasing or eliminating the possibility of the lung's retracting when the pleural space is entered.[86]

Infection of the pleural space related to the presence of a chest tube is uncommon. In one study of 1249 trauma patients, it was documented in 30 patients (2.4 per cent).[85]

Abdominal Drainage Tubes

Potentially serious complications can follow transgression of the pleural space during placement of interventional drainage catheters into the liver and upper abdomen. When carrying out this procedure, it is important not to puncture the ninth intercostal space in the midaxillary line, because in virtually all cadaver studies carried out, needles inserted through this interspace have traversed pleura.[87]

Nasogastric Tubes

Since the majority of nasogastric tubes are opaque, any malposition should be readily apparent roentgenographi-

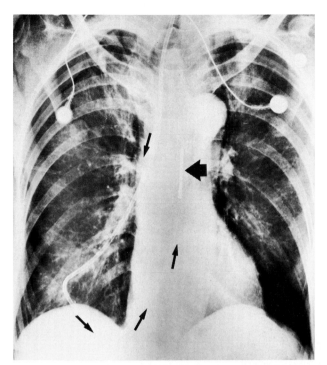

Figure 15–17. Faulty Insertion of a Dobbhoff Feeding Tube. The circuitous course taken by this Dobbhoff feeding tube *(small arrows)* can be established only partly from this anteroposterior roentgenogram. Obviously, the catheter passed into the right lower lobe, and then as it turned to the left it presumably penetrated the visceral pleura covering this lobe. It then passed superiorly either within the mediastinum or in the pleural space adjacent to the azygoesophageal recess to a point where its tip overlies the region of the tracheal carina *(large arrow)*. The patient suffered no ill effects following removal of the tube.

cally. The most common abnormality is coiling within the esophagus. A less frequent but far more important complication is related to faulty insertion of the tube into the tracheobronchial tree (Fig. 15–17). Such malposition can

be particularly hazardous if the tube is meant for hyperalimentation, because the injection of a large amount of fluid into the lungs or pleural cavity, rather than the stomach, can have disastrous consequences.[88] In addition, a patient on a positive-pressure breathing apparatus whose feeding tube has inadvertently been placed in the tracheobronchial tree close to the pleural surface is in danger of developing a large pneumothorax on removal of the tube.[89] In this situation, the feeding tube may be acting as a "finger in the dike" and insertion of a thoracostomy tube into the pleural space may be advisable before the feeding tube is withdrawn.

Endotracheal Tubes

During the first few days after insertion of an endotracheal tube, serious complications are infrequent and occur more often with emergency resuscitation than with more routine respiratory therapy.[90] The chief complication is large airway obstruction resulting from malpositioning of the tube too low in the trachea and major bronchi. In the vast majority of such cases, the tube enters the right main bronchus, and the orifice of the left main bronchus is occluded by the balloon cuff of the endotracheal tube, resulting in complete obstruction and atelectasis of the left lung (Fig. 15–18). If the tube is advanced into the bronchus intermedius, the right upper lobe bronchus may be occluded, with resultant atelectasis of this lobe as well as the left lung.

The rate at which atelectasis occurs depends on the gas content of the lung at the moment of occlusion. Total collapse requires 18 to 24 hours if the parenchyma contains air but may occur in a matter of minutes if the lung contains 100 per cent oxygen (often the case in acute respiratory emergencies). Withdrawal of the tube typically results in rapid re-expansion of the collapsed lung or lobe.

It has been recommended that with the head and neck in a neutral position, the ideal distance between the tip of

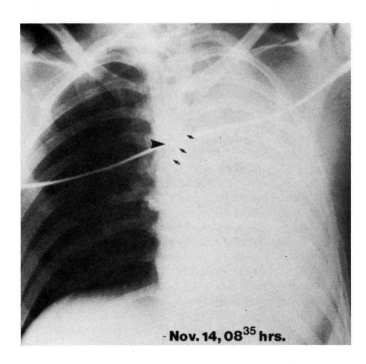

Figure 15–18. Acute Atelectasis of the Left Lung Due to Faulty Insertion of a Cuffed Tracheostomy Tube. An anteroposterior roentgenogram in the supine position reveals complete airlessness of the left lung associated with slight displacement of the mediastinum to the left. A tracheostomy tube is in position, its tip *(arrowhead)* situated in the right main bronchus just beyond the carina (the medial wall of the right main bronchus is indicated by *arrows*). This atelectasis occurred over a very brief period of time, since a high-oxygen mixture was being administered.

the endotracheal tube and the carina is 5 ± 2 cm.[91] Flexion and extension of the neck may cause a 2-cm descent and ascent, respectively, of the tip of the endotracheal tube. Thus, if the position of the neck can be established from the roentgenogram (through visualization of the mandible), the ideal distance between the tip of the endotracheal tube and the carina should be 3 ± 2 cm with the neck flexed and 7 ± 2 cm with the neck extended.[91]

Complications that result from prolonged inflation of the cuff of an endotracheal tube, such as tracheal stenosis, are discussed on page 628.

Transtracheal Catheters

The use of chronic indwelling transtracheal catheters to administer oxygen to patients with COPD has been described in several reports.[92, 93] Complications of their use include subcutaneous emphysema, localized skin infection or hemorrhage, abnormal tracheal mucus production, breakage of catheter parts into the trachea, and the formation of partly occlusive mucus or mucopurulent plugs around the catheter tip.

Percutaneous Central Venous Catheters

The use of polyethylene catheters to monitor central venous pressure and to provide a route for hyperalimentation is associated with a number of complications.[94] Some pertain to the catheterization procedure itself and relate to abnormalities in or around the catheterized vein. Others, perhaps the majority, arise from incorrect positioning of the catheter tip.

Central venous catheters can be inserted via an arm vein, a subclavian vein (by either an infraclavicular or a supraclavicular route), or an external or internal jugular vein. The majority of faulty placements are associated with arm and subclavian approaches, particularly on the right side.[95] In one review of the complications of central venous catheterization, only 186 (62 per cent) of 300 central venous lines were positioned in the subclavian or innominate veins or superior vena cava at the time of the initial chest roentgenogram obtained immediately after catheterization.[96] Of the remainder, 48 (16 per cent) were in the internal jugular vein (Fig. 15–19), 39 (13 per cent) in the right atrium or right ventricle, and 22 (7 per cent) in extrathoracic sites other than the internal jugular vein. In none of these cases was the incorrect position recognized clinically.

Apart from faulty placement, there are three major complications of central venous catheterization.

Thrombosis. Although this is probably the most common complication of venous catheterization, its incidence is difficult to establish.[97] It is more likely to occur in association with catheters left in place for long periods of time. The thrombus is typically sterile and causes no symptoms; it is attributable to reaction to the foreign material of the catheter and trauma to the vessel wall rather than to the type of fluid administered. Although often small and of no clinical consequence, the thrombus may become large enough to occlude the vessel lumen or may serve as a source of pulmonary emboli.

Perforation of a Vein. A vein can be perforated either at the time of insertion[98] or sometime later,[99] the latter

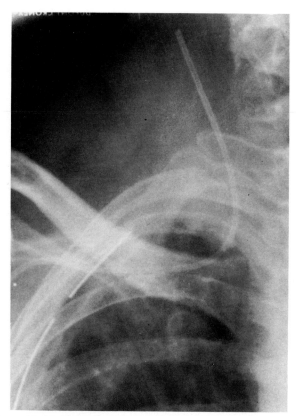

Figure 15–19. Malpositioning of a Subclavian Catheter in the Jugular Vein. The catheter occupies a correct position in the subclavian vein but then ascends the jugular vein. Such a position probably will not record true central venous pressure.

caused by gradual erosion of the vessel wall by the catheter tip propelled by cardiac and respiratory movements.[100] Depending on the vein involved, perforation can result in pneumothorax, hemothorax, hydrothorax (Fig. 15–20), mediastinal hemorrhage, or extrapleural hematoma.[94] Unilateral pneumothorax is undoubtedly the most common of these. Although it is usually evident at the time of catheter insertion or shortly thereafter, it is important to realize that it can develop slowly, particularly in association with positive pressure ventilation.[101]

Catheter Coiling, Knotting, and Breaking. Coiled catheters traumatize the vein and are much more likely to perforate, break, or embolize. They also have a much greater tendency to twist into knots. Although these sometimes can be manipulated free, this is not always possible, and thoracotomy is occasionally required for removal.

Other Complications. Miscellaneous complications of central venous catheterization include sepsis, pulmonary embolization of fragments of catheters, thoracic duct laceration,[102] and perforation of the myocardium.[103]

Indwelling Balloon-Tipped Pulmonary Arterial Catheters

Flow-directed balloon-tipped (Swan-Ganz) catheters for monitoring pulmonary arterial and left atrial pressure in critically ill patients have been used with increasing frequency since they were first described in 1970.[104] Although several types of complications occur, serious ones are un-

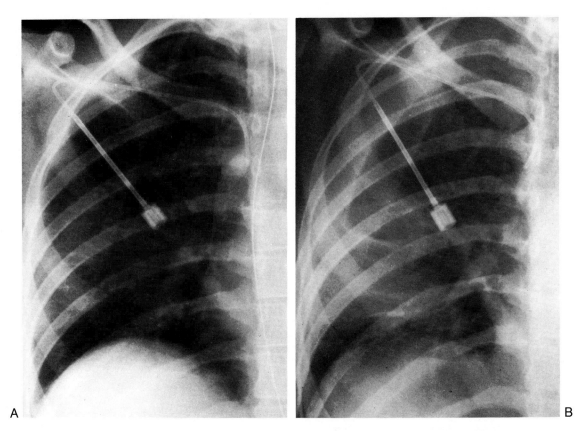

Figure 15–20. Faulty Position of Subclavian Catheter in the Pleural Space. Immediately following insertion of a right subclavian catheter, an anteroposterior roentgenogram *(A)* reveals the tip to lie in a position consistent with the superior vena cava, although it could be argued that it is more medial than usual. Following injection of several hundred milliliters of fluid for hyperalimentation, a second roentgenogram exposed in the supine position *(B)* reveals a large accumulation of fluid in the right pleural space, indicating that the tip of the catheter had perforated the vein and mediastinal parietal pleura.

common; for example, in one prospective study of 528 catheterizations, they were considered to have occurred in only 23 (4.4 per cent).[105]

Pulmonary artery occlusion, with or without infarction, is probably the most common pulmonary complication.[106] It can occur by four mechanisms: (1) irritation of the endothelium of the vena cava, right-sided heart chambers, or a major pulmonary artery by the catheter tip or inflated balloon, resulting in thrombus formation and subsequent embolization; (2) formation of thrombus around the distal end of the catheter itself, again followed by embolization; (3) prolonged inflation of the balloon for recording of wedge pressure; and (4) extension of the tip of the catheter into the lung to the point where it occludes a small peripheral artery (Fig. 15–21). The last mechanism can be avoided if the technique described by Swan and associates is strictly adhered to—the balloon should be inflated as soon as a large-caliber vein is encountered, and the catheter is permitted to float into the pulmonary artery.[107]

It has been estimated that the pulmonary artery is perforated in 0.1 to 0.2 per cent of all catheter insertions,[108] although there is autopsy evidence that it may occur more often.[108] The most common clinical situation associated with perforation is cardiac surgery, an observation attributed to one or more of three factors:[109] (1) shrinkage of heart chambers as a result of evacuation of blood with distal

migration of the catheter; (2) cooling of the perfusate and cardiovascular tissue, leading to increased rigidity of the tubing and vessel walls; and (3) manipulation of the heart, causing increased movement of the catheter. As might be expected, the usual result of pulmonary arterial perforation is hemorrhage, generally into pulmonary parenchyma but on occasion predominantly into the bronchovascular interstitium[110] or pleural space. The complication should be suspected roentgenologically when an airspace opacity develops near the tip of the catheter. The main clinical manifestation is hemoptysis,[111] which can be massive.

COMPLICATIONS OF DIAGNOSTIC BIOPSY PROCEDURES

Pleuropulmonary complications of diagnostic biopsy procedures such as transbronchial biopsy, transthoracic needle aspiration, and closed chest pleural biopsy, are well-known. Because these procedures necessarily cause tissue disruption in order to obtain material for diagnosis, infiltration of air or blood into the pleural cavity, mediastinum, lung parenchyma, or bronchovascular interstitium is, to some extent, an inevitable consequence. In most instances, the extent of this infiltration is limited, so that related clinical problems are minimal or nonexistent. Details of the inci-

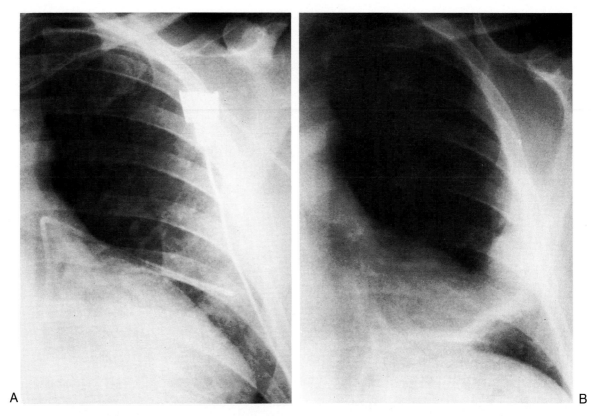

A   B

Figure 15–21. Pulmonary Infarction Associated with a Swan-Ganz Catheter. In the anteroposterior roentgenogram illustrated in *A*, a Swan-Ganz catheter is in position in the left lower lobe, its tip situated less than 2 cm from the visceral pleural surface. Several days later *(B)*, a wedge-shaped opacity had appeared in the left axillary lung zone, highly suggestive of a pulmonary infarct; its position corresponds precisely to what was undoubtedly an impacted Swan-Ganz catheter tip.

dence and type of complications with the different procedures are discussed in Chapters 2 and 3.

RADIATION INJURY OF THE LUNG

It is safe to assume that within the therapeutic range of doses usually administered, the pulmonary parenchyma reacts to ionizing radiation in virtually 100 per cent of patients. Despite this, a demonstrable abnormality on conventional roentgenograms is absent in many cases[112]; in these, CT and pulmonary function testing are more sensitive procedures for determining the presence and extent of damage. The lungs are usually affected by radiation aimed directly at the lungs, although they also can be injured when the beam is directed elsewhere in the thorax, such as at the mediastinum or chest wall. In only a relatively small number of patients, however—possibly no more than 5 to 15 per cent—does the latter type of therapy result in respiratory symptoms.[113] In addition to the effects of roentgen therapy, radiation injury to the lungs may also follow inhalation of beta-emitting radionuclides.

Several factors are important in determining whether and to what extent radiation injury of the lungs is manifested roentgenographically.

Volume of Lung Irradiated. This is considered by some investigators to be the most important factor.[114] For example, it has been estimated that a 30-Gy total dose delivered in fractions to 25 per cent of total lung volume may not produce any symptoms, whereas an identical dose delivered in the same manner to the entire volume of both lungs would probably prove fatal.[114]

Dose of Radiation. In lungs that are normal before the administration of ionizing radiation, its effects (as measured by symptoms and signs, roentgenologic changes, and physiologic tests) are probably proportionate to the amount of radiation delivered. Thus, radiation pneumonitis seldom occurs with a dose of less than 20 Gy[115]; by contrast, doses in excess of 60 Gy given over a period of 5 to 6 weeks almost invariably lead to severe radiation pneumonitis.

Time-Dose Factor. The effect of radiation on the lung is related less to the total dose than to the rate at which it is delivered, since fractionation permits repair of sublethal damage between fractions.[113] This biologic effect of relative equivalent therapy takes into account the total dose absorbed, the number of fractions, and the time elapsed between first and last treatments.[116]

Other Factors. Other variables that influence pulmonary damage include retreatment, associated chemotherapy,[117] and corticosteroid withdrawal[118]; each of these apparently increases susceptibility. There is little evidence to support the clinical impression that patients with COPD are more likely to develop radiation pneumonitis than those without.

Pathogenesis

The pathogenesis of radiation-induced pulmonary disease is complex and incompletely understood.[119] It is believed that x-rays or gamma rays exert their effects by colliding with and exciting electrons, which, in turn, generate ion pairs and a variety of free radicals. The latter are highly reactive and cause breakage of covalent bonds in both small and large molecules; such damage can be repaired in some instances but in others is irreversible, particularly in the presence of oxygen. The resulting molecular changes can then lead to significant biochemical, structural, and functional abnormalities. These abnormalities can be considered as being caused by two classes of molecules: (1) those such as DNA, that are concerned with genetic effects; and (2) a variety of "nongenetic" macromolecules contained in the cell cytoplasm, organelles, and membranes. Damage to the latter group can result in several immediate effects, such as leaky cell membranes or impaired transport of intracellular material; if sufficiently severe, these can lead directly to cell death. Such injury may be the mechanism of capillary endothelial and type I epithelial cell damage in early radiation pneumonitis.[119] Damage to both types of cells at this stage also may be related directly to an increase in capillary permeability and the accumulation of intra-alveolar fluid.[119]

Less obvious in its effect, at least in the early stages of radiation pneumonitis, is injury to DNA. This may take several forms, including breaks that are incorrectly repaired, abnormal cross-links, and chromosome rearrangements. Cells containing such abnormal DNA can remain viable and apparently unharmed until they divide, at which time the progeny may die or show functional disturbances.

These effects are most evident in cells with a rapid turnover rate and least obvious in highly differentiated cells. In the lungs, the cells most sensitive to radiation-induced chromosome abnormalities are capillary endothelial, bronchial epithelial, and alveolar type II cells. The cytologic atypia of type II pneumocytes in radiation pneumonitis presumably reflects this genetic damage.

The precise pathogenesis of the pulmonary fibrosis that occurs in long-standing irradiated lung is unclear. Although it may be caused by a direct effect of radiation on parenchymal interstitial cells, there is experimental evidence that primary endothelial damage resulting in alteration of the normal endothelial-fibroblast interaction may be responsible.[120]

Pathologic Characteristics

The initial pathologic manifestations of radiation pneumonitis have been identified only in experimental animals. One of the earliest and most consistent abnormalities is endothelial damage that is manifested initially as swelling and vacuolization of the cytoplasm, followed by necrosis and detachment from the basement membrane.[121] Platelet thrombi develop and are organized by a process of either recanalization or fibrosis. This in turn can cause significant vascular narrowing, decreased lung perfusion,[122] and pulmonary arterial hypertension.[123] Soon after irradiation, type I cells also show degenerative changes and may become necrotic.[121]

In humans, two stages of radiation damage can be recognized, an early reaction (acute radiation pneumonitis) and a late or fibrotic stage. Typically, the acute reaction is characterized by diffuse alveolar damage (Fig. 15–22) con-

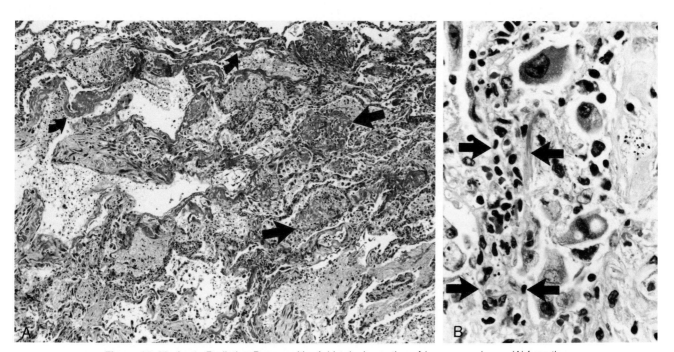

Figure 15–22. Acute Radiation Pneumonitis. A histologic section of lung parenchyma *(A)* from the upper lobe of a patient treated 3 months prior to death with radiation therapy for breast carcinoma reveals extensive airspace filling by a proteinaceous exudate *(straight arrows)*, mild interstitial thickening, and focal hyaline membrane formation *(curved arrows)*. A magnified view of a single alveolus *(B)* shows a mononuclear inflammatory infiltrate in the septal interstitium *(between arrows)* and several irregularly shaped type II pneumocytes with hyperchromatic and cytologically atypical nuclei. (*A* × 60; *B* × 400.)

sisting of an exudate of proteinaceous material in the alveolar airspaces associated with hyaline membranes. The parenchymal interstitium is thickened by congested capillaries, edema, and, with time, fibroblasts and loose connective tissue; an inflammatory cellular infiltrate is usually minimal in extent. Type II cells are hyperplastic and often have very large nuclei, sometimes bizarre in shape (see Fig. 15–22).

The late or fibrotic stage of radiation damage is characterized by parenchymal fibrosis that may be so severe that the underlying lung architecture is difficult to identify. Proliferation and fragmentation of elastic fibers are common. Although somewhat distorted by the adjacent fibrosis, airways can appear remarkably unaffected. Arterioles and arteries often show myointimal proliferation.

Roentgenographic Manifestations

Pulmonary disease is rarely, if ever, manifested either symptomatically or roentgenographically while the patient is receiving radiation therapy. In fact, changes are seldom apparent roentgenographically until at least 1 month after cessation of treatment,[124] and in many cases they take as long as 4 to 6 months to appear.[125]

Acute radiation pneumonitis is manifested by consolidation of lung parenchyma, usually associated with considerable loss of volume. Depending on the severity of the reaction, the resultant opacity may be patchy or confluent. The volume of lung affected usually, but not always, corresponds to the area irradiated, and thus there is no tendency to segmental or lobar distribution (Fig. 15–23). The margins of affected lung, in fact, usually bear a close relationship to the position of the radiation ports.[126] Loss of volume may be severe, caused either by extensive bronchiolar plugging or, more likely, by a loss of surfactant (adhesive atelectasis). Despite this, the major and segmental bronchi are more or less unaffected and an air bronchogram is almost invariably present (Fig. 15–24).[124, 125]

The late or chronic stage of radiation damage is characterized by fibrosis. The affected lung shows severe loss of volume, with obliteration of all normal architectural markings, and the peripheral parenchyma is characteristically airless and opaque as a result of replacement by fibrous tissue. It has been stated that such fibrosis generally is well established and stable 9 to 12 months after the completion of radiation therapy.[127] Dense linear opacities frequently extend from the hilum to the periphery and present an appearance suggesting severe bronchiectasis. At this stage, differentiation from lymphangitic spread of carcinoma may be impossible on the basis of a single roentgenographic study. However, the lack of progression with time and the roentgenographic demonstration of fairly severe changes in the absence of corresponding clinical symptoms should suggest the diagnosis of radiation fibrosis. CT also has been found to permit ready differentiation of radiation-induced fibrosis from recurrent pulmonary neoplasm.[128]

Pleural effusion that can be demonstrated roentgenographically is very uncommon; however, fairly extensive thickening of the pleura may be seen.[129] The presence of pleural thickening can be established with ease on CT scans.[130]

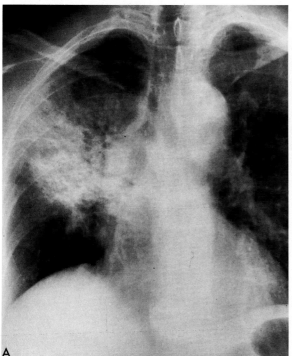
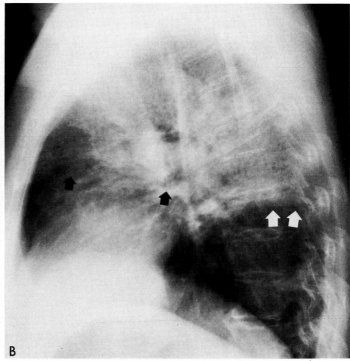

Figure 15–23. Acute Radiation Pneumonitis Illustrating "Through-and-Through" Effect. Posteroanterior (A) and lateral (B) roentgenograms reveal inhomogeneous consolidation of the upper half of the right lung associated with a prominent air bronchogram. In lateral projection (B), the lower border of the consolidation is almost a straight line (arrows), conforming precisely to the lower margin of the collimated beam of radiation. These films were of a 48-year-old woman approximately 3 months following an intensive course of cobalt therapy for primary pulmonary carcinoma.

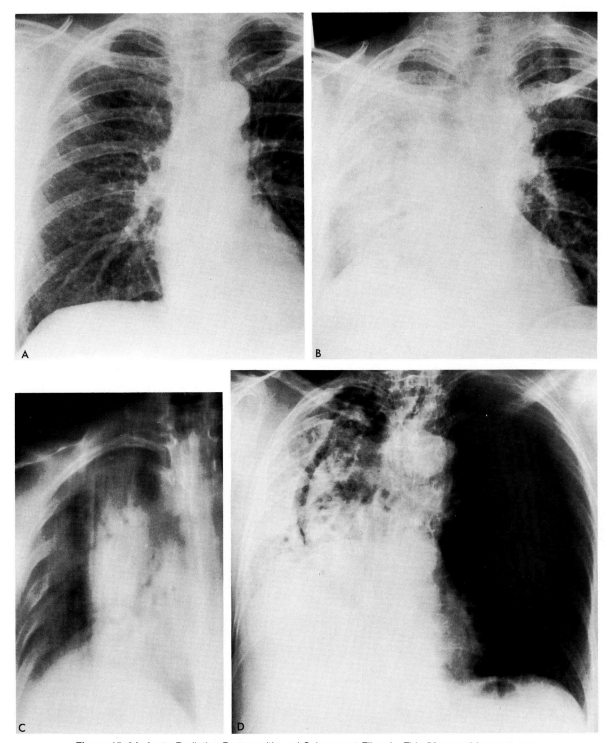

Figure 15–24. Acute Radiation Pneumonitis and Subsequent Fibrosis. This 52-year-old woman presented with a large ulcerated breast carcinoma and was treated with preoperative cobalt teletherapy to the breast and mediastinum in a dosage of approximately 30 Gy. The breast was then removed, and over a period of 6 weeks postoperative cobalt therapy was administered to the right lung in a dosage of 51 Gy, and to the mediastinum in a dosage of 35 Gy. A posteroanterior roentgenogram *(A)* at the end of the radiation therapy revealed no significant abnormalities. Three weeks later, however, the right lung *(B)* had undergone severe loss of volume (as evidenced by elevation of the hemidiaphragm and shift of the mediastinum). The underlying density is rather granular in nature, and an air bronchogram is identified within it (seen to better advantage in the anteroposterior tomogram of the right hemithorax illustrated in *C*). She was treated with corticosteroids for the following month. A posteroanterior roentgenogram approximately 1 month later *(D)* revealed severe loss of volume of the right lung. The pattern observed earlier had changed to a very coarse inhomogeneous pattern in which extensive bronchiectasis was readily apparent.

Clinical Manifestations

Many patients with roentgenographic evidence of radiation damage remain asymptomatic. When symptoms do develop, they usually have an insidious onset and consist of nonproductive cough, weakness, and shortness of breath on exertion. Cough may be very troublesome and occur in spasms. The patient may have a sensation of inability to inspire to total lung capacity (TLC) and when encouraged to do so will invariably cough. Chest pain develops occasionally,[124] but hemoptysis is rare. Fever may be a prominent finding and is usually low grade but sometimes high and spiking.[113] Dyspnea is generally mild and noted only on exertion; however, death may be caused by respiratory insufficiency. Tachycardia out of proportion to the fever may be observed. Crepitations at the height of inspiration are common, and there may be signs of lung consolidation in patients with severe pneumonitis.

Acute radiation pneumonitis may persist for up to 1 month and can either resolve completely or progress to pulmonary fibrosis. With the onset of fibrosis, symptoms of the acute pneumonitis gradually abate.

The institution of radiation therapy for an endobronchial neoplasm can induce edema and narrowing of the airway lumen. In the authors' experience and that of others,[131] this effect can have disastrous consequences if the tumor is in the trachea. This complication can be prevented by preliminary treatment with corticosteroids.[132] It is also important to note that discontinuation of corticosteroids in patients receiving combined steroid and radiation therapy can precipitate severe radiation pneumonitis.[118]

Pulmonary Function Studies

The major impairment in function is restrictive in nature; vital capacity and flow rates are decreased, the former to a proportionately greater degree. Diffusing capacity is decreased when a large volume of lung is involved. It may return to normal as the acute process subsides but more commonly remains decreased as fibrosis ensues.[133] As might be expected, the greater the amount of lung affected the more severe the diffusion defect.[134]

References

1. Kerns SR, Gay SB: CT of blunt chest trauma. Am J Roentgenol 154: 55, 1990.
2. Wagner RB, Crawford WO Jr, Schimpf PP: Classification of parenchymal injuries of the lung. Radiology 167: 77, 1988.
3. Stevens E, Templeton AW: Traumatic nonpenetrating lung contusion. Radiology 85: 247, 1965.
4. Wiot JF: The radiologic manifestations of blunt chest trauma. JAMA 231: 500, 1975.
5. Fagan CJ: Traumatic lung cyst. Am J Roentgenol 97: 186, 1966.
6. Williams JR, Bonte FJ: Pulmonary damage in nonpenetrating chest injuries. Radiol Clin North Am 1: 439, 1963.
7. Williams JR, Stembridge VA: Pulmonary contusion secondary to nonpenetrating chest trauma. Am J Roentgenol 91: 284, 1964.
8. Shirakusa T, Araki Y, Tsutsui M, et al: Traumatic lung pseudocyst. Thorax 42: 516, 1987.
9. Santos GH, Mahendra T: Traumatic pulmonary pseudocysts. Ann Thorac Surg 27: 359, 1979.
10. Baumgartner F, Sheppard B, de Virgilio C, et al: Tracheal and main bronchial disruptions after blunt chest trauma: Presentation and management. Ann Thorac Surg 50: 569, 1990.
11. Burke JF: Early diagnosis of traumatic rupture of the bronchus. JAMA 181: 682, 1962.
12. Woodring JH, Fried AM, Hatfield DR, et al: Fractures of the first and second ribs: Predictive value for arterial and bronchial injury. Am J Roentgenol 138: 211, 1982.
13. Collins JP, Ketharanathan V, McConchie I: Rupture of major bronchi resulting from closed chest injuries. Thorax 28: 371, 1973.
14. Reynolds J, Davis JT: Injuries of the chest wall, pleura, pericardium, lungs, bronchi and esophagus. Radiol Clin North Am 4: 383, 1966.
15. Harvey-Smith W, Bush W, Northrop C: Traumatic bronchial rupture. Am J Roentgenol 134: 1189, 1980.
16. Lotz PR, Martel W, Rohwedder JJ, et al: Significance of pneumomediastinum in blunt trauma to the thorax. Am J Roentgenol 132: 817, 1979.
17. Weisel W, Watson RR, O'Connor TM: Long-term follow-up study of patients with bronchial anastomosis or tracheal replacement. Chest 61: 141, 1972.
18. Felson B: Lung torsion: Radiographic findings in nine cases. Radiology 162: 631, 1987.
19. Weisbrod GL: Left upper lobe torsion following left lingulectomy. J Can Assoc Radiol 38: 296, 1987.
20. Switzer P, Pitman RG, Fleming JP: Pneumomediastinum associated with zygomatico-maxillary fracture. J Can Assoc Radiol 25: 316, 1974.
21. Fishbone G, Robbins DI, Osborn DJ, et al: Trauma to the thoracic aorta and great vessels. Radiol Clin North Am 11: 543, 1973.
22. Sanborn JC, Heitzman R, Markarian B: Traumatic rupture of the thoracic aorta: Roentgen-pathological correlations. Radiology 95: 293, 1970.
23. Eller JL, Ziter FMH Jr: Avulsion of the innominate artery from the aortic arch. An evaluation of roentgenographic findings. Radiology 94: 75, 1970.
24. Dennis LN, Rogers LF: Superior mediastinal widening from spine fractures mimicking aortic rupture on chest radiographs. Am J Roentgenol 152: 27, 1989.
25. Milne ENC, Imray TJ, Pistolesi M, et al: The vascular pedicle and the vena azygos. Part III: In trauma—the "vanishing" azygos. Radiology 153: 25, 1984.
26. Gerlock AJ Jr, Muhletaler CA, Coulam CM, et al: Traumatic aortic aneurysm: Validity of esophageal tube displacement sign. Am J Roentgenol 135: 713, 1980.
27. Peters DR, Gamsu G: Displacement of the right paraspinous interaorta. Radiology 134: 599, 1980.
28. Woodring JH, Pulmano CM, Stevens RK: The right paratracheal stripe in blunt chest trauma. Radiology 143: 605, 1982.
29. Simeone JF, Deren MM, Cagle F: The value of the left apical cap in the diagnosis of aortic rupture. A prospective and retrospective study. Radiology 139: 35, 1981.
30. Heiberg E, Wolverson MK, Sundaram M, et al: CT in aortic trauma. Am J Roentgenol 140: 1119, 1983.
31. Gundry SR, Williams S, Burney RE: Indications for aortography. Radiography after blunt chest trauma: A reassessment of the radiographic findings associated with traumatic rupture of the aorta. Invest Radiol 18: 230, 1983.
32. Marnocha KE, Maglinte DDT: Plain-film criteria for excluding aortic rupture in blunt chest trauma. Am J Roentgenol 144: 19, 1985.
33. Mirvis SE, Bidwell JK, Buddemeyer EU, et al: Value of chest radiography in excluding traumatic aortic rupture. Radiology 163: 487, 1987.
34. Mirvis SE, Bidwell JK, Buddemeyer EU, et al: Imaging diagnosis of traumatic aortic rupture. A review and experience at a major trauma center. Invest Radiol 22: 187, 1987.
35. Wilson RF, Murray C, Antonenko DR: Nonpenetrating thoracic injuries. Surg Clin North Am 57: 17, 1977.
36. Miller DC, Stinson EB, Oyer PE, et al: Operative treatment of aortic dissections. J Thorac Cardiovasc Surg 78:365, 1979.
37. Finkelmeier BA, Mentzer RM Jr, Kaiser DL, et al: Chronic traumatic thoracic aneurysm: Influence of operative treatment on natural history. An analysis of reported cases, 1950–1980. J Thorac Cardiovasc Surg 84: 257, 1982.
38. Heystraten FM, Rosenbusch G, Kingma LM, et al: Chronic posttraumatic aneurysm of the thoracic aorta: Surgically correctable occult threat. Am J Roentgenol 146: 303, 1986.
39. Stanbridge RDeL: Tracheo-oesophageal fistula and bilateral recurrent laryngeal nerve palsies after blunt chest trauma. Thorax 37: 548, 1982.
40. Ebert PA, Gaertner RA, Zuidema GD: Traumatic diaphragmatic hernia. Surg Gynecol Obstet 125: 59, 1967.
41. Bernatz PE, Burnside AF Jr, Clagett OT: Problem of the ruptured diaphragm. JAMA 168: 877, 1958.
42. Marchand P: Traumatic hiatus hernia. Br Med J 1: 754, 1962.

43. Holm A, Bessy PQ, Aldrete JS: Diaphragmatic rupture due to blunt trauma: Morbidity and mortality in 42 cases. South Med J 81: 956, 1988.

44. Ammann AM, Brewer WH, Maull KI, et al: Traumatic rupture of the diaphragm: Real-time sonographic diagnosis. Am J Roentgenol 140: 915, 1983.

45. Aronchick JM, Epstein DM, Gefter WB, et al: Chronic traumatic diaphragmatic hernia: The significance of pleural effusion. Radiology 168: 675, 1988.

46. Salomon NW, Zukoski CF: Rupture of the right hemidiaphragm with eventration of the liver. JAMA 241: 1929, 1979.

47. Albers JE, Rath RK, Glaser RS, et al: Severity of intrathoracic injuries associated with 1st rib fractures. Ann Thorac Surg 33: 614, 1982.

48. Wynn-Williams N, Young RD: Cough fracture of the ribs. Including one complicated by pneumothorax. Tubercle 40: 47, 1959.

49. Sebba L, Baigelman W: Postsurgical lung hernia. Am J Med Sci 284: 40, 1982.

50. Bhalla M, Leitman BS, Forcade C, et al: Lung hernia: Radiographic features. Am J Roentgenol 154: 51, 1990.

51. Dubeau L, Fraser RS: Long-term effects of pulmonary shrapnel injury. Report of a case with carcinoma and residual shrapnel tract. Arch Pathol Lab Med 108: 407, 1984.

52. Oparah SS, Mandal AK: Penetrating gunshot wounds of the chest in civilian practice: Experience with 250 consecutive cases. Br J Surg 65: 45, 1978.

53. Goodman LR: Review: Postoperative chest radiograph. II. Alterations after major intrathoracic surgery. Am J Roentgenol 134: 803, 1980.

54. Carter AR, Sostman HD, Curtis AM, et al: Thoracic alterations after cardiac surgery. Am J Roentgenol 140: 475, 1983.

55. Hamilton W: Atelectasis, pneumothorax, and aspiration as postoperative complications. Anesthesiology 22: 708, 1961.

56. Gamsu G, Singer MM, Vincent HH, et al: Postoperative impairment of mucus transport in the lung. Am Rev Respir Dis 114: 673, 1976.

57. Templeton AW, Almond CH, Seaber A, et al: Postoperative pulmonary patterns following cardiopulmonary bypass. Am J Roentgenol 96: 1007, 1966.

58. Serry C, Bleck PC, Javid H, et al: Sternal wound complications. Management and results. J Thorac Cardiovasc Surg 80: 861, 1980.

59. Goodman LR, Kay HR, Teplick SK, et al: Complications of median sternotomy: Computed tomographic evaluation. Am J Roentgenol 141: 225, 1983.

60. Williams NS, Lewis CT: Bronchopleural fistula: A review of 86 cases. Br J Surg 63: 520, 1976.

61. Heater K, Revzani L, Rubin JM: CT evaluation of empyema in the postpneumonectomy space. Am J Roentgenol 145: 39, 1985.

62. Smiell J, Widmann WD: Bronchopleural fistulas after pneumonectomy. A problem with surgical stapling. Chest 92: 1056, 1987.

63. Peters JC, Desai KK: CT demonstration of postpneumonectomy tumor recurrence. Am J Roentgenol 141: 259, 1983.

64. Tschersich HU, Skopara V Jr, Fleming WH: Acute cardiac herniation following pneumonectomy. Radiology 120: 546, 1976.

65. Shepard JO, Grillo HC, McLoud TC, et al: Right-pneumonectomy syndrome: Radiologic findings and CT correlation. Radiology 161: 661, 1986.

66. Poe RH, Kallay MC, Dass T, et al: Can postoperative pulmonary complications after elective cholecystectomy be predicted? Am J Med Sci 295: 29, 1988.

67. Olsen GN, Bolton JW, Weiman DS, et al: Stair climbing as an exercise test to predict the postoperative complications of lung resection. Two years' experience. Chest 99: 587, 1991.

68. Hodgkin JE, Dines DE, Didier EP: Preoperative evaluation of the patient with pulmonary disease. Mayo Clin Proc 48: 114, 1973.

69. Block AJ, Olsen GN: Preoperative pulmonary function testing. JAMA 235: 257, 1976.

70. Markos J, Mullan BP, Hillman DR, et al: Preoperative assessment as a predictor of mortality and morbidity after lung resection. Am Rev Respir Dis 139: 902, 1989.

71. Rehder K, Sessler AD, Marsh HM: General anesthesia and the lung. Am Rev Respir Dis 112: 541, 1975.

72. Tokics L, Strandberg A, Brismar B, et al: Computerized tomography of the chest and gas exchange measurements during ketamine anaesthesia. Acta Anaesthesiol Scand 31: 684, 1987.

73. Bartlett RH, Gazzaniga AB, Geraghty TR: Respiratory maneuvers to prevent postoperative pulmonary complications. JAMA 224: 1017, 1973.

74. Byrd RB, Burns JR: Cough dynamics in post-thoracotomy state. Chest 67: 654, 1975.

75. Yamazaki S, Ogawa J, Shohzu A, et al: Intrapleural cough pressure in patients after thoracotomy. J Thorac Cardiovasc Surg 80: 600, 1980.

76. Ali MK, Mountain C, Miller JM, et al: Regional pulmonary function before and after pneumonectomy using [133]xenon. Chest 68: 288, 1975.

77. Begin P, Deschamps C, Gauthier JJ, et al: Functional effects of pneumonectomy and bilobectomy for lung cancer. Respiration 46: 8, 1984.

78. Gaensler EA, Weisel RD: The risks in abdominal and thoracic surgery in COPD. Postgrad Med 54: 183, 1973.

79. Hall JC, Tarala RA, Hall JL, et al: A multivariate analysis of the risk of pulmonary complications after laparotomy. Chest 99: 923, 1991.

80. Goodman LR: Review: Postoperative chest radiograph: I. Alterations after abdominal surgery. Am J Roentgenol 134: 533, 1980.

81. Ravin CE, Putman CE, McLoud TC: Hazards of the intensive care unit. Am J Roentgenol 126: 423, 1976.

82. Daly RC, Mucha P, Pairolero PC, et al: The risk of percutaneous chest tube thoracostomy for blunt thoracic trauma. Ann Emerg Med 14: 865, 1985.

83. Miller KS, Sahn SA: Chest tubes. Indications, technique, management and complications. Chest 91: 258, 1987.

84. Webb WR, LaBerge JM: Radiographic recognition of chest tube malposition in the major fissure. Chest 85: 81, 1984.

85. Milikan JS, Moore EE, Steiner E, et al: Complications of tube thoracostomy for acute trauma. Am J Surg 140: 738, 1980.

86. Fraser RS: Lung perforation complicating tube thoracostomy: Pathologic description of three cases. Hum Pathol 19: 518, 1988.

87. Nichols DM, Cooperberg PL, Golding RH, et al: The safe intercostal approach? Pleural complications in abdominal interventional radiology. Am J Roentgenol 141: 1013, 1984.

88. Wendell GD, Lenchner GS, Promisloff RA: Pneumothorax complicating small-bore feeding tube placement. Arch Intern Med 151: 599, 1991.

89. Miller WT: Inadvertent tracheobronchial placement of feeding tubes. Letter to the editor. Radiology 167: 875, 1988.

90. Twigg HL, Buckley CE: Complications of endotracheal intubation. Am J Roentgenol 109: 452, 1970.

91. Conrardy PA, Goodman LR, Laing F, et al: Alteration of endotracheal tube position—flexion and extension of the neck. Crit Care Med 4: 7, 1976.

92. Heimlich HJ, Carr GC: Transtracheal catheter technique for pulmonary rehabilitation. Ann Otol Rhinol Laryngol 94: 502, 1985.

93. Fletcher EC, Nickeson D, Costarangos-Galarza C: Endotracheal mass resulting from a transtracheal oxygen catheter. Chest 93: 438, 1988.

94. Scott WL: Complications associated with central venous catheters. A survey. Chest 94: 1221, 1988.

95. Yerdel MA, Karayalcin K, Aras N, et al: Mechanical complications of subclavian vein catheterization. A prospective study. Int Surg 76: 18, 1991.

96. Langston CS: The aberrant central venous catheter and its complications. Radiology 100: 55, 1971.

97. Walters MB, Stanger HAD, Rotem CE: Complications with percutaneous central venous catheters. JAMA 220: 1455, 1972.

98. Schorlemmer GR, Khouri RK, Murray GF, et al: Bilateral pneumothoraces secondary to iatrogenic buffalo chest. An unusual complication of median sternotomy and subclavian vein catheterization. Ann Surg 199: 372, 1984.

99. Ellis LM, Vogel SB, Copeland EM III: Central venous catheter vascular erosions. Diagnosis and clinical course. Ann Surg 209: 475, 1989.

100. Tocino IM, Watanabe A: Impending catheter perforation of superior vena cava: Radiographic recognition. Am J Roentgenol 146: 487, 1986.

101. Cronen MC, Cronen PW, Arino P, et al: Delayed pneumothorax after subclavian vein catheterization and positive pressure ventilation. Br J Anaesth 67: 480, 1991.

102. McGoon MD, Benedetto PW, Greene BM: Complications of percutaneous central venous catheterization. A report of two cases and review of the literature. Johns Hopkins Med J 145: 1, 1979.

103. Hunt R, Hunter TB: Cardiac tamponade and death from perforation of the right atrium by a central venous catheter [letter to the editor]. Am J Roentgenol 151: 1250, 1988.

104. Swan HJC, Ganz W, Forrester J, et al: Catheterization of the heart in man with use of a flow-directed balloon-tipped pulmonary arterial catheter. N Engl J Med 283: 447, 1970.
105. Boyd KD, Thomas SJ, Gold J, et al: A prospective study of complications of pulmonary artery catheterizations in 500 consecutive patients. Chest 84: 245, 1983.
106. Katz JD, Cronau LH, Barash PG, et al: Pulmonary artery flow-guided catheters in the perioperative period. Indications and complications. JAMA 237: 2832, 1977.
107. Chun GMH, Ellestad MH: Perforation of the pulmonary artery by a Swan-Ganz catheter. N Engl J Med 284: 1041, 1971.
108. Fraser RS: Catheter-induced pulmonary artery perforation: Pathologic and pathogenic features. Hum Pathol 18: 1246, 1987.
109. Stone JG, Khambatta HJ, McDaniel DD: Catheter-induced pulmonary arterial trauma: Can it always be averted? J Thorac Cardiovasc Surg 86: 146, 1983.
110. Rosenblum SE, Ratliff NB, Shirey EK, et al: Pulmonary artery dissection induced by a Swan-Ganz catheter. Cleve Clin Q 51: 671, 1984.
111. Pellegrini RV, Marcelli GD, DiMarco RF, et al: Swan-Ganz catheter–induced pulmonary hemorrhage. J Cardiovasc Surg 28: 646, 1987.
112. Cooper G Jr, Guerrant JL, Harden AG, et al: Some consequences of pulmonary irradiation. Am J Roentgenol 85: 865, 1961.
113. Gross NJ: Pulmonary efects of radiation therapy. Ann Intern Med 86: 81, 1977.
114. Rubin P, Casarett GW: Clinical Radiation Pathology. Vol I. Philadelphia, WB Saunders, 1968.
115. Jennings FL, Arden A: Development of radiation pneumonitis. Time and dose factors. Arch Pathol 74: 351, 1962.
116. Wara WM, Phillips TL, Margolis LW, et al: Radiation pneumonitis: A new approach to the derivation of time-dose factors. Cancer 32: 547, 1973.
117. Trask CWL, Joannides T, Harper PG, et al: Radiation-induced lung fibrosis after treatment of small cell carcinoma of the lung with very high-dose cyclophosphamide. Cancer 55: 57, 1985.
118. Pezner RD, Bertrand M, Cecchi GR, et al: Steroid withdrawal radiation pneumonitis in cancer patients. Chest 85: 816, 1984.
119. Gross NJ: The pathogenesis of radiation-induced lung damage. Lung 159: 115, 1981.
120. Adamson IYR, Bowden DH: Endothelial injury and repair in radiation-induced pulmonary fibrosis. Am J Pathol 112: 224, 1983.
121. Adamson IYR, Bowden DH, Wyatt JP: A pathway to pulmonary fibrosis: An ultrastructural study of mouse and rat following radiation to the whole body and hemithorax. Am J Pathol 58: 481, 1970.
122. Teates CD: The effects of unilateral thoracic irradiation on pulmonary blood flow. Am J Roentgenol 102: 875, 1968.
123. Schreiner BF Jr, Michaelson SM, Yuile CL: The effects of thoracic irradiation upon cardiopulmonary function in the dog. Am Rev Respir Dis 99: 205, 1969.
124. Lichtenstein H: X-ray diagnosis of radiation injuries of the lung. Dis Chest 38: 294, 1960.
125. Smith JC: Radiation pneumonitis. A review. Am Rev Respir Dis 87: 647, 1963.
126. Polansky SM, Ravin CE, Prosnitz LR: Pulmonary changes after primary irradiation for early breast carcinoma. Am J Roentgenol 134: 101, 1980.
127. Libshitz HI, Southard ME: Complications of radiation therapy: The thorax. Semin Roentgenol 9: 41, 1974.
128. Bourgouin P, Cousineau G, Lemire P, et al: Differentiation of radiation-induced fibrosis from recurrent pulmonary neoplasm by CT. J Can Assoc Radiol 38: 23, 1987.
129. Lougheed MN, Maguire GH: Irradiation pneumonia in the treatment of carcinoma of the breast. J Can Assoc Radiol 11: 1, 1960.
130. Srinivasan G, Kurtz DW, Lichter AS: Pleural-based changes on chest x-ray after irradiation for primary breast cancer: Correlation with findings on computerized tomography. Int J Radiat Oncol Biol Phys 9: 1567, 1983.
131. Cameron SJ, Grant IWB, Lutz W, et al: The early effect of irradiation on ventilatory function in bronchial carcinoma. Clin Radiol 20: 12, 1969.
132. Cameron SJ, Grant IWB, Pearson JG, et al: Prednisolone and mustine in prevention of tumour swelling during pulmonary irradiation. Br Med J 1: 535, 1972.
133. Kanagami H, Baba K, Ogata K, et al: Clinical aspects of radiation fibrosis of the lung with emphasis on respiratory function. Jap J Chest Dis (Nippon Kyobu Rinsho) 21: 682, 1962.
134. Brady LW, Germon PA, Cander L: The effects of radiation therapy on pulmonary function in carcinoma of the lung. Radiology 85: 130, 1965.

16

METABOLIC PULMONARY DISEASE

PULMONARY ALVEOLAR PROTEINOSIS

This rare but fascinating disease (also known as alveolar lipoproteinosis) is characterized by the deposition of amorphous granular material, high in protein and lipid content, within the airspaces of the lung. Although the condition occurs predominantly in patients between the ages of 20 and 50 years, very young children also are susceptible.[1] There is a male-to-female predominance[2] of about 2:1 to 3:1.

Etiology and Pathogenesis

In both humans and experimental animals, pulmonary alveolar proteinosis (PAP) is seen in a variety of settings,

suggesting that multiple factors are involved in the pathogenesis. These settings include the following:

1. An immunocompromised state, especially lymphopenia, thymic aplasia, or immunoglobulin deficiency in infants and children[3] and lymphoma or leukemia in adults.[2] Occasional cases also have been reported in patients with acquired immunodeficiency syndrome (AIDS)[4] or autoimmune connective tissue diseases.[5] Although it has been suggested that the drugs used in the therapy of some of these conditions may be responsible for the proteinosis,[6] a more attractive hypothesis is that the underlying immunodeficiency is reflected in malfunction of alveolar macrophages[2] that, in turn, leads to the accumulation of the abnormal intra-alveolar material (*see* later on).

2. Rarely, in infants and young children without evi-

dence of underlying systemic disease. Some of these individuals have been siblings.[7] In at least two instances, a history of consanguinity was obtained, strongly suggesting the possibility of a genetic factor in some cases. However, in the majority of patients no family history of the disease can be elicited.

3. In experimental animals following exposure to a variety of airborne dusts, including aluminum powder, quartz,[8] and fiberglass,[9] and in humans exposed to a high concentration of silicon dioxide (acute silicoproteinosis, see page 708).[10]

Ultrastructural,[11] immunohistochemical,[12] and biochemical[13] observations suggest that the material that accumulates in the alveoli in PAP is derived from type II pneumocytes and that it represents surfactant or a component thereof. There is still considerable uncertainty, however, about the cause of its accumulation. Although it is possible that overproduction of surfactant by hyperplastic or abnormally stimulated type II pneumocytes may be responsible, experimental studies have failed to detect any enhancement of lipid synthesis.[14] It seems likely, therefore, either that the removal of alveolar phospholipid is impaired or that its degradation is defective. In fact, several experiments have provided evidence of abnormal macrophage function, including impaired phagocytosis and defective antimicrobial activity.[15] In addition, analysis of bronchoalveolar lavage (BAL) fluid from affected patients has shown a significant reduction in macrophage number.[16]

The basis for the macrophage dysfunction is unclear. It has been suggested that an underlying immunodeficiency state may be involved[2]; however, the rarity of alveolar proteinosis in comparison with the relatively common occurrence of an immunodeficiency state clearly indicates that other factors must be involved. It is possible that by altering macrophage function some inhaled inorganic dusts may be responsible. Although this mechanism has been most clearly implicated in silicoproteinosis, there is evidence that patients with PAP but without a history of occupational dust exposure have increased amounts of particulate material in their lungs.[17] An understanding of the underlying cause of macrophage dysfunction is made more difficult by in vitro studies in which the phagocytic function of alveolar macrophages has been shown to be suppressed by the lipoproteinaceous debris itself.[18] This suggests that once the condition is established, a positive feedback mechanism acts to sustain it, and possibly to enhance it.

PAP may be complicated by infection with a variety of microorganisms, especially Nocardia, Aspergillus and Cryptococcus species.[2] Although it has been suggested that the organisms themselves may be the cause of the proteinosis,[2] it seems more likely that their presence is secondary and is the result of either an abnormality of macrophage function[19] or the presence of a favorable growth environment provided by the intra-alveolar proteinaceous material.

Pathologic Characteristics

Pathologically, the alveoli are filled with granular, proteinaceous material that is rich in lipids and that stains eosinophilic with hematoxylin and eosin and purple with periodic acid–Schiff (Fig. 16–1). Acicular crystals and laminated bodies that stain with varying intensity and are believed to be cellular fragments also can be seen. Intact and apparently degenerating macrophages are present within

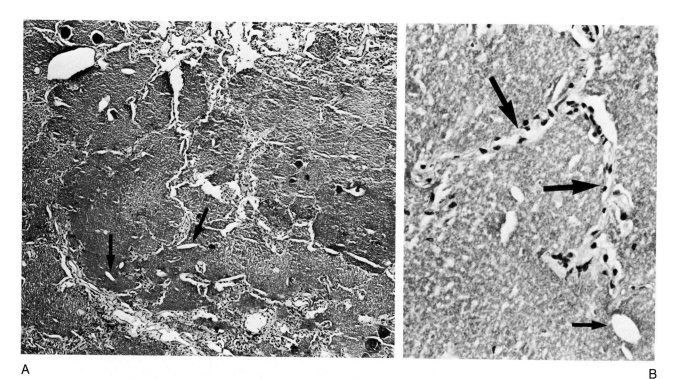

A

B

Figure 16–1. Pulmonary Alveolar Proteinosis. A histologic section of lung parenchyma *(A)* shows the airspaces to be almost completely filled by amorphous, finely granular, PAS-positive material (seen to better advantage at greater magnification in *B*). Scattered oval or elongated crystal-like spaces *(small arrows)* and mononuclear cells (lymphocytes and macrophages) are present within the material. The alveolar septa *(larger arrows in B)* are normal. (*A* × 50; *B* × 250; both PAS.)

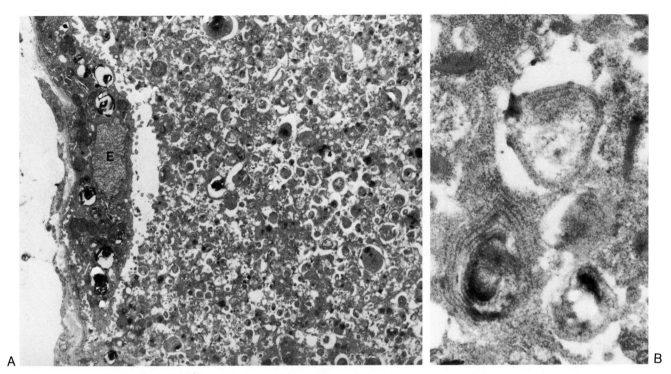

Figure 16–2. Pulmonary Alveolar Proteinosis. A transmission electron micrograph *(A)* shows a type II pneumocyte (E) and adjacent alveolar airspace filled with numerous, variably electron-dense bodies, some of which *(B)* show distinct lamellations resembling those seen in the normal type II cell osmiophilic body. *(A* × 9500; *B* × 56,000.)

the granular material but are usually not abundant except focally at the border between normal and affected lung. Alveolar septa are usually normal or at most slightly thickened by a lymphocytic infiltrate.

Ultrastructural examination shows the intra-alveolar material to consist of amorphous granular debris containing numerous, relatively discrete osmiophilic granules or lamellar bodies, some of which resemble tubular myelin (Fig. 16–2).[11]

Roentgenographic Manifestations

With rare exceptions, the roentgenographic pattern is bilateral and symmetric[20] and is identical in both distribution and character to that of pulmonary edema (Fig. 16–3). Since the process is one of airspace consolidation, the basic lesion is the acinar shadow. Confluence of acinar shadows is the rule, with the production of irregular, rather poorly defined, patchy opacities scattered widely throughout the lungs. In many cases, the shadows are distributed in a "butterfly" or "bat's wing" pattern that is sometimes seen with pulmonary edema and is commonly, but erroneously, attributed to uremia.[21] Differentiation from pulmonary edema of cardiac origin may be difficult, but the absence of other signs of pulmonary venous hypertension should be of considerable help: there is no tendency to cardiac enlargement, there are usually no signs of interstitial edema, and there is no evidence of upper lobe vessel distention.

Occasionally, the roentgenographic pattern simulates diffuse interstitial lung disease despite pathologic confirmation of its predominantly alveolar location,[22] a paradox that also

has been observed on computed tomography (CT) (Fig. 16–4).[23] This may be caused by patchy, incomplete alveolar filling wherein irregular subacinar, rather than acinar, shadows project as a reticulonodular pattern. Similarly, the development of Kerley B lines has been reported[24] and probably is related to lymphatic obstruction. These appearances render differential diagnosis even more difficult.

Resolution usually is complete roentgenographically but can occur asymmetrically and in a spotty fashion. Occasionally, new foci of airspace consolidation develop in areas not previously affected.[21, 24] The formation of denser nodules and linear streaks have been described and may represent pulmonary fibrosis.[21] Resolution may be associated with manifestations of bronchial obstruction, including segmental atelectasis and "obstructive overinflation."[21] Neither lymph node enlargement nor pleural effusion occurs at any stage of the disease.

Clinical Manifestations

Approximately one third of patients are asymptomatic. The remainder manifest a variety of symptoms, the most frequent being shortness of breath on exertion that is usually progressive in severity and unassociated with orthopnea. Cough is often present and usually is dry. Fatigue, weight loss, and pleuritic pain may be present,[25] and a low-grade fever is said to develop at the onset of the illness in 50 per cent of patients.[26] Fine or coarse rales sometimes can be heard on auscultation. Clubbing of the fingers and toes is not uncommon.

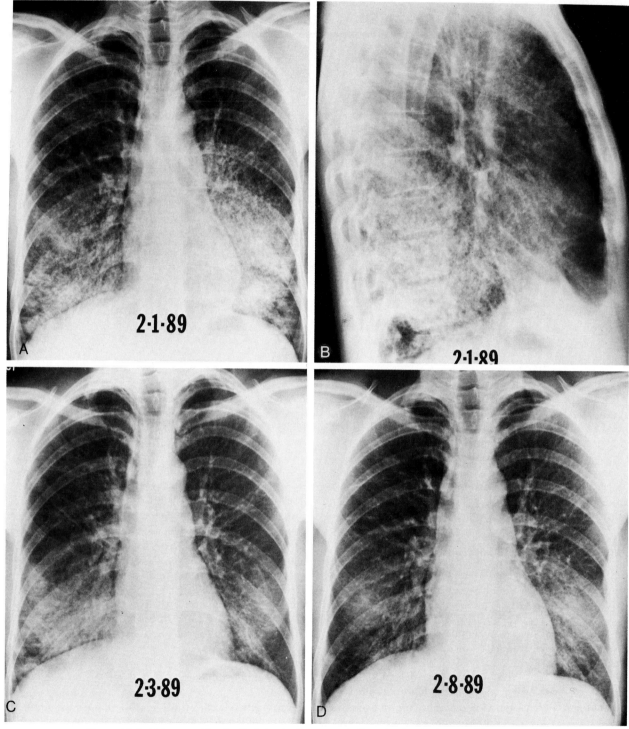

Figure 16–3. Pulmonary Alveolar Proteinosis: Response to Bronchoalveolar Lavage. Posteroanterior (A) and lateral (B) roentgenograms of the chest of this 29-year-old woman with known alveolar proteinosis reveal extensive bilateral patchy airspace opacities with middle and lower zonal predominance. Approximately 1 month later, repeat roentgenograms 24 hours following left (C) and right (D) lung lavage show almost complete clearing of the opacities.

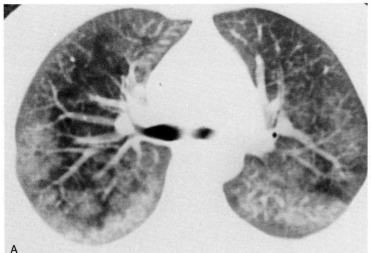

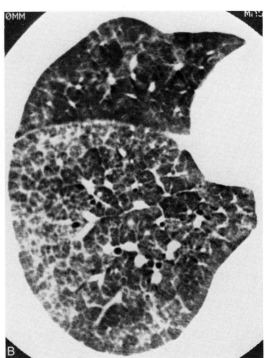

Figure 16–4. Pulmonary Alveolar Proteinosis: CT Manifestations in Two Patients. In the first patient, a CT scan with 10-mm collimation *(A)* reveals extensive bilateral airspace opacities with marked peripheral anatomic predominance, at least in the right lung. This appearance is consistent with virtually any diffuse airspace-filling process, including alveolar proteinosis. In the second patient, a high-resolution CT scan with 1.5-mm collimation *(B)* shows a rather coarse reticulation consistent with thickening of interlobular septa; multiple polygonal lines can be identified, creating what some would consider a honeycomb pattern.

Laboratory Findings

Laboratory investigation reveals a normal or slightly elevated white cell count. Polycythemia is common.[27] In a few patients, IgA levels have been decreased in serum and IgG, IgA, and IgM levels increased in BAL fluid.[28] Hyperlipidemia and an increase in the level of serum lactate dehydrogenase (LDH) have been observed in some cases.[25]

Pulmonary function studies can be completely normal or can reveal a reduction in diffusing capacity, vital capacity, and pulmonary compliance. Hypoxemia is caused by ventilation-perfusion inequality and intrapulmonary shunt[29] and may result in pulmonary hypertension that can be relieved by breathing oxygen.[30] The results of follow-up function studies of patients treated successfully with BAL correlate well with clinical improvement.[31]

The diagnosis can be confirmed by BAL. With PAP the fluid shows the following characteristics: (1) a grossly opaque effluent, a milky effluent, or both; (2) very few alveolar macrophages; (3) large acellular eosinophilic bodies in a diffuse background of eosinophilic granules; and (4) PAS staining of the proteinaceous material. The measurement of apoprotein A in sputum may prove helpful in diagnosis[32]; however, in many cases the diagnosis must be confirmed by examination of tissue obtained by transbronchial or open lung biopsy.

Prognosis

PAP is fatal in about one third of cases. Death results either from respiratory failure caused by the proteinosis or from superimposed infection.[33] Spontaneous remission without treatment has been reported in 25 per cent of patients in some series.[1] Irrigation of the tracheobronchial tree by BAL is an effective therapeutic procedure that can

be life saving and has greatly improved the prognosis of the disease.[34] Some patients do not require more than one or two BALs, but a few require whole-lung lavage repeated semiannually or annually.[1]

AMYLOIDOSIS

Because of its great variety of clinical and pathologic manifestations, amyloidosis has been classified in several ways.[35] The traditional division has been into four major groups that reflect the underlying clinical features: (1) a *primary* type, in which no associated disease is recognized or in which there is an underlying plasma cell disorder (most commonly multiple myeloma); (2) *secondary* amyloidosis, in which there is an associated chronic disease such as tuberculosis, cystic fibrosis, bronchiectasis, rheumatoid disease, syphilis, or Hodgkin's disease; (3) a relatively uncommon *familial* form that can be localized to a single tissue such as nerve; and (4) a so-called *senile* form that affects many organs and tissues (including the lungs), most often of persons older than 70 years.

Recently it was proposed that amyloidosis can be better classified on the basis of the specific protein of which the amyloid is composed.[36] Following this concept, the most important forms are (1) *amyloid L* (AL), associated with the deposition of immunoglobulin light chains and usually seen in association with such conditions as multiple myeloma and macroglobulinemia; (2) *amyloid A* (AA), associated with the deposition of a protein derived from an acute serum phase reactant (SAA) and occurring in association with chronic inflammatory diseases, certain neoplasms, and familial Mediterranean fever; and (3) amlyoid associated with the deposition of transthyretin (prealbumin) such as occurs in the heart and pulmonary vessels in "senile" amyloidosis.

Although these classifications are helpful in understanding the pathogenesis of amyloidosis, from the point of view of diagnosis and the clinical consequences of pulmonary disease, it is more useful to classify amyloidosis according to its anatomic location. According to this concept, there are three principal forms of amyloid deposition in the trachea and lungs—tracheobronchial mucosal, nodular parenchymal, and diffuse parenchymal. Although these forms can occur in combination, in most cases the amyloid is deposited predominantly in one pattern. In addition to the trachea and lungs, amyloidosis can also involve the pleura,[37] pulmonary arteries,[38] respiratory muscles,[39] and hilar and mediastinal lymph nodes,[40, 41] either alone or in combination with airway or parenchymal disease; deposition in pulmonary neuroendocrine tumors occurs occasionally.[42]

In considering a diagnosis of thoracic amyloidosis, it must be remembered that pulmonary diseases such as chronic fibrocaseous tuberculosis, bronchiectasis, lung abscess, and cystic fibrosis[43] can themselves result in amyloidosis. Although rare, this secondary phenomenon can occasionally alter the course or roentgenographic appearance of the underlying pulmonary abnormality.

Pathogenesis

A detailed description of the basic pathogenetic features of amyloidosis is beyond the scope of this text. However, certain specific features related to localized pulmonary disease deserve mention. With the exception of "senile" amyloid, most localized deposits in the lungs consist of AL.[44] In the great majority of these cases, there is no evidence of systemic disease (including multiple myeloma and Waldenström's macroglobulinemia), and, in the few cases that have been studied,[44, 45] no serologic immunoglobulin abnormality. Thus, it has been speculated that local immunoglobulin deposition, possibly related to either overproduction or impaired clearance secondary to a chronic inflammatory process, may be responsible for the accumulation.[44]

Pathologic Characteristics

Airway involvement occurs most commonly in the trachea and proximal bronchi. Although there is overlap, it is usually manifested in one of two ways: a localized nodule or (more commonly) multiple discrete or confluent intramural plaques that distort the airway wall and cause stenosis of its lumen.[44, 45] Histologically, the amyloid is situated in the subepithelial interstitial tissue and often surrounds tracheobronchial gland ducts and acini, some of which may show atrophy (Fig. 16–5).

The parenchymal nodules of localized pulmonary amyloid can be solitary or multiple and are usually fairly well-defined and 2 to 4 cm in diameter. Amyloid is often identifiable in the alveolar interstitium at the periphery of the nodule; however, in the central region, the normal parenchymal architecture is usually obscured by a more or less solid mass of amyloid, typically containing fairly numerous multinucleated giant cells and variable numbers of lymphocytes and plasma cells. Calcification and ossification are not uncommon.

In diffuse interstitial disease, amyloid is present in the media of small blood vessels and in the parenchymal inter-

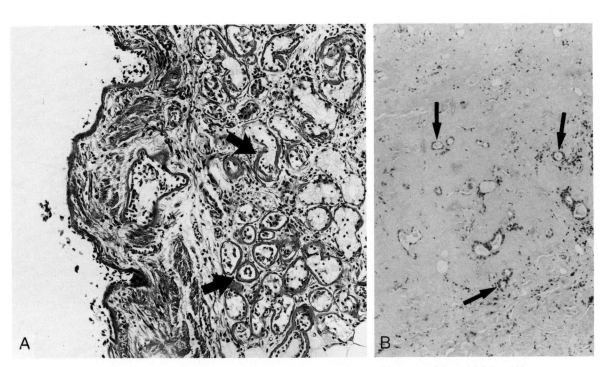

Figure 16–5. Amyloidosis: Tracheobronchial. A histologic section *(A)* shows mild amyloid deposition in relation to a bronchial gland duct and acini *(arrows)*, representing an early stage of bronchial wall amyloidosis. A section of a more advanced lesion *(B)* shows virtual complete replacement of airway interstitial tissue by amyloid, with separation and atrophy of bronchial gland acini *(arrows)*. (A × 100; B × 60.)

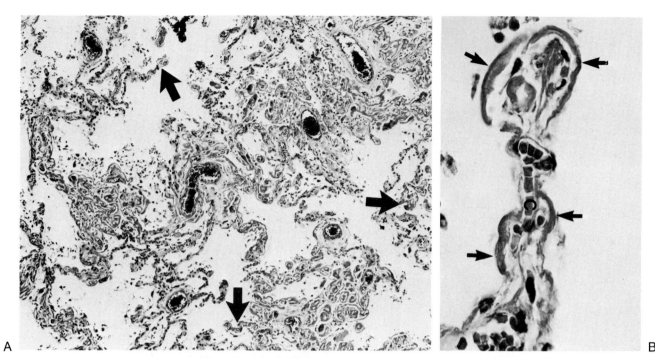

A   B

Figure 16–6. Amyloidosis: Diffuse Interstitial. A histologic section of lung parenchyma *(A)* shows amyloid in the interstitium around small vessels, transitional airways, and alveolar septa *(arrows)*. A magnified view of one septum *(B)* shows thin deposits between the capillary lumen (C) and overlying alveolar epithelium *(arrows)*. *(A × 60; B × 600.)*

stitium (Fig. 16–6). In the latter site, it is typically located adjacent to endothelial and epithelial basement membranes and can appear in a uniform and more or less linear pattern or as multiple small nodules.[46] Inflammatory cells and ossification or calcification are typically absent.

Roentgenographic Manifestations

In the tracheobronchial form, roentgenographic features range from general accentuation of bronchovascular markings associated with overinflation to the effects of more severe bronchial obstruction such as atelectasis or obstructive pneumonitis. The latter may involve a segment, a lobe, or an entire lung (Fig. 16–7).[47] The nodular parenchymal form is manifested by solitary or multiple masses (Fig. 16–8), in some cases with cavitation.[45, 48] Calcification or ossification may be seen,[49] particularly on computed tomography images (Fig. 16–9).[50]

Diffuse parenchymal amyloidosis can be manifested by a nodular pattern that simulates miliary tuberculosis, silicosis, or sarcoidosis, a manifestation that can be exquisitely demonstrated by high-resolution CT.[51] Such disease is relatively uncommon in *secondary* or "senile" amyloidosis[45, 52] and tends to be of slight or moderate severity. It is much more frequent in generalized *primary* disease,[35] with 35 to 70 per cent of patients showing roentgenographic evidence of this pattern of deposition.[53]

Hilar[40] and mediastinal[41] lymph node involvement may be apparent roentgenographically as enlargement that can be massive and associated with dense calcification. Pleural effusion is uncommon.[37]

Clinical Manifestations

The plaquelike form of tracheobronchial amyloidosis can cause symptoms that simulate bronchial asthma; hemoptysis is common, as are recurrent bronchitis and pneumonia.[47, 54] Discrete tracheal and endobronchial nodules seldom cause symptoms and are usually discovered incidentally at bronchoscopy; however, they can be large enough to cause airway obstruction, atelectasis, and bronchiectasis.[55] Other symptoms and signs depend on the volume of lung affected and whether infection is present.

The nodular parenchymal form of amyloidosis usually provokes no symptoms[56] and is discovered on a screening chest roentgenogram. New lesions occasionally have been reported to appear following surgical excision of nodules,[57] but whether this represents the effect of inadequate resection or the development of independent lesions is unclear. Progressive dyspnea and respiratory insufficiency are frequent in diffuse interstitial disease.[45, 58]

Circulating and tissue-bound monoclonal light chains, more often lambda than kappa, are frequently present in patients with primary amyloidosis.[58, 59] In other patients, including those with secondary amyloidosis, nonspecific immunoglobulin abnormalities may be observed, with serum levels of IgA, IgG, and IgM being either increased or decreased. Biopsy of rectal tissue or of subcutaneous abdominal fat may be required to confirm the diagnosis. When disease is localized to the lungs, transbronchial biopsy, open lung biopsy, or transthoracic needle aspiration usually yields diagnostic tissue.

The prognosis in the nodular parenchymal type of amyloidosis is good; in most cases the nodules remain stationary

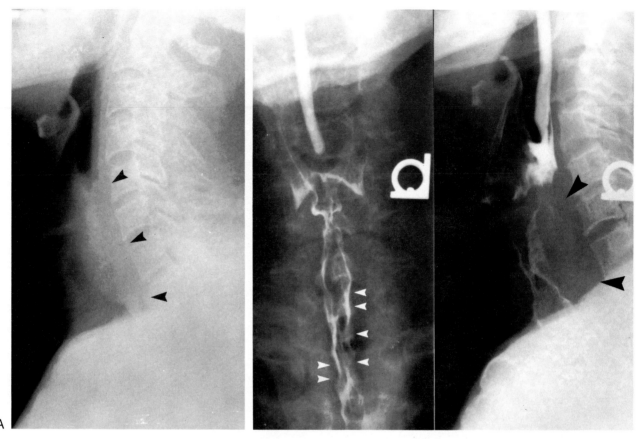

Figure 16–7. Laryngotracheal Amyloidosis. A lateral view of the neck *(A)* shows a posteriorly located laryngotracheal soft tissue mass *(arrowheads)*. Faint stippled calcification is suggested within the lesion. Detail views of the larynx and trachea from a laryngotracheogram in anteroposterior and lateral projections *(B)* confirm the presence of an intraluminal soft tissue mass *(large black arrowheads)* encroaching on the sagittal diameter of the tracheal air column; note the more diffuse nodular coronal narrowing of the proximal and middle parts of the trachea *(small white arrowheads)*. A biopsy of the proximal mass disclosed amyloidosis.

in size or grow slowly, if at all, and cause no symptoms. By contrast, patients with diffuse interstitial disease often die from respiratory insufficiency.[56] Patients with tracheobronchial disease may require surgical excision of a lobe or entire lung, particularly if there are chronic changes related to airway obstruction.

LIPID STORAGE DISEASE

Gaucher's Disease

Gaucher's disease is an autosomal recessive abnormality characterized by a deficiency of beta-glucosidase, the enzyme that catabolizes glucosylceramide. This deficiency results in an accumulation of this substance, predominantly in reticuloendothelial cells (Gaucher's cells) of the liver, spleen, lymph nodes, bones, and, in the infantile form of the disease, brain. The majority of patients are female and more than 95 per cent are Jews.

Pulmonary involvement is uncommon.[60] Histologically, Gaucher's cells are found predominantly in the alveolar interstitium and adjacent airspaces. Roentgenographic

manifestations consist of a reticulonodular or miliary pattern affecting both lungs diffusely.[61] Lytic lesions are occasionally seen in the ribs. Clinically significant pulmonary involvement is usually manifested by dyspnea, and sometimes by pulmonary hypertension and respiratory failure.[62] Elevated levels of serum angiotensin-converting enzyme have been described.[63]

Niemann-Pick Disease

Niemann-Pick disease is caused by an inherited defect in the production of sphingomyelinase, a deficiency that results in the deposition of sphingomyelin in the liver, spleen, lung, bone marrow, and brain. Five clinical variants have been described that depend on the age of onset and predominant organs affected. Many patients die in infancy or childhood; however, some survive into adulthood, occasionally presenting with the first manifestations of their disease at that time.[64]

Pathologically, aggregates of large multivacuolated "foam" cells are present in the parenchyma of many organs, including the lungs. Roentgenographic manifestations consist of a diffuse reticulonodular pattern (Fig. 16–10).[65, 66]

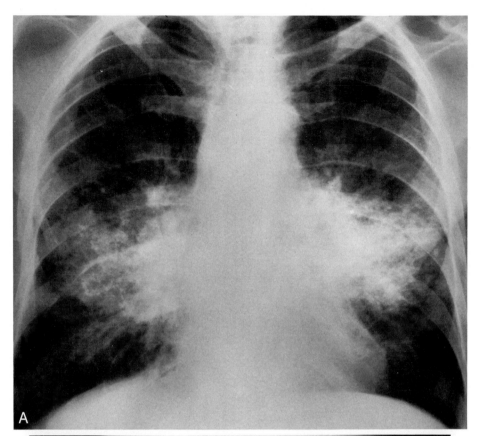

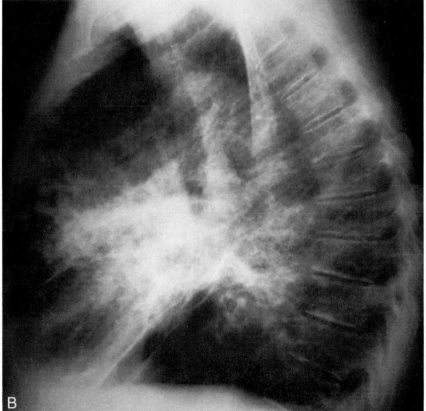

Figure 16–8. Parenchymal Amyloidosis. Posteroanterior *(A)* and lateral *(B)* roentgenograms reveal fairly large, poorly defined inhomogeneous opacities in the medial and central portions of both lungs that possess a "butterfly" distribution. The lungs are otherwise normal. Possible hilar lymph node enlargement cannot be evaluated because of contiguity of the parenchymal disease.

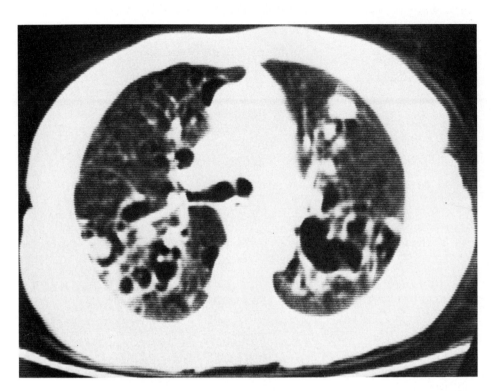

Figure 16–9. Amyloidosis: Nodular Parenchymal. A CT scan at the level of the carina reveals multiple nodules and thick, irregular linear opacities throughout both lungs. A number of air-containing "cystic" spaces probably represent bullae. (Courtesy of Dr. Micheal O'Donovan, Montreal General Hospital, Montreal, Quebec.)

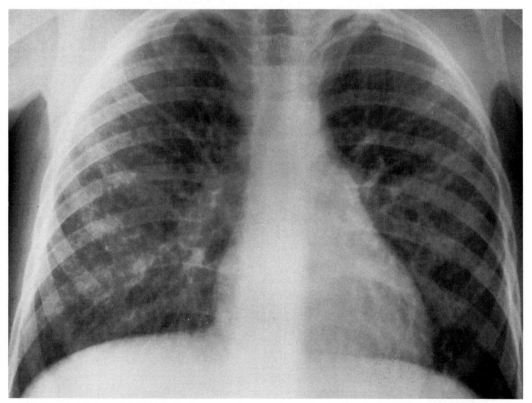

Figure 16–10. Niemann-Pick Disease. A posteroanterior roentgenogram reveals a coarse reticular pattern throughout both lungs without anatomic predominance. The pattern indicates diffuse interstitial lung disease. There are no associated findings such as lymph node enlargement or pleural effusion. (Courtesy of Dr. J. S. Dunbar.)

The nodules are 1 to 2 mm in diameter and may be associated with linear shadows, creating a honeycomb pattern.[66] Hepatomegaly and peripheral lymph node enlargement are common; pulmonary involvement can cause respiratory failure.

Hermansky-Pudlak Syndrome

The Hermansky-Pudlak syndrome is an autosomal recessive condition characterized by tyrosinase-positive oculocutaneous albinism, a storage pool platelet defect, and the accumulation of ceroid pigment in macrophages throughout the body. The disease is uncommon, approximately 200 cases[67] having been reported by 1985. It most often affects persons from Puerto Rico or Holland.

Involvement of the pulmonary interstitium has been documented in a number of reports.[68, 69] Histologically, there is mild to severe parenchymal and peribronchial fibrosis associated with variable numbers of ceroid-laden macrophages. Roentgenographic manifestations consist of a reticulonodular pattern associated with bullae and bronchiectasis, sometimes with considerable upper zonal predominance of the latter changes.[70]

Patients complain of progressive dyspnea and appear to be susceptible to infection and to have a bleeding tendency. Pulmonary function studies reveal a restrictive pattern; hypoxemia at rest is characteristic.

GLYCOGEN STORAGE DISEASE

Involvement of thoracic structures other than the heart is seen only rarely in glycogen storage disease. However, aggregates of intra-alveolar foamy macrophages containing glycogen-like material have been noted in some cases,[71] and these can cause respiratory dysfunction and roentgenographic abnormalities. *Pompe's disease* (acid maltase deficiency) is a type II glycogen storage disease characterized by the accumulation of glycogen in skeletal muscle and a variety of visceral organs. Although the condition usually affects infants and is fatal, occasional cases of adult onset have been reported.[72] Involvement of the diaphragm and respiratory muscles of the chest wall in these individuals can cause dyspnea and respiratory failure (*see* Chapter 21).

MUCOPOLYSACCHARIDE STORAGE DISEASE

Deficient activity of lysosomal enzymes involved in the catabolism of glycosaminoglycans causes disease that predominantly affects the skeletal, cardiovascular, and central nervous systems. Patients with some of these metabolic disorders die in childhood or adolescence, whereas others with conditions such as Hurler's, Hunter's, or Morquio's syndrome survive into adulthood. Respiratory complications include kyphoscoliosis, respiratory failure, susceptibility to pulmonary infection, and airway obstruction, sometimes accompanied by sleep apnea.[73]

HERITABLE DISEASES OF CONNECTIVE TISSUE

More than 100 distinct heritable disorders of connective tissue exist, each presumed to be caused by a mutation in a single gene that controls the structure or metabolism of one or more macromolecules. Several of these disorders are complicated by abnormalities of the thoracic cage and pleuropulmonary interstitium.[74]

Marfan's Syndrome

The underlying biochemical defect of Marfan's syndrome is unknown. The syndrome is defined and diagnosed clinically on the strength of cardinal features in the skeletal, ocular, and cardiovascular systems. The predominant intrathoracic abnormalities are emphysema[75] and scoliosis; the latter can be very deforming and may result in cor pulmonale. Other manifestations include bullae (usually apical), upper lobe fibrosis, frequent respiratory infections, bronchial hyper-reactivity,[76] bronchiectasis, dissecting aneurysm of the pulmonary artery[77] and pneumothorax.[78] Although the sudden onset of chest pain in a patient with Marfan's syndrome may indicate this last complication, dissecting aneurysm of the aorta should also be considered in the differential diagnosis, particularly during pregnancy.[79]

Ehlers-Danlos Syndrome

The Ehlers-Danlos syndrome consists of a group of inherited disorders of connective tissue divided into different types on the basis of clinical, genetic, and biochemical features. Pleuropulmonary and thoracic skeletal abnormalities, including bullae, pneumothorax, and scoliosis, are very similar to those of Marfan's syndrome.[80] Easy bruisability is a prominent feature, especially in type 4 disease, and rupture of vessels, including those of the pulmonary circulation, can be life threatening. Some cases have been reported in which involvement of the bronchial tree resulted in weakness of the walls and subsequent bronchiectasis.

PULMONARY ABNORMALITIES IN SYSTEMIC ENDOCRINE DISEASE

Diabetes Mellitus

Although the most common and serious pulmonary complication of diabetes mellitus is infection, a variety of other abnormalities occur occasionally, including pneumothorax, aspiration pneumonia (secondary to gastroparesis), airway mucus plugs, and disordered breathing during sleep.[81] In addition, studies of the alveolar epithelial and capillary basal laminae have shown both to be significantly greater in thickness in diabetics than in control subjects (although the increase in thickness is much less than that observed in the basal laminae of muscle and renal tubules).[82] These changes may be reflected in the mild, duration-related reduction in lung elastic recoil, pulmonary diffusing capacity, and pulmonary capillary blood volume that are observed in some patients with insulin-dependent diabetic mellitus.[83] The threshold for cough reflex response to inhaled citric acid has been found to be higher in diabetics with autonomic neuropathy than in control diabetic patients who have no neuropathy, suggesting impairment of the vagal innervation of the bronchial tree.[84]

Hypopituitarism and Acromegaly

Both experimental[85] and physiologic[86] investigations suggest that growth hormone exerts an important influence on lung structure and growth. Patients with hypopituitarism have a restrictive type of ventilatory impairment, total lung capacity being approximately 75 per cent of normal.[86] By contrast, patients with acromegaly tend to have large lungs with a total lung capacity approximately 25 per cent greater than that of matched controls.[87]

Other disorders associated with acromegaly include abnormal small airway function[88] and an increased prevalence of sleep apnea.[89] In addition, death from respiratory causes (predominantly upper airway obstruction) has been reported to be three times more common in acromegalic patients than in the general population.[90]

Hypothyroidism

An abnormal accumulation of fluid can occur in the pericardial and pleural spaces in patients with myxedema in the absence of cardiovascular, renal, or other causes of fluid retention.[91] Patchy airspace disease has been described as well and in one study was presumed to be edema, although there was no dyspnea or cardiomegaly; the disease cleared on treatment of myxedema.[92] Hypoxemia can also occur in patients with myxedema. Although it is usually seen in association with obesity and hypoventilation and often with coma,[93] some patients are not obese and their blood gas values have been shown to return to normal with thyroid therapy, despite little or no change in body weight.[94]

Hyperparathyroidism

Hypercalcemia associated with hyperparathyroidism can result in metastatic calcification of the lungs. Usually detectable only by histologic examination, it is sometimes severe enough to be visible roentgenographically, especially with CT or dual-energy digital radiography.[95] Parathyroid hormone undoubtedly plays a role in the ectopic calcium deposition that occurs in patients with kidney[96] and liver[97] transplants and in those with chronic renal failure, especially when undergoing maintenance hemodialysis.[98]

Klinefelter's Syndrome

This inherited syndrome is characterized classically by small firm testes, azoospermia, gynecomastia, elevated urinary gonadotropins, and often eunuchoid skeletal proportions. Patients are said to be prone to bronchitis, bronchiectasis, and asthma.[99]

PULMONARY ABNORMALITIES IN NON-NEOPLASTIC HEMATOLOGIC DISORDERS

Sickle-Cell Disease

An "acute chest syndrome" characterized by the abrupt onset of fever, chest pain, and leukocytosis occurs in patients with homozygous sickle cell anemia and hemoglobin sickle cell disease. It is very common and has been attributed to pneumonia, particularly when it affects children. However, although there is little doubt that these patients are more susceptible to pneumococcal, *Haemophilus*, and *Mycoplasma* pneumonia, most studies indicate that infection is a relatively uncommon cause of the syndrome.[100, 101] Instead, it is likely that most episodes result when sickling leads to obstruction in the pulmonary vessels.[102] Patients with sickle cell anemia also are prone to the development of pnemococcal septicemia[103] and pulmonary thrombosis and thromboembolism.[102, 104]

Thalassemia Major

This inherited disorder of beta globulin synthesis is manifested largely by anemia and osteoporosis. It can be associated with a restrictive respiratory defect with low PaO_2 and reduced static compliance, findings that may be explained by a decrease in the growth of airspaces relative to the vascular bed and major airways during childhood.[105]

References

1. Kariman K, Kylstra JA, Spook A: Pulmonary alveolar proteinosis: Prospective clinical experience in 23 patients for 15 years. Lung 162: 223, 1984.
2. Bedrossian CWM, Luna MA, Conklin RH, et al: Alveolar proteinosis as a consequence of immunosuppression. A hypothesis based on clinical and pathologic observations. Hum Pathol 11: 527, 1980.
3. Colon AR, Lawrence RD, Mills SD, et al: Childhood pulmonary alveolar proteinosis (PAP). Am J Dis Child 121: 481, 1971.
4. Ruben FL, Talamo TS: Secondary pulmonary alveolar proteinosis occurring in two patients with acquired immune deficiency syndrome. Am J Med 80: 1187, 1986.
5. Samuels MP, Warner J: Pulmonary alveolar lipoproteinosis complicating juvenile dermatomyositis. Thorax 43: 939, 1988.
6. Aymard J-P, Gyger M, Lavallee R, et al: A case of pulmonary alveolar proteinosis complicating chronic myelogenous leukemia. Cancer 53: 954, 1984.
7. Teja K, Cooper PH, Squires JE, et al: Pulmonary alveolar proteinosis in four siblings. N Engl J Med 305: 1390, 1981.
8. Corrin B, King E: Pathogenesis of experimental pulmonary alveolar proteinosis. Thorax 25: 230, 1970.
9. Lee KP, Barras CE, Griffith FD, et al: Pulmonary response to glass fiber by inhalation exposure. Lab Invest 40: 123, 1979.
10. Buechner HA, Ansari A: Acute silico-proteinosis. A new pathologic variant of acute silicosis in sandblasters, characterized by histologic features resembling alveolar proteinosis. Dis Chest 55: 274, 1969.
11. Gilmore LB, Talley FA, Hook GE: Classification and morphometric quantitation of insoluble materials from the lungs of patients with alveolar proteinosis. Am J Pathol 133: 252, 1988.
12. Singh G, Katyal SL: Surfactant apoprotein in nonmalignant pulmonary disorders. Am J Pathol 101: 51, 1980.
13. Satoh K, Arai H, Yoshida T, et al: Glycosaminoglycans and glycoproteins in bronchoalveolar lavage fluid from patients with pulmonary alveolar proteinosis. Inflammation 7: 347, 1983.
14. Ramirez J, Harlan WR Jr: Pulmonary alveolar proteinosis. Nature and origin of alveolar lipid. Am J Med 45: 502, 1968.

15. Golde DW, Territo M, Finley TN, et al: Defective lung macrophages in pulmonary alveolar proteinosis. Ann Intern Med 85: 304, 1976.
16. Milleron BJ, Costabel U, Teschler H, et al: Bronchoalveolar lavage cell data in alveolar proteinosis. Am Rev Respir Dis 144: 1330, 1991.
17. McEuen DD, Abraham JL: Particulate concentrations in pulmonary aveolar proteinosis. Environ Res 17: 334, 1978.
18. Nugent KM, Pesanti EL: Macrophage function in pulmonary alveolar proteinosis. Am Rev Respir Dis 127: 780, 1983.
19. Carre PC, Didier AP, Pipy BR, et al: The lavage fluid from a patient with alveolar proteinosis inhibits the in vitro chemiluminescence response and arachidonic acid metabolism of normal guinea pig alveolar macrophages. Am Rev Respir Dis 142: 1068, 1990.
20. Mendenhall E Jr, Solu S, Easom HF: Pulmonary alveolar proteinosis. Am Rev Respir Dis 84: 876, 1961.
21. Greenspan RH: Chronic disseminated alveolar diseases of the lung. Semin Roentgenol 2: 77, 1967.
22. Miller PA, Ravin CE, Smith GJW, et al: Pulmonary alveolar proteinosis with interstitial involvement. Am J Roentgenol 137: 1069, 1981.
23. Godwin JD, Müller NL, Rakasugi JE: Pulmonary alveolar proteinosis: CT findings. Radiology 169: 609, 1988.
24. Ramirez J: Pulmonary alveolar proteinosis. A roentgenologic analysis. Am J Roentgenol 92: 571, 1964.
25. Rogers RM, Levin DC, Gray BA, et al: Physiologic effects of bronchopulmonary lavage in alveolar proteinosis. Am Rev Respir Dis 118: 255, 1978.
26. Kroeker EJ, Korfmacher S: Pulmonary alveolar proteinosis. Report of case with application of a special sputum examination as an aid to diagnosis. Am Rev Respir Dis 87: 416, 1963.
27. Ray RL, Salm R: A fatal case of pulmonary alveolar proteinosis. Thorax 17: 257, 1962.
28. Bell DY, Hook GER: Pulmonary alveolar proteinosis: Analysis of airway and alveolar proteins. Am Rev Respir Dis 119: 979, 1979.
29. Fraimow W, Cathcart RT, Taylor RC: Physiologic and clinical aspects of pulmonary alveolar proteinosis. Ann Intern Med 52: 1177, 1960.
30. Oliva PB, Vogel JHK: Reactive pulmonary hypertension in alveolar proteinosis. Chest 58: 167, 1970.
31. Yeh SD, White DA, Stover-Pepe DE, et al: Abnormal gallium scintigraphy in pulmonary alveolar proteinosis (PAP). Clin Nucl Med 12: 294, 1987.
32. Masuda T, Shimura S, Sasaki H, et al: Surfactant apoprotein-A concentration in sputum for diagnosis of pulmonary alveolar proteinosis. Lancet 337: 580, 1991.
33. Davidson JM, MacLeod WM: Pulmonary alveolar proteinosis. Br J Dis Chest 63: 13, 1969.
34. DuBois RM, McAllister WA, Branthwaite MA: Alveolar proteinosis: Diagnosis and treatment over a 10-year period. Thorax 38: 360, 1983.
35. Amyloid and the lower respiratory tract [editorial]. Thorax 38: 84, 1983.
36. Kisilevsky R: Biology of disease. Amyloidosis: A familiar problem in the light of current pathogenetic developments. Lab Invest 49: 381, 1983.
37. Knapp MJ, Roggli VL, Kim J, et al: Pleural amyloidosis. Arch Pathol Lab Med 112: 57, 1988.
38. Smith RRl, Hutchins GM, Moore GW, et al: Type and distribution of pulmonary parenchymal and vascular amyloid. Correlation with cardiac amyloidosis. Am J Med 66: 96, 1979.
39. Santiago RM, Scharnhorst D, Ratkin G, et al: Respiratory muscle weakness and ventilatory failure in AL amyloidosis with muscular pseudohypertrophy. Am J Med 83: 175, 1987.
40. Hsiu J-G, Stitik FP, D'Amato NA, et al: Primary amyloidosis presenting as a unilateral hilar mass. Report of a case diagnosed by fine needle aspiration biopsy. Acta Cytol 30: 55, 1986.
41. Melato M, Antonutto G, Falconieri G, et al: Massive amyloidosis of mediastinal lymph nodes in a patient with multiple myeloma. Thorax 38: 151, 1983.
42. Gordon HW, Miller R Jr, Mittman C: Medullary carcinoma of the lung with amyloid stroma: A counterpart of medullary carcinoma of the thyroid. Hum Pathol 4: 431, 1973.
43. Michalsen H, Storrøsten OT, Lindboe CF: Generalized amyloidosis in cystic fibrosis. Eur J Respir Dis 66: 306, 1985.
44. DaCosta P, Corrin B: Amyloidosis localized to the lower respiratory tract: Probable immunoamyloid nature of the tracheobronchial and nodular pulmonary forms. Histopathology 9: 703, 1985.
45. Cordier JF, Loire R, Brune J: Amyloidosis of the lower respiratory

tract. Clinical and pathologic features in a series of 21 patients. Chest 90: 827, 1986.
46. Monreal FA: Pulmonary amyloidosis: Ultrastructural study of early alveolar septal deposits. Hum Pathol 15: 388, 1984.
47. Rubinow A, Celli BR, Cohen AS, et al: Localized amyloidosis of the lower respiratory tract. Am Rev Respir Dis 118: 603, 1978.
48. Jimenez C, Vital C, Merlio JP, et al: Plasmacytoma and gastric amyloidosis associated with nodular pulmonary amyloidosis. Ann Pathol 8: 155, 1988.
49. Bhate DV: Case of the spring season: Diffuse primary amyloidosis with nodular calcified lung lesions. Semin Roentgenol 14: 81, 1979.
50. Savader SJ, Nokes SR, Chappel G: Case report and review: Computed tomography of multiple nodular pulmonary amyloidosis. Comput Radiol 11: 111, 1987.
51. Graham CM, Stern EJ, Finkbeiner WE, et al: High-resolution CT appearance of diffuse alveolar septal amyloidosis. Am J Roentgenol 158: 265, 1992.
52. Westermark P, Pitkanen P, Benson L, et al: Serum prealbumin and retinol-binding protein in the prealbumin-related and familial forms of systemic amyloidosis. Lab Invest 52: 314, 1985.
53. Briggs GW: Amyloidosis. Ann Intern Med 55: 943, 1961.
54. Hodge DS, Anderson WR, Tsai SH: Primary diffuse bronchial amyloidosis. Arch Pathol Lab Med 101: 615, 1977.
55. Flemming AFS, Fairfax AJ, Arnold AG, et al: Treatment of endobronchial amyloidosis by intermittent bronchoscopic resection. Br J Dis Chest 74: 183, 1980.
56. Lee S-C, Johnson HA: Multiple nodular pulmonary amyloidosis. A case report and comparison with diffuse alveolar-septal pulmonary amyloidosis. Thorax 30: 178, 1975.
57. Laden SA, Cohen ML, Harley RA: Nodular pulmonary amyloidosis with extrapulmonary involvement. Hum Pathol 15: 594, 1984.
58. Hui AN, Koss MN, Hochholzer L, et al: Amyloidosis presenting in the lower respiratory tract. Clinicopathologic, radiologic, immunohistochemical and histochemical studies on 48 cases. Arch Pathol Lab Med 110: 212, 1986.
59. Hardy TJ, Myerowitz RL, Bender BL: Diffuse parenchymal amyloidosis of lungs and breast. Its association with diffuse plasmacytosis and kappa-chain gammopathy. Arch Pathol Lab Med 103: 583, 1979.
60. Wolson AH: Pulmonary findings in Gaucher's disease. Am J Roentgenol 123: 712, 1975.
61. Jackson DC, Simon G: Unusual bone and lung changes in a case of Gaucher's disease. Br Med J 38: 698, 1965.
62. Schneider EL, Epstein CJ, Kaback MJ, et al: Severe pulmonary involvement in adult Gaucher's disease. Report of three cases and review of the literature. Am J Med 63: 475, 1977.
63. Lieberman J, Beutler E: Elevation of serum angiotensin-converting enzyme in Gaucher's disease. N Engl J Med 294: 1442, 1976.
64. Long RG, Lake BD, Pettit JE, et al: Adult Niemann-Pick disease. Its relationship to the syndrome of the sea-blue histiocyte. Am J Med 62: 627, 1977.
65. Crocker AC, Farber S: Niemann-Pick disease: A review of eighteen patients. Medicine 37: 1, 1958.
66. Lachman R, Crocker A, Schulman J, et al: Radiological findings in Niemann-Pick disease. Radiology 108: 659, 1973.
67. Schinella RA, Greco MA, Garay SM, et al: Hermansky-Pudlak syndrome: A clinicopathologic study. Hum Pathol 16: 366, 1985.
68. Garay SM, Gardella JE, Fazzini EP, et al: Hermansky-Pudlak syndrome. Pulmonary manifestations of a ceroid storage disorder. Am J Med 66: 737, 1979.
69. DePinho RA, Kaplan KL: The Hermansky-Pudlak syndrome. Report of three cases and review of pathophysiology and management considerations. Medicine 64: 192, 1985.
70. Leitman BS, Balthazar EJ, Garay SM, et al: The Hermansky-Pudlak syndrome: Radiographic features. J Can Assoc Radiol 37: 41, 1986.
71. Caplan H: A case of endocardial fibro-elastosis with features of glycogen-storage disease. J Pathol Bact 76: 77, 1958.
72. Lightman NI, Schooley RT: Adult-onset acid maltase deficiency. Case report of an adult with severe respiratory difficulty. Chest 72: 250, 1977.
73. Semenza GL, Pyeritz RE: Respiratory complications of mucopolysaccharide storage disorders. Medicine 67: 209, 1988.
74. Pyeritz RE: Connective tissue in the lung. Lessons from the Marfan syndrome. Ann Intern Med 103: 289, 1985.
75. Bolande RP, Tucker AS: Pulmonary emphysema and other cardio-

respiratory lesions as part of the Marfan abiotrophy. Pediatrics 33: 356, 1964.

76. König P, Boxer R, Morrison J, et al: Bronchial hyperreactivity in children with Marfan syndrome. Pediatr Pulmonol 11: 29, 1991.

77. Shilkin KB, Low LP, Chen BTM: Dissecting aneurysm of the pulmonary artery. J Pathol 98: 25, 1969.

78. Wood JR, Bellamy D, Child AH, et al: Pulmonary disease in patients with Marfan syndrome. Thorax 39: 780, 1984.

79. Pyeritz RE: Maternal and fetal complications of pregnancy in the Marfan syndrome. Am J Med 71: 784, 1981.

80. Smit J, Alberts C, Balk AG: Pneumothorax in the Ehlers-Danlos syndrome: Consequence or coincidence? Scand J Respir Dis 59: 239, 1978.

81. Hansen LA, Prakash UB, Colby TV: Pulmonary complications in diabetes mellitus. Mayo Clin Proc 64: 791, 1989.

82. Vracko R, Thorning D, Huang TW: Basal lamina of alveolar epithelium and capillaries: Quantitative changes with aging and in diabetes mellitus. Am Rev Respir Dis 120: 973, 1979.

83. Sandler M, Bunn AE, Stewart RI: Cross-section study of pulmonary function in patients with insulin-dependent diabetes mellitus. Am Rev Respir Dis 135: 223, 1987.

84. Vianna LG, Gilbey SG, Barnes NC, et al: Cough threshold to citric acid in diabetic patients with and without autonomic neuropathy. Thorax 43: 569, 1988.

85. Brody JS, Buhain WJ: Hormonal influence on post-pneumonectomy lung growth in the rat. Respir Physiol 19: 344, 1973.

86. De Troyer A, Desir D, Copinschi G: Regression of lung size in adults with growth hormone deficiency. Q J Med (New Series 49) 195: 329, 1980.

87. Trotman-Dickenson B, Weetman AP, Hughes JM: Upper airflow obstruction and pulmonary function in acromegaly: Relationship to disease activity. Q J Med 79: 527, 1991.

88. Siafakas NM, Sigalas J, Filaditaki B, et al: Small airway function in acromegaly. Bull Eur Physiopathol Respir 23: 329, 1987.

89. Grunstein RR, Ho KY, Sullivan CE: Sleep apnea in acromegaly. Ann Intern Med 115: 527, 1991.

90. Murrant NJ, Gatland DJ: Respiratory problems in acromegaly. J Laryngol Otol 104: 52, 1990.

91. Brown SD, Brashear RE, Schnute RB: Pleural effusion in a young woman with myxedema. Arch Intern Med 143: 1458, 1983.

92. Sadiq MA, Davies JC: Unusual lung manifestations of myxoedema. Br J Clin Pract 31: 224, 1977.

93. Wilson WR, Bedell GN: The pulmonary abnormalities in myxedema. J Clin Invest 39: 42, 1960.

94. Domm BM, Vassalo CL: Myxedema coma with respiratory failure. Am Rev Respir Dis 107: 842, 1973.

95. Sanders C, Frank MS, Rostand SG, et al: Metastatic calcification of the heart and lungs in end-stage renal disease: Detection and quantification by dual-energy digital chest radiography. Am J Roentgenol 149: 881, 1987.

96. Breitz HB, Sirotta PS, Nelp WB, et al: Progressive pulmonary calcification complicating successful renal transplantation. Am Rev Respir Dis 136: 1480, 1987.

97. Raisis IP, Park CH, Yang SL, et al: Lung uptake of technetium-99m phosphate compounds after liver transplantation. Clin Nucl Med 13: 188, 1988.

98. Jolles H, Johnson AC, Ell SR: Subcutaneous calcifications masquerading as pulmonary lesions in long-term hemodialysis. Review of nodular pulmonary opacities in the population undergoing hemodialysis. Chest 88: 234, 1985.

99. Huseby JS, Petersen D: Pulmonary function in Klinefelter's syndrome. Chest 80: 31, 1981.

100. Poncz M, Kane E, Gill FM: Acute chest syndrome in sickle cell disease: Etiology and clinical correlates. J Pediatr 107: 861, 1985.

101. Powers D, Weidman JA, Odom-Maryon T, et al: Sickle cell chronic lung disease: Prior morbidity and the risk of pulmonary infection. Medicine 67: 66, 1988.

102. Haupt HM, Moore GW, Bauer TW, et al: The lung in sickle cell disease. Chest 81: 332, 1982.

103. Gray A, Anionwu EN, Davies SC, et al: Patterns of mortality in sickle cell disease in the United Kingdom. J Clin Pathol 44: 459, 1991.

104. Israel RH, Salipante JS: Pulmonary infarction in sickle cell trait. Am J Med 66: 867, 1979.

105. Cooper DM, Mansell AL, Weiner MA, et al: Low lung capacity and hypoxemia in children with thalassemia major. Am Rev Respir Dis 121: 639, 1980.

17

PULMONARY DISEASE OF UNKNOWN ORIGIN

SARCOIDOSIS

Sarcoidosis is a disorder of unknown etiology characterized pathologically by non-necrotizing granulomatous inflammation, and clinically and radiologically by bilateral hilar lymph node enlargement, with or without interstitial pulmonary or systemic disease.[1]

There is considerable variation in the reported incidence of the disease in different countries and continents. As a rule, it is more frequent in countries with temperate climates such as Sweden and, to a lesser extent, Norway and Finland[2] than in countries with tropical climates.[3] Although it is rarely seen in African[4] or South American blacks or mulattoes,[5] it is unusually common in the black population of the United States, particularly women. A disproportion-ately high incidence also has been observed in Puerto Ricans living in the United States[6] and in West Indians in the United Kingdom.[7] The disease appears to be more prevalent in rural areas.

Sex incidence is equal in young persons but shows a definite female predominance in middle-aged and elderly persons.[2] Although the disease may occur at any age, more than 50 per cent of patients are between the ages of 20 and 40 years.[4, 8]

Etiology and Pathogenesis

The almost invariable presence of granulomatous inflammation in the thorax, has led to speculation that an inhaled foreign material such as a microorganism is responsible for the disease. The most likely agents to come under suspicion are mycobacteria[4] and, to a lesser extent, gram-negative bacteria such as *Yersinia enterocolitica.*[9] Experimental evidence implicating a transmissible agent such as a microorganism emanates from several sources. Granulomas have been produced in the footpads or viscera of mice by inoculating homogenates of human sarcoid tissue[10] and in the skin of patients with sarcoidosis injected intracutaneously with autologous bronchoalveolar lavage (BAL) cells.[11] In addition, investigations of granulomas from patients with sarcoidosis have revealed tadpole-shaped structures resembling bacteria by electron microscopy.[12] Despite these observations, culture of affected tissue in sarcoidosis is invariably sterile, microorganisms are not seen with special tissue stains, and search for mycobacterial deoxyribonucleic acid (DNA) in sarcoid granulomas using the polymerase chain reaction has been positive in only a few cases.[13] In addition, there is no evidence of human-to-human transmission of the disease.

Although the pathogenesis of sarcoidosis is also poorly understood and undoubtedly complex (Fig. 17–1), there is abundant evidence that some abnormality of immune function is important. Much of the work confirming this hypothesis has been derived from analysis of cells and immune mediators obtained by BAL. In normal, nonsmoking individuals, a typical BAL cell population consists of about 90 per cent macrophages, 9 per cent lymphocytes, and fewer than 1 per cent polymorphonuclear leukocytes. Of the lymphocytes, more than 90 per cent are T cells, of which approximately 50 per cent are helper (CD4) cells and 25 per cent suppressor (CD8) cells; fewer than 10 per cent

are B cells. By contrast, the BAL fluid of patients with active sarcoidosis contains approximately 60 per cent macrophages and 40 per cent lymphocytes.[14] This increase in lymphocytes is caused almost entirely by an increase in the CD4 subset, the proportion of helper to suppressor T cells generally ranging from about 6:1[15] to 10:1.[16] Proliferation of lymphocytes and an increased CD4/CD8 ratio also have been described in other pulmonary interstitial diseases; however, proportions greater than 2.5:1 are seldom encountered.[17] The reason for the specific expansion of activated CD4 cells is unclear; however, it does not appear to be caused by an alteration in the suppressor function of CD8 cells.[18]

Interestingly, the blood does not show the same CD4 cell proliferation and increased CD4/CD8 ratio as in BAL fluid. In fact, the blood of patients with active sarcoidosis shows lymphopenia, a decrease in the number of CD4 cells, and a decrease in the CD4/CD8 ratio.[16, 19] In addition, *in vitro* assessment of cell-mediated immune function using recall antigens has shown that peripheral blood T cells from patients with active sarcoidosis show little or no response.[20] This *in vitro* anergy could explain the negative delayed hypersensitivity skin reactions to various antigens seen in sarcoidosis. Several studies[21] suggest that an inhibitor of interleukin 1 (very likely a prostaglandin) produced by bronchoalveolar inflammatory cells[22] may leak into the peripheral circulation and be responsible for these alterations in systemic immune reactivity.

Although T-cell abnormalities are the most obvious feature of sarcoidosis, the proportions and types of a variety of other cells in BAL fluid are also altered. For example,

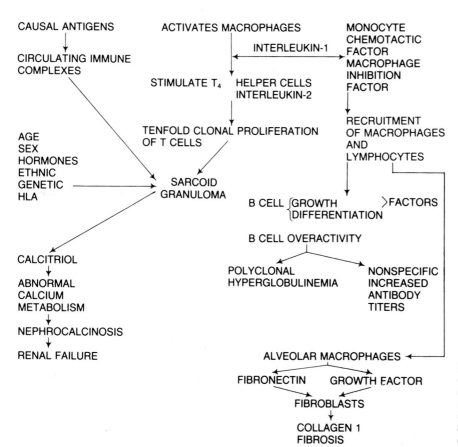

Figure 17–1. Factors Contributing to Sarcoid Granuloma Formation and to Sarcoidosis. (Reprinted with permission from James DG: Definition and classification of granulomatous disorders. Seminars in Respiratory Medicine 8:1, July 1986, p 2, Thieme Medical Publishers, Inc.)

subpopulations of alveolar macrophages in patients with active sarcoidosis differ from those of normal subjects.[23, 23a] Many are immature, probably because they are recently recruited from blood monocytes.[24] In addition, the density of HLA-DR antigen expression is increased, a finding that appears to be linked to a combination of lymphocytosis, T-lymphocyte subtype distribution, and the production of chemical mediators. There is also an increase in the number of killer and natural killer lymphocytes,[25] HLA-DR antigen–bearing lymphocytes,[26] and mast cells,[27] many of which show ultrastructural features of "activation."[28]

Activated CD4 lymphocytes appear to play a role in the activation of B lymphocytes, with resultant hypergammaglobulinemia.[29] In the peripheral blood, B-lymphocyte overactivity is reflected in increased levels of immunoglobulins and of kappa and lambda chains, sometimes accompanied by circulating immune complexes. These manifestations of altered humoral immunity are usually seen in patients with more extensive organ involvement and are less common in those with hilar lymph node enlargement only.[30] The exception appears to be patients presenting with erythema nodosum, in whom an abrupt rise in immunoglobulins is associated with a rapidly developing alveolitis.[31] Immune complexes are found more often in patients with a combination of erythema nodosum, arthralgia, and uveitis; these patients also show an increased incidence of the histocompatibility antigen HLA-B8.[32]

In addition to the cellular abnormalities of BAL fluid, a variety of immune mediators are present in the supernatant of CD4 cells grown in culture, mediators that are undoubtedly present *in vivo* as well and that are important in the pathogenesis of the disease. These include monocyte chemotactic factor, migration inhibition factor, leukocyte inhibitory factor, a polyclonal activator of B cells that causes production of immunoglobulins, a fibroblast growth factor, interleukin-2, and gamma interferon.[29, 33] Pulmonary T lymphocytes obtained by BAL from patients with active sarcoidosis (but not those from normal subjects or patients with fibrosing alveolitis) secrete an amount of chemotactic factor for monocytes estimated to be 25 times more than that produced by peripheral blood T lymphocytes,[34] thus establishing a gradient between lung and blood that results in a virtually continuous supply of the cells that eventually become the epithelioid cells of pulmonary granulomas. Other substances that are found in the BAL fluid of patients with active sarcoidosis include fibronectin, hyaluronin, and procollagen peptide.[35]

Although immunologic abnormalities are the most consistently demonstrated and perhaps the most important in the pathogenesis of sarcoidosis, other factors also have been investigated. Familial clustering has suggested the possibility of a genetic factor.[36] However, such clustering often occurs in nonconsanguineous relatives[37] and in close acquaintances,[38] thus supporting the concept of common exposure to the etiologic agent. Some investigators have found a higher incidence of disease in nonsmokers,[39] suggesting that cigarette smoking might have a "protective" effect; however, the mechanism of such an effect is unknown.

The pathogenesis of the fibrosis in the lungs of patients with sarcoidosis is probably multifactorial.[33] A variety of substances produced by alveolar macrophages and lymphocytes, such as gamma interferon, interleukin-1, fibronectin, alveolar macrophage–derived growth factor, and platelet-derived growth factor, have been described as playing roles.[40–43] Prostaglandin E_2 may act both as an inhibitor of fibroblast proliferation and as a modulator of the fibrotic response. Alveolar macrophages from patients with sarcoidosis produce increased amounts of the initial enzymes of both coagulation and fibrinolytic pathways, suggesting that they may regulate the formation of a fibrin matrix in which fibrosis subsequently can develop.[44] There is also reason to believe that oxygen radicals, proteinases, cationic proteins, and various other substances released from injured cells may contribute to the lung destruction and subsequent fibrosis.[45]

Pathologic Characteristics

The pathologic hallmark of sarcoidosis is the granuloma, which, in its early stages, is identical to that caused by many other etiologic agents—a well-defined collection of epithelioid histiocytes often containing multinucleated giant cells (Fig. 17–2). Lymphocytes, occasionally plasma cells, and rarely neutrophils and eosinophils can be intermingled. The majority of granulomas are non-necrotizing; however, some contain small foci of necrosis, the presence of which does not exclude the diagnosis.[46] Such necrosis typically occurs in the central portion of the granuloma and appears as

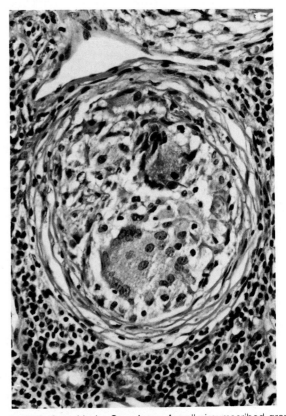

Figure 17–2. Sarcoidosis: Granuloma. A well-circumscribed granuloma contains two multinucleated giant cells, epithelioid histiocytes, and scattered small mononuclear cells. A distinct zone of collagen possessing a clear-cut lamellated appearance can be seen at the periphery. (*A* and *B* × 300.)

amorphous eosinophilic material often associated with degenerated, hyperchromatic nuclei.

Fibroblasts are present in considerable numbers at the periphery of more "mature" granulomas,[47] and it appears that the fibrosis begins at this site. In this circumstance, concentric lamellae of collagen can be seen to separate the histologically "active" central portion of the granuloma from the adjacent tissue (*see* Fig. 17–2). With time, the fibrosis proceeds inward until the entire granuloma is converted into a scar. This pattern of peripheral lamellar fibrosis is characteristic of healing sarcoidosis and is itself strong evidence in favor of the diagnosis.

It should be emphasized that the finding of non-necrotizing granulomas does not in itself constitute absolute evidence of sarcoidosis, since such lesions are by no means specific. Local or diffuse non-necrotizing granulomas can be found in the lungs and in other organs in association with a wide variety of conditions, including infections (par-

ticularly mycobacterial and fungal), extrinsic allergic alveolitis, neoplasms (including pulmonary carcinoma), pneumoconiosis (particularly that caused by beryllium), drugs, and foreign bodies. In some cases, ancillary procedures such as culture of biopsied material, special stains for mycobacteria or fungi, and polarization microscopy may clarify the etiology of the granulomatous process. However, even negative results of these and other investigations do not exclude all specific etiologic agents, and it is necessary to make a careful distinction between the pathologic finding of non-necrotizing granulomatous inflammation and the clinical-roentgenographic disease known as sarcoidosis.

Pulmonary involvement in sarcoidosis is characteristically most prominent in the peribronchovascular, interlobular septal, and pleural interstitial tissue (Fig. 17–3). In the early stages, granulomas are discrete and histologically active; as the disease progresses, however, they often become confluent and undergo fibrosis, resulting in more or less

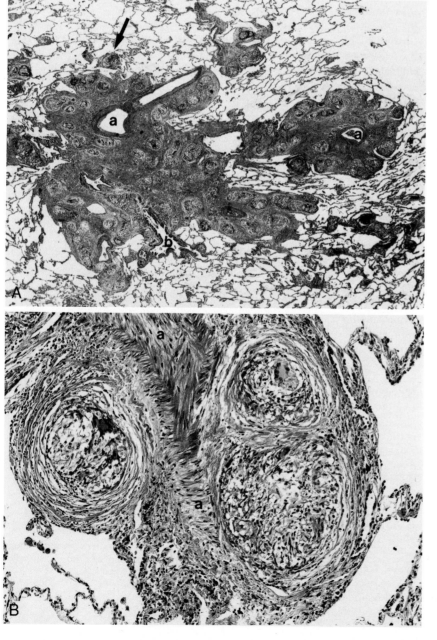

Figure 17–3. Pulmonary Sarcoidosis. A low-magnification histologic section of lung parenchyma *(A)* shows numerous granulomas associated with a moderate amount of collagen; both granulomas and fibrous tissue are located predominantly in the interstitium adjacent to pulmonary arteries (a) and bronchioles (b). Only an occasional granuloma appears to be located within parenchymal interstitium *(arrow)*. A magnified view *(B)* shows three granulomas with a peripheral rim of lamellated fibrous tissue adjacent to a tangentially sectioned pulmonary artery (a). (*A* × 15; *B* × 120.)

diffuse interstitial thickening. The parenchymal interstitium is also affected, although typically less than in peribronchovascular, septal, and pleural locations. In the early stage of the disease, this is manifested by nonspecific pneumonitis comprised largely of an infiltrate of lymphocytes and histiocytes in alveolar septa.[47] Subsequently, typical granulomas develop. Individual foci of disease are usually microscopic but can conglomerate to form relatively discrete masses 4 cm in diameter or larger, an appearance sometimes referred to as "nodular sarcoidosis."

Possibly because of the prominent peribronchovascular and septal location of the granulomatous inflammation, involvement of pulmonary arteries and veins is common in sarcoidosis.[48] Although this inflammation can be associated with disruption of the elastic laminae, necrosis usually does not occur. (Nevertheless, there is evidence that at least some cases of necrotizing sarcoid granulomatosis may represent a variant of sarcoidosis [see page 415]). Granulomas are also common in airway mucosa, particularly in small bronchi.[49]

The gross appearance of pulmonary sarcoidosis depends on the stage and severity of disease. In the early, milder forms in which inflammation is most prominent in relation to peribronchovascular, interlobular, and pleural connective tissue, the appearance can resemble lymphangitic carcinomatosis. As disease progresses, involvement of the parenchymal interstitium becomes more evident and large portions of lung can become consolidated and eventually fibrotic. This process is usually most severe in the apical portion of the upper lobes, where it can take the form of more or less solid areas of fibrous tissue associated with bronchiectasis (Fig. 17–4). The latter can be severe enough to result in the formation of large "cavities" that are frequently the site of aspergilloma formation.[50]

Lymph node involvement in sarcoidosis is characterized by more or less diffuse replacement of the node by granulomas (Fig. 17–5), often with a variable histologic appearance.[51] Initially, the granulomas are discrete and appear "active"; as in pulmonary disease, however, they tend to become confluent and undergo progressive fibrosis over time. In advanced disease, this can result in completely fibrotic nodes in which granulomas are difficult to recognize.

Roentgenographic Manifestations

The roentgenographic changes in thoracic sarcoidosis can be usefully classified for descriptive purposes into five groups or stages.

Stage 0. No demonstrable abnormality.
Stage 1. Hilar and mediastinal lymph node enlargement not associated with pulmonary abnormality.
Stage 2. Hilar and mediastinal lymph node enlargement associated with pulmonary abnormality.
Stage 3. Diffuse pulmonary disease not associated with node enlargement.
Stage 4. Pulmonary fibrosis.

Lymph Node Enlargement Without Pulmonary Abnormality

Conventional roentgenography reveals evidence of lymph node enlargement in 75 to 85 per cent of patients with sarcoidosis, in approximately equal numbers with and without diffuse parenchymal disease.[52] It is usually localized to the hilar, tracheobronchial, and paratracheal groups and typically is bilaterally symmetric. The contour of the outer borders of enlarged hila usually is lobulated, particularly on the right side (Fig. 17–6); enlargement of right paratracheal nodes obscures the right tracheal stripe and creates a smooth or slightly lobulated contour. As might be expected, computed tomography (CT) can reveal enlargement of lymph nodes in locations not suspected on conventional roentgenograms, such as the anterior mediastinum, axilla, internal mammary chain, and infradiaphragmatic area.[53]

Unilateral hilar lymph node enlargement is uncommon, being reported in no more than 5 per cent of proved cases.[54] Occasionally, enlarged hilar and carinal nodes can compress the major bronchi or pulmonary arteries (Fig. 17–7), resulting in atelectasis or a reduction in pulmonary perfusion. The prevalence of calcification of hilar lymph nodes in thoracic sarcoidosis has been reported to range from 5 to 20 per cent.[55, 56] It is usually a late manifestation and is almost invariably associated with advanced disease.

Paratracheal node enlargement seldom, if ever, occurs without concomitant enlargement of hilar nodes. This bilaterally symmetric hilar and paratracheal lymph node enlargement contrasts sharply with the node enlargement that characterizes the lymphomas. In Hodgkin's disease, for example, enlargement tends to occur predominantly in the anterior mediastinal and paratracheal groups; when it involves the hilar nodes, it is predominantly unilateral and asymmetric. As indicated earlier, although retrosternal node enlargement is uncommon in sarcoidosis, there are individual case reports[55] of anterior mediastinal lymph node enlargement evident on conventional roentgenograms, and there is no doubt that the incidence is considerably higher on CT scans, perhaps as high as 10 per cent.[57] Thus, the possibility of sarcoidosis should not be dismissed when such node enlargement is present, particularly when it is associated with enlargement of hilar nodes. Enlargement of posterior mediastinal nodes in sarcoidosis is very uncommon.[58]

It is important to appreciate the fact that, as in other interstitial diseases, the lungs can be involved in the absence of a demonstrable abnormality on the chest roentgenogram.[59, 60] One group of investigators found the prevalence of pathologically proven pulmonary sarcoidosis in stage 0 to be slightly greater than 9 per cent, a rate that must reflect liberal use of biopsy.[59] Similarly, in a report of 21 consecutive patients with stage 1 disease who underwent open lung biopsy,[61] typical sarcoid granulomas were found in all; however, the extent of granulomatous inflammation and fibrosis was significantly less than that seen in open lung biopsies of patients with roentgenographic evidence of diffuse lung involvement. Similar results have been obtained in studies in which CT scans were compared with conventional roentgenograms in patients with sarcoidosis: focal pulmonary parenchymal abnormalities have been identified on CT in most patients with stage 0 or stage 1 disease.[62] Pulmonary function impairment also can be present in the absence of roentgenographically apparent lung abnormality,[63] as can abnormalities in BAL fluid such as lymphocytosis and the presence of activated alveolar macrophages.[64]

Seventy to eighty per cent of patients with hilar lymph node enlargement, with or without visible pulmonary in-

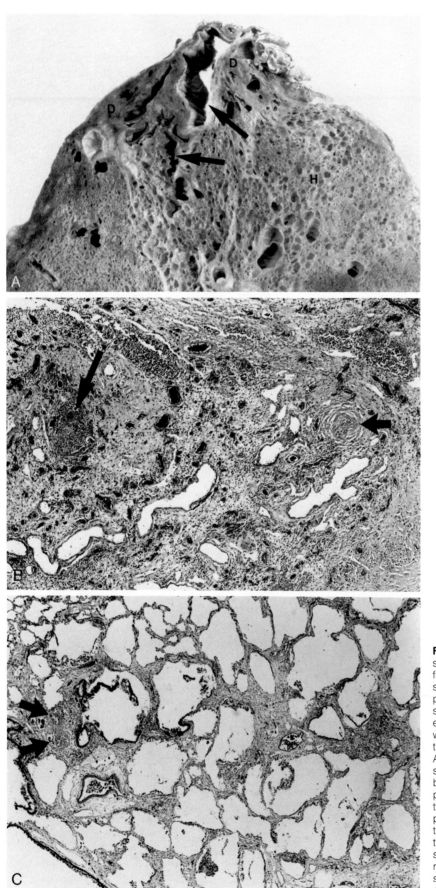

Figure 17–4. Sarcoidosis: Interstitial Fibrosis. A section of the apical portion of an upper lobe *(A)* from a patient with long-standing sarcoidosis shows foci of dense fibrosis in which the lung parenchyma is completely destroyed (D); extensive but less severe fibrosis with an early "honeycomb" appearance (H) is also present in areas where the parenchyma is still evident. Bronchi in the region of severe fibrosis are ectatic *(arrows).* A histologic section from the area of dense fibrosis *(B)* shows replacement of lung parenchyma by collagen and scattered aggregates of lymphocytes. The only evidence of sarcoidosis is two granulomas, one *(short arrow)* almost completely fibrosed and the other *(long arrow)* containing a single multinucleated giant cell. A section from the area of early "honeycombing" *(C)* shows less extensive fibrosis and numerous irregular cystic spaces representing dilated transitional airways. Two largely fibrosed granulomas are present *(arrows).* (*B* × 40; *C* × 20.)

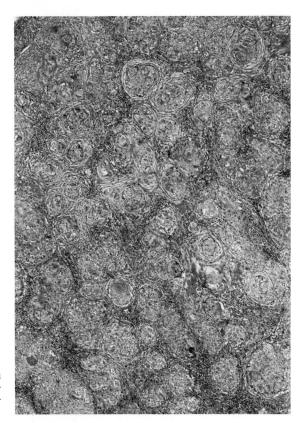

Figure 17–5. Sarcoidosis: Lymph Node Involvement. A histologic section of a mediastinal lymph node shows numerous discrete and focally confluent granulomas that virtually obliterate the normal nodal architecture. There is no necrosis. (× 40.)

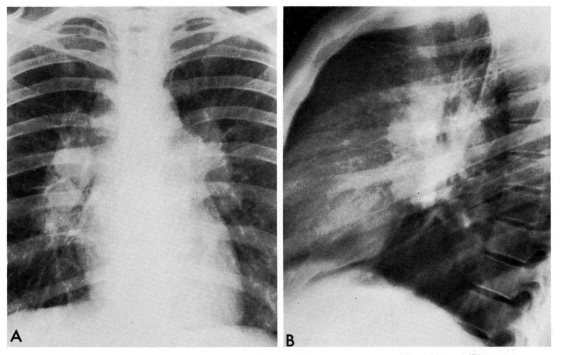

Figure 17–6. Sarcoidosis: Lymph Node Involvement Alone. Posteroanterior *(A)* and lateral *(B)* roentgenograms of a 32-year-old asymptomatic woman demonstrate marked enlargement of both hila, the lobulated contour being typical of lymph node enlargement. Nodes are also enlarged in the right paratracheal and aortopulmonary regions. The lungs are clear.

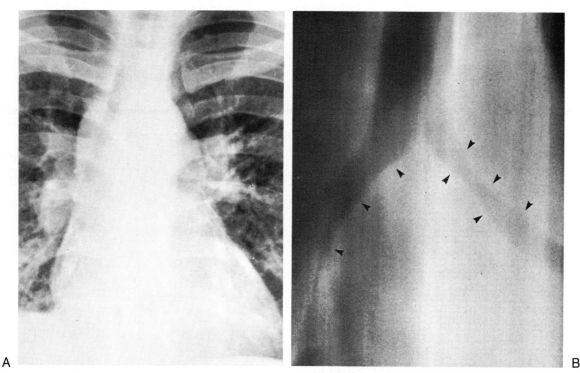

Figure 17–7. Sarcoidosis: Lymph Node Enlargement with Bronchial Compression. A posteroanterior roentgenogram *(A)* of this asymptomatic man in his 20s reveals marked enlargement of hilar and paratracheal lymph nodes bilaterally. On the original roentgenogram, there was highly suggestive evidence of blunting of the carina and narrowing of the left main bronchus. An anteroposterior tomogram *(B)* confirms the presence of upward displacement of the medial wall of the right main bronchus and marked narrowing of the lumen of the left main bronchus *(arrowheads)*. (Courtesy of Dr. James McCort, Santa Clara Valley Medical Center, San Jose, California.)

volvement, eventually show complete roentgenographic resolution without residua.[65] Occasionally, enlarged hilar and mediastinal nodes regress to normal size, only to enlarge once again later.[66] On the other hand, hilar and paratracheal node enlargement can persist unchanged for 15 years or more.[67]

Diffuse Pulmonary Disease With or Without Lymph Node Enlargement

In one follow-up study of 66 patients who initially presented with roentgenologic evidence of only enlarged hilar lymph nodes,[68] the subsequent development of pulmonary disease was documented in 21 patients (32 per cent). On the other hand, approximately 15 per cent[52] to 25 per cent[65, 69] of patients with pulmonary sarcoidosis present with pulmonary disease without hilar lymph node enlargement (Fig. 17–8). In the majority of cases the pulmonary abnormality is diffuse and evenly distributed throughout the lungs, although sometimes there is upper zonal predominance, particularly during the fibrotic stage. Occasionally the disease is asymmetric, and, in fact, it may be unilateral.[70] Although there is no question that conventional CT employing 10-mm sections can reveal parenchymal disease in the absence of abnormality on conventional roentgenograms, when roentgenograms display disease the extent and profusion of opacities are little different from those revealed by CT.[63] However, it has now been well established that high-resolution CT is superior to conventional roentgenography in revealing diagnostic abnormalities.[71]

When diffuse pulmonary disease and lymph node enlargement coexist, their roentgenographic appearance is no different from that of separate involvement. Diffuse disease usually appears when hilar node enlargement is present, although the latter may be regressing. Node enlargement may disappear and be replaced by diffuse pulmonary involvement, either concurrently or several years later, or it may remain and diffuse pulmonary involvement may be superimposed on it. So far as the authors are aware, there has been no report to indicate that hilar lymph node enlargement may develop subsequent to pulmonary parenchymal disease; however, in long-standing sarcoidosis, retraction secondary to fibrosis may produce sufficient hilar deformity to suggest lymph node enlargement.

Three basic patterns of disease can be recognized on conventional roentgenograms: the reticulonodular pattern, the acinar pattern, and large nodules.

The Reticulonodular Pattern. This pattern can range from purely nodular to purely reticular but is usually a combination of the two.[52, 69] The reticulation may be a very fine or a very coarse network and was observed in 70 of 150 patients (46 per cent) in one study.[52] A so-called miliary pattern is very rare. A linear pattern has been described as being relatively common on CT scans[53]; alternatively, a reticular pattern on a conventional roentgenogram can be manifested by a nodular pattern on CT. In fact, nodules are the most frequent CT manifestation of sarcoidosis (Fig. 17–9). In one study using high-resolution CT, they were identified in all 44 patients[72]; in this series, nodules were seen occasionally in the absence of abnormality on conven-

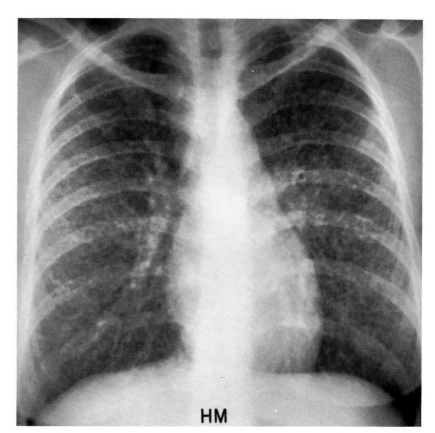

Figure 17–8. Sarcoidosis: The Diffuse Reticulo-nodular Pattern. A posteroanterior roentgenogram reveals a rather coarse reticulonodular pattern throughout both lungs with some mid-zonal pre-dominance. There is no evidence of hilar or me-diastinal lymph node enlargement.

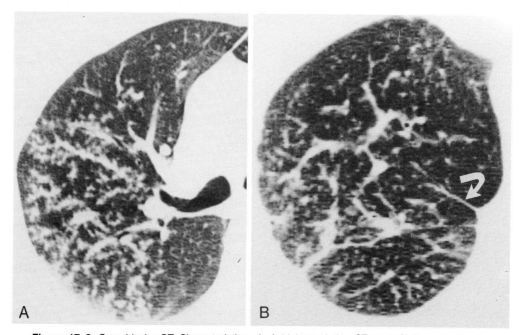

Figure 17–9. Sarcoidosis: CT Characteristics. *A,* A high-resolution CT scan (1.5 mm collimation reconstructed using a high-frequency resolution algorithm) targeted to the right lung at the level of the right upper lobe bronchus shows irregular nodular thickening of the bronchovascular bundles. *B,* In another patient, a high-resolution CT scan (1.5 mm collimation reconstructed using high-frequency resolution algorithm) through the upper lobes shows a reticulonodular pattern. The linear opacities are caused by thickening of the interlobular septa *(curved arrow).* (Courtesy of Dr. Nestor Müller, University of British Columbia, Vancouver.)

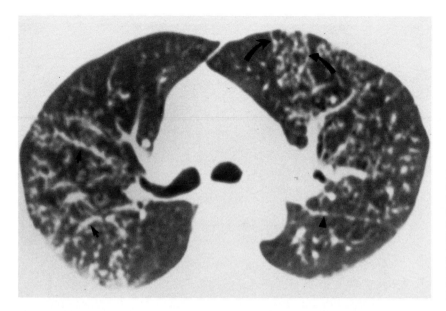

Figure 17–10. Sarcoidosis: CT Manifestations. A CT scan at a level just distal to the tracheal carina with 1.5-mm collimation shows numerous small nodules bilaterally. The majority of nodules are associated with bronchovascular bundles, giving them a beaded appearance *(arrows).* Nodular thickening of interlobular septa is also apparent *(curved arrows)* as well as nodular thickening of the left major fissure *(arrowhead).* (Courtesy of Dr. Nestor L. Müller, University of British Columbia, Vancouver.)

tional roentgenograms. Nodules tend to be related to pulmonary vessels, giving them a beaded appearance (Fig. 17–10). Both linear and nodular opacities can be seen to decrease in size on sequential CT scans.[72a]

The "Acinar" Pattern. This pattern consists chiefly of indistinctly defined opacities measuring up to 6 or 7 mm in diameter and, thus, possessing features of acinar shadows (Fig. 17–11). They may be discrete or coalescent, and in the latter circumstance may be associated with an air bronchogram. In the study of 150 patients cited above,[52] this was the predominant pattern in 32 patients (20 per cent) but was frequently associated with a reticulonodular pattern

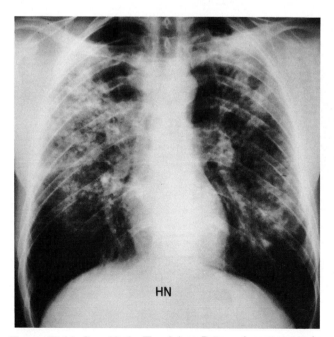

Figure 17–11. Sarcoidosis: The Acinar Pattern. A posteroanterior roentgenogram reveals patchy opacities in both lungs, situated predominantly in central regions. This pattern simulates patchy airspace consolidation. There is evidence of enlargement of lymph nodes in both hila and the right paratracheal region.

elsewhere in the lungs. Sometimes, confluence of acinar shadows can produce large areas of consolidation or scattered, hazy areas of consolidation with irregular borders (Fig. 17–12). In patients in whom the disease is confined largely to the upper lung zones, the pattern may mimic postprimary tuberculosis.[73]

Approximately one third of patients eventually show complete roentgenographic resolution of their pulmonary disease, the remainder showing either persistence of the acinar pattern for the duration of follow-up or progression to pulmonary fibrosis.[52]

Large Nodules. An occasional case of sarcoidosis shows large, dense, sharply marginated nodules or masses simulating metastatic neoplasm (Fig. 17–13)[74]; rarely, they are solitary.[75]

Miscellaneous Abnormalities. Unusual manifestations of thoracic sarcoidosis appear to be particularly common in older individuals.[77] Cavitation is very uncommon and usually occurs in patients with the more chronic debilitating form of the disease; aspergillomas develop in some cases.

Atelectasis occurs in about 1 per cent of cases[78] and is caused by extrinsic compression by enlarged lymph nodes, by endobronchial inflammation, or perhaps most commonly by a combination of the two. Occasionally, enlarged hilar and carinal nodes can compress and narrow major bronchi without causing atelectasis (*see* Fig. 17–7).[79]

Pleural effusion is also uncommon, although probably not to the extent that was once thought. In one study of 227 patients with biopsy-proved sarcoidosis in which evidence of pleural involvement was specifically sought,[80] pleural effusion was found in 15 (7 per cent) and pleural thickening in 8 (3 per cent). All of the patients with effusion manifested moderately advanced pulmonary sarcoidosis, and non-necrotizing granulomas were identified on pleural biopsy in 7 of the 15 cases. Pleural effusion tended to clear in 4 to 8 weeks but in some cases progressed to chronic pleural thickening. Despite these observations, pleural effusion in association with pulmonary sarcoidosis must be carefully differentiated from tuberculosis,[81] coincidental pneumonia, or heart failure.[67]

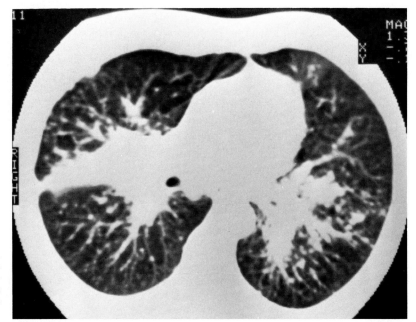

Figure 17–12. Acinar Sarcoidosis: CT Characteristics. A CT scan employing 10-mm collimation reveals extensive consolidation of lung parenchyma in the medial and central portions of both lungs. A few nodules can be identified in the periphery, most of which relate to bronchovascular bundles.

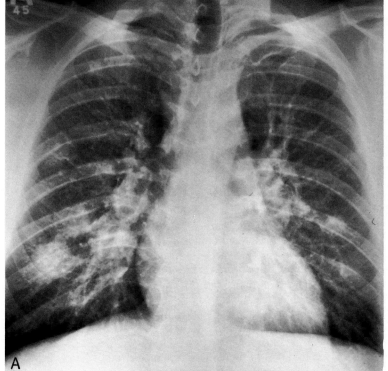

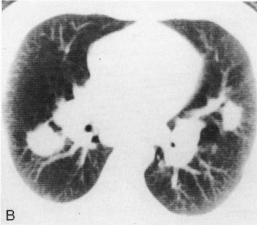

Figure 17–13. Sarcoidosis: Large Nodules. A posteroanterior roentgenogram (A) reveals several opacities in both lungs ranging in diameter from about 1 to 2 cm. The opacities have ill-defined margins but are homogeneous in density. Hilar node enlargement is present bilaterally, and there is also suggestive evidence of mild enlargement of paratracheal nodes. A CT scan through the lower portion of the thorax (B) reveals homogeneous masses in both lungs and bilateral hilar node enlargement. The resolution of the image is insufficient to permit evaluation of lung parenchyma generally.

Sarcoidosis is complicated by spontaneous pneumothorax in about 1 to 2 per cent of cases.[82] Bullae tend to develop in the upper lobes in advanced fibrotic disease, and they have been said to rupture in approximately 5 per cent of cases.[83]

Osseous involvement is said to occur in approximately 10 to 40 per cent of cases, as judged roentgenologically,[84] the incidence being much greater in blacks.[85] Characteristically, the small bones of the hands are predominantly involved, the pattern being chiefly lytic and consisting of cystic lesions and a lacy trabecular pattern. However, a number of reports have found the predominant bone reaction to be osteosclerosis rather than osteolysis and the primary involvement to occur in the skull, axial skeleton, and proximal bones of the extremities.[86, 87] Scintigraphy may be valuable for early detection of these lesions.[88]

Pulmonary Fibrosis

Although there is disagreement as to what percentage of patients with pulmonary sarcoidosis develop irreversible pulmonary changes, an incidence of 20 per cent probably is reasonably accurate.[65, 89] When changes have been present for 2 years or longer, resolution is the exception rather than the rule. Scarring usually is rather coarse and in the form of irregular linear strands extending outward from the hila toward the periphery (Fig. 17–14). Commonly more uneven in its distribution than the reticulonodular pattern characteristic of the active stage, pulmonary fibrosis often shows considerable upper zone predominance. It is usually associated with well-defined structural changes in the lungs, including bulla formation, bronchiectasis, and emphysema.[89, 90] CT can be useful in evaluating the extent of disease (Fig. 17–15) and sometimes reveals evidence of fibrosis not discernible on conventional roentgenograms.[72] When fibrosis and emphysema are severe, changes in the heart and pulmonary vasculature are those of pulmonary hypertension and cor pulmonale of any cause.

Clinical Manifestations

Symptoms develop in approximately 50 per cent of patients, the remainder being identified in asymptomatic indivduals on screening chest roentgenograms.[4] Patients with roentgenographic evidence of hilar and paratracheal lymph node enlargement alone are almost always asymptomatic. The importance of this constellation of findings to diagnosis was exemplified in one series of 100 patients with bilateral hilar node enlargement:[91] of the 30 who were asymptomatic all had sarcoidosis; by contrast, all 11 patients whose node enlargement was a result of neoplasia were symptomatic.

Constitutional symptoms such as weight loss, fatigue, weakness, and malaise often are associated with multisystem involvement and usually develop insidiously. Fever occurs in about 15 to 20 per cent of cases.[8] The acute onset of symptoms, usually with erythema nodosum, is particularly common in Scandinavian women.[92] A predilection for erythema nodosum also has been reported in Irish women in London and Puerto Ricans in New York City.[93]

Symptoms of pulmonary involvement—most commonly dry cough and shortness of breath—develop in 20 to 30 per cent of patients.[8, 94] Hemoptysis is rare and is usually attributable to a complicating aspergilloma.[95] Chest pain can be caused by excessive coughing and rarely is pleuritic.[96] Auscultatory signs usually are absent in the early stages of the disease, although rhonchi may be audible in patients with endobronchial involvement. With the development of pulmonary fibrosis, crepitations can become widespread and the breath sounds can become bronchial.

Involvement of the upper respiratory passages is uncommon. The epiglottis is most frequently affected and can be associated with serious obstruction.[97] Laryngeal granulomas have been identified in 1 to 3 per cent of patients.[98] Symptoms include dyspnea, cough, and hoarseness. Hoarseness can also result from the extension of the inflammatory process into the recurrent laryngeal nerve from contiguous lymph nodes.[99]

The cardiovascular system can be affected directly or indirectly. Indirect involvement results in pulmonary arterial hypertension and cor pulmonale and can be caused by extensive parenchymal fibrosis or (rarely) direct compression of the pulmonary arteries[100] or veins[101] by enlarged lymph nodes. Although direct involvement of the myocardium occurs in approximately 25 per cent of cases at autopsy,[102] it is recognized clinically in only a minority. It can be manifested by sudden death, paroxysmal arrhythmias, left ventricular failure, and ventricular aneurysm. Electrocardiographic abnormalities occur more frequently in patients with sarcoidosis than in matched controls[103]; in fact, the presence of arrhythmias in a young person should suggest the possibility of myocardial sarcoidosis.

Enlargement of peripheral lymph nodes is said to be clinically evident in about 75 per cent of cases.[8] However, it is probable that nodal involvement occurs at some time in every case of sarcoidosis whether nodes are palpable or not; lymph node biopsies from regions such as the scalene area are positive in 80 per cent of cases, even when they are not palpable.[104] Palpable lymph nodes are found most frequently in the cervical region but may also be felt in the axilla, epitrochlear regions, and groin.[4]

The incidence of ocular involvement in sarcoidosis is probably about 20 to 30 per cent.[4, 8] The characteristic lesion is uveitis; involvement of the conjunctiva, sclera, retina, and lens also may occur and result in cataracts or glaucoma.

Cutaneous disease is also thought to occur in about 20 to 30 per cent of patients and may take several forms.[105] In contrast to other forms of nonpulmonary involvement, skin lesions are not uncommonly the only clinical manifestation of disease. They are particularly frequent in blacks and consist most commonly of slightly raised, often purplish nodules that usually occur on the face, neck, shoulders, or digits (lupus pernio). Large plaques resembling psoriasis also may develop over the trunk or extremities. Both abnormalities usually are associated with a chronic persistent course. Erythema nodosum—transitory, raised, slightly painful erythematous lesions, usually on the skin of the lower extremities—occurs in 5 to 25 per cent of patients. Acute onset of sarcoidosis characterized by fever, arthralgia, hilar lymph node enlargement, and erythema nodosum (Löfgren's syndrome) is a fairly common mode of presentation in Europe.[106] The infiltration of cutaneous scars by granulomatous inflammatory tissue is well recognized.[107]

Granulomas can be identified in the liver or spleen in

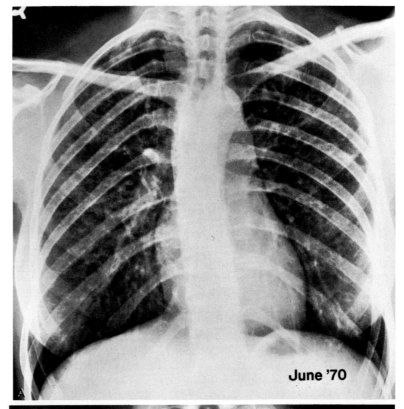

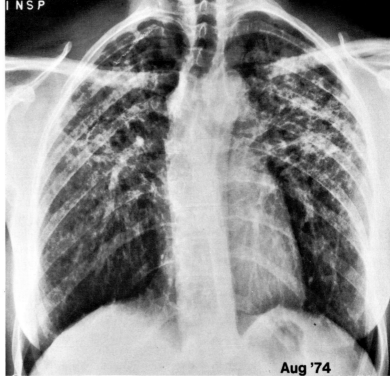

Figure 17–14. Diffuse Pulmonary Sarcoidosis with Progressive Fibrosis. The initial chest roentgenogram *(A)* of this 37-year-old woman reveals a rather coarse reticular pattern throughout both lungs with definite upper-zonal predominance. There is no evidence of hilar or mediastinal lymph node enlargement. Four years later *(B)*, the reticulation had become more marked, and there had occurred an upward displacement and flaring of lower zone vessels, indicating the fibrotic nature of the upper zone disease. Note that despite the fibrosis, there had occurred no overall reduction in lung volume, chiefly because of overinflation of lower zone parenchyma.

B

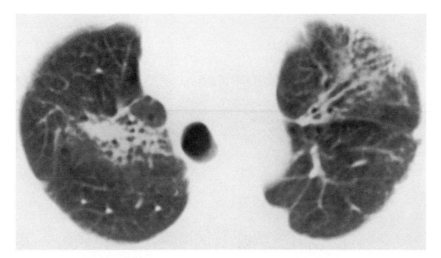

Figure 17–15. Sarcoidosis: CT Manifestations of Fibrosis. A CT scan at the level of the aortic arch with 10-mm collimation reveals irregular, poorly defined opacities in both lungs extending outward from the mediastinum. The opacities appear to radiate along bronchovascular bundles, particularly on the left side, and are accompanied by appreciable bronchiectasis. A few subpleural nodules can be seen bilaterally. (Courtesy of Dr. Nestor L. Müller, University of British Columbia, Vancouver.)

approximately 70 per cent of cases at necropsy[94]; however, these organs are clinically palpable in only about 25 per cent of patients. Although the degree of liver involvement is seldom sufficient to impair its function, it is not rare for enlargement of the spleen to be so severe as to cause hypersplenism.[108]

Symptomatic involvement of the gastrointestinal tract is very rare[109] and must be distinguished from the much more common Crohn's disease. The incidence of celiac disease in patients with sarcoidosis is greater than can be explained by chance[110]; in fact, a study of the incidence of humoral sensitivity to dietary proteins has revealed that about 40 per cent of patients with sarcoidosis show a specific sensitization to alpha-gliadin.[111]

Three forms of joint involvement have been described:[112] (1) migratory "polyarthritis" associated with erythema nodosum, fever, and hilar lymph node enlargement; (2) single or recurrent episodes of polyarticular or monarticular arthritis; and (3) persistent arthritis. The first is the most common and is an arthralgia rather than an arthritis, with a tendency to involve the larger joints, particularly the ankles, wrists, elbows, and knees. Symptoms range in duration from a few days to several weeks, and the patient typically is free from disability. True arthritis is uncommon and usually is seen in patients with chronic pulmonary disease.[113] Although the arthritis is usually transient, it can persist for as long as a year. Hypertrophic pulmonary osteoarthropathy occurs rarely.[114] The arthropathies that occur in adults with cystic fibrosis[115] and that are associated with fever and erythema nodosum strangely resemble those of sarcoidosis.

Involvement of minor salivary glands has been found in almost 60 per cent of random lip biopsies.[116] The combination of parotid gland involvement, uveitis, and pyrexia is called uveoparotid fever.

Renal disease can be caused by several mechanisms. Granulomas have been found in about 10 to 20 per cent of necropsied patients,[117] although they rarely cause functional impairment. When renal insufficiency does develop, it is usually the result of hypercalcemia, nephrocalcinosis, and nephrolithiasis. The association of membranous glomerulonephritis and sarcoidosis[118] appears to be more than coincidental. Systemic hypertension can be caused by granulomatous inflammation and stenosis of the renal artery.

The nervous system is involved in about 5 per cent of patients.[119] Although any cranial nerve can be affected, those most commonly involved are the seventh and second, presumably as a result of extension of disease from underlying basal granulomatous meningitis or from nasal lesions.[119] Unilateral or bilateral facial palsy is sometimes associated with uveoparotid fever. Cerebral lesions can result in grand mal seizures and can simulate metastatic carcinoma.[120] Patients with sarcoidosis appear to be at risk for infection with the papovavirus that causes progressive multifocal leukoencephalopathy.[121] Psychiatric presentations include delirium, depression, personality changes, and psychosis.[122]

Granulomatous inflammation also can affect the hypothalamus and pituitary gland.[119] Affected patients often complain of polyuria and polydipsia. Involvement of other endocrine glands is relatively uncommon,[123] although there appears to be an unexplained association between sarcoidosis and either Hashimoto's thyroiditis or hyperthyroidism.[124]

Some patients with multiorgan non-necrotizing granulomas have overlap syndromes with various connective tissue diseases, including CREST syndrome[125] and Sjögren's syndrome.[126] Despite some reports linking sarcoidosis with malignancy,[127] it is most likely that the association is purely coincidental, with the possible exception of testicular carcinoma.[128] Sarcoidosis has developed years before and years after the appearance of the testicular neoplasm; in at least some cases,[129] orchiectomy was the only treatment for the testicular tumor, thus eliminating radiotherapy and chemotherapy as precipitating causes.

Pulmonary Function Tests

There is poor correlation between the degree of pulmonary disease as seen on conventional chest roentgenograms and the severity of pulmonary function abnormaliites.[130] The extent and pattern of pulmonary disease on CT scans shows a somewhat better agreement.[63] According to one study, 80 per cent of patients without roentgenographic evidence of parenchymal abnormality had a normal vital capacity (VC) and 70 per cent a normal diffusing capacity[131]; by contrast, 35 per cent of those with roentgenographic evidence of parenchymal disease had a normal VC and 34 per cent a normal DLCO. The diffusing capacity can remain reduced after symptoms have disappeared and the chest roentgenogram has returned to normal; in such cases, lung biopsy usually reveals interstitial granulomatous or fibrotic disease.[132] Disturbances in blood-air gas transfer have been attributed to ventilation-perfusion (V̇/Q̇) inequality rather than to a diffusion defect.[133] Some reduction in pulmonary compliance, diffusing capacity, and gas transfer can be present on exercise, even in asymptomatic patients.[134] In patients with significant restrictive pulmonary function, exercise testing detects failure of the right ventricular ejection fraction to show an expected rise.[135] Although the majority of patients with sarcoidosis show a restrictive deficiency in function, some can manifest an obstructive deficit as well; in fact, in a small percentage of cases the pattern is solely obstructive.[136]

Laboratory Investigation

Laboratory techniques that have been employed to support a diagnosis of sarcoidosis, to assess the likelihood of response to treatment, to monitor response to treatment, and to evaluate prognosis include differential cell counts of BAL fluid, measurement of a variety of substances that BAL fluid contains, measurement of levels of BAL and serum angiotensin-converting enzyme (ACE) and lysozyme, and assessment of gallium-67 uptake by the lungs. Innumerable attempts have been made to correlate the findings of these tests with each other and with clinical manifestations, roentgenographic stage, and the results of pulmonary function tests. Unfortunately, there are so many variables to take into consideration that the conclusions of the various studies not only differ in many respects but in some instances are actually contradictory. Thus, the usefulness in diagnosis of any of these laboratory techniques is open to question.

Many reports suggest that there is good correlation between the percentage of lymphocytes found in BAL fluid of patients with sarcoidosis and the degree of positivity of gallium-67 scintiscans.[137] However, although the sensitivity of gallium-67 scintigraphy in detecting inflammatory lesions has been estimated to range from 80 per cent to more than 90 per cent, the specificity is closer to 50 per cent.[138] Its most useful function may be in the detection of pulmonary parenchymal disease in patients with normal chest roentgenograms and stage 0 or I disease.[139]

The concentration of ACE in BAL fluid has been found to be elevated in patients with active sarcoidosis,[140] but since levels of albumin in BAL fluid are also elevated, this could simply reflect nonspecific increased permeability of the alveolocapillary membrane.[141] The level of serum ACE (SACE) also is often increased in sarcoidosis.[142] Although its measurement has potential value in confirming the diagnosis, it must be remembered that false positives—values that are two standard deviations above the control mean— occur in healthy individuals[143] and in patients with many other diseases, including tuberculosis, fungal infection, silicosis, berylliosis, hypersensitivity pneumonitis, idiopathic pulmonary fibrosis, and even chronic obstructive pulmonary disease and asthma.[144, 145] Despite this, patients with sarcoidosis are much more likely to have higher values than patients with these conditions.

Serial measurements of SACE levels in patients with sarcoidosis show variations that appear to correlate with the clinical course. Gradual falls have coincided with spontaneous improvement, whereas rapid falls to normal levels have been recorded by several investigators in patients receiving corticosteroid therapy.[146] On the other hand, changes in the SACE levels have been observed during periods of disease stability, as reflected by unchanging chest roentgenograms and pulmonary function tests.[147] In addition, SACE levels do not correlate with the usually accepted criteria for alveolitis,[148] such as the number of lymphocytes found in BAL fluid or the gallium-67 scan, and in fact are often normal when these markers are present.[149]

Serum lysozyme levels also have been proposed as a useful index of activity, particularly in the early stages of the disease in patients with erythema nodosum.[150] However, like SACE, lysozyme levels can be raised in many pulmonary diseases that are included in the differential diagnosis of sarcoidosis.[151]

Approximately 2 per cent of unselected patients with sarcoidosis have hypercalcemia.[152] However, in patients with disseminated disease who are seen as referrals, hypercalciuria is present in approximately 30 per cent and hypercalcemia in 15 per cent, both usually in association with the chronic form of the disease.[123] In addition, many patients with normal blood calcium levels can be shown by special studies to have abnormal calcium metabolism.[153] Although the majority of patients show only a slight elevation of the calcium level, in a small number the levels pose a threat to life.[123] The most significant effect is on the kidneys, in which nephrocalcinosis and nephrolithiasis can develop and can impair renal function.[154] In most patients, the abnormal metabolism probably is related to increased absorption of calcium from the gastrointestinal tract as a result of increased sensitivity to vitamin D or increased conversion of 25-hydroxycholecalciferol to 1,25-dihydroxycholecalciferol.[155]

In one review of 75 patients with active pulmonary sarcoidosis,[156] one or more hematologic abnormalities were identified in almost 90 per cent; anemia was present in 21 patients (28 per cent), in 17 of whom bone marrow examination revealed granulomas. Leukopenia and lymphocytopenia are common, white cell counts below 5000 per mL being observed in approximately 30 per cent of patients. Eosinophilia greater than 5 per cent is present in about one third of cases.

Diagnosis and Differential Diagnosis

In our experience with the predominantly white population of Montreal, Quebec, about 50 per cent of patients are asymptomatic when first seen. The disease is discovered on a screening chest roentgenogram that reveals bilateral symmetric hilar and paratracheal lymph node enlargement. Patients with metastatic malignancy, especially of renal origin, or lymphoma[157] can also present with such a pattern but usually are symptomatic. Even when the hilar node enlargement is asymmetric, sarcoidosis is almost certainly the diagnosis if the patient is asymptomatic. The syndrome of bilateral hilar lymph node enlargement, fever, arthralgia, and erythema nodosum has been accepted as diagnostic of sarcoidosis, in the author's opinion not requiring pathologic confirmation.

Although the clinical picture in sarcoidosis usually is non-specific, the diagnosis can be made with confidence in most cases when a tissue specimen reveals non-necrotizing granulomas, usually obtained by transbronchial biopsy. Biopsies of bronchial mucosa alone are also useful[158]—in fact, the diagnosis in specimens obtained by transbronchial biopsy is often made on the fragments of bronchial wall invariably present in these specimens. The reported yield with trans-bronchial biopsy varies considerably, depending on the stage of the disease and the number of biopsy specimens obtained; however, as a general rule, positive specimens are obtained in about 90 to 95 per cent of patients when 4 to 10 sites are sampled.[159, 160] Mediastinoscopic lymph node biopsy is positive in 95 to 100 per cent of cases.[161] Transthoracic needle biopsy provides a low yield in diffuse pulmonary disease but can be valuable in cases with large nodules.[162] Because of the high yield from transbronchial biopsies, biopsy of various other tissues of the body such as labial glands and muscle is usually not justified in view of the low positive yield (about 50 per cent).

Prognosis

The assessment of prognosis in patients with sarcoidosis varies considerably in published reports, largely as a result of the selection of patients; for example, when pathologic proof is required for entry into a study or when patients are chosen from a referred practice in which more difficult clinical problems are seen, it is only to be expected that the overall outcome from the disease will be somewhat worse.

Despite these statements, several generalizations appear reasonable. African-Americans appear to be more susceptible to the disease, and in some,[163] but not all,[164, 165] series have a poorer prognosis. The incidence of severe disability appears to be increased in the elderly[166] and in patients with clinical or roentgenographic evidence of extrathoracic involvement,[167] especially those with persistent skin lesions, bone lesions, hepatomegaly, or hypercalcemia.[168] Disability tends to be more severe in young children.[169] Onset of the disease with erythema nodosum, arthralgia and bilateral hilar lymph node enlargement (with or without low-grade fever) almost invariably indicates a favorable prognosis.

Most observers agree that prognosis is strongly related to the roentgenographic stage of disease on presentation: stage 1 patients fare better than stage 2, and stage 2 patients better than stage 3.[166, 170] An absence of improvement in the chest roentgenogram over a 1-year period is a bad prognostic sign, whereas roentgenographic resolution that lasts for 2 years can be regarded as a cure.[166] Clearing of the chest roentgenogram is usually associated with a return to normal function,[170] although in some patients there can be a persistent diffusion defect.[171] The risk of developing abnormal pulmonary function when the initial assessment of function is normal appears small.[172] The prognosis for patients who manifest airflow obstruction on routine pulmonary function tests does not appear to differ from that of the nonobstructed group.[173]

Many attempts have been made to use the various markers of activity in sarcoidosis to indicate prognosis, to predict which patients will respond to therapy, and to monitor therapeutic management. Although the results of some studies have suggested that the cellular composition of BAL fluid—such as the number of lymphocytes[174] or the ratio of CD4 to CD8 lymphocytes[175]—can help predict outcome, no definitive criteria have emerged. Although gallium-67 scanning appears to be a useful indicator of activity, it is not a reliable predictor of prognosis. As discussed previously, serial measurement of SACE levels also is a good method of monitoring activity; levels fall and rise with clinical[176] and functional[177] change, even when the initial values are within the normal range. However, evidence that measurement of SACE levels can play a role in predicting prognosis or the outcome of therapy is not convincing.[33] Serial chest roentgenograms, pulmonary function tests, and measurements of SACE levels are less invasive and cheaper than BAL and gallium-67 scanning, and are probably just as accurate in assessing disease activity.[178]

The reported overall mortality rate ranges from 5 to 10 per cent; in patients followed for many years, it is probably closer to 10 per cent.[172, 179] However, these figures undoubtedly reflect a referred patient population with advanced disease; if the relatively more numerous asymptomatic patients were all included in analysis, the measured mortality rate would probably be closer to 1 per cent. Pregnancy and the immediate postpartum period have been associated with an increased mortality rate.[180] Most patients who die have cardiac decompensation as a result of cor pulmonale secondary to pulmonary fibrosis. Sudden death can result from cardiac arrhythmias, central nervous system disease, or hemorrhage caused by complicating aspergilloma.

FIBROSING ALVEOLITIS

The subject of chronic interstitial pneumonitis and fibrosis is complex, both because of the multitude of terms that have been employed to describe the condition (e.g., fibrosing alveolitis, chronic interstitial pneumonia, interstitial pulmonary fibrosis, usual interstitial pneumonia [UIP], desquamative interstitial pneumonia [DIP]) and because of the numerous etiologies with which it has been associated. One of the most important papers to address these issues was published by Liebow and Carrington in 1969.[181] In this paper, these authors recognized five subgroups of interstitial pneumonitis, distinguishable predominantly by histologic criteria:

1. Classic interstitial pneumonia or UIP, characterized by thickening of the alveolar interstitium by fibrous tissue and mononuclear inflammatory cells, typically varying in severity from one focus to another.

2. DIP, in which a striking accumulation of macrophages in the alveolar airspaces is associated with relatively mild but uniform interstitial thickening by mononuclear inflammatory cells.

3. A diffuse lesion similar to UIP but with superimposed bronchiolitis obliterans (BIP).

4. Lymphoid interstitial pneumonia (LIP), in which there is marked infiltration of interstitium by lymphocytes in a pattern that sometimes is difficult to distinguish from lymphoma.

5. Giant cell interstitial pneumonia (GIP), consisting of an interstitial infiltrate of mononuclear cells associated with large numbers of multinucleated giant cells.

Each of these histologic patterns can be regarded as a tissue reaction to a variety of etiologic agents rather than as a manifestation of a specific disease process. For example, in addition to cases in which no etiology is apparent, BIP can be seen in connective tissue disorders such as rheumatoid disease and following aspiration of gastric contents, GIP is associated with viral infection (especially measles) and with exposure to heavy metals such as tungsten carbide, and LIP can be seen in Sjögren's syndrome and the acquired immunodeficiency syndrome (AIDS).

Although there is some histologic overlap among the five forms of interstitial pneumonitis, the last three (BIP, LIP, and GIP) are fairly characteristic and are considered in appropriate sections elsewhere in this book. By contrast, there has been considerable debate about the distinctiveness of DIP and UIP. Liebow and Carrington[181] suggested that the different pathologic, roentgenographic, and clinical features of the two varieties and the usual favorable response of DIP to corticosteroid therapy might be related to differences in etiology and pathogenesis and that distinction between the two was justified. According to Scadding and Hinson, however, the distinguishing features are not as clear as Liebow and Carrington suggested:[182] in their study of 16 patients with diffuse interstitial pulmonary disease, they found considerable histologic overlap in tissue from different patients and suggested that the patterns of UIP and DIP reflected different stages of one disease process that they termed "diffuse fibrosing alveolitis." We concur with this view and consider it preferable to use the latter term to refer to each of these stages of disease. Despite this, it seems reasonable to identify those cases in which the histologic pattern of DIP is present, since there is some indication that prognosis and response to therapy are more favorable than for UIP.

Etiology and Pathogenesis

Investigations into the etiology and pathogenesis of fibrosing alveolitis have focused on several areas, including immunologic abnormalities, genetic abnormalities, viral infection, mediator cells, and lung collagen.

Immunolgic Abnormalities. There is abundant evidence that some abnormality of immune function is involved in the pathogenesis of fibrosing alveolitis. Many patients with interstitial pneumonitis and fibrosis pathologically identical to that of idiopathic fibrosing alveolitis present with clinical and serologic evidence of autoimmunity. In some of these patients, the diagnosis of a specific connective tissue disorder, such as rheumatoid disease or progressive systemic sclerosis, can be made.[183] In other individuals, the pneumonitis is associated with tissue or organ involvement not included under the umbrella of connective tissue disorders, but in which an abnormality of immune function is implicated, such as myasthenia gravis,[184] chronic active hepatitis,[185] and hemolytic anemia.[186] Serologic abnormalities also are common in persons who have no clinical evidence of extrapulmonary disease; for example, it has been estimated that about one third of patients with fibrosing alveolitis have antinuclear antibodies, and one third rheumatoid factor, albeit usually in low titers.[187] Immune complexes, both circulating and bound to lung tissue, are found in a minority of patients.[188]

Some pathologic and experimental animal studies also provide evidence for an immune mechanism in the pathogenesis of fibrosing alveolitis. For example, the intravenous administration of Freund's adjuvant to rabbits can result in pneumonitis with a pattern similar to DIP[189] and the intratracheal instillation of hapten to previously immunized hamsters causes interstitial fibrosis.[190]

Genetic Abnormalities. A genetic factor has been documented in a minority of patients with fibrosing alveolitis; in some of these, there is evidence for an association between inheritance and disturbed immune reactivity.[191] The disease has been described in monozygotic twins,[192] and a review of the literature in 1983[193] revealed 73 definite cases in 19 families. Transmission appears to occur by an autosomal dominant mechanism with reduced penetrance. Designated "familial fibrocystic pulmonary dysplasia" by some authors,[194] this condition possesses pathologic and roentgenographic characteristics identical to those of the nonfamilial form of fibrosing alveolitis.

Attempts to identify a specific gene responsible for fibrosis have not been successful; however, several studies have demonstrated abnormalities of HLA loci. Of particular interest in this regard was the observation in one study of an increased frequency of HLA-DR2 antigen in patients with fibrosing alveolitis,[193] an alloantigen that has been associated with disorders of altered immunoreactivity such as systemic lupus erythematosus and rheumatoid disease.

Viral Infection. Although the diagnosis of fibrosing alveolitis often coincides with recognition of a viral-type syndrome,[195] it is rare to document a *specific* viral infection that terminates in pathologically proven interstitial fibrosis.[196] Intranuclear inclusion bodies have been described,[197] particularly in patients with DIP, but it is believed that they represent the products of nuclear degeneration rather than bodies of viral origin.[198] One group of investigators documented specific immunoglobulins for Epstein-Barr virus (EBV) in 10 of 13 patients with fibrosing alveolitis,[199] a finding that could either reflect nonspecific depression of cell-mediated immunity or indicate that EBV plays a part in the production of the disease. A possible etiologic association with hepatitis C virus has also been reported.[199a]

Mediator Cells. The inflammatory cell population of the lung parenchyma in fibrosing alveolitis, as revealed by both BAL and open lung biopsy, consists of alveolar macrophages, neutrophils, eosinophils, and lymphocytes.[200] The precise role(s) of each of these cells in the pathogenesis of disease is unclear. In normal nonsmokers, neutrophils make up less than 1 per cent of the total number of cells obtained by BAL, whereas in patients with fibrosing alveolitis, the percentage of neutrophils rises to 10 to 20 per cent.[201] The accumulation of these cells has been attributed to the release of a chemotactic factor by alveolar macrophages[202] that have been activated by immune complexes deposited in lung tissue.[203] Since the neutrophil carries such a potent armamentarium of inflammatory mediators as well as oxygen radicals and proteases, it is possible that this cell is chiefly responsible for the alveolar derangement that occurs in fibrosing alveolitis.[204] In fact, some investigators have shown a positive correlation between the percentage of neutrophils and the amount of oxygen free radicals in BAL fluid.[205] (Despite this, other workers feel that the increased presence of oxygen free radicals is more likely to be related to immature macrophages,[206] which are also increased in number).

The role played by T cells and cell-mediated immunity in the pathogenesis of fibrosing alveolitis is also unclear. Some investigators have found that most of the lymphocytes in the alveolar septa are B lymphocytes.[207] There is evidence that this may be related to an imbalance of T lymphocyte subsets leading to an increased release of lymphokine B-cell growth factor.[208]

Lung Collagen. There is considerable evidence that a variety of processes can initiate fibrogenesis, chief among which are the secretions of various enzymes from alveolar macrophages and polymorphonuclear leukocytes. Activated alveolar macrophages from patients with fibrosing alveolitis have been shown to produce growth-promoting factors for lung fibroblasts, including fibronectin[42] and platelet-derived growth factor.[209] In addition, prostaglandin E_2 secreted by alveolar macrophages, pulmonary epithelial and endothelial cells, or fibroblasts themselves may play a role by suppressing interstitial mesenchymal cell proliferation.[210]

There are several differences between the collagen fibers in lungs involved by fibrosing alveolitis and in normal lungs. In contrast to the regular arrangement of parallel cross-banded fibers characteristic of normal lung tissue, the collagen fibers in fibrosing alveolitis are randomly oriented, twisted, and frayed. Assays of lung collagen show an increase in the ratio of type 1 to type 3 fibers[211]; since type 1

fibers are less compliant than type 3 fibers, this may have important physiologic implications.

The increase in the collagen content of the lung in pulmonary fibrotic diseases could result from either increased synthesis or decreased degradation. Studies of collagen synthesis in lung biopsy specimens from patients with and without pulmonary fibrosis have found no differences[211, 212]; however, it is possible that an increase in collagen synthesis occurs early in the course of the disease when tissue is not obtained, or that *in vitro* synthesis does not reflect *in vivo* synthesis. An alternative explanation for increased lung collagen could be decreased degradation; some investigators have found less collagenolytic activity in samples of homogenized lung tissue from patients with fibrosing alveolitis than in lung tissue from normal subjects.[212]

Pathologic Characteristics

Histologically, fibrosing alveolitis is typically a condition of variable severity; areas of normal and severely diseased lung are often present in different areas of the same lobe and even in a single tissue fragment. In the least affected areas, a mild degree of alveolar septal thickening is present, caused predominantly by an infiltrate of inflammatory cells (Fig. 17–16); lymphocytes are usually the most numerous, although plasma cells, mast cells, histiocytes, eosinophils, and polymorphonuclear leukocytes are also encountered.

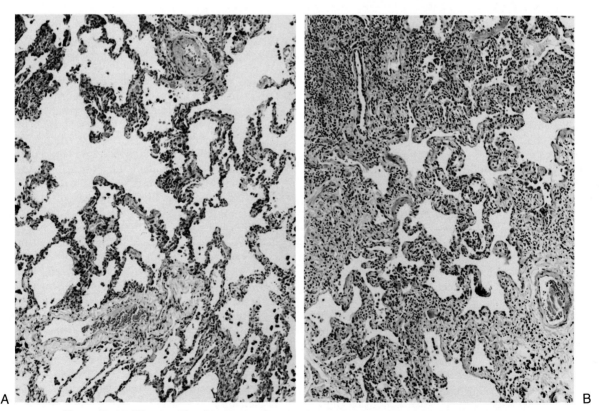

A   B

Figure 17–16. Fibrosing Alveolitis: Varying Severity. An early stage *(A)* shows mild interstitial thickening, caused predominantly by an infiltrate of lymphocytes. More advanced disease *(B)* is characterized by moderate thickening of the interstitium; although there are still abundant lymphocytes, these are now associated with appreciable fibrous tissue. *(A* and *B* × 80.)

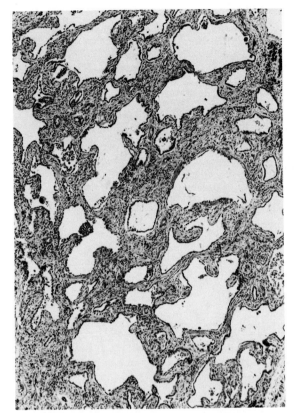

Figure 17–17. Fibrosing Alveolitis: "Honeycomb" Change. The majority of the lung parenchyma has been replaced by fibrous tissue, accompanied by a moderate infiltrate of lymphocytes. Irregularly shaped cystic spaces derived from transitional airways (representing the cells of the "honeycomb") are present at regular intervals within the fibrotic lung parenchyma. (× 35.)

In more advanced disease, the interstitial thickening is greater and is usually associated with some degree of fibrosis. Most often this consists of mature collagen; however, foci of loose fibroblastic tissue indicating active fibrogenesis can also be found. In the most severely affected areas, interstitial thickening is so marked that alveoli can be completely obliterated, resulting in the loss of lung parenchyma and coalescence and dilatation of transitional airways (Fig. 17–17), an appearance that corresponds to the classic honeycomb pattern so characteristic of the gross appearance of advanced disease (*see* later). Other common abnormalities include type II cell hyperplasia and an increased number of macrophages in the alveolar airspaces (although these are typically less abundant and distributed less evenly than in DIP [*see* later]).

A small number of patients with a history of asbestos exposure and the histologic pattern of fibrosing alveolitis are misdiagnosed as having asbestosis; such cases can be recognized pathologically by a lack of asbestos bodies and the absence of asbestos fibers by analytic electron microscopy.[213] On the other hand, a lack of asbestos bodies on optical microscopy may lead to a diagnosis of fibrosing alveolitis in the occasional patient in whom asbestos fibers can be recognized only by scanning electron microscopy and energy-dispersive x-ray analysis.[214]

Grossly, the early stages of fibrosing alveolitis consist of only a slight coarseness of the normal parenchyma. As dis-

ease progresses, clear-cut areas of fibrosis alternating with small cystic spaces 1 to 2 mm in diameter appear. Eventually, a whole lobe can be affected, resulting in innumerable 5- to 10-mm cystic spaces separated by a variable amount of firm, gray fibrous tissue (so-called honeycomb lung) (Fig. 17–18). These changes almost invariably affect the lower lobes predominantly, particularly in the subpleural region. The external surface of affected lung typically has a coarse, nodular appearance—likened by some investigators to cirrhosis[215]—that is caused by bulging of the cysts and retraction of the adjacent scarred parenchyma.

Unlike the variable appearance of fibrosing alveolitis as described above, the histologic pattern of DIP is distinctly uniform: all portions of lung on a tissue section appear more or less similar (Fig. 17–19). The alveolar interstitium is usually mildly to moderately thickened by an infiltrate of mononuclear inflammatory cells and a small amount of collagen. Type II cell hyperplasia is prominent and again fairly uniform. Alveolar airspaces are filled with numerous mononuclear cells, originally believed to be desquamated type II cells but now known to be predominantly alveolar macrophages. It is important to recognize that this histologic pattern can be seen focally in association with otherwise typical cases of fibrosing alveolitis and can also occur with other conditions such as tuberculosis, eosinophilic granuloma, and rheumatoid disease.[216] Thus, a diagnosis of DIP that is based on a small amount of tissue, such as that obtained by transbronchial biopsy, should be made with caution.

Roentgenographic Manifestations

As might be expected, the roentgenographic appearance varies with the stage of disease. Though the classic pattern of DIP as described in early investigations consists of symmetric "ground-glass" opacification predominantly at the lung bases,[217] this pattern has uncommonly been identified in subsequent studies.[218] The more frequent appearance is one of nonspecific irregular opacities that are most numerous in the lung bases.

It is probable that the earliest roentgenographic changes in fibrosing alveolitis consist of a fine reticulation with lower zone predominance. Some observers have also described a pattern suggesting combined airspace and interstitial involvement (Fig. 17–20), representing the desquamative phase of the disease.[219] At this stage, patients may be asymptomatic even though pulmonary function may be greatly impaired. On the other hand, an occasional patient with biopsy-proven disease is symptomatic yet shows no abnormality on conventional roentgenograms,[217, 220] particularly when disease is relatively early and confined to the alveolar interstitium. In many such patients, however, CT scans (particularly with high resolution) may show changes highly suggestive of the desquamative phase (Fig. 17–21).

More advanced disease is characterized by a coarse reticular or reticulonodular pattern throughout the lungs. Thick-walled cystic spaces 3 to 10 mm in diameter are present and create a honeycomb pattern (Fig. 17–22). The severe disorganization of lung architecture usually can be much better appreciated on CT scans than on conventional roentgenograms (Fig. 17–23).[221]

The authors have been repeatedly impressed by the

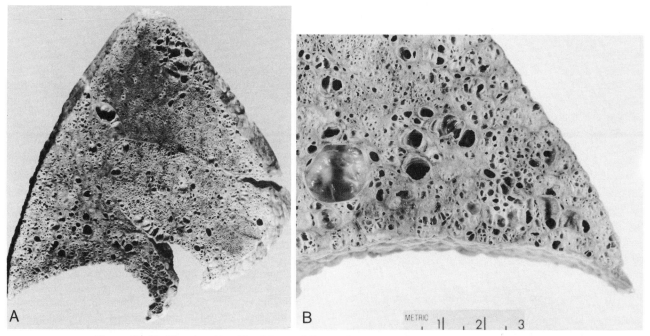

Figure 17–18. Fibrosing Alveolitis: Advanced Stage. A sagittal section of a right lung *(A)* shows advanced interstitial fibrosis with extensive "honeycomb" change. Note the relative sparing of the central portion of the upper lobe. A magnified view of the basal aspect of a lower lobe from another patient *(B)* shows severe interstitial fibrosis with virtually no remaining normal parenchyma. Note the nodular appearance of the pleural surface caused by alternating areas of fibrosis and cyst formation, sometimes referred to as pulmonary "cirrhosis."

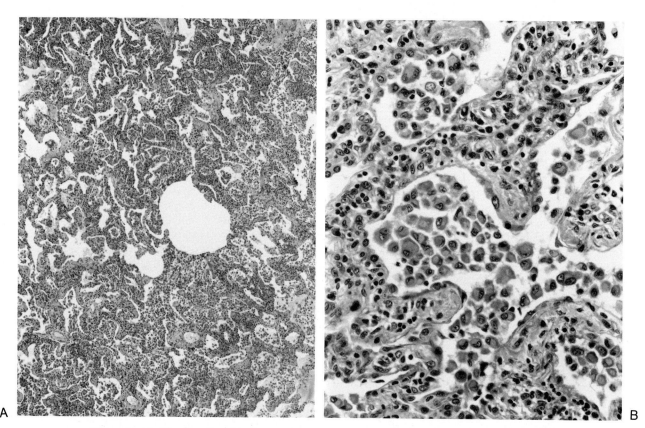

Figure 17–19. Fibrosing Alveolitis: Desquamative Pattern. A low-magnification histologic section of lung parenchyma *(A)* shows moderately severe, fairly uniform disease affecting all the tissue. At higher power *(B)*, interstitial thickening can be seen to be caused by a combination of mononuclear inflammatory cells (predominantly lymphocytes) and fibrous tissue; the adjacent airspaces contain numerous macrophages. *(A × 40; B × 250.)* (Courtesy of Dr. Claude Auger, Jean Talon Hospital, Montreal.)

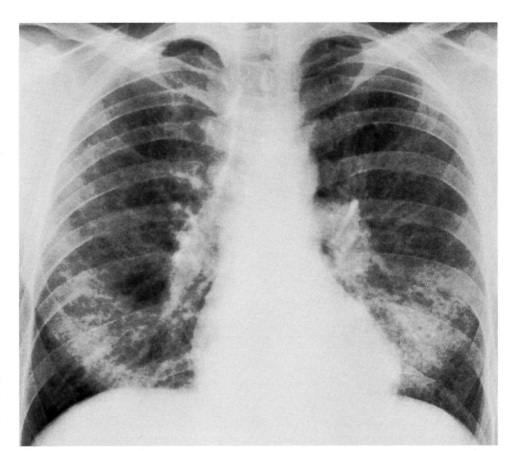

Figure 17–20. Fibrosing Alveolitis: Desquamative Phase. A posteroanterior roentgenogram reveals diffuse involvement of both lungs by a rather coarse reticular pattern, which is slightly more prominent in the bases than elsewhere, thus simulating airspace disease. Hilar lymph nodes appear slightly enlarged.

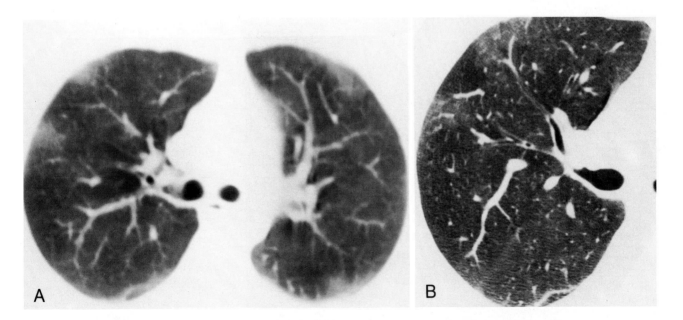

Figure 17–21. Fibrosing Alveolitis: CT Manifestations of the Desquamative Phase. A CT scan at the level of the right upper lobe bronchus with 10-mm collimation (A) shows patchy, ill-defined areas of airspace opacification (a ground-glass pattern) situated predominantly in subpleural lung regions bilaterally. A high-resolution scan at the same level with 1.5-mm collimation (B) shows the areas of airspace opacification to be sharply demarcated from contiguous normal parenchyma. Note that these opacities do not obscure the underlying vascular markings. (Reproduced with permission from Müller NL, Staples CA, Miller RR, et al: Disease activity in idiopathic pulmonary fibrosis: CT and pathologic correlation. Radiology 165:731, 1987.)

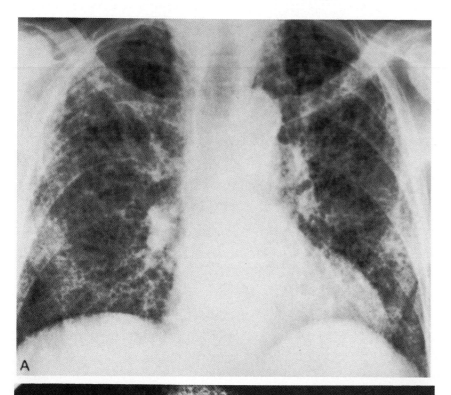

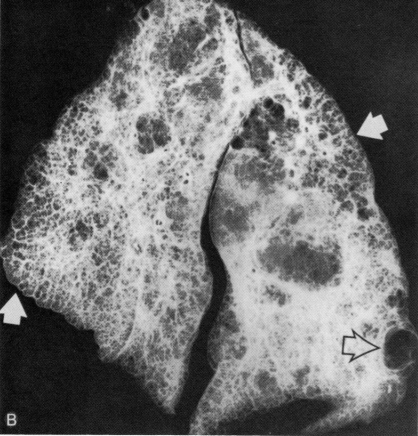

Figure 17–22. Advanced Fibrosing Alveolitis with Honeycombing. A posteroanterior roentgenogram *(A)* reveals a coarse reticular pattern without anatomic predominance. Honeycomb changes are present in several areas. A roentgenogram of a 1-cm thick slice of left lung removed at autopsy *(B)* shows the honeycombing well *(solid arrows)* and also reveals a large subpleural bulla in the lower lobe *(open arrow)*.

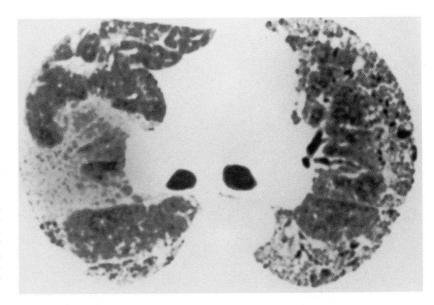

Figure 17–23. Fibrosing Alveolitis: CT Manifestations. A CT scan at the level of the bronchus intermedius reveals extensive bilateral pulmonary disease consisting predominantly of a reticular pattern. On the left side particularly, the fibrosis involves the subpleural lung regions predominantly. (Courtesy of Dr. Nestor L. Müller, University of British Columbia, Vancouver.)

striking loss of lung volume apparent on serial roentgenographic studies over a period of several years (Fig. 17–24) and consider that a diffuse reticulonodular pattern accompanied by progressive elevation of the diaphragm—signs that occur much less frequently in other forms of diffuse interstitial disease—strongly suggests the diagnosis of either fibrosing alveolitis or progressive systemic sclerosis. In the occasional patient in whom no loss of volume is evident, high-resolution CT may reveal upper lobe emphysema.[222] Although hilar and mediastinal lymph node enlargement is seldom evident on conventional roentgenograms, CT scans have been shown to reveal such enlargement not infrequently.[223] Pleural effusion is rare and its presence should suggest other diagnoses or complications. Pneumothorax is uncommon.[224]

In two studies in which CT findings were correlated with pathologic,[225] clinical, functional, and conventional roentgenographic[226] manifestations, the following findings were observed: (1) disease activity on CT scans—judged by the presence or absence of airspace opacification (ground-glass attenuation)—correlated well with the presence or absence of pathologic evidence of intra-alveolar and interstitial cellularity[225]; (2) changes were seen to better advantage on 1.5-mm than on 10-mm collimation scans; (3) scans gave a better estimate of disease extent and showed more extensive honeycombing than did conventional roentgenograms (Fig. 17–25)[227]; (4) a significant correlation was found between the extent of disease as assessed with CT and the severity of dyspnea and impairment of gas exchange (diffusing capacity)[226]; and (5) correlation between disease severity

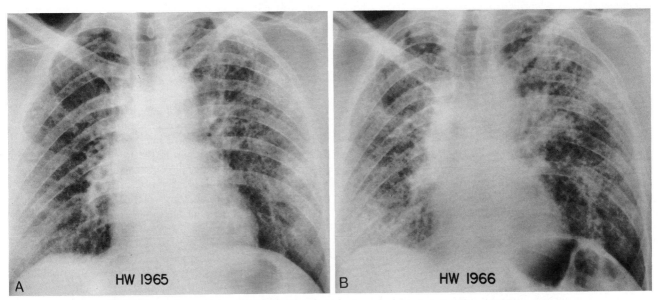

Figure 17–24. Fibrosing Alveolitis: Rapid Progression. A posteroanterior roentgenogram (A) reveals a coarse reticular pattern without anatomic predominance; 1 year later (B), lung volume had reduced appreciably, and the reticular opacities had worsened.

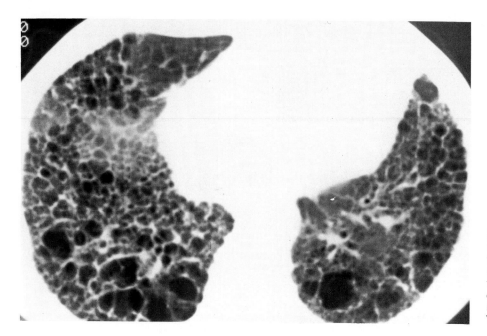

Figure 17–25. End-Stage Fibrosing Alveolitis: CT Manifestations. A CT scan through the base of both lungs reveals extensive honeycombing extending from the visceral pleura to the mediastinum on both sides. (Courtesy of Dr. Nestor L. Müller, University of British Columbia, Vancouver.)

as assessed on conventional roentgenograms and clinical and functional variables was poor.

In addition to establishing a diagnosis, CT may be useful in evaluating response to therapy.[228] For example, in one high-resolution CT study it was shown that the extent of ground-glass attenuation was significantly correlated with improvement in diffusing capacity, forced VC and forced expiratory volume in 1 second (FEV$_1$) after steroid therapy.[229] Proton magnetic resonance imaging also has been advocated for early diagnosis and for evaluating response to treatment.[230] Published results are encouraging, particularly with respect to sensitivity.

Although fibrosing alveolitis is primarily a disease of the lung parenchyma, abnormalities of the large airways also can be seen in some cases. For example, in one autopsy study of 12 patients with advanced pulmonary fibrosis, bronchiectasis was identified in 9 patients.[231] Its confinement to areas of advanced fibrosis suggested that its cause was traction by the fibrous tissue. The bronchiectasis was much better depicted on CT scans than on conventional roentgenograms; on the latter it was thought to contribute to the appearance of honeycombing. Tracheomegaly also has been reported to occur in an appreciable number of patients.[232]

Clinical Manifestations

Fibrosing alveolitis probably affects men slightly more often than women, and most patients are between the ages of 40 and 70 years.[233] Symptoms include progressive dyspnea, nonproductive cough, weight loss, and fatigue. Clubbing is common, and its presence can antedate symptoms and other signs of pulmonary disease. It occurs equally as often in the "desquamative" stage of the disease as in the advanced fibrotic stage.

In the early stages, findings on examination of the chest can be within normal limits, but as the disease progresses, diffuse crepitations of a very superficial quality are frequently heard, predominantly over the lung bases. These

are mostly inspiratory, but can be mid- and late-expiratory,[234] and have been termed "Velcro rales" because of their resemblance to the sound produced by tearing apart mated strips of Velcro adhesive.[235] Cyanosis and signs of pulmonary hypertension and cor pulmonale are late manifestations of the disease. Other infrequent clinical findings include sexual impotence, presumably caused by suppression of the hypothalamic-pituitary-testicular axis by hypoxia,[236] and hyponatremia associated with the syndrome of inappropriate secretion of antidiuretic hormone.[237] Arthralgia and myalgia have been described in patients with DIP.[197]

When clinical findings and the roentgenographic pattern suggest interstitial lung disease, the diagnostic possibilities are numerous. Although the combination of clubbing, slowly progressive dyspnea, serial reduction in pulmonary function, and roentgenographic evidence of progressive loss of lung volume strongly suggest the diagnosis, in most cases fibrosing alveolitis is a diagnosis of exclusion. Nevertheless, it is rare for biopsy to reveal a different diagnosis when a careful history, physical examination, and laboratory investigation have reasonably excluded other diagnostic possibilities.

Autoimmune connective tissue diseases are usually readily recognized by their clinical manifestations and specific autoantibodies. Error is most likely to arise during the early stages of polymyositis when muscle weakness may be overlooked or may be ascribed to nonspecific manifestations of the pulmonary disability or to corticosteroid therapy.[238] The diagnosis of a pneumoconiosis or drug reaction usually requires little more than a searching clinical history regarding occupation and medications, a step that is often neglected in the former instance until such a possibility is suggested by the roentgenographic pattern. Similarly, a history of exposure to birds or moldy hay should raise the possibility of extrinsic allergic alveolitis. Eosinophilic granuloma generally presents with normal or increased lung volume, in contrast to the classic shrunken lungs of fibrosing alveolitis, and characteristically affects the upper lung zones more than the lower.

Open lung biopsy, thoracoscopic biopsy, and, in some hands, trephine biopsy[239] are the only procedures that yield sufficient tissue to support a diagnosis of fibrosing alveolitis. The last procedure particularly is not without risk, however, and is performed relatively rarely. Transbronchial biopsy often does not result in a specific diagnosis,[240] although the absence of granulomas is helpful in excluding a diagnosis of sarcoidosis.

Pulmonary Function Tests

Vital capacity, diffusing capacity,[241] gas transfer, and pulmonary hemodynamics[242] appear to be more severely affected in fibrosing alveolitis than in other interstitial diseases. In morphologic-physiologic correlation studies based on biopsies, lung function does not appear to discriminate between fibrosis and infiltration of the lung by inflammatory cells.[243] Patients with fibrosing alveolitis who smoke cigarettes show a greater degree of functional impairment than nonsmoking patients. This appears to be related to associated emphysema, since physiologic correlates of airflow obstruction are not reduced,[244] and their pressure-volume curves are shifted upward and to the left.[245]

It is probable that values of PaO_2 and $P(A - a)O_2$ on exercise are the most sensitive means of assessing disability in patients with fibrosing alveolitis.[246] Hypoxemia is caused chiefly by $\dot{V}/\dot{Q}$ inequality,[247] although approximately 20 per cent of the hypoxemia observed during exercise can be attributed to a diffusion defect.[248] Most patients show normal or even increased expiratory flow rates when related to absolute lung volume.

Prognosis

In the great majority of patients with fibrosing alveolitis, deterioration is gradual and inexorable with increasing shortness of breath and, in many individuals, the development of cor pulmonale. Overall mean survival is probably less than 5 years.[249] Occasional patients have acute fulminant disease that ends in early death from respiratory failure, a variant often referred to as Hamman-Rich syndrome.[250] Although approximately 20 per cent of patients die from cardiac complications, most succumb to respiratory failure, often precipitated by infection.[251] The incidence of lung cancer is increased in patients with fibrosing alveolitis, an association between parenchymal scarring (regardless of etiology) and pulmonary neoplasia that has been discussed previously (*see* page 449).

Many attempts have been made to define criteria that relate to prognosis and response to treatment of fibrosing alveolitis. There appears to be general agreement that patients fare better who have a shorter duration of symptoms before presentation[252] or are younger (except for infants younger than 1 year of age).[219] Pregnancy has been linked to rapid deterioration.[253] Patients whose lung biopsy specimens show a histologic pattern of desquamative interstitial pneumonitis usually pursue a relatively benign course.[219, 220]

There is some indication that prognosis can be improved by corticosteroid or immunosuppressive therapy or both[252, 254]; however, although 50 per cent of patients are said to improve symptomatically with corticosteroid therapy,[239] only half of them show roentgenographic[239] or functional[252] improvement. As might be expected, pulmonary function tests performed before and after corticosteroid therapy can reveal a beneficial effect during the early stages of the disease, but typically show a negligible response when the roentgenographic stage of honeycombing has been reached.[255]

LYMPHANGIOLEIOMYOMATOSIS

Lymphangioleiomyomatosis (lymphangiomyomatosis, myomatosis) is an uncommon pulmonary abnormality characterized pathologically by a diffuse proliferation of smooth muscle within the airway walls, parenchymal interstitium, and lymphatics. It is a disease primarily of young and middle-aged women, the average age at presentation being about 35 years.

Although the precise nature of the condition is not known, it is possible that it represents a developmental (hamartomatous) abnormality. The similarity of both pathologic and clinical features to those of tuberous sclerosis, a condition well characterized as a disease of disordered development, supports this hypothesis; in fact, there is persuasive evidence that pulmonary lymphangioleiomyomatosis represents simply a *forme fruste* of tuberous sclerosis.[256] Since the disease is seen almost always in women during the reproductive years, it is logical to suggest that there may be some association with abnormal hormone secretion or tissue response to hormones. Supporting this hypothesis are reports of exacerbations of disease during pregnancy[257] and following the administration of exogenous estrogens[258]; in addition, cytosolic[257] and immunohistochemical[259] studies have documented the presence of receptors for estrogen and progesterone in tissue biopsies. There is also evidence that progesterone therapy may be associated with amelioration of signs and symptoms in some patients.

Pathologic Characteristics

Grossly, the lungs in advanced lymphangioleiomyomatosis show numerous cystic spaces of variable size (usually 0.2 to 2.0 cm in diameter) separated by thickened interstitial tissue (Fig. 17–26). Microscopically,[260] the most striking abnormality is the presence of numerous interlacing fascicles of smooth muscle that form the walls of the cystic spaces observed grossly. Increased smooth muscle also can be identified within otherwise normal parenchymal interstitium and in the walls of airways, pulmonary veins, and lymphatics. Smooth muscle proliferation is often observed in the thoracic duct, which may be totally obliterated, and in lymph nodes in the mediastinum and retroperitoneum. Involvement of these structures causes some degree of disturbance in lymph flow and may result in the development of chylothorax, chyloperitoneum, and, occasionally, chylopericardium.[261]

Roentgenographic Manifestations

The appearance of the lungs in lymphangioleiomyomatosis as seen on conventional roentgenograms is indistinguishable from that of fibrosing alveolitis, with the exception of the effects on lung volume: characteristically,

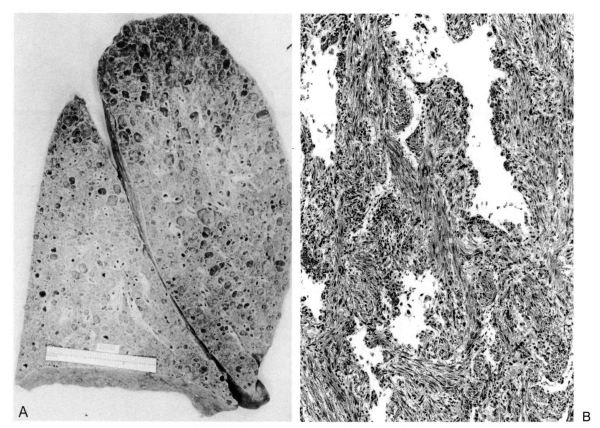

Figure 17–26. Lymphangioleiomyomatosis. A sagittal slice through the middle portion of the left lung *(A)* shows numerous cystic spaces of variable size throughout both lobes. A histologic section *(B)* reveals moderate to marked thickening of the parenchymal interstitium caused by a proliferation of uniform spindle cells consistent with smooth muscle. (*B* × 100.)

alveolitis manifests progressive loss of lung volume, whereas in lymphangioleiomyomatosis volume tends to be increased.[262] The basic pattern is coarse reticulonodular and tends to be generalized, although in some patients it is more prominent in the lung bases (Fig. 17–27). The late pattern is one of honeycombing. These conventional roentgenographic findings are relatively nonspecific. High-resolution CT scans, however, can reveal abnormalities that are characteristic (Fig. 17–28), consisting of well-defined cystic spaces ranging in diameter from a few millimeters to 5 cm and distributed diffusely throughout both lungs[263–265]; the walls of the cystic spaces tend to be uniformly thin.

Pleural effusion (chylothorax) may be unilateral or bilateral and typically is large and recurrent. It may occur in the absence of lung involvement. Spontaneous pneumothorax is common. Mediastinal lymph node enlargement, sometimes not apparent on conventional chest roentgenograms, also can be identified in some patients.

Clinical Manifestations

The presenting complaint is usually shortness of breath, sometimes in association with pneumothorax or a history of repeated hemoptysis. Unilateral or bilateral chylothorax is a common manifestation. Occasionally, chyle is coughed up (chyloptysis) or passed in the urine (chyluria).

The pulmonary function pattern is one of obstruction; VC is reduced and FRC and RV are increased. Detection of the increase in total lung capacity may require plethysmographic measurement of lung volumes.[260] FEV_1 and mid–expiratory phase forced expiratory flow ($FEF_{25\%-75\%}$) are considerably decreased, and FEV_1/FVC is usually well below the predicted normal. DLCO is reduced, and hypoxemia is common and may be severe. PCO_2, however, is almost invariably decreased.[262, 266] These impairments in mechanics have been reported to be related to airway narrowing or obstruction rather than to a loss of elastic recoil.

Reports from the 1970s and 1980s suggested a poor prognosis; the majority of patients died from respiratory failure within 10 years.[262] A recent review of 32 patients, however, documented a much more favorable course: almost 80 per cent were alive an average of 8 years after the onset of symptoms.[267]

TUBEROUS SCLEROSIS

Tuberous sclerosis (Bourneville's disease) is an autosomal dominant familial disorder that affects males and females equally and is characterized classically by the triad of mental retardation, epilepsy, and adenoma sebaceum. Pulmonary involvement is very uncommon,[268] occurring in only 0.1 to 1 per cent of patients.

Although the pathologic characteristics of tuberous sclerosis and lymphangioleiomyomatosis have been generally regarded as being similar if not identical, some authors have

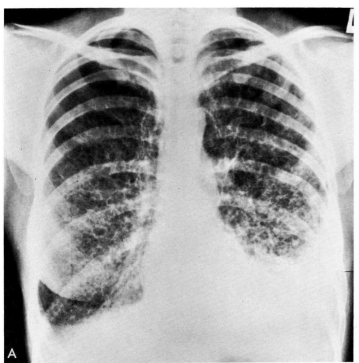
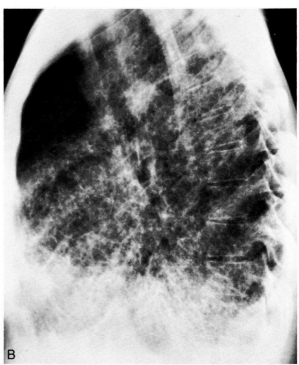

Figure 17–27. Pulmonary Lymphangioleiomyomatosis. Roentgenograms in posteroanterior *(A)* and lateral *(B)* projections reveal a coarse reticulation throughout both lungs, with considerable basal and midzone predominance. In the lower lung zones particularly, there are multiple thick-walled cystic spaces ranging from 5 to 10 mm in diameter, the basic pattern of "honeycomb lung." There are bilateral pleural effusions, larger on the left. The heart is not enlarged. (Courtesy of Dr. Melvin Figley, University of Washington Hospital, Seattle.)

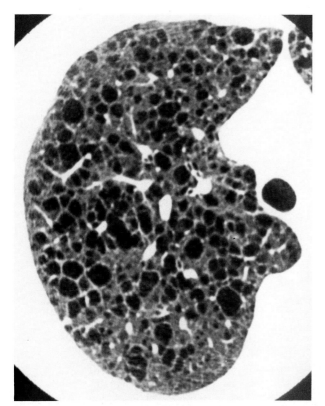

Figure 17–28. Lymphangioleiomyomatosis: CT Manifestations. A high-resolution CT scan through the right upper lobe with 1.5-mm collimation reveals a multitude of cystic spaces ranging in diameter from 5 to 20 mm. For the most part the cyst walls are very thin. Lung parenchyma between cysts is normal. (Courtesy of Dr. Nestor L. Müller, University of British Columbia, Vancouver.)

found differences in the composition and distribution of the lesions.[262] For example, lymphangioleiomyomatosis has been said to be characterized by intranodal and extranodal involvement of the lymphatics of the central part of the body, whereas tuberous sclerosis has been regarded as a more generalized mesodermal disorder with a special tendency to involve the smooth muscle of blood vessels.

Despite these possible differences, the roentgenographic manifestations of thoracic involvement in tuberous sclerosis are very similar to those of lymphangioleiomyomatosis except for the pleura. Although pneumothorax occurs, chylous effusions are rarely observed in tuberous sclerosis.[269] The identification of numerous sclerotic lesions (or sometimes cystic rarefactions[270]) throughout the skeleton, together with the other typical changes, should establish the diagnosis beyond reasonable doubt. Further confirmation may be obtained by the roentgenologic demonstration of renal enlargement secondary to angiomyolipomas or of intracranial calcifications.[270]

Respiratory symptoms and pulmonary function abnormalities are similar to those of lymphangioleiomyomatosis and are usually first noted between the ages of 18 and 34 years.[271]

NEUROFIBROMATOSIS

Neurofibromatosis (von Recklinghausen's disease) is a relatively common familial disorder with a frequency of about 1 in 3000. There is no sex predominance. Although it is inexorably progressive, it shows markedly variable expressivity,[272] and only about 20 per cent of affected patients develop disabling disease. The most prominent manifestations are cutaneous *café au lait* spots and neurofibromas of the cutaneous and subcutaneous peripheral nerves and nerve roots. Neurofibromas of viscera and blood vessels innervated by the autonomic nervous system are also seen.[272]

Thoracic disease in neurofibromatosis can be manifested in several ways, the most common of which is undoubtedly the cutaneous and subcutaneous neurofibromas. Roentgenographically, these can be seen in profile as nodules on the chest wall or projected over the lungs (Fig. 17–29). Other chest wall abnormalities include kyphoscoliosis[272] and ribbon deformity of the ribs.

Pulmonary manifestations occur in 5 to 10 per cent of patients[273, 274] and consist of diffuse interstitial fibrosis and bullae, either alone or in combination (*see* Fig. 17–29). The interstitial fibrosis characteristically involves both lungs symmetrically with some basal predominance, whereas the bullae usually are asymmetric and tend to develop in the upper lobes.[273] Pathologically, the interstitial fibrosis is similar to that of fibrosing alveolitis.

Thoracic neoplasms, predominantly neurogenic in type, also are not uncommon. They can arise in the intercostal nerves (in which case they may be associated with rib destruction and a chest wall mass), in the mediastinum (often with characteristic CT manifestations[275]), and, occasionally, in the lungs themselves.[276]

Pulmonary disease typically does not become evident until the patient reaches adulthood. Respiratory symptoms are usually mild, the most common complaint being dysp-

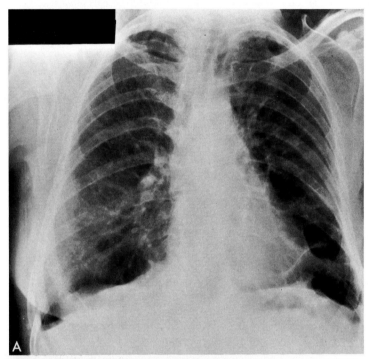

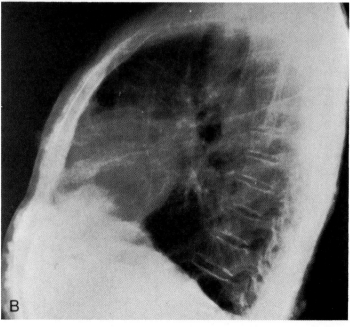

Figure 17–29. Neurofibromatosis: Pulmonary and Cutaneous Manifestations. Posteroanterior *(A)* and lateral *(B)* views of the chest reveal numerous bullae in the lower portion of both lungs. A background of diffuse reticulation is present, suggesting interstitial pulmonary fibrosis. Along the lateral chest wall in *A* and on the anterior and posterior chest walls in lateral projection *(B)* are numerous nodular opacities representing cutaneous neurofibromas.

nea on exertion.[277] Pulmonary function tests usually reveal evidence of obstruction, although a restrictive pattern may be dominant. Diffusing capacity is often decreased.[277]

EOSINOPHILIC GRANULOMA

Eosinophilic granuloma is the adult form of histiocytosis X (the infantile and childhood varieties being known as Letterer-Siwe disease and Hand-Schüller-Christian disease, respectively). Although it can be widely disseminated throughout the body, it is more commonly localized to the lungs or bones or both. It occurs most frequently in whites and has been described only rarely in blacks.[278] Although it was originally thought to be more common in young adult males, recent reports have described a significant number of cases in middle-aged women.[279]

The etiology and pathogenesis of the varieties of histiocytosis are unknown and may, in fact, be multiple: some cases may reflect a primary mononuclear phagocytic abnormality and others a disorder of suppressor T-lymphocyte control of cytotoxic cells.[280] Some investigators have found circulating immune complexes in patients whose lung biopsies show active cellular histology[281] and elevated levels of immunoglobulin G in BAL fluid.[282] In some series,[283] an association with tobacco smoke has been described, a history of smoking being identified in more than 90 per cent of patients with eosinophilic granuloma and in fewer than 50 per cent of matched control subjects.

Pathologic Characteristics

Grossly, the lungs in the early stage of eosinophilic granuloma show multiple nodules measuring up to a few millimeters in diameter. With time, these relatively discrete nodular lesions become confluent, and irregularly shaped areas of fibrosis result. In long-standing disease, the appearance is similar to that of advanced fibrosing alveolitis, with normal parenchyma being replaced by fibrous tissue and multiple cysts of variable size. The only distinguishing feature is that eosinophilic granuloma, unlike fibrosing alveolitis, tends to be more severe in the upper lobes.[284]

Microscopically, abnormalities in the early stage are located predominantly in the interstitial connective tissue around small bronchioles and adjacent arteries, and consist mainly of a cellular infiltrate. In more advanced disease, this infiltrate extends into the adjacent alveolar interstitium and the central portion of the lesion undergoes fibrosis, resulting in more or less discrete, stellate nodules (Fig. 17–30). As the disease progresses, individual foci of disease

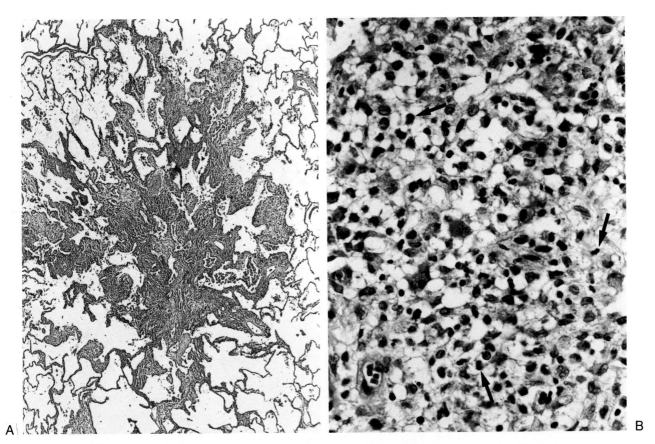

Figure 17–30. Eosinophilic Granuloma. A histologic section of lung parenchyma at low magnification *(A)* shows a vaguely stellate-shaped focus of interstitial thickening caused by cellular infiltration and mild fibrosis. A magnified view of the infiltrate *(B)* shows it to be composed of numerous histiocytes and scattered, bilobed eosinophils *(arrows)*. *(A × 32; B × 400.)*

coalesce, the fibrous tissue becomes more and more prominent, and an ever increasing amount of lung is destroyed.

The cellular portion of the stellate lesions contains a variety of inflammatory cells, the proportion being variable from area to area. The predominant cells are large mononuclear cells (so-called Hx cells) that react with an antibody to protein S-100[285] and have characteristic cytoplasmic inclusions (Langerhans' granules) that can be identified by electron microscopy.[286] Admixed among the Hx cells are fairly numerous eosinophils and smaller numbers of neutrophils, plasma cells, and lymphocytes. Despite the designation of eosinophilic granuloma, true granulomas do not form. Although the identification of Hx cells in BAL fluid[287] by ultrastructural or immunohistochemical examination is suggestive of eosinophilic granuloma, these cells also can be identified in cases of pulmonary fibrosis of other etiology.[285, 288]

Roentgenographic Manifestations

The roentgenographic pattern in the lungs varies with the stage of the disease. Involvement is characteristically diffuse and bilaterally symmetric; unlike many other diffuse diseases of the lungs, however, eosinophilic granuloma tends to upper zone predominance. The early, active stage of the disease is manifested by a nodular pattern with individual lesions ranging from 1 to 10 mm in diameter. These are assumed to represent largely cellular foci with minimal fibrosis[289] and may regress or even completely resolve.[290] In later stages, the pattern may become reticulonodular. The end stage is characterized by a very coarse reticular pattern that, in the upper lung zones particularly, often assumes a cystic appearance characteristic of the honeycomb pattern (Fig. 17–31). These cysts usually are about 1 cm in diameter but may measure up to 3 cm, especially in the periphery. This pattern and distribution are highly suggestive of the diagnosis.[291]

The typical CT manifestations consist of thin-walled cysts, usually less than 10 mm in diameter, that may be the sole finding or may be accompanied by multiple nodules (usually less than 5 mm in diameter) (Fig. 17–32).[292] Occasionally, multiple nodules themselves are the sole abnormality. Other findings include cavitated nodules, thick-walled cysts, reticulation, and ground-glass opacities.[293] It has been hypothesized that the evolution of the changes observed on CT consist first of nodules, followed by cavitation with the formation of thick-walled cysts, then progression to thin-walled cysts and finally to confluence of cysts.[293]

In our experience and that of others,[279, 294] the progressive loss of lung volume that is so characteristic of fibrosing alveolitis is seldom seen in eosinophilic granuloma. Perhaps the tendency for the development of cysts and bullae counteracts the cicatricial effect of the diffuse fibrosis. In fact, dynamic ultrafast high-resolution CT during forced expiration has been shown to reveal focal and diffuse air trapping.[295]

Hilar and mediastinal lymph node enlargement and pleural effusion are rare in adults,[289, 294] although node enlargement is a recognized manifestation of the disease in children.[296] Spontaneous pneumothorax has been identified in 10 to 15 per cent of patients[279, 294]; it may be the first indicator of the disease and occasionally occurs in the absence of roentgenographic abnormality in the lungs.[296] Although concomitant involvement of bones and lungs has been reported,[297] it is probably rare in adults.

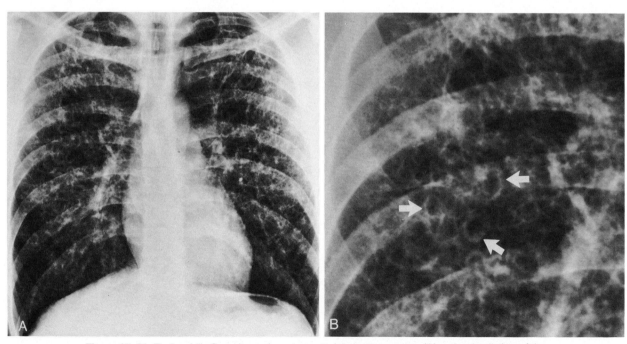

Figure 17–31. Eosinophilic Granuloma. A posteroanterior roentgenogram *(A)* and a detail view of the middle portion of the right lung *(B)* reveal a rather coarse reticulonodular pattern throughout both lungs with some upper-zonal predominance. In several areas, ring shadows are visible, measuring 7 to 10 mm in diameter and characterized by a central radiolucency surrounded by a wall of variable thickness. This honeycomb pattern is well demonstrated in the magnified view *(arrows)*.

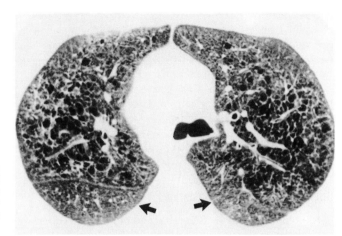

Figure 17–32. Eosinophilic Granuloma: CT Manifestations. A high-resolution CT scan (1.5-mm collimation) at the level of the tracheal carina demonstrates bilateral cystic spaces with thin walls. These cystic spaces involve most of the visualized portions of the upper lobes, while the superior segments of the lower lobes *(arrows)* are virtually normal.

Clinical Manifestations

When first seen, 20 to 25 per cent of patients are asymptomatic,[279] the disease often being discovered on a screening chest roentgenogram. Somewhat less than one third of patients have nonspecific constitutional symptoms such as fatigue, weight loss, and fever. Respiratory symptoms are present in approximately two thirds of patients and usually consist of dry cough and dyspnea. Chest pain can be caused by pneumothorax. Hemoptysis is uncommon.[298] Physical findings are of little help in diagnosis; occasionally, rales may be heard over the lungs or there is local tenderness over a bony lesion. Finger clubbing is extremely rare.

The association of diffuse lung disease with diabetes insipidus should strongly suggest the diagnosis, although this combination occasionally occurs in histoplasmosis and sarcoidosis. Reports in the literature[298] indicate that hypothalamic involvement is detected in 10 to 25 per cent of patients, an incidence much higher than the authors would have expected judging from our referred patient population as pulmonologists.

Pulmonary function studies show both restrictive and obstructive patterns of insufficiency, the former being manifested by decreased VC, normal residual volume, and normal flow rates.[279] Patients tend to hyperventilate, and the combination of low diffusing capacity[299] and increased physiologic dead space indicates the presence of ventilation-perfusion inequality. Despite a distinct roentgenographic abnormality, function may be within the normal predicted range, a state of affairs that seldom occurs in cryptogenic fibrosing alveolitis.[300]

The prognosis is generally good.[294] In one series of 60 patients,[279] 16 patients were initially asymptomatic and remained so, 17 had complete remission and 11 partial remission of symptoms, 11 remained stable but symptomatic, 4 showed progression with increasing disability, and 1 patient died. An additional factor that worsens the prognosis is the development of both epithelial[301] and lymphoreticular[280] neoplasms.

PULMONARY ALVEOLAR MICROLITHIASIS

Pulmonary alveolar microlithiasis is a rare disease characterized by the presence within alveolar airspaces of nu-

merous tiny calculi ("calcispherytes").[302, 303] In Japan, the peak incidence occurs between the ages of 4 and 9 years,[304] but in western countries the majority of reported cases have been in patients between the ages of 30 and 50 years.[305]

Etiology and Pathogenesis

The etiology and pathogenesis of alveolar microlithiasis are unknown. Hypothetical mechanisms that have been proposed include an inborn error of metabolism, an unusual response to an unspecified pulmonary insult, an immune reaction to various irritants,[306] and an acquired abnormality of calcium or phosphorus metabolism.

Familial occurrence has been noted in more than half the reported cases[303]; however, disease in this situation has been restricted almost completely to siblings, suggesting that environmental rather than genetic factors may be more important. Despite this, no common history of inhalation exposure or occupation has been discovered.

Theories based on an acquired metabolic disturbance have been proposed but are difficult to substantiate in view of the consistently normal serum calcium and phosphorus levels in reported series.[307] However, several isolated case reports suggest that such a disturbance occasionally may be a factor. For example, although the microliths are almost invariably confined to the lungs, one patient also had multiple urinary calculi[308]; in addition, there is one report of a patient with milk-alkali syndrome in whom microliths appeared to form secondary to mineralization of desquamated epithelial cells.[309] Since calcium salts are more soluble in an acid medium and are more easily precipitated from alkaline solutions, it has been postulated that microlithiasis may result from some undefined alteration in the alveolar lining membrane or in alveolar secretions that promotes alkalinity at the alveolar interface and thus predisposes to the deposition or precipitation of calcium phosphate within the alveoli.[307]

Pathologic Characteristics

Microliths range from 0.01 to 3.0 mm in diameter[302] and are located almost invariably within alveolar airspaces. Despite this, there is evidence suggesting that they are formed in the alveolar walls, possibly in relation to type II cells, and are extruded into the adjacent airspaces.[310] Individual microliths are round, oval, or irregular in shape and have a concentric laminated appearance.[311] Chemical analysis and energy-dispersive x-ray microanalysis have shown them to be composed of calcium phosphate.[302]

In the early stages of the disease, the alveolar walls appear perfectly normal[305]; later on, interstitial fibrosis results in alveolar wall thickening, sometimes associated with giant cell formation. Blebs and bullae often develop, particularly in the lung apices. How these relate to the presence of microliths is unclear.

Roentgenographic Manifestations

Although there is considerable variation from patient to patient depending on the severity of affliction, the fundamental pattern is one of a very fine sandlike micronodulation diffusely involving both lungs (Fig. 17–33). Regardless of the effect of superimposition or summation of shadows,

individual deposits are usually identifiable, particularly with magnification roentgenography. Very sharply defined, they measure less than 1 mm in diameter and are so discrete as to give the impression that one could pick out individual microliths with a pair of fine tweezers. The overall density is greater over the lower than the upper zones, probably because of increased thickness of lung rather than selectively greater involvement. The opacities may be so numerous as to appear confluent, in which circumstance a normally exposed chest roentgenogram shows the lungs as almost uniformly white, often with total obliteration of the mediastinal and diaphragmatic contours. However, employment of an overexposed roentgenographic technique with stationary or moving grid usually reveals the underlying pattern to better advantage.

Pleural thickening has been described,[312] although it is probable that this roentgenographic appearance is caused not by actual thickening of the pleura itself but by a visual effect produced by an exceptionally heavy concentration of

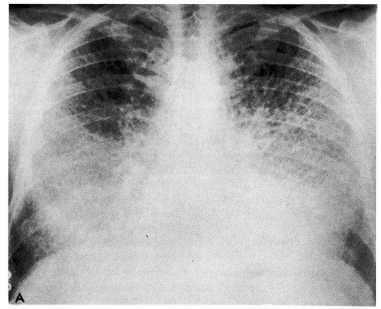

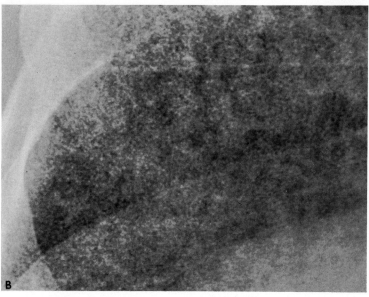

Figure 17–33. Alveolar Microlithiasis. A posteroanterior roentgenogram (A) of this 40-year-old asymptomatic man reveals a remarkably uniform opacification of both lungs. On close scrutiny (B), this can be seen to be produced by a multitude of tiny, discrete opacities of calcific density (B is a detail view of the right lower zone from a two-to-one primary magnification image).

microliths in the subpleural parenchyma.[305] In fact, the contrast between the extreme density of the lung parenchyma on one side of the pleura and the ribs on the other may create the illusion of a black pleural line. Spontaneous pneumothorax may result from rupture of apical bullae or blebs.[313]

Scintigraphy with technetium-99m–diphosphonate has shown uptake of the tracer by microliths,[314] indicating the presence of active metabolic exchange across the alveolo-capillary membrane.

Clinical Manifestations

The majority of patients are asymptomatic when alveolar microlithiasis is first discovered. The diagnosis is made on the basis of the typical pattern on a screening chest roentgenogram or in the investigation of persons whose siblings are known to have the disease. In no other condition is the lack of association between roentgenologic and clinical findings so striking as in pulmonary alveolar microlithiasis: symptoms may be completely absent even when the chest roentgenogram reveals the lungs to be almost solid and white, with little visible air-containing parenchyma.

The first symptom to develop in advanced cases is dyspnea on exertion. Cough and expectoration are uncommon, but occasionally produce diagnostic microliths.[314] As the disease progresses, respiratory insufficiency may develop, with cyanosis, clubbing of the fingers, and clinical signs of cor pulmonale. Physical signs usually are absent, except in the late stages when breath sounds may be decreased, particularly at the bases.

Chemical analysis of blood is invariably within the normal range.[305] In the late stages, right ventricular strain may become apparent electrocardiographically, and secondary polycythemia may develop. Microliths can sometimes be identified in BAL fluid.[315]

Pulmonary function studies vary considerably from case to case, depending on both the extent of replacement of alveolar air by concretions and the presence or absence of interstitial fibrosis. In one series of eight patients,[302] most values for lung volumes were on the low side of predicted normal; however, other investigations[316] have documented an increase in residual volume, associated with a decrease in maximal breathing capacity and a decrease in diffusing capacity.

The prognosis appears to be variable. It has been suggested that in many patients the microliths continue to form and perhaps increase in size as the disease progresses.[305] However, there is no doubt that the disease may become "arrested," and the deposition of microliths may cease. In fact, the authors have followed two patients in whom extensive roentgenographic change did not progress for 30 years.

References

1. James DG, Turiaf J, Hosoda Y, et al: Description of sarcoidosis: Report of the subcommittee on classification and definition. Ann NY Acad Sci 278: 742, 1976.
2. Milman N, Selroos O: Pulmonary sarcoidosis in the Nordic countries 1950–1982. Epidemiology and clinical picture. Sarcoidosis 7: 50, 1990.
3. DaCosta JL: Geographic epidemiology of sarcoidosis in Southeast Asia. Am Rev Respir Dis 108: 1269, 1973.
4. Scadding JG: Sarcoidosis. London, Eyre and Spottiswoode, 1967.
5. Purriel P, Navarrete E: Epidemiology of sarcoidosis in Uruguay and other countries of Latin America. Am Rev Respir Dis 84: 155, 1961.
6. Keller AZ: Anatomic sites, age attributes, and rates of sarcoidosis in U.S. veterans. Am Rev Respir Dis 107: 615, 1973.
7. Honeybourne D: Ethnic differences in the clinical features of sarcoidosis in south-east London. Br J Dis Chest 74: 63, 1980.
8. Mayock RL, Bertrand P, Morrison CE, et al: Manifestations of sarcoidosis. Analysis of 145 patients, with a review of nine series selected from the literature. Am J Med 35: 67, 1963.
9. Agner E, Larsen JH: *Yersinia enterocolitica* infection and sarcoidosis. A report of seven cases. Scand J Respir Dis 60: 230, 1979.
10. Mitchell DN, Rees RJW: The nature and physical characteristics of a transmissible agent from human sarcoid tissue. Ann NY Acad Sci 278: 233, 1976.
11. Holter JF, Park HK, Sjoerdsma KW, et al: Nonviable autologous bronchoalveolar lavage cell preparations induce intradermal epithelioid cell granulomas in sarcoid patients. Am Rev Respir Dis 145: 864, 1992.
12. Dewar A, Corrin B, Turner-Warwick M: Tadpole-shaped structures in a further patient with granulomatous lung disease. Thorax 39: 466, 1984.
13. Bocart D, Lecossier D, de Lassence A, et al: A search for mycobacterial DNA in granulomatous tissues from patients with sarcoidosis using the polymerase chain reaction. Am Rev Respir Dis 145: 1142, 1992.
14. Keogh BA, Crystal RG: Alveolitis: The key to the interstitial lung disorders. Thorax 37: 1, 1982.
15. Ginns LC, Goldenheim PD, Burton RC, et al: T-lymphocyte subsets in peripheral blood and lung lavage in idiopathic pulmonary fibrosis and sarcoidosis: Analysis by monoclonal antibodies and flow cytometry. Clin Immunol Immunopathol 25: 11, 1982.
16. Hunninghake GW, Crystal RG: Pulmonary sarcoidosis: A disorder mediated by excess helper T-lymphocyte activity at sites of disease activity. N Engl J Med 305: 429, 1981.
17. Robinson BW, Rose AH, Thompson PJ, et al: Comparison of bronchoalveolar lavage helper/suppressor T-cell ratios in sarcoidosis versus other interstitial lung diseases. Aust NZ J Med 17: 9, 1987.
18. Lecossier D, Valeyre D, Loiseau A, et al: T-lymphocytes recovered by bronchoalveolar lavage from normal subjects and patients with sarcoidosis are refractory to proliferative signals. Am Rev Respir Dis 137: 592, 1988.
19. Groman GS, Castele RJ, Altose MD, et al: Lymphocyte subpopulations in sarcoid pleural effusion. Ann Intern Med 100: 75, 1984.
20. Lecossier D, Valeyre D, Loiseau A, et al: Antigen-induced proliferative response of lavage and blood T-lymphocytes. Comparison of cells from normal subjects and patients with sarcoidosis. Am Rev Respir Dis 144: 861, 1991.
21. Baughman RP, Gallon LS, Barcelli U: Prostaglandins in the bronchoalveolar lavage fluid. Possible block of immunoregulation in sarcoidosis. Ann NY Acad Sci 465: 41, 1986.
22. Baughman RP, Gallon LS, Barcelli U: Prostaglandins and thromboxanes in the bronchoalveolar lavage fluid: Possible immunoregulation in sarcoidosis. Am Rev Respir Dis 130: 933, 1984.
23. Campbell DA, Poulter LW, du Bois RM: Immunocompetent cells in bronchoalveolar lavage reflect the cell populations in transbronchial biopsies in pulmonary sarcoidosis. Am Rev Respir Dis 132: 1300, 1985.
23a. Spiteri MA, Clarke SW, Poulter LW: Alveolar macrophages that suppress T-cell responses may be crucial to the pathogenetic outcome of pulmonary sarcoidosis. Eur Respir J 5: 394, 1992.
24. Hoogsteden HC, van Dongen JJ, van Hal PT, et al: Phenotype of blood monocytes and alveolar macrophages in interstitial lung disease. Chest 95: 574, 1989.
25. James DG, Williams WJ: Immunology of sarcoidosis. Am J Med 72: 5, 1982.
26. Costabel U, Bross KJ, Ruhle KH, et al: Ia-like antigens on T-cells and their subpopulations in pulmonary sarcoidosis and in hypersensitivity pneumonitis. Analysis of bronchoalveolar and blood lymphocytes. Am Rev Respir Dis 131: 337, 1985.
27. Flint KC, Leung KB, Hudspith BN, et al: Bronchoalveolar mast-cells in sarcoidosis: Increased numbers and accentuation of mediator release. Thorax 41: 94, 1986.
28. Danel C, Dewar A, Corrin B, et al: Ultrastructural changes in bronchoalveolar lavage cells in sarcoidosis and comparison with the tissue granuloma. Am J Pathol 112: 7, 1983.

29. Gerli R, Darwish S, Broccucci L, et al: Helper/inducer T cells in the lungs of sarcoidosis patients. Chest 95: 811, 1989.

30. Saint-Remy J-MR, Mitchell DN, Cole PJ: Variation in immunoglobulin levels and circulating immune complexes in sarcoidosis. Correlation with extent of disease and duration of symptoms. Am Rev Respir Dis 127: 23, 1983.

31. Valeyre D, Saumon G, Georges R, et al: The relationship between disease duration and noninvasive pulmonary explorations in sarcoidosis with erythema nodosum. Am Rev Respir Dis 129: 938, 1984.

32. Smith MJ, Turton CWG, Mitchell DN, et al: Association of HLA-B8 with spontaneous resolution in sarcoidosis. Thorax 36: 296, 1981.

33. Thomas PD, Hunninghake GW: Current concepts of the pathogenesis of sarcoidosis. Am Rev Respir Dis 135: 747, 1987.

34. Hunninghake GW, Gadek JE, Young RC Jr, et al: Maintenance of granuloma formation in pulmonary sarcoidosis by T-lymphocytes within the lung. N Engl J Med 302: 594, 1980.

35. Blaschke E, Eklund A, Hernbrand R: Extracellular matrix components in bronchoalveolar lavage fluid in sarcoidosis and their relationship to signs of alveolitis. Am Rev Respir Dis 141: 1020, 1990.

36. Brennan NJ, Crean P, Long JP, et al: High prevalence of familial sarcoidosis in an Irish population. Thorax 39: 14, 1984.

37. Edmondstone WM, Wilson AG: Temporal clustering of familial sarcoidosis in nonconsanguineous relatives. Br J Dis Chest 78: 184, 1984.

38. Stewart IC, Davidson NM: Clustering of sarcoidosis. Thorax 37: 398, 1982.

39. Valeyre D, Soler P, Clerici C, et al: Smoking and pulmonary sarcoidosis: Effect of cigarette smoking on prevalence, clinical manifestations, alveolitis, and evolution of the disease. Thorax 43: 516, 1988.

40. Bitterman PB, Adelberg S, Crystal RG: Mechanism of pulmonary fibrosis: Spontaneous release of the alveolar macrophage-derived growth factor in the interstitial lung disorders. J Clin Invest 72: 1801, 1983.

41. Cantin AM, Boileau R, Begin R: Increased procollagen III aminoterminal peptide–related antigens and fibroblast growth signals in the lungs of patients with idiopathic pulmonary fibrosis. Am Rev Respir Dis 137: 572, 1988.

42. Yamauchi K, Martinet Y, Crystal RG: Modulation of fibronectin gene expression in human mononuclear phagocytes. J Clin Invest 80: 1720, 1987.

43. Martinet Y, Rom WN, Grotendorst GR, et al: Exaggerated spontaneous release of platelet-derived growth factor by alveolar macrophages from patients with idiopathic pulmonary fibrosis. N Engl J Med 317: 202, 1987.

44. Chapman HA, Allen CL, Stone OL: Abnormalities in pathways of alveolar fibrin turnover among patients with interstitial lung disease. Am Rev Respir Dis 133: 437, 1986.

45. Calhoun WJ, Salisbury SM, Chosy LW, et al: Increased alveolar macrophage chemiluminescence and airspace cell superoxide production in active pulmonary sarcoidosis. J Lab Clin Med 112: 147, 1988.

46. Mitchell KN, Scadding JG, Heard BE, et al: Sarcoidosis: Histopathological definition and clinical diagnosis. J Clin Pathol 30: 395, 1977.

47. Rosen Y, Athanassiades TJ, Moon S, et al: Nongranulomatous interstitial pneumonitis in sarcoidosis. Relationship to development of epithelioid granulomas. Chest 74: 122, 1978.

48. Rosen Y, Moon S, Huang C-T, et al: Granulomatous pulmonary angiitis in sarcoidosis. Arch Pathol Lab Med 101: 170, 1977.

49. Rossman MD, Daniele RP, Dauber JH: Nodular endobronchial sarcoidosis: A study comparing blood and lung lymphocytes. Chest 79: 427, 1981.

50. Wollschlager C, Khan F: Aspergillomas complicating sarcoidosis. A prospective study in 100 patients. Chest 86: 585, 1984.

51. Maarsseveen ACM, Veldhuizen RW, Stam J, et al: A quantitative histomorphologic analysis of lymph node granulomas in sarcoidosis in relation to radiological stage I and II. J Pathol 134: 441, 1983.

52. Kirks DR, McCormick VD, Greenspan RH: Pulmonary sarcoidosis. Roentgenologic analysis of 150 patients. Am J Roentgenol 117: 777, 1973.

53. Kuhlman JE, Fishman EK, Hamper UM, et al: The computed tomographic spectrum of thoracic sarcoidosis. RadioGraphics 9: 449, 1989.

54. Spann RW, Rosenow EC III, DeRemee RA, et al: Unilateral hilar or paratracheal adenopathy in sarcoidosis: A study of 38 cases. Thorax 26: 296, 1971.

55. Rabinowitz JG, Ulreich S, Soriano C: The usual unusual manifestations of sarcoidosis and the "hilar haze"—a new diagnostic aid. Am J Roentgenol 120: 821, 1974.

56. Israel HL, Lenchner G, Steiner RM: Late development of mediastinal calcification in sarcoidosis. Am Rev Respir Dis 124: 302, 1981.

57. Rockoff SK, Rohatgi PK: Unusual manifestations of thoracic sarcoidosis. Am J Roentgenol 144; 513, 1985.

58. Bein ME, Putman CE, McCloud TC, et al: A re-evaluation of intrathoracic lymphadenopathy in sarcoidosis. Am J Roentgenol 131: 409, 1978.

59. Epler GR, McLoud TC, Gaensler EA, et al: Normal chest roentgenograms in chronic diffuse infiltrative lung disease. N Engl J Med 298: 934, 1978.

60. Schlossberg O, Sfedu E: Disseminated sarcoidosis. Sarcoidosis 4: 149, 1987.

61. Rosen Y, Amorosa JK, Moon S, et al: Occurrence of lung granulomas in patients with stage I sarcoidosis. Am J Roentgenol 129: 1083, 1977.

62. Austin JHM: Pulmonary sarcoidosis: What are we learning from CT? Radiology 171: 603, 1989.

63. Müller NL, Mawson JB, Mathieson JR, et al: Sarcoidosis: Correlation of extent of disease at CT with clinical, functional, and radiographic findings. Radiology 171: 613, 1989.

64. Wallaert B, Ramon P, Fournier EC, et al: Activated alveolar macrophage and lymphocyte alveolitis in extrathoracic sarcoidosis without radiological mediastinopulmonary involvement. Ann NY Acad Sci 465: 201, 1986.

65. Scadding JG: Prognosis of intrathoracic sarcoidosis in England. A review of 136 cases after five years' observation. Br Med J 2: 1165, 1961.

66. Baughman RP: Sarcoidosis. Usual and unusual manifestations (clinical conference). Chest 94: 165, 1988.

67. Stone DJ, Schwartz A: A long-term study of sarcoid and its modification by steroid therapy. Lung function and other factors in prognosis. Am J Med 41: 528, 1966.

68. Smellie H, Hoyle C: The hilar lymph nodes in sarcoidosis: With special reference to prognosis. Lancet 2: 66, 1957.

69. Ellis K, Renthal G: Pulmonary sarcoidosis: Roentgenographic observations on course of disease. Am J Roentgenol 88: 1070, 1962.

70. Mesbahi SJ, Davies P: Unilateral pulmonary changes in the chest x-ray in sarcoidosis. Clin Radiol 32: 283, 1981.

71. Grenier P, Valeyre D, Cluzel P, et al: Chronic diffuse interstitial lung disease: Diagnostic value of chest radiography and high-resolution CT. Radiology 179: 123, 1991.

72. Brauner MW, Grenier P, Mompoint D, et al: Pulmonary sarcoidosis: Evaluation with high-resolution CT. Radiology 172: 467, 1989.

72a. Murdoch J, Müller NL: Pulmonary sarcoidosis: Changes on follow-up CT examination. Am J Roentgenol 159: 473, 1992.

73. Teirstein AS, Siltzbach LE: Sarcoidosis of the upper lung fields simulating pulmonary tuberculosis. Chest 64: 303, 1973.

74. Rubinstein I, Solomon A, Baum GL, et al: Pulmonary sarcoidosis presenting with unusual roentgenographic manifestations. Eur J Respir Dis 67: 335, 1985.

75. Rose RM, Lee RG, Costello P: Solitary nodular sarcoidosis. Clin Radiol 36: 589, 1985.

76. Rakower J: Sarcoidal bilateral hilar lymphoma (Löfgren's syndrome): A review of 31 cases. Am Rev Respir Dis 87: 518, 1963.

77. Conant EF, Glickstein MF, Mahar P, et al: Pulmonary sarcoidosis in the older patient: Conventional radiographic features. Radiology 169: 315, 1988.

78. Freundlich IM, Libshitz HI, Glassman LM, et al: Sarcoidosis. Typical and atypical thoracic manifestations and complications. Clin Radiol 21: 376, 1970.

79. Henry DA, Kiser PE, Scheer CE, et al: Multiple imaging evaluation of sarcoidosis. RadioGraphics 6: 75, 1986.

80. Wilen SB, Rabinowitz JG, Ulreich S, et al: Pleural involvement in sarcoidosis. Am J Med 57: 200, 1974.

81. Knox AJ, Wardman AG, Page RL: Tuberculosis pleural effusion occurring during corticosteroid treatment of sarcoidosis. Thorax 41: 651, 1986.

82. Gomm SA: An unusual presentation of sarcoidosis: Spontaneous haemopneumothorax. Postgrad Med J 60: 621, 1984.

83. Whitcomb ME, Hawley PC, Domby WR, et al: The role of fiberoptic bronchoscopy in the diagnosis of sarcoidosis. Clinical conference in pulmonary disease from Ohio State University, Columbus. Chest 74: 205, 1978.

84. Murray RO, Jacobson HG: The Radiology of Skeletal Disorders. Baltimore, Williams & Wilkins, 1971.

85. McBrine CS, Fisher MS: Acrosclerosis in sarcoidosis. Radiology 115: 279, 1975.

86. Lin S-R, Levy W, Go EB, et al: Unusual osteosclerotic changes in sarcoidosis, simulating osteoblastic metastases. Radiology 106: 311, 1973.

87. Weston M, Duffy P: Osteosclerosis in sarcoidosis. Australas Radiol 19: 191, 1975.

88. Yaghmai I: Radiographic, angiographic and radionuclide manifestations of osseous sarcoidosis. RadioGraphics 3: 375, 1983.

89. McCort JJ, Paré JAP: Pulmonary fibrosis and cor pulmonale in sarcoidosis. Radiology 62: 496, 1954.

90. Miller A: The vanishing lung syndrome associated with pulmonary sarcoidosis. Br J Dis Chest 75: 209, 1981.

91. Winterbauer RH, Belic N, Moores KD: A clinical interpretation of bilateral hilar adenopathy. Ann Intern Med 78: 65, 1973.

92. Rudberg-Roos I: The course and prognosis of sarcoidosis as observed in 296 cases. Acta Tuberc Scand 52(Suppl): 1, 1962.

93. Siltzbach LE, James DG, Neville E, et al: Course and prognosis of sarcoidosis around the world. Am J Med 57: 847, 1974.

94. Longcope WT, Freiman DG: A study of sarcoidosis. Based on a combined investigation of 160 cases including 30 autopsies from The Johns Hopkins Hospital and Massachusetts General Hospital. Medicine 31: 1, 1952.

95. Israel HL, Lenchner GS, Atkinson GW: Sarcoidosis and aspergilloma: The role of surgery. Chest 82: 430, 1982.

96. Liss HP: Pleuropericarditis in sarcoidosis. South Med J 79: 258, 1986.

97. Fogel TD, Weissberg JB, Dobular K, et al: Radiotherapy in sarcoidosis of the larynx: Case report and review of the literature. Laryngoscope 94: 1223, 1984.

98. Firooznia H, Young R, Lee T: Sarcoidosis of the larynx. Radiology 95: 425, 1970.

99. el-Kassimi FA, Ashour M, Vijayaraghavan R: Sarcoidosis presenting as recurrent left laryngeal nerve palsy. Thorax 45: 565, 1990.

100. Damuth TE, Bower JS, Cho K, et al: Major pulmonary artery stenosis causing pulmonary hypertension in sarcoidosis. Chest 78: 888, 1980.

101. Hoffstein V, Ranganathan N, Mullen JB: Sarcoidosis simulating pulmonary veno-occlusive disease. Am Rev Respir Dis 134: 809, 1986.

102. Silverman KJ, Hutchins GM, Buckley BH: Cardiac sarcoid: A clinicopathologic study of 84 unselected patients with systemic sarcoidosis. Circulation 58: 1204, 1978.

103. Thunell M, Bjerle P, Stjernberg N: ECG abnormalities in patients with sarcoidosis. Acta Med Scand 213: 115, 1983.

104. Lillington GA, Jamplis RW: Scalene node biopsy. Ann Intern Med 59: 101, 1963.

105. Olive KE, Kataria YP: Cutaneous manifestations of sarcoidosis. Relationships to other organ system involvement, abnormal laboratory measurements, and disease course. Arch Intern Med 145: 1811, 1985.

106. Löfgren S, Lundbäck H: The bilateral hilar lymphoma syndrome. I. A study of the relation to age and sex in 212 cases. II. A study of the relation to tuberculosis and sarcoidosis in 212 cases. Acta Med Scand 142: 259, 1952.

107. James DG: Dermatological aspects of sarcoidosis. Q J Med 28: 109, 1959.

108. Kataria YP, Whitcomb ME: Splenomegaly in sarcoidosis. Arch Intern Med 140: 35, 1980.

109. Sprague R, Harper P, McClain S, et al: Disseminated gastrointestinal sarcoidosis. Case report and review of the literature. Gastroenterology 87: 421, 1984.

110. Douglas JG, Gillon J, Logan RF, et al: Sarcoidosis and coeliac disease: An association? Lancet 2: 13, 1984.

111. McCormick PA, Feighery C, Dolan C, et al: Altered gastrointestinal immune response in sarcoidosis. Gut 29: 1628, 1988.

112. Kaplan H: Sarcoid arthritis: A review. Arch Intern Med 112: 924, 1963.

113. Perruquet JL, Harrington TM, Davis DE, et al: Sarcoid arthritis in a North American Caucasian population. J Rheumatol 11: 521, 1984.

114. Rahbar M, Sharma OP: Hypertrophic osteoarthropathy in sarcoidosis. Sarcoidosis 7: 125, 1990.

115. Dixey J, Redington AN, Butler RC, et al: The arthropathy of cystic fibrosis. Ann Rheum Dis 47: 218, 1988.

116. Nessan VJ, Jacoway JR: Biopsy of minor salivary glands in the diagnosis of sarcoidosis. N Engl J Med 301: 922, 1979.

117. King BP, Esparza AR, Kahn SI, et al: Sarcoid granulomatous nephritis occurring as isolated renal failure. Arch Intern Med 136: 241, 1976.

118. Taylor RG, Fisher C, Hoffbrand BI: Sarcoidosis and membranous glomerulonephritis: A significant association. Br Med J 284: 1297, 1982.

119. Delaney P: Neurologic manifestations in sarcoidosis. Review of the literature, with a report of 23 cases. Ann Intern Med 87: 336, 1977.

120. Karnik AS: Nodular cerebral sarcoidosis simulating metastatic carcinoma. Arch Intern Med 142: 385, 1982.

121. Rosenbloom MA, Uphoff DF: The association of progressive multifocal leukoencephalopathy and sarcoidosis. Chest 83: 572, 1983.

122. Stoudemire A, Linfors E, Houpt JL: Central nervous system sarcoidosis. Gen Hosp Psychiatry 5: 129, 1983.

123. Winnacker JL, Becker KL, Katz S: Endocrine aspects of sarcoidosis. N Engl J Med 278: 427, 1968.

124. Rubinstein I, Baum GL, Hiss Y, et al: Sarcoidosis and Hashimoto's thyroiditis: A chance occurrence? Respiration 48: 136, 1985.

125. Sharma OP, Ahamad I: The CREST syndrome and sarcoidosis. Another example of an overlap syndrome. Sarcoidosis 5: 71, 1988.

126. Deheinzelin D, de Cavalho CR, Tomazini ME, et al: Association of Sjögren's syndrome and sarcoidosis. Report of a case. Sarcoidosis 5: 68, 1988.

127. Swen JS, Forse MS, Hyland RH, et al: The malignancy-sarcoidosis syndrome. Chest 98: 1300, 1990.

128. Van Hoef ME, Schornagel JH: Testicular cancer with enlarged mediastinal lymph nodes: A diagnostic pitfall. Neth J Med 37: 202, 1990.

129. Urbanski SJ, Alison RE, Jewett MAS, et al: Association of germ cell tumours of the testis and intrathoracic sarcoid-like lesions. Can Med Assoc J 137: 416, 1987.

130. Keogh BA, Crystal RG: Pulmonary function testing in interstitial pulmonary disease: What does it tell us? Chest 78: 856, 1980.

131. Winterbauer RH, Hutchinson JF: Use of pulmonary function tests in the management of sarcoidosis. Chest 78: 640, 1980.

132. Young RC Jr, Carr C, Shelton TG, et al: Sarcoidosis: Relationship between changes in lung structure and function. Am Rev Respir Dis 95: 224, 1967.

133. Divertie MB, Cassan SM, O'Brien PC, et al: Fine structural morphometry of diffuse lung diseases with abnormal blood-air gas transfer. Mayo Clin Proc 51: 42, 1976.

134. Bärdvik I, Wollmer P, Blom-Bülow B, et al: Lung mechanics and gas exchange during exercise in pulmonary sarcoidosis. Chest 99: 572, 1991.

135. Baughman RP, Gerson M, Bosken CH: Right and left ventricular functions at rest and with exercise in patients with sarcoidosis. Chest 85: 301, 1984.

136. Sharma OP, Johnson R: Airway obstruction in sarcoidosis. A study of 123 nonsmoking black American patients with sarcoidosis. Chest 94: 343, 1988.

137. Line BR, Hunninghake GW, Keogh BA, et al: Gallium-67 scanning to stage the alveolitis of sarcoidosis: Correlation with clinical studies, pulmonary function studies and bronchoalveolar lavage. Am Rev Respir Dis 123: 440, 1981.

138. Ebright JR, Soin JS, Manoli RS: The gallium scan: Problems and misuse in examination of patients with suspected infection. Arch Intern Med 142: 246, 1982.

139. Klech H, Kohn H, Kummer F, et al: Assessment of activity in sarcoidosis. Sensitivity and specificity of 67 gallium scintigraphy, serum ACE levels, chest roentgenography, and blood lymphocyte populations. Chest 82: 732, 1982.

140. Perrin-Fayolle M, Pacheco Y, Harf R, et al: Angiotensin-converting enzyme in bronchoalveolar lavage fluid in pulmonary sarcoidosis. Thorax 36: 790, 1981.

141. Mordelet-Dambrine MS, Stanislas-Leguern GM, Huchon GJ, et al: Elevation of the bronchoalveolar concentration of angiotensin-I converting enzyme in sarcoidosis. Am Rev Respir Dis 126: 472, 1982.

142. Fanburg BL, Schoenberger MD, Bachus B, et al: Elevated serum angiotensin-I converting enzyme in sarcoidosis. Am Rev Respir Dis 114: 525, 1976.

143. Rohatgi PK, Ryan JW, Lindeman P: Value of serial measurement of serum angiotensin-converting enzyme in the management of sarcoidosis. Am J Med 70: 44, 1981.

144. Rohatgi PK: Serum angiotensin-converting enzyme in pulmonary disease [review]. Lung 160: 287, 1982.
145. Baur X, Fruhmann G, Dahlheim H: Follow-up of angiotensin-converting enzyme in serum of patients with sarcoidosis. Respiration 41: 133, 1981.
146. Yotsumoto H: Longitudinal observations of serum angiotensin-converting enzyme activity in sarcoidosis with and without treatment. Chest 82: 556, 1982.
147. Selroos O, Gronhagen-Riska C: Angiotensin-converting enzyme. III. Changes in serum level as an indicator of disease activity in untreated sarcoidosis. Scand J Respir Dis 60: 328, 1979.
148. Schoenberger CI, Line BR, Keogh BA, et al: Lung inflammation in sarcoidosis: Comparison of serum angiotensin-converting enzyme with bronchoalveolar lavage and gallium-67 scanning assessment of the T-lymphocyte alveolitis. Thorax 37: 19, 1982.
149. Rossman MD, Dauber JH, Cardillo ME, et al: Pulmonary sarcoidosis: Correlation of serum angiotensin-converting enzyme with blood and bronchoalveolar lymphocytes. Am Rev Respir Dis 125: 366, 1982.
150. Gronhagen-Riska C, Selroos O: Angiotensin-converting enzyme. IV. Changes in serum activity and in lysozyme concentrations as indicators of the course of untreated sarcoidosis. Scand J Respir Dis 60: 337, 1979.
151. Turton CWG, Grundy E, Firth G, et al: Value of measuring serum angiotensin-I converting enzyme and serum lysozyme in the management of sarcoidosis. Thorax 334: 57, 1979.
152. Goldstein RA, Israel HL, Becker KL, et al: The infrequency of hypercalcemia in sarcoidosis. Am J Med 51: 21, 1971.
153. Reiner M, Sigurdsson G, Nunziata V, et al: Abnormal calcium metabolism in normocalcaemic sarcoidosis. Br Med J 2: 1473, 1976.
154. Löfgren S, Snellman B, Lindgren AGH: Renal complications in sarcoidosis. Functional and biopsy studies. Acta Med Scand 159: 295, 1957.
155. Meyrier A, Valeyre D, Bouillon R, et al: Different mechanisms of hypercalciuria in sarcoidosis. Correlations with disease extension and activity. Ann NY Acad Sci 465: 575, 1986.
156. Lower EE, Smith JT, Martelo OJ, et al: The anemia of sarcoidosis. Sarcoidosis 5: 51, 1988.
157. Bogaerts Y, Van Der Straeten M, Tasson J, et al: Sarcoidosis or malignancy: A diagnostic dilemma. Eur J Respir Dis 64: 541, 1983.
158. Mitchell DM, Mitchell DN, Collins JV, et al: Transbronchial lung biopsy through fibreoptic bronchoscope in diagnosis of sarcoidosis. Br Med J 280: 679, 1980.
159. Mitchell DM, Mitchell DN, Collins JV, et al: Transbronchial lung biopsy through fibreoptic bronchoscope in diagnosis of sarcoidosis. Br J Dis Chest 74: 320, 1980.
160. Roethe RA, Fuller PB, Byrd RB, et al: Transbronchoscopic lung biopsy in sarcoidosis: Optimal number and sites for diagnosis. Chest 77: 400, 1980.
161. Mikhail JR, Mitchell DN, Drury RAB, et al: A comparison of the value of mediastinal lymph node biopsy and the Kveim test in sarcoidosis. Am Rev Respir Dis 104: 544, 1971.
162. Vernon SE: Nodular pulmonary sarcoidosis. Diagnosis with fine needle aspiration biopsy. Acta Cytologica 29: 473, 1985.
163. Johns CJ, Schonfeld SA, Scott PP, et al: Longitudinal study of chronic sarcoidosis with low-dose maintenance corticosteroid therapy. Outcome and complications. Ann NY Acad Sci 465: 702, 1986.
164. Reich JM, Johnson RE: Course and prognosis of sarcoidosis in a nonreferral setting. Analysis of 86 patients observed for 10 years. Am J Med 78: 61, 1985.
165. Young RC Jr, Titus-Dillon PY, Schneider ML, et al: Sarcoidosis in Washington, D.C. Clinical observations in 105 black patients. Arch Intern Med 125: 102, 1970.
166. Management of pulmonary sarcoidosis [editorial]. Lancet 1: 890, 1982.
167. Israel HL, Karlin P, Menduke H, et al: Factors affecting outcome of sarcoidosis. Influence of race, extrathoracic involvement, and initial radiologic lung lesions. Ann NY Acad Sci 465: 609, 1986.
168. Neville E, Walker AN, James DG: Prognostic factors predicting the outcome of sarcoidosis: An analysis of 818 patients. Q J Med 52: 525, 1983.
169. Kendig EL, Brummer DL: The prognosis of sarcoidosis in children. Chest 70: 351, 1976.
170. Huhti E, Poukkula A, Lilja M: Prognosis for sarcoidosis in a defined geographical area. Br J Dis Chest 81: 381, 1987.
171. Johnston RN: Pulmonary sarcoidosis after ten to twenty years. Scott Med J 31: 72, 1986.
172. McLoud TC, Epler GR, Gaensler EA, et al: A radiographic classification for sarcoidosis: Physiologic correlation. Invest Radiol 17: 129, 1982.
173. Meier-Sydow J, Rust MG, Kappos A, et al: The long-term course of airflow obstruction in obstructive variants of the fibrotic stage of sarcoidosis and of idiopathic pulmonary fibrosis. Ann NY Acad Sci 465: 515, 1986.
174. Keogh BA, Hunninghake GW, Line BR, et al: The alveolitis of pulmonary sarcoidosis. Evaluation of natural history and alveolitis-dependent changes in lung function. Am Rev Respir Dis 128: 256, 1983.
175. Costabel U, Bross KJ, Guzman J, et al: Predictive value of bronchoalveolar T cell subsets for the course of pulmonary sarcoidosis. Ann NY Acad Sci 465: 418, 1986.
176. Ueda E, Kawabe T, Tachibana T, et al: Serum angiotensin-converting enzyme activity as an indicator of prognosis in sarcoidosis. Am Rev Respir Dis 121: 667, 1980.
177. Weaver LJ, Solliday NH, Celic L, et al: Serial observations of angiotensin-converting enzyme and pulmonary function in sarcoidosis. Arch Intern Med 141: 931, 1981.
178. Okada M, Takahashi H, Nukiwa T, et al: Correlative analysis of longitudinal changes in bronchoalveolar lavage, 67 gallium scanning, serum angiotensin-converting enzyme activity, chest x-ray, and pulmonary function tests in pulmonary sarcoidosis. Jpn J Med 26: 360, 1987.
179. Israel HL: Prognosis of sarcoidosis. Ann Intern Med 73: 1038, 1970.
180. Haynes de Regt R: Sarcoidosis and pregnancy. Obstet Gynecol 70: 369, 1987.
181. Liebow AA, Carrington CB: The interstitial pneumonias. In Simon M, Potchen EJ, LeMay M (eds): Frontiers of Pulmonary Radiology. New York, Grune & Stratton, 1969, p 102.
182. Scadding JG, Hinson KFW: Diffuse fibrosing alveolitis (diffuse interstitial fibrosis of the lungs). Thorax 22: 291, 1967.
183. Chapman JR, Charles PJ, Venables PJW, et al: Definition and clinical relevance of antibodies to nuclear ribonucleoprotein and other nuclear antigens in patients with cryptogenic fibrosing alveolitis. Am Rev Respir Dis 130: 439, 1984.
184. McFadden RG, Craig ID, Paterson NAM: Interstitial pneumonitis in myasthenia gravis. Br J Dis Chest 78: 187, 1984.
185. Turner-Warwick M: Fibrosing alveolitis and chronic liver disease. Q J Med 37: 133, 1968.
186. Williams AJ, March J, Stableforth DE: Cryptogenic fibrosing alveolitis, chronic active hepatitis, and autoimmune haemolytic anaemia in the same patient. Br J Dis Chest 79: 200, 1985.
187. Scadding JG: Diffuse pulmonary alveolar fibrosis. Thorax 29: 271, 1974.
188. Nagaya H, Elmore M, Ford CD: Idiopathic interstitial pulmonary fibrosis. An immune complex disease. Am Rev Respir Dis 107: 826, 1973.
189. Deodhar SD, Bhagwat AG: Desquamative interstitial pneumonia–like syndrome in rabbits. Arch Pathol 84: 54, 1967.
190. Stein-Streilein J, Lipscomb MF, Fisch H, et al: Pulmonary interstitial fibrosis induced in hapten-immune hamsters. Am Rev Respir Dis 136: 119, 1987.
191. Barzo P: Familial idiopathic fibrosing alveolitis. Eur J Respir Dis 66: 350, 1985.
192. Solliday NH, Williams JA, Gaensler EA, et al: Familial chronic interstitial pneumonia. Am Rev Respir Dis 108: 193, 1973.
193. Libby DM, Gibofsky A, Fotino M, et al: Immunogenetic and clinical findings in idiopathic pulmonary fibrosis. Association with the B-cell alloantigen HLA-DR2. Am Rev Respir Dis 127: 618, 1983.
194. Koch B: Familial fibrocystic pulmonary dysplasia: Observations in one family. Can Med Assoc J 92: 801, 1965.
195. Campbell EJ, Harris B, Avioli LV: Idiopathic pulmonary fibrosis. Arch Intern Med 141: 771, 1981.
196. Pinsker KL, Schneyer B, Becker N, et al: Usual interstitial pneumonia following Texas A2 influenza infection. Chest 80: 123, 1981.
197. Patchefsky AS, Banner M, Freundlich IM: Desquamative interstitial pneumonia: Significance of intranuclear viral-like inclusion bodies. Ann Intern Med 74: 322, 1971.
198. McNary WF Jr, Gaensler EA: Intranuclear inclusion bodies in desquamative interstitial pneumonia. Ann Intern Med 74: 404, 1971.
199. Vergnon JM, Vincent M, de The G, et al: Cryptogenic fibrosing

alveolitis and Epstein-Barr virus: An association? Lancet 2: 768, 1984.

199a. Ueda T, Ohta K, Suzuki N, et al: Idiopathic pulmonary fibrosis and high prevalence of serum antibodies to hepatitis C virus. Am Rev Respir Dis 146: 266, 1992.

200. Haslem PL, Turton CWG, Heard B, et al: Bronchoalveolar lavage in pulmonary fibrosis: Comparison of cells obtained with lung biopsy and clinical features. Thorax 35: 9, 1980.

201. O'Donnell K, Keogh B, Cantin A, et al: Pharmacologic suppression of the neutrophil component of the alveolitis in idiopathic pulmonary fibrosis. Am Rev Respir Dis 136: 288, 1987.

202. Ozaki T, Hayashi H, Tani K, et al: Neutrophil chemotactic factors in the respiratory tract of patients with chronic airway diseases or idiopathic pulmonary fibrosis. Am Rev Respir Dis 145: 85, 1992.

203. Hunninghake GW, Gadek JE, Lawley TJ: Mechanisms of neutrophil accumulation in the lungs of patients with idiopathic pulmonary fibrosis. J Clin Invest 68: 259, 1981.

204. Keogh BA, Bernardo J, Hunninghake GW, et al: Effect of intermittent high dose parenteral corticosteroids on the alveolitis of idiopathic pulmonary fibrosis. Am Rev Respir Dis 127: 18, 1983.

205. Behr J, Maier K, Krombach F, et al: Pathogenetic significance of reactive oxygen species in diffuse fibrosing alveolitis. Am Rev Respir Dis 144: 146, 1991.

206. Kiemle-Kallee J, Kreipe H, Radzun HJ, et al: Alveolar macrophages in idiopathic pulmonary fibrosis display a more monocyte-like immunophenotype and an increased release of free oxygen radicals. Eur Respir J 4: 400, 1991.

207. Campbell DA, Poulter LW, Janossy G, et al: Immunohistological analysis of lung tissue from patients with cryptogenic fibrosing alveolitis suggesting local expression of immune hypersensitivity. Thorax 40: 405, 1985.

208. Emura M, Nagai S, Takeuchi M, et al: In vitro production of B cell growth factor and B cell differentiation factor by peripheral blood mononuclear cells and bronchoalveolar lavage T lymphocytes from patients with idiopathic pulmonary fibrosis. Clin Exp Immunol 82: 133, 1990.

209. Vignaud JM, Allam M, Martinet N, et al: Presence of platelet-derived growth factor in normal and fibrotic lung is specifically associated with interstitial macrophages, while both interstitial macrophages and alveolar epithelial cells express the c-sis proto-oncogene. Am J Respir Cell Mol Biol 5: 531, 1991.

210. Ozaki T, Moriguchi H, Nakamura Y, et al: Regulatory effect of prostaglandin E_2 on fibronectin release from human alveolar macrophages. Am Rev Respir Dis 141: 965, 1990.

211. Fulmer JD, Bienkowski RS, Cowan MJ, et al: Collagen concentration and rates of synthesis in idiopathic pulmonary fibrosis. Am Rev Respir Dis 122: 289, 1980.

212. Selman M, Montaño M, Ramos C, et al: Concentration, biosynthesis and degradation of collagen in idiopathic pulmonary fibrosis. Thorax 41: 355, 1986.

213. Gaensler EA, Jederlinic PJ, Churg A: Idiopathic pulmonary fibrosis in asbestos-exposed workers. Am Rev Respir Dis 144: 689, 1991.

214. Monosó I, Tura JM, Pujadas J, et al: Lung dust content in idiopathic pulmonary fibrosis: A study with scanning electron microscopy and energy dispersive x-ray analysis. Br J Ind Med 48: 327, 1991.

215. Kuisk H, Sanchez JS: Diffuse bronchiolectasis with muscular hyperplasia ("muscular cirrhosis of the lung"): Relationship to chronic form of Hamman-Rich syndrome. Am J Roentgenol 96: 979, 1966.

216. Bedrossian CWM, Kuhn C III, Luna MA, et al: Desquamative interstitial pneumonia-like reaction accompanying pulmonary lesions. Chest 72: 166, 1977.

217. Liebow AA, Steer A, Billingsley J: Desquamative interstitial pneumonia. Am J Med 39: 369, 1965.

218. Feigin DS, Friedman PJ: Chest radiography in desquamative interstitial pneumonitis: A review of 37 patients. Am J Roentgenol 134: 91, 1980.

219. Stilwell PC, Norris DG, O'Connell EJ, et al: Desquamative interstitial pneumonitis in children. Chest 77: 165, 1980.

220. Carrington CB, Gaensler EA, Coutu RE, et al: Natural history and treated course of usual and desquamative interstitial pneumonia. N Engl J Med 298: 801, 1978.

221. Nishimura K, Mitaichi M, Izumi T, et al: Usual interstitial pneumonia: Histologic correlation with high-resolution CT. Radiology 182: 337, 1992.

222. Wiggins J, Strickland B, Turner-Warwick M: Combined cryptogenic

fibrosing alveolitis and emphysema: The value of high resolution computed tomography in assessment. Respir Med 84: 365, 1990.

223. Bergin C, Castellino RA: Mediastinal lymph node enlargement on CT scans in patients with usual interstitial pneumonitis. Am J Roentgenol 154: 251, 1990.

224. Picado C, Gomez de Almeida R, Xaubet A, et al: Spontaneous pneumothorax in cryptogenic fibrosing alveolitis. Respiration 48: 77, 1985.

225. Müller NL, Staples CA, Miller RR, et al: Disease activity in idiopathic pulmonary fibrosis: CT and pathologic correlation. Radiology 165: 731, 1987.

226. Staples CA, Müller NL, Vedal S, et al: Unusual interstitial pneumonia: Correlation of CT with clinical, functional, and radiologic findings. Radiology 162: 377, 1987.

227. Terriff BA, Kwan SY, Chan-Yeung MM, et al: Fibrosing alveolitis: chest radiography and CT as predictors of clinical and functional impairment at follow-up in 26 patients. Radiology 184: 445, 1992.

228. Müller NL, Staples CA, Miller RR, et al: Disease activity in idiopathic pulmonary fibrosis: CT and pathologic correlation. Radiology 165: 731, 1987.

229. Lee JS, Im J-G, Ahn JM, et al: Fibrosing alveolitis: Prognostic implication of ground-glass attenuation at high-resolution CT. Radiology 184: 451, 1992.

230. McFadden RG, Carr TJ, Wood TE: Proton magnetic resonance imaging to stage activity of interstitial lung disease. Chest 92: 31, 1987.

231. Westcott JL, Cole SR: Traction bronchiectasis in end-stage pulmonary fibrosis. Radiology 161: 665, 1986.

232. Woodring JH, Barrett PA, Rehm SR, et al: Acquired tracheomegaly in adults as a complication of diffuse fibrosis. AJR 152: 743, 1989.

233. Crystal RG, Fulmer JD, Roberts WC, et al: Idiopathic pulmonary fibrosis. Ann Intern Med 85: 769, 1976.

234. Walshaw MJ, Nisar M, Pearson MG, et al: Expiratory lung crackles in patients with fibrosing alveolitis. Chest 97: 407, 1990.

235. DeRemee RA, Harrison EG Jr, Andersen HA: The concept of classic interstitial pneumonitis-fibrosis (CIP-F) as a clinicopathologic syndrome. Chest 61: 213, 1972.

236. Semple PD, Beastall GH, Brown TM, et al: Sex hormone suppression and sexual impotence in hypoxic pulmonary fibrosis. Thorax 39: 46, 1984.

237. Snell NJC, Coysh HL: Persistent hyponatremia complicating fibrosing alveolitis. Thorax 33: 820, 1978.

238. Webb DR, Currie GD: Pulmonary fibrosis masking polymyositis. JAMA 222: 1146, 1972.

239. Wright PH, Heard BE, Steel SJ, et al: Cryptogenic fibrosing alveolitis: Assessment by graded trephine lung biopsy. Histology compared with clinical, radiographic, and physiological features. Br J Dis Chest 745: 61, 1981.

240. Chuang MT, Raskin J, Krellenstein DJ, et al: Bronchoscopy in diffuse lung disease: Evaluation by open lung biopsy in nondiagnostic transbronchial lung biopsy. Ann Otol Rhinol Laryngol 96: 654, 1987.

241. Epler GR, Saber FA, Gaensler EA: Determination of severe impairment (disability) in interstitial lung disease. Am Rev Respir Dis 121: 647, 1980.

242. Weitzenblum E, Ehrart M, Rasaholinjanahary J, et al: Pulmonary hemodynamics in idiopathic pulmonary fibrosis and other interstitial pulmonary diseases. Respiration 44: 118, 1983.

243. Chinet T, Jaubert F, Dusser D, et al: Effects of inflammation and fibrosis on pulmonary function in diffuse lung fibrosis. Thorax 45: 675, 1990.

244. Schwartz DA, Merchant RK, Helmers RA, et al: The influence of cigarette smoking on lung function in patients with idiopathic pulmonary fibrosis. Am Rev Respir Dis 144: 504, 1991.

245. Hanley ME, King TE Jr, Schwarz MI, et al: The impact of smoking on mechanical properties of the lungs in idiopathic pulmonary fibrosis and sarcoidosis. Am Rev Respir Dis 144: 1102, 1991.

246. Risk C, Epler GR, Gaensler EA: Exercise alveolar-arterial oxygen pressure difference in interstitial lung disease. Chest 85: 69, 1984.

247. McCarthy D, Cherniack RM: Regional ventilation-perfusion and hypoxia in cryptogenic fibrosing alveolitis. Am Rev Respir Dis 107: 200, 1973.

248. Agustí AG, Roca J, Gea J, et al: Mechanisms of gas-exchange impairment in idiopathic pulmonary fibrosis. Am Rev Respir Dis 143: 219, 1991.

249. Turner-Warwick M, Burrows B, Johnson A: Cryptogenic fibrosing alveolitis: Clinical features and their influence on survival. Thorax 35: 171, 1980.

250. Olson J, Colby TV, Elliot CG: Hamman-Rich syndrome revisited. Mayo Clin Proc 65: 1538, 1990.
251. Stack BHR, Choo-Kang YFJ, Heard BE: The prognosis of cryptogenic fibrosing alveolitis. Thorax 27: 535, 1972.
252. Tukiainen P, Taskinen E, Holsti P, et al: Prognosis of cryptogenic fibrosing alveolitis. Thorax 38: 349, 1983.
253. Prichard MG, Musk AW: Adverse effect of pregnancy on familial fibrosing alveolitis. Thorax 39: 319, 1984.
254. Raghu G, Depaso WJ, Cain K, et al: Azathioprine combined with prednisone in the treatment of idiopathic pulmonary fibrosis: A prospective double-blind, randomized, placebo-controlled clinical trial. Am Rev Respir Dis 144: 291, 1991.
255. Chester EH, Fleming GM, Montenegro H: Effect of steroid therapy on gas exchange abnormalities in patients with diffuse interstitial lung disease. Chest 69: 269, 1976.
256. Capron F, Ameille J, Leclerc P, et al: Pulmonary lymphangioleiomyomatosis and Bourneville's tuberous sclerosis with pulmonary involvement: The same disease? Cancer 52: 851, 1983.
257. Hughes E, Hodder RV: Pulmonary lymphangiomyomatosis complicating pregnancy. A case report. J Reprod Med 32: 553, 1987.
258. Shen A, Iseman MD, Waldron JA, et al: Exacerbation of pulmonary lymphangioleiomyomatosis by exogenous estrogens. Chest 91: 782, 1987.
259. Berger U, Khaghani A, Pomerance A, et al: Pulmonary lymphangioleiomyomatosis and steroid receptors. An immunocytochemical study. Am J Clin Pathol 93: 609, 1990.
260. Carrington CB, Cugell DW, Gaensler EA, et al: Lymphangioleiomyomatosis. Physiologic-pathologic-radiologic correlations. Am Rev Respir Dis 116: 977, 1977.
261. Jenner RE, Oo HLA: Isolated chylopericardium due to mediastinal lymphangiomatous hamartoma. Thorax 30: 113, 1975.
262. Corrin B, Liebow AA, Friedman PJ: Pulmonary lymphangiomyomatosis. Am J Pathol 79: 347, 1975.
263. Müller NL, Chiles C, Kullnig P: Pulmonary lymphangiomyomatosis: Correlation of CT with radiographic and functional findings. Radiology 175: 335, 1990.
264. Lenoir S, Grenier P, Brauner MW, et al: Pulmonary lymphangiomyomatosis and tuberous sclerosis: Comparison of radiographic and thin-section CT findings. Radiology 175: 329, 1990.
265. Aberle DR, Hansell DM, Brown K, et al: Lymphangiomyomatosis: CT, chest radiographic, and functional correlations. Radiology 176: 381, 1990.
266. McCarty KS Jr, Mossler JA, McLelland R, et al: Pulmonary lymphangiomyomatosis responsive to progesterone. N Engl J Med 303: 1461, 1980.
267. Taylor JR, Ryu J, Colby TV, et al: Lymphangioleiomyomatosis. Clinical course in 32 patients. N Engl J Med 323: 1254, 1990.
268. Slingerland JM, Grossman RF, Chamberlain D, et al: Pulmonary manifestations of tuberous sclerosis in first degree relatives. Thorax 44: 212, 1989.
269. Foresti V, Casati O, Zubani R, et al: Chylous pleural effusion in tuberous sclerosis. Respiration 57: 398, 1990.
270. Lagos JC, Gomez MR: Tuberous sclerosis: Reappraisal of a clinical entity. Mayo Clin Proc 42: 26, 1967.
271. Dwyer JM, Hickie JB, Garvan J: Pulmonary tuberous sclerosis. Report of three patients and a review of the literature. Q J Med 40: 115, 1971.
272. Riccardi VM: von Recklinghausen neurofibromatosis. N Engl J Med 3205: 1617, 1981.
273. Massaro D, Katz S: Fibrosing alveolitis: Its occurrence, roentgenographic and pathologic features in von Recklinghausen's neurofibromatosis. Am Rev Respir Dis 93: 934, 1966.
274. Burkhalter JL, Morano JU, McCay MB: Diffuse interstitial lung disease in neurofibromatosis. South Med J 79: 944, 1986.
275. Bourgouin PM, Shepard JO, Moore EH, et al: Plexiform neurofibromatosis of the mediastinum: CT appearance. Am J Roentgenol 151: 461, 1988.
276. Unger PD, Geller SA, Anderson PJ: Pulmonary lesions in a patient with neurofibromatosis. Arch Pathol Lab Med 108: 654, 1984.
277. Webb WR, Goodman PC: Fibrosing alveolitis in patients with neurofibromatosis. Radiology 122: 289, 1977.
278. Dunmore LA Jr, El-Khoury SA: Eosinophilic granuloma of the lung. A report of three cases in Negro patients. Am Rev Respir Dis 90: 789, 1964.
279. Friedman PJ, Liebow AA, Sokoloff J: Eosinophilic granuloma of lung:

Clinical aspects of primary pulmonary histiocytosis in the adult. Medicine 60: 385, 1981.
280. Greenberger JS, Crocker AC, Vawter G, et al: Results of treatment of 127 patients with systemic histiocytosis (Letterer-Siwe's syndrome, Schuller-Christian syndrome and multifocal eosinophilic granuloma). Medicine 60: 311, 1981.
281. King TE Jr, Schwarz MI, Dreisin RE, et al: Circulating immune complexes in pulmonary eosinophilic granuloma. Ann Intern Med 91: 397, 1979.
282. Weinberger SE, Kelman JA, Elson NA, et al: Bronchoalveolar lavage in interstitial lung disease. Ann Intern Med 89: 459, 1978.
283. Hance AJ, Basset P, Saumon G, et al: Smoking and interstitial lung disease. The effect of cigarette smoking on the incidence of pulmonary histiocytosis X and sarcoidosis. Ann NY Acad Sci 465: 643, 1986.
284. Colby TV, Lombard C: Histiocytosis X in the lung. Human Pathol 14: 847, 1983.
285. Webber D, Tron V, Askin F, et al: S-100 staining in the diagnosis of eosinophilic granuloma of lung. Am J Clin Pathol 84: 447, 1985.
286. Ide F, Iwase T, Saito I, et al: Immunohistochemical and ultrastructural analysis of the proliferating cells in histiocytosis X. Cancer 53: 917, 1984.
287. Verea-Hernando H, Fontan-Bueso J, Martin-Egana MT, et al: Langerhans' cells in bronchoalveolar lavage in the late stages of pulmonary histiocytosis X. Chest 81: 130, 1982.
288. Flint A, Lloyd RV, Colby TV, et al: Pulmonary histiocytosis X. Immunoperoxidase staining for HLA-DR antigen and S100 protein. Arch Pathol Lab Med 110: 930, 1986.
289. Arnett NL, Schulz DM: Primary pulmonary eosinophilic granuloma. Radiology 69: 224, 1957.
290. Kittredge RD, Geller A, Finby N: The reticuloendothelioses in the lung. Am J Roentgenol 100: 588, 1967.
291. McLetchie NGB, Reynolds DP: Histiocytic reticulosis and honeycomb lungs. Can Med Assoc J 71: 44, 1954.
292. Moore ADA, Godwin JD, Müller NL, et al: Pulmonary hystiocytosis X: Comparison of radiographic and CT findings. Radiology 172: 249, 1989.
293. Brauner MW, Grenier P, Mouelhi MM, et al: Pulmonary histiocytosis X: Evaluation with high-resolution CT. Radiology 172: 255, 1989.
294. Lacronique J, Roth C, Battesti J-P, et al: Chest radiological features of pulmonary histiocytosis X: A report based on 50 adult cases. Thorax 37: 104, 1982.
295. Stern EJ, Webb WR, Golden JA, et al: Cystic lung disease associated with eosinophilic granuloma and tuberous sclerosis: Air trapping at dynamic ultrafast high-resolution CT. Radiology 182: 325, 1992.
296. Carlson RA, Hattery RR, O'Connell EJ, et al: Pulmonary involvement by histiocytosis X in the pediatric age group. Mayo Clin Proc 51: 542, 1976.
297. Favara BE, McCarthy RC, Mierau GW: Histiocytosis X. Hum Pathol 14: 663, 1983.
298. Lewis JG: Eosinophilic granuloma and its variants with special reference to lung involvement. A report of 12 patients. Q J Med 33: 337, 1964.
299. Basset F, Corrin B, Spencer H, et al: Pulmonary histiocytosis X. Am Rev Respir Dis 118: 811, 1978.
300. Bates DV, Macklem PT, Christie RV: Respiratory Function in Disease: An introduction to the Integrated Study of the Lung. 2nd ed. Philadelphia, WB Saunders, 1971.
301. Tomashefski JF, Khiyami A, Kleinerman J: Neoplasms associated with pulmonary eosinophilic granuloma. Arch Pathol Lab Med 115: 499, 1991.
302. Prakash UBS, Barham SS, Rosenow EC III, et al: Pulmonary alveolar microlithiasis. A review including ultrastructural and pulmonary function studies. Mayo Clin Proc 58: 290, 1983.
303. Miro JM, Moreno A, Coca A, et al: Pulmonary alveolar microlithiasis with an unusual radiological pattern. Br J Dis Chest 76: 91, 1982.
304. Kino T, Kohara Y, Tsuji S: Pulmonary alveolar microlithiasis. A report of two young sisters. Am Rev Respir Dis 105: 105, 1972.
305. Sosman MC, Dodd GD, Jones WD, et al: The familial occurrence of pulmonary alveolar microlithiasis. Am J Roentgentol 77: 947, 1957.
306. Barnard NJ, Crocker PR, Blainey AD, et al: Pulmonary alveolar microlithiasis. A new analytical approach. Histopathology 11: 639, 1987.
307. O'Neill RP, Cohn JE, Pellegrino ED: Pulmonary alveolar microlithiasis–a family study. Ann Intern Med 67: 957, 1967.

308. Badger TL, Gottlieb L, Gaensler EA: Pulmonary alveolar microlithiasis, or calcinosis of the lungs. N Engl J Med 253: 709, 1955.

309. Portnoy LM, Amadeo B, Hennigar GR: Pulmonary alveolar microlithiasis. An unusual case (associated with milk-alkali syndrome). Am J Clin Pathol 41: 194, 1964.

310. Bab I, Rosenmann E, Ne'eman Z, et al: The occurrence of extracellular matrix vesicles in pulmonary alveolar microlithiasis. Virchows Arch [A] 391: 357, 1981.

311. Hawass ND, Noah MS: Pulmonary alveolar microlithiasis. Eur J Respir Dis 69: 199, 1986.

312. Chalmers AG, Wyatt J, Robinson PJ: Computed tomographic and pathological findings in pulmonary alveolar microlithiasis. Br J Radiol 59: 408, 1986.

313. Waters MH: Microlithiasis alveolaris pulmonum. Tubercle 41: 276, 1960.

314. Brown ML, Swee RG, Olson RJ, et al: Pulmonary uptake of ^{99m}Tc diphosphonate in alveolar microlithiasis. Am J Roentgenol 131: 703, 1978.

315. Palombini BC, Porto NS, Wallau CV, et al: Bronchopulmonary lavage in alveolar microlithiasis [letter]. Anaesth Intensive Care 6: 265, 1978.

316. Oka S, Shiraishi K, Ogata K, et al: Pulmonary alveolar microlithiasis. Report of three cases. Am Rev Respir Dis 93: 612, 1966.

18

THE PLEURA

PLEURAL EFFUSION

Effusion* is one of the most important pleural abnormalities observed in thoracic disease. It can occur without other changes in the thorax or can be associated with abnormalities of the lungs, mediastinum, or chest wall. In the

---

*The character of fluid in the pleural space—transudate, exudate, pus, blood, chyle, or any combination of these—is seldom, if ever, discernible by conventional roentgenologic techniques (although magnetic resonance imaging [MRI][1] and sonography[1a] hold some promise in this respect). Strictly speaking, therefore, "increase in pleural fluid" rather than "pleural effusion" is the correct term for reporting the abnormality. Because it is in common usage, however, "pleural effusion" is used here to refer to the presence of an abnormal amount of fluid, regardless of its character. Where appropriate, the precise terms "hydrothorax" (for serous effusions, either transudate or exudate), "empyema," "hemothorax," and "chylothorax" are employed.

former circumstance, diagnosis may prove exceedingly difficult, even with bacteriologic, biochemical, and pathologic investigations. When effusion occurs as part of a complex of roentgenographic changes, however, it may provide an important diagnostic clue. Often its cause is immediately apparent; for example, when it accompanies enlargement of the heart and is the result of cardiac decompensation or when it occurs as a hemothorax in association with multiple rib fractures following trauma. Just as often, however, an effusion constitutes one facet of a complex of roentgenologic signs that tries the diagnostic skills of the physician.

When considering the etiology of an effusion, it is clear that *any* abnormality on the chest roentgenogram besides the fluid must be taken into account. For example, an elevated hemidiaphragm (not to be confused with infrapulmonary effusion) constitutes a significant finding in that it may indicate an acute subphrenic abscess. It is important to remember, however, that underlying pulmonary or mediastinal disease is not always detectable on the first available roentgenograms: large effusions may mask parenchymal shadows or mediastinal masses, and these may become evident only when fluid has been removed or when roentgenography in the supine or lateral decubitus position renders the underlying lung or mediastinal contour visible. However, computed tomography (CT) can aid in distinguishing pleural fluid from pulmonary abnormalities in many cases, even before thoracentesis.

The following section briefly describes the general clinical, pulmonary function, and laboratory features of pleural effusion; roentgenographic manifestations are discussed in Chapter 4 (see page 243).

Clinical Manifestations

Pleural pain is a frequent manifestation of "dry" pleurisy but often diminishes when effusion develops. In some cases, the pain is not accentuated by breathing and is felt as a dull ache. Since the parietal pleura is innervated by branches of the intercostal nerves, the pain usually is well localized, although it may be referred to the abdomen. When the phrenic nerve endings are irritated by inflammation of the diaphragmatic pleura, pain may be felt in the shoulder. Dyspnea is common; if it is severe and associated with decreased respiratory reserve, immediate thoracentesis may be required for relief. The mediastinal displacement that occurs in tension hydrothorax can cause respiratory distress, dysphagia, engorged neck veins, a tender liver, and edema of the lower extremities[2]; thoracentesis characteristically produces immediate relief of symptoms and signs.

Physical examination reveals dullness or flatness on percussion and a decrease or absence of breath sounds. When dullness on percussion is shifting, this sign by itself is diagnostic. Breath sounds may persist even when the effusion is large and may sound distant and be bronchial in type. The explanation for this discrepancy is not always apparent.

Pulmonary Function Studies

In the absence of underlying pulmonary disease, the effects of pleural effusion on pulmonary function reflect the combination of a space-occupying process and a reduction in lung volume as a consequence of relaxation atelectasis. The space-occupying process reduces all subdivisions of lung volume, although ventilatory ability may be little impaired when the other lung is normal and no pleural pain inhibits chest movement.[3] Depending on the amount of fluid, diffusing capacity may be moderately diminished, although it often remains within the predicted normal range. Arterial oxygen saturation usually is unaffected, even with a major degree of atelectasis, since perfusion adjusts downward in response to the reduction in ventilation. $PaCO_2$ may decrease if unilateral pulmonary collapse results in hyperventilation, but otherwise it remains unaffected.

The slight but significant increase in PaO_2 and lung volumes and the decrease in $P(A-a)O_2$ that occur in some patients following thoracentesis are insufficient to explain the relief of dyspnea that is commonly experienced. It has been suggested instead that this results from a reduction in the size of the thoracic cage that allows the inspiratory

muscles to operate on a more advantageous portion of their length-tension curve.[4] In some patients, thoracentesis results in hypoxemia, presumably as a result of the development of pulmonary edema (see page 615).[5]

Laboratory Procedures

When clinical and roentgenographic findings fail to indicate the etiology of a pleural effusion, it is usually necessary to perform invasive diagnostic procedures, initially thoracentesis (with hematologic, cytologic, and biochemical analysis of fluid, Table 18–1), with or without closed pleural biopsy. If these fail to yield a diagnosis, thoracoscopic or open biopsy may be necessary. When considering the use of these latter procedures, however, it is important to remember that as many as 25 to 30 per cent of pleural effusions do not recur and are found on follow-up to have a benign cause.[6]

Specific Causes of Pleural Effusion
Infection

Pleural infections usually produce an exudative effusion (i.e., with protein content greater than 3 g per 100 mL). By far the most common etiologic agents are bacteria; fungi, viruses, and parasites are much less frequent.

Mycobacterium Tuberculosis. Tuberculous pleural effusion occurs most commonly in young adults, although there is some evidence that the average age is increasing.[7] Although it may complicate established pulmonary tuberculosis—in which case it invariably indicates activity of the pulmonary disease—it can also present as uncomplicated "pleurisy with effusion." In fact, in many developing countries, tuberculosis remains the most common cause of pleural effusion in the absence of demonstrable pulmonary disease.[8] Nontuberculous mycobacteria rarely cause pleural effusion, either in the form of primary disease or as a complication of pulmonary involvement.[9]

The effusion has been hypothesized to develop initially secondary to rupture of subpleural foci of necrotic tissue into the adjacent pleural space, resulting in a delayed hypersensitivity reaction.[10] Supporting this hypothesis are observations of the presence in tuberculous pleural fluid of T lymphocytes that are specifically sensitized to PPD[11] as well as high levels of interleukin-2 (IL-2) and IL-2 receptors.[12] This delayed hypersensitivity reaction can occur in the pleura of some patients who fail to react to cutaneous PPD, a fact that may be explained by the presence in the circulation of suppressor cells that inhibit response in the skin; these suppressor cells are apparently lacking in the pleural fluid.[13] The small foci of necrotic lung that spill their contents into the pleural space usually cannot be seen on conventional chest roentgenograms but have been documented with CT.[14]

Tuberculous effusion is almost invariably unilateral and seldom massive. Thoracentesis typically yields clear, straw-colored fluid containing more than 3 g protein per 100 mL. If the aspirate is bloody, serosanguineous, or even pink, a tuberculous etiology is unlikely. Lymphocytes predominate, amounting to more than 70 per cent of the total white blood cell count; on preparations examined cytologically, they can appear to be the only cell type, a finding that may

Table 18–1. **CHARACTERISTICS OF PLEURAL EFFUSIONS OF DIFFERENT CAUSES**

Feature	Transudate	Malignancy	Tuberculosis	Nontuberculous Parapneumonic	Rheumatoid Disease
Clinical	Signs and symptoms of congestive heart failure, cirrhosis or nephrosis (hypoproteinemia)	Older patient; poor health prior to effusion; known primary malignancy	Younger patient, good health prior to effusion; known exposure	Signs and symptoms of respiratory infection	History of arthritis ± subcutaneous rheumatoid nodules ±
Gross appearance	Clear, straw-colored ("serous")	Serous → often sanguineous	Serous → occasionally sanguineous	Serous → sanguineous turbid (pus)	Serous → turbid or yellow green
Microscopic examination	0	Cytology positive in about 50%; higher with multiple samples, cell block	Cholesterol crystals	May or may not be + for organisms	Occasionally amorphous granular material and multinucleated giant cells
Cell count + differential	85% < 10,000 RBC/mL; majority WBC count < 1000 mL	40% > 100,000 RBC/mL; WBC 1000 to 10,000/mL, usually mononuclears predominate	In majority small lymphocytes predominate. Polymorphonuclear leukocytes may predominate initially. Rarely > 5% mesothelial cells	Polymorphonuclears predominate; 10,000/mL and left shift	Mononuclear cells predominate
Culture	0	0	Positive 20–25%; 10–15% sputum +/or gastric washings +	May or may not be positive	0
Protein	75% < 3 g; pleural fluid–serum protein ratio < 0.5	90% > 3 g; pleural fluid–serum protein ratio > 0.5	90% > 3 g; pleural fluid–serum protein ratio > 0.5	> 3 g; pleural fluid–serum protein ratio > 0.5	> 3 g; pleural fluid–serum protein ratio > 0.5
Lactic acid dehydrogenase (LDH)	Pleural fluid–serum LDH ratio < 0.6	Pleural fluid–serum LDH ratio > 0.6	Pleural fluid–serum LDH ratio > 0.6	Pleural fluid–serum LDH ratio > 0.6; LDH level greater than 1000 IU/mL suggests complicated effusion (empyema)	Pleural fluid–serum LDH ratio > 0.6
Glucose	> 60 mg/dL	May be < 60 mg/dL; lower levels associated with poor prognosis	May be < 60 mg/dL	May be < 60 mg/dL; lower levels suggest complicated effusion (empyema)	85% < 50 mg/dL; 65% < 20 mg/dL
pH	Equal to or higher than blood pH	15% have pH < 7.20; low pH associated with poor prognosis	May be < 7.20	May be < 7.20; lower pH suggests complicated pleural effusion (empyema)	May be < 7.20
Other	Most common with biventricular heart failure	Pleural biopsy positive in 30–50%	Tuberculin skin test usually positive. Adenosine deaminase level > 30 IU/L may be specific. Pleural biopsy + for granuloma in 60 to 80%	Foul-smelling fluid with anaerobic organisms	Reduced complement; high rheumatoid factor (higher than serum titer); may have high cholesterol level

Table 18–1. **CHARACTERISTICS OF PLEURAL EFFUSIONS OF DIFFERENT CAUSES** *Continued*

Systemic Lupus Erythematosus	Pulmonary Embolism	Fungal Infection	Traumatic	Chylous	Chyliform
Known SLE ± young women	Predisposing factors: postoperative, immobilization, venous disease	Exposure in endemic area	History of trauma–fractured ribs	History of trauma (25%) or malignancy (50%)	Usually chronic effusion
Serous → occasionally sanguineous	Serous → often sanguineous	Serous → occasionally sanguineous	Sanguineous	Turbid whitish; turbid supernatant with centrifugation, does not clear with ethyl alcohol	Turbid whitish; turbid supernatant with centrifugation, clears with ethyl alcohol
Occasionally LE cells	0	May or may not be + for organism	0	Fat droplets	Cholesterol crystals
Mononuclear or polymorphonuclear cells predominate	Mononuclear or polymorphonuclear cells predominate; RBC < 10,000/mL in 30%, RBC > 100,000/mL in 20%	Mononuclear or polymorphonuclear cells predominate	RBC predominate	Mononuclear cells predominate	Variable
0	0	May or may not be positive	0	0	0
> 3 g; pleural fluid–serum protein ratio > 0.5 Pleural fluid–serum LDH ratio > 0.6	> 3 g; pleural fluid–serum protein ratio > 0.5 Pleural fluid–serum LDH ratio > 0.6	> 3 g; pleural fluid–serum protein ratio > 0.5 Pleural fluid–serum LDH ratio > 0.6	> 3 g; pleural fluid–serum protein ratio > 0.5 Pleural fluid–serum LDH ratio > 0.6	> 3 g; pleural fluid–serum protein ratio > 0.5 Pleural fluid–serum LDH ratio > 0.6	> 3 g; pleural fluid–serum protein ratio > 0.5 Pleural fluid–serum LDH ratio > 0.6
> 60 mg/dL	> 60 mg/dL	> 60 mg/dL	> 60 mg/dL	> 60 mg/dL	May be < 60 mg/dL depending on etiology
> 7.20	> 7.20	?	May be < 7.20 with hemothorax	> 7.20	May be < 7.20 depending on etiology
Reduced complement and presence of antinuclear antibody	Source of emboli may or may not be apparent, but venogram or impedance plethysmography usually positive	Skin and serologic tests may be helpful. Sulfur granules with actinomycosis	—	Pleural fluid triglyceride usually > 110 mg/dL	—

result in a mistaken diagnosis of lymphoma.[15] Although polymorphonuclear leukocytes can be fairly numerous during the early stages, it is reasonable to assume that effusions containing more than 50 per cent of these cells are of nontuberculous etiology. Eosinophils rarely are present in significant numbers unless there is an associated pneumothorax, a complication that may have been caused by an earlier thoracentesis.

Pleural fluid glucose content can be low in tuberculous effusion; however, this finding does not help differentiate it from that caused by other bacteria, rheumatoid disease, or carcinoma. In fact, the majority of patients with effusions of tuberculous etiology have pleural fluid glucose levels above 60 mg per 100 mL.[16] Most investigators have found the level of adenosine deaminase to be greater in tuberculous pleural effusions than in effusions of other etiologies,[17] although some have reported overlap in activity, particularly in rheumatoid disease.[18] Simultaneous determination of adenosine deaminase and of pleural fluid lysozyme–serum lysozyme ratio has been recommended as a more sensitive and specific biochemical approach to diagnosis.[19]

A *presumptive* diagnosis of tuberculous pleural effusion can be made with a combination of a positive tuberculin test and a predominantly lymphocytic response in the pleural fluid. However, a negative PPD reaction does not exclude the diagnosis, and the skin test should be repeated when any patient suspected of having tuberculosis has a negative initial reaction. In about 60 to 80 per cent of patients with proven tuberculosis, pleural biopsy specimens reveal granulomas.[20] Although this finding is virtually diagnostic, *definitive* diagnosis still requires the identification of acid-fast organisms in the tissue specimen or a positive culture of pleural fluid or tissue. The rate of positive culture from pleural fluid is surprisingly low—only 20 to 25 per cent of proven cases. Cultures of biopsy specimens are positive in 55 to 80 per cent of patients.[21, 22]

Bacteria Other Than Mycobacterium Tuberculosis. Parapneumonic pleural effusion has been reported to occur in about 40 per cent of cases,[23] but it is likely that the recorded incidence would increase sharply if roentgenograms were obtained with patients in the lateral decubitus position or if computed tomography (CT) were performed in all cases of pneumonia.[24] Typically, there is a predominance of polymorphonuclear leukocytes. In a few patients, the fluid becomes grossly cloudy or frankly purulent (empyema).

Although some cases of parapneumonic effusion resolve with antibiotic therapy alone,[25] drainage is usually required when empyema develops or when a serous effusion becomes loculated.[26] According to Light,[27] there are four main indications for tube drainage: (1) the presence of gross pus; (2) the demonstration of organisms on Gram staining; (3) a glucose level in the pleural fluid less than 40 mg per 100 mL; and (4) pleural fluid pH less than 7.00 (a criterion that applies only when parapneumonic effusions are collected anaerobically and only when the pH of the pleural fluid is at least 0.15 units lower than a simultaneously measured arterial blood pH).

The management of parapneumonic effusions also can be based on the amount of fluid present. Patients in whom the thickness of pleural fluid on a decubitus roentgenogram is less than 10 mm often have spontaneous resolution of their effusions.[23] If the fluid measures more than 10 mm in depth, however, thoracentesis is probably indicated, and the decision to insert a tube is based on the criteria previously enunciated. In about one third of patients with empyema, tube drainage proves inadequate, and pleural decortication or open drainage with rib resection is required.[25]

The specific bacteria responsible for empyema vary with the host's health. In patients who acquire infection in the community, the most frequent organisms are *Staphylococcus aureus* and *Haemophilus influenzae*. The latter is a common cause of empyema in children[28] and is accompanied by pleural effusion in approximately 50 per cent of adults with pneumonia.[29] Parapneumonic effusion or empyema occurs in roughly one half of adult patients with staphylococcal pneumonia; in infants and young children, empyema develops in almost every case.[30] In hospitalized patients, gram-negative organisms are the principal agents of empyema.[31] As in bacterial pneumonia, cultures in any case of empyema may reveal multiple organisms, sometimes consisting of a combination of aerobic and anaerobic bacteria.[32]

Not uncommonly, pus aspirated from the pleural cavity of patients with empyema is sterile on culture, a finding that may reflect the administration of antimicrobial drugs before admission. In such circumstances, the responsible organism may be determined by counterimmunoelectrophoresis, since soluble bacterial antigens can persist in body fluids after organisms no longer can be isolated.[33] Perhaps more often, negative results are caused by a failure to culture pleural fluid anaerobically.[32]

Roentgenography has a limited but sometimes important role in the investigation of bacterial effusion. In the vast majority of cases of empyema it cannot identify a specific etiology; however, infections caused by *Clostridium perfringens* and *Bacteroides fragilis* can be associated with the presence of gas in the soft tissues of the chest wall or in the pleural space (pyopneumothorax), permitting a presumptive diagnosis. Contrast-enhanced CT may show pleural and extrapleural changes suggestive of empyema and help differentiate this complication from simple effusion.[34] Ultrasonography can also be helpful in detecting empyema[1a] and, as with CT, may be essential for positioning a catheter for adequate drainage.[35]

Uncomplicated pleural effusions—those that clear spontaneously—do not alter the prognosis of pneumonia. By contrast, pleural effusions that require drainage or thoracotomy are associated with increased morbidity and mortality.[36] Prognosis also varies with the age of the patient, the presence or absence of underlying disease, and the cause of the empyema. Empyema in children usually responds to simple closed drainage, whereas hospital-acquired empyema in the elderly is associated with considerable morbidity and a high mortality rate.[37]

Other Organisms
Actinomyces Israelii *and* Nocardia Species. Pulmonary involvement is an invariable accompaniment of pleural disease caused by these organisms, usually in the form of acute airspace pneumonia, homogeneous in density and nonsegmental in distribution. Abscess formation is common. The infection extends into the pleura, producing empyema, and subsequently may transgress the parietal pleura to involve the chest wall, with rib destruction and subcutaneous abscess formation (empyema necessitatis).[38]

Fungi. Histoplasmosis is rarely complicated by pleural effusion at the time of primary infection; when it occurs, pleural disease can be caused by direct infection by *Histoplasma* organisms or by a reaction to antigen that diffuses into the pleural space from a histoplasmoma. Effusions caused by *Blastomyces dermatitidis* and *Cryptococcus neoformans* are also very uncommon and are usually associated with acute airspace pneumonia.[39]

Effusion occurs in about 5 per cent of symptomatic patients with primary coccidioidomycosis; it may be associated with erythema nodosum and peripheral blood eosinophilia (rarely with pleural fluid eosinophilia).[40] In addition, hydropneumothorax can develop when a coccidioidal cavity ruptures into the pleural space, which is said to occur in 1 to 5 per cent of patients with chronic cavitary coccidioidomycosis.[16]

Pleural invasion by *Aspergillus* species occurs in three situations: (1) as a late complication of thoracoplasty for tuberculosis, often in association with a bronchopleural fistula[41]; (2) as a complication of resection surgery[42]; or (3) perhaps most commonly, as a complication of invasive pulmonary aspergillosis.

Viruses and **Mycoplasma Pneumoniae.** Pleural effusion can be demonstrated in as many as 20 per cent of patients with pneumonia caused by these organisms, although roentgenography in the lateral decubitis position may be required.[43] Effusion, large in some cases, also is said to be a common accompaniment of the acute pneumonia of "atypical measles."[44]

Parasites. Pleuropulmonary involvement in amebiasis is almost invariably secondary to liver abscess, with transmission of the infection into the thorax by direct extension through the diaphragm. It is said to occur in 15 to 20 per cent of patients with liver involvement.[45] The effusion usually is serofibrinous. When the infestation extends into lung parenchyma, however, the pulmonary lesion may cavitate, providing communication between the bronchial tree and the liver abscess; in this situation, fluid of typical "chocolate sauce" appearance may be seen on thoracentesis.

Pleural effusion is uncommon in hydatid disease.[46] It occurs when a pulmonary hydatid cyst ruptures into the pleural space; since air also is present in most cases, the roentgenographic appearance is that of hydropneumothorax. Daughter cysts floating on the surface of the fluid may produce irregularities of the fluid surface, creating the "water lily" sign. Scolices or hooklets may be identified in fluid obtained by thoracentesis.

Connective Tissue Disease

Of the connective tissue diseases, only systemic lupus erythematosus (SLE) and rheumatoid disease are important causes of pleural effusion. In patients with progressive systemic sclerosis, dermatomyositis, and Sjögren's syndrome, effusion probably results from other causes (e.g., heart failure) rather than immune-mediated disease of the pleura. Effusion is said to occur fairly frequently in Wegener's granulomatosis,[47] but its presence in other pulmonary vasculitides and in Goodpasture's syndrome is very uncommon and likely related to extrapulmonary disease.

Systemic Lupus Erythematosus. The reported incidence of pleural effusion in SLE varies from 33 per cent of cases[48] to as much as 75 per cent.[49] In one series, the effusion occurred as an isolated abnormality in 12 per cent of patients and in combination with cardiac enlargement and pulmonary abnormalities in 20 per cent.[49] Effusions are bilateral in about half the cases and when unilateral are predominantly left sided. They are usually small.

The fluid usually possesses no diagnostic biochemical findings. The protein concentration is variable: when the effusion is attributable to direct pleural involvement, it is probable that inflammation, possibly mediated by immune complexes,[50] causes increased capillary permeability, resulting in pleural effusion with a relatively high protein concentration. By contrast, when the effusion results from the nephrotic syndrome secondary to SLE, it is a transudate. The glucose concentration is approximately equal to that in the blood, in contrast to the low levels characteristic of rheumatoid disease. Also in contrast to rheumatoid pleural effusion, the pH is greater than 7.35 and levels of rheumatoid factor are not significantly elevated.[51] LE cells, a high antinuclear antibody (ANA) titer, and a low complement level can be present.[52]

The most common associated roentgenologic finding is enlargement of the cardiovascular silhouette, which is said to occur in 35 to 50 per cent of all cases.[48, 49] This is usually nonspecific in character and minimal to moderate in degree. Variation in heart size usually takes place over a period of weeks but may occur with startling abruptness. The combination of bilateral pleural effusion with enlargement of the cardiovascular silhouette should suggest the diagnosis, particularly in young women.

Rheumatoid Disease. Pleural disease probably is the most frequent manifestation of rheumatoid disease in the thorax. For unexplained reasons, it has a distinct male predominance, despite the fact that rheumatoid arthritis occurs more often in women. Middle-aged patients are usually affected. Clinically, the effusion is often unsuspected because it is asymptomatic and is found by chance during roentgenographic examination. In some patients, however, it develops abruptly and is associated with pain, fever, or dyspnea.[53] Although the effusion usually appears sometime after the clinical onset of rheumatoid arthritis and is often associated with episodic exacerbations of it, it may antedate both signs and symptoms of joint disease. It occurs in a significantly greater number of patients with subcutaneous nodules than in those without and tends to occur independently of pulmonary rheumatoid disease.

The effusions are usually unilateral, slightly more often on the right side. The only distinctive roentgenographic characteristic is a tendency to remain relatively unchanged for many months or even years.

The fluid is typically an exudate, usually turbid and greenish yellow, with a predominance of lymphocytes and a paucity of mesothelial cells. In some cases polymorphonuclear leukocytes are found in abundance.[54] Cytologic examination of filter specimens may reveal the presence of multinucleated giant cells and clumps of amorphous granular material, an appearance that is caused by rupture of a subpleural necrobiotic nodule into the pleural space and is diagnostic of the rheumatoid etiology of the effusion.[55] So-called rheumatoid arthritis cells—mostly polymorphonuclear leukocytes with cytoplasm containing minute black granules believed to be lipids—also can be found in some effusions, although their presence is not specific for rheumatoid disease.[56]

Characteristically, the glucose content of rheumatoid pleural effusion is very low; in fact, it has been estimated that glucose levels below 30 mg per 100 mL are found in 70 to 80 per cent of patients.[57] Typically, a low pleural fluid glucose level is associated with a normal blood level and does not rise following intravenous infusion of glucose (in contrast to tuberculous effusion, in which the level rises following intravenous loading with glucose).

Rheumatoid factor is frequently present in the effusion, typically when it is also elevated in the serum. Its presence, however, is not diagnostic of a rheumatoid etiology, since elevated levels also have been described in parapneumonic, carcinomatous, and tuberculous effusions.[58] The pH of the fluid is also reduced, usually below 7.20; when accompanied by low glucose and complement levels and a high rheumatoid factor level, this finding is virtually diagnostic of rheumatoid pleural effusion.[59]

Asbestos

Pleural effusion is probably more common in individuals with a history of asbestos exposure than is generally recognized.[60] The likelihood of its developing appears to be dose related. The latency period is shorter than for other asbestos-related disorders; in fact, it is the most common abnormality during the first 20 years after exposure. Most effusions are small and about 30 per cent recur. Approximately two thirds of patients are asymptomatic; chest pain is the most common symptom and some patients have fever, suggesting a viral infection.

In most, if not all, cases, the fluid is a serous or blood-tinged exudate. The differential diagnosis must include tuberculosis and mesothelioma. Large effusions are more likely to be caused by mesothelioma than to have a benign origin[61]; however, painful and bloody effusions are just as likely to have a benign cause as a malignant one.

Drugs

Some drugs, such as bromocriptine, methysergide, dantrolene sodium, and nitrofurantoin, appear to affect the pleura almost selectively.[62] Effusions tend to have a predominance of lymphocytes in the first two and of eosinophils in the others.

Neoplasms

The most common cause of exudative pleural effusion is malignancy,[63] the major sources being the lungs, breast, stomach, ovaries, and lymph nodes (lymphoma). Primary lung and metastatic breast malignancies head the list.[64] The importance of cancer as a cause of pleural effusion is also reflected in the etiology of bilateral effusions associated with normal heart size. In one series of 78 such cases, 35 cases (45 per cent) were caused by cancer, of which 13 (37 per cent) showed no roentgenographic abnormality of the thorax other than the bilateral pleural effusions.[65]

It is likely that in most cases the pathogenesis of pleural effusion in malignancy is multifactorial. Possible mechanisms include (1) tumor invasion of the pleura, stimulating an inflammatory reaction associated with capillary leakage; (2) tumor invasion of the pulmonary or pleural lymphatics and bronchopulmonary, hilar, or mediastinal lymph nodes,

hindering the return of lymphatic fluid to the systemic circulation; (3) bronchial obstruction, creating an increased negative intrapleural pressure, thus increasing transudation; (4) hypoproteinemia, leading to increased transudation; (5) infection in association with obstructive pneumonitis, resulting in a parapneumonic effusion; and (6) deposition of immune complexes related to circulating tumor antigens, causing increased pleural capillary permeability.[50]

The diagnosis of carcinoma as the etiology of pleural effusion may be strongly suspected from the chest roentgenogram, the manifestation being one of either primary pulmonary cancer or diffuse nodular or linear opacities characteristic of metastatic carcinoma. Most investigators have found the majority of effusions to be on the same side as the primary lesions.[66] Bronchoscopy can occasionally yield the diagnosis even in patients whose chest roentgenograms reveal nothing more than pleural effusion, particularly if there is a history of hemoptysis. In such cases, however, thoracentesis and pleural biopsy are more likely to prove fruitful.[67] The incidence of positive cytologic examination of malignant pleural effusion ranges from 30 to almost 85 per cent, with most series reporting about 50 per cent. Such examination gives a higher yield than needle biopsy, although these procedures are complementary.[68] When pleural fluid persists and cytology is negative for malignant cells, thoracoscopic or open pleural biopsy may be required for diagnosis.

Pleural effusions associated with malignancy are almost invariably exudates; those that meet exudative criteria by the lactic dehydrogenase (LDH) level but not by the protein level are usually malignant.[16] Although lymphocytes predominate, polymorphonuclear leukocytes are usually prominent. A minority are grossly bloody. The great majority have normal glucose levels and pH above 7.30[66]; those with glucose levels below 60 mg per 100 mL and a pH below 7.30 are more likely to be large, to have a positive cytology, and to carry a poor prognosis.[69]

There have been numerous reports of attempts to distinguish between benign and malignant effusions by using a variety of tumor markers in pleural fluid.[70] In the great majority, however, considerable overlap has been found in the levels of these markers, so at the time of this writing it is likely that they serve little practical purpose.

Pulmonary Carcinoma. Pleural involvement in primary pulmonary carcinoma is common. By the time patients first seek medical attention, effusion is observed in about 5 to 15 per cent,[66, 71] and during the course of the disease at least 50 per cent of patients with disseminated cancer develop the complication.[16] Such effusions are nearly always associated with a roentgenographically demonstrable pulmonary abnormality. Occasionally, however, the primary lesion is so small as to be almost invisible roentgenologically except with such special techniques as CT.

The identification of malignant cells in pleural fluid or tissue of patients with proved pulmonary carcinoma is generally regarded as evidence of inoperability. If cells are not found and if a reasonable explanation exists for fluid formation without direct neoplastic involvement, thoracotomy with intent to resect is probably justified. Pleural effusion with proved carcinomatous involvement has a very poor prognosis; in one series of 96 patients,[66] 54 per cent were dead within 1 month and 84 per cent within 6 months.

Lymphoma. Because of the almost invariable involvement of mediastinal lymph nodes in lymphoma affecting the thorax, it is often difficult to say if a specific case of pleural effusion is related to central lymphatic obstruction or to neoplastic pleural disease.[72, 72a] Reflecting this uncertainty is the observation that the fluid may be serous or serosanguineous and have the characteristics of either a transudate or exudate.

The cytologic diagnosis of lymphoma in pleural fluid specimens can be difficult, particularly in the small lymphocytic (well-differentiated) form. Atypical lymphocytes can be virtually the only cell in tuberculous effusions, resulting in an appearance that can be mistaken for lymphoma.[15] Despite this, some investigators report a high degree of accuracy in diagnosis and, to some extent, even in classification of types of lymphoma by cytologic examination.[73] Immunohistochemical analysis can be particularly helpful in difficult cases.[74]

Leukemia. As a roentgenographic abnormality of thoracic leukemia, effusion is second in frequency only to mediastinal lymph node enlargement and is identified in as many as 25 per cent of patients.[75] It is probably caused by leukemic infiltration of the pleura in no more than 5 per cent, the majority of cases being related to obstructed lymphatics, cardiac failure, or infection. Cytochemical and immunocytochemical studies of cells obtained from the fluid may be helpful in diagnosis.[76]

Multiple Myeloma. Pleural effusion in multiple myeloma is uncommon[77] but can be associated with other roentgenographic changes in the ribs and soft tissues of the chest wall that are sufficiently distinctive to permit a strongly presumptive diagnosis. A high level of the specific immunoglobulin produced by the myeloma cells can sometimes be identified in pleural fluid. In many cases, the exudate is probably caused by direct infiltration of the pleura by myeloma cells.[78]

Metastatic Carcinoma. The major sites of origin of malignant pleural effusion from extrathoracic neoplasms are breast, ovary, and stomach, of which the breast is the most common. In this tumor, the effusion is usually unilateral, in some studies almost as frequently on the contralateral as the ipsilateral side[79] and in others with a clear ipsilateral predominance.[80] Most cases probably occur by lymphatic spread; direct extension across the chest wall to the parietal pleura is rare. Although bilateral effusion is uncommon in patients with breast carcinoma,[79] it is one of the major causes of this manifestation of pleural disease. There is evidence that it represents secondary metastases from the liver.[81]

Thromboembolism

As a roentgenographic manifestation of thromboembolic disease, pleural effusion is as common as parenchymal consolidation. In our experience, it nearly always indicates infarction, although the parenchymal shadow may be diminutive or hidden by the fluid, confusing the diagnostic possibilities to such an extent that an embolic episode will be suggested only if there is a high index of suspicion. The amount of pleural fluid is frequently small, but it may be abundant and is most often unilateral.[82] Fluid usually develops and is absorbed synchronously with the infarct, but sometimes it appears later and clears sooner.[83]

Light[16] has stated categorically that analysis of the pleural fluid in pulmonary thromboembolism is not helpful in diagnosis, since it can have the features of either a transudate or an exudate and in only a minority of cases is it grossly bloody. The authors concur that transudates can occur but suspect that in most, if not all, such cases they are caused by clinically unrecognized heart failure. The authors also feel that in a patient suspected on clinical grounds of having pulmonary embolism, a bloody pleural effusion is strong confirmatory evidence for associated infarction.

Cardiac Decompensation

One of the most common forms of pleural effusion is that associated with increase in hydrostatic pressure in the venous circulation, either pulmonary or systemic (or both). It occurs most commonly with cardiac decompensation but may be seen also with constrictive pericarditis or obstruction of the superior vena cava or azygos vein.

The mechanisms whereby the effusions develop are complex and are related to increased hydrostatic pressure, altered capillary permeability (secondary to hypoxia), and reduced lymphatic drainage. Although there is some difference of opinion, in our view right-sided or left-sided cardiac failure in relatively "pure" form seldom leads to hydrothorax, decompensation of both sides of the heart being required. This hypothesis is supported by experiments in which dogs were subjected to an increase in pulmonary or systemic venous pressure or both[84]; in this model, the largest accumulation of pleural fluid occurred when both venous pressures were elevated.

Pleural effusion associated with cardiac decompensation is usually bilateral. Occasionally, however, it is unilateral, in which case it is more likely to be right-sided. In fact, if an effusion is confined to the left hemithorax the possibility of an etiology other than heart failure should be seriously considered. Associated clinical and roentgenologic evidence of cardiac enlargement, with or without pulmonary venous hypertension, makes the diagnosis obvious in most cases.

The fluid, usually clear and light yellow, is a transudate with low protein and LDH content and a specific gravity of 1.015 or less. When it is subjected to serial assays while a patient is undergoing treatment, however, it can develop the characteristics of an exudate.[85]

Trauma

Pleural effusion is a common manifestation of penetrating and nonpenetrating trauma and may develop from a variety of causes (Table 18–2) (see also Chapter 15). Hemothorax may result from laceration of the parietal or visceral pleura by fractured ribs, but it can also occur in closed chest trauma without evidence of fracture. It commonly complicates traumatic rupture of the aorta, in which case it is almost invariably left-sided and must not be attributed erroneously to left-sided rib fracture.

Pleural effusion or hydropneumothorax, again almost always left-sided, frequently develops following esophageal perforation, usually as a complication of esophagoscopy or gastroscopy.[86] In these circumstances, identification of ingested material such as milk in pleural fluid is diagnostic. The level of pleural fluid amylase (derived from the salivary glands) is raised in most patients.[87] In the majority of cases, the site of rupture must be identified precisely (and some-

Table 18–2. **TRAUMATIC CAUSES OF PLEURAL EFFUSION**

Etiology	Nature of the Fluid	Selected Reference
Penetrating or nonpenetrating trauma		
Lung	Blood	—
Aorta	Blood	210
Esophagus	Oral or gastric contents	87
Thoracic duct	Chyle	211
Diaphragm	Blood	212
Thoracotomy	Serosanguineous, empyema if infected	—
Vascular catheters	Blood, hyperalimentation fluid	213, 214
Subarachnoid-pleural fistula	Cerebrospinal fluid	215
Radiation	Serous	216

times with considerable difficulty) by roentgenographic evidence of extravasation of ingested contrast material.

Malpositioning of central venous and Swan-Ganz catheters[88] can cause perforation of a vessel, either at the time of insertion or sometime later as a result of gradual erosion of a relatively thin-walled intrathoracic vessel by the catheter tip. Depending on the vessel involved, the result may be mediastinal hemorrhage, hemothorax, pneumothorax, massive hydrothorax, or extrapleural hematoma. In patients receiving hyperalimentation, the infusion of potentially toxic solutions obviously increases the hazard.

Pleural Effusion Secondary to Disease Below the Diaphragm

A variety of intra-abdominal and pelvic disorders are associated with pleural effusion. The pathogenesis of the effusion is complex and can be related to secondary effects on cardiac function, changes in plasma oncotic pressure, or the production of ascitic fluid that is transferred through the diaphragm into the pleural space. Experimental work has shown that in the presence of ascites, carbon particles or radioiodinated serum albumin instilled into the peritoneal space passes into the pleural cavity and that flow is always from the peritoneum to the pleura, never in the opposite direction.[89] Although it seems probable that most such fluid transfer occurs by way of diaphragmatic lymphatic channels, it is possible that defects in the diaphragm also may permit passage in some patients.[90]

Pancreatitis. Acute or chronic pancreatitis is sometimes associated with pleural effusion, often without roentgenographic evidence of other intrathoracic abnormality. They are left-sided in 60 to 70 per cent of cases, right-sided in 10 to 30 per cent, and bilateral in 10 to 30 per cent.[91] In the majority of patients with acute pancreatitis, symptoms suggest an acute upper abdominal disorder; in some, however, the clinical presentation can be confused with a parapneumonic effusion.[92] A minority of patients develop a pancreatic abscess[93] that becomes apparent only 2 to 3 weeks after the acute episode; the abscess itself can be responsible for the pleural effusion.

Chronic pancreatitis is associated with pleural effusion even more often than the acute disease.[94, 95] The effusion is often recurrent, and symptoms frequently direct attention to the thorax rather than the abdomen. In many cases, the patient has a history of heavy alcohol consumption that was responsible for the pancreatitis. Duct disruption can lead to the creation of a pancreaticopleural fistula, with or without pseudocyst formation.

The pleural fluid in both acute and chronic pancreatitis has the characteristics of an exudate and is sometimes serosanguineous and occasionally bloody. In acute pancreatitis, the effusion is more likely to be slight or moderate in amount and bloody, whereas in chronic pancreatitis it tends to be serous and massive. The amylase content is characteristically very high and is almost invariably greater than that of the serum. With proper patient positioning, the pancreaticopleural fistula in either acute or chronic pancreatitis can be demonstrated with contrast medium by endoscopic retrograde cholangiopancreatography (ERCP) or CT.[96]

Sequela of Abdominal Surgery. The development of small pleural effusions is common after abdominal surgery, particularly in the upper abdomen.[97] Most resolve spontaneously.

Subphrenic Abscess. Small pleural effusions are often found in cases of acute subphrenic infection.[98] Associated findings include elevation and restriction of movement of the ipsilateral hemidiaphragm and basal discoid atelectasis or pneumonitis. This combination of findings should strongly suggest the diagnosis, especially in the postoperative period after laparotomy or following rupture of a hollow abdominal viscus (*see* page 949).

Meigs-Salmon Syndrome. This syndrome is associated with a variety of ovarian neoplasms, including fibroma, thecoma, granulosa cell tumor, and even adenocarcinoma. Occasionally, extraovarian pelvic tumors such as uterine leiomyomas have been implicated.[99] It is believed that the tumor size, rather than the specific histologic type, is the most important factor leading to the formation of sufficient fluid to cause ascites and accompanying pleural effusion.[16]

The effusions vary widely in volume and may be massive; they occur more frequently on the right but may be left-sided or bilateral. Although the fluid is usually a transudate, it occasionally contains blood.[99] Removal of the pelvic tumor is usually followed by disappearance of the ascites and hydrothorax.

Dialysis. Since ascites may be associated with pleural effusion, it might be reasonably anticipated that peritoneal dialysis would sometimes lead to hydrothorax, and several such cases have been reported.[100] Patients receiving regular maintenance hemodialysis may also develop pleural effusion[101]; the fluid is often serosanguineous as a consequence of the use of heparin during hemodialysis. Because such patients are uremic, it may not be possible to distinguish effusion complicating hemodialysis from that associated with uremia itself (*see* later).

Hydronephrosis and Urinothorax. The majority of investigators attribute the source of urine collection in the thorax to retroperitoneal collections of urine (urinomas). These form as a result of extravasation of urine from the urinary tract secondary to obstruction in the renal pelvis, ureters, bladder, or urethra. The diagnosis of urinothorax is made by the demonstration of a level of creatinine in pleural fluid that is higher than that in the blood.[102] Surgical drainage of the urinoma results in rapid clearing of the effusion.

Nephrotic Syndrome. Pleural effusion is common in the nephrotic syndrome and is typically a transudate. The main influence in its formation is diminution in the plasma osmotic pressure, thereby upsetting the fine balance that normally keeps the pleural space "dry." The nephrotic syndrome is one of the few disorders associated with a high incidence of atypical location of pleural effusion, commonly in the infrapulmonary space.[103] The reasons underlying this high incidence are obscure.

Cirrhosis. There are at least three possible mechanisms for the development of pleural effusion in patients with cirrhosis: hypoproteinemia, azygos hypertension, and transfer of peritoneal fluid to the pleural cavity via lymphatics or diaphragmatic defects. It is probable that the last one is the most important, although hypoproteinemia is likely a contributing factor in some cases since effusion has been documented in the absence of ascites.[104] In most reports, the effusion is right-sided.[105]

Acute Glomerulonephritis. The incidence of pleural effusion in association with acute glomerulonephritis in children is fairly high.[106] It is postulated that it is caused by an alteration in extracellular fluid volume, although the evidence that it is not infectious in origin has not been clearly documented.

Uremic Pleuritis. Both the pericardium and pleura may become inflamed in patients with uremia. In some patients, the fluid is an exudate containing high levels of protein and LDH, suggesting that there must be some disruption of the pleural membrane.[107] Affected patients sometimes complain of pain, and friction rubs frequently are heard on auscultation.[108] If the patient is receiving regular maintenance hemodialysis the effusion usually clears slowly. The fluid frequently contains blood, possibly as a result of the anticoagulation associated with hemodialysis.[101]

Miscellaneous Causes

Myxedema. Abnormal accumulations of pleural fluid are known to occur in patients with myxedema even in the absence of cardiovascular, renal, or other causes of fluid retention. Most often, the effusion occurs in the pericardium, but it may develop in the pleural space.[109] It has no distinctive roentgenographic characteristics.

Lymphatic Hypoplasia. Pleural effusion may develop as a result of hypoplasia of the lymphatic system. In some instances, the clinical presentation is that of Milroy's disease,[110] a form of congenital lymphedema of the legs caused by lymphatic obstruction. In others, the effusion is associated with lymphedema of an extremity, yellow nails, and bronchiectasis (see page 687). The pleural fluid characteristically has a high protein content.

Dressler's Syndrome. The postpericardiectomy or postmyocardial infarction syndrome, known eponymously as Dressler's syndrome, is characterized by chest pain, fever, and pericardial and pleural effusion. It has been estimated to occur in 3 to 4 per cent of patients following myocardial infarction,[111] and it is probable that the incidence is even higher following surgical procedures involving the pericardium.[16] The pathogenesis is suspected to be a form of immune reaction. Symptoms appear 2 to 3 weeks after the infarct or pericardial surgery. Analysis of fluid in one series revealed a bloody exudate with a pH greater

than 7.40. The syndrome can recur several years after the initial episode.[112]

Familial Paroxysmal Polyserositis. This disease (known also as familial Mediterranean fever and recurrent hereditary polyserositis[113]) is a rare cause of paroxysmal attacks of pleurisy that occurs predominantly in Sephardic Jews, Arabs, Turks, and Armenians. Although there appears to be a genetic factor in its etiology, the incidence of the disease in the same racial population at risk apparently is considerably less in North America than in the Mediterranean area. The actual precipitant of attacks is unknown.

In one large study of 175 Arabs with the disease,[113] the most common manifestation was peritonitis (94 per cent), followed by arthritis (34 per cent) and pleurisy (32 per cent). Most attacks of pleurisy are associated with arthritis and arthralgia, usually involving the large joints. Fever, sometimes as high as 104°F, persists for 12 to 48 hours. Remissions may last for months to years. Despite the recurrent disability, the prognosis is apparently excellent in most cases.

CHYLOTHORAX

Chylothorax is an increase in pleural fluid that is rich in lipids. The fluid is characteristically milky in appearance, although not all milky effusions are truly chylous and not all chylous effusions are milky.[114] The effusions can be divided into those that are *chylous* (caused by the escape of chyle into the pleural space as a result of obstruction or laceration of the thoracic duct) and those that are *chyliform* (caused by degeneration of malignant and other cells in pleural fluid). Chylous effusion is high in neutral fat and fatty acid but low in cholesterol, whereas chyliform effusions are low in neutral fat and high in cholesterol and lecithin and may contain triglycerides.[115]

The lymphatic drainage of the small intestine (chyle) is carried entirely by the thoracic duct; thus, chylothorax can occur only with obstruction or laceration of this duct, obstruction of the right lymphatic duct or pulmonary lymphatics causing pleural effusion but never chylothorax. Even when the duct is blocked by neoplasm, chylous effusion tends to be very uncommon, probably as a result of the presence of collaterals between the thoracic duct and the right posterior intercostal lymphatics and of the opening up of pre-existing lymphovenous channels.[116] In order for chylothorax to occur, therefore, there must be an additional deficiency of one or both of these channels of communication. Chyle may reflux from an obstructed thoracic duct by two routes—the left posterior intercostal lymphatics to the parietal pleural lymphatics, and the left bronchomediastinal trunk to lymphatics of the pulmonary parenchyma and visceral pleura. From either the visceral or the parietal lymphatics, chyle then is extravasated into the pleural cavity.

The most common causes of chylothorax are neoplasms, particularly lymphoma, and trauma (see page 791),[121] the former being responsible twice as often as the latter.[16] Occasionally, it occurs spontaneously.[117] The effusion is often bilateral and is usually accompanied by chylous ascites. Although patients with chyliform effusions are often asymptomatic, sometimes a history of disease indicates the cause of the effusion; rheumatoid disease and tuberculosis are the most common.[118] Miscellaneous causes of chylothorax include sclerosing mediastinitis,[119] Gorham's syndrome,[120] and lymphangioleiomyomatosis (see page 853).

Lymphangiography is said to play an important role in the investigation of patients with chylothorax.[122] It has been pointed out, however, that roentgenographic visualization of intrapulmonary and pleural lymphatics following lymphangiography, while usually associated with chylothorax, can occasionally occur without it.[123]

The prognosis of chylothorax is generally good, except when the cause is a neoplasm, in which case it is usually a late manifestation of disease. Considerable difference of opinion exists as to when surgical intervention is indicated; however, many authorities report success with conservative management, including aspiration or drainage, restriction of oral fat intake, and intravenous replacement.

PNEUMOTHORAX

Air in the pleural space—pneumothorax—is one of the more common forms of thoracic disease. It is caused most often by trauma, either accidental or iatrogenic (see page 785). In the absence of such a history, it is traditionally referred to as *spontaneous*, in which case it can be either *primary* (not associated with clinical or roentgenographic evidence of significant pulmonary disease) or *secondary* (when such disease is present). Pneumothorax can also occur as a complication of pneumomediastinum, when air tracks from that location into the pleural space via the mediastinal pleura. In this situation, there is evidence that the most likely sites of rupture are small areas just above the root of the left lung and at the junction with the pericardium.[124]

Primary spontaneous pneumothorax occurs most commonly in the third and fourth decades of life and shows a distinct male predominance, ranging from 2 to 1[125] to as high as 15 to 1.[126]

Etiology and Pathogenesis

A hereditary factor in at least some cases of spontaneous pneumothorax is suggested by the observation of an increased incidence of the disorder in some families.[127] The risk of developing the complication has been related to specific HLA haplotypes and alpha$_1$-antiprotease phenotypes. The anatomic basis for this increased incidence is uncertain; however, it is possible that some inherited abnormality of connective tissue is involved.[128]

The details of the pathogenesis of spontaneous pneumothorax are not clear. The primary form appears to be caused in many cases by rupture of a bleb or a bulla immediately deep to the visceral pleura. The mechanisms behind the formation of each of these are themselves ill understood. In the case of blebs, the pathogenesis usually is attributed to dissection of air from a ruptured alveolus through interstitial tissue into the thin vascular layer of visceral pleura, where it accumulates in the form of a "cyst." (Such dissection may also lead directly to pneumothorax without the formation of a bleb, in which case there may be concomitant extension of air proximally into the

mediastinum with the development of pneumomediastinum (see page 903).

The mechanisms behind the formation of bullae are also uncertain. Most speculation has centered about the possibility of regional damage to the apical portion of the lung, related either to ischemia or to the greater distensive forces on apical alveoli caused by more negative pleural pressure.[129] In support of both of these mechanisms is the pathologic and roentgenologic identification of apical bullae in many individuals with spontaneous pneumothorax and the well-documented clinical observation that primary spontaneous pneumothorax occurs predominantly in tall, thin men.[130] An intrinsic abnormality of connective tissue resulting in an increased tendency to bulla or bleb formation is probably also important in occasional individuals with connective tissue disorders such as Marfan's syndrome.[131]

The immediate cause of rupture of a bleb or bulla is often unknown. It is not necessarily related to exertional effort, since the majority of patients are at rest when the pneumothorax occurs.[132] Blebs and bullae distend with decreasing atmospheric pressure (e.g., with increasing altitude during flight and with rapid surfacing after diving[133]), and this mechanism is probably important in some cases. It has also been postulated that the increased mechanical stress to which the apex of the lung is subjected in taller patients causes rupture of apical blebs in addition to acting as a mechanism in their formation.[134] Increased pressure during the Valsalva maneuver appears to be an important mechanism in some cases, particularly during emesis, bouts of coughing,[135] and, perhaps most commonly, pregnancy and labor.[136] The increasing incidence of marijuana and cocaine smoking in recent years and the use of a prolonged Valsalva's maneuver to augment the "high" also have been associated with pneumothorax in drug users.[135, 137]

The pathogenesis of secondary pneumothorax is multifactorial. Many cases are associated with the presence of bullae in diffuse emphysema or subpleural cystic spaces in diffuse interstitial fibrosis. Rupture of one of these is likely the immediate cause of pneumothorax in many cases. Since patients with secondary pneumothorax by definition have underlying pulmonary disease, local airway obstruction caused by pneumonia, mucus plugs, or physiologic abnormalities may be important in promoting bulla or cyst rupture. In addition, many episodes occur during artificial ventilation used as therapy for the underlying disease, and this is undoubtedly a factor in some cases (see later). Two situations associated with pneumothorax deserve specific comment.

Catamenial Pneumothorax. This is an uncommon condition in which recurrent pneumothorax is associated with menstrual periods.[138] It usually occurs in the fourth decade in women who are otherwise healthy, except perhaps for endometriosis. Several mechanisms have been proposed to explain the mechanism by which air enters the pleural space in these patients:

1. Migration of air through the vagina, uterus, and fallopian tubes into the peritoneal cavity and thence through diaphragmatic defects into the pleural space.[139] Such defects have been found in about one third of patients with pneumothorax associated with pleural endometriosis and have been considered to represent both developmental

anomalies and acquired lesions secondary to endometriosis itself.

2. Necrosis of endometrial tissue at sites of visceral pleural endometriosis during menses, resulting in an air leak between lung and pleura. Although this is an attractive hypothesis, it is nevertheless unusual to find foci of endometriosis at thoracotomy, either grossly or microscopically.

3. Rupture of apical blebs, possibly related to some unidentified factor associated with menses.[140]

Iatrogenic Pneumothorax. With the increasing use of invasive diagnostic procedures, this complication has become an important cause of pneumothorax, although most episodes are minor in degree and of little clinical significance. A variety of such procedures can be complicated by pneumothorax, the most common being transbronchial biopsy,[141] transthoracic needle aspiration, central venous catheterization, and faulty feeding tube insertion.[142]

Patients being assisted by artificial ventilation are at special risk for the development of pneumothorax, particularly when volume-cycled machines and positive end-expiratory pressure (PEEP) are used. The incidence of pneumothorax in these situations has been estimated to be between 0.5 and 15 per cent, depending on the duration of ventilation, the nature of the underlying disease, and the use of PEEP.[143] Pneumothorax is more likely to occur when very high peak inspiratory pressures are employed to ventilate patients with severely obstructed airways or noncompliant lungs; in such circumstances, it is sometimes associated with pneumomediastinum or pneumoperitoneum and may be a terminal event.

Pathologic Characteristics

In our experience, the most common abnormality in lung excised from individuals with primary spontaneous pneumothorax is a bulla, usually 0.5 to 1.5 cm in diameter and located adjacent to fibrotic pleura (Fig. 18–1). True blebs (i.e., entirely intrapleural cystic spaces) are relatively uncommon. Pathologic findings in secondary spontaneous pneumothorax depend on the nature of the underlying disease. Emphysematous bullae and cystic spaces associated with interstitial fibrosis are the most common.

Histologic examination of pleura excised at thoracotomy for therapy of pneumothorax often reveals characteristic changes termed "eosinophilic pleuritis" that are believed to represent a reaction to the presence of air.[144] These consist of a fibrinous exudate within which are large numbers of eosinophils and mononuclear cells (probably a combination of macrophages and mesothelial cells) and occasional multinucleated giant cells.

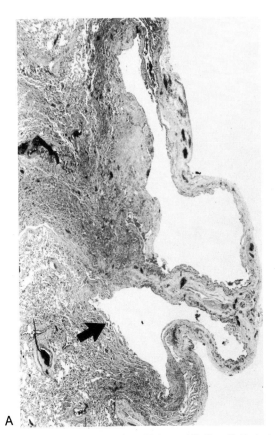
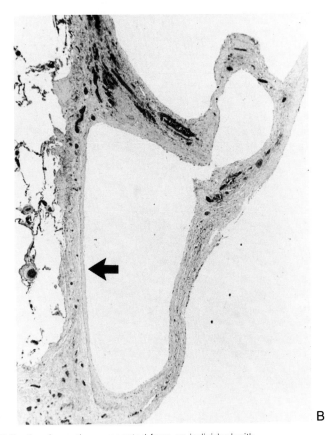

A   B

Figure 18–1. Blebs and Bullae: Pathologic Distinction. Lung tissue resected from an individual with spontaneous pneumothorax (A) shows two cystic spaces lined by fibrous tissue. Although these spaces appear to be largely within the pleura, one (arrow) is in direct contact with lung parenchyma, indicating that it represents a bulla. A section of lung from another patient (B) shows similar cystic spaces but in this instance completely surrounded by pleura (arrow), indicating that they are true blebs. (A × 12; B × 18.)

Roentgenographic Manifestations

As previously discussed (*see* page 250), the roentgenologic diagnosis of pneumothorax is made by identification of the visceral pleural line (Fig. 18–2), although this can be very difficult on roentgenograms exposed at total lung capacity. Even in the presence of pneumothorax, blebs or bullae are sometimes not identifiable on conventional chest roentgenograms,[145] although their visualization may be facilitated by roentgenography in expiration or at the time of maximal pulmonary collapse. Tomography, both conventional and computed, may reveal small blebs or bullae that are invisible on plain roentgenograms. One CT study showed that the number and size of blebs correlates with the incidence of recurrence.[146]

Pleural effusion coincident with pneumothorax appears to occur less frequently than might be anticipated. For example, one study of 72 patients found fluid in only 19 (26 per cent) before diagnostic or therapeutic manipulation.[147] Of the 15 effusions aspirated, 11 were serous and 4 were bloody. Eosinophilia is common in the fluid.[148]

Clinical Manifestations

Chest pain and dyspnea, either alone or in combination, are the classic symptoms of spontaneous pneumothorax. The latter can be severe but may disappear within 24 hours, regardless of whether the collapsed lung undergoes partial re-expansion. The major physical sign suggesting pneumothorax is a decrease in or absence of breath sounds despite normal or increased resonance on percussion. Even with a small pneumothorax, the relative difference in breath sounds between the two hemithoraces should suggest the diagnosis. However, in patients with emphysema whose breath sounds are already greatly reduced and in whom percussion is normal or increased, the presence of pneumothorax may be very difficult to recognize by physical signs. Hamman's sign (*see* page 147), originally considered to be caused by pneumomediastinum, is now thought to be associated much more frequently with left pneumothorax. Bilateral pneumothorax is uncommon[149] and should suggest the possibility of intravenous drug injection into neck veins.

Occasionally, inspired air becomes trapped in a pleural

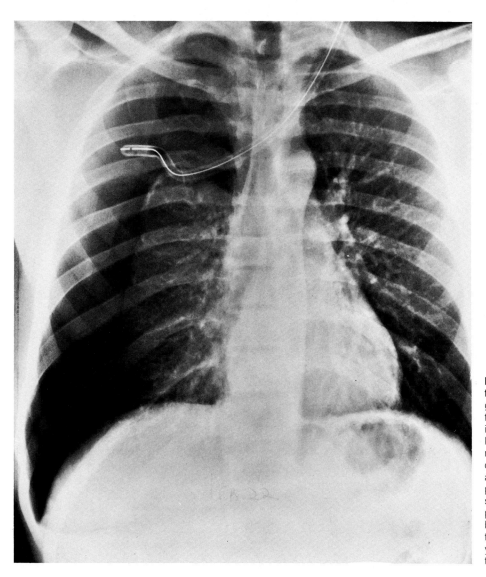

Figure 18–2. Spontaneous Pneumothorax. A posteroanterior roentgenogram reveals a large right pneumothorax. A chest tube has been introduced, but the lung is still collapsed to less than 50 per cent of its normal volume. It is important to recognize two facts revealed by this examination: (1) the density of right lung parenchyma is approximately the same as that of the left despite its 50 per cent reduction in volume (caused by hypoxic vasoconstriction); and (2) the right chest wall has expanded beyond its normal position as a result of the loss of the elastic recoil of the lung.

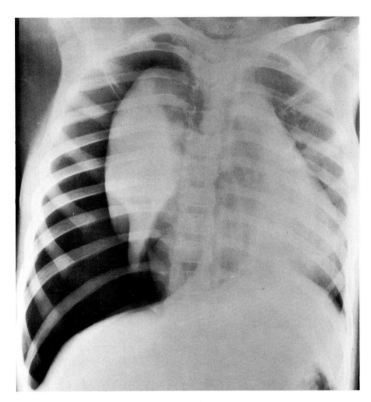

Figure 18–3. Spontaneous Pneumothorax Associated with Massive Pneumonia. This 6-year-old girl was admitted to the hospital following a 2-day history of acute respiratory illness and the abrupt onset 2 hours before of severe right-sided chest pain and shortness of breath. An anteroposterior roentgenogram on admission reveals a massive right pneumothorax associated with marked shift of the mediastinum to the left, an appearance consistent with the presence of "tension." Despite this, the volume of the airless right lung is obviously greater than could be accounted for by relaxation atelectasis alone, shown later to be caused by right upper lobe pneumonia of probable staphylococcal etiology. (Courtesy of St. Joseph's General Hospital, Blind River, Ontario.)

space, presumably on the basis of a bronchopleural check-valve mechanism, leading to tension pneumothorax (Fig. 18–3) (*see* page 254). Immediate recognition of this complication is essential, since these patients may rapidly become hypoxic and acidotic, not uncommonly with fatal outcomes.[2]

The frequency of recurrence of spontaneous pneumothorax on the same side is surprisingly high, amounting to about 30 per cent in most reported series. In approximately 10 per cent of cases, it develops subsequently on the contralateral side.

PLEURAL FIBROSIS

After effusion, fibrosis is undoubtedly the most common pleural abnormality. Like effusion, it has numerous causes and is the outcome of many primary diseases of the pleura, as well as a potential complication of virtually every inflammatory condition that affects the lungs. In the majority of cases, the fibrosis is localized to a single relatively small area, in which situation clinical and functional abnormalities are absent and the condition is recognized on a screening roentgenogram, during the investigation of other intrathoracic disease, or at necropsy. Less commonly, the fibrosis is more or less diffuse in one or both pleural cavities, in which case functional abnormalities may be apparent. Because of this important difference, the two forms are discussed separately. Roentgenographic signs of pleural fibrosis are described on page 250.

Local Pleural Fibrosis

Healed Pleuritis

The most common cause of localized pleural fibrosis is organized fibrinous or fibrinopurulent pleuritis secondary to pneumonia. The usual roentgenographic abnormality is blunting of the posterior and lateral costophrenic sulcus, in some cases associated with line shadows in the adjacent lung. Thickening of the pleural line may extend for a variable distance up the lateral and posterior thoracic walls, diminishing gradually toward the apex and seldom amounting to more than 1 to 2 mm in width. Obliteration of the costophrenic sulcus often has a roentgenographic appearance difficult to differentiate from that of a small pleural effusion; however, in fibrosis the posterior costophrenic angle is usually sharp and not blunted, thus effectively excluding effusion as the cause.

The "Apical Cap"

Somewhat similar to fibrosis secondary to healed pleuritis but in a different location are curved shadows of unit density situated at the apex of one or both hemithoraces in the concavity formed by the first and second ribs (*see* Fig. 4–94, page 252). Such apical caps occur with equal frequency in men and women and are more common and larger in older persons.[150]

Pathologically, the abnormality consists of a combination of pleural and pulmonary parenchymal fibrosis, the latter usually predominating (Fig. 18–4).[151] Although the pathogenesis of the abnormality has been ascribed to tuberculosis, evidence of prior granulomatous inflammation and necrosis suggestive of this disease is invariably absent. It is perhaps more likely that the relative ischemia in the apical portion of the lung is responsible.

The physician must not fail to recognize apparent apical pleural thickening as a possible early manifestation of much more serious disease—apical pulmonary cancer or Pancoast's tumor. Early apical carcinoma of the Pancoast type can closely mimic pleural thickening; suspicion should be

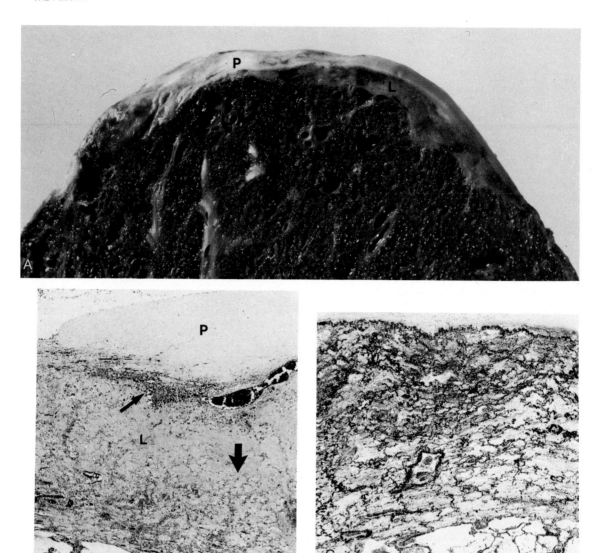

Figure 18–4. Apical Pleural Cap. A magnified view of the apex of the right upper lobe *(A)* shows a mild degree of fibrosis affecting both the pleura (P) and the underlying lung parenchyma (L). A histologic section *(B)* reveals fibrosis within the pleura (P) and lung (L) associated with focal chronic inflammation *(thin arrow)*. Despite the parenchymal fibrosis, the underlying lung architecture is clearly preserved as demonstrated in sections stained with hematoxylin-eosin *(large arrow in B)* and with elastic tissue stain *(C)*. (B × 25; C Verhoeff–van Gieson × 25.)

enhanced when the abnormality is predominantly unilateral.

Pleural Plaques

Four types of roentgenographic changes occur in the pleura of patients exposed to asbestos or talc—plaque formation, calcification, diffuse pleural thickening, and pleural effusion. Plaque formation is by far the most common and is discussed on pages 720 and 723.

General Pleural Fibrosis (Fibrothorax)

Like local pleural fibrosis, fibrothorax has several causes, including asbestos exposure,[152] uremia,[107] and some connective tissue diseases. Healing of a massive hemothorax or empyema particularly may be associated with deposition of

a layer of dense fibrous tissue that may be 2 cm thick around a whole lung, resulting in marked decrease in volume of the hemithorax. In some patients, the fibrosis is associated with significant clinical and functional abnormalities. Calcification occurs frequently on the *inner* aspect of the fibrous peel and provides an indicator by which its thickness can be accurately measured (Fig. 18–5).

The degree to which unilateral fibrothorax impairs ventilation of the underlying lung can be roughly gauged by assessing pulmonary vascularity. If the pulmonary vessels of the affected lung are smaller than those of the opposite side, it can be assumed that the reduction in perfusion has occurred in response to reduced ventilation, presumably as a result of hypoxic vasoconstriction (Fig. 18–6). By contrast, if the vascularity of the two lungs is roughly symmetric, it is reasonable to assume that reflex vasoconstriction has not occurred and that ventilation is therefore preserved. The

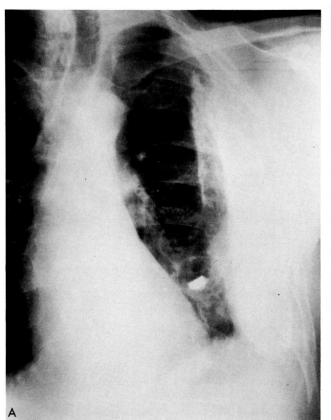

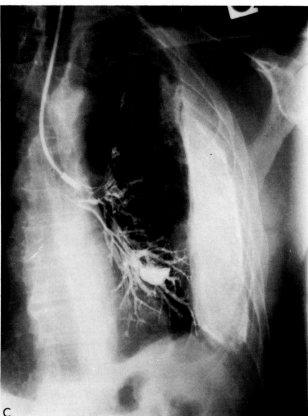

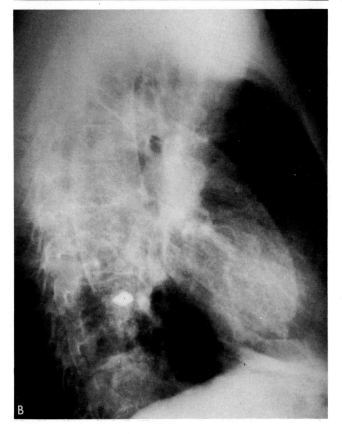

Figure 18–5. Long-Term Follow-up of Shrapnel Wound of the Left Lower Lobe and Pleura. Posteroanterior (A) and lateral (B) roentgenograms reveal moderate loss of volume of the left hemithorax associated with marked thickening of the pleura over the whole of the left lung (fibrothorax). A thick calcific plaque covers the axillary portion of the lung. A metallic foreign body is situated in the midportion of the left lower lobe, associated with a poorly defined cystic space. In view of a history of chronic productive cough, a bronchogram was performed (C). Contrast medium entered the cystic space and completely obscured the metallic foreign body, thus confirming the suspicion that the fragment of shrapnel lay within the cystic space. The calcific fibrothorax was the result of traumatic hemothorax.

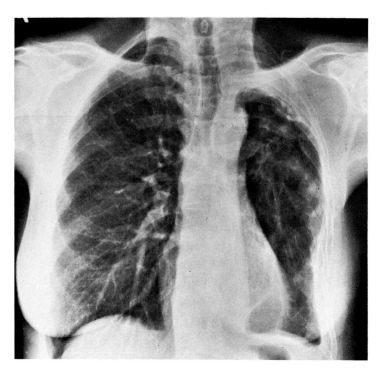

Figure 18–6. Unilateral Fibrothorax Leading to Hypoventilation and Reflex Vasoconstriction. A posteroanterior roentgenogram of this 73-year-old asymptomatic woman reveals moderate thickening of the pleura over the whole of the left lung. The pleura is calcified over the lower axillary lung zone. The volume of the left lung is moderately reduced, and its vessel markings diminutive. The volume of the left lung showed little change from inspiration to expiration, indicating hypoventilation.

authors have frequently been impressed by the fact that the degree of pleural thickening does not bear a close relationship to reduced ventilation and perfusion. In other words, a thick pleural peel does not necessarily imply reduced ventilation and perfusion any more than a thin peel.

PRIMARY NEOPLASMS OF THE PLEURA

Localized Fibrous Tumor

Localized (solitary) fibrous tumor (fibrous or benign mesothelioma) is an uncommon neoplasm of the pleura that is believed to be derived from a submesothelial mesenchymal cell that possesses the capacity for fibroblastic differentiation. It is probably less common than diffuse malignant mesothelioma, although more than 350 cases had been documented in the literature by 1980[153] and an additional 223 cases were reported from the files of the Armed Forces Institute of Pathology (AFIP) in 1989.[154] It occurs slightly more often in women than in men, and the mean age at presentation is about 50 years.[153] The etiology is unknown, but there is no association with asbestos exposure.

Pathologic Characteristics

Most localized fibrous tumors arise from the visceral pleura and grow into the pleural space, compressing the adjacent lung to a variable degree (Fig. 18–7). Occasionally, tumors arising in the medial pleura extend into the mediastinum[155] and those in a fissure into the pulmonary parenchyma.[154] The majority are spherical or oblong in shape and well defined or encapsulated; many are attached to the pleura by a short vascular pedicle. They can grow to huge size, examples up to 36 cm in diameter having been re-

ported.[153] Cysts, hemorrhage, necrosis, and calcification can be present, especially in the larger tumors.

Histologically, the tumors consist of haphazardly arranged or interlacing fascicles of spindle cells with a variable amount of intervening collagen (Fig. 18–8). Small vascular channels may be prominent. Immunohistochemical studies have generally shown a negative reaction for keratin,[156] in contrast to the sarcomatous form of diffuse malignant mesothelioma in which the reaction is often positive.

Roentgenographic Manifestations

Roentgenologically, localized fibrous tumors are typically sharply defined, somewhat lobulated masses of homogene-

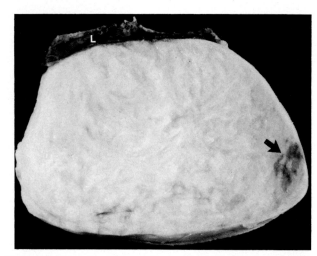

Figure 18–7. Localized Fibrous Tumor of the Pleura. A cut section of a pleural tumor shows a well-defined, lobulated mass compressing a small amount of attached lung parenchyma (L). There is focal hemorrhage *(arrow)* but no necrosis.

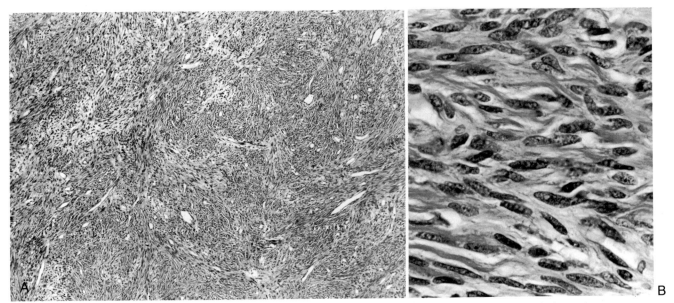

Figure 18–8. Localized Fibrous Tumor of the Pleura. A histologic section *(A)* shows interlacing fascicles of spindle cells with little intercellular collagen. A magnified view *(B)* demonstrates minimal pleomorphism of cell nuclei. *(A × 60; B × 600.)*

ous density ranging in diameter from 2 to 14 cm. In one series of 17 cases,[157] there was no predilection for either side, but only two lesions were in the upper half of the chest. Characteristically, the tumors form an obtuse angle with the chest wall or mediastinum, a finding important to the establishment of the extrapulmonary origin of a thoracic mass (Fig. 18–9). When a tumor is very large, however, the site of origin is frequently difficult or impossible to establish on conventional roentgenograms and even on CT. In such circumstances, determination of the blood supply of the mass by arteriography may be of help.[158] Should the tumor opacify following injection of the inferior phrenic, intercostal, or internal mammary arteries, its extrapulmonary origin may be considered to be reasonably (although perhaps not conclusively) established.

Of considerable diagnostic value is the tendency for a

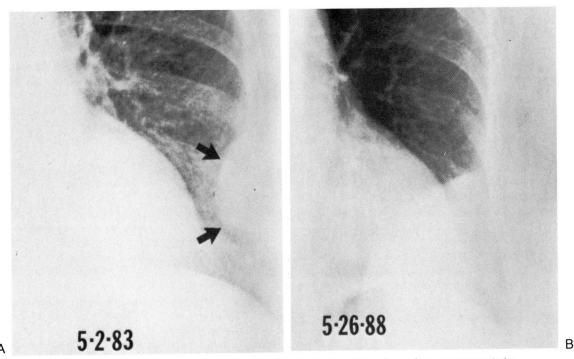

Figure 18–9. Localized Fibrous Tumor Showing Growth. A view of the left lung from a posteroanterior roentgenogram *(A)* reveals a sharply defined opacity in the axillary region inferiorly *(arrows)*. The mass is homogeneous and possesses a broad pleural base. Note the obtuse angle the mass makes with the pleural surface, indicating its extrapulmonary location. Five years later *(B)*, the tumor had undergone remarkable growth.

lesion to change position with respiration or needling,[159] regardless of its site of origin. Movement is detected by relating the position of the tumor to contiguous ribs or mediastinal structures. Calcification was evident in 7 per cent of cases reviewed in the AFIP series,[154] and pleural effusion was demonstrated in 17 per cent.

The CT findings have been described in one series of nine patients, for all of whom pathologic correlation was available.[160] The only distinctive feature was intense increased attenuation on contrast-enhanced scans attributable to the marked vascularity of the tumors.

Clinical Manifestations

Many patients with localized fibrous tumors are asymptomatic; cough, chest pain, and dyspnea occur occasionally, especially with larger tumors.[161] One particularly common finding is hypertrophic osteoarthropathy,[153] an association that is much stronger than with pulmonary carcinoma. In fact, its presence in a patient with a large intrathoracic mass should suggest the diagnosis. Another interesting association is symptomatic hypoglycemia, a complication that occurs in about 5 per cent of patients.[161] In the AFIP series, it was somewhat more common with malignant than with benign tumors and three times more frequent in women than in men.[154]

The majority of localized fibrous tumors behave in a benign fashion, growing slowly and compressing rather than invading contiguous structures. Surgical excision usually results in complete cure, particularly when the tumor possesses a well-defined pedicle; however, local recurrence can occur and death caused by extensive intrathoracic disease has been reported in 10 to 15 per cent of patients.[153] Prediction of an aggressive or benign behavior can be difficult. In the AFIP series,[154] a considerably greater proportion of malignant tumors was associated with pleural effusion and arose in the parietal pleura. Chest wall invasion was present in almost half the cases. Histologic appearances are not predictive in individual cases: cellular pleomorphism and a high mitotic rate do not necessarily imply a bad prognosis and occasional tumors with a bland histologic appearance ultimately recur.[153, 154] Extrathoracic metastases are rare.

Diffuse Malignant Mesothelioma

Diffuse mesothelioma is an uncommon, but increasingly recognized, malignant neoplasm of the pleura. In the 1970s, the incidence in England and the United States was estimated to be 2.2 cases per million per year,[162] but more recently this estimate was increased to 7 to 13 per million.[163] The neoplasm is important not only because it is almost always lethal, usually within a short time after diagnosis, but also because of the potential economic impact of litigation and workers' compensation.

Etiology and Pathogenesis

Asbestos. There is good evidence that the etiologic agent in the majority of cases of diffuse mesothelioma is asbestos. This evidence can be summarized under three categories.

Epidemiologic Studies and Clinical Experience Showing a Strong Relationship Between Asbestos Ex- *posure and Mesothelioma.* A history of exposure to asbestos is obtained from more than 50 per cent of subjects in most series of patients with mesothelioma[164, 165]; in some reports,[166] the prevalence is as high as 85 per cent. Epidemiologic studies show a high incidence of the tumor in persons involved in both the mining and the production of asbestos and in the numerous secondary occupations associated with its use (*see* page 720); the risk appears to be greater in manufacturing and secondary uses than in mining and milling.[167] Some occupations, such as shipbuilding, are especially hazardous.[168]

There is also good evidence that contact with asbestos secondarily related to occupation can be hazardous; for example, mesothelioma has been reported in wives of workers in asbestos plants (who are probably exposed while laundering workers' clothes)[169] and in persons who reside near factories that process asbestos,[170] presumably as a result of contact with asbestos in the atmosphere. Nonoccupational environmental contact with asbestos in soil has also been related to an increased risk of mesothelioma.[171]

Studies of Asbestos Fiber Burden in the Lungs of Patients with Mesothelioma. There is clearly an association between a large number of asbestos fibers in lung tissue and the presence of mesothelioma. For example, in one investigation of the lung tissue of 100 patients with mesothelioma,[172] 88 had a history of asbestos exposure. In all but one of these patients, light microscopy showed more than 20,000 coated and uncoated asbestos fibers per gram of dried lung. By contrast, of the 7 patients in the group who could confidently deny exposure to asbestos, 6 had a fiber count below 20,000. Despite these observations, some workers[173] have reported that the number of asbestos fibers in patients with mesothelioma is intermediate between that in the general population and that in patients with asbestosis. Patients whose fiber count overlaps those of the general population tend to be unable to identify an occupational exposure.[174]

Experimental Studies in Animals Showing the Development of Mesothelioma After Asbestos Exposure. Diffuse mesothelioma morphologically similar to that seen in humans has been shown to develop following instillation of asbestos fibers into the pleural space[163] or trachea[175] of various animals.

The likelihood of developing mesothelioma varies considerably with the type of asbestos. The majority of evidence indicates that the risk is greatest with the amphiboles crocidolite and amosite, that it is substantially less with chrysotile, and that it is virtually nonexistent with anthophyllite. The relative importance of chrysotile has been the subject of some debate:[163] although the bulk of evidence suggests that exposure to this variety does increase the risk of mesothelioma, it is possible that this is related to the presence of contaminating amphiboles, particularly tremolite.[176]

The variable pathogenicity of the different types of asbestos may be related to their different physicochemical characteristics. Long, straight fibers, such as those of the amphiboles, tend to be transported in the center of the airway lumen to the periphery of the lung; by contrast, the irregular, curly shape of the chrysotile fibers predisposes them to deposition in the more central airways.[163] Thus, amosite and crocidolite tend to accumulate in relatively large numbers in the peripheral portions of the lung close to the pleura. There is also evidence that chrysotile fibers fragment with time and are transported out of the lung via the mucociliary escalator or lymphatics.[163] Amphiboles, on the other hand, are relatively stable and remain either constant in number in an individual who is no longer exposed or continue to accumulate over the lifetime of an individual who is continually exposed. Finally, there is experimental evidence that chrysotile and crocidolite fibers interact differently with chromosomes of mesothelial cells,[177] possibly reflecting a different carcinogenic potential.

The pathogenesis of asbestos-related mesothelioma is far from clear. Experimental studies have shown that the size and shape of the fibers are important determinants of carcinogenicity. For example, it is possible to prepare samples of chrysotile that are long and straight (in contrast to their natural state) and that are at least as carcinogenic as amosite.[178] In addition to amphiboles, other fibers such as fiberglass and certain metals[163] can induce cancer when introduced directly into the pleural space of animals; however, inhalation of these substances by humans does not appear to be associated with an increased risk of mesothelioma. This suggests that factors associated with deposition or clearance of these particles may be at least as important as their physical properties.

Other Etiologic Agents. Despite the presence of a large asbestos burden in the lungs of many individuals with mesothelioma, there are some patients in whom the burden is relatively light and, in fact, overlaps that of the general population,[174] suggesting that other etiologic agents may be important. Because the pathogenesis of asbestos-related mesothelioma appears to be intimately associated with its fibrous nature, attention has been directed to the possibility that other minerals with the same physical characteristics as asbestos also may be pathogenic. The most clearly implicated of these is erionite, a nonasbestos mineral of the zeolite group found in the soil of central Turkey and the western United States (*see* page 729). Strong epidemiologic[179] and experimental[180] evidence has accumulated that implicates this substance in the production of both pleural plaques and mesothelioma.

It is probable that radiation is also responsible for occasional cases of mesothelioma.[181] In fact, experimental evidence suggests that the risk is significantly increased when radiation is combined with asbestos exposure.[182] A familial occurrence of mesothelioma has been documented in several studies[183]; although this may be largely explained by shared exposure to asbestos dust brought into the home or to another common source of exposure, it is also possible that there is a degree of genetic susceptibility. The risk of developing mesothelioma appears to be independent of cigarette smoking.[165]

Pathologic Characteristics

In the vast majority of cases, malignant mesothelioma appears as a diffuse, plaquelike thickening that more or less encases the entire lung, at least in autopsy specimens (Fig. 18–10). Extension of the neoplasm along fissures and into adjacent tissues, such as the chest wall, diaphragm, and pericardium, is not uncommon. Despite this, the border between the tumor and underlying lung parenchyma is usually well defined, although nodular expansions occasionally project from the thickened pleura into the lung itself.

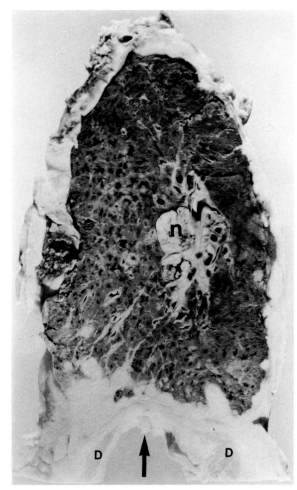

Figure 18–10. Diffuse Mesothelioma. A sagittal section of left lung shows mild to moderate thickening of the pleura over almost its entire surface; the lung parenchyma is unremarkable. The tumor has extended into the adjacent hemidiaphragm (D) to involve the peritoneum *(arrow)*. Metastases are evident in peribronchial lymph nodes (n).

Histologically, mesothelioma is usually classified in three forms—*epithelial, mesenchymal* (sarcomatous), and *biphasic* (mixed). The epithelial form is the most common and has a variable appearance, cells being organized in papillary projections, tubular or acinar clusters, and solid sheets (Fig. 18–11). An elongated, slitlike space lined on either side by a single layer of neoplastic cells is characteristic. Typically, the tumor cells are cuboidal and possess a moderate amount of cytoplasm and nuclei that are often rather uniform in size and shape. The mesenchymal form typically consists of spindle cells that are arranged either in a fascicular or storiform pattern. Interstitial collagen may be apparent, suggesting fibroblastic differentiation. Occasionally this tissue is abundant, leading to the designation "desmoplastic" mesothelioma.[184]

There are two major practical problems in the pathologic diagnosis of mesothelioma: (1) distinguishing mesothelial hyperplasia from neoplasia; and (2) distinguishing mesothelioma from metastatic carcinoma, especially adenocarcinoma. Both of these problems are particularly troublesome with the small tissue fragments commonly obtained by closed chest pleural biopsy.

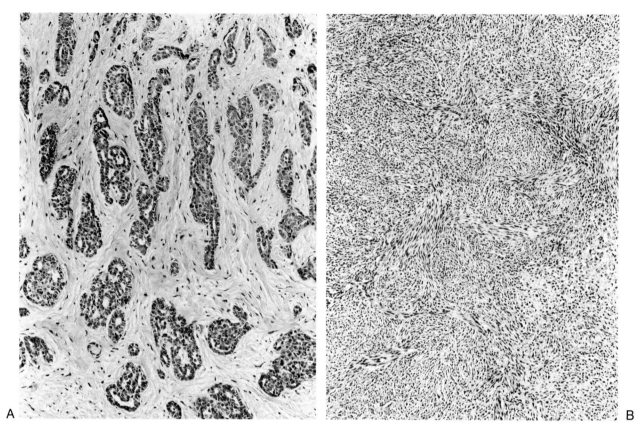

Figure 18–11. Diffuse Mesothelioma: Histologic Types. Section from the epithelial subtype of mesothelioma *(A)* reveals nests of cells separated by a fibroblastic stroma and associated with round or elongated slitlike spaces. *B,* Section from the mesenchymal form shows fascicles of spindle-shaped cells arranged in an interdigitating pattern. *(A × 100; B × 120.)*

Mesothelial Hyperplasia versus Neoplasia. Mesothelial cells commonly react to pleural injury by proliferating, sometimes to a marked degree. This proliferation can result in a variety of morphologic appearances, occasionally with features suggesting neoplasia such as mitotic activity, cytologic atypia, and entrapment of mesothelial cell clusters in underlying fibrous tissue, simulating invasion.[185] Since these features also can be present in mesothelioma, the distinction between a reactive and a neoplastic process can be extremely difficult. Although histologic criteria[186] and various ancillary techniques such as flow cytometry,[187] morphometry,[188] and identification of tumor suppressor genes[188a] have been proposed to aid in such differentiation, in some cases it may be impossible to be definitive.

Mesothelioma versus Metastatic Carcinoma. The second major problem in the pathologic diagnosis of mesothelioma lies in distinguishing it from metastatic carcinoma. As with hyperplasia and neoplasia, a variety of ancillary studies have been employed to aid in the solution of this problem. Of some differential diagnostic value is the reaction to PAS with diastase, which is positive in many adenocarcinomas and almost never in mesothelioma. The demonstration of acid mucopolysaccharides, specifically hyaluronic acid, within tumor cells is also quite suggestive of mesothelioma.[189]

Numerous studies have been performed to document the immunohistochemical features of mesothelioma and adenocarcinoma in an attempt to find consistent differences between the two. Many investigators have reported a positive reaction of adenocarcinoma for CEA (in 60 to 100 per cent of cases), whereas the reaction in mesothelioma is almost always negative.[190, 191] It can be reasonably concluded, therefore, that a clearly positive reaction for CEA argues greatly against the diagnosis of mesothelioma; however, since as many as 40 per cent of adenocarcinomas show a negative reaction for this substance, the lack of a reaction does not establish the diagnosis of mesothelioma. The reaction to Leu-M1, a sugar linked to membranes in intercellular proteins and lipids, also has been found to be almost always negative in mesothelioma and often positive in adenocarcinoma.[192] Studies of other antibodies used in attempts to differentiate mesothelioma and adenocarcinoma generally have given results of unproved or equivocal value.

The ultrastructural features of the better differentiated epithelial forms of mesothelioma include[193] (1) the absence of microvillus core rootlets, glycocalyceal bodies, and secretory granules (three structures that are characteristic of adenocarcinoma); and (2) the presence of intercellular desmosomes and junctional complexes, intracytoplasmic lumina, intermediate filaments (often aggregated in a perinuclear location), and microvilli (Fig. 18–12). Of all these features, the appearance of the microvilli is the most important diagnostically: in mesothelioma they are numerous

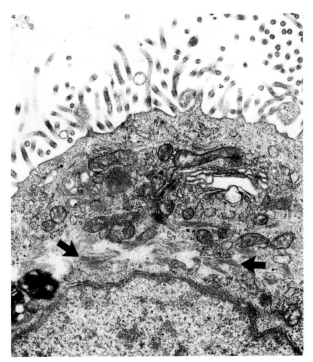

Figure 18–12. Diffuse Mesothelioma: Ultrastructure. An electron micrograph of a single cell from a well-differentiated epithelial mesothelioma shows perinuclear clusters of intermediate filaments (arrows) and long, thin surface microvilli. (× 21,700.)

and are characteristically long and thin, whereas in adenocarcinoma they are typically much less frequent and are usually short and stubby.

As with histochemical detection of hyaluronic acid in mesothelioma cells, the demonstration of this substance in tissue fragments by digestion and electrophoresis is evidence in favor of the diagnosis of mesothelioma.[194] A second glycosaminoglycan, chondroitin sulfate, is also elaborated by some mesotheliomas and is sometimes the principal substance present[195]; it is also suggestive of the diagnosis.

Roentgenographic Manifestations

The most common roentgenographic presentation of malignant mesothelioma is irregular, nodular opacities around the periphery of the lung, either over the convexity or along the mediastinum or diaphragm (Fig. 18–13). Such opacities may or may not be associated with pleural effusion; when present, it frequently obscures the underlying neoplasm (Fig. 18–14). In contrast to other forms of pleural effusion, that associated with mesothelioma is frequently not accompanied by significant shift of the mediastinum to the contralateral side, a peculiarity that has two possible explanations: (1) the formation of a large pleural "peel" acts in a restrictive capacity and prevents inflation of the lung on full inspiration, thus reducing volume; and (2) less likely, local invasion of the medial aspect of the lung by the neoplasm occludes bronchi and results in atelectasis. This pattern of massive pleural effusion unassociated with mediastinal shift can also occur with primary pulmonary carcinoma accompanied by obstructive atelectasis and pleural metastases, and it is obviously important to differentiate these two causes.

Computed tomography is generally superior to conventional roentgenograms in determining the extent of the neoplasm (Fig. 18–15). For example, in one study in which CT and conventional radiography were compared,[196] although the major pathologic features of both metastatic carcinoma and mesothelioma were well documented by both modalities, CT demonstrated the findings more frequently and in greater detail. Nodular involvement of the pleural fissures, pleural effusion, and ipsilateral volume loss are features that predominate in mesothelioma.

Calcification occasionally can be identified in both the primary tumor and metastases on conventional roentgenograms and CT.[197, 198] In the former, it probably reflects incorporation of calcified pleural plaques into the neoplasm, whereas in metastases it is likely caused by osseous differentiation of the mesenchymal form of the tumor. The diagnosis of mesothelioma may be suggested by the finding of parenchymal fibrosis or pleural plaques (or both), but these clues are often absent.

Clinical Manifestations

Patients with diffuse pleural mesothelioma can present with either vague chest or shoulder ache or true pleuritic pain.[199] As the disease progresses, shortness of breath, weight loss, and dry hacking cough can develop. Physical examination often reveals clubbing, retraction of the thorax, and dullness on percussion. Occasionally, the neoplasm invades the chest wall along a needle track established at thoracentesis or biopsy; in this situation, a localized tumor may be palpated at the puncture site, a finding highly suggestive of the diagnosis. Cardiac abnormalities are common; in one series of 64 patients, electrocardiographic abnormalities were present in 55 patients (89 per cent) and consisted of arrhythmia (60 per cent) and a conduction abnormality (37 per cent).[200] Although metastases outside the thorax are not uncommonly identified at autopsy,[201] they are infrequently detected clinically.

An occupational history of asbestos exposure may suggest the diagnosis, although some patients give a history of minimal exposure, and careful questioning may be necessary to elicit evidence of the asbestos association. Compounding this difficulty is a latent period between exposure and the development of clinical signs that usually exceeds 20 years and sometimes is as long as 40 years or more.

Pleural effusion may be either straw-colored or serosanguineous. A low level, if any, of carcinoembryonic antigen (less than 12 mg/mL) in aspirated fluid has been found to be characteristic of mesothelioma, whereas values greater than 15 mg/mL are indicative of metastatic carcinoma.[201a]

Cytologic features of malignant mesothelioma cells in pleural fluid have been described in several reports[202]; as with histologic diagnosis, problems are encountered in distinguishing reactive from neoplastic mesothelial cells and mesothelioma from metastatic adenocarcinoma. Although a variety of ancillary procedures have been investigated in an attempt to overcome these problems[203] and although some observers report a high degree of accuracy in the cytologic diagnosis of mesothelioma,[204] the authors and others [203] find that a diagnosis based on cytology alone can be quite difficult and that examination of pleural tissue specimens obtained at thoracoscopy or thoracotomy is usually necessary to confidently establish a diagnosis.

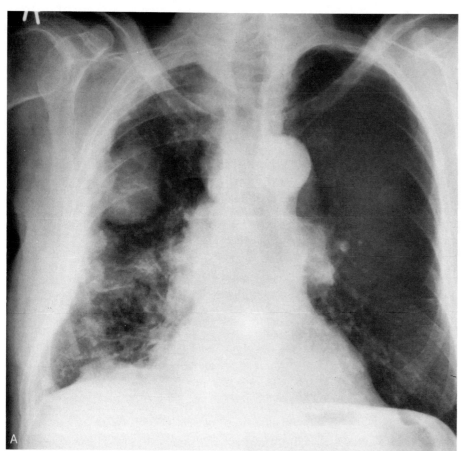

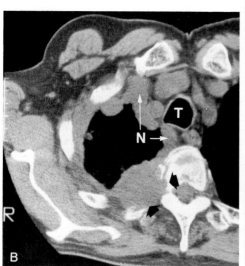

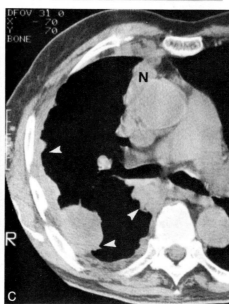

Figure 18–13. Diffuse Mesothelioma. An overpenetrated posteroanterior chest roentgenogram *(A)* shows a reduction in volume of the right hemithorax. There is marked thickening of the pleura over the whole of the right lung, including its mediastinal surface. The thickening is very irregular and nodular and is associated with a large mass in the upper axillary region. High-resolution CT scans through the upper *(B)* and middle *(C)* thorax confirm the extensive right pleural thickening *(arrowheads)* and demonstrate extrapleural extension of the neoplasm in and around the ribs and vertebra *(closed arrows)* and within some of the mediastinal lymph nodes (N). The diagnosis of mesothelioma was confirmed at autopsy several months later.

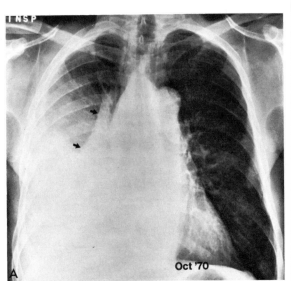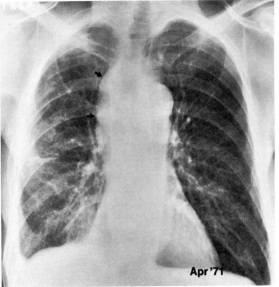

Figure 18–14. Malignant Mesothelioma Presenting with a Massive Pleural Effusion. The initial roentgenogram of this 56-year-old man *(A)* reveals a massive right pleural effusion whose upper configuration is somewhat atypical, suggesting the presence of pulmonary disease underlying the effusion. In addition, there is an unusual opacity in the medial portion of the right hemithorax contiguous to the mediastinum *(arrows)*. Thoracotomy was performed, and a large paramediastinal mesothelioma removed. This was followed by a course of antineoplastic drug therapy. Six months later, a roentgenogram *(B)* reveals a smooth, sharply defined mass in the right paramediastinal zone *(arrows)*; there is still a small pleural effusion.

Prognosis

The prognosis of diffuse pleural mesothelioma is extremely poor; many patients die within a year after the onset of symptoms, and there is almost no long-term survival.[205] It has been suggested that prognosis tends to be somewhat better in patients whose neoplasm possesses an epithelial morphology rather than a mesenchymal one.[206]

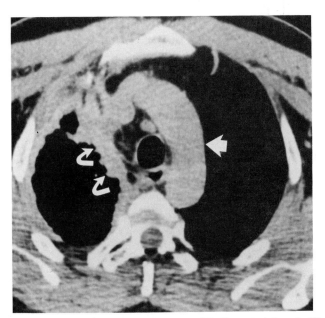

Figure 18–15. Malignant Mesothelioma: CT Characteristics. A CT scan at the level of the aortic arch *(straight arrow)* demonstrates circumferential right pleural thickening, maximal over the mediastinum *(curved arrows)*; the thickening is somewhat nodular. Note also the decreased volume of the right hemithorax.

Extrapleural pneumonectomy, consisting of *en bloc* excision of parietal pleura, lung, pericardium, diaphragm, and attached tumor, has been said to offer some benefit in selected patients.[207] As might be expected, however, operative deaths and serious postoperative complications are not uncommon.

Miscellaneous Pleural Tumors

In addition to localized fibrous tumors, a variety of soft tissue neoplasms have been reported to develop in the pleura. Although some of these are probably derived from the submesothelial mesenchymal cells of the pleura itself and thus indeed arise in this location, it is likely that others originate in the chest wall and simply expand into the pleural space. The most common of these is lipoma, a tumor that is usually small but can become large enough to erode contiguous ribs.[208] The shape of these lesions may change during respiration, presumably as a result of the relatively fluid nature of their content.

Intrathoracic splenosis is a rare condition in which tissue from a traumatized spleen crosses an injured diaphragm and proliferates in the left pleural space, creating nodular opacities.[209] Once the diagnosis is suspected it can be easily confirmed by radionuclide imaging.

References

1. Davis SD, Henschke CI, Yankelevitz DF, et al: MR imaging of pleural effusions. J Comput Assist Tomogr 14: 192, 1990.
1a. Targhetta R, Bourgeois JM, Chavagneux R, et al: Ultrasonographic approach to diagnosing hydropneumothorax. Chest 101: 931, 1992.
2. DeSouza R, Lipsett N, Spagnolo SV: Mediastinal compression due to tension hydrothorax. Chest 72: 782, 1977.

3. Gilmartin JJ, Wright AJ, Gibson GJ: Effects of pneumothorax or pleural effusion on pulmonary function. Thorax 40: 60, 1985.
4. Estenne M, Yernault JC, De Troyer A: Mechanism of relief of dyspnea after thoracocentesis in patients with large pleural effusions. Am J Med 74: 813, 1983.
5. Brandstetter RD, Cohen RP: Hypoxemia after thoracentesis. A predictable and treatable condition. JAMA 242: 1060, 1979.
6. Ryan CJ, Rodgers RF, Unni KK, et al: The outcome of patients with pleural effusion of indeterminate cause at thoracotomy. Mayo Clin Proc 56: 145, 1981.
7. Seibert AF, Haynes J Jr, Middleton R, et al: Tuberculous pleural effusion. Twenty-year experience. Chest 99: 883, 1991.
8. Sinzobahamvya N, Bhakta HP: Pleural exudate in a tropical hospital. Eur Respir J 2: 145, 1989.
9. Pfeutze K: Pulmonary disease caused by photochromogenic mycobacteria. Gen Practitioner 35: 85, 1967.
10. Stead WW, Eichenholz A, Stauss HK: Operative and pathologic findings in twenty-four patients with syndrome of idiopathic pleurisy with effusion, presumably tuberculous. Am Rev Respir Dis 71: 473, 1955.
11. Fujiwara H, Tsuyuguchi I: Frequency of tuberculin-reactive T-lymphocytes in pleural fluid and blood from patients with tuberculous pleurisy. Chest 89: 530, 1986.
12. Ito M, Kojiro N, Shirasaka T, et al: Elevated levels of soluble IL-2R receptors in tuberculous pleural effusions. Chest 97: 1141, 1990.
13. Ellner JJ: Pleural fluid and peripheral blood lymphocyte function in tuberculosis. Ann Intern Med 89: 932, 1978.
14. Hulnick DH, Naidich DP, McCauley DI: Pleural tuberculosis evaluated by computed tomography. Radiology 149: 759, 1983.
15. Spieler P: The cytologic diagnosis of tuberculosis in pleural effusions. Acta Cytol 23: 374, 1979.
16. Light RW: Pleural Diseases. Philadelphia, Lea & Febiger, 1983.
17. Banales JL, Pineda PR, Fitzgerald JM, et al: Adenosine deaminase in the diagnosis of tuberculous pleural effusions. A report of 218 patients and review of the literature. Chest 99: 355, 1991.
18. Ocaña I, Ribera E, Martiniz-Vázquez JM, et al: Adenosine deaminase activity in rheumatoid pleural effusion. Ann Rheum Dis 47: 394, 1988.
19. Fontan Bueso J, Verea Hernando H, Garcia-Buela JP, et al: Diagnostic value of simultaneous determination of pleural adenosine deaminase and pleural lysozyme/serum lysozyme ratio in pleural effusions. Chest 93: 303, 1988.
20. Scerbo J, Keltz H, Stone DJ: A prospective study of closed pleural biopsies. JAMA 218: 377, 1971.
21. Klockars M, Pettersson T, Riska H, et al: Pleural fluid lysozyme in tuberculous and non-tuberculous pleurisy. Br Med J 1: 1381, 1976.
22. Levine H, Metzger W, Lacera D, et al: Diagnosis of tuberculous pleurisy by culture of pleural biopsy specimen. Arch Intern Med 126: 269, 1970.
23. Light RW: Management of parapneumonic effusions. Arch Intern Med 141: 1339, 1981.
24. Light RW, Girard WM, Jenkinson SG, et al: Parapneumonic effusions. Am J Med 69: 507, 1980.
25. Berger HA, Morganroth ML: Immediate drainage is not required for all patients with complicated parapneumonic effusions. Chest 97: 731, 1990.
26. Potts DE, Levin DC, Sahn SA: Pleural fluid pH in parapneumonic effusions. Chest 70: 325, 1976.
27. Light RW: Management of parapneumonic effusions. Chest 70: 325, 1976.
28. McLaughlin FJ, Goldmann DA, Rosenbaum DM, et al: Empyema in children: Clinical course and long-term follow-up. Pediatrics 73: 587, 1984.
29. Berk SL, Holtsclaw SA, Wiener SL, et al: Nontypeable *Haemophilus influenzae* in the elderly. Arch Intern Med 134: 537, 1982.
30. Hendren WH III, Haggerty RJ: Staphylococcal pneumonia in infancy and childhood: Analysis of seventy-five cases. JAMA 168: 6, 1958.
31. Benefield GFA: Recent trends in empyema thoracis. Br J Dis Chest 75: 358, 1981.
32. Varkey B, Rose HD, Kutty CPK, et al: Empyema thoracis during a 10-year period: Analysis of 72 cases and comparison to a previous study (1952 to 1967). Arch Intern Med 141: 1771, 1981.
33. Coonrod JD, Wilson HD: Etiologic diagnosis of intrapleural empyema by counterimmunoelectrophoresis. Am Rev Respir Dis 113: 637, 1976.
34. Waite RJ, Carbonneau RJ, Balikian JP, et al: Parietal pleural changes in empyema: Appearances at CT. Radiology 175: 145, 1990.
35. van Sonnenberg E, Nakamoto SK, Mueller PR, et al: CT- and ultrasound-guided catheter drainage of empyemas after chest-tube failure. Radiology 151: 349, 1984.
36. Muskett A, Burton NA, Karwande SV, et al: Management of refractory empyema with early decortication. Am J Surg 156: 529, 1988.
37. Mayo P: Early thoracotomy and decortication for nontuberculous empyema in adults with and without underlying disease. A twenty-five year review. Am Surg 51: 230, 1985.
38. Murray JF, Finegold SM, Froman S, et al: The changing spectrum of nocardiosis. A review and presentation of nine cases. Am Rev Respir Dis 83: 315, 1961.
39. Conces DJ Jr, Vix VA, Tarver RD: Pleural cryptococcosis. J Thorac Imaging 5: 84, 1990.
40. Lonky SA, Catanzaro A, Moser KM, et al: Acute coccidioidal pleural effusion. Am Rev Respir Dis 114: 681, 1976.
41. Case records of the Massachusetts General Hospital. Weekly clinicopathological exercises. Case 38-1983. Empyema 40 years after a thoracoplasty. N Engl J Med 309: 715, 1983.
42. Meredith HC, Corgan BM, McLaulin B: Pleural aspergillosis. Am J Roentgenol 130: 164, 1978.
43. Fine NL, Smith LR, Sheedy PF: Frequency of pleural effusions in *Mycoplasma* and viral pneumonias. N Engl J Med 283: 790, 1970.
44. Gokeirt JG, Beamish WE: Altered reactivity to measles virus in previously vaccinated children. Can Med Assoc J 103: 724, 1970.
45. Webster BH: Pleuropulmonary amebiasis. A review with an analysis of ten cases. Am Rev Respir Dis 81: 683, 1960.
46. Rakower J, Miwidsky H: Hydatid pleural disease. Am Rev Respir Dis 90: 623, 1964.
47. Pinching AJ, Lockwood CM, Pussell BA, et al: Wegener's granulomatosis. Observations on 18 patients with severe renal disease. Q J Med 52: 435, 1983.
48. Bulgrin JG, Dubois EL, Jacobson G: Chest roentgenographic changes in systemic lupus erythematosus. Radiology 74: 42, 1960.
49. Gould DM, Daves ML: A review of roentgen findings in systemic lupus erythematosus. (SLE). Am J Med Sci 235: 596, 1958.
50. Andrews BS, Arora NS, Shadforth MF, et al: The role of immune complexes in the pathogenesis of pleural effusions. Am Rev Respir Dis 124: 115, 1981.
51. Halla JT, Schronhenloher RE, Volanakis JE: Immune complexes and other laboratory features of pleural effusions. Ann Intern Med 92:748, 1980.
52. Good JT Jr, King TE, Antony VB, et al: Lupus pleuritis: Clinical features and pleural fluid antinuclear antibodies. Chest 84: 714, 1983.
53. Torrington KG: Rapid appearance of rheumatoid pleural effusion. Chest 73: 409, 1978.
54. Campbell GD, Ferrington E: Rheumatoid pleuritis with effusion. Dis Chest 53: 521, 1968.
55. Engel U, Aru A, Francis D: Rheumatoid pleurisy. Acta Pathol Microbiol Immunol Scand 94: 53, 1986.
56. Faurschou P, Faarup P: Granulocytes containing cytoplasmic inclusions in human tuberculous pleuritis. Scand J Respir Dis 54: 341, 1973.
57. Lillington GA, Carr DT, Mayne JG: Rheumatoid pleurisy with effusion. Arch Intern Med 128: 764, 1971.
58. Laboratory features of pleural effusions. Br Med J 281: 763, 1980.
59. Pettersson T, Klockars M, Hellström P-E: Chemical and immunological features of pleural effusion: Comparison between rheumatoid arthritis and other diseases. Thorax 37: 354, 1982.
60. Epler GR, McCloud TC, Gaensler EA: Prevalence and incidence of benign asbestos pleural effusion in a working population. JAMA 247: 617, 1982.
61. Mysterious pleural effusion [editorial]. Lancet 1: 1226, 1982.
62. Jurivich DA: Iatrogenic pleural effusions. South Med J 81: 1417, 1988.
63. Storey DD, Dines DE, Coles DT: Pleural effusion. A diagnostic dilemma. JAMA 236: 2183, 1976.
64. Johnston WW: The malignant pleural effusion. A review of cytopathologic diagnoses of 584 specimens from 472 consecutive patients. Cancer 56: 905, 1985.
65. Rabin CB, Blackman NS: Bilateral pleural effusion. Its significance in association with a heart of normal size. J Mt Sinai Hosp 24: 45, 1957.
66. Chernow B, Sahn SA: Carcinomatous involvement of the pleura: An analysis of 96 patients. Am J Med 63: 695, 1977.
67. Chang SC, Perng RP: The role of fiberoptic bronchoscopy in evaluating the causes of pleural effusions. Arch Intern Med 149: 855, 1989.

68. Irani DR, Underwood RD, Johnson EH, et al: Malignant pleural effusions. A clinical cytopathologic study. Arch Intern Med 147: 1133, 1987.

69. Sahn SA, Good JT Jr: Pleural fluid pH in malignant effusions. Diagnostic, prognostic, and therapeutic implications. Ann Intern Med 108: 345, 1988.

70. Tamura S, Nishigaki T, Moriwaki Y, et al: Tumor markers in pleural effusion diagnosis. Cancer 61: 298, 1988.

71. Cohen S, Hossain MS-A: Primary carcinoma of the lung. A review of 417 histologically proved cases. Dis Chest 49: 67, 1966.

72. Stolberg HO, Patt NL, MacEwen KF, et al: Hodgkin's disease of the lung: Roentgenologic-pathologic correlation. Am J Roentgenol 92: 96, 1964.

72a. Fisher AMH, Kendall B, Van Leuven BD: Hodgkin's disease: A radiological survey. Clin Radiol 13: 115, 1962.

73. Spriggs AI, Vanhegan RI: Cytological diagnosis of lymphoma in serous effusions. J Clin Pathol 34: 1311, 1981.

74. Spieler P, Kradolfer D, Schmid U: Immunocytochemical characterization of lymphocytes in benign and malignant lymphocyte-rich serous effusions. Virchows Arch (Pathol Anat) 409: 211, 1986.

75. Hartweg H: Das Röntgenbild des Thorax bei den chronischen Leukosen. (The roentgenogram of the thorax in chronic leukoses.) Fortschr Roentgenstr 92: 477, 1960.

76. Yam LT: Granulocytic sarcoma with pleural involvement. Identification of neoplastic cells with cytochemistry. Acta Cytol 29: 63, 1985.

77. Shoenfeld Y, Pick AI, Weinberger A, et al: Pleural effusion—presenting sign in multiple myeloma. Respiration 36: 160, 1978.

78. Kapadia SB: Cytological diagnosis of malignant pleural effusion in myeloma. Arch Pathol Lab Med 101: 534, 1977.

79. Fentiman IS, Millis R, Sexton S, et al: Pleural effusion in breast cancer: A review of 105 cases. Cancer 47: 2087, 1981.

80. Raju RN, Kardinal CG: Pleural effusion in breast carcinoma: Analysis of 122 cases. Cancer 48: 2524, 1981.

81. Meyer PC: Metastatic carcinoma of the pleura. Thorax 21: 437, 1966.

82. Fleischner FG: Roentgenology of the pulmonary infarct. Semin Roentgenol 2: 61, 1967.

83. Figley MM, Gerdes AJ, Ricketts HJ: Radiographic aspects of pulmonary embolism. Semin Roentgenol 2: 389, 1967.

84. Mellins RB, Levine OR, Fishman AP: Effect of systemic and pulmonary venous hypertension on pleural and pericardial fluid accumulation. J Appl Physiol 29: 564, 1970.

85. Roth BJ, O'Meara TF, Cragun WH: The serum-effusion albumin gradient in the evaluation of pleural effusions. Chest 98: 546, 1990.

86. Traumatic perforation of oesophagus. Br Med J 1: 524, 1972.

87. Abbott OA, Mansour KA, Logan WD Jr, et al: Atraumatic so-called "spontaneous" rupture of the esophagus. A review of 47 personal cases with comments on a new method of surgical therapy. J Thorac Cardiovasc Surg 59: 67, 1970.

88. Hart U, Ward DR, Gillilian R, et al: Fatal pulmonary hemorrhage complicating Swan-Ganz catheterization. Surgery 91: 24, 1982.

89. Johnston RF, Loo RV: Hepatic hydrothorax. Studies to determine the source of the fluid and report of thirteen cases. Ann Intern Med 61: 385, 1964.

90. Lieberman FL, Hidemura R, Peters RL, et al: Pathogenesis and treatment of hydrothorax complicating cirrhosis with ascites. Ann Intern Med 64: 341, 1966.

91. Kaye MD: Pleuropulmonary complications of pancreatitis. Thorax 23: 297, 1968.

92. Belfar HL, Radecki PD, Friedman AC, et al: Pancreatitis presenting as pleural effusions: Computed tomography demonstration of pleural space extension of pancreatitis exudate. J Comput Tomogr 11: 184, 1987.

93. Falk A, Gustafsson L, Gamklou R: Silent pancreatitis. Report of 4 cases of acute pancreatitis with atypical symptomatology. Acta Chir Scand 150: 341, 1984.

94. Dewar NA, Kinney WW, O'Donohue WJ Jr: Chronic massive pancreatic pleural effusion. Chest 85: 497, 1984.

95. Izbicki JR, Wilker DK, Waldner H, et al: Thoracic manifestation of internal pancreatic fistulas: Report of five cases. Am J Gastroenterol 84: 265, 1989.

96. McCarthy S, Pellegrini CA, Moss AA, et al: Pleuropancreatic fistula: Endoscopic retrograde cholangiopancreatography and computed tomography. Am J Roentgenol 142: 1151, 1984.

97. Light RW, George RB: Incidence and significance of pleural effusion after abdominal surgery. Chest 69: 621, 1976.

98. Miller WT, Talman EA: Subphrenic abscess. Am J Roentgenol 101: 961, 1967.

99. Handler CE, Fray RE, Snashall PD: Atypical Meigs' syndrome. Thorax 37: 396, 1982.

100. Rudnick MR, Coyle JF, Beck LH, et al: Acute massive hydrothorax complicating peritoneal dialysis, report of 2 cases and a review of the literature. Clin Nephrol 12: 38, 1979.

101. Galen MA, Steinberg SM, Lowrie EG, et al: Hemorrhagic pleural effusion in patients undergoing chronic hemodialysis. Ann Intern Med 82: 359, 1975.

102. Stark DD, Shanes JG, Baron RL, et al: Biochemical features of urinothorax. Arch Intern Med 142: 1509, 1982.

103. Dunbar JS, Favreau M: Infrapulmonary pleural effusion with particular reference to its occurrence in nephrosis. J Can Assoc Radiol 10: 24, 1959.

104. Kirsch CM, Chui DW, Yenokida GG, et al: Case report: hepatic hydrothorax without ascites. Am J Med Sci 302: 103, 1991.

105. Verrault J, Lepage S, Bisson G, et al: Ascites and right pleural effusion: Demonstration of a peritoneopleural communication. J Nucl Med 27: 1706, 1986.

106. Kirkpatrick JA Jr, Fleisher DS: The roentgenographic appearance of the chest in acute glomerulonephritis in children. J Pediatr 64: 492, 1964.

107. Gilbert L, Ribot S, Frankel H, et al: Fibrinous uremic pleuritis—surgical entity. Chest 67: 53, 1975.

108. Nidus BD, Matalon R, Cantacuzino D, et al: Uremic pleuritis—a clinicopathological entity. N Engl J Med 281: 255, 1969.

109. Schneierson SJ, Katz M: Solitary pleural effusion due to myxedema. JAMA 168: 1003, 1958.

110. Hurwitz PA, Pinals DJ: Pleural effusion in chronic hereditary lymphedema (Nonne, Milroy, Meige's disease). Report of two cases. Radiology 82: 246, 1964.

111. Sahasranam KV, Chandra P, Ravindran KN: Early onset Dressler's syndrome—a study of fifteen cases. Indian J Chest Dis Allied Sci 32: 153, 1990.

112. Domby WR, Whitcomb ME: Pleural effusion as a manifestation of Dressler's syndrome in the distant post-infarction period. Am Heart J 96: 243, 1978.

113. Barakat MH, Karnik AM, Majeed HW, et al: Familial Mediterranean fever (recurrent hereditary polyserositis) in Arabs—a study of 175 patients and review of the literature. Q J Med 60: 837, 1986.

114. Staats BA, Ellefson RD, Budahn LL, et al: The lipoprotein profile of chylous and nonchylous pleural effusions. Mayo Clin Proc 55: 700, 1980.

115. Latner AL: Cantarow and Trumper Clinical Biochemistry. 7th ed. Philadelphia, WB Saunders, 1975.

116. Schulman A, Fataar S, Dalrymple R, et al: The lymphographic anatomy of chylothorax. Br J Radiol 51: 420, 1978.

117. Garcia Restoy E, Bella Cueto F, Espejo Arenas E, et al: Spontaneous bilateral chylothorax: Uniform features of a rare condition. Eur Respir J 1: 872, 1988.

118. Hillerdal G: Chyliform (cholesterol) pleural effusion. Chest 88: 426, 1985.

119. Bristo LD, Mandal AK, Oparah SS, et al: Bilateral chylothorax associated with sclerosing mediastinitis. Int Surg 68: 273, 1983.

120. Pedicelli G, Mattia P, Zorzoli AA, et al: Gorham syndrome. JAMA 252: 1449, 1984.

121. Dulchavsky SA, Ledgerwood AM, Lucas CE: Management of chylothorax after blunt chest trauma. J Trauma 28: 1400, 1988.

122. Sachs PB, Zelch MG, Rice TW, et al: Diagnosis and localization of laceration of the thoracic duct: Usefulness of lymphangiography and CT. Am J Roentgenol 157: 703, 1991.

123. Grant T, Levin B: Lymphangiographic visualization of pleural and pulmonary lymphatics in a patient without chylothorax. Radiology 113: 49, 1974.

124. Riemann R, Jake R: Pneumothorax nach Mediastinalemphysem über den Ort und den Mechanismus der Pleuraruptur. Acta Anat 128: 115, 1986.

125. Primrose WR: Spontaneous pneumothorax: A retrospective review of aetiology, pathogenesis and management. Scott Med J 29: 15, 1984.

126. Chan TB, Tan WC, Tech PC: Spontaneous pneumothorax in medical practise in a general hospital. Ann Acad Med Singapore 14: 457, 1985.

127. Lenler-Petersen P, Grunnet N, Jesperen TW, et al: Familial spontaneous pneumothorax. Eur Respir J 3: 342, 1990.

128. Yellin A, Shriner RJ, Lieberman Y: Familial multiple bilateral pneumothorax associated with Marfan syndrome. Chest 100: 577, 1991.
129. Spontaneous pneumothorax and apical lung disease. Br Med J 4: 573, 1971.
130. Kawakami Y, Irie T, Kamishima K: Stature, lung, height, and spontaneous pneumothorax. Respiration 43: 35, 1982.
131. Hall JR, Pyeritz RE, Dudgeon DL, et al: Pneumothorax in the Marfan syndrome: Prevalence and therapy. Ann Thorac Surg 37: 500, 1984.
132. Bense L, Wiman LG, Hedenstierna G: Onset of symptoms in spontaneous pneumothorax: Correlations to physical activity. Eur J Respir Dis 71: 181, 1987.
133. Saywell WR: Submarine escape training, lung cysts and tension pneumothorax. Br J Radiol 62: 276, 1989.
134. Vawter DL, Matthews FL, West JB: Effect of shape and size of lung and chest wall on stresses in the lung. J Appl Physiol 39: 9, 1975.
135. Birrer RB, Calderon J: Pneumothorax, pneumomediastinum, and pneumopericardium following Valsalva's maneuver during marijuana smoking. NY State J Med 84: 619, 1984.
136. Farrell SJ: Spontaneous pneumothorax in pregnancy: A case report and review of the literature. Obstet Gynecol 62(3 Suppl): 43s, 1983.
137. Bush MN, Rubenstein R, Hoffman I, et al: Spontaneous pneumomediastinum as a consequence of cocaine use. NY State J Med 84: 618, 1984.
138. Slasky BS, Siewers RD, Lecky JW, et al: Catamenial pneumothorax: The roles of diaphragmatic defects and endometriosis. Am J Roentgenol 138: 639, 1982.
139. Maurer ER, Schaal JA, Mendez FL: Chronic recurrent spontaneous pneumothorax due to endometriosis of the diaphragm. JAMA 168: 2013, 1958.
140. Spontaneous pneumothorax and menstruation [editorial]. Br Med J 1: 269, 1969.
141. Frazier WD, Pope TL Jr, Findley LJ: Pneumothorax following transbronchial biopsy. Low diagnostic yield with routine chest roentgenograms. Chest 97: 539, 1990.
142. Scholten DJ, Wood TL, Thompson DR: Pneumothorax from nasoenteric feeding tube insertion. A report of five cases. Am Surg 52: 381, 1986.
143. Albelda SM, Gefter WB, Kelley MA, et al: Ventilator-induced subpleural air cysts: Clinical, radiographic, and pathologic significance. Am Rev Respir Dis 127: 360, 1983.
144. McDonnell TJ, Crouch EC, Gonzalez JG: Reactive eosinophilic pleuritis. A sequela of pneumothorax in pulmonary eosinophilic granuloma. Am J Clin Pathol 91: 107, 1989.
145. Inouye WY, Berggren RB, Johnson J: Spontaneous pneumothorax—treatment and mortality. Dis Chest 51: 67, 1967.
146. Warner BW, Bailey WW, Shipley RT: Value of computed tomography of the lung in the management of primary spontaneous pneumothorax. Am J Surg 162: 39, 1991.
147. Lindskog GE, Halasz NA: Spontaneous pneumothorax. A consideration of pathogenesis and management with review of seventy-two hospitalized cases. Arch Surg 75: 693, 1957.
148. Adelman M, Albelda SM, Gottlieb J, et al: Diagnostic utility of pleural fluid eosinophilia. Am J Med 77: 915, 1984.
149. Donovan PJ: Bilateral spontaneous pneumothorax: A rare entity. Ann Emerg Med 16: 1277, 1987.
150. Renner RR, Markarian B, Pernice NJ, et al: The apical cap. Radiology 110: 569, 1974.
151. Butler C II, Kleinerman J: The pulmonary apical cap. Am J Pathol 60: 205, 1970.
152. McLoud TC, Woods BO, Carrington CB, et al: Diffuse pleural thickening in an asbestos-exposed population: Prevalence and causes. Am J Roentgenol 144: 9, 1985.
153. Briselli M, Mark EJ, Dickerson GR: Solitary fibrous tumors of the pleura: Eight new cases and review of 360 cases in the literature. Cancer 47: 2678, 1981.
154. England DM, Hochholzer L, McCarthy MJ: Localized benign and malignant fibrous tumors of the pleura. A clinicopathologic review of 223 cases. Am J Surg Pathol 13: 640, 1989.
155. Witkin GB, Rosai J: Solitary fibrous tumor of the mediastinum. A report of 14 cases. Am J Surg Pathol 13: 547, 1989.
156. El-Naggar AK, Ro JY, Ayala AG, et al: Localized fibrous tumor of the serosal cavities. Immunohistochemical, electron-microscopic, and flow-cytometric DNA study. Am J Clin Pathol 92: 561, 1989.
157. Hutchinson WB, Friedenberg MJ: Intrathoracic mesothelioma. Radiology 80: 937, 1963.

158. Hahn PF, Novelline RA, Mark EJ: Arteriography in the localization of massive pleural tumors. Am J Roentgenol 139: 814, 1982.
159. Soulen MC, Greco-Hunt VT, Templeton P: Migratory chest mass. Invest Radiol 25: 209, 1990.
160. Lee KS, Im J-G, Choe KO, et al: CT findings in benign fibrous mesothelioma of the pleura: Pathologic correlation in nine patients. Am J Roentgenol 158: 983, 1992.
161. Kniznik DO, Roncoroni AJ, Rosenberg M, et al: Giant fibrous pleural mesothelioma associated with myocardial restriction and hypoglycemia. Respiration 37: 346, 1979.
162. Legha SS, Muggia FM, Pleural mesothelioma: Clinical features and therapeutic implications. Ann Intern Med 87: 613, 1977.
163. Craighead JE: Current pathogenetic concepts of diffuse malignant mesothelioma. Hum Pathol 18: 544, 1987.
164. Solomons K: Malignant mesothelioma—clinical and epidemiological features. A report of 80 cases. S Afr Med J 66: 407, 1984.
165. Muscat JE, Wynder EL: Cigarette smoking, asbestos exposure, and malignant mesothelioma. Cancer Res 51: 2263, 1991.
166. Churg A: Malignant mesothelioma in British Columbia in 1982. Cancer 55: 672, 1985.
167. Churg A, Wiggs B: Fiber size and number in amphibole asbestos-induced mesothelioma. Am J Pathol 115: 437, 1984.
168. Sheers G, Coles RM: Mesothelioma risks in a naval dockyard. Arch Environ Health 35: 276, 1980.
169. Epler GR, FitzGerald MX, Gaensler EA, et al: Asbestos-related disease from household exposure. Respiration 39: 229, 1980.
170. Fischbein A, Rohl AN: Pleural mesothelioma and neighborhood asbestos exposure. Findings from micro-chemical analysis of lung tissue. JAMA 252: 86, 1984.
171. Constantopoulos SH, Malamou-Mitsi VD, Goudevenos JA, et al: High incidence of malignant pleural mesothelioma in neighbouring villages of Northwestern Greece. Respiration 51: 266, 1987.
172. Davies D: Are all mesotheliomas due to asbestos? [Editorial]. Br Med J 289: 1164, 1984.
173. Roggli VL, McGavran MH, Subach J, et al: Pulmonary asbestos body counts and electron probe analysis of asbestos body cores in patients with mesothelioma: A study of 25 cases. Cancer 50: 2423, 1982.
174. Mowé G, Gylseth B, Hartveit F, et al: Occupational asbestos exposure, lung-fiber concentration and latency time in malignant mesothelioma. Scand J Work Environ Health 10: 293, 1984.
175. Humphrey EW, Ewing SL, Wrigley JV, et al: The production of malignant tumors of the lung and pleura in dogs from intratracheal asbestos instillation and cigarette smoking. Cancer 47: 1994, 1981.
176. McDonald JC, Armstrong B, Case B, et al: Mesothelioma and asbestos fiber type. Evidence from lung tissue analysis. Cancer 63: 1544, 1989.
177. Wang NS, Jaurand MC, Magne L, et al: The interactions between asbestos fibers and metaphase chromosomes of rat pleural mesothelial cells in culture. A scanning and transmission electron microscopic study. Am J Pathol 126: 343, 1987.
178. Amosite asbestos and mesothelioma [editorial]. Lancet 2: 1397, 1981.
179. Ozesmi M, Hillerdal G, Svane B, et al: Prospective clinical and radiologic study of zeolite-exposed Turkish immigrants in Sweden. Respiration 57: 325, 1990.
180. Wagner JC, Skidmore JW, Hill RJ, et al: Erionite exposure and mesotheliomas in rats. Br J Cancer 51: 727, 1985.
181. Lerman Y, Learman Y, Schachter P, et al: Radiation associated malignant pleural mesothelioma. Thorax 46: 463, 1991.
182. Warren S, Brown CE, Chute RN, et al: Mesothelioma relative to asbestos, radiation, and methylcholanthrene. Arch Pathol Lab Med 105: 305, 1981.
183. Hammar SP, Bockus D, Remington F, et al: Familial mesothelioma: A report of two families. Hum Pathol 20: 107, 1989.
184. Cantin R, Al-Jabi M, McCaughey WTE: Desmoplastic diffuse mesothelioma. Am J Surg Pathol 6: 215, 1982.
185. McCaughey WTE, Al-Jabi M: Differentiation of serosal hyperplasia and neoplasia in biopsies. Pathol Annu 1: 271, 1986.
186. Tuder RM: Malignant disease of the pleura: A histopathological study with special emphasis on diagnostic criteria and differentiation from reactive mesothelium. Histopathology 10: 851, 1986.
187. Frierson HF, Mills SE, Legier JF: Flow cytometric analysis of ploidy in immunohistochemically confirmed examples of malignant epithelial mesothelioma. Am J Clin Pathol 90: 240, 1988.
188. Gavin FM, Gray C, Sutton J, et al: Morphometric differences between cytologically benign and malignant serous effusions. Acta Cytol 32: 175, 1988.

188a. Kafiri G, Thomas DM, Shepherd NA, et al: p53 expression is common in malignant mesothelioma. Histopathology 21: 331, 1992.

189. Arai H, Kang K-Y, Sato H, et al: Significance of the quantification and demonstration of hyaluronic acid in tissue specimens for the diagnosis of pleural mesothelioma. Am Rev Respir Dis 120: 529, 1979.

190. Corson JM, Pinkus GS: Mesothelioma: Profile of keratin proteins and carcinoembryonic antigen. An immunoperoxidase study of 20 cases and comparison with pulmonary adenocarcinomas. Am J Pathol 108: 80, 1982.

191. Holden J, Churg A: Immunohistochemical staining for keratin and carcinoembryonic antigen in the diagnosis of malignant mesothelioma. Am J Surg Pathol 8: 277, 1984.

192. Ordóez NG: The immunohistochemical diagnosis of mesothelioma. Differentiation of mesothelioma and lung adenocarcinoma. Am J Surg Pathol 13: 276, 1989.

193. Coleman M, Henderson DW, Mukherjee TM: The ultrastructural pathology of malignant pleural mesothelioma. Pathol Annu 24: 303, 1989.

194. Nakano T, Fujii J, Tamura S, et al: Glycosaminoglycan in malignant pleural mesothelioma. Cancer 57: 106, 1986.

195. Iozzo RV, Goldes JA, Chen W-J, et al: Glycosaminoglycans of pleural mesothelioma: A possible biochemical variant containing chondroitin sulfate. Cancer 48: 89, 1981.

196. Rabinowitz JG, Efremidis SG, Cohen B, et al: A comparative study of mesothelioma and asbestosis using computed tomography and conventional chest radiography. Radiology 144: 453, 1982.

197. Nichols DM, Johnson MA: Calcification in a pleural mesothelioma. J Can Assoc Radiol 34: 311, 1983.

198. Campbell GD, Greenberg SD: Pleural mesothelioma with calcified liver metastases. Chest 79: 229, 1981.

199. Pillgram-Larsen J, Urdal L, Smith-Meyer R, et al: Malignant pleural mesothelioma. A clinical review of 19 patients. Scand J Thorac Cardiovasc Surg 18: 69, 1984.

200. Wadler S, Chahinian P, Slater W, et al: Cardiac abnormalities in patients with diffuse malignant pleural mesothelioma. Cancer 58: 2744, 1986.

201. Krumhaar D, Lange S, Hartmann C, et al: Follow-up study of 100 malignant pleural mesotheliomas. J Thorac Cardiovasc Surg 33: 272, 1985.

201a. Whitaker D, Shilkin KB, Stuckey M, et al: Pleural fluid CEA levels in the diagnosis of malignant mesothelioma. Pathology 18: 328, 1986.

202. Triol JH, Conston AS, Chandler SV: Malignant mesothelioma. Cytopathology of 75 cases seen in a New Jersey community hospital. Acta Cytol 28: 37, 1984.

203. Dardick I, Butler EB, Dardick AM: Quantitative ultrastructural study of nuclei from exfoliated benign and malignant mesothelial cells and metastatic adenocarcinoma cells. Acta Cytol 30: 379, 1986.

204. Whitaker D, Shilkin KB: Diagnosis of pleural malignant mesothelioma in life—a practical approach. J Pathol 143: 147, 1984.

205. Chailleux E, Dabouis G, Pioche D, et al: Prognosis factors in diffuse malignant pleural mesothelioma. A study of 167 patients. Chest 93: 159, 1988.

206. Griffiths MH, Riddell RJ, Xipell JM: Malignant mesothelioma: A review of 35 cases with diagnosis and prognosis. Pathology 12: 591, 1980.

207. DaValle MJ, Faber P, Kittle CF, et al: Extrapleural pneumonectomy for diffuse, malignant mesothelioma. Ann Thorac Surg 42: 612, 1986.

208. Ten Eyck EA: Subpleural lipoma. Radiology 74: 295, 1960.

209. Yousem SA: Thoracic splenosis. Ann Thorac Surg 44: 411, 1987.

210. Williams JR, Bonte FJ: The Roentgenologic Aspect of Nonpenetrating Chest Injuries. Springfield, IL, Charles C Thomas, 1961.

211. Reynolds J, Davis JT: Injuries of the chest wall, pleura, pericardium, lungs, bronchi and esophagus. Radiol Clin North Am 4: 383, 1966.

212. Wolfe CA, Peterson MW: An unusual cause of massive pleural effusion in pregnancy. Thorax 43: 484, 1988.

213. Usselman JA, Seat SG: Superior caval catheter displacement causing bilateral pleural effusions. Am J Roentgenol 133: 738, 1979.

214. Carbone K, Gimenez LF, Rogers WH, et al: Hemothorax due to vena caval erosion by a subclavian dual-lumen dialysis catheter. South Med J 80: 795, 1987.

215. Qureshi MM, Roble DC, Gindin RA, et al: Subarachnoid-pleural fistula. Case report and review of the literature. J Thorac Cardiovasc Surg 91: 238, 1986.

216. Whitcomb ME, Schwarz MI: Pleural effusion complicating intensive mediastinal radiation therapy. Am Rev Respir Dis 103: 100, 1971.

19

DISEASES OF THE MEDIASTINUM

Conditions that predominantly or solely affect the mediastinum constitute only a small proportion of thoracic diseases, but diagnosis is often difficult because of a common roentgenographic manifestation, widening of the mediastinal silhouette. The majority have an insidious onset and may be present for a long time without causing symptoms or signs. Occasionally, as in the acute mediastinitis that follows esophageal rupture, disease is abrupt in onset and alarming in acuity. Between these two extremes of clinical presentation are those patients who complain of a mild sensation of pressure in the retrosternal area or who seek medical aid because of symptoms resulting from compression of the air-, blood-, or food-conducting passages within the narrow mediastinal confines. Although a history of such symptoms is of differential diagnostic value, knowledge of the precise roentgenographic location of a lesion within a mediastinal compartment may be more important, and an understanding of the normal mediastinal anatomy is essential (*see* page 73). For readers interested in delving more deeply into diseases of the mediastinum, particularly with regard to radiologic correlations with anatomy and pathology, the monograph by Heitzman is highly recommended.[1]

MEDIASTINITIS

Mediastinitis is most often due to infection. Acute disease usually is caused by bacteria and is associated with signs and symptoms; many cases are fulminating and lethal. By contrast, chronic disease is most often the result of tuberculous or fungal infection and characteristically does not cause symptoms and is insidious in onset. In addition to cases of infectious origin, there is a group of mediastinopathies of unknown cause characterized by the accumulation of dense fibrous tissue, sometimes associated with similar deposits elsewhere in the body, notably the retroperitoneal space.[2]

Acute Mediastinitis

In the majority of patients, acute infectious mediastinitis results from esophageal perforation by a primary carcinoma, an impacted foreign body, or diagnostic or therapeutic instrumentation (the last-named during procedures such as esophagoscopy, balloon dilatation,[3] variceal sclerotherapy,[4] or insertion of an esophageal prosthesis[5]). Spontaneous perforation (Boerhaave's syndrome) occurs most frequently after episodes of severe vomiting but also can develop during labor, a severe asthma attack, or strenuous exercise. The usual site of rupture is the lower 8 cm of the esophagus, particularly adjacent to the gastroesophageal junction. Typically, the tear is vertical and involves the left posterolateral wall.[6] Acute mediastinitis also can develop following surgery involving mediastinal structures, especially cardiac surgery[7] and colonic interposition,[8] or as a result of direct extension of infection from adjacent tissues such as the retropharyngeal space, lungs, or mediastinal lymph nodes.

The main roentgenographic manifestation, widening of the mediastinum, usually is more evident superiorly and typically possesses a smooth, sharply defined margin. When

infection has resulted from esophageal rupture, air may be visible within the mediastinum as well as in the soft tissues of the neck. Pneumothorax or hydropneumothorax also may develop; when the perforation occurs in the distal esophagus, these tend to occur on the left, whereas midesophageal perforation tends to cause pleural changes on the right.[9] Multiple abscesses may develop (Fig. 19–1). The diagnosis is readily confirmed by demonstration of extravasation of ingested contrast material into the mediastinum or pleural space. Although we consider barium sulfate to be the medium of choice in this examination, others[10] believe that water-soluble contrast medium should be administered first, followed by barium sulfate if the water-soluble medium does not demonstrate a perforation and the clinical picture is suggestive. Regardless of the contrast substance employed, it is important that the examination be performed as soon as possible after the suspected perforation.[11]

The diagnosis should be suspected when severe retrosternal pain develops abruptly and radiates to the neck in a person whose history points to one of the etiologies described. Chills and high fever are common, and the effects of obstruction of the superior vena cava may be apparent. Physical examination of a patient whose esophagus has perforated commonly reveals subcutaneous emphysema in the soft tissues of the neck or a loud crunching or clicking sound synchronous with the heartbeat on auscultation over the apex of the heart (Hamman's sign).

When the diagnosis is not suspected initially and treatment is not instituted promptly, the infection can progress to an abscess that, in turn, can rupture into the esophagus, a lung, a bronchus, or the pleural cavity. The prognosis in such cases is poor.[12]

Chronic Sclerosing Mediastinitis

Chronic sclerosing mediastinitis (fibrosing mediastinitis, granulomatous mediastinitis, or idiopathic mediastinal fibrosis) is a rare condition characterized pathologically by chronic inflammation and fibrosis of mediastinal soft tissues. The process is often progressive and can occur either focally or more or less diffusely throughout the mediastinum. It can cause compression and sometimes obliteration of vessels, airways, and the esophagus and can result in a variety of functional and roentgenographic manifestations and occasionally death.

Etiology and Pathogenesis

Infection—as evidenced by either positive culture of mediastinal tissue or the identification of organisms within granulomatous inflammation on histologic examination—is probably the most common etiology of chronic sclerosing mediastinitis. In the majority of cases, the causative organism is *Histoplasma capsulatum*[13] or *Mycobacterium tuberculosis*. The precise pathogenesis of the progressive mediastinal fibrosis in these cases probably varies. In some, it may be related to slowly progressive tissue invasion and destruction by microorganisms; in others, especially those caused by *H. capsulatum*, it may represent an idiosyncratic hypersensitivity reaction to the presence of organisms or associated degenerated material.[13]

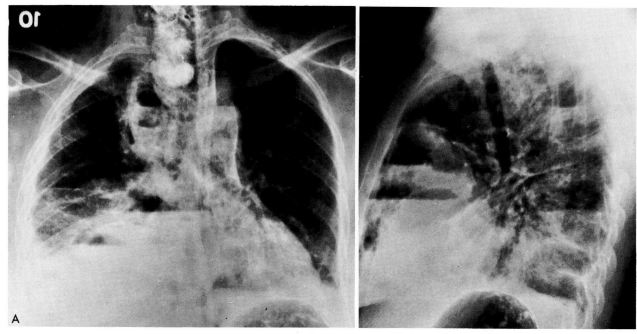

Figure 19–1. Acute Perforation of the Esophagus with Acute Mediastinitis and Mediastinal Abscesses. Three days before the roentgenograms illustrated, this 41-year-old woman swallowed a fork and shortly thereafter developed severe retrosternal pain and fever. Posteroanterior *(A)* and lateral *(B)* roentgenograms taken with the patient in the erect position reveal an irregularly widened upper mediastinum and multiple air-fluid levels within the mediastinum anteriorly and posteriorly. There are bilateral pleural effusions and probable bilateral lower lobe pneumonia. Barium administered by mouth opacified the whole of the esophagus but showed a large sinus tract extending into the mediastinum posteriorly.

A second group of cases (sometimes designated idiopathic mediastinal fibrosis) shows no cultural and little histologic evidence of an infectious etiology. Although some of these cases (perhaps the majority) likely represent the end stage of chronic infection in which the organism is difficult to identify, in others the etiology is undoubtedly not infection. Evidence for this derives from the occasional patient in whom a similar fibrotic process can be identified elsewhere, including the retroperitoneal space (retroperitoneal fibrosis), the orbit (orbital pseudotumor), and the thyroid (Riedel's struma).[2] The pathogenesis of this variety of mediastinitis is also likely to be multifactorial. Immunologic factors seem to be involved in some cases, as evidenced by the reports of both mediastinal and retroperitoneal fibrosis in cases of systemic lupus erythematosus or rheumatoid disease.[14] Methysergide, a drug used to alleviate headache, also has been clearly associated in occasional cases.[15]

Pathologic Characteristics

Pathologically, disease tends to affect the upper half of the mediastinum predominantly, anterior to the trachea and around the hilum (Fig. 19–2); more extensive lesions can extend from the brachiocephalic veins to the base of a lung.[16] Compression of vessels (especially the superior vena cava and pulmonary veins), airways, and the esophagus may be apparent. Histologically, the tissue "mass" varies in appearance depending on the etiology. In cases in which an infectious organism is identified, there is often clear-cut

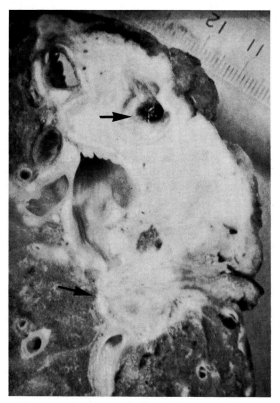

Figure 19–2. Chronic Sclerosing Mediastinitis. A poorly circumscribed mass of fibrous tissue is situated in the mediastinum and hilum enveloping branches of the pulmonary artery *(upper arrow)* and vein *(lower arrow)*, which are partly or completely obstructed.

necrotizing granulomatous inflammation. In others, the granulomatous component is relatively minimal in extent or absent altogether, the abnormal tissue being composed predominantly of mature fibrous tissue containing scattered lymphocytes.

Because the fibrosing process tends to compress vessels and airways in the hilar region, secondary effects on the lung itself are relatively common. In lobes in which the draining veins are affected, parenchymal interstitial fibrosis and vascular changes consistent with pulmonary hypertension may be seen.[17] Occasionally, venous or arterial thrombi in various stages of organization can be identified,[18] sometimes accompanied by parenchymal infarcts.

Roentgenographic Manifestations

The most common roentgenographic manifestation is general widening of the upper half of the mediastinum (Fig. 19–3) caused by a somewhat lobulated paratracheal mass that usually projects more to the right than to the left.[19] In a minority of patients, parenchymal disease or bronchopulmonary lymph node enlargement indicates the pulmonary origin of the mediastinal disease. In some cases, the mediastinal silhouette is normal, and the roentgenographic manifestations result from narrowing of the trachea or major bronchi (Fig. 19–4), obstruction of pulmonary veins or arteries (Fig. 19–5), or narrowing of the esophagus.[19]

Computed tomography (CT) manifestations include a mediastinal or hilar mass, calcification within the mass or in associated lymph nodes, and narrowing of the tracheobronchial tree (Fig. 19–6). In one study of seven patients, CT demonstrated abnormalities that were not evident on conventional roentgenograms in six.[20] Magnetic resonance imaging (MRI) also can be of value in assessing vascular patency without the need for contrast media.[21]

When mediastinal and retroperitoneal fibrosis coexist, the two are remote anatomically, the latter being situated in the lower abdomen and pelvis in the region of the common iliac vessels. Such disease is evidenced by medial displacement of the ureters and unilateral or bilateral hydronephrosis.[22, 23] When the fibrosis is methysergide induced, the roentgenographic abnormalities may disappear following withdrawal of the drug.[15]

Clinical Manifestations

Symptoms and signs of chronic sclerosing mediastinitis are quite variable, depending on the extent of the fibrosis and the particular structures in the mediastinum that are affected. Involvement of the superior vena cava is probably the most common cause of clinical abnormalities[16] and results in the typical manifestations of the superior vena cava syndrome. Obstruction of large central pulmonary veins can cause signs of pulmonary venous hypertension and edema, sometimes with associated pulmonary arterial hypertension. Other complications result from involvement of the tho-

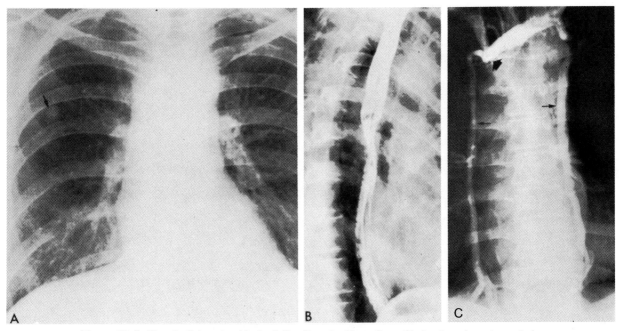

Figure 19–3. Chronic Sclerosing Mediastinitis: Superior Vena Cava Obstruction. A posteroanterior roentgenogram *(A)* shows a somewhat widened upper mediastinum possessing a smooth contour. A partly calcified nodule can be identified in the upper portion of the right lung *(arrow)*. This 51-year-old man presented with a typical picture of obstruction of the superior vena cava. In addition to the symptoms and signs referable to the head and neck and upper extremities, the patient complained of "hemoptysis," which on further questioning and examination was found to arise from the esophagus rather than the lungs and to be caused by "downhill" esophageal varices *(B)*. A roentgenogram of the thorax following the rapid injection of contrast medium into an antecubital vein *(C)* reveals complete obstruction of the superior vena cava just proximal to the junction of the right and left innominate veins *(thick arrow)*. Filling of the internal mammary veins can be identified on both sides *(thin arrows)*, representing part of the extensive collateral circulation.

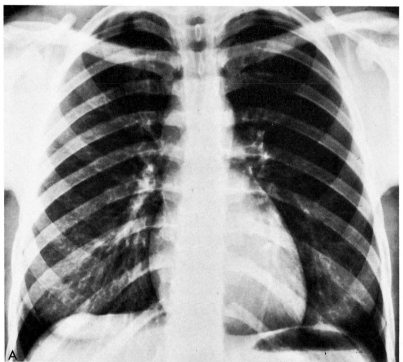

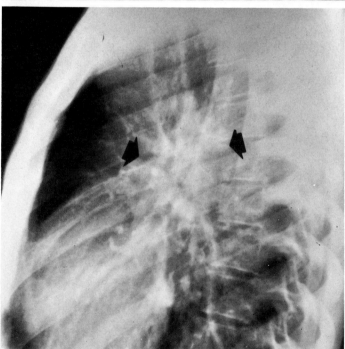

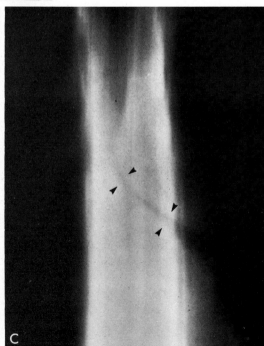

Figure 19–4. Chronic Sclerosing Mediastinitis with Involvement of Major Airways. Roentgenograms of the chest in posteroanterior *(A)* and lateral *(B)* projections reveal diffuse oligemia of the left lung; lung volume is normal. A smooth, well-defined, homogeneous mass is seen in the right tracheobronchial angle, obscuring the shadow of the azygos vein. In lateral projection, the aortic window is not visualized and has apparently been obliterated. In addition, there is a suggestion of narrowing of the air column of the main bronchi. A tomogram of the carinal region in anteroposterior projection *(C)* reveals a severe degree of stenosis of the whole length of the left main bronchus *(arrowheads)*. The lower 2 cm of the trachea and right main bronchus are similarly, but less severely, affected. At right thoracotomy, a diffuse mass with ill-defined edges was found extending from the posterior wall of the superior vena cava over the trachea, into the mediastinum behind the trachea, and downward around the right upper lobe bronchus and into the mediastinum. (Courtesy of St. Boniface General Hospital, St. Boniface, Manitoba.)

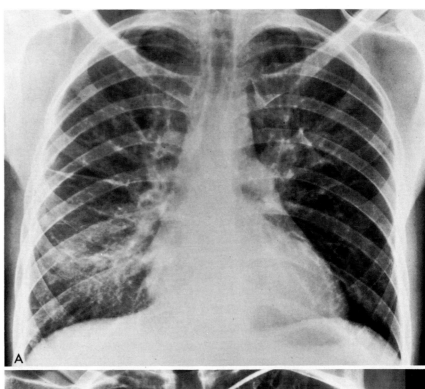

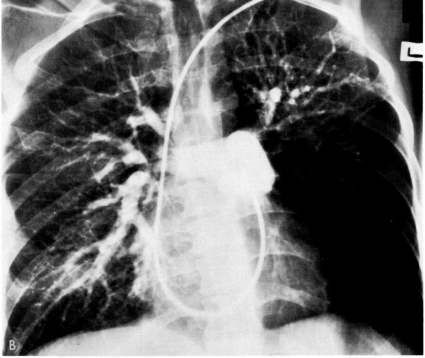

Figure 19–5. Chronic Sclerosing Mediastinitis: Encasement of Pulmonary Arteries and Veins. A posteroanterior roentgenogram *(A)* reveals interstitial edema throughout the right lung and left upper zone and oligemia of the lower half of the left lung. A pulmonary arteriogram *(B)* shows almost complete occlusion of the left interlobar artery with virtually no perfusion of the left lower lobe and lingula. Although there appears to be good opacification of the arteries of the right lung, the truncus anterior and interlobar arteries show concentric narrowing medial to the hilum. The venous phase of the angiogram is not available, but it is almost certain that the pulmonary veins are affected in the same manner, resulting in venous hypertension and the interstitial edema apparent on the plain roentgenogram. (Courtesy of Dr. M.J. Palayew, Jewish General Hospital, Montreal.)

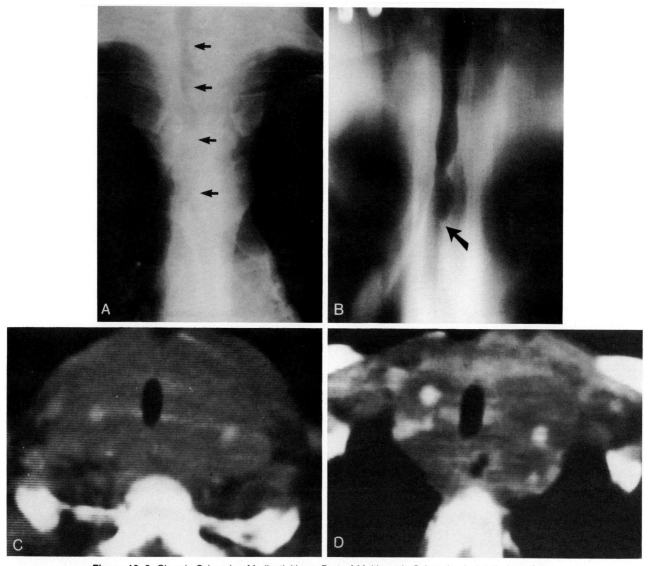

Figure 19–6. Chronic Sclerosing Mediastinitis as Part of Multicentric Sclerosis. A detail view of the upper half of the thorax from a posteroanterior roentgenogram *(A)* reveals mild, uniform widening of the mediastinum. The air column of the trachea *(arrows)* is irregularly narrowed from the larynx to the carina, narrowing that was also observed in the sagittal plane on the lateral view *(not illustrated)*. The coronal narrowing is demonstrated to better advantage on a conventional tomogram *(B)*; an *arrow* points to the carina. A CT scan through the neck just below the larynx *(C)* demonstrates a large, homogeneous soft tissue mass surrounding the trachea and narrowing it from side to side. A CT scan through the upper mediastinum *(D)* reveals a large amount of tissue of inhomogeneous density widely separating opacified vessels and causing narrowing of the trachea in a coronal plane. Following resection, the neck mass proved to be caused by Riedel's struma. There was also radiographic evidence of retroperitoneal fibrosis. (Courtesy of Dr. Nancy Hickey and the Ottawa General Hospital.)

racic duct (chylothorax), the recurrent laryngeal nerve (hoarseness),[16] and the esophagus (dysphagia).[24]

Precise diagnosis usually requires histologic examination of tissue removed at mediastinoscopy or thoracotomy. In addition to routine morphologic examination, such tissue should be cultured for mycobacteria and other organisms.

PNEUMOMEDIASTINUM

Pneumomediastinum (mediastinal emphysema) connotes the presence of gas in the mediastinal space. It is most common in newborn infants and rare in adults, in whom it occurs predominantly following trauma or spontaneously during the second and third decades of life.[25]

Etiology and Pathogenesis

Gas in the mediastinum almost always originates from one of four sites: lung, mediastinal airways, esophagus, or neck.[26]

Lung Parenchyma. Extension of gas from the airspaces of the pulmonary parenchyma into the interstitial tissues and thence into the mediastinum is undoubtably the most common mechanism of pneumomediastinum in both neonates and adults. In most patients, the initial event is probably related to an incident that causes an abrupt rise in alveolar pressure, often accompanied by airway narrowing. This results in rupture of marginally situated alveoli whose bases are adjacent to airways or to pulmonary arteries or veins; gas then passes into and along the perivascular or peribronchial interstitial tissue to the hilum and the mediastinum.[27] Gas can also extend peripherally in the interstitial tissue toward the visceral pleura and rupture into the pleural space to cause pneumothorax (*see* page 878).

In some patients a precipitating event for pneumomediastinum cannot be identified, and the diagnosis is made following the discovery of subcutaneous emphysema in the soft tissues of the neck or from a chest roentgenogram obtained because of retrosternal discomfort.[28] In most patients, however, the abnormality can be clearly related to an incident that results in a sudden rise in alveolar pressure or to a disease process in which such an event is likely to occur. Such incidents or diseases include deep respiratory maneuvers (e.g., those that occur during strenuous exercise[29]), the Valsalva maneuver (e.g., those that occur during parturition[30]), asthma (particularly in children but also in adults[31]), vomiting of any cause,[32] artificial ventilation (particularly in patients with obstructive pulmonary disease and in those being maintained on positive end-expiratory pressure [PEEP][33]), closed chest trauma (in which shearing forces directly disrupt alveolar walls), or a sudden drop in atmospheric pressure (such as occurs during the rapid ascent of a scuba diver or a pilot[34]).

Mediastinal Airways. Rupture of the trachea or proximal mainstem bronchi inevitably results in pneumomediastinum. Such rupture is most often caused by trauma, usually accidental but occasionally following diagnostic instrumentation such as bronchoscopic biopsy.

The Esophagus. Rupture of the esophagus occurs most frequently during episodes of severe propulsive vomiting[6] or extended or iatrogenic trauma (*see* page 897); however,

it can also develop as a result of labor, a severe asthma attack, or strenuous exercise. It must be remembered that each of the last three events can cause pneumomediastinum in the absence of esophageal injury. Because of the almost inevitable development of mediastinitis following esophageal rupture, it is obviously vital to distinguish pneumomediastinum secondary to this injury from that caused by less ominous abnormalities.[6]

The Neck. Occasionally, air tracks into the mediastinum along deep fascial planes as a result of trauma to the neck or following surgical procedures or dental extraction.[35]

Roentgenographic Manifestations

Roentgenographic signs of pneumomediastinum are usually easy to detect. In posteroanterior projection, the mediastinal pleura is displaced laterally, creating a longitudinal line shadow parallel to the heart border and separated from the heart by gas.[36] This shadow is usually more evident on the left side (Fig. 19–7). A longitudinal gas shadow also may be identified adjacent to the thoracic aorta and sometimes around the pulmonary artery ("ring around the artery" sign) (Fig. 19–8).[37] Dissection of air into the neck and over the thoracic wall is much less common in infants than in adults. The consequent buildup in pressure in such infants often gives rise to unilateral or bilateral pneumothorax, a less common complication in adolescents and adults.

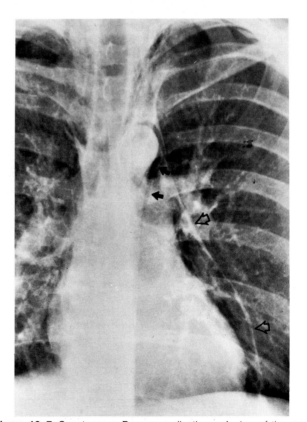

Figure 19–7. Spontaneous Pneumomediastinum. A view of the mediastinum from a posteroanterior roentgenogram reveals a long linear opacity roughly paralleling the left heart border (*open arrows*), representing the laterally displaced mediastinal pleura. In addition, considerable gas is present around the aortic arch and proximal descending thoracic aorta (*solid arrows*).

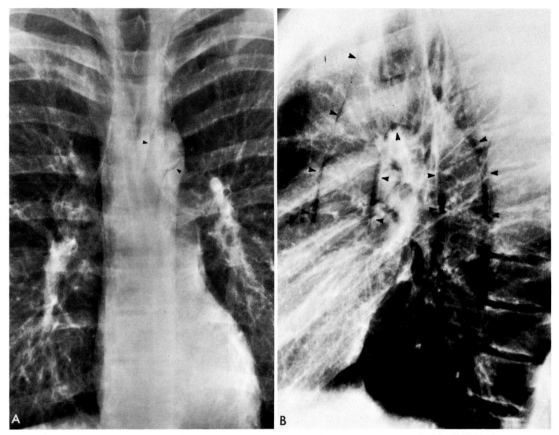

Figure 19–8. Spontaneous Pneumomediastinum. Posteroanterior *(A)* and lateral *(B)* roentgenograms reveal linear and curvilinear shadows of air density outlining almost all portions of the aortic arch in both projections *(arrowheads)*. In lateral projection, the gas outlining the anterior wall of the ascending aorta extends superiorly and relates to the right innominate artery.

When gas becomes interposed between the heart and the diaphragm, it permits identification of the central portion of the diaphragm in continuity with the lateral portions by creating what has been termed the "continuous diaphragm sign."[38] When it is not clear whether a collection of gas is within the pericardial sac or the mediastinal space, differentiation is readily established by demonstrating a change in the position of pericardial gas on roentgenograms exposed with the patient in different positions.[36]

Clinical Manifestations

The symptoms and signs resulting from pneumomediastinum depend largely on the amount of air in the mediastinal space and on the presence or absence of associated infection. The diagnosis may be suggested by a history of abrupt onset of retrosternal pain radiating to the shoulders and down both arms, usually preceded by some event such as a spasm of vomiting that resulted in excessive increase in intrathoracic pressure. The pain usually is aggravated by respiration and sometimes by swallowing. Dyspnea may be severe. Physical examination generally reveals air in the subcutaneous tissues of the neck or over the thoracic wall. Hamman's sign has been estimated to occur in approximately 50 per cent of cases *(see page 147)*.

MEDIASTINAL HEMORRHAGE

The majority of cases of mediastinal hemorrhage result from severe trauma such as that associated with an automobile accident or vigorous cardiopulmonary resuscitation. Less common causes include rupture of an aortic aneurysm, perforation of a vein by faulty insertion of a central venous line, and extension of blood from the retropharyngeal soft tissues secondary to trauma or to spontaneous hemorrhage associated with coagulation disorders. Undoubtedly, the majority of cases are unrecognized because the amount of bleeding is insufficient to produce symptoms and signs.

Roentgenologically, hemorrhage typically results in uniform, symmetric widening of the upper half of the mediastinum *(see* Fig. 15–6, page 789). Local accumulation of blood in the form of a hematoma is manifested by a homogeneous mass that can project to one or both sides of the mediastinum and may be situated in any compartment.

MEDIASTINAL MASSES

The diseases of the mediastinum that have been described to this point show little or no predilection for a specific anatomic zone in the mediastinum. By contrast, a variety of lesions that present as masses show a strong predilection for one of the three mediastinal compartments. Thus, it is logical to classify these masses on the basis of anatomic location. Despite the usefulness of such a classification, it should be clear that overlap is bound to occur, and all that the classification implies is that lesions occur *predominantly* in one or another compartment.

The normal anatomy of the mediastinum was described in detail in Chapter 1 according to the Heitzman classification.[1] This method was employed because we felt that it provides a logical subdivision of spaces within the mid-mediastinum that emphasizes the importance of major vascular channels. However, the authors feel that this classification is not particularly appropriate for a logical analysis of mediastinal masses, for which the more traditional classification of anterior, middle, and posterior is preferred.

The wide variety of tissues within the mediastinum is reflected in the many forms of neoplastic, developmental, and inflammatory masses that can be seen. In a 1971 review of 1064 cases identified over a 40-year period at the Mayo Clinic,[39] neurogenic neoplasms, thymomas, and benign cysts constituted about 60 per cent; lymphomas, teratomas, granulomas, and intrathoracic goiters 30 per cent; and miscellaneous types of benign or malignant mesenchymal tumors 10 per cent. In this series, the great majority of patients were adults (only 8 per cent were younger than 15 years of age at diagnosis), and there was no sex predominance. Almost half of all mediastinal masses do not produce symptoms and are discovered on a screening chest roentgenogram.[39, 40]

MEDIASTINAL MASSES SITUATED PREDOMINANTLY IN THE ANTERIOR COMPARTMENT

The anterior mediastinal compartment is bounded anteriorly by the sternum and posteriorly by the pericardium, aorta, and brachiocephalic vessels. It is the site of most thymomas and a variety of other thymic abnormalities as well as almost all mediastinal germ cell tumors and hyperplastic and neoplastic abnormalities of thyroid and ectopic parathyroid tissue. The CT and MRI characteristics of anterior mediastinal masses were recently reviewed.[41]

Tumors and Tumorlike Conditions of the Thymus

Thymic Hyperplasia

True thymic hyperplasia, as opposed to the lymphoid hyperplasia that is associated with myasthenia gravis (*see* later on), is distinctly uncommon. It can be defined as an increase in the size of the thymus gland associated with intact gross architecture and a normal histologic appearance. In practice, the diagnosis can be confirmed either by noting a significant increase in the weight of the thymus compared to that expected for age or by detecting an increase in the size of a histologically normal gland on serial roentgenograms. In most patients, the cause of the hyperplasia is unknown; however, some cases have been reported following chemotherapy for malignant neoplasms, in which

situation it has been suggested that the hyperplasia may represent a rebound phenomenon.[42] Most patients are infants or children.[43] Symptoms are usually absent.

The term "thymic hyperplasia" also has been used to describe a distinctive histologic reaction in the thymus of patients with myasthenia gravis. In approximately two thirds of these individuals, the thymic cortex is the site of multiple well-defined lymphoid follicles, many containing germinal centers. Since the weight of the thymus gland in these cases is usually within normal limits,[44] the designation "thymic hyperplasia" is, strictly speaking, a misnomer. The large number of cases of myasthenia gravis associated with "thymic hyperplasia" and the favorable response to thymectomy in many patients suggest a pathogenetic association between the two conditions[45]; however, the details of this relationship remain unclear.

Thymolipoma

Thymolipomas are uncommon anterior mediastinal tumors consisting of an admixture of fat and thymic epithelial and lymphoid tissue.[46] No sex predilection is evident, and the tumor can occur at any age, although young men appear to be particularly susceptible.

The precise nature of the tumor is unknown.[47] It has been considered to represent no more than a lipoma occurring within the thymus gland; however, since the thymic tissue itself appears to be increased in amount[47] this hypothesis appears unlikely. It is also possible that the tumor begins as true thymic hyperplasia (i.e., an increase in the amount of normal thymic tissue) that subsequently regresses and is replaced by adipose tissue.

Grossly, thymolipomas are typically yellow, soft, and roughly bilobate, somewhat resembling the normal thymus gland. They are often large and can grow to huge proportions: in about two thirds of reported cases they have weighed more than 500 g, and in one quarter more than 2000 g.[46] Histologically, the tumor consists of mature adipose tissue interspersed with areas of normal thymic tissue.[46]

When thymolipomas are small they present no roentgenographic features that distinguish them from other anterior mediastinal masses. When they are large, however, they tend to slump toward the diaphragm as a result of their soft, pliable consistency. They thus adapt themselves to the diaphragmatic contour by becoming largely inferior in position, leaving the superior mediastinal space relatively clear (Fig. 19–9).[46] Their fat content serves to distinguish them from other mediastinal masses on a CT scan.[48]

Thymolipoma characteristically causes few or no symptoms even when very large; thus, the lesion is usually discovered on a screening roentgenogram. The behavior is typically benign.

Thymic Cysts

Thymic cysts are uncommon mediastinal lesions that account for only 2 to 3 per cent of all tumors in the anterior compartment.[49] It has been suggested that there may be two pathogenetically distinct forms:[50] one that is unilocular and thin-walled and may be derived from remnants of the

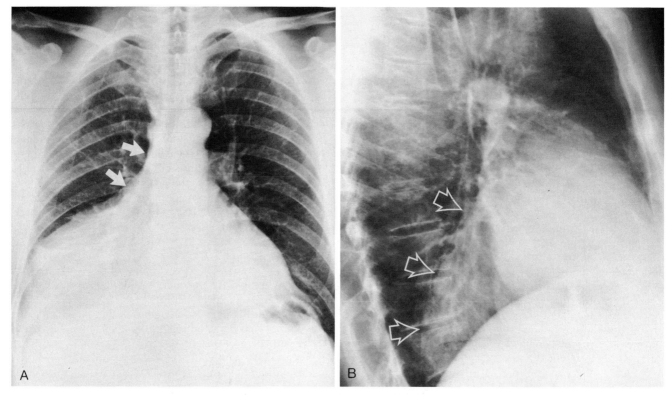

Figure 19–9. Thymolipoma. Posteroanterior (A) and lateral (B) roentgenograms demonstrate a large mass situated in the lower half of the right hemithorax. The obtuse angle the mass creates with the mediastinum (arrows in A) indicates its origin from that structure. In lateral projection, note that the mass extends almost the whole anteroposterior depth of the thorax, obscuring most of the right hemidiaphragm (the posterior margin of the mass is indicated by open arrows in B). The anterior mediastinum looks "empty." (Courtesy of Dr. R. Hedvigi, Montreal Chest Hospital.)

fetal thymopharyngeal duct and a second multilocular, thick-walled form that may represent an acquired abnormality following thymic inflammation (Fig. 19–10). Histologically, the cyst wall is lined by squamous, respiratory, or simple cuboidal epithelium; underlying fibrosis, chronic inflammation, and evidence of remote hemorrhage (hemosiderin-laden macrophages and cholesterol clefts) are almost invariable in the multilocular form.

The appearance of thymic cysts on conventional roentgenograms is in no way characteristic or diagnostic,[49] although their cystic nature should be readily apparent on CT or MR images (see Fig. 19–10). Most patients are asymptomatic.

An important point in the pathologic differential diagnosis is the observation that some malignant tumors, particularly thymoma, Hodgkin's disease, and seminoma, can show prominent cystic changes, occasionally associated with neoplastic tissue that is relatively small in amount. Consequently, every thymic "cyst" must be thoroughly sampled to exclude the possibility of neoplasia, especially if the cyst wall is thickened by fibrous tissue.[51]

Thymoma

Thymomas are neoplasms of thymic epithelium that can behave in either a benign or a malignant fashion and that characteristically consist of rather uniform cells with a variable amount of admixed lymphocytes. (Thymic epithelial neoplasms composed of cells with significant cytologic atypia and a high mitotic rate are more appropriately termed "thymic carcinoma" and are discussed separately later.) The tumor is probably the second most common primary neoplasm (after lymphoma) to affect the mediastinum, accounting for about 10 per cent of all cases in one literature review.[52] Most are discovered in middle-aged adults and they are rare in individuals younger than 20 years of age. The etiology and pathogenesis are uncertain; however, one study from Hong Kong suggested an association with Epstein-Barr virus.[53]

Pathologic Characteristics

Grossly, the majority of tumors present as well-encapsulated, round or slightly lobulated masses.[54] Most measure 5 to 10 cm in diameter, although they tend to be somewhat smaller in individuals with myasthenia gravis, presumably because of the presence of symptoms at an earlier stage. Cut sections reveal a firm, gray or tan tumor that typically is subdivided into lobules by variably thick fibrous bands (Fig. 19–11). One or more cysts are frequent. Infiltration of adjacent structures, particularly the pleura and lung, occurs in 10 to 15 per cent of cases; however, it is important to recognize that the tumor can be adherent to adjacent structures without actually invading them.[54]

The cellular composition of thymoma and the appearance of the tumor cells are highly variable, both within a single tumor and between different tumors. The neoplastic

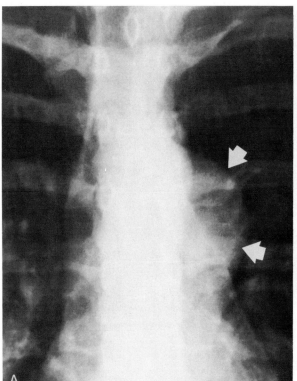

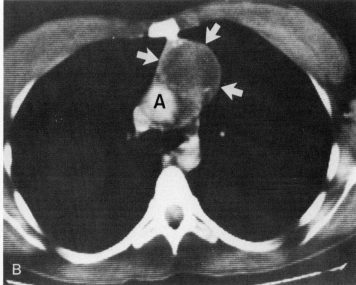

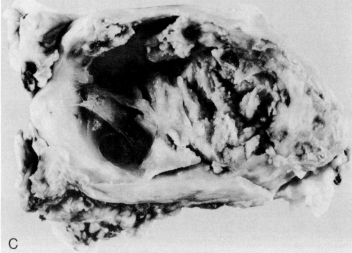

Figure 19–10. Thymic Cyst. A detail view of the mediastinum from a posteroanterior roentgenogram *(A)* reveals a sharply defined homogeneous opacity extending to the left at the level of the aortopulmonary window *(arrows)*. A CT scan at the same level *(B)* shows the lesion to be a fluid-filled cyst *(arrows)* relating to the anterior aspect and left side of the ascending aorta *(A)*. The excised specimen *(C)* shows the cyst to contain abundant friable material, reflecting prior hemorrhage.

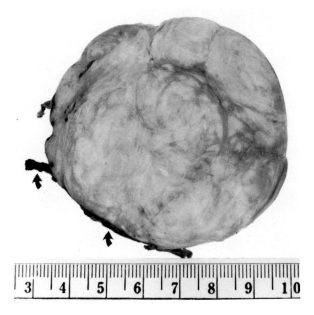

Figure 19–11. Thymoma. A cut section of an anterior mediastinal mass shows a well-circumscribed tumor possessing a distinctly lobulated appearance. There is no necrosis or hemorrhage. A small amount of compressed lung is adherent to the tumor *(arrows)* but is not invaded.

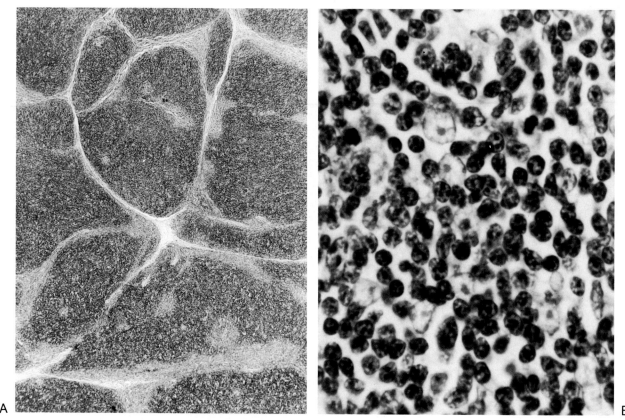

A   B

Figure 19–12. Thymoma: Lymphocyte Predominant. A low-power view of a predominantly lymphocytic thymoma *(A)* shows it to be divided by thin, fibrous bands into numerous lobules of variable size
and shape. *B*, A magnified view shows the lobules to consist of neoplastic thymic epithelial cells with
vesicular nuclei separated by numerous lymphocytes. (*A* × 40; *B* × 1000.)

epithelial cells vary from polygonal to distinctly spindle in
shape, and the associated lymphocytic infiltrate can be absent or can be so marked as to almost completely obscure
the presence of the epithelial cells themselves (Fig. 19–
12).[54, 55] Such histologic variability has given rise to several
morphologic "subtypes" of thymoma, the most common
classification consisting of (1) a predominantly lymphocytic
form (20 to 25 per cent of cases); (2) a mixed lymphoepi-
thelial form (45 to 50 per cent); and (3) a predominantly
epithelial form (Fig. 19–13; 25 to 30 per cent).[54–56] The last-
named itself is sometimes divided into polygonal and spindle cell varieties. This classification is useful for descriptive
and occasionally for diagnostic purposes, but it should be
borne in mind that there is a histologic continuum between
each of these categories. Thus, although there is some evidence of different clinical behavior in some variants (*see*
later), it is unlikely that any one represents a specific entity
in itself.

Classification of thymomas based solely on epithelial cell
morphology also has been proposed.[57] According to this
schema, tumors are divided into cortical, medullary, and
mixed forms, depending on the shape of the neoplastic
epithelial cells, without consideration for the number of
admixed lymphocytes. Since there are morphologic, immunohistochemical, and perhaps functional differences[58] between the cortical and the medullary regions of the normal
thymus, such a classification has some theoretical merit;
however, its usefulness in predicting clinical behavior has
not been established (*see* later).

Roentgenographic Manifestations

Most thymomas are situated near the junction of the
heart and great vessels. Roentgenologically, they are round
or oval and their margins smooth or lobulated.[59] They can
protrude to one or both sides of the mediastinum and, if
large enough, can displace the heart and great vessels posteriorly. In some cases, calcification is apparent at the periphery of the lesion or throughout its substance. When
very large, their site of origin can be exceedingly difficult to
establish without arteriography (Fig. 19–14).

CT is clearly the examination of choice for definitive
diagnosis.[60, 61] In a Mayo Clinic study of 69 cases,[60] although
CT did not reveal any lesions that were not suspected from
other roentgenographic studies, it clarified significant anatomic relationships and, perhaps more important, demonstrated adherence and invasion to best advantage. None of
the imaging techniques, however, was accurate in predicting malignancy. CT is also the examination of choice in the
investigation of patients with myasthenia gravis.[62] For example, in one radiologic-pathologic correlative study of 57
patients with this condition,[63] 14 of 16 cases of thymoma
were either suspected or definitely diagnosed on CT evidence. In another study of 154 consecutive patients who
were subjected to thymectomy for myasthenia gravis,[64] it
was concluded that for patients 21 years of age and older
CT should be used routinely; for younger patients, CT
should be employed only when symptoms, signs, or conventional roentgenographic findings suggest a thymic abnormality. Recent studies have suggested that MRI can be

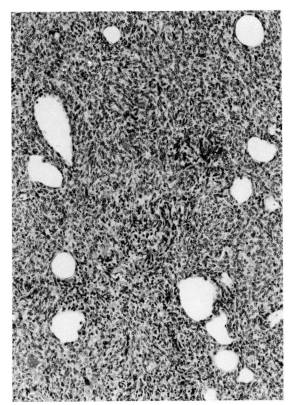

Figure 19–13. Thymoma: Predominantly Epithelial. In contrast to the pattern illustrated in Figure 19–12, this tumor consists almost entirely of uniform polygonal to round epithelial cells with only occasional admixed lymphocytes. (× 120.)

helpful in determining the benign or malignant nature of thymoma.[65, 66]

Clinical Manifestations

Although some patients with thymoma are asymptomatic when the tumor is discovered, the majority manifest symptoms related to local compression or invasion of thoracic structures or to systemic autoimmune disease, or to both. Hematologic abnormalities, especially red cell hypoplasia,[67] and, less commonly, aplastic anemia are also present in some patients. The effects of local compression or invasion, seen in about one third of patients, consist predominantly of chest pain, shortness of breath, and cough.[54] Myasthenia gravis is by far the most common autoimmune disease associated with thymoma. Approximately 15 per cent of patients with myasthenia have this tumor,[54] and about 35 per cent (range 5 to 55 per cent) of patients with thymoma have myasthenia.[39, 40, 54] The tumor is sometimes occult, the resected thymus being of normal size or only minimally enlarged.[56]

Prognosis

The majority of thymomas are slow-growing, encapsulated neoplasms, and surgical excision results in cure. Some, however, are locally aggressive and are unresectable or recur following apparently complete excision. Histologic features are not predictive of the behavior of any one tumor. Thus, local invasion, recurrence after excision, and intrathoracic metastases can occur with different tumors

that possess the same histologic appearance. Despite this, several studies have reported that predominantly epithelial tumors tend to be more aggressive.[54] Although a number of investigators have shown that the cortical type of thymoma is more likely to be associated with invasion than the medullary form,[57, 58, 68] one relatively large investigation documented no predictive difference between the two with respect to relapse-free survival.[69] Despite these pathologic observations, there is little question that the best criterion of malignancy is local invasion, a state that is usually established by the surgeon at the time of thoracotomy.

Recurrence is the rule with invasive tumors because complete resection is usually impossible. Since such tumors may grow slowly, however, residual disease can be associated with long survival. Recurrence usually occurs in the mediastinum or pleural space; extrathoracic metastases are very uncommon.[54]

Thymic Neuroendocrine Neoplasms

This term encompasses several varieties of thymic neoplasm, all of which have in common histologic, ultrastructural, immunohistochemical, and occasionally clinical features of neuroendocrine function. The tumors are believed to be derived from neuroendocrine cells analogous to intestinal Kulchitsky's cells or thyroid C cells, whose presence has been documented in normal thymus.[70] These tumors are uncommon: only about 100 cases had been reported by 1984.[71] Most occur in young men.

Pathologically, the most common histologic subtype of thymic neuroendocrine neoplasm is carcinoid tumor. Like their pulmonary counterparts, these may be well differentiated (so-called "typical" carcinoid tumor) or show features suggestive of a more aggressive nature (moderately differentiated or "atypical" carcinoid tumor).[70] Grossly, the tumors are usually bulky and somewhat lobulated. About half are encapsulated, and the remainder show invasion of adjacent pleura, pericardium, diaphragm, or mediastinum.[70] The histologic pattern is similar to that of pulmonary carcinoid tumor. Silver stains show intracytoplasmic argyrophilic granules in some cases; ultrastructural examination reveals the presence of neurosecretory granules in virtually all.[70, 72]

Roentgenographic features of thymic carcinoid tumors are nonspecific, generally consisting of a lobulated anterior mediastinal mass. Calcification can be identified in some cases.[72] The tumors associated with Cushing's syndrome tend to be smaller and may be identifiable only with CT.[72] As with metastatic carcinoid tumors from other sites, skeletal metastases tend to be osteoblastic.

Clinically, many mediastinal carcinoid tumors produce no symptoms and are discovered on screening chest roentgenograms. Signs and symptoms caused by compression or invasion of mediastinal structures include chest or shoulder pain, dyspnea, cough, and superior vena cava syndrome.[70] Clinical findings of paraneoplastic disease are also present in some patients and include Cushing's syndrome,[73] inappropriate secretion of antidiuretic hormone,[70] carcinoid syndrome,[74] and hyperparathyroidism.[75] Ten to fifteen per cent of cases have been associated with the syndrome of multiple endocrine neoplasia.[71]

As might be expected, complete excision of well-differentiated, encapsulated carcinoid tumors of the thymus is

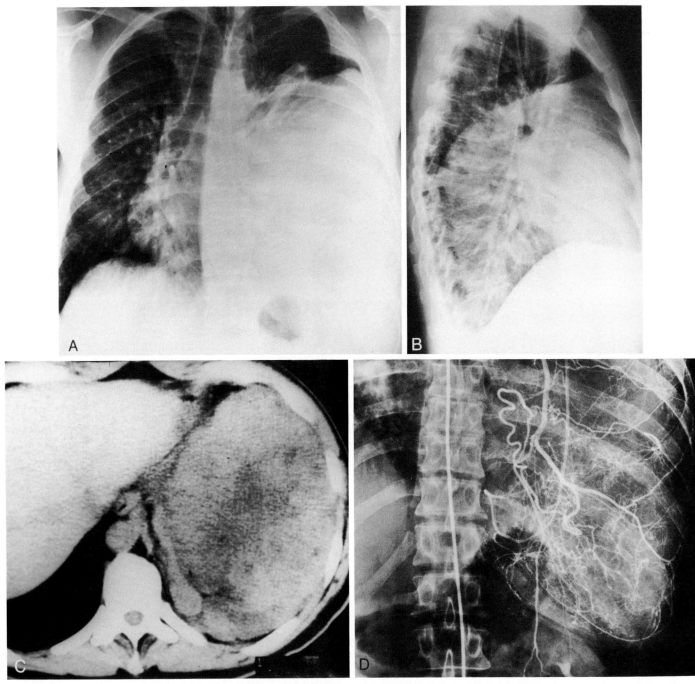

Figure 19–14. Huge Thymoma of the Mediastinum. Posteroanterior *(A)* and lateral *(B)* roentgeno-grams reveal a large homogeneous mass occupying much of the left hemithorax, displacing the mediastinum markedly to the right and depressing the left hemidiaphragm (note the position of the gastric air bubble). A CT scan *(C)* through the base of the thorax shows the left hemithorax to be filled with a mass of inhomogeneous density. At this stage, the precise origin of the mass was disputed, and a left internal mammary arteriogram *(D)* was performed in an attempt to discover the tissue of origin. This study showed that much of the mass was supplied by this vessel, indicating its origin from either the mediastinum or the chest wall.

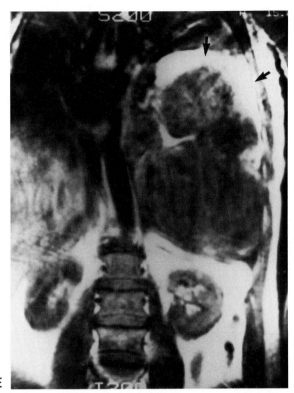

E

Figure 19–14 *Continued* A T₁-weighted coronal reconstruction magnetic resonance image *(E)* shows the mass to be situated above the left hemidiaphragm and to be relatively inhomogeneous in density. A considerable amount of fat is near the mass superiorly *(arrows)*.

associated with a good prognosis,[70] even in the few patients who have regional lymph node metastases. The prognosis for patients with "atypical" forms is guarded; death is caused in many by local extension of disease or metastases.[70, 72] The overall 5-year survival rate is said to be 65 per cent.[71]

Thymic Carcinoma

A proportion of thymomas that show histologic features consistent with a benign neoplasm are found to invade adjacent mediastinal tissues and lung and occasionally metastasize. Although this behavior indicates that such tumors are malignant and hence might be called carcinomas, this term is usually reserved for the rare neoplasm that possesses the traditional histologic and cytologic features of malignancy.[76, 77]

Pathologically, thymic carcinomas are usually bulky masses that range from 5 to 15 cm in diameter[78] and often invade adjacent structures at the time of diagnosis. Histologically, a remarkable variety of patterns has been reported, the most common being squamous cell carcinoma (many cases resembling so-called lymphoepithelioma of the nasopharynx).[76, 77]

Clinically, most patients are symptomatic at the time of diagnosis, the most common complaints being chest pain and cough; systemic findings such as fever, weight loss, fatigue, and night sweats are fairly common. No association with myasthenia gravis and other autoimmune disorders has been described. CT or MRI should be capable of revealing invasion of the mediastinum or lung; despite this, it is important to realize that absence of invasion does not exclude the diagnosis (Fig. 19–15).

The prognosis is poor; in the majority of patients, local intrathoracic growth and extrathoracic metastases result in death in 1 to 3 years.[76, 77]

Thymic Lymphoma

The thymus is a fairly frequent site of involvement by lymphoma, particularly in Hodgkin's disease,[79] in which the histologic type is almost always nodular sclerosis. The tumor has a tendency to cystic degeneration, particularly following radiation therapy.[80] Lymphoblastic lymphoma, a neoplasm that frequently shows features of T-cell lineage, also commonly affects the thymus and, in fact, is believed by many investigators to be derived from thymic lymphocytes.[81]

The roentgenographic features of lymphoma confined to the thymus gland are not in any way specific; however, should mediastinal or hilar lymph nodes be enlarged in association with a mass in the region of the thymus, the diagnosis should be seriously considered. The CT and sonographic manifestations of thymic involvement in Hodgkin's disease have recently been described.[82]

Germ Cell Neoplasms

This term encompasses a group of tumors histologically identical to certain testicular and ovarian neoplasms, all of

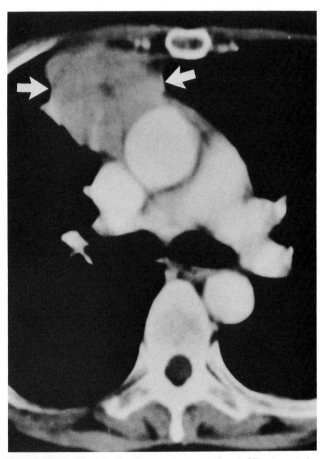

Figure 19–15. Thymic Carcinoma. A conventional CT scan at the level of the pulmonary artery reveals a homogeneous mass measuring 5 cm in diameter *(arrows)*. The sharp line of definition with the aorta suggests an absence of local invasion. Despite this, histologic examination revealed a clearly malignant neoplasm.

which are believed to be derived from primitive germ cell elements. It includes benign and malignant teratoma, seminoma, endodermal sinus (yolk sac) tumor, choriocarcinoma, and embryonal carcinoma. Although many tumors are histologically "pure," combined forms are not infrequent. The most common form is benign teratoma, particularly the cystic variety.[40] The most frequent malignant tumor is seminoma.[83]

Mediastinal germ cell tumors are generally considered to arise from cells whose journey along the urogenital ridge to the primitive gonad is interrupted in the mediastinum.[84] Occasionally, pathologic examination of a testicle reveals a viable tumor mass, focal scarring consistent with regressed tumor,[85] or carcinoma in situ,[86] implying that the mediastinal neoplasm represents metastasis. However, the relatively large number of negative pathologic examinations of the testes at autopsy[85] and the usual lack of emergence of a gonadal primary lesion during prolonged clinical follow-up indicate that this is, in fact, a rare event. Helpful findings that favor a primary mediastinal origin are the absence of retroperitoneal lymph node involvement (testicular carcinoma almost always affects this site before the mediastinum[86]) and the presence of diploid or nearly tetraploid features on flow cytometry (in contrast to testicular neoplasms which are usually hyper- or hypotriploid).[87]

A relationship between mediastinal germ cell neoplasms and Klinefelter's syndrome has been documented in a number of reports. In one review of the literature, 21 of 272 tumors (7.7 per cent) showed this association.[88] The reason for the increased risk of germ cell neoplasia in these patients is unclear, but it may be related to the abnormal androgen and gonadotropin secretion that is characteristic of the syndrome or to intrinsically abnormal germ cell tissue.

Because mediastinal germ cell neoplasms have a varied histologic appearance, pathologic diagnosis can be difficult, especially when the amount of tissue submitted for examination is small.[89] Although this diagnostic problem may not be very important in relation to specific typing of the tumors, particularly since many of the neoplasms have mixed histologic features in any event, current advances in chemotherapy make the distinction from metastatic carcinoma of some significance. It seems reasonable to suggest, therefore, that the possibility of a primary germ cell neoplasm be considered in any young patient with an anterior mediastinal mass in whom a diagnosis of metastatic carcinoma is made in the absence of an obvious primary focus.

In the majority of cases, mediastinal germ cell neoplasms are manifested in adolescence or early adulthood. The age incidence of benign and malignant tumors is similar.[39] For unexplained reasons, benign lesions are more common in females, and malignant tumors in males.[39, 83] The vast majority of tumors are located in the anterior compartment (about 95 per cent in one series[39]), the remainder posteriorly.

Teratoma

The majority of mediastinal teratomas are cystic and benign; the relatively uncommon solid forms are usually malignant. Pathologically, tumors can be divided into three types.

Mature teratomas, the most common variety, are usually well delimited from surrounding mediastinal structures and are unicystic or multicystic. Solid forms occur occasionally (Fig. 19–16). Histologically, they are composed of irregularly arranged but well-differentiated adult tissues (*see* Fig. 19–16). Ectodermal elements, particularly epidermis and skin appendages, predominate[90]; other relatively common tissues include cartilage, fat, smooth muscle, pancreatic tissue, and respiratory mucosa.

Immature teratomas consist of the same adult tissues as the mature variety but in addition contain foci of primitive, less well-organized tissue resembling that seen in the developing fetus.

Teratomas with malignant transformation contain areas of frankly malignant tissue in addition to the fetal and well-differentiated adult tissues that are found in the immature and mature varieties. Adenocarcinoma is the most common type of neoplasm associated with mature teratoma; a soft tissue sarcoma, usually angio- or rhabdomyosarcoma, is the most frequent in immature teratomas.[91] Teratomas with malignant transformation tend to be larger than their benign counterparts and not infrequently show invasion of contiguous structures at the time of diagnosis.

Roentgenologically, the majority of mediastinal teratomas occur in the anterior compartment close to the origin of the major vessels from the heart. Benign lesions are round or oval and smooth in contour, whereas the malignant forms tend to be lobulated and to extend superiorly, inferiorly, and laterally, often asymmetrically. On average, they are considerably larger than thymomas. Calcification may be present in the periphery of the lesion, particularly in mature cystic teratomas, but since such calcification also occurs in thymomas, this finding is of no diagnostic value. The diagnosis of mature teratoma can be made with a reasonable degree of confidence on a standard roentgenogram in the occasional case when mature bone or a tooth is demonstrated in the lesion. Occasionally, a cystic teratoma contains fat that may be apparent roentgenographically as a zone of relative radiolucency that creates a fat-fluid level in the cystic mass. This manifestation can be exquisitely demonstrated by CT (Fig. 19–17).[92, 93]

Teratomas of the mediastinum usually cause no symptoms and are discovered on a screening chest roentgenogram. Those that grow to large size can cause shortness of breath, cough, and a sensation of pressure or pain in the retrosternal area. Large lesions, particularly the malignant forms, may obstruct the superior vena cava. Although these tumors can grow rapidly, it is important to recognize that a rapid increase in size does not necessarily indicate malignancy: hemorrhage into the cyst of a mature teratoma can also result in an abrupt increase in size and can cause severe retrosternal pain or discomfort. Occasionally, a cystic tumor ruptures and spills its contents into the mediastinum or pleural cavity, with resultant mediastinitis or empyema, respectively. When communication occurs with the airways, the contents of the cyst may be expectorated. If this material contains hair (trichoptysis), the diagnosis of teratoma can be made clinically with certainty.

Hematologic malignancies, most commonly nonlymphocytic leukemia and occasionally malignant histiocytosis, have been associated with mediastinal germ cell neoplasms, particularly immature teratomas.[94] Many are diagnosed

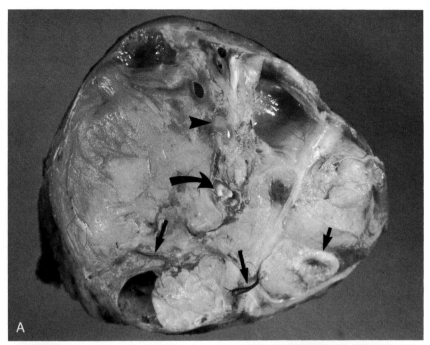

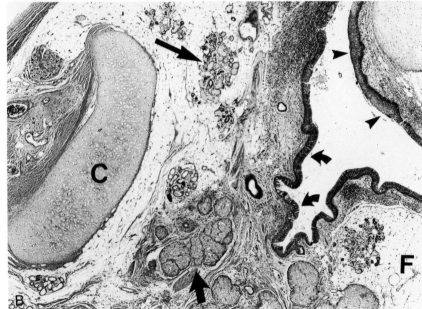

Figure 19–16. Mature Teratoma. A section through this well-circumscribed mediastinal tumor *(A)* shows mostly solid tissue containing several small cystic spaces. In addition to the relatively nondescript fleshy areas of tumor, there are scattered foci that possess specific differentiation, including hair *(long straight arrows)*, skin *(short straight arrow)*, mucus *(arrowhead)*, and bone *(curved arrow)*. A histologic section *(B)* shows multiple foci of cytologically mature, but architecturally disorganized tissue including fat (F), cartilage (C), sebaceous glands *(short arrow)*, salivary or bronchial type glands *(long arrow)*, and squamous *(arrowheads)* and respiratory *(curved arrows)* epithelium. (× 25.)

after recognition of the mediastinal tumor (not infrequently after chemo- or radiotherapy), but some appear to develop before or along with it. The pathogenetic basis of this relationship is unclear.

The prognosis for benign cystic teratomas is excellent, resection resulting in cure in virtually all patients. The behavior of an immature teratoma is somewhat dependent on the age of the patient. Tumors that present in infancy or early childhood are often treated successfully by surgical excision, whereas those that present later frequently follow an aggressively malignant course.[95, 96] Teratomas with malignant transformation are usually highly aggressive and cause death within a few months of diagnosis as a result of local spread or metastases, or both.

Seminoma

Seminoma is the next most frequent mediastinal germ cell tumor after teratoma. Like the malignant form of the latter neoplasm, seminoma occurs almost exclusively in men whose average age at presentation is about 30 years.[97] Pathologically, the tumor is composed of nests of clear or vacuolated cells separated by a variably thick fibrovascular stroma containing numerous lymphocytes.

Roentgenographically, seminoma usually appears as a lobulated noncalcified mass that cannot be distinguished from other malignant germ cell tumors. It can protrude from one or both sides of the mediastinum.[98]

Clinically, approximately 30 per cent of patients are

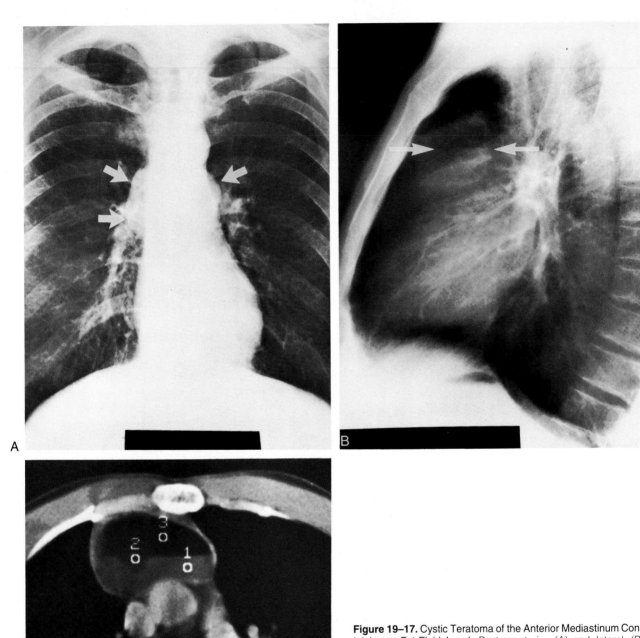

Figure 19–17. Cystic Teratoma of the Anterior Mediastinum Containing a Fat-Fluid Level. Posteroanterior *(A)* and lateral *(B)* roentgenograms reveal a mass of moderate size situated in the anterior mediastinum. The mass is somewhat lobulated and projects to both sides of the mediastinum *(arrows in A)*. In lateral projection, a fluid level is suggested within the mass *(arrows in B)*. A CT scan at the level of the left pulmonary artery *(C)* reveals the mass to excellent advantage, its posterior aspect being indented by the ascending aorta. A prominent fluid level is visible in the center of the mass, the surface of the level being deformed slightly just to the left of its center by a small addition defect. Measurement of attenuation coefficients revealed the following determinations of Hounsfield units: 1 = 16; 2 = 78; and 3 = − 139. (Reprinted with permission, slightly modified from Fulcher AS, Proto AV, and Jolles H: Cystic teratoma of the mediastinum: Demonstration of fat/fluid level. Am J Roentgenol 154: 259, 1990.)

asymptomatic at the time of initial diagnosis. When present, symptoms usually derive from pressure or invasion of vascular structures within the mediastinum. The prognosis for patients with pure seminomas is considerably better than that for patients with mixed or nonseminomatous germ cell tumors, the 5-year survival rate ranging from 50 to 75 per cent.[97, 99] Characteristically, the tumors are exquisitely radiosensitive.[100]

Endodermal Sinus Tumor

Endodermal sinus tumors are highly malignant germ cell neoplasms believed to show differentiation toward yolk sac endoderm. The mediastinal form is rare: only 38 cases of the pure form had been reported in the English language literature by 1986.[101] Pathologically, the neoplasm is quite variable in appearance, showing reticular, tubulopapillary, cystic, and solid patterns. Immunohistochemical studies have shown a positive reaction for alpha-fetoprotein and alpha$_1$-antitrypsin in most cases.[101]

Most endodermal sinus tumors present in young men, the mean age being about 20 years.[101] Roentgenographic findings are nonspecific, consisting of an anterior mediastinal mass. Symptoms related to local mediastinal compression or invasion are present in most patients at the time of diagnosis. Systemic symptoms (anorexia, weight loss, and fever) and symptoms related to metastases are also often present.[101] Serum levels of alpha-fetoprotein are elevated in virtually all patients and can be a useful indicator of disease progression or remission with therapy. Although the prognosis is generally poor, prolonged survival and even cure have been documented in some patients who were treated aggressively.[102]

Choriocarcinoma

Choriocarcinoma is a rare variety of mediastinal germ cell neoplasm that is usually seen in combination with other forms, especially embryonal carcinoma.[103] The incidence peaks between age 20 and 30 years, and like other malignant germ cell tumors, most choriocarcinomas occur in males. Pathologically, the tumor is typically a bulky lobulated mass associated with prominent necrosis and hemorrhage. Histologically, sheets of cells with vesicular nuclei and abundant eosinophilic cytoplasm (cytotrophoblasts) are located adjacent to large multinucleated giant cells (syncytiotrophoblasts). The latter show a positive immunohistochemical reaction for beta–human chorionic gonadotropin (HCG).

The roentgenographic appearance is not distinctive, consisting of an anterior mediastinal mass with a somewhat lobulated contour expanding the mediastinum to one or both sides. In comparison with other germ cell tumors, growth tends to be extremely rapid.

At the time of presentation, mediastinal choriocarcinoma is usually associated with signs and symptoms, including dyspnea, hemoptysis, hoarseness, stridor, dysphagia, and Horner's syndrome.[84] Gynecomastia is reported to occur in about two thirds of cases[104] and is invariably associated with elevated serum levels of HCG. In the past, the prognosis was extremely poor, most patients dying within 4 to 6 weeks to months of diagnosis. With modern therapy, however, remission and even cure can be expected in some patients.

Tumors of Thyroid Tissue

Although extension of thyroid tissue into the thorax is seen in only 1 to 3 per cent of patients subjected to thyroidectomy,[105] such tissue nevertheless constitutes a significant percentage of anterior mediastinal masses. About 75 per cent of tumors arise from a lower pole or the isthmus and extend into the anterior mediastinum in front of the trachea. Most of the remainder arise from the posterior aspect of either lobe and extend into the posterior mediastinum behind the trachea, innominate vein, and innominate or subclavian arteries.[106] In the latter site, they are almost always on the right side.[107] Most patients are in the fifth decade of life; there is a female-to-male predominance of 3 or 4 to 1.[108]

Pathologically, the vast majority of tumors are multinodular goiters that measure 6 to 10 cm in diameter and often show areas of hemorrhage, fibrosis, cyst formation, and calcification. Carcinoma occurs in 2 to 3 per cent of cases.[108]

Roentgenographically, the appearance is that of a sharply defined, smooth or lobulated mass of homogeneous density (Fig. 19–18). Anterior goiters displace the trachea posteriorly and laterally, whereas those in the posterior mediastinum displace the trachea anteriorly and the esophagus posteriorly and laterally. Calcification within the mass is fairly common. Displacement and obstruction of the brachiocephalic vessels may be demonstrated by angiography or MRI,[109] procedures that also permit differentiation of the mass from a vascular aneurysm.

Radioactive isotope studies are usually diagnostic and should constitute the first line of investigation once the possibility of a thyroid origin of a mediastinal mass is considered on the basis of conventional roentgenographic studies. However, false-negative radionuclide examinations do occur, in which case CT should be performed, as it is the next most definitive procedure for diagnosis. One review of the CT characteristics of 10 intrathoracic goiters listed five signs:[110] (1) clear continuity with the cervical thyroid gland; (2) well-defined borders; (3) punctate, coarse, or ringlike calcifications; (4) inhomogeneity, often with discrete, nonenhancing, low-density areas; and (5) precontrast attenuation values at least 15 H greater than adjacent muscles and more than 25 H after contrast enhancement.

Many patients with intrathoracic goiter are asymptomatic,[108] the abnormality being discovered on a screening chest roentgenogram. When present, symptoms include respiratory distress (which can be exacerbated by certain movements of the neck) and hoarseness. Hoarseness is usually caused by compression of the recurrent laryngeal nerve and does not necessarily indicate invasion[111]; however, its presence should raise the possibility of malignancy. Posterior mediastinal goiters can cause dysphagia, whereas those in the anterior and middle compartment can cause a superior vena cava syndrome as a result of obstruction of brachiocephalic vessels.[112] Physical examination usually reveals evidence of a goiter ascending into the neck when the patient swallows; inspiratory and expiratory stridor may be apparent. Thyrotoxicosis is present in some patients.[113]

Tumors of Parathyroid Tissue

Parathyroid tumors constitute a rare cause of an anterior mediastinal mass. Their presence within the mediastinum

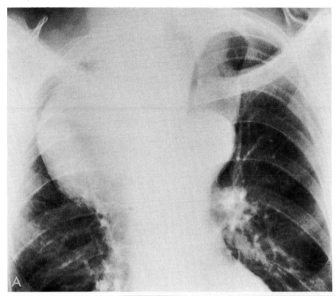

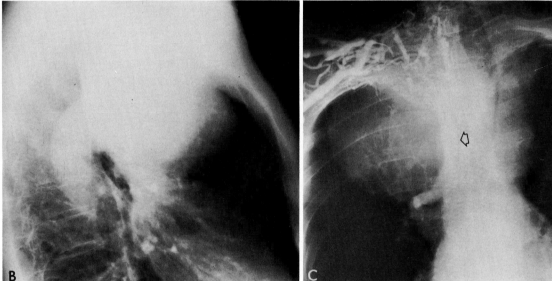

Figure 19–18. Mediastinal (Retrosternal) Goiter. Posteroanterior *(A)* and lateral *(B)* roentgenograms demonstrate a huge mass situated in the upper mediastinum, projected chiefly to the right of the midline. It is homogeneous and sharply defined and shows no evidence of calcification. It displaces the trachea markedly to the left and slightly posteriorly. Scanning revealed no evidence of iodine uptake. A venous angiogram *(C)* demonstrates complete obstruction of the subclavian vein, opacification of the superior vena cava *(arrow)* being obtained by numerous collateral channels in the lower portion of the neck (there were no symptoms of venous obstruction).

is best explained on the basis of the normal migration of parathyroid glands with the thymus during embryonic development. Although they usually separate and remain in the neck, occasionally they proceed distally, most often in direct continuity with thymic tissue. The tumors are usually situated in the upper or mid portion of the anterior mediastinum. Most are adenomas or are hyperplastic; rarely, they are malignant.[114]

Roentgenographically, parathyroid tumors occasionally are sufficiently large to widen the mediastinal silhouette, usually unilaterally.[115] In the majority of patients, however, they are so small as to be invisible. They rarely calcify. In cases of known hyperparathyroidism, evidence to date indicates that selective arteriography is the procedure of choice for identifying mediastinal glands.[116] In fact, opacification of the whole gland with contrast medium can result

in eventual ablation (Fig. 19–19). Neither CT nor nonselective digital arteriography has proved effective in the initial investigation of these elusive glands[116]; however, for reasons that are unclear, CT can be very useful in patients in whom previous explorations have failed.[117]

Unlike most other mediastinal masses, parathyroid tumors usually can be diagnosed on the basis of clinical and laboratory findings. Since most tumors are functioning, patients present with signs and symptoms of hyperparathyroidism. The masses are seldom large enough to cause symptoms or signs of local compression.

Soft Tissue Tumors and Tumorlike Conditions

Soft tissue tumors account for about 5 per cent of all mediastinal masses and include benign and malignant neo-

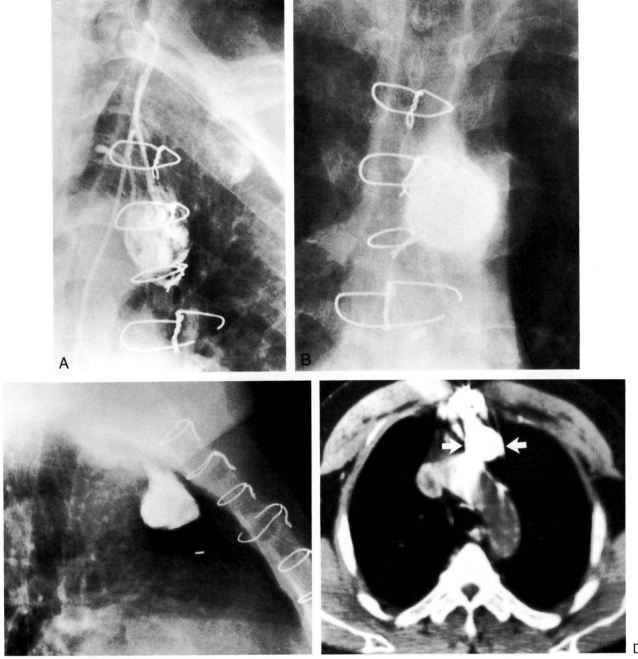

Figure 19–19. Solitary Mediastinal Parathyroid Gland: Opacification and Subsequent Ablation by Arteriography. This middle-aged man had severe secondary hyperparathyroidism as a result of end-stage renal disease. Exploration of the neck resulted in removal of three parathyroid glands, but the fourth was not evident. Conventional roentgenograms revealed no abnormality, although a contrast-enhanced CT scan showed a mass adjacent to the aortic arch (not reproduced). Injection of the left internal mammary artery with 76 per cent Renografin *(A)* resulted in extensive opacification of a mediastinal gland situated contiguous with the arch of the aorta. Twenty-four hours later, detail views of the upper half of the mediastinum from posteroanterior *(B)* and lateral *(C)* roentgenograms reveal persistent dense opacification of the gland. A CT scan at the level of the aortic arch *(D)* also shows the uniformly opacified parathyroid gland *(arrows)*. Subsequent follow-up revealed reversal of the severe secondary hyperparathyroidism.

plasms of fat, fibrous tissue, smooth and striated muscle, blood and lymphatic vessels, bone, and neural tissue. In addition, several developmental and acquired abnormalities composed predominantly of mesenchymal tissue (such as hemangioma and lipomatosis) can present as mediastinal masses. Each of these can occur in any mediastinal compartment; however, tumors of neural tissue are most common posteriorly (*see* page 934), whereas the others are usually located anteriorly.

Tumors of Adipose Tissue

Lipoma. Although infrequent compared with other neoplasms, lipoma is probably the most common mesenchymal tumor to occur in the mediastinum.[118] By contrast, liposarcomas are rare.[119]

Certain roentgenographic features of mediastinal lipomas can aid in their diagnosis. Since fat is less dense than other soft tissues, the roentgenographic density of lipomas is often less than that of other mediastinal masses, particularly if the mass happens to be surrounded by mediastinal tissue of unit density. In some patients, the masses have an hourglass shape, part of the lesion lying outside the thorax in either the neck or the chest wall.[120] Usually they project from only one side of the mediastinum.[59] When doubt exists as to the true nature of a mediastinal mass of this type, CT is diagnostic in the majority of patients. When the CT number of a fatty lesion is approximately −45 H units, intervention is usually unnecessary[121]; however, when the CT numbers range from −10 to −20 H units, intervention may be necessary in order to rule out liposarcoma.

Perhaps because of their pliability, mediastinal lipomas usually do not cause symptoms, even when they are massive.[118] By contrast, liposarcomas are often locally invasive at the time of diagnosis, resulting in dyspnea, wheezing, chest pain, or cough.[119] The prognosis of mediastinal lipoma is excellent: surgical excision is curative in virtually all cases. The behavior of liposarcomas is variable; for low-grade, encapsulated forms cure usually can be expected, whereas for locally invasive or high-grade forms recurrence and death are common.

Lipomatosis. Lipomatosis is an unusual non-neoplastic abnormality of mediastinal adipose tissue characterized by the excessive accumulation of fat in normal locations. It is most commonly seen in conditions associated with hypercortisolism, such as Cushing's syndrome,[122] ectopic adrenocorticotropic hormone (ACTH) production,[123] and long-term corticosteroid therapy.[122] In these situations corticosteroids mobilize and redistribute reserve fatty tissue, resulting in the excessive deposition of fat in the upper mediastinum and in both pleuropericardial angles (Fig. 19–20). The condition also can occur in obese patients without hypercortisolism. Patients are invariably asymptomatic.

Roentgenographically, mediastinal widening tends to be smooth and symmetric, although margins can be lobulated if the accumulation is very large. The widening usually extends from the thoracic inlet to the hila bilaterally. Increasing size of the pleuropericardial fat pads may be evident on serial roentgenographic studies. If evidence provided by conventional roentgenograms is equivocal, CT[124] or MRI[125] is almost always diagnostic.

Tumors of Vascular Tissue

Vascular tumors of the mediastinum are uncommon and include hemangioma, angiosarcoma (hemangioendothelioma), hemangiopericytoma, and lymphangioma. The first of these is the most common and the remainder are rare.[126]

Hemangioma. Hemangiomas have been estimated to comprise about 0.5 per cent of all mediastinal tumors.[127] The majority are discovered in young persons. They can be isolated or can occur as part of a multifocal hemangiomatous malformation affecting several organs (Osler-Weber-Rendu syndrome).[127] Like their pulmonary counterparts, many if not all probably represent developmental malformations rather than true neoplasms.

Pathologically, hemangiomas are often encapsulated. Occasionally, they extend into adjacent tissues, making surgical excision difficult.[128, 129] Histologically, the tumors are composed of thin- or thick-walled vessels of large, small, or mixed size, corresponding to cavernous, capillary, or mixed hemangiomas, respectively.

Roentgenographically, hemangiomas tend to be smooth in outline but are sometimes lobulated. Most are located in the upper portion of the anterior mediastinum. Phleboliths may be identified within them,[126] a virtually diagnostic sign. CT is helpful in delineating the extent of local tissue infiltration.[128] Clinically, many patients are asymptomatic, although chest pain and dyspnea can occur. Superior vena cava and Horner's syndromes have been reported.[129]

Angiosarcoma. Most angiosarcomas (hemangioendotheliomas) of the mediastinum occur in the anterior compartment and have no obvious source.[129] Patients usually have chest pain at the time of diagnosis and die within 3 years.

Hemangiopericytoma. Like its pulmonary counterpart, hemangiopericytoma of the mediastinum is believed to be derived from the vascular pericyte.[129] The tumor can be locally infiltrative and aggressive or can be encapsulated and apparently benign; histologic features of the two varieties are virtually identical. Roentgenographic and clinical manifestations are nonspecific.

Lymphangioma. Mediastinal lymphangiomas occur in two forms: (1) a cavernous or cystic variety that typically extends from the neck into the mediastinum and usually occurs in infants (cystic hygroma) (Fig. 19–21);[130] and (2) a more or less well-defined variety that occurs later in life and is usually located in the lower anterior mediastinum remote from the neck[131] and, occasionally, more posteriorly (Fig. 19–22). Like hemangiomas, these uncommon tumors probably represent developmental anomalies rather than true neoplasms. Pathologically, both forms consist of thin-walled, usually multilocular "cysts" lined by endothelial cells and containing clear yellow fluid.[39]

CT examination typically reveals a well-defined lesion of low attenuation that molds to the mediastinal contours.[132] Because of their soft, yielding consistency, the tumors seldom cause symptoms even when large. A soft tissue mass may be palpable or visible in the neck.

Tumors of Muscle

The origin of mediastinal smooth muscle neoplasms, other than those that arise in the esophagus or trachea, is

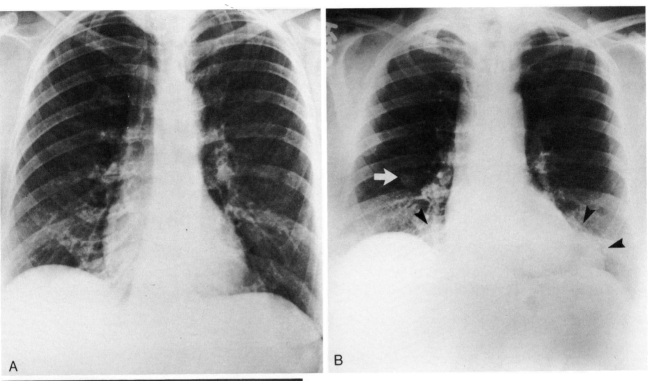

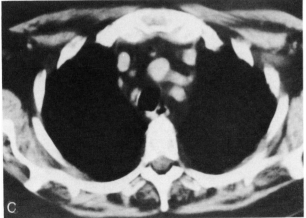

Figure 19–20. Mediastinal Lipomatosis Secondary to Paraneoplastic Cushing's Syndrome. A posteroanterior roentgenogram *(A)* of this 68-year-old woman is normal. Two years later, during which time the patient had gained a great deal of weight, a repeat posteroanterior roentgenogram *(B)* reveals considerable widening of the upper half of the mediastinum and appreciable enlargement of the pleuropericardial fat pads bilaterally *(arrowheads).* In addition, a solitary pulmonary nodule measuring 12 mm in diameter had appeared in the lower portion of the right lung *(arrow).* A CT scan through the upper half of the mediastinum *(C)* reveals the presence of a large amount of fat separating the numerous vessels in the upper mediastinum. Following resection, the solitary pulmonary nodule proved to be a carcinoid tumor. (Courtesy of Dr. Anthony Proto, Virginia Commonwealth University, Medical College of Virginia, Richmond, Virginia.)

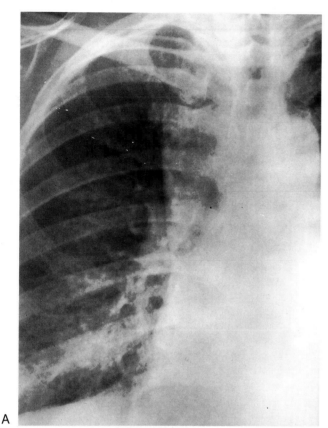

A

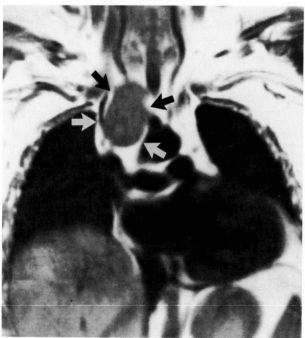

B

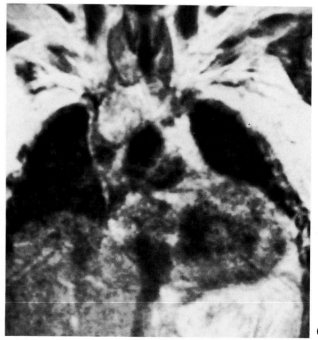

C

Figure 19–21. Cystic Hygroma of the Anterior Mediastinum. A view of the right lung and mediastinum (A) of this asymptomatic 48-year-old woman reveals an opacity in the paramediastinal region, extending superiorly from the upper portion of the right hilum. A T₁-weighted magnetic resonance image (B) reveals a sharply defined, homogeneous opacity extending from just above the thoracic inlet downward into the right side of the mediastinum (arrows). A T₂-weighted image (C) shows an alteration in the density of the mass consistent with the presence of fluid.

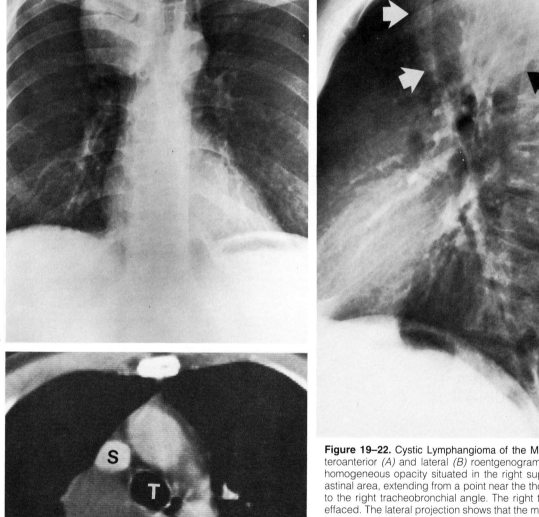

Figure 19–22. Cystic Lymphangioma of the Mediastinum. Posteroanterior *(A)* and lateral *(B)* roentgenograms reveal a large homogeneous opacity situated in the right superior paramediastinal area, extending from a point near the thoracic inlet down to the right tracheobronchial angle. The right tracheal stripe is effaced. The lateral projection shows that the mass is situated in both the middle and the posterior mediastinal compartments *(arrows)*. Note that the conventional roentgenograms reveal the mass to extend down to the level of the azygos arch, beyond which it cannot pass. A CT scan at the level of the aortopulmonary window *(C)* shows that the mass is of water density and that it possesses a sharp interface with contiguous lung parenchyma. It relates intimately to the posterior surface of the superior vena cava (S) and the right posterolateral wall of the trachea (T), which is slightly indented. On other CT scans, the mass was seen to begin just below the level of the thoracic inlet, thus possessing no communication with the neck.

often not clear, and it has been suggested that the majority are derived from the walls of small mediastinal blood vessels.[133] Pathologic findings are those of a spindle cell neoplasm with varying degrees of nuclear atypia and mitotic rate. Roentgenographic and clinical features are nonspecific.[134]

The origin of primary mediastinal rhabdomyosarcoma also is unclear,[118] although the well-documented occurrence of rhabdomyosarcoma in association with immature teratoma[135] suggests that at least some may be derived from this neoplasm.

Fibrous and Fibrohistiocytic Tumors

The precise incidence of primary mediastinal fibromas and fibrosarcomas is difficult to determine because of the relative rarity of well-documented cases.[118] For example, it is possible that some neoplasms reported as fibroma or fibrosarcoma may instead represent neurogenic neoplasms or pleural tumors that have extended into the mediastinum. In fact, some of these tumors are histologically identical to fibrous tumor of the pleura (*see* page 884).[136] There are no distinctive roentgenographic features. The majority of patients are asymptomatic even when the tumors are very large. Pleural effusion can occur with both malignant and benign lesions.[137]

Benign fibrous histiocytoma of the mediastinum is a rare tumor whose precise nature is uncertain, particularly with respect to its inflammatory or neoplastic character. Pathologically, the tumors are usually well encapsulated[118] and are composed of a variable number of intermingled fibroblasts, histiocytes, and multinucleated giant cells. Malignant fibrous histiocytoma of the mediastinum is exceedingly rare, only five cases having been documented by 1986.[138]

MEDIASTINAL MASSES SITUATED PREDOMINANTLY IN THE MIDDLE COMPARTMENT

The middle mediastinal compartment contains the heart, pericardium, all the major vessels leaving and entering this organ, the trachea and main bronchi, paratracheal and tracheobronchial lymph nodes, the phrenic nerves, and the upper portions of the vagus nerves.

Lymph Node Enlargement

Lymph node enlargement is undoubtedly the most common mediastinal abnormality and is caused most often by lymphoma, metastatic carcinoma, sarcoidosis, infection (particularly due to *H. capsulatum* or *M. tuberculosis*), or hyperplasia. Only two conditions—primary mediastinal lymphoma and angiofollicular lymph node hyperplasia (Castleman's disease)—are considered in detail here. With the exception of Hodgkin's disease, in which the anterior mediastinal and retrosternal nodes are most often affected, the anatomic distribution of lymph node enlargement in all these diseases is predominantly midmediastinal.

Primary Mediastinal Lymphoma

Hodgkin's disease is undoubtedly the most common lymphoma to present in the mediastinum, lymph node enlargement being evident on the initial roentgenogram of approximately 60 per cent of patients.[139] An anterior mediastinal mass involving the thymus is also common.[75] Nodular sclerosis is by far the most common histologic subtype. Roentgenographic features of nodal involvement are described in Chapter 8 (*see* page 492).

About 60 per cent of primary mediastinal non-Hodgkin's lymphomas are classified as lymphoblastic,[140] and approximately 50 per cent of patients with this neoplasm have a prominent mass in the mediastinum at the time of presentation.[141] The majority of patients are children or young adults; immunologic studies show that most tumors have features of immature T cells. Prognosis is poor; widespread dissemination (especially to bone marrow and the central nervous system) and leukemic transformation occur in many patients.

The remaining 40 per cent of primary mediastinal non-Hodgkin's lymphomas are composed of different histologic subtypes, the most common of which is the large cell (histiocytic) variety.[141] Grossly, the tumors tend to be large (averaging about 12 cm in diameter[142]) and frequently invade the contiguous mediastinal structures, chest wall, or lung at the time of presentation.[142] Histologically, the majority of tumors are diffuse and are composed of large cleaved or noncleaved cells. Sclerosis is often a prominent feature. Most tumors appear to be of B-cell origin. Pathologic differentiation from other mediastinal neoplasms, particularly thymoma and germ cell tumors, can be difficult, especially with small tissue samples. The majority of these tumors occur in young adults. Symptoms referable to the thorax, particularly dyspnea and pain, are present in the majority of patients. Superior vena cava syndrome also occurs in many.[142] With aggressive chemotherapy and radiation therapy, a 50 to 60 per cent 5-year survival can be expected.

Angiofollicular Lymph Node Hyperplasia

Angiofollicular lymph node hyperplasia (Castleman's disease, giant lymph node hyperplasia) is an unusual condition of unknown etiology and pathogenesis that may be localized or generalized and that may show two histologic patterns.

The more common histologic type (74 of 81 cases in one study[143]), termed the *hyaline vascular type,* is characterized histologically by the presence of multiple germinal centers separated by a polymorphous lymphoreticular infiltrate containing numerous capillaries.[143] This form of disease usually is not associated with symptoms and is discovered as a mass in the mediastinum or perihilar region on a screening chest roentgenogram.

The second histologic variant, termed the *plasma cell type,* shows numerous plasma cells between the germinal centers and the relatively few capillaries. In contrast to the hyaline vascular type, this variant tends to produce systemic manifestations, including fever, anemia, weight loss, and hypergammaglobulinemia.[143]

Both histologic types of the localized form of the disease

tend to occur in young adults and are associated with a good prognosis following surgical excision.[144] Systemic manifestations usually resolve, and typically there is no tendency to recurrence or development of new disease.

The lesions described by Castleman and colleagues[143] were usually solitary and in the majority of patients (70 of 81) affected the mediastinum or hilum. More recently, patients have been described who have histologically similar tumors that are multifocal and tend to affect superficial lymph node groups rather than the mediastinum. Sometimes termed "multicentric Castleman's disease" or "multicentric lymph node hyperplasia,"[145] this condition tends to affect individuals older than those with the solitary form and to be associated with signs and symptoms of systemic disease such as hepatosplenomegaly, anemia, hypergammaglobulinemia, altered liver function tests, renal disease, skin rash, and central nervous system manifestations.[146] Some patients have concomitant HIV infection[147] or Kapo-

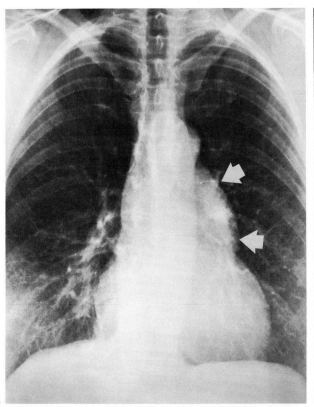

A

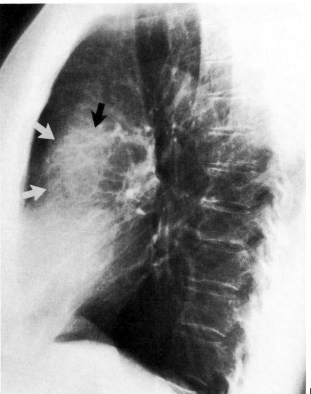

B

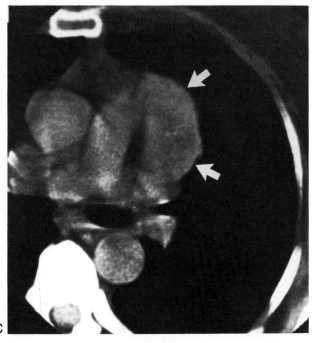

C

Figure 19–23. Giant Lymph Node Hyperplasia (Castleman's Disease). Posteroanterior *(A)* and lateral *(B)* roentgenograms reveal a well-defined opacity protruding to the left from the region of the main pulmonary artery *(arrows* in *A)*. In lateral projection, an ill-defined opacity can be identified in the anterior mediastinum *(arrows)*. A CT scan at the level of the main pulmonary artery *(C)* reveals a well-defined, homogeneous mass *(arrows)* contiguous with the left side of the mediastinum and protruding into the left hemithorax.

si's sarcoma. The prognosis is distinctly poorer than that of the solitary form, many patients having a tendency to develop serious infectious complications or lymphoma.

The roentgenographic appearance of the localized form of giant lymph node hyperplasia is a solitary mass with a smooth or lobulated contour (Fig. 19–23), in any of the three mediastinal compartments but most commonly in the middle or posterior one.[39] Calcification is uncommon.[148] Both angiography and contrast-enhanced CT scans characteristically reveal hypervascularity.[148]

Aorticopulmonary Paraganglioma (Chemodectoma)

The extra-adrenal paraganglionic system consists of minute macroscopic or microscopic collections of neuroendocrinelike cells in intimate association with the autonomic nervous system.[149] In the thorax, they occur in two distinct locations: (1) the perivascular adventitial tissue in the aortopulmonary window (aorticopulmonary paraganglia); and (2) in association with the segmental ganglia of the sympathetic chain in the posterior mediastinum (aorticosympathetic paraganglia). Paragangliomas derived from the first group thus occur in the middle mediastinum in relation to the aorta and pulmonary artery, whereas those in the second group arise in the posterior mediastinum in a paravertebral location (see page 934).

Pathologically,[149] the tumors can be either discrete, encapsulated nodules or more diffusely spreading growths encompassing and invading adjacent vascular structures. Histologic features are characteristic and consist of multiple loosely arranged cellular nests separated by a prominent fibrovascular stroma. Intracytoplasmic granules can be identified with silver stain, and electron microscopic examination reveals dense core intracytoplasmic neurosecretory granules.

Roentgenographic features are those of a mass in the aortopulmonary window. The precise localization of the tumors is aided by the use of angiography,[150, 151] iodine-131 scintigraphy, two-dimensional echocardiography, and of course CT.

The mean age at diagnosis is about 50 years, and there is a slight female predominance.[150] Clinically, most tumors do not occasion symptoms and are discovered on a screening chest roentgenogram;[150] however, they can sometimes compress or invade local structures and cause symptoms such as cough, chest pain, hoarseness, dysphagia, and superior vena cava syndrome. Clinical evidence of endocrine function by the tumors is rare. Some patients, especially young females, also develop gastric leiomyoblastomas and pulmonary chondromas, either synchronously or metachronously (Carney's triad, see page 516).

The prognosis for aorticopulmonary paragangliomas must be somewhat guarded. Because of their location and intrinsic vascularity, the operative mortality rate is high.[150] In addition, complete excision frequently cannot be achieved; although recurrence is the rule in these patients, the growth rate is often slow. Metastases have been documented in about 10 to 15 per cent of reported patients.[150]

Masses Situated in the Anterior Cardiophrenic Angle

Although they are situated anteriorly, masses in the vicinity of the cardiophrenic angle on either side relate to the heart and therefore are truly in the middle mediastinum. The differential diagnosis of such masses is extensive and includes lesions arising within the lung parenchyma, in the visceral or parietal pleura or pleural space, within the space between the pericardium and the mediastinal pleura (usually but not invariably fat), within the pericardium or contiguous myocardium (e.g., cardiac aneurysm), within the diaphragm, and even from beneath the diaphragm (hernia). Lesions arising in any of these anatomic regions can conceivably produce roentgenographic shadows of a similar nature, although CT can be employed to advantage in their differential diagnosis.[152] Only three are considered here—pleuropericardial fat, mesothelial cysts, and enlargement of diaphragmatic lymph nodes.

Pleuropericardial Fat

Accumulations of adipose tissue normally occupy the cardiophrenic angles. Such pleuropericardial fat pads are always bilateral but may be asymmetric, that on the right usually being the larger (Fig. 19–24). They can increase considerably in size over time, either from simple obesity or from hyperadrenocorticism (e.g., Cushing's syndrome), and as such can cause a potentially confusing roentgenographic opacity. Variations in the CT[153] and MR[125] images of fat around the heart have been reviewed.

Mesothelial Cysts

The vast majority of mesothelial cysts (pericardial or pleuropericardial) are probably congenital and result from aberrations in the formation of the coelomic cavities. Grossly, they are spherical or oval in shape, thin-walled, and often translucent. Almost all are unilocular[39] and most contain clear or straw-colored fluid (however, see later). Microscopically, the cyst wall is composed of a thin layer of fibrous tissue lined by a single layer of flattened or cuboidal cells resembling mesothelial cells.

Roentgenographically, the great majority of mesothelial cysts are smooth in contour and round or oval. Most are situated on the right.[39] Lateral projection may reveal a teardrop configuration caused by insertion of the cyst into the interlobar fissure between the middle and lower lobes. In most cases they range in diameter from 3 to 8 cm. The cystic nature of these masses can be confirmed by CT or ultrasonography, thus obviating thoracotomy. Like bronchial cysts, however, mesothelial cysts may manifest CT numbers in the range of 30 to 40, suggesting the possibility of a solid neoplasm.[154] The cause of the elevated CT numbers is undoubtedly the viscous, mucoid secretion that some cysts contain.

Symptoms are almost invariably absent, and most cysts are discovered on a screening chest roentgenogram. Occasionally, a very large cyst can give rise to a sensation of retrosternal pressure or to dyspnea.[155]

Hernia Through the Foramen of Morgagni

Contents of a hernia through a foramen of Morgagni include omentum, liver, and small or large bowel, each of which may be manifested as a mass in the anterior cardiophrenic angle (Fig. 19–25) (see page 949).

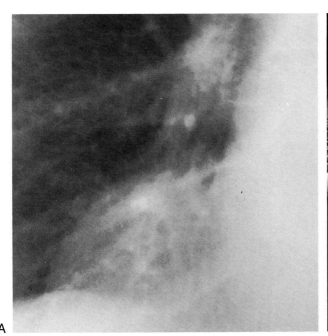
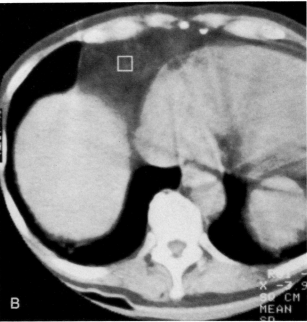

Figure 19–24. Right Cardiophrenic Angle Mass: Fat Pad. A view of the lower portion of the right hemithorax from a posteroanterior roentgenogram *(A)* reveals a sharply defined opacity of homogeneous density obscuring the medial portion of the right hemidiaphragm and the right border of the heart. The density of the mass is roughly equivalent to that of the pulmonary artery several centimeters above. A CT scan at the level of the right hemidiaphragm *(B)* reveals the mass to be of fat density, possessing a mean attenuation of − 105 Hounsfield units.

Enlargement of Diaphragmatic Lymph Nodes

The diaphragmatic group of parietal lymph nodes normally is not visualized on chest roentgenograms because of their small size and their investment with fat and other connective tissue. When these lymph nodes are enlarged, however, they displace the pleura laterally and produce a smooth or lobulated mass projecting out of the cardiophrenic angle. In patients with Hodgkin's disease particularly, enlargement of these nodes causes opacities that simulate enlarged pleuropericardial fat pads (*see* Fig. 8–39, page 495). Although such enlargement may be apparent on conventional roentgenograms, CT is obviously a superior method of assessment.[156] This abnormality can be the initial presentation in patients with Hodgkin's disease, although it has been said to occur more often during relapse of the disease.[157]

Dilatation of the Main Pulmonary Artery

The main pulmonary artery may be so greatly dilated as to suggest a mediastinal mass. Although the great majority of cases are associated with either pulmonary arterial hypertension or left-right shunt, some are poststenotic and related to pulmonary valve stenosis.[158] A few cases are idiopathic. Roentgenographic manifestations depend on the cause of dilatation. Differentiation of the idiopathic and poststenotic varieties may be difficult, although fluoroscopic examination usually reveals increased amplitude of arterial pulsation in the latter condition and not in the former.

Dilatation of the Major Mediastinal Veins

Superior Vena Cava

The great majority of cases of dilatation of the superior vena cava (SVC) are the result of raised central venous pressure, commonly from cardiac decompensation and less often from tricuspid valve stenosis or cardiac tamponade. The roentgenographic appearance is distinctive and consists of a smooth, well-defined widening of the right side of the mediastinum. The azygos vein is almost always dilated as well, a finding that is a more dependable sign of systemic hypertension because the diameter of the vein in the right tracheobronchial angle can be precisely measured (*see* later).

The superior vena cava syndrome is caused by obstruction of the vena cava, either by external compression or, more often, by intraluminal thrombosis or neoplastic infiltration. Frequently, a combination of all three processes is involved. The etiology is malignancy in at least 95 per cent of cases.[159] Pulmonary carcinoma is the cause in 80 to 85 per cent, and lymphoma and metastatic carcinoma of nonpulmonary origin in 5 to 10 per cent. Of the pulmonary carcinomas, small cell carcinoma is the most common subtype.[160] The most frequent benign lesion is chronic sclerosing mediastinitis.[161]

The usual symptoms are dyspnea and a feeling of fullness in the head. Physical findings include dilatation of the veins of the neck and chest wall, and edema of the face, neck, upper extremities, and thorax. The diagnosis is usually apparent clinically but can be made by CT in some patients

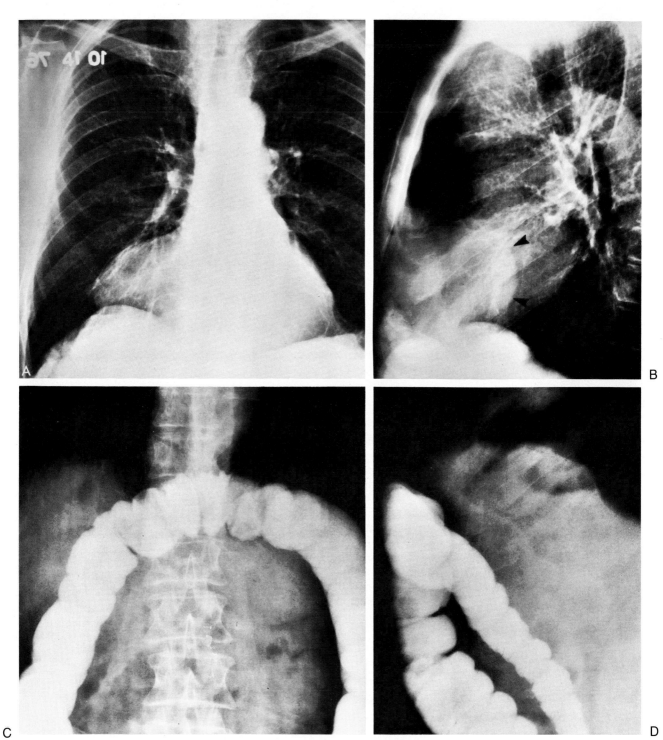

Figure 19–25. Hernia of Omentum Through the Foramen of Morgagni. Posteroanterior *(A)* and lateral *(B)* roentgenograms of this 73-year-old asymptomatic man reveal a large, fairly sharply defined mass in the right cardiophrenic angle *(arrowheads in B)*. Anteroposterior *(C)* and lateral *(D)* projections of the abdomen following barium enema reveal moderate elevation of the transverse colon, whose superior aspect lies contiguous to the diaphragm anteriorly. This deformity of the colon is character-istic of herniation of omentum through the foramen of Morgagni, which was proved at thoracotomy.

with an upper mediastinal mass before the characteristic clinical signs are manifested.[162] In most cases, a mass can be readily detected roentgenographically, widening the mediastinum to the right.

Persistence of a left SVC is an uncommon anomaly that occurs in 0.3 per cent of normal subjects and in about 5 per cent of patients with congenital heart disease.[163] The right SVC develops partly from the right anterior cardinal vein, whereas the left anterior cardinal vein normally regresses. Persistence of the latter results in a left SVC. In such circumstances, a straight-edged shadow is present on the left side of the mediastinum that overlies the aortic arch and proximal descending aorta.[164] Although the diagnosis of this anomalous vessel may be suggested from plain roentgenographic findings, CT is virtually diagnostic.[163]

Azygos and Hemiazygos Veins

There are many causes of dilatation of the azygos and hemiazygos veins: intrahepatic and extrahepatic portal vein obstruction, anomalous pulmonary venous drainage, acquired occlusion of the inferior or superior vena cava, azygos continuation (infrahepatic interruption) of the inferior vena cava (Fig. 19–26),[165, 166] persistence of the left superior vena cava, hepatic vein obstruction (Budd-Chiari syndrome or hepatic veno-occlusive disease), and (by far the most common) elevated central venous pressure as a result of cardiac decompensation, tricuspid valvular lesions, acute pericardial tamponade, or constrictive pericarditis.

Roentgenographically, dilatation of the azygos vein is evidenced by a round or oval shadow in the right tracheobronchial angle more than 10 mm in diameter on standard roentgenograms exposed with the patient in the erect position.[167] For supine films, the critical number is 14 mm.[168] Measurements exceeding these figures indicate increase in either pressure or flow.

A dilated azygos vein can be differentiated from an enlarged azygos lymph node fairly easily by comparing the diameter of the shadow on roentgenograms exposed in the erect and supine positions. When the vein is responsible, there is a noticeable difference in size. When the nature of such a shadow is in doubt, CT provides definitive information. Similarly, the CT appearance of azygos and hemiazygos continuation of the inferior vena cava is so characteristic that angiography is seldom indicated for diagnosis.[169-171] This anomaly is often associated with a congenital cardiac malformation, with errors in abdominal situs, or with asplenia or polysplenia.[165] Most patients are asymptomatic.

Left Superior Intercostal Vein

Dilatation of the left superior intercostal vein generally possesses the same etiologic significance as that of dilatation of the azygos vein, although roentgenographic visualization of this vein is not nearly as frequent as that of the azygos. The normal left superior intercostal vein originates from a confluence of the second, third, and fourth left intercostal veins. As it passes anteriorly from the spine, it relates intimately to some portion of the aortic arch and in this location is seen end-on as the aortic "nipple," a local protuberance that is identifiable in about 10 per cent of normal subjects.[172] On erect posteroanterior chest roentgenograms,

the maximum diameter of the aortic nipple in normal subjects is 4.5 mm.[173] A diameter greater than this is a useful sign of circulatory abnormalities, the most common of which is cardiac decompensation; other causes include azygos continuation of the inferior vena cava, hypoplasia of the left innominate vein, cardiac decompensation, portal hypertension, Budd-Chiari syndrome, obstruction of the superior or inferior vena cava,[173] and congenital absence of the azygos vein.[174]

Dilatation of the Aorta or Its Branches

Aneurysms of the Thoracic Aorta

The most common cause of a thoracic aortic aneurysm is atherosclerosis. The manifestations depend largely on the location. Those of the ascending aorta may be saccular or fusiform, the former usually extending anteriorly and to the right. Aneurysms of the transverse arch produce a mass in the middle mediastinum that characteristically obliterates the aortic window. Aneurysms of the descending aorta characteristically project from the posterolateral aspect of the aorta on its left side and may erode the vertebral column. Calcification of the walls of an aneurysm due to complicated atherosclerosis is relatively common at all three locations (Fig. 19–27).

Traumatic aneurysms of the thoracic aorta typically involve the posterior portion of the descending arch just beyond the origin of the left subclavian artery (Fig. 19–28) and tend to project to the left (see page 789).

Dissecting aneurysms can occur at any site in the thoracic aorta but originate most often in the ascending arch. They are most often associated with idiopathic systemic hypertension but are also seen in Marfan's syndrome, in aortic coarctation, and during pregnancy. So-called cystic medial necrosis is identifiable histologically in the aortic wall in many cases. Whereas CT with bolus injection of contrast medium was formerly considered the procedure of choice in the initial investigation of most patients with suspected aortic dissection (Fig. 19–29),[175, 176] experience with MRI in recent years strongly suggests that this procedure is superior (Fig. 19–30).[177, 178] However, it is possible that aortography remains the examination of choice for defining vascular anatomy, especially when surgical intervention is anticipated.[179]

The clinical manifestations of aortic aneurysms vary according to the size and location of the dilatation. Although aneurysms of the ascending portion often do not cause symptoms, when large enough they can erode the sternum and give rise to a prominent thumping pulsation over the anterior chest wall—thus the designation "aneurysm of signs." Aneurysms of the transverse arch tend to compress contiguous structures, resulting in a brassy cough, hemoptysis, hoarseness, and cyanosis of the face and upper extremities, and thus are sometimes referred to as the "aneurysm of symptoms." Aneurysms of the descending portion can become very large without causing symptoms. Dissecting aneurysms usually cause severe retrosternal pain that radiates through to the back and may suggest the diagnosis of myocardial infarction or pulmonary embolism. Sometimes there is syncope. Physical examination may reveal evidence of acute peripheral arterial occlusion, aortic insuf-

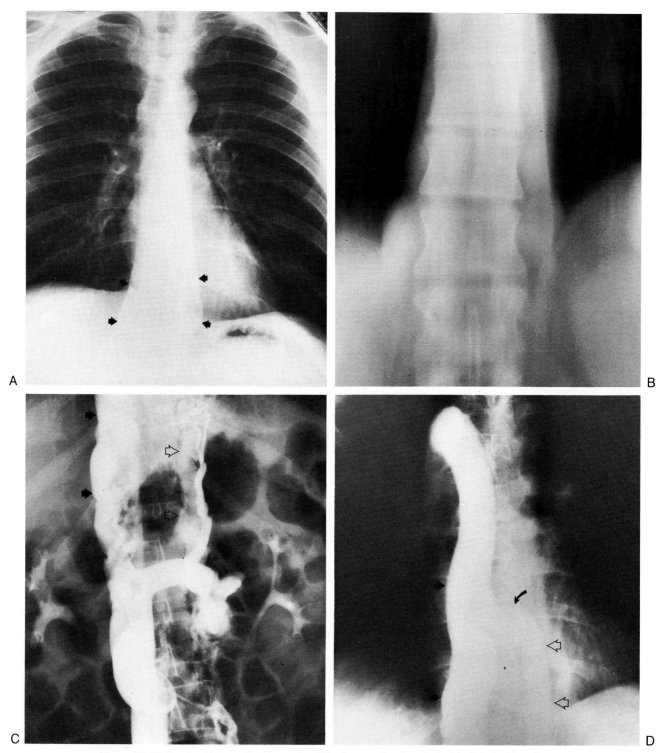

Figure 19–26. Proximal Interruption (Azygos and Hemiazygos Continuation) of the Inferior Vena Cava. A screening chest roentgenogram *(A)* of this 31-year-old asymptomatic man reveals an increased width of the paraspinal soft tissues in the lower thoracic region bilaterally *(arrows)*. The shadow of the azygos vein in the right tracheobronchial angle measured 10 mm, the upper limits of normal. An anteroposterior tomogram of the lower thoracic spine in the supine position *(B)* shows the bilateral opacities to be greater in width than on the erect study and to be somewhat lobulated in contour. With the patient in the recumbent position, the diameter of the azygos vein had increased to 24 mm, a marked degree of dilatation. Following insertion of a catheter into the inferior vena cava, contrast medium was injected *(C)*. Excellent opacification of the inferior vena cava was observed up to the level of the renal veins, but flow proximal to that point was by way of markedly dilated azygos *(solid arrows)* and hemiazygos *(open arrows)* veins. Within the thorax *(D)*, the hemiazygos vein *(open arrows)* passed across the midline to join the azygos *(solid arrows)* at the level of T-8 *(curved arrow)*. The markedly dilated azygos then continued cephalad to terminate in the superior vena cava at its familiar location in the right tracheobronchial angle.

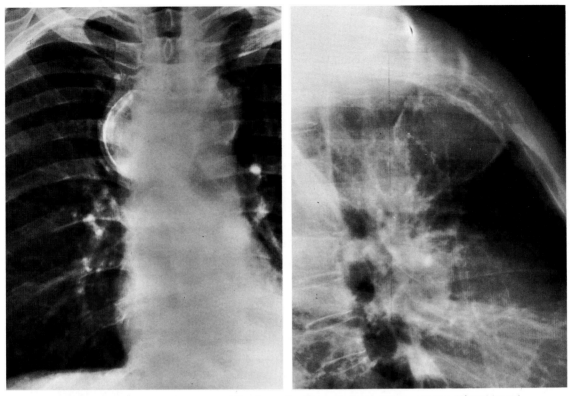

A

B

Figure 19–27. Saccular Aneurysm of the Ascending Thoracic Aorta. Posteroanterior *(A)* and lateral *(B)* roentgenograms of this 52-year-old asymptomatic man reveal a well-defined opacity situated in the anterior mediastinum and projecting entirely to the right. Its wall is densely calcified. The etiology of the aneurysm was not established.

ficiency, or bruits over the affected portion of aorta.[180] Many patients who reach the hospital have distal aortic dissections that tend to be confused clinically with renal colic or pancreatitis.[181]

Buckling and Aneurysm of the Innominate Artery

Both of these conditions are evident roentgenographically as a smooth, well-defined opacity in the right superior paramediastinal area, extending upward from the aortic arch. Buckling is a relatively common condition that occurs in 15 to 20 per cent of patients with hypertension or atherosclerosis or both.[182] The following pathogenesis has been proposed:[183] the innominate artery is about 5 cm long and is firmly fixed proximally at its origin from the aorta and distally by the subclavian and carotid arteries. When the thoracic aorta elongates and dilates as a result of atherosclerosis, the arch moves cephalad, carrying with it the origin of the innominate artery. Because of its fixation superiorly, the innominate artery buckles to the right.

Buckling seldom occasions symptoms and is usually innocuous; however, its presence in patients younger than 30 years should suggest the possibility of coarctation of the aorta.[183] Aneurysms can cause pain, cough, dyspnea, hoarseness, dysphagia, Horner's syndrome, and clubbing of the fingers of the right hand. They may be evidenced by a pulsatile mass at the base of the neck.[182]

Congenital Anomalies of the Aorta

Although the majority of cases of congenital malformations of the aortic arch become manifest during the first year of life, occasionally they are not recognized until adulthood.[184] A congenital aortic vascular ring results from persistence of the two aortic arches or of the right aortic arch and left ductus arteriosus. In a minority of patients the right subclavian artery, also of anomalous origin, arises from the descending aorta. The roentgenographic diagnosis may be made by the demonstration of a double aortic knob and of a vessel posterior to the esophagus. Symptoms result from compression of the trachea or esophagus and include frequent respiratory infections, shortness of breath and, in some cases, dysphagia.

Other congenital anomalies that result in abnormalities of mediastinal contour include (1) pseudocoarctation of the aorta (Fig. 19–31), in which a left paramediastinal "mass" is visible just above the aortic knob, caused by simple elongation and buckling of the aorta[185]; (2) the cervical aortic arch, a rare congenital anomaly in which the aortic arch extends into the soft tissues of the neck before turning downward on itself to become the descending aorta[186]; (3) the three types of aortic diverticula[187]; and (4) by far the most common, the three types of right aortic arch.[188] A right aortic arch can occasionally compress the trachea sufficiently to cause a clinical picture suggesting asthma.[189]

Text continued on page 934

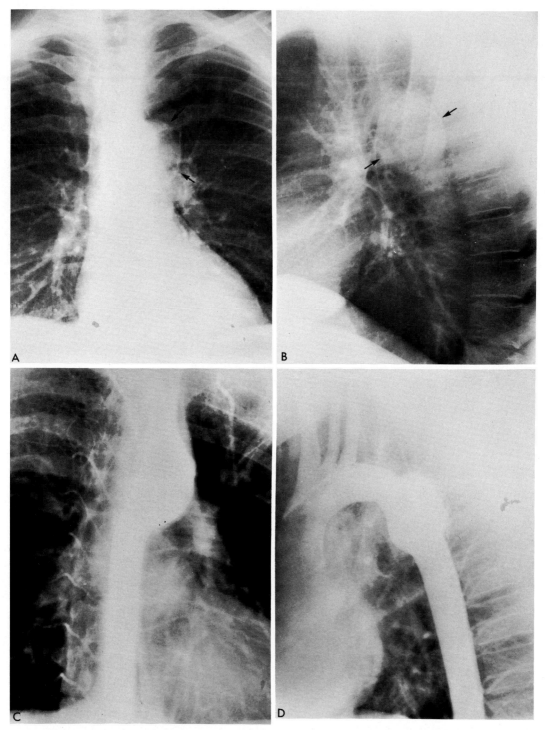

Figure 19–28. Traumatic Aneurysm of the Aorta. Two years before these roentgenographic studies, this 43-year-old airline pilot was involved in a serious car accident in which he suffered severe trauma to his chest and multiple rib fractures. A chest roentgenogram (not illustrated) shortly before the accident was reported as being normal. Roentgenograms of the chest in posteroanterior (A) and lateral (B) projections 2 years after the accident (at which time the patient was asymptomatic) demonstrated a smooth, well-defined soft tissue mass situated in relation to the posterior portion of the arch of the aorta (*arrows* in both projections). Aortography in anteroposterior (C) and lateral (D) projections shows the mass to opacify with contrast medium and to be situated approximately 3 cm beyond the origin of the left subclavian artery. The aneurysm is symmetric, involving the whole circumference of the aorta.

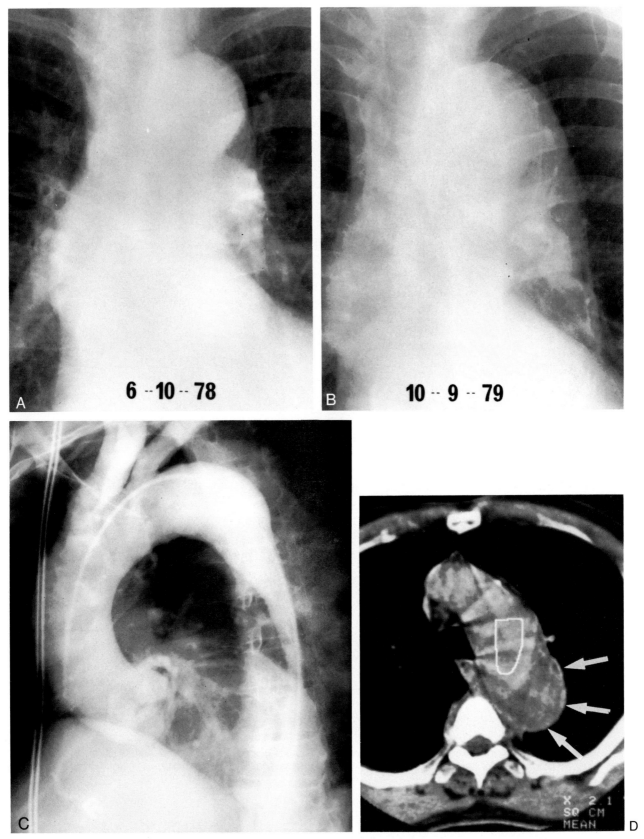

Figure 19–29. Dissecting Aneurysm of the Descending Thoracic Aorta. A view of the upper mediastinum from a posteroanterior roentgenogram *(A)* reveals marked elongation of the thoracic aorta consistent with atherosclerosis. Approximately 1 year later, shortly following the abrupt onset of severe pain in the back, a repeat roentgenogram *(B)* reveals a marked widening of the mediastinum in the region of the aorta that possesses a configuration consistent with acute dissection. An aortogram in left anterior oblique projection *(C)* shows an abrupt narrowing of the lumen of the aorta at the beginning of the descending arch. The false lumen of this dissection did not opacify. A CT scan through the arch *(D)* reveals the nonopacified false channel situated posterolaterally *(arrows).*

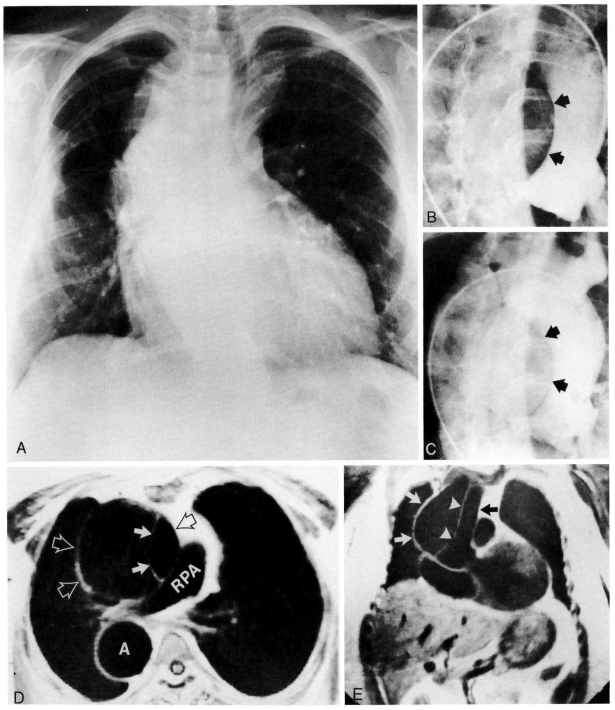

Figure 19–30. Dissecting Aneurysm of the Ascending Aorta in a Patient with a Right Aortic Arch. A posteroanterior roentgenogram *(A)* reveals evidence of a former right thoracotomy that had been performed many years previously for repair of a coarctation and aortic valvotomy. The trachea is deviated markedly to the left by a right-sided aortic arch. The width of the aorta at the point of maximal tracheal displacement is obviously wider than normal. Because of the concern over the possibility of a dissecting aneurysm in this 27-year-old woman with Turner's syndrome, an aortogram was performed: an early phase following injection of contrast medium *(B)* reveals opacification of the true aortic lumen. Two or three seconds later *(C)*, there has occurred opacification of a structure situated posteromedial to the true arch *(arrows)*, indicating partial opacification of a false channel. (Compare the density indicated by *arrows* in *B* with that indicated by *arrows* in *C*.) A T$_1$-weighted magnetic resonance image *(D)* at the level of the right pulmonary artery (RPA) shows a markedly dilated ascending aorta *(open arrows)*. Situated within it is a curvilinear shadow *(arrows)* representing the intimal flap, the smaller area to the left of the flap representing the true lumen, and the larger area to the right representing the false lumen of the dissection. Note that the descending aorta *(A)* at this level is still on the right side. A coronal reconstruction *(E)* again reveals the markedly dilated ascending aorta *(arrows)* containing the intimal flap *(arrowheads)*. Again the true lumen is on the left, and the false lumen on the right.

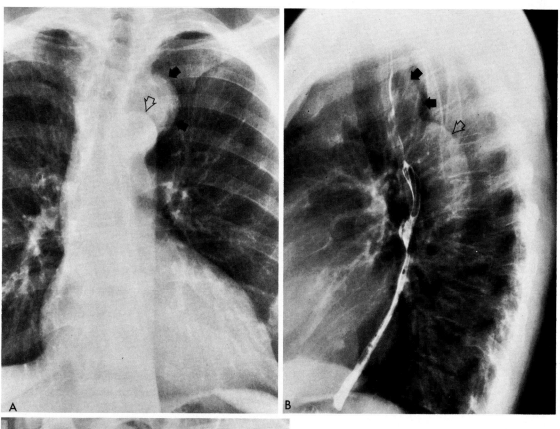

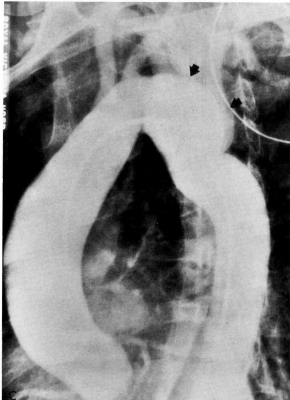

Figure 19–31. Pseudocoarctation of the Aorta. A posteroanterior view *(A)* of the chest of this 63-year-old asymptomatic woman reveals a homogeneous soft tissue opacity *(solid arrows)* projected above the shadow of the aortic knob *(open arrow)*. In lateral projection *(B)*, the posterior aspect of the "mass" is again identified by *solid arrows,* and the posterior portion of the aortic arch by an *open arrow.* Although these findings were thought to be compatible with pseudocoarctation of the aorta, an aortogram was performed for confirmation. This study in oblique projection *(C)* confirms the fact that the abnormal opacity observed on the plain roentgenogram is due to an unusually high aortic arch *(solid arrows)* that buckled in its descending portion so as to produce a prominent notch on its posterior and left lateral aspects.

MEDIASTINAL MASSES SITUATED PREDOMINANTLY IN THE POSTERIOR COMPARTMENT

The posterior mediastinal compartment lies between the pericardium and the anterior aspect of the vertebral column. It contains the descending aorta, the esophagus, the thoracic duct, the lower portion of the vagus nerves, and the posterior group of mediastinal lymph nodes. Since the posterior limit of the mediastinum, by definition, is formed by the anterior surface of the vertebral column, the paravertebral zones and posterior gutters are anatomically excluded. However, since these areas contain structures of importance in the histogenesis of posterior mediastinal masses, including the sympathetic nerve chains and peripheral nerves, these zones customarily are included in a discussion of masses in the posterior mediastinum.

Tumors and Tumorlike Conditions of Neural Tissue

Neoplasms of neural tissue have been said to constitute almost 20 per cent of mediastinal tumors.[50] There are two basic types: those arising from the peripheral nerves and those originating from sympathetic ganglia. Tumors arising from paraganglionic tissue and developmental anomalies of the spinal canal are also considered under this heading.

Tumors Arising from Peripheral Nerves

This group includes neurofibroma, neurilemmoma (schwannoma), and neurogenic sarcoma (malignant schwannoma), the vast majority of which arise from one of the intercostal nerves. Pathologically, most tumors are encapsulated, roughly spherical masses projecting from the chest wall into the paravertebral space. Occasionally, a tumor extends through a spinal foramen and grows in a dumbbell fashion in both spinal canal and mediastinum. Although malignant tumors (about one tenth as common as the benign form[50]) can show invasion of contiguous structures at the time of diagnosis, they also can be encapsulated.

Roentgenographic features of the three forms of tumor are similar and consist of a sharply defined, round or oval shadow of homogeneous density in the paravertebral zone on one side or the other. Tumors that originate in a nerve root within the spinal canal can expand the intervertebral foramen. Special procedures that may be helpful in certain cases include CT, MRI, and myelography (to determine whether a neurofibroma is of intraspinal origin). Neurilemmomas have been shown to have a mixed attenuation on CT, attributable to confluent areas of hypocellularity adjacent to densely cellular or collagenous regions, xanthomatous change, or regions of cystic degeneration.[190]

Most tumors occur in young adults. Usually, they do not cause symptoms and are discovered on a screening chest roentgenogram. In a minority of patients, compression of intercostal nerves or tracheobronchial airways gives rise to pain or dyspnea, respectively. Mediastinal neurofibromas can be associated with neurofibromas and other neoplasms elsewhere in the body (usually in the setting of von Recklinghausen's neurofibromatosis).

Provided complete surgical excision can be achieved, the prognosis of benign peripheral nerve tumors of the mediastinum is excellent. By contrast, the malignant neoplasms are usually aggressive, the average survival time from the time of diagnosis being only 2 years.[50]

Tumors Arising from Sympathetic Ganglia

The principal tumors in this category are ganglioneuroma, ganglioneuroblastoma, and neuroblastoma. Pathologically, they represent a continuum of histologic appearances from mature, fully differentiated neural tissue in the first to immature tissue in the last. Because of this, distinguishing between these neoplasms is to some extent arbitrary[191] and sometimes can be difficult.

The roentgenographic appearance of these tumors is similar to that of the peripheral nerve tumors described above, consisting of a sharply defined homogeneous opacity in the paravertebral zone (Fig. 19–32). It has been said that ganglioneuromas may have an elongated, flattened, or triangular configuration with a broad base toward the mediastinum, thus being somewhat less defined than nerve sheath tumors, especially in lateral projection.[39, 192] Calcification is relatively common,[193] and its identification can be an important aid in differentiating it from other mediastinal tumors. Calcification is not a reliable indicator of whether the lesion is benign or malignant.[192] The ribs or vertebrae are eroded in some cases, just as often by benign as by malignant forms.

Neuroblastomas and ganglioneuroblastomas occur most commonly in infants and children, whereas ganglioneuromas tend to occur in adolescents and young adults.[191] About half the patients are asymptomatic; the remainder have nonspecific respiratory symptoms. Ganglioneuromas are benign neoplasms, and complete excision typically results in cure. By contrast, neuroblastomas are aggressive tumors for which the 2-year survival rate is usually 45 to 50 per cent.[191] The prognosis of ganglioneuroblastoma is less predictable and depends to some extent on the age at diagnosis (younger age being associated with a better outcome), stage, and the histologic growth pattern.[191]

Aorticosympathetic (Paravertebral) Paraganglioma

Intrathoracic paragangliomas in the posterior mediastinum develop in relation to the aorticosympathetic paraganglia.[194] The average age at the time of diagnosis is about 30 years and there is a male-to-female predominance of 2 to 1. The pathologic features are identical to those of tumors in an aorticopulmonary location.

Roentgenographically, most aorticosympathetic paragangliomas are sharply defined, round or oval masses in the paravertebral area and are indistinguishable from other neurogenic neoplasms.

Clinically, about 50 per cent of patients are asymptomatic. About half of the reported patients have shown signs and symptoms related to excess catecholamine production, including headache, sweating, tachycardia, palpitations, dyspnea, and nausea. Hypertension is present in most, as are increased levels of plasma and urine catecholamines.[195] Many patients have adrenal and other extrathoracic paraganglionic tumors that can present either synchronously or metachronously.[196]

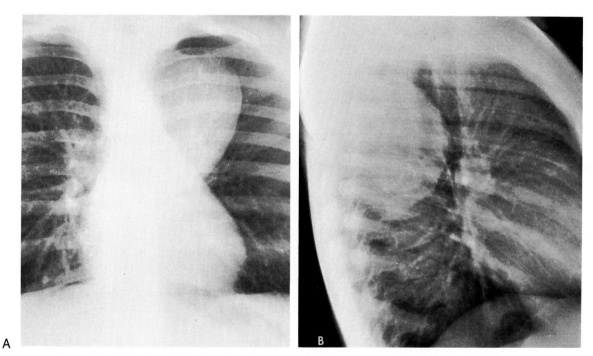

A

B

Figure 19–32. Posterior Mediastinal Ganglioneuroma. Roentgenograms of the thorax in posteroanterior *(A)* and lateral *(B)* projections reveal a smooth, sharply defined mass situated in the left paravertebral gutter superiorly. The mass contains numerous speckled deposits of calcium throughout its substance. (Courtesy of Montreal Children's Hospital.)

The prognosis of aorticosympathetic paragangliomas is better than that of those in the aorticopulmonary region.[196] In many cases, complete surgical excision and cure are possible.

Meningocele and Meningomyelocele

These rare anomalies of the intrathoracic spinal canal consist of herniation of the leptomeninges through an intervertebral foramen. (A meningocele contains cerebrospinal fluid only; a meningomyelocele also contains nerve elements.) The lesion is solitary in the large majority of patients[197] and can be situated anywhere between the thoracic inlet and the diaphragm. It is usually detected in middle age.[197]

On conventional roentgenograms, these lesions show no specific features that distinguish them from solid neurogenic neoplasms. However, CT examination should prove diagnostic, especially if associated with metrizamide myelography, which usually reveals passage of contrast medium into the meningocele.[137] Kyphoscoliosis is frequent; the meningocele usually is situated at the apex of the curvature on its convex side. An association with vertebral and rib anomalies is also fairly frequent and should suggest the diagnosis.[198] Enlargement of the intervertebral foramen and an association with generalized neurofibromatosis are common, although the latter is of little differential value, since neurogenic neoplasms are also part of von Recklinghausen's disease.

Posterior Mediastinal Cysts

Gastroenteric (Neurenteric) Cyst

Gastroenteric (neurenteric) cysts are believed to develop as a result of incomplete separation of endoderm from the notochord during early fetal life.[199, 200] Histologically, the cysts are lined by a variety of types of epithelium, including gastric, small intestinal, duodenal, and respiratory.[199] The first type can be functional and associated with peptic ulceration.

The roentgenographic appearance is that of a sharply defined, lobulated opacity of homogeneous density situated in a paravertebral location. Because of their fluid content, they tend to mold themselves to surrounding structures. The cysts are often connected by a stalk to the meninges and commonly also to a portion of the gastrointestinal tract. If attachment is to the esophagus, communication is rare; however, if it is to the gastrointestinal tract, in most cases communication permits gas to enter the cyst. In fact, the cyst may opacify with barium during examination of the upper gastrointestinal tract. Some cases are associated with congenital defects of the thoracic spine[200, 201]; in these, myelography occasionally reveals a patent stalk communicating with the spinal subarachnoid space.[201] Very large cysts may be associated with scoliosis.

Gastroenteric cysts typically produce symptoms and therefore become obvious early in life.[202] They can grow very large and cause compression atelectasis, thereby leading to respiratory distress. Peptic ulceration can cause pain.

Esophageal Cyst

Esophageal (esophageal duplication) cysts[203] are believed to represent a failure of complete vacuolation of the originally solid esophagus to produce a hollow tube.[199] They are lined by nonkeratinizing squamous or ciliated columnar epithelium; a double layer of smooth muscle in their walls and absence of cartilage are necessary findings to exclude a diagnosis of bronchial cyst. The cysts are usually located within or adjacent to the wall of the esophagus. Many patients are asymptomatic, although esophageal compression can cause dysphagia.[199]

Thoracic Duct Cyst

A rare type of posterior mediastinal mass, thoracic duct cyst can occur anywhere from the thoracic inlet to the diaphragm and can communicate with the thoracic duct either superiorly or inferiorly.[204, 205] It may be large enough to displace the mediastinum to the opposite side. Patients are most often asymptomatic but sometimes complain of dysphagia or back pain.

Diseases of the Esophagus

Esophageal lesions that may present roentgenographically as mediastinal masses or as diffuse mediastinal widening include neoplasms, diverticula, esophageal hiatus hernia, and megaesophagus. The manifestations of esophageal disease on conventional chest roentgenograms have recently been reviewed.[206]

Neoplasms

Although barium examination and esophagoscopy are the two definitive procedures in the diagnosis of primary carcinoma of the esophagus, conventional roentgenograms of the chest can provide several clues to its presence. The most frequent abnormalities are an abnormal azygoesophageal recess interface, a widened mediastinum, posterior tracheal indentation or mass, a widened retrotracheal stripe, and tracheal deviation (Fig. 19–33).[207, 208] Although thickening of the esophageal wall is the earliest CT manifestation of esophageal carcinoma, it is by no means diagnostic of that condition. Other causes are reflux and monilial esophagitis, esophageal varices, and postirradiation scarring.[209]

Benign neoplasms of the esophagus (principally leiomyomas, fibromas, and lipomas) can grow large and present as a rounded mass projecting to one or both sides of the posterior mediastinum (Fig. 19–34).[210]

Diverticula

Zenker's diverticulum originates between the transverse and oblique fibers of the inferior pharyngeal constrictor muscle and thus is a pharyngeal rather than an esophageal diverticulum. It may become large enough to be identified in the superior mediastinum on plain roentgenograms, where it is situated posterior to the trachea and esophagus and frequently contains an air-fluid level. Barium studies

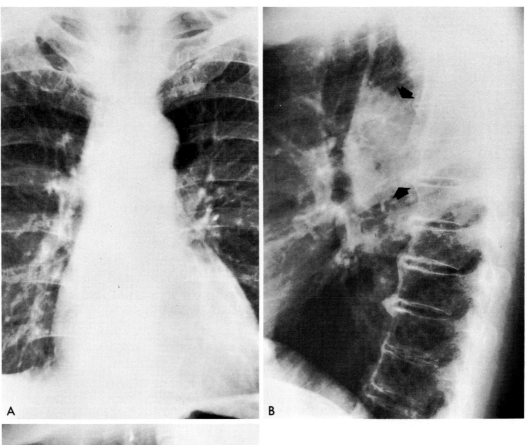

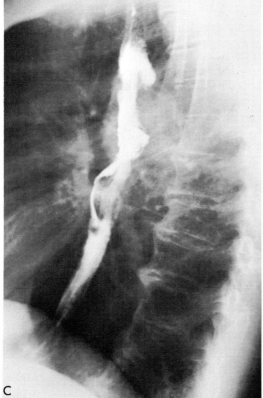

Figure 19–33. Posterior Mediastinal Mass Caused by Carcinoma of the Esophagus. A posteroanterior roentgenogram *(A)* reveals no significant abnormalities of the mediastinal silhouette, but in lateral projection *(B)*, there is evidence of a poorly defined increase in density in the posterior mediastinum, obliterating the aortic window and causing slight anterior displacement of the trachea *(arrows)*. A lateral view of the thorax following ingestion of barium *(C)* reveals severe deformity of the esophageal contour characteristic of primary esophageal cancer. The neoplasm had invaded the adjacent mediastinal soft tissues and had metastasized to regional posterior mediastinal nodes.

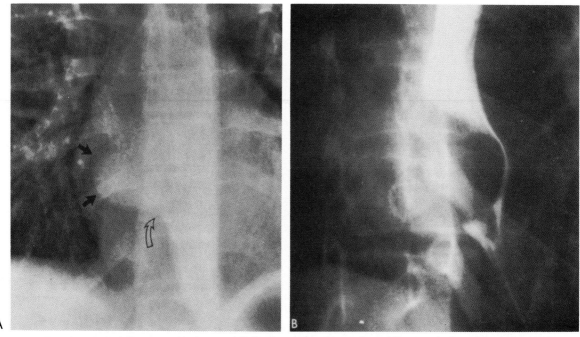

Figure 19–34. Esophageal Leiomyoma Deforming the Azygoesophageal Recess. A view of the mediastinum from a posteroanterior roentgenogram *(A)* reveals a smooth, sharply defined mass *(solid arrows)* displacing the azygoesophageal recess to the right. Note the obtuse angle formed by the mass and the recess *(open arrow)*. Barium opacification of the esophagus *(B)* reveals a sharply defined deformity of the barium column in a configuration typical of an extramucosal intramural lesion.

not only clearly outline the sac but also reveal the degree of anterior displacement of the proximal esophagus. Symptoms include dysphagia, chronic cough due to aspiration and, in some patients, recurrent pneumonia.

Diverticula arising from the lower third of the esophagus are almost always congenital in origin and present as round, cystlike structures to the right of the midline just above the diaphragm. An air-fluid level is present in most cases. Barium studies are diagnostic.[211]

Megaesophagus

Of the several causes of dilatation of the esophagus— inflammatory stenosis (secondary to mediastinitis or reflux esophagitis), progressive systemic sclerosis (PSS), carcinoma, and achalasia—the last causes the most severe generalized dilatation. The abnormality is apparent as a shadow projecting entirely to the right side of the mediastinum. Since it is behind the heart, it does not cause a silhouette sign with that structure. The trachea may bulge anteriorly, and an air-fluid level may be observed in the dilated esophagus, most frequently in achalasia and seldom in PSS. On conventional chest roentgenograms, air also may be identified in the esophagus in some patients postoperatively[212] and in laryngectomy patients who employ esophageal speech.[213] Symptoms of achalasia include dysphagia, pain on swallowing, and chronic cough and recurrent pneumonia due to aspiration.

Tracheoesophageal and Bronchoesophageal Fistulae

Fistulae between the esophagus and the airways can be congenital *(see* page 268) or acquired. The most common cause of the latter type is carcinoma of the esophagus, in which case the fistula may be precipitated by irradiation therapy.[214] Once this complication has developed, the prognosis is extremely bad, most patients dying within weeks to months. Acquired nonmalignant tracheoesophageal fistulae can be caused by cuffed endotracheal tubes, surgical trauma, blunt injuries, and foreign bodies.[215] Diagnosis is usually made by endoscopic or barium examination.

Mediastinal Masses Due to Transdiaphragmatic Herniation of Abdominal Contents

Herniation of abdominal contents, most often the stomach, liver, or omentum, occurs occasionally through a variety of defects in the diaphragm and may be manifested as a mediastinal mass. They are discussed in Chapter 20 *(see* page 947).

Diseases of the Thoracic Spine
Neoplasms

Metastatic carcinoma as well as a wide variety of primary neoplasms of bone and cartilage can involve the thoracic spine and posterior rib cage. In a few cases, the major roentgenographic finding is an extraosseous soft tissue mass, and identification of the primary bone lesion requires careful roentgenographic study. Lymphoma, particularly Hodgkin's disease, may be manifested roentgenologically as a fusiform paraspinal soft tissue mass produced by enlargement of the posterior parietal group of lymph nodes; in such cases, contiguous vertebrae may be eroded by extranodal invasion.

Infectious Spondylitis

Tuberculous or nontuberculous spondylitis is often associated with inflammation and abscess formation in contiguous soft tissues. Commonly, roentgenograms show a bilateral fusiform mass in the paravertebral zone that is widest at the point of major bone destruction.

Fracture with Hematoma Formation

Fractures of thoracic vertebral bodies can result in extraosseous hemorrhage and the development of unilateral or bilateral paraspinal masses. Although the fracture is usually visible roentgenographically, the major evidence of its presence may be deformity of the contiguous paraspinal soft tissues.

Extramedullary Hematopoiesis

Extramedullary hematopoiesis occurs as a compensatory phenomenon in various diseases in which there is inadequate production or excessive destruction of blood cells. The majority of cases are associated with congenital hemolytic anemia (usually hereditary spherocytosis) or thalassemia (usually thalassemia major or intermedia).[216] Occasional cases also have been reported in association with sickle cell disease.[217]

The most common sites are the liver and spleen, but foci can also occur in many other organs and tissues, including the paravertebral areas of the thorax.[216] The origin of extramedullary hematopoiesis in the the latter site is unclear; however, it has been postulated that it represents extension of hyperplastic marrow from adjacent bone or lymph nodes[218] or that it develops from embryonic nests of primitive hematopoietic tissue.[219] Pathologically, foci of extramedullary hematopoiesis appear as one or more soft, reddish nodules that can resemble hematomas.[216] Histologically, all marrow elements can be identified, usually with marked erythroid hyperplasia.

The characteristic roentgenographic finding is multiple masses, smooth or lobulated in contour and of homogeneous density, situated in the paravertebral regions, either unilaterally or bilaterally.[59] Most often, they are located below the level of the seventh thoracic vertebra. A presumptive diagnosis usually can be made when this roentgenographic finding is present in patients with severe anemia and splenomegaly. The masses seldom cause symptoms.

References

1. Heitzman ER: The Mediastinum. Radiologic Correlations with Anatomy and Pathology. St. Louis, CV Mosby, 1977.
2. Comings DE, Skubi K-B, Eyes JV, et al: Familial multifocal fibrosclerosis. Findings suggesting that retroperitoneal fibrosis, mediastinal fibrosis, sclerosing cholangitis, Riedel's thyroiditis, and pseudotumor of the orbit may be different manifestations of a single disease. Ann Intern Med 66: 884, 1967.
3. LaBerge JM, Kerlan RK Jr, Pogany AC, et al: Esophageal rupture: Complication of balloon dilatation. Radiology 157: 56, 1985.
4. Zeller FA, Cannan CR, Prakash UB: Thoracic manifestations after esophageal variceal sclerotherapy. Mayo Clin Proc 66: 727, 1991.
5. Chavy AL, Rougier M, Pieddeloup C, et al: Esophageal prostheses for neoplastic stenosis. A prognostic study of 77 cases. Cancer 57: 1426, 1986.
6. Rogers LF, Puig AW, Dooley BN, et al: Diagnostic considerations in mediastinal emphysema: A pathophysiologic-roentgenologic approach to Boerhaave's syndrome and spontaneous pneumomediastinum. Am J Roentgenol 115: 495, 1972.
7. Rutledge R, Applebaum RE, Kim BJ: Mediastinal infection after open heart surgery. Surgery 97: 88, 1985.
8. Larson TC III, Shuman LS, Sibshitz HI, et al: Complications of colonic interposition. Cancer 56: 681, 1985.
9. Han SY, McElvein RB, Aldrete JS, et al: Perforation of the esophagus: Correlation of site and cause with plain film findings. Am J Roentgenol 145: 537, 1985.
10. Dodds WJ, Stewart ET, Vlymen WJ: Appropriate contrast media for evaluation of esophageal disruption. Radiology 144: 439, 1982.
11. Appleton DS, Sandrasagra FA, Flower CDR: Perforated oesophagus: Review of twenty-eight consecutive cases. Clin Radiol 30: 493, 1979.
12. Craddock DR, Logan A, Mayell M: Traumatic rupture of the oesophagus and stomach. Thorax 23: 657, 1968.
13. Loyd JE, Tillman BF, Atkinson JB, et al: Mediastinal fibrosis complicating histoplasmosis. Medicine 67: 295, 1988.
14. Dozois RR, Bernatz PE, Woolner LB, et al: Sclerosing mediastinitis involving major bronchi. Mayo Clin Proc 43: 557, 1968.
15. Graham JR, Suby HI, LeCompte PR, et al: Fibrotic disorders associated with methysergide therapy for headache. N Engl J Med 274: 359, 1966.
16. Schowengerdt CG, Suyemoto R, Main FB: Granulomatous and fibrous mediastinitis—a review and analysis of 180 cases. J Thorac Cardiovasc Surg 57: 365, 1969.
17. Katzenstein ALA, Mazur MT: Pulmonary infarct: An unusual manifestation of fibrosing mediastinitis. Chest 77: 521, 1980.
18. Sobrinho-Simões MA, Vaz Saleiro J, Wagenvoort CA: Mediastinal and hilar fibrosis. Histopathology 5: 53, 1981.
19. Feigin DS, Eggleston JC, Siegelman SS: The multiple roentgen manifestations of sclerosing mediastinitis. Johns Hopkins Med J 144: 1, 1979.
20. Weinstein JB, Aronberg DJ, Sagel SS: CT of fibrosing mediastinitis: Findings and their utility. Am J Roentgenol 141: 247, 1983.
21. Rholl KS, Levitt RG, Glazer HS: Magnetic resonance imaging of fibrosing mediastinitis. Am J Roentgenol 145: 255, 1985.
22. Morgan AD, Loughridge LW, Calne RY: Combined mediastinal and reproperitoneal fibrosis. Lancet 1: 67, 1966.
23. Salmon HW: Combined mediastinal and reproperitoneal fibrosis. Thorax 23: 158, 1968.
24. Ramakantan R, Shah P: Dysphagia due to mediastinal fibrosis in advanced pulmonary tuberculosis. Am J Roentgenol 154: 61, 1990.
25. Bodey GP: Medical mediastinal emphysema. Ann Intern Med 54: 46, 1961.
26. Cyrlak D, Milne EN, Imray TJ: Pneumomediastinum: A diagnostic problem. CRC Crit Rev Diagn Imaging 23: 75, 1984.
27. Macklin MT, Macklin CC: Malignant interstitial emphysema of the lungs and mediastinum as an important occult complication in many respiratory diseases and other conditions. An interpretation of the clinical literature in the light of laboratory experiment. Medicine 23: 281, 1944.
28. Munsell WP: Pneumomediastinum: A report of 28 cases and review of the literature. JAMA 202: 689, 1967.
29. Morgan EJ, Henderson DA: Pneumomediastinum as a complication of athletic competition. Thorax 36: 155, 1981.
30. Dudley DK, Patten DE: Intrapartum pneumomediastinum associated with subcutaneous emphysema. Can Med Assoc J 139: 641, 1988.
31. Dattwyler RJ, Goldman MA, Bloch KJ: Pneumomediastinum as a complication of asthma in teenage and young adult patients. J Allergy Clin Immunol 63: 412, 1979.
32. Girard DE, Carlson V, Natelson EA, et al: Pneumomediastinum in diabetic ketoacidosis: Comments on mechanism, incidence, and management. Chest 60: 455, 1971.
33. Altman AR, Johnson TH: Pneumoperitoneum and pneumoretroperitoneum. Consequences of positive end-expiratory pressure therapy. Arch Surg 114: 208, 1979.
34. Norman JC, Rizzolo PJ: Subcutaneous, mediastinal and probable subpericardial emphysema treated with recompression. N Engl J Med 261, 169, 1959.
35. Sandler CM, Libshitz HI, Marks G: Pneumoperitoneum, pneumomediastinum and pneumopericardium following dental extraction. Radiology 115: 539, 1975.
36. Felson B: The mediastinum. Semin Roentgenol 4: 40, 1969.

37. Landay MJ, Cohen DJ, Deaton CW Jr: Another look at the "ring-around-the-artery" in pneumomediastinum. J Can Assoc Radiol 36: 343, 1985.

38. Levin B: The continuous diaphragm sign. A newly recognized sign of pneumomediastinum. Clin Radiol 24: 337, 1973.

39. Wychulis AR, Payne WS, Clagett OT, et al: Surgical treatment of mediastinal tumors. A 40-year experience. J Thorac Cardiovasc Surg 62: 379, 1971.

40. Benjamin SP, McCormack LJ, Effler DB, et al: Critical review—"primanry tumours of the mediastinum." Chest 62: 297, 1972.

41. Brown LR, Aughenbaugh GL: Masses of the anterior mediastinum: CT and MR imaging. Am J Roentgenol 157: 1171, 1991.

42. Düe W, Dieckmann K-P, Stein H: Thymic hyperplasia following chemotherapy of a testicular germ cell tumor. Immunohistological evidence for a simple rebound phenomenon. Cancer 63: 446, 1989.

43. Judd RL: Massive thymic hyperplasia with myoid cell differentiation. Hum Pathol 18: 1180, 1987.

44. Levine GD, Rosai J: Thymic hyperplasia and neoplasia: A review of current concepts. Hum Pathol 9: 495, 1978.

45. Clark RE, Marbarger JP, West PN, et al: Thymectomy for myasthenia gravis in the young adult: Long-term results. J Thorac Cardiovasc Surg 80: 696, 1980.

46. Teplick JG, Nedwich A, Haskin ME: Roentgenographic features of thymolipoma. Am J Roentgenol 117: 873, 1973.

47. Rosai J, Levine GD: Atlas of Tumor Pathology: Tumors of the Thymus. Second Series, Fascicle 13. Washington, DC, Armed Forces Institute of Pathology, 1976.

48. Yeh H-C, Gordon A, Kirschner PA, et al: Computed tomography and sonography of thymolipoma. Am J Roentgenol 140: 1131, 1983.

49. McCafferty MH, Bahnson HT: Thymic cyst extending into the pericardium: A case report and review of thymic cysts. Ann Thorac Surg 33: 503, 1982.

50. Suster S, Rosai J: Multiocular thymic cyst: An acquired reactive process. Study of 18 cases. Am J Surg Pathol 15: 388, 1991.

51. Leong AS-Y, Brown JH: Malignant transformation in a thymic cyst. Am J Surg Pathol 8: 471, 1984.

52. Ingels GW, Campbell DC, Giampetro AM, et al: Malignant schwannomas of the mediastinum. Cancer 27: 1190, 1971.

53. McGuire LJ, Huang DP, Teoh R, et al: Epstein-Barr virus genome in thymoma and thymic lymphoid hyperplasia. Am J Pathol 131: 385, 1988.

54. Lewis JE, Wick MR, Scheithauer BW, et al: Thymoma. A clinico-pathologic review. Cancer 60: 2727, 1987.

55. Hofmann W, Möller P, Manke H-G, et al: Thymoma. A clinicopathologic study of 98 cases with special reference to three unusual cases. Pathol Res Pract 179: 337, 1985.

56. Maggi G, Giaccone G, Conadio M, et al: Thymomas. A review of 169 cases, with particular reference to results of surgical treatment. Cancer 58: 765, 1986.

57. Marino M, Müller-Hermelink H-K: Thymoma and thymic carcinoma. Relation of thymoma epithelial cells to the cortical and medullary differentiation of thymus. Virchows Arch [A] 407: 119, 1985.

58. Lee D, Wright DH: Immunohistochemical study of 22 cases of thymoma. J Clin Pathol 41: 1297, 1988.

59. Leigh TF, Weens HS: Roentgen aspects of mediastinal lesions. Semin Roentgenol 4: 59, 1969.

60. Brown LR, Muhm JR, Gray JE: Radiographic detection of thymoma. Am J Roentgenol 134: 1181, 1980.

61. Baron RL, Lee JKT, Sagel SS, et al: Computed tomography of the abnormal thymus. Radiology 142: 127, 1982.

62. Brown LR, Muhm JR, Sheedy PF II, et al: The value of computed tomography in myasthenia gravis. Am J Roentgenol 140: 31, 1983.

63. Fon GT, Bein ME, Mancuso AA, et al: Computed tomography of the anterior mediastinum in myasthenia gravis. A radiologic-pathologic correlative study. Radiology 142: 135, 1982.

64. Ellis K, Austin JHM, Ill AJ: Radiologic detection of thymoma in patients with myasthenia gravis. Am J Roentgenol 151: 873, 1988.

65. Sakai F, Sone S, Kiyono I, et al: MR imaging of thymoma: radiologic-pathologic correlation. Am J Roentgenol 158: 751, 1992

66. Molina PL, Siegel MJ, Glazer HS: Thymic masses on MR imaging. Am J Roentgenol 155: 495, 1990.

67. Masaoka A, Hashimoto T, Shibata K, et al: Thymomas associated with pure red cell aplasia. Histologic and follow-up studies. Cancer 64: 1872, 1989.

68. Nomori H, Ishihara T, Torikata C: Malignant grading of cortical and medullary differentiated thymoma by morphometric analysis. Cancer 64: 1694, 1989.

69. Kornsstein MJ, Curran WJ Jr, Turrisi AT, et al: Cortical versus medullary thymomas: A useful morphologic distinction? Hum Pathol 19: 1335, 1988.

70. Rosai J, Levine G, Weber WR, et al: Carcinoid tumors and oat cell carcinomas of the thymus. Pathol Ann 11: 201, 1976

71. Viebahn R, Hiddemann W, Klinke F, et al: Thymus carcinoid. Pathol Res Pract 180: 445, 1985

72. Wick MR, Bernatz PE, Carney JA, et al: Primary mediastinal carcinoid tumors. Am J Surg Pathol 6: 195, 1982.

73. Brown LR, Aughenbaugh GL, Wick MR, et al: Roentgenologic diagnosis of primary corticotropin-producing carcinoid tumors of the mediastinum. Radiology 142: 143, 1982

74. Lowenthal RM, Gumpel JM, Kreel L, et al: Carcinoid tumour of the thymus with systemic manifestations: A radiological and pathological study. Thorax 29: 553, 1974.

75. Birnberg FA, Webb WR, Selch MT, et al: Thymic carcinoid tumors with hyperparathyroidism. Am J Roentgenol 139: 1001, 1982.

76. Truong LD, Mody DR, Cagle PT, et al: Thymic carcinoma. A clinicopathologic study of 13 cases. Am J Surg Pathol 14(2): 151, 1990.

77. Kuo T-T, Chang J-P, Lin F-J, et al: Thymic carcinomas: Histopathological varieties and immunohistochemical study. Am J Surg Pathol 14(1): 24, 1990.

78. Snover DC, Levine GD, Rosai J: Thymic carcinoma. Five distinctive histological variants. Am J Surg Pathol 6: 451, 1982.

79. Keller AR, Castleman B: Hodgkin's disease of the thymus gland. Cancer 33: 1615, 1974.

80. Kim HC, Nosher J, Haas A, et al: Cystic degeneration of thymic Hodgkin's disease following radiation therapy. Cancer 55: 354, 1985.

81. Yousem SA, Weiss LM, Warnke RA: Primary mediastinal non-Hodgkin's lymphomas: A morphologic and immunologic study of 19 cases. Am J Clin Pathol 83: 676, 1985

82. Wernecke K, Vassallo P, Rutsch F, et al: Thymic involvement in Hodgkin disease: CT and sonographic findings. Radiology 181: 375, 1991.

83. Knapp RH, Hurt RD, Payne WS, et al: Malignant germ cell tumors of the mediastinum. J Thorac Cardiovasc Surg 89: 82, 1985.

84. Wenger ME, Dines DE, Ahmann DL, et al: Primary mediastinal choriocarcinoma. Mayo Clin Proc 43: 570, 1968.

85. Luna MA, Valenzuela-Tamariz J: Germ-cell tumors of the mediastinum, postmortem findings. Am J Clin Pathol 65: 450, 1976.

86. Daugaard G, von der Masse H, Olsen J, et al: Carcinoma-in-situ testis in patients with assumed extragonadal germ-cell tumours. Lancet 2: 528, 1987.

87. Oosterhuis JW, Rammeloo RHU, Cornelisse CJ, et al: Ploidy of malignant mediastinal germ-cell tumors. Hum Pathol 21: 729, 1990.

88. Lachman MF, Kim K, Koo B-C: Mediastinal teratoma associated with Klinefelter's syndrome. Arch Pathol Lab Med 110: 1067, 1986.

89. Richardson RL, Schoumacher BS, Fer MF, et al: The unrecognized extragonadal germ cell cancer syndrome. Ann Intern Med 94: 181, 1981.

90. Pachter MR, Lattes R: "Germinal" tumors of the mediastinum: A clinicopathologic study of adult teratomas, teratocarcinomas, choriocarcinomas and seminomas. Dis Chest 45: 301, 1964.

91. Manivel C, Wick MR, Abenoza P, et al: The occurrence of sarcomatous components in primary mediastinal germ cell tumors. Am J Surg Pathol 10: 711, 1986.

92. Fulcher AS, Proto AV, Jolles H: Cystic teratoma of the mediastinum: Demonstration of fat/fluid level. Am J Roentgenol 154: 259, 1990.

93. Weinberg B, Rose JS, Stavros C, et al: Posterior mediastinal teratoma (cystic dermoid): Diagnosis by computerized tomography. Chest 77: 694, 1980.

94. deMent SH: Association between mediastinal germ cell tumors and hematologic malignancies: An update. Hum Pathol 21: 699, 1990.

95. Carter D, Bibro M, Touloukian RJ: Benign clinical behavior of immature mediastinal teratoma in infancy and childhood: Report of two cases and review of the literature. Cancer 49: 398, 1982.

96. Harms D, Jènig U: Immature teratomas of childhood. Report of 21 cases. Pathol Res Pract 179: 388, 1985.

97. Polansky SM, Barwick KW, Ravin CE: Primary mediastinal seminoma. Am J Roentgenol 132: 17, 1979.

98. Shin MS, Ho KJ: Computed tomography of primary mediastinal seminomas. J Comput Assist Tomogr 7: 990, 1983.

99. Hurt RD, Bruckman JE, Farrow GM, et al: Primary anterior mediastinal seminoma. Cancer 49: 1658, 1982.

100. Raghavan D, Barrett A: Mediastinal seminomas. Cancer 46: 1187, 1980.

101. Truong LD, Harris L, Mattioli C, et al: Endodermal sinus tumor of

the mediastinum. A report of seven cases and review of the literature. Cancer 58: 730, 1986.

102. Sham JST, Fu KH, Chiu CSW, et al: Experience with the management of primary endodermal sinus tumor of the mediastinum. Cancer 64: 756, 1989.

103. Knapp RH, Fritz SR, Reiman HM: Primary embryonal carcinoma and choriocarcinoma of the mediastinum. Arch Pathol Lab Med 106: 507, 1982.

104. Primary mediastinal choriocarcinoma. Br Med J 2: 135, 1969.

105. Lahey FH: Intrathoracic goiters. Surg Clin North Am 25: 609, 1945.

106. Fragomeni LS, Ceratti de Zambuja P: Intrathoracic goitre in the posterior mediastinum. Thorax 35: 638, 1980.

107. Reitz K-A, Werner B: Intrathoracic goiter. Acta Chir Scand 119: 379, 1960.

108. Katlic MR, Wang C, Grillo HC: Substernal goiter. Ann Thorac Surg 39: 391, 1985.

109. Hansen ME, Spritzer CE, Sostman HD: Assessing the patency of mediastinal and thoracic inlet veins: Value of MR imaging. Am J Roentgenol 155: 1177, 1990.

110. Bahist B, Ellis K, Gold RP: Computed tomography of intrathoracic goiters. Am J Roentgenol 140: 455, 1983.

111. Dontas NS: Intrathoracic goitre. Br J Tuberc 52: 154, 1958.

112. Hershey CO, McVeigh RC, Miller RP: Transient superior vena cava syndrome due to propylthiouracil therapy in intrathoracic goiter. Chest 79: 356, 1981.

113. Samanta A, Jones GR, Burden AC, et al: Thoracic inlet compression due to amiodarone induced goitre. Postgrad Med J 61: 249, 1985.

114. Murphy MN, Glennon PG, Diocee MS, et al: Nonsecretory parathyroid carcinoma of the mediastinum. Light microscopic, immunocytochemical, and ultrastructural features of a case, and review of the literature. Cancer 58: 2468, 1986.

115. Braxel C, Haemers S, van der Straeten M: Mediastinal parathyroid adenoma, detected on a routine chest X-ray. Scand J Respir Dis 60: 367, 1979.

116. Krudy AG, Doppman JL, Miller DL, et al: Detection of mediastinal parathyroid glands by nonselective digital arteriography. Am J Roentgenol 142: 693, 1984.

117. Krudy AG, Doppman JL, Brennan MF, et al: The detection of mediastinal parathyroid glands by computed tomography, selective arteriography and venous sampling. An analysis of 17 cases. Radiology 140: 739, 1981.

118. Pachter MR, Lattes R: Mesenchymal tumors of the mediastinum. I. Tumors of fibrous tissue, adipose tissue, smooth muscle, and striated muscle. Cancer 16: 1963.

119. Standerfer RJ, Armistead SH, Paneth M: Liposarcoma of the mediastinum: Report of two cases and review of the literature. Thorax 36: 693, 1981.

120. Hodge J, Aponte G, McLaughlin E: Primary mediastinal tumors. J Thorac Surg 37: 730, 1959.

121. Mendez G Jr, Isikoff MB, Isikoff SK, et al: Fatty tumors of the thorax demonstrated by CT. Am J Roentgenol 133: 207, 1979.

122. Price JE, Rigler LG: Widening of the mediastinum resulting from fat accumulation. Radiology 66: 497, 1970.

123. Drasin GF, Lynch T, Temes GP: Ectopic ACTH production and mediastinal lipomatosis. Radiology 127: 610, 1978.

124. Streiter ML, Schneider HJ, Proto AV: Steroid-induced thoracic lipomatosis: Paraspinal involvement. Am J Roentgenol 139: 679, 1982.

125. Kriegshauser JS, Julsrud PR, Lund JT: MR imaging of fat in and around the heart. Am J Roentgenol 155: 271, 1990.

126. Davis JM, Mark GJ, Greene R: Benign blood vascular tumors of the mediastinum. Radiology 126: 581, 1978.

127. Gindhart TD, Tucker WY, Choy SH: Cavernous hemangioma of the superior mediastinum. Report of a case with electron microscopy and computerized tomography. Am J Surg Pathol 3: 353, 1979.

128. Cohen AJ, Sbaschnig RJ, Hochholzer L, et al: Mediastinal hemangiomas. Ann Thorac Surg 43: 656, 1987.

129. Pachter MR, Lattes R: Mesenchymal tumors of the mediastinum. II. Tumors of blood vascular origin. Cancer 16: 95, 1963.

130. Woods D, Young JEM, Filice R, et al: Late-onset cystic hygromas: The role of CT. J Can Assoc Radiol 40: 159, 1989.

131. Feng Y-F, Masterson JB, Riddell RH: Lymphangioma of the middle mediastinum as an incidental finding on a chest radiograph. Thorax 35: 955, 1980.

132. Pilla TJ, Wolverson MK, Sundaram M, et al: CT evaluation of cystic lymphangiomas of the mediastinum. Radiology 144: 841, 1982.

133. Sunderrajan EV, Luger AM Rosenholtz MJ, et al: Leiomyosarcoma in the mediastinum presenting as superior vena cava syndrome. Cancer 53: 2553, 1984.

134. Rasaretnam R, Panabokke RG: Leiomyosarcoma of the mediastinum. Br J Dis Chest 69: 63, 1975.

135. Ulbright TM, Loehrer PJ, Roth LM, et al: The development of nongerm cell malignancies within germ cell tumors. Cancer 54: 1824, 1984.

136. Witkin GB, Rosai J: Solitary fibrous tumor of the mediastinum. A report of 14 cases. Am J Surg Pathol 13: 547, 1989.

137. Leigh TF: Mass lesions of the mediastinum. Radiol Clin North Am 1: 377, 1963.

138. Natsuaki M, Yoshikawa Y, Itoh T, et al: Xanthogranulomatous malignant fibrous histiocytoma arising from posterior mediastinum. Thorax 41: 322, 1986.

139. Colby TV, Hoppe RT, Warnke RA: Hodgkin's disease: A clinicopathologic study of 659 cases. Cancer 49: 1848, 1981.

140. Waldron JA Jr, Dohring EF, Farber LR: Primary large cell lymphomas of the mediastinum: An analysis of 20 cases. Semin Diagn Pathol 2: 281, 1985.

141. Trump DL, Mann RB: Diffuse large cell and undifferentiated lymphomas with prominent mediastinal involvement. A poor prognostic subset of patients with non-Hodgkin's lymphoma. Cancer 50: 277, 1982.

142. Perrone T, Frizzera G, Rosai J: Mediastinal diffuse large-cell lymphoma with sclerosis. A clinicopathologic study of 60 cases. Am J Surg Pathol 10: 176, 1986.

143. Keller AR, Hochholzer L, Castleman B: Hyaline-vascular and plasma-cell types of giant lymph node hyperplasia of the mediastinum and other locations. Cancer 29: 670, 1972.

144. Maier HC, Sommers SC: Mediastinal lymph node hyperplasia, hypergammaglobulinemia, and anemia. J Thorac Cardiovasc Surg 79: 860, 1980.

145. Weisenburger DD, Nathwani BN, Winberg CD, et al: Multicentric angiofollicular lymph node hyperplasia. Hum Pathol 16: 162, 1985.

146. Frizzera G: Castleman's disease: More questions than answers. Hum Pathol 16: 202, 1985.

147. Lowenthal DA, Filippa DA, Richardson ME, et al: Generalized lymphadenopathy with morphologic features of Castleman's disease in an HIV-positive man. Cancer 60: 2454, 1987.

148. Breatnach E, Meyers JD, McElvein RB, et al: Unusual cause of a calcified anterior mediastinal mass. Chest 89: 113, 1986.

149. Glenner GG, Grimley PM: Atlas of Tumor Pathology. Second Series. Fascicle 9. Tumors of the Extra-Adrenal Paraganglion System (Including Chemoreceptors). Washington, DC, Armed Forces Institute of Pathology, 1974.

150. Lack EE, Stillinger RA, Colvin DB, et al: Aorticopulmonary paraganglioma. Report of a case with ultrastructural study and review of the literature. Cancer 43: 269, 1979.

151. Drucker EA, McLoud TC, Dedrick CG, et al: Mediastinal paraganglioma: Radiologic evaluation of an unusual vascular tumor. Am J Roentgenol 148: 521, 1987.

152. Modic MT, Janicki PC: Computed tomography of mass lesions of the right cardiophrenic angle. J Comput Assist Tomogr 4: 521, 1980.

153. Paling MR, Williamson BRJ: Epipericardial fat pad: CT findings. Radiology 165: 335, 1987.

154. Brunner DR, Whitley NO: A pericardial cyst with high CT numbers. Am J Roentgenol 142: 279, 1984.

155. Daniel RA Jr, Diveley WL, Edwards WH, et al: Mediastinal tumors. Ann Surg 151: 783, 1960.

156. Cho CS, Blank N, Castellino RA: CT evaluation of cardiophrenic angle lymph nodes in patients with malignant lymphoma. Am J Roentgenol 143: 719, 1984.

157. Castellino RA, Blank N: Adenopathy of the cardiophrenic angle (diaphragmatic) lymph nodes. Am J Roentgenol 114: 509, 1972.

158. Buckingham WB, Sutton GC, Meszaros WT: Abnormalities of the pulmonary artery resembling intrathoracic neoplasms. Dis Chest 40: 698, 1961.

159. Davies PF, Shevland JE: Superior vena caval obstruction: An analysis of seventy-six cases, with comments on the safety of venography. Angiology 36: 354, 1985.

160. Shimm DS, Logue GL, Rigsby LC: Evaluating the superior vena cava syndrome. JAMA 245: 951, 1981.

161. Doty DB: Bypass of superior vena cava: 6 years' experience with spiral vein graft for obstruction of superior vena cava due to benign and malignant disease. J Thorac Cardiovasc Surg 83: 326, 1982.

162. Bechtold RE, Wolfman NT, Karstaedt N, et al: Superior vena caval obstruction: Detection using CT. Radiology 157: 485, 1985.
163. Webb WR, Gamsu G, Speckman JM, et al: Computed tomographic demonstration of mediastinal venous anomalies. Am J Roentgenol 139: 157, 1982.
164. Fleming JS, Gibson RV: Absent right superior vena cava as an isolated anomaly. Br J Radiol 37: 696, 1964.
165. van der Horst RL, Hastreiter AR: Congenital interruption of the inferior vena cava. Chest 80: 638, 1981.
166. Bernal-Ramirez M, Hatch HB Jr, Bower PJ: Interruption of the inferior vena cava with azygos continuation. Chest 65: 469, 1974.
167. Preger L, Hooper TI, Steinbach HL, et al: Width of azygos vein related to central venous pressures. Radiology 93: 521, 1969.
168. Doyle FH, Read AT, Evans KT: The mediastinum in portal hypertension. Clin Radiol 12: 114, 1961.
169. Breckenridge JW, Kinlaw WB: Azygos continuation of inferior vena cava: CT appearance. J Comput Assist Tomogr 4: 392, 1980.
170. Takasugi JE, Godwin JD: CT appearance of the retroaortic anastomoses of the azygos system. Am J Roentgenol 154: 41, 1990.
171. Dudiak CM, Olson MC, Posniak HV: CT evaluation of congenital and acquired abnormalities of the azygos system. Radiographics 11: 233, 1991.
172. Ball JB Jr, Proto AV: The variable appearance of the left superior intercostal vein. Radiology 144: 445, 1982.
173. Friedman AC, Chambers E, Sprayregen S: The normal and abnormal left superior intercostal vein. Am J Roentgenol 131: 599, 1978.
174. Hatfield MK, Vyborny CJ, MacMahon H, et al: Congenital absence of the azygos vein: A cause for "aortic nipple" enlargement. Am J Roentgenol 149: 273, 1987.
175. Thorsen MK, San Dretto MA, Lawson TL, et al: Dissecting aortic aneurysm accuracy of computed tomographic diagnosis. Radiology 148: 773, 1983.
176. Posniak HV, Olson MC, Demos TC, et al: CT of thoracic aortic aneurysms. Radiographics 10: 839, 1990.
177. Kersting-Sommerhoff BA, Higgins CB, White RD, et al: Aortic dissection: Sensitivity and specificity of MR imaging. Radiology 166: 651, 1988.
178. Wolff KA, Herold CJ, Tempany CM, et al: Aortic dissection: Atypical patterns seen at MR imaging. Radiology 181: 489, 1991.
179. Petasnick JP: Radiologic evaluation of aortic dissection. Radiology 180: 297, 1991.
180. Charrette EJ, Winton TL, Salerno TA: Acute respiratory insufficiency from an aneurysm of the descending thoracic aorta. J Thorac Cardiovasc Surg 85: 467, 1983.
181. Talbot S: Clinical features and prognosis of dissecting aneurysm and ruptured saccular aneurysms. Chest 66: 252, 1974.
182. Green RA: Enlargement of the innominate and subclavian arteries simulating mediastinal neoplasm. Am Rev Tuberc 79: 790, 1959.
183. Schneider HJ, Felson B: Buckling of the innominate artery simulating aneurysm and tumor. Am J Roentgenol 85: 1106, 1961.
184. Idbeis B, Levinsky L, Srinivasan V, et al: Vascular rings: Management and a proposed nomenclature. Ann Thorac Surg 31: 255, 1981.
185. Gaupp RJ, Fagan CJ, Davis M, et al: Pseudocoarctation of the aorta. Case report. J Comput Assist Tomogr 5: 571, 1981.
186. Kennard DR, Spigos DG, Tan WS: Cervical aortic arch: CT correlation with conventional radiologic studies. Am J Roentgenol 141: 295, 1983.
187. Salomonowitz E, Edwards JE, Hunter DW, et al: The three types of aortic diverticula. Am J Roentgenol 142: 673, 1984.
188. Shuford WH, Sybers RG, Edwards FK: The three types of right aortic arch. Am J Roentgenol 109: 67, 1970.
189. Bevelaqua F, Schicchi JS, Haas F, et al: Aortic arch anomaly presenting as exercise-induced asthma. Am Rev Respir Dis 140: 805, 1989.
190. Cohen LM, Schwartz AM, Rockoff SD: Benign schwannomas: Pathologic basis for CT inhomogeneities. Am J Roentgenol 147: 141, 1986.
191. Adam A, Hochholzer L: Ganglioneuroblastoma of the posterior mediastinum. A clinicopathologic review of 80 cases. Cancer 47: 373, 1981.
192. Reed JC, Hallet KK, Feigin DS: Neural tumors of the thorax: Subject review from the AFIP. Radiology 126: 9, 1978.
193. Schweisguth O, Mathey J, Renault P, et al: Intrathoracic neurogenic tumors in infants and children: A study of forty cases. Ann Surg 150: 29, 1959.
194. Odze R, Bégin LR: Malignant paraganglioma of the posterior mediastinum. A case report and review of the literature. Cancer 65: 564, 1990.
195. Ogawa J, Inoue H, Koide S, et al: Functioning paraganglioma in the posterior mediastinum. Ann Thorac Surg 33: 507, 1982.
196. Gallivan MVE, Chun B, Rowden G, et al: Intrathoracic paravertebral malignant paraganglioma. Arch Pathol Lab Med 104: 46, 1980.
197. Miles J, Pennybacker J, Sheldon P: Intrathoracic meningocele. Its development and association with neurofibromatosis. J Neurol Neurosurg Psychiatry, 32: 99, 1969.
198. Cabooter M, Bogaerts Y, Javaheri S, et al: Intrathoracic meningocele. Eur J Respir Dis 63: 347, 1982.
199. Salyer DC, Salyer WR, Eggleston JC: Benign developmental cysts of the mediastinum. Arch Pathol Lab Med 101: 136, 1977.
200. Madewell JE, Sobonya RE, Reed JC: Neurenteric cyst. RPC from the AFIP. Radiology 109: 707, 1973.
201. Ochsner JL, Ochsner SF: Congenital cysts of the mediastinum: 20-year experience with 42 cases. Ann Surg 163: 909, 1966.
202. Benton C, Silverman FN: Some mediastinal lesions in children. Semin Roentgenol 4: 91, 1969.
203. Kirwan WO, Walbaum PR, McCormack RJM: Cystic intrathoracic derivatives of the foregut and their complications. Thorax 28: 424, 1973.
204. Hori S, Harada K, Morimoto S, et al: Lymphangiographic demonstration of thoracic duct cyst. Chest 789: 652, 1980.
205. Morettin LB, Allen TE: Thoracic duct cyst: Diagnosis with needle aspiration. Radiology 161: 437, 1986.
206. Stark P, Thordarson S, McKinney M: Manifestations of esophageal disease on plain chest radiographs. Am J Roentgenol 155: 729, 1990.
207. Lindell MM Jr, Hill CA, Libshitz HI: Esophageal cancer: Radiographic chest findings and their prognostic significance. Am J Roentgenol 133: 461, 1979.
208. Daffner RH, Postlethwait RW, Putman CE: Retrotracheal abnormalities in esophageal carcinoma: Prognostic implications. Am J Roentgenol 130: 719, 1978.
209. Reinig JW, Stanley JH, Schgabel SI: CT evaluation of thickened esophageal walls. Am J Roentgenol 140: 931, 1983.
210. Cohen AM, Cunat JS: Giant esophageal leiomyoma as a mediastinal mass. J Can Assoc Radiol 32: 129, 1981.
211. Jalundhwala JM, Shah RC: Epiphrenic esophageal diverticulum. Chest 57: 97, 1970.
212. Blomquist G, Mahoney PS: Noncollapsing air-filled esophagus in diseased and postoperative chests. Acta Radiol 55: 32, 1961.
213. Schabel SI, Stanley JH: Air esophagram after laryngectomy. Am J Roentgenol 136: 19, 1981.
214. Sumbas PN, McKeown PP, Hatcher CR Jr, et al: Tracheoesophageal fistula from carcinoma of the esophagus. Ann Thorac Surg 38: 382, 1984.
215. Hilgenberg AD, Grillo MC: Acquired nonmalignant tracheoesophageal fistula. J Thorac Cardiovasc Surg 85: 492, 1983.
216. Verani R, Olson J, Moake JL: Intrathoracic extramedullary hematopoiesis. Report of a case in a patient with sickle cell disease–β-thalassemia. Am J Clin Pathol 73: 133, 1980.
217. Gumbs RV, Higginbotham-Ford EA, Teal JS, et al: Thoracic extramedullary hematopoiesis in sickle cell disease. Am J Roentgenol 149: 889, 1987.
218. Ross P, Logan W: Roentgen findings in extramedullary hematopoiesis. Am J Roentgenol 106: 604, 1969.
219. Da Costa JL, Loh YS, Hanam E: Extramedullary hemopoiesis with multiple tumor-simulating mediastinal masses in hemoglobin E–thalassemia disease. Chest 65: 210, 1974.

DISEASES OF THE DIAPHRAGM AND CHEST WALL

The thoracic cage, including the chest wall and diaphragm, serves the dual purpose of enclosing and protecting the contents of the thorax and of producing the movements that result in the changes in pleural pressure necessary for respiration. This chapter is concerned with the diseases and anomalies that involve these structures and that can affect either or both of these major functions. The effects of trauma are discussed in Chapter 15.

THE DIAPHRAGM

Roentgenologic assessment of diaphragmatic motion is best accomplished fluoroscopically, particularly when subtle changes are sought; for example, the relatively minor degrees of restriction of motion that may be associated with acute subphrenic inflammation. Although major asymmetry of diaphragmatic excursion may be evidenced on roentgen-

ograms exposed at total lung capacity (TLC) and residual volume (RV), minor degrees of asymmetry may become evident only when the motion of both hemidiaphragms is observed simultaneously. Fluoroscopic examination should be carried out not only in posteroanterior (PA) projection but also in various degrees of oblique projection, to reveal any disturbance in motion of portions of the diaphragm that may not be present at other sites. For example, a subphrenic abscess localized to the posterior subphrenic space on the right side may produce local restriction posteriorly without concomitant disturbance in the excursion of the anterior portion. Diaphragmatic motion should be observed during breathing at tidal volume, while the patient breathes deeply and preferably rapidly, and while he or she sniffs. In many cases, the last-named procedure reveals restriction or paradoxical motion not clearly apparent during either tidal or deep breathing (*see* later).

The roentgenographic appearances of the normal and

diseased diaphragm have been the subject of two excellent reviews.[1, 2] Additional aspects of the pathophysiology of the diaphragm are discussed in Chapter 21, particularly with respect to diaphragmatic paralysis and alveolar hypoventilation.

Abnormalities of Diaphragmatic Position or Motion

Unilateral Diaphragmatic Paralysis

Paralysis of a hemidiaphragm usually results from interruption of transmission of nerve impulses through the phrenic nerve. Although invasion of the nerve by a neoplasm, usually of pulmonary origin, is the most frequent etiology, a variety of benign conditions also can be responsible (Table 20–1).[3] The second most common category is paralysis of unknown etiology; in these idiopathic cases, the paralysis is almost invariably right-sided and usually occurs in males. The use of cold topical cardioplegia has been suggested as a possible etiology of diaphragmatic paralysis after coronary artery bypass surgery.[4] During this procedure, ice slush cooled to subfreezing temperatures by the addition of salt is packed into the pericardial cavity around the heart. Since the left phrenic nerve runs immediately within the posterior pericardium on the left side, cold-induced injury can occur and may lead to paralysis.[5]

There are four cardinal signs of unilateral diaphragmatic paralysis:[6] (1) elevation of a hemidiaphragm above the normal range; (2) diminished, absent, or paradoxical motion during respiration; (3) paradoxical motion under conditions of augmented load such as sniffing; and (4) mediastinal swing during respiration.

Characteristically, a paralyzed hemidiaphragm presents an accentuated dome configuration in both PA and lateral projections (Fig. 20–1). Since the peripheral points of attachment of the diaphragm are fixed, costophrenic and costovertebral sulci tend to appear deepened, narrowed, and sharpened. If the paralysis is left-sided, the stomach and splenic flexure of the colon relate to the inferior surface of the elevated hemidiaphragm and usually contain more gas than normal.

The most reliable roentgenographic maneuver to confirm hemidiaphragmatic paralysis is the sniff test. This is accomplished by having the subject produce a rapid inspiration, usually through the nostrils; diaphragm position and movement are observed fluoroscopically. Normally, both hemidiaphragms descend sharply during a sniff, but with unilateral diaphragmatic paralysis there is paradoxical upward motion of the affected side. Although significant paradoxical motion provides strong evidence for diaphragmatic paralysis or eventration, it should be remembered that sniffing by normal subjects may produce paradoxical excursion of one hemidiaphragm[6]; such a finding can be regarded as pathologic only if the excursion exceeds 2 cm and if it involves the whole hemidiaphragm as seen in oblique or lateral projection. In addition, false-negative results can be recorded if the subject uses the abdominal musculature to elevate the diaphragm during the expiratory phase of breathing (see later).

Most patients with a paralyzed hemidiaphragm are asymptomatic, although some complain of dyspnea on effort.[7] The severity of symptoms relates to the rapidity of development of the paralysis and to the presence or absence of underlying pulmonary disease. Physical examination may reveal decreased breath sounds over the affected side and decreased diaphragmatic excursion. Examination of the anterior abdominal wall of some individuals in the supine position may reveal paradoxical inward movement of the ipsilateral abdominal wall (see Fig. 21–2, page 975).

Pulmonary function tests typically show mild restrictive insufficiency. Total lung capacity is usually about 85 per cent of predicted, whereas vital capacity is reduced to 75 per cent; functional residual capacity and the ratio of FEV_1 to forced vital capacity are usually normal.[8] Maximal inspiratory pressures, measured either at the mouth (Pimax) or across the diaphragm (Pdimax), are only mildly reduced and values are similar whether the paralysis is right-sided or left-sided.[9] Hypoxemia is usually absent or mild, although it may develop when patients assume a supine position.[10] Plication of the paralyzed hemidiaphragm can improve lung volumes and arterial blood gases, presumably by stiffening the paralyzed side and preventing paradoxical motion.[11]

A definitive diagnosis of phrenic nerve dysfunction as the cause of hemidiaphragmatic paralysis can be obtained by employing the technique of cervical phrenic nerve stimulation.[12] Felt-tipped electrodes are placed over the phrenic nerve in the neck, and the stimulation voltage is increased in a step-wise fashion while the compound action potential of the ipsilateral hemidiaphragm is recorded using surface electrodes placed on the anterolateral aspect of the chest in the eighth and ninth intercostal spaces. Phrenic nerve latency is the interval from stimulation of the nerve to the first detection of the compound action potential. When the nerve is completely interrupted or is significantly demyelinated, the compound action potential of the hemidiaphragm will be absent or will show prolonged latency.

Bilateral Diaphragmatic Paralysis

Bilateral diaphragmatic paralysis is less common than the unilateral form but shares some of its etiologies (Table 20–2). The roentgenographic appearance consists of elevated hemidiaphragms in both PA and lateral projections.[6] Horizontal linear opacities, possibly caused by discoid atelectasis, may be present at the lung bases. Paradoxical upward

Table 20–1. **CAUSES OF UNILATERAL DIAPHRAGMATIC PARALYSIS**

Cause	Reference
Neoplasms	
Idiopathic	
Surgical section or stretch	
Phrenic thermal injury	4
Cervical manipulation	109
Cervical spondylosis	110
Cervical venipuncture	111
Birth injury	112
Brachial neuritis	113
Neuralgic amyotrophy	114
Mediastinal lymph node enlargement	115
Aortic aneurysm	
Substernal thyroid	
Herpes zoster	116
Vasculitis (mononeuritis multiplex)	
Multiple sclerosis	117
Diabetes mellitus	

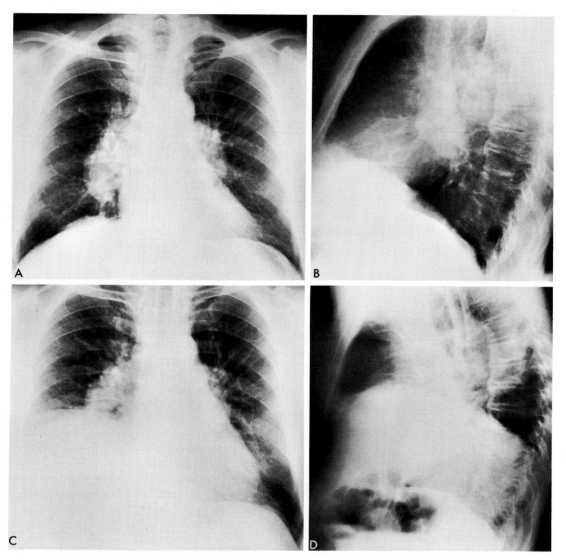

Figure 20–1. Iatrogenic Paralysis of the Right Hemidiaphragm. Posteroanterior *(A)* and lateral *(B)* roentgenograms reveal marked enlargement of the hilar lymph nodes bilaterally. No other intrathoracic abnormality is evident. Note the normal position of both hemidiaphragms. As part of the investigation, a right scalene node biopsy was performed, during which the right phrenic nerve was accidentally severed. Ten days later roentgenograms of the chest in posteroanterior *(C)* and lateral *(D)* projections demonstrate marked elevation of the right hemidiaphragm. (Courtesy of Montreal Chest Hospital Center.)

Table 20–2. **CAUSES OF BILATERAL DIAPHRAGMATIC PARALYSIS**

Cause	Reference
Birth injury	118
Infantile spinomuscular atrophy	119
Neuralgic amyotrophy	114
Arnold-Chiari malformation	120
Syringomyelia	121
Peripheral neuropathy	122
Brachial neuritis	123
Multiple sclerosis	124
Cervical disc surgery	125
Paraneoplastic neuritis	126
Blunt chest trauma	127
Phrenic thermal injury	128
Idiopathic	129

motion of both hemidiaphragms during an inspiratory effort or sniff is usually observed on fluoroscopic examination. It should be remembered, however, that recruitment of abdominal expiratory muscles can cause a false-negative sniff test:[13] some patients with bilateral diaphragmatic paralysis actively expire to a lung volume below the true resting functional residual capacity and then use the elastic recoil forces of the abdominothoracic structures to assist the next inspiration passively; the sudden downward motion of the diaphragm coincident with abdominal muscle relaxation may be misinterpreted as diaphragmatic contraction when viewed fluoroscopically. Diaphragmatic motion also can be monitored by ultrasonography.[14]

Most patients with bilateral diaphragmatic paralysis or significant weakness eventually develop ventilatory respiratory failure and hypercapnia. Some present with evidence of cor pulmonale and right ventricular failure. Dyspnea on exertion and on assuming the supine position is a characteristic complaint. Dyspnea during recumbency is particularly distressing, since it can interfere with adequate sleep and result in daytime hypersomnolence. The inadequate inspiratory effort also predisposes to atelectasis and respiratory tract infections.

On physical examination, percussion reveals dullness at both bases and decreased or absent diaphragmatic excursion owing to the elevated resting position of the diaphragm. Patients are usually tachypneic and are clearly using the accessory inspiratory muscles. A characteristic physical finding, readily detectable in the supine position, is a paradoxical inward motion of the anterior abdominal wall on inspiration (see Fig. 21–3, page 976). This is caused by upward movement of the flaccid diaphragm during inspiration as a result of the negative intrathoracic pressure generated by the normally contracting external intercostal and accessory muscles. The functional effects of bilateral diaphragmatic paralysis are discussed further on page 974).

Bilateral diaphragmatic paralysis can be confirmed by measuring transdiaphragmatic pressure swings during tidal breathing and maximal inspiratory efforts.[13] Transdiaphragmatic pressure is measured by recording gastric and esophageal pressures. During inspiration, gastric pressure normally becomes positive and esophageal pressure negative. In the presence of diaphragmatic paralysis or weakness, the diaphragm acts as a flaccid membrane, with the result that the negative intrathoracic pressure is transmitted to the

abdominal cavity so that transdiaphragmatic pressure does not change. Even with maximal inspiratory effort, no transdiaphragmatic pressure develops, although maximal expiration may be associated with some transdiaphragmatic pressure as the diaphragm is passively stretched near residual volume.[15]

Bilateral diaphragmatic paralysis causes quite severe lung restriction. TLC and FRC typically are between 55 and 65 per cent of the predicted value, and vital capacity is in the range of 45 to 50 per cent predicted.[16] The FEV_1 usually is decreased in proportion to the forced vital capacity, so FEV_1/FVC is normal. Maximal inspiratory mouth pressure is reduced to well below the normal range. Blood gas measurements show arterial hypoxemia—which is related to ventilation-perfusion mismatch at the lung bases and is exacerbated in the supine position[17]—and, in some cases, hypercarbia.

Eventration

Eventration is a congenital anomaly consisting of failure of muscular development of part or all of one or both hemidiaphragms.[18] Despite the apparent developmental nature of the condition, there is evidence that its incidence increases with age,[19] suggesting that acquired factors may also be involved in pathogenesis. In some cases, it may be difficult or impossible to distinguish the abnormality from diaphragmatic paralysis. In fact, there is a tendency to use the terms "eventration" and "diaphragmatic paralysis" interchangeably.

Partial eventration is somewhat more common than total eventration and is usually present in the anteromedial portion of the right hemidiaphragm.[20] It occurs with equal frequency in men and women.[21] Total eventration occurs almost exclusively on the left side.

The roentgenologic signs of eventration are identical to those described for diaphragmatic paralysis (Fig. 20–2). A confident diagnosis can be established by liver scan[22] or, in questionable cases, by computed tomography (CT).[23]

Characteristically, eventration in the adult does not cause symptoms and is discovered on a screening chest roentgenogram. Occasionally, gastrointestinal symptoms develop with increasing obesity and consequent increased intra-abdominal pressure. Respiratory embarrassment and cardiac distress also have been attributed to this anomaly,[24] particularly in neonates.

Restriction of Diaphragmatic Motion

A great variety of diseases of the lungs, pleura, abdominal organs, and the diaphragm itself may lead to restriction of diaphragmatic motion. In some, the limitation of motion is imposed by the character of the disease itself; for example, the severe pulmonary overinflation and air trapping that characterize diffuse emphysema prevent normal ascent of the diaphragm during expiration. In others, local irritation causes "splinting" of a hemidiaphragm that is manifested not only by reduced excursion but also by elevation. Such splinting can be caused by acute lower lobe pneumonia or infarction, acute pleuritis, rib fractures, or acute intra-abdominal inflammatory processes such as subphrenic abscess, cholecystitis, and peritonitis.

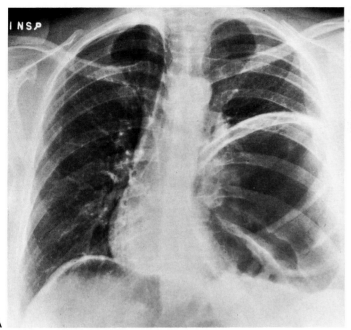
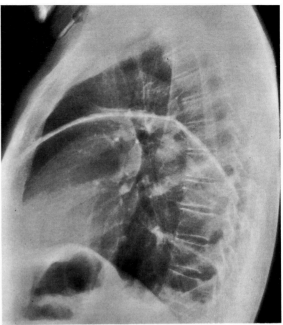

A   B

Figure 20–2. Eventration of the Left Hemidiaphragm Associated with Severe Colonic Dilatation Secondary to Sigmoid Volvulus. Posteroanterior *(A)* and lateral *(B)* roentgenograms reveal a remarkable degree of elevation of the left hemidiaphragm. Severely dilated loops of colon are situated beneath this hemidiaphragm and, to a lesser extent, beneath the right one. The mediastinum is displaced considerably into the right hemithorax.

While other skeletal muscle groups react to irritation or injury by spasm, the diaphragm appears to react by relaxation. This is the only way of explaining the elevation that characteristically accompanies local inflammation. The mechanism by which the diaphragm "splints" in the postoperative period is thought to be neural inhibition of diaphragmatic activation,[25, 26] possibly caused by stimulation of diaphragmatic or splanchnic afferents. Such diaphragmatic dysfunction is maximal 8 hours after surgery, and function improves over the subsequent 2 to 7 days.[25] The decreased diaphragmatic activation is not directly related to pain; in one study, narcotic analgesia did not improve the deficit in transdiaphragmatic pressure generation.[26] Similarly, postoperative diaphragmatic dysfunction is not caused by a decrease in diaphragmatic contractility, since direct stimulation of the phrenic nerve can result in normal transdiaphragmatic pressure.[27]

Diaphragmatic Hernias

Herniation of abdominal or retroperitoneal organs or tissues into the thorax can occur through congenital or acquired weak areas in the diaphragm or through rents resulting from traumatic rupture *(see* page 791). Nontraumatic herniation occurs at three sites: the esophageal hiatus, the foramen of Bochdalek, and the foramen of Morgagni.

Hernia Through the Esophageal Hiatus

This is the most common form of diaphragmatic hernia in the adult. Although a congenital weakness of the esophageal hiatus may be partly responsible for the development of this type of hernia, there is little doubt that acquired

factors play a significant role, the most important being obesity and pregnancy.

The effects of a hiatus hernia relate almost entirely to the gastrointestinal tract, although sometimes its presence is manifested by changes in the chest roentgenogram. When this does occur, plain roentgenograms typically show a mass in the posteroinferior mediastinum, usually containing an air-fluid level (Fig. 20–3). In cases in which most of the stomach has herniated through the hiatus, the stomach may undergo volvulus and present as a large mass, sometimes containing a double fluid level. Incarceration of such hernial contents is frequent. When the diagnosis is in doubt on the basis of evidence provided by plain roentgenograms, barium opacification usually is confirmatory.

The majority of patients with esophageal hiatus hernias are asymptomatic, the abnormality being discovered during a barium study of the upper gastrointestinal tract or on a screening examination of the chest or upper gastrointestinal tract. When present, symptoms consist of retrosternal "burning" and pain, typically occurring after meals and accentuated when the patient lies down. They are relieved by ingestion of antacids. Symptoms of anemia caused by blood loss may predominate.[28] Occasionally, patients with an incarcerated hernia complain of retrosternal chest pain that is difficult to distinguish from that of myocardial or pericardial origin. However, pain from esophageal disease is often precipitated by changes in posture, such as lying down or bending over, and there may be the additional complaint of dysphagia.

The development of acute upper gastrointestinal tract symptoms in a patient with a herniated stomach that has undergone volvulus should immediately raise the suspicion of strangulation,[29] a life-threatening complication that necessitates immediate surgical intervention.

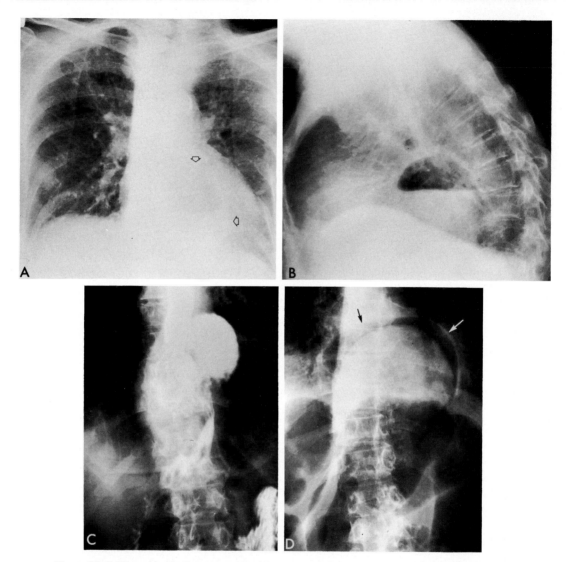

Figure 20–3. Hiatus Hernia. Posteroanterior *(A)* and lateral *(B)* roentgenograms of the chest reveal a large soft tissue mass containing a prominent air-fluid level occupying the posteroinferior portion of the mediastinum *(arrows in A)*. An anteroposterior roentgenogram of the lower mediastinum and upper abdomen following the ingestion of barium *(C)* confirms the presence of herniation of a large portion of stomach into the posterior mediastinum. The patient had no symptoms referable to this hernia. Somewhat later, the patient developed an acute abdomen, with severe abdominal distention and signs of peritonitis. An anteroposterior roentgenogram *(D)* revealed a double density in the posterior mediastinum, the hernial sac being outlined by gas *(arrows)*, and the central portion of the sac containing a homogeneous mass representing a fluid-filled gastric fundus. A hollow abdominal viscus had perforated, releasing gas into the peritoneal space; some of the gas had passed through the esophageal hiatus, outlining the sac.

Hernia Through the Foramen of Bochdalek

Herniation through the pleuroperitoneal hiatus (foramen of Bochdalek) is caused by a deficiency of the pleuroperitoneal membranes (*see* page 96). In infants, it is not only the most common form of diaphragmatic hernia but also by far the most serious: when large, it is associated with a high death rate unless surgically corrected. Between 80 and 90 per cent of Bochdalek hernias detected on conventional roentgenograms occur on the left side,[30] partly because defects in the right hemidiaphragm are protected by the liver. However, on CT scans, left-sided hernias show a preponderance of only 2:1 over right-sided hernias.[31]

The size of the defect varies widely and, as might be expected, is clearly related to the severity of complications. When the defect is large, as with complete or almost complete absence of a hemidiaphragm, virtually the entire abdominal contents may be in the left hemithorax, thereby interfering with normal lung development and resulting in hypoplasia.[32] In most cases of large hernia, there is no peritoneal sac, and communication between the pleural and the peritoneal cavities is wide open. When the defect is small, a portion of the spleen or kidney, or omentum, may be the sole hernial content. This form of limited herniation is the type usually found by chance in asymptomatic adults, either roentgenographically or at necropsy.

Although Bochdalek defects are most commonly situated posterolaterally, they may occur anywhere along the posterior aspect of the diaphragm, even in the vicinity of the costovertebral junction. The roentgenographic manifestations depend almost entirely on hernial contents and thus on the size of the defect. In infants in whom the defect is large, the roentgenographic appearance is characteristic (Fig. 20–4): the ipsilateral hemidiaphragm is partly or completely obscured; multiple radiolucencies representing gas-containing loops of intestine, some containing fluid levels, are seen within the hemithorax; the heart and mediastinum are shifted into the opposite hemithorax; the ipsilateral lung is compressed and airless; and there is little or no intestinal gas in the abdomen.[30] In adults with a relatively small defect, the roentgenographic appearance may consist of no more than a "bump" on the superior aspect of the diaphragm posteriorly. Occasionally, herniation occurs into the mediastinum.[33] Barium examination of the gastrointestinal tract, CT, and ultrasonography can be useful in confirming the diagnosis.[34] The abnormality also can be diagnosed by fetal ultrasonography.[35]

The roentgenographic presentation of congenital right diaphragmatic hernia may be delayed for several days after birth; the hernial content is usually liver.[36] Radionuclide scintigraphy using technetium-99m–sulfur colloid to outline the liver can aid in diagnosis.[37]

Hernia Through the Foramen of Morgagni

The foramina of Morgagni are small clefts bounded by diaphragmatic muscle fibers originating from the sternum medially and from the seventh costal cartilages laterally. They are triangular, the base being formed by the anterior thoracic wall and the apex being directed posteriorly. The clefts contain the mammary vessels and normally are filled with loose areolar connective tissue and fat. Since the left foramen relates to the heart, the majority of herniations occur on the right. The abnormality is an uncommon form of diaphragmatic hernia, constituting fewer than 10 per cent in most series.[38] Affected patients are usually overweight, middle-aged women.

Although these defects are developmental in origin, it is probable that herniation requires the additional presence of obesity, at least in adults.[38] In contrast to Bochdalek hernias, a peritoneal sac is present in most cases. The content of the hernial sac is usually omentum, but sometimes liver or bowel.

Roentgenographically, the typical appearance is that of a smooth, well-defined opacity in the right cardiophrenic angle (Fig. 20–5). When the hernial sac is filled with liver, the roentgenographic shadow is homogeneous and usually indistinguishable from a large pleuropericardial fat pad. Occasionally, it is inhomogeneous as a result of either an air-containing loop of bowel or the predominantly fatty nature of the hernial contents. In the latter situation, the hernia is likely to contain omentum, and a barium enema study will reveal the transverse colon to be situated high in the abdomen with a peak situated anteriorly and superiorly (*see* Fig. 19–25, page 926), a finding that is virtually diagnostic. Ultrasonography can be a valuable addition to roentgenography by helping to define the size of the defect and the contents of the hernial sac.[39]

The majority of hernias through the foramen of Morgagni do not give rise to symptoms. Occasionally, there is epigastric or lower sternal pressure and discomfort.[38] When the sac contains portions of the gastrointestinal tract, strangulation and obstruction may occur.

Subphrenic Abscess

Subphrenic abscesses develop most commonly after perforation of a hollow viscus or as a complication of abdominal surgery. In the past, they occurred predominantly in young patients with appendicitis and developed chiefly in the posterior subphrenic space on the right; however, there is evidence suggesting that they now occur as frequently after abdominal surgery, that the incidence on the two sides is approximately equal, and that they involve the anterior and posterior subphrenic spaces equally as often. It is probable that in many patients, postoperative antibiotic therapy prevents the development of subphrenic suppuration, although in some it may only suppress the acute symptoms and thus permit the development of chronic, low-grade infection that is difficult to recognize.[40]

The pathogenesis of abscess formation differs somewhat, depending on whether it occurs on the right or left side of the abdomen. Meyers[41] has shown that the main pathway by which infection spreads to and from the upper and lower peritoneal compartments is the right paracolic gutter. Further, he states that it is probable that hydrostatic pressure differences between the lower and the upper abdomen are capable of helping convey infected peritoneal fluid from the lower abdomen to the subhepatic and subphrenic regions, even in the erect position. Superiorly, the right paracolic gutter is continuous with the subhepatic space and its posterosuperior extension, Morison's pouch, and from there with the right subphrenic space.[41] Thus, an abscess in the right subhepatic space often spreads to the right subphrenic space.

Abscesses located in the left upper quadrant occur pre-

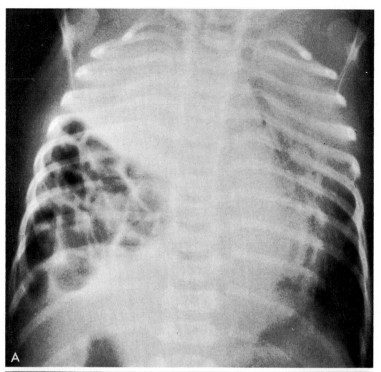

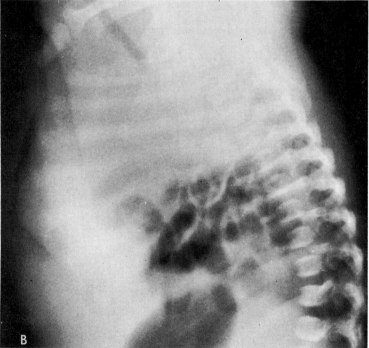

Figure 20–4. Diaphragmatic Hernia Through the Foramen of Bochdalek. This newborn baby boy was referred for roentgenography of the chest when it was noted in the nursery that he was cyanotic and showed chest retraction, subcostal indrawing, and grunting respiration. These roentgenograms in anteroposterior *(A)* and lateral *(B)* projections demonstrate numerous loops of air-filled bowel in the posteroinferior portion of the right hemithorax. The right lung above the hernia contents is airless, and the mediastinum is displaced considerably to the left. Only the lower portion of the left lung appears to be air-containing. At thoracotomy, the right hemithorax was found to contain the liver, stomach, small intestine, kidneys, and adrenal gland; the right lung was severely hypoplastic. The hernial contents were returned to the abdomen, and a large right pleuroperitoneal foramen was closed. The infant died 2 days later.

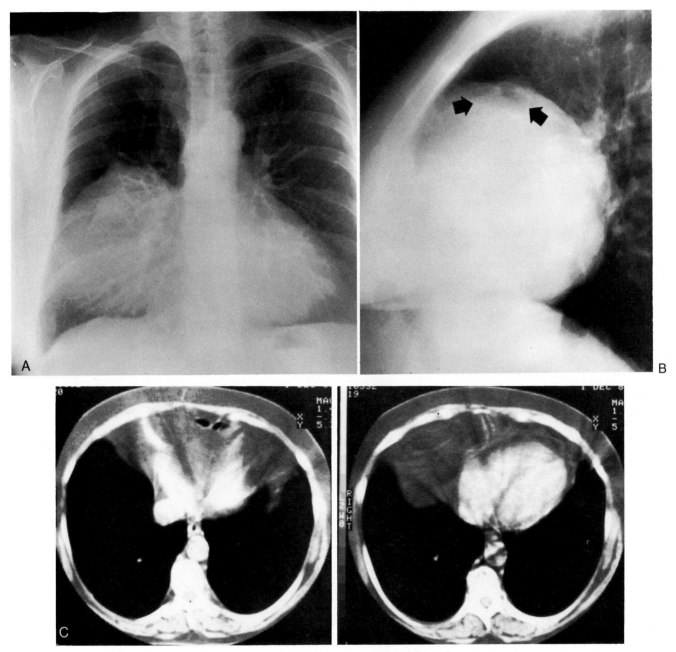

Figure 20–5. Herniation of Omentum and Bowel Through the Foramen of Morgagni. Posteroanterior *(A)* and lateral *(B)* roentgenograms reveal a large mass situated in the inferior portion of the right hemithorax, lying chiefly anteriorly and obliterating the right border of the heart. Its density is homogeneous except for a small radiolucency situated in its most superior portion *(arrows in B)*. Serial CT scans through the lower mediastinum *(C)* reveal a large mass of fat density (mean attenuation, – 120 Hounsfield units) situated in the region of the right cardiophrenic angle and extending around the anterior aspect of the heart. In the left scan, two small loops of bowel can be readily identified.

dominantly in two anatomic locations—the left anterior subphrenic space and the lesser sac. Both extend to the right of the midline,[42] the former compartment being bounded on the right by the falciform ligament, while the lesser sac extends to the right coronary ligament and foramen of Winslow. Therefore, abscesses arising in either of these locations can extend across the midline into the right upper quadrant. Abscesses in the left anterior subphrenic space and in the lesser sac can be differentiated by the fact that the former is immediately subdiaphragmatic, whereas the latter usually is not contiguous with the diaphragm. Subphrenic abscesses on the left side usually result from perforated gastric or duodenal ulcers[41] and tend to cause a characteristic CT appearance.[42]

Roentgenologic signs of subphrenic abscess include abnormalities in the lung, the pleural space, the subphrenic space, and the diaphragm itself (Fig. 20–6). One analysis of the signs in 48 cases documented the following findings:[43]

Elevation of the ipsilateral diaphragm	44/47	94%
Restriction of diaphragmatic motion	33/36	92%
Fixation of the hemidiaphragm	19/36	53%
Pleural effusion	37/47	79%
Basal pulmonary opacity (pneumonitis or atelectasis or both)	33/47	70%

Gas in the abscess cavity was identified in 30 per cent of patients, and displacement of intra-abdominal viscera in 35 per cent. The gas may be derived from gas-forming organisms or a perforated abdominal viscus or may represent a residuum of "air" after laparotomy.

Procedures of value in confirming the diagnosis include barium examination of the gastrointestinal tract (particularly for abscesses situated on the left), CT (especially for differentiating abscess and pleural effusion[44]), gallium scanning,[45] and ultrasonography (particularly useful for subphrenic abscesses on the right[46]).

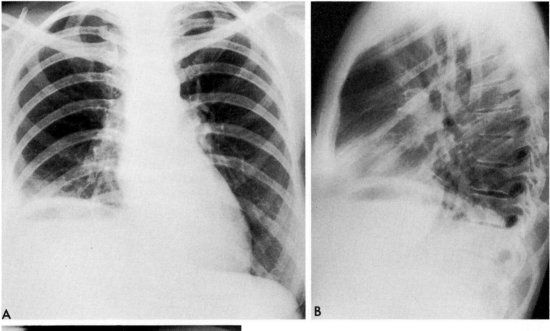

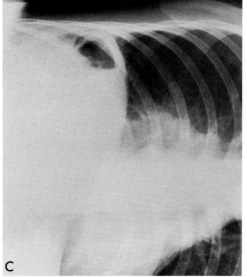

Figure 20–6. Subphrenic Abscess. Two weeks prior to this roentgenographic examination, this 34-year-old woman had had an appendectomy for acute, gangrenous appendicitis. Her only complaint on admission was a vague discomfort in the upper right abdomen. Posteroanterior *(A)*, lateral *(B)*, and lateral decubitus *(C)* roentgenograms reveal a large accumulation of gas and fluid beneath a moderately elevated right hemidiaphragm; there was a small right pleural effusion. Focal areas of increased density in the right lung base represent inflammatory reaction in the contiguous lung.

The clinical manifestations include chronic fever, vague upper abdominal pain, loss of weight and, sometimes, chills and anemia.[40] The physical findings include elevation and fixation of the affected hemidiaphragm and tenderness on pressure over the twelfth rib posteriorly (if the abscess is in the posterior space) or along the lateral and anterior costal margin (if the abscess is anteriorly situated).

Neoplasms of the Diaphragm

Primary neoplasms of the diaphragm are very uncommon.[47] Most develop from the tendinous or anterior muscular portion. Benign and malignant forms occur with relatively equal frequency,[48] the former including lipoma (the most common), neurogenic tumors, and leiomyoma, and the latter fibrosarcoma (the most common), malignant fibrous histiocytoma, hemangiopericytoma, and leiomyosarcoma. Various non-neoplastic abnormalities that form localized tumors, such as lymphangioma, endometriosis, and hydatid cyst (Fig. 20–7), are also occasionally found.

Roentgenographically, most diaphragmatic tumors present as smooth or lobulated soft tissue masses protruding into the inferior portion of the lung. In many cases, malignant tumors involve much of one hemidiaphragm and thus simulate diaphragmatic elevation; associated pleural effusion is common. The precise location of the mass and its extent can be established most easily by CT.[49]

Characteristically, benign neoplasms occasion no symptoms. By contrast, the majority of patients with primary malignant tumors complain of epigastric or lower chest pain, cough, dyspnea, and gastrointestinal discomfort.[47]

Secondary neoplastic involvement of the diaphragm is common. It occurs most frequently by direct extension of neoplasm from the basal pleura in cases of pulmonary carcinoma or mesothelioma; however, any neoplasm that metastasizes to the pleura or that involves the basal lung, liver, or subphrenic peritoneum can involve the diaphragm. Roentgenographic features and clinical manifestations are usually related to the presence of neoplasm in contiguous structures rather than in the diaphragm itself.

THE CHEST WALL

Abnormalities of the Pectoral Girdle and Adjacent Structures

With few exceptions, congenital anomalies of the pectoral girdle cause no serious disabilities.[50] The most important anomaly of the clavicle is cleidocranial dysostosis, a syndrome characterized by incomplete ossification of the clavicle and defective development of the pubic bones, vertebral column, and long bones. The chief anomaly of the scapula is Sprengel's deformity, in which the scapula fails to descend normally so that its superior angle lies on a plane higher than the neck of the first rib. This is frequently associated with fusion of two or more cervical vertebrae, resulting in a short, wide neck with considerably limited movement (Klippel-Feil deformity).

Poland's syndrome consists of hypoplasia or aplasia of the pectoralis major muscle and ipsilateral syndactyly.[51] Other anomalies that may be associated include absence of the pectoralis minor muscle, absence or atrophy of ipsilateral ribs two to five, aplasia of the ipsilateral breast or nipple, and simian crease of the affected extremity.[51] Absence of the pectoralis muscles results in unilateral hypertranslucency on the chest roentgenogram, not to be confused with the Swyer-James syndrome (however, *see* Fig. 11–40, page 676).

Cervical lung hernia results from excessive excursion of the dome of the pleura, which permits protrusion of the apex of the lung into the cervical region during periods of increased intrathoracic pressure. The herniation usually occurs between the anterior scalene and the sternocleidomastoid muscles. Typically, it follows severe trauma; in some cases, however, it is associated with chronic obstructive pulmonary disease.[52]

Abnormalities of the Ribs

Congenital Anomalies

Congenital anomalies of the ribs, including fusion of two or more ribs and various types of bifid ribs, are relatively common and are of little or no clinical significance. Of potentially greater importance is an anomalous accessory rib ("Eve's rib," cervical rib) that usually arises from the seventh cervical vertebra and occurs in about 0.5 per cent of the population. Both the anomaly and the symptoms that derive therefrom are said to be more common in women.[53] In about 90 per cent of cases, cervical ribs do not cause symptoms; however, when they compress subclavian vessels or the brachial plexus, the patient may complain of pain and weakness of the arm or swelling of the hand. Variation in the intensity of the pulses in the two arms may be present when the affected extremity is in certain positions. This syndrome may be mimicked by other conditions in which structures at the cervicothoracic inlet are compressed, including the scalenus anticus, costoclavicular, hyperabduction, subcoracoid, pectoralis minor, and first thoracic rib syndromes.[54] In most of these situations, arteriography can be of considerable assistance in evaluation and is essential in some patients for diagnosis and preoperative assessment.[55]

Notching and Erosion

Pathologic notching of ribs may occur on the inferior or superior aspect; it is most frequent in the former location and has many causes (Table 20–3).[56] By far the most common cause is coarctation of the aorta, which typically produces notching several centimeters lateral to the costovertebral junction on the inferior aspect of ribs three to nine (Fig. 20–8). The notches result from erosion by pulsating, dilated intercostal arteries taking part in collateral arterial flow. These arteries may become extremely tortuous and may even extend to and erode the superior aspects of contiguous ribs. The abnormality can be seen in patients before the age of 6 or 7 years but usually is not well developed until the early teens.[57]

Notching or erosion of the superior aspects of the ribs usually is considered to be much less common than that of the inferior aspects; however, the authors suspect that it may be present more often than is generally recognized because of its more subtle roentgenologic appearance. The defects have been classified into three main etiologic

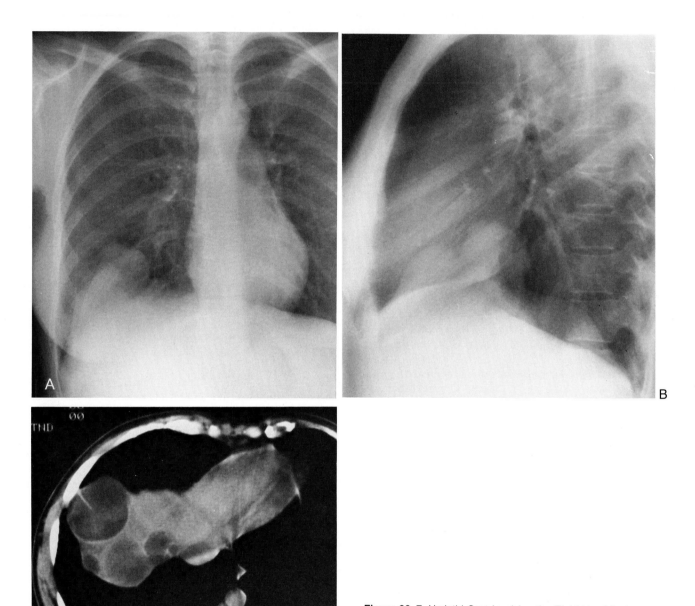

Figure 20–7. Hydatid Cyst Involving the Right Hemidiaphragm. Posteroanterior *(A)* and lateral *(B)* chest roentgenograms reveal a lobulated mass extending from the right hemidiaphragm into the inferior aspect of the right middle lobe. A CT scan through the dome of the right hemidiaphragm *(C)* shows several cystic lesions. At surgery, the patient was found to have hydatid disease of the liver that extended through the diaphragm and into the lung. (Courtesy of Dr. Nestor Müller, Vancouver General Hospital, Vancouver, British Columbia.)

Table 20–3. CAUSES OF INFERIOR RIB NOTCHING

Arterial
A. Aortic obstruction
  1. Coarctation of the aortic arch
  2. Thrombosis of the abdominal aorta
B. Subclavian artery obstruction
  1. Blalock-Taussig operation
  2. Takayasu's arteritis
C. Widened arterial pulse pressure
D. Decreased pulmonary blood flow
  1. Tetralogy of Fallot
  2. Pulmonary atresia (pseudotruncus)
  3. Ebstein's malformation
  4. Pulmonary valve stenosis
  5. Unilateral absence of the pulmonary artery
  6. Pulmonary emphysema

Venous
A. Superior vena cava obstruction

Arteriovenous
A. Pulmonary arteriovenous fistula
B. Intercostal arteriovenous fistula

Neurogenic
A. Intercostal neurinoma

Osseous
A. Hyperparathyroidism

Idiopathic

groups (Table 20–4).[58] Formerly, the most common cause of notching or erosion of the superior aspects of the ribs undoubtedly was chronic paralytic poliomyelitis. However, the rarity with which this disease is now seen places it far down on the differential diagnosis list, and it is likely that

quadriplegia as a result of cervical cord injury is now the most common etiology.[59] In both of these situations, the erosions are probably caused by an absence of the normal "stress stimulus" provided by repetitive contraction of the intercostal muscles. Roentgenographic manifestations typically consist of localized shallow indentations ranging from 1 to 4 cm in length on the superior margins of ribs three to nine posterolaterally.[58]

Inflammatory Diseases

Primary osteomyelitis of the ribs is rare and may be difficult to appreciate roentgenologically until bone destruction is advanced. More commonly, it is secondary to infectious processes in the lung (usually of tuberculous or fungal etiology) or to empyema (empyema necessitatis). Tuberculous osteitis was formerly the most common inflammatory lesion of a rib and occasionally was the first manifestation of the disease.[60] It may begin as a chondritis or osteitis, the roentgenographic manifestations being characterized by destructive lesions associated with a periosteal reaction and a soft tissue mass. Disease in either location can be confused with malignancy.[61] Rib lesions of this and other types often can be detected by bone scanning before they are apparent on chest roentgenograms.[62]

Costochondral osteochondritis (Tietze's syndrome) is characterized by painful, nonsuppurative swelling of one or more costochondral or sternochondral joints.[63] In the majority of patients, the condition is an isolated finding, although in some it is associated with a systemic arthritic disorder or psoriasis.[64] The etiology is unknown, and involved cartilage is said to be histologically normal.[65] It al-

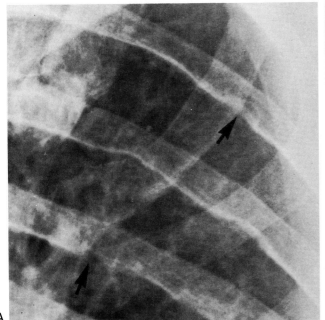 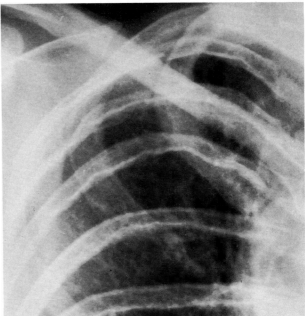

Figure 20–8. Rib Notching: Two Causes. A magnified view of the left upper ribs (A) of a patient with coarctation of the aorta demonstrates numerous defects of the inferior surfaces of ribs 4 to 8 bilaterally (several are indicated by arrows). In another patient (B), a detail view of the right upper ribs also demonstrates extensive rib notching, affecting not only the inferior surface of the ribs, as in A, but also in some areas the superior surface. Many years previously, this patient had had a bilateral Blalock-Taussig anastomosis for tetralogy of Fallot.

Table 20–4. CAUSES OF SUPERIOR RIB NOTCHING

Disturbance of Osteoblastic Activity (Decreased or Deficient Bone Formation)
1. Quadriplegia
2. Autoimmune connective tissue diseases (rheumatoid arthritis, progressive systemic sclerosis, lupus erythematosus, Sjögren's syndrome)
3. Localized pressure (rib retractors, chest tubes, multiple hereditary exostoses, neurofibromatosis, coarctation of the aorta)
4. Osteogenesis imperfecta
5. Marfan's syndrome
6. Radiation damage
7. Paralytic poliomyelitis (bulbar or spinal)

Disturbance of Osteoclastic Activity (Increased Bone Resorption)
1. Hyperparathyroidism
2. Hypervitaminosis D

Idiopathic

most invariably becomes manifest in the second to fourth decades of life.

The majority of affected patients undoubtedly manifest no roentgenologic changes. In some, however, there is hypertrophy and excess calcification of the costal cartilages, best demonstrated by tangential roentgenography.[63] The second ribs are the most commonly involved. The affected ribs may show evidence of periosteal reaction (usually along the superior aspects) and increased size and density anteriorly. In addition, there may be enlargement and alteration of the trabecular pattern of the anterior portion of the first ribs, which may become extremely dense. CT can sometimes help distinguish the swelling of Tietze's syndrome from more sinister causes of chest wall masses.[66]

The clinical picture consists of painful swelling of one or more upper rib cartilages, without apparent cause; in some cases, it alternates between remission and exacerbation. The pain may antedate or coincide with the swelling and is accentuated by movement, deep respiration, and cough. Multiple sites are involved in approximately one third of cases.[63] The disease is usually self-limited, although months may elapse before the swelling and pain disappear.

Abnormalities of the Sternum

Pectus Excavatum

This common deformity, also known as "funnel chest," consists of depression of the sternum so that the ribs on each side protrude farther anteriorly than the sternum itself. It is generally believed that it is a genetically determined abnormality of the sternum and related portions of the diaphragm that can occur either sporadically or via a dominant pattern of inheritance.[67] It is frequently associated with other congenital connective tissue disorders, such as Marfan's syndrome, Poland's syndrome, scoliosis, and Pierre Robin syndrome.[68]

The roentgenographic manifestations are easily recognized (Fig. 20–9).[69] In posteroanterior projection, the heart is seen to be displaced to the left and rotated in a way suggestive of a "mitral configuration." The parasternal soft tissues of the anterior chest wall, which are seen in profile rather than *en face*, are apparent as increased density over the inferomedial portion of the right hemithorax and should not be mistaken for disease of the right middle lobe, even though the right heart border is obscured by a silhouetting

effect. The degree of sternal depression is easily seen on lateral roentgenograms. The severity of the defect is best quantified by CT, the "pectus index" being derived by dividing the transverse diameter of the chest by the anteroposterior diameter. The normal value of this index is about 2.55 (± 0.35 SD), and it has been suggested that patients with a ratio of 3.25 or greater require surgical correction.[70]

The vast majority of patients with pectus excavatum are symptom-free, except possibly for the anxiety occasioned by the physical deformity. However, cardiac[71, 72] and respiratory[73] symptoms occasionally have been attributed to the abnormality. A heart murmur is also fairly common,[71] often simulating pulmonic stenosis and probably resulting from kinking of the pulmonary artery. Increased splitting of the second heart sound is observed frequently. In association with the pulmonic murmur, it may suggest an atrial septal defect.

Considerable controversy surrounds the usefulness and advisability of surgical correction of pectus excavatum. Although the majority of studies have found little or no functional benefit from surgical correction,[73] the occasional patient with lung restriction can show considerable improvement.[68]

Pectus Carinatum

The reverse of pectus excavatum is pectus carinatum, or "pigeon breast," a congenital or acquired deformity in which the sternum protrudes anteriorly more than normal. It occurs more often in boys than in girls, and is associated with a family history of chest wall deformity in about 25 per cent of affected individuals and of scoliosis in 10 per cent.[74] The most common congenital variety consists of simple anterior protrusion of the sternum and costal cartilages that develops with growth.[75] The most frequent acquired cause is congenital atrial or ventricular septal defect[76]; approximately 50 per cent of patients with uncorrected defects develop the deformity. Another acquired cause is prolonged and severe asthma dating from early childhood.[77] The great majority of patients with congenital pectus carinatum are asymptomatic. Surgery can satisfactorily correct the cosmetic deformity but is rarely indicated for functional abnormalities.[74]

Inflammatory Diseases

Inflammatory diseases affecting the sternum and sternal articulations are uncommon and nowadays occur most frequently in patients whose sternum has been "split" for surgical procedures on the mediastinum. Osteomyelitis causes localized pain, swelling, and redness and may be detectable on a lateral chest roentgenogram or on conventional or computed tomograms. Heroin addicts are unusually prone to developing septic arthritis of the sternoclavicular and sternochondral joints, the most common causative organisms being *Pseudomonas aeruginosa* and *Staphylococcus aureus*.[78]

Abnormalities of the Thoracic Spine

Kyphoscoliosis

Abnormalities of curvature of the thoracic spine may be predominantly lateral (scoliosis), predominantly posterior

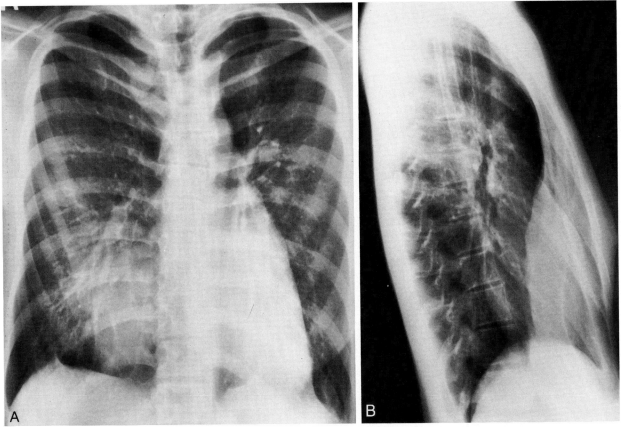

Figure 20–9. Severe Pectus Excavatum. Posteroanterior *(A)* and lateral *(B)* roentgenograms of the chest reveal a fairly large opacity projected over the lower portion of the right hemithorax contiguous with the shadow of the thoracic spine. The pulmonary arteries to the right lower lobe are displaced laterally, and the heart is displaced to the left. The severe deformity of the sternum can be readily identified in lateral projection and is of sufficient degree to displace the heart posteriorly such that the contour of the left ventricle is projected over the thoracic vertebral bodies.

(kyphosis), or a combination of the two (kyphoscoliosis). Although such abnormalities are common, particularly scoliosis, deformity of sufficient degree to cause symptoms and signs of cardiac or pulmonary disease is rare. When they do occur, there is almost invariably a severe degree of kyphoscoliosis rather than simple scoliosis or kyphosis.

The abnormalities can be divided into three groups, depending on the etiology: (1) *congenital*, including anomalies of the thoracic spine such as hemivertebrae, and various hereditary disorders in which spinal deformity constitutes only a part of the clinical picture, such as neurofibromatosis, Friedreich's ataxia, muscular dystrophy, Morquio's syndrome, and Marfan's syndrome[77]; (2) *paralytic*, the majority of cases being secondary to poliomyelitis, muscular dystrophy, or cerebral palsy; and (3) *idiopathic*, which includes approximately 80 per cent of patients with severe disease (Fig. 20–10). The last-named variety shows a female predominance of 4:1.

The principal pathophysiologic effect of severe kyphoscoliosis is restrictive lung disease that in turn results in pulmonary arterial hypertension and cor pulmonale. The major influence in their development is probably chronic hypoxic vasoconstriction caused by alveolar hypoventilation, although mechanical factors such as compression of small intraparenchymal vessels due to low lung volumes may also

contribute. In addition, pulmonary vessels may fail to develop fully when the deformity occurs during the growth period of childhood.[79]

In the great majority of cases, the scoliosis is convex to the right, and there is generally good correlation between the degree of curvature and the presence and severity of cardiopulmonary disease. The angle of scoliosis is best determined by the Cobb method.[80] Lines are drawn parallel to the upper border of the highest and the lower border of the lowest vertebral bodies of the curvature as seen on an anteroposterior roentgenogram of the spine, and the angle is measured at the intersection point of lines drawn perpendicular to these. Assessment of cardiac size and the state of the pulmonary parenchyma and vasculature can be exceedingly difficult because of the severe deformity of the thoracic cage.

Most children with kyphoscoliosis are asymptomatic,[81] and the presence of cardiac abnormalities in these individuals should suggest primary heart disease independent of the spinal deformity. It is the combination of the kyphotic and scoliotic defects that determines the severity of symptoms and the likelihood of developing ventilatory respiratory failure:[82] lesser degrees of scoliosis cause more severe impairment in the presence of severe kyphosis, and *vice versa*. In general, adults whose scoliotic angle is 100 de-

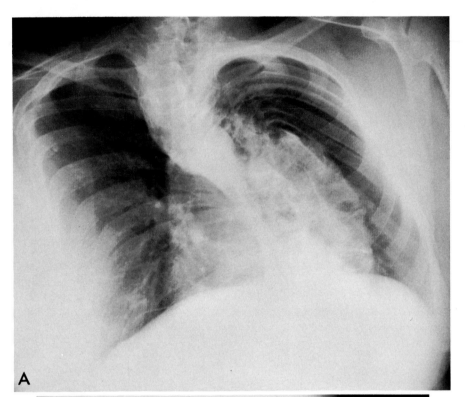

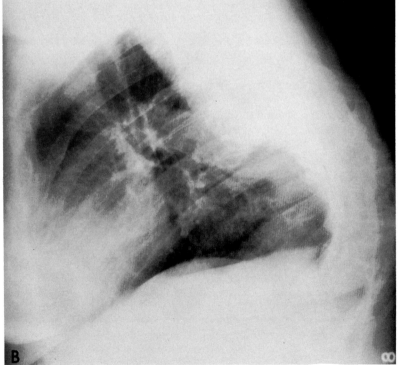

Figure 20–10. Kyphoscoliosis. Posteroanterior *(A)* and lateral *(B)* roentgenograms reveal severe deformity of the thoracic skeleton, the spine possessing a marked scoliosis to the left in the midthoracic region and a severe kyphos in the middle and lower regions. Deformity of the rib cage is as might be anticipated from the thoracic curvature.

grees or more will develop respiratory failure, although usually not until the fourth or fifth decade.

Tests of pulmonary function characteristically reveal a decrease in VC and TLC and normal or increased values of RV.[81] In patients with cor pulmonale, TLC may be reduced to as little as 2 L.[83] Predicted values for lung volumes are based at least partly on height, however, and it has been suggested that it is more accurate to use arm span in predicting values in patients with kyphoscoliosis.[84] Flow is reduced only in proportion to the reduction in VC, and direct measurement of airway resistance reveals normal values.[83] In patients with mild or moderate lung restriction, measurement of steady-state diffusing capacity[85] reveals relatively normal values for gas transfer corrected for the reduction in alveolar volume. In patients who are hypercapnic and in heart failure, however, the values are decreased out of proportion to the reduced lung volumes.

Arterial blood gas values are almost invariably abnormal in adults with kyphoscoliosis and occasionally in adolescents.[81] In the more advanced cases, it is common to find both hypoxemia and hypercarbia, a combined form of respiratory failure that can be attributed to alveolar hypoventilation secondary to shallow respiration and to $\dot{V}/\dot{Q}$ imbalance. Studies with radioactive xenon have shown defects in both ventilation and perfusion.[86] Although the arterial hypoxemia associated with severe kyphoscoliosis can be ascribed to both gas exchange impairment and hypoventilation, the relative contribution of the former is much less than in patients who have similar degrees of alveolar hypoventilation secondary to chronic obstructive pulmonary disease.[85] In fact, even in the presence of advanced disease associated with arterial hypertension and cor pulmonale, the majority of the arterial hypoxemia is caused by alveolar hypoxia rather than $\dot{V}/\dot{Q}$ mismatch or shunt. Patients with kyphoscoliosis can be particularly susceptible to ventilatory depression and oxygen desaturation during sleep[87]; desaturation is particularly profound during rapid eye movement sleep.

Compliance of both the chest wall and the lung is decreased in kyphoscoliosis. The decrease in chest wall compliance, particularly, may be profound and correlates significantly with the angle of scoliosis.[88] The mechanism by which lung compliance is reduced is unclear; theoretically, however, it could be caused by either small foci of atelectasis or an increase in the surface tension resulting from failure of the lung to inflate because of the chest wall restriction (or both).

Once respiratory and cardiac failure are manifested, the clinical course may be rapidly downhill; repeated episodes of failure often are precipitated by pulmonary infection. Recent studies, however, suggest that the prognosis may be considerably improved by the use of intermittent mechanical ventilation.[89] Either cuirass-type or positive-pressure ventilation applied during the nocturnal hours can result in a prolonged interim improvement in pulmonary gas exchange and lung mechanics and a reduction in pulmonary artery pressures and the severity of symptoms.

Ankylosing Spondylitis

Involvement of the thoracic spine by ankylosing spondylitis results in fixation of the chest cage in an inspiratory position and leads to the paradoxical combination of hyper-

inflation (increased FRC) and lung restriction (decreased TLC and VC). The disorder is strongly associated with HLA-B27. Approximately 90 per cent of patients with ankylosing spondylitis have this histocompatibility antigen,[90] and about 20 per cent of HLA-B27–positive individuals will develop the disease.[91] Although peripheral joint involvement develops eventually in about 15 to 25 per cent of cases, there is little question that ankylosing spondylitis is an entity distinct from rheumatoid arthritis.[92]

Pathologically, ankylosing spondylitis consists of synovitis, chondritis, and juxta-articular osteitis of the sacroiliac, apophyseal, and costovertebral articulations. Progression of the disease is marked by erosion of subchondral bone, destruction of cartilage, and eventually ankylosis.

In addition to the characteristic changes in the thoracic skeleton, approximately 1 to 2 per cent of patients develop pleuropulmonary manifestations,[93] most commonly in the form of upper lobe fibrobullous disease similar to that seen occasionally in rheumatoid disease (see page 398).[94] These lesions sometimes contain fungus balls and are associated with pneumothorax in about 10 per cent of patients. In one series,[93] an unexpected number of patients manifested evidence of pleuritis and pleurisy with effusion.

The typical patient with ankylosing spondylitis is a young male with a history of onset of symptoms early in the third decade of life. The clinical picture is characterized by intermittent or continuous low back pain, sometimes associated with constitutional symptoms such as fatigue, weight loss, anorexia, and low-grade fever. The pain can be distinguished from that of a mechanical or nonspecific type by its insidious onset, its duration (usually more than 3 months before the patient seeks medical help), its association with morning stiffness, and its improvement with exercise.[91] As the disease progresses upward and involves the thoracic spine, the patient may complain of chest pain that is sometimes accentuated during respiration.[95] After the spine has fused, the kyphotic curvature gradually increases and chest expansion progressively diminishes. Few patients complain of dyspnea.

The pattern of pulmonary function is one of restriction and overinflation, the result of fixation of the thorax in an expanded position. VC is reduced, often to 70 per cent or less of predicted values; RV and FRC are usually, but not always, increased.[96]

Neoplasms and Non-neoplastic Tumors of the Chest Wall

Although they are uncommon, many types of benign and malignant primary neoplasms originate in the chest wall.[97, 98] Many can be detected on plain roentgenograms of patients who complain of chest pain or swelling. However, for more specific information concerning the origin of a tumor and its extent of spread, CT or magnetic resonance imaging (MRI) is an essential investigative procedure (Fig. 20–11).[99]

Neoplasms and Non-neoplastic Tumors of Soft Tissues

In adults, the most common benign tumor of the chest wall is lipoma; the most common malignant neoplasms are fibrosarcoma and malignant fibrohistiocytoma. In children, the most frequent malignant tumors are primitive neuroec-

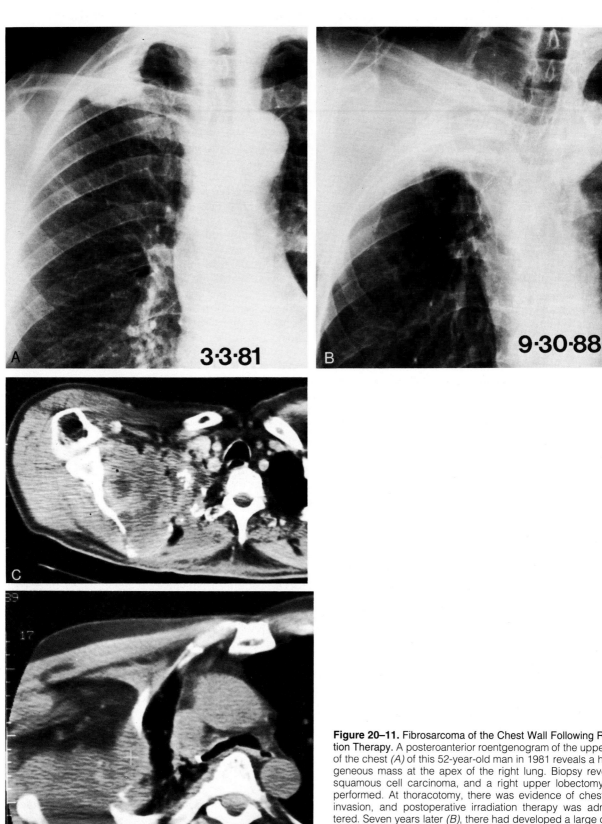

Figure 20–11. Fibrosarcoma of the Chest Wall Following Radiation Therapy. A posteroanterior roentgenogram of the upper half of the chest *(A)* of this 52-year-old man in 1981 reveals a homogeneous mass at the apex of the right lung. Biopsy revealed squamous cell carcinoma, and a right upper lobectomy was performed. At thoracotomy, there was evidence of chest wall invasion, and postoperative irradiation therapy was administered. Seven years later *(B)*, there had developed a large opacity in the right apical region associated with extensive destruction of ribs. CT scans just below the thoracic inlet *(C)* and at the level of the main bronchi *(D)* reveal an almost complete absence of the ribs in the apical region and extensive invasion of the soft tissues of the chest wall. The scapula has been partly destroyed, seen to best advantage in *D (arrow)*. (Courtesy of Dr. Jim Wilson, Montreal Chest Hospital.)

todermal tumor,[100] rhabdomyosarcoma, and extraosseous Ewing's sarcoma ("malignant small cell tumor of thoraco-pulmonary region," Askin's tumor).[101]

The point of origin of a lipoma in the chest wall establishes its mode of presentation. When it originates adjacent to the parietal pleura, it causes a soft tissue mass that indents the lung and possesses a contour characteristic of its extrapulmonary origin. When it arises outside the rib cage, it presents as a palpable soft tissue mass that may be visualized roentgenographically if viewed in profile or, if it is large enough, even *en face*. Most lipomas that arise between the ribs have a dumbbell or hourglass configuration, part projecting inside and part outside the thoracic cage. The density of lipomas is intermediate between that of air and that of soft tissue. Therefore, when a lipoma relates to lung parenchyma, it may not be readily distinguishable roentgenographically from other soft tissue masses, whereas when it relates to the soft tissues of the chest wall the contrast with contiguous soft tissues usually permits its identification as fat.[102] As a result of the specificity of CT in identifying fat-containing structures, this technique is especially valuable in these tumors.[103]

Other benign tumors of the soft tissues of the chest wall include desmoid tumor,[104] neurogenic neoplasms of the intercostal nerves, and fibromas and angiofibromas of the intercostal muscles. Non-neoplastic tumors, such as abscesses, various granulomas, and echinococcal cysts, also must be considered in the differential diagnosis of a chest wall mass.[105]

Neoplasms and Non-neoplastic Tumors of Bone

The majority of neoplasms of the thoracic skeleton occur in the ribs. Of the 134 cases reported in one series,[106] 72 involved the ribs, 26 the scapulae, 15 the thoracic vertebrae, 14 the clavicles, and 7 the sternum. The following characteristics were noted: (1) rib lesions were most commonly metastatic, chiefly from the lung and breast; (2) the majority of lesions arising in the sternum were malignant, most often chondrosarcoma; (3) involvement of the clavicles was most often by metastatic neoplasm; (4) primary neoplasms in the scapulae were more numerous than metastatic ones, with the majority benign; (5) involvement of the thoracic vertebrae almost invariably represented metastasis.

Of the cartilaginous and osteogenic neoplasms and non-neoplastic tumors, osteochondroma is the most common benign type, rarer varieties being enchondroma, osteoblastoma, and endostoma ("bone islands"). The most common malignant neoplasm is chondrosarcoma[107]; osteogenic sarcoma, malignant fibrohistiocytoma, hemangiopericytoma, and fibrosarcoma are less frequent.[98, 106]

The most frequent non-neoplastic tumor of the thoracic skeleton is fibrous dysplasia (Fig. 20–12); eosinophilic granuloma, hemangioma, and aneurysmal bone cyst occur less frequently.[106] Involvement of the rib cage by Paget's disease has a typical roentgenographic appearance similar to that in any other bone (Fig. 20–13). Myeloma and (occasionally) solitary plasmacytoma are the most frequent malignant

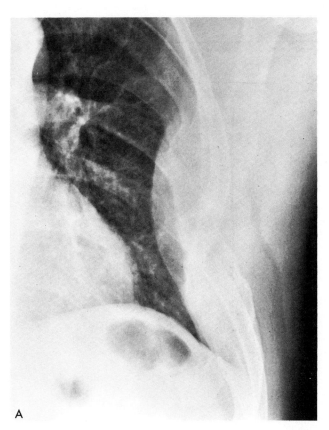
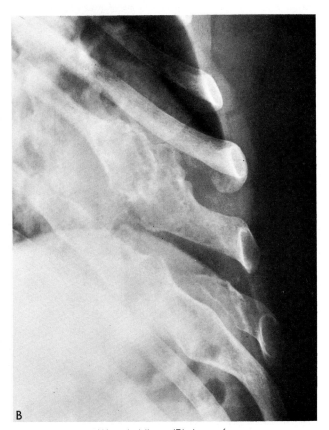

A

B

Figure 20–12. Fibrous Dysplasia of the Left Rib Cage. Posteroanterior *(A)* and oblique *(B)* views of the left rib cage reveal considerable expansion and distortion of ribs along the lower axillary lung zone (one rib has been removed).

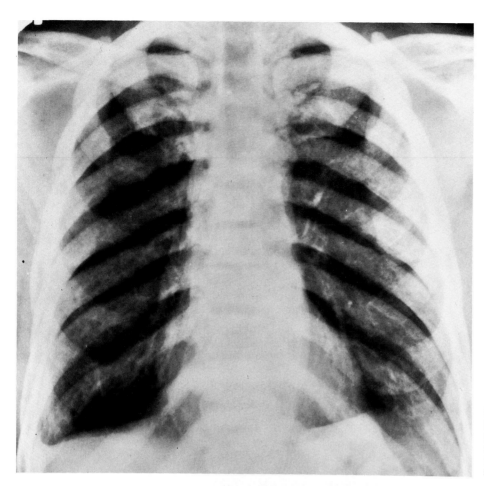

Figure 20–13. Paget's Disease of the Rib Cage. A posteroanterior roentgenogram reveals a marked increase in density and uniform expansion of all ribs bilaterally. The clavicles are involved in a similar process.

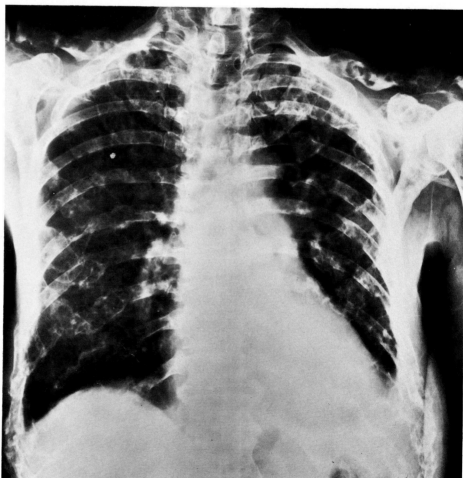

Figure 20–14. Multiple Myeloma of the Rib Cage. A posteroanterior roentgenogram reveals extensive destruction of virtually all ribs bilaterally. Note that several of the ribs have been expanded, a common feature in multiple myeloma of ribs.

neoplasms of reticuloendothelial origin, followed by Hodgkin's disease and large-cell lymphoma.[106] In older patients, particularly men, the association of a destructive lesion of one or more ribs with a soft tissue mass that protrudes into the thorax and indents the lung is highly suggestive of myeloma (*see* Fig. 8–51, page 506).[108] However, a similar appearance can be created by primary lung carcinoma invading the chest wall and by metastatic carcinoma. Advanced myelomatosis of the rib cage may be associated with expansion of bone (Fig. 20–14).

The majority of benign neoplasms of the thoracic skeleton occasion no symptoms and usually are detected in asymptomatic subjects on a screening chest roentgenogram. Malignant neoplasms may cause pain and, if extensive, respiratory insufficiency. Roentgenologic assessment may be of value in suggesting the diagnosis, but definitive diagnosis requires close correlation between the pathologic and the roentgenologic appearances of the neoplasm.

References

1. Panicek DM, Benson CB, Gottlieb RH, et al: The diaphragm: Anatomic, pathologic, and radiologic considerations. Radiographics 8: 385, 1988.
2. Naidich DP, Zerhouni FA, Siegelman SS (eds): Diaphragm. *In* Computed Tomography of the Thorax. New York, Raven Press, 1984.
3. Riley EA: Idiopathic diaphragmatic paralysis. A report of eight cases. Am J Med 32: 404, 1962.
4. Wilcox P, Baile EM, Hards J, et al: Phrenic nerve function and its relationship to atelectasis after coronary artery bypass surgery. Chest 93: 693, 1988.
5. Rousou JA, Parker T, Angelman RM, et al: Phrenic nerve paresis associated with the use of iced slush and the cooling jacket for topical hypothermia. J Thorac Cardiovasc Surg 89: 921, 1985.
6. Alexander C: Diaphragm movements and the diagnosis of diaphragmatic paralysis. Clin Radiol 17: 79, 1966.
7. Ridyard JB, Stewart RM: Regional lung function in unilateral diaphragmatic paralysis. Thorax 31: 438, 1976.
8. Easton PA, Fleetham JA, De la Rocha A, et al: Respiratory function after paralysis of the right hemidiaphragm. Am Rev Respir Dis 127: 1125, 1983.
9. Lisboa C, Paré PD, Pertuze J, et al: Inspiratory muscle function in unilateral diaphragmatic paralysis. Am Rev Respir Dis 134: 488, 1986.
10. Clague HW, Hall DR: Effect of posture on lung volume, airway closure and gas exchange in hemidiaphragmatic paralysis. Thorax 34: 523, 1979.
11. Wright CD, Williams JG, Ogilvie CM, et al: Results of diaphragmatic plication for unilateral diaphragmatic paralysis. J Thorac Cardiovasc Surg 90: 195, 1985.
12. Shochina M, Ferber I, Wolf E: Evaluation of the phrenic nerve in patients with neuromuscular disorders. Int J Rehabil Res 6: 455, 1983.
13. Newsom Davis J, Goldman M, Loh L, et al: Diaphragm function and alveolar hypoventilation. Q J Med 45: 87, 1976.
14. Diament MJ, Boechat MI, Kangarloo H: Real-time sector ultrasound in the evaluation of suspected abnormalities of diaphragmatic motion. J Clin Ultrasound 13: 539, 1985.
15. Kreitzer SM, Feldman NT, Saunders NA, et al: Bilateral diaphragmatic paralysis with hypercapnic respiratory failure. Am J Med 65: 89, 1978.
16. Molho M, Katz I, Schwartz E, et al: Familial bilateral paralysis of the diaphragm. Chest 91: 464, 1987.
17. Loh L, Hughes JBM, Newsom Davis J: Gas exchange problems in bilateral diaphragm paralysis. Bull Eur Physiopathol Respir 15: 137, 1979.
18. Bhattacharya SK, Singh SK, Lahiri TK: Eventration of diaphragm. J Indian Med 84: 15, 1986.
19. Okuda K, Nomura F, Kawai M, et al: Age-related gross changes of the liver and right diaphragm, with special reference to partial eventration. Br J Radiol 52: 870, 1979.
20. Vogl A, Small A: Partial eventration of the right diaphragm (congenital diaphragmatic herniation of the liver). Ann Intern Med 43: 61, 1955.
21. Tarver RD, Godwin JD, Putman CE: The diaphragm. Radiol Clin North Am 22: 615, 1984.
22. Spencer RP, Spackman TJ, Pearson HA: Diagnosis of right diaphragmatic eventration by means of liver scan. Radiology 99: 375, 1971.
23. Rubinstein ZJ, Solomon A: CT findings in partial eventration of the right diaphragm. J Comput Assist Tomogr 5: 719, 1981.
24. Chin EF, Lynn RB: Surgery of eventration of the diaphragm. J Thorac Surg 32: 6, 1956.
25. Ford GT, Whitelaw WA, Rosenal TW, et al: Diaphragm function after upper abdominal surgery in humans. Am Rev Respir Dis 127: 431, 1983.
26. Simonneau G, Vivien A, Sartene R, et al: Diaphragm dysfunction induced by upper abdominal surgery—role of postoperative pain. Am Rev Respir Dis 128: 899, 1983.
27. Bertrand D, Viires N, Cantineau J-P, et al: Diaphragmatic contractility after upper abdominal surgery. J Appl Physiol 61: 1775, 1986.
28. Felder SL, Masley PM, Wolff WI: Anemia as a presenting symptom of esophageal hiatal hernia of the diaphragm. Arch Intern Med 105: 873, 1960.
29. Menuck L: Plain film findings of gastric volvulus herniating into the chest. Am J Roentgenol 126: 1169, 1976.
30. Reed JO, Lang EF: Diaphragmatic hernia in infancy. Am J Roentgenol 82: 437, 1959.
31. Gale ME: Bochdalek hernia: Prevalence and CT characteristics. Radiology 156: 449, 1985.
32. Page DV, Stocker JT: Anomalies associated with pulmonary hypoplasia. Am Rev Respir Dis 125: 216, 1982.
33. deNoronha LL, deCosta, MF, Godinho MTM: Thoracic kidney. Am Rev Respir Dis 109: 678, 1974.
34. Curley FJ, Hubmayr RD, Raptopoulos V: Bilateral diaphragmatic densities in a 72-year-old woman. Chest 86: 915, 1986.
35. Chinn DH, Filly RA, Callen PW, et al: Congenital diaphragmatic hernia diagnosed prenatally by ultrasound. Radiology 148: 119, 1983.
36. Kirchner SG, Burko H, O'Neill JA, et al: Delayed radiographic presentation of congenital right diaphragmatic hernia. Radiology 115: 155, 1975.
37. Yeung SC, Park C, Kramer N: Diaphragmatic herniation of the liver in a newborn demonstrated by liver scan. Clin Nucl Med 9: 729, 1984.
38. Betts RA: Subcostosternal diaphragmatic hernia, with report of five cases. Am J Roentgenol 75: 269, 1956.
39. Merten DF, Bowie JD, Kirks DR, et al: Anteromedial diaphragmatic defects in infancy: Current approaches to diagnostic imaging. Radiology 142: 361, 1982.
40. Rosenberg M: Chronic subphrenic abscess. Lancet 2: 379, 1968.
41. Meyers MA: The spread and localization of acute intraperitoneal effusions. Radiology 95: 547, 1970.
42. Halvorsen RA, Jones MA, Rice RP, et al: Anterior left subphrenic abscess: Characteristic plain film and CT appearance. Am J Roentgenol 139: 283, 1982.
43. Miller WT, Talman EA: Subphrenic abscess. Am J Roentgenol 101: 961, 1967.
44. Alexander ES, Proto AV, Clark RA: CT differentiation of subphrenic abscess and pleural effusion. Am J Roentgenol 140: 47, 1983.
45. Briggs RC: Combined liver-lung scanning in detecting subdiaphragmatic abscess. Semin Nucl Med 2: 150, 1972.
46. Fataar S, Schulman A: Subphrenic abscess: The radiological approach. Clin Radiol 32: 147, 1981.
47. Anderson LS, Forrest JV: Tumors of the diaphragm. Am J Roentgenol 119: 259, 1973.
48. Ochsner A, Ochsner A Jr: Tumors of the diaphragm. *In* Spain D (ed): Diagnosis and Treatment of Tumors of the Chest. New York, Grune & Stratton, 1960, p 240.
49. Müller NL: CT features of cystic teratoma of the diaphragm. J Comput Assist Tomogr 10: 325, 1986.
50. Goldenberg DB, Brogdon BG: Congenital anomalies of the pectoral girdle demonstrated by chest radiography. J Can Assoc Radiol 18: 472, 1967.
51. Pearl M, Chow TF, Friedman E: Poland's syndrome. Radiology 101: 619, 1976.
52. Lightwood RG, Cleland WP: Cervical lung hernia. Thorax 29: 349, 1974.
53. Fisher MS: Eve's rib [letters]. Radiology 140: 841, 1981.

54. Rasmussen P, Simonsen NG: The scalenus anticus syndrome. II. Results of operative treatment in 20 cases, including 16 with costa · cervicalis syndrome. Nord Med 62: 1572, 1959.

55. Dick R: Arteriography in neurovascular compression at the thoracic outlet, with special reference to embolic patterns. Am J Roentgenol 110: 141, 1970.

56. Boone ML, Swenson BE, Felson B: Rib notching: Its many causes. Am J Roentgenol 91: 1075, 1964.

57. Ferris RA, LoPresti JM: Rib notching due to coarctation of the aorta: Report of a case initially observed at less than one year of age. Br J Radiol 47: 357, 1974.

58. Sargent EN, Turner AF, Jacobson G: Superior marginal rib defects. An etiologic classification. Am J Roentgenol 106: 491, 1969.

59. Wignall BK, Williamson BRJ: The chest x-ray in quadriplegia: A review of 119 patients. Clin Radiol 31: 81, 1980.

60. Wolstein D, Rabinowitz JG, Twersky J: Tuberculosis of the rib. J Can Assoc Radiol 25: 307, 1974.

61. Ip M, Chen NK, So SY, et al: Unusual rib destruction in pleuropulmonary tuberculosis. Chest 95: 242, 1989.

62. Fogelman I: Lesions in the ribs detected by bone scanning. Clin Radiol 31: 317, 1980.

63. Skorneck AB: Roentgen aspects of Tietze's syndrome. Painful hypertrophy of costal cartilage and bone—osteochondritis? Am J Roentgenol 83: 748, 1960.

64. Jurik AG, Graudal H: Sternocostal joint swelling—clinical Tietze's syndrome. Scand J Rheumatol 17: 33, 1988.

65. Ausubel H, Cohen BD, LaDue JS: Tietze's disease of eight years' duration. N Engl J Med 261: 190, 1959.

66. Edelstein G, Levitt RG, Slaker DP, et al: CT observation of rib abnormalities: Spectrum of findings. J Comput Assist Tomogr 9: 65, 1985.

67. Leung AKC, Hoo JJ: Familial congenital funnel chest. Am J Med Genet 26: 887, 1987.

68. Shamberger RC, Welch KJ: Surgical repair of pectus excavatum. J Pediatr Surg 23: 615, 1988.

69. Backer Ole G, Brünner S, Larsen V: Radiologic evaluation of funnel chest. Acta Radiol 55: 249, 1961.

70. Haller JA, Kramer SS, Lietman SA: Use of CT scans in selection of patients for pectus excavatum surgery: A preliminary report. J Pediatr Surg 22: 904, 1987.

71. Guller B, Hable K: Cardiac findings in pectus excavatum in children: Review and differential diagnosis. Chest 66: 165, 1974.

72. Skinner EF: Xiphoid horn in pectus excavatum. Thorax 24: 750, 1969.

73. Fink A, Rivin A, Murray JF: Pectus excavatum. An analysis of twenty-seven cases. Arch Intern Med 108: 427, 1961.

74. Schamberger RC, Welch KJ: Surgical correction of pectus carinatum. J Pediatr Surg 22: 48, 1987.

75. Lester CW: Pectus carinatum, pigeon breast and related deformities of the sternum and costal cartilages. Arch Paediatr 77: 399, 1960.

76. Davies H: Chest deformities in congenital heart disease. Br J Dis Chest 53: 151, 1959.

77. Zorab PA: Chest deformities. Br Med J 1: 1155, 1966.

78. Goldin RH, Chow AW, Edwards JE Jr, et al: Sternoarticular septic arthritis in heroin users. N Engl J Med 289: 616, 1973.

79. Reid L: Autopsy studies of the lungs in kyphoscoliosis. In Zorab PA (ed): Proceedings of a Symposium on Scoliosis. London, National Fund for Research in Poliomyelitis and Other Crippling Diseases, 1966, p 71.

80. James JIP: Scoliosis. Baltimore, Williams & Wilkins, 1968.

81. Weber B, Smith JP, Briscoe WA, et al: Pulmonary function in asymptomatic adolescents with idiopathic scoliosis. Am Rev Respir Dis 111: 389, 1975.

82. Bergofsky EH, Turino GM, Fishman AP: Cardiorespiratory failure in kyphoscoliosis. Medicine 38: 263, 1959.

83. Bates DV, Macklem PT, Christie RV: Respiratory Function in Disease: An Introduction to the Integrated Study of the Lung. 2nd ed. Philadelphia, WB Saunders, 1971.

84. Hepper NGG, Black LF, Fowler WS: Relationships of lung volume to height and arm span in normal subjects and in patients with spinal deformity. Am Rev Respir Dis 91: 356, 1965.

85. Bergofsky EH: Respiratory failure in disorders of the thoracic cage. Am Rev Respir Dis 119: 643, 1979.

86. Bake B, Bjure J, Kasalichy J, et al: Regional pulmonary ventilation and perfusion distribution in patients with untreated idiopathic scoliosis. Thorax 27: 703, 1972.

87. Sawicka EH, Branthwaite MA: Respiration during sleep in kyphoscoliosis. Thorax 42: 801, 1987.

88. Kafer E: Idiopathic scoliosis. Mechanical properties of the respiratory system and the ventilatory response to carbon dioxide. J Clin Invest 55: 1153, 1975.

89. Hoeppner V, Cockcroft D, Dosman J, et al: Nighttime ventilation improves respiratory failure in secondary kyphoscoliosis. Am Rev Respir Dis 129: 240, 1984.

90. Schlosstein L, Terasaki PI, Bluestone R, et al: High association of an HLA antigen, W27, with ankylosing spondylitis. N Engl J Med 288: 704, 1973.

91. Calin A, Porta J, Fried JF, et al: Clinical history as a screening test for ankylosing spondylitis. JAMA 237: 2613, 1977.

92. Boland EW: Ankylosing spondylitis. In Hollander JL (ed): Arthritis and Allied Conditions. 7th ed. Philadelphia, Lea & Febiger, 1966, pp 633–655.

93. Rosenow EC III, Strimlan CV, Muhm JR, et al: Pleuropulmonary manifestations of ankylosing spondylitis. Mayo Clin Proc 52: 641, 1977.

94. Jessamine AG: Upper lobe fibrosis in ankylosing spondylitis. Can Med Assoc J 98: 25, 1968.

95. Good AE: The chest pain of ankylosing spondylitis. Its place in the differential diagnosis of heart pain. Ann Intern Med 58: 926, 1963.

96. Franssen MJ, van Herwaarden CL, van de Putte LB: Lung function in patients with ankylosing spondylitis. A study of the influence of disease activity and treatment with nonsteroidal anti-inflammatory drugs. J Rheumatol 13: 936, 1986.

97. Pairolero PC, Arnold PG: Chest wall tumors: Experience with 100 consecutive patients. J Thorac Cardiovasc Surg 90: 367, 1985.

98. King RM, Pairolero PC, Trastek VF, et al: Primary chest wall tumors: Factors affecting survival. Ann Thorac Surg 41: 597, 1986.

99. Jafri SZH, Roberts JL, Bree RL, et al: Computed tomography of chest wall masses. Radiographics 9: 51, 1989.

100. Gonzalez-Crussi F, Wolfson SL, Misugi K, et al: Peripheral neuroectodermal tumors of the chest wall in childhood. Cancer 54: 2519, 1984.

101. Linnoila RI, Tsokos M, Triche TJ, et al: Evidence for neural origin and PAS-positive variants of the malignant small cell tumor of thoracopulmonary region ("Askin tumor"). Am J Surg Pathol 10: 124, 1986.

102. Rosenberg RF, Rubinstein BM, Messinger NH: Intrathoracic lipomas. Chest 60: 507, 1971.

103. Castillo M, Shirkhoda A: Computed tomography of diaphragmatic lipoma. J Comput Assist Tomogr 9: 167, 1985.

104. Klein DL, Gamsu G, Gant TD: Intrathoracic desmoid tumor of the chest wall. Am J Roentgenol 129: 524, 1977.

105. Rami-Porta R, Bravo-Bravo JL, Aroca-Gonzalez MJ, et al: Tumours and pseudotumours of the chest wall. Scand J Thorac Cardiovasc Surg 19: 97, 1985.

106. Ochsner A Jr, Lucas GL, McFarland GB Jr: Tumors of the thoracic skeleton. Review of 134 cases. J Thorac Cardiovasc Surg 52: 311, 1966.

107. Marcove RC, Huvos AG: Cartilaginous tumors of the ribs. Cancer 27: 794, 1971.

108. Wolfel DA, Dennis JM: Multiple myeloma of the chest wall. Am J Roentgenol 89: 1241, 1963.

109. Heffner JE: Diaphragmatic paralysis following chiropractic manipulation of the cervical spine. Arch Intern Med 145: 562, 1985.

110. Buszek MC, Szymke TE, Honet JC, et al: Hemidiaphragmatic paralysis: An unusual complication of cervical spondylosis. Arch Phys Med Rehabil 64: 601, 1983.

111. Hadeed HA, Braun TW: Paralysis of the hemidiaphragm as a complication of internal jugular vein cannulation: Report of a case. J Oral Maxillofac Surg 46: 409, 1988.

112. Smith CD, Sade RM, Crawford FA, et al: Diaphragmatic paralysis and eventration in infants. J Thorac Cardiovasc Surg 91: 490, 1986.

113. Biberstein MP, Eisenberg H: Unilateral diaphragmatic paralysis in association with Erb's palsy. Chest 75: 209, 1979.

114. Graham AN, Martin PD, Haas LF: Neuralgic amyotrophy with bilateral diaphragmatic palsy. Thorax 40: 635, 1985.

115. Shin MS, Ho K-J: Computed tomographic evaluation of the pathologic lesion for the idiopathic diaphragmatic paralysis. J Comput Assist Tomogr 6: 257, 1982.

116. Dervaux L, Lacquet LM: Hemidiaphragmatic paralysis after cervical herpes zoster. Thorax 37: 870, 1982.

117. Balbierz JM, Ellenberg M, Honet JC: Complete hemidiaphragmatic

paralysis in a patient with multiple sclerosis. Am J Phys Med Rehabil 67: 161, 1988.

118. Bowman ED, Murton LJ: A case of neonatal bilateral diaphragmatic paralysis requiring surgery. Aust Paediatr J 20: 331, 1984.

119. McWilliam RC, Gardner-Medwyn D, Doyle D, et al: Diaphragmatic paralysis due to spinal muscular atrophy. Arch Dis Child 60: 145, 1985.

120. Montserrat JM, Picado CF, Agusti-Vidal A: Arnold-Chiari malformation and paralysis of the diaphragm. Respiration 53: 128, 1988.

121. Mier A, Brophy C, Green M: Diaphragm weakness and syringomyelia. J R Soc Med 81: 59, 1988.

122. Goldstein RL, Hyde RW, Lapham LW, et al: Peripheral neuropathy presenting with respiratory insufficiency as the primary complaint. Am J Med 56: 443, 1974.

123. Walsh NE, Dumitru D, Kalantri A, et al: Brachial neuritis involving the bilateral phrenic nerves. Arch Phys Med Rehabil 68: 46, 1987.

124. Cooper CB, Trend PJ, Wiles CM: Severe diaphragm weakness in multiple sclerosis. Thorax 40: 633, 1985.

125. Spiteri MA, Mier AK, Brophy CJ, et al: Bilateral diaphragm weakness. Thorax 40: 631, 1985.

126. Thomas NE, Passamonte PM, Sunderrajan EV, et al: Bilateral diaphragmatic paralysis as a possible paraneoplastic syndrome from renal cell carcinoma. Am Rev Respir Dis 129: 507, 1984.

127. Sandham JD, Shaw DT, Guenter CA: Acute supine respiratory failure due to bilateral diaphragmatic paralysis. Chest 72: 97, 1977.

128. Cabrera MR, Edsall JR: Bilateral diaphragm paralysis associated with topical cardiac hypothermia. NY State J Med 87: 514, 1987.

129. Camfferman F, Bogaard JM, van der Meche FGA, et al: Idiopathic bilateral diaphragmatic paralysis. Eur J Respir Dis 66: 65, 1985.

21

RESPIRATORY DISEASE ASSOCIATED WITH A NORMAL CHEST ROENTGENOGRAM

There is little doubt that significant pulmonary and pleural disease, sometimes of life-threatening severity, can exist in the presence of a normal chest roentgenogram. This limitation of roentgenographic visibility exists not only in the early stages of various alveolar and interstitial diseases but also during the healing stages, when an acute inflammatory exudate has been replaced by organization tissue or mature fibrous tissue. Although this discrepancy is sometimes confusing in diagnosis, in many cases it constitutes a significant, positive diagnostic feature, excluding those diseases in which respiratory symptoms and signs are commonly associated with roentgenographic abnormalities.

In addition to cases in which the roentgenogram is undoubtedly normal, from time to time a roentgenographic pattern is encountered in the "gray area"—at the outer range of normal but not unequivocally abnormal. An example of such a problem is deciding whether one or both hemidiaphragms are elevated beyond the normal range; although a high diaphragm is often a reflection of suboptimal inspiration, it can be an important indication of small lung volume.

Both the equivocal and the unequivocal situations are most easily discussed in terms of whether disease is localized or generalized. In each instance, a repeat roentgenogram or comparison with previous roentgenograms may resolve the problem. It should also be empasized that the following discussion relates specifically to conventional roentgenography, since computed tomography (CT), particularly high-resolution, is clearly capable of revealing abnormalities not identifiable by standard techniques.

DISEASES OF THE LUNG PARENCHYMA

Local Diseases

Acute airspace disease such as that caused by bacterial infection or alveolar hemorrhage characteristically produces roentgenographic shadows at a very early stage. By contrast, acute local disease confined largely to the interstitium of the lung (e.g., viral or *Mycoplasma* pneumonia) can cause symptoms that antedate roentgenographic signs by 48 hours or longer. Localized abnormalities of the pulmonary vascular system, particularly acute pulmonary embolism, also frequently show no roentgenographic abnormalities in the chest. Even when embolism results in an infarct, an opacity is seldom visible until 12 to 24 hours after the embolic episode.

Chronic pulmonary disease also may be present and active for months or even years before it becomes roentgenographically visible. It has been estimated, for example, that a focus of active tuberculosis is not roentgenologically detectable until 2 or 3 months after initial infection.[1] Similarly, most pulmonary carcinomas are present for years before they become visible. A solitary uncalcified lesion less than 6 mm in diameter is rarely appreciated and then usually only in retrospect when the lesion has grown and is detected on subsequent roentgenograms. In fact, nodules as large as 2 cm in diameter may be overlooked, particularly if they are situated over the convexity of the lung or in the paramediastinal area where the rib cage, large vessels, or mediastinal contents tend to obscure their image.

General Diseases

In contrast to localized pulmonary tuberculosis, in which symptoms and signs may not appear for many weeks after the chest roentgenogram has become abnormal, in miliary tuberculosis fever, general malaise, and headaches may develop some weeks before a roentgenologic abnormality is visible.

In diseases such as sarcoidosis, eosinophilic granuloma, fibrosing alveolitis, and allergic alveolitis no lesions may be roentgenographically visible even when symptoms and disturbances of pulmonary function indicate involvement of the lung interstitium. Among the connective tissue diseases, progressive systemic sclerosis is frequently associated with a lowered diffusing capacity and arterial partial pressure of oxygen (PO_2) despite a normal chest roentgenogram.[2] By contrast, pulmonary involvement in rheumatoid disease typically is detectable roentgenologically before pulmonary function becomes impaired.[3] In systemic lupus erythematosus, there may be a significant reduction in vital capacity (VC) despite a normal chest roentgenogram; however, when serial roentgenographic studies are available, a progressive loss of lung volume may be evidenced by diaphragmatic elevation.[3]

Diffuse pulmonary vascular disease also may be quite severe without producing roentgenographic manifestations; for example, the extensive obstruction of the vasculature in thromboembolic disease and the vasculopathy of progressive systemic sclerosis.

DISEASES OF THE PLEURA

The chest roentgenogram may be normal in cases of acute pleuritis; however, "dry pleurisy" often is associated with diaphragmatic elevation and reduction in diaphragmatic excursion. As discussed previously (*see* page 243), effusions as large as 300 mL may not be visible on standard posteroanterior and lateral chest roentgenograms exposed with the patient erect; films exposed in the lateral decubitus position, however, can reveal effusions of 100 mL or less, and special roentgenographic techniques may show as little as 5 to 15 mL, an amount that may be visible even in healthy subjects.

DISEASES OF THE AIRWAYS

Many patients with diseases of the conducting airways have normal chest roentgenograms. In fact, in uncomplicated chronic bronchitis, this is the rule rather than the exception. Although the majority of patients who experience acute asthmatic attacks show evidence of pulmonary overinflation on pulmonary function testing, roentgenographic evidence of its presence is seldom convincing, except in children and adolescents with early-onset asthma. However, the presence of overinflation during an attack can sometimes be appreciated by comparing current films with films obtained during remission.

Approximately 5 to 10 per cent of patients with bronchiectasis fail to show evidence of this disease on standard chest roentgenograms.[4] Patients with mild to moderate emphysema also may have completely normal films. For example, in one study of 696 patients in which the accuracy of the roentgenologic diagnosis of emphysema was assessed on the basis of paper-mounted whole-lung sections made following necropsy,[5] only 41 per cent of the patients with moderately severe emphysema were correctly diagnosed from roentgenograms.

Patients with various types of endobronchial tumors that only partly obstruct an airway can have normal chest roentgenograms (Fig. 21–1), at least when films are exposed at full inspiration. More commonly, however, the volume of lung parenchyma distal to the partial obstruction is *smaller* than normal. In such circumstances, a roentgenogram exposed following full expiration, preferably forced, will reveal air trapping distal to the partial obstruction. When the obstruction is in the trachea or a major bronchus, dyspnea and generalized wheezing may suggest the diagnosis of asthma.

ALVEOLAR HYPOVENTILATION

The term "alveolar hypoventilation" (ventilatory respiratory failure) is used to designate a deficiency in ventilation

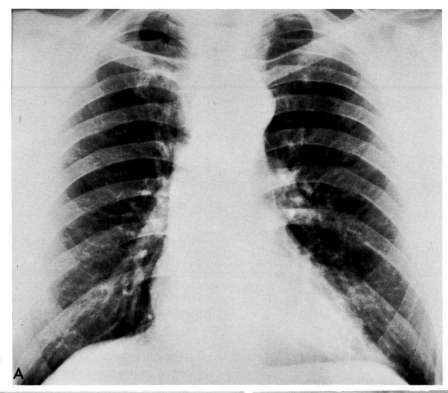

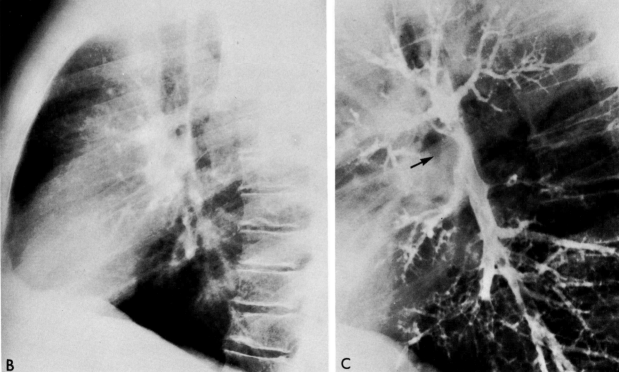

Figure 21–1. Bronchogenic Carcinoma with a Normal Chest Roentgenogram. This 56-year-old man was admitted to the hospital with a 2-month history of right-sided wheeze; he had had one episode of hemoptysis. Posteroanterior (A) and lateral (B) roentgenograms reveal a normal appearance of the lungs and mediastinum. In view of abnormal findings on bronchoscopy, a right bronchogram was performed (C) and showed an irregular mass arising from the anterior wall of the intermediate stem bronchus (arrow). It is probable that roentgenography of the chest in expiration would have shown evidence of air trapping in the right middle and lower lobes. This was proved squamous cell carcinoma.

Table 21-1. **NONPULMONARY CAUSES OF RESPIRATORY FAILURE WITH HYPERCAPNIA**

Disorders of Ventilatory Control	Disorders of the Respiratory Pump
Cerebral Dysfunction	***Neuromuscular Disease***
Infection (encephalitis), trauma, vascular accident	Anterior horn cells
Status epilepticus	Poliomyelitis
Narcotic and sedative overdose	Amyotrophic lateral sclerosis
Respiratory dyskinesia	Peripheral nerves
Respiratory Center Dysfunction	Landry–Guillain-Barré syndrome
Impaired brain stem controller	Acute intermittent porphyria
Primary alveolar hypoventilation (Ondine's curse)	Toxic dinoflagellate poisoning
Obesity hypoventilation syndrome	Neurotoxic shellfish poisoning (*Ptychodiscus brevis*)
Myxedema	Paralytic shellfish poisoning (*Protogonyaulax catenella*
Metabolic alkalosis (compensatory)	and *Protogonyaulax tamarensis*)
Sudden infant death syndrome	Ciguatera fish poisoning (*Gambierdiscus toxicus*)
Parkinson's syndrome	Puffer fish poisoning (tetrodotoxin)
Tetanus	Myoneural junction
Ablation of afferent and efferent spinal pathways	Myasthenia gravis
Bilateral high cervical cordotomy	Myasthenia-like syndromes (medications, particularly
Cervical spinal cord trauma	antibiotics, and associated neoplasm)
Transverse myelitis	*Clostridium botulinum* poisoning
Multiple sclerosis	Respiratory muscles
Parkinson's disease	Muscular dystrophies
Peripheral Receptor Dysfunction	Acid maltase deficiency
Carotid body destruction (bilateral carotid endarterectomy	Nemaline myopathy
and carotid body resection for asthma)	Polymyositis
Bilateral damage to afferent nerves	Hypokalemia (in treatment of diabetes with insulin, renal
Arnold-Chiari syndrome with syringomyelia	tubular acidosis)
Familial dysautonomia	Hypophosphatemia
Diabetic neuropathy	Hypermagnesemia
Tetanus	Idiopathic rhabdomyolysis (myoglobinuria)
	Chest Cage Disorders
	Flail chest
	Kyphoscoliosis
	Thoracoplasty

that is sufficient to raise the arterial carbon dioxide pressure above 45 mm Hg. Although regional underventilation can result in ventilation-perfusion mismatch and arterial hypoxemia, it does so without causing hypercapnia,° and the term "hypoventilation" should not be utilized in this situation but should instead be reserved for cases in which there is a generalized decrease in ventilation characterized by the presence of hypercapnia. It is emphasized that the diagnosis of alveolar hypoventilation requires measurement of blood gases and cannot be made by clinical examination or by measurement of minute ventilation alone.

Respiratory failure associated with hypercapnia occurs in two groups of disorders—those of pulmonary origin and those of nonpulmonary origin (Table 21–1). The latter conditions are dealt with more extensively in this chapter, since they are frequently associated with a normal chest roentgenogram. For purposes of clarity, these disorders are themselves considered under two headings—those that result from defective ventilatory control and those caused by an inadequate respiratory pump.

Although the chest roentgenogram is within normal limits in most cases of hypoventilation resulting from central nevous system disturbances or neuromuscular disease, it is important to realize that this is not always the case. In those instances in which hypoventilation is caused by respiratory muscle weakness or paralysis, the diaphragm is often elevated, although this finding is frequently ignored on the

supposition that the chest roentgenogram was exposed at a position of incomplete inspiration. More important are the complications of prolonged alveolar underventilation. Patients who hypoventilate, particularly those with a raised diaphragm, are subject to atelectasis and pneumonia,[6] and in fact such complications may be responsible for bringing the primary disease to the attention of the physician. In addition, severe and prolonged hypoventilation can result in pulmonary hypertension and cor pulmonale, reflected in the chest roentgenogram by diminution of the peripheral vasculature and enlargement of the cardiac silhouette.

Disorders of Ventilatory Control

Disorders of the Central Nervous System

Cerebral Dysfunction

Many disorders that affect cerebral function are associated with respiratory depression. In some, the depression is a direct effect of cerebral dysfunction, whereas in others it is secondary to the effects on the brainstem of increased intracranial pressure. Narcotic, analgesic, and sedative agents in prescribed amounts frequently produce hypoventilation and respiratory failure in patients with underlying chronic pulmonary disease; in individuals with normal lungs, drug-induced hypoventilation usually occurs in adults following suicide attempts and in children following accidental ingestion. Drugs that result in respiratory depression include the barbiturates, glutethimide, the phenothiazines and benzodiazepines, the tricyclic antidepressants, ethchlorvynol, diphenhydramine, and meprobamate.

Cerebral damage resulting from infection, trauma, or vascular accidents can also cause hypoventilation, usually

---

°The shapes of the dissociation curves for carbon dioxide and oxygen are the explanation for the respiratory system's ability to compensate for regional hypercapnia and its inability to compensate for regional hypoxia (*see* page 48).

following an initial period of hyperventilation. In many patients with these abnormalities, it is probable that increased intracranial pressure, caused at least partly by edema, plays a role in the hypoventilation.

The disorders associated with respiratory dyskinesia can also influence respiration and sometimes cause respiratory depression. This abnormality is characterized by irregular contraction of inspiratory and expiratory muscles and simultaneous contraction of opposing muscles acting on the rib cage and upper airway. It occurs most often in patients with neuroleptic-induced tardive dyskinesia in association with a generalized choreiform movement disorder.[7]

Primary Alveolar Hypoventilation

Alveolar hypoventilation that occurs predominantly as a result of an abnormality of central neurogenic control has been termed "primary alveolar hypoventilation of the non-obese" (Ondine's curse, central sleep apnea). It is a condition in which gas exchange and lung function are normal or almost so when the patient is awake and operating under voluntary ventilatory control, but in which respiratory failure and even death may ensue during sleep. The typical physiologic feature is a decrease in the sensitivity of the central nervous system to carbon dioxide; occasionally, a similar decrease in the ventilatory response to hypoxemia is also seen.[8] Characteristically, patients can voluntarily increase their ventilation and lower their PCO_2 to within the normal range.

The disorder can be caused by a specific congenital (sometimes familial[9]) defect in the respiratory center or can be acquired as a consequence of a variety of diseases that affect the central nervous system. The former becomes manifest within minutes or hours of birth in the form of cyanosis and respiratory acidosis that require prolonged mechanical ventilation.[10] In adults, the abnormality occurs equally as often in association with another primary disease as it does in an isolated fashion. In one review of 31 cases,[11] the syndrome was more common in men than in women in a ratio of 5:1. The patients' ages ranged from 20 to 50 years, and approximately 50 per cent had a history of central nervous system disease, usually encephalitis, Parkinson's disease, syringomyelia, or neurosyphilis. The other 50 per cent had no associated neurologic disorder. Alveolar hypoventilation during sleep and wakefulness is also a sequela of western equine encephalitis,[12] radiation therapy,[13] high percutaneous cordotomy for relief of chronic pain,[14] and (transiently) after bilateral carotid endarterectomy.[15] (In the last two conditions, the apnea and hypoventilation are secondary to an interruption of afferent input into the respiratory center rather than to a disturbance of the respiratory center itself.)

Since upper or lower airway obstruction and neuromuscular disorders must be excluded before the diagnosis is accepted, primary alveolar hypoventilation represents a diagnosis of exclusion. Suggested criteria include arterial PCO_2 greater than 45 mm Hg, a history of respiratory arrest or apnea during sleep, normal or nearly normal tests of ventilatory capacity, and a marked decrease in the ventilatory response to carbon dioxide. There are also several clinical features that help distinguish patients with upper airway obstruction from those with central neurogenic hypoventilation. In the latter, the apneic episodes are usually

of shorter duration and are associated with less bradycardia than occurs in patients with obstruction. In addition, patients with primary alveolar hypoventilation complain more of insomnia and less of daytime hypersomnolence.[16]

There is a clinical spectrum of severity in patients with primary alveolar hypoventilation. In some patients, hypoventilation occurs only at night, and arterial blood gas tensions become normal during waking hours, whereas in others, the hypoventilation persists throughout the day. As might be expected, the latter patients have the worse prognosis.[17]

Obesity Hypoventilation Syndrome

Considerable uncertainty exists in the literature as to the precise meaning of the term "obesity hypoventilation syndrome." The authors suggest that it be reserved for hypoventilation by obese persons whose findings do not fit the criteria for obstructive sleep apnea. In some of these patients, there may be a primary hypothalamic defect that causes both obesity and hypoventilation. Alternatively, affected individuals may be those whose ventilatory response to carbon dioxide and hypoxemia are at the low end of the wide normal range. When challenged by the increased work of breathing associated with obesity, these individuals may hypoventilate in much the same way that so-called blue bloaters hypoventilate when faced with the increased work of breathing associated with chronic obstructive pulmonary disease.[18]

The inter-relationships among obesity, obstructive sleep apnea, and depressed central respiratory drive are complex.[19] Although it is likely that differences in central drive to breathe are principally responsible for the hypoventilation, there is evidence that patients who hypoventilate have a lower thoracic compliance, an increased work of breathing, an increased V_D/V_T, and decreased respiratory muscle efficiency compared with equally obese subjects who do not hypoventilate.[20] Frequently, patients also have additional respiratory problems because of heavy smoking, asthma, or recurrent pulmonary emboli. In fact, it is possible that the combination of cigarette smoke–induced abnormalities of airflow and ventilation-perfusion matching plus the mechanical effects of obesity causes respiratory failure in many patients. Obesity also markedly increases the incidence of obstructive sleep apnea (see page 632), probably because of narrowing of the oropharyngeal airway by increased fat deposition. In addition, by altering lung volumes, it influences ventilation-perfusion matching and arterial blood gas tensions.

Despite this rather impressive array of potential pathogenetic mechanisms of disease, the vast majority of patients with morbid obesity do not suffer from obstructive sleep apnea or the obesity hypoventilation syndrome.[21]

Myxedema

Although a decrease in central neurogenic drive to breathe is a contributing factor in the hypoventilation sometimes observed in patients with myxedema,[22] other factors are also involved in some individuals. Obstructive sleep apnea[23] is common in patients with myxedema and is possibly caused by narrowing of the upper airway by macroglossia secondary to deposition of mucopolysaccharides in the pharynx and tongue. Patients with hypothyroidism also demonstrate significant respiratory muscle weakness that improves following thyroid replacement therapy.[22]

Metabolic Alkalosis

Metabolic alkalosis as a result of repeated episodes of vomiting can be associated with hypoxemia, carbon dioxide retention, and an increase in serum bicarbonate. These changes appear to represent compensatory mechanisms that permit a rise in serum bicarbonate, thereby enabling the acid-base balance to return toward normal.

Sudden Infant Death Syndrome

Considerable evidence has accumulated to suggest that disturbed regulation of ventilation may be responsible for at least some cases of sudden infant death syndrome (SIDS). Much of this evidence has come from studies of infants who are considered to have had "near misses." These patients show an abnormal breathing pattern characterized by an excessive number of apneic episodes that may be both central and obstructive. In addition, some infants hypoventilate at rest and show decreased ventilatory responses to hypoxia and hypercapnia.[24] In some studies, parents of infants who die of SIDS demonstrate decreased ventilatory responses to carbon dioxide and hypoxemia as well as decreased inspiratory muscle recruitment in response to added loads.[25] The basis for the hypothesized disturbance in ventilatory regulation in individuals with SIDS is unclear.

Parkinson's Syndrome

Patients with Parkinson's syndrome can suffer respiratory insufficiency for several reasons.[26] In some, the hypoventilation and hypoxemia appear to be related to central hypoventilation. In others, they are caused by intrinsic pulmonary disease such as aspiration pneumonia and atelectasis, both of which are frequent complications in this condition. In still others, decreased maximal expiratory flow and oscillatory fluctuations in expiratory flow are believed to be related to tremor involving the upper airway[27] or expiratory muscles.[28]

Tetanus

Tetanus is now more often found in developing countries, where hygiene is poor and there is increased likelihood of wound contamination on bare feet by soil or feces containing *Clostridium tetani*. In relatively developed countries, the overall incidence has decreased considerably; however, in certain large cities such as New York, where drug addiction is a major problem, the disease has undergone a resurgence.

Tetanus toxin causes blockade of inhibitory synapses at both the cortical and the spinal cord levels and is frequently associated with symptoms and signs of autonomic dysfunction, suggesting that involvement of the afferent inputs to the respiratory center contributes to the respiratory failure. However, the remarkable improvement that occurs in patients with severe tetanus following the administration of muscle-paralyzing agents and the institution of artificial ventilation[29] indicates that direct ventilatory muscle dysfunction plays a significant role in the disease.

Respiratory problems are common in tetanus. Even patients with mild disease manifest hypoxemia and hyperventilation associated with metabolic acidosis and a restrictive pattern of pulmonary function.[30] In severe cases, death from respiratory failure may ensue.

Disorders of the Spinal Cord

Patients who suffer spinal cord injury at the level of C-5 or lower have preserved diaphragm function but paralyzed intercostal muscles. In these circumstances, diaphragmatic contraction during inspiration results in exaggerated protrusion of the abdomen and in-drawing of the sternum and lower ribs. On expiration the diaphragm relaxes and ascends, with the abdomen flattening and the lower chest expanding as a result of the elasticity of the rib cage.[31] This pattern, termed "chest wall paradox," tends to decrease with time following the development of quadriplegia, presumably because the denervated intercostal muscles develop spasticity. As a result, pulmonary function tends to improve 6 to 12 months after the injury.[32]

Although hypoventilation following spinal cord injury is caused mainly by inspiratory muscle dysfunction, involvement of expiratory muscles is of great clinical significance as well, since it interferes with effective clearance of pulmonary secretions.[33]

Cervical cordotomy can interfere with respiratory control and result in a reduction in vital capacity, maximal breathing capacity, minute ventilation, and tidal volume, particularly if the operation is bilateral. Although such findings can be attributed to section of efferent pathways to the phrenic nerve nuclei, there is evidence that respiratory control mechanisms are also disturbed, probably as a result of ablation of reticular formation spinal tracts.[34] The major clinical manifestations consist of hypoventilation, diminished carbon dioxide response, and irregular breathing. Sleep-induced apnea and even sudden death can occur.

Disorders of the Peripheral Chemoreceptors

Bilateral carotid endarterectomy or removal of both carotid bodies—a therapeutic "procedure" that has been advocated without proven benefit for relief of bronchial asthma[35]—can abolish compensatory hyperventilation when patients become hypoxemic and can cause a decreased ventilatory response to exercise.[36] Sleep apnea also has been reported as a complication following bilateral excision of carotid body tumors.[37]

The syndromes of autonomic dysfunction represent a heterogeneous group of congenital and acquired disorders usually characterized by orthostatic hypotension, hypohidrosis, a relatively fixed heart rate, and bladder and sexual dysfunction.[38] In patients with such syndromes, there may also be abnormalities of peripheral chemoreceptor and mechanoreceptor input to the respiratory center, resulting in respiratory difficulty. For example, in one large review, 5 per cent of 297 patients with autonomic dysfunction had a history of respiratory arrest.[38] Children with familial dysautonomia (Riley-Day syndrome) are relatively unresponsive to hypoxia and hypercapnia,[39] and the breathing of hypoxic mixtures by these patients results in a dramatic fall in arterial oxygen saturation.

Diabetics with severe autonomic neuropathy have been

reported to have unexplained cardiac arrest that appears to be primarily respiratory in origin.[40] The complication occurs following anesthesia, bronchopneumonia, or the administration of depressant drugs, and the sequence of events has suggested the possibility that the chemoreceptors are unable to respond to hypoxia.[40]

Disorders of the Respiratory Pump

For the purposes of this discussion, the respiratory pump is considered to include not only the rib cage and muscles of respiration but also their electrical connections. Thus, disturbances of the respiratory pump can result from disease of the anterior horn cells, the phrenic and intercostal nerves, the myoneuronal junctions, or the respiratory muscles themselves.

Disorders of the Anterior Horn Cells

A variety of disorders of the anterior horn cells that subserve the respiratory muscles can result in acute or chronic respiratory failure. Although poliomyelitis associated with respiratory failure has been almost eradicated in the developed countries by immunization, occasional cases are still seen and affected patients can develop unexpected life-threatening hypoventilation.[41] Some patients also develop a state of chronic hypoventilation that may result in secondary polycythemia.[42] Others can exhibit late-onset respiratory failure secondary to kyphoscoliosis.

Amyotrophic lateral sclerosis (motor neuron disease) can also result in ventilatory respiratory failure. Although in most patients, respiratory muscle involvement develops after the diagnosis has been well established, respiratory failure may be the initial mode of presentation, resulting in a difficult diagnostic problem.[43] In addition to ventilatory respiratory failure caused by destruction of the anterior horn cells that innervate the inspiratory muscles, involvement of the neurons supplying the abdominal expiratory muscles and the muscles of the upper airway can result in abnormalities of expiratory flow.[44]

As in many forms of neuromuscular disease that cause ventilatory respiratory failure, patients with spinal cord degeneration may benefit from intermittent assisted ventilation, particularly at night. Such assistance can stabilize or temporarily improve the respiratory status.[45] The exact mechanism by which such ventilation improves interim lung function remains speculative. Possibilities include the reversal of chronic respiratory muscle fatigue, resetting of central chemoreceptors, and improvement in pulmonary mechanics.

Disorders of the Peripheral Nerves

Landry–Guillain-Barré Syndrome

Acute polyneuritis (Landry–Guillain-Barré syndrome) is probably the most common of all neuromuscular diseases that cause respiratory failure[46] and can be associated with either acute or subacute hypoventilation. Although in some respects it is a diagnosis of exclusion, an accepted clinical presentation includes symmetric ascending paralysis and a lack of cellular response in the cerebrospinal fluid. The disease shows a striking predilection for patients younger than 25 years of age of either sex. A second, smaller peak occurs between the ages of 45 and 60 years. Cases tend to show a seasonal clustering, almost half the patients being afflicted during late summer and autumn.[47]

Between 15 per cent[48] and 60 per cent[49] of patients develop respiratory muscle paralysis severe enough to require mechanical ventilation. In these patients, there is a slow but progressive improvement in respiratory muscle strength, although assisted ventilation may be required for a period of 2 months or longer. The need for assisted ventilation can be assessed by repeated measurements of VC or, preferably, maximal inspiratory pressure; however, serial measurements of phrenic nerve conduction velocity may be a more sensitive method of assessing the severity of the disease and of predicting impending ventilatory failure.[50]

Porphyria

Each of the hereditary hepatic porphyrias—acute intermittent porphyria, porphyria variegata, and hereditary coproporphyria—can be associated with ascending paralysis and respiratory failure. Some patients also manifest symptoms of bulbar involvement and experience difficulty in clearing bronchial secretions. The diagnosis is supported when it is learned that other members of the family are afflicted, and confirmation can be obtained by the discovery of porphyrin precursors, such as aminolevulinic acid and porphobilinogen, in the urine.[51] Exacerbations of the disease can be prolonged and require artificial ventilation.

Fish and Shellfish Poisoning

At least four different species of toxic dinoflagellates can cause fish and shellfish poisoning; the respiratory muscles can be involved with each type.[52] The syndrome known as *neurotoxic shellfish poisoning* is caused by the ingestion of clams or oysters contaminated with the toxins (brevetoxins, "red tide" toxins) of *Ptychodiscus brevis*.[53] The syndrome typically consists of nausea, diarrhea, abdominal pain, and circumoral paresthesia. Onset can occur a few minutes to 3 hours after ingestion of the clams or oysters. In addition to the problems associated with ingestion of the toxin, respiratory symptoms can also develop following inhalation of the toxin generated by whitecaps and breaking waves and liberated as an odorless aerosol. People exposed to the toxin on beaches can develop nonproductive cough, shortness of breath, lacrimation, sneezing, and rhinorrhea.[52]

A second syndrome, *paralytic shellfish poisoning*, is caused by the ingestion of mussels, clams, scallops, and oysters that have concentrated saxitoxin, the neurotoxin present in *Protogonyaulax catenella* and *Protogonyaulax tamarensis*. The symptoms are similar to those associated with the ingestion of brevetoxins.[54]

Ciguatera fish poisoning results from eating fish contaminated with toxins derived from the organism *Gambierdiscus toxicus*. Symptoms usually develop within 12 hours of ingestion and include gastrointestinal and cerebellar symptoms, sensory disturbances, and motor paralysis. The paralysis can develop up to 1 week after the onset of the illness. Although this syndrome occurs primarily in the tropics, isolated cases have been reported in temperate climates in people who have eaten fish imported from tropical areas.[55]

Severe neuromuscular paralysis with rapid respiratory

failure can also occur after ingestion of puffer fish. The responsible neurotoxin, tetrodotoxin, blocks sodium channels in the peripheral nerves and originates in the fish itself (in contrast to the poisons derived from ingested dinoflagellates, as described earlier). The case-fatality rate is approximately 50 per cent, death occuring as a result of respiratory muscle paralysis.[56]

Disorders of the Myoneural Junction

Myasthenia Gravis

Exacerbations of respiratory muscle weakness and the development of respiratory failure in patients with myasthenia gravis can be precipitated by surgery, infection, or the parenteral administration of radiographic contrast media.[57] Prior to the onset of hypoventilation, patients usually manifest paresthesia, diplopia, dysphagia, ptosis, generalized weakness, and dyspnea. The administration of acetylcholinesterase inhibitors results in an immediate increase in respiratory muscle strength and lung volume,[58] although it can also cause a transient increase in airway resistance and a decrease in maximal expiratory flow, presumably because of an accentuation of cholinergic tone in the airway smooth muscle.[59] In the authors' experience, respiratory failure usually necessitates ventilatory support for days to weeks and sometimes for months.

Drug-Induced Respiratory Paralysis

Respiratory paralysis caused by antibiotics has been reported with neomycin, streptomycin, dihydrostreptomycin, viomycin, kanamycin, polymyxin B, and colistin (polymyxin E). Affected patients usually have renal disease or myasthenia gravis.[60] Ventilatory muscle depression develops within 1 to 24 hours after the administration of the drug. In most cases, it is of short duration, and spontaneous ventilation is resumed within 24 hours[61]; however, it can be very prolonged.[62]

Botulism

Respiratory involvement in botulism can occur after ingestion of food contaminated with the toxin[63] or as a result of wound infection by *Clostridium botulinum*.[64] Peripheral muscle weakness and bulbar symptoms secondary to cranial nerve involvement usually appear within 18 to 36 hours after ingestion of contaminated food. Patients complain of blurred vision, weakness, dizziness, dysphonia, dysphagia, respiratory difficulty, and urine retention. Characteristically, the pupils are dilated and nonreactive, and there is marked dryness of the mouth and tongue.

Respiratory failure secondary to ventilatory muscle weakness occurs in 30 to 60 per cent of affected patients and is the primary cause of mortality[65]; in one study, the development of full-blown third nerve palsy was predictive of this complication.[65a] Although recovery of muscle strength is usually slow, but eventually complete, respiratory failure may be very prolonged. Despite this, a number of patients continue to complain of fatigability and exertional dyspnea several years after the initial ingestion of toxin.

Disorders of the Respiratory Muscles

Muscular Dystrophy

Duchenne type muscular dystrophy causes death from respiratory failure in at least 80 per cent of affected individuals.[66] The failure typically develops insidiously and, like other forms of respiratory failure related to muscle weakness, is aggravated during sleep.[67] Respiratory failure also develops in approximately 10 per cent of patients with myotonic muscular dystrophy.[68] The respiratory difficulties relate not only to weakness but also to increased impedance of the respiratory system secondary to myotonia of the abdominal and chest wall muscles.[69] The increased tone is caused by inappropriate electrical activity of the muscles during the respiratory cycle.[70]

Acid Maltase Deficiency

Acid maltase deficiency is a recessively inherited type 2 glycogen storage disease in which glycogen accumulates in intracellular vacuoles in muscle and other organs; it is caused by a deficiency of the enzyme acid maltase. The condition occurs in three forms, depending on the age at onset: (1) an infantile form, in which patients usually die before the age of 2 years; (2) a childhood form, characterized by variable muscle and organ involvement and usually by slow progression to respiratory failure; and (3) an adult form, in which specific muscle groups can be involved and the course is even more insidiously progressive.[71] In the last-named variety, respiratory failure may be the presenting feature and is an inevitable development in the majority of patients.[72]

Myopathy in Connective Tissue Disease

Although the usual cause of respiratory problems in polymyositis and dermatomyositis is interstitial pneumonitis or aspiration of gastric contents secondary to pharyngeal muscle paralysis, some patients have sufficient involvement of the diaphragm to cause acute or chronic hypoventilation. In fact, respiratory muscle dysfunction is sometimes not recognized because of undue attention directed to associated pulmonary disease. In such cases, withdrawal of corticosteroid therapy may uncover the underlying respiratory muscle weakness. Some patients with bilateral diaphragmatic paralysis or myopathy appear to have associated blunting of respiratory drive, which may be attributable to resetting of central sensitivity to carbon dioxide because of intermittent hypercapnia during sleep-induced hypoventilation.[73] Muscle weakness also occurs in systemic lupus erythematosus[74] and has been postulated to be the mechanism that causes "shrinking" of the lungs in some patients.[75]

Miscellaneous Myopathic Processes

Respiratory muscle weakness and resulting respiratory failure also have been reported in patients with hyperthyroidism or myoglobinuria,[76] in asthmatics following parenteral administration of large doses of steroids,[77] and in patients with a variety of metabolic abnormalities, such as hypophosphatemia,[78] hypokalemia,[79] and hypermagnesemia.[80]

Respiratory Muscle Weakness and Fatigue

Muscle fatigue is defined as the inability of a muscle continuously to generate a predetermined force. Factors that may be responsible include depletion of nutrient stores in the muscle, decreased delivery of oxygen or nutrients in the blood stream, the accumulation of metabolic end products that inhibit or reduce muscle contraction, and actual damage to respiratory muscle fibers. Clinically, fatigue can be precipitated by an increased load on the respiratory muscles, like that which occurs with airway obstruction or pulmonary fibrosis, or with normal loads if the muscles are sufficiently weakened.

Ultimately, respiratory muscle fatigue occurs when an imbalance exists between the energy demand of the contracting muscle and the energy supply. The latter is determined by several variables; for example, malnutrition can deplete muscle substrate stores and decreased blood flow can decrease the supply of oxygen. Respiratory muscle efficiency is also profoundly affected by muscle length: when there is hyperinflation, muscles are relatively short, resulting in the generation of less force for a given amount of neural activation and substrate metabolism. Fatigue inevitably develops when respiratory muscles are forced to continuously generate pressure greater than 40 to 50 per cent of that of which they are maximally capable.[81]

Respiratory muscle weakness or fatigue can be suspected from the clinical history and physical examination and from characteristic abnormalities on pulmonary function testing. In addition, there are specific tests to assess respiratory muscle strength and endurance and to delineate whether the underlying abnormality is primarily neural or muscular (see page 160).

Patients with respiratory failure secondary to neuromuscular abnormalities complain of anxiety, lethargy, headache, dyspnea, and sometimes a feeling of suffocation. When ventilation is severely restricted, confusion, coma, and death can ensue rapidly. Cyanosis may or may not be present, depending on the degree of hypoventilation. Appreciation of the degree of alveolar ventilation clinically is unreliable except when apnea has occurred,[82] and by that time the patient is severely cyanotic.

Since the diaphragm is the principal muscle of inspiration, evidence on physical examination of diaphragmatic weakness or paralysis is important in establishing a neuromuscular cause for respiratory failure. When it contracts, the diaphragm not only pushes down on the abdominal viscera and displaces the abdominal wall outward but also lifts and expands the rib cage. The latter action is dependent on the acute angle of insertion of diaphragmatic muscle fibers into the ribs and results in an increase in the diameter of the chest in both its anteroposterior and lateral axes.

When one hemidiaphragm is paralyzed or weakened, its movement is paradoxical (Fig. 21–2): the development of negative intrapleural pressure secondary to rib cage expansion and the normal descent of the nonparalyzed hemidiaphragm suck the paralyzed hemidiaphragm into the thoracic cavity. Although the resulting inward motion of the anterior abdominal wall on the paralyzed side can be detected clinically, paradoxical motion is much more apparent on fluoroscopic examination: on inspiration, the paralyzed hemidiaphragm moves upward coincident with expansion

of the rib cage and descent of the normal hemidiaphragm, a motion that can be appreciated to better advantage when the patient sniffs.

When both hemidiaphragms are paralyzed, as in bilateral phrenic nerve palsy or a neuropathic or myopathic disorder, abdominal paradox is even more apparent. With each inspiratory effort of the external intercostal and accessory muscles of respiration, the rib cage expands, lowering intrapleural pressure and sucking the diaphragm into the thorax—a most inefficient form of breathing (Fig. 21–3A through D). This upward movement of the diaphragm results in equal reduction of both abdominal and pleural pressures, so that the transdiaphragmatic pressure difference remains zero. The fall in abdominal pressure induces in-drawing of the abdominal wall that is readily apparent clinically. In patients who have incipient diaphragmatic fatigue, abdominal paradox can develop during or after a period of increased respiratory muscle activity, such as when they are being "weaned" from ventilatory support.

When assessing diaphragmatic weakness clinically, it should be remembered that recruitment of abdominal expiratory muscles can mask these characteristic signs of paradoxical breathing.[83] During expiration, the abdominal wall muscles contract and force the flaccid diaphragm into the thoracic cavity. At the onset of inspiration, the sudden relaxation of these muscles causes rapid diaphragmatic descent and apparent outward movement of the abdomen (see Fig. 21–3E, F). Recruitment of expiratory abdominal muscles during tidal breathing can be detected by palpation of the anterior abdominal wall. Abdominal muscle contraction can restore an apparently normal pattern of movement to the anterior abdominal wall (Fig. 21–3G through J). This pattern of expiratory muscle recruitment may be responsible for the false-negative results of fluoroscopic examination of the diaphragm in some patients with bilateral diaphragmatic paralysis or weakness.[84]

When the lung parenchyma is normal and patient cooperation is complete, a decrease in total lung capacity or an increase in residual volume—thus a decrease in vital capacity—may indicate respiratory muscle weakness.[85] Abnormalities of arterial blood gas tensions are late findings in patients with primary neuromuscular disease. Initially, patients may hyperventilate,[86] but hyperventilation is inevitably succeeded by hypoventilation as the disease progresses.

In patients with severe weakness or complete paralysis of the diaphragm, assumption of the supine posture causes further deterioration in gas exchange. The explanation for this lies in a change of gravitational forces. The weight of the abdominal organs displaces the flaccid diaphragm upward into the thoracic cavity, further reducing the effectiveness of the remaining inspiratory muscles.[87] In addition, a further drop in Pa_{O_2} and a rise in Pa_{CO_2} often occur during sleep, when breathing control is solely automatic.[88]

VENOARTERIAL SHUNTS

Extrapulmonary Venoarterial Shunts

Oxygen transport to the tissues may be inadequate despite normal structure and function of the lung parenchyma, airways, and respiratory pump. In these circumstances, the hypoxemia is caused by shunting of venous

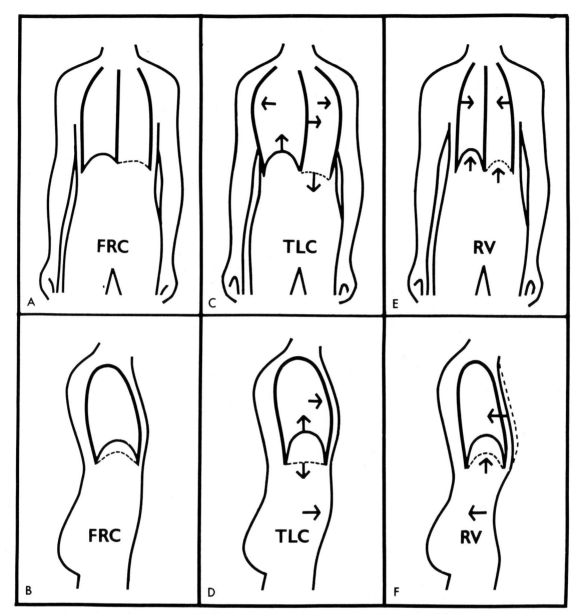

Figure 21–2. Schematic Depiction of Chest Cage and Diaphragmatic Movements Throughout the Respiratory Cycle: Right Hemidiaphragmatic Paralysis. At FRC *(A* and *B)*, the right hemidiaphragm is elevated. On full inspiration to TLC *(C* and *D)*, the left hemidiaphragm contracts and descends, whereas the flaccid right hemidiaphragm passively elevates in response to the more negative intrapleural pressure. On full expiration to RV *(E* and *F)*, a rise in intra-abdominal pressure evokes an even greater elevation of the paralyzed right hemidiaphragm.

blood into arterial channels, and blood gas analysis reveals a reduced PO_2 and a normal or reduced PCO_2.

One form of extrapulmonary venoarterial shunting is found in some patients with advanced cirrhosis. These patients usually have normal chest roentgenograms, and evidence of shunting lies in the results of arterial blood gas analyses that reveal mild to moderate hypoxemia and respiratory alkalosis.[89] The lowered PCO_2 is balanced by a proportional decrease in bicarbonate, indicating that a prolonged state of hyperventilation has resulted in compensation through renal excretion of bicarbonate. In this condition, blood from the portal system reaches the left side of the heart through anastomoses with pulmonary veins.

Pulmonary Venoarterial Shunts

Patients with cirrhosis can also experience intrapulmonary shunting, sometimes in the presence of a normal chest roentgenogram.[90] Studies employing quantitative perfusion scintigraphy have revealed indirect evidence for pulmonary arteriovenous communications that are too small to be detected angiographically and that may be responsible for the hypoxemia.[91] Despite this, the response of the shunt to the breathing of 100 per cent oxygen is greater than would be expected in a true anatomic shunt. Thus, it is probable that the shunt in these cases actually represents a unique form of diffusion impairment in which there is failure of equili-

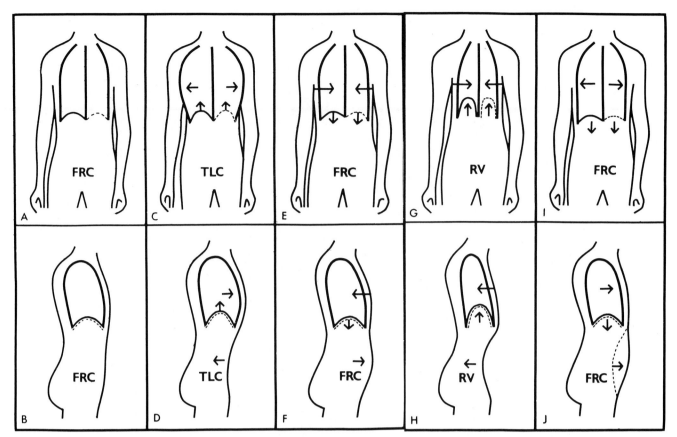

Figure 21–3. Schematic Depiction of Chest Cage and Diaphragmatic Movements Throughout the Respiratory Cycle: Bilateral Diaphragmatic Paralysis. On inspiration to TLC from FRC *(A to D)*, the increased negative intrapleural pressure "sucks" the diaphragm up and draws the abdominal wall in. On expiration to FRC *(E and F)*, the diaphragm descends and the abdomen protrudes. With a deeper expiration to RV accompanied by active contraction of the abdominal muscles *(G and H)*, the diaphragm rises. Subsequently, during the first part of inspiration to FRC *(I and J)*, abdominal muscle recoil is associated with descent of the flaccid diaphragm, creating the false impression of active contraction.

bration between alveolar gas and capillary blood as a result of the large diameter of the vessels and a very rapid red blood cell transit time through the vessels. Ventilation-perfusion mismatch caused by increased airway closure or hypoxic vasoconstriction at the lung bases probably also contributes to the hypoxemia.[92, 93]

The hypoxemia observed in patients with hepatic cirrhosis is more severe in the erect than in the recumbent position,[94] a phenomenon that is termed "orthodeoxia" and that is attributable to the increased blood flow through the lung bases where most shunts are found. When orthodeoxia is severe, the patient may complain of increased dyspnea when in the erect position (platypnea).[95] Occasionally, the hypoxemia is sufficiently severe to cause secondary polycythemia.[96]

In addition to patients with cirrhosis whose hypoxemia is caused by pulmonary arteriovenous shunts, there are some patients in whom blood is shunted from pulmonary artery to pulmonary vein during the postoperative period but whose chest roentgenograms are within normal limits. When hypoxemia persists for several days after surgery, impairment of ventilation-perfusion ratios may be demonstrable.[97]

METHEMOGLOBINEMIA

Methemoglobin is hemoglobin in which ferrous iron has been oxidized to the ferric form. Its accumulation in the blood—methemoglobinemia—can be either hereditary or acquired. The latter is most often caused by nitrates, which can be introduced into the body in several ways, including ingestion of well water containing a high concentration of nitrate,[98] use of topically applied nitrate in the treatment of burns,[99] ingestion of meat to which nitrates had been applied as preservatives,[100] and use of topical anesthetic containing Cetacaine,[101] benzocaine, or lidocaine.[102] Two types of hereditary methemoglobinemia have been described, one caused by enzymatic deficiency and the other associated with an abnormal type of hemoglobin (hemoglobin M).

Blood turns a chocolate brown color when approximately 15 per cent of hemoglobin is oxidized to methemoglobin; the result is cyanosis that is unresponsive to oxygen therapy.[103] Patients usually present with symptoms and signs caused by tissue anoxia, including headache, nausea, dizziness, pounding pulse, and listlessness. In most cases a diffuse, persistent, grayish cyanosis is present, although it may not be obvious. The chest roentgenogram is normal. The congenital variety of the disease is associated with mental retardation.[104]

CARBON MONOXIDE POISONING

Carbon monoxide is an odorless, colorless gas whose affinity for the hemoglobin binding site is 200 times greater than the affinity of oxygen. When carboxyhemoglobin levels reach 20 per cent of total hemoglobin, affected individuals develop headache, nausea, and vomiting, and decreased manual dexterity. When levels reach 50 per cent, convulsions, coma, and death rapidly ensue.[105] Acute poisoning can cause death as a result of either cerebral anoxia or a condition resembling adult respiratory distress syndrome (ARDS), the pulmonary edema possibly being caused by a direct effect of carbon monoxide on the permeability of the alveolocapillary membrane (*see* page 775).[106, 107]

ALVEOLAR HYPERVENTILATION

Normally, alveolar ventilation is proportional to the metabolic requirements of the tissues. In response to fever, exertion, or thyrotoxicosis, the demand for oxygen at the tissue level increases, as does carbon dioxide production. As a result, alveolar ventilation increases, but since the increase is appropriate, arterial PCO_2 remains within the normal range. When ventilation increases to a point at which it is greater than that required to maintain PCO_2 between 35 and 40 mm Hg, hyperventilation is said to occur. This can result from both pulmonary and extrapulmonary causes; however, in the majority of patients, it is of psychogenic origin.

It is important to emphasize that the clinical appraisal of ventilation with respect to blood gas abnormalities is notoriously inaccurate[82]; as a result, assessment of the adequacy of ventilation requires either direct analysis of the carbon dioxide tension in the blood or measurement of the mixed venous PCO_2 by the rebreathing technique.

Organic Pulmonary Disease

Hyperventilation may occur in patients with asthma, pneumonia, pulmonary embolism, or diffuse granulomatous or fibrotic interstitial disease. Hypocapnia is usually associated with hypoxemia, although the PO_2 of some patients with diffuse pulmonary fibrosis may be normal at rest and fall only during exercise. Diffuse interstitial disease sometimes engenders dyspnea on exertion, but by itself hyperventilation at rest seldom causes symptoms.

If the hyperventilation is of recent origin, bicarbonate levels remain relatively elevated in proportion to the PCO_2, and this is reflected in a lower hydrogen ion concentration. If overventilation is of longer duration, renal compensation for the lowered PCO_2 results in increased urinary excretion of bicarbonate and a lowered serum bicarbonate level; the hydrogen ion concentration is maintained within normal limits. In some patients with chronic destructive pulmonary disease or asthma, the minute ventilation may be greatly increased over the estimated normal value, and yet the

PCO_2 may be normal or higher than normal because of severe $\dot{V}/\dot{Q}$ inequality.

Extrapulmonary Disorders

Central Nervous System Disorders

Central nervous system disorders that cause hyperventilation include cerebrovascular accidents, brain trauma, meningitis, and encephalitis. The mechanism by which hyperventilation develops has not been established. It has been suggested that in some cases a breakdown product in the brain may be responsible for a rise in hydrogen ion concentration of cerebrospinal fluid that directly stimulates the respiratory center to cause a state of hyperventilation.[108]

In many patients with organic brain disease, hypoxemia and hypercapnia develop as a result of compression of the respiratory center by increasing intracranial pressure. During the initial stage, blood gas analysis may indicate respiratory alkalosis. Later, when the hydrogen ion concentration begins to rise as a result of hypoventilation and carbon dioxide retention, respiratory acidosis may develop.

Cheyne-Stokes Breathing

Cheyne-Stokes breathing is a form of hyperventilation recognizable clinically by the contrast between periods of hyperventilation and apnea. Tidal volume increases progressively during the phase of hyperpnea and subsequently decreases without change in respiratory rate.[109] This cyclic form of breathing is caused by instability of the ventilatory control system, in which circulation time, controller sensitivity, and the damping characteristics of the oxygen and carbon dioxide stores play important roles.[110] Instability of the automatic control systems occurs when the activity of the controller is excessive, either because of a delay in the feedback signal or because the controller is too sensitive or responds to stimulation in a nonlinear fashion.[111] In contrast to the change in blood gases that occurs during voluntary hyperventilation and breath-holding, the stage of hyperventilation in Cheyne-Stokes respiration is associated with a decreased PaO_2 and increased $PaCO_2$, probably because of the delay in feedback signal. During the apneic phase, PaO_2 and pH are increased and $PaCO_2$ is decreased.[112]

Cheyne-Stokes breathing occurs in patients with left ventricular failure or impaired cerebrovascular circulation. In the former, it develops particularly during sleep, and its presence is a poor prognostic sign.[113]

Psychogenic Hyperventilation

By far the most common cause of hyperventilation is a psychological phenomenon. According to one definition,[114] the resulting "hyperventilation syndrome" is characterized by "a variety of somatic symptoms induced by physiologically inappropriate hyperventilation and usually reproduced in whole or in part by voluntary hyperventilation." The abnormality varies in degree and clinical presentation in different patients, ranging from those who complain of dyspnea at rest and who require frequent deep respiratory efforts to the hysterical patient who overbreathes to the extent of inducing coma or tetany. Occasionally, the condition is epidemic.[115] The syndrome also has been closely related to a psychiatric condition termed "panic disorder," which is characterized by the sudden onset of extreme fear for which there is no known cause.[116] In this disorder, the hyperventilation syndrome can develop during the attack, or attacks can be precipitated by voluntary hyperventilation.

The symptoms of psychogenic hyperventilation are primarily neurologic and cardiorespiratory. The former includes giddiness or light-headedness, paresthesias, loss of consciousness and visual disturbances, and the latter dyspnea and palpitations.[117] Dyspnea is usually noted at rest, but when associated with exertion it characteristically occurs following, rather than during, effort. Two types of pain have been described:[118] one is a sharp pain considered to be caused by distention of the stomach, and the other is a dull, aching tightness in the chest. The aching is the more common of the two and probably results from overuse of the intercostal muscles.

The mechanism for the neurologic symptoms in the hyperventilation syndrome is probably a combination of cerebral hypoxia and metabolic alkalosis. By producing hypocapnia, hyperventilation decreases cerebral blood flow and causes a shift in the oxygen dissociation curve to the left, decreasing unloading of oxygen at the tissue level.[119]

Although in many patients psychogenic hyperventilation is readily diagnosed from the characteristics of psychoneurosis, in some the symptoms closely simulate organic diseases, such as transient ischemic attacks, multiple sclerosis, and myasthenia gravis.[120] Hyperventilation can also precipitate migraine headaches[121] or seizure disorders.[122] Spirometry often confirms the diagnosis when it is suspected on clinical grounds. The characteristic pattern is highly irregular breathing punctuated by deep inspiration. In the majority of cases, arterial blood gas analysis shows a reduction in the PCO_2, usually with a proportional reduction in bicarbonate levels.

Although hyperventilation is usually a benign disturbance readily reversible by suggestion or reassurance, in some patients the overbreathing can have serious consequences. For example, it is probable that maternal hyperventilation during labor can sometimes result in severe fetal hypoxia and metabolic acidosis.[117]

Metabolic Acidosis

Hyperventilation in primary metabolic acidosis results from stimulation of the respiratory center and carotid bodies by an increase in hydrogen ion concentration. The major causes of this type of hyperventilation are the ketosis associated with uncontrolled diabetes and the metabolic acidosis of renal failure. In contrast to other disorders that cause hyperventilation, blood gas analysis reveals acidosis, the hydrogen ion concentration being increased and the bicarbonate level reduced; PO_2 is within normal limits, and PCO_2 reduced. Many patients who overventilate as a result of central nervous system lesions or metabolic acidosis are semicomatose; the hyperventilation is obviously an inconsequential feature of a much more complex problem.

Salicylate Ingestion

The ingestion of salicylates in sufficiently large quantities to provoke hyperventilation usually occurs accidentally in children, but such ingestion sometimes is deliberate, as in suicide attempts by young adults or abuse of prescribed medications by the elderly.[123] Salicylates probably act by increasing the sensitivity of the respiratory center to the existing level of PCO_2. The acid-base disorder usually consists of mixed respiratory alkalosis and anion gap–type metabolic acidosis, although occasionally it is uncomplicated respiratory alkalosis or pure metabolic acidosis.[123]

Salicylate intoxication in young individuals is generally considered to be a benign condition with a low mortality rate, but such is not the case in the elderly, in whom the clinical presentation is often confusing and may suggest cardiopulmonary disease or encephalopathy.[123] Permeability pulmonary edema (ARDS) is a frequent complication and is associated with a high mortality rate.

References

1. Rigler LG: Roentgen examination of the chest. Its limitations in the diagnosis of disease. JAMA 142: 773, 1950.
2. Ritchie B: Pulmonary function in scleroderma. Thorax 19: 28, 1964.
3. Huang CT, Lyons HA: Comparison of pulmonary function in patients with systemic lupus erythematosus, scleroderma and rheumatoid arthritis. Am Rev Respir Dis 93: 865, 1966.
4. Gudbjerg CE: Bronchiectasis: Radiological diagnosis and prognosis after operative treatment. Acta Radiol (Suppl) 143, 1957.
5. Thurlbeck WM, Simon G: Radiographic appearance of the chest in emphysema. Am J Roentgenol 130: 429, 1978.
6. Wathen CG, Capewell SJ, Heath JP, et al: Recurrent lobar pneumonia associated with idiopathic Eaton-Lambert syndrome. Thorax 43: 574, 1988.
7. Chiang E, Pitts WM, Rodriguez-Garcia M: Respiratory dyskinesia: Review and case reports. J Clin Psychiatry 46: 232, 1985.
8. Farmer WC, Glenn WW, Gee JB: Alveolar hypoventilation syndrome. Studies of ventilatory control in patients selected for diaphragm pacing. Am J Med 64: 39, 1978.
9. Manon-Espaillat R, Gothe B, Adams N, et al: Familial "sleep apnea plus" syndrome: Report of a family. Neurology 38: 190, 1988.
10. Yasuma F, Nomura H, Sotobata I, et al: Congenital central alveolar hypoventilation (Ondine's curse): A report and review of the literature. Eur J Pediatr 146: 81, 1987.
11. Mellins RB, Balfour HH Jr, Turino GM, et al: Failure of automatic control of ventilation (Ondine's curse): Report of an infant born with this syndrome and review of the literature. Medicine 49: 487, 1970.
12. White DP, Miller F, Erickson RW: Sleep apnea and nocturnal hypoventilation after western equine encephalitis. Am Rev Respir Dis 127: 132, 1983.
13. Udwadia ZF, Athale S, Misra VP: Radiation necrosis causing failure of automatic ventilation during sleep with central sleep apnea. Chest 92: 567, 1987.
14. Polatty RC, Cooper KR: Respiratory failure after percutaneous cordotomy. South Med J 79: 897, 1986.
15. Beamish D, Wildsmith JA: Ondine's curse after carotid endarterectomy. Br Med J 2: 1607, 1978.
16. Kryger MH: Central apnea. Arch Intern Med 142: 1793, 1982.
17. Bradley TD, McNicholas WT, Rutherford R, et al: Clinical and physiologic heterogeneity of the central sleep apnea syndrome. Am Rev Respir Dis 134: 217, 1986.
18. Ahmad M, Cressman M, Tomashefski JF: Central alveolar hypoventilation syndromes. Arch Intern Med 140: 29, 1980.
19. Lopata M, Onal E: Mass loading, sleep apnea, and the pathogenesis of obesity hypoventilation. Am Rev Respir Dis 126: 640, 1982.
20. Sugerman HJ: Pulmonary function in morbid obesity. Gastroenterol Clin North Am 16: 225, 1987.
21. Sugerman HJ, Baron PL, Fairman RP, et al: Hemodynamic dysfunction in obesity hypoventilation syndrome and the effects of treatment with surgically induced weight loss. Ann Surg 207: 604, 1988.
22. Weiner M, Chausow A, Szidon P: Reversible respiratory muscle weakness in hypothyroidism. Br J Dis Chest 80: 391, 1986.
23. Skatrud J, Iber C, Ewart R, et al: Disordered breathing during sleep in hypothyroidism. Am Rev Respir Dis 124: 325, 1981.

24. Shannon DC, Kelly DH: SIDS and near-SIDS (second of two parts). N Engl J Med 306: 1022, 1982.
25. Schiffman PL, Remolina C, Westlake RE, et al: Ventilatory response to isocapnic hypoxia in parents of victims of sudden death syndrome. Chest 81: 707, 1982.
26. Lilker ES, Woolf CR: Pulmonary function in Parkinson's syndrome: The effect of thalamotomy. Can Med Assoc J 99: 752, 1968.
27. Vincken WG, Gauthier FG, Dollfuss RE, et al: Involvement of upper airway muscles in extrapyramidal disorders: A cause of air flow limitation. N Engl J Med 3311: 438, 1984.
28. Estenne M, Hubert M, De Troyer A: Respiratory-muscle involvement in Parkinson's disease. N Engl J Med 311: 1516, 1984.
29. Adams EB, Holloway R, Thambiran AK, et al: Usefulness of intermittent positive-pressure respiration in the treatment of tetanus. Lancet 2: 1176, 1966.
30. Femi-Pearse D: Blood gas tensions, acid-base status, and spirometry in tetanus. Am Rev Respir Dis 110: 390, 1974.
31. Sandor F: Diaphragmatic respiration: A sign of cervical cord lesion in the unconscious patient ("horizontal paradox"). Br Med J 1: 465, 1966.
32. Udwadia FE, Lall A, Udwadia ZF, et al: Tetanus and its complications: Intensive care and management experience in 150 Indian patients. Epidemiol Infect 99: 675, 1987.
33. Goswami U, Channabasavanna SM: On the lethality of acute respiratory component of tardive dyskinesia. Clin Neurol Neurosurg 87: 99, 1985.
34. Kuperman AS, Krieger AJ, Rosomoff HL: Respiratory function after cervical cordotomy. Chest 59: 128, 1971.
35. Lugliani R, Whipp BJ, Seard C, et al: Effect of bilateral carotid-body resection on ventilatory control at rest and during exercise in man. N Engl J Med 285: 1105, 1971.
36. Honda Y, Myojo S, Hasegawa S, et al: Decreased exercise hyperpnea in patients with bilateral carotid chemoreceptor resection. J Appl Physiol 46: 908, 1979.
37. Zikk D, Shanon E, Rapoport Y, et al: Sleep apnea following bilateral excision of carotid body tumors. Laryngoscope 93: 1470, 1983.
38. Hines S, Houston M, Robertson D: The clinical spectrum of autonomic dysfunction. Am J Med 70: 1091, 1981.
39. Bartels J, Mazzia VDB: Familial dysautonomia. JAMA 212: 318, 1970.
40. Page MM, Watkins PJ: Cardiorespiratory arrest and diabetic autonomic neuropathy. Lancet 1: 14, 1978.
41. Saxton GA Jr, Rayson GE, Moody E, et al: Alveolar-arterial gas tension relationships in acute anterior poliomyelitis. Am J Med 30: 871, 1961.
42. Cherniak RM, Ewart WB, Hildes JA: Polycythemia secondary to respiratory disturbances in poliomyelitis. Ann Intern Med 46: 720, 1957.
43. Mayrignac C, Poirer J, Degos JD: Amyotrophic lateral sclerosis presenting with respiratory insufficiency as the primary complaint. Clinicopathological study of a case. Eur Neurol 24: 115, 1985.
44. Kreitzer SM, Saunders NA, Tyler HR, et al: Respiratory muscle function in amyotrophic lateral sclerosis. Am Rev Respir Dis 117: 437, 1978.
45. Braun SR, Sufit RL, Giovannoni R, et al: Intermittent negative pressure ventilation in the treatment of respiratory failure in progressive neuromuscular disease. Neurology 37: 1874, 1987.
46. O'Donohue WJ, Baker JP, Bell GM, et al: Respiratory failure in neuromuscular disease management in a respiratory intensive care unit. JAMA 235: 733, 1976.
47. Dowling PC, Menonna JP, Cook SD: Guillain-Barré syndrome in greater New York-New Jersey. JAMA 238: 317, 1977.
48. Gracey DR, McMichan JC, Divertie MB, et al: Respiratory failure in Guillain-Barré syndrome: A 6-year experience. Mayo Clin Proc 57:P 742, 1982.
49. Hu-Sheng W, Qi-Fen Y, Tian-Ci L, et al: The treatment of acute polyradiculoneuritis with respiratory paralysis. Brain Develop 10: 147, 1988.
50. Gourie-Devi M, Ganapathy GR: Phrenic nerve conduction time in Guillain-Barré syndrome. J Neurol Neurosurg Psychiatry 48: 245, 1985.
51. Becker DM, Kramer S: The neurological manifestations of porphyria: A review. Medicine 56: 411, 1977.
52. Sakamoto Y, Lockey RF, Krzanowski JJ: Shellfish and fish poisoning related to the toxic dinoflagellates. South Med J 80: 866, 1987.
53. Ellis S: Introduction to symposium—Brevetoxins: Chemistry and pharmacology of "red tide" toxins from Ptychodiscus brevis (formerly Gymnodinium breve). Toxicon 23: 469, 1985.
54. Hughes JM, Merson MH: Fish and shellfish poisoning. N Engl J Med 295: 1117, 1976.
55. Tatnall FM, Smith HG, Welsby PD, et al: Ciguatera poisoning. Br Med J 281: 948, 1980.
56. Mills AR, Passmore R: Pelagic paralysis. Lancet 1: 161, 1988.
57. Chagnac Y, Hadani M, Goldhammer Y: Myasthenic crisis after intravenous administration of iodinated contrast agent. Neurology 35: 1219, 1985.
58. Radwan L, Strugalska M, Koziorowski A: Changes in respiratory muscle function after neostigmine injection with myasthenia gravis. Eur Res J 1: 119, 1988.
59. Shale DJ, Lane DJ, David CJF: Air-flow limitation in myasthenia gravis—The effect of acetylcholinesterase inhibitor therapy on airflow limitation. Am Rev Respir Dis 128: 618, 1983.
60. Antibiotic-induced myasthenia [Editorial]: JAMA 204: 164, 1968.
61. Lindesmith LA, Baines D Jr, Bigelow DB, et al: Reversible respiratory paralysis associated with polymyxin therapy. Ann Intern Med 68: 318, 1968.
62. Foldes FF, Lunn JN, Benz HG: Prolonged respiratory depression caused by drug combinations. Muscle relaxants and intraperitoneal antibiotics as etiologic agents. JAMA 183: 672, 1963.
63. Wilcox P, Andolfatto G, Fairbarn MS, et al: Long term follow-up of symptoms, pulmonary function, respiratory muscle strength and exercise performance after botulism. Am Rev Respir Dis 139: 157, 1988.
64. Lewis SW, Pierson DJ, Cary JM, et al: Prolonged respiratory paralysis in wound botulism. Chest 75: 59, 1979.
65. Schmidt-Nowara WW, Samet JM, Rosario PA: Early and late pulmonary complications of botulism. Arch Intern Med 143: 451, 1983.
65a. Terranova W, Palumbo JN, Breman JG: Ocular findings in botulism type B. JAMA 241: 475, 1979.
66. Begin R, Bureau M, Lupien L, et al: Control of breathing in Duchenne's muscular dystrophy. Am J Med 69: 227, 1980.
67. Skatrud J, Iber C, McHugh W, et al: Determinants of hypoventilation during wakefulness and sleep in diaphragmatic paralysis. Am Rev Respir Dis 121: 587, 1980.
68. Gillam PMS, Heaf PJD, Kaufman L, et al: Respiration in dystrophia myotonica. Thorax 19: 112, 1964.
69. Begin R, Bureau MA, Lupien L, et al: Pathogenesis of respiratory insufficiency in myotonic dystrophy—The mechanical factors. Am Rev Respir Dis 125: 312, 1982.
70. Jammes Y, Pouget J, Grimaud C, et al: Pulmonary function and electromyographic study of respiratory muscles in myotonic dystrophy. Muscle Nerve 8: 586, 1985.
71. Rosenow EC, Engel AG: Acid maltase deficiency in adults presenting as respiratory failure. Am J Med 64: 485, 1978.
72. Trend PS, Wiles CM, Spencer GT, et al: Acid maltase deficiency in adults. Diagnosis and management in five cases. Brain 108: 845, 1985.
73. Newsom Davis J, Goldman M, Loh L, et al: Diaphragm function and alveolar hypoventilation. Q J Med 45: 87, 1976.
74. Isenberg DA, Snaith ML: Muscle disease in systemic lupus erythematosus: A study of its nature, frequency and cause. J Rheumatol 8: 917, 1981.
75. Gibson GJ, Edmonds JP, Hughes GRV: Diaphragm function and lung involvement in systemic lupus erythematosus. Am J Med 63: 926, 1977.
76. Taverner D, Zardawi IM, Walls J: Acute ventilatory failure and myoglobinuria. Neurology 34: 369, 1984.
77. Williams TJ, O'Hehir RE, Czarny D, et al: Acute myopathy in severe acute asthma treated with intravenously administered corticosteroids. Am Rev Respir Dis 137: 460, 1988.
78. Aubier M, Murcino D, Legocquic Y, et al: Effect of hypophosphatemia on diaphragmatic contractility in patients with acute respiratory failure. N Engl J Med 31: 420, 1985.
79. Dorin RI, Crapo LM: Hypokalemic respiratory arrest in diabetic ketoacidosis. JAMA 257: 1517, 1987.
80. Ferdinandus J, Pederson JA, Whang R: Hypermagnesemia as a cause of refractory hypotension, respiratory depression, and coma. Arch Intern Med 141: 669, 1981.
81. Roussos C: The failing ventilatory pump. Lung 160: 59, 1982.

82. Mithoefer JC, Bossman OG, Thibault DW, et al: The clinical estimation of alveolar ventilation. Am Rev Respir Dis 98: 868, 1968.

83. Grinman S, Whitelaw WA: Pattern of breathing in a case of generalized respiratory muscle weakness. Chest 84: 770, 1983.

84. Miller A, Granada M: In-hospital mortality in the Pickwickian syndrome. Am J Med 56: 144, 1974.

85. Derenne JP, Macklem PT, Roussos CL: The respiratory muscles: Mechanics, control and pathophysiology. 1. Am Rev Respir Dis 118: 119, 1978.

86. Harrison BDW, Collins JV, Brown KGE, et al: Respiratory failure in neuromuscular disease. Thorax 26: 579, 1971.

87. Spitzer SA, Korczyn AD, Kalaci J: Transient bilateral diaphragmatic paralysis. Chest 64: 355, 1973.

88. Newsom Davis J, Goldman M, Loh L, et al: Diaphragm function and alveolar hypoventilation. Q J Med 45: 87, 1976.

89. Rodman T, Sobel M, Close HP: Arterial oxygen unsaturation and the ventilation-perfusion defect of Laennec's cirrhosis. N Engl J Med 263: 73, 1960.

90. Bank ER, Thrall JH, Dantzker DR: Radionuclide demonstration of intrapulmonary shunting in cirrhosis. AJR 140: 967, 1983.

91. Wolfe JD, Taskin DP, Holly FE, et al: Hypoxemia of cirrhosis. Detection of abnormal small pulmonary vascular channels by a quantitative radionuclide method. Am J Med 63: 746, 1977.

92. Mélot C, Naeije R, Dechamps P, et al: Pulmonary and extrapulmonary contributors to hypoxemia in liver cirrhosis. Am Rev Respir Dis 139: 632, 1989.

93. Schaefer JW, Reeves JT: The lung and the liver. Chest 80: 526, 1981.

94. Robin ED, Horn B, Goris ML, et al: Detection, quantitation and pathophysiology of lung "spiders." Trans Assoc Am Physicians 88: 202, 1975.

95. Robin ED, Laman D, Horn BR, et al: Platypnea related to orthodeoxia caused by true vascular shunts. N Engl J Med 294: 941, 1976.

96. Brownstein MH, Ballard HS: Hepatoma associated with erythrocytosis. Report of eleven new cases. Am J Med 40: 204, 1966.

97. Diament ML, Palmer KNV: Postoperative changes in gas tensions of arterial blood and in ventilatory function. Lancet 2: 180, 1966.

98. Comly HH: Cyanosis in infants caused by nitrates in well water. JAMA 129: 112, 1945.

99. Strauch B, Buch W, Grey W, et al: Successful treatment of methemoglobinemia secondary to silver nitrate therapy. N Engl J Med 281: 257, 1969.

100. Finch CA: Methemoglobinemia and sulfhemoglobinemia. N Engl J Med 239: 470, 1948.

101. Douglas WW, Fairbanks VF: Methemoglobinemia induced by a topical anesthetic spray (Cetacaine). Chest 71: 587, 1977.

102. O'Donohue WJ, Moss LM, Angelillo VA: Acute methemoglobinemia induced by topical benzocaine and lidocaine. Arch Intern Med 140: 1508, 1980.

103. Harris JC, Rumack BH, Peterson RG, et al: Methemoglobinemia resulting from absorption of nitrates. JAMA 242: 2869, 1979.

104. Jaffé ER: Hereditary methemoglobinemias associated with abnormalities in the metabolism of erythrocytes. Am J Med 41: 786, 1966.

105. Jackson DL, Menges H: Accidental carbon monoxide poisoning. JAMA 243: 772, 1980.

106. Fein A, Grossman RF, Gareth Jones J, et al: Carbon monoxide effect on alveolar epithelial permeability. Chest 78: 726, 1980.

107. Hopkinson JM, Pearce PJ, Oliver JS: Carbon monoxide poisoning mimicking gastroenteritis. Br Med J 281: 214, 1980.

108. Froman C, Smith AC: Hyperventilation associated with low pH of cerebrospinal fluid after intracranial haemorrhage. Lancet 1: 780, 1966.

109. Morse SR, Chandrasekhar AJ, Cugell DW: Cheyne-Stokes respiration redefined. Chest 66: 345, 1974.

110. Cherniak NS, Longobardo GS: Cheyne-Stokes breathing: An instability in physiologic control. N Engl J Med 288: 952, 1973.

111. Cherniak NS: Commentary: Abnormal breathing patterns, their mechanisms and clinical significance. JAMA 230: 57, 1974.

112. Gotoh F, Meyer JS, Takagi Y: Cerebral venous and arterial blood gases during Cheyne-Stokes respiration. Am J Med 47: 534, 1969.

113. Findley LJ, Zwillich CW, Ancoli-Israel S, et al: Cheyne-Stokes breathing during sleep in patients with left ventricular heart failure. South Med J 78: 11, 1985.

114. Lewis RA, Howell JBL: Definition of the hyperventilation syndrome. Bull Eur Physiopathol Respir 22: 201, 1986.

115. Moss PD, McEvedy CP: An epidemic of overbreathing among schoolgirls. Br Med J 2: 1295, 1966.

116. Ley R: Panic disorder and agoraphobia: Fear of fear or fear of the symptoms produced by hyperventilation? J Behav Ther Exp Psychiatry 18: 305, 1987.

117. Motoyama EK, Rivard G, Acheson F, et al: Adverse effect of maternal hyperventilation on the foetus. Lancet 1: 286, 1966.

118. Rice RL: Symptom patterns of the hyperventilation syndrome. Am J Med 8: 691, 1950.

119. Nisam M, Albertson TE, Panacek E, et al: Effects of hyperventilation on conjunctival oxygen tension in humans. Crit Care Med 14: 12, 1986.

120. Coyle PK, Sternman AP: Focal neurologic symptoms in panic attacks. Am J Psychiatry 143: 648, 1986.

121. Blau JN, Dexter SL: Hyperventilation in migraine attacks. Br Med J 280: 1254, 1980.

122. Magarian GJ, Olney RK: Absence spells. Hyperventilation syndrome as a previously unrecognized cause. Am J Med 76: 905, 1984.

123. Anderson RJ, Potts DE, Gabow PA, et al: Unrecognized adult salicylate intoxication. Ann Intern Med 85: 745, 1976.

Index

Note: Page numbers in *italics* refer to illustrations; page numbers followed by t refer to tables.